COMMUNITY & PUBLIC HEALTH NURSING

Promoting the Public's Health

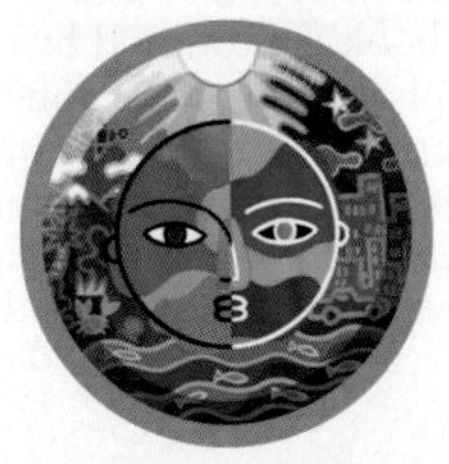

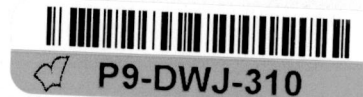

8th EDITION

Judith Ann Allender, EdD, MSN, MEd, RN
Professor Emeritus
Department of Nursing, College of Health and Human Services
California State University
Fresno, California

Cherie Rector, PhD, RN, PHN
Professor Emeritus
Department of Nursing
California State University, Bakersfield
Bakersfield, California

Kristine D. Warner, PhD, MPH, RN
Professor
School of Nursing
Director ASBSN Program
California State University, Stanislaus
Stockton, California

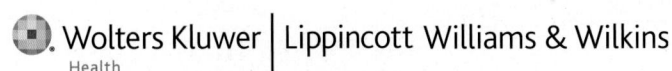

Philadelphia • Baltimore • New York • London
Buenos Aires • Hong Kong • Sydney • Tokyo

Acquisitions Editor: Christina C. Burns
Product Manager: Katherine Burland
Production Project Manager: David Orzechowski
Editorial Assistant: Dan Reilly
Design Coordinator: Holly McLaughlin
Illustration Coordinator: Brett MacNaughton
Manufacturing Coordinator: Karin Duffield
Prepress Vendor: SPi Global

8th edition

9 8 7 6 5 4 3

Printed in China

Library of Congress Cataloging-in-Publication Data

Community and public health nursing: promoting the public's health / [edited by] Judith A. Allender, Kristine D. Warner, Cherie Rector. — 8th ed.
p. ; cm.
Rev. ed. of: Community health nursing / Judith A. Allender, Cherie Rector, Kristine D. Warner. 7th ed. c2010.
Includes bibliographical references and index.
ISBN 978-1-60913-688-8 (alk. paper)
I. Allender, Judith Ann. II. Warner, Kristine D. III. Rector, Cherie L. IV. Allender, Judith Ann. Community health nursing.
[DNLM: 1. Community Health Nursing—United States. 2. Public Health Nursing—United States. 3. Health Promotion—United States. WY 108]
610.73'43—dc23

2012039468

LWW.com

In memory of my husband, Gilbert F. Allender (1937–2009)—in my heart and thoughts forever.
—Judy Allender

To my husband—my greatest supporter—and to my children and grandchildren, who make it all worthwhile. This book is dedicated to them and to my parents, who always encouraged me to keep learning and growing.
—Cherie Rector

To my son Sean and his family, my daughters Erin and Kathleen Whalen, and the best mom in the world Dolores Warner—thank you for your unwavering love and support.
—Kris Warner

ACKNOWLEDGEMENTS

We are grateful for the feedback we have received from nursing faculty and students, and have worked to incorporate many of your suggestions into this new edition. For the most part, feedback has been positive, but we appreciate all comments and suggestions. We hope that this textbook meets your needs, and we encourage your continued feedback.

We appreciate the efforts of many people who have assisted us in writing this textbook. We are grateful to have such talented contributors and thank them for sharing their knowledge and expertise. We also want to acknowledge the work of former contributors whose work may remain, in part.

To our hardworking editors, Katherine Burland, Hillarie Surrena, and Christina Burns, along with other staff at Lippincott Williams & Wilkins (Wolters Kluwer), we express our thanks.

We are indebted to our family and friends who provided support throughout this experience.

We look forward to the new generation of public health nurses, and hope that this book may inspire students to consider this exciting nursing specialty!

ABOUT THE AUTHORS

Dr. Judith A. Allender has been a nurse since 1963. For 30 years she taught nursing—first at Good Samaritan Hospital in Cincinnati, Ohio, and later at California State University, Fresno, where she retired as a Professor Emeritus. Her nursing practice experiences were varied. She worked with surgical patients, in intensive care units, as a school nurse, in-patient hospice, home care, and community health nursing. She has authored five nursing textbooks in addition to this one. During her long career, she received several awards. The fourth edition of this textbook received a Robert Wood Johnson award for the end-of-life care content in 2001. She was voted RN of the Year in Education for the Central Valley of California in 1998. In 2005 she was inducted into the Central San Joaquin Valley Nursing Hall of Fame. Presently, Dr. Allender consulted for a nonprofit immigrant and refugee center called Stone Soup of Fresno until 2010. She wrote a weekly health column for a local newspaper from 2002 to 2010. Her undergraduate nursing degree is from the State University of New York in Plattsburgh, master's in guidance and counseling from Xavier University in Cincinnati, Ohio, master's in nursing from Wright State University, Dayton, Ohio, and a doctorate in education from the University of Southern California. When not busy at home, she can be found traveling around the world. She and her late husband have a blended family with 7 children, 14 grandchildren, and 3 great grandsons.

Dr. Cherie Rector is a native Californian who is an Emeritus Professor at California State University, Bakersfield, Department of Nursing. She served as lead faculty in community health nursing, Director of the School Nurse Credential Program and the RN to BSN Program there, and formerly was the Coordinator of the School Nurse Credential Program at California State University, Fresno, where she also taught community health nursing, health teaching, and leadership. She has served as the Director of Allied Health and the Disabled Students Program at College of the Sequoias. She has consulted with school districts and hospitals in the areas of child health, research, and evidence-based practice, and has practiced community health and school nursing as well as neonatal nursing in the acute care setting. She currenty consults with a local Magnet hospital on evidence-based practice and research. She has taught graduate-level courses in community health, vulnerable populations, research, family theories, interprofessional development, and school nursing. Her grants, research, publications, and presentations have focused largely on child and adolescent health, school nursing, public health nursing, nursing education, and disadvantaged students. She earned an associate degree in nursing from College of the Sequoias over 40 years ago and, later, a bachelor of science in nursing degree from the Consortium of the California State Universities, Long Beach. She completed a master's degree in nursing (Clinical Nurse Specialist, Community Health) and a school nurse credential from California State University, Fresno. Her PhD in educational psychology is from the University of Southern California. She is an active member of the American Public Health Association, the Western Institute of Nursing, and the Association of Community Health Nursing Educators. Dr. Rector and her husband have three grown sons, seven grandsons, and two granddaughters.

Dr. Kristine Warner, also a native Californian, is a Professor at California State University, Stanislaus, with a specialization in Public/Community Health Nursing. With over three decades in the field of Public/Community Health, she has taught in nursing programs in both Pennsylvania and California. Undergraduate and graduate courses she has taught include community health nursing, nursing research, program planning and development, and health policy. Her nursing career began in adult and pediatric acute care, and she has practiced home care and public health in rural and urban settings. Her current professional interests include evidence-based practice, nursing education, emergency preparedness, and health needs of vulnerable populations. Her grants, research, publications, and presentations have focused on emergency preparedness, poverty, chronic illness, and nutrition. Dr. Warner is a retired Navy Nurse Corps Captain, ending a 29-year career of both active and reserve service in 2002. She was recalled to active duty and stationed in the Saudi Arabian desert during the First Gulf War as Assistant Charge Nurse of a 20-bed medical unit. She received her BSN from Harris College of Nursing, Texas Christian University, MPH (Community Health Nursing) and MS (Community Health Nursing & Nursing Education) from the University of South Florida, and PhD in Nursing from the University of Pennsylvania. Dr. Warner has three grown children and two grandchildren.

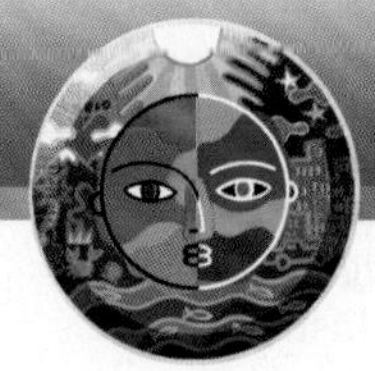

CONTRIBUTORS

Sheila Adams-Leander, RN, PhD
Assistant Professor
Coordinator, Accelerated BSN Program
St. Louis University
St. Louis, Missouri
Chapter 5

Elizabeth M. Andal, PhD, MSN, APRN-BC, FAAN
Mental Health Service Consultant
Las Vegas, Nevada
Chapter 27

Margaret Avila, PhD, PHN, RN/NP
Assistant Professor
School of Nursing
California State University, Los Angeles
Los Angeles, California
Chapter 29

Barbara Blake, RN, PhD, ACRN
Associate Professor
WellStar School of Nursing
Kennesaw State University
Kennesaw, Georgia
Chapter 23

Lydia C. Bourne, BSN, RN, MA, PHN
Principal, Bourne & Associates
Legislative Advocate
El Macero, California
Chapter 13

Bonnie Callen, PhD, RN, C/PHCNS-BC
Associate Professor
College of Nursing
University of Tennessee, Knoxville
Knoxville, Tennessee
Chapter 24

Janna L. Deickmann, PhD, RN
Clinical Associate Professor
University of North Carolina, Chapel Hill
Chapel Hill, North Carolina
Chapter 26

Paula Dorhout, RN, MSN, APHN-BC
Southeast Region Nursing Director
Children's Medical Services
West Palm Beach, Florida
Chapter 10

Mary Ann Drake, PhD, RN
Professor
Webster University
St. Louis, Missouri
Chapter 18

Naomi E. Ervin, PhD, RN, PHCNS-BC, FAAN
Professor (Retired)
School of Nursing
Eastern Michigan University
Ypsilanti, Michigan
Chapter 25

Marie P. Farrell, EdD, MPH, RN, ACC
Professor
Human and Organizational Development
Fielding Graduate University
Santa Barbara, California
Chapter 16

Sheila Holcomb, EdD, RN, MSN, PHN
School Nurse
Walnutwood High School
Rancho Cordova, California
Chapter 20

Katherine Laux Kaiser, PhD, RN, APHN, BC
Associate Professor
Department of Community-Based Health
University of Nebraska Medical Center, College of Nursing
Omaha, Nebraska
Chapter 21

Mary Lashley, PhD, RN, PHCNS-BC
Professor
Towson University
Towson, Maryland
Chapter 28

Roberta Lavin, PhD, APRN
Chair and Professor
Department of Nursing
Clarke University
Dubuque, Iowa
Captain (Retired)
US Public Health Service
Washington, District of Columbia
Chapter 17

Jeanne M. Leffers, PhD, RN, APHN
Professor
University of Massachusetts, Dartmouth
North Dartmouth, Massachusetts
Chapter 9

Karin Lightfoot, MSN, RN-BC, PHN
Lecturer
Community/Public Health Nursing
California State University, Chico
Chico, California
Chapter 14

Barbara B. Little, DNP, MPH, RN, APHN-BC
Associate in Nursing
Florida State University, College of Nursing
Tallahassee, Florida
Chapter 10

Eileen Lukes, PhD, RN, COHN-S, CCM, FAAOHN
Health Services Manager
Boeing Company
Mesa, Arizona
Chapter 31

Erin D. Maughan, RN, PhD, APHN-BC
Director of Research
National Association of School Nurses
Silver Spring, Maryland
Chapter 30

Mary Ellen Miller, PhD, RN
Assistant Professor
DeSales University
Center Valley, Pennsylvania
Chapter 31

Debra J. Millar, MSN, PHN
Program Manager
Public Health Institute
Center for Health Leadership and Practice
Oakland, California
Chapter 11

Barbara J. Polivka, PhD, RN
Professor and Shirley B. Powers Endowed Chair in Nursing Research
University of Louisville School of Nursing
Louisville, Kentucky
Chapter 4

Cherie Rector, PhD, RN, PHN
Professor Emeritus
Department of Nursing
California State University, Bakersfield
Bakersfield, California
Chapters 1, 4, 5, 6, 10, 15, 21, 22, 24, 25, and 29

Bassam M. Salemeh, PhD
Instructor
Microbiology and Biology
Antelope Valley College
Lancaster, California
Chapter 7

Phyllis G. Salopek, MSN, FNP
Assistant Professor
California State University, Chico
Chico, California
Chapter 19

Joann E. Smith, PhD, RN, APHN, CNE
Assistant Professor
College of Nursing and Allied Health Sciences
College of Medicine, Community and Family Medicine
Howard University
Washington, District of Columbia
Chapter 22

Karen Smith-Sayer, MSN, RN, PHN
Public Health Nurse
CA Department of Corrections
Pelican Bay State Prison
Crescent City, California
Chapter 8

Sharon S. Strand, MSN, PHN, RN-BC
Health Specialist
Mountain States Early Head Start
Coeur d'Alene, Idaho
Chapter 29

Mary E. Summers, PhD, MSN, RN, PHN
Professor Emeritus
Sacramento State University
Sacramento, California
Chapter 12

Gloria Ann Jones Taylor, DSN, RN
Professor
WellStar School of Nursing
Kennesaw State University
Kennesaw, Georgia
Chapter 23

Rose Utley, PhD, RN, CNE
Professor
Missouri State University
Springfield, Missouri
Chapter 31

Kristine D. Warner, PhD, MPH, RN
Professor
School of Nursing
Director ASBSN Program
California State University, Stanislaus
Stockton, California
Chapters 2, 3, 7, 11, 12, 14, 19, and 32

Joyce Zerwekh, EdD, RN
Emeritus Professor of Nursing
Concordia University
Portland, Oregon
Chapter 32

REVIEWERS

Jo Ann Abegglen, DNP, APRN, PNP
Associate Professor of Nursing
Brigham Young University College of Nursing
Provo, Utah

Marie H. Ahrens, MS, RN
Assistant Clinical Professor
The University of Tulsa
Tulsa, Oklahoma

Mary T. Bouchaud, MSN, CNS, RN, CRRN
Community Clinical Coordinator and Nursing Faculty
Thomas Jefferson University School of Nursing
Philadelphia, Pennsylvania

Carolyn Braudaway, MS, RN
Assistant Professor, Nursing
Columbia Union College (as of July 1, Washington Adventist University)
Takoma Park, Maryland

Angeline Bushy, PhD, RN, FAAN
Professor and Bert Fish Chair
University of Central Florida, College of Nursing
Daytona Beach, Florida

Karen J. Egenes, RN, EdD
Associate Professor
Loyola University Chicago, Niehoff School of Nursing
Chicago, Illinois

Susan L. Fogarty, BSN, MSN
Associate Professor
Ferris State University
Big Rapids, Michigan

Sue K. Goebel, RN, MS, NP, SANE
Associate Professor of Nursing
Mesa State College
Grand Junction, Colorado

Margaret Leahy Hopkins, MS, RN
Associate Professor
Elmira College
Elmira, New York

Katherine Howard, MS, RN-BC
Nursing Instructor
Middlesex County College
Edison, New Jersey

Kimberly Lacey, DNSc, MSN, BSN, CNS
Assistant Professor of Nursing
Southern CT State University
New Haven, Connecticut

Susan Primm Lehmann, MSN, RN
Clinical Assistant Professor
University of Iowa College of Nursing
Iowa City, Iowa

Ruth Elizabeth McShane, PhD, APRN, MAPS
Faculty Member (Part-time)
Marquette University
Milwaukee, Wisconsin

Valerie Evans Minor, RN, BSN, MSN
Associate Professor of Nursing
Alderson-Broaddus College
Philippi, West Virginia

Deborah Yoder Miranda, BSN, MSN, PhD, RNC-OB
Assistant Professor
Mississippi University for Women
Columbus, Mississippi

Judith Mouch, RSM, MSN, MA
Associate Professor
University of Detroit Mercy
Detroit, Michigan

Nadine F. Nelson, BSN, MN
Lecturer II
School of Nursing
University of Michigan
Ann Arbor, Michigan

C. Virginia Palmer, PhD, RN
Professor of Nursing
Millersville University
Millersville, Pennsylvania

Rosemary Ricks-Saulsby, RN, BS, MSN, MA, PhD
Assistant Professor of Nursing
Chicago State University
Chicago, Illinois

Carol Sapp, RN
Associate Professor
Georgia College & State University
Milledgeville, Georgia

Candide Sloboda, BN, MEd
Faculty Lecturer
University of Alberta, Faculty of Nursing
Edmonton, Alberta, Canada

Linda Spencer, PhD, RN
Director
Public Health Nursing Leadership Program
Emory School of Nursing
Atlanta, Georgia

Julie Bertelson St. Clair, RN, MSN
Instructor
University of Southern Indiana
Evansville, Indiana

Sharon J. Thompson, PhD, RN, MPH
Associate Professor of Nursing
Gannon University/Villa Maria School of Nursing
Erie, Pennsylvania

Joy E. Wachs, PhD, RN, PHCNS-BC, FAAOHN
Professor
East Tennessee State University
Johnson City, Tennessee

Barbara Wind, MSN, RN
Instructor
Community Health Nursing
Frankford Hospital School of Nursing at Aria Health
Philadelphia, Pennsylvania

OTHER REVIEWERS

Janet Alexander
Samford University
Birmingham, Alabama

Grace E. Ayton
Missouri Southern State University
Joplin, Missouri

Dot Baker
Wilmington University
Georgetown, Delaware

Cynthia Banks
Sentara College of Health Sciences
Chesapeake, Virginia

Mary Bannon
University of North Carolina at Greensboro
Jamestown, North Carolina

Sue Bell
Minnesota State University, Mankato
Mankato, Minnesota

Carolanne Bianchi
University of Rochester School of Nursing
Rochester, New York

Elizabeth H. Bicknell
University of Maine
Orono, Maine

Kelley Blackburn
University of Iowa
Urbandale, Iowa

Debbie Bomgaars
Northwestern College
Orange City, Iowa

Anne Bongiorno
State University of New York, Plattsburgh
Plattsburgh, New York

Cindy Bork
Winona State University
Winona, Minnesota

Mary Lou Bost
Carlow University
Pittsburgh, Pennsylvania

Bonnie Bowie
Seattle University
Seattle, Washington

Jeri Brandt
Nebraska Wesleyan University
Lincoln, Nebraska

Brandy Brown
Union University
Michie, Tennessee

Mary Bruun
University of Mary
Bismarck, North Dakota

Kathleen Buck
Huntington University
Huntington, Indiana

Angeline Bushy
University of Central Florida College of Nursing
Daytona Beach, Florida

Minnie Campbell
School of Nursing – Kean University
Union, New Jersey

Sharon Canclini
Texas Christian University
Fort Worth, Texas

Susan M. Cherry
University of Texas at Arlington
Arlington, Texas

Jane Christianson
University of Cincinnati
Cincinnati, Ohio

Barbara Cornett
Otterbein University
Westerville, Ohio

Ben Crandall
Indiana Wesleyan University
Marion, Indiana

Elizabeth Crusse
Towson University
Towson, Maryland

Sarah Coulter Danner
Castleton State College
Castleton, Vermont

Becky Davis
BryanLGH College of Health Sciences
Lincoln, Nebraska

Jean DeDonder
Emporia State University
Emporia, Kansas

Glenda Dexter-Brown
Indiana University Northwest
Gary, Indiana

Debra Dickman
Blessing-Rieman College of Nursing
Quincy, Illinois

Kim Dinsey-Read
Northern Kentucky University
Highland Heights, Kentucky

Norma Hannigan
Columbia University
New York, New York

Barbara Harrison
College of Virginia Beach—Nursing
Virginia Beach, Virginia

Frances Long
Coastal Carolina University
College of Science
Conway, South Carolina

Juan Carlos Ramirez, BSN, DHS, MBA
Professional Training Centers
Miami, Florida

Cheryl Schlamb
West Chester University of Pennsylvania
West Chester, Pennsylvania

Amy Spurlock
Troy University
Troy, Alabama

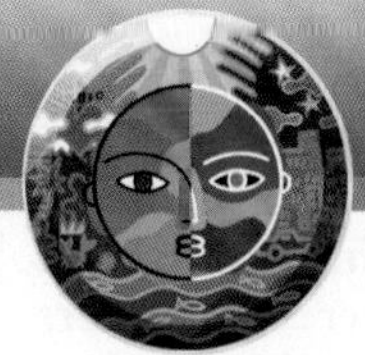

PREFACE

Continuing a rich tradition initiated by Barbara Spradley with the first edition of this book in 1981, the eighth edition of *Community and Public Health Nursing: Promoting the Public's Health* introduces undergraduate nursing students to population-focused nursing in community settings (e.g., public health agencies, schools, and other community health organizations). We are passionate about public health nursing and the immense power for good it can bring about for individuals, families, and communities. We recognize that most nursing students remain focused on acute care and will seek employment in hospital settings. To that end, throughout the book, we have endeavored to provide students with examples and information that will broaden their knowledge of their patients and enable them to provide more effective nursing care wherever they may be. When a patient is discharged, it is important for the nurse to understand the patient's unique circumstances and how to best work with the patient and the family to prevent further illness and promote better health. Population-focused tools and interventions are needed in acute care, as infection rates continue to rise and nurse-sensitive outcome indicators are closely monitored. In the process of learning about public health nursing, we hope to light a spark in those nursing students interested in this nursing specialty and its rich history. Public health nurses often work in a more autonomous practice setting and can have a real impact on the general health status of their communities through large-scale interventions and political advocacy. Nurses working in the community are important role models for social justice and are on the front line of communicable disease prevention and control.

The book is designed to give students a basic grounding in the principles of public health nursing and introduce them to key populations they may engage while working in the community setting. Entry-level public health nurses may also find it a helpful resource as they begin to familiarize themselves with their unique practice settings and target populations. The nexus of public health nursing lies in the utilization of public health principles along with nursing science and skills in order to promote health, prevent disease, and protect at-risk populations. Throughout this book, we use the term *community health nurse* interchangeably with *public health nurse* to describe the practitioner who does not simply "work in the community" (physically located outside the hospital setting, in the community), but rather one who has a focus on nursing and public health science that informs their community-based, population-focused nursing practice.

ABOUT THE EIGHTH EDITION

We have continued to try to keep this textbook user-friendly for nursing students, who are entering the world of public health nursing for the first time. We strive to write in an accessible style with little use of jargon or long passages of dry narrative. Also, we seek to have a more conversational quality and highlight student, practitioner, and instructor perspectives on common issues and problems. We use pertinent examples and case studies to convey real-life situations and interventions in order to aid students in applying the concepts and principles of public health nursing practice. Storytelling has been shown to be very effective in nursing education. We feel that these client stories can greatly influence learning, as the student strives to grasp the art and skill of working with clients in a community setting. Our goal is also to provide the most accurate, pertinent, and current information for students and nursing faculty. We have sought out experts in various fields and specialty areas of public health nursing in order to provide a balanced and complete product. With the addition of over 30 contributors from across the country and countless reviewers, the content reflects a broad spectrum of views and expertise. But, we have also carefully edited material to make this a cohesive textbook with a common voice.

ORGANIZATION OF THE TEXT

For the eighth edition, we have strongly emphasized *Healthy People 2020* goals and objectives throughout the text, and have also included more examples of evidence-based practice. We have added more visual interest, with photos and graphics highlighting written content. We have maintained the changes made to chapter and unit organization in the seventh edition, but have added more emphasis on population health and prevention/health promotion strategies.

Unit I, Foundations of Community Health Nursing, covers fundamental principles and background about public health nursing. Chapter 1 discusses basic public health concepts of health, illness, wellness, community, aggregate, population, and levels of prevention. Leading Health Indicators are introduced in this chapter, along with *Healthy People 2020* goals and objectives. In Chapter 2, public health nursing's rich and meaningful history is examined, along with social influences that have shaped our current practice. Educational preparation, and the roles and functions of public health nursing, are discussed in both Chapters 2 and 3. Core

Public Health Functions are described in Chapter 3, and common settings for public health nursing are introduced. Chapter 4 considers values, ethical principles, and decision making unique to this nursing specialty. Evidence-based practice and research principles relating to community health nursing are also discussed, along with the nurse's role in utilizing current research. Community-based participatory research is highlighted. Cultural principles are defined and the importance of cultural diversity and sensitivity in public health nursing are explained in Chapter 5 as well as cultural assessment and folk remedies.

Unit II, Public Health Essentials for Community Health Nursing, covers the structure of public health within the health system infrastructure, and introduces the basic public health tools of epidemiology, communicable disease control, and environmental health. Chapter 6 examines the economics of health care and compares U.S. outcomes with those of other countries, while also introducing the Affordable Care Act (health care reform). It also examines official health agencies and landmark legislation related to public health, as well as basic information on different types of health insurance. Different methods of epidemiologic investigation and research are explored in Chapter 7, along with population-focused communicable disease control in Chapter 8. The concepts vital to environmental health are covered in Chapter 9, along with public health nursing's role in researching and intervening to promote a healthier environment for all. Prevention is emphasized and an ecological approach used to address issues of environmental health and safety.

Unit III, Community Health Nursing Tool Box, includes tools used by the public health nurse to ensure effectiveness in his or her practice. Chapter 10 covers communication and collaboration, as well as contracting with clients. Incorporating technology and social media to promote population health and prevent disease, important for all nurses, are also included in this chapter. Health promotion is the focus of Chapter 11, with an emphasis on helping clients and aggregates achieve behavioral change through the application of educational and theoretical models. In Chapter 12, the focus is on planning and developing community health programs including the contribution of the Quality and Safety Education for Nurses (QSEN) project to community/public health nursing practice. Designing interventions and evaluating outcomes, along with social marketing approaches and grant funding, are examined. Chapter 13 concludes this unit with an explanation of the public health nurse's role in political advocacy and policy making, highlighting examples of successful political action campaigns and client empowerment strategies.

Unit IV, The Community as Client, further expands the focus of the public health nurse. Chapter 14 examines common theories and models used in public health nursing practice, and Chapter 15 applies the well-known nursing process to communities as clients (contrasted to its use with individual patients, as done in acute care settings). Different types of assessments are discussed, along with sources of data, community diagnoses, and community development. Global health and international nursing are considered in Chapter 16. International agencies and health problems/practices are discussed, highlighted by real-life case examples and perspectives. Preparedness is examined in Chapter 17, with a closer look at disasters and terrorism. The public health nurse's role in emergency preparedness, disaster management, preventive measures against terrorism, and *Healthy People 2020* objectives are also included in this chapter.

Unit V, The Family as Client, introduces the family as an aggregate, and Chapter 18 provides theoretical frameworks that promote better family health and provide a means for nurses to better understand and work with families experiencing dysfunction. Applying the nursing process to families and family assessment are covered in Chapter 19. Helpful tools are provided, and case studies help to emphasize concepts. In Chapter 20, family violence, child and spousal abuse, and effective interventions are examined, along with educational strategies and resources.

Unit VI, Promoting and Protecting the Health of Aggregates with Developmental Needs, provides information about client groups as often aggregated by public health departments. Chapter 21 covers common issues, concerns, and interventions for maternal child clients and their infants. Health problems affecting children and adolescents are examined in Chapter 22, and the prevention concerns of adult women and men are highlighted in Chapter 23. Unique issues facing the older client can be found in Chapter 24. These chapters build upon the content presented in Unit V, and can be very helpful in tailoring public health nursing efforts for these select population groups.

Unit VII, Promoting and Protecting the Health of Vulnerable Populations, deals with how to best address the needs of the most vulnerable clients. In Chapter 25, the concept of vulnerability is addressed along with theoretical frameworks and effective methods of working with vulnerable clients and populations. In Chapter 26, clients with chronic illnesses and disabilities are discussed, and Chapter 27 covers clients and populations with behavioral health problems, such as mental health issues and substance abuse. The homeless population is addressed in Chapter 28, along with factors contributing to homelessness and the role of the community health nurse. Chapter 29 addresses the unique challenges of rural and urban populations. It also explores issues of social justice, migrant populations, and frontier nursing.

Unit VIII, Settings for Community Health Nursing, examines public (Chapter 30) and private (Chapter 31) settings in more depth. Practice options in government-sponsored agencies, such as state and local public health departments, public schools, or prisons, are described. Nurse-managed clinics, faith-based nursing, and occupational health are included in the chapter on private organizations. These chapters provide overviews of a number of practice options available to both new and experienced nurses. Finally, the important roles of home health and hospice nursing are discussed in Chapter 32. With the aging of our population, these nursing roles will continue to be in demand.

KEY FEATURES

The eighth edition of *Community and Public Health Nursing: Promoting the Public's Health* includes key features from previous editions as well as new features.

Features continued from previous editions include:

- **Evidence-Based Practice**—this feature incorporates current research examples and how they can be applied to public/community health nursing practice to achieve optimal client/aggregate outcomes.
- **From the Case Files**—presentation of a scenario/case study with student-centered, application-based questions. Emphasizing nursing process, students are challenged to reflect on assessment and intervention in typical, yet challenging examples.
- **Perspectives**—this feature is included in most chapters and provides stories (viewpoints) from a variety of sources. The perspective may be from a nursing student, a novice or experienced public health nurse, a faculty member, a policy maker, or a client. These short features are designed to promote critical thinking, reflect on commonly held misconceptions about public/community health nursing, or to recognize the link between skills learned in this specialty practice and other practice settings, especially acute care hospitals.
- A **Summary** of highlights at the end of each chapter provides an overview of material covered and serves as a review for study.
- **References** at the end of each chapter provide you with classic sources, current research, and a broad base of authoritative information for furthering knowledge on each chapter's subject matter.
- **Learning Objectives** and **Key Terms** sharpen the reader's focus and provide a quick guide for learning the chapter content.
- **Activities to Promote Critical Thinking** at the close of each chapter are designed to challenge students, promote critical-thinking skills, and encourage active involvement in solving community health problems. They include Internet activities.
- **Levels of Prevention Pyramid** boxes enhance understanding of the levels of prevention concept, basic to community health nursing. Each box addresses a chapter topic, describes nursing actions at each of the three levels of prevention, and is unique to this text in its complexity and comprehensiveness.
- Additional assessment tools are provided throughout the chapters. They are added to enhance assessment skills with individuals, families, or aggregates/populations.

FEATURES NEW TO THIS EDITION

- *Healthy People 2020*—highlights pertinent goals and objectives to promote health and is applied to specific populations or problems noted in each of the chapters. Evaluation of select *Healthy People 2010* goals and objectives is also provided.
- Enhanced art program to appeal to today's learner.

RESOURCES FOR INSTRUCTORS

A set of tools to assist you in teaching your course is available on *thePoint* at thepoint.lww.com/allender8e. *thePoint* is a Web-based system that allows you to manage your course and content and provides every resource instructors need in one easy-to-use site.

Available resources include:

- Audio Podcasts covering key points from each chapter
- Videos on Vulnerable Populations
- Guided Lecture Notes and PowerPoint Presentations
- Student Quiz Bank
- Journal Articles
- Assignments, Discussion Topics, Case Studies, and Pre-Lecture Quizzes
- Test Generator
- Learning Objectives
- Image Bank
- Selected Readings and Internet Resources

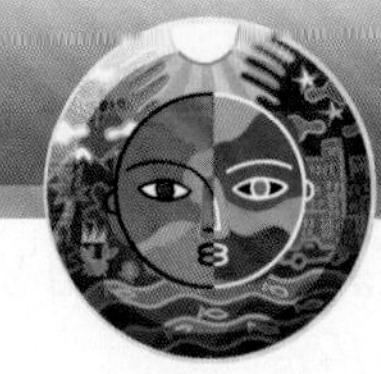

CONTENTS

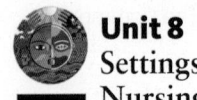

UNIT 1

FOUNDATIONS OF COMMUNITY HEALTH NURSING

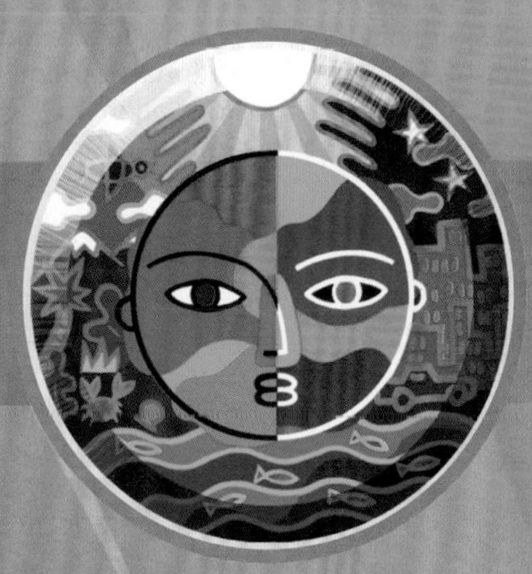

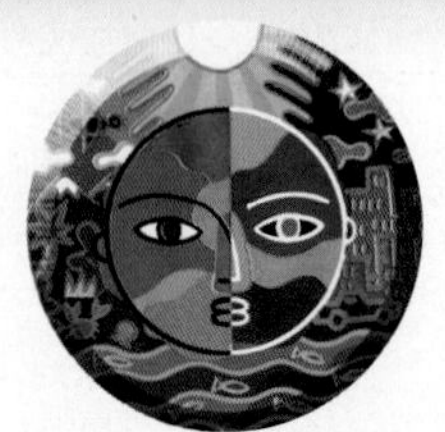

CHAPTER 1

The Journey Begins: Introduction to Community Health Nursing

"For a community to be whole and healthy, it must be based on people's love and concern for each other."

—*Millard Fuller* (1935 to 2009) Founder, Habitat For Humanity

KEY TERMS

Aggregate
Collaboration
Community
Community health
Community health nursing
Continuous needs
Epigenetics
Episodic needs
Genomics
Geographic community
Global health
Health
Health continuum
Health literacy
Health promotion
Illness
Leading health indicators
Pharmacogenomics
Population
Population-focused
Primary prevention
Public health
Public health nursing
Secondary prevention
Self-care
Self-care deficit
Tertiary prevention
Wellness

LEARNING OBJECTIVES

Upon mastery of this chapter, you should be able to:

- Define community health and distinguish it from public health.
- Explain the concept of community.
- Diagram the health continuum.
- Name 3 of the 10 leading health indicators.
- Discuss ways that public health nursing (PHN) practice is linked to acute care nursing practice.
- Discuss the two main components of community health practice (health promotion and disease prevention).
- Differentiate among the three levels of prevention.
- Describe the eight characteristics of community health nursing.

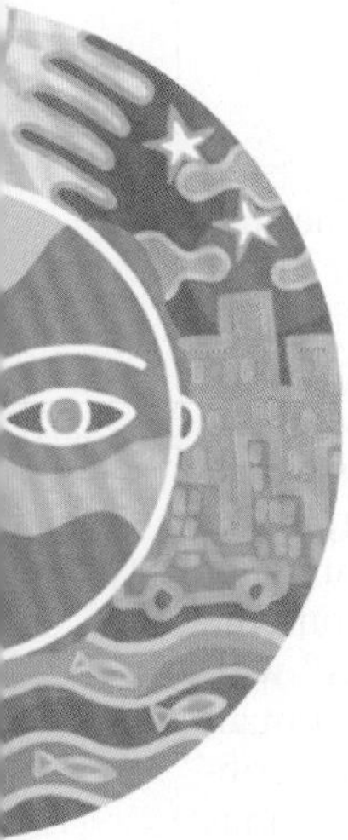

Opportunities and challenges in nursing are boundless and rapidly changing. You have spent a lot of time and effort learning how to care for individual patients in medical–surgical and other acute-care–oriented nursing specialties. Now you are entering a unique and exciting area of nursing–community/public health.

As one of the oldest specialty nursing practices, public health nursing offers unique challenges and opportunities. A nurse entering this field will encounter the complex challenge of working with populations rather than just individual clients and the opportunity to carry on the heritage of early public health nursing efforts with the benefit of modern sensibilities. There is the challenge of expanding nursing's focus from the individual and family to encompass communities and the opportunity to affect the health status of populations. There also is the challenge of determining the needs of populations at risk and the opportunity to design interventions to specifically address their needs. There is the challenge of learning the complexities of a constantly changing health care system and the opportunity to help shape service delivery. Public health nursing is community-based and, most importantly, it is population-focused. Operating within an environment of rapid change and increasingly complex challenges, this nursing specialty holds the potential to shape the quality of community health services and improve the health of the general public.

You have provided nursing care in familiar acute care settings for the very ill, both young and old, but always with other professionals at your side. You have worked as part of a team, in close proximity, to welcome a new life, reestablish a client's health, or comfort someone toward a peaceful death. Now, you are being asked to leave that familiar acute care setting and go out into the community—into homes, schools, recreational facilities, work settings, parishes, and even street corners that are commonplace to your clients and unfamiliar to you. Here, you will find few or no monitoring devices, charts full of laboratory data, or professional and allied health workers at your side to assist you. You will be asked to use the nontangible skills of listening, assessing, planning, teaching, coordinating, evaluating, and referring. You will also draw on the skills you have learned throughout your acute care setting experiences (e.g., behavioral health nursing; women's, children's, adult health nursing), and begin to "think on your feet" in new and exciting situations. Often, your practice will be solo, and you will need to combine creativity, ingenuity, intuition, and resourcefulness along with these skills. You will be providing care not only to individuals but also to families and other groups in a variety of settings within the community. Talk about boundless opportunities and challenges! (see "Perspectives: Student Voices.")

You may feel that this is too demanding. You may be anxious about how you will perform in this new setting. But perhaps, just perhaps, you might find that this new area is a rewarding kind of nursing—one that constantly challenges you, interests you, and allows you to work holistically with clients of all ages, at all stages of illness and wellness; one that absolutely demands the use of your critical-thinking skills. And you may decide, when you finish your public health nursing course, that you have found your career choice. Even if you are not drawn away from acute care nursing, your community health nursing experience will give you a deeper understanding of the people for whom you provide care—where and how they live, the family and cultural dynamics at play, and the problems they will face when discharged from your care. You will also discover myriad community agencies and resources to better assist you in providing a continuum of care for your clients. Finding out begins with understanding the concepts of community and health.

This chapter provides an overview of the basic concepts of community and health, the components of public health practice, and the salient characteristics of contemporary public health nursing practice, so that you can enter this specialty area of nursing in concert with its intentions. The opportunities and challenges of community health nursing will become even more apparent as the chapter progresses. The discussion of the concepts and theories that make public health nursing an important specialty within nursing begins with the broader field of community health, which provides the context for public health nursing practice.

COMMUNITY HEALTH

Human beings are social creatures. All of us, with rare exception, live out our lives in the company of other people. An Eskimo lives in a small, tightly knit community of close relatives; a rural Mexican may live in a small village with hardly more than 200 members. In contrast, someone from New York City might be a member of many overlapping communities, such as professional societies, a political party, a religious group, a cultural society, a neighborhood, and the city itself. Even those who try to escape community membership always begin their lives in some type of group, and they usually continue to depend on groups for material and emotional support. Communities are an essential and permanent feature of the human experience.

The communities in which we live and work have a profound influence on our collective health and well-being (Edwards & Tsouros, 2008). And, from the beginning, people have attempted to create healthier communities. Here are three recent examples:

- Before the historic Surgeon General's *Report on Smoking and Health*, it was common to see people smoking on television, at work, in restaurants, and even in physician offices (*Morbidity and Mortality*

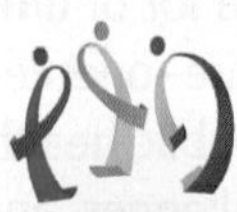

PERSPECTIVES STUDENT VOICE

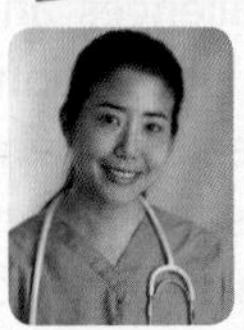

I was really terrified when I got to my community health rotation and found that I had to go to people's homes and knock on their doors! I was going to graduate in a few months, and I felt really comfortable in the hospital.... I knew the routines and the machines well. Now, I had to actually find houses and apartments in an area of the city I would normally never venture into! And, it wasn't clear to me what I was supposed to do! I didn't have much equipment—a baby scale, a blood pressure cuff, a stethoscope, a thermometer, and a paper tape measure—that was all! I was told to go visit this 16-year-old mother who had a 4-month-old baby, and to monitor the baby's progress. I don't even have children! What can I tell her? And, besides, she is a teenager who "knows it all." My clinical instructor told me to "build a relationship with her" and to "gain trust and rapport." That is hard to do when you are scared to death! I was afraid of her responses, of being out in that part of the city alone, and of trying to answer questions without anyone there to turn to. But, I wanted to get through nursing school, so I drove over there and knocked on her door. I was shocked to see the condition of the apartment building in which she lived. Peeling paint, loud music, trash everywhere, and strange characters at every turn. When she answered the door, she seemed uninterested—or maybe a little defensive. I told her who I was and why I was there, and she motioned me inside and pointed toward the baby, propped up on the tattered couch. I spent the next 15 weeks visiting Anna and her baby: weighing and measuring the baby, doing a Denver II and sharing the results with Anna, helping her schedule appointments for immunizations, listening to Anna's story of abuse and abandonment, and realizing that what I was doing was actually exciting and rewarding. By the end of my rotation, I was truly going to miss Anna and little José! He always smiled at me, and I enjoyed "playing" with him as I instructed her about baby-proofing her apartment, finding resources for food and clothing, and getting birth control. We even talked about how she could finish high school. I thought about Anna and José occasionally, when young mothers would bring their babies into the emergency department, where I worked after graduation. I learned from my community health nursing rotation that I needed to look beyond the bravado of a teenage mother and try to "connect" with her in order to assure that she would follow through with the antibiotics and antipyretics we were prescribing for her baby's dangerously high fever and serious infection. A year and a half after I graduated, one day when it had been particularly hectic but was now calming down, I glanced up to see Anna and José. She looked so relieved to see me! She was frantic with worry about the serious burn José had on his right hand. The other nurses were mumbling about "child abuse" and how "irresponsible teen mothers always were." I learned that Anna had left José with a neighbor for an hour while she visited a nearby high school to see about getting her GED. The older neighbor was not used to dealing with a busy toddler, and she had left the handle of a pan of refried beans where José could reach it. The team treated José's burn, and I gave Anna instructions for follow-up care. The bond we had developed was still there. She trusted me, and I knew that she would follow through with the instructions. I also knew that the other nurses who were making comments about her did not know Anna's circumstances. I feel that I am a more effective ER nurse because of the things I learned in community health. Someday, when I get tired of the hospital, I may try working as a Public Health Nurse. You never know!

Courtney, Age 25

Weekly Report [MMWR], 2004). Since that report linked tobacco to disease and death more than 40 years ago, much has changed in our living spaces. In most states, it is now uncommon to see smoking in public places, and smokers are often relegated to outdoor smoking areas. With the assistance of the Master Settlement Agreement negotiated by state attorneys general and the tobacco industry in 1999, $206 billion has been given to states to promote smoking cessation; create smoke-free environments in the workplace, restaurants, and bars; and develop antismoking public information campaigns (Curley, 2010; *Milestones in Public Health*, 2006). Along with policy changes and settlements, public awareness has been raised about the harmful effects of secondhand smoke (Public Health Institute, 2010a). However, smoking still causes around 443,000 deaths annually in the United States, and over 46 million Americans continue to smoke cigarettes (Curley, 2010). Smoking has been shown to triple the risk of dying from heart disease among middle-aged men and women (Centers for Disease Control & Prevention [CDC], 2009). While total U.S. consumption of tobacco products has dropped, states with the lowest incidence of smoking (around 14%), like California, New Jersey, and Maryland, have been successful in implementing strategies suggested by the CDC (e.g., raising prices of tobacco products, enacting laws for smoke-free public spaces, limiting tobacco advertising while utilizing antismoking campaigns, limiting access to tobacco vending machines or sales to minors, smoking cessation programs) (Curley, 2010). California has documented fewer deaths from heart disease and incidences of lung cancer since implementing these strategies (Curley, 2010). Other states that have not uniformly implemented these strategies, like West Virginia, Kentucky, and Missouri, have smoking rates between 25% and 26% (Curley, 2010). Even though only 22% of Americans now report that they are current smokers, as a whole, they generally oppose an outright ban on smoking (81% per a 2009 Gallup poll), leaving a toehold for tobacco companies to promote the individual's right to choose smoking over the public's right to the health benefits of banning tobacco (Gallup, 2011).

- More than 20 million American children and adults live with asthma (Asthma & Allergy Foundation of America [AAFA], n.d.). Evidence of a connection between asthma attacks and community environments has been demonstrated both in the United States and abroad. In Harlem, 25% of the children were reported to have asthma—twice the expected rate. Public health officials note chronic environmental factors as a possible cause for increased asthma cases: pollution from high-traffic areas, secondhand smoke in homes, as well as poor living conditions characterized by dust mites, mold, industrial air pollution, mouse and cockroach droppings, and animal dander (Krisberg, 2006; Wisnivesky et al., 2008). For 2010, the city named "asthma capital" of the United States was Richmond, Virginia (AAFA, 2010, p. 1). Over half of the asthma capitals were in the South, largely due to the lack of smoke-free legislation in many tobacco-producing states, along with poor air quality and high pollen counts. To further make the case for a connection between environment and asthma, in Atlanta, the 1996 Olympics brought an unexpected benefit: a 42% reduction in asthma-related emergency room visits. With the Olympic congestion downtown, Atlanta restricted traffic and thus improved air quality. The same outcomes were experienced with the Beijing Olympics. Internationally, Singapore also noticed a reduction in emergency room visits for asthma after it restricted automobile traffic in its central business district (Li, Wang, Zhang, Lin, & Yang, 2011; *Milestones in Public Health*, 2006).
- In a local effort to address the problem of childhood obesity, Santa Clara county—where one in four children are obese or overweight—passed an ordinance that sets standards for toys included with children's restaurant meals. It simply requires that the meals that include the toys meet basic nutritional standards. It does not ban toys (Baxter, 2010). However, the fast food industry has opposed this effort, as they spend over $360 million on toys that encourage kids and parents to purchase 1.2 billion kid's meals annually. Second only to television advertising targeted to children, the toys given away with kid's meals are a substantial expenditure by the fast food industry. And, interestingly, 10 of 12 meals with the highest calorie levels were found to include toys—indicating that these toys are used to market meals to children that may promote obesity (Public Health Institute, 2010c). So, lawmakers counter that toys should only be used as an incentive for kids to purchase meals with lower sugar, sodium, fat, and calories (Baxter, 2010). The community of Santa Clara, California took a stand to improve their environment in order to address a serious health problem that is affecting their population.

Systems theory, advanced by biologist Ludwig von Bertalanffy in the 1940s and modified by Ross Ashby in the 1950s, proposes that systems are "open to and interact with their environments" (Heylighen & Joslyn, 1992, para. 1). As systems theory reminds us that a whole is greater than the sum of its parts, the health of a community is more than the sum of the health of its individual citizens. A community that achieves a high level of wellness is composed of healthy citizens, functioning in an environment that protects and promotes health. Public health, as a specialty of nursing practice, seeks to provide organizational structure, a broad set of resources, and the collaborative activities needed to accomplish the goal of an optimally healthy community.

When you work in hospitals or other acute care settings, your primary focus is the individual patient. Patients' families are often viewed as ancillary. Public health, however, broadens the view to focus on families, aggregates (see p. 8), populations, and the community at large. The community becomes the recipient of service, and health becomes the product. Viewed from another perspective, public health is concerned with the interchange between population groups and their total environment, and with the impact of that interchange on collective health. The narrow view of the solitary patient, so common in acute care nursing, is expanded to encompass a much wider vista.

Although many believe that health and illness are individual issues, evidence indicates that they are also community issues, and that the world is a community. The spread of the human immunodeficiency virus (HIV) pandemic, nationally and internationally, is a dramatic and tragic case in point, having spread across the globe with 2.7 million new infections annually (Hitt, 2010). Other community, national, and global concerns include the rising incidence and prevalence of tuberculosis (Poltzer, 2008), the "critical and urgent international public health problem" of cardiovascular disease (McDermott, 2007, p. 1254), the rise in antibiotic resistance that has led to calls for global treaties to combat resistant strains (Anomaly, 2010), terrorism, and pollution-driven environmental hazards. While the United States and other developed nations fight rising rates of obesity, many countries in Africa battle malnutrition and starvation. Communities can influence the spread of disease, provide barriers to protect members from health hazards, organize ways to combat outbreaks of infectious disease, and promote practices that contribute to individual and collective health (American Nurses Association [ANA], 2007; Institute of Medicine [IOM], 2002; County Health Rankings, 2010).

Many different professionals work in community health to form a complex team. The city planner designing an urban renewal project necessarily becomes involved in community health. The social worker providing counseling about child abuse or working with adolescent substance abusers is involved in public or community health. A physician treating clients affected by a sudden outbreak of hepatitis and seeking to find the source is engaged in public health practice. Prenatal clinics, meals for the elderly, genetic counseling centers, and educational programs for the early detection of cancer all are part of the public health effort.

The professional nurse is an integral member of this team, a linchpin and a liaison between physicians, social workers, government officials, and law enforcement officers. Public health nurses work in every conceivable kind of community agency, from a state public health department to a community-based advocacy group. Their duties range from examining infants in a well-baby clinic, to teaching elderly stroke victims in their homes, to carrying out epidemiologic research or engaging in health policy analysis and decision making. Despite its breadth, however, public health nursing is a specialized practice. It combines all of the basic elements of professional clinical nursing with public health and community practice. Together, we will examine the unique contribution made by community health nursing to our health care system.

Community health and public health share many features. Both are organized community efforts aimed at the promotion, protection, and preservation of the public's health. Historically, as a practice specialty, public health has been associated primarily with the efforts of official or government entities—for example, federal, state, or local tax-supported health agencies that target a wide range of health issues. In contrast, private health efforts or nongovernmental organizations (NGOs), such as those of the American Lung Association or the American Cancer Society, work toward solving selected health problems. The latter augments the former. Currently, community health practice encompasses both approaches and works collaboratively with all health agencies and efforts, public or private, which are concerned with the public's health. In this text, community health practice refers to a focus on specific, designated communities. It is a part of the larger public health effort and recognizes the fundamental concepts and principles of public health as its birthright and foundation for practice.

In the IOM's landmark publication, *The Future of the Public's Health* (1998), the mission of public health is defined simply as "fulfilling society's interest in assuring conditions in which people can be healthy" (p. 7). (See "Perspectives: Public Health Nursing Instructor.") Winslow's classic 1920 definition of **public health** still holds true and forms the basis for our understanding of community health in this text:

> Public health... is the science and art of preventing disease, prolonging life, and promoting health and efficiency through organized community efforts for the sanitation of the environment, the control of communicable infections, the education of the individual in personal hygiene, the organization of medical and nursing services for the early diagnosis and preventive treatment of disease, and the development of the social machinery to insure everyone a standard of living adequate for the maintenance of health (Clinton County Health Department, n.d., p. 1).

PERSPECTIVES
PUBLIC HEALTH NURSING INSTRUCTOR

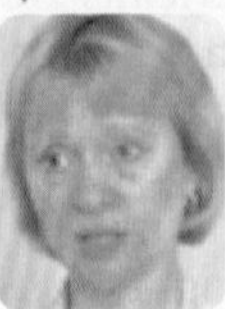

When I first introduce the topic of public health, I ask students "Why do people end up in the hospital?" Many of them give the usual answers—"They need surgery," "They get in accidents," and the like. Then I tell them the *Story of Jason*:

"Why is Jason in the hospital? (Because he has a bad infection in his leg.)

But why does he have an infection? (Because he has a cut on his leg and it got infected.) But why does he have a cut on his leg? (Because he was playing in the junkyard next to his apartment building and there was some sharp, jagged steel there that he fell on.)

But why was he playing in a junkyard? (Because his neighborhood is kind of run-down. A lot of kids play there, and there is no one to supervise them.)

But why does he live in that neighborhood? (Because his parents can't afford a nicer place to live.)

But why can't his parents afford a nicer place to live? (Because his Dad is unemployed and his Mom is sick.)

But why is his Dad unemployed? (Because he doesn't have much education and he can't find a job.) But why...?" (Public Health Agency of Canada, 1999. *Toward a Healthy Future: Second Report on the Health of Canadians*, p. vii.)

And, they suddenly become more aware of the complex social and economic issues that affect health.

More recent and concise definitions of public health include "an effort organized by society to protect, promote, and restore the people's health" (Trust for America's Health, 2006, p. 27) and "the health of the population as a whole rather than medical health care, which focuses on treatment of the individual ailment" (Public Health Data Standards Consortium, 2006, p. 120). A Web site sponsored by the Association of Schools of Public Health with support from Pfizer Public Health, *What is Public Health?* (www.whatispublichealth.org, n.d.), provides some interesting videos and a quiz about this topic and also proffers this definition:

> Public health is the science and art of protecting and improving the health of communities through education, promotion of healthy lifestyles, and research for disease and injury prevention.
>
> Public health helps improve the health and wellbeing of people in local communities and across our nation.
>
> Public health helps people who are less fortunate to achieve a healthier lifestyle.
>
> Public health works to prevent health problems before they occur.
>
> Public health professionals achieve true job satisfaction by knowing they are making the world a better place (para. 1).

The core public health functions have been delineated as assessment, policy development, and assurance. These are discussed in more detail in Chapter 3.

Given this basic understanding of public health, the concept of community health can be defined. **Community health** is the identification of needs, along with the protection and improvement of collective health, within a geographically defined area.

One of the challenges public health practice faces is to remain responsive to the community's health needs. As a result, its structure is complex; numerous health services and programs are currently available or will be developed. Examples include health education, family planning, accident prevention, environmental protection, immunization, nutrition, early periodic screening and developmental testing, school programs, mental health services, occupational health programs, and the care of vulnerable populations. The Department of Homeland Security, for example, is a community health and safety agency developed in the aftermath of the terrorist attacks on New York City and Washington, DC, on September 11, 2001.

Community health practice, a part of public health, is sometimes misunderstood. Even many health professionals think of community health practice in limiting terms such as sanitation programs, health clinics in poverty areas, or massive public awareness campaigns to prevent communicable disease. Although these are a part of its ever-broadening focus, community health practice is much more. To understand the nature and significance of this field, it is necessary to more closely examine the concept of community and the concept of health.

THE CONCEPT OF COMMUNITY

The concepts of community and health together provide the foundation for understanding community health. Broadly defined, a community is a collection of people who share some important feature of their lives. In this text, the term **community** refers to a collection of people who interact with one another and whose common interests or characteristics form the basis for a sense of unity or belonging. It can be a society of people holding common rights and privileges (e.g., citizens of a town), sharing common interests (e.g., a community of farmers), or living under the same laws and regulations (e.g., a prison community). The function of any community includes its members' collective sense of belonging and their shared identity, values, norms, communication, and common interests and concerns (Anderson & McFarlane, 2012). Some communities—for example, a tiny village in Appalachia—are composed of people who share almost everything. They live in the same location, work at a limited type and number of jobs, attend the same churches, and make use of the sole health clinic with its visiting physician and nurse. Other communities, such as members of Mothers Against Drunk Driving (MADD) or the community of professional nursing organizations, are large, scattered, and composed of individuals who share only a common interest and involvement in a certain goal. Although most communities of people share many aspects of their experience, it is useful to identify three types of communities that have relevance to community health practice: geographic, common interest, and health problem or solution.

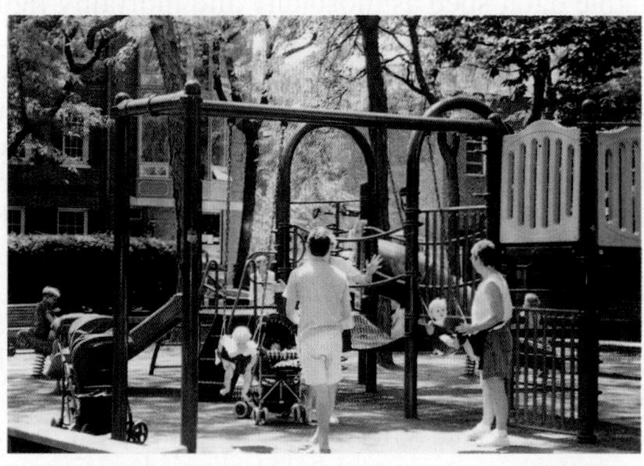

Geographic Community

A community often is defined by its geographic boundaries and thus is called a **geographic community**. A city, town, or neighborhood is a geographic community. Consider the community of Hayward, Wisconsin. Located in northwestern Wisconsin, it is set in the north woods environment, far removed from any urban center and in a climatic zone characterized by extremely harsh winters. With a population of approximately 2,200, it is considered a rural community. The population has certain identifiable characteristics, such as age and sex ratios, and its size fluctuates with the seasons: summers bring hundreds of tourists and seasonal residents. Hayward is a social system as well as a geographic location. The families, schools, hospital, churches, stores, and government institutions are linked in a complex network. This community, like others, has an informal power structure. It has a communication system that includes gossip, the newspaper, the "co-op" store bulletin board, and the radio station. In one sense, then, a community consists of a collection of people located in a specific place and is made up of institutions organized into a social system.

Local communities such as Hayward vary in size. A few miles south of Hayward lie several other communities, including Northwoods Beach and Round Lake; these three, along with other towns and isolated farms, form a larger community called Sawyer County. If a nurse worked for a health agency serving only Hayward, that community would be of primary concern; however, if the nurse worked for the Sawyer County Health Department, this larger community would be the focus. A public health nurse employed by the State Health Department in Madison, Wisconsin, would have an interest in Sawyer County and Hayward, but only as part of the larger community of Wisconsin.

Frequently, a single part of a city can be treated as a community. Cities are often broken down into *census tracts*, or neighborhoods. In Seattle, for example, the district near the waterfront forms a community of many transient and homeless people. In New York City, the neighborhood called Harlem is a community, as is the Haight-Ashbury district of San Francisco.

In community health, it is useful to identify a geographic area as a community. A community demarcated by geographic boundaries, such as a city or county, becomes a clear target for the analysis of health needs. Available data, such as morbidity and mortality figures, can augment assessment studies to form the basis for planning health programs. Media campaigns and other health education efforts can readily reach intended audiences. Examples include distributing educational information on safe sex, self-protection, the dangers of substance abuse, or where to seek shelter from abuse and violence. A geographic community is easily mobilized for action. Groups can be formed to carry out intervention and prevention efforts that address needs specific to that community. Such efforts might include more stringent policies on day care, shelters for battered women, work site safety programs in local hazardous industries, or improved sexuality education in the schools. Furthermore, health actions can be enhanced through the support of politically powerful individuals and resources present in a geographic community.

On a larger scale, the world can be considered as a global community. Indeed, it is very important to view the world this way. Borders of countries change with political upheaval. Communicable diseases are not aware of arbitrary political boundaries. A person can travel around the world in <24 hours, and so can diseases. Children starving in Africa affect persons living in the United States. Political uprisings in the Middle East have an impact on people in Western countries. Floods or tsunamis in Southeast Asia or volcano eruptions in Iceland have meaning for other national economies. The world is one large community that needs to work together to ensure a healthy today and a healthier and safer tomorrow. **Global health** has become a dominant phrase in international public health circles. Globalization raises an expectation of health for all, for if good health is possible in one part of the world, the forces of globalization should allow it elsewhere (Skolnik, 2008). Governments need to work together to develop a broader base for international relations and collaborative strategies that will place greater emphasis on global health security. We learn more about global health issues and the global community in Chapter 16.

Common-Interest Community

A community also can be identified by a common interest or goal. A collection of people, even if they are widely scattered geographically, can have an interest or goal that binds the members together. This is called a *common-interest community*. The members of a church in a large metropolitan area, the members of an international nursing professional organization, and women who have had mastectomies are all common-interest communities. Sometimes, within a certain geographic area, a group of people may develop a sense of community by promoting their common interest. Disabled individuals scattered throughout a large city may emerge as a community through a common interest in promoting adherence to federal guidelines for wheelchair access, parking spaces, toilet facilities, elevators, or other services for the disabled. The residents of an industrial community may develop a common interest in air or water pollution issues, whereas others who work but do not live in the area may not share that interest. Communities form to protect the rights of children, stop violence against women, clean up the environment, promote the arts, preserve historical sites, protect endangered species, develop a smoke-free environment, or provide support after a crisis. The kinds of shared interests that lead to the formation of communities vary widely.

Common-interest communities whose focus is a health-related issue can join with community health agencies to promote their agendas. A group's single-minded commitment is a mobilizing force for action. Many successful prevention and health promotion efforts, including improved services and increased community awareness of specific problems, have resulted from the work of common-interest communities. MADD is one example. In 1980, after a repeat drunk-driving offender killed her 13-year-old daughter Cari, Candace Lightner gathered with a group of outraged mothers at a restaurant in Sacramento, California. Across the country, another mother was soon touched by a similar tragedy. Cindi Lamb's five-and-a-half-month-old infant daughter became a quadriplegic at the hands of a repeat drunk driver. Within a short time, the two women joined forces to form MADD, and 2 years later, President Ronald Reagan organized a Presidential Task Force on drunk driving and invited MADD to participate. With media attention and perseverance, MADD quickly grew to over 100 chapters across the United States and Canada and worked to establish a federal legal minimum drinking age and standard blood alcohol levels of 0.08%, as well as to defend sobriety checkpoints before the Supreme Court. The National Highway Transportation and Safety Administration credited MADD when they released the 1994 figures showing a 30-year low in alcohol-related traffic deaths. Even though our U.S. numbers have dropped considerably, still, every 45 minutes someone is killed by a drunk driver, and every minute of every day, one person is injured (Morris, 2010). MADD now claims more than 3 million members worldwide, and is one of the largest and most successful common-interest organizations (*Milestones in Public Health*, 2006; Morris, 2010).

Community of Solution

A type of community encountered frequently in community health practice is a group of people who come together to solve a problem that affects all of them. The shape of this community varies with the nature of the problem, the size of the geographic area affected, and the number of resources needed to address the problem. Such a community has been called a *community of solution*. For example, a water pollution problem may involve several counties whose agencies and personnel must work together to control upstream water supply, industrial waste disposal, and city water treatment. This group of counties forms a community of solution focusing on a health problem. In another instance, several schools may collaborate with law enforcement and health agencies, as well as legislators and policy makers, to study patterns of substance abuse among students and

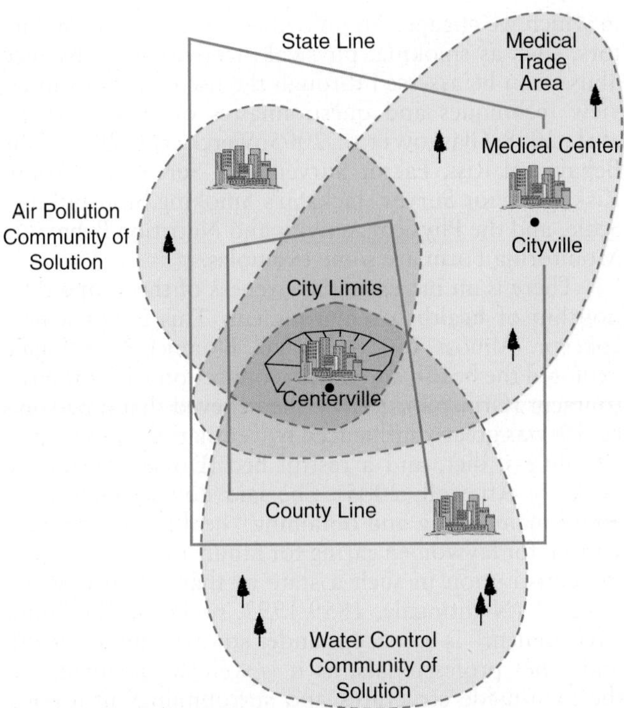

FIGURE 1-1. A city's communities of solution. State, county, and city boundaries (*solid lines*) may have little or no bearing on health solution boundaries (*dashed lines*).

design possible preventive approaches. The boundaries of this community of solution form around the schools, agencies, and political figures involved. Figure 1-1 depicts some communities of solution related to a single city.

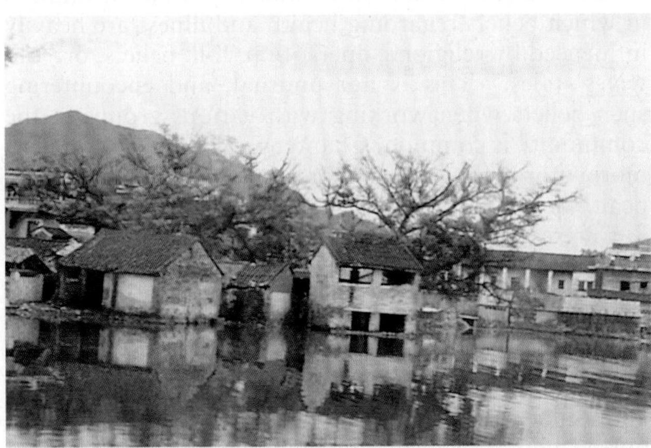

In recent years, communities of solution have formed in many cities to attack the spread of HIV/AIDS, and have worked with community members to assess public safety and security and create plans to make the community a safer place in which to live. Public health agencies, social service groups, schools, and media personnel have banded together to create public awareness of dangers that are present and to promote preventive behaviors (e.g., childhood obesity). Former President Bill Clinton organized the Alliance for a Healthier Generation in partnership with the American Heart Association, and they recently announced an agreement with beverage companies such as Coca-Cola and PepsiCo. Vending machines that once stocked calorie-laden sodas now have supplies of low-calorie soft drinks and sports drinks, juices with no added sugar, tea, low or fat-free milk, and water (American Cancer Society, 2008). The American Academy of Pediatrics issued a policy statement about the health effects of soft drink consumption and urged school districts to restrict sales in 2004, reaffirming it in 2009 (Committee on School Health, 2009). Although soft drinks are not the only culprit in the childhood obesity epidemic, this is an important step in helping kids make healthier choices (Engelhard, Garson, & Dorn, 2009; Public Health Institute, 2010b). And the efforts are bearing fruit. In 2008, 63% of schools limited carbonated soft drinks—up from 38% in 2006. The amount of sodas purchased by students dropped from 12 to 8 ounces a week (Reuters, 2010). A community of solution is an important conduit for change in community health.

Populations and Aggregates

The three types of communities just discussed underscore the meaning of the concept of community: in each instance, a collection of people chose to interact with one another because of common interests, characteristics, or goals. The concept of population has a different meaning. In this text, the term **population** refers to all of the people occupying an area, or to all of those who share one or more characteristics. In contrast to a community, a population is made up of people who do not necessarily interact with one another and do not necessarily share a sense of belonging to that group. A population may be defined geographically, such as the population of the United States or a city's population. This designation of a population is useful in community health for epidemiologic study and for collecting demographic data for purposes such as health planning. A population also may be defined by common qualities or characteristics, such as the elderly population, the homeless population, or a particular racial or ethnic group. In community health, this meaning becomes useful when a specific group of people (e.g., homeless individuals) is targeted for intervention; the population's common characteristics (e.g., the health-related problems of homelessness) become a major focus of the intervention.

In this text, the term **aggregate** refers to a mass or grouping of distinct individuals who are considered as a whole, and who are loosely associated with one another. It is a broader term that encompasses many different-sized groups. Both communities and populations are types of aggregates. The aggregate focus, or a concern for groupings of people in contrast to individual health care, becomes a distinguishing feature of community health practice. Community health nurses may work with aggregates such as pregnant and parenting teens, elderly adults with diabetes, or gay men with HIV/AIDS. Unit 6 discusses public health nursing with aggregates and Unit 7 discusses vulnerable populations.

Most registered nurses (RNs) in the United States work in hospitals, and although that number had dropped, a 6% jump was noted between 2004 and 2008. These nurses most often work with individuals, not aggregates or communities. However, over 14% of RNs work in public or community health and home health settings (Health Resources & Services Administration [HRSA], 2010) and have a greater focus on families and communities. With the recent health care reform legislation, the nursing workforce in public health, home visitation programs, and nurse-managed health centers will be expanded (American Nurses Association [ANA], 2010). Dr. David Satcher, former U.S. Surgeon General, has remarked:

> Nurses have always been ahead of their time in their focus on prevention and health promotion. As we move toward a more balanced health system with more focus and support for health promotion and disease prevention, the role of nurses will be more significant than ever before (Robert Wood Johnson Foundation, 2009, p. 2).

Because of public health nursing's focus on communities, aggregates, and families, new nursing and health care delivery systems may be developed that are more gainful and effective in preventing health problems that require expensive hospitalizations.

Community health workers, including community health nurses, need to define the community targeted for study and intervention: Who are the people who comprise the community? Where are they located, and what are their characteristics? A clear delineation of the community or population must be established before the nurse can assess needs and design interventions. The complex nature of communities also must be understood. What are the characteristics of the people in terms of age, gender, race, socioeconomic level, and health status? How does the community interact with other communities? What is its history? What are its resources? Is the community undergoing rapid change, and, if so, what are the changes? These questions, as well as the tools needed to assess a community for health purposes, are discussed in detail in Chapter 15.

THE CONCEPT OF HEALTH

Health, in the abstract, refers to a person's physical, mental, and spiritual state; it can be positive (as being in good health) or negative (as being in poor health). Optimal health is defined as "a dynamic balance of physical, emotional, social, spiritual, and intellectual health" (O'Donnell, 2009, p. iv). In a classic article from 1997, Sarrachi describes health as a "basic and universal human right" (p. 1409). The World Health Organization (WHO) defines health positively as "a state of complete physical, mental, and social wellbeing and not merely the absence of disease or infirmity" (Ustin & Jakob, 2005, p. 802). Our understanding of the concept of health builds on this classic definition. **Health**, in this text, refers to a holistic state of wellbeing, which includes soundness of mind, body, and spirit. Community health practitioners place a strong emphasis on **wellness**, which includes this definition of health, but also incorporates the capacity to develop a person's potential to lead a fulfilling and productive life—one that can be measured in terms of *quality of life*. Today, our health is greatly affected by the lifestyles we lead and the risk behaviors in which we engage. An individual's behavioral risk factors, such as smoking, physical inactivity, or substance abuse, can be assessed through the use of various interview techniques and questionnaires or surveys (Aspy et al., 2008; Glasgow et al., 2005; Werch et al., 2007). The Behavioral Risk Factor Surveillance Survey, the Youth Risk Behavior Survey, Jackson's Smoking Susceptibility Scale, and the Physical Activity and Nutrition Behaviors Monitoring Form are some examples.

There is an increasing awareness of the strong relationship of health to environment. This is not a new concept. Almost 150 years ago, Florence Nightingale explored the health and illness connection with the environment (Grinspun, 2010). She believed that a person's health was greatly influenced by ventilation, noise, light, cleanliness, diet, and a restful bed (Dossey, Selanders, Beck, & Attewell, 2005). She laid down simple rules about maintaining and obtaining "health," which were written for laywomen caring for family members to "put the constitution in such a state as that it will have no disease" (Nightingale, 1859/1992, preface). The "built environment" is a concept under study by public health and other professionals, as it is well documented that the man-made structures and surroundings in a community (e.g., highways and bike paths, parks and open spaces, public buildings, and housing developments) have an impact on the health of individuals and populations (CDC, 2011; Perera, 2008; Rauh, Frank, Engelke, & Washington, 2003). Environment's relationship to health is discussed in more detail in Chapter 9.

In some cultures, health is viewed differently. Some see it as the freedom from and absence of evil. Illness may be seen as punishment for being bad or doing evil (Galanti, 2008). Many individuals come from families in which beliefs regarding health and illness are heavily influenced by religion, superstition, folk beliefs, or "old wives' tales." This is not unusual, and encountering such beliefs when working with various groups in the community is common. Chapter 5 explores these beliefs more thoroughly for a better understanding of how health beliefs influence every aspect of a person's life.

Prerequisites for health were outlined in the Ottawa Charter (WHO, 2010b) as "peace, shelter, education, food, income, a stable eco-system, sustainable resources, social justice, and equity" (para. 4). Although health is widely accepted as desirable, the nature of health is often ambiguous. Consumers and providers often define health and wellness in different ways. To clarify the concept for nurses who are considering community health practice, the distinguishing features of health are briefly characterized here; the implications of this concept for professionals in the field can then be examined more fully.

The Health Continuum: Wellness–Illness

Society suggests a polarized or "either/or" way of thinking about health: people either are well or they are ill. Yet wellness is a relative concept, not an absolute, and **illness** is a state of being *relatively* unhealthy. The study of factors affecting health and illness is known as epidemiology, and it is discussed in Chapter 7. There are many levels and degrees of wellness and illness, from a robust 70-year-old woman who is fully active and functioning at an optimal level of wellness, to a 70-year-old man with end-stage renal disease whose health is characterized as frail. Someone recovering from pneumonia may be mildly ill, whereas a teenaged boy with functional limitations because of episodic depression may be described as mildly well.

The continuum, however, can change. The Human Genome Project, begun in 1990 and completed in 2000, and the genomic era of health care it generated may skew the health continuum toward the healthy end (*Milestones in Public Health*, 2006; National Human Genome Research Institute, 2009). **Genomics**, the identification and plotting of human genes and the study of the interaction of genes with each other and the environment, will alter how we view and treat disease (National Human Genome Research Institute, 2009). Intervention services can be individually designed based on genetic findings, and client lifestyle modifications may be recommended from birth—a very powerful type of preventive health care. **Pharmacogenomics** will permit the design of drugs tailored to a person's genetic makeup or to a targeted disease. Already, over 350 biotech products are in clinical trials. The capacity for this kind of health care will be a reality over the next decade, and we must guard against limiting access to this type of care and permitting further disenfranchisement of vulnerable populations (National Human Genome Research Institute, 2009; Ray, 2010). Other innovations in **epigenetics**, the study of human gene activity changes not involving alterations in DNA that can be passed from one generation to the next, may be even more astounding. Epigenetic marks can turn genes off and on and help explain why "environmental factors like diet, stress, and prenatal nutrition can make an imprint on genes… passed from one generation to the next" (Cloud, 2010, para. 8). Lifestyle choices like overeating, smoking, and drug use may influence genes that affect obesity and longevity, for instance, to be more strongly or weakly expressed. Drugs have already been developed for some epigenetic marks (e.g., blood malignancies, tumors), and this area of science holds promise in discovering why, for instance, autism is more frequently found in boys or why one twin develops asthma when the other does not. The Human Epigenome Project has begun, but will take much more time and technological advances in order to achieve success than the Human Genome Project (Cloud, 2010).

Because health involves a range of degrees from optimal health at one end to total disability or death at the other (Fig. 1-2), it often is described as a continuum. This **health continuum** applies not only to individuals, but also to families and communities. A nurse might speak of a

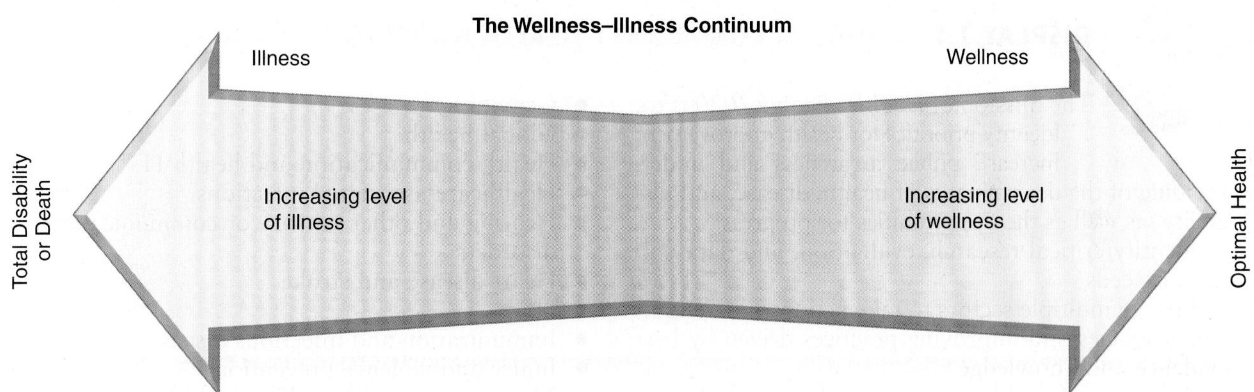

The level (degree) of illness increases as one moves toward total disability or death; the level of wellness increases as one moves toward optimal health. This continuum shows the relative nature of health. At any given time a person can be placed at some point along the continuum.

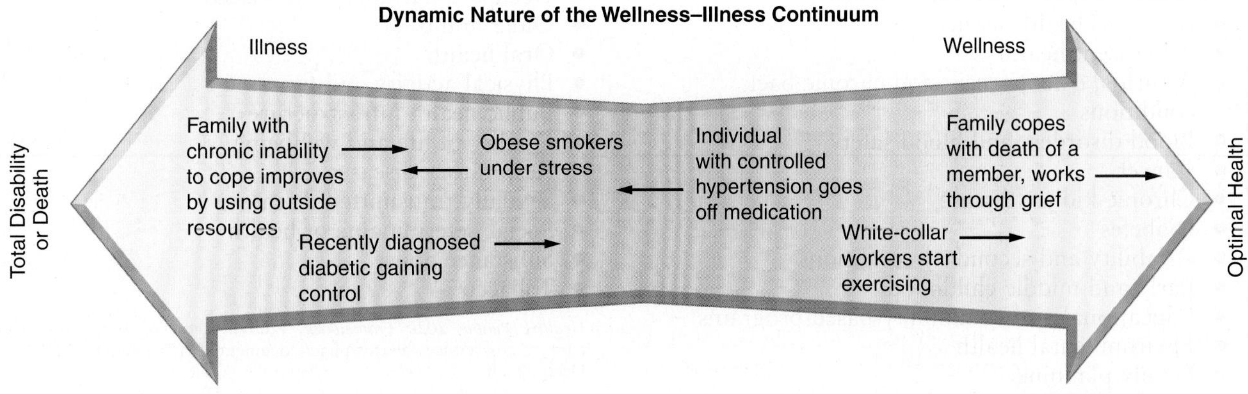

A person's relative health is usually in a state of flux, either improving or deteriorating. This diagram of the wellness-illness continuum shows several examples of people in changing states of health.

FIGURE 1-2. The health continuum.

dysfunctional family, meaning one that is experiencing a relative degree of illness or altered functioning; or, a healthy family might be described as one that exhibits many wellness characteristics, such as effective communication and conflict resolution, as well as the ability to effectively work together and use resources appropriately. More information on families is included in Unit 5. Likewise, a community, as a collection of people, may be described in terms of degrees of wellness or illness. The health of an individual, family, group, or community moves back and forth along this continuum throughout the lifespan. Healthy people make healthy communities and a healthy society. The Declaration of Alma Ata, which took place in 1978, noted that health is a "fundamental human right" and that the level of health must be raised for all countries in order for any society to improve their health (WHO, 2010a, para. 2).

By thinking of health relatively, as a matter of degree, the scope of nursing practice can be broadened to focus on preventing illness or disability and promoting wellness. Traditionally, most health care has focused on treatment of acute and chronic conditions at the illness end of the continuum. Gradually, the emphasis is shifting to focus on the wellness end of the continuum, as outlined in the government document, *Healthy People 2020* (U.S. Department of Health and Human Services [USDHHS], 2011). This effort aims to improve the health of American citizens by establishing objectives and benchmarks that can be monitored over time. There have been Healthy People objectives for 2000, 2010, and now for 2020. The four overarching goals of *Healthy People 2020* are to:

- Attain high-quality, longer lives free of preventable disease, disability, injury, and premature death
- Achieve health equity, eliminate disparities, and improve the health of all groups
- Create social and physical environments that promote good health for all
- Promote quality of life, healthy development and healthy behaviors across all life stages (para. 5)

These goals overarch the 42 topics and objectives (see Display 1.1). The objectives are stated in measurable terms that specify targeted incidence and prevalence changes and address age, gender, and culturally vulnerable groups along with improvement in public health systems. Progress toward the *Healthy People 2010* objectives has been mixed, with preliminary data showing over 70% of objectives either met or some progress demonstrated (Koh, 2010). While our life

DISPLAY 1.1 ISSUES IN COMMUNITY HEALTH NURSING

The mission of *Healthy People 2020* is to:

Identify priorities for health improvement

Increase public awareness and understanding of the determinants of health, disease, and disability (as well as the opportunities for progress)

Identify critical research, evaluation, and data collection needs

Engage multiple sectors to take actions in strengthening policies and improving practices driven by best evidence and knowledge

Provide measurable objectives and goals applicable at the national, state and local levels (*Healthy People 2020* Framework, 2009, para.1).

Healthy People 2020 Topic Areas

- Access to health services
- Adolescent health
- Arthritis, osteoporosis, and chronic back conditions
- Blood disorders and blood safety
- Cancer
- Chronic kidney disease
- Diabetes
- Disability and secondary conditions
- Early and middle childhood
- Educational and community-based programs
- Environmental health
- Family planning
- Food safety
- Genomics
- Global health
- Health communication and health IT
- Healthcare-associated infections
- Hearing and other sensory or communication disorders
- Heart disease and stroke
- HIV
- Immunization and infectious diseases
- Injury and violence prevention
- Maternal, infant, and child health
- Medical product safety
- Mental
- Nutrition and weight status
- Occupational safety and health
- Older adults
- Oral health
- Physical activity and fitness
- Public health infrastructure
- Quality of life and wellbeing
- Respiratory diseases
- Sexually transmitted diseases
- Social determinants of health
- Substance abuse
- Tobacco

Healthy People 2020 Framework. (2009). Retrieved from http://www.cdph.ca.gov/services/boards/phac/Documents/PHAC-Summary-HP2020-Oct2009.pdf

expectancy has improved and childhood immunization rates have risen, with advancement toward reducing racial and ethnic disparities, our rates of obesity and diabetes have risen well beyond baseline levels from the previous decade (Koh, 2010). The **leading health indicators** for *Healthy People 2020*, an outcomes metric for measuring progress toward national public health goals, are found in Display 1.2.

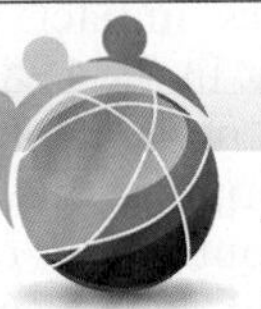

DISPLAY 1.2 LEADING HEALTH INDICATORS

The leading health indicators are used to measure the health of the nation. There are 26 indicators arranged under 12 general topics. Each of the leading health indicators has one or more objectives from *Healthy People 2010* associated with it. As a group, the leading health indicators reflect the major health concerns in the United States, and progress toward the goals derived from these will be assessed during the 2010–2020 time period. The leading health indicators were selected on the basis of their ability to motivate action, the availability of data to measure progress, and their importance as public health issues. The Federal consumer health information Web site, www.healthfinder.gov, is a good starting point for more information on these topics.

Access to Health Services

- Increase the proportions of persons with health insurance (AHS-1).
- Increase the proportion of persons who have a specific source of care (AHS-5).

Clinical Preventive Services

- Increase the proportion of adults who receive a colorectal cancer screening based on the most recent guidelines (C-16).
- Increase the proportion of adults with hypertension whose blood pressure is under control (HDS-12).
- Reduce the proportion of the diabetic population with an A1c value >9% (D-5.1).
- Increase the proportion of children aged 19 to 35 months who receive the recommended doses of DTaP, polio, MMR, Hib, hepatitis B, varicella, and PCV vaccines (IID-8).

Environmental Quality

- Reduce the number of days the Air Quality Index (AQI) exceeds 100 (EH-1).
- Reduce the proportion of children aged 3 to 11 years exposed to secondhand smoke (TU-11.1).

Injury and Violence

- Reduce fatal and nonfatal injuries (IVP-1.1).
- Reduce homicides (IVP-29).

Maternal, Infant, and Child Health

- Reduce all infant deaths (within 1 year) (MICH-1.3).
- Reduce total preterm births (MICH-9).

Mental Health

- Reduce the suicide rate (MHMD-1).
- Reduce the proportion of adolescents aged 12 to 17 years who experience major depressive episodes (MDEs) (MHMD-41).

Nutrition, Physical Activity, and Obesity

- Increase the proportion of adults who meet the objectives for aerobic physical activity and for muscle-strengthening activity (PA-2.4).
- Reduce the proportion of adults who are obese (NWS-10.4).
- Reduce the proportion of children and adolescents aged 2 to 19 years who are considered obese (NWS-10.4).
- Increase the contribution of total vegetables to the diets of the population aged 2 years and older (NWS-15.1).

Oral Health

- Increase the proportion of children, adolescents, and adults who used the oral health care system in the past 12 months (OH-7).

Reproductive and Sexual Health

- Increase the proportion of sexually active females aged 15 to 44 years who received reproductive health services in the past 12 months (FP-7.1).
- Increase the proportion of persons living with HIV who know their serostatus (HIV-13).

Social Determinants

- Increase the proportion of students who graduate with a regular diploma 4 years after starting 9th grade (AH-5.1).

Substance Abuse

- Reduce the proportion of adolescents reporting use of alcohol or any illicit drugs during the past 30 days (SA-13.1).
- Reduce the proportion of persons engaging in binge drinking during the past 30 days—adults aged 18 years and older (SA-14.3).

Tobacco

- Reduce cigarette smoking by adults (TU-1.1).
- Reduce adolescent cigarette use (past 30 days) (TU-2).

Healthy People 2020. (2011). *Leading health indicators*. Retrieved from http://www.healthypeople.gov/2020/LHI/default.aspx

Community health practice ranges across the entire health continuum; it always works to improve the degree of health in individuals, families, groups, and communities. In particular, community health practice emphasizes the promotion and preservation of wellness and the prevention of illness or disability. *Healthy People 2010* and *Healthy People 2020* emphasize that the health of an individual is linked to the health of the larger community, and that this larger community's health is related to the health of the corresponding state, and ultimately our nation (Koh, 2010).

Community characteristics of health have been described by the Centers for Disease Control as health-related quality of life indicators. Early descriptions included such things as rates of poverty and unemployment, levels of high school education and severe work disability, mortality rates, and the proportion of adolescent births (*Morbidity and Mortality Weekly Report* [*MMWR*], 2000). However, even what most people would consider lifestyle choices (e.g., dietary patterns leading to obesity, reduced levels of physical activity, smoking, alcohol consumption) have been shown to be strongly influenced by environmental factors. Canada has examined such factors as life stress, body mass index (BMI) and dietary practices, smoking and alcohol use, unemployment rate, leisure-time physical activity, number of health professionals, as well as the total health expenditures in their list of health indicators (Bambra et al., 2010; Canadian Institute for Health Information, 2009). The *Community Health Status Indicators Project* provides county-level reports related to such things as infectious and chronic diseases, health-related quality of life, behavioral risk factors, vulnerable populations, causes of death, births, and summary measures of health and health disparities (Metzler et al., 2008). How does the United States compare to other developed countries on population health indicators? (see Chapter 6 for details). *Healthy Communities* is one program sponsored by the Centers for Disease Control and Prevention (CDC, 2010). *Pioneering Healthier Communities* and *Racial and Ethnic Approaches to Community Health (REACH)* are also under the auspices of the CDC. All serve to provide resources and support for local communities to address the preventable risk factors related to chronic disease, such as poor diet, tobacco use, excessive use of alcohol, and physical inactivity (Giles, Holmes-Chavez, & Collins, 2009). A healthy community is defined as one that "continuously creates and improves both its physical and social environments, helping people to support one another in aspects of daily life and to develop to their fullest potential" (CDC, 2009, para. 1).

Another description of a healthy community, first described by Cottrell (1976) as a *competent community*, is one in which the various organizations, groups, and aggregates of people making up the community do at least four things:

1. They collaborate effectively in identifying the problems and needs of the community.
2. They achieve a working consensus on goals and priorities.
3. They agree on ways and means to implement the agreed-on goals.
4. They collaborate effectively in the required actions.

Healthy communities and healthy cities impact the health of their populations and vice versa. In the 1980s, the WHO initiated the *Healthy Cities* movement to improve the health status of urban populations. A healthy city is defined as "one that is continually creating and improving those physical and social environments and expanding those community resources that enable people to mutually support each other in performing all functions of life and in developing their maximum potential" (WHO, 2009, para. 1). The 10 key components of a healthy city are listed in Display 1.3. How many of these are found in your city or community?

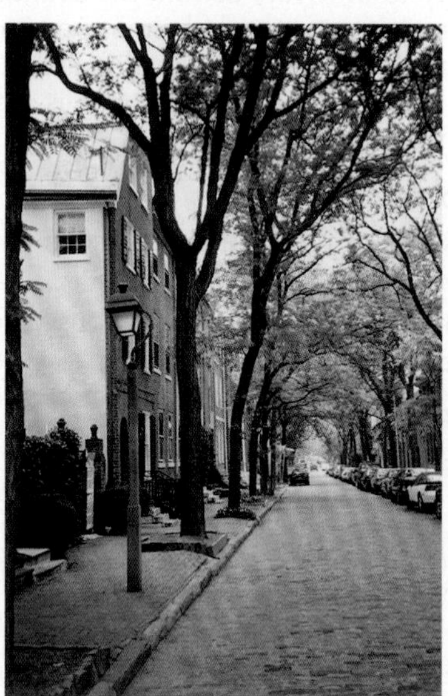

Health as a State of Being

Health refers to a state of being, including many different qualities and characteristics. An individual might be described in terms such as energetic, outgoing, enthusiastic, beautiful, caring, loving, and intense. Together, these qualities become the essence of a person's existence; they describe a state of being. Similarly, a specific geographic community, such as a neighborhood, has many characteristics. It might be characterized by the terms congested, deteriorating, unattractive, dirty, and disorganized. These characteristics suggest diminishing degrees of vitality. A third example might be a population, such as workers involved in a massive layoff, who band together to provide support and share resources to effectively seek new employment. This community shows signs of healthy adaptation and positive coping.

Health involves the total person or community. All of the dimensions of life affecting everyday

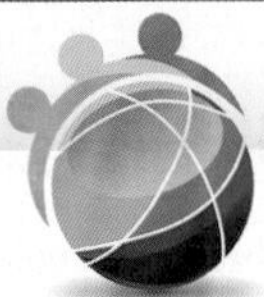

DISPLAY 1.3 WHAT ARE THE QUALITIES OF A HEALTHY CITY?

- A clean, safe physical environment of a high quality (including housing quality)
- An ecosystem that is stable now and sustainable in the long term
- A strong mutually supportive and nonexploitative community
- A high degree of participation in and control by the citizens over the decisions affecting their lives, health, and wellbeing
- The meeting of basic needs (food, water, shelter, income, safety, and work) for all the city's people
- Access by the people to a wide variety of experiences and resources, with the chance for a wide variety of contact, interaction, and communication
- A diverse, vital, and innovative economy
- The encouragement of connectedness with the past, with the cultural and biologic heritage of city dwellers, and with other groups and individuals
- A form that is compatible with and enhances the preceding characteristics
- An optimum level of appropriate public health and sickness care services, accessible to all, and high health status (high levels of positive health and low levels of disease)

Retrieved May 20, 2010 from http://www.euro.who.int/healthy-cities/introducing/20050202_4?PrinterFriendly=1&.

functioning determine an individual's or a community's health, including physical, psychological, spiritual, economic, and sociocultural experiences. All of these factors must be considered when dealing with the health of an individual or community. The approach should be holistic. A client's placement on the health continuum can be known only if the nurse considers all facets of the client's life, including not only physical and emotional status, but also the status of home, family, and work.

When considering an aggregate or group of people in terms of health, it becomes useful for intervention purposes to speak of the "health of a community." With aggregates as well as individuals, health as a state of being does not merely involve that group's physical state but also includes psychological, spiritual, and socioeconomic factors. As an example, the health of the Gulf Coast region is yet to be fully determined after a massive oil drilling spill in the Gulf of Mexico, but early estimates note that as much as $1.6 billion annually may be lost in fishing, tourism, and wetlands storm protection (Broder & Zeller, 2010) as a result of the "worst oil spill in U.S. history" (Lavelle, 2010, para. 1). The true impact—including long-term health effects—will not be known for years. It is another serious blow to this region affecting population health. This oil spill comes 5 years after hurricane Katrina made landfall on the Gulf Coast in August 2005. Widespread damage occurred after the deadliest hurricane since the 1920s, and then, only 26 days later, hurricane Rita (the fourth most intense Atlantic hurricane on record) hit near the Texas–Louisiana border. The Centers for Disease Control (CDC) estimated that more than 200,000 people converged on evacuation centers, and the country watched in anguish as the Federal Emergency Management Agency (FEMA) struggled to meet the emergency needs of the survivors. At the same time, over 1,000 deaths were attributed to Katrina, and the survivors were left with many physical, emotional, and social difficulties. The CDC estimated that almost 2 months after Katrina made landfall, more than 20% of houses did not have water, almost 56% of households had at least one member with a chronic health condition, and almost half of the adults had a level of emotional distress indicating a need for mental health services (*MMWR*, March 10, 2005; January 19, 2006). In 2009, it was estimated that more than 16,000 families were still housed in apartments provided by government assistance and almost 3,500 families were living in temporary housing or trailers (Dewan, 2009). A deadly tornado hit Joplin, Missouri in 2011 killing 159 people, destroying 7,000 homes, displacing 5,000 workers, and leaving almost 2 million cubic yards of debris (Zagier, 2011). To make matters worse, the CDC identified a necrotizing fungal soft-tissue wound infection, cutaneous mucormycosis, in 13 of the injured survivors (*MMWR*, 2011). As this community struggles to rebuild, some community members are moving out of the path of future tornados.

Prior to these recent disasters, on September 11, 2001, thousands of lives were lost in New York City's World Trade Center towers, in the Pentagon in Washington, DC, and in an airliner that crashed in Somerset County, Pennsylvania. The trauma of these events left our nation shaken. The health of many communities was dangerously poor. A surprising health effect related to these attacks was more recently reported. Researchers found that "widespread social and economic disruption" from 9/11 led to "high levels of stress and anxiety" and a statistically significant drop in male births and higher miscarriage rates. This phenomenon has been found in previous studies in other countries after natural disasters and economic downturns (Park, 2010, para. 14). We examine disaster and bioterrorism as it relates to community health nursing in Chapter 17.

Subjective and Objective Dimensions of Health

Health involves both *subjective* and *objective* dimensions; that is, it involves both how people feel (subjective) and how well they can function in their environment (objective). Subjectively, a healthy person is one who feels well and who experiences the sensation of a vital, positive state. Healthy people are full of life and vigor, capable of physical and mental productivity. They feel minimal discomfort and displeasure with the world around them. Again, people experience varying degrees of vitality and wellbeing. The state of feeling well fluctuates. Some mornings we wake up feeling more energetic and enthusiastic than we do on other mornings. How people feel varies day by day, even hour by hour; nonetheless, how they feel overall is a strong indicator of their overall state of health.

PERSPECTIVES
VOICES FROM THE COMMUNITY

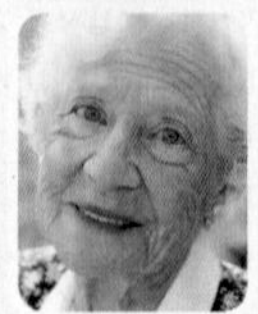

"I never thought much about being healthy or not, now that you ask. I keep busy, I cook like I'm expecting company, I have a good appetite. I really think all these so-called healthy things people suggest are fads, just so someone can get rich—like tofu and low fat this and that. Don't give me margarine, only butter, ... and skim milk, it's like drinking water! I work in my garden, I read, and I eat fresh foods, and don't talk to me about my smoking, it's the one pleasure I have left."

—Bettie, age 81

Health also involves the objective dimension of ability to function. A healthy individual or community carries out necessary activities and achieves enriching goals. Unhealthy people not only feel ill, but they are limited, to some degree, in their ability to carry out daily activities. Indeed, levels of illness or wellness are measured largely in terms of ability to function (Chan, 2010). A person confined to bed is labeled sicker than an ill person managing self-care. A family that meets its members' needs is healthier than one that has poor communication patterns and is unable to provide adequate physical and emotional resources. A community actively engaged in crime prevention or policing of industrial wastes shows signs of healthy functioning. The degree of functioning is directly related to the state of health (see Perspectives: Voices from the Community).

The ability to function can be observed. A man dresses and feeds himself and goes to work. Despite financial exigencies, a family nourishes its members through a supportive emotional climate. A community provides adequate resources and services for its members. These performances, to some degree, can be regarded as indicators of health status.

The actions of an individual, family, or community are motivated by their values. Some activities, such as walking and taking care of personal needs, are functions valued by most people. Other actions, such as bird watching, volunteering to help a charity, or running, have more limited appeal. In assessing the health of individuals and communities, the community health nurse can observe people's ability to function, but also must know their values, which may contrast sharply with those of the professional. The influence of values on health is examined more closely in Chapter 4.

The subjective dimension (feeling well or ill) and the objective dimension (functioning) together provide a clearer picture of people's health. When they feel well and demonstrate functional ability, they are close to the wellness end of the health continuum. Even those with a disease, such as arthritis or diabetes, may feel well and perform well within their capacity. These people can be considered healthy or closer to the wellness end of the continuum. Figure 1-3 depicts the relationships between the subjective and objective views of health.

Continuous and Episodic Health Care Needs

Community health practice encompasses populations in all age groups with birth to death developmental

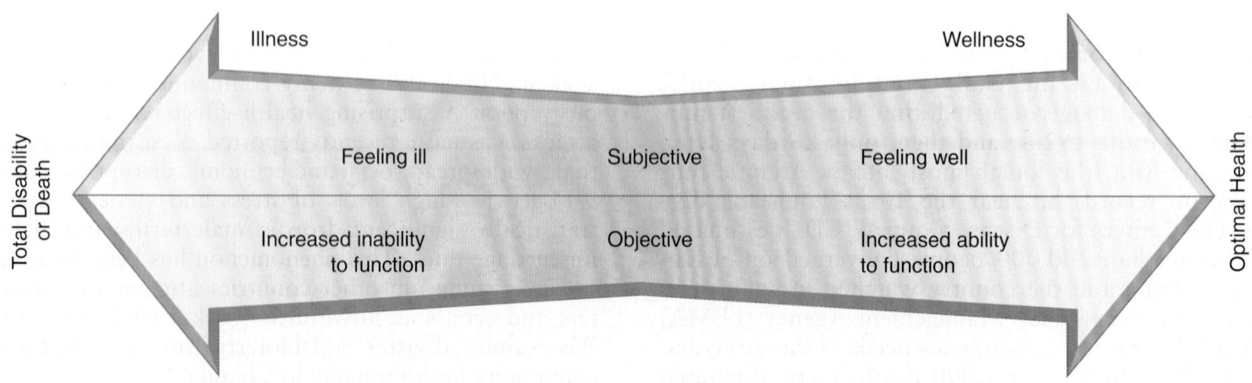

FIGURE 1-3. Subjective and objective views of the wellness–illness continuum.

health care needs. These **continuous needs** may include, for example, assistance with providing a toddler-proof home or establishing positive toilet-training techniques, help in effectively dealing with the progressive emancipation of preteens and teenagers, anticipatory guidance for reducing and managing the stress associated with retirement, or help coping with the death of an aged parent. These are developmental events experienced by most people, and they represent typical life occurrences. The community health nurse has the skills to work at the individual, family, and group level to meet these needs. On an individual and family level, a home visit may be the appropriate place for intervention. If the nurse sees that the community has many young and growing families, and several families have similar developmental issues, a class for mothers and babies, parents and teenagers, or preretirement adults may be formed to meet weekly at the library or health clinic waiting room. In these instances, the nurse works with groups ranging from small to large.

In addition, populations may have a one-time, specific, negative health event, such as an illness or injury that is not an expected part of life. These **episodic needs** might derive from the birth of an infant with Down's syndrome, a head injury incurred from an automobile crash, or a diagnosis of HIV/AIDS, tuberculosis, or another communicable disease (see Chapter 8).

In a given day, the community health nurse may interact with clients having either continuous or episodic health care needs, or both. For example, when can parents expect a child with Down's syndrome to begin toilet training? How do middle-aged adults, planning their retirement and preparing for the death of an aged parent, deal with their adult child's AIDS diagnosis? Complex situations such as these may be positively influenced by the interaction with and services of the community health nurse.

COMPONENTS OF COMMUNITY HEALTH PRACTICE

Community health practice can best be understood by examining two basic components—promotion of health and prevention of health problems. The levels of prevention are a key to community health practice.

Promotion of Health

Promotion of health is recognized as one of the most important components of public health and community health practice (DiClemente, Crosby, & Kegler, 2009). **Health promotion** includes all efforts that seek to move people closer to optimal well-being or higher levels of wellness. Nursing, in particular, has a social mandate for engaging in health promotion (Pender, Murdaugh & Parsons, 2011). Health promotion programs and activities include many forms of health education—for example, teaching the dangers of drug use, demonstrating healthful practices such as regular exercise, and providing more health-promoting options such as heart-healthy menu selections. Community health promotion, then, encompasses the development and management of preventive health care services that are responsive to community health needs. Wellness programs in schools and industry are examples. Demonstration of such healthful practices as eating nutritious foods and exercising more regularly often is performed and promoted by individual health workers. In addition, groups and health agencies that support a smoke-free environment, encourage physical fitness programs for all ages, or demand that food products be properly labeled underscore the importance of these practices and create public awareness.

The goal of health promotion is to raise levels of wellness for individuals, families, populations, and communities. Community health efforts accomplish this goal through a three-pronged effort to

1. Increase the span of healthy life for all citizens
2. Reduce health disparities among population groups
3. Achieve access to preventive services for everyone

Specifically, in the 1980s, the U.S. Public Health Service published the Surgeon General's report, *Healthy People*, and continued with *Promoting Health, Preventing Disease: 1990 Health Objectives for the Nation* and *Healthy People 2000*. The third set of health objectives for the nation, *Healthy People 2010* (2006; USDHHS, 2000), built on the previous two decades of success in Healthy People initiatives. These documents provide guidance for promoting health as a nation. *Healthy People 2020* will continues in this tradition.

The Surgeon General's report provided vision and an agenda for significantly reducing preventable death and disability nationwide, enhancing quality of life, and greatly reducing disparities in the health status of populations. It emphasized the need for individuals to assume personal responsibility for controlling and improving their own health destiny. It challenged society to find ways to make good health available to vulnerable populations whose disadvantaged state placed them at greater risk for health problems. Finally, it called for an intensified shift in focus from treating preventable illness and functional impairment to concentrating resources and targeting efforts that promote health and prevent disease and disability. The Institute of Medicine's 2001 report, *The Future of the Public's Health in the 21st Century*, notes that the majority of health care spending, "as much as 95%," focuses on "medical care and biomedical research," whereas evidence suggests that "behavior and environment are responsible for over 70% of avoidable mortality" and that health care is only one of many "determinants of health" (p. 2).

The implications of this national agenda for health have far-reaching consequences for persons engaged in health care. For centuries, health care has focused on the illness end of the health continuum, but health professionals can no longer justify concentrating most of their efforts exclusively on treating the sick and injured. We now live in an age when it is not only possible to promote health and prevent disease and disability, but it is our mandate and responsibility to do so. (For more on health promotion, see Chapter 11).

Prevention of Health Problems

Prevention of health problems constitutes a major part of community health practice. Prevention means anticipating and averting problems or discovering them as early as possible in order to minimize potential disability and impairment. It is practiced on three levels in community health: primary prevention, secondary prevention, and tertiary prevention (Pacala, 2007; Wallace, n.d.). These concepts recur throughout the chapters of this text, in narrative format and in the Levels of Prevention Pyramids, because they are basic to community health nursing. Once the differences among the levels of prevention are recognized, a sound foundation on which to build additional community health principles can be developed.

Primary prevention obviates the occurrence of a health problem; it includes measures taken to keep illness or injuries from occurring. It is applied to a generally healthy population and precedes disease or dysfunction. Examples of primary prevention activities by a public health nurse include providing childhood vaccinations; encouraging elderly people to install and use safety devices (e.g., grab bars by bathtubs, hand rails on steps) to prevent injuries from falls; teaching young adults healthy lifestyle behaviors, so that they can make them habitual behaviors for themselves and their children; or working through a local health department in consultation with a school district to help control and prevent communicable diseases such as rubeola, poliomyelitis, or varicella by providing regular immunization programs and vaccine oversight.

Primary prevention involves anticipatory planning and action on the part of community health professionals, who must project themselves into the future, envision potential needs and problems, and then design programs to counteract them, so that they never occur. A community health nurse who instructs a group of overweight individuals on how to follow a well-balanced diet while losing weight is preventing the possibility of nutritional deficiency (see Levels of Prevention Pyramid). Educational programs that teach safe-sex practices or the dangers of smoking and substance abuse are other examples of primary prevention. In addition, when the community health nurse serves on a fact-finding committee exploring the effects of a proposed toxic waste dump on the outskirts of town, the nurse is concerned about primary prevention. The concepts of primary prevention and planning for the future are foreign to many social groups, who may resist on the basis of conflicting values. The Parable of the Dangerous Cliff (Display 1.4) illustrates such a value conflict. How often does our nation put an ambulance at the bottom of the cliff?

Secondary prevention involves efforts to detect and treat existing health problems at the earliest possible stage, when disease or impairment is already present. Hypertension and cholesterol screening programs in many communities help to identify high-risk individuals and encourage early treatment to prevent heart attacks or stroke. Other examples are encouraging breast and testicular self-examination, regular mammograms, and Pap smears for early detection of possible cancers and providing skin testing for tuberculosis (in infants at 1 year of age and periodically throughout life, with increasing frequency for high-risk groups). Secondary prevention attempts to discover a health problem at a point when intervention may lead to its control or eradication. This is the goal behind testing of water and soil samples for contaminants and hazardous chemicals in the field of community environmental health. It also prompts community health nurses to watch for early signs of child abuse in a family, emotional disturbances among widows, or alcohol and drug abuse among adolescents.

Tertiary prevention attempts to reduce the extent and severity of a health problem to its lowest possible level, so as to minimize disability and restore or preserve function. Examples include treatment and rehabilitation of persons after a stroke to reduce impairment, postmastectomy exercise programs to restore functioning, and early treatment and management of diabetes to reduce problems or slow their progress. The individuals involved have an existing illness or disability whose impact on their lives is lessened through tertiary prevention. In community health, the need to reduce disability and restore function applies equally to families, groups, communities, and individuals. Many groups form for rehabilitation and offer support and guidance for those recuperating from some physical or mental disability. Examples include Alcoholics Anonymous, halfway houses for psychiatric patients discharged from acute care settings, ostomy clubs, and drug rehabilitation programs. In broader community health practice, tertiary prevention is used to minimize the effects of an existing unhealthy community condition. Examples of such prevention are insisting that businesses provide wheelchair access, warning urban residents about the dangers of a chemical spill, and recalling a contaminated food or drug product. When a community experiences a disaster such as an earthquake, a fire, a hurricane, or even a terrorist attack, preventing injuries among the survivors and volunteers during rescue is another example of tertiary prevention—eliminating additional injury to those already experiencing a tragedy.

Health assessment of individuals, families, and communities is an important part of all three levels of preventive practice. Health status must be determined to anticipate problems and select appropriate preventive measures. Community health nurses working with young parents who themselves have been victims of child abuse can institute early treatment for the parents to prevent abuse and foster adequate parenting of their children. If the assessment of a community reveals inadequate facilities and activities to meet the future needs of its growing senior population, agencies and groups can collaborate to develop the needed resources.

Health problems are most effectively prevented by maintenance of healthy lifestyles and healthy environments. To these ends, community health practice directs many of its efforts to providing safe and satisfying living and working conditions, nutritious food, and clean air and water. This area of practice includes the field of preventive medicine, which is a population-focused,

LEVELS OF PREVENTION PYRAMID

SITUATION: Poor nutritional habits and inactivity are leading to obesity among children and adults and greater incidence of type 2 diabetes.

GOAL: Using the three levels of prevention, negative health conditions are avoided, or promptly diagnosed and treated, and population health is improved.

TERTIARY PREVENTION		
Rehabilitation	**Primary Prevention**	
	Health Promotion & Education	*Health Protection*
• If diabetic, encourage weight, blood pressure, and cholesterol maintenance, along with good glucose control to prevent complications of diabetes. • Reassess data to determine effectiveness of interventions.	• Teach children and families the importance of maintaining a healthy weight through proper diet and exercise. Promote awareness of dangers of obesity and diabetes through use of PSAs and billboards.	• Provide weight loss support. • Provide access to periodic health care to check A_1C levels, foot and eye exams.

SECONDARY PREVENTION	
Early Diagnosis	**Prompt Treatment**
• Encourage weight loss in obese populations to prevent development of type 2 diabetes. Provide screening programs for high-risk groups • Refer clients with high glucose or other problems (e.g., hypertension, high cholesterol) to primary care provider or diabetes clinics	• Initiate educational and incentive programs to improve dietary practices • Teach clients (individuals or families) on a one-to-one basis to modify dietary practices and activity levels

PRIMARY PREVENTION	
Health Promotion and Education	**Health Protection**
• Provide nutrition educational programs to promote awareness at schools, work sites, etc. • Encourage restaurants and schools to offer healthy menu items • Recommend nutrition classes offered at neighborhood centers or health care facilities	• Promote physical fitness, nutritional and wellness activities • Work with local entities to reduce easy access to sodas, tax high calorie foods, and provide easier access to fresh fruits and vegetables, as well as provide bike paths and walking clubs.

or community-oriented, branch of medical practice that incorporates public health sciences and principles (American Board of Medical Specialties, n.d.).

CHARACTERISTICS OF COMMUNITY HEALTH NURSING

As a specialty field of nursing, community health nursing adds public health knowledge and skills that address the needs and problems of communities and aggregates and focuses care on communities and vulnerable populations. Public health nursing is grounded in both public health science and nursing science, which makes its philosophical orientation and the nature of its practice unique. It has been recognized as a subspecialty of both fields. Recognition of this specialty field continues with a greater awareness of the important contributions made by community health nursing to improve the health of the public.

Knowledge of the following elements of public health is essential to community health nursing (ANA, 2007; Quad Council, 2003; Williams, 1977):

- Priority of preventive, protective, and health-promoting strategies over curative strategies
- Means for measurement and analysis of community health problems, including epidemiologic concepts and biostatistics (see Chapter 7)
- Influence of environmental factors on aggregate health (see Chapter 9)
- Principles underlying management and organization for community health, because the goal of public

DISPLAY 1.4 PARABLE OF THE DANGEROUS CLIFF

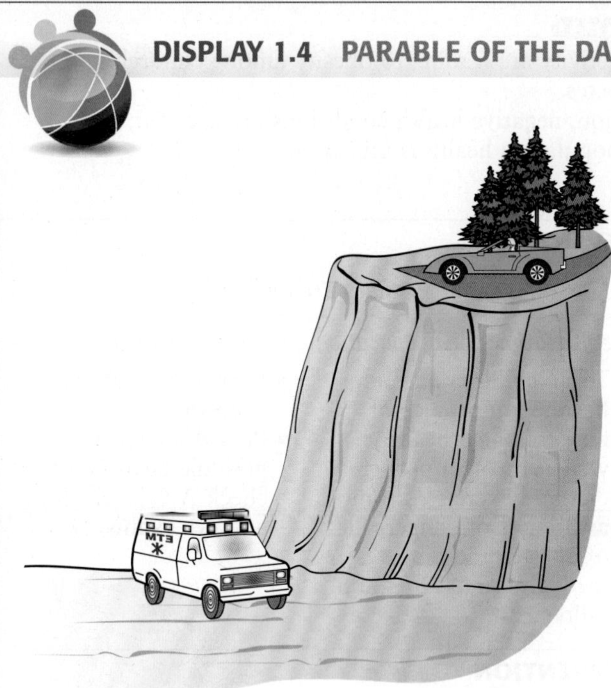

Twas a dangerous cliff, as they freely confessed,
Though to walk near its crest was so pleasant;
But over its terrible edge there has slipped
A duke, and full many a peasant.
The people said something would have to be done
But their projects did not at all tally.
Some said, "Put a fence around the edge of the cliff";
Some, "an ambulance down in the valley."
The lament of the crowd was profound and was loud,
As their hearts overflowed with their pity;
But the cry of the ambulance carried the day
As it spread through the neighboring city.
A collection was made to accumulate aid
And the dwellers in highway and alley
Gave dollars or cents not to furnish a fence
But "an ambulance down in the valley."
"For the cliff is all right if you're careful," they said.
"And if folks ever slip and are dropping,
It isn't the slipping that hurts them so much
As the shock down below when they're stopping."
So for years (we have heard), as these mishaps occurred,
Quick forth the rescuers sally,
To pick up the victims who fell from the cliff,
With the ambulance down in the valley.
Said one in his plea, "It's a marvel to me
That you'd give so much greater attention
To repairing results than to curing the cause;
You had much better aim at prevention.
For the mischief, of course, should be stopped at its source,
Come neighbors and friends, let us rally.
It is far better sense to rely on a fence
Than an ambulance down in the valley."
"He is wrong in his head," the majority said;
"He would end all our earnest endeavor.
He's a man who would shirk this responsible work,
But we will support it forever.
Aren't we picking up all, just as fast as they fall, and giving them care liberally?
A superfluous fence is of no consequence,
If the ambulance works in the valley."
The story looks queer as we've written it here,
But things oft occur that are stranger.
More humane, we assert, than to care for the hurt,
Is a plan for removing the danger.
The very best plan is to safeguard the man,
And attend to the thing rationally;
To build up the fence and try to dispense
With the ambulance down in the valley.
Better still! Cut down the hill!

Adapted from Joseph Malins' (1895) *A Fence or an Ambulance?* Retrieved from www.startwithyourheart.com/taskforce/philosophy.aspx

health is accomplished through organized community efforts (see Chapter 15)

- Public policy analysis and development, along with health advocacy and an understanding of the political process (see Chapter 13)

Confusion over the meaning of "community health nursing" arises when it is defined only in terms of where it is practiced. Because health care services have shifted from the hospital to the community, many nurses in other specialties now practice in the community. Examples of these practices include home health care, community mental health, geriatric nursing, long-term care, and occupational health. Although community health nurses today practice in the same or similar settings, the difference lies in applying the public health principles to large groups and communities of people—or having a population focus (Fig. 1-4). For nurses moving into this field of nursing, it requires a shift in focus—from individuals to aggregates and populations. Nursing and other theories undergird its practice (see Chapter 14), and the nursing process (incorporated in Chapters 15 and 19) is one of its basic tools (see the levels of prevention discussed earlier).

Community health nursing, then, as a specialty of nursing, combines nursing science with public health science to formulate a community-based and population-focused practice (Anderson & McFarlane, 2012). "Public health nursing is the practice of promoting and protecting the health of populations using knowledge from nursing, social, and public health sciences" (ANA, 2007, p. 5) (see Display 1.5). For instance, community health nurses are nursing when their concern for homeless individuals sleeping in a park leads to

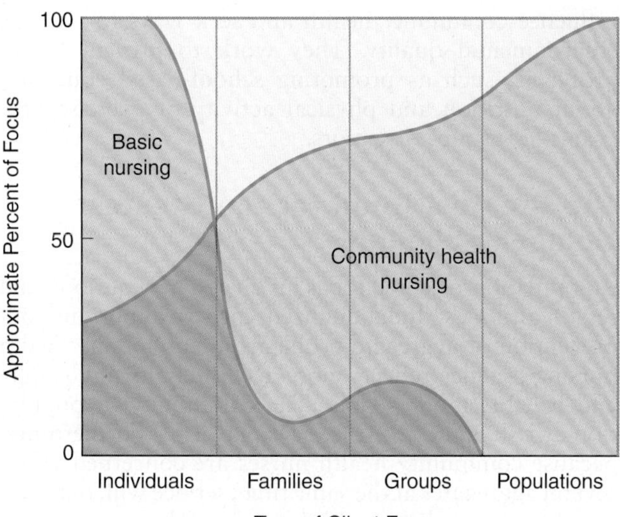

FIGURE 1-4. Difference in client focus between basic nursing and community health nursing

development of a program providing food and shelter for this population. Community health nurses are nursing when they collaborate to institute an AIDS education curriculum in the local school system. When they assess the needs of elderly people in retirement homes to ensure necessary services and provide health instruction and support, they are, again, nursing.

During the first 70 years of the 20th century, community health nursing was known as **public health nursing**. The PHN section of the American Public Health Association's definition of a public health nurse is a "nursing professional with educational, preparation in public health and nursing science with a primary focus on population-level outcomes" and notes the primary focus for public health nursing is to "promote health and prevent disease for entire population groups" (1996, p. 2). The later title of community health nursing was adopted to better describe where the nurse practices. As used in this text, the terms are interchangeable.

Eight characteristics of community health nursing are particularly salient to the practice of this specialty (ANA, 2007, pp. 8–9):

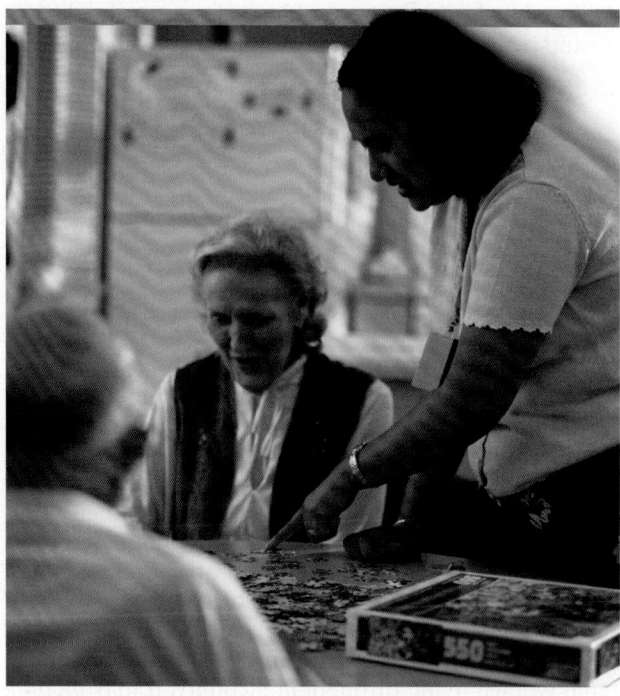

1. The client or "unit of care" is the population.
2. The primary obligation is to achieve the greatest good for the greatest number of people or the population as a whole.

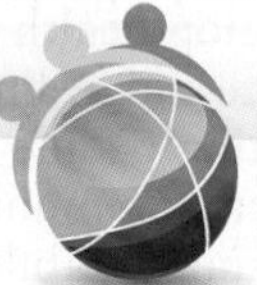

DISPLAY 1.5 THE ROLE OF PUBLIC HEALTH NURSES

Public health nurses integrate community involvement and knowledge about the entire population with personal, clinical understandings of the health and illness experiences of individuals and families within the population. They translate and articulate the health and illness experiences of diverse, often vulnerable individuals and families in the population to health planners and policy makers, and assist members of the community to voice their problems and aspirations. Public health nurses are knowledgeable about multiple strategies for intervention, from those applicable to the entire population, to those for the family, and the individual. Public health nurses translate knowledge from the health and social sciences to individuals and population groups through targeted interventions, programs, and advocacy. Public health nursing may be practiced by one public health nurse or by a group of public health nurses working collaboratively. In both instances, public health nurses are directly engaged in the interdisciplinary activities of the core public health functions of assessment, assurance, and policy development. Interventions or strategies may be targeted to multiple levels, depending on where the most effective outcomes are possible. They include strategies aimed at entire population groups, families, or individuals. In any setting, the role of public health nurses focuses on the prevention of illness, injury, or disability; the promotion of health; and the maintenance of the health of populations.

Public Health Nursing Section, American Public Health Association [1996]. The definition and role of public health nursing. Washington, DC: APHA.

3. The processes used by public health nurses include working with the client as an equal partner.
4. Primary prevention is the priority in selecting appropriate activities.
5. Public health nursing focuses on selecting strategies that create healthy environmental, social, and economic conditions in which populations may thrive.
6. A public health nurse is obligated to actively identify and reach out to all who might benefit from a specific activity or service.
7. Optimal use of available resources to assure the best overall improvement in the health of the population is a key element of the practice.
8. Collaboration with a variety of other professions, organizations, and other stakeholder groups is the most effective way to promote and protect the health of people.

Population-Focused

The central mission of public health practice is to improve the health of population groups. Community health nursing shares this essential feature: it is **population-focused**, meaning that it is concerned for the health status of population groups and their environment. A population may consist of the elderly living throughout the community or of Southeast Asian refugees clustered in one section of a city. It may be a scattered group with common characteristics, such as people at high risk of developing heart disease or battered women living throughout a county. It may include all people living in a neighborhood, district, census tract, city, state, or province. Community health nursing's specialty practice serves populations and aggregates of people.

Working with individuals and families as aggregates has been common for community health nursing; however, such work must expand to incorporate a population-oriented focus, a feature that distinguishes it from other nursing specialties. Basic nursing focuses on individuals, and community health nursing focuses on aggregates, but the many variations in community needs and nursing roles inevitably cause some overlap.

A population-oriented focus requires the assessment of relationships. When working with groups and communities, the nurse does not consider them separately but rather in context—that is, in relationship to the rest of the community. When an outbreak of hepatitis occurs, for example, the community health nurse does more than just work with others to treat it. The nurse tries to stop the spread of the infection, locate possible sources, and prevent its recurrence in the community. As a result of their population-oriented focus, community health nurses seek to discover possible groups with a common health need, such as expectant mothers or groups at high risk for development of a common health problem (e.g., obese children at risk for type 2 diabetes, victims of child abuse). Community health nurses continually look for problems in the environment that influence community health and seek ways to increase environmental quality. They work to prevent health problems, such as promoting school-based education about nutrition and physical activity or exercise programs for groups of seniors.

The Greatest Good for the Greatest Number of People

A population-oriented focus involves a new outlook and set of attitudes. Individualized care is important, but prevention of aggregate problems in community health nursing practice reflects more accurately its philosophy and benefits more people. The community or population at risk is the client (see Display 1.6). Furthermore, because community health nurses are concerned about several aggregates at the same time, service will, of necessity, be provided to multiple and overlapping groups. The ethical theory of *utilitarianism* promotes the greatest good for the greatest number. Further discussion of ethical principles in community health nursing can be found in Chapter 4.

Clients as Equal Partners

The goal of public health, "to increase quality and years of healthy life and eliminate health disparities" (USDHHS, 2000, para. 3), requires a partnership effort. Just as learning cannot take place in schools without student participation, the goals of public health cannot be realized without consumer participation. Community health nursing's efforts toward health improvement go only so far. Clients' health status and health behavior will not change unless people accept and apply the proposals (developed in collaboration with clients) presented by the community health nurse.

Public health nurses can encourage individuals' participation by promoting their autonomy rather than permitting a dependency. For example, elderly persons attending a series of nutrition or fitness classes can be encouraged to take the initiative and develop health or social programs on their own. Independence and feelings of self-worth are closely related. By treating people as independent adults, with trust and respect, community health nurses help promote self-reliance and the ability to function independently. Autonomy is an important objective of public health, as is equality (Brulde, 2008; Munthe, 2008).

Frequently, consumers are intimidated by health professionals and are uninformed about health and health care. They do not know what information to seek and are hesitant to act assertively. For example, a migrant worker brought her 2-year-old son,who had symptoms resembling those of scurvy, to a clinic. Recognizing a vitamin C deficiency, the physician told her to feed the boy large quantities of orange juice but gave no further explanation. Several weeks later, she returned to the clinic, but the child was much worse. After questioning her, the nurse discovered that the mother had been feeding the child large amounts of an orange soft drink, not knowing the difference between that beverage and

DISPLAY 1.6 PARABLE OF THE TREES: POPULATION-FOCUSED PRACTICE

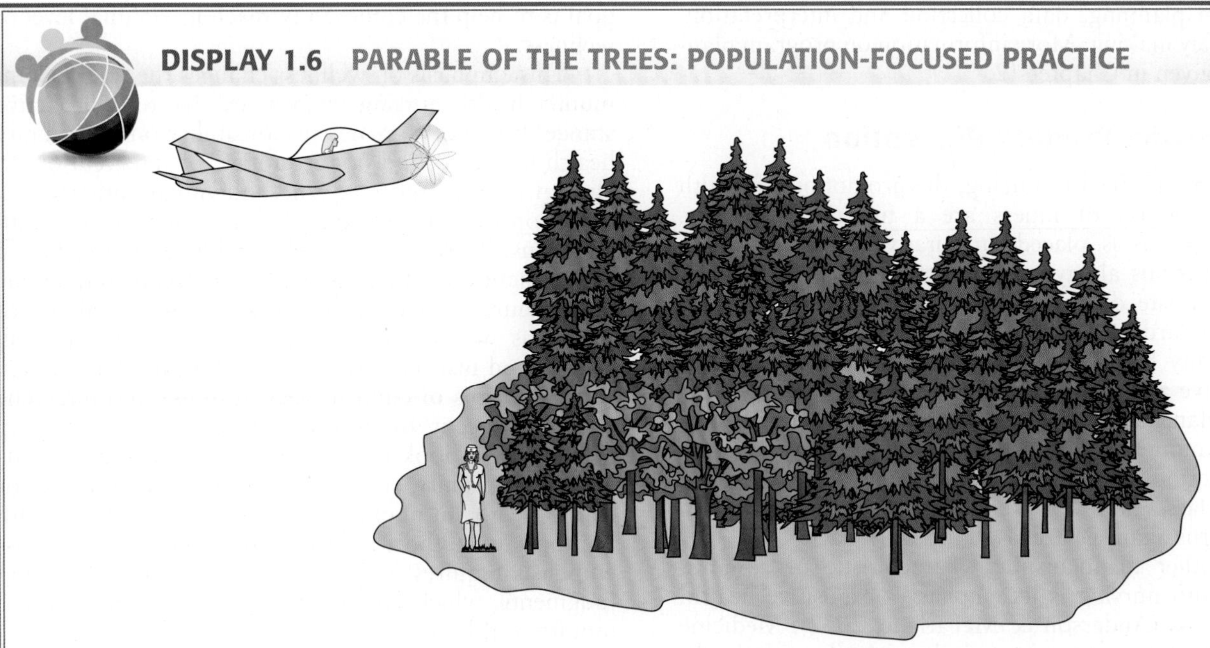

There were once two sisters who inherited a large tract of heavily forested land from their grandmother. In her will, the grandmother stipulated that they must preserve the health of the trees. One sister studied tree surgery and became an expert in recognizing and treating diseased trees. She also was able to spot conditions that might lead to problems and prevent them. Her work was invaluable in keeping single or small clusters of trees healthy. The other sister became a forest ranger. In addition to learning how to care for individual trees, she studied the environmental conditions that affected the wellbeing of the forest. She learned the importance of proper ecologic balance between flora and fauna and the impact of climate, geography, soil conditions, and weather. Her work was to oversee the health and growth of the whole forest. Although she spent time walking through the forest assessing conditions, her aerial view from their small plane was equally important for spotting fires, signs of disease, or other potential problems. Together, the sisters preserved a healthy forest.

Nursing also has tree surgeons and forest rangers. Various nursing specialties, like the tree surgeons, serve the health needs of individuals and families. Community health nurses, like the forest rangers, study and address the needs of populations. Both are needed and must work together to ensure healthy communities.

orange juice. Obviously, the quality of care is affected when the consumer does not understand and cannot participate in the health care process. **Health literacy**, or the ability to "obtain, process, and understand basic health information and services needed to make appropriate health decisions," is an important concept that is discussed more fully in Chapter 10 (Glassman, 2010, para. 1).

When people believe that their health, and that of the community, is their own responsibility, not just that of health professionals, they will take a more active interest in promoting it. The process of taking responsibility for developing one's own health potential is called **self-care**. As people maintain their own lives, health, and wellbeing, they are engaging in self-care. Some examples of self-care activities at the aggregate level include building safe playgrounds, developing teen employment opportunities, and providing senior exercise programs.

When people's ability to continue self-care activities drops below their need, they experience a **self-care deficit**. At this point, nursing may appropriately intervene. However, nursing's goal is to assist clients to return to or reach a level of functioning at which they can attain optimal health and assume responsibility for maintaining it (Hanucharurnkul, 2009; Orem, 2001). To this end, community health nurses foster their clients' sense of responsibility by treating them as adults capable of managing their own affairs. Nurses can encourage people to negotiate health care goals and practices, develop their own programs, contact their own resources (e.g., support groups, transportation services), identify and implement lifestyle changes that promote wellness, and learn ways to monitor their own health.

When planning for the health of communities, for example, partnerships must be established and the values and priorities of the community incorporated into program planning, data collection and interpretation, and policy making. More information on program planning is given in Chapter 12.

Prioritizing Primary Prevention

In community health nursing, the promotion of health and prevention of illness are a first-order priority. Less emphasis is placed on curative care. Some corrective actions always are needed, such as cleanup of a toxic waste dump site, stricter enforcement of day care standards, or home care of the disabled; however, community health best serves its constituents through preventive and health-promoting actions (Anderson & MacFarlane, 2012; USDHHS, 2000). These include services to mothers and infants, prevention of environmental pollution, school health programs, senior citizens' fitness classes, and "workers' right-to-know" legislation that warns against hazards in the workplace.

Another distinguishing characteristic of community health nursing is its emphasis on positive health, or wellness (Anderson & McFarlane, 2012). Medicine and acute care nursing have dealt primarily with the illness end of the health continuum. With the potentials of genomics and epigenetics becoming reality, the wellness end of the continuum will come into greater focus. In contrast, community health nursing always has had a primary charge to prevent health problems from occurring and to promote a higher level of health. For example, although a community health nurse may assist a population of new mothers in the community with postpartum fatigue and depression, the nurse also works to prevent such problems among women of child-bearing age by developing health education programs, establishing prenatal classes, and encouraging proper rest and nutrition, adequate help, and stress reduction.

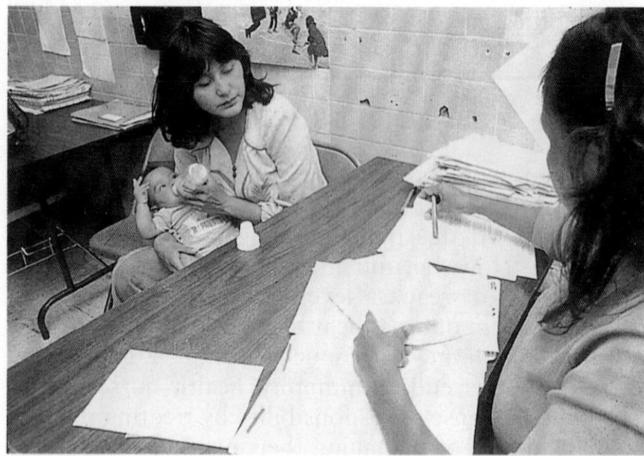

Community health nurses concentrate on the wellness end of the health continuum in a variety of ways. They teach proper nutrition or family planning, promote immunizations among preschool children, encourage regular physical and dental checkups, assist with starting exercise classes or physical fitness programs, and promote healthy interpersonal relationships. Their goal is to help the community reach its optimal level of wellness.

This emphasis on wellness changes the role of community health nursing from a reactive to a proactive stance. It places a greater responsibility on community health nurses to find opportunities for intervention. In clinical nursing and medicine, individual patients seek out professional assistance because they have health problems. They present their problems to the health care practitioner for diagnosis and treatment. Public health nurses, in contrast, seek out potential health problems in the community. They identify high-risk groups and institute preventive programs. They watch for early signs of child neglect or abuse and intervene when any occur, often long before a request for help is made. They look for possible environmental hazards in the community, such as smoking in public places or lead-based paint in older housing units, and work with appropriate authorities to correct them. A wellness emphasis requires taking initiative and making sound judgments, which are characteristics of effective community health nursing.

Selecting Strategies That Create Healthy Conditions in Which Populations May Thrive

With our population focus, it is prudent for community health nurses to design interventions for the whole community, not limiting it "to those who seek service, are poor, or otherwise vulnerable," but "directed toward the entire populations within a community" and the systems that could potentially affect or are affecting the health of those individuals, families, and populations (ANA, 2006, p. 5). Advocacy for our clients (individuals, families, aggregates, communities, or populations) is an essential function of public health nursing. We want to create healthy environments for our clients, so that they can thrive and not simply survive, and we do this by having a proactive stance toward "social and health-care trends, changing concerns, and policy and legislative activities" (ANA, 2006, p. 6). More about health advocacy and policy making is given in Chapter 13.

Actively Reaching Out

We know that some clients are more prone to develop disability or disease because of their vulnerable status (e.g., poverty, no access to health care, homeless). Outreach efforts are needed to promote the health of these clients and to prevent disease. In acute care and primary health care settings, like emergency rooms or physician offices, clients come to you for service. However, in community health, nurses must focus on the whole population—not just those who come to us for services—and seek out clients wherever they may be (ANA, 2006). Like Lillian Wald and her Henry Street Settlement, community health nurses must learn about the populations they serve and be willing to search out those most at risk. You can learn more about the rich history of community/public health nursing in Chapter 2. Chapters 25 through 29 will cover vulnerable populations.

Optimal Use of Available Resources

It is our duty to wisely use the resources we are given. For most public health agencies, budgets are critically stressed. Tertiary health care uses up the greatest percentage of our health care dollar, leaving decreased funds for primary and secondary services (Ginsburg, 2008; IOM, 2002), and challenging economic times lead to deep budget cuts at state and local levels. The use of documented evidence as a basis for community health nursing practice promotes "efficient, effective, and cost-beneficial strategies in promoting the public's health" (ANA, 2006, p. 7). It is vital that community health nurses ground their practice in research (see Chapter 4), and use that information to educate policy makers about best practices. Utilizing personnel and resources effectively and prudently will pay off in the long run.

Interprofessional Collaboration

Community health nurses must work in cooperation with other team members, coordinating services and addressing the needs of population groups. This interprofessional **collaboration** among health care workers, other professionals and organizations, and clients is essential for establishing effective services and programs. Individualized efforts and specialized programs, when planned in isolation, can lead to fragmentation and gaps in health services. For example, without collaboration, a well-child clinic may be started in a community that already has a strong Early and Periodic Screening and Developmental Testing (EPSDT) program, yet community prenatal services may be nonexistent. Interprofessional collaboration is important in individualized practice, because nurses need to plan with the client, family, physician, social worker, physical therapist, teacher, or counselor, and must keep them informed of the client's health status; however, it is an even greater necessity when working with population groups, especially those from vulnerable or at-risk segments.

Effective collaboration requires team members who are strong individuals, with various areas of expertise and who can make a commitment to team goals. Community health nurses who think and act interdependently make a great contribution to the team effort. In appropriate situations, community health nurses also function autonomously, making independent judgments. Collaboration involves working with members of other professions on community advisory boards and health planning committees to develop needs assessment surveys and to contribute toward policy development efforts. In addition to partnering with the population, other groups the public health nurse collaborates with include:

- Members of the public health team (e.g. epidemiologists, social workers, nutritionists, environmental health workers, and health educators)
- Local, state, and federal public health organizations
- Healthcare providers
- Community organizations and coalitions
- Community service agencies (e.g., schools, law enforcement and emergency response)
- Faith-based organizations;
- Businesses and industries
- Academic and research institutions (ANA, 2006, pp. 5–6)

Interprofessional collaboration requires clarification of each team member's role, a primary reason for community health nurses to fully understand the nature of their practice. When planning a city-wide immunization program with a community group, for example, community health nurses need to explain the ways in which they might contribute to the program's objectives. They can offer to contact key community leaders, with whom they have established relationships, to build community acceptance of the program. They can share their knowledge of the public's preference about times and locations for the program. They can meet with various local agencies and organizations (e.g., health insurance companies, local hospitals) to gain financial support. They can help to organize and give immunizations, and they can influence planning for follow-up programs. Another component includes development of policies to promote and protect the health of clients. Meeting with local legislators and providing testimony to local, state, and national bodies are common methods of ensuring enactment of effective health policies. Public health nurses can join with others to promote legislation to mandate helmets for cyclists, ban sugar-laden beverages in school vending machines, or provide funding for specific community-based programs. Collaboration is discussed further in Chapter 10.

Client participation is promoted when people serve as partners on the health care team. An aim of community health nursing is to collaborate *with* people, rather than do things *for* them. As consumers of health services are treated with respect and trust, confidence and skill in self-care are gained. Thus, promoting their own health and that of their community as their contribution to health programs becomes increasingly valuable. The consumer perspective in planning and delivering health services makes those services relevant to consumer needs. Community health nurses encourage the involvement of health care consumers by soliciting their ideas and opinions, by inviting them to participate on health boards and committees, and by finding ways to promote their participation in decisions affecting their collective health. By assessing the needs of community, based partly upon the population's perceptions, the public health nurse can discover the most pressing health needs and work toward more effective interventions. Community assessment and intervention are explored in depth in Chapter 15.

SUMMARY

Community health nursing has opportunities and challenges to keep the nurse interested and involved in a community-focused career for a lifetime. Community health is more than environmental programs and large-scale efforts to control communicable disease. It is defined as the identification of needs and the protection and improvement of collective health within a geographically defined area. To comprehend the nature and significance of community health and to clarify it's meaning for the specialty practice of community health nursing, it is important to understand the concepts of community and of health.

A *community*, broadly defined, is a collection of people who share some common interest or goal. Three types of communities were discussed in this chapter: geographic, common-interest, and health problem-solving communities. Sometimes, a community such as a neighborhood, city, or county is formed by geographic boundaries. At other times, a community may be identified by its common interest; examples are a religious community, a group of migrant workers, or citizens concerned about air pollution. A community also is defined by a pooling of efforts by people and agencies toward solving a health-related problem.

Health is an abstract concept that can be understood more clearly by examining its distinguishing features. First, people are neither sick nor well in an absolute sense, but have levels of illness or wellness. These levels may be plotted along a continuum ranging from optimal health to total disability or death. This is known as the *health continuum*. A person's state of health is dynamic, varying from day to day and even hour to hour.

Second, health is a state of being that includes all of the many characteristics of a person, family, or community, whether physical, psychological, social, or spiritual. These characteristics often indicate the degree of wellness or illness of an individual or community and suggest the presence or absence of vitality and wellbeing.

Third, health has both subjective and objective dimensions: the subjective involves how well people feel; the objective refers to how well they are able to function. Most often, functional performance diminishes dramatically toward the illness end of the health continuum.

Fourth, health care needs can be either continuing, as in developmental concerns that occur over a person's lifetime, or episodic, occurring unexpectedly once or twice in a lifetime. Community health nursing deals with continuing needs, whereas episodic needs are more often managed in acute care settings.

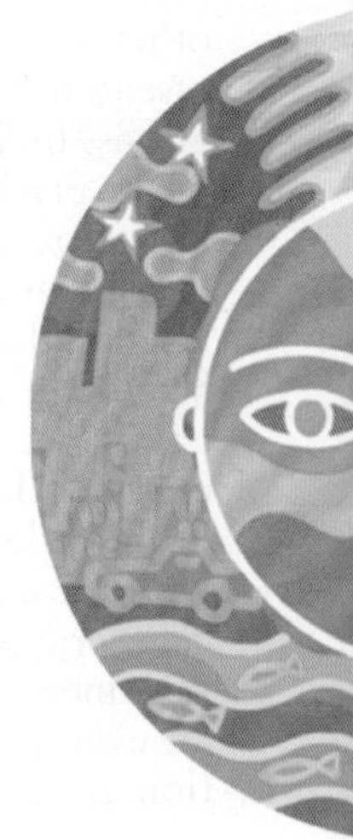

Community health practice incorporates the elements of promotion of health and prevention of health problems.

The eight important characteristics of community health practice are the client is the population; the primary obligation is to achieve the greatest good for the greatest number of people; working with clients as equal partners is the key process used by PHNs; primary prevention is the priority; focus on strategies that create healthy environmental, social and economic conditions; reach out to all who might benefit; make optimal use of available resources; and collaborate with a variety of professions, populations, organizations, and other stakeholders "to promote and protect the health of the people" (ANA, 2006, pp. 8–9).

ACTIVITIES TO PROMOTE **CRITICAL THINKING**

1. Identify a community of people about whom you have some knowledge. What makes it a community? What characteristics do this group of people share? Work on this activity in a group of peers or family members. Do they think as you do? Is there a difference between the views of family members and those of nursing student peers?
2. Select three populations for whom you have some concern, and place each group on the health continuum. What factors influenced your decision?

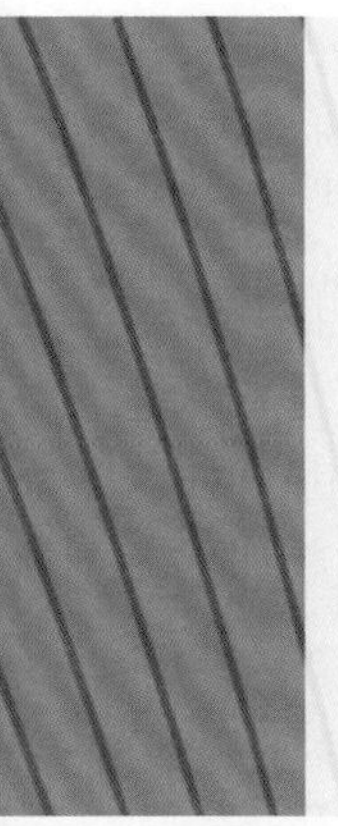

3. Describe three preventive actions (one primary, one secondary, and one tertiary) that might be taken to move each of your selected populations closer to optimal wellness.
4. Select a current health problem and identify the three levels of prevention and corresponding activities in which you as a community health nurse would engage at each level.
5. Discuss how you might implement one health-promotion effort with each of your selected populations.
6. Browse the Internet for community health nursing research articles that focus on levels of prevention. Find one focusing on each level. For those involved in the articles focusing on secondary and tertiary prevention, what could you as a community health nurse have done to keep the clients at the primary level of prevention?
7. Place yourself on the health continuum. What factors influenced your decision?
8. Using the eight characteristics of community health nursing outlined in this chapter, give examples of how a community health nurse might demonstrate meeting each characteristic.

REFERENCES

American Board of Medical Specialties. (n.d.). *Preventive medicine*. Author. Retrieved from http://www.abms.org/Who_We_Help/Consumers/About_Physician_Specialties/preventive.aspx

American Cancer Society. (2008). *Schools move to limit 'junk' foods*. Retrieved August 2, 2008, from http://www.cancer.org/docroot/SPC/content/SPC_1_Schools_Move_to_Expel_Junk_ Foods.asp

American Nurses Association (ANA). (2007). *Public health nursing: Scope and standards of practice*. Silver Springs, MD: Author.

American Nurses Association (ANA). (2010). *Health care reform: Key provisions related to nursing*. Silver Springs, MD: Author.

American Public Health Association (APHA) Public Health Nursing Section. (1996). *The definition and role of public health nursing*. Washington, DC: APHA.

Anderson, E. T., & McFarlane, J. (2012). *Community as partner: Theory and practice in nursing* (6th ed.). Philadelphia, PA: Lippincott Williams & Wilkins.

Anomaly, J. (2010). Combating resistance: The case for a global antibiotics treaty. *Public Health Ethics, 3*(1), 13–22.

Aspy, C. B., Mold, J., Thompson, D., Blondell, R., Landers, P., Reilly, K., et al. (2008). Integrating screening and interventions for unhealthy behaviors into primary care practices. *American Journal of Preventive Medicine, 35*(Suppl. 5), S373–S380.

Asthma & Allergy Foundation of America (AAFA). (n.d.). *Asthma facts and figures*. Retrieved May 18, 2010, from http://www.aafa.org/display.cfm?id=8&sub=42

Asthma & Allergy Foundation of America (AAFA). (2010). *2010 asthma capitals: The most challenging places to live with asthma*. Landover, MD: Author.

Bambra, C., Gibson, M., Sowden, A., Wright, K., Whitehead, M., & Petticrew, M. (2010). Tackling the wider social determinants of health and health inequalities: Evidence from systematic reviews. *Journal of Epidemiology and Community Health, 64*, 284–291.

Baxter, S. (2010, May 6). *Santa Clara county ban on toys with unhealthy meals is a first*. Retrieved from http://www.mercurynews.com/almaden/ci_15035487

Broder, J. M., & Zeller, T. (2010, May 4). Gulf oil spill is bad, but how bad? *New York Times*, p. A1.

Brulde, B. (2008). Inequity, inequality, and the distributive goals of public health. *International Journal of Public Health, 53*, 5–6.

Canadian Institute for Health Information. (2009). *Health indicators: 2009*. Ottawa, ON: Author.

Centers for Disease Control & Prevention (CDC). (2009). *Tobacco-related mortality*. Retrieved from http://www.cdc.gov/tobacco/data_statistics/fact_sheets/health_effects/tobacco_related_mortality/

Centers for Disease Control & Prevention (CDC). (2010). *Investments in communities: CDC's role in activating local change*. Retrieved from http://www.cdc.gov/healthycommunitiesprogram/communities/

Centers for Disease Control & Prevention (CDC). (2011). *Designing and building healthy places*. Retrieved from http://cdc.gov/healthyplaces/

Chan, C. (2010, March 1). New guidelines for treating depression emphasize everyday ability to function. *Epoch Times*. Retrieved from http://www.theepochtimes.com/n2/index2.php?option=com_content&task=view&id=30532&pop=1&page=0&Itemid=1

Clinton County Health Department. (n.d.). *A definition of public health*. Retrieved May 15, 2010, from www.co.clinton.ny.us/Departments/Health/print_page/aboutus.pdf

Cloud, J. (2010, January 6). Why DNA isn't your destiny. *Time*. Retrieved from http://www.time.com/time/printout/0,8816,1951968,00.html#

Committee on School Health. (2009). AAP publications retired and reaffirmed. Policy statement: Soft drinks in schools. *Pediatrics, 123*(5), 1421–1422.

Cottrell, L. S. (1976). The competent community. In B. H. Kaplan, R. N. Wilson, & A. H. Leighton (Eds.), *Further explanations in social psychiatry* (pp. 195–209). New York: Basic Books.

County Health Rankings. (2010). *County health rankings and roadmaps: A healthier nation, county by county.* Retrieved from http://www.countyhealthrankings.org/

Curley, A. (2010). *CDC urges 50-state anti-smoking effort*. Retrieved from http://www.cnn.com/2014/HEALTH/04/22/cdc.smoking.report/index.html

Dewan, S. (2009, June 3). Katrina victims will not have to vacate trailers. *The New York Times*. Retrieved from http://www.nytimes.com/2009/06/04/us/04trailers.html?_r=1

DiClemente, R. J., Crosby, R. A., & Kegler, M. (Eds.). (2009). *Emerging theories in health promotion practice and research*. San Francisco, CA: Jossey-Bass.

Dossey, B., Selanders, L., Beck, D., & Attewell, A. (2005). *Florence Nightingale today*. Silver Springs, MD: American Nurses Association.

Edwards, P. & Tsouros, A. D. (2008). *A healthy city is an active city: A physical activity planning guide*. Copenhagen, Denmark: World Health Organization.

Engelhard, C. L., Garson, A., & Dorn, S. (2009). *Reducing obesity: Policy strategies from the tobacco wars*. Retrieved from http://www.Urban.org/UploadedPDF/411926_reducing_obesity.pdf

Galanti, G. (2008). *Caring for patients from different cultures* (4th ed.). Philadelphia, PA: University of Pennsylvania Press.

Gallup Poll. (2011). *For first time, majority in U.S. supports public smoking ban: Little support for making smoking illegal, however.* Retrieved from http://www.gallup.com/poll/148514/first-time-majority-supports-public-smoking-ban.aspx

Giles, W., Homes-Chavez, A., & Collins, J. (2009). Cultivating healthy communities: The CDC perspective. *Health Promotion Practice, 10*, 86S–87S.

Ginsburg, P. B. (October, 2008). High and rising health care costs: Demystifying U.S. health care spending. The Robert Wood Johnson Foundation. *Research Synthesis Report No. 16*. Retrieved from http://www.rwjf.org/files/research/101508.policysynthesis.costdrivers.rpt.pdf

Glasgow, R. E., Ory, M. G., Klesges, L. M., Cifuentes, M., Fernald, D., & Green, L. A. (2005). Practical and relevant self-report measures of patient health behaviors for primary care research. *Annals of Family Medicine, 3*, 73–81.

Glassman, P. (2010). *Health literacy*. National Network of Libraries of Medicine. Retrieved from http://nnlm.gov/outreach/consumer/hlthlit.html

Grinspun, D. (2010). Commentary on "Expanding our Nightingale horizon: Seven recommendations for 21st-century nursing practice". *Journal of Holistic Nursing, 28*(4), 327–330.

Hanucharurnkul, S. (2009). Self-care deficit nursing theory in research and practice in Thailand. *Self-Care, Dependent-Care, and Nursing, 17*(1), 16–21.

Health Resources & Services Administration (HRSA). (2010). *The registered nurse population: Initial findings from the 2008 national sample survey of registered nurses*. Retrieved from http://bhpr.hrsa.gov/healthworkforce/rnsurveys/rnsurveyinitial2008.pdf

Healthy People 2020. (2011). *Leading health indicators*. Retrieved from http://www.healthypeople.gov/2020/LHI/default.aspx

Heylighen, F. & Joslyn, C. (1992). What is systems theory? In F. Heylighen, C. Joslyn, & V. Turchin (Eds.), *Principia cybrnetica web*. Retrieved from http://pespmc1.vub.ac.be/systheor.html

Hitt, E. (2010, May 4). Ending the HIV/AIDS epidemic still the goal, Fauci says. *Medscape Medical News*. Retrieved from http://www.medscape.com/viewarticle/721253

Institute of Medicine. (1998). *The future of public health*. Washington, DC: National Academy Press.

Institute of Medicine. (2002). *The future of the public's health in the 21st century*. Washington, DC: National Academy Press.

Koh, H. K. (2010, May 6). A 2020 vision for healthy people. *New England Journal of Medicine, 362*(18), 1653–1656.

Krisberg, K. (April, 2006). Safer housing conditions mean healthier lives for children. *The Nation's Health, 1*, 22–23.

Lavelle, M. (2010, May 27). *Gulf oil spill worst in U.S. history: Drilling postponed. National Geographic*. Retrieved from http://news.nationalgeographic.com/news/2010/05/100527-energy-nation-gulf-oil-spill-top-kill-obama/

Li, Y., Wang, W., Zhang, X., Lin, W., & Yang, Y. (2011). Impact of air pollution control measures and weather conditions on asthma during the 2008 Summer Olympic Games in Beijing. *International Journal of Biometerology, 53*(4), 547–554.

McDermott, M. M. (2007). The international pandemic of chronic cardiovascular disease. *The Journal of American Medical Association, 297*(11), 1253–1255.

Metzler, M., Kanarek, N., Highsmith, K., Bialek, R., Straw, R., Auston, I., et al. (2008). Community health status indicators project: The development of a national approach to community health. *Preventing Chronic Disease, 5*(3), 1–8.

Milestones in Public Health: Accomplishments in public health over the last 100 years. (2006). New York: Pfizer, Inc.

Morbidity and Mortality Weekly Report (MMWR). (2011, July 29). Notes from the field: Fatal fungal soft-tissue infections after a tornado—Joplin, Missouri, 2011. *Morbidity and Mortality Weekly Report (MMWR), 60*(29), 992.

Morbidity and Mortality Weekly Report (MMWR). (March 10, 2006). Public health response to hurricanes Katrina and Rita: United States, 2005.

Morbidity and Mortality Weekly Report (MMWR). (January 19, 2006). Assessment of health-related needs after hurricane Katrina: Orleans and Jefferson Parishes, New Orleans area, Louisiana, October 17–22, 2005.

Morbidity and Mortality Weekly Report (MMWR). (January 30, 2004). 40th anniversary of the First Surgeon General's Report on Smoking and Health/Prevalence of cigarette use among 14 racial/ethnic populations: United States, 1999–2001.

Morbidity and Mortality Weekly Report (MMWR). (April 7, 2000). Community indicators of health-related quality of life: United States, 1993–1997.

Morris, E.A. (2010, April 27). Drunk driving: Is the glass half-empty? *The New York Times*. Retrieved from http://www.freakonomics.blogs.nytimes.com/2010/04/27/drunk-driving-is-the-glass-half-empty/?pagemode=print

Munthe, C. (2008). The goals of public health: An integrated, multidimensional model. *Public Health Ethics, 1*(1), 39–52.

National Human Genome Research Institute. (2009). *The human genome project completion: Frequently asked questions*. U.S. Department of Health & Human Services. National Institutes of Health. Retrieved from http://www.genome.gov/pf.cfm?pageID=11006943

Nightingale, F. (1859/1992). *Notes on nursing: What it is, and what it is not* [Commemorative edition]. Philadelphia, PA: Lippincott Williams & Wilkins.

O'Donnell, M. P. (2009). Definition of health promotion 2.0: Embracing passion, enhancing motivation, recognizing dynamic balance, and creating opportunities. *American Journal of Health Promotion, 24*(1), iv.

Orem, D. (2001). *Nursing concepts of practice* (6th ed.). St. Louis, MO: Mosby-Year Book.

Pacala, J. (2007). *Tools of prevention*. Merck Manuals Online Library. Retrieved from http://www.merck.com/mmhe/sec01/ch005/ch005b.html

Park, M. (2009, May 25). Distress of 9/11 may have led to miscarriages, research says. *CNN*. Retrieved from http://www.cnn.com/2010/HEALTH/05/25/9.11.miscarriage.bereavement/index.html

Pender, N. J., Murdaugh, C., & Parsons, M. A. (2011). *Health promotion in nursing practice* (6th ed.). Upper Saddle River, NJ: Prentice-Hall.

Perera, F. P. (2008). Children are likely to suffer most from our fossil fuel addiction. *Environmental Health Perspectives, 116*(8), 987–990.

Poltzer, P. (2008, November, 17). *Tuberculosis: A new pandemic?* Retrieved from http://www.cnn.com/2008/HEALTH/11/17/tb.pandemic/index.html

Public Health Data Standards Consortium. (2006). Public Health Data Standards tutorial: Glossary of terms. Retrieved June 27, 2008 from www.phdatastandards.info/knowresources/tutorials/glossary.html

Public Health Institute. (2010a). *Tobacco control. Milestones in public health*. Retrieved from http://www.phi.org/public_health_101/milestones_in_public_health.html

Public Health Institute. (2010b, January 22). *Huffington Post article mentions PHI's online tool Dialogue4Health*. Retrieved from http://www.phi.org/news_events/news-viewRelease.cfm?pressReleaseID=184&year=2010

Public Health Institute. (2010c, May 7). *Santa Clara county toy law allows incentives for healthy food*. Retrieved from http://www.phi.org/news_events/news-viewRelease.cfm?pressReleaseID=196&year=2010

Quad Council. (2003). *Public health nursing competencies*. Retrieved June 27, 2008, from www.astdn.org/downloadablefiles/PHB%20competencies%20final%20comb.pdf

Rauh, V., Frank, L., Engelke, P., & Washington, T. (2003). *Health and community design: The impact of the built environment on physical activity*. Washington, DC: Island Press.

Ray, T. (2010, February 12). CDC official urges Healthy People 2020 effort to expand genomic targets. *Pharmacogenomics Reporter*. Retrieved from http://www.genomeweb.com/dxpgx/cdc-official-urges-healthy-people-2020-effort-expand-genomic-targets

Reuters. (2010, March 8). *Ban on sugary drinks in school appears to work*. Retrieved from http://www.msnbc.msn.com/id/35764878/ns/health-diet_and_nutrition/#storyContinued

Robert Wood Johnson Foundation. (2009, March). Nursing's prescription for a reformed health system. *Charting Nursing's Future, 9*, 1–8.

Sarrachi, R. (1997). The World Health Organization needs to reconsider its definition of Health. *British Medical Journal, 314*, 1409–1410.

Skolnik, R. L. (2008). *Essentials of global health*. Sudbury, MA: Jones & Bartlett Publishers.

Trust for America's Health. (2006). Ask the epidemiologist: Glossary of terms. Retrieved June 27, 2008, from http://healthyamericans.org/docs/?DocID=96

U.S. Department of Health and Human Services (USDHHS). (2011). *Healthy people 2020: About healthy people*. Retrieved from http://healthypeople.gov/2020/about/default.aspx

Ustin, B., & Jakob, R. (2005). Calling a spade a spade: Meaningful definitions of health conditions. *Bulletin of the World Health Organization, 83*, 802.

Wallace, R. B. (n.d.). Disease prevention. *Encyclopedia of Public Health*. Retrieved from http://www.enotes.com/public-health-encyclopedia/disease-prevention

Werch, C. E., Blan, H., Moore, M., Ames, S., DiClemente, C., & Weller, R. (2007). Brief multiple behavior interventions in a college student health care clinic. *Journal of Adolescent Health, 41*(6), 577–585.

What is Public Health? (n.d.). *Definition of public health*. Retrieved from http://www.whatispublichealth.org/

Williams, C. (1977). Community health nursing: What is it? *Nursing Outlook, 25*(4), 250–254.

Wisnivesky, J., Lorenzo, J., Lyn-Cook, R., Newman, T., Aponte, A., Kiefer, E., et al. (2008). Barriers to adherence to asthma management guidelines among inner-city primary care providers. *Annals of Allergy, Asthma, and Immunology, 101*(3), 264–270.

World Health Organization (WHO). (2009, June 25). *What are the qualities of a healthy city?* Retrieved from http://www.euro.who.int/healthy-cities/introducing/20050202_4?PrinterFriendly=1&

World Health Organization (WHO). (2010a). *WHO called to return to the Declaration of Alma Ata*. Retrieved from http://www.who.int/social_determinants/tools/multimedia/alma_ata/en/index.html

World Health Organization (WHO). (2010b). *The Ottawa Charter for health promotion*. Retrieved from http://www.who.int/healthpromotion/conferences/previous/ottawa/en/

Zagier, A. S. (2011, July 23). Joplin tornado restoration begins two months later. *The Huffington Post*. Retrieved from http://www.huffingtonpost.com/2011/07/23/joplin-tornado-restoration_n_907816.html

thePoint: Everything You Need to Make the Grade!

thePoint Visit http://thePoint.lww.com/Allender8e for selected readings, study aids for all learning styles, and more!

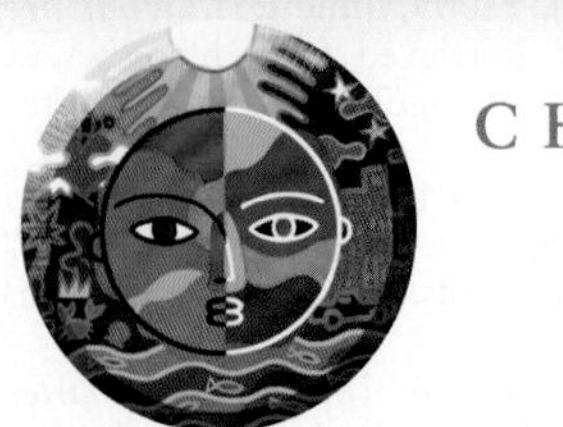

CHAPTER

2

History and Evolution of Community Health Nursing

"Our basic idea was that the nurse's peculiar introduction to the patient and her organic relationship with the neighborhood should constitute the starting point for a universal service to the region. we considered ourselves best described by the term 'public health nurses.'"

—***Lillian Wald*** **(1867–1940), pioneer of public health nursing**

KEY TERMS

Causal thinking
Community-based nursing
District nursing
Frontier nursing service
Henry street settlement
Industrial nursing
Nightingale model
Visiting nurse association

LEARNING OBJECTIVES

Upon mastery of this chapter, you should be able to:

- Describe the four stages of community health nursing's development.
- Recognize the contributions of selected nursing leaders throughout history to the advancement of community health nursing.
- Analyze the impact of societal influences on the development and practice of community health nursing.
- Explore the academic and advanced professional preparation of community health nurses.

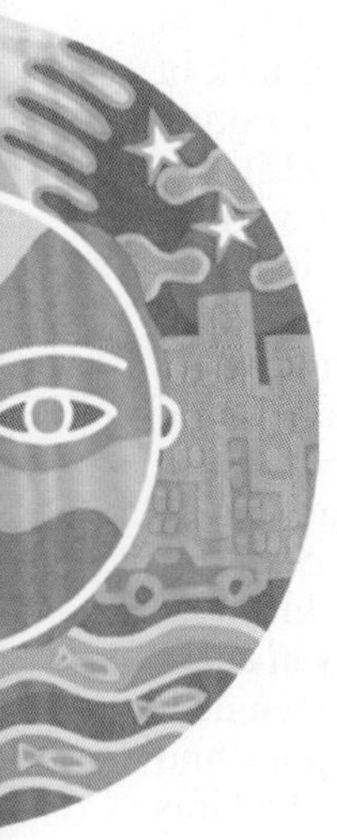

You just left the home of a long-time client who is concerned about a new family who just moved into the building where she lives. The family of six lives in an apartment with barely enough room for two. After years in this neighborhood, you are well aware of the high rents charged for apartments with peeling paint, rodents, and garbage all around the buildings. Your client is concerned that the young mother looks "worn out" and coughs all the time. She said she tried to help, but the family doesn't speak much English. She describes four young children all under the age of about 5. She's never seen the husband, but you know that most of the men in this neighborhood leave early in the morning to try to get some day work, so you are not surprised. You assure your client that you will do what you can to help her new neighbors and thank her for being such a kind person. Thinking about how you will prepare for the visit to the family who doesn't even expect you, your thoughts are racing. At the top of your list is trying to find someone who speaks their language; you only know a few words. You suspect without even seeing the mother what the cough means, although you hope you are wrong. Then you think about the four young children living so close together and creating so much work for a woman who isn't well. The husband may want to help his wife more, but if he doesn't work, they can't get by. You wonder if he has the cough too.

As you read this scenario, what picture did you have in your mind? What language did this family speak? What disease did this young mother likely have? Now, think about when this event might have occurred. If you thought it was now, it certainly could be, but this scenario was actually set in the early 1900s. This family emigrated from Greece and had not yet mastered the English language. The mother likely had consumption (the old name for tuberculosis). Because birth control information was not available to most women, she had no idea how to space out her pregnancies. The filthy and overcrowded housing, often called *tenement housing*, was typical of the time. The husband found work as he could. Few social services were available; no work, no food for the family, and no money to pay the rent. The family came to America with the hope of a new start, but what they found was in many ways worse than what they had left. At least at home in Greece, they had family and friends to count on; here, they were alone. There were others from Greece who lived nearby, but it wasn't the same. Life was hard, and they worried most about their children, wondering what the future could hold for them.

Community health nurses in the early 20th century had to deal with many of the same issues we face today. We thought for a long time that tuberculosis was a disease of the past; now clients with multidrug-resistant strains are becoming alarmingly more common. Poverty, communicable diseases, poor housing, lack of social services, and limited access to family planning information remain as challenges to improving the health of our populations. As a community health nurse, you will be facing similar challenges to those faced by nurses of the past. History is not always exciting, but without it we often fail to see where we need to go next. The often misquoted saying by George Santayana (1863–1952), "Those who cannot remember the past are condemned to repeat it," serves to caution us not to "forget" our heritage (Kaplin, 1992, p. 588). As you read through this chapter, think about how your practice has been shaped by the hard work of the nurses who went before.

This chapter examines the international roots of community health nursing as a specialty, exploring the historical and philosophical foundations that undergird the dynamic nature of its practice. The chapter traces community health nursing's historical development, highlighting the contributions of several nursing leaders and examining the global societal influences that shaped early and evolving community health nursing practice. The final section of the chapter describes the academic and advanced professional preparation required of community health nurses today. Nursing's past influences its present and both guide the future of community health nursing in the 21st century.

HISTORICAL DEVELOPMENT OF COMMUNITY HEALTH NURSING

Before the nature of community health nursing can be fully grasped or its practice defined, it is necessary to understand its roots and the factors that shaped its growth over time. Community health nursing is the product of centuries of responsiveness and growth. Its practice has adapted to accommodate the needs of a changing society, yet it has always maintained its initial goal of improved community health. Community health nursing's development, which has been influenced by changes in nursing, public health, and society, can be traced through several stages. This section examines these stages.

The history of public health nursing, since its recognized inception in Europe, and more recently in America, encompasses continuing change and adaptation (Hein, 2001). The historical record reveals a professional nursing specialty that has been on the cutting edge of innovations in public health practice and has provided leadership to public health efforts. A summary of public health nursing made in the early 1900s still holds true:

> It is precisely in the field of the application of knowledge that the public health nurse has found her great opportunity and her greatest usefulness. In the nationwide campaigns for the early detection of cancer and mental disorders, for the elimination of venereal disease, for the training of new mothers, and the teaching of the

> principles of hygiene to young and old; in short, in all measures for the prevention of disease and the raising of health standards, no agency is more valuable than the public health nurse. (Central Hanover Bank and Trust Company, 1938, p. 8)

In tracing the development of public health nursing and, later, community health nursing, the leadership role has been clearly evident throughout its history. Nurses in this specialty have provided leadership in planning and developing programs, in shaping policy, in administration, and in the application of research to community health.

Four general stages mark the development of community health/public health nursing: (1) the early home-care nursing stage, (2) the district nursing stage, (3) the public health nursing stage, and (4) the community health nursing stage. It is well worth referring to the Chapter 1 discussion of the interchangeable terms *public health nurse* and *community health nurse*. In the course of the historical evolution of this specialty, there was a definite shift in thinking about the focus of practice, resulting in the broader use of the term *community health nurse*. However, the discussion that follows is about the practice emphasis, not the title. There are nurses in practice who use the title public health nurse, in addition to those called community health nurses; more recently, the term community/public health nurse has been widely accepted as depicting the generalist practice in this specialty (Callen et al., 2010). Whether by custom, preference, or established employment title, nurses call themselves by many professional titles. It is important to recognize that the work of the nurse is, as it always has been, to improve the health of the community.

Early Home-Care Nursing (Before Mid-1800s)

The prototype of **community-based nursing** can be seen within the historical development of home-care nursing. For many centuries, the sick were tended at home by female family members and friends. In fact, in 1837, Farrar (p. 57) reminded women, "You may be called upon at any moment to attend upon your parents, your brothers, your sisters, or your companions." The focus of this care was to reduce suffering and promote healing.

The Origins of Early Nursing

The early roots of home-care nursing began with religious and charitable groups. Even emergency care was provided. In 1244, a group of monks in Florence, Italy, known as the Misericordia provided first-aid care for accident victims on a 24-hour basis. Another example is the Knights Hospitalers, who were warrior monks in Western Europe. They protected and cared for pilgrims on their way to Jerusalem (Men, monasteries, wars, and wards, 2001). During the 1500s, the Spanish nurse Bernardino de Obregon and his congregation provided both care of the ill and specialized nursing training at "houses of approval" (Jesús & Martínez, 2010). These and other men's contributions to the early practice of nursing have been long overlooked. Further, the lack of attention to these early works "perpetuates the notion of men nurses as anomalies" (Evans, 2004, p. 321).

Medieval times saw the development of various institutions devoted to the sick, including hospitals and nursing orders. In England, the Elizabethan Poor Law, written in 1601, provided medical and nursing care to the poor and disabled. St. Frances De Sales organized the Friendly Visitor Volunteers in the early 1600s in France. This association was directed by Madame de Chantel and assisted by wealthy women who cared for the sick poor in their homes (Dolan, 1978). In 1617, St. Vincent de Paul started the Sisters of Charity in Paris, an organization composed of nuns and lay women dedicated to serving the poor and needy. The ladies and sisters, under the supervision of Mademoiselle Le Gras in 1634, promoted the goal of teaching people to help themselves as they visited the sick in their homes. In their emphasis on preparing nurses and supervising nursing care, as well as determining causes and solutions for clients' problems, the Sisters of Charity laid a foundation for modern community health nursing (Bullough & Bullough, 1978).

Unfortunately, the years that followed these accomplishments marked a serious setback in the status of nursing and care of the sick. From the late 1600s to the mid-1800s, the social upheaval after the Reformation caused a decline in the number of religious orders, with subsequent curtailing of nursing care for the sick poor. Babies continued to be delivered at home by self-declared midwives, most of whom had little or no training. Concern over high maternal mortality rates prompted efforts to better prepare midwives and medical students. One midwifery program was begun in Paris in 1720 and another in London by Dr. William Smellie in 1741 (Bullough & Bullough, 1978).

The Industrial Revolution created additional problems; among them were epidemics, high infant mortality, occupational diseases and injuries, and increasing mental illness in both Europe and America. Hospitals were built in larger cities, and dispensaries were developed to provide greater access to physicians. However, disease was rampant; mortality rates were high; and institutional conditions, especially in prisons, hospitals, and "asylums" for the insane, were deplorable. The sick and afflicted were kept in filthy rooms without adequate food, water, cover, or care for their physical and emotional needs (Bullough & Bullough, 1978). Reformers such as John Howard, an Englishman who investigated the spread of disease in hospitals in 1789 (Kalisch & Kalisch, 2004), revealed serious needs that would not be addressed until much later (Bullough & Bullough, 1978). It would take another 64 years and the seminal work of John Snow with the London cholera epidemic of 1853 to link a water pump and the transmission of the disease (Ramsey, 2006) and the germ theory proposed by Louis Pasteur in 1862, to dispel many myths of the time, including the miasmic theory of disease (Fealy, McNamara & Geraphty, 2010). The term miasma referred to "bad air" and was attributed as the cause of illness not "germs." The work of these early scientists would bring attention to the need for changes in the care of the sick as well as the prevention of illness.

During this same period, Dorothea Dix brought attention to the plight of the mentally ill from abuse and neglect in US jails and almshouses. In what was arguably one of the first social research efforts in the United States, she presented her firsthand accounts of the terrible situations she found to the legislatures of Massachusetts, New York, New Jersey, and Pennsylvania (Reddi, 2005). Through her efforts there was an almost 10-fold increase in the number of mental institutions and the overall care of the mentally ill improved. Although not trained as a nurse, Dix would in later years oversee the Union Army female nurses prior to resuming her efforts with the mentally ill.

Both Catholic and Anglican religious nursing orders, although few in number, continued the work of caring for the sick poor in their homes. For example, in 1812, the Sisters of Mercy organized in Dublin to provide care for the sick at home. With the status of women at an all-time low, often only the least respectable women pursued nursing. In 1844, in his novel *Martin Chuzzlewit*, Charles Dickens (1910) portrayed the nurse Sairy Gamp as an unschooled and slovenly drunkard, reflecting society's view of nursing at the time. It was in the midst of these deplorable conditions and in response to them that Florence Nightingale began her work.

The Early Nightingale Years

Much of the foundation for modern community health nursing practice was laid through Florence Nightingale's remarkable accomplishments (Fig. 2-1). She has been referred to as a reformer, a reactionary, and a researcher (Palmer, 2001). Born in 1820 into a wealthy English family, her extensive travel, excellent education—including training at the first school for nurses in Kaiserwerth, Germany—and determination to serve the needy resulted in major reforms and improved status for nursing. Her work during the Crimean War (1854–1856) with the wounded in Scutari is well documented (Florence Nightingale Museum Trust, 1997; Woodham-Smith, 1951). Conditions in the military hospitals during the war were unspeakable. Thousands of sick and wounded men lay in filth, without beds, clean coverings, food, water, or laundry facilities. Florence Nightingale organized competent nursing care and established kitchens and laundries that resulted in hundreds of lives being saved. Her work further demonstrated that capable nursing intervention could prevent illness and improve the health of a population at risk—precursors to modern community health nursing practice. Her subsequent work for health reform in the military was supported by implementing another public health strategy: the use of biostatistics. Through meticulously gathered data and statistical comparisons, Miss Nightingale demonstrated that military mortality rates, even in peacetime, were double those of the civilian population because of the terrible living conditions in the barracks. This work led to important military reforms.

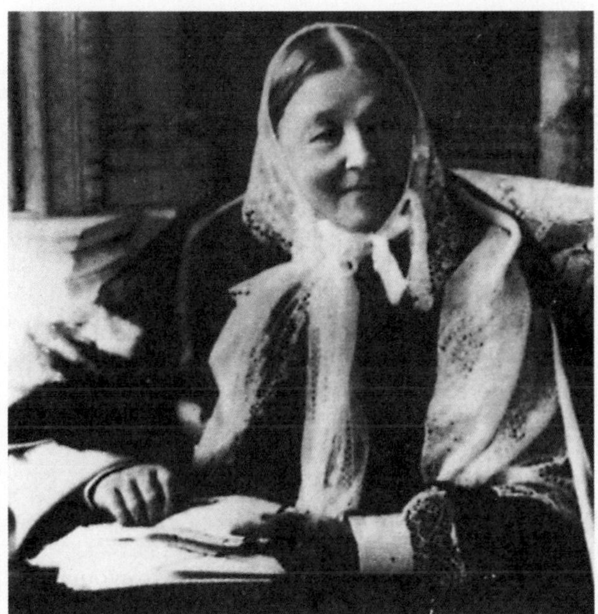

FIGURE 2-1. Florence Nightingale's concern for populations at risk, as well as her vision and successful efforts at health reform, provided a model for community health nursing today.

Miss Nightingale's concern for populations at risk included a continuing interest in the population of the sick at home. Her book, *Notes on Nursing: What It Is, and What It Is Not,* published in England in 1859, was written to improve nursing care in the home. It was also during this period that Nightingale clarified nursing as a woman's occupation (Evans, 2004). This gender distinction in nursing was due more to the culture of the times than as a direct exclusion of men from the practice; it was consistent with social norms of that period.

Florence Nightingale also became a skillful lobbyist for health care reform. Her exemplary influence on English politics and policy improved the quality of existing health care and set standards for future practice. Furthermore, she demonstrated how population-focused nursing works.

In her work to help establish the first nonreligious school for nurses in 1860 at St. Thomas Hospital in London, she promoted a standard for proper education and supervision of nurses in practice, known as the **Nightingale Model**. Principles she wrote about in *Notes on Nursing* relate directly to her early education and the notions held by Hippocrates in ancient Greece, which she had studied for years. Specifically, her concern with the environment of patients, the need for keen observation, the focus on the whole patient rather than the disease, and the importance of assisting nature to bring about a cure all reflect Hippocrates' teachings (Nightingale, 1859/1969; Palmer, 2001).

Another great nurse and healer in her own right was Mary Seacole (1805–1881), who has been called the "Black Nightingale." She was the daughter of a well-respected "doctress" who practiced Creole or Afro-Caribbean medicine in Jamaica, and began helping her mother at an early age. Spending many years developing her skills, she helped populations who experienced tropical diseases, especially cholera, in Central America, Panama, and the Caribbean. She attempted, through many formal channels, to join Florence Nightingale in Scutari, but was rejected again and again. Undaunted, she went to the Crimea on her own to open a hotel for sick and convalescing soldiers, where she met Miss Nightingale and many of the troops she had cared for in Jamaica. Many of the military commanders sought her out for her knowledge of healing, and she was affectionately known by the troops as "Mother Seacole." After the war and into her old age, she continued to provide nursing care in London and when visiting Jamaica. She focused her caregiving among high-risk clients of the day and did so in an innovative, entrepreneurial manner unique for women, especially for women of color in the 1800s (Florence Nightingale Museum Trust, 1997). Her autobiography *Wonderful Adventures of Mrs. Seacole in Many Lands* was published in 1857 and became a best seller, providing much needed financial support for Mary Seacole (Stanley, 2007). W. H. Russell Esq. wrote in the introduction "…I trust that England will not forget one who nursed her sick, who sought out her wounded to aid and succour them, and who performed the last offices for some of her illustrious dead" (Seacole, 1857) (see Display 2.1).

District Nursing (Mid-1800s to 1900)

Nightingale's Continued Influence

The next stage in the development of community health nursing was the formal organization of visiting nursing, or **district nursing**. In 1859, William Rathbone, an English philanthropist, became convinced of the value of home nursing as a result of private care given to his wife. He employed Mary Robinson, the nurse who had cared for his wife, to visit the sick poor in their homes and teach them proper hygiene to prevent illness. The need was so great that it soon became evident that more nurses were needed. In 1861, with Florence Nightingale's help and advice, Rathbone opened a training school for nurses connected with the Royal Liverpool Infirmary and established a visiting nurse service for the sick poor in Liverpool. Florence Lees, a graduate of the Nightingale School, was appointed first Superintendent-General of the District Nursing System (Mowbray, 1997). As the service grew, visiting nurses were assigned to districts in the city—hence the name, district nursing. Subsequently, other British cities also developed district nursing training and services. An example is the Nurse Training Institution for district nurses, founded in Manchester in 1864 and the work done by Ellen Ranyard and others in London (Prochaska, 1980/2003). Privately financed, the nurses were trained and then "dispensed food and medicine" to the sick poor in their homes; they were "closely supervised by various middle and upper class women who collected the necessary supplies" (Bullough & Bullough, 1978, p. 143).

Although Florence Nightingale is best remembered for her professionalization of nursing, she had a full understanding of the need for community health nursing. This was documented in her writings and recorded conversations:

> Hospitals are but an intermediate stage of civilisation. At present hospitals are the only place where the sick poor can be nursed, or, indeed often the sick rich. But the ultimate object is to nurse all sick at home. (Nightingale, 1876)
>
> The aim of the district nurse is to give first-rate nursing to the sick poor at home. (Nightingale, 1876 [cited in Mowbray, 1997, p. 24])
>
> The health visitor must create a new profession for women. (conversation with Frederick Verney, 1891 [cited in Mowbray, 1997, p. 25])

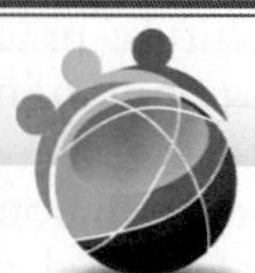

DISPLAY 2.1 TWENTY YEARS IN HISTORY: 1845 TO 1865

1845	Dorothea Dix addresses the New Jersey and Pennsylvania legislatures regarding abuse and neglect of the mentally ill
1848	The first women's rights convention in the United States is held in Seneca Falls, New York
1849	Harriet Tubman escapes from slavery and will lead many slaves to freedom through the Underground Railroad
1850	Florence Nightingale begins nursing training at the Institute of St. Vincent de Paul in Alexandria, Egypt
1854	Florence Nightingale cares for the injured in the Crimean War
1855	Mary Seacole establishes a boarding house to care for sick and injured soldiers in the Crimea
1857	Ellen Ranyard pioneers the first district nursing program in England
1860	Florence Nightingale's *Notes on Nursing—What it is and what is not* is published
1861	Civil War embroils the country until 1865; Harriet Tubman serves as an unpaid nurse to wounded civilians and soldiers; Dorothea Dix is placed in charge of all female nurses in Union military hospitals
1865	Sojourner Truth serves as a nurse for the Freedman's Relief Association during Reconstruction in Washington, DC.

For years, Miss Nightingale studied the social and economic conditions of India (Nightingale, 1864). The plight of the poor and ill in India led her to become involved with Frederick Verney in a pioneering "health at home" project in England in 1892. She wrote a series of papers on the need for "home missioners" and "health visitors," endorsing the view that prevention was better than cure (Mowbray, 1997).

Home Visiting Takes Root

In the United States, the first community health nurse, Frances Root, hired by the Women's Branch of the New York Mission in 1877, pioneered home visits to the poor in New York City. District nursing associations were founded in Buffalo in 1885 and in Boston and Philadelphia in 1886 (Display 2.2). These district associations served the sick poor exclusively, because patients with enough money had private home nursing care. However, the English model with its standards for visiting nurses' education and practice, established in 1889 under Queen Victoria, was not followed in the United States. Instead, visiting nursing organizations sprang up in many cities without common standards or administration. Twenty-one such services existed in the United States in 1890 (Bullough & Bullough, 1978; Kalisch & Kalisch, 2004).

Although district nurses primarily cared for the sick, they also taught cleanliness and wholesome living to their patients, even during that early period. For example, the Boston program, founded by the Women's Educational Association, "emphasized the teaching of hygiene and cleanliness, giving impetus to what was called instructive district nursing" (Bullough & Bullough, 1978, p. 144). This early emphasis on prevention and "health" nursing became one of the distinguishing features of district nursing and, later, of public health nursing as a specialty.

The work of district nurses in the United States focused mostly on the care of individuals. District nurses recorded temperatures and pulse rates and gave simple treatments to the sick poor under the immediate direction of a physician. They also instructed family members in personal hygiene, diet and healthful living habits, and the care of the sick. The problems of early home-care patients in the United States were numerous and complex. Thousands of European and eastern European immigrants filled tenement housing in the poorest and most crowded slums of the large coastal cities during the late 1800s. Inadequate sanitation, unsafe and unhealthy working conditions, and language and cultural barriers added to poverty and disease. Nursing educational programs at that time did not prepare district nurses to cope with their patients' multiple health and social problems.

The sponsorship of district nursing changed over time. Early district nursing services in both England and the United States were founded by religious organizations. Later, sponsorship shifted to private philanthropy. Funding came from contributions and, in a few instances, from fees charged to patients on an ability-to-pay basis. Finally, visiting nursing began to be supported by public money. An early example occurred in Los Angeles where, in 1898, a nurse was hired as a city employee, making Los Angeles the first city in the United States to establish "municipal nursing" (Brainard, 1922). Although one form of funding dominated, all three types of financing continued to exist, as they still do. Although the government was beginning to assume more responsibility for the public's health, most district nursing services during this time remained private.

In England, the establishment of "health visitors" in poor areas of London began early in the 19th century. These health care providers enhanced the English model of health visitor/district nurse/midwife as the backbone of the primary health care system in the second half of the 1800s. "The impact of early health visiting was clearly shown by the halving of infant mortality in the areas within two years" (Beine, 1996, p. 59). The main focus of the health visitor's work was giving advice to poor mothers and teaching hygiene to prevent infant diarrhea (Beine, 1996).

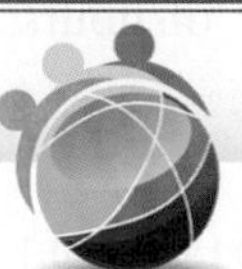

DISPLAY 2.2 TWENTY YEARS IN HISTORY: 1873 TO 1893

1873	First Nightingale-model nursing school established in the United States at Bellevue Hospital
1877	Francis Root—First Public Health Nurse hired by the Women's Branch of the New York Mission
1878	Woman Suffrage Amendment is introduced in the U.S. Congress
1879	Mary Eliza Mahoney becomes the first African-American to graduate from an American nursing school
1881	American Red Cross established by Clara Barton and associates becoming its first president
1885	Visiting Nurse Association established in Buffalo, New York
1886	Visiting Nurse Associations established in Philadelphia and Boston
1893	Lillian Wald and Mary Brewster organize a visiting nurses service for the poor in New York, which would be named the Henry Street Settlement in 1906; *American Society of Superintendents of Training Schools for Nursing* founded by Isabel Adams Hampton Robb (later renamed the National League for Nursing)

Public Health Nursing (1900 to 1970)

By the beginning of the 20th century, district nursing had broadened its focus to include the health and welfare of the general public, not just the poor. This new emphasis was part of a broader consciousness about public health. Robert Koch's demonstration that tuberculosis was communicable led the Johns Hopkins Hospital to hire a nurse, Reba Thelin, in 1903, to visit the homes of tuberculosis patients. Her job was to ensure that patients followed prescribed regimens of rest, fresh air, and proper diet and to prevent possible infection (Sachs, 1908). A growing sense of urgency about the interrelatedness of health conditions and the need to improve the health of all people led to an increased number of private health agencies. These agencies supplemented the often-limited work of government health departments. By 1910, new federal laws made states and communities accountable for the health of their citizens.

Nurses Making a Difference

Three years before Reba Thelin began her work with Johns Hopkins Hospital, Jessie Sleet was hired by the Charity Organization Society's (COS) tuberculosis committee as a temporary district nurse in New York City (Mosley, 2007). Her position called for her to visit the city's black community, which was ravaged by the disease. Jessie Sleet had been trained at the Provident Hospital in Chicago (a hospital for black patients), which had a nurse's training program for black women. Credited as the first black public health nurse, Ms. Sleet was not eagerly accepted by the COS membership, but they agreed in hope that she would be accepted by the black community. She was so successful in her efforts that, 1 year later, the society hired her as a permanent employee (Mosley, 2007). Jessie Sleet was a pioneer in early community health nursing practice and forged the way for many. Display 2.3 outlines other historical events during those intervening years.

As specialized programs such as infant welfare, tuberculosis clinics, and venereal disease control were developed, there was an increased demand for nurses to work in these areas (Fig. 2-2). As Bullough and Bullough (1978, p. 143).commented, "Although the hospital nursing school movement emphasized the care of the sick, a small but growing number of nurses were finding employment in preventive health care." In 1900, there were an estimated 200 public health nurses. By 1912, that number had grown to 3,000 (Gardner, 1936). "This development was important: it brought health care and health teaching to the public, gave nurses an opportunity for more independent work, and helped to improve nursing education" (Bullough & Bullough, 1978, p. 143).

The role of the district nurse expanded during this stage. Lillian D. Wald (1867–1940), a leading figure in this expansion, first used the term *public health nursing* to describe this specialty (Bullough & Bullough, 1978). District nurses, while caring for the sick, had pioneered in health teaching, disease prevention, and promotion of good health practices. Now, with a growing recognition of familial and environmental influences on health, public health nurses broadened their practice even more. Nurses working outside of the hospital increased their knowledge and skills in specialized areas such as tuberculosis, maternal and child health, school health, and mental disorders.

Lillian Wald's contributions to public health nursing were enormous. A graduate of the New York Hospital Training School, she started teaching home nursing but

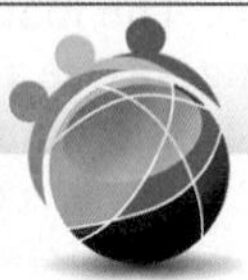

DISPLAY 2.3 TWENTY YEARS IN HISTORY: 1894 TO 1914

1894	Mary Adelaide Nutting appointed Superintendent of the Johns Hopkins School of Nursing—under her leadership, the curriculum was expanded from 2 to 3 years and limited the number of hours students could work
1895	Vermont Marble Company forms the Industrial Nursing Service to care for sick employees and their families
1897	First meeting of the *Nurses Associated Alumnae of the United States and Canada* that in 1911 would be renamed the American Nurses Association
1898	Spanish American War leads to outbreak of Yellow Fever among solders
1900	Jessie Sleet Scales becomes the first African-American public health nurse in United States
1902	New York City Board of Education hires Lina Rogers Struthers as a school nurse and begins the first public school nurse program in the county
1905	American Red Cross receives Congressional Charter
1909	Metropolitan Life Insurance Company provides first insurance reimbursement for visiting nursing care
1910	Public Health Nursing program instituted at Teacher's College, Columbia University
1912	National Organization for Public Health Nursing formed, with Lillian Wald as first President
1914	Margaret Sanger publishes the monthly newsletter *The Woman Rebel* to promote contraception and is charged with distributing illegal "birth control' information

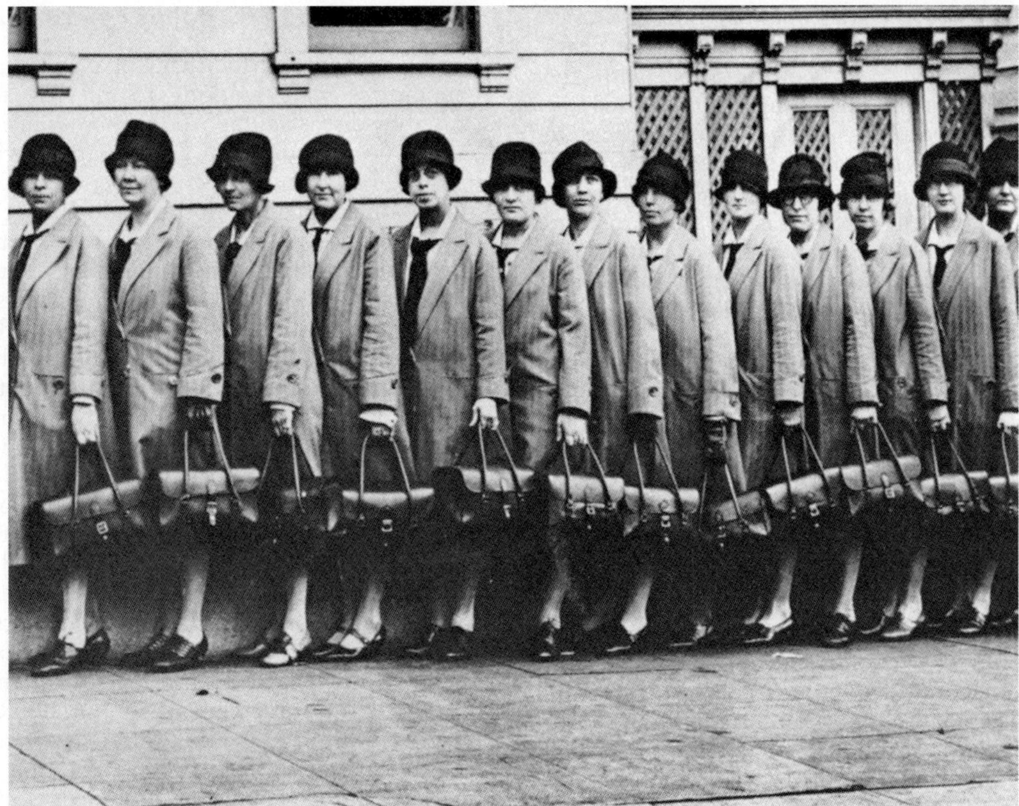

FIGURE 2-2. Public health nurses—uniforms and symbols. (Photograph courtesy of Visiting Nurses and Hospice of San Francisco.)

quickly changed to a career of social reform and nursing activism (Christy, 1970). Appalled by the conditions of an immigrant neighborhood in New York's Lower East Side, she and a nurse-friend, Mary Brewster, started the Henry Street Settlement in 1893 to provide nursing and welfare services. Her books, *The House on Henry Street* (1915) and *Windows of Henry Street* (1934), portray her work and views on public health nursing. Nursing visits conducted through her organization were supervised by nurses, in contrast to earlier models, in which nursing services were administered by lay boards and actual care was supervised by lay persons. It was during these early years that Wald asked Jessie Sleet to recommend another black nurse for service at the settlement (Mosley, 2007). Miss Sleet recommended her schoolmate Miss Elizabeth Tyler, a graduate of the Freedmen's Hospital Training School for Nurses (Washington, DC). In 1906, Miss Tyler became the first black nurse hired at the Henry Street Settlement; she would not be the last. This was no small event in the progress of public health nursing and was a clear demonstration of Miss Wald's commitment to social change.

Wald's Growing Influence

The work done at the Henry Street Settlement showed clearly that nursing could reduce illness-caused employee absenteeism. She demonstrated this in her early work with the city of New York. She would use this success to address the issue of childhood illness and school absenteeism (Bullough & Bullough, 1978). In the early 1900s, approximately 15 to 20 children per day were sent home from each school in New York City for health-related reasons. Wald suggested that placing nurses in the schools would allow for follow-up on recurring cases and home visits during the periods of exclusion. She argued that the nurses could supplement the work done by local physicians, who occasionally examined the children. Offering the services of one nurse for 1 month, Wald hoped to demonstrate how effective a school nurse could be. The work done by this first school nurse, Lina Rogers Struthers, was a resounding success (Kalisch & Kalisch, 2004). One year after this initial experiment, the number of children sent home from the New York City schools had dropped dramatically. By September 1903, only 1,000 children needed to be excluded (compared with 10,000 1 year earlier); a nearly 10-fold reduction. As a result, the New York Board of Health hired dozens of nurses to work at the schools becoming the first school nursing program in the country (Vessey & McGowen, 2006). Lina Rogers Struthers would go on to author the first textbook for school nurses *The School Nurse: A Survey of the Duties and Responsibilities of the Nurse in the Maintenance of Health and Physical Perfection and the Prevention of Disease Among School Children (1917).*

Just 6 years after her efforts with the New York City schools, Wald embarked on another visionary path. In

1909, she convinced the Metropolitan Life Insurance Company that nurse intervention could reduce death rates (Hamilton, 2007). In collaboration with the Henry Street Settlement, the company organized the Visiting Nurse Department and provided services to policy holders in a section of Manhattan (see Display 2.3). The success of this program resulted in expansion to other parts of the city and to 12 other eastern cities within 1 year. By 1912, the company had organized 589 Metropolitan nursing centers and, when possible, contracted with local **Visiting Nurses Associations**, although they also hired their own nurses (Kalisch & Kalisch, 2004).

The legendary accomplishments of Lillian Wald reflect her driving commitment to serve needy populations. Through her efforts, the New York City Bureau of Child Hygiene was formed in 1908, and the Children's Bureau at the federal level in 1912. Wald's emphasis on illness prevention and health promotion through health teaching and nursing intervention, as well as her use of epidemiologic methodology, established these actions as hallmarks of public health nursing practice. She promoted rural nursing and family-focused nursing and encouraged improved coursework at the Teachers College of Columbia University (New York) to prepare public health nurses for practice. Through her work and influence with the legislature to establish health and social policies, improvements were made in child labor and pure food laws, tenement housing, parks, city recreation centers, immigrant handling, and teaching of mentally handicapped children. In 1912, she helped to found and was first president of the National Organization for Public Health Nursing (NOPHN), an organization that set standards and guided public health nursing's further development and impact on public health (Christy, 1970). Her exemplary accomplishments truly reflect a concern for populations at risk. They further demonstrate how nursing leadership, involvement in policy formation, and use of epidemiology led to improved health for the public.

Another Nurse—Another Problem

During the same period that Lillian Wald and her contemporaries were working to alleviate the suffering caused by disease and poverty, another nurse, Margaret Sanger, began a different battle. Sanger, who was born in 1879, had seen her own mother die at the age of 48 after a long struggle with tuberculosis. Her 18 pregnancies undoubtedly contributed to her both contracting the disease and eventually succumbing to it. After her mother's death, she was accepted at White Plains Hospital as a nursing probationer (Ruffing-Rahal, 1986). Later, as a visiting nurse, Sanger was prevented by the Comstock Act of 1873 from providing any information on contraception to the women she cared for (Draper, 2006). She knew, as did many at the time, that the affluent and educated in American society were the only ones to have reliable contraception. Even discussing the topic was prohibited, placing increased pressure on the poor and uneducated women who were most in need of this basic information. In 1912, Sanger watched helplessly as a 28-year-old mother of three died from abortion-induced septicemia. "A few months earlier, during a similar crisis, this woman had begged Sanger for the 'secret' of preventing future pregnancy" (Ruffing–Rahal, 1986, pp. 247–248). In 1916, Sanger openly offered birth control information in the Brownsville section of Brooklyn. Ten days after opening the first birth control clinic in America, Sanger was arrested and the clinic was closed. This was not the first, nor would it be her last encounter with the legal system (see Display 2.4). Her open defiance of a law that she saw as unjust eventually resulted in the formation of the International Planned Parenthood Federation.

The Profession Evolves

By the 1920s, public health nursing was acquiring a more professional stature, in contrast to its earlier association with charity. Nursing as a whole was gaining professional status as a science, in addition to being an

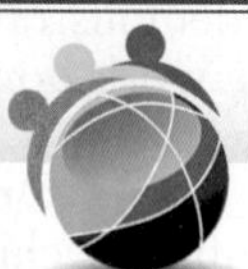

DISPLAY 2.4 TWENTY YEARS IN HISTORY: 1917 TO 1937

1917	United States entry into World War I; 18th Amendment passed by Congress (Prohibition)
1918	U.S. Public Health Service establishes Division of Public Health Nursing to aid the war effort; World War I Armistice; Worldwide influenza epidemic begins; Frances Reed Elliott becomes the first African-American nurse accepted into the American Red Cross Nursing Service
1919	19th Amendment passed by Congress
1920	Women vote for the first time in a presidential election
1921	Margaret Sanger founds the American Birth Control League to distribute contraception information
1925	Frontier Nursing Service established
1929	Stock Market Crash
1933	18th Amendment repealed (Prohibition)
1935	Passage of Social Security Act
1937	Birth control information legal in all but two states (Massachusetts and Connecticut)

art. National nursing organizations began to form during this stage and contributed to nursing's professional growth. The first of these emphasized establishing educational standards for nursing. Called the American Society of Superintendents of Training Schools for Nurses in the United States and Canada, it was started by Isabel Hampton Robb in 1893, and later became known as the National League of Nursing Education in 1912. This was the forerunner of the National League for Nursing (NLN), which was established in 1952 (Ellis & Hartley, 2000). In 1890, a meeting of nursing leaders at the World's Fair in Chicago initiated an alumnae organization of 10 schools of nursing to form the National Associated Alumnae of the United States and Canada in 1896, which was created to promote nursing education and practice standards. In 1899, the group was renamed the Nurses' Associated Alumnae of the United States and Canada. Canada was excluded from the title in 1901, because New York, where the organization was incorporated, did not allow representation from two countries. In 1911, the organization went through a final name change to the American Nurses' Association (ANA), while Canadian nurses formed their own nursing organization (Ellis & Hartley, 2000). The previously mentioned NOPHN, founded by Lillian Wald and Mary Gardner, merged with the NLN in 1952. These three organizations, in particular, strengthened ties between nursing groups and improved nursing education and practice.

As nursing education became increasingly rigorous, collegiate programs began to include public health as essential content in basic nursing curricula. The first collegiate program with public health content to be accredited by the NLN began in 1944 (National Organization for Public Health Nursing, 1944) (Display 2.5). Previously, only postgraduate courses in public health nursing had been offered for nurses choosing this specialty. The first such course had been developed by Adelaide Nutting in 1912, at Teachers College in New York, in affiliation with the Henry Street Settlement. A group of agencies met in 1946 to establish guidelines for public health nursing, and by 1963, public health content was required for NLN accreditation in all baccalaureate nursing programs. The nurse practitioner (NP) movement, starting in 1965 at the University of Colorado, was initially a part of public health nursing and emphasized primary health care to rural and underserved populations. The number of educational programs to prepare NPs increased, with some NPs continuing in public health and others moving into different clinical areas.

During this period of public health nursing, as a result of the influence of Lillian Wald and other nursing leaders, the family began to emerge as a unit of service (Fig. 2-3). The multiple problems faced by many families impelled a trend toward nursing care generalized enough to meet diverse needs and provide holistic services. Public health nurses gradually gained more autonomy in such areas as home care and instruction of good health practices to families and community groups. Their collaborative relationships with other community health providers grew as the need to avoid gaps and duplication of services became apparent. Public health nurses also began keeping better records of their services.

Industrial nursing, another form of public health nursing, also expanded during the early 1900s. The first known industrial nurse, Philippa Flowerday Reid, was hired in Norwich, England, by J. and J. Colmans in 1878. Her job was to assist the company physician and to visit sick employees and their families in their homes.

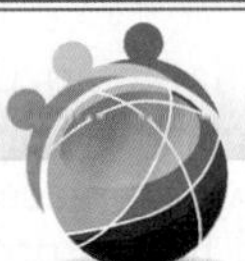

DISPLAY 2.5 TWENTY YEARS IN HISTORY: 1941 TO 1961

1941	United States entry into World War II
1943	Cadet Nursing Corps Program established, providing federal funding for academic nursing education in exchange for work in "essential nursing services"
1944	First basic program in nursing accredited as including sufficient public health content; Public Health Service Act authorizes qualified nurses to be commissioned in the U.S. Public Health Service
1945	World War II ends; United Nations votes to establish the World Health Organization
1946	Hill-Burton Act approved—shift to hospital based care with federal funding of hospitals and medical centers: Communicable Disease Center established (forerunner of the Centers for Disease Control and Prevention)
1949	Lucile Petry Leone becomes the Chief Nurse Officer of the Public Health Service, the first nurse and the first woman to achieve flag rank in the Public Health Service or military
1950	United States involvement in Korean Conflict (ends in 1953)
1954	Brown versus Board of Education—Landmark Supreme Court decision prohibits racial segregation in public schools
1955	Introduction of the Salk Polio Vaccine
1956	Health Amendments Act provided funds to support public health nurse advanced training
1961	Peace Corps is founded; United States entry into the Vietnam War

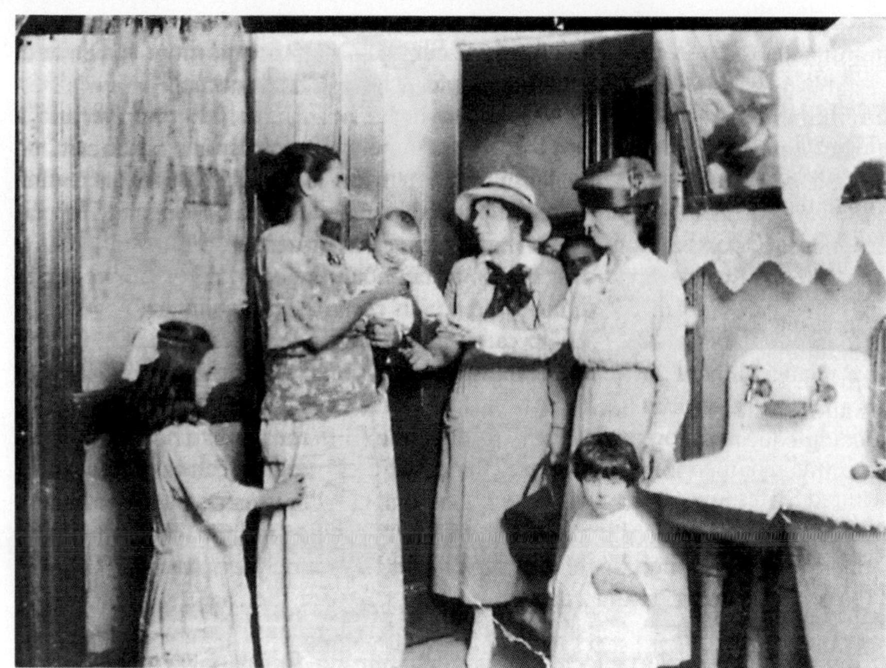

FIGURE 2-3. The public health nurse, carrying her bag of equipment and supplies, makes regular home visits to provide physical and psychological care, as well as health lessons to families.

In the United States, the Vermont Marble Company was first to begin a nursing service in 1895; other companies followed soon after. By 1910, 66 firms in the United States employed nurses. During World War I, the number of industrial nurses greatly increased with the recognition that nursing service reduced worker absenteeism (Bullough & Bullough, 1978). Early industrial nursing was the forerunner of modern occupational and environmental health nursing.

During this stage, the institutional base for much of public health nursing shifted to the government. By 1955, 72% of the counties in the continental United States had local health departments. Public health nursing constituted the major portion of these local health services and emphasized health promotion, as well as care for the ill at home (Scutchfield & Keck, 2009). Some of the district nursing services, known as ***visiting nurse associations*** (VNAs), remained privately funded and administered, offering their own home nursing care. In some places, city or county health departments joined administratively and financially with VNAs to provide a combination of services, such as home care of the sick and health promotion to families.

Rural public health nursing, which had already been organized around 1900 in Great Britain, Germany, and Canada, also expanded in the United States (see Chapter 29). Initially, starting in 1912, rural nursing was privately financed and largely administered through the Red Cross and the Metropolitan Life Insurance Company, but responsibility had shifted to the government by the 1940s (Bullough & Bullough, 1978). An innovative example of rural nursing was the **Frontier Nursing Service**, which was started by Mary Breckenridge (1881–1965) in 1925, to serve mountain families in Kentucky. From six outposts, nurses on horseback visited remote families to deliver babies and provide food and nursing services. Over the years, the service has expanded to provide medical, dental, and nursing care. The Frontier Nursing Service continues today, with its remarkable accomplishments of reducing mortality rates and promoting health among this disadvantaged population, as the parent holding company for the Frontier School of Midwifery and Family Nursing. It is the largest nurse–midwifery program in the United States. In addition, Mary Breckinridge Healthcare, Inc. consists of a home health agency, two outpost clinics, one primary care clinic, and the Kate Ireland Women's Healthcare Clinic (Simpson, 2000).

The public health nursing stage was characterized by service to the public, with the family targeted as a primary unit of care. Official health agencies, which placed greater emphasis on disease prevention and health promotion, provided the chief institutional base.

Community Health Nursing (1970 to the Present)

The emergence of the term *community health nursing* heralded a new era. By the late 1960s and early 1970s, while public health nurses continued their work, many other nurses who were not necessarily practicing public health were based in the community. Their practice settings included community-based clinics, doctors' offices, work sites, and schools. To provide a label that encompassed all nurses in the community, the ANA and others called them community health nurses. Display 2.6 provides examples of significant events in mid-60s to early 1980s.

This term was not universally accepted, however, and many people—including nurses and the general public—had difficulty distinguishing community health

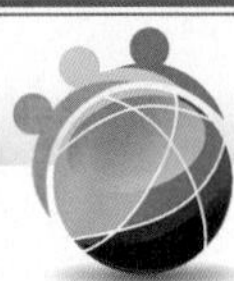

DISPLAY 2.6 TWENTY YEARS IN HISTORY: 1965 TO 1985

1965	Medicare and Medicaid established
1972	Social Security Administration allows Medicare coverage for those <65 years with long-term chronic disease and end stage renal disease
1973	U.S. military troops leave S. Vietnam; Roe versus Wade—Landmark Supreme Court decision legalizes abortion
1977	Global smallpox eradication achieved
1978	Drug resistant TB reported in Mississippi
1979	*Healthy People: The Surgeon General's Report on Health Promotion and Disease Prevention* released
1985	Red Cross Blood Services begin testing for HIV antibody

nursing from public health nursing. For example, nursing education, recognizing the importance of public health content, required course work in public health for all baccalaureate students. This meant that graduates were expected to incorporate public health principles such as health promotion and disease prevention into nursing practice, regardless of their sphere of service. Consequently, some questioned whether public health nursing retained any unique content. Although leaders such as Carolyn Williams clearly stated that community health nursing's specialized contribution lay in its focus on populations (Williams, 1977), this concept did not appear to be widely understood or practiced.

Confusion also arose regarding the question of whether community health nursing was a generalized or a specialized practice. Graduates from baccalaureate nursing programs were inadequately prepared to practice in public health; their education had emphasized individualized and direct clinical care and provided little understanding of applications to populations and communities. By the mid-1970s, various community health nursing leaders had identified knowledge and skills needed for more effective community health nursing practice (Roberts & Freeman, 1973). These leaders valued promoting the health of the community, but both education and practice continued to emphasize direct clinical care to individuals, families, and groups in the community (de Tornyay, 1980). Reflecting this view, the ANA's Division of Community Health Nursing developed *A Conceptual Model of Community Health Nursing* in 1980. This document distinguished generalized community health nursing preparation at the baccalaureate level and specialized community health nursing preparation at the masters or postgraduate level. The generalist was described as one who provides nursing service to individuals and groups of clients while keeping "the community perspective in mind" (American Nurses Association, 1980, p. 9).

To distinguish the domains of community and public health nursing, in 1984, the U.S. Department of Health and Human Services, Bureau of Health Professionals, Division of Nursing, convened a Consensus Conference on the Essentials of Public Health Nursing Practice and Education in Washington, DC (U.S. Department of Health and Human Services [USDHHS], Division of Nursing, 1984). This group concluded that *community health nursing* was the broader term, referring to all nurses practicing in the community, regardless of their educational preparation. *Public health nursing*, viewed as a part of community health nursing, was described as a generalist practice for nurses prepared with basic public health content at the baccalaureate level and a specialized practice for nurses prepared in public health at the master's level or beyond.

Finally, confusion also arose regarding the changing roles and functions of community health nurses. Accelerated changes in health care organization and financing, technology, and social issues made increasing demands on community health nurses to adapt to new patterns of practice. Many new kinds of community health services appeared. Hospital-based programs reached into the community. Private agencies proliferated, offering home care and other community-based services. Other community health professionals assumed responsibilities that traditionally had been the domain of public health nursing. For example, some school counselors in Oregon began coordinating home visits previously done by school nurses, and health educators (who were part of a more recently developed discipline) took over large segments of client education. Social workers, too, provided services that overlapped with community health nursing roles. Health educators, counselors, social workers, epidemiologists, and nutritionists working in community health came prepared with different backgrounds and emphases in their practice. Their contributions were and still are important. Their presence, however, forced community health nurses to reexamine their own contribution to the public's health and incorporate stronger interdisciplinary and collaborative approaches into their practice (see "Levels of Prevention Pyramid").

The debate over these areas of confusion continued through the 1980s, and some issues are yet unresolved. Still, the direction in which public health and community health nursing must move remains clear: to care *for*, not simply *in*, the community. Public health nursing continues to mean the synthesis of nursing and the public health sciences applied to promoting and protecting

LEVELS OF PREVENTION PYRAMID

GOAL: Clarify and enhance the community health nurse's role to promote impact

TERTIARY PREVENTION

- Promote increasing influence of the nurse through an expanded role in service delivery
- Minimize the impact of community misunderstandings of the nurse's role through education

SECONDARY PREVENTION

- Promote aggregate-level interventions
- Foster nurse involvement on community boards and other political groups

PRIMARY PREVENTION

- Participate in policy formation
- Be politically active
- Assist in acquiring funding for community health programs
- Conduct research on health and nursing outcomes to enhance evidence-based practice
- Collaborate with the news media to publicize current public health issues

the health of populations. Community health nursing, for some, refers more broadly to nursing in the community. In this text, the term *community health nursing* is used synonymously with *public health nursing* and refers to specialized, population-focused nursing practice, which applies public health science and nursing science. A possible distinction between the two terms might be to view community health nursing as a beginning level of specialization and public health nursing as an advanced level. Clarification and consensus on the meaning of these terms may help to avoid misconceptions and misuse, and are explored more fully in Chapter 3. Whichever term is used to describe this specialty, the fundamental issues and defining criteria remain the same: (1) Are populations and communities the target of practice? and (2) Are the nurses prepared in public health and engaging in public health practice?

As community health nursing continues to evolve, many signs of positive growth are evident. Community health nurses are carving out new roles for themselves in primary health care. Collaboration and interdisciplinary teamwork are recognized as crucial to effective community nursing. Practitioners work through many kinds of agencies and institutions, such as senior citizen centers, ambulatory services, mental health clinics, and family planning programs. Community needs assessment, documentation of nursing outcomes, program evaluation, quality improvement, public policy formulation, and community nursing research are high priorities. This field of nursing is assuming responsibility as a full professional partner in community health.

Internationally, community nursing services are well established in England, Scandinavia, the Netherlands, and Australia. Services, however, are relatively underdeveloped in France and Ireland. Furthermore, relatively few professional nurses are working in the community in central and eastern Europe and in the former Union of Soviet Socialist Republics (USSR). Ivanov and Paganpegara (2003) note that changes have occurred in nursing education subsequent to the collapse of the Soviet Union, but they have not included content in public health nursing. Moreover, the concepts of health promotion and health education are not well understood, with the vast majority of health care provided at the tertiary level. It is concerning that modernization in many countries has not included expansion of public health services in general and community health nursing more specifically. In many of the most populated regions of the world—such as China, Africa, and India—volunteers, lay providers, and paraprofessionals provide the bulk of community health services.

In 1978, a joint World Health Organization (WHO) and the United Nations Children's Fund International Conference in Alma-Ata, in the Soviet Union, adopted a declaration on primary health care as the key to attaining the goal of health for all by the year 2000. At this conference, delegations from 134 governments agreed to incorporate the concepts and principles of primary health care in their health care systems to reach this goal (WHO, 1978; 1998). This was adopted by the World Health Assembly and endorsed by the United Nations General Assembly in 1981. On paper, at least, everyone acknowledged the crucial need for nurses to be involved in reaching this goal. In practice, support has not been forthcoming in many countries. Policy makers and the public still need to be educated to realize that nursing's

Table 2.1 Development of Community Health Nursing

Stages	Focus	Nursing Orientation	Service Emphasis	Institutional Base (Agencies)
Early home care (Before mid-1800s)	Sick poor	Individuals	Curative	Lay and religious orders
District nursing (1860–1900)	Sick poor	Individuals preventive	Curative; beginning of	Voluntary; some government
Public health nursing (1900–1970)	Needy public	Families	Curative; preventive	Government; some voluntary
Emergence of community health nursing (1970–present)	Total community	Populations illness prevention	Health promotion; practice	Many kinds; some independent

most effective contributions to the overall health of the population are based in the community.

Table 2-1 summarizes the most important changes that have occurred during community health nursing's four stages of development. It shows these changes in terms of focus, nursing orientation, service emphasis, and institutional base.

SOCIETAL INFLUENCES ON THE DEVELOPMENT OF COMMUNITY HEALTH NURSING

Many factors have influenced the growth of community health nursing. To better understand the nature of this field, the forces that began and continue to shape its development must be recognized. Six are particularly significant: advanced technology, progress in causal thinking, changes in education, demographic changes and the role of women, the consumer movement, and economic factors.

Advanced Technology

Advanced technology has contributed in many ways to shaping the practice of community health nursing. For example, technologic innovation has greatly improved health care, nutrition, and lifestyle and has caused a concomitant increase in life expectancy. Consequently, community health nurses direct an increasing share of their effort toward meeting the needs of the elderly population and addressing chronic conditions. The advances in technology in the home can be life-altering. For example, the use of social media can enable the community health nurse to reach an even broader audience. The implications for this use are supported by the 2010 findings of the Pew Research Center that social networking among users 50 to 64 years had increased from 25% to 42%. For those over 65 years of age, the percentage doubled from 13% to 26% (Pew Research Center, 2010). While these figures still represent a smaller percentage than users <50 years of age, the potential of this medium cannot be overemphasized. Despite the benefits, with any type of information sharing there is always the risk of inaccurate information being disseminated. Online access to health information can provide a critical link to information for all elderly persons, but it is important to recognize that not all websites are reputable. An increasing number of online websites catering to the elderly provide inaccurate information and, in some cases, are designed to defraud (Moore, 2005) or possibly harm those who access the website. It is critical for the community health nurse to check carefully any websites that are recommended for clients. It is important for clients to access only reputable sites and participate in discussion groups that utilize a facilitator or moderator (Moore, 2005). To further stress the importance of reliable and accurate health information, the Pew Research Center (2011) reported that 80% of adult internet users have looked for health information online and 17% of cell phone owners have likewise used their phones to access health or medical information.

Advanced technology has been a strong force behind industrialization, large-scale employment, and urbanization. We are now primarily an urban society, with approximately 75% of the world's population living in urban or suburban areas. Population density leads to many health-related problems, particularly the spread of disease and increased stress. Community health nurses are learning how to combat these urban health problems. In addition, changes in transportation and high job mobility have affected the health scene. As people travel and relocate, they are separated from families and traditional support systems; community health nurses design programs to help urban populations cope with the accompanying stress. New products, equipment, methods, and energy sources in industry have also increased environmental pollution and industrial hazards. Community health nurses have become involved in related research, occupational health, and preventive education. Technologic innovation has promoted complex medical diagnostic and treatment procedures, making illness-oriented care more dramatic and desirable, as well as more costly. Community health nurses face a challenge to demonstrate the physical and economic value of technology for wellness-oriented care.

Finally, innovations in communications and computer technology have shifted America from an industrial society to an "information economy." Our economy is built on information—the production and marketing of knowledge—making it global and active around-the-clock. Community health nurses now are in the business of information distribution, and they use computer technologies to enhance the efficiency and effectiveness of their services. Geographic Information Systems (GISs) is an example of emerging computer technology that the community health nurse can use to design and evaluate population-focused programs (Callen et al., 2010). GIS technology can be a valuable tool for many purposes, including examining health disparities and outbreaks of disease and for determining health priorities within a community (Riner, Cunningham, & Johnson, 2004). Telenursing, telehealth, and nursing informatics are part of our professional activities as community health nurses. We communicate by e-mail, use computer-based applications to enhance education among peers and with clients, and comfortably use the computers that are found in all areas where nurses function. As we move deeper into the 21st century, we move to "mobile care," using handheld, wireless technology tools that are nurse-friendly and compatible with the nurse's role. We have the ability to remotely visit our clients, and we regularly use smaller and smaller laptop computers and even have the ability to video conference on cell phones and other handheld computers. We can even take a "bird's-eye" view of the distribution of service providers and chronic disease clusters in a community through the use of GIS technology. Access to information is increasing, and the use of the information is limitless. The emerging difficulty is how to manage the sheer volume of information and still meet the needs of our communities.

Progress in Causal Thinking

Relating disease or illness to its cause is known as **causal thinking** in the health sciences. Progress in the study of causality, particularly in epidemiology, has significantly affected the nature of community health nursing (Fos & Fine, 2000; Thomas & Weber, 2001). The *germ theory* of disease causation, established in the late 1800s, was the first real breakthrough in control of communicable disease. At that time, it was established that disease could be spread or transmitted from patient to patient or from nurse to patient by contaminated hands or equipment. Nurses incorporated the teaching of cleanliness and personal hygiene into basic nursing care.

A second advance in causal thinking was initiated by the tripartite view that called attention to the interactions among a causative agent, a susceptible host, and the environment. This information offered community health nurses new ways to control and prevent health disorders. For example, nurses could decrease the vulnerability of individuals (hosts) by teaching them healthier lifestyles. They could instigate measles vaccination programs as a means of preventing the organism (agent) from infecting children. They could promote proper disinfection of a neighborhood swimming pool (environment) to prevent disease.

Further progress in causal thinking led to the recognition that not just one single agent but many factors—a multiple causation approach—contribute to a disease or health disorder. A food poisoning outbreak that is associated with a restaurant might be caused not only by the *Salmonella* organism but also by improper food handling and storage, lack of adherence to minimum food preparation standards, and lack of adequate health department supervision and enforcement (see Chapter 7). A chronic condition such as coronary heart disease can be related to other kinds of multicausal factors such as heredity, diet, lack of exercise, smoking, and personal and work stress.

Community health nurses can control health problems by examining all possible causes and then attacking strategic causal points. Efforts to prevent acquired immunodeficiency syndrome (AIDS) provide a dramatic case in point. Contact reporting, condom use, protection of health workers serving patients infected with the human immunodeficiency virus (HIV), screening for HIV infection, and public education about AIDS are examples of a multifaceted approach.

Current causal thinking has led to a broader awareness of unhealthy conditions; in addition to disease, problems such as accidents and environmental pollution are major targets of concern. Work-related stress, environmental hazards, chemical food additives, and alcohol and nicotine consumption during pregnancy are all examples of concerns in community health nursing practice.

Nursing's contribution to public health adds a further application to causal thinking. That is, nursing seeks to identify and implement the causes, or contributing factors, of wellness. Community health nurses do more than prevent illness; they seek to promote health. By conducting research and applying research findings, community health nurses promote health-enhancing behaviors. Nurses promote healthier lifestyle practices such as eating low-fat diets, exercising, and maintaining social support systems; promote healthy conditions in schools and work sites; and design meaningful activities for adolescents and the elderly.

Changes in Education

Changes in education, especially those in nursing education, have had an important influence on community health nursing practice. Education, once an opportunity for a privileged few, has become widely available; it is now considered a basic right and a necessity for a vital society. When people's understanding of their environment grows, an increased understanding of health usually is involved. For the community health nurse, health teaching has steadily assumed greater importance in practice. For the learner, education has led to more responsibility. As a result, people believe that they have a right to know and question the reasons behind the care they receive. Community health nurses have shifted from planning for clients to collaborating with clients.

Education has had other effects. Scientific inquiry, considered basic to progress, has created a dramatic increase in knowledge. The wealth of information relevant to community health nursing practice means that nursing students have more content to assimilate, and practicing community health nurses have to make greater efforts to keep abreast of knowledge in their field. In contrast to earlier times, when nurses were trained to work as apprentices in hospitals or health agencies and to follow orders perfunctorily, today's educational programs, including continuing education, prepare nurses to think for themselves in the application of theory to practice. Community health nursing has always required a fair measure of independent thinking and self-reliance; now, community health nurses need skills in such areas as population assessment, policy making, political advocacy, research, management, collaborative functioning, global health, human diversity, as well as information and health care technology (Callen et al., 2010). As the result of expanding education, community health nurses have had to reexamine their practice, sharpen their knowledge and skills, and clarify their roles.

Demographic Changes and the Role of Women

The changing demographics in the United States and the changing role of women have profoundly affected community health nursing. In the 20th century, the Women's Rights movement made considerable progress; women achieved the right to vote and gained greater economic independence by moving into the labor force (see Displays 2.2 and 2.4). Today, 152 million people are employed in nonfarm positions in the United States, representing 58.5% of women and 69.3% of men (U.S. Department of Labor, 2011b). In the decade between 1998 and 2008, the number of women in the labor force increased by 15%, compared with 10% for men. In the same decade, the percentage of workers aged 45 years or older increased from approximately 33% to 40% of the workforce (USDHHS, 2006).

Women nurses are aging in a predominantly female profession. In 1996, the average age of a registered nurse (RN) was 42.3 years. By 2004, the average age had increased to 46.8 years. Looking back just 25 years, a dramatic shift has occurred in the ratio of younger to older RNs. In 1980, 40.5% of RNs were under the age of 35. By 2004, only 16.4% of RNs fit into that demographic age group (USDHHS, 2006). Although most nursing schools remain full and many have a waiting list, the number of nurses staying active in their profession is dwindling. Those remaining in the profession are "graying" and retiring. Added to this is the aging population of nursing faculty, which raises concern over meeting the increased demand for nurses in the coming decade.

Salaries for nurses compare favorably with those for other workers who have 4 years of education in fields other than health care, such as education, human services (social work), and business. When compared with other workers in the health care field, however, nurses generally do not fare as well. For example, among the 2,655,020 practicing RNs in the United States in 2010, the average salary was $67,720. In comparison, the average salary for physical therapists was $77,990; for dental hygienists, it was $68,680, and for occupational therapists, it was $73,380.

Changing demographics, such as shifting patterns in immigration, varying numbers of births and deaths, and a rapidly increasing population of elderly persons, affect community health nursing planning and programming efforts. Monitoring these changes is essential for relevant and effective nursing services. Equally important is a diverse and representative workforce in nursing. The 2004 findings of the National Sample Survey of Registered Nurses indicated that the vast majority of nurses (81.8%) specifying a racial background selected White (non-Hispanic). With 7.5% of nurses not specifying a racial background, that left 10.7% in one or more of the groups identified in the survey. Because of a change in the form of questioning, these figures are difficult to compare with earlier surveys. It is concerning, however, that in 2000, 12.3% of the RNs identified themselves as being non-White, whereas the 2004 estimate was only 10.7%; clearly, this is a move in the wrong direction if the 2004 estimate is correct. The 2004 data also showed the racial background of the nurses surveyed to be 4.2% Black/African-American; 3.1% Asian/Pacific Islander; 1.7% Hispanic; 0.3% American-Indian/Alaskan Native; and a further 1.4% indicated two or more racial backgrounds (USDHHS, 2006). Increased racial and ethnic representation in community health nursing is essential and remains one of the major challenges facing the profession in the coming years.

Although the diversity of career options and employment opportunities for women has been a positive social factor, these gains have impacted the number of women entering nursing. As a profession, nursing's contributions and status have improved, but its ability to compete with careers offering higher pay and status remains problematic. Changes resulting from the women's movement continue. Nurses still struggle for equality—equality of recognition, respect, and autonomy, as well as job selection, equal pay for equal work, and equal opportunity for advancement in the health field. If community health nurses are to influence the field of community health, they need status and authority equal to that of their colleagues. This step requires nurses to demonstrate their competence and learn to be assertive in assuming roles as full professional partners. It is worth noting that, in 2002, men held more than one-third of the nursing administrative positions (U.S. Department of Labor, 2002). This is significant because, in that same year, men represented only 5.4% of the total RN population. Despite efforts to recruit more men into nursing, the 2004 data suggest only minimal improvement to 5.8% of RNs (USDHHS, 2006). The high proportion of leadership positions held by the men may in part reflect a larger proportion of women in nursing who have less than full-time careers. The women's movement has contributed to community health nursing's gains in assuming leadership roles, but a need for greater influence and involvement remains for all nurses.

Consumer Movement

The consumer movement has also affected the nature of community health nursing. Consumers have become more aggressive in demanding quality services and goods; they assert their right to be informed about goods and services and to participate in decisions that affect them regardless of sex, race, or socioeconomic level. This movement has stimulated some basic changes in the philosophy of community health nursing. Health care consumers are viewed as active members of the health team rather than as passive recipients of care. They may contract with the community health nurse for family care or group services, represent the community on the local health board, or act as ombudsmen by serving as representatives or advocates for their community constituents (e.g., to investigate complaints and report findings to protect the quality of care in a local nursing home). This assumption of consumers' responsibility for their own health means that the community health nurse often supplements clients' services, rather than primarily supervising them.

The consumer movement has also contributed to increased concern for the quality of health services, including a demand for more humane, personalized health care. Dissatisfied with fragmented services offered by an array of health workers, consumers seek more comprehensive, coordinated care. For example, senior citizens in a high-rise apartment building need more than a series of social workers, nutritionists, recreational therapists, nurses, and other callers ascertaining a variety of specific needs and starting a variety of separate programs. Community health nurses seek to provide holistic care by collaborating with others to offer more coordinated, comprehensive, and personalized services—a case-management approach. One example of the current attention given to the opinions of consumers is exemplified by the 2010 Gallup Poll discussed in Display 2.7. In this poll, nursing is the most highly rated profession with respect to honesty and ethics, not a bad position to be in.

Economic Forces

Myriad economic forces have affected the practice of community health nursing. Unemployment and the rising cost of living, combined with mounting health care costs, have resulted in numerous people carrying little or no health insurance. With limited or no access to needed health services, these populations are especially vulnerable to health problems and further economic stress. Other economic forces affecting community health nursing are changing health care financing patterns (including prospective payment and diagnosis-related groups); decreased federal, state, and local subsidies of public health programs; pressures for health care cost containment through managed care; and increased competition and managed competition among providers of health services (see Chapter 6) (Display 2.8).

Global economic forces also influence community health nursing practice. As the United States experiences increasing interdependence with foreign countries for trade, investment, and production of goods, the population has experienced a growing mobility and increased immigration, particularly among Hispanic and Asian groups. Under these conditions, the spread of communicable diseases poses a serious threat, as do problems associated with unemployment and poverty. Furthermore, the fastest-growing sector of the job market is in technical fields, which require new or retrained workers, and these jobs frequently are accompanied by health problems related to the stresses of ever-changing technology and financial and competitive pressures to produce.

Community health nursing has responded to these economic forces in several ways. One is by assuming new roles, such as health educators in industry or case managers for government and privately sponsored programs for the elderly. Another is by directly competing with other community health service providers, particularly in such areas as ambulatory care or home care. Still another is by developing new programs and service emphases.

DISPLAY 2.7 NURSES RANK HIGH IN HONESTY AND ETHICAL STANDARDS

Nurses are again at the top of the list, according to a Gallup Poll taken in 2010. When asked how they would rate the honesty and ethical standards of members of various professions, Americans rated nurses highest. Each year, a random sample of Americans rates select professions on a five-point scale ranging from "very high" to "very low." Since being added to the list in 1999, nurses have been at the top of the list each year except 2001, when firefighters took the No. 1 spot. Here are the results for the top scoring professions:

Nurses	81%
Military Officers	73%
Pharmacists	71%
Grade School Teachers	67%
Medical Doctors	66%
Policemen	57%
Clergy	53%

Source: Gallup. (2011). *Nurses Top Honesty and Ethics List for 11th Year.* Washington, DC: Author. Retrieved from http://www.gallup.com/poll/145043/nurses-top-honesty-ethics-list-11-year.aspx

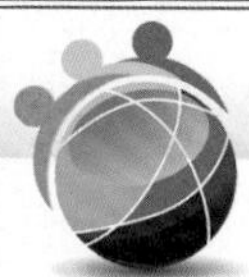

DISPLAY 2.8 TWENTY YEARS IN HISTORY: 1986 TO 2006

1986	*Standards of Community Health Nursing Practice* published by ANA; National Center for Nursing Research created at the National Institutes of Health
1990	*Healthy People 2000: National Health Promotion and Disease Prevention Objectives*
1991	Elizabeth Dole becomes the first woman president of the American Red Cross since Clara Barton
1993	National Center for Nursing Research becomes the National Institute of Nursing Research;
1996	*Health Insurance Portability and Accountability Act* (HIPPA) signed into law
1999	*Scope and Standards of Public Health Nursing Practice* published by ANA
2000	*Healthy People 2010: Understanding and Improving Health*
2001	September 11 attacks result in over 3,000 deaths in New York City, Washington, and Pennsylvania
2003	War in Iraq begins; Worldwide epidemic of Severe Acute Respiratory Syndrome (SARS)
2006	Medicare Part D Prescription Drug benefit implemented; *Public Health Nursing: Scope and Standards of Practice* published by ANA

Elder day care, respite care, senior fall-prevention programs, teen pregnancy and drug prevention projects, and programs for the homeless are a few examples of the response by community health nursing to the changing community needs created by demographic and economic forces. Yet another community health nursing response has been to develop new revenue-generating services, such as workplace wellness or health screening programs, to augment depleted budgets.

Economic factors continue to play a significant role in shaping community health nursing practice. Limited dollars for health promotion services and a continued need for home care have drawn some public health agencies into more illness-oriented rather than wellness-oriented services. Yet, community health nurses continue to be resourceful in finding ways to foster the community's optimal health while adapting to changing economic conditions.

PREPARATION FOR COMMUNITY HEALTH NURSING

The demands of community health nursing practice are significant, as described in Chapter 1, and are elaborated elsewhere in this textbook. The daily routine of the community health nurse may include organizing a flu clinic for seniors in the community, making home visits, giving a presentation on playground safety at a parent–teacher meeting, participating in a team meeting in the health department office, answering telephone calls, and charting. All of the skills learned in a basic baccalaureate nursing program are needed to effectively manage this type of day. Furthermore, this day may not represent the bigger picture of the community health nurse's role in community advisory panels, grant writing for new programs, or participation in or presentation of in-service programs. Academic preparation for this role is necessary, as is continuous professional development, and this training must meet the requirements of both employers and, in many instances, state regulations.

Academic Preparation

The minimum preparation for community health nurses in many states has been graduation from a baccalaureate-level nursing program, a nursing major built on 2 years of liberal arts and sciences courses (Ellis & Hartley, 2000). This can be achieved in a variety of ways. Some students enter a baccalaureate program as their initial higher educational experience after high school or later. Others with existing degrees in other fields have opted for 12 to 15 month accelerated programs to complete the baccalaureate in nursing degree. Still others complete an associate degree program in nursing and continue on to a university to receive the baccalaureate degree. This requires additional courses in liberal arts and sciences, along with selected nursing courses, usually one or more courses in public health nursing, nursing research, and leadership-management courses. In some programs designed to extend an RN to a Bachelor of Science in Nursing (BSN), nurses with years of experience in acute care nursing can "challenge" the previously mentioned courses by taking a test to demonstrate clinical expertise or by presenting a portfolio of experience, or a combination of these. Nevertheless, whatever the initial entry into practice, a comprehensive nursing education that is rich in leadership, management, research, health maintenance and promotion, disease prevention, and community health nursing experience is needed to meet the demands of this specialty.

In some states, meeting criteria for entry into practice as a public health nurse is required by some employers. Published in 1986, 1999, and again in 2006, the ANA has set standards of practice for community health nurses that serve as a framework for entry level and more recently advanced public health nursing practice (ANA, 2006). Building on the ANA standards, the Association of Community Health Nursing Educators published the *Essentials of Baccalaureate Nursing Education for Entry Level Community/Public Health Nursing* (Callen et al., 2010) to provide clarity for educators and employers on the professional role and

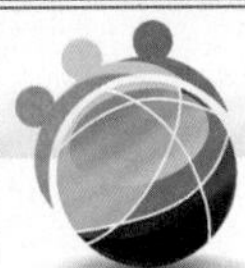

DISPLAY 2.9 TWENTY YEARS IN HISTORY: 2008 AND BEYOND

2008	Barack Obama elected President; first African-American to hold this position
2009	*Essentials of Baccalaureate Nursing Education for Entry Level Community/Public Health Nursing* published by the Association of Community Health Nursing Educators, Education Committee; H1N1 swine outbreak declared a national emergency with over 22 million American's contracting the disease and 4,000 deaths
2010	*Patient Protection and Affordable Care Act* signed and includes federal funding for nurse–family home visitation programs such as the Nurse Family Partnership to improve maternal/child health; Institute of Medicine publishes the *Future of Nursing: Leading Change, Advancing Health*
2011	*Healthy People 2020* released

responsibilities of public health nurses (Display 2.9). The ability to work as a public health nurses varies from state to state. Meeting minimum qualifications in the state of California, for example, the State Board of Registered Nursing (BRN), has established specific criteria including completion of specific coursework (e.g., child abuse and prevention information), which must be documented in undergraduate classes. On graduation, a school transcript, application, and fee are sent to the BRN to receive the public health nursing certificate. After passing the RN license examination (NCLEX), these nurses can sign "RN, PHN" after their names. Only those who have completed a baccalaureate nursing program can apply for this certificate, and only individuals with the certificate can take jobs as public health nurses. In California, this means that employment as an RN in settings such as health departments, schools, and Native American health services requires a PHN certificate.

Professional Development

Completion of a baccalaureate education may not be sufficient educational preparation for the more demanding community health nursing settings. Furthermore, to maintain licensure in most states, it is mandated that nurses participate in continuing education programs and receive continuing education units (Ellis & Hartley, 2000). In the United States, courses on specific topics are offered by employers, nursing associations, nursing journals, and private programs that travel to various cities. These help nurses to remain current on topics covered by the courses; however, a community health nurse may consider more lengthy and formal professional development opportunities such as advanced nursing practice (eg. NP) programs or certification opportunities.

To someone who is just finishing an undergraduate nursing program, the thought of continuing in school may be overwhelming. However, within a few months or years after graduation, continuing in higher education may seem right. It can take time and experience to find a particular focus in nursing and to decide on specializing at an advanced level. When that time comes, a variety of course work and degree options are available. For example, short-term certificate programs specialize in a narrow focus of health care, such as early recognition and prevention of child abuse, research, grant writing, or team management. These may or may not be offered for university credit, but the content enhances a nurse's role in an agency.

Matriculation in an NP program or a master's degree program in nursing is a longer commitment and gives the nurse greater marketability. In some health departments, NPs run well-child clinics, and a school nurse with an NP license can direct a school-based clinic. Advanced practice in community health nursing can open doors into leadership positions in community health agencies. A master's degree in business, public health, education, or epidemiology can lead to management positions, private community health agency ownership, agency teaching, or research positions. A doctoral program may be the next educational step for those wanting tenure-track university teaching, research, or upper-level administrative positions. Options for those seeking doctoral degrees include the PhD, the educational doctorate, as well as the Doctor of Nursing Practice degree.

The American Nurses Credentialing Center (ANCC, 2011) provides other opportunities by offering nurses certification in six specialty areas. Currently, only one specialty is available in community health nursing: Advanced Public Health Nurse. A generalist certificate in public/community health nursing had been available but was suspended in 2006 and the Clinical Nurse Specialist exam in Public Health Nursing is likewise no longer available. Related certifications in nursing informatics or nurse executive also exist. Each certificate is awarded after completion of a certain number of years of practice in the specialty, payment of a fee, and passage of an ANCC Certification Examination. Many employers reward the initiative required for certification with promotion or a higher salary, accompanied by additional responsibilities and opportunities. It is important to note that of the 168,546 national certified nurses in 2004, <1% (0.3 %) held a certification in Community Health Nursing. Clearly, this specialty has far to go in terms of increasing the number of certified nurses and determining the reasons for the low percentage.

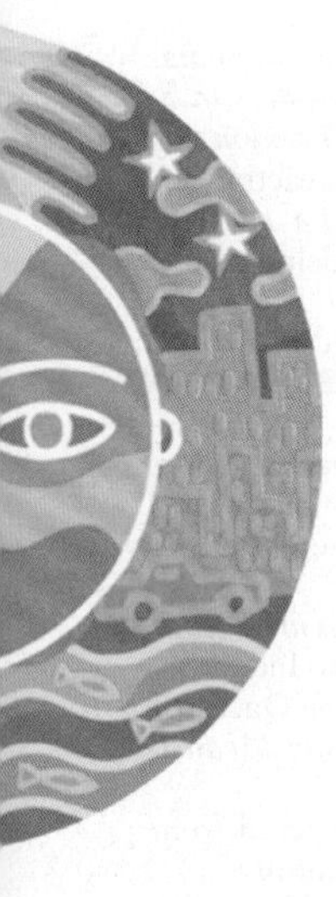

SUMMARY

The specialty of community health nursing developed historically through four stages. The early home-care stage (before the mid-1800s) emphasized care to the sick poor in their homes by various lay and religious orders. The district nursing stage (mid-1800s) included voluntary home nursing care for the poor by specialists or "health nurses" who treated the sick and taught wholesome living to patients. The public health nursing stage (1900–1970) was characterized by an increased concern for the health of the general public. The community health nursing stage (1970 to the present) includes increased recognition of community health nursing as a specialty field, with focus on communities and populations.

Six major societal influences have shaped the development of community health nursing. They are advanced technology, progress in causal thinking, changes in education, the changing demographics and role of women, the consumer movement, and economic factors such as health care costs, access, limited funds for public health, and increased competition among health service providers.

Academic preparation for community health nursing begins at the baccalaureate level. However, students beginning at the diploma or associate degree level can advance to a BSN completion program and are then prepared to enter this challenging specialty in nursing. The demands of community health nursing require additional courses in liberal arts and science, along with courses in community health nursing practice at the student level. Once students achieve an undergraduate degree, completion of additional educational programs is required to keep current and, in most states, to maintain licensure, advance in practice opportunities, or branch out into administration, teaching, or research.

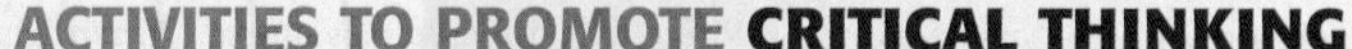

ACTIVITIES TO PROMOTE **CRITICAL THINKING**

1. Select one societal influence on the development of community health nursing and explore its continuing impact. What other events are occurring today that shape community health nursing practice? Support your arguments with documentation. Use the Internet to find your documentation.
2. Using the Internet, seek out information about a historical public health nursing leader. Using this information, determine how this practitioner might deal with current population-based issues such as AIDS, sexually transmitted diseases, or child neglect and abuse.
3. Assume that you have been asked to make a home visit to a 75-year-old man, living alone, whose wife recently died. Besides assessing his individual needs, what additional factors should you consider for assessment and intervention that would indicate an aggregate or population-focused approach? What self-care practices might you encourage or teach?
4. Interview a community health nursing director to determine what population-based programs are offered in your locality. Explore nursing's role in the assessment, development, implementation, and evaluation of these programs. Discuss with the director how community health nurses might expand their population-focused interventions.
5. Go to your university, nursing college, or school and locate brochures for advanced degrees in nursing and related areas. Peruse them and see whether any of the programs appeals to you. Request more information from at least one of these programs through the mail or the Internet.

REFERENCES

American Nurses Association. (2006). *Public health nursing: Scope and standards of practice*. Silver Spring, MD: Author.

American Nurses Association, Community Health Nursing Division. (1980). *A conceptual model of community health nursing* (Publication No. CH-10 2M 5/80). Kansas City, MO: Author.

American Nurses Credentialing Center (ANCC). (2011). *ANCC Certification Center*. Retrieved from http://www.nursecredentialing.org/certification.aspx#specialty

Beine, J. (1996). Changing with the times. *Nursing Times, 92*(48), 59–62.

Brainard, A. M. (1922). *The evolution of public health nursing*. Philadelphia, PA: W. B. Saunders Company.

Bullough, V., & Bullough, B. (1978). *The care of the sick: The emergence of modern nursing*. New York: Neale, Watson.

Callen, B., Block, D., Joyce, B., Lutz, J., Brown-Schott, N., Smith, C. M. (2010). Essentials of Baccalaureate Nursing Education for Entry-Level Community/Public Health Nursing. *Public Health Nursing, 27*, 371–382. Doi: 10.000/j.1525–1446.2010.00867.x.

Central Hanover Bank and Trust Company, Department of Philanthropic Information. (1938). *The public health nurse*. New York: National Organization for Public Health Nursing.

Christy, T. W. (1970). Portrait of a leader: Lillian D. Wald. *Nursing Outlook, 18*(3), 50–54.

de Tornyay, R. (1980). Public health nursing: The nurse's role in community-based practice. *Annual Review of Public Health, 1*, 83.

Dickens, C. (1910). *Martin Chuzzlewit*. New York: Macmillan.

Dolan, J. A. (1978). *Nursing in society: A historical perspective*. Philadelphia, PA: W.B. Saunders.

Draper, L. (2006). Working women and contraception: History, health, and choices. *AAOHN Journal, 54*, 317–324.

Ellis, J. R., & Hartley, C. L. (2000). *Nursing in today's world: Challenges, issues, and trends* (7th ed.). Philadelphia, PA: Lippincott Williams & Wilkins.

Evans, J. (2004). Men nurses: A historical and feminist perspective. *Journal of Advanced Nursing, 47*, 321–328.

Farrar, E. W. (1837). *The young lady's friend—By a lady* (p. 57). Boston, MA: American Stationer's Co.

Fealy, G. M., McNamara, M. S., & Geraghty, R. (2010). The health of hospitals and lessons from history: Public health and sanitary reform in the Dublin hospitals, 1858–1898. *Journal of Clinical Nursing, 19*, 3468–3476. Doi: 10.1111/j.1365–2702.2010.03475.x.

Florence Nightingale Museum Trust. (1997). *The Florence Nightingale Museum's School Visit Pack*. London: Author.

Fos, P. J., & Fine, D. J. (2000). *Designing health care for populations: Applied epidemiology in health care administration*. San Francisco, CA: Jossey-Bass.

Gardner, M. S. (1936). *Public health nursing* (3rd ed.). New York: Macmillan.

Hamilton, D. (2007). The cost of caring: The Metropolitan Life Insurance Company's Visiting Nurse Service, 1909–1953. In P. D'Antonio, E. D. Baer, S. D. Rinker, & J. E. Lynaugh (Eds.), *Nurses' work: Issues across time and place* (pp. 141–164). New York: Springer Publishing Company.

Hein, E. C. (2001). *Nursing issues in the 21st century: Perspectives from the literature*. Philadelphia, PA: Lippincott Williams & Wilkins.

Ivanov, L. L., & Paganpegara, G. (2003). Public health nursing education in Russia. *Journal of Nursing Education, 42*, 292–295.

Jesús, M., & Martínez, A. C. (2010). The houses of approval of the nurses Obregones in the Spain of the 16th century: Precedents of our schools of nursing. *Abstract presented at the International Perspectives in the History of Nursing*, Royal College of Nursing.

Kalisch, P. A., & Kalisch, B. J. (2004). *American nursing: A history* (4th ed.). Philadelphia, PA: Lippincott Williams & Wilkins.

Kaplin, J. (Ed). (1855/1992). *Bartlett's familiar quotations* (16th ed.). New York: Little, Brown and Company.

Men, monasteries, wars, and wards. (2001). *Nursing Times, 97*(44), 25–26.

Mosley, M. O. P. (2007). Satisfied to carry the bag: Three black community health nurses' contributions to health care reform, 1900–1937. In P. D'Antonio, E. D. Baer, S. D. Rinker, & J. E. Lynaugh (Eds.), *Nurses' work: Issues across time and place* (pp. 65–78). New York: Springer Publishing Company.

Mowbray, P. (1997). *Florence Nightingale museum guidebook*. London: The Florence Nightingale Museum Trust.

National Organization for Public Health Nursing. (1944). Approval of Skidmore College of Nursing as preparing students for public health nursing. *Public Health Nursing, 36*, 371.

Nightingale, F. (1859/1969). *Notes on nursing: What it is, and what it is not*. London: Harrison.

Nightingale, F. (1864). *How people may live and not die in India*. London: Longman, Green, Longman, Roberts, & Green.

Nightingale, F. (1876). [Letter to the editor]. *The Times (London)*.

Palmer, I. S. (2001). Florence Nightingale: Reformer, reactionary, researcher. In E. C. Hein, *Nursing issues in the 21st century: Perspectives from the literature* (pp. 26–38). Philadelphia, PA: Lippincott Williams & Wilkins.

Pew Research Center. (2010). *Older adults and social media*. Retrieved from http://www.pewinternet.org/Reports/2010/Older-Adults-and-Social-Media.aspx

Pew Research Center. (2011). *Who doesn't gather health information online*? Retrieved from http://www.pewinternet.org/Commentary/2011/October/Who-Doesnt-Gather-Health-Information-Online.aspx

Prochaska, F. K. (1980/2003). *Women and philanthropy in nineteenth century England*. New York: Oxford University Press, Inc.

Ramsey, M. A. (2006). John Snow, MD: Anaesthetist to the Queen of England and pioneer epidemiologist. *Baylor University Medical Center Proceedings, 19*(1), 24–28.

Reddi, V. (2005). Dorothea Lynde Dix (1802–1887). Retrieved from http://www.truthaboutnursing.org/press/pioneers/dix.html

Riner, M. E., Cunningham, C., & Johnson, A. (2004). Public health education and practice using geographic information system technology. *Public Health Nursing, 21*, 57–65.

Roberts, D., & Freeman, R. (Eds.). (1973). *Redesigning nursing education for public health: Report of the conference* (Publication No. HRA 75–75). Bethesda, MD: U.S. Department of Health, Education, and Welfare.

Ruffing-Rahal, M. (1986). Margaret Sanger: Nurse and feminist. *Nursing Outlook, 34*, 246–249.

Sachs, T. B. (1908). The tuberculosis nurse. *American Journal of Nursing, 8*, 597.

Scutchfield, F. D., & Keck, C. W. (2009). *Principles of public health practice*. Florence, KY: Cengage Learning.

Seacole, M. (1857). *Wonderful adventures of Mrs. Seacole in many lands*. London, England: James Blackwood Paternoster Row. Retrieved from http://digital.library.upenn.edu/women/seacole/adventures/adventures.html

Simpson, M. S. (2000). Nurses and models of practice: Then and now. *American Journal of Nursing, 100*(2), 82–83.

Stanley, D. (2007). Lights in the shadows: Florence Nightingale and others who made their mark. *Contemporary Nurse, 24*(1), 45–51.

Struthers, L. R. (1917). *The School Nurse: A survey of the duties and responsibilities of the nurse in the maintenance of health and physical perfection and the prevention of disease among school children*. New York: G. P. Putman's Sons.

Thomas, J. C., & Weber, D. J. (2001). *Epidemiologic methods for the study of infectious diseases*. Oxford, UK: Oxford University Press.

U.S. Department of Health and Human Services, Division of Nursing. (1984). *Consensus conference on the essentials of public health nursing practice and education: Report of the conference*. Rockville, MD: Author.

U.S. Department of Health and Human Services, Health Resources and Service Administration. (2006). The *Registered nurse population: Findings* from the *2004 National Sample Survey of Registered Nurses*. Retrieved from http://bhpr.hrsa.gov/healthworkforce/rnsurveys/rnsurvey2004.pdf

U.S. Department of Health and Human Services, National Center for Health Statistics. (2002). *Health, United States, 2002 with chartbook on trends in the health of America* (DHHS Publication No. 1232). Washington, DC: Author.

U.S. Department of Labor, Bureau of Labor Statistics. (2002). Retrieved from http://www.dol.gov.

U.S. Department of Labor, Bureau of Labor Statistics. (2011a). *Occupational Employment Statistics*. Retrieved from http://www.bls.gov/oes/oes_dl.htm#2002

U.S. Department of Labor, Bureau of Labor Statistics. (2011b). *Economic news release*. Retrieved from http://www.bls.gov/news.release/work.nr0.htm

Vessey, J. A., & McGowen, K. A. (2006). A successful public health experiment: School nursing. *Pediatric Nursing, 32*, 213, 255–258.

Wald, L. D. (1915). *The house on Henry Street*. New York: Holt.

Wald, L. D. (1934). *Windows of Henry Street*. Boston, MA: Little Brown.

Williams, C. A. (1977). Community health nursing: What is it? *Nursing Outlook, 25*, 250–254.

Woodham-Smith, C. (1951). *Florence Nightingale*. New York: McGraw-Hill.

World Health Organization. (1978). *Primary health care: Report of the International Conference on Primary Health Care, Alma-Ata, USSR*. Geneva: Author.

World Health Organization. (1998). *The world health report: 1998*. Geneva: Author.

thePoint: Everything You Need to Make the Grade!

thePoint Visit http://thePoint.lww.com/Allender8e for selected readings, study aids for all learning styles, and more!

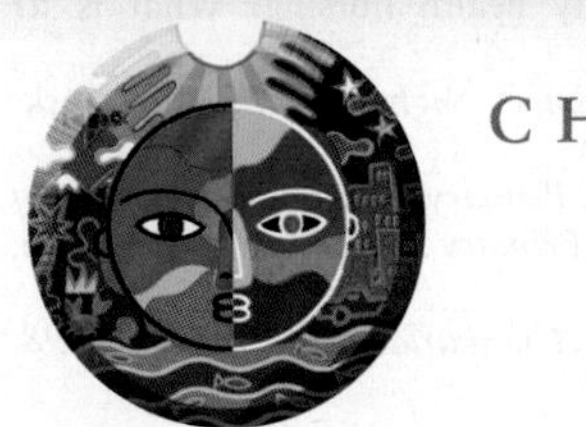

CHAPTER 3

Setting the Stage for Community Health Nursing

"One good community nurse will save a dozen policemen."

—Herbert Hoover

KEY TERMS

Advocate
Assessment
Assurance
Case management
Clinician
Collaborator
Educator
Leader
Manager
Policy development
Researcher

LEARNING OBJECTIVES

Upon mastery of this chapter, you should be able to:

- Identify the three core public health functions basic to community health nursing.
- Describe and differentiate among seven different roles of the community health nurse.
- Discuss the seven roles within the framework of public health nursing functions.
- Explain the importance of each role for influencing people's health.
- Identify and discuss factors that affect a nurse's selection and practice of each role.
- Describe seven settings in which community health nurses practice.
- Discuss the nature of community health nursing, and the common threads basic to its practice, woven throughout all roles and settings.
- Identify principles of sound nursing practice in the community.

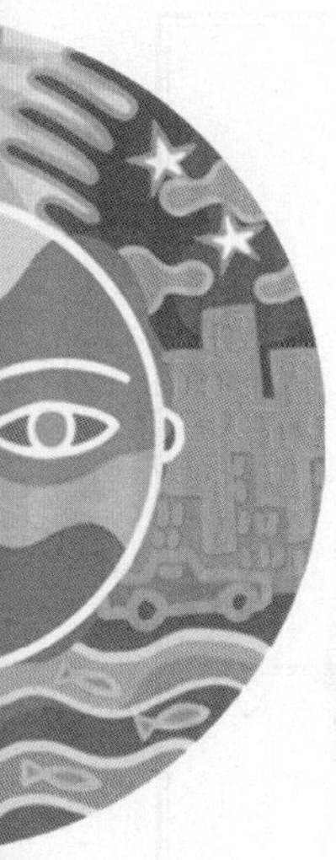

Historically, community health nurses have engaged in many professional roles. Nurses in this professional specialty have provided care to the sick, taught positive health habits and self-care, advocated on behalf of needy populations, developed and managed health programs, provided leadership, and collaborated with other professionals and consumers to implement changes in health services. Although the practice settings may have differed, the essential goal of the community health nurse has always been a healthier community. The home certainly has been one site for practice, but so too have public health clinics, schools, factories, and other community-based locations. Today, the roles and settings of community health nursing practice have expanded even further, offering a wide range of professional opportunities.

This chapter examines how the conceptual foundations and core functions of community health practice are integrated into the various roles and settings of community health nursing. It provides an opportunity to gain greater understanding about how and where community health nursing is practiced. Moreover, it will expand awareness of the many existing and future possibilities for community health nurses to improve the public's health. As you read through this chapter, think about client populations that you may have encountered in the acute care setting and consider your role with these same populations in a community setting. Perhaps you may discover a community health nursing specialty area that you never even considered.

CORE PUBLIC HEALTH FUNCTIONS

Community health nurses work as partners within a team of professionals (in public health and other disciplines), nonprofessionals, and consumers to improve the health of populations. The various roles and settings for practice hinge on three primary functions of public health: assessment, policy development, and assurance (Institute of Medicine, 1988). These functions are foundational to all roles assumed by the community health nurse and are applied at three levels of service: to individuals, to families, and to communities (see Display 3.1). Regardless of the role or setting of choice, these three essential responsibilities direct the work of all community health nurses.

Assessment

An essential first function in public health, **assessment**, means that the community health nurse must gather and analyze information that will affect the health of the people to be served. As described in Display 3.1, assessment is *the systematic collection, assembly, analysis, and dissemination of information about the health of a community*. The nurse and others on the health team need to determine health needs, health risks, environmental conditions, political agendas, and financial and other resources, depending on the individuals, community, or population targeted for intervention. Data may be gathered in many ways; typical methods include interviewing people in the community, conducting surveys, gathering information from public records (many of which are available online), and using research findings.

The community health nurse is typically both trusted and valued by clients, agencies, and private providers. Trust placed in the community health nurse can often be attributed to consistency, honesty, dependability, and an ongoing presence in the community. Although securing and maintaining the trust of others is pivotal to all nursing practice, it is even more critical when working in the community. Trust can afford a nurse access to client populations that are difficult to engage, to agencies, and to health care providers. In the capacity of trusted professional, community health nurses gather relevant client data that enable them to identify strengths, weaknesses, and needs. It is important to recognize that as difficult as it may be for the nurse to gain the trust and respect of the community, if ever lost, these attributes can be difficult if not impossible to regain.

At the community level, assessment is done both formally and informally as nurses identify and interact with key community leaders. With families, the nurse can evaluate family strengths and areas of concern in the immediate living environment and in the neighborhood. At the individual level, people are identified within the family who are in need of services, and the nurse evaluates the functional capacity of these individuals through the use of specific assessment measures and a variety of tools. Assessment of communities and families as the initial step in the nursing process is discussed more fully in Chapters 15 and 19.

Policy Development

Policy development (defined in Display 3.1) is enhanced by the synthesis and analysis of information obtained during assessment. At the community level, the nurse provides leadership in convening and facilitating community groups to evaluate health concerns and develop a plan to address those concerns. Typically, the nurse recommends specific training and programs to meet identified health needs of target populations. This is accompanied by raising the awareness of key policy makers about factors such as health regulations and budget decisions that negatively affect the health of the community (see Chapter 13). With families, the nurse recommends new programs or increased services based on identified needs. Additional data may be needed to identify trends in groups or clusters of families, so that effective intervention strategies can be used with these families. At the individual level, the nurse assists in the development of standards for individual client care,

DISPLAY 3.1 PUBLIC HEALTH NURSING WITHIN THE CORE PUBLIC HEALTH FUNCTIONS MODEL

The model includes assessment, policy development, and assurance surrounding the individual, family, and community. *Assessment* is the systematic collection, assembly, analysis, and dissemination of information about the health of a community. *Policy development* uses the scientific information gathered during assessment to create comprehensive public health policies. *Assurance* is the pledge to constituents that services necessary to achieve agreed-upon goals are provided by encouraging actions of others (private or public), requiring action through regulation, or providing service directly.

From The Institute of Medicine. (1988). *The future of public health*. Retrieved from *http://www.iom.edu/Reports/1988/The-Future-of-Public-Health.aspx*

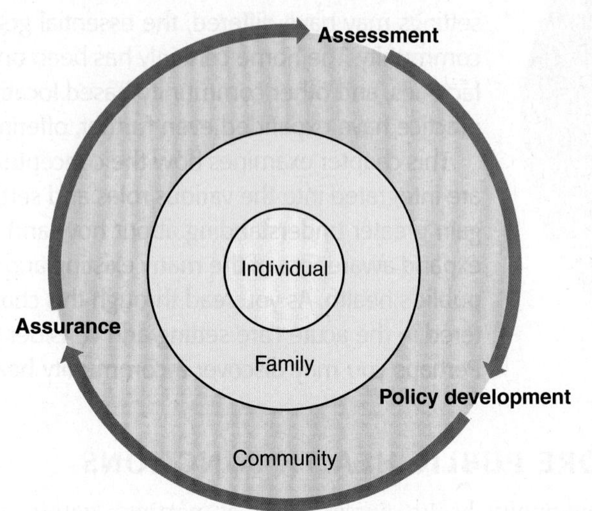

recommends or adopts risk-classification systems to assist with prioritizing individual client care, and participates in establishing criteria for opening, closing, or referring individual cases.

Assurance

Assurance activities—activities that make certain that services are provided—often consume most of the community health nurse's time. Community health nurses perform the assurance function at the community level when they provide services to target populations, improve quality assurance activities, maintain safe levels of communicable disease surveillance and outbreak control, and collaborate with community leaders in the preparation of a community emergency preparedness plan. In addition, they participate in outcome research, provide expert consultation, promote evidence-based practice, and provide services within the community based on standards of care.

Essential Services

To more clearly articulate the services that are linked to the core functions of assessment, policy development, and assurance, a list of 10 essential services was developed in 1994 by the Public Health Functions Steering Committee (U.S. Department of Health and Human Services [USDHHS], 1997) (see Display 3.2). This initial effort to define the service components of the core functions provided an organized service delivery plan for public health providers across the country. A model

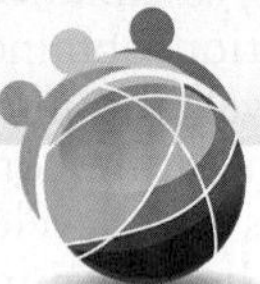

DISPLAY 3.2 TEN ESSENTIAL SERVICES OF PUBLIC HEALTH

1. *Monitor* health status to identify and solve community health problems.
2. *Diagnose and investigate* health problems and health hazards in the community.
3. *Inform*, *educate*, and *empower* people about health issues.
4. *Mobilize* community partnerships and action to identify and solve health problems.
5. *Develop policies and plans* that support individual and community health efforts.
6. *Enforce* laws and regulations that protect health and ensure safety.
7. *Link* people to needed personal health services and assure the provision of health care when otherwise unavailable.
8. *Ensure* competent public and personal health care workforces.
9. *Evaluate* effectiveness, accessibility, and quality of personal and population-based health services.
10. *Research* for new insights and innovative solutions to health problems.

From USDHHS. (2010b). *Healthy People 2020: Public health infrastructure*. Retrieved from http://healthypeople.gov/2020/topicsobjectives2020/overview.aspx?topicid=35

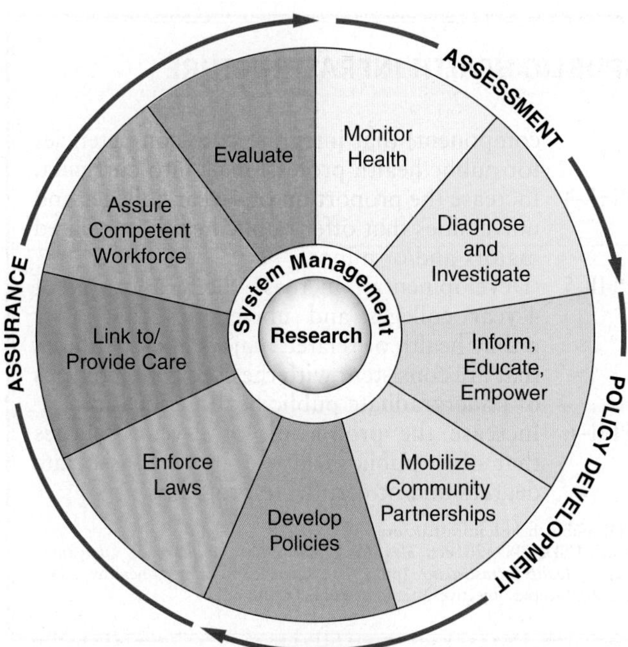

FIGURE 3-1. The core functions and 10 essential services of public health. (From US Department of Health and Human Services, Office of Disease Prevention & Health Promotion. (1999). Retrieved from http://www.health.gov/phfunctions/public.htm)

depicting the relationships between the core functions and the essential services was eventually developed (USDHHS, 1999). The model (Fig. 3-1) shows the types of services necessary to achieve the core functions of assessment, policy development, and assurance. It also emphasizes the circular or ongoing nature of the process. The placement of research at the center of the model is a clear indication of the high priority placed on providing scientific evidence in all areas of service delivery. Research is essential to evidence-based practice and is vital to achieving healthy communities. As you review this model, think about what types of services might be provided in each category, depending on whether you are focusing on an individual, a family, or a community. It is not necessary that the community health nurse provide each of the listed services. Working in collaboration with an interdisciplinary team, the community nurse can support the efforts of others to achieve improved health in the community. What is important is that the team members all recognize their respective roles and are working toward the same goal.

STANDARDS OF PRACTICE

In 2008, the American Association of Colleges of Nursing (AACN) published the revised *The Essentials of Baccalaureate Education for Professional Nursing Practice*. Building on the 1998 version, this document was a major step in providing clear guidelines as to what constitutes professional nursing education. Roles of beginning professional nursing practice were grouped into three broad roles: "provider of care; designer/manager/coordinator of care; and member of a profession" (AACN, 2008, p. 3). Although this document describes educational preparation in all areas of nursing practice, the link to community health nursing is quite evident. The document outlines the knowledge, skills, and attitudes seen as vital to the education of the baccalaureate nurse. Practice-focused outcomes typically associated with community health nursing are emphasized in Essential Seven: Clinical Prevention and Population Health, stressing that "health promotion and disease prevention at the individual and population level are necessary to improve population health and are important components of baccalaureate generalist nursing practice" (AACN, 2008, p. 4). This document clearly articulates the growing need to prepare nurses to assume a variety of roles in the community emphasizing that the baccalaureate nurse "is prepared to practice with patients, including individuals, families, groups, communities, and populations across the lifespan and across the continuum of healthcare environments" (AACN, 2008, p. 4).

Community health nursing practice is further defined by specific standards developed under the auspices of the American Nurses Association (ANA) in collaboration with the Quad Council of Public Health Nursing Organizations (ANA, 2007c). The Quad Council is composed of representatives from the ANA—Council on Nursing Practice and Economics; the American Public Health Association—Public Health Nursing Section; the Association of Community Health Nursing Educators; and the Association of Public Health Nurses. These four organizations represent academics and professional practitioners, providing a broad spectrum of views regarding professional practice in the field of community health nursing. *Public Health Nursing: Scope and Standards of Practice* (ANA, 2007c) provides guidance as to what constitutes public health nursing and how it can be differentiated from other nursing specialties. Standards of care are consistent with the nursing process and include assessment, population diagnosis and priorities, outcomes identification, planning, implementation, and evaluation. This document is an important reference for all those practicing in the community. It provides the basis for evaluating an individual's performance in this field, and is used by many employers to assess job performance.

In addition to their work on the practice standards, the Association of Community Health Nursing Educators (ACHNE) published the updated *Essentials of Baccalaureate Nursing Education for Entry-level Community/Public Health Nursing* in 2010 (Education Committee of ACHNE). This document builds on previous versions and is consistent with both the *Essentials* document (AACN, 2008) and the scope and standards of public health nursing practice (ANA, 2007c). This document describes core professional values as well as knowledge and basic competencies. Core values of professional behavior emphasize community/population as client, prevention, partnership, healthy environment, and diversity. Building on these common values, 15 essential concepts and their related

DISPLAY 3.3 *HEALTHY PEOPLE 2020*—PUBLIC HEALTH INFRASTRUCTURE

Workforce Objectives

PHI–1 Increase the proportion of federal, tribal, state, and local public health agencies that incorporate core competencies for public health professionals into job descriptions and performance evaluations.

PHI–2 (Developmental) Increase the proportion of tribal, state, and local public health personnel who receive continuing education consistent with core competencies for public health professionals.

PHI–3 Increase the proportion of Council on Education for Public Health (CEPH) accredited schools of public health, CEPH accredited academic programs, and schools of nursing (with a public health or community health component) that integrate core competencies for public health professionals into curricula.

PHI–4 Increase the proportion of 4-year colleges and universities that offer public health or related majors and/or minors.

PHI–5 (Developmental) Increase the proportion of 4-year colleges and universities that offer public health or related majors and/or minors that are consistent with the core competencies of undergraduate public health education.

PHI–6 Increase the proportion of 2-year colleges that offer public health or related associate degrees and/or certificate programs.

PHI, public health infrastructure.
From USDHHS. (2010c). *Healthy People 2020 Summary of Objectives: Public Health Infrastructure* (pp. 1–10). Retrieved from http://healthypeople.gov/2020/topicsobjectives2020/pdfs/PublicHealth.pdf

competencies are delineated including 3 newly defined essentials; communication; social justice; and emergency preparedness, response, and recovery (ACHNE, Education Committee, 2010). It is also important to recognize that an emphasis of *Healthy People 2020* is to create and support a competent public and personal health care workforce including professional competencies required for sound practice (see Display 3.3) (USDHHS, 2010a).

The community health nurse provides nursing services based on other standards developed by the ANA, such as the *Code of Ethics for Nurses with Interpretive Statements* (2001), *Nursing's Social Policy Statement* (2010b), and *Nursing: Scope and Standards of Practice* (2nd ed.) (2010a). Each of these documents provides essential information regarding sound general nursing practice. When combined with *Public Health Nursing: Scope and Standards of Practice* (ANA, 2007c), they provide the community health nurse with a clear understanding of accepted practice in this nursing specialty. With specific standards of practice and clear competencies to achieve, the community health nurse can integrate the core functions of assessment, policy development, and assurance throughout all of the various roles and community settings of practice.

ROLES OF COMMUNITY HEALTH NURSES

Just as the health care system is continually evolving, community health nursing practice evolves to remain effective with the clients it serves. Over time, the role of the community health nurse has broadened. This breadth is reflected in the description of public health nursing from the American Public Health Association, Public Health Nursing Section (2012):

> Public health nurses integrate community involvement and knowledge about the entire population with personal, clinical understandings of the health and illness experiences of individuals and families within the population. They translate and articulate the health and illness experiences of diverse, often vulnerable individuals and families in the population to health planners and policy makers, and assist members of the community to voice their problems and aspirations. Public health nurses are knowledgeable about multiple strategies for intervention, from those applicable to the entire population, to those for the family, and the individual. Public health nurses translate knowledge from the health and social sciences to individuals and population groups through targeted interventions, programs, and advocacy.

Community health nurses wear many hats while conducting day-to-day practice. At any given time, however, one role is primary. This is especially true for specialized roles, such as that of full-time manager. This chapter examines seven major roles: clinician, educator, advocate, manager, collaborator, leader, and researcher. It also describes the factors that influence the selection and performance of those roles.

Clinician Role

The most familiar role of the community health nurse is that of clinician or care provider. The provision of nursing care, however, takes on new meaning in the context of community health practice. The **clinician** role in community health means that the nurse ensures health services are provided not just to individuals and families, but also to groups and populations. Nursing service is still designed for the special needs of clients; however, when those clients comprise a group or population, clinical practice takes different forms. It requires different skills to assess collective needs and tailor service accordingly. For instance, one community health nurse might visit elderly residents in a seniors' high-rise apartment building. Another might serve as the clinic nurse in a rural prenatal clinic that serves migrant farm workers. These are opportunities to assess the needs of entire aggregates and design appropriate services.

For community health nurses, the clinician role involves certain emphases that are different from those of basic nursing. Three clinician emphases, in particular, are useful to consider here: holism, health promotion, and skill expansion.

Holistic Practice

Most clinical nursing seeks to be broad and holistic. In community health, however, a holistic approach means considering the broad range of interacting needs that affect the collective health of the "client" as a larger system (Dossey & Keegan, 2013). Holistic nursing care encompasses the comprehensive and total care of the client in all areas, such as physical, emotional, social, spiritual, and economic. All are considered and cared for when the client is a large system, just as they should be with individual clients. The client is a composite of people whose relationships and interactions with each other must be considered in totality. Holistic practice must emerge from this systems perspective.

For example, when working with a group of pregnant teenagers living in a juvenile detention center, the nurse would consider the girls' relationships with one another, their parents, the fathers of their unborn children, and the detention center staff. The nurse would evaluate their ages, developmental needs, and peer influences, as well as their knowledge of pregnancy, delivery, and issues related to the choice of keeping or giving up their babies. The girls' reentry into the community and their future plans for school or employment would also be considered. Holistic service would go far beyond the physical condition of pregnancy and childbirth. It would incorporate consideration of pregnant adolescents in this community as a population at risk. What factors contributed to these girls' situations, and what preventive efforts could be instituted to protect other teenagers or these teens from future pregnancies? The clinician role of the community health nurse involves holistic practice from an aggregate perspective.

Focus on Wellness

The clinician role in community health also is characterized by its focus on promoting wellness. As discussed in Chapter 1, the community health nurse provides service along the entire range of the health continuum, but especially emphasizes promotion of health and prevention of illness. Effective services include seeking out clients who are at risk for poor health and offering preventive and health-promoting services, rather than waiting for them to come for help after problems arise. The community health nurse identifies people, programs, and agencies interested in achieving a higher level of health, and works with them to accomplish that goal and to sustain the expected changed behavior (Pender, Murdaugh, & Parsons, 2011). The nurse may help employees of a business learn how to live healthier lives or work with a group of people who want to quit smoking. The community health nurse may hold seminars with a men's group on enhancing fathering skills or assist a corporation with the implementation of a health promotion program. Groups and populations are identified that may be vulnerable to certain health threats, and preventive and health-promoting programs can be designed in collaboration with the community (Pender et al., 2011). Examples include immunization of preschoolers, family planning programs, cholesterol screening, and prevention of behavioral problems in adolescents. Protecting and promoting the health of vulnerable populations is an important component of the clinician role and is addressed extensively in the chapters in Unit VII on vulnerable aggregates.

Expanded Skills

Many different skills are used in the role of the community health clinician. In the early years of community health nursing, emphasis was placed on physical care skills. With time, skills in observation, listening, communication, and counseling became integral to the clinician role as it grew to encompass psychological and sociocultural factors. Recently, environmental and community-wide considerations—such as problems caused by pollution, violence and crime, drug abuse, unemployment, poverty, homelessness, and limited funding for health programs—have created a need for stronger skills in assessing the needs of groups and populations and intervening at the community level. The clinician role in population-based nursing also requires skills in collaboration with consumers and other professionals, use of epidemiology and biostatistics, community organization and development, research, program evaluation, administration, leadership, and effecting change (ANA, 2007c). These skills are addressed in greater detail in later chapters.

Educator Role

A second important role of the community health nurse is that of **educator** or health teacher. Health teaching, a widely recognized part of nursing practice, is legislated through nurse practice acts in a number of states and is one of the major functions of the community health nurse (ANA, 2007c).

The educator role is especially useful in promoting the public's health for at least two reasons. First, community clients are usually not acutely ill and can absorb and act on health information. For example, a class of expectant parents, unhampered by significant health problems, can grasp the relationship of diet to fetal development. They understand the value of specific exercises to the childbirth process, are motivated to learn, and are more likely to perform those exercises. Thus, the educator role has the potential for finding greater receptivity and providing higher-yield results.

Second, the educator role in community health nursing is significant because a wider audience can be reached. With an emphasis on populations and aggregates, the educational efforts of community health nursing are appropriately targeted to reach many people. Instead of limiting teaching to one-on-one or small groups, the nurse has the opportunity and mandate to develop educational programs based on community needs that seek a community-wide impact. Community-wide antidrug campaigns, dietary improvement programs, and improved hand washing efforts among children provide useful models for implementation of the educator role at the population level and demonstrate its effectiveness in reaching a wide audience (Redman, 2007).

One factor that enhances the educator role is the public's higher level of health consciousness. Through plans ranging from the President's Council on Fitness, Sport and Nutrition (2012) to local antismoking campaigns, people are recognizing the value of health and are increasingly motivated to achieve higher levels of wellness. When a middle-aged man, for example, is discharged from the hospital after a heart attack, he is likely to be more interested than before the attack in learning how to prevent another. He can learn how to reduce stress, develop an appropriate and gradual exercise program, and alter his eating habits. Families with young children often are interested in learning about children's growth and development; most parents are committed to raising happy, healthy children. Health education can affect the health status of people of all ages (Pender et al., 2011). Today, in more businesses and industries, nurses promote the health of employees through active wellness-education and injury-prevention programs. The companies recognize that improving the health of their workers, which includes earning a living wage, means less absenteeism and higher production levels, in addition to other benefits (Baker et al., 2008; Kowlessar, Goetzel, Carls, Tabrizi, & Guindon, 2011). Some companies even provide exercise areas and equipment for employees to use and pay for the cost of their participation or allow paid time off for exercise.

Whereas nurses in acute care teach patients with a one-on-one focus about issues related to their hospitalization, community health nurses go beyond these topics to educate people in many areas. Community-living clients need and want to know about a wide variety of issues, such as family planning, weight control, smoking cessation, and stress reduction. Aggregate-level concerns also include such topics as environmental safety, sexual discrimination and harassment at school or work, violence, and drugs. What foods and additives are safe to eat? How can people organize the community to work for reduction of violence on television? What are health consumers' rights? Topics taught by community health nurses extend from personal and family health to environmental health and community organization.

As educators, community health nurses seek to facilitate client learning. Information is shared with clients both formally and informally. Nurses act as consultants to individuals or groups. Formal classes may be held to increase people's understanding of health and health care. Established community groups may be used in the nurse's teaching practice. For example, a nurse may teach parents and teachers at a parent–teacher meeting about signs of mood-modifying drug and alcohol abuse, discuss safety practices with a group of industrial workers, or give a presentation on the importance of early detection of child abuse to a health planning committee considering funding a new program. At times, the community health nurse facilitates client learning through referrals to more knowledgeable sources or through use of experts on special topics. Client self-education is facilitated by the nurse; in keeping with the concept of self-care, clients are encouraged and helped to use appropriate health resources and to seek out health information. The emphasis throughout the health teaching process continues to be placed on illness prevention and health promotion. Health teaching as a tool for community health nursing practice is discussed in detail in Chapter 11.

Advocate Role

The issue of clients' rights is important in health care. Every patient or client has the right to receive just, equal, and humane treatment. The role of the nurse includes client advocacy, which is highlighted in the ANA *Code of Ethics for Nurses with Interpretive Statements* (2001) and *Nursing's Social Policy Statement* (2010b). Our current health care system is often characterized by fragmented and depersonalized services, and many clients—especially the poor, the disadvantaged, those without health insurance, and people with language barriers—frequently are denied their rights. They become frustrated, confused, degraded, and unable to cope with the system on their own. The community health nurse often acts as an **advocate** for clients, pleading their cause or acting on their behalf. Clients may need someone to explain which services to expect and which services they ought to receive, to make referrals as needed, and to write letters to agencies or health care providers for them. They need someone to guide them through the complexities of the system, and assure the satisfaction of their needs. This is particularly true for minorities and disadvantaged groups (McCann, 2010; Traeger, Thompson, Dickson, & Provencio, 2006).

Advocacy Goals

Client advocacy has two underlying goals. One is to help clients gain greater independence or self-determination. Until they can research the needed information and access health and social services for themselves, the community health nurse acts as an advocate for the clients by showing them what services are available, those to which they are entitled, and how to obtain them. A second goal is to make the system more responsive and relevant to the needs of clients. By calling attention to inadequate, inaccessible, or unjust care, community health nurses can influence change.

Consider the experience of the Merrill family. Gloria Merrill has three small children. Early one Tuesday morning, the baby, Tony, suddenly started to cry. Nothing would comfort him. Gloria went to a neighbor's apartment, called the local clinic, and was told to come in the next day. The clinic did not take appointments and was too busy to see any more patients that day. Gloria's neighbor reassured her that "sometimes babies just cry." For the rest of the day and night, Tony cried almost incessantly. On Wednesday, Gloria and her children made the 45-minute bus ride to the clinic, and waited 3 hours in the crowded reception room; the wait was punctuated by interrogations from clinic workers. Gloria's other children were restless, and the baby was crying. Finally, they saw the physician. Tony had an inguinal hernia that could have strangulated and become gangrenous. The doctor admonished Gloria for waiting so long to bring in the baby. Immediate surgery was necessary. Someone at the clinic told Gloria that Medicaid would pay for it. Someone else told her that she was ineligible. At this point, all of her children were crying. Gloria had been up most of the night. She was frantic, confused, and felt that no one cared. This family needed an advocate.

Advocacy Actions

The advocate role incorporates four characteristic actions: being assertive, taking risks, communicating and negotiating well, and identifying resources and obtaining results.

First, advocates must be assertive. Fortunately, in the Merrill's dilemma, the clinic had a working relationship with the City Health Department and contacted Tracy Lee, a community health nurse liaison with the clinic, when Gloria broke down and cried. Tracy took the initiative to identify the Merrill's needs and find appropriate solutions. She contacted the Department of Social Services and helped the Merrills to establish eligibility for coverage of surgery and hospitalization costs. She helped Gloria to make arrangements for the baby's hospitalization and the other children's care.

Second, advocates must take risks—go "out on a limb" if need be—for the client. The community health nurse was outraged by the kind of treatment received by the Merrill family: the delays in service, the impersonal care, and the surgery that could have been planned as elective rather than as an emergency. She wrote a letter describing the details of the Merrill's experience to the clinic director, the chairman of the clinic board, and the nursing director. This action resulted in better care for the Merrill family and a series of meetings aimed at changing clinic procedures and providing better telephone screening.

Third, advocates must communicate and negotiate well by bargaining thoroughly and convincingly. The community health nurse helping the Merrill family stated the problem clearly and argued for its solution.

Finally, advocates must identify and obtain resources for the client's benefit. By contacting the most influential people in the clinic and appealing to their desire for quality service, the nurse caring for the Merrill family was able to facilitate change.

Advocacy at the population level incorporates the same goals and actions. Whether the population is homeless people, battered women, or migrant workers, the community health nurse in the advocate role speaks and acts on their behalf. The goals remain the same: to promote clients' self-determination and to shape a more responsive system. Advocacy for large aggregates, such as the millions with inadequate health care coverage, means changing national policies and laws (see Chapter 13). Advocacy may take the form of presenting public health nursing data to ensure that providers deliver quality services. It may mean conducting a needs assessment to demonstrate the necessity for a shelter and multiservice program for the homeless. It may mean testifying before the legislature to create awareness of the problems of battered women and the need for more protective laws. It may mean organizing a lobbying effort to require employers of migrant workers to provide proper housing and working conditions. In each case, the community health nurse works with representatives of the population to gain their understanding of the situation and to ensure their input.

Manager Role

Community health nurses, like all nurses, engage in the role of managing health services. As a **manager**, the nurse exercises administrative direction toward the accomplishment of specified goals by assessing clients' needs, planning and organizing to meet those needs, directing and leading to achieve results, and controlling and evaluating the progress to ensure that goals are met. The nurse serves as a manager when overseeing client care as a case manager, supervising ancillary staff, managing caseloads, running clinics, or conducting community health needs assessment projects. In each instance, the nurse engages in four basic functions that make up the management process. The management process, like the nursing process, incorporates a series of problem-solving activities or functions: planning, organizing, leading, and controlling and evaluating. These activities are sequential, yet also occur simultaneously for managing service objectives (Cherry & Jacob, 2011). While performing these functions, community health nurses most often are participative managers; that is, they participate with clients, other professionals, or both to plan and implement services.

Nurse as Planner

The first function in the management process is planning. A planner sets the goals and direction for the organization or project and determines the means to achieve them. Specifically, planning includes defining goals and objectives, determining the strategy for reaching them, and designing a coordinated set of activities for implementing and evaluating them. Planning may be strategic, which tends to include broader, more long-range goals (Cherry & Jacob, 2011; USDHHS, 2010a). An example of *strategic planning* is setting 2-year agency goals to reduce teenage pregnancies in the county by 50%. Planning may be operational, which focuses more on short-term planning needs. An example of *operational planning* is setting 6-month objectives to implement a new computer system for client record keeping.

The community health nurse engages in planning as a part of the manager role when supervising a group of home health aides working with home care clients. Plans of care must be designed to include setting short-term and long-term objectives, describe actions to carry out the objectives, and design a plan for evaluating the care given. With larger groups, such as a program for a homeless mentally ill population, the planning function is used in collaboration with other professionals in the community to determine appropriate goals for shelter and treatment and to develop an action plan to carry out and evaluate the program (Burke, 2005). The concepts of planning with communities and families are discussed further in Chapters 15 and 19, respectively.

Nurse as Organizer

The second function of the manager role is that of organizer. This involves designing a structure within which people and tasks function to reach the desired objectives. A manager must arrange matters so that the job can be done. People, activities, and relationships have to be assembled to put the plan into effect. Organizing includes deciding on the tasks to be done, who will do them, how to group the tasks, who reports to whom, and where decisions will be made (Cherry & Jacob, 2011). In the process of organizing, the nurse manager provides a framework for the various aspects of service, so that each runs smoothly and accomplishes its purpose. The framework is a part of service preparation. When a community health nurse manages a well-child clinic, for instance, the organizing function involves making certain that all equipment and supplies are present, required staff are hired and are on duty, and that staff responsibilities are clearly designated. The final responsibility as an organizer is to evaluate the effectiveness of the clinic. Is it providing the needed services? Are the clients satisfied? Do the services remain cost-effective? All of these questions must be addressed by the organizer.

Nurse as Leader

In the manager role, the community health nurse also must act as a **leader**. As a leader, the nurse directs, influences, or persuades others to effect change that will positively impact people's health and move them toward a goal. The leading function includes persuading and motivating people, directing activities, ensuring effective two-way communication, resolving conflicts, and coordinating the plan. Coordination means bringing people and activities together, so that they function in harmony while pursuing desired objectives.

Community health nurses act as leaders when they direct and coordinate the functioning of a hypertension screening clinic, a weight control group, or a three-county mobile health assessment unit. In each case, the leading function requires motivating the people involved, keeping open clear channels of communication, negotiating conflicts, and directing and coordinating the activities established during planning, so that the desired objectives can be accomplished.

Nurse as Controller and Evaluator

The fourth management function is to control and evaluate projects or programs. A controller monitors the plan and ensures that it stays on course. In this function, the community health nurse must realize that plans may not proceed as intended and may need adjustments or corrections to reach the desired results or goals. Monitoring, comparing, and adjusting make up the controlling part of this function. At the same time, the nurse must compare and judge performance and outcomes against previously set goals and standards—a process that forms the evaluator aspect of this management function.

An example of the controlling and evaluating function was evident in a program started in several preschool day care centers in a city in the Midwest. The goal of the project was to reduce the incidence of illness among the children through intensive physical and emotional preventive health education with staff, parents, and children. The two community health nurses managing the project were pleased with the progress of the classes and monitored the application of the prevention principles in day-to-day care. However, staff became busy after several weeks, and some plans were not being followed carefully. Preventive activities, such as ensuring that the children coughed into their shirt sleeve and washed their hands after using the bathroom and before eating, were not being closely monitored. Several children who were clearly sick had not been kept at home. Including the quiet or reserved children in activities was often overlooked. The nurses worked with staff and parents to motivate them and get the project back on course. They held monthly meetings with the staff, observed the classes periodically, and offered one-on-one instruction to staff, parents, and children. One activity was to establish competition between the centers for the best health record, with the promise of a photograph of the winning center's children and an article in the local newspaper. Their efforts were successful.

Management Behaviors

As managers, community health nurses engage in many different types of behaviors. These behaviors or parts of the manager role were first described by Mintzberg (1973). He grouped them into three sets of behaviors: decision-making, transferring of information, and engaging in interpersonal relationships.

Decision-Making Behaviors

Mintzberg identified four types of decisional roles or behaviors: entrepreneur, disturbance handler, resource allocator, and negotiator. A manager serves in the entrepreneur role when initiating new projects. Starting a nurse-managed center to serve a homeless population is an example. Community health nurses play the disturbance-handler role when they manage disturbances and crises—particularly interpersonal conflicts among staff, between staff and clients, or among clients (especially when being served in an agency). The resource-allocator role is demonstrated by determining the distribution and use of human, physical, and financial resources. Nurses play the negotiator role when negotiating, perhaps with higher levels of administration or a funding agency, for new health policy or budget increases to support expanded services for clients.

Transfer of Information Behaviors

Mintzberg described three informational roles or behaviors: monitor, information disseminator, and spokesperson. The monitor role requires collecting and processing information, such as gathering ongoing evaluation data to determine whether a program is meeting its goals. In the disseminator role, nurses transmit the collected information to people involved in the project or organization. In the spokesperson role, nurses share information on behalf of the project or agency with outsiders.

Interpersonal Behaviors

While engaging in various interpersonal roles, the community health nurse may function as a figurehead, a leader, and a liaison. In the figurehead role, the nurse acts in a ceremonial or symbolic capacity, such as participating in a ribbon-cutting ceremony to mark the opening of a new clinic or representing the project or agency for news media coverage. In the leader role, the nurse motivates and directs people involved in the project. In the liaison role, a network is maintained with people outside the organization or project for information exchange and project enhancement.

Management Skills

What types of skills and competencies does the community health nurse need in the manager role? Three basic management skills are needed for successful achievement of goals: human, conceptual, and technical. *Human skills* refer to the ability to understand, communicate, motivate, delegate, and work well with people (Cherry & Jacob, 2011). An example is a nursing supervisor's or team leader's ability to gain the trust and respect of staff and promote a productive and satisfying work environment. A manager can accomplish goals only with the cooperation of others. Therefore, human skills are essential to successful performance of the manager role. *Conceptual skills* refer to the mental ability to analyze and interpret abstract ideas for the purpose of understanding and diagnosing situations and formulating solutions. Examples are analyzing demographic data for program planning and developing a conceptual model to describe and improve organizational function. Finally, *technical skills* refer to the ability to apply special management-related knowledge and expertise to a particular situation or problem. Such skills performed by a community health nurse might include implementing a staff development program or developing a computerized management information system.

Case Management

Case management has become the standard method of managing health care in the delivery systems in the United States, and managed care organizations have become an integral part of community-oriented care. **Case management** is a systematic process by which a nurse assesses clients' needs, plans for and coordinates services, refers to other appropriate providers, and monitors and evaluates progress to ensure that clients' multiple service needs are met in a cost-effective manner. Managed care, the broader umbrella under which case management exists, is a cost-containing system of health care administration (Cohen & Cesta, 2005). Managed care, as an approach to delivering health care, is discussed in detail in Chapter 6. As clients leave hospitals earlier, as families struggle with multiple and complex health problems, as more elderly persons need alternatives to nursing home care, as competition and scarce resources contribute to fragmentation of services, and as the cost of health care continues to increase, there is a growing need for someone to oversee and coordinate all facets of needed service (Cohen & Cesta, 2005). Through case management, the nurse addresses this need in the community.

The activity of case management often follows discharge planning as a part of continuity of care. When applied to individual clients, it means overseeing their transition from the hospital back into the community and monitoring them to ensure that all of their service needs are met. Case management also applies to aggregates (Kneipp et al., 2011). In this context, it involves overseeing and ensuring that group or population health-related needs are met, particularly for those who are at high risk of illness or injury. For example, the community health nurse may work with battered women who come to a shelter. First, the nurse must ensure that their immediate needs for safety, security, food, finances, and child care are met. Then, the nurse must work with other professionals to provide more permanent housing, employment, ongoing counseling, and financial and legal resources for this group of women. Whether applied to families or aggregates, case management, like other applications of the manager role, uses the three sets of management behaviors and engages the community health nurse as planner, organizer, leader, controller, and evaluator.

Collaborator Role

Community health nurses seldom practice in isolation. They must work with many people, including clients, other nurses, physicians, teachers, health educators, social workers, physical therapists, nutritionists, occupational therapists, psychologists, epidemiologists, biostatisticians, attorneys, secretaries, environmentalists, city planners, and legislators. As members of the health team, community health nurses assume the role of **collaborator**, which means working jointly with others in a common endeavor, cooperating as partners. Successful community health practice depends on this multidisciplinary collegiality and leadership (Clark-McMullen, 2010; Powell, Gilliss, Hewitt, & Flint, 2010). Everyone on the team has an important and unique contribution to make to the health care effort. As on a championship ball team, the better all members play their individual positions and cooperate with other members, the more likely the health team is to win.

The community health nurse's collaborator role requires skills in communicating, in interpreting the nurse's unique contribution to the team, and in acting assertively as an equal partner. The collaborator role also may involve functioning as a consultant.

The following examples show a community health nurse functioning as collaborator. Three families needed to find good nursing homes for their elderly grandparents. The community health nurse met with the families, including the elderly members; made a list of desired features, such as a shower and access to walking trails; and then worked with a social worker to locate and visit several homes. The grandparents' respective physicians were contacted for medical consultation, and in each case, the elderly member made the final selection. In another situation, the community health nurse collaborated with the city council, police department, neighborhood residents, and the manager of a senior citizens' high-rise apartment building to help a group of elderly people organize and lobby for safer streets. In a third example, a school nurse noticed a rise in the incidence of drug use in her schools. She initiated a counseling program after joint planning with students, parents, teachers, the school psychologist, and a local drug rehabilitation center.

Leadership Role

Community health nurses are becoming increasingly active in the leadership role, separate from leading within the manager role mentioned earlier. The leadership role focuses on effecting change (see Chapter 11); thus, the nurse becomes an agent of change. As leaders, community health nurses seek to initiate changes that positively affect people's health. They also seek to influence people to think and behave differently about their health and the factors contributing to it. The leader recognizes the complex set of factors contributing to health outcomes and works to address those myriad factors in affecting needed change. The role of social determinants of health (e.g., availability of health services and the physical environment) are discussed in Chapter 11 in relation to health promotion of individuals and communities.

At the community level, the leadership role may involve working with a team of professionals to direct and coordinate such projects as a campaign to eliminate smoking in public areas or to lobby legislators for improved child day care facilities. When nurses guide community health decision-making, stimulate an industry's interest in health promotion, initiate group therapy, direct a preventive program, or influence health policy, they assume the leadership role. For example, a community health nurse started a rehabilitation program that included self-esteem building, career counseling, and job placement to help women in a halfway house who had recently been released from prison.

The community health nurse also exerts influence through health planning. The need for coordinated, accessible, cost-effective health care services creates a challenge and an opportunity for the nurse to become more involved in health planning at all levels: organizational, local, state, national, and international. A community health nurse needs to exercise leadership responsibility and assert the right to share in health decisions (Cherry & Jacob, 2011). One community health nurse determined that there was a need for a behavioral health program in his district. He planned to implement it through the agency for which he worked, but certain individuals on the health board were opposed to adding new programs because of the cost. The nurse's approach was to gather considerable data to demonstrate the need for the program and its cost-effectiveness. He invited individual, key board members to lunch to convince them of the need. He prepared written summaries, graphs, and charts, and at a strategic time, he presented his case at a board meeting. The behavioral health program was approved and implemented.

A broader attribute of the leadership role is that of visionary. A leader with *vision* develops the ability to see what can be and leads people on a path toward that goal. A leader's vision may include long- and short-term goals. In one instance, it began as articulating the need for stronger community nursing services to an underserved population in an inner-city neighborhood served by a community health nurse. In this densely populated, tenant-occupied neighborhood, drugs, crime, and violence were commonplace. One summer, an 8-year-old boy was shot and killed. The enraged immigrant families in the neighborhood felt helpless and hopeless. Several families were visited by the nurse, and they shared their concerns with him. The nurse felt strongly about this blighted community and offered to work with the community to effect change. He gathered volunteers from neighborhood churches, and together they began to discuss the community's concerns. Together they prioritized their needs and began planning to make theirs a healthy community. The nurse organized his work week to provide health screening and education to families in the basement of a church on one morning each week. Initially, only a few families accessed this new service. In a matter of months, it became recognized as a valuable community service, and it expanded to a full day; the expanding volunteer group soon outgrew the space. The community health nurse worked closely with influential community members and the families being served. They determined that many more services were needed in this neighborhood, and they began to broaden their outreach and think of ways to provide the needed services.

Within a year, the group had written several grants to the city and to a private corporation in an effort to expand the voluntary services. The funding that they obtained allowed them to rent vacant storefront space, hire a part-time nurse practitioner, contract with the health department for additional community health nursing services, and negotiate with the local university to have medical, nursing, and social work students placed on a regular basis. The group, under the visionary leadership of the community health nurse, planned to add a one-on-one reading program for children, a class in English as a second language for immigrant families, a mentoring program for teenagers, and dental services. Even the police department had opened a substation in the neighborhood, making their presence more visible. This community health nurse's vision filled an immediate, critical need in the short term and developed into a comprehensive community center in the long term. Violence and crime diminished, and the neighborhood became a place where children could play safely.

Researcher Role

In the **researcher** role, community health nurses engage in the systematic investigation, collection, and analysis of data for solving problems and enhancing community health practice. But how can research be combined with practice? Although research technically involves a complex set of activities conducted by persons with highly developed and specialized skills, research also means applying that technical study to real-practice situations. Community health nurses base their practice on the evidence found in the literature to enhance and change practice as needed. For example, the work of researchers over two decades supports the value of intensive home visiting to high-risk families (Eckenrode et al., 2010; Olds et al., 2010). The outcomes of this research are changing practice protocol to high-risk families in many health departments today.

Research is an investigative process in which all community health nurses can become involved in asking questions and looking for solutions. Collaborative practice models between academics and practitioners combine research methodology expertise with practitioners' knowledge of problems to make community health nursing research both valid and relevant. The ongoing need for evidence-based practice is supported by *Healthy People 2020*, which stresses that the "emerging field of public health systems and services research is playing an important role in the development of this evidence base; its role should be supported and expanded over the decade, with a strong focus on translating research into practice" (USDHHS, 2010b).

The Research Process

Community health nurses practice the researcher role at several levels. In addition to everyday inquiries, community health nurses often participate in agency and organizational studies to determine such matters as practice activities, priorities, and education of public health nurses (Meagher-Stewart et al., 2010). Some community health nurses participate in more complex research on their own or in collaboration with other health professionals (Butterfield, Hill, Postma, Butterfield, & Odom-Maryon, 2011; Wieland et al., 2011). The researcher role (at all levels) helps to determine needs, evaluate effectiveness of care, and develop a theoretic basis for community health nursing practice. Chapters 4 and 12 will explain community health research in greater detail.

Research literally means to *search again*—to investigate, discover, and interpret facts. All research in community health, from the simplest inquiry to the most complex epidemiologic study, uses the same fundamental process. Simply put, the research process involves the following steps: (1) identify an area of interest, (2) specify the research question or statement, (3) review the literature, (4) identify a conceptual framework, (5) select a research design, (6) collect and analyze data, (7) interpret the results, and (8) communicate the findings (see Chapter 4).

Investigation builds on the nursing process, that essential dynamic of community health nursing practice, using it as a problem-solving process (Burns & Grove, 2011). In using the nursing process, the nurse identifies a problem or question, investigates by collecting and analyzing data, suggests and evaluates possible solutions, and either selects a solution or rejects them all and starts the investigative process over again. In a sense, the nurse is gathering data for health planning—investigating health problems to design wellness-promoting and disease-preventing interventions for community populations.

Attributes of the Researcher Role

A questioning attitude is a basic prerequisite for good nursing practice. A nurse may have revisited a patient many times and noticed some change in her condition, such as restlessness or pallor; consequently, the nurse wonders what is causing this change and what can be done about it. In everyday practice, numerous situations challenge the nurse to ask questions. Consider the following examples:

- The local newspaper reports that another group of children has been arrested for using illegal drugs. Is there an increase in the incidence of illegal drug use in the community?
- Children attending a day care center appear to have excessive bruises on their arms and legs. What is the incidence of reported child abuse in this community? What could be done to promote earlier detection and improved reporting?
- Elderly persons are living alone and without assistance in a neighborhood. How prevalent is this situation, and what are this population's needs?
- While driving through a particular neighborhood, the nurse notices not a single playground. Where do the kids play?

Each of these questions places the nurse in the role of investigator. They demonstrate the fundamental attitude of every researcher: a spirit of inquiry.

A second attribute, careful observation, is also evident in the examples just given. The nurse needs to develop a sharpened ability to notice things as they are, including deviations from the norm and subtle changes suggesting the need for nursing action. Coupled with observation is open-mindedness, another attribute of the researcher role. In the case of the bruises seen on day care children, a community health nurse's observations suggest child abuse as a possible cause. However, open-mindedness requires consideration of other alternatives, and, as a good investigator, the nurse explores these possibilities as well.

Analytic skills also are used in this role. In the example of illegal drug use, the nurse already has started to analyze the situation by trying to determine its cause-and-effect relationships. Successful analysis depends on how well the data have been collected. Insufficient information can lead to false interpretations, so it is important to seek out the needed data. Analysis, like a jigsaw puzzle, involves studying the pieces and fitting them together until the meaning of the whole picture can be described.

Finally, the researcher role involves tenacity. The community health nurse persists in an investigation until facts are uncovered and a satisfactory answer is found. Noticing an absence of playgrounds and wondering where the children play is only a beginning. Being concerned about the children's safety and need for recreational outlets, the nurse gathers data about the location and accessibility of play areas, as well as expressed needs of community residents. A fully documented research report may result. If the data support a need for additional play space, the report can be brought before the proper authorities.

SETTINGS FOR COMMUNITY HEALTH NURSING PRACTICE

The previous section examined community health nursing from the perspective of its major roles. The roles can now be placed in context by viewing the settings in which they are practiced. The types of places in which community health nurses practice are increasingly varied and include a growing number of nontraditional settings and partnerships with non-health groups. Employers of community health nurses range from state and local health departments and home health agencies to managed care organizations, businesses and industries, and nonprofit organizations. For this discussion, these settings are grouped into seven categories: homes, ambulatory service settings, schools, occupational health settings, residential institutions, faith communities, and the community at large (domestic and international). This section provides a brief overview of the various settings. Chapters 30 and 31 will provide much more detail on specific roles and settings, including both public and private practice settings.

Homes

Since Lillian Wald and the nurses at the Henry Street Settlement first started their practice at the beginning of the last century, the most frequently used setting for community health nursing practice was the home. In the home, all of the community health nursing roles are performed to varying degrees. Clients who are discharged from acute care institutions, such as hospitals or behavioral health facilities, are regularly referred to community health nurses for continued care and follow-up. Here, the community health nurse can see clients in a family and environmental context, and service can be tailored to the clients' unique needs.

For example, Mr. White, 67 years of age, was discharged from the hospital with a colostomy. Doreen Levitz, the community health nurse from the county public health nursing agency, immediately started home visits. She met with Mr. White and his wife to discuss their needs as a family and to plan for Mr. White's care and adjustment to living with a colostomy. Practicing the clinician and educator roles, she reinforced and expanded on the teaching started in the hospital for colostomy care, including bowel training, diet, exercise, and proper use of equipment. As part of a total family care plan, Doreen provided some forms of physical care for Mr. White as well as counseling, teaching, and emotional support for both Mr. White and his wife. In addition to consulting with the physician and social service worker, she arranged and supervised visits from the home health aide, who gave personal care and homemaker services. She thus performed the manager, leader, and collaborator roles.

The home is also a setting for health promotion. Many community health nursing visits focus on assisting families to understand and practice healthier living behaviors. Nurses may, for example, instruct clients on parenting, infant care, child discipline, diet, exercise, coping with stress, or managing grief and loss.

The character of the home setting is as varied as the clients served by the community health nurse. In one day, the nurse may visit a well-to-do widow in her luxurious home, a middle-income family in their modest bungalow, an elderly transient man in his one-room fifth-story walk-up apartment, and a teen mother and her infant living in a group foster home. In each situation, the nurse can view the clients in perspective and, therefore, better understand their limitations, capitalize on their resources, and tailor health services to meet their needs. In the home, unlike in most other health care settings, clients are on their own "turf." They feel comfortable and secure in familiar surroundings and often are better able to understand and apply health information. Client self-respect can be promoted, because the client is host and the nurse is a guest.

Sometimes, the thought of visiting in clients' homes can cause anxiety for the nurse. This may be the nurse's first experience outside the acute care, long-term care, or clinic setting. Visiting clients in their own environment can make the nurse feel uncomfortable. The nurse may be asked to visit families in unfamiliar neighborhoods, and she must walk through those neighborhoods to locate the clients' homes. Frequently, fear of the unknown is the real fear—a fear that often has been enhanced by stories from previous nurses. This may be the same feeling as that experienced when caring for your first client, first entering the operating room, or first having a client in the intensive care unit. However, in the community, more variables exist, and basic safety measures should be used by all people when out in public. General guidelines for safety and making home visits are covered in detail in Chapter 19. Nevertheless, the specific instructions given during the clinical experience should be followed, and everyday, common-sense safety precautions should be used.

Changes in the health care delivery system, along with shifting health economics and service delivery (discussed in Chapter 6), are changing community health nursing's use of the home as a primary setting for practice. Many local health departments are finding it increasingly difficult to provide widespread home visiting by their public health nurses. Instead, many agencies are targeting populations that are most in need of direct intervention. Examples include families of children with elevated blood lead levels, low-birth-weight babies, clients requiring directly observed administration of tuberculosis medications, and families requiring ongoing monitoring due to identified child abuse or neglect. With limited staff and limited financial resources, the highest-priority clients or groups are targeted.

With skills in population-based practice, community health nurses serve the public's health best by focusing on sites where they can have the greatest impact. At the same time, they can collaborate with various types of home care providers, including hospitals, other nurses, physicians, rehabilitation therapists, and durable medical equipment companies, to ensure continuous and holistic service. The nurse continues to supervise home care services and engage in case management. The increased demand for highly technical acute care in the home requires specialized skills that are best delivered by nurses with this expertise. Chapter 32 further examines the nurse's role in the home health and hospice settings. The ANA documents *Home Health Nursing: Scope and Standards of Practice* (2007b) and *Hospice and Palliative Nursing: Scope and Standards of Practice* (ANA/Hospice and Palliative Nurses Association, 2007) offer additional insight on these specialty areas.

Ambulatory Service Settings

Ambulatory service settings include a variety of venues for community health nursing practice in which clients come for day or evening services that do not include overnight stays. A community health center is an example of an ambulatory setting. Sometimes, multiple clinics offering comprehensive services are community based or are located in outpatient departments of hospitals or medical centers. They also may be based in comprehensive neighborhood health centers. A single clinic, such as a family planning clinic or a well-child clinic, may be found in a location that is more convenient for clients, perhaps a church basement or empty storefront. Some kinds of day care centers, such as those for the physically disabled or adults with behavioral health issues, use community health nursing services. Additional ambulatory care settings include health departments (city, county, or state) and community health nursing agencies, where clients may come for assessment and referral or counseling. An increasing number of nurse-managed health centers have also been formed over the past decade, often as a community service component of schools of nursing. The mission of these centers varies, but they are typically used to enhance student clinical experiences while providing identified community needs in the areas of primary health care and health promotion (see Chapter 31).

Offices are another type of ambulatory care setting. Some community health nurses provide service in conjunction with a medical practice; for example, a community health nurse associated with a health maintenance organization sees clients in the office and undertakes screening, referrals, counseling, health education, and group work. Others establish independent practices by seeing clients in community nursing centers as well as making home visits.

Another type of ambulatory service setting includes places where services are offered to selected groups. For example, community health nurses practice in migrant camps, on tribal lands, at correctional facilities, in children's day care centers, through faith communities, and in remote mountain and coal-mining communities. In each ambulatory setting, all of the community health nursing roles are used to varying degrees (see Perspectives: Student Voices).

Schools

Schools of all levels make up a major group of settings for community health nursing practice. Nurses from community health nursing agencies frequently serve private schools at elementary and intermediate levels. Public schools are served by the same agencies or by community health nurses hired through the public school system. The community health nurse may work with groups of students in preschool settings, such as Montessori schools, as well as in vocational or technical schools, junior colleges, and college and university settings. Specialized schools, such as those for the developmentally disabled, are another setting for community health nursing practice.

Community health nurses' roles in school settings are changing. School nurses, whose primary role initially was that of clinician, are widening their practice to include more health education, interprofessional collaboration, and client advocacy. For example, one school had been accustomed to using the nurse as a first-aid provider and record keeper. Her duties were handling minor problems, such as headaches and cuts, and keeping track of such events as immunizations. This nurse sought to expand her practice and, after consultation and preparation, collaborated with a health educator

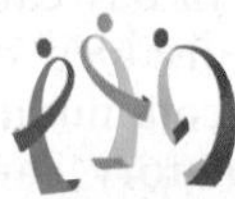

PERSPECTIVES STUDENT VOICE

A Graduating Student Viewpoint on Postgraduation Employment

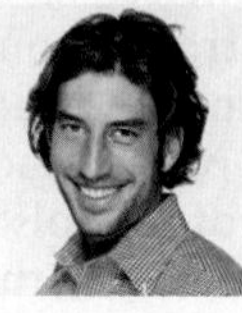

Before entering nursing school, I spent 6 years on active duty as a corpsman in the Navy. I remembered seeing some nurses who visited our hospital wearing what looked like Navy uniforms, but was told that they worked for the federal government and weren't in the Navy. I didn't think much of it until I was looking up information on the US Public Health Service and the Surgeon General. Only then did it dawn on me that those nurses were part of the Commissioned Corps of the Public Health Service. I didn't even know they existed, much less what they did, so I looked around the section of the Web site dealing with nursing. It turns out that they do quite a bit—respond to disasters, provide health services to Native Americans, and even work with the federal prisons. It surprised me to find out that they hire new graduates for many of their positions. I still haven't decided what I want to do after I graduate, but I may seriously consider this option. They even have an extern program available while I'm still in school—who knows, I may be in uniform again.

Matt, Age 24

and some of the teachers to offer a series of classes on personal hygiene, diet, and sexuality. She started a drop-in health counseling center in the school and established a network of professional contacts for consultation and referral.

Community health nurses in school settings also are beginning to assume managerial and leadership roles and to recognize that the researcher role should be an integral part of their practice. The nurse's role with school-age and adolescent populations is discussed in detail in Chapter 22. The ANA *School Nursing: Scope and Standards of Practice* (2011) provides additional information on this important specialty.

Occupational Health Settings

Business and industry provide another group of settings for community health nursing practice. Employee health has long been recognized as making a vital contribution to individual lives, the productivity of business, and the wellbeing of the entire nation. Organizations are expected to provide a safe and healthy work environment, in addition to offering insurance for health care. More companies, recognizing the value of healthy employees, are going beyond offering traditional health benefits to supporting health promotional efforts. Some businesses, for example, offer healthy snacks, such as fruit at breaks, and promote jogging during the noon hour. A few larger corporations have built exercise facilities for their employees, provide health education programs, and offer financial incentives for losing weight or staying well.

Community health nurses in occupational health settings practice a variety of roles. The clinician role predominated for many years, as nurses continued to care for sick or injured employees at work. However, recognition of the need to protect employees' safety and, later, to prevent their illness led to the inclusion of health education in the occupational health nurse role. Occupational and environmental health nurses also act as employee advocates, assuring appropriate job assignments for workers and adequate treatment for job-related illness or injury. They collaborate with other health care providers and company management to offer better services to their clients. They act as leaders and managers in developing new health services in the work setting, endorsing programs such as hypertension screening and weight control. Occupational health settings range from industries and factories, such as an automobile assembly plant, to business corporations and even large retail sales systems. The field of occupational health offers a challenging opportunity, particularly in smaller businesses, where nursing coverage usually is not provided. Chapter 31 more fully describes the role of the nurse serving the working adult population. The American Association of Occupational Health Nurses sets the standards for this specialty and is the exclusive publisher of the *Standards of Occupational and Environmental Health Nursing* (2012).

Residential Institutions

Any facility where clients reside can be a setting in which community health nursing is practiced. Residential institutions can include a halfway house in which clients live temporarily while recovering from drug addiction or an inpatient hospice program in which terminally ill clients live. Some residential settings, such as hospitals, exist solely to provide health care; others provide a variety of services and support. Community health nurses based in a community agency maintain continuity of care for their clients by collaborating with hospital personnel, visiting clients in the hospital, and planning care during and after hospitalization. Some community health nurses serve one or more hospitals on a regular basis by providing a liaison with the community, consultation for discharge planning, and periodic in-service programs to keep hospital staff updated on community services for their clients. Other community health nurses with similar functions are based in the hospital and serve the hospital community.

A continuing care center is another example of a residential site providing health care that may use community health nursing services. In this setting, residents usually are elderly; some live quite independently, whereas others become increasingly dependent and have many chronic health problems. The community health nurse functions as advocate and collaborator to improve services. The nurse may, for example, coordinate available resources to meet the needs of residents and their families and help safeguard the maintenance of quality operating standards. Chapter 24 discusses the community health nurse's role with elders aging in place. Chapter 32 discusses nursing services needed by clients after hospitalization through home care services or by families and clients in hospice programs. Sheltered workshops and group homes for mentally ill or developmentally disabled children and adults are other examples of residential institutions that serve clients who share specific needs.

Community health nurses also practice in settings where residents are gathered for purposes other than receiving care, where health care is offered as an adjunct to the primary goals of the institution. For example, many nurses work with camping programs for children and adults offered by religious organizations and other community agencies, such as the Boy Scouts, Girl Scouts, or the YMCA. Other camp nurses work with children and adults who have chronic or terminal illnesses, through disease-related community agencies such as the American Lung Association, American Diabetes Association, and American Cancer Society. Camp nurses practice all available roles, often under interesting and challenging conditions.

Another often overlooked practice setting is the correctional institution. Inmates may be incarcerated both short and long term and have the same health care needs as the general public. Due to the unique nature of this population, there are typically additional health and social service needs for this population, often stemming from the reason for the incarceration in the first place (drug abuse) and that place them at increased risk for select health problems (AIDS, tuberculosis, poor nutrition, etc.). The challenge to the nurse in this setting is to provide health care in an unbiased and nonjudgmental manner within the realities of the setting. Chapter 30 discusses the role of the nurse in the correctional setting, and the ANA's *Corrections Nursing: Scope and Standards of Practice* (2007a) offers insight into this practice specialty.

Residential institutions provide unique settings for the community health nurse to practice health promotion. Clients are more accessible, their needs can be readily assessed, and their interests can be stimulated. These settings offer the opportunity to generate an environment of caring and optimal-quality health care provided by community health nursing services.

Faith Communities

Faith community nursing finds its beginnings in an ancient tradition. The beginnings of community health nursing can be traced to religious orders (see Chapter 2), and for centuries, religious and spiritual communities were important sources of health care. In faith community nursing today, the practice focal point remains the faith community and the religious belief system provided by the philosophical framework. Faith community nursing may take different names such as church-based health promotion, parish nursing, or primary care parish nursing practice. Whatever the service is called, it involves a large-scale effort by the church community to improve the health of its members through education, screening, referral, treatment, and group support.

In some geopolitical communities, faith community nurses are the most acceptable primary care providers. The role of the nurse can be broad, being defined by the needs of the members and the philosophy of the religious community. However, the goal is to enhance and extend services available in the larger community, not to duplicate them.

The ANA has published standards of care for faith community nursing practice in collaboration with the Health Ministries Association, Inc. (ANA, 2012). The standards act as guidelines for faith communities that plan to offer or are offering faith community nursing services. This specialty area of practice is guided by a variety of standards set up by several groups. Together, these standards provide guidance and direction for caregiving within the faith community.

When community health nurses work as faith community nurses, they enhance accessibility to available health services in the community while meeting the unique needs of the members of that religious community, practicing within the framework of the tenets of that religion. A nurse working within a faith community must be cognizant of the basic principles and practices of the religious group served. In most situations, the nurse is a practitioner of the same religious belief system. Chapter 31 provides more detailed information about this specialty area of practice.

Community at Large

Unlike the six settings already discussed, the seventh setting for community health nursing practice is not confined to a specific philosophy, location, or building. When working with groups, populations, or the total community, the nurse may practice in many different places (Display 3.4). For example, a community health nurse, as clinician and health educator, may work with a parenting group in a church or town hall. Another nurse, as client advocate, leader, and researcher, may study the health needs of a neighborhood's elderly population by collecting data throughout the area and meeting with resource people in many places. Also, a nurse may work with community-based organizations such as an AIDS organization or a support group for parents experiencing the violent death of a child. Again, the community at large becomes the setting for practice for a nurse who serves on health care planning committees, lobbies for

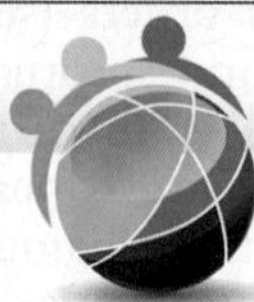

DISPLAY 3.4 INNOVATIVE COMMUNITY HEALTH NURSING PRACTICE

In some community health nursing courses, students do not have access to an established agency such as a health department or community center from which to establish a client base. Student nurses and practicing community health nurses can provide outreach services and do case-finding in innovative settings such as these:

Settings	*Clients*	*Roles of the Community Health Nurse*
1. Senior centers when flu shots are given or commodities are distributed	Older adults	Educator, clinician, advocate
2. Outside of grocery stores, department stores, movie theaters, large pharmacies	People of all ages and families	Educator, clinician, advocate
3. At parent-teacher association (PTA) meetings, sporting events, dances, and school registration (in collaboration with school nurses)	Young adults, children, and teenagers	Educator, clinician, advocate
4. Outside of concerts, plays, the circus, etc.	People of all ages	Educator, clinician, advocate
5. Other public gatherings: farmers markets, neighborhood yard sales, etc.	People of all ages	Educator, clinician, advocate
6. Conferences or seminars	People of all ages	Leader, educator, clinician
7. "On the street"	Homeless persons, passersby, transients, low-income urban dwellers	Educator, clinician, advocate
8. Truck stops	Predominantly employed men	Educator, clinician, advocate

Leader's role initiate, plan, strategize, collaborate, and cooperate with community groups to present programs that are focused on specific population's needs.

Educator's role—teach nutrition, stress management, safety, exercise, prevention of sexually transmitted diseases, and other men and women's health issues, child home/school/play and stranger safety, and child growth and development, and provide anticipatory guidance. Have pamphlets available to support verbal information on health and safety topics, specific diseases, social security, Medicare, and Medicaid.

Clinician's role—perform blood pressure screening, height, weight, blood testing for diabetes and cholesterol, occult blood test, hearing and vision tests, scoliosis measurements, and administration of immunizations.

Advocate's role—provide information regarding community resources as needed, cut "red tape" for those who need it, answer questions, and guide people to additional resources, such as Internet Web sites and "800" phone numbers.

health legislation at the state capital, runs for a school board position, or assists with flood relief in another state or another country.

Although the term "setting" implies a place, remember that community health nursing practice is not limited to a specific site. Community health nursing is a specialty of nursing that is defined by the nature of its practice, not its location, and it can be practiced anywhere. As you read through this chapter, perhaps an area of practice or a particular population captured your attention. If you are interested in tribal health, you might consider working as a US Public Health Service nurse, or if you find that you are more interested in providing comprehensive health promotion programs to rural individuals, a nurse-managed health center may be of interest. Opportunities for community health nursing include the American Red Cross, state and local health departments, the Peace Corps, and various international aid groups. Both private and public health agencies are actively seeking nurses with an interest in improving the health of their communities. Take some time to read over Chapters 30 and 31; perhaps you will find an opportunity that supports your professional goals.

SUMMARY

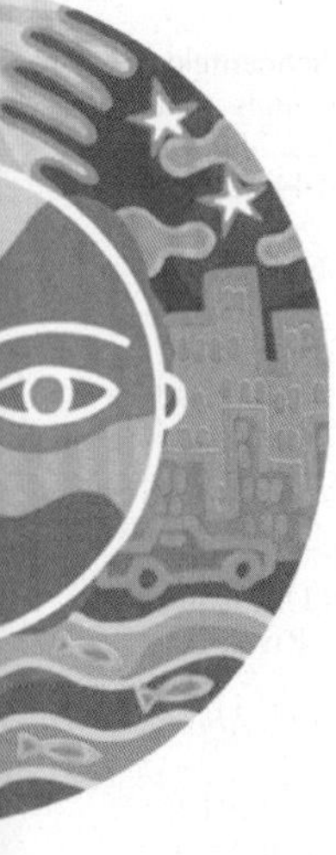

Community health nurses play many roles, including that of clinician, educator, advocate, manager, collaborator, leader, and researcher. Each role entails special types of skills and expertise. The type and number of roles that are practiced vary with each set of clients and each specific situation, but the nurse should be able to successfully function in each of these roles as the particular situation demands. The role of manager is one that the nurse must play in every situation, because it involves assessing clients' needs, planning and organizing to meet those needs, directing and leading clients to achieve results, and controlling and evaluating the progress to ensure that the goals and clients' needs are met. A type of comprehensive management of clients that has become known as *case management* is an integral part of community health nursing practice.

As a part of the manager role, the nurse must engage in three crucial management behaviors: decision-making, transferring information, and relationship building. Nurses must also use a comprehensive set of management skills: human skills that allow them to understand, communicate, motivate, and work with people; conceptual skills that allow them to interpret abstract ideas and apply them to real situations to formulate solutions; and technical skills that allow them to apply special management-related knowledge and expertise to a particular situation or problem.

There also are many types of settings in which the community health nurse may practice and in which these roles are enacted. "Setting" does not necessarily refer to a specific location or site but rather to a particular situation. These situations can be grouped into seven major categories: homes; ambulatory service settings, where clients come for care but do not stay overnight; schools; occupational health settings, which serve employees in business and industry; residential institutions such as hospitals, continuing care facilities, halfway houses, or other institutions in which people live and sleep; faith communities, where care is based on the philosophy of the religious organization; and the community at large, which encompasses a variety of expected and innovative locations.

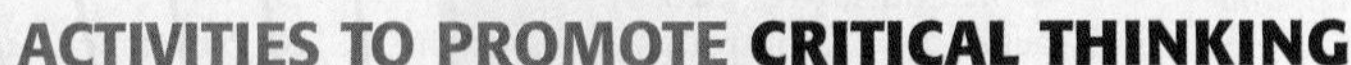

ACTIVITIES TO PROMOTE **CRITICAL THINKING**

1. Discuss ways for a community health nurse to make service holistic and focused on wellness with
   a. preschool-age children in a day care setting.
   b. a group of chemically dependent adolescents.
   c. a group of elders living in a senior high-rise building.
2. Select one community health nursing role and describe its application in meeting the needs of your friend or next-door neighbor.
3. Describe a hypothetical or real situation in which you, as a community health nurse, would combine the roles of leader, collaborator, and researcher (investigator). Discuss how each of these roles might be played.
4. If your community health nursing practice setting is the community at large, will your practice roles be any different from those of the nurse whose practice setting is the home? Why? What determines the roles played by the community health nurse?
5. Interview a practicing community health nurse and determine which roles are part of the nurse's practice during 1 month of caregiving. Describe the ways in which each role is enacted. How many instances of this nurse's practice were aggregate focused? In which of the settings does the nurse mostly practice? If you were a public health consultant, what suggestions might you make to expand this nurse's role into aggregate-level practice?
6. Search the Internet or go to the library and find two sources of health-related information for consumers. Was the information accurate?
7. Search the Internet or go to the library and find two research articles on community health nursing. In what settings did the research take place? Did the nursing authors collaborate with interdisciplinary team members on this research? If so, how do you think this collaboration helped the research? If you were to conduct research in the community, would you conduct it with only nurses on the team, or would your team be interdisciplinary? Why? What would be the benefits or limits of each approach?

REFERENCES

American Association of Colleges of Nursing. (2008). *The essentials of baccalaureate education for professional nursing practice*. Washington, DC: Author.

American Association of Occupational Health Nurses. (2012). *Standards of occupational and environmental health nursing*. Pensacola, FL: Author.

American Nurses Association. (2001). *Code of ethics for nurses with interpretive statements*. Silver Spring, MD: Nursesbooks.org.

American Nurses Association. (2007a). *Corrections nursing: Scope and standards of practice*. Silver Springs, MD: Nursesbooks.org.

American Nurses Association. (2007b). *Home health nursing: Scope and standards of practice*. Silver Spring, MD: Nursesbooks.org.

American Nurses Association. (2007c). *Public health nursing: Scope and standards of practice*. Silver Spring, MD: Nursesbooks.org.

American Nurses Association. (2010a). *Nursing: Scope and standards of practice* (2nd ed.). Silver Spring, MD: Nursesbooks.org.

American Nurses Association. (2010b). *Nursing's social policy statement: The essence of the profession*. Silver Spring, MD: Nursesbooks.org.

American Nurses Association. (2011). *School nursing: Scope and standards of practice* (2nd ed.). Silver Spring, MD: Nursesbooks.org.

American Nurses Association. (2012). *Faith community nursing: Scope and standards of practice* (2nd ed.). Silver Spring, MD: Nuresesbooks.org.

American Nurses Association/Hospice and Palliative Nurses Association. (2007). *Hospice and palliative nursing: Scope and standards of practice*. Silver Spring, MD: Nursesbooks.org.

American Public Health Association. (2012). *A Statement of APHA Public Health Nursing Section*. Retrieved from http://www.apha.org/extranet/phn/default.htm

Association of Community Health Nursing Educators, Education Committee. (2010). Essentials of Baccalaureate nursing education for entry-level community/public health nursing. *Public Health Nursing, 27*, 371–382. doi: 10.1111/j.1525-1446.2010.00867.x

Baker, K. M., Goetzel, R. Z., Pei, X., Weiss, A. J., Bowen, J., Tabrizi, M. J., et al. (2008). Using a return-on-investment estimation model to evaluate outcomes from an obesity management worksite health promotion program. *Journal of Occupational and Environmental Medicine, 50*, 981–990.

Burke, J. (2005). Educating the staff at a homeless shelter about mental illness and anger management. *Journal of Community Health Nursing, 22*, 65–76.

Burns, N., & Grove, S. K. (2011). *Understanding nursing research: Building an evidence-based practice* (5th ed.). St. Louis, MO: Saunders.

Butterfield, P. G., Hill, W., Postma, J., Butterfield, P. W., & Odom-Maryon, T. (2011). Effectiveness of a household environmental health intervention delivered by rural public health nurses. *American Journal of Public Health, 101*, S262–S270. doi:10.2105/AJPH.2001.300164.

Cherry, B., & Jacob, S. R. (2011). *Contemporary nursing: Issues, trends, and management* (5th ed.). St. Louis, MO: Mosby.

Clark-McMullen, D. M. (2010). Evaluation of a successful fetal alcohol spectrum disorder coalition in Ontario, Canada. *Public Health Nursing, 27*, 240–247. doi: 10.1111/j.1525-1446.2010.00849.x

Cohen, E. L., & Cesta, T. G. (2005). *Nursing case management: From essential to advanced practice applications* (4th ed.). Philadelphia, PA: Mosby.

Dossey, B. M., & Keegan L. (2013). *Holistic nursing: A handbook for practice* (6th ed.). Sudbury, MA: Jones & Bartlett Publishers.

Eckenrode, J., Campa, M., Luckey, D. W., Henderson, C. R., Cole, R., Kitzman, H., et al. (2010). Long-term effects of prenatal and infancy nurse home visitation on the life course of youths: 19-year follow-up of a randomized trial. *Archives of Pediatrics and Adolescent Medicine, 164*, 9–15.

Institute of Medicine. (1988). *The future of public health*. Washington, DC: National Academy Press.

Kneipp, S. M., Kairalla, J. A., Lutz, B. J., Pereira, D., Hall. A. G., Flocks, J., et al. (2011). Public health nurse case management for women receiving Temporary Assistance of Needy Families: A randomized controlled trial using community-based participatory research. *American Journal of Public Health, 101*, 1759–1768. doi:10.2105.AJPH.2011.300210.

Kowlessar, N. M., Goetzel, R. Z., Carls, G. S., Tabrizi, M. J., & Guindon, A. (2011). The relationship between 11 health risks and medical and productivity costs for a large employer. *Journal of Occupational and Environmental Medicine, 53*, 468–477.

McCann, E. (2010). Building a community-academic partnership to improve health outcomes in an underserved community. *Public Health Nursing, 27*, 32–40. doi: 10.1111/j.1525-1446.2009.00824.x.

Meagher-Stewart, D., Underwood, J., MacDonald, M., Schoenfeld, B., Blyth, J., Knibbs, K., et al. Organizational attributes that assure optimal utilization of public health nurses. *Public Health Nursing, 27*, 433–441. doi: 10.1111/j.1525-1446.2010.00876.x.

Mintzberg, H. (1973). *The nature of managerial work*. New York: Harper & Row.

Olds, D. L., Kitzman, H. J., Cole, R. E., Hanks, C. A., Arcoleo, K. J., Anson, E. A., et al. (2010). Enduring effects of prenatal and infancy home visiting by nurses on maternal life course and government spending: Follow-up of a randomized trial among children at age 12 years. *Archives of Pediatrics and Adolescent Medicine, 164*, 419–424.

Pender, N. J., Murdaugh, C. L., & Parsons, M. A. (2011). *Health promotion in nursing practice* (6th ed.). Upper Saddle River, NJ: Prentice Hall.

President's Council on Fitness, Sports and Nutrition. (2012). *About us*. Retrieved from http://fitness.gov

Powell, D., Gilliss, C. L., Hewitt, H. H., & Flint, E. P. (2010). Application of a partnership model for transformative and sustainable international development. *Public Health Nursing, 27*, 54–70. doi: 10.1111/j.1525-1446.2009.00827.x.

Redman, B. K. (2007). *The practice of patient education* (10th ed.). St. Louis, MO: Mosby.

Traeger, M., Thompson, A., Dickson, E., & Provencio, A. (2006). Bridging disparity: A multidisciplinary approach for influenza vaccination in an American Indian community. *American Journal of Public Health, 96*, 921–925.

U.S. Department of Health and Human Services. (1997). *The public health workforce: An agenda for the 21st century*. Washington, DC: U.S. Government Printing Office.

U.S. Department of Health and Human Services, Office of Disease Prevention & Health Promotion. (1999). *Public Health Functions Project*. Retrieved from http://www.health.gov/phfunctions/public.htm

U.S. Department of Health and Human Services. (2010a). *Healthy People 2020*. Washington, DC: U.S. Government Printing Office.

U.S. Department of Health and Human Services. (2010b). *Healthy People 2020: Public health infrastructure*. Retrieved from http://healthypeople.gov/2020/topicsobjectives2020/overview.aspx?topicid=35

U.S. Department of Health and Human Services. (2010c). *Healthy People 2020 Summary of Objectives: Public Health Infrastructure* (pp. 1–10). Retrieved from http://healthypeople.gov/2020/topicsobjectives2020/pdfs/PublicHealth.pdf

Wieland, M. L., Weis, J. A., Olney, M. W., Aleman, M., Sullivan, S., Millington, K., et al. (2011). Screening for tuberculosis at an adult education center: Results of a community-based participatory process. *American Journal of Public Health, 101*, 1264–1267. doi:10.2105/AJPH.2010.300024.

thePoint: Everything You Need to Make the Grade!

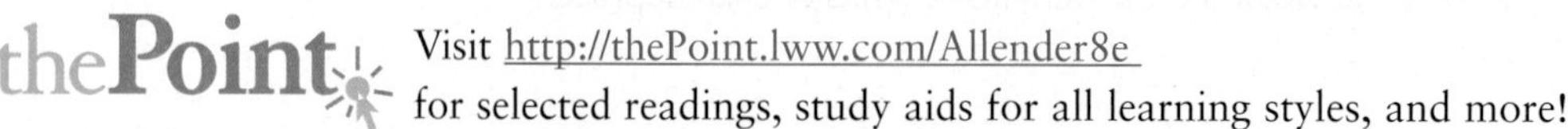

Visit http://thePoint.lww.com/Allender8e for selected readings, study aids for all learning styles, and more!

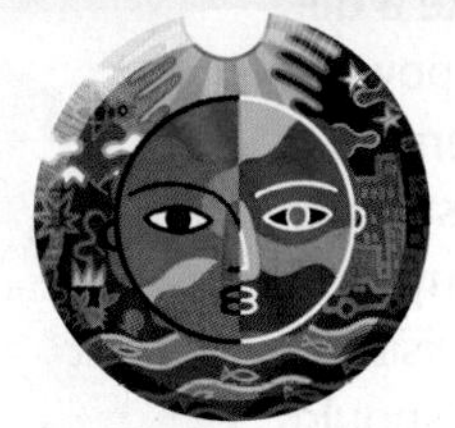

CHAPTER

4

Evidence-Based Practice and Ethics in Community Health Nursing

"Research is formalized curiosity. It is poking and prying with a purpose."

—**Zora Neale Hurston**

"We must not see any person as an abstraction. Instead, we must see in every person a universe with its own secrets, with its own treasures, with its own sources of anguish, and with some measure of triumph."

—**Elie Wiesel** from *The Nazi Doctors and the Nuremberg Code*

KEY TERMS

Research/Evidence-Based Practice
- Community-based participatory research (CPBR)
- Conceptual model
- Control group
- Descriptive statistics
- Evidence-based practice
- Experimental design
- Experimental group
- Generalizability
- Health policy evaluation
- Inferential statistics
- Instrument
- Integrative review
- Meta-analysis
- Mixed methods
- Nonexperimental design
- Qualitative research
- Quantitative research
- Quasi-experiment
- Randomization
- Randomized control trial (RCT)
- Reliability
- Research
- Research utilization
- Systematic review
- True experiment
- Validity

Ethics
- Autonomy
- Beneficence
- Bioethics
- Distributive justice
- Egalitarian justice
- Equity
- Ethical decision making
- Ethical dilemma
- Ethics
- Fidelity
- Instrumental values
- Justice
- Moral
- Moral evaluations
- Nonmaleficence
- Respect
- Restorative justice
- Self-determination
- Self-interest
- Social justice
- Terminal values
- Value
- Value systems
- Values clarification
- Veracity
- Wellbeing

LEARNING OBJECTIVES

Upon mastery of this chapter, you should be able to:

- Discuss the concept of evidence-based practice (EBP).
- List the necessary steps in the process of EBP.
- Explain the difference between quantitative research and qualitative research.
- List the nine steps of the research process.
- Analyze the potential impact of research on community health nursing practice.
- Identify the community health nurse's role in conducting research and using research findings to improve his or her practice.
- Describe the nature of values and value systems and their influence on community health nursing.
- Articulate the impact of key values on professional decision making.
- Discuss the application of ethical principles to community health nursing decision making.
- Use a decision-making process with and for community health clients that incorporates values and ethical principles.

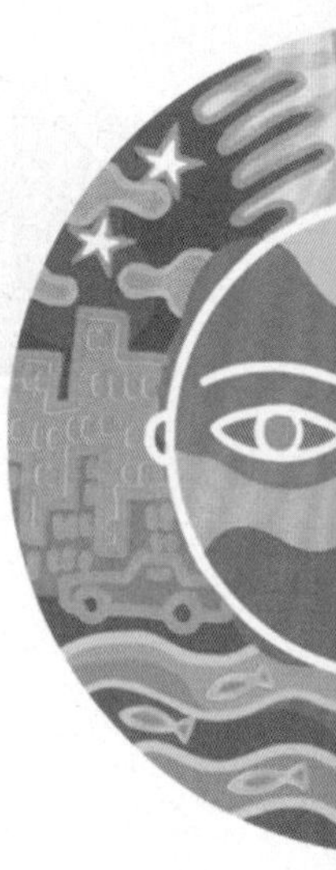

As a new student in community health nursing, you may ask, "Can I really do something to make a difference in the lives of my clients?" You may often feel shocked and discouraged by the crushing poverty and overwhelming sense of helplessness experienced by many of your clients and by the continual recurrence of substance abuse, domestic violence, job failure, and criminal activity. For the first time, you may truly confront the inequalities and injustices of our health care system. You will face many ethical dilemmas in community health nursing. You may ask, "Why should I bother to make home visits to pregnant teens? Why should I offer smoking cessation classes at the local homeless shelter? Why should I teach clients about the importance of taking their antituberculosis medications? Will it really matter?"

Recent community health nursing research validates that nursing care *does* matter and that you really *can* make a difference in the lives of your clients. For example, Nurse–Family Partnership (NFP) programs, based on research conducted by David Olds and his colleagues, are reaping results in many communities across the United States (Child Welfare Information Gateway, 2010; Nurse–Family Partnership, 2010). In a classic longitudinal study by Olds and his research team (1997), conducted with a primarily White sample in a semirural setting over a 15-year period, regular visits by public health nurses (PHNs) to poor, unmarried women and their first-born children resulted in dramatic differences when compared with similar mothers and children in a control group. Many of the women in the study were younger than 19 years of age, and nurses made an average of 9 prenatal visits and 23 child-related visits (up to age 2 years). The effects of the intervention continued for up to 15 years after the birth of the first child.

Statistically significant differences were noted in the following outcomes:

- Fewer subsequent pregnancies and increased percentage of live births
- Longer intervals between first and second births
- Fewer incidences of reported child abuse and neglect
- Fewer months on public assistance and food stamps
- Fewer arrests and convictions of mothers
- Less impairment from alcohol or other drug use reported by mothers

This is powerful evidence noting the effectiveness of a program of regular community/PHN visits to this vulnerable group. A related study by the Olds research team studying pregnancy outcomes, childhood injuries, and repeated childbearing (Kitzman et al., 1997) was recognized as one of ten landmark nursing research studies by the National Institute of Nursing Research (National Institutes of Health, 2006).

The NFP model is based on theory and research. Olds and his colleagues have conducted repeated randomized control trials (RCTs) with different populations living in a variety of settings and contexts, over varying lengths of time, and have consistently found that the NFP program (Eckenrode et al., 2010; Kitzman et al., 2010; Olds, 2007; Olds et al., 2010):

- Improves prenatal health
- Reduces rates of subsequent pregnancies/births
- Increases intervals between first and second pregnancies/births
- Reduces mothers' use of welfare
- Reduces childhood injuries
- Reduces children's mental health problems
- Reduces the proportion of female children who enter the criminal justice system
- Increases school readiness and academic achievement for children
- Reduces government and society costs (NFP, 2010, p. 1).

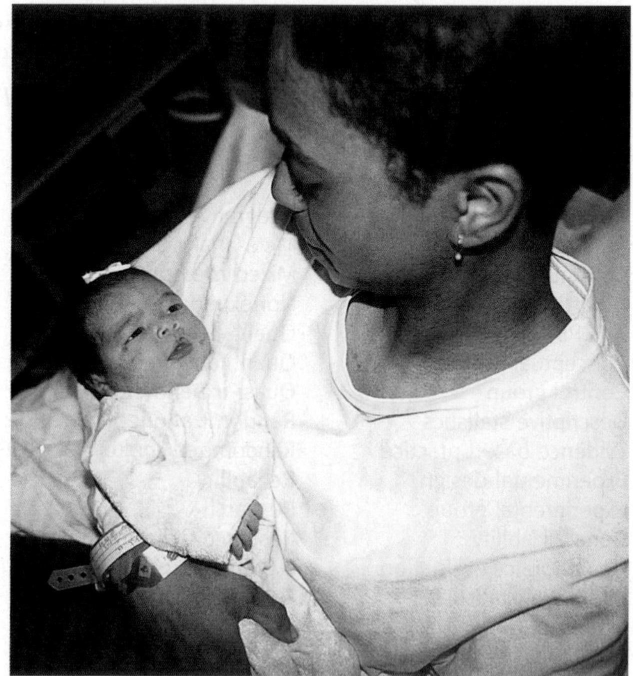

Mother–infant bonding

In a time of tight budgets, number crunchers may ask if community health nurses really make the difference, or can less expensive health care workers also get results? Olds et al. (2004) examined differences between nurse and paraprofessional (e.g., home aides) visitation in a large, randomized study of mostly Mexican American low-income first-time mothers. At the beginning of the study, no statistical differences were noted between control and paraprofessional subjects. Two years after the end of the program, participants visited by paraprofessionals had fewer low-birth-weight babies and better results than control subjects on measures of mastery and mental health, and their home environments were conducive to early learning. However, these benefits were only noticeable 2 years after the visits ended. On the other hand, mothers visited by nurses showed immediate as well as long-term benefits. They had longer intervals between first and second births, there were fewer incidences of domestic violence, and their home environments were found to be conducive to early learning. Children of those mothers had better behavioral adaptation during testing, more advanced language scores, and better executive functioning. Others have reported similar findings (Isaacs, 2008). Olds and his fellow researchers are convinced that public/community health nurses are the key to success!

In tough budget times, state and local agencies may be hesitant to expand programs. But the costs of community health nurse visits are more than offset by the large savings in both dollars and human suffering. Over the years, several policy and think tank groups have done cost-benefit analyses of the program, all concluding that this program reaps large returns on investment. The RAND Corporation estimated that programs of this type "generate a return to society ranging from $1.80 to $17.07 for each dollar spent" (2005, p. 1). Bartik (2009) cited a $15,000 state and local benefit for each NFP case. A Washington state policy group noted that there is a $17,000 return on investment accrued over the life of each child enrolled (Aos, Lieb, Mayfield, Miller, & Pennucci, 2004). RAND also noted that "stronger impacts" occurred when a nurse provided home visits "as opposed to a paraprofessional or lay professional home visitor" (2005, p. 2). A Brookings Institute report recommended, among other things, that the government invest $14 billion for nurse home-visiting programs to promote prenatal care and child development (Isaacs, 2007). When H.R. 3590 (The Patient Protection & Affordable Care Act—"health care reform") was passed in 2010, early childhood home visitation programs were singled out as effective practices and new grant funding to states was made available to promote these programs (U.S. Congress, 2010). The value of this program that provides PHNs to visit at-risk mothers and children in their homes has been validated. So, community/PHNs really *do* make a difference!

This evidence about the effectiveness of public health nursing visits could be gleaned only by conducting formal nursing research. Research in nursing is not a new phenomena; Florence Nightingale is considered the earliest nurse researcher. She collected and analyzed data on the soldiers she cared for during the Crimean War (1859). She also employed principles of evidence-based practice (EBP) because she sought to enhance their care by using evidence to improve her nursing practice and patient outcomes. **Research** is the systematic collection and analysis of data related to a particular problem or phenomenon. Research that is properly conducted and analyzed has the potential to yield valuable information that can affect the health of large groups of people. Indeed, it should guide our practice of community health nursing, and it often serves as the basis for changes in health care policies and programs. The Quad Council PHN Competencies include analytic assessment skills, basic public health science skills, and policy development/program planning skills that include research and EBP (2003). In the current national atmosphere of managed care and obstinately rising health care costs, the importance of valid research on how health care dollars can be spent to benefit the greatest number of people is vitally important.

EVIDENCE-BASED PRACTICE

Across many different settings, from acute to community-based care, implementation of EBP guidelines or practices has been shown to improve nursing practice and client outcomes, as well as reduce costs and standardize care (Davies, Edwards, Ploeg, & Virani, 2008; Doren et al., 2010; Markham & Carney, 2008; McGinty & Anderson, 2008). But how did this more recent paradigm shift toward EBP occur? Dr. Archie Cochrane, a British epidemiologist, is widely regarded as the force behind evidence-based clinical practice in medicine (The Cochrane Collaboration, 2008). As health care has become more and more complex, we have developed "superspecialists" and increasingly advanced technology (Gawande, 2010, p. 31). Even though we often cling to "the way we've always done it," we certainly have ample evidence of the need for a shift to EBP in health care: the Institute of Medicine (IOM) has been studying the issues of health care quality and effectiveness over the past decade and has called for widespread and systematic changes through their reports—*To Err Is Human: Building a Safer Health System* (2000), *Crossing the Quality Chasm: A New Health System for the 21st Century* (2001), and *Priority Areas for National Action: Transforming Health Care Quality* (2003). These reports draw attention to the fact that we spend billions of dollars each year researching new treatments, and more than a trillion dollars are spent annually on health care, but "we repeatedly fail to translate that knowledge and capacity into clinical practice" (IOM, 2003, p. 2). In response, the federal Agency for Healthcare Research and Quality (AHRQ) has established EBP centers across the United States and Canada. Schools of nursing, such as Arizona State University, the University of Texas Health Science Center at San Antonio, Case Western Reserve, and the University of Rochester, also have established centers for EBP.

The Future of Nursing highlights the need for nursing to work with other health professionals in "redesigning health care" by "conducting research" and improving practices through evidence-based means (IOM, 2011, pp. 7, 11). According to Melnyk and Fineout-Overholt (2011), **evidence-based practice** in nursing means just that—systematically searching for and critically appraising and synthesizing evidence (or research findings), along with consideration of expert clinical nursing judgment and patients' wishes, in making decisions about how to care for patients or clients (see Display 4.1, Steps of Evidence-Based Practice and Fig. 4.1). Rebar, Gersch, Macnee, and McCabe (2011, p. 6) further clarify it as:

- Reviewing the best available evidence, most often the results of research
- Using the nurse's clinical expertise
- Determining the values and cultural needs of the individual
- Determining the preferences of the individual, family, and community

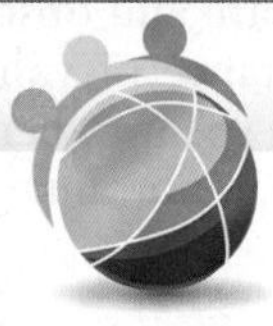

DISPLAY 4.1 THE STEPS OF EVIDENCE-BASED PRACTICE PROCESS

0. Cultivate a spirit of inquiry.
1. Ask the burning clinical question in PICOT format.
2. Search for and collect the most relevant best evidence.
3. Critically appraise the evidence (i.e., rapid critical appraisal, evaluation, and synthesis)
4. Integrate the best evidence with one's clinical expertise and patient preferences and values in making a practice decision or change.
5. Evaluate outcomes of the practice decision or change based on evidence.
6. Disseminate the outcomes of the evidence-based practice decision or change.

From Melnyk, B., & Fineout-Overholt, E. (2011). *Evidence-based practice in nursing and healthcare: A guide to best practice* (2nd ed., p. 11), Philadelphia, PA: Lippincott Williams & Wilkins, with permission.

LEVELS OF EVIDENCE
High
Low
Evidence Strength
Systematic Reviews From non-peer reviewed low to peer-reviewed (e.g., Cochrane, Joanna Briggs) high
Level I
Experimental Research Studies
Meta-analysis of RCTs
Level II
Quasi-experimental studies (an intervention, with either no control group or no randomization)
Level III
Non-experimental studies [case-control, cross-sectional, cohort studies]
Qualitative studies (phenomenological, etc.)
Meta-synthesis of qualitative studies; secondary analysis of existing quantitative data
Descriptive or comparative survey research
Level IV
Expert consensus on evidence findings, clinician expertise, and patient preferences
Clinical practice guidelines
Level V
Opinions of experts recognized on a national level. Includes literature reviews, case studies, experience (not based on empirical evidence).
Organizational experience (internal program evaluations/external (e.g., national health surveys) reports)
Financial reports; cost/benefit studies
Quality improvement studies; local data (e.g., immunization rates, morbidity stats)

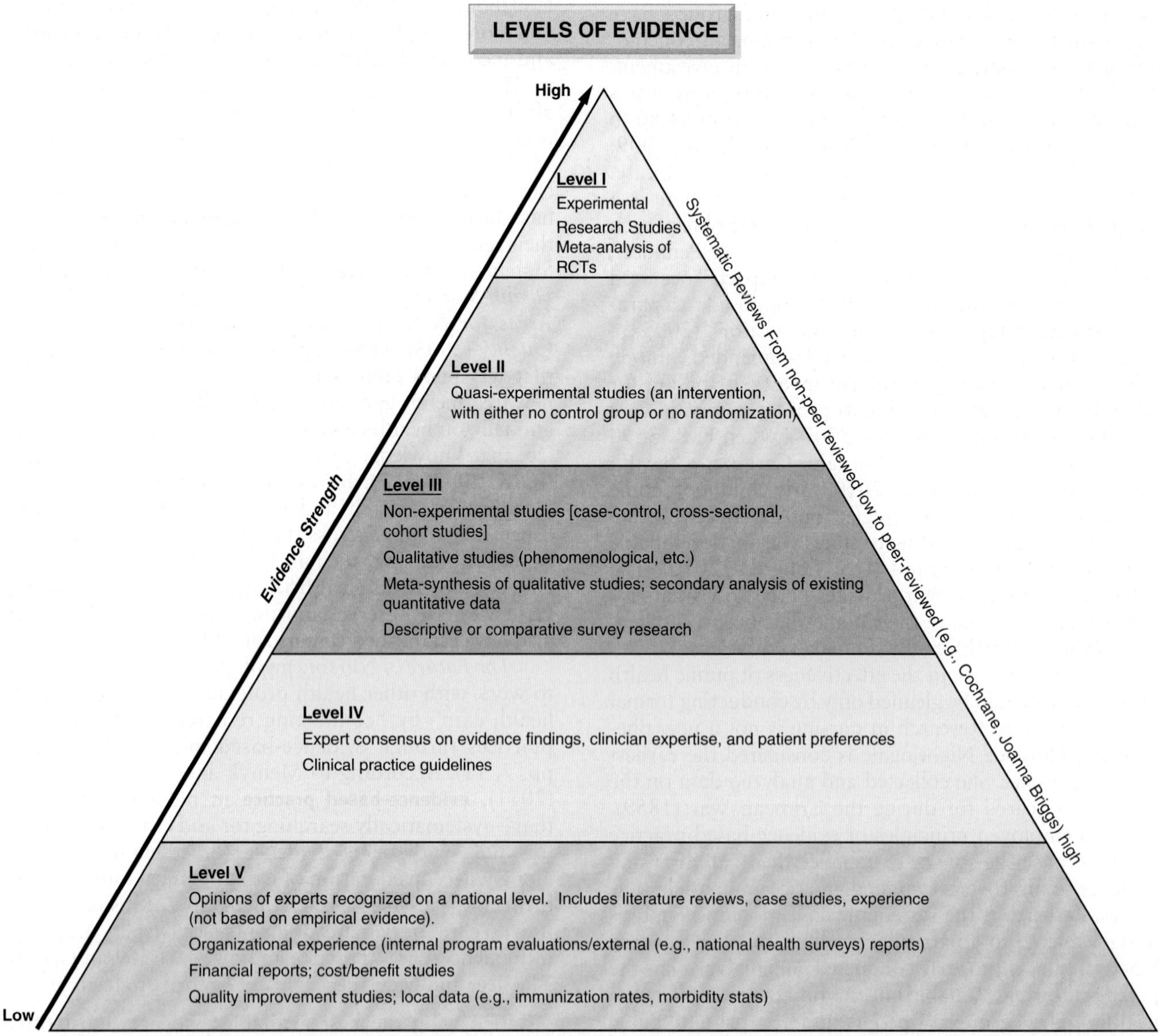

Adapted from: Newhouse, R.P., Dearholt, S., Poe, S., Pugh, L., & White, K. (2007) *Johns Hopkins Nursing Evidence-Based Practice Model & Guidelines.* Indianpolis, IN: Sigma Theta Tau International; Olson keller, L., & Strohschein, S. (2011, June1). *show me the; Evidence-based public health nursing practice. Webinar. Handouts retrieved* from http://publichealthnurses.org/images/uploads/Webinar_I_Slides_Updated.pdf; Olson Keller, L., & Strohschein, S. (2011, June 15). *Innovations in translating evidence into practice.* Webinar. Handouts retrieved from http://publichealthnurses.org/images/uploads/Web_II_Handout_(1).pdf

FIGURE 4-1. Levels of evidence.

Olson Keller and Strohschein (2011, June 1) note that, in public health, the best available evidence includes not only that from clinical research but also from health data (e.g., immunization rates, mortality rates, health status surveys) and practice (e.g., program evaluations, reports from expert panels). Clinical reasoning is an important component in EBP. Bonner (2007) reiterates that the practice knowledge of expert clinical nurses is vital to the process. For Porter-O'Grady (2010), EBP is the "integration of the best possible research" evidence with clinical knowledge and expertise, along with patient preferences and needs (p. 1). Thinking critically about practice problems is an important component of EBP. Reflecting on why we do things a particular way and critically thinking through a problem in a purposeful, systematic way are vital steps in the process. For instance, Porter O'Grady (2010) finds commonalities between EBP and critical thinking:

- Explore a problem.
- Address a purpose or goal.
- Make assumptions about the problem derived from an assessment of the problem and its elements.
- Clarify the problem around central concepts or indicators.
- Access data, evidence, information, and sources to better explain the problem.
- Interpret accumulated evidence about the specific situation or problem.
- Use reasoning, processing, defining, planning, and documenting to guide subsequent actions in addressing the issue.
- Act on the problem, consistent with protocols and parameters, and assess its effect and impact, as well as the process.
- Evaluate, adjust, generalize, and apply to a broader problem set (indicative of a successful problem-solving process).

STEPS OF THE EVIDENCE-BASED PRACTICE PROCESS

The effective practitioner utilizes his or her clinical judgment and expertise to reflect on the practice of community health nursing and determine if safe, effective, quality, and cost-efficient care is being delivered. Problems or situations that need clarification can then be identified, and current research can be reviewed to guide needed changes in practice. Although acknowledged barriers exist, they can be overcome utilizing available resources (Van Hook, 2009). Melnyk and Fineout-Overholt (2011, pp. 10–11) outline the steps of the EBP process as, as seen in Display 4.1:

0. Cultivate a spirit of inquiry.
1. Ask the burning clinical question in PICOT format (see below).
2. Search for and collect the most relevant best evidence.
3. Critically appraise the evidence for its validity, reliability and applicability, then synthesize that evidence.
4. Integrate the best evidence with one's clinical expertise and patient preferences and values in making a practice decision or change.
5. Evaluate outcomes of the practice decision or change based on evidence.
6. Disseminate the outcomes of the EBP decision or change.

These steps will be explored in more detail, as well as available resources and implications for public health nursing practice.

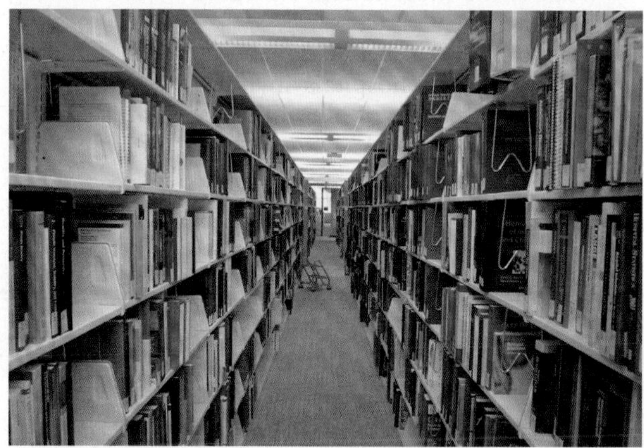

Finding evidence can be daunting in this era of information overload. (Photo courtesy of CDC Public Health Image Library.)

CULTIVATING A SPIRIT OF INQUIRY

The importance of this initial step cannot be overstated. In order for effective change to occur, current practices must be continually examined, questioned, and challenged. Individuals and organizations must be open to this cultural shift from the status quo, and it should be reflected in the agency's mission and philosophy (Melnyk & Fineout-Overholt, 2011). "Ongoing curiosity about the best evidence to guide clinical decision making—and a culture that supports it"—are the foundation of this step (Melnyk, Fineout-Overholt, Stillwell, & Williamson, 2009, p. 49). Asking questions like "Why are we doing this?" and "Is there evidence to support this practice?" demonstrates this spirit of inquiry. Agencies that provide access to systematic reviews, evidence-based journals, and research consultants also demonstrate a commitment to this step.

ASKING THE QUESTION

What if you or your colleagues doubt the effectiveness of some method in your current nursing practice and want to find out if there is new research or evidence that may convince you to make a change? How do you begin your journey to evidence-based practice? Melnyk and others suggest that the first step to solving the problem is "asking the burning clinical question" (2011, p. 10). This question may be about client care or effective interventions, such as:

- What methods are most effective in ensuring client medication compliance with tuberculosis (TB) protocols?
- What is the best information I can give new mothers about preventing sudden infant death syndrome (SIDS)?

It could also be about systems approaches to population health:

- What is the most effective method of immunizing toddlers?
- How can PHNs better collaborate with families, physicians, and hospitals in preventing complications of high levels of bilirubin in newborns coming home within 24 to 48 hours after birth?

The PICOT question (see Display 4.2) is one way to develop an answerable, searchable EBP question. First, the population or problem must be specified. The Association of Women's Health, Obstetric, and Neonatal Nurses (AWHONN) asked a "burning clinical question" when they wanted to find a scientific basis for the development of standards of practice for their members regarding counseling pregnant women on smoking cessation. The project, *Setting Universal Cessation Counseling, Education, and Screening Standards* (SUCCESS), was an attempt to integrate best practices in primary care settings where women of childbearing age receive care. They did extensive searches in the Cumulative Index on Nursing and Allied Health Literature (CINAHL) and MEDLINE for research studies relating to low-birth-weight infants, effects of prenatal smoking on infants, and effects of smoking cessation intervention on premature labor and birth weight with both pregnant women and those seeking care prior to conception (Albrecht et al., 2006; Maloni, Albrecht, Thomas, Halleran, & Jones, 2006). They critically analyzed 98 articles, and found evidence of a higher incidence of many complications, including preterm labor, premature rupture of membranes, lower

DISPLAY 4.2 PICOT: COMPONENTS OF AN ANSWERABLE, SEARCHABLE QUESTION

Term	*Definition*	*Specific Example*
Patient Population/problem	The patient population or problem of interest, for example: • Age • Gender • Ethnicity • With certain disorder (e.g., hepatitis A)	For example: • Adolescent females, ages 12–20
Intervention	The intervention or range of interventions of interest, for example: • Exposure to disease • Risk behavior (e.g., smoking) • Education	For example: • Sexuality education program
Comparison intervention or issue of interest	What you want to compare the intervention against, for example: • No disease • Absence of risk factor (e.g., smoking) • Placebo or no intervention	For example: • Current practice or no intervention
Outcome	Outcome of interest, for example: • Risk of disease • Rate of occurrence of adverse outcome (e.g., death) • Accuracy of diagnosis	For example: • Unplanned pregnancies
Time	The time involved for the intervention to demonstrate an outcome, for example: • Time it takes for intervention to achieve the outcome • Time interval selected to observe the population or problem/condition	For example: • One school year (to implement curriculum)

Adapted from Melnyk, B., & Fineout-Overholt, E. (2011). *Evidence-based practice in nursing and healthcare: A guide to best practice* (2nd ed., p. 30). Philadelphia, PA: Lippincott Williams & Wilkins. Used with permission.

birth weight and length, spontaneous abortion, and placenta previa or abruption in women using tobacco. Infants and children exposed to secondhand smoke had a higher risk for ear infections, asthma and other respiratory problems, SIDS, and learning disorders. Significant evidence suggested that this was a problem that needed to be addressed. They also concluded "office-based assessment, client-specific tobacco counseling, skill development, and support programs serve as an effective practice guideline" for their members, so they developed protocols and began piloting them in 13 states (Albrecht et al., 2006, p. 298). They continue to collect evaluation research to determine the effectiveness of the protocols.

Finding the Evidence

Melnyk and Fineout-Overholt (2011) stress the importance of systematically searching for all relevant research on a clinical question of interest and critically analyzing the evidence. They argue that this is not merely **research utilization**, in which new interventions may be tried based on the results of one or two good studies, but "the synthesis of evidence from multiple studies" (e.g., systematic reviews of randomized control trials [RCTs]) and critical reviews of both quantitative and qualitative studies pertinent to a particular question of interest (p. 4). While doing this, the nurse must keep in mind the unique needs and wants of the clients served, as well as current practice standards, guidelines, and ethical considerations. National clinical practice guidelines should be reviewed (e.g., National Guideline Clearinghouse at www.guideline.gov), and expert clinicians may be interviewed for their opinions on the problem at hand (Cassey, 2007). However, Spenceley, Leary, Chizawsky, Ross, and Estabrooks (2008) note that nurses rely on RN peers most often, along with other "interactive and informal sources" (p. 954), and this can result in "basing practice decisions on inadequate information" (p. 965). A solid understanding of the evidence is needed.

Although expert nurses may be a good starting point in seeking evidence, clinically relevant research that is both medically sound and patient centered must be reviewed. Excellent places to begin are **integrative** or **systematic reviews** that compile all recent studies and summarize what is known about the problem or situation. The Cochrane Collaboration (www.cochrane.org) lists systematic reviews on various topics of interest to both physicians and nurses. For instance, a community health nurse working with a group of adults who have diabetes might be interested in the systematic review on the importance of exercise for clients with type 2 diabetes. This Cochrane review is based on 14 RCTs that compared the use of exercise in a group of 377 participants over periods of between 8 weeks and 12 months. When compared with those who got no exercise intervention, the results indicated decreased body fat and triglyceride levels and improved blood sugar control for those exercising (even for those who did not lose any weight). Although a community health nurse may certainly have a "hunch" that exercise is good for his or her clients, this systematic review of current studies provides solid evidence on which to base specific recommendations (Thomas, Elliott, & Naughton, 2006). Another review on promoting adherence to antiretroviral therapy for human immunodeficiency virus (HIV)/acquired immune deficiency syndrome (AIDS) clients might be helpful to a PHN supervisor in designing an AIDS case management program utilizing PHNs. Over 2,159 participants in 19 RCTs were part of this Cochrane review, which found that interventions such as "practical medication management skills ... administered to individuals versus groups and ... delivered over 12 weeks or more" led to improved medication adherence (Rueda et al., 2006, para. 6). From this evidence, a community health nurse case manager may conclude that medication compliance can be effectively ensured through development of a nurse–client relationship based on the nurse's consistent availability to the client—through home visits or individual appointments at clinics—and focused patient education on medication management skills. Another source of systematic reviews includes the Campbell Collaboration (http://www.campbellcollaboration.org) covering education and social welfare research that may be of interest to PHNs examining, for instance, effective group or individual interventions such as parenting programs for teens (Barlow et al., 2011).

The AHRQ EBP centers also provide evidence reports that are easily accessible online (www.ahrq.gov-clinic/epcindex.htm). Searching may be done by use of a topical index, clinical area, or health care services (e.g., bioterrorism) and technical areas (e.g., community-based participatory research [CBPR]). Other sources for systematic or integrative reviews include:

- Cochrane Nursing Care Field podcasts (http://cncf.cochrane.org/podcasts)
- Cochrane Public Health Group (http://ph.cochrane.org/welcome)
- *Worldviews on Evidence-Based Nursing* from Sigma Theta Tau International (www.nursingsociety.org)
- *Evidence-Based Nursing*, a British online journal (www.ebn.bmjjournals.com)
- Joanna Briggs Institute, an Australian nursing research organization (http://www.joannabriggs.edu.au/about/home.php)
- The Community Guide, a CDC site for research on population health promotion (http://www.thecommunityguide.org/index.html)
- Health-Evidence Canada, a Canadian website for promoting evidence-based decision making (http://health-evidence.ca/)
- RAND (Research And Development) Corporation research briefs (www.rand.org)

Critical Appraisal of the Evidence

Collection and critical analysis of the best evidence in the literature, like that done by AWHONN above, comprise the second and third steps in the EBP process.

Systematic reviews should be carefully examined to determine validity (Schlosser, 2007). You can do this by asking these types of questions:

- What was the review question? (Specific population, intervention, etc.)
- Were search strategies explained and are they reasonable?
- What were exclusion criteria/were any important, relevant studies overlooked?
- Were the studies in the review properly designed and executed (findings valid)?
- Were there similar results found in all studies?
- How reliable are the results (minimal bias)?
  - Were sample sizes large enough?
  - Were results statistically significant?
  - Were there confounding factors (outside influences that make you doubt the results; differences between groups in intervention or outcome assessment, high attrition)?

It is also helpful to compare the results with previous research and clinical practice (Melnyk & Fineout-Overholt, 2011). Grids outlining levels and quality of evidence in public health nursing can be found at www.publichealthnurses.org. Qualitative research (see below) can also be evaluated by asking questions about the study participants (How were they chosen?), the data (Is it accurate and complete?), and the results (Is it plausible? Is it logical, consistent, and relevant?) (Melnyk & Fineout-Overholt, 2011).

What if no systematic reviews are available in your area of interest? Where can you find the necessary evidence needed in order to make good practice decisions? You can look for RCTs, meta-analysis research, program evaluation studies, systematic literature reviews, or practice guidelines (see Fig. 4.1, Levels of Evidence), keeping in mind that several studies (or one or two large-scale, tightly controlled studies) are preferred.

Integrating the Evidence

Fourth, it is important to make a decision, based on your clinical expertise and knowledge of your clients' values and preferences, about incorporating this information into your practice. You can do this by asking:

- How can I apply these results to my community health nursing practice?
- Will it benefit my clients?
- Are my clients similar to the population studied?
- Do I have the necessary resources?
- Does this go against my client's values or preferences?

Evidence has shown that PHNs have been effective with different client populations in ameliorating postpartum depression, promoting awareness and use of folic acid by women of childbearing age, and have consistently demonstrated multiple benefits of the NFP for children, mothers, and families (Amitai et al., 2008; Glavin, Smith, Sorum, & Ellefsen, 2010; NFP, 2010; Olds, 2007). Newer research outside of public health nursing may also be applied in the community, depending upon clinical expertise and knowledge of our clients. For instance, a new area of research about low levels of vitamin D associated with cognitive decline in the elderly might spark an interest for community health nurses to counsel adult clients attending yearly flu clinics to include this supplement in their daily regimen, especially in areas where exposure to sunlight is less prevalent (Annweiler et al., 2009, 2010; Buell et al., 2010; Evatt, 2010; Llewellyn et al., 2010; Slinin et al., 2010).

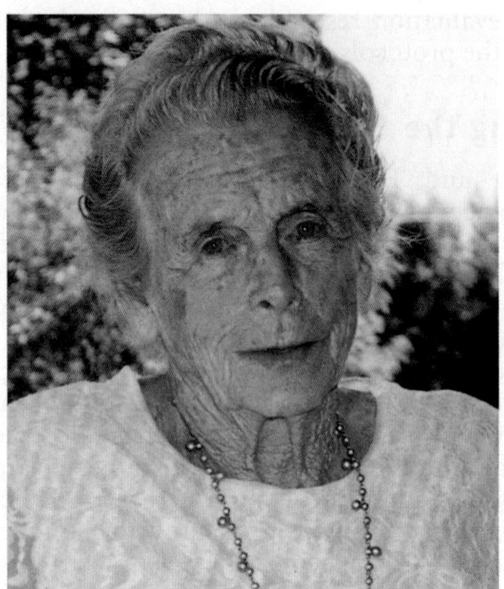

New research examines if the elderly may benefit from vitamin D supplementation.

An example of a systematic review of interest to PHNs is from the Cochrane Nursing Care Field and concerns smoking cessation. Young and Skorga (2011) produced a synopsis of a Cochrane review done by Lindson et al. in 2010 that examined 10 clinical trials for differences in success rates and adverse events between participants who abruptly quit smoking and those who utilized a more gradual reduction in smoking. Findings revealed no statistical differences between the two groups for smoking abstinence, despite types of interventions used (e.g., self-help therapy, pharmacotherapy, behavioral support). However, some of the study results were inadequate, making it impossible to conclude if there were any differences in adverse effects. Because smoking cessation is often advised for community health clients, PHNs could utilize this information to encourage either method of smoking cessation. When examining population-based strategies, The Community Guide provides task force recommendations based on systematic reviews, along with additional resources on the topic of interest. For instance, when searching the term "dental caries," community water fluoridation is recommended, as are school-based/linked sealant delivery programs. However, state or community sealant promotion programs are not recommended due to insufficient evidence.

Evaluating Outcomes

The final step of the EBP process is to evaluate any practice change. For instance, if you decide to implement findings from the systematic review on HIV/AIDS medication compliance cited above, a standardized protocol of home visits and patient education by PHNs would need to be established and both baseline and postintervention data collected in order to deduce any potential positive change noted. Results can vary based on specific environment, population, implementation, and other factors. Evidence can lead you to choose a course, but evaluation of your outcomes is necessary to ensure that you have achieved the best results.

The design of an evidence-based research project represents the overall plan for carrying out the study. The overall plan guides the conduct of the study and, depending on its effectiveness, can influence investigators' confidence in their results. A major consideration in selecting a particular design is to try to control as much as possible those factors that are not included in the study but can influence the results. For example, in a classic study by Douglas, Mallonee, and Istre (1999), researchers wanted to discover the percentage of homes with functioning smoke alarms. They initially conducted a telephone survey, a commonly used method of survey research in community health, and found that 71% of households reported functioning smoke alarms. Concerned that this might be an inflated number, they conducted an on-site survey to confirm the results. After face-to-face interviews, they found that only 66% of householders reported having functioning alarms. However, when researchers actually tested the smoke alarms in those homes, only 49% were fully functioning. By having researchers actually test the smoke alarms, this design controlled for inflated results of the more commonly conducted, convenient, and economical telephone survey. Is self-report always unreliable? A small study of working middle-aged women revealed that self-reported weekly physical activity was strongly associated with pedometer data, indicating in this case self-report yielded reasonably reliable data (Speck & Looney, 2006). This provides evidence that the community health nurse must determine the most efficacious method of obtaining necessary data.

In another example, researchers themselves controlled the variables to ensure true results. Flynn, Budd, and Modelski (2008) knew from their review of the literature and practical experience that pregnant teens are a vulnerable population who often receive no prenatal care (between "33% and 55%," p. 141). Their inadequate use of resources and risk-taking behaviors often lead to premature delivery and low-birth-weight infants at a rate two to three times higher than older mothers. They noted that "inadequate use of resources and adverse birth outcomes" warranted development of a pilot program of home visitation—the Teen Parent Partnership Program (p. 141). The goals of the program were to improve resource utilization (e.g., prenatal visits, WIC [Womens, Infants, & Children] and Medicaid enrollment) and improve health outcomes (e.g., low birth weight). They employed a quasi-experimental design (see below) and recruited teens 18 years or younger who were pregnant with their first child. A total of 83 participants were admitted to the program at least 3 months before delivery, and they were visited a minimum of six times (three each by a PHN and three each by a medical social worker). Researchers compiled 216 records of teens who also met the criteria for the study, but who were not visited. Data were collected from these records and the two groups were matched on age at delivery, race/ethnicity, number of prenatal visits, infant birth weight, infant gender, and gestational age. When results were analyzed, the group participating in the home visitation program had statistically significant increases over the control group (no visits) in the number of pregnant teens who had a prenatal care provider, made/kept prenatal appointments, enrolled in the WIC program and received WIC nutritional supplements, and were enrolled and utilizing Medicaid. All teens in the intervention group received some form of prenatal care. No significant difference was found between groups in the number of low-birth-weight infants, although researchers feel that this might be found if there are larger numbers of participants in future research studies.

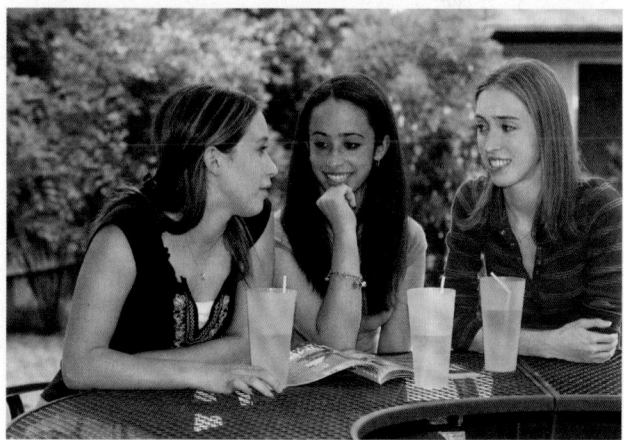

Pregnant teens

Once an intervention is developed, further research can evaluate its appropriateness and, ultimately, its effectiveness. Beyond EBP implementation, other lines of clinically based research can also be designed. The choice of research design influences the ability to generalize the results, and the attention given to the details of the study affects the value of the knowledge derived. Research done with larger numbers of participants drawn from a geographically diverse area is more complete than small scale, exploratory studies done in an isolated area with a small, homogeneous sample. Valid tools or instruments and appropriately applied statistical methods lead to greater confidence in the results of the study.

Disseminating Outcomes

We need to share our results in order to improve the body of knowledge in public health nursing and provide studies that can be used in future systematic reviews. Often, community health nurses are required to report results to stakeholders (e.g., grant-funding agencies, local or county governing bodies). Formal reports are often required, or scorecards may be used that compare local results to state and national data. We can also share outcomes information with our colleagues locally, through informal networking, blogs, listservs, etc. However, when EBP outcomes are shared at state and national professional meetings or through publication in peer-reviewed journals, a wider audience is reached and our knowledge based is exponentially increased.

DIFFERENCES BETWEEN EBP IMPLEMENTATION, QUALITY IMPROVEMENT, AND RESEARCH

If you have worked as a student in an acute care hospital, you have been introduced to quality or performance improvement (QI/PI) initiatives. QI/PI became even more important to health care after the IOM reports cited earlier. These approaches involve a systematic analysis of data and processes with the aim of improving the delivery of health care. Over the last decade, the National Quality Forum has endorsed over 600 quality measures, and hospitals are now required to publicly report certain quality data indicators. The Centers for Medicare and Medicaid Services (CMS) began to financially penalize hospitals by not paying for services when certain quality indicators were not met (e.g., pressure ulcers) (Lindenauer et al., 2007). Accrediting bodies for acute care hospitals first mandated quality care initiatives, but these are now spreading to "ambulatory and other care settings" (Chassin, Loeb, Schmaltz, & Wachter, 2010, p. 683). With the push for accreditation in public health agencies, this issue will become even more pertinent to PHNs (Olson Keller & Strohschein, 2011, June 15).

The differences between QI/PI, EBP implementation, and clinical research are sometimes unclear. Melnyk and Fineout-Overholt (2011) note that generalizability of findings is often not part of EBP implementation because representative samples are not used. Rather, convenience samples of inpatients or clients are used to test initiatives for practice improvement. However, that distinction alone does not release nurses from gaining ethical approval (e.g., Institutional Review Board [IRB], Human Subjects Committee [HSC]). This is certainly required when disseminating results through publication or national presentations. Informed consent is another area where clear distinctions are also problematic. If you change your practice to benefit your clients, based on the best evidence and your clinical judgment/knowledge of your clients, it would be cumbersome to ask for written consent from every patient before implementing changes. It is not feasible, and it is expected that professional practice changes will be made over time without consulting clients. However, some clinical management oversight is expected in order to ensure that client rights are not violated.

One example of a QI project (or arguably an EBP implementation project) that was halted due to questions raised by the federal oversight agency for human subjects research protection is a large-scale study (67 intensive care units [ICUs] in Michigan) implementing EBP procedures to reduce catheter infection rates. The outcomes were "stunning," as it was estimated that over 1,500 lives were saved over the 18 months of the QI initiative (Gawande, 2010; Miller & Emanuel, 2008). However, the federal agency criticized the hospital that organized the study for dismissing the need for patient consent (waived because their IRB saw it as QI and exempt). Researchers published the phenomenal results, bringing it to the attention of federal overseers. Protection of human subjects remains vitally important, and Baily (2008) acknowledges this fact along with the concern about additional layers of oversight that make health care improvement "more difficult and expensive, and....more likely to harm than to help" (p. 769). Practical rules, infrastructure, and supervision within organizations can ensure that QI activities are appropriately reviewed and differentiated from clinical research (Lynn et al., 2007).

To effectively practice EBP implementation, community health nurses must know how to correctly compose a clinical question, find an appropriate database to search for systematic reviews or other evidence, critically review the evidence, consult practice guidelines and expert practitioners, and work with their clients to develop an appropriate plan of action. A clear understanding of basic research principles is needed to apply the principles of EBP and integrate the latest research into community health nursing practice. Evidence, in the form of systematic reviews, is most often drawn from quantitative research studies, but some public health nursing researchers also advocate the use of qualitative research in making evidence-based public health practice decisions (Flemming, 2007; Jack, 2006).

QUANTITATIVE AND QUALITATIVE RESEARCH

Scientific inquiry through research is generally pursued by means of two different approaches: quantitative research and qualitative research. Both can be part of research and EBP. **Quantitative research** concerns data that can be quantified or measured objectively. This could be as simple as counting the number of children receiving vaccination for varicella in immunization clinics during the past month and noting the number of reported cases of postvaccination complications. Another example of a rather simple quantitative study uses telephone survey methods to determine the use of complementary and alternative health care (e.g., acupuncture, herbal remedies) by older rural women. Shreffler-Grant, Hill, Weinert, Nichols, and Ide (2007) picked a random sample of 156 older adult women from rural communities in two states and found that 25.4% had used complementary and alternative medicine (CAM) in the recent past. Those most likely to use CAM were currently unmarried, older, and "fairly well educated" (p. 28). This has implications for nurses working with rural older adults, who may think that this population is not interested in alternative forms of health care, thus risking the potential for possible drug interactions or side effects of these treatments in their clients. Also, educational opportunities on safe use of these therapies may be missed.

More variables can be added to quantitative studies. An example is a study by Larsen and Reif (2011). Because the United States is becoming increasingly diverse (see Chapter 5), the researchers wanted to find an effective method of training nursing students to more successfully work with diverse clients. They utilized the common approach of classes on culture, but added a 2- to 3-week immersion experience (living in another country/culture) for those in the intervention group. A control group did not participate in an immersion experience, but both groups were tested at baseline and again after the intervention group returned from their immersion experiences. Those who had both the classes and the immersion experience showed statistically significant posttest scores on transcultural self-efficacy and change, leading them to recommend that all nursing students be encouraged to participate in "immersion experiences to enhance transcultural competence" (p. 1). By adding the variable of immersion experiences, a greater level of transcultural effectiveness was reached.

Quantitative research is helpful in identifying a problem or a relationship between two or more variables, such as type of treatment (e.g., cultural immersion experiences) and an outcome (greater levels of transcultural self-efficacy). In so doing, quantitative studies tend to examine isolated parts of problems or phenomena and do not generally pay attention to the larger context or overall health of individuals. Quantitative research involves a reductionistic tendency (focusing on the parts rather than the whole) and, if used exclusively, can limit nursing knowledge, because many of the important aspects of client services (e.g., quality of life, grieving, spirituality) cannot be measured objectively.

A more subjective or qualitative approach is needed to study those areas that need a broader focus or those that do not lend themselves to objective measurement. **Qualitative research** emphasizing subjectivity asks "how" or "why." An example of this research examined the factors that influence the disclosure of abuse by women of Mexican descent by Montalvo-Liendo, Wardell, Engebretson, and Reininger (2009). This is an area that has not been extensively studied, so a nurse researcher "from the same cultural heritage" (p. 361) wanted to learn more about why some women do not readily report abuse. This information is helpful to community health nurses, as client caseloads often include women who may be victims of domestic violence and may not know what help is available to them. The researchers recruited 26 women from two sites in south Texas: a temporary emergency shelter for abuse victims and an outreach office for those seeking assistance for sexual assaults or domestic violence. All women were of Mexican descent and over age 18, but 19 of the 26 participants were immigrants with low scores on a tool used by researchers to measure level of acculturation. Researchers found that these women tended to remain in abusive relationships longer (some for 10 to 20 years) before seeking formal assistance, when compared to Mexican American women. Reasons given for not disclosing abuse included "coercive control by their abusive partners," fear of the police or losing their children due to immigrant status, and not wanting to tell family members because they didn't want them to worry or they had seen their own mothers endure abuse (p. 363). In some cases, they reported that their mothers were not supportive, and in other cases they simply wanted to avoid the embarrassment associated with others knowing about the abuse. Sometimes, women lied or denied abuse "for the sake of their family" or because of their love for the abusive partner (p. 363). Other reasons for denying abuse were the fear of the unknown or the cyclical nature of the abuse (it sometimes got better). Some women talked to friends about the abuse but did not want advice, only someone to listen. Sadly, the women reported not often being asked by health care providers about domestic violence.

It is not uncommon to find research studies in which both quantitative and qualitative approaches are used. When both types of data are collected and analyzed (and inferences are drawn from both), this is known as **mixed methods** research (Polit & Beck, 2012). A study examining the experiences and perceptions of nurses working with elderly stroke victims at adult daycare facilities (Park & Han, 2010) used both a questionnaire and a focus group to determine the importance of services provided (skilled nursing services, functional recovery, heath counseling, referral, and supporting personal care) and the nurses' work experiences. While the survey questionnaire elicited important information about perceptions of the importance of their work, the focus group allowed nurses to more specifically discuss challenges and concerns that would not have otherwise been revealed. Concerns about policies that promoted standardized, rather than individualized, care, along with role confusion due to the nurse's work sometimes conflicting with the duties of social workers, and the need for better education for families to provide continuity of care outside the daycare facility were some of the themes noted by researchers. This mixed method study provides a broader picture of the gaps between identified areas of "key services" and the reality of issues that need to be resolved in order to facilitate better nursing care and client outcomes (p. 267). Mixed methods are also helpful in program evaluation, and can provide a more holistic vision (Polit & Beck, 2010).

Another method of analyzing research in community health uses a statistical procedure known as **meta-analysis** to evaluate the results of many similar quantitative research studies in an attempt to integrate the findings and combine the sample sizes of many small studies to obtain a single-effect measure, or "summary statistic" (Melnyk & Fineout-Overholt, 2011, p. 13). By combining the results of many similar studies, meta-analysis affords greater statistical power and can give the researcher a more complete general perspective, especially when research on a certain issue may seem inconclusive. An example of this type of nursing research can be found in the Cochrane Database. A meta-analysis done by Rice and Stead (2008) analyzed

42 randomized control trials (RCTs) examining the effectiveness of nurses as smoking cessation interventionists. Often, physicians assume this role during office visits, but community health nurses often have more intense contact with clients. The meta-analysis included both brief and more extensive interventions (i.e., advice given at a single visit lasting less than about 10 minutes, a longer initial visit with follow-up visits that included additional strategies or materials). Through complex statistical measurements, the authors found that "the potential benefits of smoking cessation advice and/or counseling given by nurses to patients" was an effective intervention (para. 10). The statistical effect was found across studies, although it was weaker with the lower intensity (briefer) interventions. Interventions for both hospitalized and nonhospitalized patients showed evidence of some benefit. The moral of this meta-analysis is that even short discussions with your public health clients about smoking cessation, along with information on accessing support groups or other resources, may prove beneficial when you are perceived as someone whose main role is to promote health (e.g., PHNs).

UNDERSTANDING RESEARCH BASICS TO PROMOTE EVIDENCE-BASED PRACTICE

In order to fully integrate the principles of EBP, it is important to have a basic understanding of the research process. More in-depth information on this subject is available in nursing research texts (e.g., Polit & Beck, 2010, 2012), but a brief synopsis is provided here (see Display 4.3). EBP methods are encouraged over basic

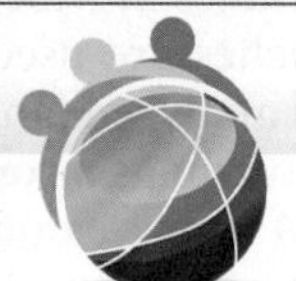

DISPLAY 4.3 STEPS IN THE RESEARCH PROCESS

All effective research follows a series of predetermined, highly specific steps, building on the previous one and providing the foundation for the eventual discussion of research findings. It is important to understand basic research principles in order to effectively implement evidence-based practice (EBP).

1. Identify an area of interest.
2. Formulate a research question or statement.
3. Review the literature.
4. Select a conceptual model.
5. Choose a research design.
6. Obtain Institutional Review Board or Human Subjects Committee approval.
7. Collect and analyze data.
8. Interpret results.
9. Communicate findings.

Identify an Area of Interest

- The problem of interest needs *specificity* (i.e., it must be specific enough to direct the formulation of a research question). For example, concern about child safety is too broad a problem; instead, the focus could be on a narrower subject, such as the use of child restraints and car seat availability and use in a particular community.
- The problem must also be *feasible*. Feasibility concerns whether the area of interest can be examined, given available resources. For example, a statewide study of the needs of pregnant adolescents might not be practical if time or funding is limited, but a study of the same group in a given school district could be more easily accomplished.
- The *meaning* of the project and its *relevance* to nursing must also be considered, such as exploring the implications for nursing practice in the study of pregnant adolescents. The nurse's specialty influences the selection of a problem for study and also the particular perspective or approaches used. Community health nurses think in terms of the broader community; their research efforts are developed with the needs of the community or specific populations in mind.

Formulate a Research Question or Statement

- Just like the PICOT question in EBP, the research question or statement reflects the kind of information desired and provides a foundation for the remainder of the project. The manner in which the question or statement is phrased suggests the research design for the project. For example, the question "What are nurses' attitudes toward pregnant women who use methamphetamine?" determines that the design will be simple, nonexperimental, and exploratory (see later discussion). In contrast, the question "What is the effect of an educational program on nurses' attitudes toward drug-abusing pregnant women?" suggests an experiment that will evaluate changes in nurses' attitudes toward pregnant women who abuse drugs after receiving an educational intervention. The first research question suggests a broad, open-ended conversation with nurse participants, asking them to discuss their attitudes toward pregnant women who abuse drugs, such as methamphetamine. From the data obtained, general themes and patterns will emerge, leading the researcher to some overall conclusions. The second question examines the effects that an educational program may have on nurses' attitudes about pregnant women who abuse crack cocaine, for instance. This is most likely a quantitative, evaluative study that may involve pretesting to determine the nurses' attitudes, conducting one

(continued)

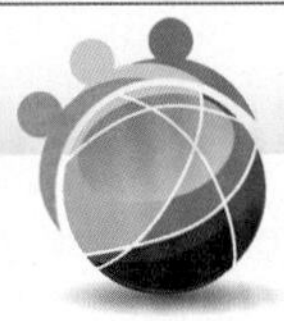

DISPLAY 4.3 STEPS IN THE RESEARCH PROCESS *(Continued)*

or more classes, and then posttesting to determine whether any change occurred in attitude or beliefs.

- Good examples of research questions addressed recently by community health nurses include:
  - Are there differences in how rural and urban families [*population of interest*] view death and end-of-life care [*variables*] for their elderly family members with dementia residing in nursing homes (Gessert, Elliott, & McAlpine, 2006)?
  - What are the barriers to mask wearing for Influenza-type illnesses [*variable*] among urban Hispanic households [*population of interest*] (Ferng, Wong-McLoughlin, Barrett, Currie, & Larson, 2011)?
  - Are there intentions to reduce the risk of falling again [*variable*] among older homebound women [*population of interest*] (Porter, Matsuda, & Lindbloom, 2010)?
  - Are parents of low-income Ohio toddlers [*population of interest*] receiving information on lead poisoning prevention [*variable*], and how would they prefer to receive this information [*variable*] (Polivka, 2006)?
  - What are the levels of psychological and physical abuse [*variables*] among pregnant women in a Medicaid-sponsored prenatal program [*population of interest*], (Raffo, Meghea, Zhu, & Roman, 2010)?

Review the Literature

- A traditional review of the literature consists of two phases. The first phase consists of a cursory examination of available publications related to the area of interest. Although several nursing research journals publish studies reflecting all areas of nursing practice, most specialty areas have dedicated journals. *Public Health Nursing, Family and Community Health, Journal of Community Health Nursing, American Journal of Public Health, Journal of School Health, Nursing and Health Sciences*, and *Journal of School Nursing* are some of the journals that publish studies of particular interest to community health nurses. In this phase, the investigator develops knowledge about the area of interest that is somewhat superficial but sufficient to make a decision about the value of pursuing a given topic.
- The second phase of the literature review involves an in-depth, critically evaluated search of all publications relevant to the topic of interest. The goal of this phase is to narrow the focus and increase depth of knowledge. Journal articles describing research conducted on the topic of interest provide the most important kind of information, followed by clinical opinion articles (information on the topic described by experts in the field) and books. Journal articles provide more up-to-date information than do books, and systematic investigations provide a foundation for other studies. Prior research that has already been done on the topic of interest provides a solid foundation for later replication studies.
- Criteria for compiling a good review of the literature include (a) using articles that closely relate to the topic of interest (relevancy); (b) using current articles that provide up-to-date and recent information—usually within the past 5 years (although earlier articles may be included based on their importance to the area of interest); and (c) using both primary and secondary sources. A *primary source* is a publication that appears in its original form. A *secondary source* is an article in which one author writes about another author's work; EBP systematic reviews fall into this category.
- The conclusions from the literature review become the basis for the new study's assumptions and methodology. Rather than making a "leap of knowledge," the hypothesis or research question must be created by basing assumptions on previous research studies.

Select a Conceptual Model

- In relation to research, a **conceptual model** is a framework of ideas for explaining and studying a phenomenon of interest. A conceptual model conveys a particular perception of the world; it organizes the researcher's thinking and provides structure and direction for research activities. Models are like a framework on which to "hang" concepts or variables, and they should be used to guide the design and methods for collecting research data.
- All fields of study identify their major areas of concerns or boundaries. Nursing, since the early work of Florence Nightingale, is concerned with the interaction between humans and the environment in relation to health (Blais & Hayes, 2011). Betty Neuman's Systems Model (Neuman, & Reid, 2007) has often been used as an organizing framework for research studies in community health and acute-care nursing, as well as curriculum design (Neuman Systems Model, 2008). Although nurse investigators frequently and successfully use conceptual models developed within other fields, the advantage of using nursing models is that they provide an understanding of the world in terms of nursing's major concerns (see Chapter 14).

Choose a Research Design

Complete descriptions of various research designs and specific methodologies are available in basic nursing research texts. For the purposes of this chapter, a few important considerations underlying design

(continued)

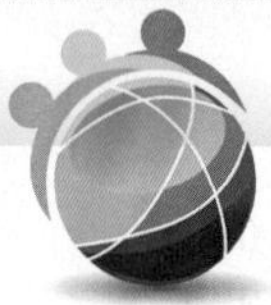

DISPLAY 4.3 STEPS IN THE RESEARCH PROCESS *(Continued)*

selection are described. First, quantitative approaches use two major categories of research design: experimental and nonexperimental (or descriptive).

- **Experimental design** requires that the investigators institute an intervention and then measure its consequences. Investigators hypothesize that a change will occur as a result of their intervention, and then they attempt to test whether their hypothesis was accurate. Experimental design requires investigators to randomly assign subjects to an **experimental group** (those receiving the intervention) and a **control group** (those not receiving the intervention). This process, called **randomization**, is the systematic sorting of research subjects, so that each one has an equal probability of selection.
- Another important distinction made within the experimental category of research is between true experiments and quasi-experiments. **True experiments** are characterized by instituting an intervention or change, assigning subjects to groups in a specific manner (randomization), and comparing the group of subjects who experience the manipulation to the control group (those not receiving the intervention). **Randomized control trials (RCTs)** are generally considered the gold standard of experimental research—they are commonly used to determine the safety and efficacy of new medications or to test the effectiveness of one intervention over another, and they are a foundation of EBP (Melnyk & Fineout-Overholt, 2011).
- **Quasi-experiments** lack one of these elements, such as the randomization of subjects. Community health nurses conduct quasi-experiments more often than true experiments because it is often difficult (and sometimes impossible) to use randomization. For instance, a nurse may conduct a nutrition education intervention with fifth grade students at a particular school. Although the nurse can have one classroom participate in the intervention and another remain the control group, he or she cannot randomly assign the children to classrooms (i.e., intervention or control). Therefore, this research would be characterized as quasi-experimental in nature.
- **Nonexperimental designs** (also called *descriptive designs*) are used in research to describe and explain phenomena or examine relationships among phenomena. Examples of this approach include examining the relationship between gender and smoking behaviors among adolescents, describing the emotional needs of families of clients with Alzheimer disease, and determining the attitudes of parents in a given community toward sex education in the schools. In each of these instances, the focus of the research is on the relationships observed or the description of what exists. Such nonexperimental designs are often the precursors of experiments.

Obtain Institutional Review Board Approval (see p. 16)

Collect and Analyze Data (see p. 16)

Interpret Results

The explanation of the findings of a study flows from the previously formulated research plan. The findings need to be a logical conclusion, based upon the building blocks of the literature review, conceptual framework, research question, and methodology (Polit & Beck, 2012). You can't jump to a conclusion for which you have not laid a foundation. Findings need to make sense, to be reasonable and logical.

Communicate Findings

- The findings of nursing research projects need to be shared with other nurses, regardless of the studies' outcomes. Negative as well as positive findings can make a valuable contribution to nursing knowledge and influence nursing practice. Whether or not the hypothesis was verified is not the most important part of research; it is equally important to know about results that are inconclusive or not statistically significant, because this information is also necessary to build the science of nursing. For instance, in an early Nurse–Family Partnership (see beginning of this chapter) study by Eckenrode et al. (2000, 2001), researchers found that participants who received nurse home visitation during pregnancy and through the child's second birthday had significantly fewer child maltreatment reports with the mother as perpetrator or the study child as subject than did participants not receiving nurse home visitation. However, for mothers reporting more than 28 incidents of domestic violence, no significant reductions were noted. This is important information, because ongoing domestic violence may limit the effectiveness of these types of programs. A review of current evidence on perinatal home visiting and intimate partner violence (Sharps, Campbell, Baty, Walker, & Bair-Merritt, 2008) concluded that those programs that add "specific intimate partner violence interventions" may be able to demonstrate reductions in violence along with improvements in infant and maternal health (p. 480). In future work, researchers need to elicit more information about domestic violence when trying to evaluate the effectiveness of this type of intervention.
- The research report should include the key elements of the research process. The research problem, methodology used, results of the study, and the investigators' conclusions and recommendations are presented. Whether investigators are presenting their findings verbally or writing for publication, they need to discuss the implications of their findings for nursing practice (Polit & Beck, 2012).

research, especially for practicing PHNs. Doctorally prepared nurses and public health professionals, in conjunction with practicing PHNs or health department staff, more often conduct traditional research studies. Problems recently identified and studied within community health nursing include:

- Perception of barriers to immunization among parents of Hmong origin (Baker, Dang, Ly, & Diaz, 2010).
- TB transmission and use of methamphetamines (Pevzner et al., 2010).
- Addressing asthma management challenges in a multisite, urban Head Start program (Garwick, Seppelt, & Riesgraf, 2010).
- Perception of childhood obesity on the Texas-Mexico border (Bayles, 2010).
- Outcomes of a breast health project for Hmong women and men (Kagawa-Singer, Tanjasiri, Valdez, Yu, & Foo, 2009).
- Low-income African American and Non-Hispanic White mothers' self-efficacy, "picky eater" perception, and toddler fruit and vegetable consumption (Horodynski, Stommel, Brophy-Herb, Xie, & Weatherspoon, 2010).
- Factors influencing mothers' abilities to engage in a comprehensive parenting intervention program (Domian, Baggett, Carta, Mitchell, & Larson, 2010).
- Population health surveillance practices of PHNs (Meagher-Stewart, Edwards, Aston, & Young, 2009).
- Policy implications of hospital nurse staffing and public health emergency preparedness (McHugh, 2010).
- Development and validation of a mass casualty conceptual model (Culley & Effken, 2010).

Each of these problem areas provides direction for the formulation of related research questions. Clear research questions, thorough review of the literature, human subjects protection, and a sound research design are factors to consider when evaluating the results of studies for incorporation into your practice.

A research question is a starting point for both traditional research and EBP methods. While somewhat similar in purpose (to answer a question), there are fewer steps in the EBP process (see Display 4.1). Formulation of a PICOT question in EBP is a similar process to the research question outlined in the steps of the research process, especially in its specificity (see Display 4.2).

While EBP steps outlined by Melnyk and Fineout-Overholt (2012) end with evaluation and dissemination, it is generally recognized that the final steps in the research process also apply to EBP. Most EBP research requires human subjects approval and dissemination of findings is very important in order to advance the science of nursing and provide effective outcomes for our clients. These steps will be examined in more detail here.

Obtain Institutional Review Board or Human Subjects Committee Approval

Whenever research is to be conducted that involves human subjects, prior approval must be gained from either an IRB or a HSC. This can be true for research studies or when measuring client outcomes elicited from EBP-implemented changes in nursing interventions (unless, perhaps, this is a quality improvement effort that affects all clients equally and involves only one setting). The reason for this approval is to safeguard the rights of prospective study participants. Each health department should have a committee or a gatekeeper, such as the health officer, who understands the federal guidelines for protecting subjects involved in research studies.

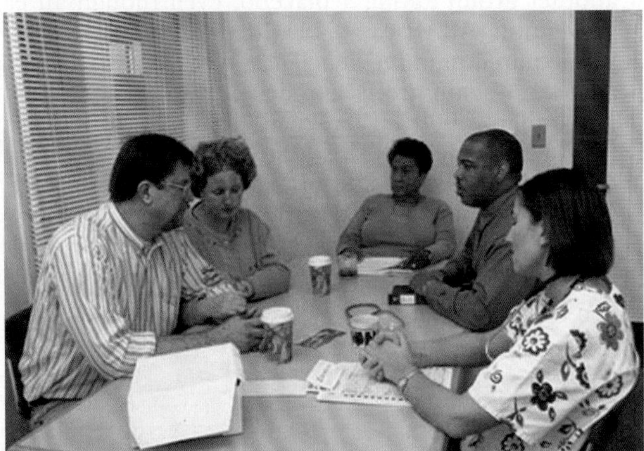

The purpose of an Institutional Review Board is to protect the rights of human subjects and ensure compliance with federal laws.

Sadly, one of the most egregious examples of exploitation of human subjects was a study carried out by the U. S. Public Health Service. The Tuskegee study, begun in 1932 and ended in 1972, sought to learn more about syphilis and to justify treatment services for Blacks in Alabama (Centers for Disease Control and Prevention [CDC], 2009). The 399 men with syphilis who participated in the study had agreed to be examined and treated. However, they were misled about the exact purpose of the study and were not given all of the facts; therefore, they were unable to truly give informed consent. Even after penicillin became the drug of choice for treatment of syphilis in 1947, the researchers failed to offer this treatment to the infected participants. Because of earlier Nazi atrocities, the Nuremberg Code and the Declaration of Helsinki were adopted by the world scientific community, then revised in 1975, as a means of ensuring ethical research practices; and the President's Council on Bioethics was established in 2001 after President Clinton apologized on behalf of the nation to the Tuskegee participants and their families in 1997 (Blais & Hayes, 2011; CDC, 2009) (see Evidence-Based Practice: Ethics in Action).

The following ethical principles are widely viewed as basic protections for research participants (U.S. Department of Health & Human Services, n.d.-a). Freedom from harm or exploitation encompasses several aspects. First, no research can be done that may inflict permanent or serious harm. Second, the research study must be stopped if it becomes evident that harm may come to participants. Debriefing, or allowing participants to ask questions of the researcher at the conclusion of the study, as a means of protecting them from any unseen psychological harm, is also a component. There should be some identified benefits from

EVIDENCE-BASED PRACTICE

Ethics in Action

Today, safeguards are in place to ensure that studies are stopped when either potential harm or insufficient benefit are noted. In April 2011, a drug trial examining daily use of an antiretroviral medication as a means of pre–human immunodeficiency virus (HIV) exposure prophylaxis was found to be ineffective in preventing HIV infection. No difference in rates of infection was noted for women taking the medication and another group taking a placebo, even though an earlier drug study with men showed some promise in HIV prevention (AllAfrica, 2011). In an earlier drug trial, a major international study of a drug-conserving protocol for acquired immune deficiency syndrome (AIDS) medication was stopped because those who were in the on-again, off-again group got sicker than those taking continuous medication therapy (Associated Press, 2006). More than 5,000 HIV patients in 33 countries participated in this study, which was halted by the National Institutes of Health. This large-scale study was initiated after several smaller studies had suggested a possible benefit from the on-and-off medication strategy. It was hoped that this strategy of only taking medications when immune cell levels dropped would not only cut costs, it would decrease medication side effects for patients. What researchers found was that this episodic strategy actually increased side effects related to the heart, liver, and kidney. Researchers say that the results are difficult to explain, but because of patient safety, it was best to stop the clinical trial.

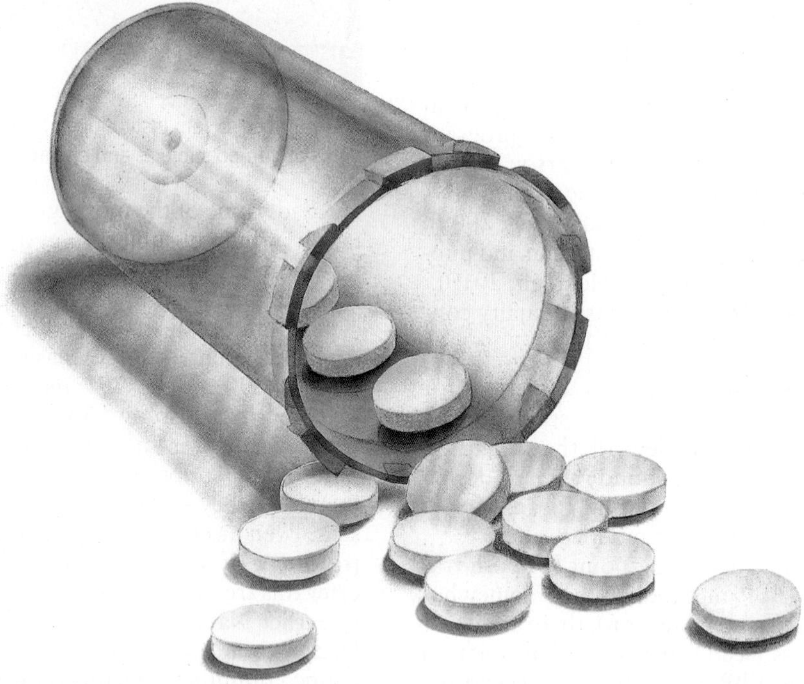

Drug safety was also questioned in a study of Avandia®, a drug used by some people with type 2 diabetes. In the summer of 2010, the Food and Drug Administration (FDA) ordered researchers to stop enrolling new participants in a trial of this drug because of heart risks and to notify the more than 1,300 participants already in the study of these risks (Wilson, 2010). In fall of 2010, they significantly restricted access to this drug, and in spring 2011 cardiovascular risk warnings were added to the label and the drug could only now be given to patients enrolled in a special FDA program (FDA, 2011).

What ethical principles are involved? Is there an ethical dilemma? Consider the rights of a few versus the rights of many. Apply Iserson's (1999) three tests (see p. 30 of this text).

participation in the research study, and any costs or risks should be clearly outlined, so that participants can more easily determine the cost–benefit ratio (referred to as *full disclosure*). Subjects should also be told that they are able to withdraw from the study at any time without prejudice or penalty (known as *self-determination*). Consent forms should include full disclosure of the nature of the study, the time and commitment required of subjects, the researcher's contact information, and a pledge of confidentiality (or *assurance of privacy*).

Vulnerable subjects, as determined by federal guidelines, include children, mentally or emotionally disabled people, physically disabled people, institutionalized people (e.g., prisoners), pregnant women, and the terminally ill. Special care must be taken to ensure protection of vulnerable subjects. Once approval has been obtained from the proper entities, data collection can begin (U.S. Department of Health & Human Services, n.d.-b).

Collect and Analyze Data

The value of the data collected in any research study or EBP project depends largely on the care taken when measuring the concepts of concern, or variables. The specific tool used to measure the variables in a study, often a questionnaire or interview guide, is called an **instrument**. The accuracy of the instrument used and the appropriateness of the choice of instruments can clearly influence the results. For instance, Spielberger's State-Trait Anxiety Inventory is a well-researched questionnaire used in studying anxiety levels in adults. It has been shown to accurately measure state anxiety and the more stable tendency toward anxious personality—*trait anxiety*. Because of this evidence, one could infer that more accurate measurements of anxiety could be found using this instrument than a researcher-developed questionnaire that has never been tested for validity and reliability.

Validity and Reliability

Two tests are used to evaluate instrument accuracy: validity and reliability. **Validity** is the assurance that an instrument measures the variables it is supposed to measure. If a written questionnaire is being used in the study, the questions included would be evaluated to make certain that they are appropriate to the subject (content validity) and that the variable of interest is actually being measured (construct validity).

Reliability refers to how consistently an instrument measures a given research variable within a particular population. Test–retest reliability ensures that similar results are obtained using the same instrument with the same population at two separate testing times. If similar results are obtained on two separate occasions, the test can be considered reliable.

Statistical tests and measurements are often used to analyze subjects' responses to questionnaires to evaluate internal consistency. A questionnaire is internally consistent to the extent that all of its subparts measure the same characteristic. Cronbach's alpha (α) is often cited as a measure of internal consistency and is reported as a correlation coefficient, so that the closer the value is to +1.0, the greater the degree of internal consistency. Results higher than 0.7 are generally regarded as desirable.

Within the area of community health nursing research, instruments appropriate to the measurement of nursing concepts may not be available. Researchers may use questionnaires that have been designed and tested by other investigators, or they may begin the tedious task of developing their own. Both approaches to measuring the variables of interest are acceptable; however, using available instruments of known reliability and validity saves considerable time.

Methods of Collecting Data

A variety of methods can be used to collect data, including self-report (subjects report their own experience verbally or in written form), observation (investigators observe subjects and document their observations), physiologic assessment (investigators use measures of physical evidence, such as blood pressure or impaired mobility), and document analysis (investigators review and analyze written materials, such as health records). For example, using these four methods, investigators examining the stress level of the caregiver when a family member chooses to die at home might do the following:

1. Design or use an existing written questionnaire or interview schedule (self-report).
2. Outline a schema, such as a list of potential stress-induced behaviors, for observing caregivers as they function in the home (observation).
3. Measure various physiologic indicators of stress, such as hypertension, insomnia, or poor diet (physiologic assessment).
4. Ask caregivers to keep a diary of their activities and feelings for 2 weeks, and analyze the diaries for evidence of stress (document analysis).

In most instances, the nature of the data to be collected dictates the best method of collection. One or more methods may be appropriate, given the topic of concern. In the example mentioned, a combination of the first three methods would probably be appropriate, or the diary could be substituted for the questionnaire.

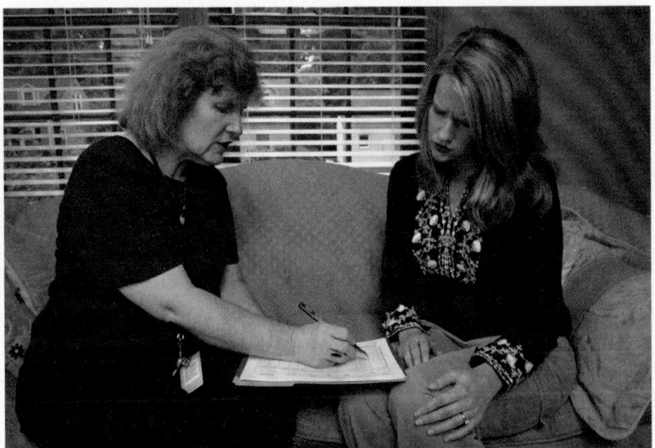

Surveys are common methods of collecting data. (Photo courtesy of CDC Public Health Image Library)

Methods of Analyzing Data

Once collected, data must be analyzed so that a meaningful interpretation can be made. Statistical procedures reduce great amounts of information to smaller chunks that can be easily interpreted. When deciding on an appropriate statistical procedure, it is helpful to consider the two major categories of statistical analysis: descriptive and inferential statistics.

Descriptive statistics portray the data collected in quantitative or mathematical terms. Commonly used descriptive statistical methods include calculating the average number (or *mean*) of a particular set of occurrences and calculating *standard deviations* (how much each score on the average deviates from the mean) and percentages. For example, an investigator analyzing data collected from 50 clients with chronic pain might find their mean pain score to be 4.96 (on a scale from 0 [no pain] to 10 [worst pain]), with a standard deviation of 0.83. These descriptive statistics suggest that clients are grouped around the middle of the pain scale and differ very little in the amount of pain they experience. The investigator may also report that more than 95% of the female clients experience pain rated between 4 and 6 on the 10-point pain scale. These descriptive statistics can be reported graphically (using graphs or charts) or in written form as shown in Table 4.1 for an example of both methods.

Inferential statistics involve making assumptions about features of a population based on observations of a sample. For example, the Gallup Poll, which surveys a sample of the population to determine what opinion they hold on a particular topic (e.g., favorite presidential candidate), uses inferential statistics to estimate the proportion of the total population that favors a particular candidate (McKenzie, Neiger, & Thackeray, 2009). The potential for **generalizability**, the ability to apply the research results to other similar populations, has great value to health professionals. It allows researchers to test their hypotheses on smaller groups before instituting widespread changes in methods, programs, and even national health policies.

Inferential statistics are also used to test hypotheses in research; they provide information about the likelihood that an observed difference between two or more groups could have happened just by chance or might be the result of some intervention or manipulation. These statistical procedures provide a determination of the extent to which changes or differences between sets of data are attributable to chance fluctuations and estimate the confidence with which one can make generalizations about the data.

It is appropriate to use both descriptive and inferential statistics to analyze the data from a study. For example, in a study designed to examine the effects of prenatal education on the health status of pregnant women, investigators might use inferential statistics to find a significant difference in health status between the group who experienced the educational program (experimental group) and the group who did not (control group). The investigators might also use descriptive statistics to report the percentage of women from the experimental group who attended all classes and the means and standard deviations for the women's health status scores.

Table 4.1 Pain Ratings

Value	Frequency	Percent (%)
3.00	1	2.0
4.00	11	22.0
5.00	30	60.0
6.00	6	12.0
7.00	1	2.0
8.00	1	2.0
MEAN 4.96	STANDARD DEVIATION 0.83	

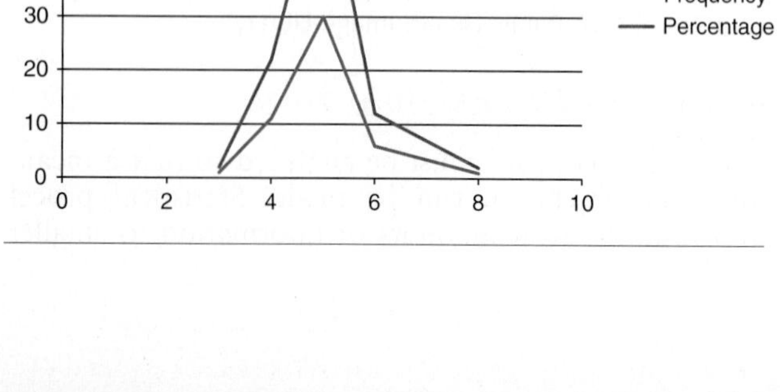

Interpret Results

The explanation of the findings of a study flows from the previously formulated research plan. The findings need to be a logical conclusion, based upon the building blocks of the literature review, conceptual framework, research question, and methodology (Polit & Beck, 2012). You can't jump to a conclusion for which you have not laid a foundation. Findings need to make sense, to be reasonable and logical. When findings support the directions developed in the research plan, their interpretation is relatively straightforward. For example, a group of community health nurse investigators might design a study to determine the effect of parenting classes on the self-esteem of single welfare mothers between 21 and 35 years of age. They could use Coopersmith's (1967) ideas on self-esteem as their conceptual model, hypothesize that self-esteem will improve as a result of the classes, and design an experiment to test their idea. If self-esteem does, in fact, increase, their finding flows logically from their framework.

If the findings do not support the hypothesis of the study, investigators question various aspects of the research to develop an explanation. In this instance, a number of questions could be posed. Coopersmith posited that self-esteem would relate to feelings of success in a given endeavor. Can that position be inaccurate? Could the parenting classes have been ineffective? Perhaps they did not enhance feelings of success. Could the intervention have been too weak to show a statistical difference (not enough sessions)? Were there problems with the methodology used: were there too few subjects, or intervening, confounding factors that affected the results? All of these questions and more should be considered in an attempt to explain the results.

If the study is descriptive in nature (i.e., one that was designed to describe particular characteristics of a population), the direction of the findings is not a concern. A detailed, accurate report of the results and their implications alone is appropriate. Given either an experimental or a descriptive design, the importance of accuracy cannot be overemphasized. Leaps of faith when reporting the results of a study are not appropriate unless labeled as such. For example, one could not conclude from the study on parenting classes that these classes develop expert parenting skills, given that parenting skills were not assessed.

A valuable contribution can be made to the advancement of nursing knowledge when investigators use their results to make suggestions for future research. The investigators' knowledge of a particular area and their experience in conducting a specific study give them an excellent background for identifying future research possibilities. As in EBP, results should be disseminated through publication, presentation, or other means.

IMPACT OF RESEARCH ON COMMUNITY HEALTH AND NURSING PRACTICE

Research has the potential to have a significant impact on community health nursing in three ways, by affecting public policy and the community's health, the effectiveness of community health nursing practice, and the status and influence of nursing as a profession. Community health nurses have been involved in research addressing all three of these dimensions.

Public Policy and Community Health

Research, with policy implications for addressing the health needs of aggregates, has been conducted on numerous topics. Many studies done by nurses and others have examined issues related to prevention, lifestyle change, quality of life, and health needs of specific at-risk populations (see Evidence-Based Practice: A Change of Position).

Often both quantitative and qualitative methods are useful when conducting **health policy evaluation** studies to determine whether existing health services are appropriate and accessible, as well as effective. Researchers at the University of California Los Angeles (UCLA) Center for Health Policy Research found that older adults in rural California had higher rates of obesity/overweight, food insecurity, and lower rates of physical activity than their urban or suburban counterparts (Durazo et al., 2011). Utilizing data from the California Health Interview Survey, they noted that these conditions are risk factors for diabetes, heart disease, and repeated falls. Barriers to transportation and health care access, along with financial constraints and social and physical isolation make this a complex issue that should be addressed on local, state, and national levels. They recommended policies to improve access to healthy food and adequate numbers of health care providers, as well as access to Internet and transportation, as a means of addressing the disparities. PHNs can use this type of research to advocate for resources, apply for grant funding, and negotiate collaborative agreements.

The results of health policy studies can influence public policy, the quality of services, and, in turn, the public's health: This is the conclusion of a Robert Wood Johnson initiative (Giovino, 2009). This change began in a few states and has spread, to some degree, across all 50 states. As an example, several studies conducted by a researcher at the University of Miami led to further policy changes regarding cigarette smoking. One study examined the projected health benefits and cost savings of raising the legal age for smoking in the United States to 21 (Ahmad, 2005a). Using a computer simulation model, the researcher concluded that changing the policy would net total savings of $212 billion in the United States and reduce the prevalence of cigarette smoking substantially. A similar study, looking only at the state of California, found that raising the legal smoking age to 21 would yield an 82% drop in prevalence in teen smoking and would save $24 billion over 50 years' time (Ahmad, 2005b). Taxes are another disincentive for smokers. California raised excise taxes on cigarettes in 1999, but Ahmad (2005c) used another computer simulation to reveal that an additional "20% tax-induced cigarette price increase would reduce smoking prevalence from 17% to 11.6% ... and reduce smoking-related medical costs by $188 billion" (p. 276). Raising cigarette taxes again would both decrease the number of smokers and increase the tax revenue that could be used to further reduce smoking in California. However, other effective methods of reducing cigarette smoking may exist. Levy, Nikolayev, and Mumford (2005) noted that smoking prevalence declined between 1997 and 2003, and, although most of the change could be explained by price increases, researchers also found that clean air laws, widespread media campaigns, and more easily accessible smoking cessation interventions also played a part. They encouraged lawmakers to continue with tax increases and to strengthen clean air laws that ban smoking in public places. In a Minnesota study, smoke-free workplaces were found to be more effective than free nicotine replacement therapy (Ong & Glantz, 2005). Other researchers have found that antismoking advertising focusing on the addictive nature of cigarettes and the dangers of environmental tobacco smoke to children increased the chances of quitting among adult smokers who have children living in their homes (Netermeyer, Andrews, & Burton, 2005). Consistent and wide-ranging antismoking media campaigns that emphasize social unacceptability and easier access to smoking cessation classes were also emphasized to policy makers (Alamar & Glantz, 2006).

Community Health Nursing Practice

A primary purpose for conducting community health research is to gain new knowledge that will improve health services and promote the public's health. Consequently, most nursing research has implications for nursing practice (Cross et al., 2006). Many studies focus on a specific health need or at-risk population, and then suggest

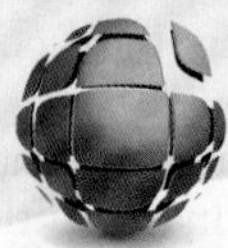

EVIDENCE-BASED PRACTICE

A Change of Position

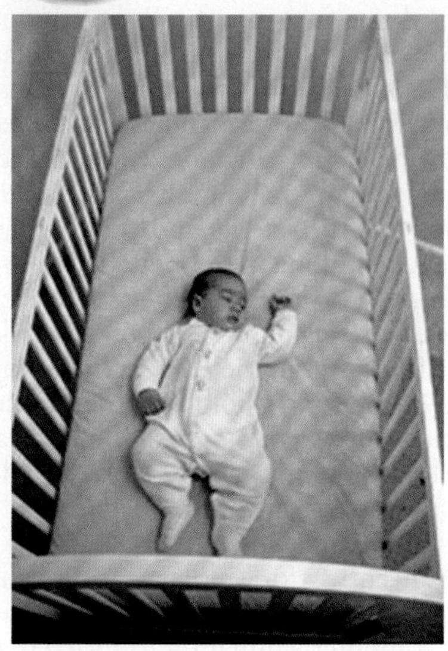

A good number of mothers today place their infants in a supine position—on their backs—to sleep. However, for most of us writing this textbook, the opposite was true—we were placed as sleeping infants in the prone position, on their stomachs. For generations, mothers were told that babies would be at risk of aspiration if they were put to sleep on their backs. Why did this change? In the late 1980s, research indicated that prone positioning of infants was related to greater incidences of sudden infant death syndrome (SIDS), according to a group at the National Institute of Child Health and Human Development (NIH) who conducted an epidemiologic study examining SIDS risk factors (Hoffman et al., 1988). In the early 1990s, an expert panel from the same institute and the American Academy of Pediatrics concluded that infant sleeping positioning was an important factor in prevention of SIDS and a recommendation was made for parents to place their infants on their backs when sleeping. The *Back to Sleep* campaign began in 1994 (National Institutes of Health, 2010). Since then, the incidence of SIDS has continued to drop steadily in the U.S.—27% between 1999 and 2007 (California Department of Public Health, 2008). Despite this, SIDS is still the leading cause of death in infants between the ages of 1 month and 1 year (CDC, 2007). More recent research has focused on an increased risk with parental use of alcohol (Phillips et al., 2010), decreased risk for breast-fed infants (Vennemann et al., 2009), and possible deficits in serotonin and tryptophan hydroxylase causing increased risk for SIDS (Duncan et al., 2010). Current recommendations from the American Academy of Pediatrics (2005, 2008) include continuing the *Back to Sleep* campaign and advising parents to:

- Place their sleeping infants in a supine position (not on side or stomach)
- Use a firm sleeping surface (no pillows or quilts under the baby)
- Keep soft objects (e.g., stuffed animals) and loose bedding (e.g., extra quilts or loose bedding) out of baby's crib
- Not smoke during pregnancy and avoid baby's exposure to secondhand smoke
- Not share the bed with baby—put baby in a separate crib or bassinet with parents in the same room
- Offer a pacifier at sleep time throughout the 1st year of life (it has been shown to reduce the risk of SIDS)
- Avoid overheating (keep room temperature comfortable for lightly clothed adults—do not overbundle babies)
- Encourage "tummy time" to avoid development of positional plagiocephaly (uneven head)
- Avoid the use of apnea monitors (not shown to be effective) and other commercial devices marketed as effective in reducing SIDS cases (not sufficient proof of efficacy)

Do your community health clients put their babies to sleep on their backs? If not, how can you convince them that it is beneficial?

nursing actions to be taken based on study findings. An example is a study examining effective approaches to take in promoting cardiovascular health in aging women (Sawatzky & Naimark, 2009). Historically, most care has focused on individual-level prevention and the treatment of risk factors such as hypertension and obesity. However, these nurse researchers found that a survey questionnaire, the Cardiovascular Health Promotion Profile, measured population-level determinants of health (i.e., income, social status, social support networks, employment and working conditions, level of education, utilization of health services, and biology and genetic factors) and could be a valuable method of promoting cardiovascular health in women. Individual-level measures are not thought to be as effective as population-based approaches in improving the health of a nation (Edelman & Mandle, 2006). Other issues that can be individual or population-based include obesity, smoking, and communicable diseases.

Nursing's Professional Status and Influence

The third way in which research has a significant impact on community health nursing is in its potential to enhance nursing's status and influence. As community health nursing research sheds light on the critical health needs of at-risk populations, exposes deficiencies in the health care system, demonstrates more efficient and cost-effective methods for delivering services, and documents the effectiveness of nursing interventions, the profession will gain a stronger voice and have a greater impact on health policy and programs. After all, PHNs have always been advocates for their clients and promoted policies that improved health.

A recent example of CBPR assessed tribal youth physical activity and programming among an American Indian tribe of 1,000 people (Perry & Hoffman, 2010). **Community-based participatory research (CPBR)** is defined as research "conducted in communities in which community members, persons affected the condition or issue under study and other key stakeholders in the community's health have the opportunity to be full participants in each phase of the work—conception, design, conduct, analysis, interpretation, conclusions, communication of results" (USDHHS, 2008, para. 2) and actively and equally share in decision-making power (Perry & Hoffman, 2010). These community health nurse researchers recognized the inherent mistrust of university researchers among tribal communities, and spent considerable time establishing relationships and discussing ideas with tribal members. Because this research involved children and adolescents, they engaged the Tribal Youth Council, as well as the adult Tribal Council, and established a Community Advisory Board to help them design their study. This board met an average of twice monthly for 8 months. They produced a data-sharing agreement that "delineated the type of data collected..., how data were collected..., and how data were to be handled to protect confidentiality...(as well as determining) who has access to data" (p. 107). They also collaborated on development of a questionnaire to collect information on favorite and least favorite exercise, motivators and barriers to exercise, and some demographic questions. They also designed two focus groups (one with 8- to 11-year-olds, and another with 15- to 18-year-olds) to determine types and amounts of daily physical activity, as well as preferences and ideas to promote physical activity among the youth. The goal of the research project was to determine tribal youths' current patterns of behavior patterns, beliefs, and preferences related to physical activity. Results showed that youth "differentiated exercise and sports" and had different barriers and motivators for each (p. 111). They saw exercise as "work" that could improve mood and health and stabilize their weight, along with improving strength and conditioning. None of the tribal youth met the national recommendations for physical activity (60 minutes of moderate to vigorous physical activity daily), and they were less active, on average, than youth in national studies. They reported spending 50% of their day in "sedentary activities" (p. 111), and cited motivators for physical activity to be coaches, friends, team, and school. Barriers were deemed to be lack of time, lack of programs, and school and/or work. The results were presented to the tribe, and much discussion ensued. The tribe began boys' and girls' basketball groups, and planned for additional baseball and wrestling teams. They are exploring other alternatives to promote physical activity (e.g., family days to teach traditional games, building walking trails), and felt that they had ownership of this research and their destiny. The researchers respected "tribal knowledge, traditions, and beliefs"—a theme of CPBR and of public health nursing—while helping to provide effective solutions to potential health problems.

Strong documentation supports the effectiveness of community health nursing interventions. Nurses in the community setting must provide empirical proof of their worth as professionals while serving the needs of their clients. This kind of information must be made visible if it is to influence legislators, planners, administrators, and other decision makers in health care (Hinshaw & Grady, 2011). As visibility increases, nursing's status and influence will increase.

THE COMMUNITY HEALTH NURSE'S ROLE IN RESEARCH

The advantages of community health nursing include a focus on health promotion and disease prevention; provision of services across the lifespan where people live, work, and learn; development of community capacity building for health; and working with partnerships, coalitions, and policy makers to promote a healthier environment. Community health nurses have two important responsibilities with respect to research in community health: to apply research findings to practice (EBP) and to conduct or participate in nursing research. Because research results provide essential information for improving health policy and the delivery of health services, community health nurses must be knowledgeable consumers of research. That is, they need to be able to critically examine research reports and apply study findings to improve the public's health.

Community health nurses have many opportunities to apply the results of other investigators' research and systematic reviews, but a necessary prerequisite is to be informed about research findings. As an essential part of their role, community health nurses must read the journals focusing on public health and community health nursing. Subscribing to some of these journals enables nurses to make a regular review of research an ongoing part of their professional practice. Nursing agencies and employment sites in community health can encourage nurses to become more knowledgeable about research findings by subscribing to journals and circulating them among staff, by holding seminars to discuss recent research results, and by promoting nurses' application of research findings in their practice.

Although the amount of health nursing research is expanding, and its quality is improving, many more community health nurses need to conduct research and participate in EBP. An increasing number of nurses have developed skill in research through advanced preparation, and they are conducting investigations related to aggregate health needs. Other community health nurses work collaboratively with trained investigators on a variety of research projects affecting community health. Whether initiated by the nurse or involving the nurse as a team member, these projects are an opportunity to influence the types of research questions that are addressed and the ways in which the research is carried out, factors that ultimately affect the community's health.

VALUES AND ETHICS IN COMMUNITY HEALTH NURSING

While the research process leads to EBP and expands nursing theory, there are other ways to develop knowledge in nursing. According to the classic treatise by Carper (1978), there is an art to nursing, which comes from our aesthetic sensibilities. Our personal history and experiences inform our practice, as well as our values and beliefs about what it means to be a good nurse. These values and beliefs support your own decisions about the right course of action to take, how to be just and fair in dealing with others, and what outcomes you deem to be right. Every profession has ethical codes that guide decision making and provide a framework for thinking about practice issues that have a moral dimension. In this chapter, we consider the philosophical background for nursing ethics and discuss some of the recent issues that you may encounter in your community health nursing experiences that will stimulate your thinking about how you define your own philosophy of nursing.

For over a decade, nurses have ranked highest in a Gallup poll for perceived honesty and ethical standards, beating out the clergy, physicians, and police officers (Jones, 2010). Clearly, the public has a favorable impression of nursing as a profession that can be trusted. Nursing has had an ethical code for practice since 1910, when Gettner published "The Nightingale Pledge." This evolved into the current "Code of Ethics for Nurses," as the American Nurses Association (ANA) has updated the code to reflect current issues and ideologies. The latest revision was approved in 2001.

The Code of Ethics for Nurses is based on respect for persons. Respect for the dignity and value of each individual encompasses our patients, our colleagues, our workplaces, and society at large. It also includes a mandate to respect the values and beliefs of each individual nurse. Since our personal experiences, our education, and our cultural and social values shape our beliefs, we have an obligation to think about those values that shape our practice. Having a greater awareness of our personal beliefs is a process called values clarification. This is an essential first step in a discussion of ethics, so that we have established moral beliefs, against which ethical dilemmas can be evaluated. As EBP is the result of the rigorous application of scientific method, our philosophy of nursing is based on clarity about our ethical code of practice, and a logical system for moral reasoning so that we are able to practice with integrity.

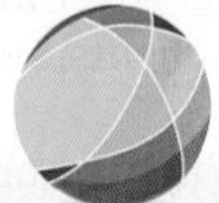

CODE OF ETHICS FOR NURSES—PROVISIONS, APPROVED AS OF JUNE 30, 2001

1. The nurse,—in all professional relationships, practices with compassion and respect for the inherent dignity, worth, and uniqueness of every individual, unrestricted by considerations of social or economic status, personal attributes, or the nature of health problems.
2. The nurse's—primary commitment is to the patient, whether an individual, family, group, or community.
3. The nurse—promotes, advocates for, and strives to protect the health, safety, and rights of the patient.
4. The nurse—is responsible and accountable for individual nursing practice and determines the appropriate delegation of tasks consistent with the nurse's obligation to provide optimum patient care.
5. The nurse—owes the same duties to self as to others, including the responsibility to preserve integrity and safety, to maintain competence, and to continue personal and professional growth.
6. The nurse—participates in establishing, maintaining, and improving health care environments and conditions of employment conducive to the provision of quality health care and consistent with the values of the profession through individual and collective action.
7. The nurse—participates in the advancement of the profession through contributions to practice, education, administration, and knowledge development.
8. The nurse—collaborates with other health professionals and the public in promoting community, national, and international efforts to meet health needs.
9. The profession of nursing, as represented by associations and their members, is responsible for articulating nursing values, for maintaining the integrity of the profession and its practice, and for shaping social policy.

For the nurse in community health, the focus is on providing care for populations within our community of concern. This is a potential source for ethical conflict, when the needs of the individual must be evaluated in light of the needs of the larger group. There are social, political, and economic issues that must be separated out from the ethical concerns. Consider the following situations:

- Imagine, for example, that you are providing health care to a population of migrant farm workers whose housing lacks adequate toilets, bathing facilities, heating, and equipment for cooking and refrigerating food. You recognize that this is a valid health and safety issue. However, when you report the situation to your supervisor, you are told to ignore the conditions because the wineries that employ the workers contribute heavily to a high-profile clinic for all low-income children in your area. What would you do?

- What if you were working in a homeless shelter and were told to evict someone who would not agree to take a tuberculin skin test. You agree that residents should comply with this demand, but would you hesitate to implement the eviction if the resident were elderly or the teenage mother of a newborn?

Within the United States, many marginalized people are failed by the public health care system or may go without any health care at all. At the same time, affluent individuals enjoy a plethora of health care options, including preventive screenings and health promotion classes. For instance, seven surgical operations are the average for an American over their lifetime, and each year approximately 5 million people will be admitted to an ICU in this country (Gawande, 2010). Community health nurses often are confronted by this disparity when making ethical decisions about client care. Social justice, human rights, and equality are hallmarks of public health nursing ethics (see more in Chapters 13, 25, and 29).

In addition to these dilemmas, progress in the United States often is linked to the exploitation of people in less-developed countries, and this contributes to widening disparities in health, wealth, and human rights. Distributive justice, or the fair allocation of goods and services, comes into play (discussed later in this chapter and in Chapter 29). Failure to respond to such global challenges only leads to greater poverty and deprivation, continuing conflict, escalating migration, and the spread of infectious disease, all further adding to our ethical dilemmas.

Advances in technology also contribute to ethical dilemmas. For example, electronic health records make client information readily accessible, thus raising issues of confidentiality, clients' rights, and informed consent (Layman, 2008). Sensitive information is now frequently stored electronically and may be accessed through unethical means (Valdez, Yoon, Quershi, Green, & Khoury, 2010). Technology also forces nurses to confront the issues of genetic testing and stem cell research, as well as assisted suicide and euthanasia (Clark, 2010; Dresser, 2010). Further ethical questions arise regarding organ, tissue, and limb transplants and the decisions about who is to receive them, as well as what happens to tissues removed during biopsy or surgery (see Display 4.4) (Ertin, Harmanci, Mahmutoglu, & Basagaoglu, 2010). Ethical issues in nursing practice have been described as a "moving picture," with challenges, values, and obligations continually being questioned (Doane, Storch, & Pauly, 2009). Underlying every issue and influencing every ethical and professional decision are *values*. Ethics and values are inextricably intertwined in professional decision making, because values are the criteria by which decisions are made.

VALUES

What are values? A **value** is something that is perceived as desirable or a personally held abstract belief "about the truth and worth of thoughts, objects, or behavior" (Guido, 2010, p. 2). A value motivates people to behave in certain ways that are personally or socially preferable. Values are usually derived from societal norms, as well as from family and/or religious beliefs. We develop our value system as a result of our experiences with others (e.g., family, peers, schools, churches, jobs). As seen in Chapter 5, a group's culture often is defined by its members' common or shared values.

STANDARDS FOR BEHAVIOR

In general, values function as standards that guide actions and behavior in daily situations or act as a code of conduct for living one's life. Once internalized by an individual, a value, such as honesty, becomes a criterion for that individual's personal conduct. Values may function as criteria for developing and maintaining attitudes toward objects and situations or for justifying a person's own actions and attitudes. Values also may be the standard by which people pass moral judgments on themselves and others.

Values have a long-term function in giving expression to human needs. Values motivate people in their work setting, in their personal lives, and in dealing with their health, as well as with the larger society. In addition, values are used as standards to guide presentation of the self to others, to ascertain personal morality and competency, and to persuade and influence others by indicating which beliefs, attitudes, and actions of others are worth trying to reinforce or change. As a practitioner, values act as a compass to direct the nurse when working with clients.

QUALITIES OF VALUES

The nature of values can be described according to five qualities: endurance, hierarchical arrangement, prescriptive–proscriptive belief, reference, and preference.

Endurance

Values remain relatively stable over time, persisting to provide continuity to personal and social existence. Enduring religious beliefs, for example, offer stability to many people. This is not to say that values are completely stable over time; values do change throughout a person's life. Certainly, the values of children are different from adults. Moral development generally follows a prescribed path, according to Lawrence Kohlberg (Colby & Kohlberg, 1987) and Carol Gilligan (1982), researchers studying changes in moral behavior and judgment from childhood to adulthood. Yet social existence in the community requires standards within the individual as well as an agreement about standards among groups of individuals (Bartels, Bauman, Skitka, & Medin, 2009). As Kluckhohn (1951, p. 400) once pointed out, without values, "the functioning of the social system could not continue to achieve group goals; individuals ... could not feel within themselves a requisite measure of order and unified purpose." A group's culture provides such a set of enduring values. By adding an element of collective purpose in social life, values most often guarantee endurance and stability in social existence.

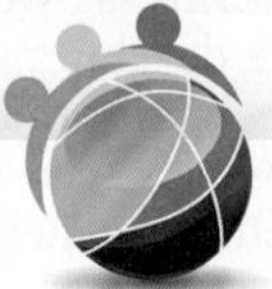

DISPLAY 4.4 IMMORTAL CELLS, ETHICAL DILEMMA

How would you feel if tissues or cells taken from you during surgery or a routine biopsy were subsequently used in health research without your knowledge or permission (or remuneration)? That happened to Henrietta

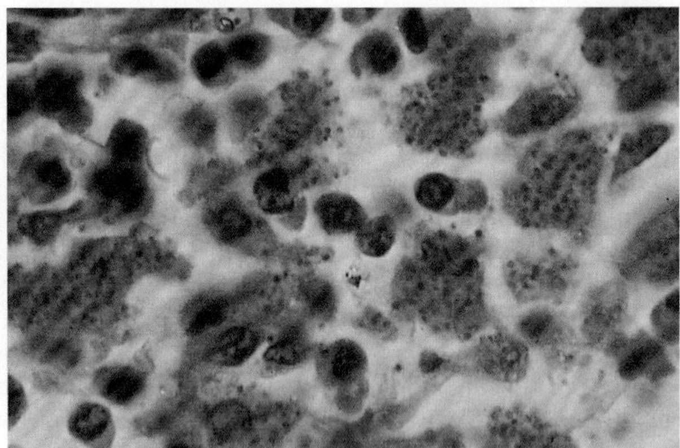

Lacks, a Black woman from Baltimore, whose cells (known as HeLa cells) were the first immortal human cells and used in the development of the field of virology. HeLa cells were tested in the first space missions to determine zero gravity's effects, and were vital to the development polio and hepatitis B vaccines, as well as chemotherapy, in vitro fertilization, cloning, and gene mapping (Skloot, 2011). These cells, taken from a biopsy of her cervix a few months before she died of cervical cancer in 1951, were useful in the development of medications for leukemia, herpes, hemophilia, and influenza. They have been used in innumerable studies around the world, to test the effects of massive radiation (e.g., nuclear blasts), hormones, vitamins, steroids, tuberculosis, salmonella, and hemorrhagic fever. HeLa cells were also instrumental in many historic scientific discoveries (e.g., cigarettes caused lung cancer, how cancer cells grew differently from normal cells, how human immunodeficiency virus infected cells), and continue to be used today in scientific research. Although this happened in the 1950s, today it is still often considered legal for a researcher to use tissues removed from your body for scientific research without your consent. It has been considered by law to be "abandoned waste" and may be used for gain without the knowledge, consent, or reimbursement to the donor.

From: Skloot, R. (2011). *The immortal life of Henrietta Lacks*. New York: Random House/Broadway Books.

Hierarchical System

Isolated values usually are organized into a hierarchical system in which certain values have more weight or importance than others. For instance, in a team sport such as baseball, values regarding individual performance, batting and running records, speed, and throwing and catching all fall into a hierarchy, with the values of team and winning being at the top. As an individual confronts social situations throughout life, isolated values learned in early childhood come into competition with other values, requiring a weighing of one value against another. Concern for others' welfare, for instance, competes with self-interest. Through experience and maturation, the individual integrates values learned in different contexts into systems in which each value is ordered relative to other values (Harris, 2010).

Prescriptive–Proscriptive Beliefs

Rokeach (1973) described values as a subcategory of beliefs. He argues that some beliefs are *descriptive* or capable of being true or false (e.g., the chair on which I am sitting will hold me up). Other beliefs are *evaluative*, involving judgments of good and bad (e.g., that was an excellent lecture). Still other beliefs are *prescriptive–proscriptive*, determining whether an action is desirable or undesirable (e.g., this music is too loud, those baseball fans shouldn't yell when the pitcher is winding up). Values, Rokeach says, are prescriptive–proscriptive beliefs. They are concerned with desirable behavior or "what ought to be." For example, parents' values about child behavior determine how they choose to discipline their children, using corporal punishment, a time-out, or a laissez-faire attitude where behavior is largely ignored. Some parents believe that their 2-year-old child has the capacity to control his bladder, and when the child wets his pants they are being "rebellious" and should be punished. Values have cognitive, affective, and behavioral components. According to Rokeach, to have a value, it is important to know the correct way to behave or the correct end state for which to strive (cognitive component); to feel emotional about it—to be affectively for or against it (affective component); and to take action based on it (behavioral component). More recent research has further delineated moral regulation within the framework of avoidance versus approach motivation (Sheikh & Janoff-Bulman, 2010). For example, proscriptive moral emotions are described as strict, duty-based, "sensitive to negative outcomes, inhibition-based" and focused on what not to do, while prescriptive moral emotions are described as abstract, discretionary, "positive outcomes, activation-based" and deal with what should be done (Janoff-Bulman, Sheikh, & Hepp, 2009, p. 521). Think about which beliefs or values (prescriptive/proscriptive) inspired you to go to nursing school.

Reference

Values also have a reference quality. That is, they may refer to end states of existence called **terminal values**, such as spiritual salvation, peace of mind, or world peace, or they may refer to modes of conduct called **instrumental values**, such as confidentiality, keeping promises, and honesty. The latter can have a moral focus or a nonmoral focus, and these values may conflict (Gecas, 2008; Johnston, 1995; Rokeach, 1973). For example, a nurse may experience a conflict between two moral values, such as whether to act honestly (tell a client about a fatal diagnosis) or to act respectfully (honor the family's request not to tell the client). Similarly, the nurse may experience conflict between two nonmoral values, such as whether to plan logically (design a traditional group intervention for mental health clients) or to plan creatively (design an innovative field experience). The nurse also may experience conflict between a nonmoral value and a moral value, such as whether to act efficiently or to act fairly when establishing priorities for funding among community health programs. Ethical reasoning in nursing develops over time, as novice nurses are exposed to various situations. One study examining ethical reasoning among nursing students found that students were "confronting the 'real world' of health care" and "lacking the confidence....to take an ethical stand" (Callister, Luthy, Thompson, & Memmott, 2009, p. 499). Even though these were adults with values adopted throughout their lives, the student nurses were still adapting to new ethical issues and reassessing their values.

Adults generally possess only a few—perhaps no more than 20—terminal values, such as peace of mind or achievement. These are influenced by complex physiologic and social factors. The needs for security, love, self-esteem, and self-actualization, proposed by Maslow (1969), are believed to be the greatest influences on terminal values. Although an individual may have only a few terminal values, the same person may possess as many as 50 to 75 instrumental values. Any single instrumental value, or several instrumental values combined, also may help to determine terminal values. For example, the instrumental values of acceptance, taking it easy, living 1 day at a time, and not being concerned about the future can shape the terminal value of peace of mind; whereas the instrumental values of hard work, driving oneself to compete, and not letting anyone get in the way can influence the terminal value of achievement. Figure 4.2 illustrates the influence of instrumental values and human needs on the development of terminal values.

Preference

A value may show preference for one mode of behavior over another, such as exercise over inactivity, or it may show a preference for one end state over another, such as physical fitness and leanness over sedentary lifestyle and obesity. The preferred end state, or mode of behavior, is located higher in the personal value hierarchy.

VALUE SYSTEMS

Value systems generally are considered organizations of beliefs that are of relative importance in guiding individual behavior (Harris, 2010; Rokeach, 1973). Instead of being guided by single or isolated values, however, behavior at any point in time (or over a period of time) is influenced by multiple or changing clusters of values. Therefore, it is important to understand how values are integrated into a person's total belief system, how values assume a place in a hierarchy of values, and how this hierarchical system changes over time.

Hierarchical System of Values

Learned values are integrated into an organized system of values, and each value has an ordered priority

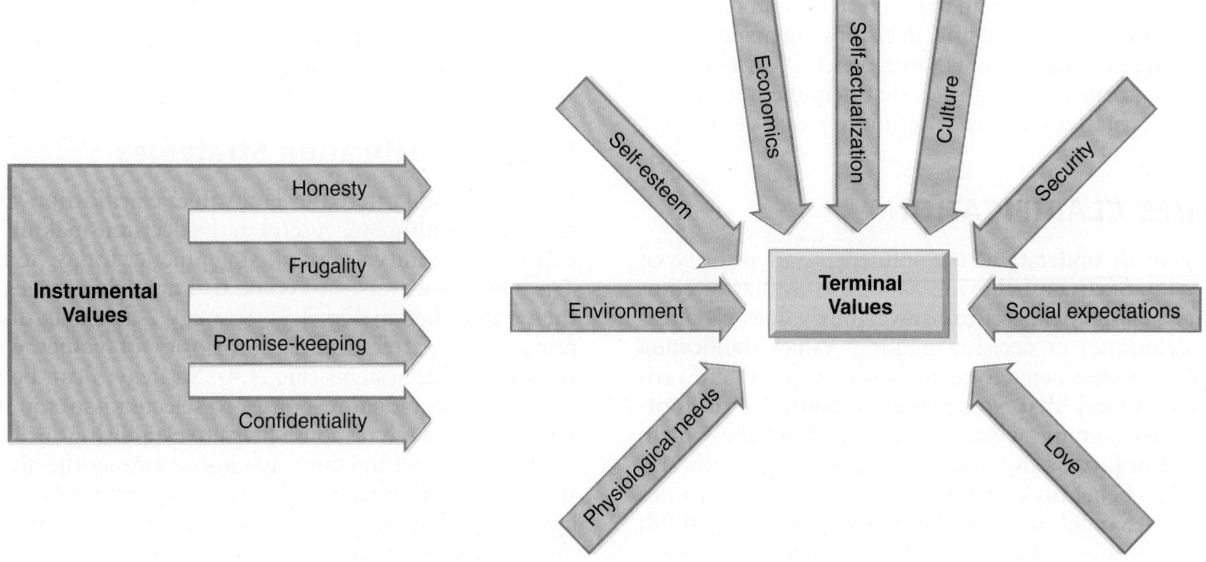

FIGURE 4-2. Factors influencing terminal values.

with respect to other values (Harris, 2010; Rokeach, 1973). For example, a person may place a higher value on physical comfort than on exercising. This system of ordered priority is stable enough to reflect the continuity of someone's personality and behavior within culture and society, yet it is sufficiently flexible to allow a reordering of value priorities in response to changes in the environment or social setting (e.g., society's emphasis on physical fitness and youth) or changes based on personal experiences (e.g., diagnosis of type 2 diabetes). Behavioral change would be regarded as the visible response to a reordering of values within an individual's hierarchical value system.

Conflict Between Values in a System

When an individual encounters a social situation, several values within the person's value system are activated, rather than just a single value. Because not all of the activated values are compatible with one another, conflict between values occurs. This conflict between values is a part of the decision-making process, and resolving these value conflicts is crucial to making good decisions. Community health nurses face conflicting values when they seek to promote the well being of certain individuals, a result that may come at the expense of the public good (Easley & Allen, 2007). Even within a single community agency, nurses may find that they prioritize client service or programming values differently.

Some values seem to consistently triumph over others, persisting as stronger directives for individual behavior; an example is the value placed on high achievement in the United States. It is this persistence on the part of some values (e.g., individualism vs. community) that makes universal coverage and other issues so controversial in health care reform (Axtell-Thompson, 2005; Kerkhoff, 2009; Schmidt, 2009). Other values lose their positions of importance in a value hierarchy (e.g., resuscitation of all hospital patients vs. do not resuscitate orders [DNRs]). It is this changing arrangement of values in a hierarchical system that determines, in part, how conflicts are resolved and how decisions are made. In this way, people's value systems function as a learned organization of principles and rules that help them to choose among alternative courses of action to reach decisions.

VALUES CLARIFICATION

One way to understand the influence and priority of values in your own behavior, as well as in that of community health clients, is to use various values clarification techniques in decision making. **Values clarification** is a process that helps to identify the personal and professional values that guide your actions, by prompting you to examine what you believe about the worth, truth, or beauty of any object, thought, or behavior and where this belief ranks compared with your other values (Allicock, Sandelowski, DeVellis, & Campbell, 2008; Feldman-Stewart, Brennenstuhl, Brundage, & Roques, 2006). Because individuals are largely unaware of the motives underlying their choices, values clarification is important for understanding and shaping the kind of decisions people make. Only by understanding your values and their hierarchy can you ascertain whether your choices are the result of rational thinking or of external influences, such as cultural or social conditioning. Values clarification by itself does not yield a set of rules for future decision making and does not indicate the rightness or wrongness of alternative actions. It does, however, help to guarantee that any course of action chosen by people is consistent and in accordance with their beliefs and values (Abhyankar, Bekker, Summers, & Velikova, 2011).

Process of Valuing

Before values clarification can take place, it must be understood how the process of valuing occurs in individuals. In 1977, Uustal listed the following seven steps, which remain useful today:

1. Choose the value freely and individually.
2. Choose the value from among alternatives.
3. Carefully consider the consequences of the choice.
4. Cherish or prize the value—feel good about the choice.
5. Publicly affirm the chosen value.
6. Incorporate the value into behavior, so that it becomes a standard or a pattern of behavior.
7. Consciously use the value in decision making.

These steps provide specific actions for the discovery and identification of people's values. They also assist the decision-making process by explicating the process of valuing itself. For example, some people may choose to value honesty in a presidential candidate. They may choose this over other values, such as knowledge of foreign affairs or public speaking ability, because, when considering the consequences, they want a leader who will deliver on promises made and who will continue to be the person represented to the public during the campaign. They prize this value of honesty, affirm it publicly, and consciously use it as a standard when deciding on whom to vote into office or to reject.

Values Clarification Strategies

In 1978, Uustal offered several values clarification strategies that are ultimately useful to the decision-making process in community health nursing practice today. Strategy 1 is a way for nurses to come to know themselves and their values better (Fig. 4.3). Strategy 2 assists in discovering value patterns and the priority of values within personal value systems (Fig. 4.4). Strategy 3 can be used to examine personal responses to selected issues in nursing practice. Each response helps to establish priorities of values by asking the nurse to choose among the alternatives presented or to indicate degree of agreement or disagreement (Fig. 4.5). Other values clarification strategies are included in the critical thinking activities at the end of this chapter to assist in understanding personal ordering

Name Tag

Take a piece of paper and write your name in the middle of it. In each of the four corners, write your responses to these four questions:

1. What two things would you like your colleagues to say about you?
2. What single most important thing do you do (or would you like to do) to make your nurse–client relationships positive ones?
3. What do you do on a daily basis that indicates you value your health?
4. What are the three values you believe in most strongly?

In the space around your name, write at least six adjectives that you feel best describe who you are.

Take a closer look at your responses to the questions and to the ways in which you described yourself. What values are reflected in your answers?

FIGURE 4-3. Values clarification strategy 1.

of values and when considering directions for change. These strategies also help the nurse to assist community health clients to become clearer about their own values.

All of these strategies can be used to analyze and understand how values are meaningful to people and ultimately influence their choices and behavior. Clarification of a person's values is the first step in the decision-making process, and it affects the ability of people to make ethical decisions. Values clarification also promotes understanding and respect for values held by others, such as community health clients and other health care providers. As pointed out by Uustal (1977, p. 10), "Nurses cannot hope to give optimal, sensitive care to any patient without first understanding their own opinions, attitudes, and values." This values clarification process provides a backdrop for next exploring the role of values in ethical decision making. Values clarification has also proven helpful with clients, as a Cochrane Collaboration Review indicates (O'Connor et al., 2009). Focused values clarification exercises, as part of a package of decision aids (e.g., pamphlets, videos), for patients making treatment or screening decisions were found to improve knowledge of options/risks/benefits and promote decision making.

Patterns

Which of the following words describe you? Draw a circle around the seven words that best describe you as an individual. Underline the seven words that most accurately describe you as a professional person. (You may circle and underline the same word.)

ambitious reserved assertive opinionated
concerned generous independent
easily hurt outgoing reliable indifferent
capable self-controlled fun-loving
suspicious solitary likable dependent
intellectual argumentative dynamic unpredictable
compromising thoughtful affectionate obedient
logical imaginative self-disciplined
moody easily led helpful slow to relate

Reflect on the following questions:

1. What values are reflected in the patterns you have chosen?
2. What is the relationship between these patterns and your personal values?
3. What patterns indicate inconsistencies in attitudes or behavior?
4. What patterns do you think a nurse should cultivate?

FIGURE 4-4. Values clarification strategy 2.

Forced Choice Ranking

How do you order the following alternatives by priority? (There is no correct set of priorities.) What values emerge in response to each question?

1. With whom on a nursing team would you become most angry? The nurse who
   ____ never completes assignments.
   ____ rarely helps other team members.
   ____ projects his or her feelings on clients.
2. If you had a serious health problem, you would rather
   ____ not be told.
   ____ be told directly.
   ____ find out by accident.
3. You are made happiest in your work when you use
   ____ your technical skills in caring for adults with complex needs.
   ____ your ability to compile data and arrive at a nursing diagnosis.
   ____ your ability to communicate easily and skillfully with clients.
4. It would be most difficult for you to
   ____ listen to and counsel a dying person.
   ____ advise a pregnant adolescent.
   ____ handle a situation of obvious child abuse.

FIGURE 4-5. Values clarification strategy 3.

ETHICS

Values are central to any consideration of ethics or ethical decision making. Yet, it is not always obvious at first what constitutes an ethical problem in health care or in the practice of community health nursing. Most nurses easily recognize the moral crisis in some kinds of decisions—for example, whether to let seriously deformed newborn infants die, whether to terminate pregnancies resulting from rape, or whether to provide universal health care coverage. However, other, less obvious moral dilemmas often found in the routine practice of community health nursing are not always considered to be ethical in nature.

What is *ethics* and what is *ethical*? The *Merriam Webster Online Dictionary* (2011) defines **ethics** as "the principles of conduct governing a group" (para. 1). Ethics may also be viewed as a set of moral principles or a theory or system of moral values. Ethics are often idealized as "what ought to be." **Ethical decision making**, then, means making a choice that is consistent with a moral code or that can be justified from an ethical perspective. Of necessity, the decision maker must exercise moral judgment. Remember that the term **moral** refers to conforming to a standard that is right and good. Community health nurses become "moral agents" by making decisions that have direct and indirect consequences for the welfare of themselves and others. **Bioethics** refers to using ethical principles and methods of decision making in questions involving biologic, medical, or health care issues (Beauchamp & Childress, 2008; Jecker, Jonsen, & Pearlman, 2007), arising out of "questions of fairness in resource allocation....(and) moral issues raised by new technologies" (Kass, 2001, p. 1777). The next section examines how a PHN makes these moral decisions.

Public Health Ethics

Protection and promotion of health are at the core of public health nursing. Ethical principles are further clarified in this speciality area. Public health ethics is defined as "a systematic process to clarify, prioritize and justify possible courses of public health action based on ethical principles, values and beliefs of stakeholders, and scientific and other information" (CDC, 2011, para. 1). Specific ethical principles apply to public health in general (e.g., advocacy for healthy communities and equitable distribution of limited resources; balance between individual rights and the collective good) and public health nursing specifically (e.g., professional ethics). Preventing disease or harm, respecting individual rights, and encouraging community input are common values, as well as empowerment of the disenfranchised and equal access to resources. Promoting health, protecting confidentiality (except where justified), and collaborating or partnering with other community agencies are viewed as universal practices. Other principles include respecting diverse values/beliefs and working effectively with different cultural groups to enhance the social and physical environment, while employing competent public health professionals. Public health is most often concerned with "public goods that can be achieved only by collective action, such as clean water, adequate housing, and public safety, and with societal regulation of shared risks" (Easley & Allen, 2007, p. 369). Because of this focus, there is sometimes an uneasy balance between individual and public interests and rights.

A framework is applied in public health ethics inquiry. Three core functions of this inquiry include:

1. Identifying and clarifying the ethical dilemma
2. Analyzing it in terms of alternative courses of action and their consequences
3. Resolving the dilemma by deciding which course of action best incorporates and balances the guiding principles and values (CDC, 2011, para. 5)

Identifying Ethical Situations

Ethics involves making evaluative judgments. To be ethically responsible in the practice of community health nursing, it is important to develop the ability to recognize evaluative judgments as they are made and implemented in nursing practice. Nurses must be able to distinguish between evaluative and nonevaluative judgments. Evaluative statements involve judgments of value, rights, duties, and responsibilities. Examples are, "Parents should never strike their children," and "It is the duty of every citizen to vote." Among the words to watch for are verbs such as *want, desire, refer, should,* or *ought* and nouns such as *benefit, harm, duty, responsibility, right,* or *obligation.*

Sometimes, the evaluations are expressed in terms that are not direct expressions of evaluations but clearly are functioning as value judgments. For example, the ANA companion text, *Guide to the Code of Ethics for Nurses: Interpretation and Application* (Fowler, 2010), refers to the obligations or duties of nurses to both patient and self and discusses nursing values in more details (see "Code of Ethics for Nurses—Provisions").

Another important step is to distinguish between moral and nonmoral evaluations. **Moral evaluations** refer to judgments that conform to standards of what is right and good. Moral evaluations assess human actions, institutions, or character traits rather than inanimate objects, such as parks or architectural structures. They are prescriptive–proscriptive beliefs having certain characteristics separating them from other evaluations such as aesthetic judgments, personal preferences, or matters of taste. Moral evaluations also have distinctive characteristics (Thompson, Melia, Boyd, & Horsburgh, 2006):

- *The evaluations are ultimate.* They have a preemptive quality, meaning that other values or human ends cannot, as a rule, override them.
- *They possess universality or reflect a standpoint that applies to everyone.* They are evaluations that everyone in principle ought to be able to make and understand, even if some individuals, in fact, do not.
- *Moral evaluations avoid giving a special place to a person's own welfare.* They have a focus that keeps others in view, or at least considers one's own welfare on a par with that of others.

Moral evaluations, like "parents should take care of their children," meet these criteria. Nonmoral evaluations, like "Mrs. X has five children," does not evoke a moral judgment of Mrs. X, but only an assessment of her family composition.

Resolving Moral Conflicts and Ethical Dilemmas

When judgments involve moral values, conflicts are inevitable. In clinical practice, the nurse may be faced with moral conflicts, such as the choice between preserving the welfare of one set of clients over that of others. For example, the nurse may have to choose whether to keep a promise of confidentiality to persons who are infected by HIV when these individuals continue to have unprotected sex with unknowing partners. Nurses may have to choose between protecting the interests of colleagues or the interests of the employing institution by reporting a nurse who makes phone visits rather than home visits, so that she can spend more time shopping online from work. They may have to decide whether to serve future clients by striking for better conditions or to serve present clients by refusing to strike. Often, nurses' values are at odds with their employers' values and procedures. The moral values of a nurse may conflict with the policies and practices of a particular bureaucracy, as nurses are taught that their clients (individuals, families, aggregates) are their focus of concern (Wright & Brajtman, 2011). Each decision involves a potential conflict between moral values and is called an **ethical dilemma**. An ethical dilemma occurs when morals conflict with one another, causing the nurse to face a choice with equally attractive or equally undesirable alternatives (Kelly, 2009; Thompson et al.2006). When you are faced with two or more values of equal importance that will lead to different actions, you are faced with an ethical dilemma. It can create a decision-making problem, even in ordinary nursing situations.

Decision-Making Frameworks

To resolve ethical dilemmas or the conflict between moral values in community health nursing practice, and to provide morally accountable nursing service, several frameworks for ethical decision making have been proposed. Among these frameworks, three key steps are considered as fundamental to choosing alternative courses of action that reflect moral reasoning: separate questions of fact from questions of value, identify both clients' and nurse's value systems, and consider ethical principles and concepts (see Figure 4.6).

The identification of clients' values and those of other persons involved in conflict situations is an important part of ethical decision making. In the example given in From the Case Files I, what are Mr. Bell's values? What are the values of neighbors who are concerned about him, but feel that they can no longer care for him? What are the nurse's values? What are the values of the nurse's employer? What are society's values?

An ethical decision-making framework referred to as the DECIDE model is a practical method of making prudent value judgments and ethical decisions (Thompson et al.2006). It includes the following steps:

D—*Define the problem (or problems).* What are the key facts of the situation? Who is involved? What are their rights and duties and your rights and duties?

E—*Ethical review.* What ethical principles have a bearing on the situation, and which principle or principles should be given priority in making a decision?

C—*Consider the options.* What options do you have in the situation? What alternative courses of action exist? What help, means, and methods do you need to use?

I—*Investigate outcomes.* Given each available option, what consequences are likely to follow from each course of action open to you? Which is the most ethical thing to do?

D—*Decide on action.* Having chosen the best available option, determine a specific action plan, set clear objectives, and then act decisively and effectively.

E—*Evaluate results.* Having initiated a course of action, assess how things progress, and when concluded, evaluate carefully whether or not you achieved your goals.

Other frameworks can be used. The framework for ethical decision making shown in Display 4.5 helps to organize thoughts and acts as a guide through the decision-making process. The steps help to determine a course of action, with heavy responsibility at the evaluation level: here the outcomes need to be judged and decisions repeated or rejected in future situations. Figure 4.6

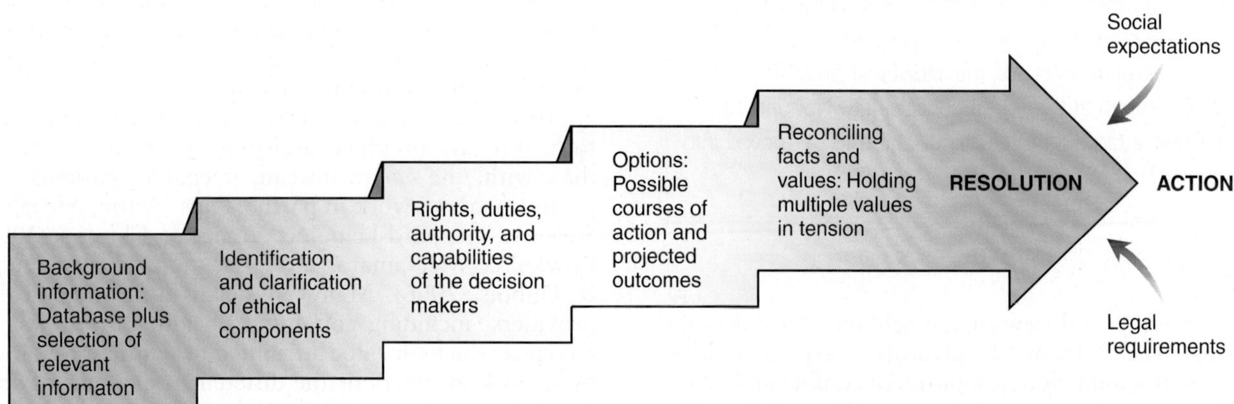

FIGURE 4-6. An ethical decision-making framework. Although legal requirements or social expectations may sway a decision one way or another, they are extrinsic to the ethical analysis and should not be confused with right and wrong. What is legal and what is expected are not necessarily right and wrong.

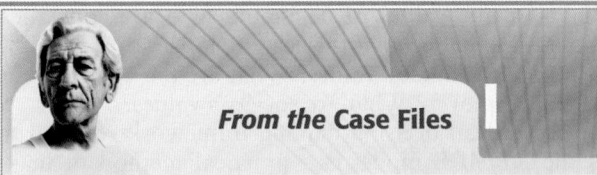

From the Case Files

Mr. Bell

Community health nurses encounter value differences every day, and value differences, in turn, create ethical problems. Consider, for example, the dilemma faced by one nurse in Seattle on her first home visit to an elderly man, Mr. Bell, referred by concerned neighbors. This 82-year-old gentleman was homebound and living alone with severe arthritis under steadily deteriorating conditions. Overgrown shrubs and vines covered the yard and house, making access impossible except through the back door. A woodburning stove in the kitchen was the sole source of heat. The kitchen, along with a corner of the dining room, constituted Mr. Bell's living quarters. The remainder of the once-lovely three-bedroom home, including the bathroom, was layered with dust, unused. His bed was a cot in the dining room; his toilet, a 2-pound coffee can sitting under the cot. Unbathed, unshaven, and existing on food and firewood brought by neighbors, Mr. Bell seemed to be living in deplorable conditions. Yet he prized his independence so highly that he adamantly refused to leave. Mr. Bell had one son living in a neighboring state, but had little contact with him.

The conflict of values between Mr. Bell's choice to live independently and the nurse's value of having him in a safer living situation raises several ethical questions. When do health practitioners or family members have the right or duty to override an individual's preferences? When do neighbors' rights (Mr. Bell's home was an eyesore and his care was a source of anxiety for his neighbors) supersede one homeowner's rights? Should the nurse be responsible when family members can help but won't take action?

In this case, the nurse entering Mr. Bell's home applied her values of respect for the individual and his right to autonomy even at the risk of public safety. Not until he fell and broke a hip did he reluctantly agree to be moved into a nursing home.

summarizes several views in the field on ethical decision making. This framework advocates keeping multiple values in tension before resolution of conflict and action on the part of the nurse. It suggests that value conflict is not capable of resolution until all possible alternative actions have been explored. Three tests may be helpful in your decision-making process (Edwards & Robey, 2010; Iserson, 1999):

- Impartiality test (e.g., Would you be willing to have this done to you? The "golden rule.")
- Universalizablity test (e.g., If every nurse in similar circumstances did the same as you, would you be comfortable with that "universal rule"?)
- Interpersonal justifiability test (e.g., Can you state a reason for your choice and justify your actions to your peers, supervisors, and society?)

Final resolution of the ethical conflict occurs through a conscious choice of action, even though some values would be overridden by other stronger, presumably moral values. The triumphant values would be those located higher in the decision maker's hierarchy of values.

Basic Values That Guide Decision Making

When applying a decision-making framework, certain values influence community health nursing decisions. Three basic human values are considered key to guiding decision making in the provider–client relationship: self-determination, wellbeing, and equity.

Self-Determination

The value of **self-determination** or individual autonomy is a person's exercise of the capacity to shape and pursue personal plans for life (Guido, 2010). Self-determination is instrumentally valued because self-judgment about a person's goals and choices is conducive to an individual's sense of wellbeing. Informed consent derives from self-determination. When one respects self-determination, it is based on the belief that better outcomes will result when autonomy is held in high regard. The outcomes that could be maximized by respecting self-determination or autonomy include enhanced self-concept, enhanced health-promoting behaviors, and enhanced quality of care. Self-determination is a major value in the United States, but does not receive the same emphasis in all societies or ethnic groups.

In health care contexts, the desire for self-determination has been of such high ethical importance in U.S. society that it overrides practitioner determinations in many situations. Client empowerment is an approach that differs from the paternalistic approach to health care in which decisions are made for, rather than with, the client; instead, it enables patients and professionals to work in partnerships (Aston, Meagher-Stewart, Sheppard-Lemoine, Vukic, & Chircop, 2006; Cawley & McNamara, 2011; Gagnon, Hibert, Dube, & Dubois, 2006). Many physicians and other health providers, including community health nurses, fail to recognize the high value attributed to self-determination by many consumers or the differences in views of self-determination among ethnic groups.

The conflict between provider and consumer may be broader. When self-determination deteriorates into self-interest, it poses a major roadblock to equitable health care. **Self-interest** is the fulfillment of one's own

DISPLAY 4.5 A FRAMEWORK FOR ETHICAL DECISION MAKING

1. *Clarify the ethical dilemma:* Whose problem is it? Who should make the decision? Who is affected by the decision? What ethical principles are related to the problem?
2. *Gather additional data:* Have as much information about the situation as possible. Be up to date on any legal cases related to the ethical question.
3. *Identify options:* Brainstorm with others to identify as many alternatives as possible. The more options identified, the more likely it is that an acceptable solution will be found.
4. *Make a decision:* Choose from the options identified and determine the most acceptable option, the one more feasible than others.
5. *Act:* Carry out the decision. It may be necessary to collaborate with others to implement the decision and identify options.
6. *Evaluate:* After acting on a decision, evaluate its impact. Was the best course of action chosen? Would an alternative have been better? Why? What went right and what went wrong? Why?

desires, without regard for the greater good. Consumers mostly have to fend for themselves when they encounter the world of for-profit health care, just as they do in other commercial markets, where "buyer beware" is the standard (Berwick, Nolan, & Whittington, 2008; Darke & Chaiken, 2005; Pugno, 2008).

When providing health care, self-determination and taking personal responsibility for health care decisions should be nurtured. This includes informing clients of options and the reasoning behind all recommendations. Yet self-determination and personal autonomy at times are impermissible or even impossible. For example, society must impose restrictions on unacceptable client choices, such as child abuse and other abusive behaviors, or situations in which clients are not competent to exercise self-determination, as is true for certain levels of mental illness or dementia. There are two situations in which self-determination should be restricted: when some objectives of individuals are contrary to the public interest or the interests of others in society (e.g., endangering others with a communicable disease), and when a person's decision making is so defective or mistaken that the decision fails to promote the person's own values or goals. When a person cannot fully comprehend the options, the consequences of actions related to the options, and the true costs and benefits, he may not have adequate capacity for making health care decisions. In these situations, self-determination is justifiably overridden on the basis of the promotion of one's own wellbeing or the wellbeing of others—another important value in health care decision making (Guido, 2010; Kelly, 2009).

Wellbeing

Wellbeing is a state of positive health. Although all therapeutic interventions by health care professionals are intended to improve clients' health and promote wellbeing, well-intended interventions sometimes fall short if they are in conflict with clients' preferences and needs. Determining what constitutes health for people and how their wellbeing can be promoted often requires knowledge of clients' subjective preferences. It is generally recognized that clients may be inclined to pursue different directions in treatment procedures based on individual goals, values, and interests. Community health nurses, who are committed not only to helping clients but also to respecting their wishes and avoiding harming them, must understand each client group's needs and develop reasonable alternatives for service from which clients may choose (see From the Case Files II). In addition, when individuals are not capable of making a choice, the nurse or other surrogate decision maker is obliged to make health care decisions that promote the value of wellbeing. This may mean that the alternatives presented by the nurse for choice are only the alternatives that will promote wellbeing. With shared decision making, the nurse not only seeks to understand clients' needs and develop reasonable alternatives to meet those needs, but also to present the alternatives in a way that enables clients to choose those they prefer. Wellbeing and self-determination are two values that are intricately related when providing community health nursing services.

Equity

The third value that is important to decision making in health care contexts is the value of **equity** or justice, which means being treated equally or fairly. The principle of equity implies that it is unjust (or inequitable) to treat people the same if they are, in significant respects, unalike. In other words, different people have different needs in health care, but all must be served equally and adequately. Equity generally means that all individuals should have the same access to health care according to benefit or needs (see Levels of Prevention Pyramid).

The major problem with this definition of equity is, of course, that it assumes that an adequate level of health care can be economically available to all citizens. In times of limited technical, human, and financial resources, however, it may be impossible to fully respect the value of equity (Franco, 2005; Hussein, 2010; Smith, Oveku, Homer, & Zuckerman, 2006). Choices must be

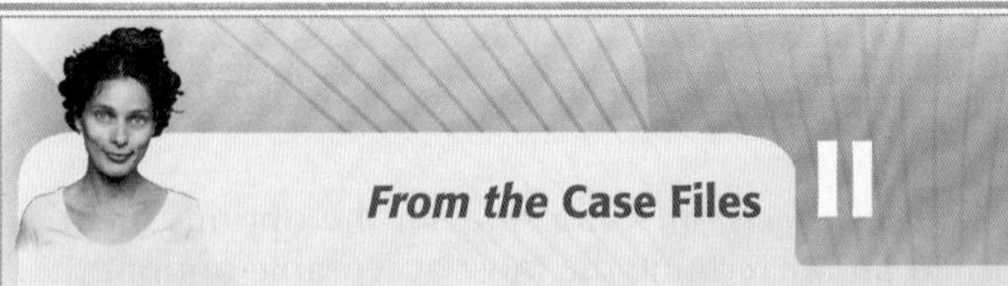

From the Case Files II

Andrea Vargas, PHN—A Family Living in Poverty

Contrasting value systems may be seen in many community health practice settings. Andrea Vargas, a community health nurse, experienced such a contrast on her first home visit to a family living in poverty. Referred by a school nurse for the children's recurring problems with head lice and staphylococcal infections, the family was living in a converted outbuilding on the outskirts of town. While basically clean and orderly, nonetheless the living conditions were cramped, inadequate, and unsafe. Three hammocks were strung, stacked one upon the other, across the far corner of the room to accommodate the three younger children (out of a total of six). The older two children slept on the couch and the floor, while the baby slept with the single mother in the small bed. There was an old gas stove for cooking, and it was currently being used to heat the room, as the wall heater did not work. The mother did not know why it was no longer working. She seemed "stuck"—unable to muster the effort to talk with the landlord about the lack of a working heater. Even though using a gas stove to heat the room was dangerous (due to carbon monoxide), it seemed to her to be the easiest way to deal with the problem. Andrea knew that landlords were sometimes slow to respond to the needs of low-income renters and she saw this as unjust. The mother's main pleasure in life was watching soap operas on television and Andrea felt that the mother seemed disinterested in trying to improve her circumstances. The nurse interpreted the situation through the framework of her own value system, in which health and safety were priorities, and justice was an instrumental value. Yet the mother, who might have shared those values in the past, appeared to prize pleasurable diversion, perhaps as a way to cope with her situation. In this instance, it is possible that environmental influences reordered the family's value system priorities. Rather than imposing her own values, Andrea chose to determine the priorities of the family, assess their needs, and begin where they were. Will she have a greater chance at success by doing this?

made and resources allotted, while the value obligations of professional practice create conflicts of values that seem impossible to resolve. Many of these conflicts are reflected in current health care reform efforts that focus on access to services, quality of services, and ways to control rising costs. However, the following list represents some of the most pressing aggregate health problems related to inequities in the distribution of and access to health and illness care facing our nation:

- *Too many women go without preventive care.* The overall rate of infant mortality (all infant deaths before 1 year of age) is 7 per 1,000 in the United States; it remains among the highest in the industrialized world (Mathews, & MacDorman, 2010). The rates for some people of color—African Americans (13.9), Native Hawaiian and other Pacific Islanders (9.6), and Native Americans (8.6) specifically—are higher than those for White, non-Hispanic (5.8) or Mexican Americans (5.4) (CDC, 2006). Forty-nine percent of pregnancies in the United States during 2001 were unintended—among White and Hispanic females 40% and 54%, respectively, were reported as unintended. But, among African American females, 69% report unintended pregnancies. Poverty is strongly related to difficulty in accessing family planning services (Finer & Henshaw, 2006), as are health care system factors (e.g., access), provider-related factors (e.g., similar culture), and patient preferences (Dehlendorf, Rodrigue, Levy, Borrero, & Steinauer, 2010).
- *Immunization rates for some diseases are at dangerously low levels.* For example, in 2004, about 82% of all children between 19 and 35 months of age had received full doses of childhood vaccines—below the 90% *Healthy People 2010* objective. By ethnicity, though, only 76% of Black children, 81% of Hispanic children, and 74% of American Indian/Alaska Native children received those immunizations. When poverty level was factored in, the total dropped to 78% for those living below the poverty level, with only 73% of Black children immunized (CDC, 2006). Vast disparities in immunization rates also exist for adults along racial and ethnic lines, as well as poverty level. Even with a number of health care encounters and socioeconomic factors controlled for in a study comparing non-Hispanic white and non-Hispanic black influenza vaccination rates, the rate for Blacks was only "70% that of Whites" (Liu, 2011).
- *The uninsured are likely to go without physician care.* Differences in access to expensive, discretionary procedures emerge according to health insurance status, race, and ethnicity, as well as other sociodemographic factors. In 2003, 17% of Americans below the age of 65 reported having no health insurance, with Black and Hispanic Americans being more likely than White non-Hispanic Americans to lack health insurance coverage. Interestingly, only 30% of those without health insurance live below the poverty level (National Center for Health Statistics, 2005). Between 2009 and 2011, an additional 9 million Americans lost health insurance due to unemployment or rising costs of coverage (Wechsler, 2011).
- *Environmental hazards threaten global health.* Global trade, travel, and changing social and cultural patterns make the population vulnerable to diseases that are endemic to other parts of the world, as well as to previously unknown diseases.

LEVELS OF PREVENTION PYRAMID

SITUATION: Provide distributive justice for battered women and children by changing a proposed state law that would eliminate funding for shelters for battered women and children to a law that preserves resources for this population.

GOAL: Using the three levels of prevention, negative health conditions are avoided, or promptly diagnosed and treated, and the fullest possible potential is restored.

TERTIARY PREVENTION		
Rehabilitation	**Primary Prevention**	
	Health Promotion & Education	*Health Protection*
If unable to stop the proposed law: • Seek volunteer services to fill the gaps in funding paid employees • Seek donations to support existing shelter buildings	• Educate the public regarding the need for lost/limited services using various forms of media and/or venues	• Seek private resources or grants to fund shelters • Propose a new bill to match private funding for shelters at the next legislative session

SECONDARY PREVENTION	
Early Diagnosis	**Prompt Treatment**
• Recognition that the proposed bill is going to pass	• Advocate for amendments to the proposed bill to preserve limited funding for shelters

PRIMARY PREVENTION	
Health Promotion & Education	**Health Protection**
• Advocacy • Active lobbying against the bill • Garnering community support in favor of the revised bill	• Community understand the impact of the potential loss • Put a "human face" on the problem

Pollution of air, water, and soil to support industry contributes to pathogen mutations and threatens public health (Selgelid, 2008).

Equity is tied to social justice (see below) and can be a difficult concept to truly grasp because we habitually have difficulty seeing "others" (those unlike us; e.g., the poor, disadvantaged) as worthy of sympathy and concern. Those close to use (more like us; e.g., family, close friends) garner our attention and consideration. True equity occurs when those who are often seen as "inferior others" are treated as "equal in worth" to the historically privileged (Anderson et al., 2009, p. 292) (see Display 4.6, Society and Individual Responsibility in Health Care).

Ethical Decision Making in Community Health Nursing

The key values of self-determination, wellbeing, and equity influence nursing practice in many ways. The value of self-determination has implications for how community health nurses regard:

- The choices of clients
- Privacy
- Informed consent
- Diminished capacity for self-determination

The value of wellbeing has implications for how community health nurses seek to:

- Prevent harm and provide benefits to client populations
- Determine effectiveness of nursing services
- Weigh costs of services against real client benefits

The value of equity has implications for community health nursing in terms of its priorities for:

- Distributing health goods (macroallocation issues)
- Deciding which populations will obtain available health goods and services (microallocation issues)

Decisions based on one value means that this value often will conflict with other values. For example, deciding primarily on the basis of client wellbeing may conflict with deciding on the basis of self-determination or

DISPLAY 4.6 SOCIETY AND INDIVIDUAL RESPONSIBILITY IN HEALTH CARE

To promote the achievement of equity, self-determination, and clients' wellbeing, certain conclusions drawn from the literature can enhance community health nursing practice (Boswell, Cannon, & Miller, 2005; Carnegie & Kiger, 2009; Des Jardin, 2001; Ellenbecker, 2010; Spenceley, Reutter, & Allen, 2006; Swiadek, 2009):

1. *Society has an ethical obligation to ensure equitable access to health care for all.* This obligation is centered on the special importance of health care and is derived from its role in relieving suffering, preventing premature death, restoring functioning, increasing opportunity, providing information about an individual's condition, and giving evidence of mutual empathy and compassion.
2. *The societal obligation is balanced by individual obligations.* Individuals ought to pay a fair share of the cost of their own health care and take reasonable steps to provide for such care when they can do so without excessive burdens.
3. *Equitable access to health care requires that all citizens can secure an adequate level of care without excessive burdens.* Equitable access also means that the burdens borne by individuals in obtaining adequate care ought not to be excessive or to fall disproportionately on particular individuals. Communities need to be empowered to address distribution problems.
4. *When equity occurs through the operation of private forces, there is no need for government involvement.* However, the ultimate responsibility for ensuring that society's obligation is met—through a combination of public and private sector arrangements—rests with the federal government.
5. *The cost of achieving equitable access to health care ought to be shared fairly.* The cost of securing health care for those who are unable to pay ought to be spread equitably at the national level and should not fall more heavily on the shoulders of particular practitioners, institutions, or residents of different localities.
6. *Efforts to contain rising health care costs are important but should not focus on limiting the attainment of equitable access for the least-served portion of the public.* Measures designed to contain health care costs that exacerbate existing inequities or impede the achievement of equity are unacceptable from a moral standpoint. Aggregates in the community should be involved in planning and problem solving to increase the distribution of resources where those resources are most needed.

equity. How community health nurses balance these values may even conflict with their own personal values or the professional values of nursing as a whole. In these situations, values clarification techniques used with an ethical decision making process may assist in producing decisions that promote the greatest wellbeing for clients without substantially reducing their self-determination or ignoring equity.

Ethical Principles

Based in utilitarianism and deontology, seven fundamental ethical principles provide guidance in making decisions regarding clients' care: respect, autonomy, beneficence, nonmaleficence, justice, veracity, and fidelity (Guido, 2010; Thompson et al. 2006).

Respect

The principle of **respect** refers to treating people as unique, equal, and responsible moral agents. This principle emphasizes one's importance as a member of the community and of the health services team. To apply this principle in decision making is to acknowledge community clients as valued participants in shaping their own and the community's health outcomes. It includes treating them as equals on the health team and holding them, as well as their views, in high regard.

Autonomy

The principle of **autonomy** means freedom of choice and the exercise of people's rights. Individualism and self-determination are dominant values underlying this principle (The William Glasser Institute, 2010). As nurses apply this principle in community health, they promote individuals' and groups' rights to and involvement in decision making. This is true, however, only so long as those decisions enhance these individuals' and groups' wellbeing and do not harm the wellbeing of others (Easley & Allen, 2007; Ebbesen & Pedersen, 2008; Franco, 2005). When applying this principle, nurses should make certain that clients are fully informed and that the decisions are made deliberately, with careful consideration of the consequences (see From the Case Files III).

Beneficence

The ethical principle of **beneficence** means doing good or benefiting others. It is the promotion of good or taking action to ensure positive outcomes on behalf of clients (Stanford Encyclopedia of Philosophy, 2008). In community health, the nurse applies the principle of beneficence by making decisions that actively promote community clients' best interests and wellbeing (Easley & Allen, 2007). Examples might encompass the development of a seniors' health program that ensures equal access to all

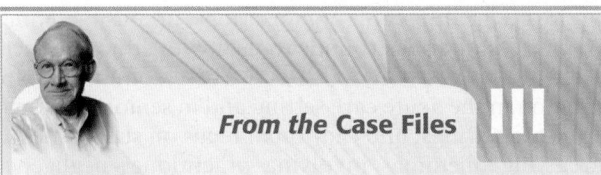

Tom Hardy, PHN—An Elderly Client Gives Up

Tom Hardy, PHN, has been assigned to monitor Mr. Jack, an elderly man who was diagnosed with tuberculosis (TB) (positive skin test, positive sputum and x-ray). Mr. Jack's wife unexpectedly died recently, and he is depressed and wants to "join her." He is not eating or sleeping much. He refuses to take TB medications, or his eight other medications for heart disease, thyroid insufficiency, type 2 diabetes, glaucoma, high cholesterol and triglycerides, and hypertension. He has consistently refused any of Tom's suggestions or assistance. He does not want to see a mental health counselor, and Tom wonders if he should continue to make home visits. He has a busy caseload and needs to focus on the most pressing cases. Mr. Jack's children feel that his depression and refusal of medications is a "temporary condition" in response to his wife's death, and have asked for Tom's assistance in keeping their father healthy. Why is this an ethical dilemma? What are the ethical principles involved? What does Mr. Jack value? What are his children's values? Tom's values? Prioritize your values. What are the possible actions you could take?

in the community who are in need, and the support of programs to encourage preschool immunizations.

Nonmaleficence

The principle of **nonmaleficence** means avoiding or preventing harm to others as a consequence of a person's own choices and actions (Stanford Encyclopedia of Philosophy, 2008). This involves taking steps to avoid negative consequences. Community health nurses can apply this ethical principle in decision making by actions such as encouraging physicians to prescribe drugs with the fewest side effects, promoting legislation to protect the environment from pollutants emitted from gasoline even if it raises prices, and lobbying for lower speed limits or gun controls to save lives.

Justice

The principle of **justice** refers to treating people fairly (Easley & Allen, 2007). It means the fair distribution of both benefits and costs among society's members. Examples might include equal access to health care, equitable distribution of services to rural as well as urban populations, not limiting the amount or quality of services because of income level, and fair distribution of resources—all of these draw on the principle of justice.

Within this principle are three different views on allocation, or what constitutes the meaning of "fair" distribution. One, **distributive justice**, says that benefits should be given first to the disadvantaged or those who need them most (see Levels of Prevention Pyramid). Decisions based on this view particularly help the needy, although it may mean withholding goods from others who may also be deserving, but less in need (e.g., food stamps). The second view, **egalitarian justice**, promotes decisions based on equal distribution of benefits to everyone, regardless of need (e.g., Medicare). The third, **restorative justice**, determines that benefits should go primarily to those who have been wronged by prior injustice, such as victims of crime or racial discrimination. Programs are in place to compensate victims for their injury or families for their loss—a beginning step to "restore justice." Another example includes the funds that were set up by several agencies, corporations, and groups to assist the families of the victims of the September 11, 2001 terrorist attacks. The principle of justice seeks to promote equity, a value that was discussed in the previous section.

Social justice refers to the fair and equitable distribution of "social benefits and burdens" (e.g., economic goods, political rights) and is tied to issues of human rights (Easley & Allen, 2007, p. 371). The National Association of Social Workers describes social justice as the "view that everyone deserves equal economic, political and social rights and responsibilities" (2011, para. 2). See Chapter 25 for more on social justice.

Veracity

The principle of **veracity** refers to telling the truth. Community clients deserve to be given accurate information in a timely manner. To withhold information or not tell the truth can be self-serving to the nurse or other health care providers and hurtful, as well as disrespectful, to clients. Truth-telling involves treating clients as equals, and it expands the opportunity for greater client involvement, as well as provides needed information for decision making (Arries, 2006).

Fidelity

The final ethical principle, **fidelity**, means keeping promises. People deserve to count on commitments being met. This principle involves the issues of trust and trustworthiness. Nurses who follow through on what they have said earn their clients' respect and trust. In turn, this influences the quality of the nurse's relationship with clients, who then are more likely to share information, which leads to improved decisions and better health. Conversely, when a promise (e.g., a commitment to institute child care during health classes) is not kept, community members may lose faith and interest in participation.

Ethical Standards and Guidelines

As the number and complexity of ethical decisions in community health increase, so too does the need for ethical standards and guidelines to help nurses make the best choices possible. The ANA's *Code for Nurses with Interpretive Statements* (2001) provides a helpful guide. Some health care organizations and community agencies, using the ANA code or a similar document, have developed their own specific standards and guidelines. For instance, the Public Healthy Leadership Society has published *Principles of the Ethical Practice of Public Health* (2002), to guide both institutions and individual practitioners as they serve the public. The guidelines encompass the ethical principles of respect, autonomy, equity, and beneficence, while also highlighting the need for fidelity and confidentiality. The Association of State and Territorial Directors of Nursing (ASTDN, n.d.), a public health nursing organization, incorporated ethical principles into their guidelines for the PHN role in eliminating health inequities (e.g., respect, beneficence, autonomy).

More health care organizations are using ethics committees or ethics rounds to deal with ethical aspects of client services (Guido, 2010). These committees are common in the acute care setting and in senior and long-term care settings, and they often focus on such issues as caregiving dilemmas involving practitioner negligence or poor client outcomes and the related health care decisions. In long-term care and home care settings, such a committee may consider conflicts in client care issues that involve family members. However, these committees also function in a variety of community health care settings. In public health agencies, cases of clients with complicated communicable disease diagnoses and health care provider concerns are discussed as they relate to policy, protocols, and the health and safety of the broader population.

SUMMARY

Implementation of EBP enables community health nurses to promote health and prevent illness among at-risk populations and to design and evaluate community-based interventions. EBP is essential to ensuring economical and effective interventions for our clients. Systematic reviews can provide direction for those who have developed a "burning clinical question." Finding accurate, complete information and critically appraising it is vital (see Evidence-Based Practice: Handwashing).

Research is defined as the systematic collection and analysis of data related to a particular problem or phenomenon. *EBP* is characterized as the use of best evidence, along with the nurse's clinical judgment and knowledge of patient's wishes, in making decisions about nursing practice and client outcomes. It encompasses the steps outlined in Display 4.1.

Systematic reviews are summaries of evidence usually compiled and analyzed by expert panels on a specific problem of interest, using predetermined criteria.

Research has a significant impact on community health and nursing practice in three ways. It provides new knowledge that helps to shape health policy, improve service delivery, and promote the public's health. It contributes to nursing knowledge and the improvement of nursing practice. And it offers the potential to enhance nursing's status and influence through documentation of the effectiveness of nursing interventions and broader recognition of nursing's contributions to health services.

Nurses must become responsible consumers of research, keeping abreast of new knowledge and applying it in practice. Nurses must learn to evaluate evidence critically, assessing the validity and applicability to their own practice. Nurses should search for current evidence and discuss EBP initiatives with colleagues and supervisors. More community health nurses must also conduct EBP implementation studies of their own or collaborate with other community health professionals in doing clinical research. A commitment to the use and conduct of research will move the nursing profession forward and enhance its influence on the health of at-risk populations.

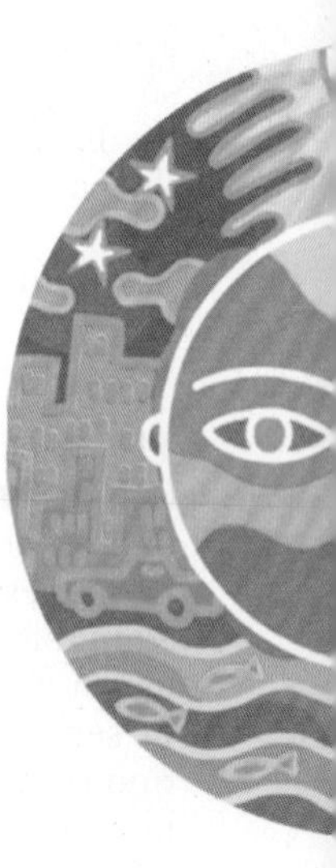

Values and ethical principles strongly influence community health nursing practice and ethical decision making. *Values* are lasting beliefs that are important to individuals, groups, and cultures. A value system organizes these beliefs into a hierarchy of relative importance that motivates and guides human behavior. Values function as standards for behavior, as criteria for attitudes, and as standards for moral judgments, and they give expression to human needs. The nature of values can be understood by examining their qualities of endurance, their hierarchical arrangement, and their function as prescriptive–proscriptive beliefs and by examining them in terms of reference and preference.

The nurse often is faced with decisions that affect client's values and involve conflicting moral values and ethical dilemmas. Understanding what personal values are and how they affect behavior

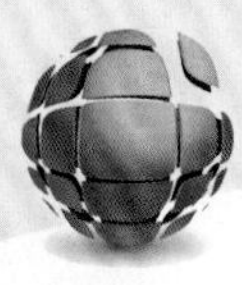

EVIDENCE-BASED PRACTICE

Handwashing

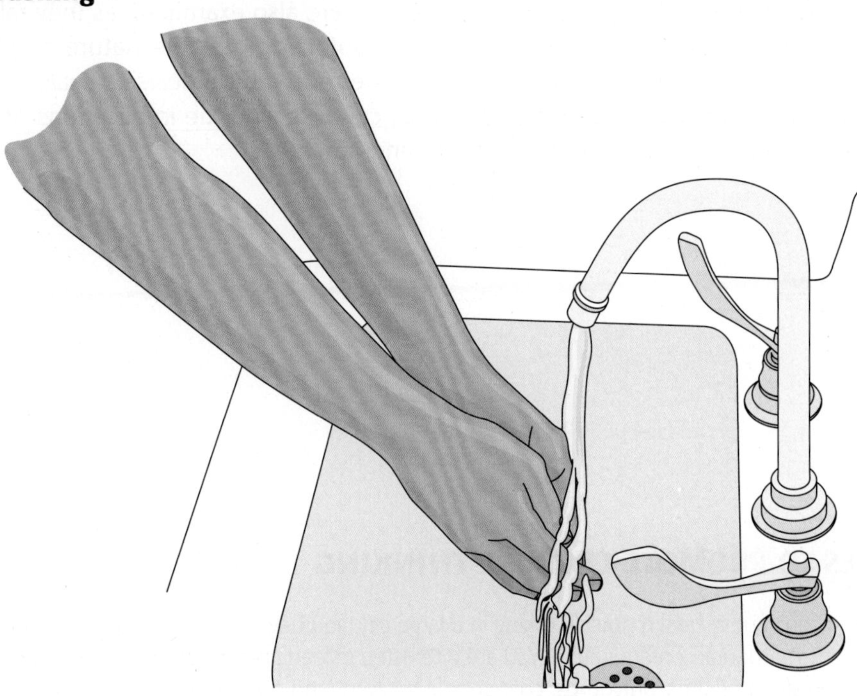

As nurses, we are taught the importance of handwashing. In nursing school, we are educated to wash our hands before and after patient care—it is often drilled into us. But, when you work in the community, you do not always have ready access to soap and water. Many public health nurses (PHNs) choose to carry small bottles of hand sanitizer as a practical alternative to handwashing. But, is this effective? Early research has shown promise. A small study of health care workers in France found that handrubbing with an alcohol-based mixture was better than handwashing with antiseptic soap when it came to reducing hand bacterial contamination for workers in intensive care settings, and a larger study examining surgical site infections showed no statistical differences between the two methods (Girou, Loyeau, Legrand, Oppein, & Brun-Buisson, 2002; Parienti, Thibon, Heller, et al., 2002). Newer research has confirmed the effectiveness of waterless alcohol-based hand sanitizers for new mothers living in areas without adequate water supplies (Pickering, Boehm, Mwanjali, & Davis, 2010). However, staff perceptions about adverse effects (e.g., dry hands) and inadequate handwashing technique (e.g., missed areas) may affect outcomes (Macdonald, McKillop, Trotter, & Gray, 2006; Stutz et al., 2009). Where would you go to find a systematic or integrative review of this subject? How would you go about presenting this information at a staff meeting to stimulate changes in policies and procedures?

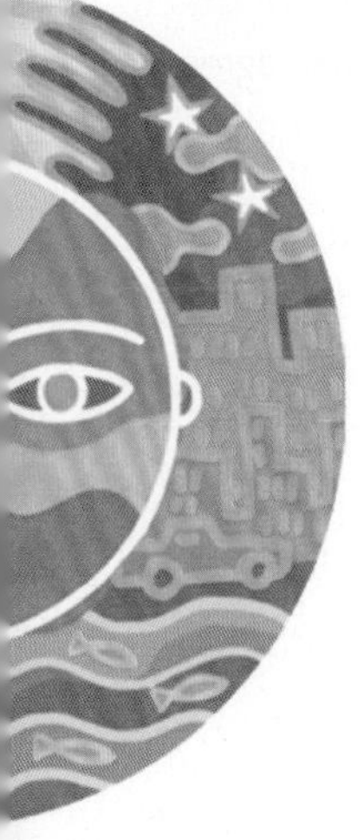

assists the nurse in making ethical evaluations and addressing ethical conflicts in practice. Various strategies can guide the nurse in making these decisions; one example is values clarification, which clarifies what values are important. Several frameworks for ethical decision making that include the identification and clarification of values impinging on the making of ethical decisions were discussed in this chapter.

Three key human values influence client health and nurse decision making: the right to make decisions regarding a person's health (self-determination), the right to health and wellbeing, and the right to equal access and quality of health care. At times, these values are affected by the value of self-interest on the part of another person or a system. Seven fundamental principles guide community health nurses in making ethical decisions: respect, autonomy, beneficence, nonmaleficence, justice, veracity, and fidelity.

This chapter discusses current research as it relates to and impacts community health nursing practice. The steps of EBP are emphasized. The chapter includes information on constructing a clinical question and incorporating client considerations and clinical guidelines, as well as helpful resources for finding and analyzing research studies. Ethics and values are also examined, as they relate to both research and community health nursing practice. This chapter explores the nature and function of values and value systems, the role of values and value systems in ethical decision making, the central values related to health care choices and their potential conflicts, and the implications of values and ethics for community health nursing decision making and practice.

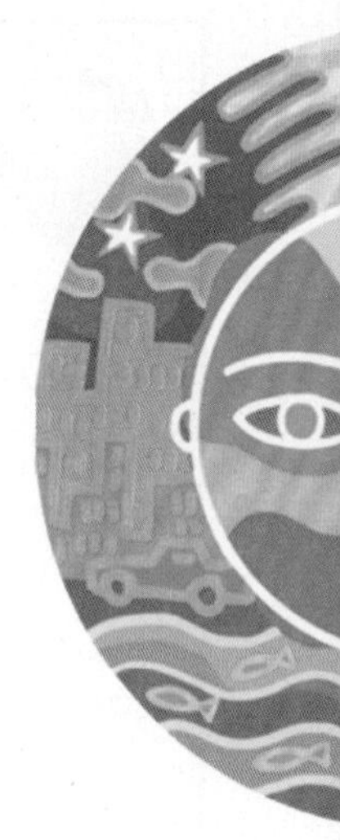

ACTIVITIES TO PROMOTE **CRITICAL THINKING**

1. As a community health nurse working in a large city, you have a large number of children with lead poisoning due to environmental contamination. You are interested in lead abatement programs. Where can you find evidence on successful programs/outcomes, cost-benefit analysis, and policies that have been implemented in other areas?
2. You want to determine whether a group of sexually active teenagers who are at risk for acquired immunodeficiency syndrome (AIDS) would be receptive to an educational program on HIV/AIDS. Where would you look for a systematic review on this topic?
3. Select a community health nursing systematic review or research article from the references listed in this chapter (or choose one of your own) and analyze its potential impact on health policy and on community health nursing practice.
4. You have just completed an evidence-based practice (EBP) implementation study on the effectiveness of a series of birth control classes in three high schools, and the results show a reduction in the number of pregnancies over the last year. Describe three ways in which you could disseminate this information to your nursing colleagues and other community health professionals.
5. You are alarmed to note that the new area to which you have been assigned has high rates of tuberculosis. Using the Internet and your college library databases to research this topic, determine the most effective forms of treatment and discuss the feasibility of implementing some newer approaches with your specific target population.
6. Take the BBC Morals–Social Responsibility Questionnaire (available at: http://www.bbc.co.uk/science/humanbody/mind/surveys/morals) and discuss your results with a trusted classmate. How similar were your responses? Why?
7. Describe where you stand on the following issues. For each statement, decide whether you strongly agree, agree, disagree, strongly disagree, or are undecided.
   a. Clients have the right to participate in all decisions related to their health care.
   b. Nurses need a system designed to credit self-study.
   c. Continuing education should not be mandatory to maintain licensure.
   d. Clients always should be told the truth.
   e. Standards of nursing practice should be enforced by state examining boards.
   f. Nurses should be required to take relicensure examinations every 5 years.
   g. Clients should be allowed to read their health record on request.
   h. Abortion on demand should be an option available to every woman.
   i. Critically ill newborns should be allowed to die.
   j. Laws should guarantee desired health care for each person in this country.
   k. Organ donorship should be automatic unless a waiver to refuse has been signed.

8. In a grid similar to the one shown, write a statement of belief in the space provided and examine it in relation to the seven steps of the process of valuing. Areas of confusion and conflict in nursing practice that should be examined are peer review, accountability, confidentiality, euthanasia, licensure, clients' rights, organ donation, abortion, informed consent, and terminating treatment. To the right of your statements, check the appropriate boxes to indicate when your beliefs reflect one or more of the seven steps in the valuing process. Is your belief a value according to the valuing process?
9. Rank in order the following 12 potential nursing actions, using "1" to indicate the most important choice in a client–community health nurse relationship and "12" to indicate the least important choice.

	Freely chosen	Alternatives	Consequences	Cherished	Affirmed	Incorporated	Employed
Statement	1	2	3	4	5	6	7

_____ Touching clients
_____ Empathetically listening to clients
_____ Disclosing yourself to clients
_____ Becoming emotionally involved with clients
_____ Teaching clients
_____ Being honest in answering clients' questions
_____ Seeing that clients conform to professionals' advice
_____ Helping to decrease clients' anxiety
_____ Making sure that clients are involved in decision making
_____ Following legal mandates regarding health practices
_____ Remaining "professional" with clients
_____ (Add an alternative of your own)

Examine your ordering of these options. What values can be identified based on your responses in this exercise? How do these values emerge in your behavior?

10. Request to attend two or three sessions of an ethics committee meeting of a community health agency or a local acute care hospital. Observe and make notes on (a) what values are evident in the discussion, (b) what ethical principles are used, (c) what decision-making framework is used, and (d) what you would have liked to contribute if you had been a member of the committee.

REFERENCES

Abhyankar, P., Bekker, H., Summers, B., & Velikova, G. (2011). Why values elicitation techniques enable people to make informed decisions about cancer trial participation. *Health Expectations, 14*(Suppl 1), 20–32.

Ahmad, S. (2005a). Closing the youth access gap: The projected health benefits and cost savings of a national policy to raise the legal smoking age to 21 in the United States. *Health Policy, 75*(1), 74–84.

Ahmad, S. (2005b). The cost-effectiveness of raising the legal smoking age in California. *Medical Decision Making, 25*(3), 330–340.

Ahmad, S. (2005c). Increasing excise taxes on cigarettes in California: A dynamic simulation of health and economic impacts. *Preventive Medicine, 41*(1), 276–283.

Alamar, B., & Glantz, S.A. (2006). Effect of increased social unacceptability of cigarette smoking on reduction in cigarette consumption. *American Journal of Public Health, 96*(8), 1359–1363.

Albrecht, S., Maloni, J., Thomas, K., Jones, R., Halleran, J., & Osborne, J. (2006). Smoking cessation counseling for pregnant women who smoke: Scientific basis for practice for WWHONN's SUCCESS project. *Journal of Obstetric, Gynecological and Neonatal Nursing*. Published online March 9, 2006, doi: 10.1177/0884217504265353

AllAfrica. (2011, April 18). *Africa: Prevention drug trial disappoints*. Retrieved from http://allafrica.com/stories/201104190163.html

Allicock, M., Sandelowski, M., DeVellis, B., & Campbell, M. (2008). Variations in meanings of the personal core value "health". *Patient Education and Counseling, 73*(2), 347–353.

American Academy of Pediatrics. (2005). Policy statement: Task force on sudden infant death syndrome. *Pediatrics, 116*(5), 1245–1255.

American Academy of Pediatrics (AAP). (2008). *A parents' guide to safe sleep: Helping you to reduce the risk of SIDS*. Retrieved from http://www.healthychildcare.org/pdf/SIDSparentsafesleep.pdf

American Nurses Association (AMA). (2001). *Code for nurses with interpretive statements*. Washington, DC: Author.

Amitai, Y., Fisher, N., Meiraz, H., Baram, N., Tounis, M., & Leventhal, A. (2008). Preconceptual folic acid utilization in Israel: Five years after the guidelines. *Preventive Medicine, 46*(2), 166–169.

Anderson, J., Rodney, P., Reimer-Kirkham, S., Browne, A., Khan, K. B., & Lynam, M. J. (2009). Inequities in health and healthcare viewed through the ethical lens of critical social justice: Contextual knowledge for the global priorities ahead. *Advances in Nursing Science, 32*(4), 282–294.

Annweiler, C., Allali, G., Allain, P., Bridenbaugh, S., Schott, A., Kressig, R., et al. (2009). Vitamin D and cognitive performance in adults: A systematic review. *European Journal of Neurology, 16*(10), 1083–1089.

Annweiler, C., Schott, A., Bridenbaugh, S., Kressig, R., Allain, P., Herrmann, F., et al. (2010). Association of vitamin D deficiency with cognitive impairment in older women. *Neurology, 74*(1), 27–32.

Aos, S., Lieb, R., Mayfield, J., Miller, M., & Pennucci, A. (2004). *Benefits and costs of prevention and early intervention programs for youth*. Olympia, WA: Washington State Institute for Public Policy.

Arries, E. (2006). Virtue ethics: An approach to moral dilemmas in nursing. *Kidney International, 69*(6), 954–955.

Associated Press. (2006). U.S. halts enrollment in major AIDS drug study. Retrieved January 18, 2006, from http//www.msnbc. msn. com/id/10907973/print/1/displaymode/1098/

Association of State and Territorial Directors of Nursing (ASTDN). (n.d.). *The public health nurse's role in achieving health equity: Eliminating inequalities in health*. Position Paper: Author. Retrieved from http://www.astdn.org/downloadablefiles/ASTDN-health-equity-11-08.pdf

Aston, M., Meagher-Stewart, D., Sheppard-Lemoine, D., Vukic, A., & Chircop, A. (2006). Family health nursing and empowering relationships. *Pediatric Nursing, 32*(1), 61–67.

Axtell-Thompson, L. M. (2005). Consumer directed health care: Ethical limits to choice and responsibility. *Journal of Medical Philosophy, 39*(2), 207–226.

Baily, M.A. (2008). Harming through protection? *New England Journal of Medicine, 358*(8), 768–769.

Baker, D., Dang, M., Ly, M., & Diaz, R. (2010). Perception of barriers to immunization among parents of Hmong origin in California. *American Journal of Public Health, 100*(5), 839–845.

Barlow, J., Smailagic, N., Bennett, C., Huband, N., Jones, H., & Coren, E. (2011). *Individual and group parenting for improving psychosocial outcomes for teenage parents and their children*. Campbell Systematic Reviews. Available at http://www.campbellcollaboration.org/library.php

Bartels, D., Bauman, C., Skitka, L., & Medin, C. (2009). *Moral judgment and decision making*. New York: Elsevier.

Bartik, T. J. (2009, June 8). *Estimated state and local fiscal effects of the Nurse Family Partnership program*. Upjohn Institute. Staff Working Paper No. 09–152. Available at: http://ssrn.com/abstract=1447868

Bayles, B. (2010). Perceptions of childhood obesity on the Texas-Mexico border. *Public Health Nursing, 27*(4), 320–328.

Beauchamp, T., & Childress, J. (2008). *Principles of biomedical ethics* (6th ed.). Oxford, UK: Oxford University Press.

Berwick, D., Nolan, T., & Whittington, J. (2008). The triple aim: Care, health, and cost. *Health Affairs, 27*(3), 759–769.

Blais, K.K., Hayes, J. S. (2011). *Professional nursing practice: Concepts and perspectives* (6th ed.). Upper Saddle River, NJ: Pearson Prentice Hall.

Bonner, A. (2007). Understanding the role of knowledge in the practice of expert nephrology nurses in Australia. *Nursing and Health Sciences, 9*(3), 161–167.

Boswell, C., Cannon, S., & Miller, J. (2005). Nurses' political involvement: Responsibility versus privilege. *Journal of Professional Nursing, 21*(1), 5–8.

Buell, J., Dawson-Hughes, B., Scott, T., Weiner, E., Dallal, G., Qui, W., et al.(2010). 25-hydroxyvitamin D dementia, and derebrovascular pathology in elders receiving home services. *Neurology, 74*, 18–26.

California Department of Public Health. (2008). *Facts about sudden infant death syndrome (SIDS): Mortality in California 2008*. Sacramento, CA: Author.

Callister, L., Luthy, K., Thompson, P., & Memmott, R. (2009). Ethical reasoning in baccalaureate nursing students. *Nursing Ethics, 16*(4), 499–510.

Carnegie, E., & Kiger, A. (2009). Being and doing politics: An outdated model or 21st century reality? *Journal of Advanced Nursing, 65*(9), 1976–1984.

Carper, B.A. (1978). Fundamental patterns of knowing in nursing. *Advances in Nursing Science, 1*(1), 13–23.

Cassey, M. A. (2007). Incorporating the National Guideline Clearninghouse into evidence-based nursing practice. *Nursing Economics, 25*(5) 302–303.

Cawley, T., & McNamara, P. M. (2011). Public health nurse perceptions of empowerment and advocacy in child health surveillance in West Ireland. *Public Health Nursing, 28*(2), 1–9.

Centers for Disease Control and Prevention (CDC). (2007). *Quickstats: Infant mortality rates for 10 leading causes of DEATH, United States, 2005*. Retrieved from http://www.cdc.gov/mmwr/preview/mmwrhtml/mm5642a8.htm

Centers for Disease Control & Prevention (CDC). (2009). *The Tuskegee timeline*. Retrieved February 28, 2011 from http://www.cdc.gov/tuskgee/timeline.htm

Centers for Disease Control & Prevention (CDC). (2011). *Public health ethics*. Retrieved from http://www.cdc.gov/od/science/integrity/phethics/

Chassin, M. Loeb, J., Schmaltz, S., & Wachter, R. (2010). Accountability measures: Using measurement to promote quality improvement. *New England Journal of Medicine, 363*(7), 683–688.

Child Welfare Information Gateway. (2010). Nurse-family partnership. Retrieved from http://www.childwelfare.gov/preventing/programs/types/nursefamily.cfm

Clark, A. P. (2010). A model for ethical decision making in cases of patient futility. *Clinical Nurse Specialist, 24*(4), 189–190.

Colby, A., & Kohlberg, L. (1987). *The measurement of moral judgment: Theoretical foundations and research validation* (Vol. 1). New York: Cambridge University Press.

Coopersmith, S. (1967). *The antecedents of self-esteem*. San Francisco, CA: Freeman & Company.

Cross, S., Block, D., Josten, L., Reckinger, D., Keller, L. O., Strohschein, S., et al.(2006). Development of the public health nursing competency instrument. *Public Health Nursing, 23*(2), 108–114.

Culley, J. M., & Effken, J. A. (2010). Development and validation of a mass casualty conceptual model. *Journal of Nursing Scholarship, 42*(1), 66–75.

Darke, P., & Chaiken, S. (2005). The pursuit of self-interest: Self-interest bias in attitude judgment and persuasion. *Journal of Personality and Social Psychology, 89*(6), 864–883.

Davies, B., Edwards, N., Ploeg, J., & Virani, T. (2008). Insights about the process and impact of implementing nursing guidelines on delivery of care in hospitals and community settings. *BMC Health Services Research, 2*(8), 29.

Dehlendorf, C., Rodriguez, M., Levy, K., Borrero, S., & Steinauer, J. (2010). Disparities in family planning. *American Journal of Obstetrics and Gynecology, 202*(3), 214–220.

Des Jardin, K. (2001). Political involvement in nursing: Politics, ethics, and strategic action. *AORN Journal, 74*(5), 614–626.

Doane, G. H., Storch, J., & Pauly, B. (2009). Ethical nursing practice: Inquiry-in-action. *Nursing Inquiry, 16*(3) 232–240.

Domian, E., Baggett, K., Carta, J., Mitchell, S., & Larson, E. (2010). Factors influencing mothers' abilities to engage in a comprehensive parenting intervention program. *Public Health Nursing, 27*(5), 399–407.

Doren, D., Haynes, R., Kushniruk, A., Straus, S., Grimshaw, J., Hall, L., et al.(2010). Supporting evidence-based practice for nurses through informational technologies. *Worldviews on Evidence-Based Practice, 7*(1), 4–15.

Douglas, M. R., Mallonee, S., & Istre, G.R. (1999). Estimating the proportion of homes with functioning smoke alarms: A comparison of telephone survey and household survey results. *American Journal of Public Health, 89*(7), 1112–1114.

Dresser, R. (2010). Stem cell research as innovation: Expanding the ethical and policy conversation. *Journal of Law and Medical Ethics, 38*(2), 332–341.

Duncan, J. R., Paterson, D. S., Hoffman, J. M., Mokler, D. J., Borenstein, N. S., Belliveau, R.A., et al. (2010). Brainstem serotonergic deficiency in sudden infant death syndrome. *Journal of the American Medical Association, 303*(5), 430–437.

Durazo E., Jones, M., Wallace, S., Van Arsdale, J., Aydin, M., & Stewart, C. (2011, June). The health status and unique health challenges of rural older adults in California. *Health Policy Brief*. Retrieved from http://www.healthpolicy.ucla.edu/pubs/files/ruralolderadultspb.pdf

Easley, C. E., & Allen, C. E. (2007). A critical intersection: Human rights, public health nursing, and nursing ethics. *Advances in Nursing Science, 30*(4), 367–382.

Ebbesen, M., & Pedersen, B. (2008). The principle of respect for autonomy: Concordant with the experience of oncology physicians and molecular biologists in their daily work? *BMC Medical Ethics, 9*(5), doi: 10.1186/1472-6939-9-5.

Eckenrode, J., Campa, M., Luckey, D., Henderson, C., Cole, R., Kitzman, H., et al. (2010). Long-term effects of prenatal and infancy nurse home visitation on the life course of youths. *Archives of Pediatrics and Adolescent Medicine, 16*(1), 9–15.

Eckenrode, J., Ganzel, B., Henderson, C., Smith, E., Olds, D. L., Powers, J., et al. (2000). Preventing child abuse and neglect with a program of nurse home visitation: The limiting effects of domestic violence. *Journal of the American Medical Association, 284*(11), 1385–1391.

Eckenrode, J., Zielinski, D., Smith, E., Marcynyszyn, L., Henderson, C., Kitzman, H., et al. (2001). Child maltreatment and the early onset of problem behaviors: Can a program of nurse home visitation break the link? *Developmental Psychopathology, 13*(4), 873–890.

Edelman, C., & Mandle, C. (2006). *Health promotion throughout the life span* (6th ed.). St. Louis, MO: Elsevier-Mosby.

Edwards, K. A., & Robey, T. (2010). Preparing for the unexpected: Teaching ER ethics. *Virtual Mentor, 12*(6), 455–458.

Ellenbecker, C. H. (2010). Preparing the nursing workforce of the future. *Policy, Politics, and Nursing Practice, 11*(2), 115–125.

Ertin, H., Harmanci, A., Mahmutoglu, F., & Basagaoglu, I. (2010). Nurse-focused ethical solutions to problems in organ transplantation. *Nursing Ethics, 17*(6), 705–714.

Evatt, M. L. (2010). Vitamin D and cognitive decline in elderly persons. *Archives of Neurology, 67*(12), 1513–1515.

Feldman-Stewart, D., Brennenstuhl, S., Brundage, M., & Roques, T. (2006). An explicit values clarification task: Development and validation. *Patient Education and Counseling, 63*(3), 3350–356.

Ferng, Y. H., Wong-McLoughlin, J., Barrett, A., Currie, L., & Larson, E. (2011). Barriers to mask wearing for influenza-like illnesses among urban Hispanic households. *Public Health Nursing, 28*(1), 13–23.

Finer, L. B., & Henshaw, S. K. (2006). Disparities in rates of unintended pregnancy in the United States, 1994 and 2001. *Perspectives on Sexual and Reproductive Health, 88*(2), 90–96.

Flemming, K. (2007). The knowledge base for evidence-based nursing: A role for mixed methods research? *Advances in Nursing Science, 30*(1), 41–51.

Flynn, L., Budd, M., & Modelski, J. (2008). Enhancing resource utilization among pregnant adolescents. *Public Health Nursing, 25*(2), 140–148.

Food and Drug Administration (FDA). (2010, September 23). *FDA significantly restricts access to the diabetes drug Avandia*. FDA News Release. Retrieved from http://www.fda.gov/newsevents/newsroom/pressannouncements/ucm226975.htm

Food and Drug Administration (FDA). (2011, May 18). *Avandia: REMS—risk of cardiovascular events*. FDA News Release. Retrieved from http://www.fda.gov/Safety/MedWatch/SafetyInformation/SafetyAlertsforHumanMedicalProducts/ucm226994.htm

Fowler, M. D. (2010). *Guide to the code of ethics for nurses: Interpretation and application* (eBook). Silver Springs, MD: American Nurses Association.

Franco, G. (2005). Ethical analysis of the decision-making process in occupational health practice. *Medical Law, 96*(5), 375–382.

Gagnon, M., Hibert, R., Dube, M., & Dubois, M. (2006). Development and validation of an instrument measuring individual empowerment in relation to personal health care: The Health Care Empowerment Questionnaire (HCEQ). *American Journal of Health Promotion, 20*(6), 429–435.

Garwick, A., Seppelt, A., & Riesgraf, M. (2010). Addressing asthma management challenges in a multisite, urban Health Start program. *Public Health Nursing, 27*(4), 329–336.

Gawande, A. (2010). *The checklist manifesto: How to get things right*. New York: Metropolitan Books.

Gecas, V. (2008). The ebb and flow of sociological interest in values. *Sociological Forum, 23*(2), 344–350.

Gessert, C., Elliott, B., & McAlpine, C. (2006). Family decision-making for nursing home residents with dementia: Rural-urban differences. *The Journal of Rural Health, 22*(1), 1–8.

Gilligan, C. (1982). *In a different voice*. Cambridge, MA: Harvard University Press.

Giovino, G. A., Chaloupka F. J., Hartman A. M., Gerlach Joyce K, Chriqui J, Orleans C T, et al. (2009). *Cigarette smoking prevalence and policies in the 50 states: An era of change—The Robert Wood Johnson Foundation impact Teen Tobacco Chart Book*. Buffalo, NY: State University of New York, 2009.

Girou, E. M., Loyeau, S., Legrand, P., Oppein, F., & Brun-Buisson, C. (2002). Efficacy of handrubbing with alcohol based solution versus standard handwashing with antiseptic soap: Randomized clinical trial. *British Medical Journal, 325*, 362–365.

Glavin, K., Smith, L., Sorum, R., & Ellefsen, B. (2010). Supportive counseling by public health nurses for women with postpartum depression. *Journal of Advanced Nursing, 66*(6), 1317–1327.

Guido, G. W. (2010). *Legal and ethical issues in nursing* (5th ed.). Upper Saddle River, NJ: Pearson-Prentice Hall.

Harris, S. (2010). *The moral landscape: How science can determine moral values*. New York: Free Press.

Hinshaw, A. S., & Grady, P. A. (Eds.). (2011). *Shaping health policy through nursing research*. New York: Springer.

Hoffman, H., Damus, K., Hillman, L., & Krongrad, E. (1988). Risk factors for SIDS. Results of the National Institute of Child Health and Human Development SIDS Cooperative

Epidemiological Study. *Annals of the New York Academy of Sciences, 533*, 13–30.

Horodynski, M., Stommel, M., Brophy-Herb, H., Xie, Y., & Weatherspoon, L. (2010). Low-income African Amerian and non-Hispanic White mothers' self-efficacy, "picky eater" perception, and toddler fruit and vegetable consumption. *Public Health Nursing, 27*(5), 408–417.

Hussein, G. M. A. (2010). When ethics survive where people do not. *Public Health Ethics, 3*(10, 72–77.

Institute of Medicine (IOM). (2000). *To err is human: Building a safer health care system*. Washington, DC: National Academies Press.

Institute of Medicine (IOM). (2001). *Crossing the quality chasm: A new health system for the 21st century*. Washington, DC: National Academies Press.

Institute of Medicine. (2003). *Priority areas for national action: Transforming health care quality*. Washington, DC: National Academies Press.

Institute of Medicine. (2011). *The future of nursing: Leading change, advancing health*. Washington, DC: National Academies Press.

Isaacs, J. B. (2007). *Cost-effective investments in children*. Washington, DC: The Brookings Institution.

Isaacs, J. B. (2008). *Impacts of early childhood programs: Nurse home visiting*. Washington, DC: The Brookings Institution.

Iserson, K. V. (1999). Ethical issues in emergency medicine. *Emergency Medicine Clinics of North America, 17*(2), 283–306.

Jack, S. M. (2006). Utility of qualitative research findings in evidence-based public health practice. *Public Health Nursing, 23*(3), 277–283.

Janoff-Bulman, R., Sheikh, S, & Hepp, S. (2009). Proscriptive versus prescriptive morality: Two faces of moral regulation. *Journal of Personality and Social Psychology, 96*(3), 521–537.

Jecker, N., Jonsen, A., & Pearlman, R. (2007). *Bioethics: An introduction to the history, methods, and practice* (2nd ed.). Sudbury, MA: Jones & Bartlett Publishers.

Johnston, C. S. (1995). The Rokeach Value Survey: Underlying structure and multidimensional scaling. *Journal of Psychology, 129*(5), 583–597.

Jones, J. (2010, December 3). *Nurses top honesty and ethics list for 11th year*. Gallup Poll. Retrieved from http://www.gallup.com/poll/145043/nurses-top-honesty-ethics-list-11-year.aspx

Kagawa-Singer M., Tanjasiri, S., Valdez, H., Yu, H., & Foo, M. (2009). Outcomes of a breast health project for Hmong women and men in California. *American Journal of Public Health, 99*(S2), S467–S473.

Kass, N. E. (2001). An ethics framework for public health. *American Journal of Public Health, 91*(11), 1776–1782.

Kelly, C. (2009). *Essentials of nursing leadership and management*. Clifton Park, NY: Delmar Cengage Learning.

Kerkhoff, T. R. (2009). Ethics and healthcare reform: Can we afford the status quo? *Journal of Head Trauma Rehabilitation, 24*(6), 475–477.

Kitzman, H., Olds, D., Henderson, C., Hanks, C., Cole, R., Arcoleo, K. J., et al. (2010). Enduring effects of prenatal and infancy home visiting by nurses on children. *Archives of Pediatrics and Adolescent Medicine, 164*(5), 412–418.

Kitzman, H., Olds, D., Henderson, C., Hanks, C., Cole, R., Tatelbaum, R, et al. (1997). Effect or prenatal and infancy home visitation by nurses on pregnancy outcomes, childhood injuries, and repeated childbearing: A randomized controlled trial. *Journal of the American Medical Association, 278*(8), 644–652.

Kluckhohn, C. (1951). Values and value-orientations in the theory of action: An exploration in definition and classification. In Parsons, T., & Shils, E.A. (Eds.), *Toward a general theory of action* (pp. 388–433). Cambridge, MA: Harvard University Press.

Larsen, R. & Reif, L. (2011). Effectiveness of cultural immersion and culture classes for enhancing nursing students' transcultural self-efficacy. *Journal of Nursing Education, 14*, 1–5.

Layman, E. J. (2008). Ethical issues and the electronic health record. *Health Care Management, 27*(2), 165–176.

Levy, D., Nikolayev, L., & Mumford, E. (2005). Recent trends in smoking and the role of public policies: Results from the SimSmoke tobacco control policy simulation model. *Addiction, 100*(10), 1526–1536.

Lindenauer, P., Remus, D., Roman, S., Rothberg, M., Benjamin, E., Ma, A., et al. (2007). Public reporting and pay for performance in hospital quality improvement. *New England Journal of Medicine, 356*(5), 486–496.

Lindson, N., Aveyard, P., & Hughes, J. (2010). Reduction versus abrupt cessation in smokers who want to quit. *Cochrane Database of Systematic Reviews, 3*. Art. No.: CD008033.

Liu, R. (2011, February 8). Startling racial disparities in vaccination persist. *Doctors for America*. Retrieved from http://www.drsforamerica.org/blog/startling-racial-disparities-in-vaccination-persist

Llewellyn, D., Lang, I., Langa, K., Muniz-Terrera, G., Phillips, C., Cherubini, A., et al. (2010). Vitamin D and risk of cognitive decline in elderly persons. *Archives of Internal Medicine, 170*(13), 1135–1141.

Lynn, J., Baily, M., Bottrell, M. Jennings, B, Levine, R., Davidoff, F., et al. (2007). The ethics of using quality improvement methods in health care. *Annals of Internal Medicine, 146*(9), 666–673.

Macdonald, D., McKillop, E., Trotter, S., & Gray, A. (2006). Improving handwashing performance—a crossover study of handwashing in the orthopaedic department. *Annals of the Royal College of Surgeons of England, 88*(3), 289–291.

Maloni, J., Albrecht, S., Thomas, K., Halleran J., & Jones, R. (2006). Implementing evidence-based practice: Reducing risk for low birth weight through pregnancy smoking cessation. *Journal of Obstetric, Gynecologic & Neonatal Nursing*. Published online March 9, 2006, doi: 10.1177/0884217503257333.

Markham, T., & Carney, M. (2008). Public health nurses and the delivery of quality nursing care in the community. *Journal of Clinical Nursing, 17*(10), 1342–1350.

Maslow, A. (1969). *Toward a psychology of being* (2nd ed.). New York: Van Nostrand.

Mathews, T. J., & MacDorman, M. F. (2010, April 30). Infant mortality statistics from the 2006 period linked birth/infant death data set. Morbidity & Mortality Weekly Reports (MMWR), 58(17), 1–32.

McGinty, J., & Anderson, G. (2008). Predictors of physician compliance with American Heart Association Guidelines for acute myocardial infarction. *Critical Care Nursing Quarterly, 31*(2) 161–172.

McHugh, M. D. (2010). Hospital nurse staffing and public health emergency preparedness: Implications for policy. *Public Health Nursing, 27*(5). 442–449.

McKenzie, J. F., Neiger, B., & Thackeray, R. (2009). *Planning, implementing and evaluating health promotion programs: A primer* (5th ed.). San Francisco, CA: Benjamin Cummings.

Meagher-Stewart, D., Edwards, N., Aston, M., & Young, L. (2009). Population health surveillance practice of public health nurses. *Public Health Nursing, 26*(6), 553–560.

Melnyk, B., & Fibneout-Overholt, E. (2011). *Evidence-based practice in nursing and healthcare: A guide to best practice* (2nd ed.). Philadelphia, PA: Lippincott Williams & Wilkins.

Melnyk, B., Fineout-Overholt, E., Stillwell, S., & Williamson, K. (2009). Igniting a spirit of inquiry: An essential foundation for evidence-based practice. *American Journal of Nursing, 109*(11), 49–52.

Merriam Webster Online Dictionary. (2011). *Ethics*. Retrieved from http://www.merriam-webster.com/medical/ethics?show=0&t=1299184335

Miller, F., & Emanuel, E. (2008). Quality-improvement research and informed consent. *New England Journal of Medicine, 358*(8), 765–767.

Montalvo-Liendo, N., Wardell, D., Engebretson, J., & Reininger, B. (2009). Factors influencing disclosure of abuse by women of Mexican descent. *Journal of Nursing Scholarship, 41*(4), 359–367.

National Association of Social Workers. (2011). *Social justice*. Retrieved from http://www.socialworkers.org/pressroom/features/issue/peace.asp

National Institutes of Health. (2006). *Ten landmark nursing research studies*. Retrieved from www.ninr.nih.gov/10landmarkstudies.htm

National Institutes of Health. (2012). *Back to Sleep public education campagin*. Retrieved from https://www.nichd.nih.gov/sids/

Netermeyer, R., Andrews, J. C., & Burton, S. (2005). Effects of antismoking advertising-based beliefs on adult smokers' consideration of quitting. *American Journal of Public Health, 95*(6), 1062–1066.

Neuman, B., & Reed, K. (2007). A Neuman systems model perspective on nursing in 2050. *Nursing Science Quarterly, 20*(2), 111–113.

Neuman Systems Model. (2008). *Neuman systems model.* Retrieved from http://neumansystemsmodel.org/index.html

Nightingale, F. (1859/1992). *Notes on nursing: What it is, and what it is not* [Commemorative ed.]. Philadelphia, PA: Lippincott.

Nurse–Family Partnership (NFP). (2010). *Evidentiary foundations of Nurse-Family Partnership.* Retrieved February 23, 2011, from http://www.nursefamilypartnership.org/assets/PDF/Policy/NFP_Evidentiary_Standards

O'Connor, A., Stacey, D, Barry, M., Col, N., Eden, K., Entwistle, V., et al. (2009). *Decision aids for people facing health treatment or screening decisions* (review). The Cochrane Collaboration. Retrieved from http://www.allhealth.org/BriefingMaterials/Connor-DecisionAidsforPeople-1939.pdf

Olds, D. L. (2007). The Family-Nurse Partnership: From trials to practice. Denver, CO; University of Colorado. Retrieved February 23, 2011, from http://www.earlychildhoodrc.org/events/presentations/olds.pdf

Olds, D., Eckenrode, J., Henderson, C., Kitzman, H., Powers, J., Cole, R., et al. (1997). Long-term effects of home visitation on maternal life course and child abuse and neglect: Fifteen-year follow-up of a randomized trial. *Journal of the American Medical Association, 278*(8), 637–643.

Olds, D., Kitzman, H., Cole, R., Hanks, C., Arcoleo, K., Anson, E., et al. (2010). Enduring effects of prenatal and infancy home visiting by nurses on maternal life course and government spending. *Archives of Pediatrics & Adolescent Medicine, 164*(5), 419–424.

Olds, D., Robinson, J., Pettitt, L., Luckey, D., Holmberg, J., Ng, R.K., et al.(2004). Effects of home visits by paraprofessionals and by nurses: Age 4 follow-up results of a randomized trial. *Pediatrics, 114*(6), 1560–1568.

Olson Keller, L., & Strohschein, S. (2011, June 1). *Show me the evidence: Evidence-based public health nursing practice.* Webinar Handouts. Retrieved from http://publichealthnurses.org/images/uploads/Webinar_I_Slides_Updated.pdf

Olson Keller, L., & Strohschein, S. (2011, June 15). *Innovations in translating evidence into practice.* Webinar. Handouts. Retrieved from http://publichealthnurses.org/images/uploads/Web_II_Handout_(1).pdf

Ong, M., & Glantz, S. A. (2005). Free nicotine replacement therapy programs vs. implementing smoke-free workplaces: A cost-effectiveness comparison. *American Journal of Public Health, 95*(1), 969–975.

Park, Y. H. & Han, H. R. (2010). Nurses' perceptions and experiences at daycare for elderly with stroke. *Journal of Nursing Scholarship, 42*(3), 262–269.

Perry, C., & Hoffman, B. (2010). Assessing tribal youth physical activity and programming using a community-based participatory research approach. *Public Health Nursing, 27*(2), 104–114.

Pevzner, E., Robison, S., Donovan, J., Allis, D., Spitters, C. Friedman, R., et al. (2010). Tuberculosis transmission and use of methamphetines in Snohomish County, WA, 1991–2006. *American Journal of Public Health, 100*(12), 2481–2486.

Phillips, D, Brwer, K., & Wadensweiler, P. (2010). Alcohol as a risk factor for sudden infant death syndrome (SIDS). *Addiction, 106*(3), 516–525.

Pickering, A., Boehm, A., Mwanjali, M., & Davis, J. (2010). Efficacy of waterless hand hygiene compared with handwashing with soap: A field study in Dar es Salaam, Tanzania. *American Journal of Tropical Medicine, 82*(2), 270–278.

Polit, D., & Beck, C. T. (2010). *Essentials of nursing research: Appraising evidence for nursing practice* (7th ed.). Philadelphia, PA: Lippincott, Williams & Wilkins.

Polit, D., & Beck, C. T. (2012). *Nursing research: Generating and assessing evidence for nursing practice* (9th ed.). Philadelphia, PA: Lippincott, Williams & Wilkins.

Polivka, B. (2006). Needs assessment and intervention strategies to reduce lead-poisoning risk among low-income Ohio toddlers. *Public Health Nursing, 23*(1), 52–58.

Porter, E., Matsuda, S., & Lindbloom, E. (2010). Intentions of older homebound women to reduce the risk of falling again. *Journal of Nursing Scholarship, 42*(1), 101–109.

Porter-O'Grady, T. (2010). A new age for practice: Creating the framework for evidence. In Malloch, K., & Porter-O'Grady, T. (Eds.), *Introduction to evidence-based practice in nursing and health care* (2nd ed., pp. 1–30). Sudbury, MA: Jones & Bartlett Publishers.

Pugno, M. (2008). Economics and the self: A formalisation of self-determination theory. *Journal of Socio-Economics, 37*(4), 1328–1346.

Quad Council. (2003, April 3). *Quad Council PHN Competencies.* Retrieved from http://www.resourcenter.net/images/ACHNE/Files/Final_PHN_Competencies.pdf

Raffo, J., Meghea, C., Zhu, Q., & Roman, L. A (2010). Psychological and physical abuse among pregnant wome in a Medicaid-sponsored prenatal program. *Public Health Nursing, 27*(5), 385–398.

Rand Corporation. (2005). *Research brief: Proven benefits of early childhood interventions.* Santa Monica, CA: Author.

Rebar, C., Gersch, C., Macnee, C., & McCabe, S. (2011). *Understanding nursing research: Using research in evidence-based practice* (3rd ed.). Philadelphia, PA: Lippincott, Williams & Wilkins.

Remler, D., & Glied, S. (2003). What other programs can teach us: Increasing participation in health insurance programs. *American Journal of Public Health, 93*(1), 67–74.

Rice, V.H. & Stead, L.F. (2008). Nursing interventions for smoking cessation. *Cochrane Database of Systematic Reviews* 2008, Issue 1. Art. No.: CD001188. DOI: 10.1002/14651858.CD001188.pub3

Rokeach, M. (1973). *The nature of human values.* New York: Free Press.

Rueda, S., Park-Wyllie, L., Bayoumi, A., Tynan, A., Anoniou, T., Rourke, S., et al. (2006). Patient support and education for promoting adherence to highly active antiretroviral therapy for HIV/AIDS. *Cochrane Database of Systematic Reviews* 2006, (3), CD001442. Retrieved from http://www.mrw.interscience.wiley.com/cochrane/clsysrev/article/CD001442/frame.html.

Sawatsky, J. V., & Naimark, B. (2009). The coronary artery bypass graft surgery trajectory: Gender differences revisited. *European Journal of Cardiovascular Nursing, 8*(4), 302–308.

Schlosser, R. W. (2007). *Appraising the quality of systematic reviews.* National Center for the Dissemination of Disability Research. Retrieved February 22, 2011, from http://www.ncddr.org/kt/products/focus/focus17/

Schmidt, H. (2009). Just health responsibility. *Journal of Medical Ethics, 35,* 21–26.

Selgelid, M. (2008). Ethics, tuberculosis and globalization. *Public Health Ethics, 1*(1), 10–20.

Sharps, P., Campbell, J., Baty, M., Walker, K., & Bair-Merritt, M. (2008). Current evidence on perinatal home visiting and intimate partner violence. *Journal of Obstetrical, Gynecological, & Neonatal Nursing, 37*(4), 480–490.

Sheikh, S., & Janoff-Bulman, R. (2010). The "shoulds" and "should nots" of moral emotions: A self-regulatory perspective on shame and guilt. *Journal of Personality & Social Psychology, 36*(2), 213–224.

Shreffler-Grant, J., Hill, W., Weinert, C., Nichols, E., & Ide, B. (2007). Complementary therapy and older rural women. *Nursing Research, 56*(1), 28–33.

Slinin, Y., Paudel, M., Taylor, B., Fink, H., Ishani, A., Canales, M., et al. (2010). 25-hydroxyvitamin D levels and cognitive performance and decline in elderly men. *Neurology, 74,* 33–41.

Smith, L., Oveku, S., Homer, C., & Zuckerman, B. (2006). Sickle cell disease: A question of equity and quality. *Pediatrics, 117*(5), 1763–1770.

Speck, B., & Looney, S. (2006). Self-reported physical activity validated by pedometer: A pilot study. *Public Health Nursing, 23*(1), 88–94.

Spenceley, S., O'Leary, K., Chizawsky, L., Ross, A., & Estabrooks, C. (2008). Sources of information used by nurses to inform practice. *International Journal of Nursing Studies, 45*(6), 954–970.

Spenceley, S., Reutter, L., & Allen, M. (2006). The road less traveled: Nursing advocacy at the policy level. *Policy, Politics, & Nursing Practice, 7*(3), 180–194.

Stanford Encyclopedia of Philosophy. (2008). *The principle of beneficence in applied ethics.* Stanford University. Retrieved from http://129.11.3.26/entries/principle-beneficence/

Stutz, N., Becker, D., Jappe, U., John, S., Ludwig, J., Spornraft-Ragaller, P., et al. (2009). Nurses' perceptions of the benefits and adverse effects of hand disinfection: Alcohol-based hand rubs vs. hygienic handwashing. A mlulticentre questionnaire study with additional patch testing by the German Contact Dermatitis Research Group. *British Journal of Dermatology, 160*(3), 565–572.

Swiadek, J. W. (2009). The impact of healthcare issues on the future of the nursing profession: The resulting increased influence of community-based and public health nursing. *Nursing Forum, 44*(1), 19–24.

The Cochrane Collaboration. (2008). *An introduction to Cochrane reviews and the Cochrane Library*. Retrieved August 2, 2008, from http://www.cochrane.org/reviews/clibintro.htm.

The William Glasser Institute. (2010). *Choice theory*. Retrieved from http://www.wglasser.com/index.php?option=com_content&task=view&id=12&Itemid=27

Thomas, E., Elliott, E., & Naughton, G. (2006). Exercise for type 2 diabetes mellitus. *Cochrane Database of Systematic Reviews 2006, 3*(CD002968). Retrieved July 4, 2008 from http://www.mrw.interscience.wiley.com/cochrane/clsysrev/articles/CD002968/frame.html

Thompson, I. E., Melia, K. M., Boyd, K. M., & Horsburgh, E. (2006). *Nursing ethics* (5th ed.). Edinburgh, UK: Churchill Livingstone.

U.S. Congress. (2010, January 5). H.R. 3590 The Patient Protection an Affordable Care Act. Retrieved February 23, 2011 from http://frwebgate.access.gpo.gov/cgi-bin/getdoc.cgi?dbname=111_cong_bills&docid=f:h3590enr.txt.pdf

U.S. Department of Health & Human Services (USDHHS). (n.d.-a). *The Belmont report: Ethical priniciples and guidelines for the protection of human subjects of research*. Retrieved February 28, 2011, from http://www.hhs.gov/ohrp/policy/belmont.html

U.S. Department of Health & Human Services (USDHHS). (n.d.-b). *Informed consent FAQs*. Retrieved February 28, 2011, from http://answers.hhs.gov/ohrp/categories/1566

U.S. Department of Health & Human Services (USDHHS). (2008). *Community-based participatory research scientific interest group*. Retrieved from http://grants.nih.gov/grants/training/esaig/cbpr_sig.htm

Uustal, D. B. (1977). The use of values clarification in nursing practice. *Journal of Continuing Education in Nursing, 8*, 8–13.

Uustal, D. B. (1978). Values clarification in nursing. *American Journal of Nursing, 78*, 2058–2063.

Valdez, R., Yoon, P., Quershi, N., Green, R., & Khoury, M. (2010). Family history in public health practice: A genomic tool for disease prevention and health promotion. *Annual Review of Public Health, 21*(31), 69–87.

Vennemann, M., Bajanowski, T., Brinkmann, B., Jorch, G., Yücesan, K., Sauerland, C., et al. (2009). Does breastfeeding reduce the risk of sudden infant death syndrome? *Pediatrics, 123*(3), e406-e410.

Wechsler, P. (2011, March 16). *Americans without health insurance rise to 52 million on job loss, expense*. Retrieved from http://www.bloomberg.com/news/print/2011–03–16/americans-without-health-insurance-rose-to-52-million-on-job-loss-expense.html

Wilson, D. (2010, July 21). Glaxo ordered to end drug trial enrollment. *The New York Times*. Retrieved from http://www.nytimes.com/2010/07/22/business/22avandia.html

Wright, D., & Brajtman, S. (2011). Relaltional and embodied knowing: Nursing ethics within the interprofessional team. *Nursing Ethics, 18*(1), 20–30.

Young, C. & Skorga, P. (2011). Reduction versus abrupt cessation in smokers who want to quit: A review summary. *Public Health Nursing, 28*(1), 54–56.

CHAPTER

5

Transcultural Nursing in the Community

"People everywhere share common biological and psychological needs, and the function of all cultures is to fulfill such needs; the nature of the culture is determined by its function."

—***Bronislaw Malinowski*** **(1884–1942), Cultural Anthropologist**

"Looking from far and above, from our high places of safety in the developed civilization, it is easy to see all the crudity and irrelevance of magic. But without its power and guidance early man could not have mastered his practical difficulties as he has done, nor could man have advanced to the higher stages of civilization."

—***Horace Miner*** **(1912–1993), Anthropologist**

KEY TERMS

Complementary therapies
Cultural assessment
Cultural diversity
Cultural relativism
Cultural self-awareness
Cultural sensitivity
Culture
Culture shock
Dominant values
Enculturation
Ethnic group
Ethnicity
Ethnocentrism
Ethnorelativism
Folk medicine
Home remedies
Integrated health care
Microculture
Minority group
Norms
Race
Subcultures
Tacit
Transcultural nursing
Value

LEARNING OBJECTIVES

Upon mastery of this chapter, you should be able to:

- Define and explain the concept of culture.
- Discuss the meaning of cultural diversity and its significance for community health nursing.
- Describe the meaning and effects of ethnocentrism on community health nursing practice.
- Identify five characteristics shared by all cultures.
- Contrast the health-related values, beliefs, and practices of selected culturally diverse populations with those of the dominant U.S. culture.
- Conduct a cultural assessment.
- Apply transcultural nursing principles in community health nursing practice.

American society values individuality, and we are a country of immigrants. Many different cultural groups and races built this nation. For example, pilgrims came here hundreds of years ago, to seek freedom to practice their religious beliefs. It took powerful independence to pioneer the West in the 1800s. Partly because of this pioneer spirit, people from all nations have sought to live in America. Some came of their own free will for adventure and opportunity. Others saw this land as a refuge from political, religious, or economic strife. Still others were brought here against their will. Consequently, we have not become the ideal *melting pot* once described, but, rather, an amalgamation of people who have different values, ideals, and behaviors.

Americans have many differences, but we also have much in common. In the Western culture, there is joy in seeing children grow and develop in unique ways. An individual's creative achievements are applauded. There is also respect for one another's personal preferences about food, dress, or personal beliefs. The right to be oneself—and thereby to be different from others—is even protected by state and federal laws.

Although individuality is a cherished American value, there are limits to the range of differences most Americans find acceptable. People whose behavior falls outside the acceptable range may be labeled as misfits. For example, the U.S. culture approves moderate social drinking, but not alcoholism. The beliefs and sanctions of the dominant or majority culture are called **dominant values.** In the United States, the majority culture is made up largely of European Americans whose dominant values include the work ethic, thrift, success, independence, initiative, privacy, cleanliness, youthfulness, attractive appearance, and a focus on the future. However, in some regions and states, European Americans are not the majority. For example, in California, 53% of the population are "people of color," and the dominant culture is no longer European American (California Pan-Ethnic Health Network, 2007, para. 3); the proportion of the population identified as White is projected to continue to fall below other ethnicities between 2010 and 2050 (U.S. Census Bureau, n.d.).

Dominant values are important to consider in the practice of community health nursing because they can shape people's thoughts and behaviors. Why are some client behaviors acceptable to health professionals and others not? Why do nurses have such difficulty persuading certain clients to accept new ways of thinking and acting? Explanations can be found by examining the concept of culture, especially its influence on health and on community health nursing practice. For example, an emphasis on the need for milk in the diet may reflect cultural blindness, considering the number of people in diverse ethnic groups who are lactose intolerant (Campbell, 2005). Regardless of their own cultural backgrounds, nurses are socialized throughout the educational process; the biomedical model is frequently the framework, and dominant social values are often involuntarily reinforced.

THE MEANING OF CULTURE

Culture refers to the beliefs, values, and behavior that are shared by members of a society and provide a design or "roadmap" for living. Culture tells people what is acceptable or unacceptable in a given situation. Culture dictates what to do, say, or believe. Culture is learned. As children grow up, they learn from their parents and others around them how to interpret the world. In turn, these assimilated beliefs and values prescribe desired behavior. We think of this as learned behavior, but can culture actually impact your neurobiology? For more on this see What Do You Think?

Anthropologists describe culture as systems of beliefs, values, and norms of behavior found in all societies (Hahn & Inhorn, 2009). This is more than simply custom or ritual; it is a way of organizing and thinking about life. It gives people a sense of security about their behavior; without having to consciously think about it, they know how to act. Culture also provides the underlying values and beliefs on which people's behavior is based. For example, culture determines the value placed on achievement, independence, work, and leisure. It forms the basis for the definitions of male and female roles. It influences a person's response to authority figures, dictates religious beliefs and practices, and shapes childrearing. According to Giger and Davidhizar (2008, p. 3), "culture is a patterned behavioral response that develops over time as a result of imprinting the mind through social and religious structures and intellectual and artistic manifestations."

Every community and social or ethnic group has its own culture. Furthermore, all of the individual members believe and act based on what they have learned within that specific culture. As anthropologist Edward Hall (1959) said a half-century ago, culture controls our lives. Even the smallest elements of everyday living are influenced by culture. For instance, culture determines the proper distance to stand from another person while talking. A comfortable talking distance for Americans is at least 2.5 feet, whereas Latin Americans prefer a shorter distance, often only 18 inches, for dialogue. Culture also influences one's perception of time. In European American culture, when someone makes an appointment, it is expected that the other person will be on time or not more than a few minutes late; to keep a person waiting (or to be kept waiting) for 45 minutes or more is considered insulting. Yet other cultural groups, including Native Americans and Hispanics, have a much more flexible response to time. Their members feel that time is much more elastic, and if someone is kept waiting, it is not considered a thoughtless act. So, as you can

What do *you* think?

CAN CULTURE AFFECT YOUR NEUROBIOLOGY?

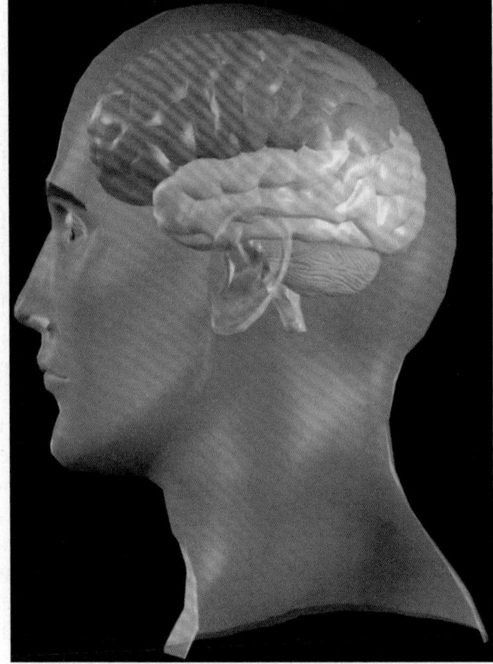

Researchers in the United States and Singapore studied brain activity through the use of functional magnetic resonance imaging (FMRI) while both young and elderly participants were shown a series of images depicting various objects on different backgrounds. For both cultures, the younger subjects demonstrated similar brain activity. But, a marked contrast was noted between the older subjects, with the neural responses of those only from the East Asian culture showing minimal activity to changes of single objects while the Americans' activity in the lateral occipital complex was continually active (Burton, 2007). Americans were more focused on the individual objects as new ones were introduced, but the East Asians maintained focus on the background information and not on new individual objects, according to earlier research. The explanation for this is that Asian culture is "less individual-oriented than Western culture" and more interdependent (p. 6). Even with Westernization, the researchers note significant differences in values between the cultures (even with educated, younger Asians when compared to Americans). They feel that these differences demonstrate that "culture is sculpting the brain at the level of perception"—evidence that culture can impact us on a biological level (p. 6).

Burton, K. W. (2007). Cultural experience affects perception. *Brain Work: The Neuroscience Newsletter, 17*(5), p. 6.

see, culture is the knowledge people use to design their own actions and, in turn, to interpret others' behavior (Spradley & McCurdy, 2009).

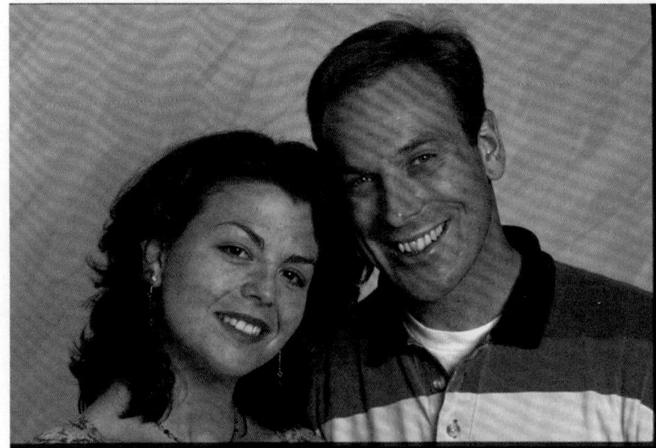

Culture influences rules about the appropriateness of public displays of affection.

Cultural Diversity

Race refers to biologically designated groups of people whose distinguishing features, such as skin color, are inherited; examples include Asian, Black, and White. An **ethnic group** is a collection of people who have common origins and a shared culture and identity; they may share a common geographic origin, race, language, religion, traditions, values, and food preferences (Spector, 2009). A person's **ethnicity** is that group of qualities that mark one's association with a particular ethnic group, or "who share cultural and/or physical characteristics including one or more of the following: history, political system, religion, language, geographical origin, traditions, myths, behaviours, foods, genetic similarities, and physical features" (Ethnicity Online, 2010, para. 1). When a variety of racial or ethnic groups join a common, larger group, cultural diversity becomes apparent. **Cultural diversity**, also called *cultural plurality*, means that a variety of cultural patterns coexist within a designated geographic area. Cultural diversity occurs not only between countries or continents, but also within many countries, including the United States (Spector, 2009). However, the term *culture*, used alone, has no single definition. We have defined it for use in this book at the beginning of this section. Others have described culture as meaning the total, socially inherited characteristics of a group, comprising everything that one generation can tell, convey, or hand down to the next. Culture has also been described as "the luggage that each of us carries around for a lifetime" (Spector, 2009, p. 21).

Immigration patterns over the years have contributed to significant cultural diversity in the United States. Early settlers came primarily from European countries through the 1800s, peaking in numbers just after the turn of the 20th century, with almost 9 million immigrants admitted in the first decade. During much of that time, especially during the late 1600s through the early 1800s, African slaves were brought to the United States against their will,

Table 5.1 Immigrants to the United States, 1901–2008

Decade	Number of Immigrants
1901–1910	8,795,386
1911–1920	5,735,611
1921–1930	4,107,209
1931–1940	528,431
1941–1950	1,035,039
1951–1960	2,515,479
1961–1970	3,322,677
1971–1980	4,493,314
1981–1990	7,338,062
1991–2000	9,095,417
2001–2008	5,192,376

Source: U.S. Department of Commerce. (2001). *Statistical abstract of the United States, 2001* (121st ed.). Washington, DC: Government Printing Office; U.S. Department of Homeland Security. (2009). *Persons naturalized by state of residence: Fiscal years 1999 to 2008*. Retrieved: http://www.dhs.gov/xlibrary/assets/statistics/yearbook/2008/table22.xls.

mostly to southern states, where they were sold to plantation owners as laborers. This "forced immigration" has had profound effects for many generations (Berlin, 2005). Immigration stayed high during the early 1900s, and then dropped sharply from 1930 to 1950. Immigration from non-European regions, such as Asia and South America, then steadily increased. The total number of immigrants from all countries in the 1990s actually exceeded the number who arrived during the first decade of the 1900s, when immigration was formerly at its peak (Table 5-1).

As shown in Table 5-2, immigrants come from all regions of the world, in greater numbers from some areas than others (U.S. Department of Homeland Security, 2009). According to the U.S. Committee for Refugees and Immigrants (USCRI, 2010), in 2008, the United States hosted 161,200 refugees and asylum seekers, a steady decline since 2001. The largest numbers of refugees are listed as coming from Cuba, China, and Myanmar.

Although the numbers of legal immigrants have dropped, illegal immigration continues to be a *hot button topic* in this country, especially after 9/11. Proposals to end the flow of illegal immigrants from Mexico include building a 700-mile fence alowng the border, and legislation that would penalize employers of undocumented workers more stiffly. The numbers of migrants losing their lives while crossing illegally into this country have risen dramatically, from 147 in 1998 to 387 in 2001; in 2005, the number climbed to 451 (Hing, 2006). Deaths on the Arizona–Mexico border from October 2009 to July 2010 numbered 139 (Unitarian Universalist Church of Tucson, 2010). What is often not considered in the debate over this issue is the economic desperation that drives people to put themselves in such jeopardy.

The population of this country continues to increase. Since the 2000 census, the population grew by more than 24.8 million; and Asians and Hispanic/Latinos showed the greatest increases (Table 5-3). Such numbers can be deceiving, however, because the 2000 census was the first one in which individuals were able to indicate two or more races or ethnic groups. Over 6 million people indicated multiple races or ethnic groups, with the number dropping to over 5 million in 2009. Approximately 50% of these people indicated Hispanic along with a second or third race or ethnic group. By 2050, the Hispanic-origin population is projected to be four times larger than its 1990 figure (U.S. Census Bureau, n.d.).

People representing more than 100 different ethnic groups—more than half of them significant in size—live in the United States. Significant minorities include Hispanic Americans, numbering more than 35 million in 2000 and over 48 million in 2009 and currently representing over 14% of the population; African Americans, numbering over 39 million, or approximately 12.9% of the population; Asian Americans, numbering more than 14 million, or approximately 4.5% of the population; and American Indians and Alaska Natives, numbering 3.1 million, or

Table 5.2 Persons Obtaining Legal Permanent Resident Status by Region of Birth, 2009

Origin	Number
All countries	1,130,818
Africa	127,050
Asia	413,312
Europe	105,398
North America	375,236
Oceania	5,578
South America	102,878

From U.S. Department of Homeland Security, *Yearbook of Immigration Statistics: 2009*. Accessed at: http://www.dhs.gov/files/statistics/publications/LPR09.shtm.

Table 5.3 U.S. Population by Race and Hispanic/Latino Origin, Census 2000 and 2010 Estimate

Origin	Census 2000 (%)	2010 estimate (%)
White	75.1	64.7
Black	12.3	12.2
American Indian/ Alaska Native	0.9	0.8
Asian	3.6	4.5
Hispanic or Latino	12.5	16.0

Sources: *Population of the United States by Race and Hispanic/Latino Origin, Census 2000 and July 1, 2005*. Accessed at: http://www.infoplease.com/ipa/A0762156.html; Kaiser Family Foundation. (2010). *Distribution of U.S. population by race/ethnicity, 2010 and 2050*. Accessed at: http://facts.kff.org/chart.aspx?ch=364.

1% of the population. In 2000, Hispanics surpassed the African American population as the largest race/ethnic group in the United States (Infoplease, 2010; U.S. Census Bureau, 2010). By 2050, the total number of Hispanic Americans is projected to double, making up 30.3% of the population; Asian–Pacific Islanders are expected to more than double their numbers, to 8.2% of the U.S. population; and the number of African Americans will increase to 15.4% of the population. The American Indian and Alaska Native population will probably stay at or near 1%. These changes, primarily resulting from immigration, are projected to result in over 50% of the U.S. population in 2050 belonging to "minority" groups, and European Americans/Whites will no longer be the majority. In some states, especially those bordering Mexico and some industrialized states in the eastern part of the country, the most current information reveals that this change already has occurred or will occur much sooner than 2050 (U.S. Census Bureau, 2006, 2009) (see Display 5.1).

Immigration patterns are strongly influenced by immigration laws established since the 1800s. The Immigration Reform and Control Act of 1986 (Public Law 99–603) and the Immigration Act of 1990 (Public Law 101–649) set new limits on the number of immigrants admitted. These laws set annual numerical ceilings on certain immigrant groups while authorizing increases for highly skilled workers or family members of aliens who have recently achieved legal status. After the terrorist attacks on September 11, 2001, President Bush suspended all immigration for 2 months. Suspicion about people from Middle Eastern countries permeated the nation—worsening the social climate for immigrants. This social climate is characterized by ambivalence about whether immigrants should be accepted and ambiguity about their status. The newcomers find an environment that is both welcoming and hostile. On the one hand, they may find tolerance of diversity in the United States—demonstrated by interest in ethnic food, cultural celebrations, and sensitivity to employees from different backgrounds. On the other hand, a backlash is demonstrated by a rise in hate crimes, national and local policies that limit services to undocumented immigrants, restriction in English as a Second Language (ESL) and bilingual education, and limits to potential class action suits challenging practices of the U.S. Citizenship and Immigration Services and Department of Homeland Security.

Although broad cultural values are shared by most large national societies, those societies contain smaller cultural groups—called subcultures. **Subcultures** are relatively large aggregates of people within a society who share separate distinguishing characteristics, such as ethnicity (e.g., African American, Hispanic American), occupation (e.g., farmers, physicians), religion (e.g., Catholics, Muslims), geographic area (e.g.,

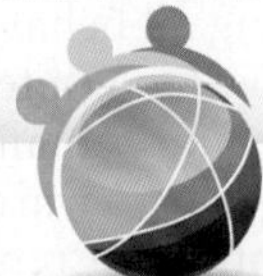

DISPLAY 5.1 HISPANIC POPULATION TREND IN THE UNITED STATES

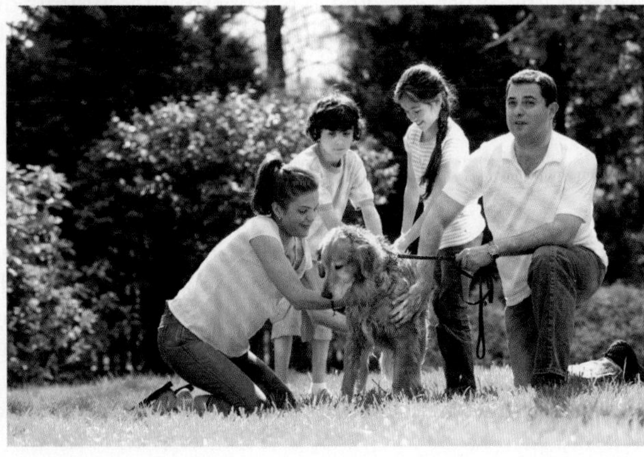

In 2008, a record number of 12.7 million Mexican immigrants lived in the United States. Currently, 32% of all immigrants living in the United States are Mexicans. It is estimated that about 11% of people born in Mexico are now residing in this country—a wholesale transfer of population. In 1970, it was estimated that only 760,000 Mexican immigrants (1.4% of Mexico's population) lived in the United States. By 1980, Mexicans became the largest foreign-born population at 2.2 million This number doubled by 1990 and grew even larger by 2000 (Pew Hispanic Center, 2009).

The current numbers of Mexican immigrants to the United States—32%—is the highest concentration of immigrants from a single country since the turn of the last century. This is not a new phenomenon. From 1850 to 1870, Irish immigrants represented a third or more of the immigrant population, and Germans comprised 26% to 30% of the foreign-born population from 1850 to 1900.

Immigrants may enter the country legally or illegally. It is estimated that 11.2 million unauthorized immigrants were living in the United States in March 2010. This number remained the same as the year before. This stabilization followed a 2-year decline from the peak of 12 million in 2007—the first significant drop in a 20-year pattern of growth. This drop is most likely due to a decrease in numbers of persons from Mexico, who remain the largest group of unauthorized immigrants at 58%. Unauthorized immigrants are estimated to make up 3.7% of the nation's 2010 population. The number of unauthorized immigrants in the United States tripled between 1990 (when it was 3.5 million) and 2007 (Pew Hispanic Center, 2011).

Pew Hispanic Center. (2011). *Unauthorized immigrant population: National and state trends, 2010.* Accessed at http://pewhispanic.org/reports/report.php?ReportID=133; Pew Hispanic Center. (2009). *Mexican immigrants in the United States, 2008.* Washington, DC: Author.

New Englanders, Southerners), age (e.g., the elderly, school-age children), gender (e.g., women), or sexual preference (e.g., gay, lesbian). Within these subcultures are even smaller groups that anthropologists call **microcultures.** Microcultures have been described as "systems of cultural knowledge characteristic of subgroups within larger societies. Members of a microculture usually share much of what they know with everyone in the greater society but possess a special cultural knowledge that is unique to the subgroup" (Spradley & McCurdy, 2009, p. 15). Examples of microcultures can range from a group of Hmong immigrants from Southeast Asia adopting selected aspects of U.S. culture to a third-generation Norwegian American community whose members share unique foods, dress, and values.

The members of each subculture and microculture retain some of the characteristics of the society from which they came or in which their ancestors lived, as noted by the eminent anthropologist Margaret Mead (1960). Some of their beliefs and practices—such as the food they eat, the language they speak at home, the way they celebrate holidays, or their ideas about sickness and healing—remain an important part of their everyday life. American Indian or Native American groups have retained some aspects of their traditional cultures. Mexican Americans, Irish Americans, Swedish Americans, Italian Americans, African Americans, Puerto Rican Americans, Chinese Americans, Japanese Americans, Vietnamese Americans, and many other ethnic groups have their own microcultures.

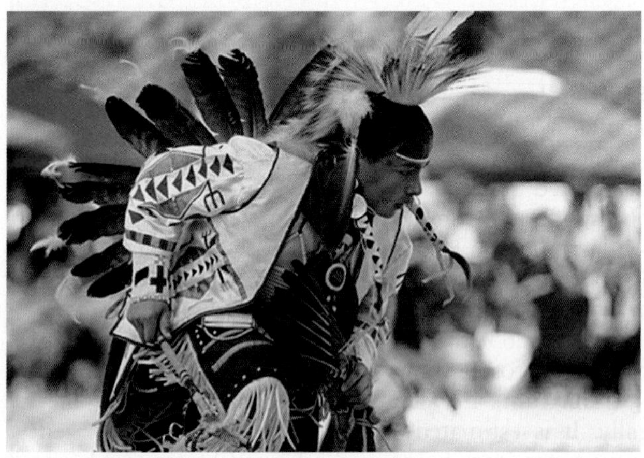

Native American groups retain some aspects of their traditional culture. (Photo courtesy USA.gov)

Furthermore, certain customs, values, and ideas are unique to the poor, the rich, the middle class, women, men, youth, or the elderly. Many deviant groups, such as narcotics abusers, transient alcoholics, gangs, criminals, and terrorist groups, have developed their own microcultures. Regional microcultures, such as that of the White and Black Appalachian people living in the hills and hollows of Kentucky or West Virginia, also have distinctive ways of defining the world and coping with life. Other microcultures, such as those of rural migrant farm workers or urban homeless families, acquire their own sets of beliefs and patterns for dealing with their environments. Many religious groups have their own microcultures. Even occupational and professional groups, such as nurses or attorneys, develop their own special languages, beliefs, and perspectives.

Ethnocentrism

There is a difference between a healthy cultural or ethnic identification and ethnocentrism. Anthropologists note "**ethnocentrism** is the belief and feeling that one's own culture is best. It reflects our tendency to judge other people's beliefs and behavior using values of our own native culture" (Spradley & McCurdy, 2009, p. 16). It causes people to believe that their way of doing things is right and to judge others' methods as inferior, ignorant, or irrational. Ethnocentrism blocks effective communication by creating biases and misconceptions about human behavior. In turn, this can cause serious damage to interpersonal relationships and interfere with the effectiveness of nursing interventions (Leininger & McFarland, 2006).

People can experience a developmental progression along a continuum from ethnocentrism, feeling one's own culture is best, to **ethnorelativism**—seeing all behavior in a cultural context (Narayanasamy & White, 2005). Some people may stop progressing and remain stagnated at one step, and others may move backward on the continuum. The left side of the continuum represents the most extreme reaction to intercultural differences: refusal or denial. On the right side is the characterization of people who show the most sensitivity to intercultural differences: incorporation (Fig. 5-1).

CHARACTERISTICS OF CULTURE

In their study of culture, anthropologists and sociologists have made significant contributions to the field of community health. Their findings shed light on why and how culture influences behavior. Five characteristics shared by all cultures are especially pertinent to nursing's efforts to improve community health: culture is learned, it is integrated, it is shared, it is tacit, and it is dynamic.

Culture Is Learned

Patterns of cultural behavior are acquired, not inherited. Rather than being genetically determined, the way

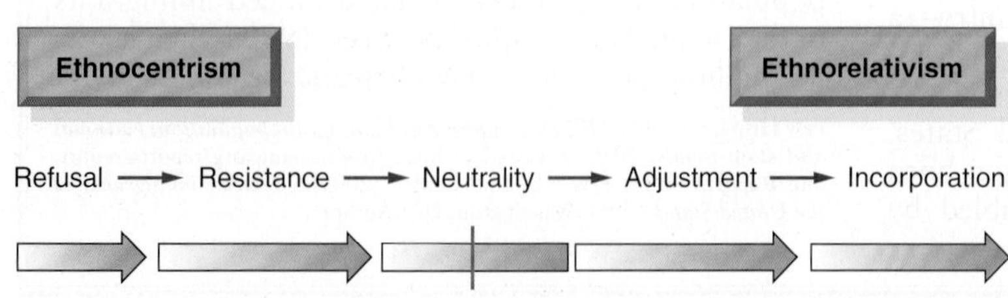

FIGURE 5-1. Cross-cultural sensitivity continuum. Being extremely ethnocentric (**left of midpoint**) and totally ethnorelative (**far right**) are reflected in the diagram. The steps toward ethnorelativism begin at the most ethnocentric view, with refusal and resistance. Neutrality is midpoint, and adjustment and incorporation bring the person to an ethnorelative perspective.

people dress, what they eat, and how they talk are all learned. Spradley and McCurdy (2009, p. 14) offered the following explanation:

> At the moment of birth, we lack a culture. We don't yet have a system of beliefs, knowledge, and patterns of customary behavior. But from that moment until we die, each of us participates in a kind of universal schooling that teaches us our native culture. Laughing and smiling are genetic responses, but as infants we soon learn when to smile, when to laugh, and even how to laugh. We also inherit the potential to cry, but we must learn our cultural rules for when crying is appropriate.

Each person learns about culture through socialization with the family or significant group, a process called **enculturation**. As a child grows up in a given society, he or she acquires certain attitudes, beliefs, and values and learns how to behave in ways appropriate to that group's definition of the female or male role; by doing so, children are learning about their culture (Spector, 2009; Spradley & McCurdy, 2009).

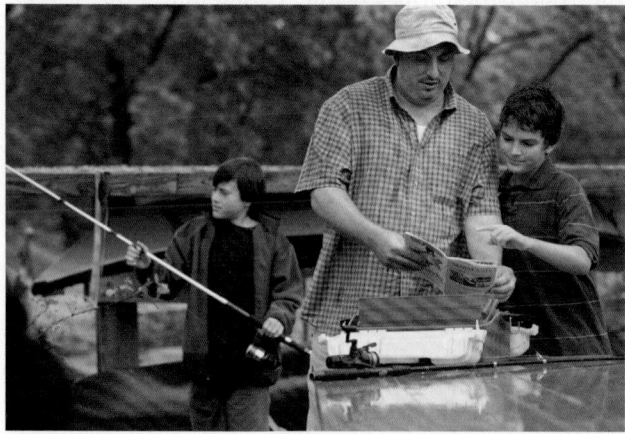

Family socialization helps acculturate children to acquire shared values and attitudes. (Photo courtesy of CDC Photo Image Library)

Although culture is learned, the process and results of that learning are different for each person. Each individual has a unique personality and experiences life in a singular way; these factors influence the acquisition of culture. Families, social classes, and other groups within a society differ from one another, and this sociocultural variation has important implications (Wang, 2006). Because culture is learned, parts of it can be relearned. People might change certain cultural elements or adopt new behaviors or values. Some individuals and groups are more willing and able than others to try new ways and thereby influence change.

Culture Is Integrated

Rather than being merely an assortment of various customs and traits, a culture is a functional, integrated whole. As in any system, all parts of a culture are interrelated and interdependent. The various components of a culture, such as its social mores or religious beliefs, perform separate functions but come into relative harmony with each other to form an operating and cohesive whole. In other words, to understand culture, single traits should not be described independently. Each part must be viewed in terms of its relationship to other parts and to the whole.

A person's culture is an integrated web of ideas and practices. For example, a nurse may promote the need for consuming three balanced meals a day, a practice tied to the beliefs that good nutrition leads to good health and that prevention is better than cure. These cultural beliefs, in turn, are related to the nurse's values about health. Health, the nurse believes, is essential for maximum energy output and productivity at work. Productivity is important because it enables people to reach goals. These values are linked to social or religious beliefs about hard work and taboos against laziness. Through such connections, these ideas and beliefs about nutrition, health, economics, religion, and family are all interrelated and work to motivate behavior.

For example, parents who are Jehovah's Witnesses may refuse a blood transfusion for their child. Their actions might seem irrational or ignorant to those who do not understand the parents' religious beliefs. However, the couple's choice represents behavior consistent with their cultural values and standards. The single behavior of refusing blood transfusions, when viewed in context, is seen to be part of a larger religious belief system and a basic component of the parents' culture. Even mothers' expectations for their children's development can vary between cultures (Damon, Lerner, Renninger, & Sigel, 2006)—something to keep in mind when we use developmental screening tools.

In some cultural groups (e.g., Muslims), modesty for women may make it uncomfortable and perhaps traumatic to be examined by a person of the opposite sex. Asking certain Native American groups to comply with rigid appointment scheduling requires them to reframe their concept of time. It also violates their values of patience and pride (Spector, 2009). Before nurses attempt to change a person's or group's behavior, they need to ask how that change will affect the people involved through its influence on other parts of their culture. Extra time and patience or different strategies may be needed if change still is indicated. Nurses often may find, however, that their own practice system can be modified to preserve clients' cultural values.

Culture Is Shared

Culture is the product of aggregate behavior, not individual habit. Certainly, individuals practice a culture, but customs are phenomena shared by all members of the group. More than 30 years ago, anthropologist G. Murdock explained (1972, p. 258):

> Culture does not depend on individuals. An ordinary habit dies with its possessor, but a group habit lives on in the survivors and is transmitted from generation to generation. Moreover, the individual is not a free agent with respect to culture. He is born and reared in a certain cultural environment, which impinges on him at every

> moment of his life. From earliest childhood his behavior is conditioned by the habits of those around him. He has no choice but to conform to the folkways current in his group.

A culture's values are among its most important elements (see Chapter 4). A **value** is a notion or idea designating relative worth or desirability. For example, some cultures place value on honesty, loyalty, and faithfulness more than other traits. Also, there may be strong values against lying, stealing, and cheating—behaviors to avoid. Each culture classifies phenomena into good and bad, desirable and undesirable, right and wrong. When people respond in favor of or against some practice, they are reflecting their culture's values about that practice. One person may eagerly anticipate eating a steak for dinner; another, who believes that eating meat is sacrilegious or unhealthful, experiences revulsion at the idea of steak for a meal. Some American subcultures think that loud, vocal expressions are a necessary way to deal with pain; others value silence and stoicism. Some have high regard for speed and efficiency, whereas others prefer patience and thoughtfulness. Either way, values serve a purpose. Shared values give people in a specific culture stability and security and provide a standard for behavior. From these values, members know what to believe and how to act (Lockwood, Marshall, & Sadler, 2005). The normative criteria by which people justify their decisions are based on values that are more deeply rooted than behaviors and, consequently, more difficult to change.

Knowing that culture is shared helps us to better understand human behavior. For example, a community health nurse tried unsuccessfully to persuade a mother to limit the amount of catnip tea she fed her infant. The infant was pacified with the tea and was not consuming a sufficient amount of infant formula, thus putting him at risk for nutritional deficiencies and developmental problems. The nurse discovered that the mother was acting in the tradition of her rural subculture, which held that catnip promoted good health (it acts as an antispasmodic, perhaps causing relaxation and resulting in a more contented infant with fewer symptoms of colic [Spector, 2009]). The fact that all of the other mothers in her small rural community also used catnip with their babies proved a powerful deterrent to the change suggested by the nurse. Other members of the same culture frequently influence health behaviors. It is difficult for one person to eliminate a cultural practice, especially if reinforced by so many other members of the group. Group acceptance and a sense of membership usually depend on conforming to these shared cultural practices (Spradley & McCurdy, 2009).

Community health nurses may need to focus on an entire group's health behavior to affect individual practices. In the example described, the pattern of consuming large amounts of catnip tea was modified after the nurse worked with the entire rural community. She began with a well-recognized cultural strategy: working through formal or informal leaders. She contacted the oldest woman in the community and discussed the cultural practice. The elder shared the group's beliefs that catnip tea is vital to the wellbeing of infants for the first 6 months. When the nurse explained her concerns about low formula intake and low weight gain, the community leader clarified that only 1 or 2 ounces of the tea a day was needed. The nurse and the community leader shared this information among the women, and, as a result, the mothers gradually reduced the amount of tea they gave their infants. Consequently, the clients' infants drank more formula and gained weight appropriately. A cultural tradition was retained while the health of the infants improved. The community health nurse could then use this new information and other supportive information from the community leader to improve the health of more infants (Spector, 2009).

Culture Is Mostly Tacit

Culture provides a guide for human interaction that is **tacit**—that is, mostly unexpressed and at the unconscious level. Members of a cultural group, without the need for discussion, know how to act and what to expect from one another. Culture provides an implicit set of cues for behavior, not a written set of rules. Spradley and McCurdy explained that culture often is "so regular and routine that it lies below a conscious level" (2009, p. 16). It is like a memory bank in which knowledge is stored for recall when the situation requires it, but this recall process is mostly unconscious. Culture teaches the proper tone of voice to use for each occasion. It prescribes how close to stand when talking with someone and how one should appropriately respond to elders. Individuals learn to make responses that are appropriate to their sex, role, and status. They know what is right and wrong. As an example, a recent study showed that cultural factors influence the desired affective state of children through their exposure to different types of storybooks (Tsai, Louie, Chen, & Uchida, 2007). All of these attitudes and behaviors become so ingrained—so tacit—that they are seldom, if ever, discussed.

Because culture is mostly tacit, realizing which of one's own behaviors may be offensive to people from other groups is difficult. It also is difficult to know the meaning and significance of other cultural practices. In some groups, such as American Indians or Islamic women, silence is valued and expected, but may make others uncomfortable. Offering food to a guest in many cultures is not merely a social gesture but an important symbol of hospitality and acceptance; to refuse it, for any reason, may be an insult and a rejection. Touching or calling someone by their first name may be viewed as a demonstration of caring by some groups, but is seen as disrespectful and offensive by others. Even how one trusts others in a group context is affected by cultural influences (Cronk, 2007). Consequently, community health nurses have a twofold task in developing cultural sensitivity: not only must we try to learn clients' cultures, but we also must try to make our own culture less tacit and more explicit. We must be more aware of our own biases and preconceived values and beliefs. Nurses bring both their professional and personal cultural history to the workplace, often developing unique values not shared with others who are not in the profession (Blais & Hayes, 2011). Cross-cultural tension can be resolved

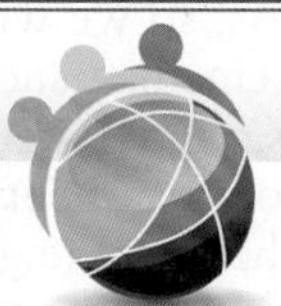

DISPLAY 5.2 CULTURE SHOCK

An increasing number of immigrants and refugees from many different countries have been assimilated into American culture in recent years. Although they quickly adapt in many respects, such as learning the language and seeking housing and employment, they continue to operate within the framework of their own cultural beliefs and behaviors. The conflict between their culture and American culture often causes **culture shock**, "a state of anxiety that results from cross-cultural misunderstanding ... and an inability to interact appropriately in the new context" (Spradley & McCurdy, 2009, p. 16). Immigrants and refugees find themselves in a strange setting with people who act in unfamiliar ways. Speaking their own language in their homes and retaining values and familiar practices all help to promote some sense of security in the new environment.

The same is true for nurses and others working in unfamiliar countries. No longer are the small but important cues available that orient a stranger to appropriate behavior. Instead, a person in a different culture may feel isolated and anxious and even become dysfunctional or ill. Immersion in the culture over time and learning the new culture are the major remedies. As adjustment occurs, old beliefs and practices that are still functional in the new setting can be retained, but others that are not functional must be replaced.

through conscious efforts to develop awareness, patience, and acceptance of cultural differences (Display 5.2).

Culture Is Dynamic

Every culture undergoes change; none is entirely static. Within every cultural group, some individuals generate innovations. More important, some members see advantages in doing things differently and are willing to adopt new practices. Each culture is an amalgamation of ideas, values, and practices from a variety of sources. This process depends on the extent of exposure to other groups. Nonetheless, every culture is in a dynamic state of adding or deleting components. Functional aspects are retained; less functional ones are eliminated.

When this adaptation does not occur, the cultural group may face serious difficulty. For example, Hmong teenagers from Southeast Asian refugee families in the United States are among the first generation to be raised in America. Their parents had high hopes for them to restore honor and pride to a displaced people, but the teens struggle to balance their American lifestyle with Hmong traditions. The stresses they feel as a result of the generational and cultural gaps between themselves and their parents are often overwhelming. Many have not been successful in balancing these stresses and have chosen gang membership or suicide as a way to relieve their frustration and depression (Lee, Jung, Su, Tran, & Bahrassa, 2009). Hmong community leaders, community health workers, school districts, law enforcement, and Hmong families have joined together to develop interventions to address these issues (see Perspectives: Voices from the Community).

Another example of problematic cultural adaptation is the case of the "one child rule" in China. In an effort to contain population growth, in 1979, China began limiting married couples to having only one child. The government strictly enforces this policy, with few exceptions. Because male offspring are more highly valued than female in the Chinese culture, there is now a significant increase in the ratio of male to female births. Couples who have a female infant may choose to place the baby in an orphanage and make her available for adoption, but, although they are considered illegal, it is thought that a large number of sex-selective abortions occur. The goal of the government's policy was to change the Chinese culture from large- to small-family preference, and recent surveys indicate that this appears to be taking place; however, there are other untoward consequences of this cultural shift (Hesketh, Lu, & Xing, 2005). "Only children" are now caring for their elderly parents, along with their own "one child," as a widespread pension system does not yet exist in China. This strain, along with the shortage of women that leads to "kidnapping and trafficking of women for marriage, and increased numbers of commercial sex workers" are issues that must still be resolved (p. 1173).

Community health nurses must remember the dynamic nature of culture for several reasons. First, cultures and subcultures do change over time. Patience and persistence are key attributes to cultivate when working toward improving health behaviors. Second, cultures change as their members see greater advantages in adopting "new ways." Discussions of these advantages need to be conducted in a language understood by members and in the context of their own cultural value system. This is an important reason for nurses to develop an understanding of their clients' culture and to deliver culturally competent care (Giger & Davidhizar, 2008; Leininger & McFarland, 2006). Third, it is important to remember that, within a culture, change may occur due to certain key individuals who are receptive to new ideas and are able to influence their peers. These key persons can adapt the change process, so that "new" practices are culturally consistent and fit with group values. Tapping into this resource becomes imperative for successful change. Finally, the health care culture is dynamic, too. Westerners are just beginning to appreciate the validity of many non-Western health care practices such as acupuncture, meditation, and the use of various therapeutic herbs and spices (e.g., turmeric, fenugreek). We can learn much from our clients and their cultures (Meuninck, 2008; Spector, 2009) (see Perspectives: Voices from the Community).

PERSPECTIVES
VOICES FROM THE COMMUNITY

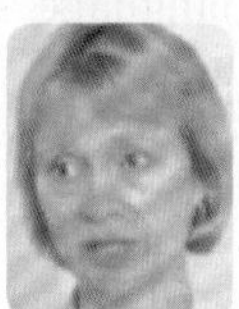

"The European immigrants who emerged from the Ford Motor Company melting pot came to the United States because they hoped to assimilate into mainstream American society. The Hmong came to the United States for the same reason they had left China in the 19th century: because they were trying to resist assimilation. What the Hmong wanted here [in the United States] was to be left alone to be Hmong: clustered in all-Hmong enclaves, protected from government interference, self-sufficient, and agrarian (p. 183)."

—Fadiman, A. (1998). The spirit catches you and you fall down: A Hmong child, her American doctors, and the collision of two cultures. New York: Farrar Straus & Giroux.

"You are talking about parents who are medieval, coming to a country that is hundreds of years ahead of theirs. They're trying to catch up, but it's hard."

—Mymee (college instructor)

"There is much research that shows people who stand in the middle of two cultures are really at risk of depression and anxiety."

—Valerie (psychologist)

"The kids are constantly living between two cultures. At some point, they may give up."

—Leng (psychologist, Southeast Asian adult services center)

"I think it's a topic that nobody wants to talk about. It's hard for me to say if the Hmong community is ready to deal with it."

—Xong (social worker, Hmong suicide task force)

"We parents think we know only one way to raise our kids. We ignore that these children are living in America and are espousing everything that is American, good and bad."

—Andy (Hmong parent)

Ellis, A. D. (2002, August 11). *Hmong Teens: Lost in America [Special report]. The Fresno Bee*, pp. 1–12.

ETHNOCULTURAL HEALTH CARE PRACTICES

Throughout history, people have relied on natural elements to treat various maladies that family, clan, tribe, or community members experience. Knowledge of culturally recognized practices or substances, such as berries, plants, barks, or rituals and incantations usually becomes the responsibility of one person in the community. This revered community leader is known as a medicine man/woman, healer, or shaman (Spector, 2009). As time passes, this person teaches the skills of recognizing and treating ailments or performing rituals to an apprentice, thereby continuing the healing knowledge and traditions.

In the following sections, we discuss how various geographic or ethnocultural groups view health care, including the biomedical, magicoreligious, and holistic views. You may encounter many distinctive ways that your clients manage their health and illness, so we will discuss selected folk medicines and home remedies, such as herbs, over-the-counter (OTC) drugs, and patent medications. In addition to these forms of treatments, there are complementary or alternative therapies (e.g., folk remedies) and various self-care practices. This section concludes with the community health nurse's role and responsibilities to provide culturally competent care in relation to caring for, respecting, teaching, and treating clients from different cultures.

The World Community

Beliefs about the causes and effects of illness, health practices, and health-seeking behaviors are all influenced by a person's, a group's, or a community's perception of what causes illness and injury and what actions can best treat or cure the health problem. The three major views in the world community are biomedical, magicoreligious, and holistic health beliefs (Spector, 2009).

Biomedical View

Western societies in general have a biomedical view of health and illness. The biomedical view relies on scientific principles and sees diseases and injuries as life events controlled by physical and biochemical processes that can be manipulated through medication, surgery, and other treatments. Examples of this view include the following beliefs:

- Elements, such as bacteria, fungi, or viruses, are causes of illness.
- Lack of certain elements, such as an adequate diet, calcium, or iron, causes other health problems, such as malnutrition, osteoporosis, or anemia.
- An accepted treatment for many physical ailments is to remove diseased organs, or to treat injuries from falls or accidents.

People living in countries where Western medicine is practiced believe that theirs is the best and, perhaps the only way, to deal with illness or injury. The dominant values presume that science is value free and not constructed by the social norms of the cultural group. The same is true, however, where Western medicine is not practiced and the social norms of the cultural group support the healing practices of that group (Leininger & McFarland, 2006; Spector, 2009). Many people, including community health nurses, are not open to other ways of looking at a person's wellness capabilities. As a result, clients may not receive culturally competent care from their caregivers. To be effective with clients, community health nurses must be knowledgeable and accepting of others' cultural practices.

Magicoreligious View

Magicoreligious themes of health and illness, which focus on the control of health and illness by supernatural forces, are prominent in some cultural groups. Diseases occur as a result of "committing sins" or "going against God's will." Good health is a gift from God, and illness is a form of punishment that affords an opportunity to be forgiven and to realign oneself with God. Prayer to God or other religious figures is used to cope with illness, seek intervention for healing, and ask for forgiveness and entrance into heaven, if death be God's will.

Some cultures mix traditional folk beliefs with organized religious practices and participate in forms of magic or voodoo. In cultures that have such beliefs, a hex or spell can be placed on another person through the use of incantations, elixirs, or an object resembling the person. For some, illness results from a look or a touch from another person considered to have special powers or intent to harm (Leininger & McFarland, 2006; Spector, 2009). Later in this chapter, we discuss some specific health beliefs and practices common to cultural groups in North America.

Religious beliefs, an individual's spirituality, and how these factors interface with feelings of wellness and specific healing practices are personal and important to clients and cannot be separated from their culture. This makes it imperative for community health nurses to be familiar with folk beliefs commonly seen in their practice. Only then can culturally competent nursing care be provided.

Holistic View

Holistic health believers come from many different cultural groups and generally view the world as being in harmonious balance. If the principles guiding natural laws to maintain order are disturbed, an imbalance in the forces of nature is created, resulting in chaos and disease. For an individual to be healthy, all facets of the individual's nature—physical, mental, emotional, and spiritual—must be in balance.

Some cultural groups believe that all things in creation or the universe have a spirit and therefore are considered equal in value, purpose, and contribution (Hill, 2006). Individuals have universal connectedness and are viewed as holistic beings. Persons are extensions of and integrated with family, community, tribe, and the universe. For example, "mother and fetus are viewed as interrelated and as affecting each other: They are one, but also they are two. In the circle of life, each individual is believed to be on a journey experiencing a process of being and becoming" (Lowe, 2002, p. 6).

Folk Medicine and Home Remedies

Many of us remember our mothers giving us hot herbal tea with lemon, or slathering on ointments and piling on blankets to lessen the effects of a mild illness. Many folk medicines and home remedies came about as a means of providing health care to family members when no medical care was available or deemed affordable.

Folk medicine is a body of preserved treatment practices that has been handed down verbally from generation to generation. It exists today as the first line of treatment for many individuals. Some clients may never plan to seek Western medical treatment but may share with you, the community health nurse, a practice they are using to treat a family member. Your response and actions may mean the difference between health and illness or injury. Some maternal–child health practices from the U.S. rural Midwest or South that may be encountered in community health nursing practice include the following (Giger & Davidhizar, 2008; Spector, 2009):

- Not reaching above your head if you are pregnant, because doing so will cause the umbilical cord to strangle the baby
- Pregnant women eating handfuls of clay, dirt, or cornstarch
- Taping coins over a newborn's umbilical area to prevent hernias
- Giving catnip tea to infants because it saves their lives
- Holding a baby upside down by the heel to "wake up the liver"
- Not letting a cat in a room with a sleeping baby, because the cat will "suck the life" out of the baby

Home remedies are individualized caregiving practices that are passed down within families. Even individuals who routinely seek the guidance of a health care practitioner for diagnosis and treatment may try home remedies before seeking professional advice. Each of us has a set of home remedies our parents used on us that we are likely to use on our own children before or instead of calling the pediatrician. Examples include using baking soda paste on a bee sting, ice on a "cold sore," or cranberry juice to prevent a urinary tract infection.

Herbalism

Textbooks have been written on the many uses of medicinal herbs (Lippincott Williams & Wilkins, 2006; Meuninck, 2008; Pizzorno, Murray, & Joiner-Bey, 2007; Thomson Healthcare, 2007). The use of some herbs has waxed and waned in favor. Some continue to be much touted, whereas others have been designated as dangerous and to be avoided (Medline Plus, 2007; Meuninck, 2008). Increasingly, the public is using herbal preparations in the form of self-selected OTC products for therapeutic or preventive purposes.

In an increasingly multicultural society, the source, form, and identity of many herbs, roots, barks, and liquid preparations become impossible for most community health nurses to distinguish. The most astute among us may be familiar with herbs used by one cultural group, whereas herbs used by another escape us. A book with pictures and descriptions, botanical form, purported indications and uses, and implications for nursing management is an important tool to keep handy when interacting with clients. *Nursing Herbal Medicine Handbook* (Lippincott Williams & Wilkins, 2006) is also available in software version for smartphones (Skyscape, 2010)—an even more efficient method of retrieving information quickly. Basic safety questions that community health nurses should answer about an herb when teaching or interacting with families include the following:

- Is the herb contraindicated with prescription medications the client is taking?
- Is the herb harmful? Does it have negative side effects?
- Is the client relying on the herb, without positive health changes, while neglecting to get effective treatment from a health care practitioner?

Herbs are not regulated as drugs and are not risk free. Dosages are not standardized and are left to the individual. Quality of the product may be suspect. For these reasons, herbs must be used only in moderation and with caution, preferably with guidance by a health care practitioner.

Prescription and Over-the-Counter Drugs

The cautions mentioned about herbs can also apply to prescription and OTC preparations. First, they are not risk free. In this country, prescription drugs are reviewed and tested by the U.S. Food and Drug Administration's (FDA's) Center for Drug Evaluation and Research (CDER), and OTC drugs go through a somewhat less-rigorous process through the CDER's Division of OTC Drug Products. Six of every ten medications bought in the United States are OTC drugs (U.S. FDA, 2007). However, many OTC drugs were once available only by prescription, and remain powerful medicines. All drugs can have major side effects, may be contraindicated in people with certain conditions, and may not be safe to use in combination with certain other drugs. Medication instruction and review is an important part of the community health nurse's role on home visits, especially with elderly clients (see Chapter 24).

Second, some new prescription medications are so expensive that clients cannot afford to take them as prescribed. Often, older, less expensive, and more frequently used drugs work as well as the newer, more expensive ones, which are heavily marketed by drug companies to health care practitioners and consumers. If you encounter clients who are unable to pay for drugs, you may need to advocate for them with health care providers to prescribe a less expensive medication or change to the generic form of the same drug, usually sold at a fraction of the cost. Some health care practitioners have samples of drugs available and may be able to use them for medically indigent clients. Many pharmaceutical companies now have low-cost prescription assistance programs for those in need (Partnership for Prescription Assistance, 2010).

Third, the efficacy of medications must be assessed. At times, the use of a new drug or an additional drug does not have the intended effect. As someone who sees the client managing their health at home over time, the community health nurse may be able to give the best information to the health care provider about the effectiveness of new medications for a particular client.

Complementary Therapies and Self-Care Practices

Complementary therapies (also called alternative medicine or alternative therapies) are practices used to complement contemporary Western medical and nursing care and are designed to promote comfort, health, and wellbeing (Snyder & Lindquist, 2010). The range of complementary therapies is broad and includes:

- Therapies (cancer diets, juice diets, fasting)
- Treatments (coffee enemas, high colonic enemas)
- Exercise activities (t'ai-chi, yoga)
- Exposure (aromatherapy, music therapy, light therapy)
- Manipulation (acupuncture, acupressure, reflexology)

Most cultural groups engage in some form of complementary therapy, either alone or in conjunction with Western medicine. **Integrated health care** is defined as the combination of complementary therapies with biomedical or Western health care (Snyder & Lindquist, 2009). Complementary therapies have become so commonplace today that many states are developing policies and guidelines for their use.

Consumers need to be well informed regarding the efficacy and safety of complementary therapies and how they can be true complements to other treatment modalities. The community health nurse should be aware of the variety of therapies available and how to get information for clients while remaining objective and supportive of the client's choices. At times, if a therapy contradicts the recommendations of the client's health care practitioner, the nurse may be in a position to provide the pros and cons of continuing the complementary therapy. On the other hand, the nurse may be able to suggest therapy forms that would complement Western medicine for the client, such as music therapy to promote relaxation and reduce stress or biofeedback for chronic pain management.

Self-care activities include complementary therapies, medications, and spiritual and cultural practices. They are uniquely individual for each person, as well as among different cultural groups. Chapter 19 includes a Self-Care Assessment Guide that may be helpful in assessing the self-care practices of families.

Role of the Community Health Nurse

When working with different cultural groups in the area of health care practices, the community health nurse can be an effective advocate for the client. First, however, the nurse must be prepared to speak knowledgeably about health care practices and choices. The nurse also must be able to assess the client or family adequately, so as to know what belief system motivates their choices. Finally, the nurse must be prepared to teach clients about the limits and benefits of cultural health care practices. The community health nurse should always individualize assessment and caregiving for the client within her culture and should not generalize about the client based on cultural group norms.

Preparation of the Community Health Nurse

To be effective when working with clients in the area of cultural health care and spirituality, the nurse must be prepared. Many ways exist for you to increase your cultural awareness and promote sensitivity to the differences among people from ethnocultural groups different from your own. You can acquire information from peers who are from the same cultural group as your clients; attend workshops or conferences on chosen cultural topics; read books on ethnocultural health care practices, herbalism, or complementary therapies; talk with clients about their views and practices and learn from them; keep an open mind and be curious about various practices; or attend community cultural events, such as Native American pow wows, ethnic food events held in some cities, or Cinco de Mayo celebrations. There are textbooks, novels, and articles about cultures in the community in which one practices. For example, the book *The Spirit Catches You and You Fall Down* (Fadiman, 1998) describes a Hmong child, her American doctors, and the collision of two cultures. Universities offer courses in transcultural nursing, ethnic studies courses or programs, and cultural events that can be valuable. The experience of Karin Urso, who worked with people from many different countries and cultures, illustrates the benefits of being open-minded (see From the Case Files I).

Assessment

When beginning to work with a group or family, it is important for you to become as familiar with them as possible. In addition to a family assessment or an individual health assessment, you can enhance your aggregate care by doing an ethnocultural or self-care assessment. Such an assessment reveals information about day-to-day living, cultural/spiritual influences, traditional/cultural health care choices and practices, and cultural taboos. Often this type of information is most useful as you work with clients on a regular basis. Useful tools include the two cultural assessment reviews at the end of this chapter and the self-care assessment tool in Chapter 19.

> ***From the* Case Files I**
>
> **Learning About Other Cultures**
>
> I was always interested in learning about other countries and cultures. But, I didn't realize that an overseas assignment would teach me so much about myself in addition to other cultures and ways of living. The lessons were sometimes difficult, but always rewarding. I knew that my expectations would not always be met and, yet it did surprise me how different the experience was from what I had imagined it would be. My job assignment, location, and team members changed frequently. Flexibility, comfort with ambiguity, a sense of humor, a deeper reliance upon my faith, patience, when results were not forthcoming, trust in others, and the ability to cross multiple cultures with some degree of ease were all skills that I developed over time. Most important to being successful at my job was to maintain the attitude of a "learner," not a "solver of problems" or the person "with all the answers." I made friends with people from all over the world who graciously accepted me into their lives, thus enriching mine. I learned that we all are different, but that every behavior has a reasonable explanation when you take the time to listen with your heart as well as with your ears. I found that I actually preferred other ways of doing and being while still maintaining those parts of my identity that were valuable to me. When I returned home, I found that my newly developed skills were still necessary–as I had changed and had to adjust to reentry into my home culture!
>
> *Karin Urso, PHN*

Teaching

As you are aware from your studies and preparation, teaching is the most important role in nursing, both in acute care settings and in the home. When working with families as a community health nurse, teaching takes a good deal of your time, because health care education is vitally important to communities, groups, and families. However, teaching that is undertaken in ways that are incomplete, culturally inappropriate, or inadequate may be frustrating and even harmful to your clients. Becoming ethnoculturally focused and prepared to teach from the client's view of the world will start you in the right direction. The suggestions in Display 5.3 offer ideas for providing culturally competent care. Chapter 11 on health promotion and education will help prepare you as well.

SELECTED CULTURAL COMMUNITIES

An examination of the meaning and nature of culture clearly underscores the need to recognize cultural differences and to understand clients in the context of their cultural backgrounds. Practically speaking, how can knowledge of cultural diversity be integrated into everyday community health nursing practice? What are the diverse cultural communities served by community health nurses? What are their differences? Do they share some features?

To provide insights and answers to these questions, this section describes 5 cultural communities, out of the more than 100 different ethnic groups living in the United States. Three are dominant in the United States; the other two represent populations native to North America and people from a Middle Eastern culture, an expanding group in the United States. These brief descriptions should not to be considered as a stand-alone guide to cultural competence; each culture is complex and unique, deserving of a more comprehensive study than is possible within the scope of this chapter. Many good references are available for nurses on cultural diversity (see References and Selected Readings).

Four of the groups highlighted represent those identified in *Healthy People 2020* (U.S. Department of Health and Human Services [U.S. DHHS], 2009a). The fifth group, Saudi Arabians, is presented because of the significant media attention people of the Middle East have received in recent years. *Healthy People 2010* (U.S. DHHS, 2009a) described significant disparities among members of some of the five groups highlighted here. Several of the disparities are given in Table 5-4. *Healthy People 2020* objectives expand on the work done through *Healthy People 2010*.

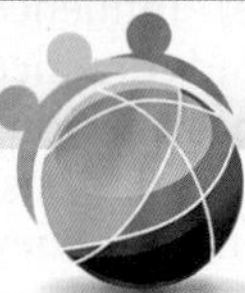

DISPLAY 5.3 DEVELOPING CULTURAL COMPETENCE

First: Know that culture is dynamic.
It is a continuous and cumulative process.
It is learned and shared by people.
Cultural behaviors and values are exhibited by people.
Culture is creative and meaningful to our lives.
It is symbolically represented through language and interaction.
Culture guides us in our thinking, feeling, and acting.

Second: Become aware of culture in yourself.
Thought processes that occur within you also occur within others but may take on a different shape or meaning.
Cultural values and biases are interpreted internally.
Cultural values are not always obvious since they are shared socially with those you meet on a daily basis and are perceived through your senses.

Third: Become aware of culture in others, especially among client groups you serve.
This is best represented by the belief that there are many cultural ways that are correct, each in its own location and context.
It is essential to build respect for cultural differences and appreciation for cultural similarities.
Develop the ability to work within others' cultural context, free from ethnocentric judgments.

Table 5.4 ***Healthy People 2010*** **and Disparities**

	Baseline Values				
Goal of *Healthy People 2010*	**White**	**Native American**	**Hispanic**	**Black**	**Asian**
Health insurance: 79% of population	89%	79%	70%	84%	83%
Cancer deaths/100,000: 158.7	202.2	131.8	125.5	262.1	127.2
End-stage renal disease/1 million: 217	218	586	N/A	873	344
Diabetes deaths/100,000: 45	68	107	86	130	62
CHD deaths/100,000: 166	214	134	151	257	125
Stroke deaths/100,000: 48	60	39	40	82	55
HIV/AIDS deaths/100,000: 0.8	2.8	2.5	8.9	26.6	0.9
Deaths from firearms/100,000: 4.9	10.4	11.4	10.7	22.9	5.0
Motor vehicle deaths/100,000: 9.0	15.8	31.5	15.2	17.0	10.6
Unintentional injury deaths/100,000: 20.8	34.3	62.7	30.1	40.9	20.9
Residential fire deaths/100,000: 0.6	1.1	2.2	0.8	3.4	0.8
Homicides/100,000: 3.2	4.3	10.4	9.9	25.2	4.1
Low-birth-weight babies: 7.6% of births	6.5	6.8	6.4	13.0	7.2
Suicides/100,000: 6.0	12.8	12.4	6.4	6.3	7.0
Drug-induced deaths/100,000:1.0	5.7	6.6	6.0	9.0	1.6
Smokers: 12% of population	25%	34%	20%	26%	16%

CHD, coronary heart disease; HIV/AIDS, human immunodeficiency virus/acquired immunodeficiency syndrome; N/A, not available.
From U.S. Department of Health and Human Services. (2011). *Healthy people 2010* (Conference edition, Vols. 1 and 2). Washington, DC: Author.

Native American Indians, Aleut, and Eskimo Communities

Native American Indians and Alaska Natives (Eskimo communities residing in Alaska), the first known settlers of this continent, form a large cluster of tribal groups whose members are descendants of the original Native Americans who inhabited this country before White Europeans settled here. The earliest European explorers were the Vikings (circa 1010 AD). Various other Europeans followed in the 16th century (Spector, 2009). Native Americans, Aleuts, and Eskimos have adopted many European American values and practices, yet they preserve many aspects of their own culture.

Population Characteristics and Culture

Native Americans and Alaska Natives are a diverse group made up of different tribes and 562 federally recognized nations that speak approximately 250 languages. Eskimos, Aleuts, and Native Americans living in Alaska are known as Alaska Natives; those living in other states are known as Native Americans or American Indians. In this chapter, the term *Native American* is used to encompass all facets of this diverse group of people. Through census estimates, these people make up just 2.4% of the U.S. population (U.S. Census Bureau, 2007). In 2007, a census report estimated that 4.5 million people are at least "part" Native American, and 2.9 million were identified only as Native American (U.S. Census Bureau, 2007). These people proudly identify themselves as being Native American, unlike in the past, when to claim Native American blood carried a social stigma. In addition to societal changes in the acceptance of Native Americans, financial incentives exist for many Americans who are recognized tribal members. Roughly 224 of the tribal governments receive revenue from gambling casinos—roughly half of all tribes have casinos in 28 states (Tribal Court Clearinghouse, n.d.; Walton, 2005). In 1988, when Congress passed the Indian Gaming Regulatory Act, casinos owned by Native Americans made $212 million; by 2000, they grossed $10 billion (Tribal Court Clearinghouse, n.d.; U.S. Department of Commerce, 2001). By 2002, native gaming revenue was $14.5 billion—or 21% of the entire gaming industry (Tribal Court Clearinghouse, n.d.). The percentage of "Indian to non-Indian employees" in these casinos is 75% to 25%, and three-quarters of gaming tribes use their revenue for "tribal government services, economic and community development....and do not give out per capita payments" (para. 19, 35). The remaining tribes pay per capita payments to tribal members (Tribal Court Clearinghouse, n.d.). Taylor and Kalt (2005) reported that real per capita income for gaming tribes increased by 36% between 1990 and 2000, while the total U.S. increase was 11%. However, even though the poverty rate fell for Native Americans overall, it is still twice the U.S. average (National Center for Education Statistics, 2008), and unemployment is nearly three times the national rate—making Native Americans among the nation's poorest groups (Native American Rights Fund, n.d.). Although gaming and other ventures have improved access to health, education, and employment for most Native Americans, access still falls behind that of other U.S. citizens.

The population of Native Americans and Alaska Natives is primarily concentrated in 26 states in the United States, including Alaska and the Aleutian Islands (Spector, 2009). Many live on reservations and in rural areas; however, more than half live in urban counties and have greater difficulty accessing the health care available to them through Indian Health Service (a federal program providing comprehensive health care to Native Americans) (Brenneman, Rhoades, & Chilton, 2006). The largest numbers live in Oklahoma, Arizona, California, New Mexico, North Carolina, and Alaska, as a result of forced westward migration (Spector, 2009). By 2050, the U.S. Census Bureau estimates about 4.5 million Native Americans will live in the United States, nearly double the number in 2000 (U.S. Department of Commerce, 2001). Some of this increase can be attributed to official recognition of persons who can provide information linking them to a tribe or nation; if they are accepted, they can then declare themselves to be Native Americans.

Each tribe or nation has its own distinct language, beliefs, customs, and rituals. The community health nurse cannot assume that knowledge of one group can be generalized to others. Knowledge of certain the various Native American cultures (Display 5.4) can assist nurses working with members of a specific tribe. For many Native American groups, large, extended family networks reinforce cultural standards and expectations and provide emotional support and practical assistance.

Health Problems

Health problems among Native Americans tend to be both chronic and socially related. One third of Native Americans live in abject poverty and experience the afflictions associated with poor living conditions, including malnutrition, tuberculosis (TB), and high maternal and infant death rates (Spector, 2009). The highest-ranking health problems in children include a postneonatal mortality rate double that of White infants (due largely to sudden infant death syndrome [SIDS], injuries, and congenital anomalies); overweight, obesity, and type 2 diabetes; and morbidity and mortality as a result of unintentional and intentional injuries (often motor vehicle injuries) (Brenneman et al., 2006). For adults, diabetes, TB, and obesity all rank higher among Native Americans than in the general population. Deaths from TB (5 times higher), alcoholism (5 times higher), diabetes (almost 2 times higher), unintentional injuries (1.5 times higher), and suicide and homicide (combined, 1.6 times higher) are higher for Native Americans than other Americans (Indian Health Services [IHS], 2010). Mortality from heart disease and cardiovascular disease is slightly higher than the general US population (269.4 per 100,000 deaths compared with 267 per 100,000 deaths [IHS, 2010]). Poor sanitation, crowded housing, and low immunization levels contribute to the prevalence of a variety of communicable diseases.

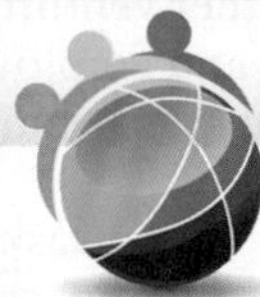

DISPLAY 5.4 SIMILARITIES AMONG NATIVE AMERICAN CULTURES

All of creation/universe has Spirit and is considered equal in value.
Everything is considered alive with energy and importance.
People have universal connectedness.
Harmony is a way of life based on cooperation and sharing.
Dignity of the individual, family, and community is valued.
Respect for advancing age is valued; elders are leaders.
There is present-time orientation, grounded in what is happening at the moment.
Symbolic arts and crafts are valued.
Life is lived in the present, with little concern for the distant future.
Generosity, harmony, and sharing are valued.
Religion is integrated into everyday life.
Herbal medicines and traditional healing practices are used.
Rituals and ceremonies are valued.
Silence is used as a way to practice presence and strength.
Thoughtful speech is valued.
Patience is valued.

Adapted from Lowe, J. (2002). Balance and harmony through connectedness: The intentionality of Native American nurses. *Holistic Nursing Practice*, 6(4), 4–11; Mehl-Madrona, L. E. (2008). *Traditional (Native American) Indian medicine treatment of chronic illness: Development of an integrated program with traditional American medicine and evaluation of effectiveness*. Retrieved January 19, 2011, from http://www.healing-arts.org/mehl-madrona/mmtraditionalpaper.htm; and Spector, R. E. (2009). *Cultural diversity in health and illness* (7th ed.). Upper Saddle River, NJ: Prentice-Hall Allied Health.

Alcoholism is the major health problem of Native Americans. Both traditional/cultural and medical explanations exist for the disproportionate number of alcohol-related health problems in Native Americans. Tribal medicine men have attributed the problems of alcoholism to losing "the opportunity to make choices," further stating that "once people return to a sense of identification within themselves they may be able to rid themselves of this problem of alcoholism" (Spector, 2009, p. 221). Medically, it appears that Native Americans have a much lower tolerance for alcohol and therefore demonstrate the effects of alcohol with lower amounts consumed. When individuals are under the influence of alcohol, other health and safety problems occur. Instances of domestic violence, child abuse and neglect, traffic injuries and deaths, and homicides are more frequent because of alcohol abuse. Along with these high rates of injuries and deaths, alcohol's destructive effects on the unborn lead to a high incidence of fetal alcohol syndrome (FAS) and fetal alcohol effects (FAE). Substance abuse is also prevalent among those living on reservations, and increasingly among youth using alcohol, tobacco, and other drugs (U.S. Substance Abuse & Mental Health Services Administration [U.S. SAMHSA], 2008).

Health Beliefs and Practices

Native Americans as a group prefer traditional healing practices and folk medicine to Western medicine. Most Native Americans today still seek out a medicine man or rely on traditional remedies before going to a health clinic. Many of their beliefs about health and illness have common traditional roots, regardless of tribe or location. Health and dietary practices are closely tied to cultural and religious beliefs. Beliefs about health reflect living in total harmony with nature. The Earth is considered a living organism that should be treated with respect, as should the body (Spector, 2009). Native Americans practice purification rituals such as immersion in water and the use of sweat lodges to maintain their harmony with nature and to cleanse the body and spirit. The basis of therapy lies in nature, with herbal teas, charms, and fetishes used as preventive and curative measures (Mehl-Madrona, 2008; Meuninck, 2008). Depending upon location, tribes use available plants or herbs to treat illnesses. For instance, those in the West often used sage (or sagebrush) tea for sore eyes, stomachache, or the pain of childbirth. It is still used in religious rituals (sweat lodges) and as a disinfectant (Meuninck, 2008).

Because of decades of racism and government paternalism, many Native Americans feel oppressed and dehumanized and carry considerable resentment and lack of trust toward Whites. As a result, many maintain a degree of separateness from overall American culture. Nurses must overcome these barriers through patience, acceptance, and respect for their clients' culture, as illustrated in the case study of the community health nurse, Sandra Josten, and her new client from a Native American community (see From the Case Files II).

Blacks or African Americans

Some of the ancestors of Black Americans, or African Americans, originally came to this continent as free settlers as early as 1619, but most of the approximately 4 million who followed came as slaves in the 17th and 18th centuries, mostly from the west coast of Africa (Byrd & Clayton, 2002). Most African Americans living today were born in the United States; some, however, have recently emigrated from African countries. Other Black Americans come from the West Indies, the Dominican Republic, Haiti, and Jamaica, often to escape poverty or political persecution. These people do not self-identify as African Americans but as Hispanics, a fact

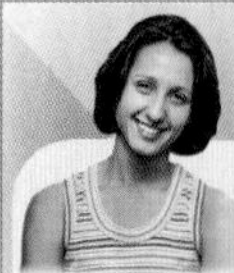

From the Case Files 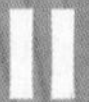

Sandra's New Clients

As she drove down the dirt road and parked her car next to the community hall, Sandra Josten felt apprehensive. The previous public health nurse had alerted her about the difficulty of working with these Native American people: "This tribe is lazy and unappreciative. You can't get anywhere with them." Only through the urging of Mrs. Brown, an Indian community aide, had a group of the women reluctantly agreed to meet with the new nurse. They would see what she had to say.

Sandra's steps echoed hollowly as she walked across the wooden floor of the large room to the far corner where a group of women sat silently in a circle. Only their eyes turned; their faces remained impassive. Mrs. Brown rose slowly, greeted the nurse, and introduced her to the group. Swallowing her fear, Sandra smiled. She told them of her background and explained that she had not worked with Indian people before. There was a long silence. No one spoke. Sandra continued, "I'd like to help you if I can, maybe with problems about care of your children when they are sick or questions about how to keep them healthy, but I don't know what you need or want." Silence fell again. She would like to learn from them, she repeated. Would they help her? Again, Sandra felt an uncomfortable silence.

Then one woman began to speak. Quietly, but with deep feeling, she described several bad experiences with the previous nurse and the county social worker. Then others spoke up: "They tell us what we should do. They don't listen. They say our way is not good." Seeing Sandra's interest and concern, the women continued. One of their main concerns was their children's health. Another was the high incidence of accidents and injuries on the reservation. They wanted to learn how to give first aid. Other concerns were expressed. The group agreed that Sandra could help them by teaching a first-aid class.

In the weeks that followed, Sandra taught several classes on first aid and emergency care. She then began a series of sessions on child health. Each time, she asked the women to choose a topic or problem for discussion and then elicited from them their accustomed ways of dealing with each problem; for example, how they handled toilet training or taught their children to eat solid foods. Her goal was to learn as much as she could about their culture and to incorporate that information into her teaching, which preserved as many of their practices as possible. Sandra also visited informally with the women in their homes and at community gatherings.

She learned about their way of life, their history, and their values. For example, patience was highly valued. It was important to be able to wait patiently, even if a scheduled meeting was delayed as much as 2 hours. It also was important for others to speak, which explained the Indian women's comfort with silences during a conversation. Other values influenced their way of life. Courage, pride, generosity, and honesty all were important determinants of behavior. These also were values by which they judged Sandra and other professionals. Sandra's honesty in keeping her promises enabled the women to trust her. Her generosity in giving her time, helping them occasionally with some household task, and arranging for childcare during classes won their respect.

The women came to accept her, and Sandra was invited to eat with them and share in tribal get-togethers. The women criticized and advised her on acceptable ways to speak and act. Her openness and patience to learn and her respect for them as a people had paved the way to improving their health. At first, Sandra felt that her progress was slow, but this slowness was an advantage. She had built a solid foundation of cross-cultural trust, and in the months that followed she saw many changes in her clients' health practices.

that may cause some difficulty for others trying to identify and accommodate to their culture. (Similarly, some people from the Philippines have Hispanic surnames and skin tones similar to those of Mexicans or other Latinos; when Filipinos—a culturally distinct group—settle in areas with large Hispanic populations, they can be similarly misidentified and misunderstood [Spector, 2009].)

Population Characteristics and Culture

The 2007 census estimated that African Americans numbered 40.7 million and constituted approximately 13.5% of the U.S. population; projections show an increase to 15.4% by the year 2050 (National Center for Health Statistics, 2007a; U.S. Census Bureau, 2007). One third of the African American population is younger than 18 years of age. Slightly more than 8% of African Americans are older than 65 years, and most of them are women; in comparison, 13% of the total population is older than 65 years. Some 58% of Black children live with their mothers only, compared with 21% of White children.

Despite improvements in the legal and social climate for African Americans, great disparities exist between them and White Americans (Byrd & Clayton, 2002). Average family income for African Americans is 63% of the income earned by White families. More than 24% of African Americans live in poverty, compared with 12.5% of Whites. Although African Americans make up only 13.5% of the population, more than 50% of prison inmates are Black.

The rate of current illicit drug use is highest for mixed race (14.7%) and Black/African American (10.1%) groups (U.S. SAMHSA, 2009). Approximately 36% of African American families in households headed by women live below the poverty level. Unemployment among African Americans is 15.6%, compared with 8.6% for Whites (U.S. Department of Labor, 2010).

Educational disparities also exist. Among people age 25 years and older, 83% of Blacks and 89% of Whites have a high school education (Infoplease, 2010). More than half of those African Americans with less than a high school education are not in the workforce, compared with 36% of Whites with a similar education. Black male college graduates were found to have twice the unemployment rate of their White counterparts, and White males generally received greater numbers of leads for high-level jobs than either women or minorities (Luo, 2009). African American women acquire more educational training than their Black male counterparts do, but their earnings are lower than those of the men, as is also the case with White and Hispanic women compared with men in those groups.

Like Native Americans and Asian Americans, African Americans do not comprise a single culture; rather, this group forms a heterogeneous community. As with other large ethnic and racial groups, many factors influence their culture, resulting in much diversity within the African American population. Among the variables determining specific microcultures within the African American community are economic level, religious background, education, occupation, social class identity, geographic origin, and residence in an integrated or segregated neighborhood. For community health nurses, this means that specific groups of African Americans have their own unique values, character, lifestyle, and health needs.

The primary language of most African Americans is English. Recent Black immigrants from Caribbean or other countries may retain the language of their country of origin, but usually learn to use English as well. Many African Americans speak nonstandard dialects of English, also called Black English, Ebonics, or African American Vernacular English. These dialects evolved from pidgin English spoken during the era of slavery, and they have become a dynamic and meaningful language of their own. For some African Americans, this dialect symbolizes racial pride and identity—it can also be used to differentiate them from the mainstream culture (Spector, 2009).

Health Problems

African Americans have much higher mortality rates than White Americans, with a life expectancy of 73.2 years (U.S. DHHS, 2009b). This number is the same as the life expectancy of Whites in 1980, revealing a 30-year lag for the Black population compared with the White population and demonstrates the inequality in mortality and life expectancy, an outcome of health care, economic, and educational disparity. A recent study compared mortality rates between Black and White males at the beginning and the end of the 20th century. No decreases were found and the 17% difference between Black and White mortality remained throughout the 20th century (Sloan, Ayyagari, Salm, & Grossman, 2010). Life expectancy for Whites in 2005 was 78.3 years. The gap for Blacks is 6.3 years for males and 4.3 years for females (U.S. DHHS, 2009b). The major health problems for Blacks include cardiovascular disease and stroke, cancer, diabetes mellitus, cirrhosis, a high infant mortality rate (twice that of Whites), homicide, accidents, and malnutrition (Display 5.5).

Stress and discrimination, poverty, lack of education, high rates of teen pregnancy, inadequate housing, and inadequate insurance for health care are among the risk factors influencing the health of this population. Female-headed households, single-parent births (most frequently among teenagers), and a limited presence of male role models have exacerbated family vulnerability. From 1980 to 1994, there was a dramatic increase in Black households headed by women, but this had declined slightly by 2000 (Joint Center Databank, 2007).

Leading causes of death for African Americans are heart disease, cancer, and stroke. As noted, infant death rates are higher in Blacks than in other groups (13.6 per 1,000 live births), leading many health departments to provide Black Infant Health programs (U.S. DHHS, 2009b). Mortality rates for communicable diseases, including acquired immunodeficiency syndrome (AIDS), also are higher for Blacks than for Whites. The incidence of TB in this population is rising, with many cases being diagnosed in conjunction with AIDS (see Chapters 8 and 26). Other infectious and parasitic diseases are three to six times more prevalent among African Americans than among Whites (U.S. DHHS, 2009b). Hypertension is a real concern in this population (37% of men and 41% of women over the age of 20 report having hypertension). In the same age group, 66% of men and 79% of women are reported as overweight (National Center for Health Statistics, 2007a). In two health-related areas, Blacks demonstrate a lower incidence than Whites: suicide is 50% less prevalent among Blacks, and the rate of chronic obstructive pulmonary disease (COPD) is 20% to 30% less. All other leading causes of death are higher for Black populations, much of which can be attributed to lifestyle and poverty (Hong, Nelson, Krohn, Mills, & Dimsdale, 2006). However, some genetic studies have shown significant differences between African Americans and Whites in those genes associated with hypertension and cardiovascular disease (Lange et al., 2006; Wang, Zhu, Dong, Treiber, & Snieder, 2006).

Blacks may have specific skin problems (e.g., keloids, melasma). In addition, sickle cell anemia occurs in Blacks, an inherited genetic trait thought to have originated in Africa as a defense against malaria (Spector, 2009).

Health Beliefs and Practices

Although African Americans have assimilated into the more dominant European American culture in the United States, some retain aspects of their ancestors' traditional values and practices. Some, for example, hold traditional African beliefs about health being a sign of harmony with nature and illness being evidence of disharmony. Evil spirits, the punishment of God, or a hex placed on the person might account for this

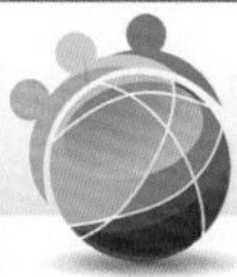

DISPLAY 5.5 EXAMPLES OF CULTURAL PHENOMENA AFFECTING HEALTH CARE AMONG BLACK OR AFRICAN AMERICANS

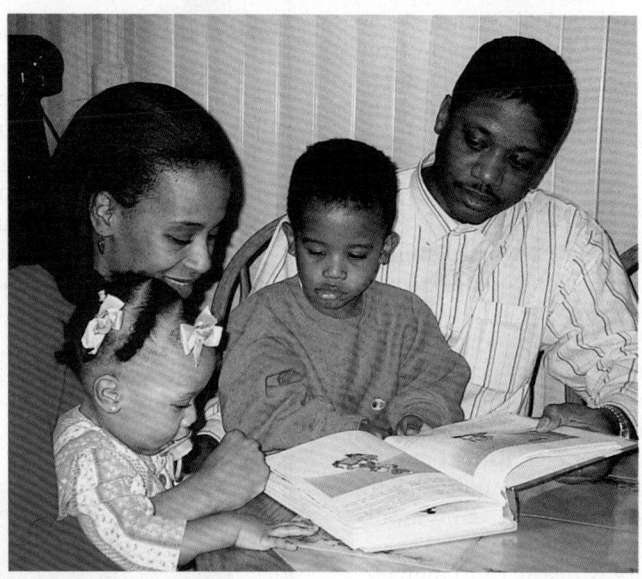

Nations of Origin	Many West African countries (as slaves) West Indian Islands The Dominican Republic, Haiti, Jamaica
Environmental Control	Traditional health and illness beliefs may continue to be observed by "traditional" people
Biological Variations	Sickle cell anemia, hypertension, cancer of the esophagus, stomach cancer, coccidioidomycosis, lactose intolerance
Social Organization	Family: many single-parent households headed by females Large, extended family networks Strong church affiliations within the community Community social organizations
Communication	National languages Dialect: Pidgin French, Spanish, Creole
Spatial Distancing	Close personal space
Time Orientation	Present over future

Adapted from Spector, R. E. (2009). *Cultural diversity in health and illness* (7th ed.). Stamford, CT: Appleton & Lange.

disharmony. Healers treat body, mind, and spirit. Prayer, laying on of hands, magic or other rituals, special diets, wearing of preventive charms or copper bracelets, ointments, and other folk remedies sometimes are practiced (Spector, 2009). African Americans have a high degree of religious involvement; 80% consider themselves to be either very or fairly religious. Higher levels of active religious participation are associated on average with less illness and better health (Taylor, Chatters, & Levin, 2004). Church attendance for African Americans is significantly associated with positive health care practices, such as blood pressure measurements, Pap smears, mammograms, and dental visits (Aaron, Levine, & Burstin, 2003) as well as decreased pain in sickle cell anemia (Harrison, Edwards, Koenig, Decastro, & Wood, 2005). Such an effect is even stronger for the chronically ill and uninsured subgroups. This is an important consideration when public health nurses plan programs targeting this population. Each African American community has its own set of health beliefs and practices that must be determined by the community health nurse before any interventions are planned.

Asian Americans

A third cultural cluster is composed of immigrants and refugees from various Pacific Rim countries, such as China, Korea, Japan, Thailand, Laos, the Philippines, Vietnam, and Cambodia (Display 5.6). Some Asian Americans have been transplanted fairly recently from their native countries and cultures to an entirely different culture, whereas others may have lived here many years or were born in America.

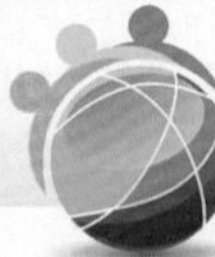

DISPLAY 5.6 ASIAN–PACIFIC POPULATIONS

Asian refers to:	*Pacific Islander refers to:*
Chinese	Polynesian
Filipino	Hawaiian
Japanese	Samoan
Asian Indian	Tongan
Korean	Micronesian
Vietnamese	Guamanian
Laotian	Melanesian
Thai	Fijian
Cambodian	Tahitian
Pakistan	Marshallese
Indonesian	Trilese
Hmong	
Mein	

Population Characteristics and Culture

In the estimated 2007 census, more than 16 million Asians and Pacific Islanders were living in the United States, representing 5.3% of the total population (U.S. Census Bureau, 2010). The largest groups were Chinese and Filipinos, with more than 1.5 million persons from each country; Vietnamese numbered a close second. Other fairly large groups came from Korea, India, Laos, and Cambodia. Each group represents a distinct culture with its own unique challenges for community health nurses, as illustrated in the case study of the Kim family (see From the Case Files III).

Whereas each Asian culture is distinct in language, values, and customs, many Asians share some general traits. Traditional Asian families tend to be patriarchal (the father is the head of the household) and patrilineal (the genealogy is carried through the male line). Male members are valued over female members. Elders are respected. The male role generally is that of provider, whereas the female role is that of homemaker. Traditional Asians value achievement because it brings honor to the family name. Saving face or preserving dignity and family pride is important. Cooperation is valued over competition (Leininger & McFarland, 2006; Spector, 2009).

Health Problems

Leading causes of death among Asians include cancer, heart disease, and stroke (U.S. DHHS, 2009b). Smoking is lower in this group (18% of males and 6% of females over age 18 smoke). Health problems for Asian Americans include malnutrition, TB, mental illness, cancer, respiratory infections, arthritis, parasitic infestations, and chronic diseases associated with aging. Suicide rates and stress-related illness are particularly high among Asian refugee groups who have had to flee their countries under stressful conditions and among teens born in the United States to Asian immigrants; many of these children have difficulty living between two cultures (Mui & Kang, 2006). However, Asians can view mental illness as shameful, and the stigma attached to it prompts them to express the mental illness as a disturbed bodily function or to hide it as long as possible (Mui & Kang, 2006; Spector, 2009).

Health Beliefs and Practices

Asian health beliefs vary among subcultures. Many Asians believe in the Chinese concepts of *yin* (cold) and *yang* (hot), which do not refer to temperature but to the opposing forces of the universe regulating normal flow of energy. A balance of yin and yang results in *qi* (pronounced *chee*), which is the desired state of harmony. Illness results when an imbalance occurs in these forces. If the imbalance is an excess of yin, then "cold" foods, such as vegetables and fruits, are avoided, and "hot" foods, such as rice, chicken, eggs, and pork, are offered. Some Asians view Western medicines as "hot" and Eastern folk medicines and herbal treatments as "cold," which explains why some groups practice both for balance. The Vietnamese have a similar hot-and-cold belief, but call it *am* and *dong*. Other Asian groups, such as the Filipinos, view illness as an act of God and pray for healing, reflecting their strong religious beliefs as Catholics or Muslims. The Khmer of Cambodia believe that illness reflects a deviation from moral standards, and the Hmong consider illness to be a visitation by spirits (Her & Culhane-Pera, 2004; Spector, 2009; Trinh-Shevri, Islam, & Rey, 2009).

Many Asian groups have traditional healers, who, depending on the culture, may include acupuncturists,

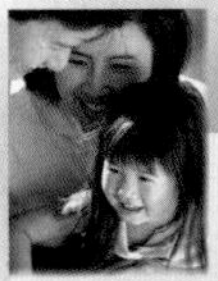

From the Case Files

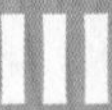

The Kim Family

Armed with enthusiasm and pamphlets on pregnancy and prenatal diet, Paula Morrow, the community health nurse, began home visits to the Kim family. Paula's initial plan was to discuss pregnancy and fetal development, teach diet, and prepare the mother for delivery. Mr. Kim, a graduate student, was present to interpret, because Mrs. Kim spoke little English. Their two children, ages 1 and 3 years, played happily on the kitchen floor. The family offered tea to the nurse and listened politely as she explained her reasons for coming and asked, "How can I be most helpful to you? What would you like from my visits?"

The Kims were grateful for this approach. Hesitant at first, they hinted at Mrs. Kim's fears of American doctors and hospitals; her first two children had been born in Korea. None of the family had any experience with Western medicine. They shared some concerns about adjustment to living in the United States. It was difficult to shop in American food stores with their overwhelming variety of foods, many of which the Kims found unfamiliar. Mrs. Kim, who had come from a family whose servants prepared the food, was an inexperienced cook. Servants also had cared for the children, and her role had been that of an aristocrat in hand-tailored silk gowns.

Listening carefully, Paula began to realize the striking differences between her own culture and that of her clients. Her care plans changed. In subsequent visits, she determined to learn about Korean culture and base her nursing intervention on that knowledge. She learned about their traditional ways of raising children, the traditional male and female roles, and practices related to pregnancy and lactation. She respected their value of "saving face" and attempted never to offend their pride or dignity. As time went on, her interest and respect for their way of life won their trust. She inquired about their cultural practices before attempting any intervention. As a result, the Kims were receptive to her suggestions. Whenever possible, Paula adapted her teaching and suggestions to comply with the Kims' culture. For example, appropriate changes were made to Mrs. Kim's diet plan to incorporate her food preferences and cultural eating patterns. Because she was not accustomed to drinking milk, she increased her calcium intake by learning to prepare custards (which disguised the milk flavor) and by eating more portions of leafy, green vegetables. After 5 months, a strong, positive relationship had been established between this family and the nurse. Mrs. Kim delivered a healthy baby girl and looked forward to continued supportive visits from the community health nurse.

herbalists, herb pharmacists, spirit and magic experts, or a shaman. Most Asian cultures also exercise traditional self-care practices, including herbal medicines and poultices, types of acupuncture, and massage (Meuninck, 2008; Spector, 2009; Trinh-Shevri et al., 2009). Southeast Asians also practice dermabrasive techniques of coining, cupping, pinching, rubbing, and burning. These methods are used to relieve symptoms such as headache, sore throat, cough, fever, and diarrhea by bringing toxins to the skin surface or compensating for heat lost. Cupping was a common medical practice in colonial America (Trinh-Shevri et al., 2009). Because these techniques leave a bruise-like lesion on the skin, they can be mistaken for physical abuse. Each client requires a careful **cultural assessment** (a detailed data-gathering about the client's cultural practices) before nursing action is implemented.

Hispanic Americans

A fourth cultural cluster comprises groups who are of Hispanic or Latino origin and have immigrated to the United States, some many generations ago. More than half come from Mexico, followed by Puerto Rico, Cuba, the Dominican Republic, and Central and South America (Spector, 2009; U.S. Census Bureau, 2006). Those with Mexican and Central American backgrounds generally are referred to as Latinos. Depending on the region of the country, socioeconomic status, immigration or citizenship status, or age, members of this large minority group refer to themselves as Mexican American, Spanish American, Chicano, Latin American, Latin, Latino, or Mexican (Eggenberger, Grassley, & Restrepo, 2006; Spector, 2009). In this chapter, for convenience, the term *Hispanic* is used to encompass this entire diverse population.

The subgroups of Hispanics vary by their patterns of geographic distribution in the United States. Of the almost 47 million Hispanics in the United States—about 15% of the population in 2008—Mexicans are the largest percentage at 66%. Central and South Americans comprise 13%, and Puerto Ricans make up 9.4% of the Hispanic population. The remaining groups include Cubans (3.9%) and Other (7.5%). The states with the largest Hispanic populations include California (13.6 million), Texas (8.9 million), New York (3.8 million), Florida (3.8 million), and Illinois (1.9 million). The Hispanic population is young, with 34.3% under the age of 18, compared to 22.3% non-Hispanic Whites (Office of Minority Health, 2009).

Population Characteristics and Culture

Hispanics are the fastest-growing and largest ethnic group in the United States, and people of Hispanic origin are predicted to number more than 73 million, or 20.1% of the population, by 2030 (U.S. Census Bureau, 2006). In 2006, this group comprised more than 44.3 million people and accounted for over 14.8% of the U.S. population (National Center for Health Statistics, 2007b; U.S. Census Bureau, 2009).

The Hispanic population uses Spanish as its common and primary language; nonetheless, its diverse cultural and linguistic backgrounds account for diversity in dialects. In 2007, about 12% of the U.S. population spoke Spanish at home (Office of Minority Health, 2009). Compared to Whites, Hispanics have lower achievement of a high school diploma (89% vs. 61%). In 2007, 21.5% of Hispanics, compared with 8.2% of Whites, lived at the poverty level (Office of Minority Health, 2009). Of particular note to public health nurses, Hispanics have the highest uninsured rates of any racial/ethnic group, with 32.1% not covered by any health insurance. White rates of uninsured were 10.4% (Office of Minority Health, 2009). Hispanic people value extended, cohesive families. Families have generally been patriarchal, with male members perceived as superior and female members seen as a family-bonding life force. These traditional family structures are changing because of migration, urbanization, women in the workforce, and social movements. Spousal roles are becoming more egalitarian (Eggenberger et al., 2006; Giger & Davidhizar, 2008; Spector, 2009). However, vestiges of the *macho* man and the self-sacrificing woman still are evident in Hispanic culture and continue to shape behavior (see From the Case Files IV).

Health Problems

Leading causes of death for the Hispanic population include heart disease, cancer, unintentional injuries (accidents), stroke, and diabetes. A large number of this population is uninsured and do not have a usual source of health care (31% for adults, almost 10% for children) (National Center for Health Statistics, 2007b). Health problems among the Hispanic population are complicated by experiences in their countries of origin, as well as by socioeconomic and lifestyle factors in this country. TB is high in this group, especially among those younger than 35 years of age. Hypertension, diabetes, and obesity are major concerns. Obesity is higher in Hispanics than Whites, and asthma, COPD, suicide, and liver disease also significantly impact Hispanics. Other problems include infectious diseases, particularly AIDS and pneumonia, parasitic infections, malnutrition,

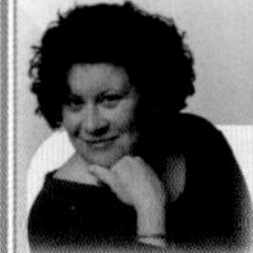

From the Case Files IV

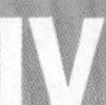

Maria Juarez

Maria Juarez, a 53-year-old Mexican American widow, was referred to a public health nursing agency by a clinic. Her married daughter reported that Mrs. Juarez was having severe and prolonged vaginal bleeding and needed medical attention. The daughter had made several appointments for her mother at the clinic, but Mrs. Juarez had refused at the last minute to keep any of them.

After two broken home visit appointments, the community health nurse made a drop-in call and found Mrs. Juarez at home. The nurse was greeted courteously and invited to have a seat. After introductions, the nurse explained that she and the others were only trying to help. Mrs. Juarez had caused a lot of unnecessary concern to everyone by not cooperating, she scolded in a friendly tone. Mrs. Juarez quickly apologized and explained that she had felt fine on the days of her broken appointments and saw no need "to bother" anyone. Questioned about her vaginal bleeding, Mrs. Juarez was evasive. "It's nothing," she said. "It comes and goes like always, only maybe a little more." She listened politely, nodding in agreement as the nurse explained the need for her to see a physician. Her promise to come to the clinic the next day, however, was not kept. The staff labeled Mrs. Juarez as unreliable and uncooperative.

Mrs. Juarez had been brought up in traditional Mexican American culture that taught her to be submissive and interested primarily in the welfare of her husband and children. She had learned long ago to ignore her own needs and found it difficult to identify any personal wants. Her major concern was to avoid causing trouble for others. To have a medical problem, then, was a difficult adjustment. The pain and bleeding had caused her great apprehension. Many Mexican Americans have a particular dread of sickness and especially hospitalization. Furthermore, Mrs. Juarez's culture had taught her the value of modesty. "Female problems" were not discussed openly. This cultural orientation meant that the sickness threatened her modesty and created intense embarrassment. Conforming to Mexican American cultural values, she had first turned to her family for support. Often, only under dire circumstances do members of this ethnic/cultural group seek help from others; to do so means sacrificing pride and dignity. Mrs. Juarez agreed to go to the clinic because refusal would have been disrespectful, but her fear of physicians and her reluctance to discuss such a sensitive problem kept her from going. Mrs. Juarez was being asked to take action that violated several deeply felt cultural values. Her behavior was far from unreliable and uncooperative. With no opportunity to discuss and resolve the conflicts, she had no other choice.

gastroenteritis, alcohol and drug abuse, unintentional injuries, and violence. Frequently, the most important health issues for Hispanics are related to the fact that the population is young and has a high birth rate (97.7 per 1,000 births) (National Center for Health Statistics, 2007b; Office of Minority Health, 2009). The rate of low-birth-weight infants is lower in Hispanics overall, but higher among Puerto Ricans, who also experience disproportionate levels of asthma, infant mortality, and HIV/AIDS. Mexicans have higher rates of diabetes; they are twice as likely as Whites to be diagnosed with diabetes. Mexican women are 130% more likely to be obese than White women (Office of Minority Health, 2009). Posttraumatic stress disorder is a major problem among refugees from Central and South America who have experienced war and physical and emotional torture.

Health Beliefs and Practices

Religion plays an important part in Hispanic culture. For most Hispanics, Catholicism is the dominant religion (e.g., 95% of Mexican Americans are Catholic), but religious beliefs often consist of a blend of Catholicism and pre-Columbian Indian beliefs and ideology, along with magicoreligious practices. Hispanics believe in submission to the will of God and that illness may be a form of *castigo*, or punishment for sins. They cope with illness through prayers and faith that God will heal them. Their religion also determines the rituals used in healing. For example, *solito*, a condition of depression in women similar to a midlife crisis seen in the American culture, is treated by having the patient lie on the floor while her body is stroked by the *curandero* (native healer) until the depression passes. Latino culture includes beliefs that witchcraft (*brujeria*) and the evil eye (*mal de ojo*) are supernatural causes of illness that cannot be treated by "Anglo" or Western medicine. *Empacho*, a stomachache in children that occurs after a traumatic event, is treated by the *curandero* with herbal mixtures made into teas. After tender loving care and a bowel movement, the child is considered healed (Table 5-5). As with Asians, Hispanics use "hot" and "cold" categories of foods to

Table 5.5 Hispanic Health Beliefs and Folk Diseases

Belief Name	Explanation/Treatment
Ataque	Severe expression of shock, anxiety, or sadness characterized by screaming, falling to the ground, thrashing about, hyperventilation, violence, mutism, and uncommunicative behavior. Is a culturally appropriate reaction to shocking or unexpected news that ends spontaneously.
Bilis	Vomiting, diarrhea, headaches, dizziness, nightmares, loss of appetite, and the inability to urinate brought on by livid rage and revenge fantasies. Believed to come from bile pouring into the bloodstream in response to strong emotions and the person "boiling over."
Bilong (hex)	Any illness may be caused by this; proper diagnosis and treatment requires consulting with a *santero* or *santera* (priest or priestess).
Caide de mollera	A condition thought to cause a fallen or sunken anterior fontanel, crying, failure to nurse, sunken eyes, and vomiting in infants. Popular home remedies include holding the child upside down over a pan of water, applying a poultice to the depressed area of the head, or inserting a finger in the child's mouth and pushing up on the palate. (Note: According to Western medicine, these symptoms are indicative of dehydration and can be life threatening. The community health nurse role is imperative—to promoting hydration and definitive health care.)
Empacho	Lack of appetite, stomachache, diarrhea, and vomiting caused by poorly digested food. Food forms into a ball and clings to the stomach, causing pain and cramping. Treated by strongly massaging the stomach, gently pinching and rubbing the spine, drinking a purgative tea (*estafiate*), or by administering *azarcon* or *greta*, medicines that have been implicated, in some cases, in lead poisoning. (Note: The community health nurse must assess family for the use of these "medicines" and initiate appropriate follow-up.)
Fatigue	Asthma-like symptoms treated with Western health care practices, including oxygen and medications.
Mal de ojo	A sudden and unexplained illness including vomiting, fever, crying, and restlessness in a well child (most vulnerable) or adult. Brought on by an admiring or covetous look from a person with an "evil eye." It can be prevented if the person with the "evil eye" touches the child when admiring him or her if the child wears a special charm. Treated by a spiritualistic sweeping of the body with eggs, lemons, and bay leaves accompanied by prayer.
Pasmo	Paralysis-like symptoms in the face and limbs treated by massage.
Susto	Anorexia, insomnia, weakness, hallucinations, and various painful sensations brought on by traumatic situations such as witnessing a death. Treatment includes relaxation, herb tea, and prayer.

Adapted from Spector, R. E. (2009). *Cultural diversity in health and illness* (7th ed.). Stamford, CT: Appleton & Lange.

influence their diet during illness. Many Hispanics tend to be present-oriented, and consequently are not as concerned as the mainstream culture about keeping to time schedules or preparing for the future (Eggenberger et al., 2006; Giger & Davidhizar, 2008; Leininger & McFarland, 2006; Spector, 2009).

Arab Populations and Muslims

The final cultural community selected for this discussion is made up of groups of people who come from Arabic countries, especially those who espouse the Muslim religion. By comparison with the groups previously mentioned, the number of people from Arabic countries in the United States is small, but because of the terrorist attacks of September 11, 2001, and the wars in the Middle East, increasing racial and religious animosity has been directed toward people from this part of the world and against those who bear physical resemblance to members of these groups. This unwarranted ostracism has led to mental anguish and distress in Arab and Muslim communities (Ahmad, 2004; Cultural Diversity in Nursing, 2008; Giger & Davidhizar, 2002). Hopefully, factual information about these groups of people will dispel myths and alleviate fear.

About 4 million people of Arab descent live in the United States. For purposes of the U.S. census, Arabs are characterized as White (Electronic Resource Center, 2007a). Los Angeles County (California), Wayne County (Michigan), and Cook County (Illinois) have the largest populations of Arab Americans, with Detroit, Los Angeles, and New York metropolitan areas reporting the largest numbers (Samhan, 2006). Arab Americans have generally done very well economically: 41% are college graduates, over 50% own their own home, 42% work as professionals or managers, and the median income for Arab American families is 4.6% higher than other Americans (Naim, 2005). Many Arab immigrants have only arrived since the 1990s, fleeing war-torn countries or repressive regimes (Naim, 2005).

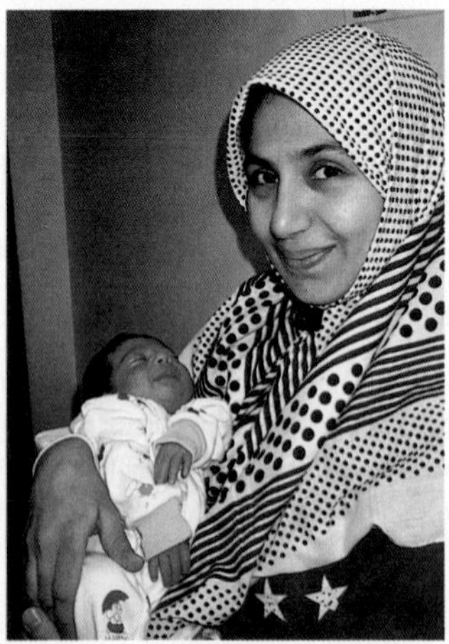

A large percentage of Arabs own their own homes, are college graduates, and work as professionals, for example, in business, medicine, nursing, and education.

A common language (Arabic) and background unite them, yet only 18% of Muslims (followers of Islam) reside in Middle Eastern countries. Arabs are largely Christian or Muslim, although some Arabs may be Jews or Druze (Electronic Resource Center, 2007b). Christian Arabs first began emigrating to the United States in the late 19th and early 20th centuries (mostly from Syria and Lebanon), but during the middle of the 20th century, Muslim Arabs began to emigrate in greater numbers (commonly from Palestine, Egypt, Iraq, and Yemen). Islam is the fastest-growing global religion, with more than 1 billion followers worldwide. Most Muslims live in Indonesia, the southern Philippines, and the United States (Electronic Resource Center, 2007c). The Council on American–Islamic Relations (2008) reports that 25% of U.S. Muslims are of Southeast Asian ancestry, while only 23% are of Arab descent. Approximately 8 million Americans are Muslim. In Britain, it is estimated that Muslim worshippers will outnumber Anglicans within a few years, and the Christian Research Organization in England projected that, if current trends continue, by 2039 Muslims will surpass all British Christians in worship attendance (Baqi-Aziz, 2001). The tenets of Islam are interpreted more liberally in some nations and more strictly in others, but all practicing Muslims adhere to the five tenets of Islam in some fashion (Table 5-6).

Population Characteristics and Culture

An Arab is generally defined as someone from one of the 22 Arab countries who speaks an Arabic dialect, and shares the values and beliefs of an Arab culture (Cultural Diversity in Nursing, 2008). Arab Americans can trace their ancestry to the North African countries of Morocco, Tunisia, Algeria, Libya, Sudan, and Egypt, as well as the Western Asian countries of Lebanon, Palestine, Syria, Jordan, Bahrain, Qatar, Oman, Saudi Arabia, Kuwait, the United Arab Emirates, and Yemen. Iran is sometimes listed in this group, although Iranians generally consider themselves to be Persian, not Arab (Arab American Institute, 2010). Assyrian/Chaldean/Syriac and sub-Saharan (Somalian and Sudanese) groups are also noted as Arab. In general, the beliefs and practices of people from such disparate and distant countries cannot be encompassed into one culture. Despite the fact that some of these countries are highly Westernized, enjoy natural resources such as crude oil and the riches that may follow, and are more liberal in following traditional cultural practices, others do not. It must also be noted that the Middle East has one of the slowest-growing levels of personal income in the world and the highest unemployment rates among developing nations (Naim, 2005).

Arabs are mostly divided into two distinct religious groups: Muslims and Christians. Arabs generally value Western medicine, trust American health care workers, and do not generally postpone seeking medical care (Electronic Resource Center, 2007d). Several practices, however, are unfamiliar to most Americans. Many Arabic women stay at home and are not in the workforce. Families impose stricter rules for girls than for boys. After menarche, teenage girls may not

Table 5.6 The Five Pillars (Tenets) of Islam

1. Faith	Declaration of faith (*shahada*) that there is no God but Allah and that Mohammad is the messenger of Allah
2. Prayer	Obligatory prayers five times a day at dawn, noon, mid-afternoon, sunset and when night falls (called *salat*) link the worshipper to God. Prayers are led by a learned man who knows the Quran, as there is no hierarchical authority in Islam (like a minister or priest).
3. Almsgiving	This is like tithing and is a very important principle as all wealth is thought to belong to God. It is called *zakat*, and each Muslim is expected to pay 2.5% of his or her wealth annually for the benefit of others in need.
4. The Fast	To abstain from food, drink, and sexual intercourse during daytime (from dawn to sunset) throughout the 9th lunar month (Ramadan). It is a means of self-purification and spirituality. The sick, elderly, or pregnant/nursing women may be permitted to break the fast.
5. The Pilgrimage	The pilgrimage to Makkah (the Hajj) once in a lifetime for those who are physically and financially able to do so. About 2 million people go to Makkah every year (located in Saudi Arabia).

socialize with boys. The adolescent female also begins to cover her head and perhaps wears a *hajab*, which takes the form of a modest dress and veil designed to diminish attractiveness and appeal to the opposite sex. Some Arab groups take this mode of dress to extremes, not even allowing a woman's eyes to show out of the *hajab*. Modesty is one of the core values for Arabs; it is expressed by both genders, although more evidently by females (Yosef, 2008).

Within the Arabic population, strict sexual taboos and social practices exist. All sexual contacts outside the marital bond are considered illegal. Those known to have been involved in such activities can be socially rejected, or in some countries even put to death. The stigma of lost honor can continue with their families for generations to come. Another social practice, at times mistakenly related to the Islamic religion, is the practice of female genital mutilation. This is practiced in a few of the Arabic countries on the African continent and has spread to southern Egypt, but it is rare or nonexistent in other Arabic countries. This horrific practice may include the removal of a young woman's labia, clitoris, or both, and it sometimes includes closing the vaginal opening by suturing (Royal College of Nursing, 2006; Yosef, 2008).

Health Problems

Health problems among Middle Easterners are most frequently lifestyle related. These include poor nutritional practices, resulting in obesity, especially among women; smoking among men; and lack of physical exercise (Yosef, 2008). In some rural areas, especially in Saudi Arabia, men and women chew tobacco, and an increase of oral cancers is seen. Major public health concerns for most Arabs are related to motor vehicle accidents, maternal–child health, TB, malaria, trachoma, typhus, hepatitis, typhoid fever, dysentery, and parasitic infections (Giger & Davidhizar, 2002; Yosef, 2008).

Most social restrictions are directed toward women and can affect their health. Pregnancy can be complicated by genital mutilation, which results in infections and difficult deliveries. Childbearing continues up until menopause, and 30% of marriages in some Arabic countries are between first cousins; both factors can contribute to the prevalence of genetically determined diseases (Giger & Davidhizar, 2002; Yosef, 2008). There is often a desire to have more sons than daughters and this may result in very large families and closely spaced pregnancies—often without the benefit of family planning. It is often debated whether birth control methods are sanctioned by Islam or not, but Akbar (2007) states that Muslims can reason for themselves, and notes that family planning is not forbidden by the beliefs of Islam. Abortion and infanticide are not accepted, however.

Health Beliefs and Practices

Traditional medicine is practiced in spite of the growth of Western medical services in some of the richer Arab nations. Traditional health care practices are much more common in the poorer Middle Eastern countries and in rural areas of all Arabic countries.

Muslims believe in predestination—that life is determined beforehand—and they attribute the occurrence of disease to the will of Allah. However, this does not prevent people from seeking medical treatment. Islamic law prohibits the use of illicit drugs, which include alcohol. Users of such substances are liable to trial, and those convicted of smuggling substances into an Arab country can be sentenced to death in some cases. *Sharaf*, or honor, is an important concept in Arab American beliefs, and drug addiction, mental illness, or unwed pregnancy of a family member brings shame to the entire family (Electronic Resource Center, 2007e). Conversely, when a member does something good or is recognized for an achievement, that honor is reflected on the family as a whole.

Cleanliness is paramount and ritualistic, especially before prayers and after sexual intercourse. The bodies of both genders are kept free of axillary and pubic hair. The left hand is used for cleaning the genitals and the right one is reserved for eating, hand shaking, and other hygienic activities. Muslims fast during Ramadan from sunrise to sunset, and this can include abstinence from all things (including medications or intravenous fluids). Illness can be an exception to this rule, but public health nurses should consult with a family elder or Muslim leader to encourage the client to continue with any necessary treatments. Also, Muslims pray several times daily, facing toward Mecca. Home visits should be planned so that prayers are not interrupted (Electronic Resource Center, 2007e).

When caring for Arabs in clinics or at home, a nurse of the same sex as the client should be assigned. It is important to note that only women may discuss many topics (e.g., menstruation, family planning, pregnancy, and childbirth); and men are not included in these discussions.

Additional guidelines for nurses working with all immigrant groups include the following:

- Make no assumptions about a client's understanding of health care issues.
- Permit more time for interviewing; allow time to evaluate beliefs and provide appropriate interventions.
- Provide educational programs to correct any misconceptions about health issues; this can occur in clinics, mosques, schools, or homes.
- Provide an appropriate interpreter to improve communication with immigrants who do not speak English well.

TRANSCULTURAL COMMUNITY HEALTH NURSING PRINCIPLES

Culture profoundly influences thinking and behavior and has an enormous impact on the effectiveness of health care. Just as physical and psychological factors determine clients' needs and attitudes toward health and illness, so too can culture. Kark emphasized over 30 years ago "culture is perhaps the most relevant social determinant of community health" (1974, p. 149). Culture determines how people rear their children, react to pain, cope with stress, deal with death, respond to health practitioners, and value the past, present, and future. Culture also influences diet and eating practices. Partly because of culturally derived preferences, dietary practices can be very difficult to change (Leininger & McFarland, 2006; Spector, 2009).

Despite its importance, the client's culture often is misunderstood or ignored in the delivery of health care (Leininger & McFarland, 2006). With the growth in non-White populations, "health care providers must be prepared for interactions with increasingly diverse health care team members and clients" (Giger & Davidhizar, 2002, p. 80). Especially in public health, the nurse must avoid ethnocentric attitudes and must attempt to understand and bridge cultural differences when working with others. It is important to develop knowledge and skill in serving multicultural clients and an ability to place clients' responses to experiences within the context of their lives, or else risk ineffectiveness in the face of a limited understanding and interpretation of client experience.

Overcoming ethnocentrism requires a concerted effort on the nurse's part to see the world through the eyes of clients. It means being willing to examine one's own culture carefully and to become aware that alternative viewpoints are possible. It also consists of attempting to understand the meaning other people derive from their culture and appreciating their culture as important and useful to them (Campinha-Bacote, 2003). Ignoring consideration of clients' different cultural origins often has negative results, as illustrated in From the Case Files IV discussion about Maria Juarez.

Culture is a universal experience. Each person is part of some group, and that group helps to shape the values, beliefs, and behaviors that make up their culture. In addition, every cultural group is different from all others. Even within fairly homogeneous cultural groups, subcultures and microcultures have their own distinctive characteristics. Further differences, based on such factors as socioeconomic status, social class, age, or degree of acculturation, can be found within microcultures. These latter differences, called *intraethnic variations*, only underscore the range of culturally diverse clients served by community health nurses.

Given such diversity, community health nurses face a considerable challenge in providing service to cross-cultural groups. This kind of practice, known as **transcultural nursing**, means providing culturally sensitive nursing service to people of an ethnic or racial background different from the nurse's (Andrews & Boyle, 2008; Leininger & McFarland, 2006). Community health nurses in transcultural practice with client groups can be guided by several principles: develop cultural self-awareness, cultivate cultural sensitivity, assess the client group's culture, show respect and patience while learning about other cultures, and examine culturally derived health practices.

Develop Cultural Self-Awareness

The first principle of transcultural nursing focuses on the nurse's own culture. Self-awareness is crucial for the nurse working with people from other cultures (Leininger & McFarland, 2006). Nurses must remember that their culture often is sharply different from the culture of their clients. **Cultural self-awareness** means recognizing the values, beliefs, and practices that make up one's own culture. It also means becoming sensitive to the impact of one's culturally based responses. The community health nurse who assisted Mrs. Juarez in the fourth Case File discussion probably thought that she was being friendly, efficient, and helpful. In terms of her own culture, this nurse's behavior was intended to reassure clients and meet their needs. Unaware of the negative consequences of her behavior, the nurse caused damage rather than met needs.

To gain skill in understanding their own culturally based behavior, nurses can complete a cultural self-assessment by analyzing their own:

- Influences related to racial background
- Verbal and nonverbal communication patterns
- Values and **norms** (expected cultural practices or behaviors)
- Beliefs and practices

Start with a detailed list of values, beliefs, and practices relative to each point. Next, enlist one or more close friends to call attention to selected behaviors, to bring them to a more conscious level. Videotaping practice interviews with colleagues and actual interviews with selected clients creates further awareness of the nurse's unconscious, culturally based responses. Finally, ask selected clients to critique nursing actions in light of the clients' own culture. Feedback from clients' perspectives can reveal many of the nurse's own cultural responses.

Because culture is mostly tacit, as discussed earlier, it takes conscious effort and hard work to bring the nurse's own cultural biases or influence to the surface. Doing so, however, rewards the nurse with a more effective understanding of self and enhanced ability to provide culturally relevant service to clients (Andrews & Boyle, 2008; Spector, 2009).

Cultivate Cultural Sensitivity

The second transcultural nursing principle seeks to expand the nurse's awareness of the significance of culture on behavior. Nurses' beliefs and ways of doing things frequently conflict with those of their clients. A first step toward bridging cultural barriers is to recognize those differences and develop cultural sensitivity. **Cultural sensitivity** requires recognizing that culturally based values, beliefs, and practices influence people's health and lifestyles and need to be considered in plans for service (Campinha-Bacote, 2003; Leininger & McFarland, 2006). Mrs. Juarez's values and health practices sharply contrasted with those of the clinic's staff. Failure to recognize these differences led to a breakdown in communication and ineffective care. Once differences in culture are recognized, it is important to accept and appreciate them. A nurse's ways are valid for the nurse; clients' ways work for them. The nurse visiting the Kim family in the third case file discussion avoided the dangerous ethnocentric trap of assuming that her way was best, and she consequently developed a fruitful relationship with her clients.

As a part of developing cultural sensitivity, nurses need to try to understand clients' points of view. They need to stand in their clients' shoes and try to see the world through their eyes. By listening, observing, and gradually learning other cultures, the nurse must add a further step of choosing to avoid ethnocentrism. Otherwise, the nurse's view of a different culture will remain distorted and perhaps prejudiced (Andrews & Boyle, 2008; Leininger & McFarland, 2006). The ability to show interest, concern, and compassion enabled one nurse to win the trust and respect of the Native American women in the second case file example and told the Kims that their nurse cared about them. These nurses attempted to understand the feelings and ideas of their clients; in this way, they established a trusting relationship and opened the door to the possibility of their clients' adopting healthier behaviors.

Assess the Client Group's Culture

A third transcultural nursing principle emphasizes the need to learn clients' cultures. All clients' actions, like one's own, are based on underlying culturally learned beliefs, values, and ideas (Andrews & Boyle, 2008; Spector, 2009). Mrs. Kim did not like milk because her culture had taught her that it was distasteful and many Asians are lactose intolerant (Swagerty, Walling, & Klein, 2002). The Native American women's response to waiting or keeping someone else waiting was influenced by their valuing patience. There usually is some culturally based reason that causes clients to engage in (or avoid) certain actions. Instead of making assumptions or judging clients' behavior, the nurse first must learn about the culture that guides that behavior (Giger & Davidhizar, 2008). During a cultural assessment, the nurse obtains health-related information about the values, beliefs, and practices of a designated cultural group. Learning the culture of the client first is critical to effective nursing practice. The Giger and Davidhizar Transcultural Assessment Model (Giger & Davidhizar, 2008) proposes six interrelated factors for assessing differences between people in cultural groups (Fig. 5-2). Understanding these phenomena is a first step toward appreciating the diversity that exists among people from different cultural backgrounds. Interviewing members of a subcultural group can provide valuable data to enhance understanding (Eggenberger et al., 2006).

To fully understand a group's culture, it should be studied in depth, as Bernal maintains (1993, p. 231):

> Although a general knowledge base and skills are applicable transculturally, immersion in a given culture is necessary to understand fully the patterns that shape the behavior of individuals within that group. Experience with one group can be helpful in understanding the concept of diversity, but each group must be understood within its own ecologic niche and for its own historical and cultural reality.

Practically speaking, however, it is not possible to study in depth all of the cultural groups that the nurse encounters. Instead, the nurse can conduct a cultural assessment by questioning key informants, observing the cultural group, and reading additional information in the literature. The data can be grouped into six categories:

1. *Ethnic or racial background*: Where did the client group originate, and how does that influence their status and identity?

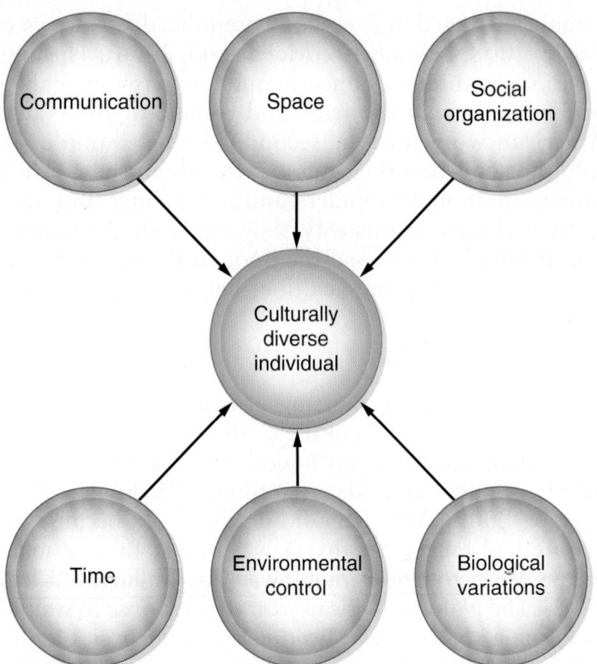

FIGURE 5-2. Components of the Giger and Davidhizar Transcultural Assessment Model showing the culturally diverse individual through communication, space, social organization, time, environmental control, and biologic variations. (Adapted from Giger, J. N., & Davidhizar, R. (2002). Culturally competent care: Emphasis on understanding the people of Afghanistan, Afghan Americans, and Islamic culture and religion. *International Nursing Review*, *49*(2), 79–86, with permission.)

2. *Language and communication patterns*: What is the preferred language spoken, and what are the group's culturally based communication patterns?
3. *Cultural values and norms*: What are the client group's values, beliefs, and standards regarding such things as family roles and functions, education, child rearing, work and leisure, aging, death and dying, and rites of passage?
4. *Biocultural factors*: Are there physical or genetic traits unique to this cultural group that predispose them to certain conditions or illnesses?
5. *Religious beliefs and practices*: What are the group's religious beliefs, and how do they influence life events, roles, health, and illness?
6. *Health beliefs and practices*: What are the group's beliefs and practices regarding prevention, causes, and treatment of illnesses?

The cultural assessment guide presented in Table 5-7 gives suggestions for more detailed data collection.

Many cultural assessment guides can be found throughout the nursing literature. Nonetheless, a thorough cultural assessment may be too time-consuming and costly. Instead, the two-phase assessment process is proposed, as outlined in Table 5-8. Categories to explore in the assessment include values, beliefs, customs, and social structure components. Two methods that have proved highly effective for in-depth study of cultural groups are ethnographic interviewing and participant observation. Spradley (1979, 1980) provides classic descriptions of these methods.

Show Respect and Patience While Learning About Other Cultures

The fourth transcultural nursing principle emphasizes key behaviors for the nurse to practice during the cultural learning process. Respect is the first behavior, and it is shown in many ways. When Sandra Josten involved the Native American women in decisions and gave them choices, she was showing respect. When the nurse gave positive recognition to the importance of the Kims' culture, she was showing respect. Attentive listening is a way to show respect and to learn about a client's culture. Within the United States, people of minority groups particularly need respect (Cowan & Norman, 2006). At times, for groups with limited English skills and a community health nurse who is not bilingual, an interpreter who can assist with communication becomes a necessity (Display 5.7).

A **minority group** is part of a population that differs from the majority and often receives different and unequal treatment. Their ways contrast with those of the dominant culture. It is difficult for them to retain pride in their lifestyles, or in themselves, when the majority culture suggests that they are inferior (Leininger & McFarland, 2006; Spector, 2009). This message may be only implied or even unintentional, as was the case for Mrs. Juarez in From the Case Files IV. The clinic's routine and the manner of the staff were not intended to show disrespect. They did, nevertheless, and Mrs. Juarez was intimidated and was unable to receive the help that she needed. Everyone needs respect to enhance pride, dignity, and self-esteem; it is an important contributor to good mental health. Showing respect also is an important means for breaking down barriers in cross-cultural communication. For community health nurses, culturally relevant care means practicing cultural relativism. **Cultural relativism** is recognizing and respecting alternative viewpoints and understanding values, beliefs, and practices within their cultural context.

In addition to respect, patience is essential. It takes time to build trust and effect cultural change. It can be difficult to establish the nurse–client relationship when it involves two different cultures. Trust must be won, and winning it may take weeks, months, or years. Time must be allowed for both nurse and clients to learn how to communicate with one another, to test one another's trustworthiness, and to learn about one another. Change in behavior (learned aspects of the culture) occurs gradually. Some aspects of both the nurse's and the clients' cultures can, and probably will, change. The Kims' nurse, Paula Morrow, for example, modified some of her usual practices and adapted them to the Kims' culture and needs. They, in turn, began to assume some American practices and values. However, the process took several months. Time, respect, and patience help to break down cultural barriers (Campinha-Bacote, 2003).

Table 5.7 Cultural Assessment Guide

Category	Sample Data
Ethnic/racial background	Countries of origin Mostly native born or U.S. born? Reasons for emigrating if applicable Racial/ethnic identity Experience with racism or racial discrimination?
Language and communication patterns	Languages of origin Languages spoken in the home Preferred language for communication How verbal communication patterns are affected by age, sex, other? Preferences for use of interpreters Nonverbal communication patterns (e.g., eye contact, touching)
Cultural values and norms	Group beliefs and standards for male and female roles and functions Standards for modesty and sexuality Family/extended family structures and functions Values regarding work, leisure, success, time Values regarding education and occupation Norms for child rearing and socialization Norms for social networks and supports Values regarding aging and treatment of elders Values regarding authority Norms for dress and appearance
Biocultural factors	Group genetic predisposition to health conditions (e.g., hypertension, anemia) Socioculturally associated illnesses (e.g., AIDS, alcoholism) Group attitudes toward body parts and functions Group vulnerability or resistance to health threats? Folk illnesses common to group? Group physical/genetic differences (e.g., bone mass, height, weight, longevity)
Religious beliefs and practices	Religious beliefs affecting roles, childbearing and child rearing, health and illness? Recognized religious healers? Religious beliefs and practices for promoting health, preventing illness, or treatment of illness Beliefs and rituals regarding conception and birth Beliefs and rituals regarding death, dying, grief
Health beliefs and practices	Beliefs regarding causes of illness Beliefs regarding treatment of illness Beliefs regarding use of healers (traditional and Western) Health promotion and illness prevention practices Folk medicine practices Beliefs regarding mental health and illness Dietary, herbal, and other folk cures Food beliefs, preparation, consumption Experience with Western medicine

Examine Culturally Derived Health Practices

The final transcultural nursing principle involves scrutiny of the client group's cultural practices, as they affect the group's health status. Once the community health nurse has assessed the culture of the client group, cultural practices affecting the health of the client group need to be examined. Are these behaviors preserving and enhancing the group's health, or are they harmful to their health? Some traditional practices, such as customary diet, birth rituals, and certain folk remedies, may promote both physical and psychological health. These can be considered healthful. Other practices may be neither harmful nor particularly health promoting but are useful in preserving the culture, security, and sense of identity of a particular ethnic group.

Table 5.8 Two-Phased Cultural Assessment Process

Phase I–Data Collection	
Stage 1	Assess values, beliefs, and customs (e.g., ethnic affiliations, religion, decision-making patterns).
Stage 2	Collect problem-specific cultural data (e.g., cultural beliefs and practices related to diet and nutrition).
Stage 3	Make nursing diagnoses.
	Determine cultural factors influencing nursing intervention (e.g., child-rearing beliefs and practices that might affect nurse teaching toilet training or child discipline).
Phase II–Data Organization	
Step 1	Compare cultural data with:
	Standards of client's own culture (e.g., client's diet compared with cultural norms)
	Standards of the nurse's culture
	Standards of the health facility providing service.
Step 2	Determine incongruities in above standards.
Step 3	Seek to modify one or more systems (client's, nurse's, or the facility's) to achieve maximum congruity.

And some traditional practices may be directly harmful to health. Examples include using herbal poultices to treat an infected wound or "burning" the abdomen to compensate for heat loss associated with diarrhea (Leininger & McFarland, 2006; Meuninck, 2008).

Cultural assessment and aggregate health assessment must go hand in hand. If the group is experiencing a high incidence of low-birth-weight babies, pregnancy complications, skin infections, mental illness, or other evidence of health problems, these can be clues to prompt an

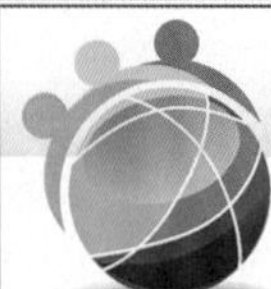

DISPLAY 5.7 INTERPRETER GUIDELINES

1. Unless the community health nurse is thoroughly effective and fluent in the client's language, an interpreter should be used.

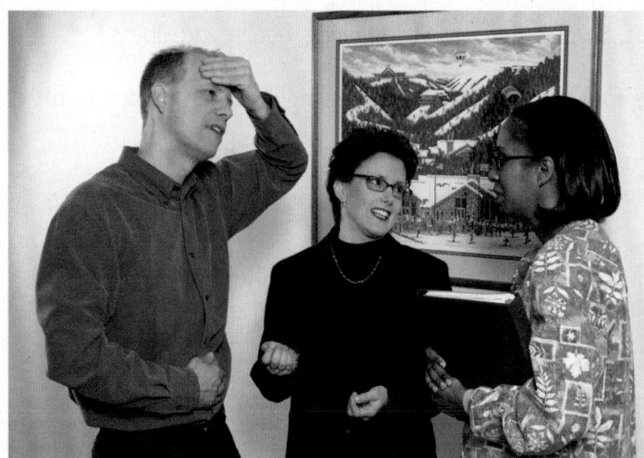

Hearing-impaired client helped by interpreter using sign language.

2. Become familiar with your interpreters. Meet with them on a regular basis, since they provide both a window and a mirror when dealing with clients.
3. The interpreter must maintain confidentiality and can divulge nothing without the full approval of the client and community health nurse.
4. Evaluate the interpreter's style, approach to clients, and ability to develop a relationship of trust and respect. Try to match the interpreter to the client.
5. Maintain eye contact with and address the client, not the interpreter. Remember that clients may understand what is being said (to some degree) even if they don't feel comfortable speaking English.
6. Be patient. Careful interpretation often requires that the interpreter use long, explanatory phrases. Confirm the client's understanding and agreement to promote improved care.
7. Interpreters must interpret everything that is said by all of the people in the interaction but should inform the community health nurse if the content might be perceived as offensive, insensitive, or harmful to the dignity and wellbeing of the client.
8. When appropriate, encourage interpreters to explain cultural differences to the client and to yourself.
9. Interpretation conveys the content and spirit of what is said, with nothing omitted or added.
10. Volunteer interpreters receive no fee. Employed interpreters usually receive their fee or salary from the hiring agency. They should not accept money or favors from clients or the community health nurse. A sincere "thank you" is the most appropriate gratuity.

Adapted from Kaufert, J. M. & Putsch, R. W. (1997). *Communication through interpreters in healthcare: Ethical dilemmas arising from differences in class, culture, language, and power.* Journal of Clinical Ethics, 8(1), 71–87. Massachusetts General Hospital. (2002). *Working with an interpreter.* Retrieved from http://www2.massgeneral.org/interpreters/working.asp Minas, M., Stankovska, M., & Ziguras, S. (2001). Working with interpreters: Guidelines for mental health professionals. The Victorian Transcultural Psychiatry Unit. Retrieved from http://www.vtpu.org.au/docs/interpreter_guidelines.pdf; Putsch, R. W. (1985). *Cross-cultural communication: The special case of interpreters in health care. JAMA,* 254(23), 3344–3348.

From the Case Files V

The Importance of Cultural Sensitivity

In Australia, well-intentioned government officials, including representatives of the health ministry, identified problems related to substandard housing among a particular aggregate of aboriginal people. To assist this community, the officials spent a great deal of time, energy, and finances planning and building homes for the Aborigines. The homes were small but modern and offered many of the conveniences that officials believed would improve the quality of life for the community.

The Aborigines were appreciative of the group's efforts and moved into their new homes. Before long, however, officials realized that one by one the community members were moving back to their "substandard" housing. When asked about their lack of appreciation for the improved lifestyle, the group informed the officials that their watering hole was their lifeline and that the houses were not only uncomfortable to them but were too far from their watering hole. Soon, all of the aboriginal families had returned to living on the land, and the homes were part of a veritable ghost town in the middle of nowhere.

Questions

- Was the aboriginal community truly "poor," as the officials seemed to think?
- Discuss your perception of the following issues: Cultural imposition, cultural poverty, dignity and spirit.
- If you were part of an international health team assigned to return to the community to try again to improve their quality of life, what steps would you take to ensure that previous mistakes are not repeated?

examination of cultural health practices. Those that are clearly damaging to health can be discussed with group leaders and healers. In this situation, knowing the group's cultural norms for authority and decision making can be helpful. Often, a cultural practice can be continued or modified while combined with Western medicine, so that respect for the culture is maintained while full treatment efficacy is accomplished (see From the Case Files V).

SUMMARY

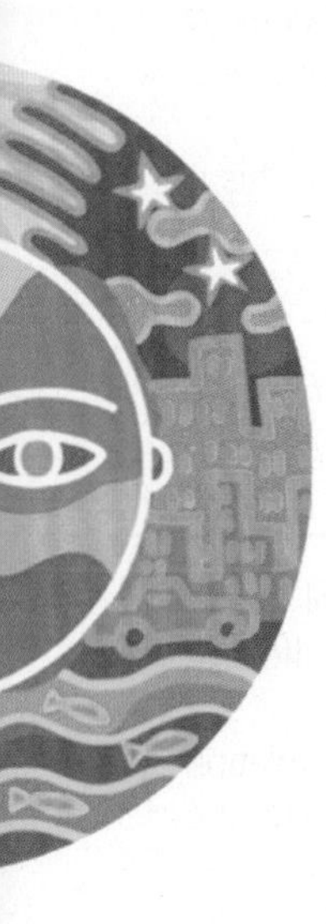

Community health clients belong to a variety of cultural groups. A culture is a design for living; it provides a set of norms and values that offer stability and security for members of a society and plays a major role in motivating behaviors. The increase in and great variety of cultural groups reinforce the need for community health nurses to understand and appreciate cultural diversity. Ethnocentrism is the bias that a person's own culture is best and others are wrong or inferior. It can create serious barriers to effective nursing care. Understanding cultural diversity and being sensitive to the values and behaviors of cultural groups often is the key to effective community health intervention.

Culture has five characteristics: it is learned from others; it is an integrated system of customs and traits; it is shared; it is tacit; and it is dynamic. Every culture preserves its integrity by deleting non-functional practices and acquiring new components that better serve the group. To gain acceptance, nurses must strive to introduce improved health practices that are presented in a manner consistent with clients' cultural values.

Five transcultural nursing principles, drawn from an understanding of the concept of culture, can guide community health nursing practice:

1. Develop cultural self-awareness.
2. Cultivate cultural sensitivity.
3. Assess the client group's culture.
4. Show respect and patience while learning other cultures.
5. Examine culturally derived health practices.

ACTIVITIES TO PROMOTE **CRITICAL THINKING**

1. Based on your own cultural background, how would you feel and what behaviors would you exhibit if you were
   a. A client sitting in a clinic waiting room in a foreign country whose language you did not know?
   b. Part of a nutrition class being told to eat foods you had never heard about before?
   c. Visited in your home by a nurse who told you to discipline your child in a way that contradicted everything you had been raised to believe about parenting?
2. Describe three tacit cultural rules that govern your own behavior. How might these affect your interactions with clients from another culture?
3. What does the term *ethnocentrism* mean to you? Have you ever experienced someone else's being ethnocentric in their attitude toward you? If so, describe that experience. Using the Cross-Cultural Sensitivity Continuum (see Fig. 4-1), explore where your own attitudes are on the continuum toward several of the cultural groups with which you regularly come in contact or from which you know people well.
4. Imagine that you are assigned to work with a Mexican American migrant population. What are the steps that you would take to gather the appropriate information to provide culturally relevant nursing service? What sources might provide that information?
5. A Hmong father who severely beat his 12-year-old son with a belt, leaving cuts and bruises, is charged with child abuse. "If I can't discipline my son, how can he be a good child?" said the father. What nursing responses would show respect for this cultural group's norms and values and yet be constructive in resolving the cultural conflict?
6. Find websites that elaborate on transcultural nursing and cross-cultural health care concerns. Print materials of interest and develop a resource file for your professional use.
7. Interprofessional communication techniques among diverse health care disciplines are imperative to effective caregiving. How comfortable are you with knowing the linguistic style, practice, and research backgrounds of social workers, pharmacists, physical therapists, educators, psychologists, and others? Seek out a colleague from a different interprofessional discipline and discuss developing a "shared language."
8. Sample exam questions for material in this chapter:
   a. A new nurse in the health department comments that the elderly Vietnamese woman was "stupid" because she could not tell the nurse how long she had been coughing up blood. What is the best response you can give to the nurse?
      (1) "Some Asians are long-time smokers and the hemoptysis is probably from smoking."
      (2) "That patient may be afraid of TB and not want to tell you. Try asking her a different way."
      (3) "That patient does not look like she understands English and I doubt it is blood, it is probably food."
      (4) "Tell her to come back in 3 weeks, when the Vietnamese interpreter is here."
   b. Your caseload includes a Columbian refugee family who witnessed the torture of their neighbors before coming to this country. The mother reports through an interpreter that her 11-year-old son is misbehaving in school, does not sleep through the night, and has lost interest in games he used to enjoy. What is your best response?
      (1) In America, boys this age focus on their peers, and often develop interests outside their family. This is normal behavior.
      (2) It sounds like he is disobedient. You should set behavioral rules and be strict with him.
      (3) He is probably tired. You should go to our clinic doctor to get sleeping medication for him.
      (4) His behavior may be related to things he saw years ago. We have a doctor at the clinic that might be able to help with that.

Key for Sample Exam Questions

a. The correct response is (2). In the response, the nurse uses clinical knowledge about potential health problems in the ethnic group. The nurse suggests that the new employee use patience to achieve effective communication with the patient.

b. The correct response is (4). In the response, the nurse is using clinical knowledge about this population and mental or physical health problems for which they may be at high risk. The nurse is addressing the mother's concerns with a referral to rule out a posttraumatic stress condition.

REFERENCES

Aaron, K. F., Levine, D., & Burstin, H. R. (2003). African American church participation and health care practices. *Journal of General Internal Medicine, 18*(18), 908–913.

Ahmad, M. (2004). *Arab American culture and health care*. Retrieved January 21, 2011, from http://www.cwru.edu/med/epidbio/mphp439/Arab-Americans.htm

Akbar, K. F. (2007). *Family planning and Islam: A review*. Retrieved July 5, 2008, from http://muslim-canada.org/family.htm

Andrews, M., & Boyle, J. (2008). *Transcultural concepts in nursing care* (5th ed.). Philadelphia, PA: Lippincott Williams & Wilkins.

Arab American Institute. (2010). *Demographics*. Retrieved August 15, 2010, from http://www.aaiusa.org/demographics/

Baqi-Aziz, M. (2001). Where does she think she is? *American Journal of Nursing, 101*(11), 11.

Berlin, I. (2005). African immigration to Colonial America. *History Now: American History Online, 3*. Retrieved March 1, 2008, from http://www.historynow.org/03_2005/historian3.html

Bernal, H. (1993). A model for delivering culture-relevant care in the community. *Public Health Nursing, 10*(4), 226–232.

Blais, K. K., & Hayes, J. S. (2011). *Professional nursing practice: Concepts and* perspectives (6th ed.). Upper Saddle River, NJ: Prentice Hall.

Brenneman, G., Rhoades, E., & Chilton, L. (2006). Forty years in partnership: The American Academy of Pediatrics and the Indian Health Service. *Pediatrics, 118*, 1257–1263.

Byrd, W. M., & Clayton, L. A. (2002). *An American health dilemma: Race, medicine, and health care in the United States 1900–2000*, Vol. II. New York: Routledge.

California Pan-Ethnic Health Network. (2007). *Racial/ethnic makeup (California, 2000)*. Retrieved July 9, 2010, from http://www.cpehn.org/demochartdetail.php?btn_viewchart=1&view_1.x=52&view_1.y=17&view_1=Get+Statistics%21

Campbell, T. C. (2005). *The China study: The most comprehensive study of nutrition ever conducted and the startling implications for diet, weight loss and long-term health*. Dallas, TX: BenBella Books.

Campinha-Bacote, J. (2003). Many faces: Addressing diversity in health care. *Online Journal of Issues in Nursing, 8*(1). Retrieved July 5, 2008, from http://www.nursingworld.org/ ojin/topic20/tpc20_2.htm

Council on American-Islamic Relations. (2008). *About Islam & American Muslims*. Retrieved August 8, 2008, from http://www.cair.com/AboutIslam/IslamBasics.aspx

Cowan, D. T., & Norman, I. (2006). Cultural competence in nursing: New meanings. *Journal of Transcultural Nursing, 17*, 82–88.

Cronk, L. (2007). The influence of cultural framing on play in the trust game: A Maasai example. *Evolution and Human Behavior, 28*(5), 352–358.

Cultural Diversity in Nursing. (2008). *Basic concepts and case studies: The Middle Eastern community*. Retrieved January 21, 2011, from http://www.cwru.edu/med/epidbio/mphp439/Arab-Americans.htm

Damon, W., Lerner, R., Renninger, K., & Sigel, I. (Eds.). (2006). *Handbook of child psychology: Child psychology in practice* (6th ed.). New York: John Wiley & Sons.

Eggenberger, S. K., Grassley, J., & Restrepo, E. (2006). Culturally competent nursing care: Listening to the voices of Mexican American women. *Online Journal of Issues in Nursing, 11*(3), 7.

Electronic Resource Center. Management Sciences for Health. (2007a). *Challenges to health and wellbeing of Arab-Americans families and communities*. Retrieved July 5, 2008, from http://erc.msh.org/mainpage.cfm? file=5.4.2k.htm&module=providers&language=English

Electronic Resource Center. Management Sciences for Health. (2007b). *Arab-Americans*. Retrieved July 5, 2008, from http://erc.msh.org/mainpage.cfm? file=5.4.2h.htm&module=providers&language=English

Electronic Resource Center. Management Sciences for Health. (2007c). *What is Islam, and who are Muslims?* Retrieved July 5, 2008, from http://erc.msh.org/mainpage.cfm? file=5.4.6a.htm&module=providers&language=English

Electronic Resource Center. Management Sciences for Health. (2007d). *Strengths and protective factors in Arab-American families and communities*. Retrieved July 5, 2008, from http://erc.msh.org/mainpage.cfm?file=5.4.2j.htm&module=providers&language=English

Electronic Resource Center. Management Sciences for Health. (2007e). *Principles for culturally competent health care for Muslim families and communities*. Retrieved July 5, 2008, from http://erc.msh.org/mainpage.cfm? file=5.4.6g.htm&module=providers&language=English

Ethnicity Online. (2010). *Cultural awareness in health care: Ethnicity is....* Retrieved July 9, 2010, from http://www.ethnicityonline.net/ethnicity_is.htm

Fadiman, A. (1998). *The spirit catches you and you fall down*. New York: Farrar, Straus, & Giroux.

Giger, J. N., & Davidhizar, R. (2002). Culturally competent care: Emphasis on understanding the people of Afghanistan, Afghanistan Americans, and Islamic culture and religion. *International Nursing Review, 49*, 79–86.

Giger, J. N., & Davidhizar, R. E. (2008). *Transcultural nursing* (5th ed.). St. Louis, MO: Elsevier.

Hahn, R. & Inhorn, M. (2009). *Anthropology and public health* (2nd ed.). New York: Oxford University Press, Inc.

Hall, E. T. (1959). *The silent language*. Garden City, NY: Doubleday.

Harrison, M., Edwards, C., Koenig, H., Decastro, L., & Wood, M. (2005). Religiosity/spirituality and pain in patients with sickle cell disease. *Journal of Nervous and Mental Disease, 193*(4), 250–257.

Her, C., & Culhane-Pera, K. (2004). Culturally responsive care for Hmong patients: Collaboration is a key treatment component. *Postgraduate Medicine, 116*(6), 39–42.

Hesketh, T., Lu, L., & Xing, Z. W. (2005). The effect of China's one-child family policy after 25 years. *New England Journal of Medicine, 353*(11), 1171–1176.

Hill, D. L. (2006). Sense of belonging as connectedness, American Indian worldview, and mental health. *Archives of Psychiatric Nursing, 20*(5), 210–216.

Hing, B. O. (2006). Immigration death trap. *San Francisco Chronicle*. Retrieved July 7, 2008, from http://www.sfgate.com/cgi-bin/article.cgi?file=/chronicle/archive/2006/01/02/ EDG5TG18EB1.DTL&type=printable

Hong, S., Nelson, R., Krohn, P., Mills, P. J., & Dimsdale, J. E. (2006). The association of social status and blood pressure with markers of vascular inflammation. *Psychosomatic Medicine, 68*(4), 517–523.

Infoplease. (2010). *African Americans by the numbers*. Infoplease.com (Pearson Education). Retrieved August 13, 2010, from http://www.infoplease.com/spot/bhmcensusl.html

Indian Health Services (IHS). (2010). *The Indian Health Services fact sheets: Facts on health disparities*. Retrieved July 30, 2010, from http://info.ihs.gov/Disparities.asp

Joint Center Databank. (2007). *Single parent families*. Retrieved January 20, 2011, from http://www.jointcenter.org/DB/factsheet/sigpatn.htm

Kark, S. L. (1974). *Epidemiology and community medicine*. New York, NY: Appleton-Century-Crofts.

Lange, L. A., Carlson, C. S., Hindorff, L. A., Lange, E. M., Walston, J., Durda, J. P., et al. (2006). Association of polymorphisms in the CRP gene with circulating C-reactive protein levels and cardiovascular events. *Journal of the American Medical Association, 296*(22), 2703–2711.

Lee, E., Jung, K., Su, J., Tran, A., & Bahrassa, N. (2009). The family life and adjustment of Hmong American sons and daughters. *Sex Roles, 60*(7–8), 549–558.

Leininger, M., & McFarland, M. (2006). *Culture, care, diversity, and universality: A theory of nursing* (2nd ed.). Boston, MA: Jones & Bartlett Publishers.

Lippincott Williams & Wilkins. (2006). *Nursing herbal medicine handbook* (3rd ed.). Philadelphia, PA: Author.

Lockwood, P., Marshall, T., & Sadler, P. (2005). Promoting success or preventing failure: Cultural differences in motivation by positive and negative role models. *Personality and Social Psychology Bulletin, 31*(3), 379–392.

Lowe, J. (2002). Balance and harmony through connectedness: The intentionality of Native American nurses. *Holistic Nursing Practice, 6*(4), 4–11.

Luo, M. (2009, November 30). In job hunt, college degree can't close racial gap. *The New York Times*. Retrieved January 19, 2011, from http://www.nytimes.com/2009/12/01/us/01race.html

Mead, M. (1960). Cultural contexts of nursing problems. In F. C. MacGregor (Ed.), *Social science in nursing* (pp. 74–88). New York, NY: Wiley.

Medline Plus. (2007). *Herbal medicine*. Retrieved July 7, 2008, from http://www.nlm.nih.gov/medlineplus/herbalmedicine.html.

Mehl-Madrona, L. E. (2008). *Traditional (Native American) Indian medicine treatment of chronic illness: Development of an integrated program with traditional American medicine and evaluation of effectiveness*. Retrieved January 19, 2011, from http://www.healing-arts.org/mehl-madrona/mmtraditionalpaper.htm

Meuninck, J. (2008). *Medicinal plants of North America: A field guide*. Guilford, CN: The Globe Pequot Press.

Mui, A., & Kang, S. (2006). Acculturation stress and depression among Asian immigrant elders. *Social Work, 51*(3), 243–255.

Murdock, G. (1972). The science of culture. In M. Freilich (Ed.). *The meaning of culture: A reader in cultural anthropology* (pp. 252–266). Lexington, MA: Xerox College Publishing.

Naim, M. (2005). *Arabs in foreign lands: What the success of Arab Americans tells us about Europe, the Middle East, and the power of culture. Foreign Policy*. Retrieved July 7, 2008, from http://www.foreignpolicy.com/story/cms.php?story_id=2781&print=1

Narayanasamy, A., & White, E. (2005). A review of transcultural nursing. *Nurse Educator Today, 25*(2), 102–111.

National Center for Health Statistics. (2006). *Health of Asian or Pacific Islander population*. Retrieved July 7, 2008, from http://www.cdc.gov/nchs/fastats/asian_health.htm

National Center for Health Statistics. (2007a). *Health of Black or African American population*. Retrieved July 7, 2008, from http://www.cdc.gov/nchs/fastats/black_health.htm

National Center for Health Statistics. (2007b). *Health of Hispanic/Latino population*. Retrieved July 7, 2008, from http://www.cdc.gov/nchs/fastats/hispanic_health.htm

National Center for Education Statistics. (2008). *Status and trends in the education of American Indians and Alaska Natives: 2008*. U.S. Department of Education, Institute of Education Sciences. Retrieved January 26, 2011, from http://nces.ed.gov/pubs2008/nativetrends/ind_1_6.asp

Native American Rights Fund. (n.d.). *Dispelling the myths about Indian gaming*. Retrieved January 12, 2011, from http://www.narf.org/pubs/misc/gaming.html

Office of Minority Health. (2009). *Hispanic/Latino profile*. U.S. Department of Health & Human Services. Retrieved January 20, 2011, from http://minorityhealth.hhs.gov/templates/browse.aspx?lvl=2&lvlID=54

Partnership for Prescription Assistance. (2010). *Prescription assistance programs*. Retrieved July 30, 2010, from www.pparx.org/

Pizzorno, J., Murray, M., & Joiner-Bey, H. (2007). *The clinician's handbook of natural medicine* (2nd ed.). London, UK: Churchill-Livingstone.

Royal College of Nursing. (2006). *Female genital mutilation: An RCN educational resource for nursing and midwifery staff*. London, UK: Author.

Samhan, H. (2006). Arab Americans. *Grolier's multimedia encyclopedia*. Retrieved from http://www.aaiusa.org/foundation/358/arab-americans

Skyscape. (2010). *RnHerbal (Nursing herbal medicine handbook 6.0.140)*. Accessed February 22, 2011, from http://www.soft32.com/download_155594.html

Sloan, F. A., Ayyagari, P., Salm, M., & Grossman, D. (2010). The longevity gap between Black and White men in the United States at the beginning and end of the 20th century. *American Journal of Public Health, 100*(21), 357–363.

Snyder, M., & Lindquist, R. (2010). *Complementary and alternative therapies in nursing* (6th ed.). New York: Springer Publishing Company.

Spector, R. E. (2009). *Cultural diversity in health and illness* (7th ed.). Upper Saddle River, NJ: Prentice-Hall Allied Health.

Spradley, J. P. (1979). *The ethnographic interview*. New York: Holt.

Spradley, J. P. (1980). *Participant observation*. New York: Holt.

Spradley, J. P., & McCurdy, D. W. (2009). *Conformity and conflict: Readings in cultural anthropology* (13th ed.). Boston, MA: Allyn & Bacon Publishing.

Swagerty, S. L., Walling, A. D., & Klein, R. M. (2002). Lactose intolerance. *American Family Physician, 65*(9), 1845–1850. Retrieved July 7, 2008, from http://www.aafp.org/afp/20020501/1845.html

Taylor, R. J., Chatters. L. M., & Levin, J. (2004). *Religion in the lives of African Americans*. Thousand Oaks, CA: Sage Publishers.

Taylor, J. B., & Kalt, J. P. (2005). *American Indians on reservations: A databook of socioeconomic change between the 1990 and 2000 censuses*. Cambridge, MA: Harvard University.

Thomson Healthcare. (2007). *Physicians desk reference for herbal medicines* (4th ed.). Montvale, NJ: Thompson Health Care.

Tribal Court Clearinghouse. (n.d.). *Native gaming resources*. Retrieved from http://www.tribal-institute.org/lists/gaming.htm

Trinh-Shevri, C., Islam, N. S., & Rey, M. J. (Eds.). (2009). *Asian American communities and health: Context, research, policy, and action*. New York: Jossey-Bass.

Tsai, J., Louie, J., Chen, E. E., & Uchida, Y. (2007). Learning what feelings to desire: Socialization of ideal affect through children's storybooks. *Personality and Social Psychology Bulletin, 33*(1), 17–30.

U.S. Census Bureau. (n.d.). *Population profile of the United States*. Retrieved from http://www.census.gov/population/www/pop-profile/natproj.html

U.S. Census Bureau. (2006). *Hispanics in the United States*. Retrieved July 22, 2010, from http://www.census.gov/population/www/socdemo/hispanic/files/Internet_Hispanic_in_US_2006.pdf

U.S. Census Bureau. (2007). *Table 3: Annual estimates of the population by sex, race, and Hispanic origin for the United States: April 1, 2000 to July 1, 2007* (NC-EST2007-03). Retrieved July 30, 2010, from http://factfinder.census.gov/home/aian/index.html

U.S. Census Bureau. (2009). *United States Population Projections: 2000 to 2050*. Retrieved July 22, 2010, from http://www.census.gov/population/www/projections/analytical-document09.pdf

U.S. Census Bureau. (2010). *Table 3. Annual estimates of the resident population by sex, race, and Hispanic origin for the United States: April 1, 2000 to July 1, 2009* (NC-EST2009-03). Retrieved July 14, 2010, from http://www.census.gov/popest/national/asrh/NC-EST2009-srh.html

U.S. Committee for Refugees and Immigrants (USCRI). (2010). *World Refugee Survey 2009*. Retrieved from http://www.refugees.org/FTP/WRS09PDFS/RefuandAsylumseek.pdf

U.S. Department of Commerce. (2001). *Statistical abstract of the United States, 2001* (121st ed.). Washington, DC: Government Printing Office.

U.S. Department of Health and Human Services (U.S. DHHS) Office of Disease Prevention and Health Promotion. (2009a). *Healthy People 2020*. Retrieved from http://www.healthypeople.gov/Default.htm

U.S. Department of Health and Human Services (U.S. DHHS) (2009b). *Health, United States, 2008*. Retrieved from http://www.cdc.gov/nchs/data/mus/hus08.pdf#026

U.S. Department of Homeland Security. (2009). *Yearbook of Immigration Statistics, 2009*. Retrieved from http://www.dhs.gov/files/stastics/publications/LPR09.shtm

U.S. Department of Labor. Bureau of Labor Statistics. (2010). *Employment statistics*. Retrieved from http://www.bls.gov/news.release/empsit.t02.htm

U.S. Food & Drug Administration (U.S. FDA). (2007). *Over-the-counter drug review process*. Retrieved from http://www.fda.gov/cder/handbook/otcpage.htm

U.S. Substance Abuse & Mental Health Services Administration (U.S. SAMHSA). (2008). *National survey on drug use and health. Substance use and substance use disorders among American Indians and Alaska Natives*. Retrieved from http://www.oas.samhsa.gov/2k7/AmIndians/AmIndians.cfm

U.S. Substance Abuse & Mental Health Services Administration (U.S. SAMHSA). (2009). *Results from the 2008 National survey on drug use and health: National findings*. Retrieved from http://oas.samhsa.gov/nsduh/2k8nsduh/2k8Results.cfm

Unitarian Universalist Church of Tucson. (2010). *No more deaths*. Retrieved from http://www.nomoredeaths.org/

Walton, M. (2005, July 6). *The business of gambling*. CNN. Retrieved from http://www.cnn.com/2005/US/07/06/cnn25.top25.gambling/index.html?iref=allsearch

Wang, Q. (2006). Culture and the development of self-knowledge. *Current Directions in Psychological Science*, *15*(4), 82–87.

Wang, X., Zhu, H., Dong, Y., Treiber, F. A., & Snieder, H. (2006). Effects of angiotensinogen and angiotensin II type I receptor genes on blood pressure and left ventricular mass trajectories in multiethnic youth. *Twin Research in Human Genetics*, *9*(3), 393–402.

Yosef, A. R. (2008). Health beliefs, practice, and priorities for health care of Arab Muslims in the United States—Implications for nursing care. *Journal of Transcultural Nursing*, *19*(3), 284–291.

thePoint: Everything You Need to Make the Grade!

thePoint Visit http://thePoint.lww.com/Allender8e
for selected readings, study aids for all learning styles, and more!

UNIT 2

PUBLIC HEALTH ESSENTIALS FOR COMMUNITY HEALTH NURSING

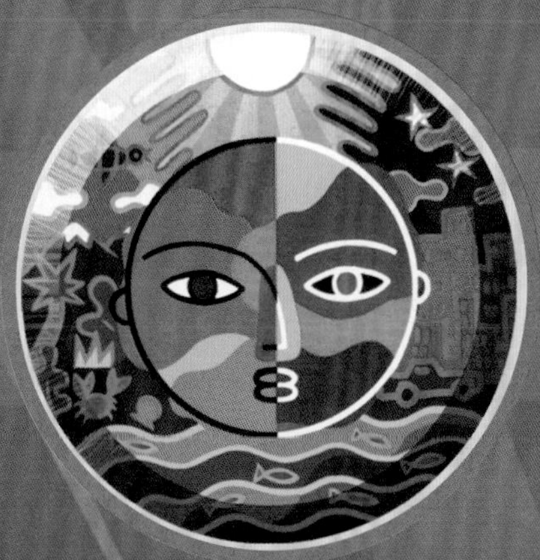

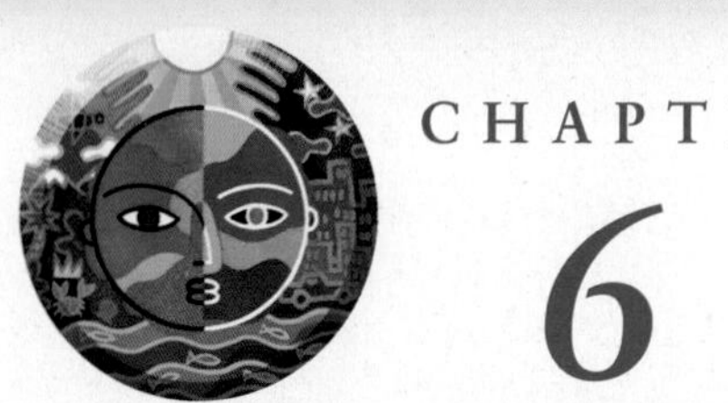

CHAPTER

6

Structure and Economics of Community Health Services

"Health care is vital to all of us some of the time, but public health is vital to all of us all of the time."

—*C. Everett Koop*, Former U.S. Surgeon General

"There are 10^{11} stars in the galaxy. That used to be a huge number. But it's only a hundred billion. It's less than the national deficit! We used to call them astronomical numbers. Now we should call them economical numbers."

—*Richard Feynman* (1918–1988)

KEY TERMS

Adverse selection
Assessment
Assurance
Capitation rates
Competition
Consumer-driven/high-deductible health plan (CDHDHP)
Core public health functions
Cost sharing
Cost shifting
Demand
Diagnosis-related groups (DRGs)
Economics
Fee-for-service
Gross domestic product (GDP)
Health care economics
Health maintenance organization (HMO)
Health savings account (HSA)
Macroeconomic theory
Managed care
Managed competition
Medicaid
Medical home
Medically indigent
Medicare
Microeconomic theory
Moral hazard
Nongovernmental organizations (NGOs)
Official health agencies
Point of service plan (POS)
Policy development
Preferred provider organization (PPO)
Proprietary health services
Prospective payment
Public Health Service
Quarantine
Rationing
Regulation
Retrospective payment
Sanitation
Shattuck Report
Single-payer system
Supply
Third-party payments
Underinsured
Uninsured
Universal coverage
Voluntary health agencies

LEARNING OBJECTIVES

Upon mastery of this chapter, you should be able to:

- Trace historic events and philosophical developments leading to today's health services delivery systems.
- Outline the current organizational structure of the public health care system.
- Examine the three core functions of public health as they apply to health services delivery.
- Differentiate between the functions of public versus private sector health care agencies.
- Examine the public health services provided by selected international health organizations.
- Explain the influence of selected legislative acts in the United States on shaping current health services policy and practice.
- Explore how the structure and functions of community health services affect community health nursing practice.
- Define the concept of health care economics.
- Describe three sources of health care financing.
- Compare and contrast retrospective and prospective health care payment systems.
- Analyze the trends and issues influencing health care economics and community health services delivery.
- Explain the causes and effects of health care rationing.
- List the pros and cons of managed competition as opposed to a single-payer system.
- Discuss health care reform and its potential impact on community health nursing.
- Explain the philosophical implications of health care financing patterns on community health nursing's mission and values.

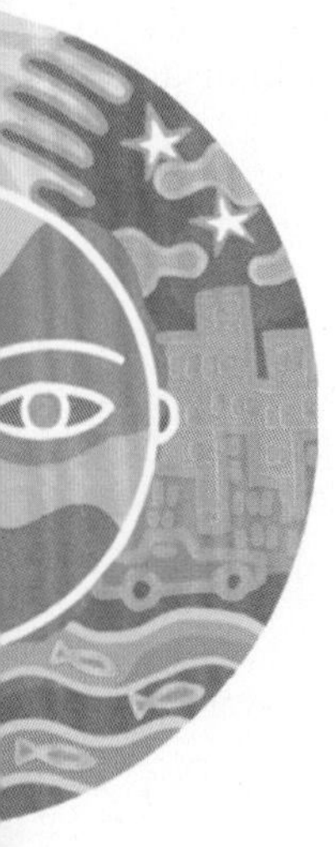

Nurses preparing for population-based practice need to be familiar with how the health care delivery system is organized and operates, because it is through this system that we are able to offer community health services (see Chapter 3). This system forms an organizing framework for the design and implementation of programs aimed at improving the health of communities and vulnerable groups. It is within this system or framework that community health nurses labor, realize the opportunity to shape future health services, and develop innovative and more effective means of improving community health.

Nurses concerned with the delivery of needed community health services also must understand how those services are financed. In an era when health care costs are rising while resources are limited and providers are competing for scarce dollars, nurses must be well informed about the issues related to health care financing and about ways to obtain funding to address identified health needs in the community. The structure and economics of community health care are intertwined. **Health care economics** is a specialized field of economics that describes and analyzes the production, distribution, and consumption of goods and services, as well as a variety of related problems such as finance, labor, and taxation (Harrington & Estes, 2008). The goal of health care economics, much like public health, is to overcome scarcity by making good choices and providing essential services.

Service delivery systems directed at restoring or promoting the public's health have evolved over centuries. The structure, function, and financing of health care systems have changed dramatically during that time in response to evolving societal needs and demands, scientific advancements, more effective methods of service delivery, new technologies, and varying approaches to resource acquisition and allocation (Kovner & Knickman, 2011). Although progress has been made toward a healthier global society, many problems remain, particularly those of controlling health care costs, assuring equitable distribution and effectiveness of health services, and assuring the quality of and access to those services (Pan American Health Organization, 2007; U.S. Department of Health and Human Services [USDHHS], 2011).

This chapter examines the current structure and functions of community health services in the United States and reviews historical and legislative events that influenced the planning for and the delivery of those services. It also provides an overview of health care economics and the ever-changing landscape of financial incentives and disincentives for enhancing the public's health.

HISTORICAL INFLUENCES ON HEALTH CARE

Despite centuries of change, some personal and community hygiene and health care practices have continued from the beginning of time. Many primitive tribes engaged in sanitary practices such as burial of excreta, removal of the dead, and isolation of members with certain illnesses. Treatment of the sick has always included using a variety of therapeutic agents administered by a "healer."

Whether health care practices were based on superstition, derived from survival needs, or primarily tied to religious beliefs is unknown. Nonetheless, records show that in Egypt and the Middle East, as early as 3000 BCE, people were building drainage systems, using toilets and systems for water flushing, and practicing personal cleanliness (Scutchfield & Keck, 2009). The Hebrew hygienic code, described in the Bible in Leviticus circa 1500 BCE, probably was the first written code in the world and was the prototype for personal and community sanitation. It emphasized bodily cleanliness, protection against the spread of contagious diseases, isolation of lepers, disinfection of dwellings after illness, sanitation of campsites, disposal of excreta and refuse, protection of water and food supplies, and maternal hygiene (Scutchfield & Keck, 2009). Even more advanced were the Athenians, circa 1000 to 400 BCE, who emphasized personal hygiene, diet, and exercise in addition to a sanitary environment, albeit for the benefit of the wealthy. Their successors, the Romans, added more community health measures, such as laws regulating environmental sanitation and nuisances and construction of paved streets, aqueducts, and a subsurface drainage system.

The Middle Ages (from about 500 to 1500 AD) were distinguished by a distinct change in health beliefs and practices in Europe, based on the philosophy that to pamper the body was evil. During this regressive period in history, health care was scarce, private, and reserved for the wealthy few, whereas public health problems were rampant, and only minimally and ineffectively addressed.

Neglected personal hygiene (e.g., infrequent bathing), improper diets, and accumulation of refuse and body wastes led to widespread epidemics and pandemics of disease, including cholera, plague, and leprosy (Hecker, 1839). Increased trade between Europe and Asia, military conquests, and Christian crusades to the Middle East furthered the spread of disease. Bubonic plague, known as the Black Death, was the most devastating of pandemics, reportedly killing more than 60 million people in the mid-1300s (Hecker, 1839). Fear of Black Death caused Venice to ban entry of infected ships and travelers—a form of quarantine.

Quarantine is a period of enforced isolation of persons exposed to a communicable disease during the incubation period of the disease, to prevent its spread should infection occur. The first known official quarantine measure was instituted in 1377, at the port of Ragusa (now Dubrovnik in Croatia, formerly Yugoslavia), where travelers from plague areas were required to wait 2 months and to be free of disease before entry.

By the 1700s, more enlightened Europeans began to challenge the prevailing beliefs and conditions (e.g., disease as a punishment for sin). Even in the 1800s, many people in the United States thought that disease and poverty were visited upon the ignorant and the dirty. We now know the cause of disease; however, stigma regarding such conditions as leprosy and tuberculosis (TB) still exists today, and some regard sexually transmitted diseases and acquired immune deficiency syndrome (AIDS) as punishment for immoral conduct. During the late 18th century, new efforts at reform were influenced by a growing emphasis on human dignity, human rights, and the search for scientific truth. These efforts continued through the 19th and 20th centuries (Scutchfield & Keck, 2009).

Despite improvement during the 17th and 18th centuries, serious problems persisted and new ones developed. Industrialization, masses of people moving to cities, and low regard for human life all contributed to deplorable living and working conditions. Hundreds of poor children died in England's abusive but socially approved workhouses and apprentice slavery system. Most European communities were characterized by unspeakable misery and filth. Householders dumped their refuse from windows or doors into the streets. Rivers and water supplies were seriously contaminated. Diseases, including cholera, typhus, typhoid, smallpox, and TB, took a tremendous toll on human life (Lindemann, 2010).

In the 16th and 17th century, London was one of the largest cities in the world, with the population tripling by the end of the 17th century (Cockayne, 2007). By the mid-18th century, noise from carriages and carts, animals, and vendors created a "hideous din" (Cockayne, 2007 p. 107). Air pollution from burning coal and wood for fuel caused Londoners to cough and spit. People "rarely washed their bodies and lived in the constant sight and smell of human feces and human urine" (Cockayne, 2007 p. 60).

Around the turn of the 19th century, England's leaders became increasingly concerned about social and sanitary reform. The term **sanitation** refers to the promotion of hygiene and prevention of disease by maintenance of health-enhancing (sanitary) conditions. The first sanitary legislation, passed in 1837, established vaccination stations in London. One of the most notable reformers, Edwin Chadwick, the father of modern public health, published his *Report on an Inquiry into the Sanitary Conditions of the Laboring Population of Great Britain* in 1842 (Richardson, 1887). His efforts resulted in passage of the English Public Health Act and establishment of a General Board of Health for England in 1848, as reported by Lewis more than a century later (1952).

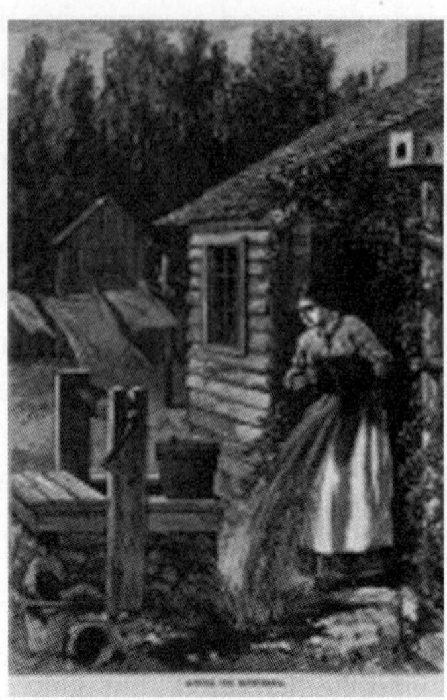

An epidemiologist and anesthetist, John Snow (1813–1858) worked on the cholera outbreak in London in 1854. His investigations of cholera outbreaks and his conclusions led to changes in the practice of sewage dumping into the Thames River, thus improving London's morbidity and mortality from cholera (see Chapter 7). His 1855 work, *On the Mode of Communication of Cholera* (2nd ed.), was a landmark public health contribution. Conditions improved, and scientific study advanced in England and, concurrently, in France, Germany, Scandinavia, and other European countries. England, however, set the pace for application of research, particularly with reference to public health measures, through steadily improved legislation. British laws subsequently became the pattern for American sanitary ordinances (Lindemann, 2010).

PUBLIC HEALTH CARE SYSTEM DEVELOPMENT IN THE UNITED STATES

The current U.S. public health care system was long in developing. Most health-related services in the United States were initially reactive, responding to the pressure of immediate needs and uncoordinated from one locality to another. Over time, events and insights contributed to a gradually improving system of programs and services, along with recognition that the health of individuals was affected by the health of the wider community (Table 6-1 highlights some of these changes). Our current public health system is not really a single entity, but more of a loosely affiliated network of federal, state, and local health agencies that have been chronically underfunded (Trust for America's Health, 2011a).

Table 6.1 Changes in Health Status and Health Care Services

Turn of the 20th Century	Turn of the 21st Century
	Morbidity and Mortality
THEN	NOW
High communicable disease and mortality	High chronic disease morbidity and mortality
Little prevention	Old and new sexually transmitted diseases
Infrequent cure	Resurgence of TB
Life span of 47 yrs.	Life span of 76 yrs.
High infant mortality	Significant infant mortality
High maternal mortality	High teenage pregnancy
Alcohol abuse	Multiple substance abuse
Many undiagnosed and untreated conditions	New strains of multidrug-resistant diseases, long-term chronic illnesses, and disability
Causes of many diseases unknown	Increased emphasis on personal responsibility (e.g., smoking, overweight)
	Access to Health Care
Access primarily for those who could pay a fee	Access for those with health insurance
No health insurance	Insurance with co-payments; costs shifting from employers to employees; health care reform
Public health clinics for poor and underserved	Free health clinics for medically indigent (especially children)
Limited treatments available	Multitude of treatments with regular new advances
	Health Care Delivery System
Extended hospital stays	Short-term, acute-care hospitalizations
Discharge on recovery	Recovery occurs at home or in a transitional setting
Extended maternal and newborn hospitalization	Short-stay maternal and newborn care
Many home deliveries with lay assistance	Few home deliveries with skilled assistance
Handwritten charts and notes	Electronic records, bar-coded medication
Home care through not-for-profit agencies	Home care through not-for-profit and proprietary agencies
PHN begun in health departments	Shifting PHN role in health departments
Health departments provide personal care	Health department's personal care services now part of managed care systems

Adapted from: Erickson, G. P. (1996). To pauperize or empower: Public health nursing at the turn of the 20th and 21st centuries. *Public Health Nursing, 13*(3), 163–169; Frist, W. H. (2005). Health care in the 21st century. *New England Journal of Medicine, 352,* 267–272.

Precursors to a Health Care System

Early health care in the American colonies consisted of private practice, with occasional (but infrequent) governmental action for the public good. Action usually was in the form of isolated local responses to specific dangers or nuisances, such as the 1647 regulation to prevent pollution of Boston Harbor or the 1701 Massachusetts law requiring ship quarantine and isolation of smallpox patients. New York City, in the late 1700s, formed a public health committee to monitor water quality, sewer construction, marsh drainage, and burial of the dead. Physicians in the early 19th century had few tools at their disposal and could do little to change the course of illness. They made house calls, as most quality care was given in the home, not in hospitals (Cutler, 2005). The U.S. Constitution, adopted in 1789, made no direct reference to public health, nor did the federal government take an active stance on health matters. It was the responsibility of each sovereign state to manage its own health affairs. The first federal intervention for health problems was the Marine Hospital Service Act of 1798. It subsidized medical and hospital care for sick and injured merchant seamen, with the first marine hospital being located in Boston.

During the early years, a scourge of epidemics, especially smallpox, cholera, typhoid, and typhus, caused deaths throughout the colonies and decimated the Native American population (Woodward, 1932). Slave trade further threatened the lives of colonists by introducing diseases, such as yaws (an infectious nonvenereal disease caused by a spirochete), yellow fever, and malaria (Klein, 2010). Local control of quarantine efforts proved ineffective. In 1837, Congress finally instituted the national port quarantine system, which was regulated and enforced by the Marine Hospital Service. Epidemics were quickly checked, causing society to recognize the benefits of uniform central government

Table 6.2 Societal Events and Situations Affecting Health Care Needs

Turn of the 20th Century	Turn of the 21st Century
Societal and Population Shifts	
THEN	NOW
Industrial society focusing on production	Postindustrial, service and information oriented
Rural to urban	Urban to suburban
Limited violence	Rampant violence and terrorism
Wide gaps between rich and poor	Widening gaps between rich and poor
Growing philanthropy	Declining support for charitable health care
Intense immigration from eastern Europe	Moderate immigration—Africa, Europe, Asia
Environment	
Overcrowded, unsanitary housing	Deteriorating inner-city neighborhoods
Unsafe workplaces, lack of worker safeguards	Environmental hazards in some workplaces
Rampant child labor	Homelessness
Poor public sanitation	Good public sanitation
Multiple health risks	Increasing environmental and behavioral risks
Skill Changes and Employment	
Farm to factory	Factory to service and information
Low wages	Improved but stagnant wages, limited benefits
Dramatic disparity in wages between men and women	Slowly resolving disparity in male/female wage differences
Not enough jobs	Downsizing, layoffs, corporate streamlining, failing companies
People Living in Poverty	
Women and children	Women, children, the aged
Immigrants—European	Immigrants—Hispanic, Caribbean, Middle Eastern, and Asian
Migration—south to north	Seasonal migration of farm workers

Adapted from: Erickson, G. P. (1996). To pauperize or empower: Public health nursing at the turn of the 20th and 21st centuries. *Public Health Nursing, 13*(3), 163–169; Frist, W. H. (2005). Health care in the 21st century. *New England Journal of Medicine, 352,* 267–272.

policy. However, improvements in public health and sanitation on a state and local level competed with other needs, such as police and fire protection (Greene, 2001; Lee, Teutsch, Thacker, & St. Louis, 2010). See Table 6-2 for examples of this.

Calls for Sanitary Reforms

The **Shattuck Report**, a landmark document, made a tremendous impact on sanitary progress. Lemuel Shattuck, a physician and legislator, chaired a legislative committee that studied health and sanitary problems in the Commonwealth of Massachusetts. In 1850, he produced the *Report of the Sanitary Commission of Massachusetts* (Shattuck., 1850) describing the public health concepts and methods that form the basis for current public health practice. Shattuck advocated the establishment of state and local boards of health, environmental sanitation, collection and use of vital statistics, systematic study of diseases, control of food and drugs, urban planning, establishment of nurses' training schools (there were none before this time), and preventive medicine.

A similar report by John Griscom on conditions of the working poor in New York City, published in 1845, concluded that illness, premature death, and poverty were directly related and were not the result of immoral or intemperate behaviors, as many public health officials advocated. He recommended sanitary reform as did others, among them Barton, Jarvis, and Martin Snow (Duffy, 1990). Almost 25 years passed before these recommendations were fully appreciated and implemented.

Recent Calls to Action

In 1988, the Institute of Medicine published *The Future of Public Health*, highlighting the state of disarray in our current public health system and calling for improvements in the public health infrastructure—largely focusing on governmental responsibilities. In 2002, the Institute issued a new publication, *The Future of the Public's Health in the 21st Century*. This report called for expanding the responsibilities of the public health system beyond governmental agencies to include private and nongovernmental entities. The report outlined how partnerships could be formed with communities, businesses, the media, universities, and other components of the health care delivery system to expand the reach of public health and achieve the *Healthy People 2010* goals (Institute of Medicine, 2002). Other needed changes included a spotlight on multiple determinants of health along with a strong population focus, transdisciplinary utilization of evidence-based practice, along with better communication and systems of accountability.

Official Health Agencies

The beginnings of an organized health care system in the United States came in the form of **official health agencies**, later called public health agencies. These were publicly funded and operated by state or local governments with a goal of providing population-based health services. Development occurred initially at the local level. Many cities established local boards of health in the late 1700s and early to middle 1800s. Among the earliest were those in Baltimore, Maryland (1798); Charleston, South Carolina (1815); and Philadelphia, Pennsylvania (1818). As their efforts expanded from handling public "nuisances" to dealing with epidemics and complex public health problems, local health boards recognized that full-time staffs were needed, and thus health departments were formed. Louisiana was first in 1855; Massachusetts followed in 1869.

Again at the national level, the Marine Hospital Service, now with a broader function, became the Public Health and Marine Hospital Service in 1902. Congress gave it a more clearly defined organizational structure and specific functions for its director, the Surgeon General. In 1912, it was renamed the U.S. Public Health Service (PHS) (Melosi, 2008; Turnock, 2011a; U.S. DHHS, 2010; Ward & Warren, 2007).

Rapidly expanding through World War I and the Great Depression, the PHS strengthened its research activity through the National Institutes of Health (NIH, founded in 1912), added demonstration projects, and initiated greater cooperation with the states. Responding to increasingly complex needs, the NIH added programs significant to public health, such as the Children's Bureau (1912); the National Leprosarium at Carville, Louisiana (1917); examination of arriving aliens (1917); the Division of Venereal Diseases (1918); the Food and Drug Administration [FDA] (1927); and the Narcotics Division (1929), which later became the Division of Mental Hygiene. Title VI of the 1935 Social Security Act promoted stronger federal support of state and local PHSs, including health workforce training (USDHHS, 2010; Ward & Warren, 2007).

As health, welfare, and educational services proliferated, the need for consolidation prompted the creation of the Federal Security Agency in 1939. In 1953, the agency was enlarged and renamed the Department of Health, Education, and Welfare (DHEW), under President Eisenhower. In 1979, education was made a separate cabinet-level department, and the DHEW was renamed the Department of Health and Human Services (DHHS). Other significant events include the establishment during World War II of the Communicable Disease Center in Atlanta, currently known as the Centers for Disease Control and Prevention (CDC), and the development after World War II of the National Office of Vital Statistics, now called the National Center for Health Statistics (NCHS) (CDC, 2011).

Voluntary Health Agencies

The private sector responded first to America's health problems and continues to complement and supplement the government's role in providing health services. By the late 1800s, **voluntary health agencies** (sometimes called private agencies or **nongovernmental organizations [NGOs]**) began to emerge. They were privately funded and operated to address specific health needs. The first of these was the Anti-Tuberculosis Society of Philadelphia, which was formed in 1892 to educate the public and the government about TB, then causing 10% of all deaths. Other agencies followed: the National Society to Prevent Blindness was formed in 1908, the Mental Health Association in 1909, the American Cancer Society in 1913, the National Easter Seal Society for Crippled Children and Adults in 1921, and the Planned Parenthood Federation of America, also in 1921. In the late 1800s, organized charities such as the Red Cross, previously denounced for promoting dependent poverty, began to be recognized for their contributions to health and welfare. Philanthropy, too, became prominent with the establishment of the Rockefeller Foundation in 1913, followed by the Carnegie-Mellon, Kellogg, and Robert Wood Johnson Foundations (Encyclopedia of Public Health, 2011).

Health-Related Professional Associations

Many health-related professional associations have influenced the quality and type of community health services delivery. Among these, the National Organization for Public Health Nursing, from 1912 to 1952, significantly influenced early preparation for and the quality of public health nursing services (Abrams, 2004). The American Public Health Association (APHA), founded in 1872, maintains a prominent role in the dissemination of public health information, influence on health policy, and advocacy for the nation's health. Other nursing and community health organizations that have promoted quality efforts in community health include the Association of State and Territorial Directors of Nursing (ASTDN), the Association of State and Territorial Health Officers (ASTHO), the National League for Nursing (NLN), the American Nurses Association (ANA), and the Association for Community Health Nursing Educators (ACHNE) (Abrams, 2004; Levin et al., 2008).

HEALTH ORGANIZATIONS IN THE UNITED STATES

Over the years, responsibility for meeting community health needs has shifted between private groups and governing institutions, each offering different viewpoints and benefits. Only within the last century have they gradually begun to work together to create a loosely structured system of health care.

Turnock (2011b) and others have noted the growing interdependence of the public and private sectors, and this partnership was encouraged by the Institute of Medicine (2002). How does that system work today? What are its strengths and weaknesses? To answer these questions, its structure must first be examined. Structure is important because it becomes the operational base for assessment, diagnosis, planning, implementation, and evaluation of services—and it provides a framework for intersystem and intrasystem communication and coordination.

Health services occur at four levels: local, state, national, and international. Like ever-widening concentric circles, these levels encompass broader populations. The organization of health services at each level can generally be classified as one of two types: public or private sector.

Public Sector Health Services

Government health agencies, the tax-supported arm of the public health effort, perform a vital function in community health practice. With their jurisdiction and types of service dictated by law, they coordinate and administer activities that often can be carried out only by group or community-wide action (e.g., proper sewage disposal, provision of sanitary water systems, or regulation of toxic wastes). Many community health activities require an authoritative legal backing to ensure enforcement—another useful function of public health agencies—in areas such as environmental pollution, highway safety practices, communicable disease control, and proper, safe handling of food. Official or public health agencies provide important record-keeping services, including the collection and monitoring of vital statistics. They also conduct research, provide consultation, and sometimes financially support other community health efforts.

Core Public Health Functions

PHSs encompass a wide variety of activities, but all can be grouped under one of three **core public health functions** (Institute of Medicine, 1988). They are assessment, policy development, and assurance (Table 6-3). As discussed in Chapters 1 and 3, public health nurses (PHNs) practice as partners with other public health professionals within these core functions.

Assessment refers to measuring and monitoring the health status and needs of a designated community or population. As a core function, it is a continuous process of collecting data and disseminating information about health, diseases, injuries, air and water quality, food safety, and available resources. This function helps to identify trends in morbidity, mortality, and causative factors. It identifies available health resources, unmet needs, and community perceptions about health issues. This is commonly done through community needs assessments.

Table 6.3 Core Public Health Functions Applied To Populations And People At Risk

Population-Wide Services
Assessment
• Health status monitoring and disease surveillance
Public Policy
• Leadership, policy, planning, and administration
Assurance
• Investigation and control of diseases and injuries
• Protection of environment, workplaces, housing, food, and water
• Laboratory services to support disease control and environmental protection
• Health education and information
• Community mobilization for health-related issues
• Targeted outreach and linkage to personal services
• Health services quality assurance and accountability
• Training and education of public health professionals
Personal Services and Home Visits for People at Risk
• Primary care for unserved and underserved people
• Treatment services for targeted conditions
• Clinical preventive services
• Payments for personal services delivered by others

Policy development is the formation of a guide for action that determines present and future decisions affecting the public's health. As a core public health function, good public policy development builds on data from the assessment function and incorporates community values and citizen input. It provides leadership and administration for the development of sound health policy and planning. This can include local ordinances, as well as statewide initiatives (e.g., water safety).

Assurance is the process of translating established policies into services. This function ensures that population-based services are provided, whether by public health agencies or private sources. It also monitors the quality of and access to those services. Training for employees, to assure current knowledge, is another assurance function. The specific functions of assessment, policy development, and assurance are described in Table 6-3.

The roles of public health agencies vary by level, with each level carrying out the core functions in different ways to form a partnership in protecting the public's health (Turnock, 2011a; Williams & Torrens, 2008). International health agencies focus on issues of global concern, setting policy, developing standards, and monitoring health conditions and programs. At the national level, government health agencies engage in similar functions aimed at regional or nationwide concerns.

The federal level provides funds (e.g., through the Medicaid program, block grants, categorical grants) and develops policy (e.g., air pollution policy, occupational safety) but depends on the states to implement them. Agencies at the federal level also develop facilities and programs for special groups, such as Native Americans, migrant workers, inmates of federal prisons, and military personnel and veterans, whose health care is not the direct responsibility of any one state or locality (Scutchfield & Keck, 2009; Turnock, 2011a). At the federal level, public health responsibilities include:

- Assuring the capacity of all levels of government to provide essential PHSs.
- Acting when health threats span many states, regions, or the whole country.
- Acting where the solution may be beyond the jurisdiction of individual states.
- Acting to assist the states when they do not have the expertise or resources to mount an effective response in a public health emergency (e.g., natural disaster, bioterrorism, or emerging disease).
- Facilitating the formulation of public health goals in collaboration with state and local governments and other relevant stakeholders (e.g., *Healthy People 2020*).
- Acting transparently and accountably for public health investments.
- Disseminating innovation and best practices from state and local public health (Trust for America's Health, 2011a, p. 9).

State government health agencies function fairly autonomously while working within federal guidelines. They assess, develop, and monitor statewide health needs and services. Historically, they have been responsible for communicable disease control, vital statistics, laboratory services, environmental sanitation and hygiene, health education and maternal–child health, with the addition of categorical programs (e.g., heart disease, migrant health) in the 1950s (Scutchfield & Keck, 2009). In the 1980s, block grants were instituted to give more flexibility to states in how funds are targeted.

At the local level, one may find a city government health agency, a county agency, or a combination of both to assess, plan, and serve the health needs of that locality. Most local health departments are under county jurisdiction, with only a small percentage of cities (usually large cities) having local health departments. Some are city–county agencies or special districts, and most local health departments report to either local government councils or boards of health (Scutchfield & Keck, 2009). In some states, local health departments also report to state public health agencies. In about 30% of the states, local health departments are operated by the state health agency, which provides services locally, without city or county oversight (Turnock, 2011b).

Unlike private organizations that tend to have a specific focus, government health agencies exist to accomplish a broad goal of protecting and promoting the health of the total population under their jurisdiction. Such a task requires a wide range of services and the combined talents of many types of professional disciplines. Among them are nurses, physicians, health educators, sanitarians, epidemiologists, statisticians, engineers, administrators, accountants, computer programmers, planners, sociologists, nutritionists, laboratory technicians, chemists, physicists, veterinarians, dentists, pharmacists, demographers, and meteorologists. Furthermore, public health agencies must function not only on an interdisciplinary basis but also on an interorganizational basis. Other government services (e.g., education) can meet their goals fairly autonomously, but public health cannot accomplish its important objectives without the collaboration of many agencies and organizations, both public and private (Turnock, 2011a; Williams & Torrens, 2008). To manage the AIDS epidemic, for example, public health agencies, educational institutions, welfare agencies, mental health programs, home care services, Medicaid, and private groups, among others, may be called upon to collaborate.

Many different government agencies contribute to the health of a community. Most obvious are the local and state health departments, which provide a variety of direct and indirect health services, including community health nursing. Other tax-supported agencies that sponsor health care or health-related services include welfare departments, departments of public works, public schools and hospitals, police departments, county agricultural services, and local housing authorities.

Local Public Health Agencies

At the grassroots level, government health agencies vary considerably in structure and function from one locality to the next. This partly results from variations in local needs and the size and resources of the community. For example, a rural community served by a county or state health department may have needs and services that differ widely from those of a densely populated urban community (see Chapter 29). Differing health care standards and regulations, as well as the type and stipulations of funding sources, also contribute to variations in the structure and function of health agencies. Nonetheless, each local governmental health agency shares some commonly held responsibilities, functions, and structural features.

The primary responsibilities of the local health department are to assess the population's health status and needs, determine how well those needs are being met, and take action toward satisfying unmet needs (Scutchfield & Keck, 2009). Specifically, local government health agencies should fulfill these core functions as follows:

- Monitor local health needs and the resources for addressing them.
- policy and provide leadership in advocating equitable distribution of resources and services, both public and private.
- Evaluate availability, accessibility, and quality of health services for all members of the community.
- Keep the community informed about how to access PHSs.

The local health agency represents a critical level of health services' provision because of its closeness to the ultimate recipients—health care consumers. The most recent survey of local health departments, reported in a classic study by Barry et al. in 1998, revealed the top three expenditure categories were enforcing laws and regulations; informing, educating, and empowering people; and ensuring the provision of care. Research on specific expenditures in local and state health departments is lacking (Sensenig, 2007).

The structure of the local health department varies in complexity with the setting. Rural and small urban agencies need only a simple organization, whereas large metropolitan agencies require more complex organizational structures to support the greater diversity and quantity of work.

Where a board of health exists, it holds the legal responsibility for the health of its citizens. About 80% of local public health departments work with a board of health, and they are more commonly found with smaller populations (Turnock, 2011b). A mayor may appoint health board members if the board of health serves a city, by a board of supervisors if the board of health serves a county, or by voters if they are publicly elected. In turn, the board of health usually appoints a health officer (about 80%)—only 15% are physicians—who directs the remaining staff of the health department, including PHNs, environmental health workers, health educators, and office personnel (Turnock, 2011b). Less than 25% of local health officers have graduate level public health training. Other public health workers, such as nutritionists, statisticians, epidemiologists, social workers, physical therapists, veterinarians, or public health dentists, may be added as needs and resources dictate. The number of staff at local health departments can range from 5 to well over 100, depending upon the size of the agency and population served (Scutchfield & Keck, 2009).

Revenues to support local health departments come from various sources. Local and county general appropriations make up the largest share of the local health department's budget—around 25%. State revenues account for about 20% of the total local budget—with additional funds provided through special levies and programs such as school health, Head Start, air pollution, toxic substance control, primary care, immunizations, fees, and private foundation grants. Federal funds provide another source of revenue (about 2% directly; 17% passed along through states) targeted at specific efforts, such as AIDS research and services, family planning, child health, environmental protection, and hypertension and nutrition programs. Medicaid and Medicare reimbursement account for about 15% of the budget. According to Turnock (2011b), fees, reimbursements, and additional miscellaneous sources, such as state laboratory revenues and food supply supplements, make up the remaining portion of the budget (between 11% and 18%). A good number of health departments bill Medicaid for personal health services rendered (e.g., prenatal care, TB treatment, well-baby care), but an increasing number of states are offering Medicaid managed care, and moving personal health care out of local health departments (Scutchfield & Keck, 2009). Figure 6-1 depicts the organization of one local health department serving a population of approximately 300,000.

State Public Health Agencies

State-level government health agencies also vary in structure and in how they carry out the core functions. Each state, as a sovereign government, establishes its own health department, which in turn determines its goals, actions, and administrative structure. The state health department is responsible for providing leadership in and monitoring of comprehensive public health needs and services in the state. It establishes statewide health policy standards, assists local communities, allocates funds, promotes state-level health planning, conducts and evaluates state-level health programs, promotes cooperation with voluntary (private) health agencies or NGOs, and collaborates with the federal government for health planning and policy development (Scutchfield & Keck, 2009). Of the various levels of government health agencies, the states recently have played the most pivotal role in health policy formation.

General functions of state health departments include (Scutchfield & Keck, 2009):

- Statewide health planning
- Intergovernmental and other agency relations
- Intrastate agency relations
- Certain statewide policy determinations
- Standards setting
- Health regulatory functions

Specifically, the Institute of Medicine (1988) described the role of state government related to health. Summarized, it includes:

- A statewide method of collecting and analyzing data to assess health needs
- Adequate statutory base for state health activities
- Statewide health objectives (holding localities accountable where power for implementation has been delegated)
- Statewide development and maintenance of essential personal, educational, and environmental health services
- Identification of problems that threaten the health of the state
- Support for local health services (when needed to achieve adequate service levels) through subsidies, technical and administrative assistance, or direct action

State public health agencies face a challenge in addressing the health-related issues confronting them. Health care reform, underinsured populations, long-term care, organ transplants and donations, AIDS, care of the **medically indigent** (those who are unable to pay for and totally lack medical services), malpractice, and certificates of need (CON) for new health services are among the problems faced by most states. Clearly, state health departments must collaborate closely with

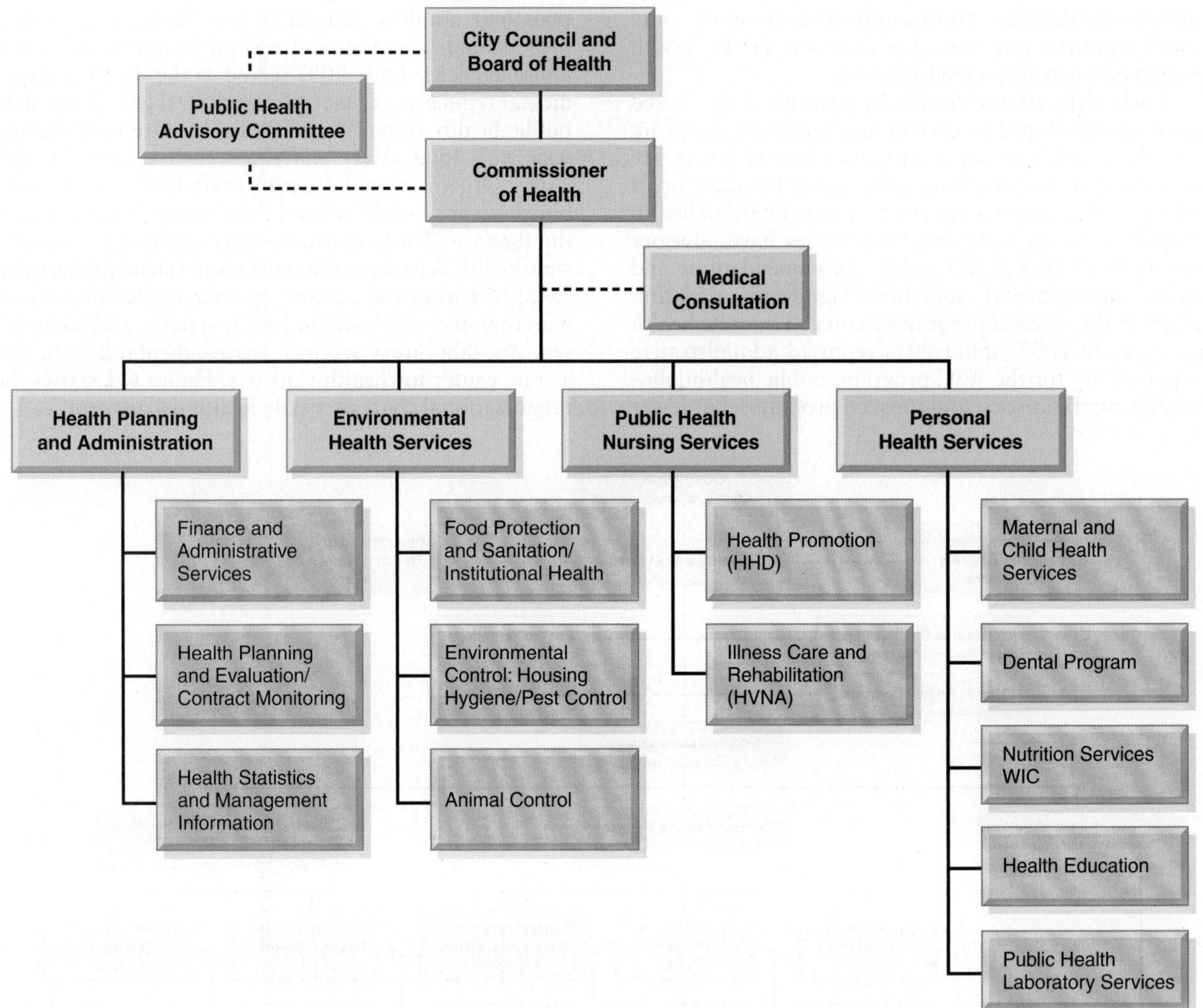

FIGURE 6-1. Organizational chart of a city public health department.

other agencies, such as social services, education, public works, the legislature, and the housing bureau, to effectively solve such problems. Thus, the solution of state health problems and delivery of health services requires the functioning of an interdependent network of organizations, many of which are not health agencies per se.

Budgetary sources for a state health department include state-generated funds, federal grants and contracts, and fees and reimbursements. A large source of federal monies to the states comes through the Department of Agriculture, which supports the Women, Infants, and Children (WIC) program, a supplemental nutrition program. State health agencies often provide grant opportunities for local health departments (often through federal grant monies awarded to states). Fragmentation of public health roles and functions among different state agencies poses problems for coordinating the core public health functions at this level (Turnock, 2011b). Funding for state public health agencies comes largely from state coffers, with less than an average of 40% coming from federal contracts and grants, and a smaller percentage generated from fees and third-party reimbursements, local taxes and funds, as well as other sources (Scutchfield & Keck, 2009). However, federal funding is characterized as "uneven from state to state" and "eroding in the face of the economic recession" (Ross, 2009, para. 1), with "budgetary shortfalls of $425 billion" since 2009 (Trust for America's Health, 2011a, p. 12). Nationally, the median level of per capita funding for public health was $30.61 in 2010, with a range between $3.61 (Nevada) and $171.30 (Hawaii) (Trust for America's Health, 2011a). The Department of Agriculture, the CDC, and Health Resources and Services Administration (HRSA) all provide substantial funding at the state level. Almost 75% of the CDC budget ($5.35 billion in 2008) is targeted to states and communities, and HRSA contributed $5.72 billion to states in 2008 (Ross, 2009). Less than 1.7% of all state expenditures go toward population health (e.g., health promotion, chronic disease control) (Milbank Memorial Fund et al., 2005). Most state public health expenditures in 2009 dealt with improving consumer health (25%), WIC programs (23%), and infectious (13%) or chronic disease (8%) control. Prevention of epidemics and communicable disease control, injury prevention, disaster preparation and response, and health infrastructure are also common public health expenditure categories (Sellers, n.d.).

Each of the 50 state health departments in the United States has developed its own unique structure. Some are strongly centralized organizations, whereas others are decentralized. In most states, the appointed director or executive of the agency reports to a state board of health or directly to the governor. Some states have advisory boards that make health policy recommendations and review departmental activities. Significant variation occurs in the types of programs managed by state health agencies—in 2007, about 90% reported administrative responsibility for the WIC program, public health laboratories, vital statistics, and tobacco programs, but fewer than half administered the state's Medicaid program, professional licensing, and mental health or substance abuse agencies. Only 20% served as the state's environmental regulatory agency (Turnock, 2011b). Many state public health agencies regulate health care facilities and deal with food safety and some environmental health issues. Organizational structures vary from state to state, but there are usually several divisions or bureaus under the director. Those divisions most commonly found in state health department organizational structures are disease prevention and control, community health services, maternal and child health, health systems and technical services, laboratory services, environmental health, and a state center for health statistics. Figure 6-2 shows the organizational chart of a state health department.

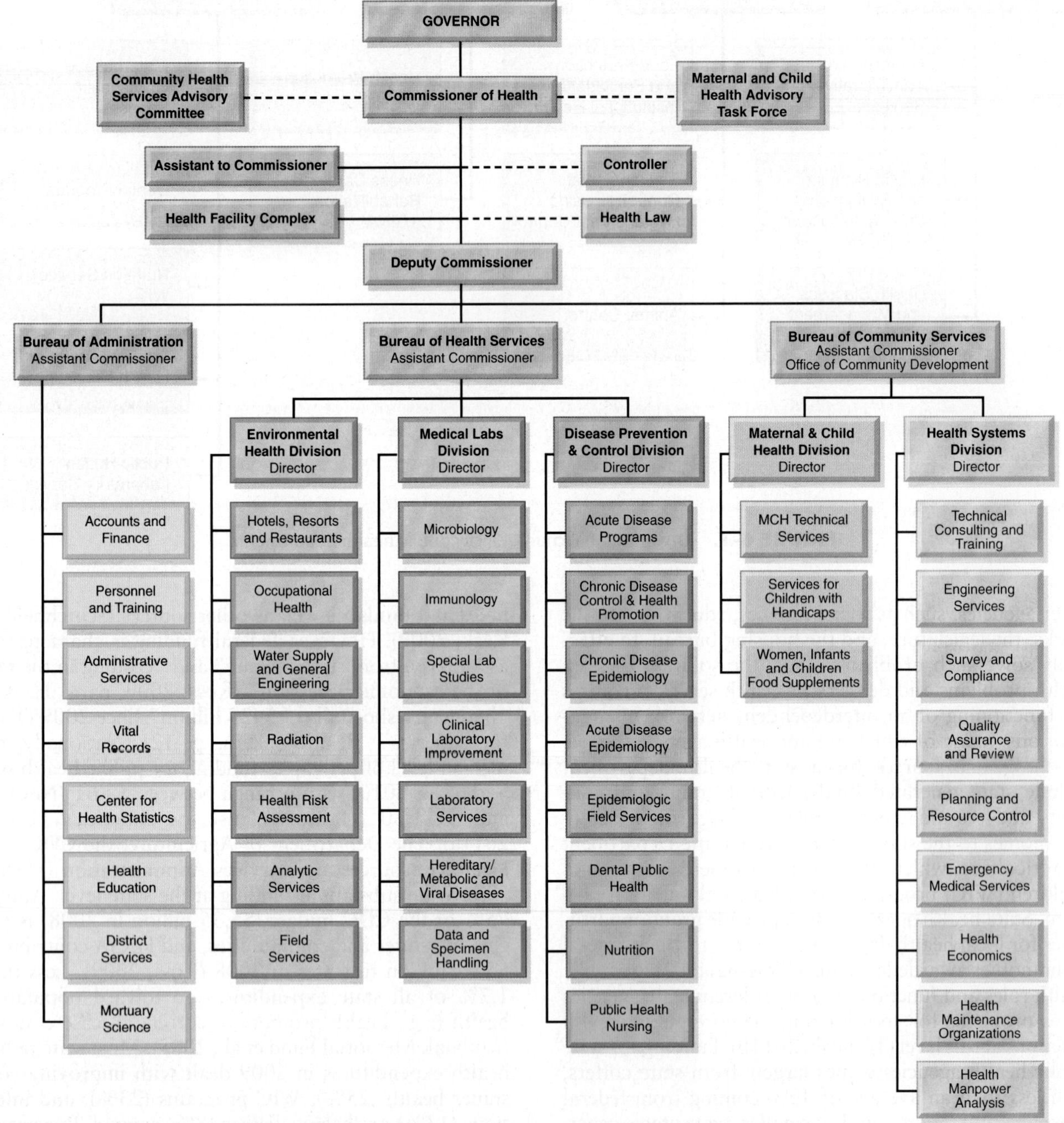

FIGURE 6-2. Organizational chart of a state public health department.

National Public Health Agencies

The national level of public health organization consists of many government agencies. They can be clustered into four groups. First and most directly focused on health is the **Public Health Service (PHS)**. It is concerned with the broad health interests of the country and is a functional (not organizational) unit of DHHS (see Chapter 30 for more on the PHS Commissioned Corps).

The Secretary of Health and Human Services (a cabinet-level position) has ultimate responsibility for the PHS. The PHS consists of the Office of Public Health and Science (headed by the Assistant Secretary for Health), and comprises the Commissioned Core (over 6,000 uniformed health professionals), the Office of the Surgeon General, and 10 regional offices across the country. The PHS is made up of 11 functional branches: the Administration for Children & Families, the Centers for Medicare & Medicaid Services, the Administration on Aging, the CDC, the FDA, the NIH, the Substance Abuse and Mental Health Services Administration (SAMHSA), HRSA, the Agency for Healthcare Research & Quality (AHRQ), the Indian Health Service, and the Agency for Toxic Substances and Disease Registry (ATSDR). One of its major functions through these 11 branches is the administration of grants and contracts with other government agencies, private organizations, and individuals. In some instances, the PHS provides hospital, clinical, and other types of health services, for example, for Native Americans and Eskimos through the Indian Health Service. Through the CDC and the NIH, it provides epidemiologic surveillance and numerous research programs. The FDA monitors the safety and usefulness of various food and drug products, as well as cosmetics, toys, and flammable fabrics (U.S. DHHS, n.d.).

Through its staff offices, the PHS offers other services. It has responsibility for the formation, planning, and evaluation of health policy; health promotion; health services management; health research and statistics; intergovernmental affairs; legislation; population affairs; and international health. It provides financial assistance to the states through grants-in-aid—monies raised by Congress through taxes for specific purposes. It also offers consultation through national advisory health councils and special advisory committees made up of lay experts. The PHS maintains 10 regional offices to make its services more readily available to the states. These offices are located in New York City, Boston, Philadelphia, Atlanta, Chicago, Kansas City, Dallas, Denver, Seattle, and San Francisco.

At the federal level, the primary agencies concerned with health are organized under the DHHS. Assistant secretaries manage offices for Health, Administration, Financial Resources, Planning and Evaluation, Preparedness and Response, Legislation, and Public Affairs. Within the DHHS, clusters of federal agencies deal with the needs of special population groups, such as the elderly (Administration on Aging), children (Administration for Children and Families), and Native Americans (Bureau of Indian Affairs), and government health insurance programs (U.S. DHHS, n.d.). Figure 6-3 is the organizational chart for U.S. DHHS.

Another cluster of service departments addresses special programs or problems. Examples are the Department of Labor, the Department of Education, the Department of Interior, the Department of Agriculture, and the Department of Transportation. A final cluster of federal agencies focuses on international health concerns of interest to the nation. Two important ones include the U.S. Agency for International Development (USAID), an independent agency, and the Office of International Health Affairs, under the Department of State (Turnock, 2011a).

Budgets and Funding for Public Health

U.S. government public health spending represented 3% of the total health spending in 2009 (Centers for Medicare & Medicaid Spending [CMS], n.d. a). The total current per capita annual health expenditure well exceeds $8,086 (CMS, n.d. b). This disproportionate funding for health continues despite estimations that a focus on population-based health promotion (e.g., public health) saves $5.60 for every dollar that is spent (Trust for America's Health, 2008).

But, in addition to health promotion, PHSs must be ready for disasters, bioterrorism, and pandemics, and evidence is mounting that the system is structurally weak and suffers from poor access and inconsistent preparation (Institute of Medicine, 2002; Roos, 2009). To meet the needs of communities and the nation, new funding is needed. The Affordable Care Act ([ACA]; health are reform legislation) created a Prevention and Public Health Fund for state and local community assistance in promoting health and preventing disease. The substantial investment—$15 billion over 10 years—also aids with early intervention to prevent later complications of illness (Healthcare.gov, 2011). Community and clinical prevention, public health infrastructure, and primary care training are also part of this fund.

Private Sector Health Services

The nongovernmental and voluntary arm of the health care delivery system includes many types of services. Privately owned, nonprofit health agencies (most hospitals and welfare agencies) make up one large group. Privately owned (proprietary), for-profit agencies are another. Private professional health care practice, composed largely of physicians in solo or group practice, forms a third group. These make up the non–tax-supported, nongovernmental dimension of community health care.

Private health services are complementary and supplementary to government health agencies. They often meet the needs of special groups, such as those with cancer or heart disease; they offer an avenue for private enterprise or philanthropy; they are less constrained than government agencies in developing innovations in health care; and they have been spurred to development, in part, by impatience or dissatisfaction with government programs. Their financial support comes from voluntary contributions, bequests, or fees (Scutchfield & Keck, 2009).

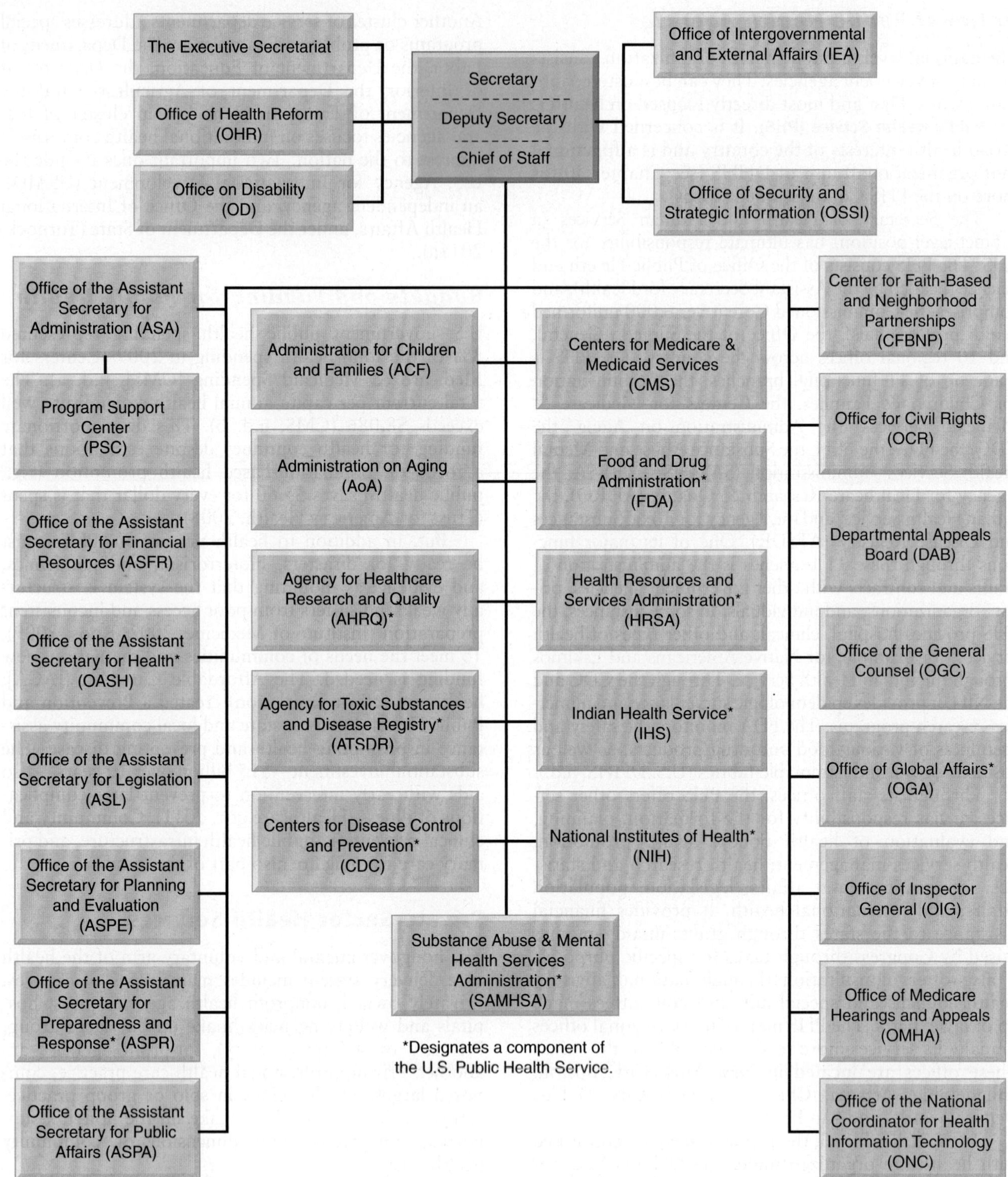

FIGURE 6-3. Department of Health and Human Services organizational chart, July 2011.

For-Profit and Not-for-Profit Health Agencies

Proprietary health services are privately owned and managed. They may be nonprofit or for-profit. Many hospitals and nursing homes offer nonprofit services, but must generate sufficient revenues to keep ahead of operating costs. Often, one or more special services offered by a hospital generate enough income to cover the drain from more expensive programs or uncompensated care. As more hospitals have merged or been integrated into larger health conglomerates, the practice in many cases has been to establish a separate, for-profit corporation that generates revenues so that the basic organization can retain its nonprofit, tax-exempt status.

Examples of for-profit health services include a wide range of private practices by physicians, nurses, social workers, psychologists, and laboratory and radiology technologists. With the greater demand for home care services since the 1980s, the number of new, for-profit services (e.g., home care agencies, nursing personnel pools, and durable medical equipment supply companies) increased dramatically. Medicare's annual costs for home care services per enrollee went from $4 in 1969 to more than $300 by the late 1990s (Tyson, 2001). Partially in response to these escalating home care costs to Medicare, the Balanced Budget Act of 1997 was passed, and payments for home health care services to the elderly dropped by 12.5% annually through the year 2000 (Meara, White, & Cutler, 2004). Even with these budget adjustments, average total Medicare expenditures grew from $5,080 per person in 1991 to $7,310 in 2001 and $9,083 in 2011 (Congressional Budget Office, 2005; Kaiser Family Foundation [KFF], 2011e). Medicare spending, like most health care spending, is skewed in that 10% of beneficiaries are responsible for 59% of total spending, representing $48,693 per capita (KFF, 2011e).

Not-for-profit private health agencies are organizations that are established and administered by private citizens for a specific health-related purpose. Often, this purpose is seen as a special need either not addressed or served inadequately by government. An example is visiting nurse associations, which were formed to provide care for the sick in their homes. The contribution of the private, not-for-profit health agency then becomes complementary to PHSs.

Three types of private, not-for-profit health agencies have specialized interests. Some, such as the American Cancer Society and the American Diabetes Association, focus on specific diseases. Others, such as the National Society for Autistic Children, Planned Parenthood Federation of America, and the National Council on Aging, focus on the needs of special populations. A third group, including agencies such as the American Heart Association and the National Kidney Foundation, are concerned with diseases of specific organs. All of these agencies are funded through private contributions. Trust for America's Health is a nonpartisan, nonprofit organization sponsored by foundation and individual support is focused on disease prevention and protection of individuals and communities.

Another group of private, not-for-profit agencies affecting health and health care includes the many foundations that support health programs, research, and professional education. Examples include the W.K. Kellogg Foundation, the Pew Charitable Trusts, the Robert Wood Johnson Foundation, and the Bill and Melinda Gates Foundation. Some agencies, such as the United Way, exist to fund other voluntary efforts.

Another group includes professional associations that work to improve the public's health through the promotion of standards, research, information, and programs. Examples are the APHA, the Association for State and Territorial Health Officials (ASTHO), the National Association of County and City Health Officials (NACCHO), the NLN, the American Nurses Association (ANA), and the American Medical Association (AMA). These organizations are funded primarily through membership dues, bequests, and contributions.

Functions of Private Sector Health Agencies

The general functions of private sector health agencies are as follows:

- Detecting unmet needs or exploring better methods for meeting needs already identified
- Piloting or subsidizing demonstration projects
- Promoting public knowledge
- Assisting official agencies with innovative programs not otherwise possible
- Evaluating official programs and assuming a public advocacy role
- Promoting health legislation
- Planning and coordinating to promote collaboration among voluntary services and between voluntary and official agencies
- Developing well-balanced community health programs that seek to make services relevant and comprehensive

Both public and private agencies are needed to maintain a viable public health system (Turnock, 2011a, 2011b). Future functions of both private and public sectors most likely will remain much the same. However, the structure of the organizations within both sectors is changing dramatically and will continue to do so as managed care organizations (MCOs) blur the lines between private and public sectors. The blurring of the private and public health care sectors has opened the doors to emerging creative health care services.

INTERNATIONAL HEALTH ORGANIZATIONS

The health of countries around the world cannot be ignored. Besides important humanitarian and moral concerns, there are pragmatic reasons for addressing health issues at the international level. Today, health—along with politics and economics—has become a global issue. Health care among most of the world's population continues to be based on traditional medicine. At the same time, technology is revolutionizing health practices via distance education, training, and telemedicine. Healthcare information technology has the potential to empower all nations, rich and poor, to enhance the health of their citizens (Hammond, 2009). The nations of the world depend on one another for goods and services, and, as in any set of interdependent systems, a problem in one nation has repercussions on others (Beaglehole & Bonita, 2009).

It may not seem possible that the health of a resident of a country 9,000 miles away can affect that of a student from the United States or vice versa; however, when boarding an international flight for a school holiday, the student will likely be seated among people from many nations. Despite close scrutiny of airline passengers for passports, visas, customs regulations, weapons, and drugs, how can anyone know whether any passenger sitting near the student has an airborne communicable disease that is resistant to known antibiotics? (See From the Case Files I.)

International cooperation in health dates back to early concerns for epidemics. In 1851, representatives from 12 countries met in Paris for the First International Sanitary Conference. They later established a more permanent organization, the Office Internationale d'Hygiene Publique, in 1907. Epidemics in the Western Hemisphere also prompted representatives from 21 American republics to meet for the First International Sanitary Conference in Mexico City in 1902. In that same year, the International Sanitary Bureau was formed and, later, renamed the Pan American Sanitary Bureau. It is now called the Pan American Health Organization (PAHO) (World Health Organization [WHO], n.d.). (See Chapter 16 for more on global health.)

From the Case Files I

Medication-Resistant Tuberculosis

In 2007, the Centers for Disease Control and Prevention (CDC) ordered federal isolation (or quarantine)—something it hadn't done since 1963—for a 31-year-old Atlanta lawyer diagnosed with tuberculosis (TB). In his initial examination, Andrew Speaker says he was told he had TB but wasn't contagious or a danger to anyone else and was not forbidden to fly to Greece and Europe for his wedding and honeymoon, but said he was told by county health officials that they preferred that he didn't fly (Ogilvie, 2007). The CDC contends that they instructed him not to travel abroad, but he ignored them (Kvinta, 2011). While he and his new wife were honeymooning, lab test results revealed that he had an extensively drug resistant (XDR) strain of TB, and the CDC warned him not to take a commercial flight home, but to turn himself over to Italian health authorities so that he could be isolated (Kvinta, 2011). However, he and his wife disregarded this admonition, flying back to Canada on Czech Air and then "sneaking" across the border to the United States. He was quarantined a day later and then sent to National Jewish Medical and Research Center in Denver, Colorado—a hospital with a long history of TB research and treatment. Several months later, new tests showed that his sputum samples were positive for multidrug-resistant (MDR) TB, with no signs of the XDR TB first noted on bronchoscopy samples. MDR TB is less resistant to antituberculosis medications and requires less intensive treatment than XDR TB. Mr. Speaker later had surgery to remove the infected lung and was subsequently diagnosed as non-contagious. At the time of the incident, the CDC recommended that fellow travelers on Mr. Speaker's transatlantic flights have TB tests to determine if they contracted the disease. This incident brought TB to the forefront and reinforced the concept of the world as a global community. It also highlighted international public health law and the need for countries to work together to protect the health of all citizens. Mr. Speaker filed suit against the CDC in 2009, claiming his privacy was invaded, but the U.S. District Court subsequently dismissed the lawsuit (Poole, 2009).

World Health Organization

The WHO, an agency of the United Nations, was developed to direct and coordinate the promotion of health worldwide. It was formed after World War II, in 1948, and assumed the functions of the League of Nation's health organization. The PAHO remained separate but became the WHO regional office for the Americas. The WHO began with 61 member nations, one of which was the United States. There are currently 194 member nations (WHO, 2011a). The mission of the WHO is to

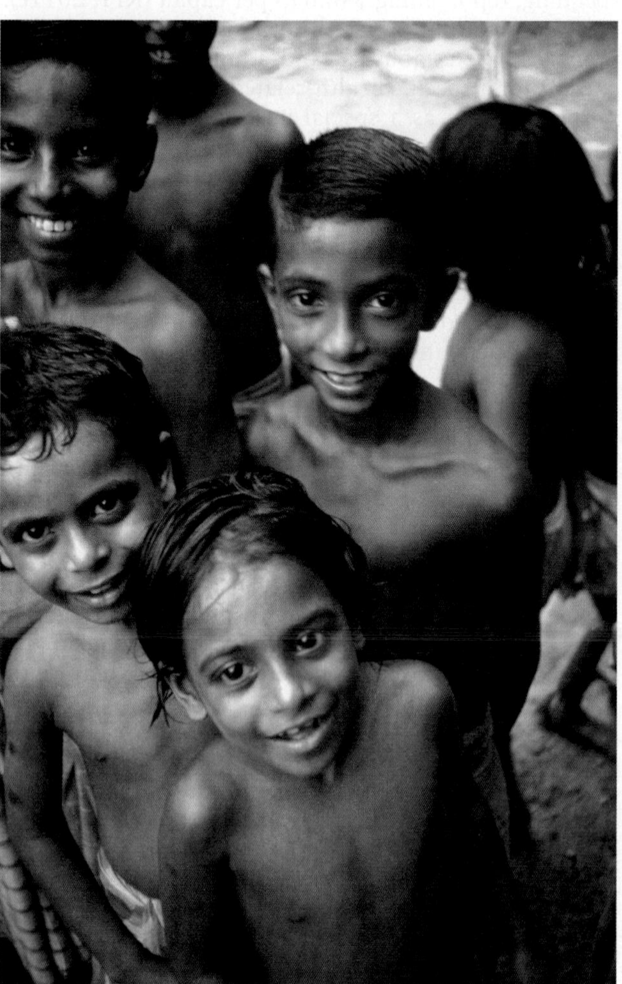

The World Health Organization helps countries improve health services and the health of their citizens, such as these Bangladeshi children examined during a smallpox search.

serve as the one directing and coordinating authority on international health. From its inception, it has influenced international thinking with its classic definition of health as "a state of complete physical, mental, and social wellbeing and not merely the absence of disease or infirmity" (Grad, 2002, p. 984). The primary function of the WHO is to help countries improve their health status and services by assisting them to help themselves and each other. To accomplish this, it provides member countries with technical services, information from epidemiology and statistics reports, advisory and consulting services, and demonstration teams.

For 20 years, the WHO had a realistic expectation that by the year 2000, no individual citizen in any country would have a level of health below an acceptable minimum, and that the global community would later adopt a new strategy to take people further toward the goal of health for all in the future (WHO, 1998). The target date of the year 2000 was intended as a challenge to the member nations, although not all goals were entirely met. Member nations renewed goals for 2015 to "combat poverty, hunger, disease, illiteracy, environmental degradation, and discrimination against women" (WHO, 2011b, para. 1). These emphases point to a change in focus from primarily reactive programs (e.g., stopping epidemics, instituting quarantines) to the more proactive promotion of health for the world community.

Headquartered in Geneva, Switzerland, the WHO has six regional offices (WHO, 2011c). The Regional Office for the Americas is located in Washington, DC. The other regional offices are in Copenhagen, Denmark (Europe); Cairo, Egypt (Eastern Mediterranean); Brazzaville, Congo (Africa); New Delhi, India (Southeast Asia); and Manila, Philippines (Western Pacific). Funding comes from member countries and from the United Nations. The WHO holds an annual World Health Assembly to discuss international health policies and programs. The organization publishes several periodicals of interest to the global community, which are available by subscription for a fee and in partial text through WHO's various Web sites www.who.int/publications/en/ and include:

Bulletin of the World Health Organization—monthly
WHO Drug Information—quarterly
Weekly Epidemiological Record—weekly
Pan American Journal of Public Health—monthly.

Pan American Health Organization

The PAHO, the central coordinating organization for public health in the Western Hemisphere, is the oldest continuously functioning international health organization in the world. Its budget comes from assessments contributed by member states, augmented by funds from WHO, the United Nations, and other sources, including private donations (PAHO, 2011a).

As WHO's regional office for the Americas, PAHO disseminates epidemiologic information, provides technical assistance, finances fellowships, and promotes cooperative research and professional education. Conferences convened by PAHO provide an opportunity for delegates from member nations to discuss issues of concern and plan strategies for addressing health needs. The most widely read journal published by PAHO is the *Pan American Journal of Public Health*, published monthly (PAHO, 2011b).

United Nations International Children's Emergency Fund

Organized in 1946, the United Nations Children's Fund, now called the United Nations International Children's Emergency Fund (UNICEF), was established initially as a temporary emergency program to assist the children of war-torn countries. That focus has broadened, and UNICEF is now a permanent agency for promoting child and maternal health and welfare globally, through a variety of programs and activities, including provision of food and supplies to underdeveloped countries, immunization programs in cooperation with the WHO, disease control (especially HIV/AIDS), creating protective environments for children, and the education of girls (UNICEF, 2011).

U.S. Agency for International Development

Since the 1960s, the USAID lists goals of improving the health, education, and wellbeing of the populations of developing countries.

> USAID invests in methods to improve the lives of those around the world by:
>
> - Investing in agricultural productivity so countries can feed their people
> - Combating maternal and child mortality and deadly diseases like HIV, malaria and tuberculosis
> - Providing life-saving assistance in the wake of disaster
> - Promoting democracy, human rights and good governance around the world
> - Fostering private sector development and sustainable economic growth
> - Helping communities adapt to a changing environment
> - Elevating the role of women and girls throughout all our work (USAID, 2012, para. 5).

Other International Health Organizations

Many other organizations deal with health concerns at the international level. The United Nations Educational, Scientific, and Cultural Organization (UNESCO) promotes quality education for all, scientific knowledge for sustainable development, cultural diversity and dialogue, information and communication, and "addressing emerging ethical challenges" (UNESCO, 2008, para. 8). The World Bank addresses health problems through funding and technical assistance. The Food and Agriculture Organization (FAO) works to improve food security, "raise levels of nutrition, improve agricultural productivity, better the lives of rural populations, and contribute to the growth of the world economy by providing information and technical assistance" (FAO, 2011, para. 2). *Medicins Sans Frontieres*, or Doctors Without Borders, is an "international medical humanitarian organization" working in over 60 countries, assisting victims of neglect, violence, or natural disasters and catastrophes (Doctors Without Borders, 2011, para. 1). Formed in France in 1971, physicians and journalists joined together recognizing a need for neutral, independent medical teams to provide quality medical care to those caught in the middle of armed conflicts or epidemics. Over 27,000 health professionals from around the world work daily to provide care operating under the "guiding principles of humanitarian action and medical ethics" (Doctors Without Borders, 2011, para. 13). Because of their close proximity to rapidly changing political situations, this group has called for action by the international community to prevent further loss of life due to atrocities and abuses. In addition to these international organizations, most developed countries have agencies that provide assistance, some in major proportions, to underdeveloped countries.

SIGNIFICANT LEGISLATION

During the past century in the United States, an ever-widening sense of responsibility for health in the public sector led to passage of an increasing amount of health-related legislation. Some acts are of particular significance to the financing and delivery of community health services (see Display 6.1). Only after World War I and the Great Depression did the U.S. government enact significant legislation that affected the health and wellbeing

(*Text continues on page 173*)

DISPLAY 6.1 LANDMARK HEALTH CARE LEGISLATION

The Shepard–Towner Act of 1921

The Shepard–Towner Act of 1921 provided federal grant-in-aid funds to the states for administration of programs to promote the health and welfare of mothers and infants. The act expired in 1929, but it set a pattern for maternal and child health programs that later was revived and strengthened through the successful and far-reaching efforts of the Children's Bureau (now known as the Maternal and Child Health Bureau), housed in the Department of Labor. Through the leadership of this bureau, many programs were instituted that enhanced children's health. Among them were services targeting prematurity, perinatal mortality, nutrition, mental retardation, audiology, rheumatic fever, cerebral palsy, epilepsy, dentistry, juvenile delinquency, and the problems of migrant workers' children (Scutchfield & Keck, 2009). The Children's Bureau maintained its impact through several administrative changes (it was moved to the Federal Security Agency in 1946 and to the Department of Health, Education, and Welfare in 1953), but was phased out in 1972, when it became the Office of Maternal and Child Health. Now under the Department of Health and Human Services, it is known as the Maternal and Child Health Bureau (Ruhl, n.d.).

The Social Security Act of 1935

The Social Security Act of 1935 had tremendous consequences for public health. In addition to its revolutionary welfare insurance and assistance programs, which particularly benefited high-risk mothers and children, Title VI of the act financially assisted states and localities in providing public health services (PHSs). These funds were and still are allocated on the basis of population public health problems, economic need, and need for training of public health personnel. Many of the grants had to be matched by the states or localities. This served to increase their knowledge of and commitment to health programs. The act strengthened local health departments and health programs in most states (Scutchfield & Keck, 2009; Social Security Online, 2007). Most commonly, this act is known for retirement benefits for those over age 65, but it also provides aid for dependent children and unemployment insurance (Social Security Administration, 2012). In 2007, over 50 million Americans will receive more than $602 billion in benefits; the vast majority of recipients are retired workers (Social Security Administration, 2012).

The Hill-Burton Act (Hospital Survey and Construction Act) of 1946

The Hill-Burton Act of 1946 was an important breakthrough in nationwide health facilities planning. It marked the first real effort to link health planning with population needs on a comprehensive basis. The act provided federal funds to states for hospital construction (about one-third of the total cost). It helped to provide access, especially in rural areas, to acute-care services, but did not address public health or preventive care. It also required participating hospitals to provide services to residents, such as "community services," regardless of "race, color, national origin, or creed" (U.S. DHHS, 2006, para. 2). Emergency services were to be provided "without regard to the person's ability to pay" (para. 1). A 1961 medical facilities bill expanded grant money to states for PHSs, nursing homes, and planning for hospitals, as well as for outpatient services for elderly and chronically ill. Expenditures for this act ended in 1975, but it has provided close to 500,000 hospital beds, and has had a lasting effect on the U.S. health care system. Few people remember that this bill was sponsored

(continued)

DISPLAY 6.1 LANDMARK HEALTH CARE LEGISLATION *(Continued)*

by the American Hospital Association in response to a proposal by President Harry Truman to add a comprehensive medical insurance program to Social Security—an effort to provide universal health coverage (Brookings Institution, 2012; Perlstadt, 1995).

The Maternal and Child Health and Mental Retardation Planning Amendments of 1963

Although the Social Security Act of 1935 provided for some services for "crippled children," the Maternal and Child Health and Mental Retardation Planning Amendments of 1963 opened the door for improved services to selected mothers and children. Recognizing the nation's high infant mortality rate and the accompanying problems of premature births, handicapping conditions, and mental retardation, Congress—through this law—authorized grants to fund projects offering comprehensive care to high-risk, low-income mothers and children. It also provided grants to states to design comprehensive programs addressing mental retardation (The ARC, 2010).

The Heart Disease, Cancer, and Stroke Amendments of 1965 (PL 89–239)

The Heart Disease, Cancer, and Stroke Amendments of 1965 are noteworthy for their establishment of regional medical programs, one of the first real efforts at comprehensive health planning. Fifty-six regions in the United States were designated, and each was charged with the responsibility to evaluate the overall health needs of its region and cooperate with other regions for program development. Although the amendments initially were categorical (limited to heart disease, cancer, and stroke), amendments in 1970 expanded the legislation's focus. The act was important for two additional reasons: it encouraged local participation in health planning, which was previously done at federal and state levels, and it funded program operations and planning (National Library of Medicine, 2003).

The Social Security Act Amendments of 1965 (PL 89–97)

The Social Security Act Amendments of 1965 addressed a concern for some version of NHI. Title XVIII, Medicare, provided federally funded health insurance for the elderly (65 years and older) and for disabled persons. Title XIX, Medicaid, is a joint federal–state welfare assistance program that serves the blind, certain families with dependent children, the disabled, and eligible elderly. These two pieces of legislation have enabled many of the poor, disabled, and elderly to receive quality health care that otherwise would not be available to them (Scutchfield & Keck, 2009; Williams & Torrens, 2008).

The Comprehensive Health Planning and Public Health Service Amendments Act (Partnership for Health Act) of 1966 (PL 89–749)

The Partnership for Health Act of 1966 promoted further advances in comprehensive health planning. It established comprehensive health planning agencies and coordinated the many categorical health and research efforts into an integrated system. It emphasized comprehensive health planning and cost containment at local, state, and regional levels. Its goals were improved efficiency and effectiveness of health care, and it also provided for some PHSs and training (Brookings Institution, 2012).

The Health Manpower Act of 1968 (PL 90–490)

The Health Manpower Act of 1968 increased the supply of health personnel by providing federal money to educational institutions for construction, training, special projects, student loans, and scholarships. This act replaced several previous acts that had similar goals but resulted in only fragmentary efforts to address the problem. Among them were the Health Amendment Acts of 1956, the Nurse Training Act (1966), and the Allied Health Professions Personnel Training Act (1966). In 1976, Congress passed the Health Professions Education Assistance Act (Pub. L. No. 94–484) to affect a better balance between the country's health needs and the supply of available health professionals. One of its major emphases was to address the problem of physician misdistribution between underserved (rural) and overserved (urban) areas through educational incentive programs (National Institutes of Health, 2007). The Health Professions Education Extension Amendments (1992) also provided educational assistance to many in the health professions (Duffy, Chen, & Sampson, 1998).

The Occupational Safety and Health Act of 1970 (PL 91–956)

The Occupational Safety and Health Act of 1970 provided protection to workers against personal injury or illness resulting from hazardous working conditions. It established the National Institute for Occupational Safety and Health (NIOSH) and OSHA—the Occupational Safety and Health Administration (U.S. Environmental Protection Agency, n.d.).

The Professional Standards Review Organization Amendment to the Social Security Act of 1972 (PL 92–603)

The Professional Standards Review Organization (PSRO) Amendment to the Social Security Act of 1972 had two goals: cost containment and improved quality of care. The PSRO legislation created autonomous organizations, external to hospitals and ambulatory health care agencies, to monitor and

(continued)

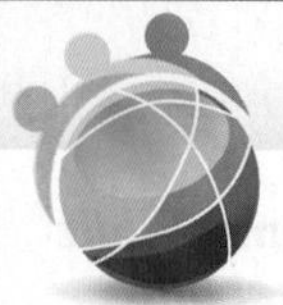

DISPLAY 6.1 LANDMARK HEALTH CARE LEGISLATION *(Continued)*

review objectively the quality of care delivered to Medicare and Medicaid patients. The PSRO review boards, composed mostly of physicians, examined such things as need for care, length of stay, and quality of care against predetermined standards developed locally. Failure to meet standards could mean denial of federal funding. In 1983, Professional Review Organizations replaced PSROs. These private organizations, employed by government agencies to review medical records and avoid excessive and inappropriate costs to taxpayers, strive to identify "best practices" (Dranove, 2000).

The Health Maintenance Organization Act of 1973 (PL 93–222)

In a cost-controlling move, the Health Maintenance Organization (HMO) Act of 1973 added federal support to the concept of prepayment for medical care. President Nixon, a proponent of wage controls, was concerned about the rising costs of health care for employers and citizens. Congress authorized funding for feasibility studies, planning, grants, and loans to stimulate growth among qualifying HMOs. In addition, this act required a business employing 25 people or more to offer an HMO health insurance option, if available locally. A subsequent law, the Employee Retirement Income Security Act (ERISA), passed in 1974, served to protect HMOs from many malpractice lawsuits, even though the intent of the law was to standardize employee benefit laws among the states (Markovich, 2003).

The National Health Planning and Resource Development Act of 1974 (PL 93–641)

The National Health Planning and Resource Development Act of 1974 was a major breakthrough in comprehensive health planning. Replacing the Partnership for Health Act, it combined Hill–Burton, comprehensive health planning agencies, and regional medical programs into a single, new program. It fostered not only comprehensive health planning, but also regulation and evaluation, and it promoted collaborative efforts among regional, state, and federal governments. An important contribution of this act was its emphasis on consumer involvement in health planning. The act was divided into two titles. Title XV, National Health Planning and Development, established national health priorities and assisted the development of area-wide and state planning through Health Systems Agencies (HSAs) and state health planning and development agencies. Title XVI, Health Resources Development, coordinated health facilities planning with health planning, replacing the Hill–Burton Act. The HSAs set targets and limited services, reviewing CON for all health care facilities seeking to expand. If a facility expanded without HSA approval, its Medicaid and Medicare reimbursements could be denied. Because many providers were members of the HSA and supported each other's projects, and others learned to "work the system," these cost-control systems failed to produce the desired results and were ended during the Reagan era (Dranove, 2000).

The National Center for Health Statistics of 1974 (PL 93–353)

The National Center for Health Statistics (NCHS), established in 1974, arose from the earlier National Office of Vital Statistics and became part of the Centers for Disease Control (CDC) under the PHS in 1987. The NCHS operates data collection systems that provide vital information for public health planning and service delivery (National Committee on Vital and Health Statistics, 2000).

The Omnibus Budget Reconciliation Act of 1981 (PL 97–35)

The Omnibus Budget Reconciliation Act (OBRA) of 1981 had a profound effect on public health. In this act, Congress halted the progress made in most of the public health laws of the previous 45 years, substantially reducing their funding authorization. To shift more power to the states and reduce the budget, the Reagan administration consolidated categorical grants into four block grants. The first block grant targeted general preventive health services; the second addressed alcohol, drug abuse, and mental health; the third focused on maternal and child health; and the fourth addressed primary care, which covered federal support for community health centers. Although block grants provide some advantages, these came with limiting restrictions on the amount and use of the funds. The result was a significant reduction in funding for state and local health programs, but states worked to better coordinate health promotion and disease prevention (Scutchfield & Keck, 2009).

The Social Security Amendments of 1983 (PL 98–21)

The Social Security Amendments of 1983 became law in response to accelerating health care costs. The act represented a major reform in health care financing from retrospective to prospective payment. It introduced a billing classification system consisting of 467 diagnosis-related groups (DRGs), with Medicare payments provided to hospitals based on a fixed rate set in advance (Social Security Online, 2007). The fixed payment could not be increased if hospital costs for care exceeded that amount. Conversely, if costs were less than the paid amount, the hospital could keep

(continued)

DISPLAY 6.1 LANDMARK HEALTH CARE LEGISLATION *(Continued)*

the difference. Thus, a positive incentive was introduced to reduce hospital costs and promote timely patient discharge (Institute of Medicine, 2001).

The Consolidated Omnibus Budget Reconciliation Act of 1985 (PL 99–272)

The Consolidated Omnibus Budget Reconciliation Act (COBRA) of 1985 extended the Medicare prospective payment system. The act also expanded Medicaid services and permitted states to offer hospice services to terminally ill recipients. It also authorized demonstration projects to determine the effectiveness of health promotion and disease prevention services for Medicare recipients. The 1990 extension of this act mandated longer-term evaluation of the demonstration projects. Results of the experimental design showed a 12% improvement in self-reported health status and better results in the areas of exercise, seat belt use, recent mammograms, and alcohol consumption (U.S. Department of Labor, n.d.).

Omnibus Budget Reconciliation Act Expansion of 1986 (PL 99–509)

The OBRA Expansion of 1986 extended the prospective payment system for hospital outpatient services, and required certain employers to provide extended (eventually up to 36 months) group-rate insurance coverage for laid-off workers and their dependents. This expense is paid by the former employee, but cannot exceed 102% of the cost for other employees. In 1989, a further OBRA expansion regulated fee schedules for physicians and mandated other measures to attempt to slow the growth in both Medicare and Medicaid (Kaiser Family Foundation, 2007b). Also, under OBRA 1989, nursing home reforms were instituted, and the Agency for Health Care Policy and Research was established to study the effectiveness of health care services.

The Medicare Catastrophic Coverage Act of 1988 (PL 100–360)

The Medicare Catastrophic Coverage Act (MCCA) of 1988 expanded Medicare benefits significantly. Coverage was extended to include a portion of outpatient prescription drug costs and greater posthospital extended care facility and home health benefits. Also, the MCCA set limits on beneficiary liability and provided increased inpatient hospital benefits, as well as set up a commission to examine the possibility of providing long-term care benefits through Medicare (Kaiser Family Foundation, 2007b). In 1989, a second MCCA rescinded the drug benefit and the limits on out-of-pocket spending, among other things.

The Family Support Act of 1988 (PL 100–485)

The Family Support Act of 1988 reformed the federal welfare system to emphasize work and child support. It established child support programs, work opportunities, and basic skill and training programs. It included a requirement that recipients seek employment and that states establish an education, training, and work program, along with the child care support. It established the Commission on Interstate Child Support to aid in locating absent parents and ensure payment of child support. It also provided for paternity testing and withholding of wages in cases in which child support was in arrears (Office of Inspector General, 1989).

The Health Objectives Planning Act of 1990 (PL 101–582)

The Health Objectives Planning Act of 1990 was significant for its support of the report by the Institute of Medicine, *Healthy People 2000,* with funding to improve the health status of the nation. Funding for health promotion and disease prevention was added in the 1991 legislative session (Centers for Disease Control & Prevention [CDC], 1991). Ten years later, *Healthy People 2010* followed.

Preventive Health Amendments of 1992 (PL 102–531)

The Preventive Health Amendments of 1992 placed a focus by the federal government on preventive health and primary prevention initiatives. It added *prevention* to the CDC. It enhanced services to Migrant Health Centers, especially in maternal and child health and community education, as well as lead poisoning prevention. It promoted international exchange programs for public health officials from around the world who have an interest in working in another country (Woolley & Peters, 2007).

Personal Responsibility and Work Opportunity Reconciliation Act of 1996 (PL 104–193)

The Personal Responsibility and Work Opportunity Reconciliation Act of 1996 is commonly known as the "Welfare Reform Bill." It amended the Social Security Act to reform the federal welfare system, imposing a 5-year lifetime limit on welfare benefits. It ended Aid to Families with Dependent Children (AFDC) and enacted Temporary Assistance to Needy Families (TANFs). It provided child care to working parents or those receiving training or education, and required unmarried minor parents to live with their parents or another responsible adult and attend school or training programs in order to receive government assistance. Finally, it restricted benefits to legal immigrants (Administration for Children & Families, 2008). As aid to children and families is usually tied to Medicaid

(continued)

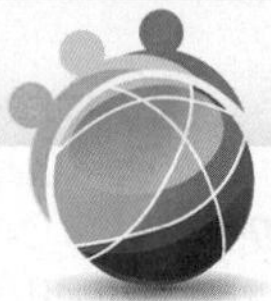

DISPLAY 6.1 LANDMARK HEALTH CARE LEGISLATION *(Continued)*

benefits, this legislation affected health by moving people off welfare rolls and onto payrolls—but often at minimum-wage jobs without insurance benefits.

Health Insurance Portability & Accountability Act (HIPAA) of 1996 (PL 104–191)

This landmark piece of legislation has two major components: one that provides protection for workers in group health insurance plans and another that protects the privacy of health records. It first became effective in 2001, with compliance dates set for 2003 and 2004 (for smaller health plans). It set national standards for protecting individually identifiable health information (including electronic health data), and limited exclusions for workers with pre-existing conditions as well as prohibited discrimination based upon health status (Office of Civil Rights, n.d.). This legislation made it easier for people to obtain or keep health insurance.

Newborns' and Mothers' Health Protection Act of 1996 (The Newborns' Act PL 104-204)

Requires that insurance plans with maternity benefits pay for a minimum 48-hour hospital stay following the birth of a child (or 96 hours following C-section birth). The physician and mother may choose an earlier discharge, but employers and insurers cannot offer incentives for shorter stays (U.S. Department of Labor, n.d.).

Nurse Reinvestment Act of 2002 (PL 107–205)

The Nurse Reinvestment Act of 2002 addresses the nation's critical shortage of nurses. Developed with support and input from female legislators, the bill is well designed to address several issues contributing to the nursing shortage. It emphasizes a media campaign to promote the nursing profession, offers scholarships for nursing students who agree to work upon graduation in an agency facing a critical shortage of nurses, cancels student loans, provides grants to hospitals and other medical facilities that are willing to offer career incentives to nurses to advance in their field and to take on larger responsibilities for organizing and directing patient care, and includes strategies to attack the burnout and frustration that are driving many people out of nursing. It also promotes career ladders, recruitment of minority students into nursing, increased interprofessional collaboration, encouragement of nurses to focus on community-based practices and to address the needs of vulnerable populations. It provides forgivable loans for new nursing faculty as well (Donley, Flaherty, Sarsfield, et al., 2003).

Medicare Prescription Drug, Improvement, and Modernization Act of 2003 (PL 108–173)

Commonly known as Medicare Part D, this voluntary program was added to Medicare Part A and Part B in 2003, and extended and improved coverage for beneficiaries beginning in January 2006 (Medicare.gov, n.d.). Participants can enroll in one of many private plans to be covered, unlike the original Medicare program that is administered through the federal government. The plans must offer the standard benefit package, or a comparable one. Beneficiaries pay 25% of the cost of covered medications up to a certain amount, at which point they reach the *coverage gap* (or "donut hole") and must pay for all covered medications above the set limit (Medicare.gov, n.d.). Changes to Medicare drug coverage are tied to the ACA of 2010. The annual enrollment period for Medicare Part D is from November 15 to December 31. Senior citizens can change plans or begin coverage during that time period.

Mental Health Parity Act of 1996 and Addiction Equity Act of 2008

Requires group health plans to provide benefits for mental illness and addiction in a manner no more restrictive than other physical health benefits. Annual and lifetime benefits for these conditions cannot be lower than for other health benefits offered through the same health plans (U.S. Department of Labor, 2009).

Patient Protection and Affordable Care Act (PL 111–148) and Health Care and Education Affordability Reconciliation Act of 2010 (PL 111–152)

President Obama's health care reform legislation was passed in 2010 and is to be incrementally instituted through 2019. It provides for expansion of Medicaid to lower-income populations, Medicare adjustments to provide better coverage and stabilize expenditures, and an individual mandate for health insurance coverage either through employers or state insurance exchanges (or a penalty is applied). It is expected that an additional 30 million Americans will gain access to health insurance coverage when the plan is fully implemented (Healthcare.gov).

of a wider range of citizens. Before that, legislation dealt with specific sectors of society (e.g., merchant seamen, mothers and infants).

In 1935, the Social Security Act ensured greater PHSs and programs and provided retirement income to participating workers age 65 years and older. The act also included aid to dependent children and unemployment insurance (Social Security Administration, 2011a). Later legislation provided federal support for expansion of hospitals; care for the mentally retarded; and research and support for heart disease, cancer, and stroke, as well as the training of health care personnel.

The landmark Medicare and Medicaid legislation moved the federal government deeper into the role of providing health care, especially for many elderly and poor people who, prior to this time, either could not get services or had to rely on charity care. More recent legislation, especially during President Reagan's term, sought to contain health care spending, ensure the quality of health care, promote national health objectives, and facilitate data collection and research (see Display 6.2). More recent laws have protected the confidentiality of health records and made it easier for workers to continue insurance coverage after being laid off.

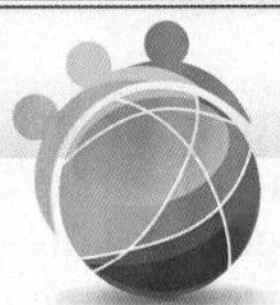

DISPLAY 6.2 DATA COLLECTION SYSTEMS

The National Center for Health Statistics Data Collection Systems

Some collection systems of the National Center for Health Statistics (NCHS) are ongoing annual systems, and others are conducted periodically. There are two major types of data systems: those based on populations (these data are collected by personal interview and examination) and those based on records, with data collected from vital and medical records.

National Health Interview Survey

The National Health Interview Survey (NHIS) is a continuous nationwide survey of illness and disability. It is the main source of data on the health of the US population (nonmilitary, noninstitutionalized). This survey, which monitors the health of the nation, has been conducted since 1957.

National Health and Nutrition Examination Survey

The National Health and Nutrition Examination Survey (NHANES) provides physical, physiologic, and biochemical data related to nutrition of national population samples. Conducted for over 40 years, NHANES provided data that led to the development of pediatric growth charts, vitamin fortification of grains and cereals, and phasing out of lead-based gasoline. It also provided information about the link between cholesterol and heart disease and information on smoking, bone density, obesity, and changes in diet over time.

National Health Care Surveys

The National Health Care Surveys (NHCS) is a series of surveys of providers that yields clear information about health care services, patients, organizations, and providers.

National Ambulatory Medical Care Survey: Gathers data from non-federal, office-based physicians giving direct patient care.

National Hospital Ambulatory Medical Care Survey (NHAMCS): Gathers data from physicians on ambulatory services by specialty and target population

NHCS: A new survey describing patterns of care delivery in hospitals and freestanding ambulatory surgery centers.

National Hospital Discharge Survey: Provides annual data on such things as length of stay, diagnosis, procedures performed, and patient use patterns

National Survey of Ambulatory Surgery (NHAMCS): Data on use and services given in hospital emergency and outpatient departments.

National Home and Hospice Care Survey: Administrators and staff are personally interviewed to retrieve information about patients and discharges

National Home Health Aide Survey: Information on home health aides employed by home health agencies and/or hospice

National Nursing Home Survey: Collects data about nursing home services, staff, and residents regarding need, level of care, costs, and use patterns

National Employer Health Insurance Survey: Provides estimates on employer-sponsored health insurance, the types of plans provided, and detailed information about the plans

National Nursing Assistant Survey (NHAMCS): Information on nursing assistants employed by nursing homes.

National Survey of Residential Care Facilities (NHAMCS): Information from a national sample of residential care facilities.

National Vital Statistics System

The National Vital Statistics System is the oldest survey and best example of public health intergovernmental data sharing. Vital statistics registries around the country provide uniform data to the national system on the following categories: births, marriages, divorces,

(continued)

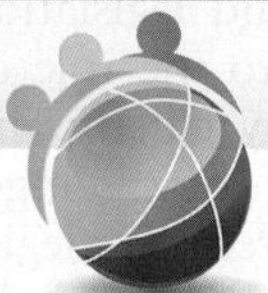

DISPLAY 6.2 DATA COLLECTION SYSTEMS *(Continued)*

deaths, and fetal deaths. Specific data are available through the following systems:

- Birth data
- Mortality data
- Fetal death data
- Linked birth/infant deaths
- National Mortality Followback Survey
- National Maternal and Infant Health Survey

National Survey of Family Growth

The National Survey of Family Growth (NSFG) assembles information on marriage and divorce, pregnancy, use of contraception, family life, infertility, and women's and men's health. The data is used to plan health programs and services.

National Immunization Survey

The National Immunization Survey (NIS) is a list-assisted random-digit-dialing survey employed to gather information on vaccination coverage rates for children between the ages of 19 and 35 months. A mailed survey follows the telephone call, and this produces timely estimates of the rates of recommended vaccine doses.

The Longitudinal Studies of Aging

The Longitudinal Studies of Aging (LSOAs) are done as a collaboration between the NCHS and the National Institute on Aging (NIA). These studies measure changes in functional status, living arrangements, health, and the utilization of health services for persons aged 70 and above. They involves two cohorts of Americans moving into old age and on to the oldest ages.

State and Local Area Integrated Telephone Survey

The State and Local Area Integrated Telephone Survey (SLAITS) collects in-depth data needed at the state and local levels to meet the needs of program planners, policymakers, and government agencies. Some of the topics researched include access to care, utilization of services, health insurance coverage, perceived health status, and measurement of child wellbeing. The same random-digit-dialing method employed by NIS is utilized on a regional basis.

From National Center for Health Statistics. Surveys and Data Collection Systems. Retrieved from http://www.cdc.gov/nchs/surveys.htm

President Clinton made an unsuccessful attempt at universal health care during his first term in office and supported legislation to reform the welfare system. But in 1997, the State Children's Health Insurance Program (SCHIP) was created to expand coverage to uninsured children at no or low cost, and this coverage was extended in 2009 under President Barak Obama (Pear, 2009). President George W. Bush added prescription drug benefits to Medicare and promoted Health Savings Accounts (HSAs). President Barak Obama signed the Patient Protection and Affordable Care Act into law in 2010. The goal of this health care reform legislation is to improve access to health care and "put consumers back in charge of their health coverage and care" (HealthReform.gov, 2010, para. 1).

Development of the Current Health Care System

In 1900, a total of 20% of infants died before they reached the age of 10, and life expectancy was about 47 years. Infectious diseases and poor sanitation and nutrition contributed to the poor outcomes. Physicians were not well trained, and the AMA had only 8,000 members (PBS, n.d.). Hospital infection rates were high, and most care was given in the home—and then only to those who could afford to pay for it or those who received charity care. (See From the Case Files II.)

As the public health system acted to improve water supplies, sanitation, and personal hygiene, the incidence of infectious disease began to diminish. Antibiotics, first widely available during World War II, and better-trained physicians began to change the health care system in the 1950s—although medical and surgical care was not at all sophisticated by today's standards. (See From the Case Files III.)

Since 1950, Americans have come to expect longer lives made possible by medications and treatments that can cure or control a wide variety of diseases and by expanding technology and services that provide a dizzying array of choices to health care consumers. These advances have come at a price, however. Health spending in 2009 was estimated at 17.6% of the U.S. **gross domestic product (GDP)**—the total amount of goods and services produced within a year. To put that in perspective, health spending in 1950 was only at 4.5% (Keehan et al., 2011). Viewed as a separate economy, U.S. health care today would be the fourth largest economy in the world and, by 2016 U.S. health spending is projected by some to exceed $4 trillion (Gardner, 2007). Others project that the share of GDP will rise to 19.8%—meaning that almost one fifth of all goods and services produced in the United States will go toward health care (Keehan et al., 2011). Clearly, to gain a deeper understanding of this phenomenon, some basic concepts must be examined. For instance, what are the economic principles behind this rapid growth in health care costs?

From the Case Files II

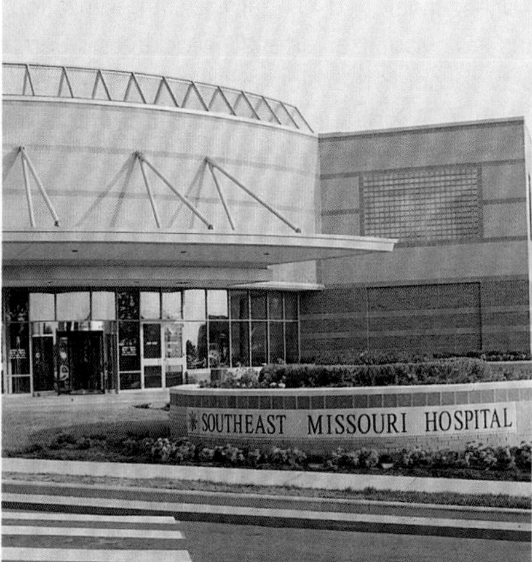

20th and 21st Century Hospital Care

At the turn of the 20th century, riots occurred in Milwaukee when a child suspected of having smallpox was ordered by a public health official to be taken by ambulance to a local hospital for isolation. One of the child's siblings had already died of smallpox in the same hospital, and his family did not want the second child to risk death at the same institution especially while upper- and middle-class children were quarantined in their own homes (not sent to isolation hospitals). A crowd of 3,000 or more people, carrying clubs, kept the ambulance attendants at bay. Why was there such concern about hospitalizing a sick child? In the 1890s, when this occurred, hospitals were rife with infection, and doctors could do little to halt its spread. Also, the inequity of how smallpox cases were handled stirred feelings of injustice and discrimination (Cutler, 2005; Solnit, 2009).

In the early 21st century, are hospitals any safer? Researchers with the Centers for Disease Control and Prevention (CDC) reported (Klevens et al., 2007) that over 1.7 million health care-related infections occur annually, resulting in almost 100,000 deaths. A more recent investigation by the Hearst media corporation estimated the number of deaths from preventable infections and medical mistakes at 200,000 (Harmon, 2009). The Society of Actuaries projected the cost of medical errors in 2008 to be almost $20 billion (2010). Can you be assured of good care when you or your loved one enters a hospital emergency room (ER)? In the case of a busy trauma center located in South Los Angeles, you might have reason for concern. Martin Luther King/Drew Medical Center was created after the 1965 Watts Riot, with a history of providing stellar neonatal care (95% of babies under 2 pounds survive) and excellent training for trauma surgeons—one-fourth of U.S. military surgeons have trained there (The Associated Press, 2004). But numerous incidents of patients in the ER going untreated and unnoticed were reported. In 2004, a 20-year-old art student entered the ER writhing in pain and vomiting. He was left alone in the crowded ER for 18 hours, while his heart rate climbed and his blood pressure fell. He was later found dead, having dropped to the floor covered in his own vomit. It was later determined that he died of gangrene of the bowel (The Associated Press, 2004). Another patient died in the ER after waiting 22 hours to be treated. The patient had a gangrenous leg, a pneumothorax, and was in kidney failure. In 2003, two patients died while on cardiac monitors, and the hospital blamed the lapse in care on the nursing shortage. Inpatient care was often no better, though, as a 46-year-old man admitted for meningitis was given chemotherapy medication for 4 days. Even after the pharmacy error was noted, nurses continued to give medications in error (at least 40 incidents). The patient subsequently lost vision in one eye. In 2007, a 43-year-old woman was admitted to the now-named Martin Luther King/Harbor Medical Center three times in 3 days complaining of intense stomach pain. Her diagnosis was listed as gallstones and she was prescribed pain medication and released each time. After the third discharge, she remained on the hospital grounds and was eventually taken to the ER by police, who were notified of a woman screaming for help. According to the police officers, the ER triage nurse refused to help the woman, and she lay on the floor in severe pain for almost an hour. She "spit up a dark-colored substance, which her boyfriend said was blood" and security cameras showed a janitor mopping around her as she lay in agony on the floor (Rosenblatt, 2007, p. 11). By fall 2007, after the federal government withdrew $200 million in annual funding, the hospital closed its doors (Ornstein, Weber, & Leonard, 2007). An urgent care center/outpatient clinic remained open. However, the community voiced concern over the closure. One recent study found "increased delays in access to care for needed medical services after the closure of Martin Luther King, Jr. Hospital" in a survey of older minority adults in South Los Angeles (Walker et al., 2011, p. 356). The Los Angeles County Board of Supervisors voted to reopen the hospital, planned for staffing by University of California physicians, and provided $50 million in start-up funding (CBS Los Angeles, 2011).

What is different about these two scenarios is the reaction of the public. In the last century, it was an angry mob trying to keep a child out of harm's way by not allowing ambulance personnel to take him to the hospital. In this century, it was the federal and local government who moved to close what was deemed an unsafe facility. Some in the community were happy to see the closure, especially those who lost loved ones to what they feel was substandard care. But many others were sad to see a much-needed neighborhood medical center close—its ER saw almost 50,000 patients in 2006—and worked with county supervisors to build a new 120-bed medical center/outpatient clinic on the site of the closed hospital (CBS Los Angeles, 2011; Ornstein, Weber, & Leonard, 2007).

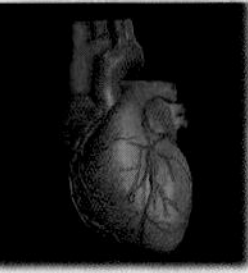

From the **Case Files** 

Care for Cardiovascular Patients

In 1950, the role that hypertension and high cholesterol levels played in heart disease was unclear. Only when someone presented with chest pain were they then monitored for blood pressure and cholesterol control. Doctors frequently recommended that their patients cut down on salt consumption and lose weight. They were also counseled to "slow down" and "rest around midday," as there were essentially no effective medications to treat these two problems (Cutler, 2005, p. 50; Jaquish, 2007). It was not until the 1960s that the Framingham Heart Study confirmed that hypertension leads to cardiovascular disease, and oral antidiuretic medications were used to control it. In the 1950s and 1960s, epidemiologist Ancel Keys' research revealed that high cholesterol intake was associated with cardiovascular disease (Jaquish, 2007). In the 1950s, cardiac patients were treated with absolute bed rest for a minimum of 6 weeks, morphine for pain, and oxygen. That was the state-of-the-art regimen prescribed for President Eisenhower after his heart attack in 1955 (Gilbert, 2008; Jaquish, 2007).

Today, bed rest is known to promote blood clots, and is ineffective in treating myocardial infarctions (MIs)—or heart attacks. Quick, intensive therapy is the standard. Aspirin, heparin, beta (β)-blockers, and thrombolytic medications help to prevent and reduce blood clots, reduce the workload on the heart, and dissolve tiny clots in cardiac vessels (Zafari, Afonso, & Aggarwal, 2011). Cardiac catheterization permits physicians to visualize arterial blockages. Percutaneous angioplasty to open the blocked arteries or coronary artery bypass graft (CABG) surgery is now routine. Well-trained emergency medical service personnel and specialized cardiac intensive care units with highly expert nurses are found in most communities. Cardiopulmonary resuscitation (CPR) is promoted and automated external defibrillators (AEDs), now commonly placed in schools, shopping malls, government buildings, and other common spaces, have saved the lives of many victims of heart disease (Zafari et al., 2011). Because of all of these advances in the last 50 years, post-MI death rates have dropped by 75%. Antihypertensive and cholesterol-lowering medications, along with healthier lifestyles that include no smoking, regular exercise, and diets low in sodium and saturated fats, have also reduced the rates of hypertension and hyperlipidemia. Compared to 1950 rates, the age-adjusted mortality rate for cardiovascular disease dropped 60% by the year 2000 (U.S. Environmental Protection Agency, 2011).

With all of these advances over the past half-century, it is reasonable to expect increased health care costs. In return, more lives have been saved and extended. But, how much can we afford to pay for future improvements in health care? How many more new advances lie ahead? And, what will we receive in return for our investment?

THE ECONOMICS OF HEALTH CARE

Economics is defined as the science of making decisions regarding scarce resources. Economics permeates our social structure—it affects and is affected by policies. Consequently, health is closely tied to economic growth and development, in that a healthy population is necessary for adequate national productivity. Ample evidence exists for a "health–income gradient," as personal income (specifically poverty) is linked to health status (Aday, 2005, p. 191; deChesnay & Anderson, 2012).

Health economics can be better understood by examining the two basic theories underlying the science of economics: microeconomics and macroeconomics. In addition, concepts of health care payment must be understood.

Microeconomics

Microeconomic theory is concerned with supply and demand. **Supply** is the quantity of goods or services that providers are willing to sell at a particular price. **Demand** denotes the consumer's willingness to purchase goods or services at a specified price (Harrington & Estes, 2008). In our free-market–driven economy, supply and demand is a key concept. Economists using microeconomic theory study the supply of goods and services as these relate to how we, as consumers, allocate and distribute our resources—as well as how markets compete. They further study how allocation and distribution affect consumer demand for these goods and services. The concepts of supply and demand are influenced by each other and, in turn, affect prices. In a simplified example, an increase in, or oversupply of, certain products usually leads to less overall consumption (decreased demand) and, usually, lowered prices. The opposite also is true. Limited availability of desired products means that supply does not meet demand, and prices usually increase. An example is the price of a gallon of gasoline. When demand for oil is high and supply begins to dwindle, the prices go up. When demand drops and supplies become more plentiful, prices go down to attract more purchasers. This occurs as long as there are no monopolies to artificially control prices, or only a few choices for goods and services that inhibit competition.

In health care, demand-side policies are enacted to reduce demand for health care (e.g., raising insurance deductibles and copayments), and supply-side policies restrict the supply of resources (e.g., preadmission screening to reduce the likelihood of insuring someone with a serious health condition, denial of coverage for specific services, utilization of preferred providers who practice within boundaries set by insurance companies) (Harrington & Estes, 2008).

Microeconomic theory is useful for understanding price determination, resource allocation, consumer income, and spending distribution at the level of individuals and organizations (Harrington & Estes, 2008). Microeconomic theory comes into play when health care competition increases, because the success of the supply-and-demand concept depends upon a competitive market. Issues such as cost containment, competition between providers, accessibility of services, quality, and need for accountability continue as targets of major concern in the 21st century.

Macroeconomics

Macroeconomic theory is concerned with the broad variables that affect the status of the economy as a whole. Economists using macroeconomics study factors influencing "aggregate consumption, production, investment and international trade, as well as inflation and unemployment" (Aday, 2005, p. 186). The focus is on the larger view of economic stability and growth. Macroeconomic theory is useful for providing a global or aggregate perspective of the variables affecting the total economic picture (Aday, 2005; Harrington & Estes, 2008). Macroeconomic theory has been useful in providing a large-scale perspective on health care financing, ultimately resulting in various proposals for national health plans, health care rationing, competition, and managed care. For instance, when the United States compares overall health spending with countries across the world, it becomes clear that we spend a large percentage of our GDP on health care—more than any other country—and we often have worse indicators of health (e.g., life expectancy, infant mortality) World Health Organization, 2011d. For example, in a study of 19 countries, the United States had "the highest rate of deaths from conditions that could have been prevented or treated successfully" (Docteur & Berenson, 2009, p. 3). The United States also had a higher prevalence of cancer, stroke and heart disease in the over-50 population than 10 European countries, while our comparison quality of care studies show mixed results; we are higher in some areas and lower in others. Some studies have indicated that we have very high (in some cases, the highest) reports of adverse events (e.g., medication errors, receiving incorrect test results) (Docteur & Berenson, 2009; Office of Inspector General, 2010; World Health Organization, 2009). While those of us with adequate health insurance report good access to services and cutting-edge care from well-trained health care professionals, many of our fellow citizens experience significant barriers to care and a fragmented, poorly staffed health care system. See Figure 6-4 for a comparison of U.S. health care expenditure and health status indicators with eight other countries.

The economics of health care encompasses both microeconomics and macroeconomics, and an intricate and complex set of interacting variables. Health care economics is concerned with supply and demand: Are available resources sufficient to meet the demand for use by consumers? Are the resources expended achieving the desired outcomes? When health care resources are scarce or insufficient to address all needs (e.g., for programs and services for at-risk populations), how should they be applied? Should there be a "public option" for healthcare or is it a "public imperative," because a healthy population promotes productivity and a more robust economy (Girouard, 2009).

Supply and Demand in Health Care Economics

When you buy textbooks, for instance, you as the purchaser are able to determine the best value for your money (generally based on price, availability, and condition of the book), and you have choices of vendors (e.g., college bookstore, online bookseller). As a health care consumer, however, can you truly be an efficient and effective purchaser of health care goods and services? How does a patient determine what services are needed, where to buy them, and how to evaluate the quality of the goods and services—much less how to coordinate all necessary services? Does health care truly represent a competitive free market, then? For instance, when purchasing a new LCD flat-screen television, consumers often rely on word-of-mouth from friends and relatives, advice from experts, past experiences with brands, and rating services like *Consumer Reports*. Also, we most often plan in advance for large purchases, like newer and bigger televisions, saving a little money each month to keep within our budget.

With health care, this is seldom the case; health care is typically unpredictable and often difficult to research. Even with the growth of health information (and sometimes misinformation) available on the Internet, physicians are still the system's main gatekeepers, and patients must trust that these care providers have the competence to appropriately diagnose and treat them, as well as coordinate necessary resources to provide quality health care. Further, they trust that physicians will put patients' interests before their own (e.g., give them accurate information about risks and benefits and not induce them to have expensive procedures to enrich the provider) (Dranove, 2008). Now, enter health insurance companies and managed care

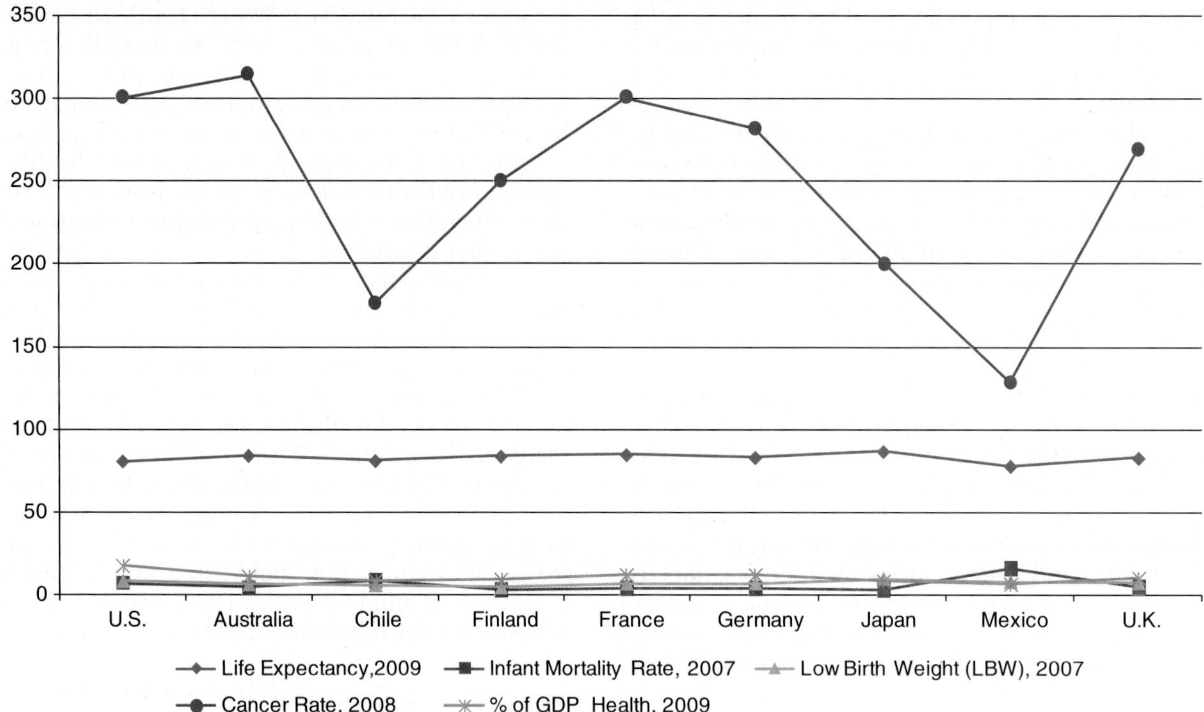

FIGURE 6-4. Comparison of United States with eight other countries on selected health status indicators and percentage or gross domestic product (GDP) spent on health.

into the mix, and you can see why health care purchases are not straightforward and easily understood. In a free-market system, competition is an important factor, but is competition truly possible with employer-based health insurance that limits the choice of plans and providers?

In 1963, economist Kenneth Arrow wrote an influential article about health care economics detailing the lack of information in the medical marketplace (reprinted as Arrow, 2004; also cited in Krugman, 2009). The main points of the article noted that risk and uncertainty prohibit a true market economy in health care because consumers:

- Do not know when or if they will become ill—but they know they will need and want medical treatment, thus the demand for health insurance
- Do not know what services will be needed and what works best for their condition—thus the need for physicians
- Do not know about the quality of health care good and services—thus the need for government regulation (e.g., licensing, certification) and malpractice lawsuits
- Have an asymmetric level of information, compared to the insurer, about the likely demand for health care services, resulting in **adverse selection** (e.g., high-risk patients are denied insurance or care) and market failure (e.g., inefficiencies and lack of appropriate competition)—although this is less severe in large group insurance plans that spread out the risk

A fundamental problem of the health care economy is that it is difficult for any person or organization (e.g., patient, physician, health plan, government) to be an effective consumer of health care goods and services (Dranove, 2008; Krugman, 2011).

One area of health care, however, that has been thought to more closely follow the free-market supply-and-demand model is LASIK eye surgery. The average cost of this surgery in 1998 was $2,200 per eye. This dropped to $1,350 in 2004 as over 3 million surgeries were performed. Many believed the drop in price was due to the lack of third-party reimbursement and the evidence of *consumer-driven purchases* in response to advertising and competition (Tabarrok, 2004). However, a study from 2007 revealed that, after stabilizing at the lower rate and with the introduction of new LASIK equipment and procedures, prices began rising once again to over $2,000 by 2005 (Tu & May, 2007). By 2010, the average price was reported at $2,150, again casting doubt on market systems in healthcare (Segre, 2011).

Health Insurance Concepts

Conventional economic theories posit that people pay small premiums monthly to offset the risk of large medical bills should they become seriously ill. This represents an *indemnity policy* (much like car or homeowners' insurance) and this is the type of health insurance first offered in the United States. In the past, patients could choose any doctor or hospital and submit the providers' bills to the insurance company for payment. **Moral hazard** is the term used by economists to explain how health insurance changes the behavior of people, resulting in more risk-taking and wasteful actions. They liken it to fire insurance without a deductible, noting that a person may be less careful about clearing brush from a house or may even resort to arson if it costs the owner nothing to have the home replaced. If a person has health insurance, many economists hypothesize, they are less likely to take good care of themselves, and if they don't pay for their health care (through premiums, co-payments, deductibles), they are more likely to misuse it or overuse it (Dranove, 2008). In other words, economists theorize that insurance has a paradoxical effect and often leads to wasteful and risk-taking behaviors. In this scenario, patients will demand expensive health care, even if it provides only the smallest benefit (Dranove, 2008). The concept of moral hazard is the reason behind larger deductibles and co-payments—it is an effort to control wasteful and excessive use of health care resources.

A newer supposition states that consumers purchase health insurance not to avoid risk, but to earn a claim for additional income (i.e., insurance paying for medical care) when they become ill and that co-payments and managed care actually work against the system by reducing the amount of income transferred to ill persons or limiting their access to needed services. Think about what would happen to you or your loved one, without health insurance coverage, if you were to suddenly need an expensive heart surgery or lengthy cancer treatment. You would want health insurance to protect against this possibility—to be able to pay medical bills without losing your assets (e.g., home, belongings). In fact, research has found that about half of the foreclosure filings in several states hardest hit by the housing crisis could be traced to a health emergency (Robertson, Egelhof, & Hoke, 2008). This substantiates the claim of a genuine risk of financial disaster when confronted with a serious medical emergency or long-term illness, and helps explain why some economists argue that our "preoccupation with moral hazard is misplaced" and has actually worked against reducing health care costs (Nyman, 2007, p. 759). Another reason that moral hazard doesn't accurately apply to health insurance is that its effects may not be as predictable as in other instances of indemnity (Whitford, 2008). The case can surely be made that even those with unlimited insurance coverage don't just "check into the hospital because it's free" (Gladwell, 2005, para. 11). Most people do not seek infinite numbers of mammograms, colonoscopies or other invasive procedures or surgeries, for instance.

Employer-Sponsored Health Insurance

Employer-sponsored health insurance is the leading source of coverage for non-elderly Americans. In a 2011 annual survey, 60% of companies offered health insurance to their workers, a 9% reduction from the previous year. However, only 79% of those workers are eligible for health coverage because of minimum work hours or mandatory waiting periods. Eighty one percent of those eligible participate in health insurance. Because not all employers offer health insurance, only about 58% of workers in the United States are covered by employer-sponsored health plans (Kaiser Family Foundation & Health Research and Educational Trust [KFF & HRET], 2011). Many small businesses do not offer employee health insurance because of the high costs. Even Wal-Mart, one of the largest U.S. employers with 1.4 million workers, offered high-premium/high-deductible plans (with 6-month waiting periods for full-time workers) that more than half of their employees could not afford—thus shifting costs to taxpayers because 60% of workers qualified for government-sponsored Medicaid (Wohl, 2011). Because of criticism over this practice, Wal-Mart expanded their insurance coverage in 2009 to over 52% of their workforce including part-time employees working <24 hours per week. However, due to rising costs and the poor economy, Wal-Mart raised 2012 premiums (some plans over 40%), and will no longer cover new part-time employees working <24 hours. For those working 24 to 33 hours per week, spouses will no longer receive coverage. Also, workers who smoke will pay extra for health care insurance (Greenhouse & Abelson, 2011).

In 2011, the average cost of group health insurance was $15,073 for a family policy and $5,429 for an individual. These figures are 9% and 8% higher, respectively, than 2010 costs. However, family coverage was 113% higher in 2011 than it was in 2001, while employee contributions increased 131% over the same time period. The average worker contributed about 28% of the premium for family coverage, and 18% for individual coverage in 2011 (KFF & HRET, 2011).

Those people whose employers do not offer health insurance coverage or who are self-employed can purchase nongroup health insurance, however; premiums are greater than the worker's share of employer group coverage and finding a suitable and affordable policy is sometimes difficult. There is also marked variation in costs. For example one large-scale survey found that in 2006 to 2007 annual premiums for family coverage ranged from $2,325 to $9,201. Coverage for one person varied depending upon age between $1,163 and $2,325 (KFF, 2008). Another large-scale analysis of individual health plans found substantial cost sharing, with 78% of enrollees having single-coverage deductibles averaging $2,117 and annual maximum out-of-pocket expenses averaging $5,271 (Whitmore, Gabel, Pickreign, & McDevitt, 2011). Cost sharing is a growing phenomenon, yet there is little evidence to prove that this will significantly reduce the overall growth in US health spending. There is, however, solid evidence that it will put those in low-income groups at greater risk for poor health outcomes, and that increased cost-sharing "disproportionately shifts financial risk to the very sick" (Swartz, 2010, p. 22).

Cost is a deterrent for many people, with only 4% to 11% of those at the lower income levels purchasing nongroup health coverage. However, although coverage levels generally increase as income rises, only 25% of those earning 10 times the poverty level purchased health insurance. The reasons for this are not clear, with one study showing that the lack of insurance may not solely be a matter of choice as some economists hypothesize (Bernard, Banthin, & Encinosa, 2009). Those who are self-employed can deduct the cost of health insurance premiums from their incomes, so rates for this group are higher (almost half of those earning 4.5 times the poverty level). But researchers have posited that lower rates of coverage are most likely due to inability to find satisfactory coverage and/or lack of affordability, however, lack of knowledge may also factor in especially for lower income families (KFF, 2008). See Figure 6-5 for trends in health insurance premium costs as compared to wages and overall inflation.

The most chilling fact is that a minimum-wage worker in 2011 earned an average of $15,000 for the year, while the average cost of an employee's share for an annual premium covering a family of four averaged $8,000 (about half of the estimated total cost of health care at over $19,000). This helps to explain the large number of working Americans who are uninsured (Kavilanz, 2011). A study commissioned by the organization, Wider Opportunities for Women (2010), found that a single worker with two young children needed an annual income of $57,756 (about $27 per hour) in order to reach economic stability (e.g., cover basic monthly expenses, save for emergencies and retirement). With a two-income household, $16 an hour per person is considered necessary.

Employers are either not offering health insurance or passing along the higher costs to employees in the form of higher employee premiums, deductibles, co-payments, and stricter enrollment requirements. Between 2006 and 2011, the percentage of covered workers enrolled in employer health plans with $1,000 or more deductible for single coverage increased from 16% to 50% (KFF & HRET, 2011).

The U.S. Census Bureau (2010) reports an increase in those reporting uninsured status. This was the first year to show an actual drop in the number of people with health insurance since tracking of this data first occurred in 1987, perhaps an indicator of the economic downturn and loss of jobs. **Uninsured** lack health

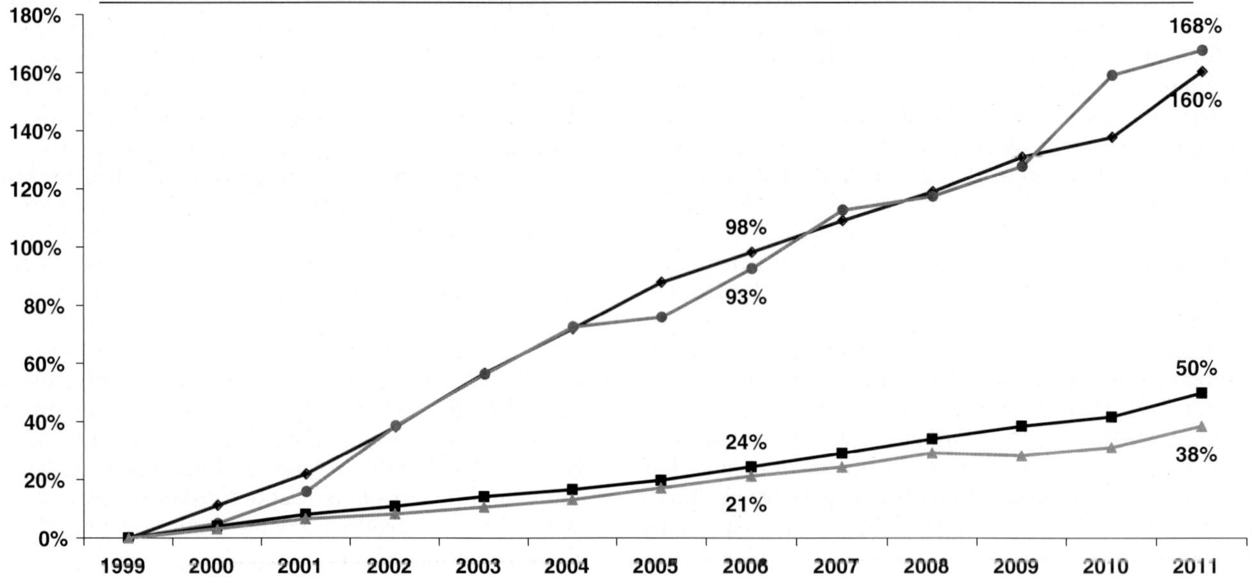

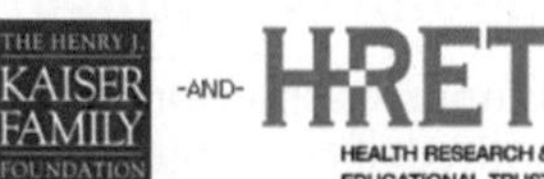

FIGURE 6-5. Increases in average annual premiums for health insurance, worker contributions, and earnings, 1999–2011. From: Kaiser Family Foundation & Health Research & Educational Trust, 2011; *Employer Health Benefits Survey 2011*. This information was reprinted with permission from the Henry J. Kaiser Family Foundation. The Kaiser Family Foundation, based in Menlo Park, California, is a nonprofit, private operating foundation focusing on the major health care issues facing the nation and is not associated with Kaiser Permanente or Kaiser Industries.

insurance coverage of any type. Over 80% of uninsured are families with at least one wage earner, and almost half are under age 30. Only 21% are legal or illegal immigrants (Henig, 2009). It is estimated that 28% of Americans are uninsured, but the **underinsured** population has increased 80% from 2003 to 2010 to around 29 million. The underinsured have some form of health insurance, but also have high deductibles or costs. They fall into one or more of three categories: (1) medical expenses totaling more than 10% of their yearly income, (2) annual income 200% of federal poverty level (FPL) with medical expenses >5% of yearly income, (3) health insurance deductibles ≥5% of their annual income (Nunley, 2008). This leaves at least 44% of U.S. adults either uninsured or underinsured (Schoen, Doty, Robertson, & Collins, 2011).

A shift has also occurred between the numbers of those insured privately (e.g., insurance provided by employers and individuals) and publicly (e.g., paid by government through Medicaid or Medicare). About half of those underinsured and 58% of those without insurance reported problems paying for medical bills, being contacted by a collection agency about unpaid medical bills, and having to pay off medical bills over time (Schoen et al., 2011). They often exhaust their savings, run up credit card debt, or else delay necessary medical care to avoid going into debt. For instance, 46% of underinsured and 63% of uninsured reported that they did not see a doctor when they were ill, did non fill a prescription, or went without a recommended medical treatment or test. This compares with only 28% those who have adequate health care coverage (Schoen et al., 2011).

SOURCES OF HEALTH CARE FINANCING: PUBLIC AND PRIVATE

Financing of health care significantly affects community health and community health nursing practice. It influences the type and quality of services offered, as well as the ways in which those services are used. Sources of payment may be grouped into three categories: third-party payments, direct consumer payment, and private or philanthropic support.

Third-Party Payments

Third-party payments are monetary reimbursements made to providers of health care by someone other than the consumer who received the care. The organizations that administer these funds are called *third-party payers* because they are a third party, or external, to the consumer–provider relationship. Included in this category are four types of payment sources: private insurance companies, independent or self-insured health plans, government health programs, and claims payment agents (Harrington & Estes, 2008).

Private Insurance Companies

Private insurance companies currently pay the majority of U.S. health care expenditures for those under age 65. They market and underwrite policies aimed at decreasing consumer risk of economic loss because of a need to use health services. Traditional indemnity health insurers have been experiencing decelerating growth for more than a decade as the result of a shift to lower-cost managed-care plans offered through employers. In a 2011 survey, only 1% of workers reported coverage by this type of plan (KFF& HRET, 2011).

There are three types of private insurers. First are commercial stock companies that sell health insurance, usually as a sideline. They are private, stockholder-owned corporations that sell insurance nationally and are responsible to these stockholders for maintaining profit margins; examples are Aetna, Travelers, and Connecticut General (CIGNA). A second type of insurer operates in the national marketplace and is owned by policyholders—a *mutual company*. Examples are Mutual of Omaha, Prudential, and Metropolitan Life. The third type, *nonprofit insurance* plans, operate under special state-enabling laws that give them an exclusive franchise to the whole state (or a part of it) and to a specific type of insurance. For example, traditionally, Blue Cross sold only hospital coverage; Blue Shield, only medical insurance; and Delta Dental, only dental insurance. Being nonprofit, companies were tax-exempt and, at the same time, subject to tighter state regulation than are the commercial health insurance companies. However, although the Blues (Blue Cross and Blue Shield) originally began as employment-based, "community-rated" (e.g., each member received the same benefits and paid the same premiums despite their age or health) nonprofit health insurers, this changed as health insurance competition became stiffer and costs soared for employer health benefits (700% when there was only a 208% increase in GDP) (Daschle, Greenberger, & Lambrew, 2008, p. 56). Unable to successfully compete with for-profit companies that employed traditional underwriting practices (e.g., charging more to those at higher risk), the "Blues" sought for-profit status so that some of their franchises could be publicly traded (e.g., sell stocks and raise capital). They often used this extra money to merge and expand market share and began adopting business strategies used by other for-profits (Ameringer, 2008). In 2004, two of these for-profit arms, Wellpoint and Anthem, merged to become the largest health insurer in the United States. This may have influenced the Blues overall—including the not-for-profit sectors—making them virtually indistinguishable as profits are now at the forefront (Varney, 2010). In 2010, Anthem Blue Cross of California announced rate hikes of up to 39%, despite its parent company, Wellpoint, reporting a first quarter profit increase of 51%. As a result of public furor, the rate hike request was withdrawn (Rogers, 2010). However, in 2011 Anthem Blue Cross California again proposed rate hikes; this time they requested 9.8%, but the California Insurance Commissioner stated they really averaged 16.4% and asked them to reduce their request. They reduced the rate hikes to 9.1%, expected to affect an estimated 600,000 policyholders. They claimed a $110 million loss in California for the year, despite the $2.9 billion profit reported by their parent company (Colliver, 2011). Combined, the nonprofit and commercial carriers have sold most of the private health insurance in the United States over the last decade (Clifton, 2009). In fact, it has been reduced to "four publicly traded corporations—Wellpoint, Inc.; United Health Group; Aetna, Inc.; and Cigna....(who cover) "almost half of all Americans with private insurance" (Nelson, 2009, p. 3). Maintaining profits for stockholders means that insurance companies must control the *medical loss ratio*, or the money paid for health services. If they can reduce the amount paid for health care services, then profits are increased and the stock is more attractive to potential buyers. Four common ways to reduce the medical loss ratio include: (1) reduce covered services, (2) raise deductibles and co-pays, (3) exclude people with pre-existing conditions, and (4) "cherry-pick" customers by using directed marketing to young, healthy populations. Also, insurers have resorted to *rescission* of coverage—or canceling coverage for failure to disclose a preexisting condition or some other means of disqualifying coverage after large medical claims have been filed (Nelson, 2009). Some of these practices will change with the enactment of the Patient Protection and Affordable Care Act in 2010—discussed in more detail later in this chapter.

A recent trend in private insurance is the move to **consumer-driven/high-deductible health plans** with savings options such as **health savings accounts (HSAs)**. Beginning in 2004, legislation provided for tax-exempt HSAs tied to high-deductible health insurance plans that can be rolled over yearly and move with the employee. The high deductibles (e.g., minimum of $1,000 for an individual and $2,000 for a family) allow for lower premiums, but the attendant HSAs can only be used on medical expenses—nothing else—or tax-exempt status is lost and a penalty is also incurred (KFF & HRET, 2011; Nelson, 2009). About 23% of employers offered this type of plan in 2011, more than the 15% in 2010. Most plans require employees to pay a percentage of their total health costs (coinsurance, e.g., 20%)—not just a small copayment per office visit or prescription as in many other plans. The average annual deductible for these plans in 2011 was $1,908 for single coverage. Some think that this improves **cost sharing**—whereby the insured assumes a greater share of health care costs, without a third-party payer intervening. Costs to employers with HDHPs are less—723 for individuals and $3,634 for families compared to average employer costs of $5,429 and $15,073 (KFF & HRET, 2011). Recent surveys have shown that this type of insurance does not result in expanded coverage for the uninsured, and may lead to more employees forgoing health insurance offered by their employers (Fronstin & MacDonald, 2008).

Employers may or may not contribute to HSAs; about 60% of employers contribute to HSAs for single coverage and 57% for family coverage. The average contribution is $885 for individuals and $1,559 for families. When employers do contribute, the cost savings in premiums are often nullified and the accounts usually cannot be moved to a new employer (KFF & HRET, 2011).

Most workers covered by their employer's health insurance also have prescription drug coverage (98%), with some cost sharing (co-payment). Only 17% are in plans that pay 100% of drug costs after a deductible is met. Often, co-payments are based on tiered systems, for example, $10 co-payment for less expensive drugs in the first-tier and $25 for slightly more expensive drugs in the second-tier (KFF & HRET, 2011). A large-scale study of the effect of cost on compliance with antihyperlipidemic (cholesterol-lowering) therapy found that for every $10 increase in prescription co-payment, patient compliance levels fell by 5% (Goldman, Joyce, & Karaca-Mandic, 2006), and later research has confirmed that patient's knowledge about their drug coverage and co-payments is limited (only 27% were correct in a survey of 932 members of a large health group). Reed, Brand, Newhouse, Selby, and Hsu (2008) also found that additional cost sharing measures (co-payments, higher caps, more tiers) correlated with greater financial burden and "cost-coping behaviors," as well as decreased adherence to medical regimens (p. 785).

Independent or Self-Insured Health Plans

Independent or self-insured health plans underwrite the remaining private health insurance in the United States. These plans have been offered through a limited number of organizations, such as large businesses, unions, school districts, consumer cooperatives, and medical groups. Employers with self-insured plans take on all or a major part of the risk for health care costs of their employees. These plans may be self-administered or utilize third-party claims administrators. Minimum premium plans are another form of self-insurance for which employers pay medical costs up to an agreed-upon limit, and insurers assume responsibility for the excess claims (Bureau of Labor Statistics, n.d.). Self-insurance plans are not subject to regulation by the states, and it is estimated that 55% of employees receiving work-related insurance benefits were part of self-insurance plans in 2008 (Employee Benefit Research Institute, 2009).

Government Health Programs

Government health programs make up the next largest source of third-party reimbursement in the United States. The government's four major health insurance programs are Medicare, Medicaid, the Federal Employees Health Benefits Plan, and the Civilian Health and Medical Program of the Uniformed Services (CHAMPUS). As a whole, the proportion of government funding of health care in the United States is less than that of 34 other developed countries (Organization for Economic Cooperation & Development [OECD], 2011). In 2011, 46% of health care spending was estimated to be paid by public sources in the United States (e.g., federal government), compared with the United Kingdom (England) at 82.4%, France at 77.7%, Japan at 80.8%, the Netherlands at 80%, Canada at 70.5%, and Mexico at 46.9% (CMS, n.d. b; Miller, 2009; Organization for Economic Cooperation & Development, 2011). Of the government's health insurance programs, Medicare and Medicaid are the largest. Estimates of public expenditures for US health spending top 56% in one study, but are closer to 46% in others (Miller, 2009; Selden & Sing, 2008). In 2011, Medicare covered some 47.5 million people, paying health care costs of $550 billion (KFF, 2011e). Spending for Medicaid in 2009 grew 9% over the previous year for a total of $373.9 billion (CMS, n.d. b). Growth was 7.4% in 2011 (Kaiser Health News, 2011). One concern about the large uninsured population is that by the time they reach age 65 and are eligible for Medicare health coverage, their health may have already been compromised and overall improvement in health status will not be possible, as one large-scale study found (Polsky et al., 2009). Another longitudinal study found that previously uninsured Medicare beneficiaries had higher annual hospitalization rates related to diabetes and cardiovascular disease complications than those who had previous insurance. This was estimated to account for almost 66% of the difference in inpatient Medicare spending (McWilliams, Meara, Zaslavsky, & Ayanian, 2009).

Medicare and Social Security Disability Insurance

Medicare, known as Title XVIII of the Social Security Act Amendments of 1965, has provided mandatory federal health insurance since July 1, 1966, for adults aged 65 years and older who have paid into the Social Security system. It also covers certain disabled persons. Medicare is administered by the Centers for Medicare and Medicaid Services (formerly the Health Care Financing Administration—HCFA) of the USDHHSs. It is the largest health insurer in the United States, covering about 45 million beneficiaries. About 85% of these are over the age of 65, and the remaining beneficiaries qualify for Medicare 24 months after they become eligible for Social Security Disability Insurance (SSDI). These recipients are younger than age 65 and permanently disabled or chronically ill, including those with end-stage renal disease (added in 1973) (CBO, 2009; CMS, 2011). The Medicare population is projected to grow to 79 million by 2030, twice the number of recipients in 2000, having a greater percentage with higher levels of education which is often associated with better general health and delayed onset of some chronic health conditions (Umans & Nonnemaker, 2009) (see Fig. 6-6).

Part A of Medicare, the hospital insurance program, covers inpatient hospitals, limited-skilled nursing facilities, home health, and hospice services to participants eligible for Social Security. The 2012 deductible per episode (not annual) for Part A is $1,156, and some coinsurance costs apply. It is financed through trust funds derived from employment payroll taxes. A total tax of 2.9% of employee wages is split between the employer and employee. These payroll taxes, along with interest earned on trust fund investments, provide the income for this program (Medicare.gov, 2011; Social Security Administration, 2011b; Umans & Nonnemaker, 2009).

Part B, the supplementary and voluntary medical insurance program, primarily covers physician services, but also covers home health care for beneficiaries not covered under Part A. There is $140 annual deductible and recipients pay 20% for services once the deductible is met. Part B is funded through enrollee monthly premiums ($99.90 in 2012). For couples earning over $170,000 annually, premiums can range from $162 to $369 (Gengler, 2011; Medicare.gov, 2011).

Part C, or Medicare Advantage, are private plans that are generously subsidized by the federal government and take the place of Part A and Part B. Some may also cover vision, dental, and prescriptions. An annual cap for out-of-pocket costs was $6,700 for 2011, and Advantage plans have provider networks that can limit the choice of physicians or hospitals. They are regional, which may be problematic for seniors who want to spend winters in Florida and summers in Montana, for instance. There were 25 plans in 2011, and seniors can change plans during open enrollment periods, or revert back to traditional Medicare Part A and Part B (Gengler, 2011).

One-third of Medicare beneficiaries have supplemental coverage through employer retiree health insurance plans—known as *Medigap* coverage—added to Medicare Part A and Part B. This supplemental coverage cannot be combined with Part C, or Medicare Advantage plans. With rising costs of health care coverage, companies are increasing premium costs for retirees, offering new options like Medicare Advantage to replace traditional health plans, or paying only a set amount for health coverage and leaving retirees to purchase their own insurance (Gengler, 2011).

Part D, the prescription benefit plan added through the Medicare Prescription Drug, Improvement and Modernization Act of 2003 cost around $26 in 2006 and over $38 in 2011 (Hoadley, Summer, Hargrave, Cubanski, & Newman, 2011). These plans are offered through private insurers, but again heavily subsidized by the federal government. Part D can be combined either with Part A/Part B or with a Medicare Advantage plan (Part C) that does not cover prescriptions. Seniors can change plans during open enrollment periods, and plans vary in coverage. Participants need to consider if their medications are covered at a low enough cost (or if only less expensive alternatives are offered), if their pharmacy is a preferred provider, or if there are quantity limits on prescriptions (Gengler, 2011). Prior to Part D coverage, more than half of seniors spent over 40% of their income on health care (after paying for essentials such as housing and food). That amount rose to 68% for those in poor health. Almost two thirds of these out-of-pocket health expenses were for premiums and medications (Briesacher et al., 2010). Even with recent improvements through health care reform, there are still large coverage gaps—known as the "Doughnut Hole." Coverage at lower levels of use is fairly good, but as use rises, participants must pay a higher share of cost. Catastrophic costs are generally covered, leaving those in the middle with a gap (the doughnut hole). As the ACA is implemented over time, the goal is to close this

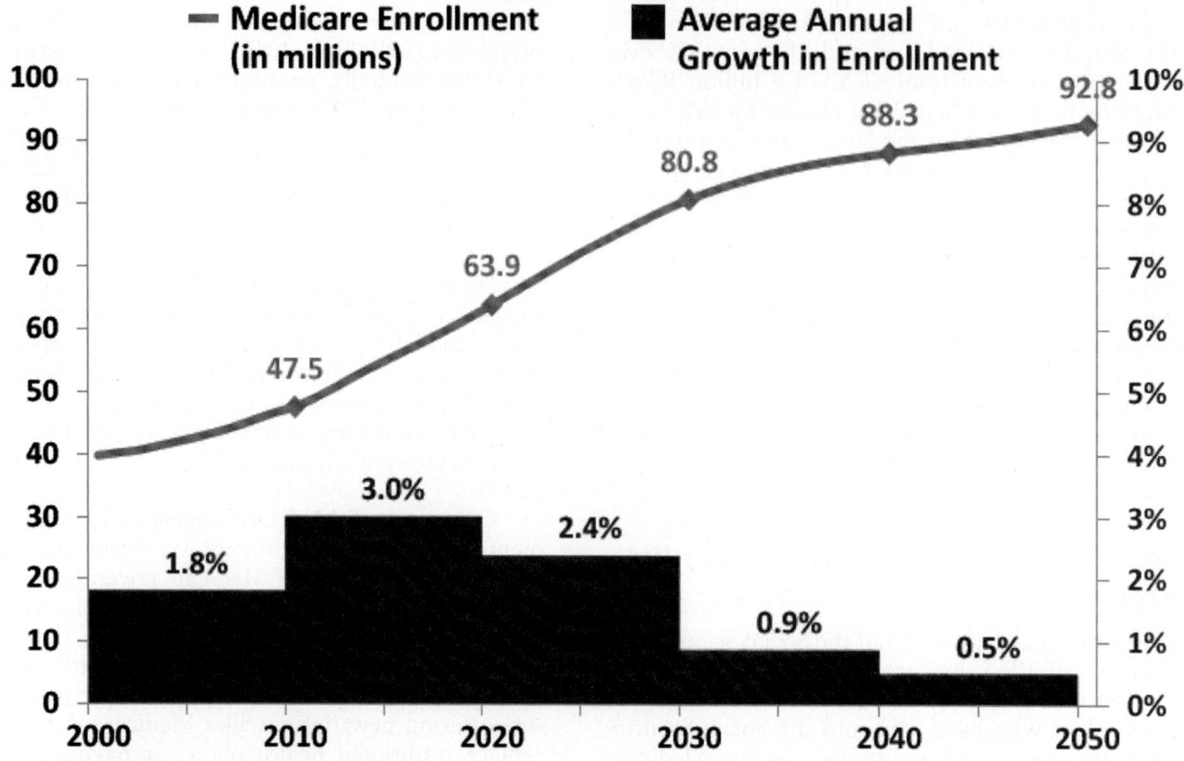

FIGURE 6-6. Projected change in medicare enrollment, 2000–2050 (depicting growth in beneficiaries and decline in ratio of workers). From: Kaiser Family Foundation, 2011, *Fact sheet: Medicare spending and financing*. This information was reprinted with permission from the Henry J. Kaiser Family Foundation. The Kaiser Family Foundation, based in Menlo Park, California, is a nonprofit, private operating foundation focusing on the major health care issues facing the nation and is not associated with Kaiser Permanente or Kaiser Industries.

gap in coverage through a combination of pharmaceutical company discounts on brand-name drugs and government rebates to participants (Hoadley et al., 2011).

The majority of elderly Medicare beneficiaries participate in both Part A and Part B, often with supplemental private insurance, or they choose a Medicare Advantage plan (Part C). Less than 9% rely solely on Medicare coverage, with over 70% having some type of supplemental insurance. Only 10% of the elderly Medicare population is over age 85. For disabled Medicare beneficiaries, roughly one third are aged 45 to 54 (Umans & Nonnemaker, 2009). Medicare was managed in the same manner for more than 30 years until August 1997, when President Clinton signed the Balanced Budget Act (PL No. 105–33). This act, which took effect in 1998, was aimed at preserving Medicare benefits for future generations and provided current Medicare beneficiaries with markedly different options with the addition of Part C (The White House, n.d.). To control Medicare costs while expanding the range of available health care options, beneficiaries were offered a program developed in an effort to accelerate the migration of patients away from Medicare's traditional and more expensive fee-for-service (FFS) program into various managed care options with a limited choice of providers. They are offered options such as joining coordinated care plans, including health maintenance organizations (HMOs), preferred provider organizations (PPOs), provider-sponsored organizations, or private FFS plans (Gengler, 2011). For more information on Medicare trends and concerns about its solvency (see Chapter 24).

A 2006 comparative analysis of administrative costs for Medicare (age 65 and over) and under age-65 private health insurance found that costs are markedly lower for Medicare at 3.3% estimated for 2010 and 1.6% by 2025. Estimated 2006 administrative costs for the hundreds of private insurers ranged from a low of 12.5% for large group markets, and a high of 30% for individual markets (Litow, 2006).

Medicaid

Medicaid, known as Title XIX of the Social Security Act Amendments of 1965, provides medical assistance for children, for pregnant women or parents with dependent children, seniors, and severely disabled persons (KFF, 2010a). In 2008, almost about 8 million people qualified for both Medicaid and Medicare making them "dual eligibles" (KFF, 2010a, p. 1). About 45% of the Medicaid goes toward these individuals, and long-term care costs comprise a large proportion of these costs. In 2008, 61% of total costs included acute-care services and 34% were for long-term care. About 5% of spending covered supplemental payments to hospitals with a high percentage of indigent patients, or disproportionate share hospitals (DSHs). Medicare premium payments for low-income dual-eligible persons encompassed 3.5% of spending (KFF, 2010a). During 2011, Medicaid covered one in three children, along with one in four poor nonelderly adults. More than one in three US births were paid for by Medicaid. Almost 9 million low-income Medicare beneficiaries and over 8 million people with disabilities were included in Medicaid coverage (KFF, 2011c). Average expenditures in 2008 totaled almost $340 billion and in 2007 included:

- $14,500 per disabled enrollee
- $12,500 per elderly enrollee
- $2,500 per nonelderly adult enrollee
- $2,100 per child (KFF, 2010a).

Medicaid is jointly funded between federal and state governments to assist the states in providing adequate medical care to eligible needy persons. The federal government pays its share (the Federal Medical Assistance Percentage—FMAP), generally around 50%, but pays a higher share to the poorest states, often near 76%, for an average cost of 57%. During the recent economic downturn, legislation increased the FMAP to between 56% and 85%, bringing the average to 66% (KFF, 2010a). The recession led to greater unemployment and poverty (15.2% for working-age adults); however, Medicaid and the SCHIP (see below) helped more than 600,000 children gain health insurance coverage from figures reported from the previous year (CBS News, 2011; Children's Defense Fund, 2011; KFF, 2011c). The states have some discretion in determining which groups their Medicaid programs will cover and the financial criteria for Medicaid eligibility, as well as the scope of services, rate of payment, and how the program will be administered (Children's Defense Fund, 2011; KFF, 2010c). To be eligible for federal funds, however, states are required to provide Medicaid coverage for most individuals who receive federally assisted income maintenance payments (welfare), as well as for related groups not receiving cash payments (especially the elderly). Healthy (non-disabled) adults without children are generally excluded from coverage, and states are forbidden from charging premiums. The states determine the type, amount, duration, and scope of services, but they are not allowed to limit enrollment or have a waiting list (KFF, 2010c).

Coverage must generally include the following:

- Outpatient and inpatient hospital services
- Physician, nurse practitioner/certified nurse midwife services
- Lab and x-ray services
- Well-child checkups up to the age of 21
- Family planning services/supplies
- Home health care and nursing home services for those over age 21
- Federally qualified health center (FQHC) and rural health clinic (RHC) services (KFF, 2010c)

Medicaid has historically reimbursed providers at a lower rate than Medicare and other insurances, and this has caused problems with access to care. Even with lower reimbursement rates, costs continue to rise. As with Medicare, Medicaid programs moved to a managed care concept, following mandates within the Balanced Budget Act of 1997. In 2008, over 70% of Medicaid enrollees received at least part of their care through a managed care plan (KFF, 2010a). The move has not been without its problems for those receiving Medicaid. Medicaid beneficiaries are economically disadvantaged, frequently reside in medically underserved areas, and often have more complex health and social needs than do Americans with higher incomes. They often must choose between multiple plans, yet fewer providers, and must often drive long distances to see specialists. One study found that California counties offering a choice of Medicaid managed care plans had more beneficiaries "delaying health plan enrollment" and that this was strongly associated with higher hospital admission rates for ambulatory-care sensitive (ACS) conditions, often nullifying the cost savings of managed care (Millett, Chattopadhyay, & Bindman, 2010, p. 2238). Another California study by Bindman, Chattopadhyay, and Auerback (2008) also noted that interruptions in Medicaid coverage were associated with higher risk of hospitalization for ACS conditions, most often diabetes, heart failure, and chronic obstructive pulmonary disease (COPD). Coverage can be interrupted due to changes in income that invalidate Medicaid eligibility or failure to enroll in a Medicaid plan.

In recent years, many people who were never before eligible for Medicaid benefits have become eligible as a result of downward national economic trends, company downsizing, and corporate mismanagement. Subsequent to these economic issues, families have lost employer-subsidized health care benefits, and some now find themselves among those eligible for Medicaid managed care programs. Medicaid's use of managed care has grown dramatically. Physicians and patient advocates often express concerns that many managed care plans are more focused on keeping their costs down (and profits up), rather than improving patient care, and thus there is wide variability in cost-effectiveness and quality. The future success of Medicaid managed care depends on the adequacy of the **capitation rates** (fixed amounts of money paid per person by the state to the health plan/providers for covered services) and the ability of state and federal governments to monitor access and quality.

Ensuring access and quality of care in a managed care environment will require fiscally solvent plans, established provider networks, education of providers and beneficiaries about managed care, and awareness of the unique needs of the Medicaid population. Access issues continue to be problematic. Primary care providers often express concern about the lack of specialists and problems with referrals (Galewitz, 2010). Even when reimbursement rates have been increased with the goal of increased physician participation, problems have remained due to delays in physician reimbursement payments and administrative burdens commonly associated with Medicaid participation (Cunningham & O'Malley, 2009). Anticipating health care reform, 17 states began *patient-centered medical home initiatives* in an effort to expand coverage and improve quality. Takach (2011) found that "expanded qualification standards along with incentive payments to address soaring costs and lagging health outcomes" had early indications of success (p. 1325). Costs, quality, and access improved, with some state per capita costs decreasing while physician participation and patient/provider satisfaction have increased. When Medicaid recipients have a regular physician (or medical home), they are more likely to get improved coordinated care and earlier interventions for chronic illness, and may decrease their use of emergency room (ER) visits.

Administrative costs for Medicaid are lower than for private health insurance, and Medicaid spending per capita has grown more slowly (4.6% annually) than both national health expenditures (5.9%) and employer-sponsored health coverage (7.7%) (KFF, 2011c).

State Children's Health Insurance Plan

Enacted as part of the Balanced Budget Act in 1997, the State Children's Health Insurance Plan (SCHIP) has provided health coverage to uninsured children under age 19 for families caught in the gap between Medicaid and affordable health insurance (FirstStep, n.d.). About $20 billion has been allocated over the first 10 years of the program (National Council of State Legislatures [NCSL], 2011). All 50 states participate, and for little or no cost provide insurance for hospitalization, physician visits, prescription drugs, and in some cases dental and vision services (FirstStep, n.d.). There are variations among the states, but SCHIP is geared to working families who may earn up to $34,100 yearly for a family of four (FirstStep, n.d.). President Obama signed into law a reauthorization and expansion of SCHIP in 2009 that expanded coverage from 7 to 11 million children by 2013 (Kritz, 2009). Authorization is extended to 2015 (NCSL, 2011).

Other Government Programs

In addition to third-party reimbursement, the government offers some direct health services to selected populations, including Native Americans, military personnel, veterans, merchant marines, and federal employees. Government support, largely through grants administered through the CDC, provides immunizations and well-child care, as well as prenatal care and other programs at the state and local level.

Payment Concepts in Health Care

Reimbursement for health care services generally has been accomplished through one of two approaches: retrospective or prospective payment. Conceptually, these approaches are polar opposites. It is helpful to understand their differences and their meaning for the financing and delivery of health services, past and present.

Retrospective Payment

A traditional form of reimbursement for any kind of service, including health care, is **retrospective payment**, which is reimbursement for a service after it has been rendered. A fee may be established in advance. However, payment of that fee occurs after the fact, or retrospectively. This is known as the **fee-for-service (FFS)** approach (Dranove, 2008).

In health care, limited accountability in the use of retrospective payment has created several problems. With third-party payers (e.g., insurance companies, the government) serving as intermediaries, neither consumers nor providers of health services were accountable for containing costs. Patients and providers alike often insisted on expensive or unnecessary tests and treatments. Because reimbursement was made retrospectively by the insuring agency, there was no incentive to keep a lid on this spending. Third-party reimbursement increased, along with other factors, to create an inflationary spiral of escalating costs. Abuse of the FFS system made it more difficult to develop retrospective payment for other health care providers, including nurses (Harrington & Estes, 2008; Nikitas, Middaugh, & Aries, 2011).

A further problem associated with the FFS concept was its tendency to encourage sickness care rather than wellness services. Physicians and other providers were rewarded financially for treating illness and for providing additional tests and services. There were few incentives for prevention or health promotion in an industry that reaped its revenues from keeping hospital beds full and caring for the sick and injured. Although retrospective payment worked well in other industries, from a cost-containment as well as a public health perspective, it was problematic in health care.

Prospective Payment

Prospective reimbursement, although not a new concept, was implemented for inpatient Medicare services in 1983, in response to the health care system's desperate need for cost containment (Dranove, 2008). It has since influenced the Medicaid program, as well as private health insurers. The prospective payment form of reimbursement has virtually eliminated the retrospective payment system (Harrington & Estes, 2008; Nikitas et al., 2011). **Prospective payment** is a payment method based on rates derived from predictions of annual service costs that are set in advance of service delivery. Providers receive payment for services according to these fixed rates, set in advance. Payments may be in the form of premiums paid before receipt of service or in response to fixed-rate (not cost) charges. To correct unlimited reimbursement patterns and counteract disincentives to contain costs, prospective payment involves four classic steps (Dowling, 1979):

1. An external authority is empowered (by statute, market power, or voluntary compliance by providers) to set provider charges, third-party payment rates, or both.
2. Rates are set in advance of the prospective year during which they will apply and are considered fixed for the year (except for major, uncontrollable occurrences).
3. Patients, third-party payers, or both pay the prospective rates rather than the costs incurred by providers during the year (or charges adjusted to cover these costs).
4. Providers are at risk for losses or surpluses.

The concept of prepayment, or consumers paying in advance of health care, has existed for many years. As far back as 1933, prepaid medical groups were advocated to reduce costs and make services more accessible (Dranove, 2008). Examples of early plans were the Health Insurance Program of Greater New York City and the Kaiser Plan (Herzlinger, 2007). The success of these two plans helped to influence the growth of the HMO, a type of managed care discussed later in this chapter.

Prospective payment imposes constraints on spending and provides incentives for cutting costs. The federal government, as mentioned earlier, enacted a prospective payment plan (Social Security Amendments Act 1983; see Landmark Health Care Legislation). The plan is a billing classification system known as **diagnosis-related groups (DRGs)**. The system is based on about 500 diagnosis and procedure groups. It provides fixed Medicare reimbursement to hospitals based on weighted formulas. Flat rates of payment are based on average national costs for a specific group, adjusted annually, with some regional variations accounting for higher wages and other costs (Dutton, 2007). This system was enacted to curb Medicare spending in hospitals and to extend the program's solvency period. The regulatory approach of DRGs changed Medicare hospital reimbursement from a cost-based retrospective payment system, in which a hospital was paid its costs, to a fixed-price prospective payment system. It was designed to create incentives for hospitals to be more efficient in delivering services.

Indeed, the prospective payment system has reduced Medicare's rate of increase in inpatient hospital spending and increased hospital productivity (Clifton, 2009). Thought to reduce hospital stays and unnecessary admissions, the system led to "DRG creep" (e.g., classifying patients into more lucrative categories) and "patient dumping" (e.g., transferring patients whose reimbursement is expected to be lower than actual costs of services) in an effort to counteract the losses in revenue to hospitals that spend more on Medicare patients than they are reimbursed (Dranove, 2003, p. 52). It also led to fierce competition among providers and mounting concern about quality of care—in hospitals, ambulatory settings, and home care. In October 2008, Medicare began withholding payments to hospitals for preventable errors in an effort to provide an incentive to prevent avoidable mistakes and improve patient care. The preventable errors include:

1. Foreign objects retained after surgery
2. Air embolism
3. Incompatible blood transfusions
4. Stage III and IV pressure ulcers
5. Injuries sustained due to falls
6. Poor blood sugar control
7. Catheter-associated urinary tract infections
8. Vascular catheter-associated infections
9. Surgical site infections
10. Deep vein thrombosis (DVT) following a total knee or hip replacement (Graham, 2008, para. 21).

These changes were instituted at the request of Congress, and initially many hospitals complained that their payments would be substantially reduced, especially for frail, complicated patients (Rosenthal, 2007). However, even though Medicare did not pay for an initial pressure ulcer, for instance, the resulting medication-resistant staph infection or sepsis resulting from that bed sore was covered (Graham, 2008). In January 2009, CMS ceased all payments (i.e., hospital and physician) for cases involving wrong surgical procedures and surgery on the wrong patient or on the wrong body part (Milstein, 2009). The days of paying physicians, who provided substandard care that resulted in subsequent procedures, hospitalizations, and thus greater income, are over (Crist, 2010). Consumers, employers, labor unions, and legislators are seeking pay for performance from providers and hospitals, as outlined in an IOM report, "Rewarding Provider Performance: Aligning Incentives in Medicare" (2007).

An expanded list of 24 *never events* for hospitals—serious incidents that could have been prevented—was approved for nonpayment by Medicaid beginning in July 2012 for all states (in 2011 about 21 states had already begun nonpayment). The goal is to reduce serious medical errors and preventable infections that should reduce costs and improve patient care. Some physician groups have objected to this move, as they state that some complications are "not entirely preventable" (Galewitz, 2011, para 6; Levinson, 2010). There are plans to expand nonpayment to other settings and possibly expand the list of conditions (see What Do You Think?).

Private insurers are also moving to nonpayment for medical errors and never events (Graham, 2008). Preventable complications within 90 days after inpatient surgery costs an average of between $11,797 and $19,480 for private insurers whose enrollees develop metabolic problems, pressure ulcers, or infections (Milstein, 2009).

What do *you* think?

What if you were to hire a glass company to replace a broken windshield in your car, and while completing the repair, they accidentally broke off your rear view mirror. Would you expect them to pay for that mistake? Or would you offer to pay for it? In the past, we the taxpayers have been paying Medicare payments to hospitals and physicians who have made serious errors that have led to adverse events, increasing costs, and resulting poor patient outcomes. Congress and others feel that this is unfair and have enacted legislation to stop paying for these types of errors or preventable events. Do you think this is fair? Can these conditions always be prevented?

A more vigorous version of prospective payment is *capitation*. As noted before, capitation refers to a fixed fee per person that is paid to a MCO for a specified package of services. Fees remain in effect until renegotiated, regardless of the number of services provided. Because profit margins are very tight, utilization, quality, and costs are carefully monitored (Nikitas et al., 2011).

The prospective payment concept has proved useful from a public health perspective. Prepaid services create incentives for providers to keep their enrollees healthy, thus reducing provider costs. A potential, indirect benefit from fixed rates and reduced costs is that more of the health care dollar is available to spend on prevention programs.

Claims Payment Agents

Claims payment agents administer the process for government third-party payments. That is, the government contracts with private fiscal agents to handle the claims payment process and function as an intermediary between them and the health care provider. More than 80% of the government's third-party payments have been handled by these private contractors, who sometimes are known as fiscal intermediaries (when processing Medicare hospital claims), carriers (when dealing with insurance under Medicare), or fiscal agents (as applied to Medicaid programs). As an example, Blue Shield and Blue Cross in addition to being private insurance companies also act as claims payment agents for Medicare (Virginia Commonwealth University, 2011).

Direct Consumer Reimbursement or Out-of-Pocket Payment

Another source of health care financing comes from direct fees paid by consumers. This refers to individual out-of-pocket payments made for several different reasons, such as payments made by individuals who have no insurance coverage (fees must be paid directly for health and medical services) or payments for limited coverage, insurance caps, and exclusions (services for which the consumer must bear the entire expense). For example, some individuals carry only major medical insurance and must pay directly for physician office visits, prescriptions, eyeglasses, and dental care. In other instances, the insurance contract may include a deductible amount that must be paid by the insured before reimbursement begins (e.g., $500 for individuals, $1,500 for a family). The contract may be established on a coinsurance basis, which determines a percentage to be paid by the insurer and the rest by the individual (e.g., 80/20 plans for which individuals pay 20% of costs after deductibles). Or, the individual may pay the remainder of a health service bill after the insurer has paid a previously agreed-on fixed amount, such as a fixed fee (known as a coverage cap) for labor and delivery, for example. About 32% of people between 19 and 64 years of age pay 10% of their income or more in out-of-pocket for health care costs; this includes those with and without health insurance (Collins, Doty, Robertson, & Garber, 2011). In comparison, for 2007, 4% of Britons, 5% of Dutch, and 12% of Canadians reported spending more than $1,000 annually out-of-pocket with Americans reporting 30% for that year (Gerencher, 2008). Seniors currently spend about 10% of their income on health care costs (U.S. News & World Report, 2010).

Another important factor for those paying directly for their health care expenses is **cost shifting**. This practice of charging different prices to different consumers most often affects those without health insurance who are paying out-of- pocket for care (Daschle et al., 2008). As health insurance plans or large companies contract with hospitals and physicians for services, they purchase these services at a reduced cost. Those without this "buying power" pay full price. For example, a $500 radiology procedure may be discounted to $225 for an insurance plan, but an individual paying out-of-pocket will pay the full price. This also occurs with government-sponsored plans. When Medicare payment changes to hospitals were instituted with the Balanced Budget Act of 1997, cost shifting to private patients in order to cover their losses became more difficult for those hospitals with large Medicare patient loads and more financial distress. Smaller hospitals with a lower proportion of Medicare patients were able to shift up to 37% of their cuts to private patients (Wu, 2010).

Private and Philanthropic Support

Private or philanthropic support, a third funding source, contributes both directly and indirectly to health care financing. Many private agencies fund programs, underwrite research, and provide benefits for people who otherwise would go without services. Charitable donations to non-profit healthcare institutions dropped 11% in 2009 from the previous year to a total of $7.64 billion (Shinkman, 2010). This is occurring at a time when Congress is debating reducing deductions for charitable donations and hospitals are providing more charitable care because of larger numbers of uninsured. The majority of contributors are individuals (70%), with about

28% of contributions coming from foundations and businesses (Shinkman, 2010). In addition, volunteerism, the efforts of numerous individuals and organizations that donate their time and services (e.g., hospital guild members), provides tremendous cost savings to health care institutions. It also enables many individuals to receive services, such as home-delivered meals or transportation to health care facilities, at no charge.

Philanthropic financing of health care has significantly decreased in the last two decades. Free medical clinics, beginning in the 1960s, have provided services to those without other sources of health care. They have helped many indigent people, but have also helped the medical profession by providing a place for medical research on chronic illness as well as a venue for teaching medical students outside the acute care setting. These clinics often rely on retired volunteer clinicians, as well as students (Reynolds, 2009). One study tracking physicians noted that over 76% offered charity care in 1996 to 1997, but that number decreased to just over 68% in 2004 to 2005, and that the charity care hours per 100 people decreased by 18% in the same time period (Cunningham & May, 2006). Surgeons were most often noted to provide free care to patients without insurance, and hospitals are required to provide emergency care to everyone. Even though some providers offer charity care, continued private support is essential, particularly when federal and state monies for health and social programs have been severely restricted (Harrington & Estes, 2008).

Further understanding of health economics and its impact on community health and community health nursing can be obtained by examining methods of health care finance, trends and issues influencing health care economics, and the effects of finance patterns on community health practice.

TRENDS AND ISSUES INFLUENCING HEALTH CARE ECONOMICS

The High Cost of Health in America

America paid over $7,538 per person for health care in 2010 (KFF, 2011d) through a combination of public tax money, individual and corporate contributions to insurance plans, and other sources. We pay the greatest amount of money for health care among the 15 participating OECD nations. Our costs are 51% higher than the second highest country, Norway. Not only do we pay almost twice the per capita expenditure of Canada and Germany and almost three times that of Japan and Italy, we have had one of the largest increases in health care spending since 1980 (KFF, 2011d). As noted earlier, health spending in 2009 was estimated at 17.6% of the U.S. GDP, while Australia and Norway spent only 8.5% of their GDP in 2008 (Keehan et al., 2011; KFF, 2011d).

Many Americans believe that we have the best health care system in the world. But what actually constitutes a good health care system? Are we truly getting our money's worth? The WHO's groundbreaking report of member countries outlined a *good health system* as one that provides good health for the whole population over the entire life cycle, responds to client's expectations for respectful treatment and a client-oriented system of health care providers, and ensures that costs are distributed according to ability to pay and provides financial protection for all (2010). A "well functioning health system responds in a balanced way to a population's needs and expectations by:

- improving the health status of individuals, families and communities
- defending the population against what threatens its health
- protecting people against the financial consequences of ill-health
- providing equitable access to people-centered care
- making it possible for people to participate in decisions affecting their health and health system" (p. 1)

The report recognizes the importance of effective leadership and governance, as well as efficient health information systems and a fair and equitable form of health care financing. Access to necessary medical technologies and products, along with a viable health workforce, is also critical. The service delivery system must be tailored to the specific country or region and should also provide methods of accountability and quality improvement for providers. The report estimates that between 20% and 40% of health care spending is the result of inefficiency and waste, and encourages all countries to provide universal coverage by improving efficiency and more effectively using resources. It notes that around the world, high costs of medical care and lack of sufficient coverage cause "150 million people (to) suffer financial catastrophe annually while 100 million are pushed below the poverty line" (WHO, 2010, p. 8).

In a global comparison of health care costs totaling over $4.1 trillion, WHO (2007) found that the United States had the highest total per person annual expenditure ($6,103), compared to total global per capita annual spending of only $639. Norway was the country with the highest government health spending per capita ($4,508). An earlier WHO (2000) study found that the U.S. health care system was the "most expensive ... in the world" largely because of high administrative costs (estimated then to range between 19.3% and 24.1%), the system of complex multiple payers, and the rising costs of prescription medications and advanced medical technology (p. 2). They also noted the shift from nonprofit to for-profit hospitals and the aging population as causative factors, along with the high proportion of uninsured people (and the attendant high cost of untreated illness). Access was a significant problem, as the United States was found to be "the only country in the developed world, except for South Africa, that does not provide health care for all of its citizens" (p. 3). In the United States, the patchwork quilt of private and public insurance—mostly tied to either employment or low-income status—makes it difficult for many people to get the care they need. The researchers noted that those without health insurance are "sicker and die younger than people with health insurance" (p. 4).

Americans believe that we have a quality health care system, and that this can make up for other deficits. The United States did rank first among all WHO countries on *responsiveness*—a construct relating to how respectfully clients are treated. However, as noted in Chapters 5 and 25, for many racial and ethnic minorities, this is not the case.

Disability-adjusted life expectancy (DALE, or the average number of healthy years expected in a population) was very low for the United States (ranked 24th), when compared with other nations of the world in the most recent WHO study (2000). The United States was ranked lowest among 14 industrialized nations and placed 54th among WHO countries on the measure of *fairness in financing* (WHO, 2000). This inequality disproportionately affects the poor, underinsured, and the uninsured, as many PHNs can corroborate. Compared to the other 190 countries studied by the WHO, the United States ranked 15th for attainment of the criteria listed above, and 37th for *performance* (a comparison of how well it *could* perform based on available resource levels). In another study of *overall efficiency* in health system performance among 191 countries, the United States ranked 37th, below Morocco, Cyprus, and Colombia (Tandon, Murray, Lauer, & Evans, n.d.).

Health-related quality of life (HRQoL—a questionnaire surveying five domains including self-care, mobility, usual activities, anxiety/depression, and pain/discomfort) was used to determine *quality-adjusted life expectancy* (QALE) across 15 countries. The US levels for males and females were lower than most other countries (e.g., Japan, the United Kingdom, Germany, Canada), but were higher than levels in Armenia, Hungary, and Slovakia (Heijink, Baal, Oppe, Koolman, & Westert, 2011).

Also, only 16% of those in the United States reported that they were *satisfied* with the health care system compared with 26% in both the United Kingdom and Canada (Klein, 2007). Even though we generally report lower wait times for elective surgery than many other countries, it is thought this may be due more to the large number of uninsured citizens who cannot access this type of medical care so there are fewer of us competing for slots. Only 30% of Americans can get a physician appointment on the same day, while 55% of Germans and 41% of Britons can be seen the same day they call for an appointment (Klein, 2007). In a Gallup poll of 30 nations, the United States was 18th in percentage of the population satisfied with their personal health (at 83%). And, only 56% of U.S. respondents stated that they were satisfied with their healthcare system compared to 68% in the other countries (Khoury, & Brown, 2009). The United States spends the most per capita and the greatest percentage of its GDP on healthcare, but the Personal Health Index score (a survey of personal health perceptions) when compared with other countries (78 compared to 86 for Ireland) was only average. Another survey showed that one third of Americans feel that the health care system needs to be completely rebuilt, while only 9% of Dutch citizens and 20% of Italians feel the same way (Gerencher, 2008).

In a survey of physicians from the United States, Australia, Canada, New Zealand, and the United Kingdom, U.S. physicians did not feel that their health care system worked well and noted inadequate resources, limitations on medications that could be prescribed, as well as quality being compromised in an effort to control costs. They were also more likely to feel that the health care system needed "complete rebuilding" than those in the other countries (Docteur & Berenson, 2009, p. 8). Fifty percent of hospital executives said they were also not satisfied with the performance of the U.S. health care system.

The Commonwealth Fund created a *National Scorecard on U.S. Health System Performance*, and defined several dimensions of a high performance health system (2011, p. 10) as on that produces:

- Long, healthy, and productive lives
- Quality
- Access
- Efficiency
- Equity

With a total possible score of 100, the United States attained 64 overall (lower than the previous two scorecards in 2006 and 2008), and only 53 on the dimension of *efficiency*. Three of the five dimensions had lower scores, but the score for quality increased from 71 to 75. The researchers also found that 51% of U.S. adults receive preventive care and all recommended screening tests (using national standards), and that 30-day hospital readmission rates averaged 20%. Only 56% of adults (ages 19 to 64) had an accessible primary care provider, and 58% of children had a medical home.

Promising improvements included an increase in the percentage of primary physicians using electronic medical records (EMRs) (i.e., from 17% to 46% between 2000 and 2009), and control of hypertension improved from 31% to 50% (although the benchmark rate is 75%). Cigarette smoking decreased from 21% to 17%, and pressure sores among short-stay nursing home residents dropped from 19% to 14%. Access to care and health insurance, along with the rising costs of care and insurance, are growing concerns. The infant mortality rate in the United States is over 35% higher than the best state level rates. These better state rates are two times higher than rates in many other industrialized nations. Childhood obesity, care for minorities, and low-income populations are also troubling. While we have made some progress, safe, effective, quality health care is still outside our reach.

In order to reach benchmark performance levels of other leading nations, the U.S. healthcare system would have to improve performance by 40% or more. If this were done, we could have:

- 91,000 fewer annual premature deaths from causes "amenable to health care"—this is twice the number of people dying in motor vehicle accidents (p. 15)
- 38 million more adults with access to a primary care provider

- 66 million more adults getting all recommended preventive care
- Savings of $1.6 to $3.1 billion in annual medical costs if we could improve control of hypertension and diabetes (reducing disease complications)
- Medicare savings of $12 billion annually if we could reduce hospital readmissions
- Savings of $55 billion if we could reduce health insurance administrative costs to the average of other countries with private–public insurance systems (The Commonwealth Fund, 2011)

Why does health care cost so much? Explanations include the following:

- Medical malpractice costs and the need to practice *defensive medicine* by ordering excessive tests and x-rays. One study found that this increased health card spending by 2.4% in 2008 (Mello, Chandra, Gawande, & Studdert, 2010), while some insiders report that lawsuits actually help improve patient care (Baker, 2005; Montini, Noble, & Stelfox, 2008).
- An aging population and the greater prevalence of chronic disease (Daschle, 2008; Dranove, 2008; Kimbuende, Ranji, Lundy, & Salganicoff, 2010)
- Advances in and the spread of medical technology; for instance, many economists project that 40% to 50% of annual health care cost increases can be traced to this major cost driver (Callahan, 2008; 2009). Others note that adopting newer technologies saves lives and improves care, arguing that costs may increase at first but will decrease as illnesses are diagnosed and treated sooner (Lichtenberg, 2009)
- Rapidly rising prescription drug and hospital costs (KFF, 2007c; WHO, 2007)
- The failure of market forces, in that health care doesn't respond to supply and demand as in other areas of the economy (Ameringer, 2008; Daschle, 2008; Dranove, 2008; Krugman, 2011)
- High costs of insurance administration—in some cases, three times that of the cost in other nations (Litow, 2006)
- Ineffective, inappropriate, and inadequate health care leading to increased morbidity and mortality and costs (Institute of Medicine, 2001)
- High proportion of uninsured—it has been estimated that 28% of Americans are uninsured. Spending on Medicare could decrease if new beneficiaries were covered by insurance during their lives, and costs of uncompensated care would also decrease with universal coverage (Hadley, Holahan, Coughlin, & Miller, 2008; Nunley, 2008)
- Americans' demand for high-tech health care and preference for freedom of choice among providers and services (Daschle, 2008; Dranove, 2008; Herzlinger, 2007)

Docteur and Berenson (2009) reported on health care comparisons across OECD countries and found that the United States was "among the worst performers" on *amenable mortality levels* (deaths prior to age 75 that may be prevented through effective, timely health care). Other indicators included:

- Life expectancy at birth—we ranked in the lower one-third of countries.
- Life expectancy at age 65 is in the average range, but women especially fare better in several other countries.
- The highest rate of deaths due to conditions that are preventable or can be treated successfully.
- Higher prevalence of 9 out of 10 conditions in the over-50 population (e.g., heart disease, stroke, cancer).
- Relatively low levels of prevention and chronic disease care, but high quality of preventive care for women (Pap smears, mammograms).
- Childhood vaccination rates below average, but above-average flu vaccination rates for seniors.

They further noted that, when compared to Canada, end-stage renal disease patients on dialysis and after kidney transplant have longer survival times in Canada. Other research comparing the two health care systems found mixed results (Guyatt et al., 2007). When compared with 17 European countries, the United States had the highest survival rates for some cancers (i.e., lung, breast, prostate, colon), and ranked in the top six for melanoma, ovarian and uterine cancers (Docteur & Berenson, 2009).

A striking example of cost differences found in different countries involves prescription drugs. For example, the Alzheimer's medication—Donepezil (Aricept)—is available in 21 countries ranging from the United States to Nigeria. One 5 mg tablet varies in price from 26 cents in India and 31 cents in Mexico to $6.64 in the United States. Researchers found similar price discrepancies for other Alzheimer's medications. Even with the lower price, many people in low-income countries still cannot afford this medication (Suh et al., 2009). However, in another study comparing seven countries on medication underuse due to cost, the US fared the worst with 20% of respondents reporting that high out-of-pocket costs and lower incomes kept them from fully utilizing their prescriptions as written. Only 3% of Dutch respondents reported underuse. Lack of patient participation in treatment decisions and younger age was also associated with underuse in the United States and four other countries (Kemp, Roughead, Preen, Glover, & Semmens, 2010).

Controlling Costs

As noted earlier, cost-control measures utilizing both supply-side and demand-side strategies have been attempted. Utilization review techniques have further enhanced utilization and cost control (Dranove, 2008). Yet, despite various public and private cost-control strategies, health care costs continue to rise. Although expenditures in the 1990s decelerated slightly from the escalation experienced during the 1970s and 1980s, in the early 2000s costs rose and have continued to rise. Many factors influenced this increase. Between 1965 and 2001, the price per day of hospitalization rose tenfold from under $200 to over $1,300; in 2009 the average was $1,853 (KFF, 2011b; KFF, n.d.). As medical care became more complex, insurance costs rose dramatically, as did costs of public health care financing through Medicare and Medicaid (Dranove, 2008). About half of the health care dollar goes to hospital and physician costs (31% and 20%, respectively) (CMS, n.d. a). The explosion of medical technology has been characterized as a "medical arms race" by some (Dranove, 2003, p. 46); a youth-oriented culture and unwillingness to accept illness and death has helped fuel this along with the growth of elective procedures, such as plastic surgery.

A focus on primary prevention demands a paradigm shift in thinking about the practice and delivery of health care (see Chapter 1). It is one that fits more closely with the mission of public health. It expects that citizens are involved in their health care, are knowledgeable about their health status, can manage self-care practices, and can modify lifestyle behaviors to promote wellness. This creates a rich environment for community health nurses to collaborate with primary care practitioners and other health care professionals to control health care costs while providing quality care focusing on primary prevention. Our focus on illness and not health promotion or prevention has proven costly. Prevention should be at the forefront of a new era in health care. Trust for America's Health (2011b) has developed 10 Top Priorities for a National Prevention Strategy:

1. Promoting Disease Prevention
2. Combating the Obesity Epidemic
3. Preventing Tobacco Use/Exposure
4. Preventing/Controlling Infectious Diseases
5. Preparing for Potential Health Emergencies/ Bioterrorism Attacks
6. Recognizing the Relationship Between Health and U.S. Economic Competitiveness
7. Safeguarding the Nation's Food Supply
8. Planning for Changing Health Care Needs of Seniors
9. Improving the Health of Low-Income/Minority Communities
10. Reducing Environmental Threats (para. 4)

Access to Health Services: The Uninsured and Underinsured

Many services, preventive or illness-focused, are not available to a large portion of our population. The U.S. Census Bureau (2010) reports that 50.7 million people (16.7% of the population) were uninsured in 2009. This was the first year to show an actual drop in the number of people with health insurance since tracking of this data first occurred in 1987. A shift has also occurred between the numbers of those insured privately (e.g., insurance provided by employers and individuals) and publicly (e.g., paid by government through Medicaid or Medicare). A growing segment of the US populace (estimated at between 18.5% and 33%) is uninsured, resulting in limited or no access to health care (Kaiser Commission on Medicaid & the Uninsured [KCMU], 2011). More than 49.1 million Americans under the age of 65, and close to 1 million over age 65, are currently without any form of health insurance coverage (KCMU, 2011). There is wide variation between states—from 6% in Massachusetts to over 25% or higher in Florida, Texas, and New Mexico—contributing to great inconsistencies in health care quality and access (KCMU, 2011).

As noted earlier, about 25% of Americans who have health insurance are underinsured, with a 60% increase in nonelderly underinsured between 2003 and 2007 (Schoen, Collins, Kriss, & Doty, 2008), and they often must chose between paying insurance and health-related expenses or foregoing needed care. The underinsured are more likely to "go without care because of costs" at a rate similar to those without health insurance, and 41% of underinsured did not fill prescriptions, while 35% reported having a problem but not visiting a physician (Schoen et al., 2008). As an example of this, one study projected that those with health insurance would pay close to $650 in out-of-pocket expenses for nonpremium medical costs in 2010—while those who were uninsured paid close to $415 (Caswell & O'Hara, 2010). In addition, many underinsured have no dental or vision coverage, and few prescription drug benefits, yet still experience higher deductibles. Credit card use to cover medical expenses is on the rise as people struggle to pay higher out-of-pocket costs (Consumer Reports, 2008).

A particularly ominous study indicates that adults in the 50- to 64-year age range—baby boomers—have unstable health insurance coverage. About 14% are uninsured, and almost one fourth of these had *never* had health insurance (Collins et al., 2007; Smolka, Purvis, & Figueiredo, 2007). More than half of these working older adults with annual incomes below $25,000 report that they have times without insurance coverage, and one third of those with incomes between $25,000 and $39,999 also experience insurance instability. People in this age group have higher rates of chronic illness (62% had at least one chronic condition, such as diabetes or hypertension) and higher medical expenses. One third of those in the study reported that they had problems paying medical bills or that they were paying off medical debt. Two thirds were concerned that they would be unable to afford medical care in the future.

Another trend includes changes in where Americans are receiving health care. Historically, they first saw their family physician when some new health concern arose. One study found that, despite insurance status, "only 42% of the 354 million annual visits for acute care (treatments for newly arising health problems) are made to patients' personal physicians" (Pitt, Carrier, Rich, & Kellerman, 2010, p. 1620). About 28% are first seen in the ED, 20% by specialists, and other outpatient departments see about 7%. Emergency physicians see one fourth of all acute-care visits and over 50% of these visits are to persons without health insurance. This number is especially high when you consider that ED physicians make up less than 5% of the total U.S. physician population.

Medical Bankruptcies

A wide variety of medical issues can lead to financial insecurity and bankruptcy. If you don't have health insurance and you need emergency surgery for appendicitis it may take a great effort to pay off your medical debt (or you may turn to high-interest credit cards). If you have health insurance but suffer from a lingering cancer, you may be hit with large out-of-pocket costs and your inability to work may lead to further financial problems. Many people have significant financial stressors but may not file for bankruptcy, due to either lack of financial resources for legal fees or other reasons. Middle income groups are more likely to file bankruptcy while lower-income groups are more often found to suffer from late payments that affect their credit scores and the subsequent ability to purchase a home or apply for credit (McCloud & Dwyer, 2011). Bankruptcy filings have been rising over the last decade—as much as 360%. In a 2001 study conducted by Harvard and Ohio University researchers, almost half of participants cited illness—sometimes with loss of work—and medical expenses as the chief cause for their bankruptcy (Himmelstein, Warren, Thorne, & Woolhandler, 2005). A large-scale follow-up study found that over 60% of bankruptcy filings were associated with medical expenses (Himmelstein, Thorne, Warren, & Woolhandler, 2009). Most of these medical debtors were middle class and educated, and 75% had health insurance. This is further evidence that the underinsured, along with those individuals without health insurance, are in danger of financial disaster when confronted with a serious medical emergency or long-term illness.

The consequences of not getting needed medical care are not trivial and can result in unnecessary hospitalization and serious health problems—along with increased costs. One of the largest groups among the uninsured have been young adults between ages 19 and 29 (Collins et al., 2007), as well as workers and their families with low incomes. Most of these families have one member working full time; some have two or more full-time workers.

Access to health care is a prime concern for the uninsured. Many have no **medical home**—defined as seeing the same health care provider for regular care. Because there is a lack of care coordination, duplicative and wasteful services are often the case (Collins, 2007). And without a reliable care provider, the uninsured tend to use ERs for nonemergency care. Recent data from a nationwide database noted that almost 20% of ED visits were from people without health insurance, and 33% of visits were from low-income persons. Rural residents accounted for about one-fifth ED visits (Kerr, 2009). Cost of uncompensated care in 2009 reached $62.1 billion, but is projected to drop after health care reform to under $47 billion in 2019 (Holahan & Garrett, 2010).

Government costs to reimburse "safety net" hospitals and other entities involved in care of the uninsured exceed $30 billion yearly—exemplifying just some of the costs to taxpayers. Because of the instability of the system, about half of the uninsured lose their health insurance coverage in a year—racking up higher administrative costs as they move between private and public insurers and change their usual sources of medical care. Interruptions in care, duplication in medical records, and verification of eligibility all lead to higher costs for everyone (Ku, MacTaggart, Pervez, & Rosenbaum, 2009).

In the private sector, numerous firms do not offer health insurance to their employees; a large number of the uninsured are employees of these firms or are their dependents and these numbers rose as unemployment rates began to jump in the mid-2000s (KCMU, 2011). Self-employed individuals also find it difficult to pay the higher costs of insurance premiums without the benefit of group rates. Consequently, many of the self-employed can access health services only by purchasing expensive individual insurance policies with high-deductibles and coinsurance or by making expensive out-of-pocket payments.

Managed Care

The term **managed care** became popular in the late 1980s. It refers to systems that contract to coordinate medical care for specific groups in order to promote provider efficiency and control costs. Although the term *managed care* is relatively new, the concept has been practiced for many years through various models of alternative health care delivery. Managed care is a cost-control strategy used in both public and private sectors of health care. Care is *managed* by regulating the use of services and levels of provider payment. This approach includes using HMOs and PPOs. In contrast to FFS models, managed care plans operate on a prospective payment basis and control costs by managing utilization and provider payments. The managed care model encourages the provision of services within fixed budgets, thus avoiding cost escalation. Because costs are tight, preventive services are generally encouraged, so that more expensive tertiary care costs can be avoided, if possible.

Health Maintenance Organizations

The HMOs and various companies' self-insured plans also are included in this category. Usually, they sell only health insurance; in some cases, they also may provide actual health services. They focus on a localized population. As a group, they generate a large amount of premium revenues; HMOs represent 17% of employer-sponsored group insurance and PPOs enroll about 55% of workers (KFF, 2011a). Consumers have often resisted the strenuous cost-containment policies of many HMOs, and prefer to have their physicians make decisions about their care—not insurance company employees. However, employers are often drawn to alternatives as a potential cost-saving method. HMO premiums have historically been lower than other types of insurance premiums, and out-of-pocket costs to consumers have also generally been lower (Gabel, Pickreign, & Whitmore, 2006; Herzlinger, 2007). However, 2011 costs for employee health coverage in 2011 is similar for HMO, PPO, and point of service (POS) plans (KFF, 2011a). Also, industry projections for HMO premium rate and cost increases vary little from other types of plans and range from 8% to 10.6%; for PPOs the range is from 5.5% to 11.1%; and, for consumer-driven/high-deductible health plans it is 10.3% to 11.9% (Managed Care Online [MCOL], 2012).

A **health maintenance organization (HMO)** is a system in which participants prepay a fixed monthly premium to receive comprehensive health services delivered by a defined network of providers. The HMOs are the oldest model of coordinated or managed care. Several HMOs have existed for decades (like Kaiser Permanente), but many have developed more recently. HMO enrollees were told that they could benefit from lower cost premiums, reduced cost sharing, and fewer administrative costs.

From 1930 to 1965, the HMO movement, supported initially by the private sector, gradually gained federal backing. Group plans were included as a part of Medicare and Medicaid legislation. The HMO Act of 1973 demonstrated stronger federal support and assistance for growth of this industry (Ameringer, 2008). Amendments to this act in 1976 lifted restrictions and further encouraged HMO growth. The skyrocketing employer health insurance costs of the 1980s and 1990s encouraged many companies to move from traditional insurance and FFS to HMOs. The number of HMO enrollees peaked in 1999 to 2000, but encompasses over 66 million in 2010 (MCOL, 2012). Enrollment in HMOs through employer-based programs numbered more than 77.7 million in 2006 (MCOL, 2007). Currently, there are numerous HMOs with a variety of configurations. The unique set of properties of HMOs include:

- A contract between the HMO and the beneficiaries (or their representative), the enrolled population
- Absorption of prospective risk by the HMO
- A regular (usually monthly) premium to cover specified (typically comprehensive) benefits paid by each enrollee of the HMO; few additional charges are levied, because the payment mechanism is not FFS
- An integrated delivery system with provider incentives for efficiency; the HMO contracts with professional providers to deliver the services due the enrollees, and the basis for reimbursing those providers varies among HMOs (Harrington & Estes, 2008)

Official encouragement, government subsidies, and the pressures for cost control spurred the growth of HMOs. Some HMOs follow the traditional model, employing health professionals (e.g., physicians, nurses), building their own hospital and clinic facilities, and serving only their own enrollees. Other HMOs provide some services while contracting for the rest. Variations of the HMO model include solo practice physicians who affiliate with hospitals (Ameringer, 2008).

HMOs have penetrated Medicare (24.2%) and Medicaid (71%) markets, as well as over half of commercial insurance markets (MCOL, 2012). They have historically been viewed as a positive alternative delivery system because of their potential for conserving costs, which results from their emphasis on prevention, health promotion, and ambulatory care; and with a concomitant reduction in hospital and medical care utilization. However, there are questions as to whether the cost savings result partly from favorable selection of enrollees. Quality concerns also have been raised about the dangers of underserving enrollees in order to stay within payment limits (Sultz & Young, 2009; Dranove, 2008; Herzlinger, 2007). Scanlon, Swaminathan, Chernew, and Lee (2006) examined longitudinal data, and found that HMO competition was related to consumer satisfaction surveys, but not necessarily to better quality of care for chronic conditions. Later research verified that increased HMO competition did not lead to improved HMO quality (Scanlon, Swaminathan, Lee, & Chernew, 2008). A study examining Medicare Advantage (Medicare managed care) plans with traditional FFS Medicare noted increased cost and scant evidence for improved management of outpatient chronic conditions (Nicholas, 2009). Also, a Cochrane review (Scott et al., 2011) found inconclusive evidence for the impact of financial incentives to primary care physicians on the quality of health care provided. A large-scale, longitudinal study of 11 quality indicators found that Medicaid-managed care enrollees received lower-quality care than managed care commercial plan enrollees (Landon et al., 2007).

These concerns about HMOs and managed care in general have not gone unattended. The Health Insurance Portability and Accountability Act (HIPAA) and the Newborns' and Mothers' Health Protection Act are both significant pieces of legislation, addressing health care concerns among the nation's citizens and official organizations, such as the APHA. HIPAA reassured people that they would not lose health care coverage if they changed jobs. In addition, for a while in the United States, insurance for labor and delivery hospitalization covered only 24 or fewer hours after birth. Infants and mothers were being sent home in unstable postdelivery conditions. Newborns would go home when younger than 1 day of age, in some cases so soon after birth that body temperature was not stabilized and the ability to suck and take breast milk or formula was not established. The Newborns' and Mothers' Health Protection Act eliminated these "drive through deliveries," ensuring that mothers and newborns would have the right to remain in the acute-care setting for at least 48 hours, covered by their insurance plan (see Landmark Health Care Legislation). In response to concerns from managed care clients, the government developed a patient bill of rights stipulating the patient's right to timely emergency services, respect and nondiscrimination, as well as participation in treatment decisions and a more consumer-friendly appeals process.

Preferred Provider Organizations

A **preferred provider organization (PPO)** is another model of managed or coordinated care that developed earlier than the HMO. A PPO is a network of physicians, hospitals, and other health-related services that contract with a third-party payer organization to provide comprehensive health services to subscribers on a fixed FFS basis. Because of contractual fixed costs, employing organizations that subscribe can offer medical services to their employees at discounted rates. In PPOs, consumer choice exists. Enrollees have a choice among providers within the plan and contracted providers out of the plan. The PPOs practice utilization review and often use formal standards for selecting providers (Dranove, 2008).

PPOs did not exist in their present form until after 1980. Enrollment in PPOs grew from about 10 plans in 1981 to more than 700 plans in the 1990s. The number of people enrolled in PPOs also increased, from an estimated 10.4% of individuals with private insurance in 1988 to 40% by the late 1990s, with the numbers leveling off as the decade came to a close. As consumers became more frustrated with limits imposed by HMOs, they began to move toward PPOs that provide more choices. In 2006, 81.3 million Americans were enrolled in a PPO, more than the number in HMOs (MCOL, 2007). In 2011, PPOs were the most common form of health insurance offered by employers—with 55% of workers choosing this type of policy (Dranove, 2008; KFF, 2011a). Early use of PPOs appeared to promote cost savings, but the long-range cost- effectiveness of this model has yet to be fully proven. PPOs have been criticized in the past for their lack of vigorous case management—more often found in HMOs—and some larger plans have moved toward this model, especially in the case of chronic diseases, such as hypertension and diabetes, or with palliative care (Porter & Teisberg, 2006; Robinson & Ginsburg, 2009; Spettell et al., 2009).

Point-of-Service Plans

A variation on the just-mentioned plans is the **point-of-service (POS) plan**, which permits more freedom of choice than a standard HMO or PPO. Enrollees choose a primary physician from within the plan (POS) who monitors their care and makes outside referrals when necessary. At an extra cost, enrollees can go outside the HMO or PPO network of contracted providers unless their primary physician has made a specific referral (Small Business Majority, 2012). It is a hybrid or combination of an HMO and PPO. This type of plan covers a small percentage of the market, estimated at around 10 million people (Dranove, 2008). In 2011, about 10% of employers utilized POS plans for their employees (KFF, 2011a). See Figure 6-7 for a look at the trend in types of health plan coverage among those employees who are covered by their employers.

Health Care Rationing

The concept of **rationing** in health care refers to limiting the provision of health care services to save costs. Sometimes, this may jeopardize the wellbeing of groups of individuals. Rationing implies that resources are fixed or limited and therefore must be used sparingly. Scheunemann and White (2011, p. 1625) state that "need is limitless and resources are not," thus there is a certain inevitability of rationing. Rationing is "the equitable, or rational, distribution of resources" according to "clinical need and effectiveness, rather than wealth or geographic location" (Saha, Coffman, & Smits, 2010, para. 1). Rationing may occur by restricting people's choices, denying access to services, or by limiting the supply of services or personnel. It may be overt, as in the oft-cited case of Britain, or more covert, as practiced by many MCOs or health plans. Often, insurers and providers of health care services make rationing decisions to contain costs. With rationing, there is a danger of compromising quality and effectiveness (Dutton, 2007).

Rationing in health care has been practiced for many years. With limited resources for health services delivery, government programs have had to establish strict eligibility levels and monitor the use of these resources to ensure the most equitable distribution. To maintain viability and some kind of profit margin, private insurers have engaged in rationing by excluding enrollees who are at greatest risk for health problems—and, thus, higher expenditures (Dranove, 2008; Dutton, 2007).

Advances in knowledge and technical capabilities through research and technology compound rationing decisions. When several individuals need an organ transplant and only one organ is available, what criteria should be used to select the recipient? Now that it is commonly accepted that certain lifestyle behaviors, such as smoking and alcohol consumption, or driving without restraints, create health risks, should people who engage in these activities pay a higher price for health care or be excluded from certain services? Should a younger person needing specialized surgery take priority over an elderly person needing similar care? There are no easy answers. Providers and insurers have struggled with these difficult policy issues for years.

With today's health care costs, the problems are even more complex. As health care spending rises, calls for rationing may intensify (Kelly & Cronin, 2011). The spending for Medicare and Medicaid has grown rapidly. Over the last 30 years, Medicare spending has grown 2.4% per year faster than the GDP, and could account for 31% of GDP in 2082 if no adjustments are made (Friedman, 2009). Technological advances have added years to life and improved national welfare, but as spending continues to consume more and more of the GDP, many will ask if the costs outweigh the benefits and may seek to limit high-cost, low-benefit health procedures, such as expensive MRIs for rare conditions or conditions with no effective treatments or cures.

Oregon began a system of rationing in 1994. The state approached the problem pragmatically and openly. In an effort to reach universal coverage, Medicaid was expanded to cover all state residents with incomes below the FPL, and then health care services rationing was planned in order to pay for the increased public coverage. Community meetings were held, and

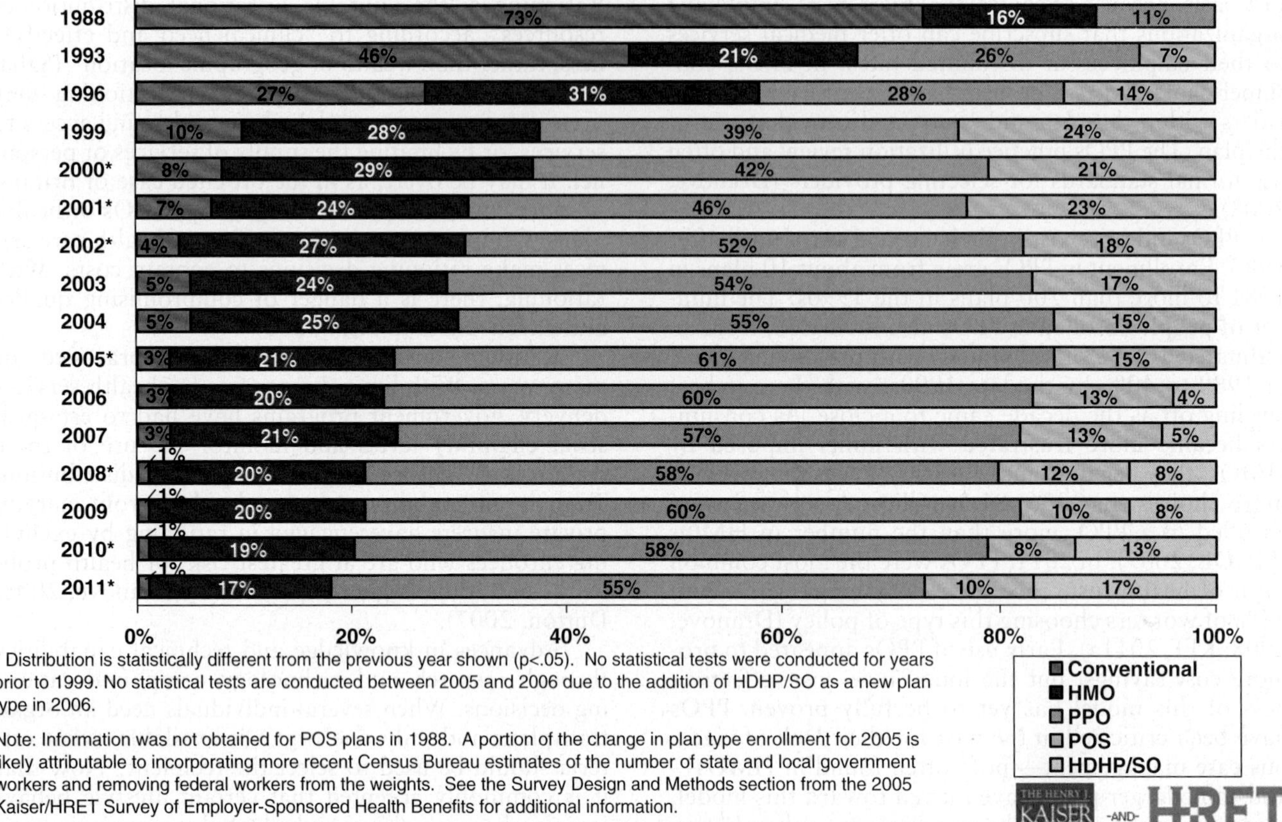

FIGURE 6-7. Distribution of health plan enrollment among covered workers, by type of plan, 1988 to 2011. From: Kaiser Family Foundation & Health Research & Educational Trust, 2011, *Employer Health Benefits Survey 2011*. This information was reprinted with permission from the Henry J. Kaiser Family Foundation. The Kaiser Family Foundation, based in Menlo Park, California, is a nonprofit, private operating foundation focusing on the major health care issues facing the nation and is not associated with Kaiser Permanente or Kaiser Industries.

over 1,000 citizens spoke out. Thirteen health-related values, under three headings: (1) value to society, (2) value to individuals at risk, and (3) essential to basic healthcare, were put forward (Landwehr, 2009). An original list of 709 medical services was decided upon. The state envisioned a plan for legislative determination of a cutoff point, depending on yearly budget allocations; the list changed yearly, and in 1995, 581 out of 745 procedures were covered (Dranove, 2008; Perry & Hotze, 2011). In 1999, Oregon's Medicaid program covered 574 of 743 conditions, but in the early part of the 2000s an economic downturn prevented further expansion of the Oregon Health Plan (OHP). Cuts were made and copays instituted that eventually led to unmet health care needs (Wright, Carlson, Allen, Holmgren, & Rustvold, 2010). In 2003, the program was divided into OHP Plus (for Medicare eligible) and OHP Standard (for those not traditionally covered by other programs). Uninsured who depended on Medicaid were allowed to choose enrollment in the plan, and many chose to not participate. In the year between 2002 and 2003, enrollment dropped more than 50% in OHP Standard, and by 2007, it was down by 75% to 77% (Perry & Hotze, 2011; Wright et al., 2010). In 2007, the prioritized list became the basis of the essential benefits package, and was divided into tiers. Lower-priority items had higher cost sharing, and value-based services got "first-dollar coverage" with incentives for healthy behaviors, management of chronic illnesses, and use of ambulatory care centers over emergency departments (EDs) (Saha et al., 2010, para. 7). Although Oregon has not been able to achieve universal coverage, this new legislation sought to cover additional children and uninsured populations. The governor has said that the goal of the OHP is not to ration care but to improve the way it is organized and delivered in order to be more cost-effective (Perry & Hotze, 2011) (see What Do You Think?).

What do *you* think?

Your physician has just given you the news—you have advanced kidney cancer and it will probably cause your death in the next 1 to 2 years. There is a drug, called Stutent, that may slow down the spread of your cancer, giving you maybe 6 more months of life. It costs $54,000. Would you choose to spend the money to extend your life? There is no guarantee about the quality of your life, just a few added months of time. Because most people would be unable to come up with this sum of money, it would be more available if covered by insurance. If this drug were available to everyone who wanted it, then all of us would share in the cost of higher insurance premiums. Do you think that is a good idea? If the drug is not covered, then is this considered rationing?

Adapted from: Singer, P. (2009, July 19). Why we must ration health care. *The New York Times*. Retrieved from http://www.med.mcgill.ca/epidemiology/courses/EPIB654/Summer2010/Policy/nytimes%20rationing%202009_07_19.pdf

Competition and Regulation

Often, competition and regulation in health economics have been viewed as antagonistic and incompatible concepts. **Competition** means a contest between rival health care organizations for resources and clients. **Regulation** refers to mandated procedures and practices affecting health services delivery that are enforced by law. In a society in which long-held values of freedom of choice and individualism reign supreme, competition provides opportunities for entrepreneurial endeavor, free enterprise, and scientific advancement. Yet, to promote the public good, oversee equitable distribution of health services, and foster community-wide participation, regulation also serves an important role.

Health care incorporates four major kinds of regulation (Ameringer, 2008; Sultz & Young, 2009):

- Laws
- Regulations
- Programs
- Policies

Laws that regulate health care include any legislation that governs financing or delivery of health services, such as legislation regulating Medicare reimbursement to hospitals. Regulations guide and clarify implementation; they are issued under the authority of law and are part of most federal health care programs. Examples include regulations governing project grants such as HMO development; formula grants, such as those provided under the Hill–Burton Act; and entitlements, such as Medicare and Medicaid. Regulatory programs are created from legislative enactments and are designed to accomplish specific goals, such as accreditation and licensing rules for hospitals, public health agencies, and other health service providers. Regulatory policies have a broader focus and involve decisions that shape the health care system by channeling the flow of resources into it and setting limits on key players' actions. Examples of regulatory policies are found by reviewing state or federal budget proposals for funding programs, such as health manpower training, research, and technology development (Ameringer, 2008).

From the 1950s through the 1970s, the federal government assumed a strong role in regulating health services. First, federal subsidy of health care costs increased, and there was greater federal control of state programs. Health services became regionalized and more comprehensive. Federal appropriations supported operational as well as capital and planning costs. Health research and the training of health professionals gained greater federal support. Group medical practice multiplied as a cost-saving measure. More than 60% of the population was covered by some form of prepaid health insurance, largely because of the effects of Medicare and Medicaid. Interagency health planning cooperation increased, and health program evaluation improved. Neighborhood health centers, community mental health centers, and other programs were developed to improve health care access for everyone. Although costs rose, the period was one of relative economic stability that emphasized quality of care, with the federal government assuming a major role in regulating the planning, use, and reimbursement of health care services (Dranove, 2008; Sultz & Young, 2009).

In the early 1980s, government cost control measures were greatly diminished as the Reagan era ushered in deregulation in many areas. The passage of the Omnibus Budget Reconciliation Act caused dramatic changes affecting health care. The federal government, having failed to contain rising health care costs, shifted responsibility for the public's health and welfare back to state and local governments. Large amounts of federal funding for health research, health manpower training, and public health programs were withdrawn. Continued escalation of health care costs prompted a concentrated effort among public and private providers alike to find cost-containment measures. From all this grew the competition-versus-regulation debate (Ameringer, 2008; Dranove, 2008; Sultz & Young, 2009).

The 1990s were marked by "merger mania" and the move from nonprofit to for-profit hospitals (Dranove, 2003, p. 115). The Clinton health plan failed to gain support, and many hospitals downsized, laying off nurses. Managed care became more popular as a means of reducing employer premiums in the early 1990s, but by the late 1990s, as they restricted benefits, fears were raised about MCOs withholding necessary care and a consumer "backlash" resulted (RAND Health, 2010). Many states and the federal government enacted benefit laws between 1990 and 2002, in response to these concerns. During this time, many smaller managed care plans merged to gain a larger market share and provide improved services. Robinson and Ginsburg (2009) note that transformation is still occurring, and "the market is generating product designs that combine elements of consumerism with elements of managed care," but with a stronger component of consumer choice and a weaker one for management of consumer choices by insurers, employers, regulators, and others (p. w272). We are still feeling the results of these changes, and one of the most obvious consequences deals with competition in health care.

Competition, its proponents say, offers wider consumer choice and positive incentives for cost containment and enhanced efficiency (Ameringer, 2008; Sultz & Young, 2009); that is, consumers are free to select among various health plans on the basis of cost, quality, and range of services. Competing providers must develop efficient production and distribution methods to stay in business, and consumers are more likely to use only necessary services, because of the required cost sharing that is part of the competition model. One downside is fragmentation of services, lack of coordination, and subsequent waste. Integrated delivery systems, such as Kaiser Permanente's fully integrated system or more loosely organized public–private partnerships, could lead to improved quality, outcomes, and reduced costs (Enthoven, 2009b).

Examples of competition have been very evident as more health plans, including HMOs and PPOs, vied with traditional insurance plans for subscribers: Currently only 1% of workers are covered by their employers through a conventional insurance plan (KFF, 2011a). However, costs have not dropped substantially. Many hospitals, too, compete aggressively for patients. Some hospitals now advertise maternity care depicting a new mother and father having a candlelight dinner in the hospital with their newborn infant in the bassinet beside them. Some surgical centers advance the "hotel guest" concept, with beautifully appointed rooms, including meals and lodging for a guest. However, some research has shown that a greater concentration of hospital markets can lead to higher prices, although prices can be lower when health plan market concentration is also high (Melnick, Shen, & Wu, 2011).

Although it appears that competition offers the best service for the least cost, regulation advocates have for almost 20 years argued that there are at least four problems associated with the competition model: (1) consumers often do not make proper health care choices because of limited knowledge of health services; (2) competition may discriminate against enrolling certain consumers, especially high-risk, high-cost patients, thus excluding those who may need services the most; (3) the competition model may not encourage enough teaching and research—expensive elements of our present system; and (4) quality may be sacrificed to keep costs down.

Regulation advocates conclude that standardization and controls are needed to guarantee quality and equal access. Leaders in the field have concluded that both competition and regulation are needed (Ameringer, 2008; Sultz & Young, 2009). With foresight, McNerney wrote in 1980, "It is rapidly becoming apparent that what we need is a proper balance between competition and regulation with more effective links [and] regulation [should be] used as a force to keep the market honest" (p. 1091).

HEALTH CARE REFORM

HMOs and PPOs have become accepted methods of delivering health care in the United States in the past 30 years. Over several generations, other methods have been considered, yet not passed by legislation and adopted as law. Health care reform became a reality in 2010, with the passage of the Patient Protection and Affordable Care Act. It is helpful to look at earlier attempts and thought processes that moved us toward this reality. Managed competition and universal coverage, as well as single-payer systems, have been part of the discussion in health care reform.

Two plans worth further review are managed competition and universal coverage, with and without a single-payer system. The benefits and drawbacks of each are important to discuss here.

Managed Competition

The idea of managed competition, as a health care delivery method, was born from the controversy regarding competition versus regulation and was driven by the need for health care reform. **Managed competition**, it was hoped, would combine with market competition to achieve cost savings with government regulation to achieve expanded coverage. This idea, whose origin is credited to economist Alain C. Enthoven of Stanford University, has played a major part in debates on health care reform. It sought to address the two fundamental issues driving reform: cost containment and universal access to health care (Enthoven, 2009a).

Managed competition has been viewed as a market-based solution that places accountability for resolving the health care crisis with the insurance industry and with consumers. Insurers would be required to accept all applicants, without excluding those at poorer risk. At the same time, the insurers must control costs. Consumers would choose among competing health insurance plans, paying above fixed amounts paid by their employers to receive the best value. But for true competition, employers must offer real choices and a wide variety of plans. To do this, Enthoven and colleagues envisioned "regional insurance exchanges" that select health plans, manage risk selection, and establish equity rules (those plans with sicker participants would be subsidized by plans with younger, healthier participants) (Arrow et al., 2009, p. 493).

Another concept of managed competition is consumer choice, and consumers must be able to access information, so that they can make responsible choices and feel that they have purchased something of value for their money (Vaiana, 2011). Other common features of managed competition proposals include regulations that prevent screening out of high-risk enrollees, penalties for companies that try to achieve better risk pools, community ratings to prevent companies from setting rates by risk pool, and guaranteed coverage for all who apply. Another critical component involves management; some standardization must be established among benefit packages and an effort must be made to dismantle health care monopolies that endeavor to gain uneven market power—in other words, a more level playing field (Enthoven and Wynand, 2007).

Proponents of managed competition cite many advantages. Managed competition would encourage insurance companies to compete on price and quality of services to attract enrollees. It would also offer consumers tax incentives to purchase the lowest-cost plans that meet minimum benefit requirements. Managed competition, although market driven, would be highly regulated to ensure quality and access. Cost-effectiveness and quality/outcomes information must be made available to consumers, although currently this information is not always easy to find or to decipher. Providers have not widely accepted systems of ranking on measures of quality. According to its proponents, managed competition, as a reform concept, would have the potential for reducing expenditures and improving access to health care coverage, and is being used successfully in other countries (Enthoven and Wynand, 2007).

Managed competition may not be beneficial for physicians, however. A study commissioned by the AMA found that, in many regions of the United States, only a few health insurance companies dominate the market, and they exert significant market power. Because physicians are often unable to exert bargaining power against these large insurers—in 64% of areas studied, one health plan had a 50% or greater market share—they have called for antitrust action by the federal government to stem the further consolidation of health plans (AMA, 2007). This example highlights some of the problems with the managed competition concept. Can market forces really work in the health care market? Similar models, such as HMOs and the Federal Employee Health Benefits Program, have failed to reign in ever-increasing health care costs (Dranove, 2008; Sultz & Young, 2009).

Another major criticism of managed competition is its potential failure to provide equitable and universal coverage. It is possible that large employers would benefit financially under managed competition, but small businesses would find the cost burden heavy, and many individuals, such as the self-employed, could remain uninsured. A basic benefits package, critics argue, must address the special concerns affecting groups such as women and elderly adults, including coverage for long-term care, home care, mental health, dental care, and prescribed drugs. Competition among providers would be inefficient in rural areas, where there are fewer provider choices, such as county nursing agencies and isolated small-town hospitals scattered over great distances.

Universal Coverage and a Single-Payer System

A different approach to health care reform emphasizes universal health insurance coverage, often through a stronger role played by government. Some proponents of this system of health care promote a **single-payer system** that would replace the health insurance companies in the United States with a single, public sector insurer that would entitle all citizens to **universal coverage** (everyone would have health insurance of some type, ensuring better access to care). Efforts to accomplish this approach have been evident for many years.

Since the time of Teddy Roosevelt in 1912, national health insurance (NHI) has been debated while its proponents have sought comprehensive health care protection, in particular, for the aged, children, and the needy. Presidents Roosevelt (both Theodore and Franklin), Truman, Nixon, Carter, and Clinton have all lobbied for some form of NHI or universal health coverage, and Senator Edward Kennedy was also a long-time supporter (Daschle, 2008). Growing concern over the cost and accessibility of health services in the 1960s and again in the mid-1970s led to a renewed focus on NHI as a solution by which health insurance coverage could be provided for all citizens through a single-payer system or a mix of public and private insurers. Numerous attempts to pass some form of NHI resulted in piecemeal legislation that added various benefits for Social Security recipients. The Kerr–Mills bill (1960) set a precedent of public financing for elderly persons who were medically needy but not receiving public assistance. Medicare (1965) was the first compulsory NHI program in the United States. By 2001, it reached some 40 million people—only 16% of the total U.S. population.

Most other developed countries offer some type of NHI or attempt to provide universal health coverage to their citizens. Other countries believe that health care is a fundamental right, and provide it as a social service, unlike the United States, which tends to view it as a commodity that is only available based on one's ability to pay (Quadagno, 2010). The APHA has long been an advocate of universal health care, initially endorsing a single-payer system. The APHA (2010) strongly endorsed passage of the current health care reform legislation.

Although many agree that insuring all Americans will improve overall national health and performance, the concept of a government-sponsored, single-payer system is controversial (Brett, 2009). Even though polls revealed that Americans were dissatisfied with the current health care system, they usually reported being satisfied with their own arrangements for health care—and they were uncomfortable with the idea of a government-controlled health plan (Blendon, Brodie, Benson, Altman, Buhr, 2006). A 2007 Gallup Poll revealed that 32% of Americans favored universal coverage (making insurance available to more people), but only 12% wanted a government-run, single-payer system (Newport, 2007). Logic indicated that single-payer plans could provide cost savings from reduced overhead and administrative costs. But, other questions remained, such as: What is the best way to provide universal coverage? Should health insurance still be linked to employment? How can the expense be funded? Should citizens become more responsible for their health outcomes?

How can quality be ensured and costs managed? These important questions spurred policy makers and health care economists to examine potential solutions (Heskett, 2007).

In testimony to Congress, experts from the Commonwealth Fund encouraged the design of a universal health care system that meets four criteria: improves access to care, has the potential to slow cost increases and improve efficiency, improves equity in the system, and has the potential to improve health care quality (Collins, 2007). Some politicians proposed expanding Medicare, Medicaid, and the SCHIP programs, or focusing more on prevention and individual responsibility. Other groups supported a system of tax credits, employer and individual taxes, and a more transparent evaluation of costs and quality.

Some states initiated legislation to extend coverage to uninsured residents. Illinois extended coverage to all children through a program called *All Kids*. Massachusetts initiated universal health coverage in 2006, and created a state agency to provide information on health insurance plans to consumers and employers. At the same time, Massachusetts required all residents above a set income level to get insurance coverage from their employer or purchase it individually; adults earning up to 150% of FPL and children of parents earning up to 300% of FPL are fully subsidized by the state. Results are mixed; more people are insured, but costs have not been curbed. Before this legislation, about 94% of residents were insured; currently 98% of residents (and 99.8%of children) are covered. The percentage of private employers providing employee health insurance rose from 70% to 77%, and companies with more than 11 full-time employees are expected to contribute to health insurance or face penalties. Increased costs to the state in the 2010 budget were only 1%, but a cost shift burden from employers to individuals is problematic. Medical bankruptcies rose by over 33% between 2007 and 2009. While most residents are supportive of the law, and 88% of physicians in a recent survey stated it improved care or didn't affect the quality of care, per capita health care spending is projected to be almost twice the current rate by 2020 (Khan, 2011).

Some have posited that universal coverage could not be attained because of the partiality toward private insurers and a lack of cost control measures and adequate provisions for low-income families (Himmelstein & Woolhandler, 2007). Proposals to build upon the current mix of public and private insurance have been more accepted. Expansion of Medicare, Medicaid, and SCHIP coverage, along with a new group insurance program with a variety of options similar to the Federal Employees Health Benefits Program (FEHBP), was envisioned, along with requirements for insurance coverage for all with income-related subsidies, as needed (Collins, 2007).

Also, even if everyone received health insurance, how could quality be assured? Some believe that the overall performance of the health care system should improve as everyone gains access to care. However, others think that a system providing incentives to *both* providers and patients to use services efficiently and effectively produces the best results (Collins, 2007). Providing information to consumers is another component of quality assurance, and this is sorely lacking. But, information is becoming more readily available. For instance, the Leapfrog Group (2007) promotes *transparency* through surveys of standard measurements and practices to enable comparisons, and reimbursement incentives to encourage quality and efficiency. Scores for local hospitals can be reviewed at the Leapfrog Web site (see Internet Resources at the end of this chapter). The quality of insurance plans, measured by the Health Plan Employer Data and Information Set (HEDIS), includes information on patient satisfaction, data on risk factor control, and procedures such as prescribing beta (β)-blockers after heart attacks, and is monitored by the National Committee for Quality Assurance (NCQA). Other systems of quality measurement, like health outcomes, the process of care, and adherence to standardized guidelines, are still required.

Health Care Reform: Making the Change

The cry for health care reform is not new. In a classic study, Perkins examined the work of the 1927 to 1932 Committee on the Costs of Medical Care. More than 75 years ago, the committee defined *costs* as the major problem and *business models of organization* as the major solution (Perkins, 1998). Today, consumers and professionals have agreed that health care reform is needed in the United States. The nexus of the disagreement has been in the form that it should take and the speed at which it should be completed. At issue is a fundamental conflict in values between advocates of the managed competition model and those seeking universal coverage or a single-payer plan. On the one hand are those who strongly value the competition model, which ensures a free market, individualism, and the right to choose the type of health care desired. On the other hand are those who propose a more regulated, statutory model.

Proponents of universal coverage argued that more comprehensive benefits were needed to include the unemployed and those who are physically or economically disadvantaged and cannot afford individual health care coverage. Furthermore, they argued that universal coverage should emphasize prevention and primary health care as key factors in reducing long-range health care costs and, more importantly, in ensuring improved levels of health for the public (Collins, 2007). In the classic position statement, *Nursing's Agenda for Health Care Reform* (2002), the American Nurses Association (ANA) supported this emphasis by promoting nurses as primary providers of health care. In 2008, ANA published its new *Health System Reform Agenda*, calling for improvements in access, quality, and costs in health care. Workforce issues were also addressed, and again the ANA called for "fundamental reform of the U.S. health care system" (p. 14).

A standard set of benefits, set by law and enjoyed by the entire population, regardless of age, health, income, and employment status, is an important health care reform element. Many countries have successfully implemented such a package under a plan called a *statutory model*. Various versions of this model have worked well in Austria, France, Belgium, Japan, Germany, Israel, Poland, the Netherlands, and Switzerland. In this model, health insurance falls under the rubric of social security, and is funded through government-mandated payroll premiums or taxes. Payment is made to private-sector health insurers, from a fund called a *sickness fund* in some countries (Frontline, 2008). Individuals select among nationwide plans and choose their doctor and hospital, and can switch plans when desired. This element of consumer choice is thought to encourage the sickness funds to respond to consumer preferences and improve efficiency in the health care system (Van de Ven, Beck, Van de Voorde, Wasem, Zmora, 2007). Reimbursement for services is made directly by insurers to providers. In Germany, a disease management program was added to the statutory health insurance plan in the 1990s; its purpose is to both promote competition and increase the quality of care (Stock, Redaelli, & Lauterbach, 2007). This statutory model eliminates the need for separate programs such as Medicaid and Medicare. It also provides uniform and comprehensive benefits (Harrington & Estes, 2008). See Display 6.3 for a comparison of health systems in five developed countries.

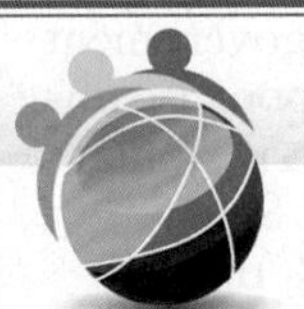

DISPLAY 6.3 HOW FIVE OTHER COUNTRIES PROVIDE HEALTH CARE

Germany

Percentage of GDP spent on health care: 10.7
Average family premium: $750 per month (depending on income).
Co-payments: 10 euros ($15) every three months; some patients exempt.

- German Statutory Health Insurance began in 1883. Germans buy insurance from private, nonprofit sickness funds (200+). Fund manager pay is based on enrollment, and there is competition for members as well as negotiations with physicians for competitive pricing.
- Single-payment system. Physician salaries are two thirds U.S. salaries, but medical school is free and malpractice insurance costs are much lower.
- Choice of physician (can see specialists first), hospital, long-term care facility; medication and dental
- The richest 10% can opt out and purchase for-profit insurance that pays physicians higher fees (so they may see patients sooner); poor Germans receive public assistance in paying sickness fund premiums

Great Britain (United Kingdom)

Percentage of GDP spent on health care: 8.3
Average family premium: Tax-funded, no additional cost.
Co-payments: None for most services; some dental and vision co-pays; 5% for prescriptions (exempt for elderly and young).

- National Health Service (NHS) since World War II (funded from general revenues). This is considered "socialized medicine" as the government both pays for and provides health care services. Hospital physicians are paid salaries from taxes, and family physicians' salaries are based on the numbers of patients seen. A few specialists work outside the NHS, seeing private-paying patients.
- Low administrative costs, no claims to review or bills to collect. Family physicians provide medical homes and make referrals to specialists. They are paid bonuses for keeping their patients well, and focusing on prevention. Well-designed system, but chronically underfunded
- Tax-based, free at point of service (covers ambulatory care, hospital, medications, long-term care, vision)
- Choice of physician, generally short waiting times for appointments, but longer waiting lists for elective referrals to specialists. Government reforms are making care more competitive and providing wider choices. Hospitals now compete for NHS funds and patients can choose where they want treatment for many procedures.

Japan

Percentage of GDP spent on health care: 8
Average family premium: $280 per month, with employers paying over 50% of this.
Co-payments: Procedures (30%), but total amount paid per month is capped per income level.

- Japan utilizes a "social insurance" system, and all citizens are mandated to have health insurance (through employers or from nonprofit, community-based plans). Public assistance is given to those unable to afford insurance. Physicians and most hospitals are in the private (not public) sector, and most health insurance is private.
- There are no gatekeepers, as in the U.K. system, and Japanese may go to any specialist as often as they wish without first seeing a family physician. The Ministry of Health negotiates with physicians on pricing every 2 years.
- Japan, perhaps partially due to diet and lifestyle, has excellent health statistics (e.g., life expectancy).

(continued)

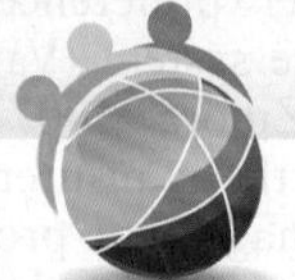

DISPLAY 6.3 HOW FIVE OTHER COUNTRIES PROVIDE HEALTH CARE *(Continued)*

- Because there is no gatekeeper, there is no incentive for patients to have a medical home. Because they have been successful in cost containment, 50% of hospitals now have budget losses.

Switzerland

Percentage of GDP spent on health care: 11.6
Average monthly family premium: $750 paid by patients, with government assistance for the poor.
Co-payments: 10% of the cost of services ($420 per year cap)

- Switzerland employs "social insurance," which began with a national referendum in 1994. At that time, 95% of their population was insured, but all citizens are now required to have health insurance. They have universal coverage, despite being a capitalistic society with large pharmaceutical and insurance industries.
- Insurance companies are forbidden from making a profit on basic care and cannot "cherry-pick" enrollees. They do make profits on supplemental insurance.
- Insurers negotiate with providers (e.g., hospitals, physicians), but the government sets prescription prices. Some, but not all, plans require physician gatekeepers; others give discounts to patients who use medical homes.
- The Swiss have the second most expensive system (still much less spent than the United States), and prices of medications are higher than in other euro countries. (Some Swiss drug companies are said to make 33% of their profits in the U.S. market.)

Taiwan

Percentage GDP spent on health care: 6.3
Average family premium: $650 per year for a family of 4
Co-payments: Prescriptions (20% of cost, up to $6.50); outpatient care ($7); dental and traditional Chinese medicine ($1.80); many exemptions apply (e.g., preventive services, major diseases, childbirth, care for poor/veterans/children).

- In 1995, Taiwan adopted the "National Insurance Model." Insurance is mandatory for all citizens, and there is one, government-run health insurer. Employers and workers split premiums, other citizens pay flat rates for insurance (with government assistance). Care for veterans and the poor is subsidized by the government. This system is similar to Canada and Medicare in the United States.
- Health insurance was extended to 40% of the uninsured population, and health care spending was actually decreased. Any physician can be seen without a referral, and smart cards are used to store medical history and for billing purposes. Public health officials are also assisted in monitoring standards, and Taiwan's administrative costs are the lowest in the world.
- Taiwan does not bring in enough money to cover all medical care provided. The parliament must approve insurance premium increases, and it has only done this once since 1995.

How do you think these systems compare with the classic U.S. health care system? How do they compare with the new health care reform (ACA)?

Adapted from: Frontline. (2010). Sick around the world: Five capitalist democracies & how they do it. Public Broadcasting System (PBS). Retrieved from http://www.pbs.org/wgbh/pages/frontline/sickaroundtheworld/countries/

Other issues include making the system more accountable, eliminating adverse risk-selection, and providing informed choices to consumers. Although reform is under way, the need continues for strong advocates of universal access and cost containment. Furthermore, health reform must focus on the central question: Is there coverage for the promotion of health and prevention of illness or simply payment for the diagnosis and treatment of those who are already ill? World Bank evaluations show that public health interventions have been found to be consistently more cost-effective than medical services, yet past health reform has often paid minimal attention to this critical issue. In addition, our frequent emphasis on medical care cost containment does not take into account the social determinants of health that need to be addressed outside the health care system. Community health nurses can play an influential role in emphasizing health promotion services as being central to future health reform efforts through political involvement and policy development.

Designers of health reform have faced a difficult challenge in reconciling these conflicting views. As a result, elements of both models have been used to shape an improved system. Recent health care reform includes an incremental plan that allows for a flexible transition and opportunities for states to experiment with approaches. With the successful passage of HR 3590 (Public Law 111–148), *The Patient Protection and Affordable Care Act,* on March 23, 2010, and the March 25 passage of HR 4872 (PL 111–152), *Health Care and Education Affordability Reconciliation Act of 2010,* amending HR 3590, the long journey toward health care system reform ended. Both pieces of legislation are referred to as the *Affordable Care Act* (ACA). While by no means a grand vision for change with its incremental implementation, it has been called "among the most consequential pieces of social policy passed since the Great Society" of Lyndon Johnson in the 1960s (Klein, 2011, para 5). The two main avenues for increasing the number of insured Americans is to expand Medicaid coverage for the poor and provide government subsidies to help others pay for private insurance, with almost equal coverage. Over 32 million additional Americans are expected to have health coverage by 2019 (Klein, 2011).

Beginning in 2010, dependent coverage for adult children was extended to age 26, and prohibition on lifetime limits on coverage and pre-existing conditions for children, along with tax credits to small employers (25 employees or less) providing health insurance began, among other things. In 2011, grants were awarded to states to investigate current tort litigations, and to small employers to establish wellness programs, as well as implementation of 50% discounts on Medicare Part D brand-name prescriptions from pharmaceutical manufacturers. An Innovation Center within CMS is also scheduled for creation, and a national quality improvement strategy developed. Small businesses have been allowed to keep insurance plans in effect—"grandfathering"—and about 72% of those with 100 or fewer workers have done so (KFF, 2012). In 2012, the Medicare Independence at Home Demonstration program will be created, other cost-cutting measures will be taken, along with enhanced collection and reporting of data. Adoption of a single set of operating rules for verification of eligibility and claims status, enrollment, premium payments, and referrals will begin in 2013, as will increased Medicaid payments to primary care providers.

More dramatic reforms will occur the following year, including the creation of an essential health benefits package and permission for states to have an option to create a Basic Health Plan for uninsured residents making between 133% and 200% of the FPL. By 2014, all U.S. citizens and legal residents will be required to have health coverage, with a phased-in penalty for those not covered. Employers with 50 or more employees who do not offer health coverage will be assessed a fine of $2,000 per full-time employee (first 30 excluded). Employers with more than 200 employees must automatically enroll all employees into health insurance plans. American Health Benefit Exchanges and Small Business Health Options Program Exchanges will be created, and deductibles for health plans in small group markets will have limits of $2,000 for individuals and $4,000 for families. Waiting periods for full coverage will be limited to 90 days, and Medicare DSHs will have payments cut 75% initially (with increases based on the percentage of uninsured population and amount of uncompensated care given). After 2015, states can form health care choice compacts and allow insurers to sell policies in any state after January 2016. Additional Medicare payment reductions for hospital-acquired infections will begin in 2015, and an excise tax on employers who offer "Cadillac health plans" (i.e., 40% on values >$10,200 for individuals and $27,500 for families) will start in 2018 (KFF, 2010b; Orszag & Emanuel, 2010). For a more complete health reform implementation schedule, see http://www.kff.org/healthreform/upload/8060.pdf.

The ACA has been described as "consumer-friendly" because applicants in each state will be screened for all available health subsidy programs and enrolled through a standardized process. Coordination and seamless transition between programs is the goal. Uniform income rules and forms, along with streamlined enrollment, will make administrative functions simpler and less costly. Paperless verification will be required through secure Web portals, where information can be securely exchanged. The goal is the help individuals better understand their choices, as well as access and maintain health coverage. Families should be able to apply online, with assistance as needed. Coordination between insurance exchanges, Medicaid, and the Children's Insurance Programs (CHIP) provide for better coverage (KFF, 2010b; Rosenbaum & Riley, 2012). Also, exchanges will have the power to remove insurers who abuse the system or provide inadequate service.

Rapidly rising health care costs will not be reigned in overnight. Projections by 2030, with health care reform, are expected to be only 0.5% lower than they would have been without reform. But the federal budget deficit is projected to be $100 billion less after the first decade of ACA and $1 trillion less in the decade beyond 2020. Total health care expenditures could even end up $600 billion less in the first decade. There is flexibility and a focus on quality improvement that should help restrain unnecessary growth in health care costs. In controlling costs, new fraud and abuse measures in both Medicare and Medicaid are being instituted, and administrative savings should occur with standardization and electronic records (Orszag & Emanuel, 2010; RAND Health, 2011). An Independent Advisory Board (comprising experts and stakeholders) will assist in controlling Medicare costs, and has the power to make changes in the system without waiting for Congress to act (Klein, 2011). As Medicare's costs per capita exceed a prescribed threshold (general inflation plus 1% after 2018), this advisory board can develop and propose new policies for reducing inflationary costs that will be implemented by U.S. DHHS, unless Congress enacts legislation resulting in similar cost savings (Orszag & Emanuel, 2010). The Patient-Centered Outcomes Research Institute will provide additional information on effectiveness of treatments and interventions, and the Innovation Center at CMS will develop, evaluate, and test new programs and policies that reduce cost and enhance care for Medicaid and Medicare patients. Improved value and quality outcomes are the proposed benefits of these three innovations (Orszag & Emanuel, 2010). ACA also increases incentives for change that will improve patient care and outcomes (e.g., hospital readmissions, hospital-acquired infections) and improve coordination of care (e.g., bundled payments to MDs and hospitals for patients with chronic illnesses, accountable care organizations, medical homes). These changes in the delivery of health care, as well as cost-control reforms suggested by economists, health policy experts, and physicians, are hoped to achieve cost reductions while providing expanded health insurance coverage (Orszag & Emanuel, 2010; RAND Health, 2011). Others note that lower payment increases to physicians seeing Medicare patients and reductions for insurers participating in Medicare, along with the increased Medicare tax on higher-income earners, will save the system money, but will be largely offset by expenditures in Medicaid expansion, small business and exchange credits, and other expenses (Klein, 2011). Only time will tell; if the reform is dynamic and flexible, as touted, perhaps we can stay a step ahead of costs.

Not everyone is convinced that health care reform is a good idea. Republican legislators have threatened repeal, but have failed to provide a viable alternative solution. As of January 2012, 19 states have passed legislation that opposes at least some elements of the ACA, and 45 states had filed over 200 measures either proposing alternative policies or opposing elements of health reform. Several lawsuits over the "individual mandate" (penalty for not purchasing health insurance) have been overturned on appeal upholding the ACA in state courts in Virginia and Ohio, as well as in the District of Columbia; the 11th Circuit in Atlanta, Georgia, ruled it unconstitutional. The U.S. Supreme Court announced in November 2011 that it plans to hear suits filed by 26 states and business organizations challenging the individual mandate provision in March 2012 (Cauchi, 2012). In June, 2012, the court ruled that that the ACA individual mandate was constitutional and constituted a tax, as those who do not obtain health insurance coverage are required to pay a penalty ("shared responsibility payment") to be collected by the IRS (p. 2). At the same time, it found the Medicaid expansion "unconstitutionally coercive of states" and ruled that the Secretary of Health and Human Services could not enforce this provision by withholding more than expansion Medicaid funding to states that choose to opt out of the Medicaid expansion outlined in the ACA (Musumeci, 2012).

EFFECTS OF HEALTH ECONOMICS ON COMMUNITY HEALTH PRACTICE

Health economics has significantly affected community health and community health practice by advancing disincentives for efficient use of resources, incentives for illness care, and conflicts with public health values.

Disincentives for Efficient Use of Resources

All of the system structures that directly or indirectly promote cost escalation and prevent cost containment contribute to disincentives for efficient use of resources. For example, retrospective financial reimbursement, with its lack of setting limits, encourages spending on nonessential tests and treatments and drives up costs. Tax-deductible employer contributions for health care coverage and nontaxable employee health benefits encourage unnecessary use of services and result in cost increases. Lack of cost sharing by consumers and of financial risk for decisions made by providers may create further disincentives to keep costs down (Daschle, 2008; Dranove, 2008).

Community health has been affected in several ways. Abuse of resources in some parts of the system leads to depletion in other areas. The trend of diminished federal and state allocations has had profound effects on community and public health programs, and severe budget cuts have affected even basic community health services. Competition from the private sector in home care and other community services, such as health education programs, has forced traditional public health agencies to reexamine their traditional programs and seek new avenues for the provision of services, along with new revenue sources (Institute of Medicine, 2002). Costs indirectly affect even appropriate use of nursing personnel in community health. Failing to recognize the differences in skill levels of community health nurses and their less-prepared counterparts, public health departments and agencies often have hired persons who are underqualified to give the high-caliber and comprehensive care required. Finally, the advent of prospective payment and limits on lengths of stay have encouraged early hospital discharge, resulting in more acutely ill people needing home care services. The immediate effect was an increase in the demand for highly skilled and more expensive home care services, which required changes in provision patterns of community health care. As acute-care nursing shortages intensified and salaries increased, the number of open, unfilled PHN positions mounted. But with the economic downturn in the late 2000s, open positions go unfilled and public health departments are often short-staffed as budgets shrink. The long-range effects of this phenomenon on family stress and caregiver health, on community health care reimbursement, and on the nature and structure of community health services, including the role of the community health nurse, have yet to be determined.

Incentives for Illness Care

The traditional American health care system tends to promote illness, because health care providers have primarily been rewarded for treating problems, not for preventing them. Hospitals derive more income when their beds are full of sick or injured people. Health insurance plans compete, not by lowering costs or increasing quality, but by avoiding the sick and seeking healthy enrollees—leaving many without access to necessary health care (Schoen et al., 2008).

The bulk of most reimbursable health services centers on treating illness or disability in hospitals, nursing homes, and ambulatory care facilities, using physicians or skilled nursing care in the home (home health services)—situations in which the individual must play the role of patient. Our disease-focused system of health care is thought by many to be the basic problem (Adams, 2006; Porter, 2009). It rewards disease by paying doctors who diagnose, treat, and refer ill patients. It does not pay them for keeping their patients healthy. Most preventive care is woefully inadequate and largely overlooked by both practitioners and patients alike: Remember, about half of all U.S. adults receive recommended health screening tests annually (Shires et al., 2012; Health promotion nursing activities, such as comprehensive prenatal, maternal, and infant care; health education; childhood immunizations; and home services to enable the elderly to live independently have not always been consistently covered by most insurers.

A system that financially supports illness care affects community health practice in several ways. The number and severity of health problems in a community increase when individuals postpone care because they cannot afford visits to the doctor or clinic. It has been more difficult to encourage community clients to assume responsibility for their own health and to engage in self-care, prevention, and active health promotion. Furthermore, such illness-oriented incentives create a basic societal valuing of illness care that, conversely, devalues wellness care. Health promotion and disease prevention efforts become second-ranked priorities in the competition for scarce resources. In communities where a greater proportion of community health practice is spent in the treatment of disorders and rehabilitation, resources are more limited for prevention and health promotion.

Prepayment methods and the growth of managed care have been positive moves in the direction of a more wellness-oriented financial incentive structure. An HMO has the incentive to offer preventive and health-promoting services, such as early detection and treatment of symptoms, regular physical examinations, and health teaching, because the HMO loses money when it must pay out for expensive tertiary care. Health care reform proposals show promise of greater recognition of the cost-saving value of prevention efforts. In the Michael Moore documentary, *Sicko*, British physicians reveal that they are awarded "bonuses" for encouraging healthy behaviors (e.g., getting patients to stop smoking) and for successful management of diseases (e.g., hypertensive patients who remain on medications to control blood pressure and cholesterol levels). Some in the United States have proposed a paradigm shift to health consultants who are paid when you stay healthy, not when you become ill. Another proposed change is from managed care to *life maintenance organizations* (LMQs) that provide life insurance and advice on needed health care—thus, having a true incentive to keep you in good health because they will be paying your life insurance claim if your life is shortened by an avoidable illness (Adams, 2006). The focus of the system would be on proper nutrition, exercise, health education, and prescription drugs to keep people healthy, not just treating disease. The MCOs have business-focused goals that are given more consideration than is the issue of equal access to health care. Perhaps, with health care reform this will change, as newer *accountable health care organizations* proliferate.

Managed Care and Public Health Values

Initially, MCOs focused on event-driven cost avoidance. Strategies included decreasing inpatient days, decreasing specialty physician use, using physician extenders, and implementing provider discounting. This evolved into a second stage, in which the principal objective was to control resource intensity and improve the delivery process. Strategies used to meet this objective included capitation of specialist costs, controls on units of service, patient-focused redesign, clinical pathways, and total quality management. But, emphasis is shifting to a focus on health promotion and population health. Community assessments are an important part of this approach, so that high-risk groups can be identified and provided early interventions. Case management of individuals with chronic illness is also a focus.

Some believe that community health assessments could become standard quality tools for not only public health interventions, but also health reform in general (Feldman, Hile, & Weinberg, 2011; Spice & Snyder, 2009). Community assessments establish the baseline health status of a community and measure changes in the health of the community over time. Community health assessments must include source information that is both primary (health status assessment surveys, focus groups, and satisfaction surveys) and secondary (data collected by public health agencies and state agencies, such as birth rates, mortality rates, and incidence of communicable diseases in the community). Health care reform legislation includes a requirement for community needs assessment every three years for state-licensed, tax-exempt health organizations such as hospitals, and imposes a $50,000 annual penalty if this is not done. Prioritization of health needs and a description of community resources are to be included, as in input from those with expertise in public health (Adams, 2011). See Chapter 15 for more on Community Assessment.

Improving the health status of a community mandates that health care agencies be actively involved in accurately assessing the community's health status and the major issues facing the community. This involves health teaching and health promotion, as well as developing community action plans to promote collaboration and focus on early intervention and treatment (Brownson, Baker, Leet, Gillespie, & True, 2011). Are these not the proposals that public health advocates have been making for more than a century?

As early as 2002, Drevdahl expressed concerns regarding the paradoxical missions of public health and managed care. One relies on partnerships for fostering health care equity and creating healthy communities and populations as it embraces a social justice mission, whereas the other "falls more along the line of market justice" (p. 163). Perhaps the incentive to keep costs down will be the motivation needed to work with clients at the primary prevention level of care. Although public health proponents have advocated preventive care as the best care for the individual, family, and community as long as the goal of community health is reached, the motivating factor becomes insignificant. If the community health approach is embraced by all, conflict with public health can be minimized and perhaps eliminated.

Competition in health care is a reality with which community health practice must cope. Although competition offers several benefits, it poses some dilemmas for community health that may be difficult to resolve. Values underlying the competition model can be in direct conflict with several basic public health values (Scutchfield & Keck, 2009). With the new focus on coordination and collaboration in health care reform, this emphasis on competition may be diminished.

Public health is committed to serving all persons in need, regardless of ability to pay. Traditionally, the competition model has focused on individuals and has been oriented to the present. Public health is concerned with aggregates and is future oriented, emphasizing prevention. Competition establishes relatively fixed limits for service, whereas public health must remain flexible if it is to respond to the health needs of the entire population. These dramatic differences are beginning to blur and, out of necessity, will continue to be less adversarial and more collegial. By shifting their focus to community health as a systems outcome, health care insurers can create several positive changes, including a safe environment, wholesome nutrition, healthy lifestyle, adequate education, sufficient income, meaningful spirituality, challenging work, recreation, and functional families (Brownson et al., 2011).

If enrollees in health insurance programs like Medicare, Medicaid, or other MCOs become empowered to assume responsibility for their own self-care and wellbeing, a cooperative and collaborative relationship can be achieved. A nurse-directed diabetes management program at a county public health clinic in Los Angeles County reflects the potential benefits of PHSs for clients of MCOs and other private health care plans. PHNs were able to significantly reduce the numbers of urgent care and ER visits, along with hospitalizations, for diabetic patients from a minority population (Davidson, Ansari, & Karlan, 2007). Working together, better health can be achieved for large numbers of patients.

Along with philosophical differences, other constraints exist, such as civil service restrictions and political influences, under which most public health agencies must operate and that make it difficult for them to compete. Likewise, MCOs have stockholders, boards of directors, employees, and state and federal regulations that they must satisfy. Public health agencies must remain committed to providing the health promotion and disease prevention services that are their public trust. This may become the commitment of MCOs as they see the cost savings and health benefits of disease prevention. Competition also may stimulate new and innovative community health services and the introduction of new roles and revenue sources for traditional public health agencies. The evolution of the reform of health care implementation may see developing public and private health care partnerships, with MCOs contracting with public health agencies for certain services and MCOs more effectively expanding the reach of public health agencies into the suburbs or rural areas. Reform will need to continue to address issues affecting the delivery of PHSs.

IMPLICATIONS FOR COMMUNITY HEALTH NURSING

The structure and functions of the health care delivery system, as well as particular legislative acts, have had a significant impact on community health nursing. Community health nurses have had to adapt to a constantly changing system. They have developed innovative modes of service delivery, such as community-based nursing centers for health education, counseling, and screening of low-income populations. They have learned to practice in a variety of settings extending beyond homes, worksites, schools, churches, clinics, and voluntary agencies. They have acquired skills in teamwork, leadership, and political activism. They have recognized the importance of outcomes research to document the value of nursing interventions with at-risk populations.

At the national, state, and local level, community health nursing has important ties to both private and public health agencies. Either type of organization may employ community and PHNs. When serving in the public sector, they often provide consultation, serve on boards, volunteer their services, or collaborate with private sector health organizations to ensure quality and access of care to the broader community. Examples include joint efforts to promote certain types of health legislation and collaboration to produce and disseminate health education materials targeting specific populations. Sometimes, community health nursing services operate within a single organization that combines public and private sector organization and funding. An example is the Metropolitan Visiting Nurse Association of Minneapolis, Minnesota, which is a combined public–private agency supported by taxes and voluntary funds.

Community health nurses also have many opportunities to serve in international health. Some work with the WHO, PAHO, or other agencies to assist in direct care projects such as famine relief, immunization efforts, or nutritional screening and education programs (see Chapter 16). Other nurses serve as health planners, assist with policy development, conduct collaborative needs assessment projects and research efforts, or engage in program development.

SUMMARY

Many factors and events have influenced the current structure, function, and financing of community health services. Understanding this background gives the community health nurse a stronger base for planning for the health of the population under her care.

Historically, health care has progressed unevenly, marked by numerous influences. Primitive practices of early centuries were replaced with more advanced sanitary measures by the Greeks and Romans. The Middle Ages saw a serious health decline in Europe, with raging epidemics leading to extensive 19th-century reform efforts in England and, later, in the United States.

Organized health care in the United States developed slowly. Public health problems, such as the need for isolation of persons with communicable diseases and control of environmental pollution, prompted the gradual development of official interventions. For example, quarantines to control the spread of communicable disease were imposed in the late 1700s. Sanitary reform was pursued more vigorously during the 1800s. Local and then state health departments were formed starting in the late 1700s. By the early 1900s, the federal government had assumed a more active role in public health, with a proliferation of health, education, and welfare services.

For years, efforts to address community health needs have been made by public agencies and private individuals. These two arms of service were not well coordinated in the past. Only gradually and recently have they begun to work together to form an emerging health care system.

The public arm of health services includes all government, tax-supported health agencies and occurs at four levels: local, state, national, and international. Each level deals with the health needs of the population encompassed within its boundaries. Each level has a different structure and set of functions. PHSs include three core public health functions: assessment, policy development, and assurance.

Private health services are the unofficial arm of the community health system. They include voluntary nonprofit agencies as well as privately owned (proprietary) and for-profit agencies. Their financial support comes from voluntary contributions, bequests, or fees. Private health organizations often supplement and complement the work of official agencies.

The delivery and financing of community health services has been significantly affected by various legislative acts. These acts have prompted such innovations as health insurance and assistance for the poor, the elderly, and the disabled; money to train health personnel and conduct health research; standards for health planning and delivery; health protection for workers on the job; and the financing of health services.

Health care economics studies the production, distribution, and consumption of health care goods and services to maximize the use of scarce resources to benefit the most people. This science underlies the financing of the health care system. It is influenced by microeconomics as well as macroeconomics.

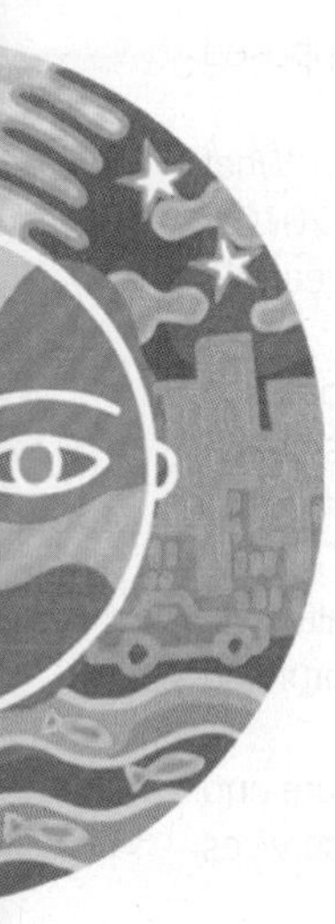

Health care is funded through public and private sources, which fall into three categories: third-party payers, direct consumer payment, and private support. Health care services have been reimbursed either retrospectively, typical of FFS plans, or prospectively, typical of most HMOs.

Several trends and issues have influenced community health care financing and delivery and are important in understanding health care economics and helping to improve community health. They include cost control, financial access, managed care, health care rationing, competition and regulation, managed competition, universal coverage, a single-payer system, and health care reform.

The changing nature of health care financing has adversely affected community health and its practice in three important ways: (1) retrospective payment without limiting costs, tax-deductible employer contributions for health care coverage, and nontaxable employee health benefits, together with a lack of consumer involvement in cost sharing, have created disincentives for efficient use of

resources; (2) because the health care system traditionally has reimbursed only for treatment of the ill or disabled, with no reward for health promotion and prevention efforts, it has promoted incentives to focus only on illness care; and (3) the competition model, which has long driven up health care costs and eliminated many from being able to afford health care services, has generated a conflict with the basic public health values of health promotion and disease prevention for all persons. Health care reform has been passed and should improve access for many Americans, but the United States remains the only industrialized nation without some type of universal health coverage. We also rank significantly lower than most other developed countries on health indicators, such as infant mortality and life expectancy.

Public health nurses can lead the effort in making health care more accessible to all citizens and encourage policies and practices that promote health, rather than reward illness.

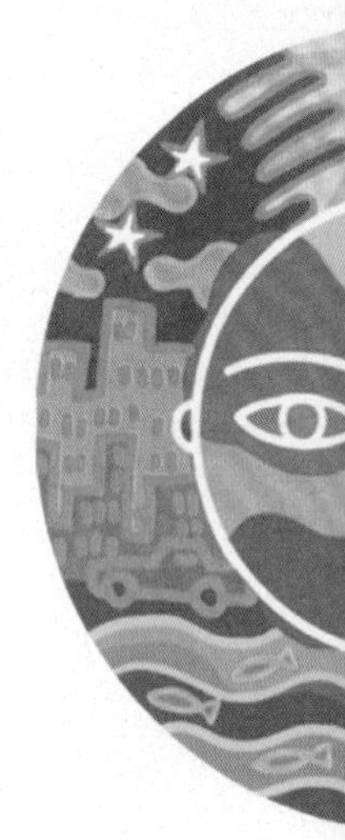

ACTIVITIES TO PROMOTE **CRITICAL THINKING**

1. If possible, interview someone at your local health department. How do the services offered compare with those listed in this chapter? How do PHNs in this agency incorporate the core public health functions?
2. Look up your state health department's Website. Compare its functions with the core public health functions described in this chapter. Identify areas where improvement may be needed.
3. If possible, conduct an interview onsite or by telephone with someone at a private health agency, voluntary agency, or community-based nongovernmental organization (or NGO). Compare the agency's functions with those listed in this chapter for private health agencies. Describe how this agency works collaboratively with public health agencies and other community organizations. What is the role of the nurse in this agency? How does the role compare to PHNs in the local public health agency?
4. Look up various international health agencies online. Explore Websites that discuss current international health care issues. What topics are of current concern? For example, are new epidemics or emerging strains of a virus being highlighted? What could (or should) a community health nurse in your local community do with this information?
5. With your classmates, debate the pros and cons of a strong federal role in health care provision, as opposed to decentralized (state and local) control.
6. Interview two consumers about their perception of the problems and strengths of our health care system. What are their thoughts and feelings about health care reform (the Affordable Care Act (ACA) enacted in 2010)? Select people who represent distinctly different age groups and life situations, such as a single 25-year-old mother of three children making minimum wage and a 75-year-old widower.
7. Form two teams and debate the advantages and disadvantages of managed competition as opposed to mandatory universal coverage. What are the advantages and disadvantages of a single-payer system? Is health care reform feasible in the United States? What is the most efficient way of ensuring universal coverage, as evidenced by other countries?
8. Locate recent articles and legislation on health care reform, strengths and weakness of the public health system, and the uninsured population. What are the most common themes on each issue? What most surprised you about your results?
9. Talk with your classmates and other students at your college or university about their access to health care and if they have some type of health insurance. Does your campus have a student health center? What services are offered there? What are the average costs to students?

REFERENCES

Abrams, S. E. (2004). From function to competency in public health nursing, 1931 to 2003. *Public Health Nursing, 21*(5), 507–510.

Adams, M. (2006). Health care economics: Diseases are too profitable to prevent or cure. *News Target*. Retrieved from http://www.newstarget.com/z019475.html

Adams, A. (2011, August 4). *Guidance issued on community health needs assessments for exempt hospitals*. Health Care Reform Insights. Retrieved from http://www.healthcarereforminsights.com/2011/08/04/guidance-issued-on-community-health-needs-assessments-for-exempt-hospitals/

Aday, L. A. (Ed.). (2005). *Reinventing public health: Policies and practices for a healthy nation*. San Francisco, CA: Jossey-Bass.

Administration for Children & Families. U.S. Department of Health & Human Services. (2008). *Office of Family Assistance (OFA): What is the Temporary Assistance for Needy Families (TANF) program?* Retrieved from http://www.acf.hhs.gov/opa/fact_sheets/tanf_factsheet.html

American Medical Association (AMA). (2007). *Competition in health insurance: A comprehensive study of U.S. markets: 2007 update*. Retrieved from http://www.ama-assn.org/ama1/pub/upload/mm/368/compstudy_52006.pdf

American Nurses Association (ANA). (2008, February). *ANA's health system reform agenda*. Retrieved from http://ana.nursingworld.org/MainMenuCategories/HealthcareandPolicyIssues/HealthSystemReform/Agenda/ANAsHealthSystemReformAgenda.aspx

American Public Health Association (APHA). (2010, March 15). *APHA strongly supports Congressional efforts to finalize comprehensive health reform this week*. Press Release. Retrieved from http://www.apha.org/about/news/pressreleases/2010/healthreform3_15.htm

Ameringer, C. F. (2008). *The health care revolution: From medical monopoly to market competition*. Berkeley, CA: University of California Press.

Arrow, K. (2004). Uncertainty and the welfare economics of medical care. *Bulletin of the World Health Organization, 82*(2), 141–149. Retrieved from http://www.who.int/bulletin/volume/82/2/PHCBP.pdf

Arrow, K., Auerbach, A., Bertko, J., Brownlee, S., Casalino, J., Cooper, F. J., et al. (2009). Toward a 21st-century health care system: Recommendations for health care reform. *Annals of Internal Medicine, 150*(7), 493–495.

Baker, T. (2005). *The medical malpractice myth*. Chicago, IL: University of Chicago Press.

Barry, M. A., Centra, L., Pratt, D., & Gioradano, L. (1998). *Where do the dollars go? Measuring local public health expenditures*. Washington, DC: National Association of County and City Health Officials.

Beaglehole, R., & Bonita, R. (Eds.). (2009). *Global public health: A new era* (2nd ed.). New York: Oxford University Press.

Bernard, D., Banthin, J., & Encinosa, W. (2009). Wealth, income, and the affordability of health insurance. *Health Affairs, 28*(3), 887–896.

Bindman, A, Chattopadhyay, A., & Auerback, G. (2008). Interruptions in Medicaid coverage and risk for hospitalization for ambulatory care-sensitive conditions. *Annals of Internal Medicine, 149*(12), 854–860.

Brett, A. S. (2009). "American values"—a smoke screen in the debate on health care reform. *New England Journal of Medicine, 361*, 440–441.

Briesacher, B. A., Ross-Degnan, D., Wagner, A., Fouayzi, H., Zhang, F., Gurwitz, J., et al. (2010). Out-of-pocket burden of health care spending and the adequacy of the Medicare Part D low-income subsidy. *Medical Care, 48*(6), 503–509.

Blendon, R., Brodie, M., Benson, J., Altman, D. E., Buhr, T. (2006). Americans' views of health care costs, access, and quality. *Millbank Quarterly, 84*(4), 623–657.

Brookings Institution. (2012). *Government's greatest achievements of the past half century*. Retrieved from http://www.brookings.edu/papers/2000/11governance_light.aspx

Brownson, R. C., Baker, E., Leet, T., Gillespie, K., & True, W. (2011). *Evidence-based public health* (2nd ed.). New York: Oxford University Press.

Bureau of Labor Statistics. (n.d.). *Definitions of health insurance terms*. Retrieved from http://www.bls.gov/ncs/ebs/sp/healthterms.pdf

Callahan, D. (2008). Healthcare costs and medical technology. *The Hastings Center*. Retrieved from http://www.thehastingscenter.org/Publications/BriefingBook/Detail.aspx?id=2178

Callahan, D. (2009). *Taming the beloved beast: How medical technology costs are destroying our health care system*. Princeton, NJ: Princeton University Press.

Caswell, K. J., & O'Hara, B. (2010). *Medical out-of-pocket expenses, poverty, and the uninsured*. SEHSD Working Paper 2010-17. Washington, DC: U.S. Census Bureau. Retrieved from http://www.census.gov/hhes/povmeas/methodology/supplemental/research/Caswell-OHara-SGE2011.pdf

Cauchi, R. (2012, January 27). *State legislation and actions challenging certain health reforms, 2011-2012*. National Conference of State Legislatures. Retrieved from http://www.ncsl.org/issues-research/health/state-laws-and-actions-challenging-aca.aspx

CBS Los Angeles. (2011, March 8). *L.A. County OKs $50M for new King-Harbor Hospital*. Retrieved from http://losangeles.cbslocal.com/2011/03/08/la-county-to-spend-50m-on-new-king-harbor-hospital/

CBS News. (2011, November 7). *Raised government estimates show new poverty high*. Retrieved from http://www.cbsnews.com/8301-201_162-57319633/revised-govt-estimates-show-new-poverty-high/

Centers for Disease Control & Prevention (CDC). (1991). Health objectives for the nation consensus set of health status indicators for the general assessment of community health status: United States. *Morbidity Mortality Weekly Report, 40*(27), 449–451.

Centers for Disease Control & Prevention (CDC). (2011). *CDC timeline*. Retrieved from http://www.cdc.gov/about/history/timeline.htm

Centers for Medicare & Medicaid Services (CMS). (2011). *History overview*. Retrieved from https://www.cms.gov/history/

Centers for Medicare & Medicaid Services (CMS). (n.d. a). *The nation's health dollar ($2.5 trillion) calendar year 2009: Where it went*. Retrieved from https://www.cms.gov/nationalhealthexpenddata/downloads/PieChartSourcesExpenditures2009.pdf

Centers for Medicare & Medicaid Services (CMS). (n.d. b). *National health expenditures 2009 highlights*. Retrieved from https://www.cms.gov/nationalhealthexpenddata/downloads/highlights.pdf

Children's Defense Fund. (2011). *Medicaid myths and facts*. Retrieved from http://www.childrensdefense.org/child-research-data-publications/data/medicaid-myths-and-facts.pdf

Clifton, G. L. (2009). *Flatlined: Resuscitating American medicine*. New Brunswick, NJ: Rutgers University Press.

Cockayne, E. (2007). *Hubbub, filth, noise stench in England 1600–1770*. New Haven, CT: Yale University Press.

Collins, S. (2007). Congressional testimony: Universal health insurance: Why it is essential to a high performing health system and why design matters. *The Commonwealth Fund*. Retrieved from http://www.commonwealthfund.org/Publications/Testimonies/2007/Nov/Congressional-Testimony–Widening-Gaps-in-Health-Insurance-Coverage-in-the-United-States–The-Need-f.aspx

Collins, S. R., Schoen, C., Davis, K., Gauthier, A. K., & Schoenbaum, S. C. (2007, October). *A roadmap to health insurance for all: Principles for reform*. The Commonwealth Fund. Retrieved from http://www.commonwealthfund.org/usr_doc/Collins_roadmaphltinsforall_1066.pdf?section=4039

Collins, S. R., Doty, M. M., Robertson, R., & Garber, T. (2011). Help on the horizon: How the recession has left missions of workers without health insurance and how health reform will bring relief. *The Commonwealth Fund*. Retrieved from http://www.commonwealthfund.org/~/media/Files/Publications/Fund%20Report/2011/Mar/1486_Collins_help_on_the_horizon_2010_biennial_survey_report_FINAL_v2.pdf

Colliver, V. (2011, March 22). *Anthem Blue Cross pulls back on planned rate hikes*. Retrieved from http://articles.sfgate.com/2011-03-22/bay-area/29173287_1_anthem-increases-rate-increases-individual-california-policyholders

Congressional Budget Office. (2005, May). *High-cost Medicare beneficiaries*. Retrieved from http://www.cbo.gov/ftpdocs/63xx/doc6332/05-03-MediSpending.pdf

Congressional Budget Office. (2009). *The long-term outlook for Medicare, Medicaid, and total health care spending.* Retrieved from http://www.cbo.gov/ftpdocs/102xx/doc10297/Chapter2.5.1.shtml#1091397

Consumer Reports. (2008, July). *New market for card companies.* Retrieved from http://www.consumerreports.org/health/insurance/cr-investigates-medical-debt/card-companies-dig-in/medical-debt-card-companies-dig-in.htm

Crist, J. (2010). Never say never: "Never events" in Medicare. *Health Matrix: Journal of Law-Medicine, 20,* 437.

Cunningham, P., & O'Malley, A. (2009). Do reimbursement delays discourage Medicaid participation by physicians? *Health Affairs, 28*(1), 1–28.

Cunningham, P. J., & May, J. H. (2006, March). A growing hole in the safety net: Physician charity care declines again. *Center for Studying Health System Change.* Tracking Report, No. 13.

Cutler, D. M. (2005). *Your money or your life: Strong medicine for America's health care system.* New York: Oxford University Press.

Davidson, M., Ansari, A., & Karlan, V. (2007). Effect of a nurse-directed diabetes disease management program on urgent care/emergency room visits and hospitalizations in a minority population. *Diabetes Care, 30*(2), 224–227.

Daschle, T., Greenberger, S., & Lambrew, J. (2008). *Critical: What we can do about the health care crisis.* New York: St. Martin's Press.

deChesnay, M., & Anderson, B. A. (2012). *Caring for the vulnerable: Perspectives in nursing theory, practice, and research* (3rd ed.). Burlington, MA: Jones & Bartlett Learning.

Docteur, E., & Berenson, R. A. (2009, August). How does the quality of U.S. health care compare internationally? *Urban Institute.* Retrieved from http://www.urban.org/uploadedpdf/411947_ushealthcare_quality.pdf

Doctors Without Borders. (2011). *About us: History and principles.* Retrieved from http://www.doctorswithoutborders.org/aboutus/?ref=main-menu

Donley, R., Flaherty, M. J., Sarsfield, E., et al. (2003). The nursing shortage: What does the Nurse Reinvestment Act mean to you? *Online Journal of Issues in Nursing, 8*(1) [manuscript 5]. Retrieved from http://www.nursingworld.org/MainMenuCategories/ANAMarketplace/ANAPeriodicals/OJIN/TableofContents/Volume82003/No1Jan2003/ArticlesPreviousTopics/NurseReinvestmentAct.html

Dowling, W. L. (1979). Prospective rate setting: Concept and practice. *Topics in Health Care Financing, 3*(2), 35–42.

Dranove, D. (2003). *What's your life worth? Health care rationing: Who lives, who dies, who decides.* Upper Saddle River, NJ: Financial Times Prentice-Hall.

Dranove, D. (2008). *Code red: An economist explains how to revive the healthcare system without destroying it.* Princeton, NJ: Princeton University Press.

Drevdahl, D. (2002). Social justice or market justice? The paradoxes of public health partnerships with managed care. *Public Health Nursing, 19*(3), 161–169.

Duffy, J. (1990). *The sanitarians: A history of American public health.* Urbana, IL: University of Illinois Press.

Duffy, R., Chen, D., & Sampson, N. (1998). History of federal legislation in health professions educational assistance in dental public health, 1956–1997. *Journal of Public Health Dentistry, 58*(S1), 84–89.

Dutton, P. V. (2007). *Differential diagnosis: A comparative history of health care problems and solutions in the United States and France.* Ithaca, NY: Cornell University Press.

Employee Benefit Research Institute. (2009). Health plan differences: Fully-insured vs. self-insured. *Fast Facts #114.* Retrieved from http://www.ebri.org/pdf/FFE114.11Feb09.Final.pdf

Encyclopedia of Public Health. (2011). Nongovernmental organizations, United States. Retrieved from http://www.enotes.com/public-health-encyclopedia/nongovernmental-organizations-united-states

Enthoven, A. C. (2009a, July 3). Building a health marketplace that works. *Health Affairs Blog.* Retrieved from http://healthaffairs.org/blog/2009/07/31/building-a-health-marketplace-that-works/

Enthoven, A. C. (2009b, December). Integrated delivery systems: The cure for fragmentation. *The American Journal of Managed Care, 15,* s284–s290.

Enthoven, A. C., & Wynand, P. M. (2007). Going Dutch: Managed-competition health insurance in the Netherlands. *New England Journal of Medicine, 357,* 2421–2423.

Feldman, M., Hile, S., & Weinberg, G. (2011). A community needs assessment to inform HIV and substance abuse prevention services for Black and Latino young men who have sex with men in New York City. *Journal of Gay Lesbian Social Services, 23*(4), 465–506.

FirstStep. (n.d.). *State Children's Health Insurance Program.* Retrieved from http://www.cms.gov/apps/firststep/content/schip-qas.html

Food and Agriculture Organization (FAO). (2011). *About FAO.* Retrieved from http://www.fao.org/about/en/

Friedman, J. N. (2009, December 3). *Predicting Medicare cost growth.* Harvard University. Retrieved from http://www.hks.harvard.edu/fs/jfriedm/medgrowth.pdf

Fronstin, P., & MacDonald, J. (2008). Consumer-driven health plans: Are they working? *The Wall Street Journal.* Retrieved from http://online.wsj.com/ad/employeebenefits-consumer_driven_plans.html

Frontline. (2008, April 15). *Sick around the world: Five capitalist democracies and how they do it.* Public Broadcasting System (PBS). Retrieved from http://www.pbs.org/wgbh/pages/frontline/sickaroundtheworld/countries/

Gabel, J. R., Pickreign, J. D., & Whitmore, H. H. (2006, December). *Behind the slow growth of employer-based consumer-driven health plans.* [Issue brief No. 107]. Retrieved from http://www.hschange.org/CONTENT/900/?PRINT=1

Galewitz, P. (2010, November 12). Medicaid managed care programs grow: so do issues. *USA Today.* Retrieved from http://www.usatoday.com/money/industries/health/2010-11-12-medicaid12_CV_N.htm

Galewitz, P. (2011, June 1). Medicaid to stop paying for hospital mistakes. *Kaiser Health News.* Retrieved from http://www.kaiserhealthnews.org/Stories/2011/June/01/medicaid-hospital-medical-error-payment-short-take.aspx

Gardner, A. (2007, February 21). US health care costs to top $4 trillion by 2016. *The Washington Post.* Retrieved http://www.washingtonpost.com/wp-dyn/content/article/2007/02/21/AR2007022100524.html

Gengler, A. (2011, November 1). *Solving the new Medicare puzzle.* CNN Money. Retrieved from http://money.cnn.com/2011/11/01/pf/medicare_plans.moneymag/

Gerencher, K. (2008, July 13). *Americans down on the U.S. health-care system.* Retrieved from http://www.marketwatch.com/story/americans-rate-us-health-care-system-lowest-among-10-nations

Gilbert, R. E. (2008). Eisenhower's 1955 heart attack: Medical treatment, political effects, and the "behind the scenes" leadership style. *Politics and the Life Sciences, 27*(1), 2–21.

Girouard, J. E. (2009, October 12). *Capitalist case for non-profit health insurance.* Retrieved from http://www.forbes.com/2009/10/12/public-health-insurance-personal-finance-financial-advisor-network-blue-shield.html

Gladwell, M. (2005, August 29). The moral-hazard myth. *The New Yorker.* Retrieved from http://www.newyorker.com/archive/2005/08/29/050829fa_fact

Goldman, D. P., Joyce, G. F., & Karaca-Mandic, P. (2006). Varying pharmacy benefits with clinical status: The case of cholesterol-lowering therapy. *The American Journal of Managed Care, 12*(1), 21–28.

Grad, F. P. (2002). The preamble of the constitution of the World Health Organization. *Bulletin of the World Health Organization, 80*(12), 981–984.

Graham, J. (2008, November 5). Medicare's "non-payment" policy for errors: A closer look. *Chicago Tribune. Triage: Making sense of health care.* Retrieved from http://newsblogs.chicagotribune.com/triage/2008/11/medicares-non-p.html

Greene, V. W. (2001). Personal hygiene and life expectancy improvements since 1850: Historic and epidemiologic associations. *American Journal of Infection Control, 29*(4), 203–206.

Greenhouse, S., & Abelson, R. (2011, October 20). Wal-Mart cuts some health care benefits. *The New York Times.* Retrieved from http://www.nytimes.com/2011/10/21/business/wal-mart-cuts-some-health-care-benefits.html?pagewanted=all

Guyatt, G., Devereaux, J., Lexchin, S., Stone, S., Yalnizyan, M., Himmelstein, D., et al. (2007). A systematic review of studies comparing health outcomes in Canada and the United States. *Open Medicine, 1*(1), e27–e36.

Hammond, W. E. (2009). Realizing the potential of healthcare information technology to enhance global health. *Studies in Health Technology Informatics, 150*, 8–13.

Hadley, J., Holahan, J., Coughlin, T., & Miller, D. (2008). Covering the uninsured in 2008: Current costs, sources of payment, and incremental costs. *Health Affairs*, doi: 10.1377/hlthaff.27.5w399.

Harmon, K. (2009, August 10). Deaths from avoidable medical error more than double in past decade, investigation shows. *Scientific American: News Blog*. Retrieved from http://www.scientificamerican.com/blog/post.cfm?id=deaths-from-avoidable-medical-error-2009-08-10

Harrington, C., & Estes, C. L. (2008). *Health policy & nursing: Crisis reform in the US healthcare delivery system* (5th ed.). Sudbury, MA: Jones & Bartlett Publishers.

Healthcare.gov. (2011). *Key features of the Affordable Care Act, by year.* Retrieved from http://www.healthcare.gov/law/timeline/full.html

HealthReform.gov. (2010, October 20). *Fact sheet: Affordable Care Act's new Patient's Bill of Rights*. Retrieved from http://www.healthreform.gov/newsroom/new_patients_bill_of_rights.html

Hecker, J. F. C. (1839). *The epidemics of the Middle Ages*. London, UK: Trubner and Company.

Heijink, R., vanBaal, P., Oppe, M., Koolman, X., & Westert, G. (2011). Decomposing cross-country differences in quality-adjusted life expectancy: The impact of value sets. *Population Health Metrics*, 9(17), 1–11.

Henig, J. (2009, March 10). *Uninsured U.S. citizens*. Retrieved from http://www.factcheck.org/2009/03/uninsured-us-citizens/

Herzlinger, R. (2007). *Who killed health care? America's $2 trillion medical problem—and the consumer-driven cure*. New York: McGraw-Hill.

Heskett, J. (2007, March 2). What is the government's role in US healthcare? *Harvard Business School (HBS) Working Knowledge for Business Leaders*. Retrieved from http://hbswk.hbs.edu/item/5645.html

Himmelstein, D., Warren, E., Thorne, D., & Woolhandler, S. (2005). Market Watch: Illness and injury as contributors to bankruptcy. *Health Affairs*. Doi: 10.1377/hlthaff.w5.63. Retrieved from http://content.healthaffairs.org/content/early/2005/02/02/hlthaff.w5.63.full.pdf+html

Himmelstein, D., & Woolhandler, S. (2007). Massachusetts' approach to universal coverage: High hopes and faulty economic logic. *International Journal of Health Services, 37*(2), 251–257.

Himmelstein, D. A., Thorne, D., Warren, E., & Woolhandler, S. (2009). Bankruptcy in the US, 2007: Results of a national study. *American Journal of Medicine, 122*(8), 741–746.

Hoadley, J., Summer, L., Hargrave, E., Cubanski, J., & Newman, T. (2011). *Analysis of Medicare prescription drug plans in 2011 and key trends since 2006*. Kaiser Family Foundation. Retrieved from http://www.kff.org/medicare/upload/8237.pdf

Holahan, J., & Garrett, B. (2010, March). *The cost of uncompensated care with and without health reform*. Urban Institute. Retrieved from http://www.urban.org/UploadedPDF/412045_cost_of_uncompensated.pdf

Institute of Medicine. (1988). *The future of public health*. Washington, DC: National Academies Press.

Institute of Medicine. (2001). *Crossing the quality chasm: A new health system for the 21st century*. Washington, DC: National Academies Press.

Institute of Medicine. (2002). *The future of the public's health in the 21st century*. Washington, DC: National Academies Press.

Jaquish, C. E. (2007). The Framingham Heart Study: On it's way to becoming the gold standard for cardiovascular genetic epidemiology? *BMC Medical Genetics, 8*, 63.

Kaiser Commission on Medicaid & the Uninsured. (2011). *The uninsured and the difference health insurance makes*. Retrieved from http://www.kff.org/uninsured/upload/1420-13.pdf

Kaiser Family Foundation (KFF). (n.d.). *Hospital adjusted expenses per patient day, 2009*. Retrieved from http://www.statehealthfacts.org/comparemaptable.jsp?yr=92&typ=4&ind=273&cat=5&sub=68&sortc=1&o=a

Kaiser Family Foundation (KFF). (2008). *How non-group health coverage varies with income*. Retrieved from http://www.kff.org/insurance/upload/7737.pdf

Kaiser Family Foundation (KFF). (2010a). *Medicaid and the uninsured*. Retrieved from http://www.kff.org/medicaid/upload/7235-04.pdf

Kaiser Family Foundation (KFF). (2010b, June). *Focus on health reform: Health reform implementation timeline*. Retrieved from http://www.kff.org/healthreform/upload/8060.pdf

Kaiser Family Foundation (KFF). (2010c, August). *Explaining health reform: Eligibility and enrollment processes for Medicaid, CHIP, and subsidies in the exchanges*. Retrieved from http://www.kff.org/healthreform/upload/8090.pdf

Kaiser Family Foundation (KFF). (2011a). *Employer health benefits, 2011 annual survey*. Retrieved from http://ehbs.kff.org/pdf/2011/8225.pdf

Kaiser Family Foundation (KFF). (2011b). *Hospital adjusted expenses per inpatient day, 2009*. Retrieved from http://www.statehealthfacts.org/comparemaptable.jsp?ind=273&cat=5

Kaiser Family Foundation (KFF). (2011c, March). *Medicaid matters: Understanding Medicaid's role in our health care system*. Retrieved from http://www.kff.org/medicaid/upload/8165.pdf

Kaiser Family Foundation (KFF). (2011d, April). *Health care spending in the United States and selected OECD countries*. Retrieved from http://www.kff.org/insurance/snapshot/OECD042111.cfm

Kaiser Family Foundation (KFF). (2011e, September). *Medicare spending and financing*. KFF Program on Medicare Policy. Retrieved from http://www.kff.org/medicare/upload/7305-06.pdf

Kaiser Family Foundation (KFF). (2012, January). *Explaining health care reform: How will the Affordable Care Act affect small businesses and their employees?* Retrieved from http://www.kff.org/healthreform/upload/8275.pdf

Kaiser Family Foundation & Health Research and Educational Trust. (2011). *Employer health benefits 2011 annual survey*. Retrieved from http://ehbs.kff.org/pdf/2011/8225.pdf

Kaiser Health News. (2011). *Chart: Change in total Medicaid spending and enrollment, 1998-2011*. Retrieved from http://www.kaiserhealthnews.org/graphics/2010/093010-change-in-total-medicaid-spending.aspx

Kavilanz, P. (2011, May 11). *Your family's health care costs: $19,393*. Retrieved from http://money.cnn.com/2011/05/11/news/economy/healthcare_costs_family/index.htm

Keehan, S., Sisko, A., Truffer, C., Poisal, J., Cuckler, G. A., Madison, A. J. et al. (2011). National health spending projections through 2020: Economic recovery and reform drive faster spending growth. *Health Affairs, 30*(8), 1594–1605.

Kelly, A. M., & Cronin, P. (2011). Rationing and health care reform: Not a question of if, but when. *Journal of the American College of Radiology, 8*(12), 830–837.

Kemp, A., Roughead, E., Preen, D., Glover, J., & Semmens, J. (2010). Determinants of self-reported medicine underuse due to cost: a comparison of seven countries. *Journal of Health Services Research & Policy, 15*(2), 106–114.

Kerr, M. (2009, July 15). Nearly one fifth of emergency department visits are by the uninsured. *Medscape Medical News*. Retrieved from http://www.medscape.com/viewarticle/705973

Khan, H. (2011, May 12). *Has Mitt Romney's Massachusetts health care law worked?* ABC News. Retrieved from http://abcnews.go.com/blogs/politics/2011/05/has-mitt-romneys-massachusetts-health-care-law-worked/

Khoury, C., & Brown, I. (2009, March 31). *Among OECD nations, U.S. lags in personal health*. Retrieved from http://www.gallup.com/poll/117205/americans-not-feeling-health-benefits-high-spending.aspx

Kimbuende, E., Ranji, U., Lundy, J., & Salganicoff, A. (2010). U.S. healthcare costs. *Kaiser Family Foundation*. Retrieved from http://www.kaiseredu.org/Issue-Modules/US-Health-Care-Costs/Background-Brief.aspx

Klein, E. (2007, November 2). Ten reasons why American health care is so bad. *The American Prospect*. Retrieved from http://prospect.org/article/ten-reasons-why-american-health-care-so-bad

Klein, E. (2011, January 11). The Affordable Care Act in one table. *The Washington Post*. Retrieved from http://voices.washingtonpost.com/ezra-klein/2011/01/the_affordable_care_act_in_one.html

Klein, H. S. (2010). *The Atlantic slave trade: New approaches to the Americas* (2nd ed.). New York: Cambridge University Press.

Klevens, R. M., Edwards, J. R., Richards, C. L., Horan, T. C., Gaynes, R. P., Pollock, D.A., et al. (2007). Estimating health care-associated infections and deaths in U.S. hospitals, 2002. *Public Health Reports, 122*, 160–166.

Kovner, A. R., & Knickman, J. R. (Eds.). (2011). *Jonas & Kovner's health care delivery in the United States* (10th ed.). New York: Springer Publishing Company.

Kritz, F. (2009, February 9). Facts about the expanded State Children's Health Insurance Program. *Los Angeles Times*. Retrieved from http://articles.latimes.com/2009/feb/09/health/he-yourmoney9

Krugman, P. (2009, July 25). Why markets can't cure healthcare. *The New York Times: The Opinion Pages*. Retrieved from http://krugman.blogs.nytimes.com/2009/07/25/why-markets-cant-cure-healthcare/

Krugman, P. (2011, September 16). Free to die. *The New York Times*, A29.

Ku, L., MacTaggart, P., Pervez, F., & Rosenbaum, S. (2009, July). *Improving Medicaid's continuity of coverage and quality of care*. Washington, DC: Association for Community Affiliated Plans.

Kvinta, B. (2011). Quarantine powers, biodefense, and Andrew Speaker. *Journal of Biosecurity, Biosafety, and Biodefense Law, 1*(1), article 5.

Landon, B., Schneider, E., Normand, S., Scholle, S., Pawlson, L. G., Epstein A. M. (2007). Quality of care in Medicaid managed care and commercial health plans. *The Journal of the American Medical Association, 298*(14), 1674–1681.

Landwehr, C. (2009). Deciding how to decide: The case of health care rationing. *Public Administration, 87*(3), 586–603.

Lee, L., Teutsch, S., Thacker, S., & St. Louis, M. (Eds.). (2010). *Principles and practice of public health surveillance* (3rd ed.). New York: Oxford University Press.

Levin, P., Cary, A., Kulbok, P., Leffers, J., Molle, M., & Polivka, B. (2008). Graduate education for advanced practice public health nursing: At the crossroads. *Public Health Nursing, 25*(2), 176–193.

Levinson, D. R. (2010, November). *Adverse events in hospitals: National incidence among Medicare beneficiaries*. Washington, DC: US Department of Health & Human Services, Office of Inspector General.

Lewis, R. A. (1952). *Edwin Chadwick and the public health movement, 1832–1854*. New York: Longman's.

Lichtenberg, F. R. (2009). *The quality of medical care, behavioral risk factors, and longevity growth* (Working Paper No. 15068). Cambridge, MA: The National Bureau of Economic Research.

Lindemann, M. (2010). *Medicine and society in early modern Europe* (2nd ed.). New York: Cambridge University Press.

Litow, M. E. (2006). Medicare vs. private health insurance: The cost of administration. *Milliman*. Retrieved from http://www.cahi.org/cahi_contents/resources/pdf/CAHIMedicareTechnicalPaper.pdf

Managed Care Online (MCOL). (2007). *National managed care enrollment, 2006*. Retrieved from http://www.mcareol.com/factshts/mcolfact.htm

Managed Care Online (MCOL). (2012). *National HMO enrollment, 2010*. Retrieved from http://www.mcareol.com/factshts/factnati.htm

Markovich, M. (2003). The rise of HMOs. RAND Dissertation. Retrieved from http://www.rand.org/pubs/rgs_dissertations/RGSD172.html

McCloud, L., & Dwyer, R. (2011). The fragile American: Hardship and financial troubles in the 21st century. *The Sociological Quarterly, 52*(1), 13–35.

McNerney, W. J. (1980). Control of health care costs in the 1980s. *The New England Journal of Medicine, 303*, 1088–1095.

McWilliams, J., Meara, E., Zaslavsky, A., & Ayanian, J. (2009). Medicare spending for previously uninsured adults. *Annals of Internal Medicine, 151*(11), 757–769.

Meara, E., White, C., & Cutler, D. (2004). Trends in medical spending by age, 1963–2000. *Health Affairs, 23*(4), 176–183.

Medicare.gov. (2011, October 27). *Medicare premiums and coinsurance rates for 2012*. Retrieved from https://questions.medicare.gov/app/answers/detail/a_id/2309/~/medicare-premiums-and-coinsurance-rates-for-2012

Medicare.gov. (n.d.). *Medicare prescription drug coverage (Part D)*. Retrieved from http://www.medicare.gov/navigation/medicare-basics/medicare-benefits/part-d.aspx#CoverageGap

Melnick, G. A., Shen, Y., & Wu, V. Y. (2011). The increased concentration of health plan markets can benefit consumers through lower hospital prices. *Health Affairs, 30*(9), 1728–1733.

Mello, M., Chandra, A., Gawande, A., & Studdert, D. (2010). National costs of the medical liability system. *Health Affairs, 29*(9), 1569–1577.

Melosi, M. (2008). *The sanitary city: Environmental services in urban America from colonial times to the present (Abridged Ed.)*. Pittsburgh, PA: University of Pittsburgh Press.

Milbank Memorial Fund, the National Association of State Budget Officers & the Reforming States Group. (2005). *2002–2003 state health care expenditure report*. Retrieved from http://www.milbank.org/reports/05NASBO/NASBO2005.pdf

Miller, T. (2009, October 6). Comparing international health care systems. *PBS News Hour*. Retrieved from http://www.pbs.org/newshour/globalhealth/july-dec09/insurance_1006.html

Millett, C., Chattopadhyay, A., & Bindman, A. (2010). Unhealthy competition: Consequences of health plan choice in California Medicaid. *American Journal of Public Health, 100*(11), 2235–2240.

Milstein, A. (2009). Ending extra payment for "never events"—stronger incentives for patients' safety. *New England Journal of Medicine, 360*(23), 2388–2390.

Montini, T., Noble, A., & Stelfox, H. T. (2008). Content analysis of patient complaints. *International Journal for Quality in Health Care, 20*(6), 412–420.

Musumeci, M. (2012, July). *A guide to the Supreme Court's Affordable Care Act decision*. Focus on Healthcare Reform. Kaiser Family Foundation, Menlo Park, CA.

National Conference of State Legislatures (NCSL). (2011). Children's health insurance program (CHIP). Retrieved from http://www.ncsl.org/default.aspx?tabid=14510

National Committee on Vital and Health Statistics (NCVHS). (2000). *NCVHS 1949–1999: A history*. Retrieved from http://www.ncvhs.hhs.gov/50history.htm

National Institutes of Health. (2007). *Health manpower act. The NIH almanac: Legislative chronology*. Retrieved from http://www.nih.gov/about/almanac/historical/legislative_chronology.htm

National Library of Medicine. (2003). *Profiles in science: Regional medical programs collection*. Retrieved from http://profiles.nlm.nih.gov/RM/A/A/U/C/

Nelson, D. I. (2009). A short history of major changes in the U.S. health care system since 1994; costs, coverage and quality. *League of Women Voters*. Retrieved from http://lwvsfc.org/files/healthcare.history_of_changes.pdf

Newport, F. (2007, April 26). *Prescription for healing healthcare from the people*. Gallup News Service. Retrieved from http://www.gallup.com/poll/27322/prescription-healing-healthcare-from-people.aspx

Nicholas, L. H. (2009). *Medicare Advantage? The effects of managed care on quality of care*. Population Studies Center Research Report 09-672. Retrieved from http://www.psc.isr.umich.edu/pubs/pdf/rr09-672.pdf

Nikitas, D. M., Middaugh, D. J., & Aries, N. (Eds.). (2011). *Policy and politics for nurses and other health professionals*. Sudbury, MA: Jones & Bartlett Publishers.

Nunley, R. M. (2008). Issues facing America: Underinsured patients. *American Academy of Orthopaedic Surgeons*. Retrieved from http://www.aaos.org/news/aaosnow/mar08/reimbursement1.asp

Nyman, J. A. (2007). American health policy: Cracks in the foundation. *Journal of Health Politics, Policy and Law, 32*(5), 759–783.

Office of Civil Rights. (n.d.). *Health information privacy*. U.S. Department of Health & Human Services. Retrieved from http://www.hhs.gov/ocr/privacy/

Office of Inspector General. (1989). *The Family Support Act of 1988: What do frontline workers know? What do they think?* Department of Health & Human Services. Retrieved from http://oig.hhs.gov/oei/reports/oei-05-89-01220.pdf

Office of Inspector General. (2010). *Adverse events in hospitals: National incidence among Medicare beneficiaries*. Department of Health & Human Services. Retrieved from http://www.mhakeystonecenter.org/documents/january2011/tab_va_nov_2010_hhs_adverse_events_study.pdf

Ogilvie, M. (2007, July 13). *TB-infected man sued by plane passengers*. Toronto Star. Retrieved from http://www.thestar.com/article/235524

Organization for Economic Cooperation & Development (OECD). (2011). Health expenditure & financing: Health expenditure by financing agent. *OECD.StatExtracts*. Retrieved from http://stats.oecd.org/index.aspx?DataSetCode=HEALTH_STAT

Ornstein, C., Weber, T., & Leonard, J. (2007, August 11). King-Harbor fails final check, will close soon. *Los Angeles Times: Archives*. Retrieved from http://pqasb.pqarchiver.com/latimes/results.html?st=advanced&QryTxt=&type=current&sortby=RELEVANCE&datetype=0&frommonth=01&fromday=01&fromyear=1985&tomonth=10&today=20&toyear=2011&By=&Title=King-Harbor+fails+final+check&at_curr=ALL&Sect=ALL

Orszag, P. R., & Emanuel, E. J. (2010). Health care reform and cost control. *New England Journal of Medicine, 363*, 601–603.

Pan American Health Organization (PAHO). (2011a). *About PAHO*. Retrieved from http://new.paho.org/hq/index.php?option=com_content&task=view&id=91&Itemid=220

Pan American Health Organization (PAHO). (2011b). *PAHO publications*. Retrieved from http://new.paho.org/hq/index.php?option=com_content&task=view&id=1245&Itemid=1497

Pan American Health Organization. (2007). *Executive Summary: Health in the Americas*. Washington, DC: Author.

PBS. (n.d.). *Healthcare crisis: Healthcare timeline*. Retrieved from http://www.pbs.org/healthcarecrisis/history.htm

Pear, R. (2009, February 4). Obama signs children's health insurance bill. *The New York Times*. Retrieved from http://www.nytimes.com/2009/02/05/us/politics/05health.html

Perry, P. A., & Hotze, T. (2011). Oregon's experiment with prioritizing public health care services. *Virtual Mentor, 13*, 4, 241–247.

Pitt, S., Carrier. E., Rich, E., & Kellerman, A. (2010). Where Americans get acute care: Increasingly, it's not at their doctor's office. *Health Affairs, 29*(9), 1620–1629.

Perkins, B. B. (1998). Economic organization of medicine and the Committee on the Costs of Medical Care. *American Journal of Public Health, 88*(11), 1721–1726.

Perlstadt, H. (1995). The development of the Hill–Burton legislation: Interests, issues and compromises. *Journal of Health Social Policy, 6*(3), 77–96.

Polsky, D., Doshi, J., Escarce, J., Manning, W., Paddock, S., Cen, L., et al. (2009). The health effects of Medicare for the near-elderly uninsured. *Health Services Research, 44*(3), 926–945.

Poole, S. M. (2009, November 23). Judge dismisses Andrew Speaker suit against CDC. *The Atlanta-Journal Constitution*. Retrieved from http://www.ajc.com/health/judge-dismisses-andrew-speaker-211263.html

Porter, M. E. (2009). A strategy for health care reform—toward a value-based system. *New England Journal of Medicine, 361*, 109–112.

Porter, M., & Teisberg, E. (2006). *Redefining health care: Creating value-based competition on results*. Cambridge, MA: Harvard Business School Press.

Quadagno, J. (2010). Institutions, interest groups, and ideology: An agenda for the sociology of health care reform. *Journal of Health and Social Behavior, 51*(2), 125–136.

RAND Health. (2010). *Managed care backlash: Did consumers vote with their feet?* Retrieved from http://www.rand.org/content/dam/rand/pubs/research_briefs/2005/RAND_RB9121.pdf

RAND Health. (2011). *How will health care reform affect costs and coverage?* Retrieved from http://www.rand.org/content/dam/rand/pubs/research_briefs/2011/RAND_RB9589.pdf

Reed, M., Brand, R., Newhouse, J., Selby, J., & Hsu, J. (2008). Coping with prescription drug cost sharing: Knowledge, adherence, and financial burden. *Health Services Research, 43*(2), 785–797.

Reynolds, H. Y. (2009). Free medical clinics: Helping indigent patients and dealing with emerging health care needs. *Academic Medicine, 84*(10), 1434–1439.

Richardson, B. W. (1887). *The health of nations: A review of the works of Edwin Chadwick,* Vol. 2. London, UK: Longmans, Green.

Robertson, C. T., Egelhof, R., & Hoke, M. (2008). Get sick, get out: The medical causes of home mortgage foreclosures. *Health Matrix, 18*, 65–72.

Robinson, J. C., & Ginsburg, P. B. (2009). Consumer-driven health care: Promise and performance. *Health Affairs, 28*(2), w272–w281.

Rogers, J. (2010, April 30). *Anthem Blue Cross withdraws California rate hike*. Retrieved from http://www.huffingtonpost.com/2010/04/29/anthem-blue-cross-withdra_n_557966.html

Roos, R. (2009, March 10). *Report says public health funding is uneven, eroding*. Center for Infectious Disease Research & Policy (CIDRAP). Retrieved from http://www.cidrap.umn.edu/cidrap/content/fs/food-disease/news/mar1009funding-jw.html

Rosenbaum, S., & Riley, T. (2012, January). *Building a relationship between Medicaid, the exchange and the individual insurance market*. National Academy of Social Insurance. Retrieved from http://www.nasi.org/sites/default/files/research/Building_A_Relationship_Between_Medicaid_the_Exchange_and_the_Individual_Insuranc

Rosenblatt, S. (2007, November 6). Family seeks $45 million in King-Harbor death; Edith Rodriguez died after writhing in pain on the hospital floor as employees ignored her. *Los Angeles Times: Archives*. Retrieved from http://pqasb.pqarchiver.com/latimes/access/1377858201.html?FMT=ABS&FMTS=ABS:FT&type=current&date=Nov+6%2C+2007&author=Susannah+Rosenblatt&pub=Los+Angeles+Times&edition=&startpage=B.6&desc=Family+seeks+%2445+million+in+King-Harbor+death%3B+Edith+Rodriguez+died+after+writhing+in+pain+on+the+hospital+floor+as+employees+ignored+her.+A+lawsuit+accuses+L.A.+County+of+negligence

Rosenthal, M. B. (2007). Nonpayment for performance? Medicare's new reimbursement rule. *The New England Journal of Medicine, 357*, 1573–1575.

Ruhl, T. (n.d.). *Children's Bureau name and hierarchy: Roots and history*. The Maternal & Child Health Library at Georgetown University. Retrieved from http://www.mchlibrary.info/history/names.html

Scanlon, D., Swaminathan, S., Chernew, M., & Lee, W. (2006). Market and plan characteristics related to HMO quality and improvement. *Medical Care Research & Review, 63*(6 Suppl.), 56–89.

Saha, S., Coffman, M. S., & Smits, A. (2010). Giving teeth to comparative-effectiveness research—the Oregon experience. *New England Journal of Medicine, 362*, e18.

Scanlon, D. P., Swaminathan, S., Chernew, M., & Lee, W. (2006). Market and plan characteristics related to HMO quality and improvement. *Medical Care Research & Review, 63*(6 Suppl), 56s–89s.

Schuenemann, L. P., & White, D. B. (2011). The ethics and reality of rationing in medicine. *Chest, 140*(6), 1625–1632.

Schoen, C., Collins, S., Kriss, J., & Doty, M. (2008). How many are underinsured? Trends among U.S. adults, 2003 and 2007. *Health Affairs, 27*(4), 298–309.

Schoen, C., Doty, M., Robertson, R., & Collins, S, (2011). Affordable Care Act reforms could reduce the number of underinsured US adults by 70 percent. *Health Affairs, 30*(9), 1762–1771.

Scott, A., Sivey, P., Ouakrim, A., Willenberg, L., Naccarella, L., Furler, J., et al. (2011, September 7). The effect of financial incentives on the quality of health care provided by primary care physicians. *Cochrane Database Systematic Review, 9*, CD008451.

Scutchfield, F. D., & Keck, C. W. (Eds.). (2009). *Principles of public health practice* (3rd ed.). Clifton Park, NY: Delmar Cengage Learning.

Segre, L. (2011). *Cost of LASIK eye surgery and other corrective procedures*. Retrieved from http://www.allaboutvision.com/visionsurgery/cost.htm

Selden, T. M., & Sing, M. (2008). The distribution of public spending for health care in the United States, 2002. *Health Affairs, 27*(5), w349–w359.

Sellers, K. (n.d.). *State public health finance: Results of the ASTHO 2010 Profile Survey*. Association of State and Territorial Health Officers (ASTHO). Retrieved from http://www.publichealthsystems.org/media/file/Sellers2D_2011.pdf

Sensenig, A. L. (2007). Refining estimates of public health spending as measured in national health expenditures accounts: The United States experience. *Journal of Public Health Management Practice, 13*(2), 103–104.

Shattuck, L. (1850). *Report of the Sanitary Commission of Massachusetts*. Cambridge, MA: Harvard University Press (Original work published by Dutton & Wentworth in 1850).

Shinkman, R. (2010, September 28). *Healthcare philanthropy plummets*. Retrieved from http://www.fiercehealthfinance.com/story/healthcare-philanthropy-takes-big-dip/2010-09-28

Shires, D. Stange, K., Divine, G., Ratliff, S., Vashi, R., Tai-Seale, M., et al. (2012). Prioritization of evidence-based preventive health services during periodic health examinations. *American Journal of Preventive Medicine, 42*(2), 164–173.

Singer, P. (2009, July 19). Why we must ration health care. *The New York Times*. Retrieved from http://www.med.mcgill.ca/epidemiology/courses/EPIB654/Summer2010/Policy/nytimes%20rationing%202009_07_19.pdf

Small Business Majority. (2012). *Reference guide: Coverage types. Point-of-service plan (POS)*. Retrieved from http://healthcoverageguide.org/reference-guide/coverage-types/point-of-service-plan-pos/

Smolka, G., Purvis, L., & Figueiredo, C. (2007, May). *Health coverage among 50- to 64-year olds*. AARP Public Policy Institute. Retrieved from http://assets.aarp.org/rgcenter/health/dd155_coverage.pdf

Snow, J. (1855). *On the mode of communication of cholera* (2nd ed.). London: John Churchill.

Social Security Administration (SSA). (2011a). *The Social Security Act—passage and development*. Retrieved from http://www.ssa.gov/history/briefhistory3.html

Social Security Administration (SSA). (2011b). *Update 2011*. Retrieved from http://ssa.gov/pubs/10003.pdf

Social Security Administration (SSA). (2012a). *SSA History*. Retrieved from http://www.ssa.gov/history/

Social Security Administration. (2012b). *Fact sheet: Social Security, 2012 Social Security changes*. Retrieved from http://www.socialsecurity.gov/pressoffice/factsheets/colafacts2012.pdf

Society of Actuaries. (2010). *The economic measurement of medical errors*. Retrieved from http://www.soa.org/files/pdf/research-econ-measurement.pdf

Solnit, R. (2009). *A paradise built in hell: The extraordinary communities that arise in disaster*. New York: Penguin Group USA (Viking).

Spettell, C., Rawlins, W., Krakauer, R., Fernandes, J., Breton, M. E., Gowdy, W, et al. (2009). A comprehensive case management program to improve palliative care. *Journal of Palliative Medicine, 12*(9), 827–832.

Spice, C., & Snyder, K. (2009). Reviewing self-reported impacts of community health assessment in local health jurisdictions. *Journal of Public Health Management & Practice, 15*(1), 18–23.

Stock, S., Redaelli, M., & Lauterbach, K. (2007). Disease management and health care reforms in Germany: Does more competition lead to less solidarity? *Health Policy, 80*(1), 86–96.

Suh, G., Wimo, A., Gauthier, S., O'Connor, D., Ikeda, M., Homma, A, et al. (2009). International price comparisons of Alzheimer's drugs: A way to close the affordability gap. *International Psychogeriatrics, 21*, 1116–1126.

Sultz, H. A., & Young, K. A. (2009). *Health care USA: Understanding its organization and delivery* (6th ed.). Sudbury, MA: Jones & Bartlett Publishers.

Swartz, K. (2010, December). *Cost-sharing: Effects on spending and outcomes*. The Synthesis Project: Research Synthesis Report No. 20. Princeton, NJ: Robert Wood Johnson Foundation.

Tabarrok, A. (2004, November 24). *Seeing is believing (in the free market)*. Retrieved from http://www.marginalrevolution.com/marginalrevolution/2004/11/seeing_is_belie.html

Takach, M. (2011). Reinventing Medicaid: State innovations to qualify and pay for patient-centered medical homes show promising results. *Health Affairs, 30*(7), 1325–1334.

Tandon, A., Murray, C., Lauer, J., & Evans, D. (n.d.). Measuring overall health system performance for 191 countries. *World Health Organization*. Retrieved from http://www.who.int/healthinfo/paper30.pdf

The ARC of Massachusetts. (2010). *A national plan to combat mental retardation*. Retrieved from http://www.arcmass.org/jfk/tabid/635/Default.aspx

The Associated Press. (2004). Crisis threatens landmark medical center: Five top administrators have been fired for ignoring problems. *MSNBC.com*. Retrieved from http://www.msnbc.msn.com/id/4780341/

The Commonwealth Fund. (2011). *Why not the best? Results from the National Scorecard on U.S. Health System Performance, 2011*. Retrieved from http://www.commonwealthfund.org/~/media/Files/Publications/Fund%20Report/2011/Oct/1500_WNTB_Natl_Scorecard_2011_web.pdf

The Leapfrog Group. (2007). *Leapfrog accomplishments*. Retrieved from http://www.leapfroggroup.org/media/file/Leapfrog_Accomplishments_3-07.pdf

The White House. (n.d.). *The Clinton-Gore administration: A record of progress*. Retrieved from http://clinton5.nara.gov/WH/Accomplishments/eightyears-03.html

Trust for America's Health. (2008). *Prevention for a healthier America: Investments in disease prevention yield significant savings, stronger communities*. Retrieved from http://healthyamericans.org/reports/prevention08/Prevention08.pdf

Trust for America's Health. (2011a). *Investing in America's health: A state-by-state look at public health funding and key health facts*. Washington, DC: Author.

Trust for America's Health. (2011b). *Ten top priorities for prevention*. Retrieved from http://healthyamericans.org/pages/?id=126

Tu, H. T., & May, J. H. (2007). Self-pay markets in health care: Consumer nirvana or caveat emptor? *Health Affairs, 26*(2), w217–w226.

Turnock, B. J. (2011a). *Public health: What it is and how it works* (5th ed.). Sudbury, MA: Jones & Bartlett Learning.

Turnock, B. J. (2011b). *Essentials of public health* (2nd ed.). Sudbury, MA: Jones & Bartlett Learning.

Tyson, L. D. (2001). Healing Medicare. In E. C. Hein (Ed.). *Nursing issues in the 21st century: Perspectives from the literature*. (pp. 459–468). Philadelphia, PA: Lippincott Williams & Wilkins.

Umans, B., & Nonnemaker, K. L. (2009). *The Medicare beneficiary population*. AARP Public Policy Institute, Fact Sheet 149. Retrieved from http://assets.aarp.org/rgcenter/health/fs149_medicare.pdf

United Nations Educational Scientific & Cultural Organization (UNESCO). (2008). *Strategic planning*. Retrieved from http://portal.unesco.org/en/ev.php-URL_ID=36920&URL_DO=DO_TOPIC&URL_SECTION=201.html

United Nations International Children's Emergency Fund (UNICEF). (2011). *Who we are*. Retrieved from http://www.unicef.org/about/who/index_introduction.html

U.S. Agency for International Development (USAID). (2012). *What we do*. Retrieved from http://www.usaid.gov/what we-do

U.S. Census Bureau. (2010, September 16). *Income, poverty and health insurance coverage in the United States: Summary of key findings*. Retrieved from http://www.census.gov/newsroom/releases/archives/income_wealth/cb10-144.html

U.S. Department of Health and Human Services. (n.d.). US Department of Health and Human Services Organizational Chart. Retrieved from http://www.hhs.gov/about/orgchart/

U.S. Department of Health & Human Services. (2011). *About Healthy People*. Retrieved from http://www.healthypeople.gov/2020/about/default.aspx

U.S. Department of Health & Human Services. (2010). *Historical highlights*. Retrieved from http://www.hhs.gov/about/hhshist.html

U.S. Department of Labor. (n.d.). *Consolidated Omnibus Budget Reconciliation Act (COBRA)*. Retrieved from http://www.dol.gov/ebsa/newsroom/fscobra.html

U.S. Department of Labor. (2009). *Fact sheet: Mental health parity and addiction equity act*. Retrieved from http://www.savingmatters.dol.gov/ebsa/regs/unifiedagenda/ebsafall2009/1210-AB30fs.html

U.S. Environmental Protection Agency. (n.d.). *Summary of the Occupational Safety and Health Act (1970)*. Retrieved from http://www.epa.gov/lawsregs/laws/osha.html

U.S. Environmental Protection Agency. (2011). *Cardiovascular disease prevalence and mortality*. Retrieved from http://cfpub.epa.gov/eroe/index.cfm?fuseaction=detail.viewInd&lv=list.listByAlpha&r=235292&subtop=381

U.S. News & World Report. (2010, April 2). *Your retiree medical bill: $197,000*. Retrieved from http://articles.moneycentral.msn.com/Insurance/InsureYourHealth/your-retiree-medical-bill-197000-dollars.aspx?page=1

Vaiana, M. E. (2011). How does growth in health care costs affect the American family? *RAND Health*. Retrieved from http://www.rand.org/pubs/research_briefs/RB9605/index1.html

Van de Ven, W., Beck, K., Van de Voorde, C., Wasem J., Zmora I. (2007). Risk adjustment and risk selection in Europe: 6 years later. *Health Policy, 83*(2–3), 162–179.

Virginia Commonwealth University. (2011). Medicare claims processing. *Work World*. Retrieved from http://www.workworld.org/wwwebhelp/medicare_claims_processing.htm

Varney, S. (2010, March 18). *Did Blue Cross' mission stray when plans became for-profit?* Morning Edition: NPR. Retrieved from http://www.npr.org/templates/story/story.php?storyId=124807720

Walker, K., Leng, M., Liang, L., Forge, N., Morales, L., Jones, L., et al. (2011). Increased patient delays in care after the closure of Martin Luther King Hospital: Implications for monitoring health system changes. *Ethnicity Disease, 21*(3), 356–360.

Ward, J., & Warren, C. (Eds.). (2007). *Silent victories: The history and practice of public health in twentieth-century America*. New York: Oxford University Press.

Whitford, A. B. (2008). The policy implications of economic reasoning: What we do not know about moral hazard in health policy. *Evidence Policy, 4*(1) 69–73.

Whitmore, J., Gabel, J., Pickreign, J., & McDevitt, R. (2011). The individual insurance markets before reform: Low premiums and low benefits. *Medicare Care Research Review*. Advance online publication. Doi: 10.1177/1077558711399767.

Wider Opportunities for Women. (2010). *The basic economic security tables™ for the United States 2010*. Retrieved from http://www.wowonline.org/documents/BESTIndexforTheUnitedStates2010.pdf

Williams, S. J., & Torrens, P. R. (2008). *Introduction to health services* (7th ed.). Clifton Park, NY: Delmar Thomson Learning.

Wohl, J. (2011, October 21). *Wal-Mart trims some U.S. health coverage*. Reuters. Retrieved from http://www.reuters.com/article/2011/10/21/us-walmart-idUSTRE79K43Z20111021

Woodward, S. B. (1932). The story of smallpox in Massachusetts. *New England Journal of Medicine, 206*, 1181.

Woolley, J., & Peters, G. (2007). *George Bush: Statement on signing the Preventive Health Amendments of 1992. The American Presidency Project*. Retrieved from http://www.presidency.ucsb.edu/ws/index.php?pid=21681

World Health Organization (WHO). (n.d.). *History of WHO and international cooperation in public health*. Retrieved from https://apps.who.int/aboutwho/en/history.htm

World Health Organization (WHO). (1998). *Health for all policy for the twenty-first century* (Resolution WHA51.7). Geneva, Switzerland: Author.

World Health Organization (WHO). (2000). *The world health report 2000. Health systems: Improving performance*. Retrieved from http://www.who.int/whr/2000/en/index.html

World Health Organization (WHO). (2007). *Spending on health: A global overview*. Retrieved from http://www.who.int/mediacentre/factsheets/fs319.pdf

World Health Organization (WHO). (2009). *World health statistics, 2009*. Retrieved from http://www.who.int/whosis/whostat/2009/en/index.html

World Health Organization (WHO). (2010). *Executive summary: The world health report*. Retrieved from http://www.who.int/whr/2010/10_summary_en.pdf

World Health Organization (WHO). (2011a). *Countries*. Retrieved from http://www.who.int/countries/en/

World Health Organization (WHO). (2011b). *Millennium development goals (MDGs)*. Retrieved from http://www.who.int/topics/millennium_development_goals/en/

World Health Organization (WHO). (2011c). *WHO—It's people and offices*. Retrieved from http://www.who.int/about/structure/en/index.html

World Health Organization (WHO). (2011d). *Key components of a well functioning health care system*. Retrieved from http://www.who.int/healthsystems/EN_HSSkeycomponents.pdf

Wright, B., Carlson, M., Allen, H., Holmgren, A., & Rustvold, D. L. (2010). Raising premiums and other costs for Oregon Health Plan enrollees drove many to drop out. *Health Affairs, 29*(12), 2311–2316.

Wu, V. (2010). Hospital cost shifting revisited: New evidence from the balanced budget act of 1997. *International Journal of Health Care Finance and Economics, 10*(1), 61–83.

Zafari, A. M., Afonso, L. C., & Aggarwal, K. (2011, October 11). Myocardial infarction treatment & management. *Medscape: Reference*. Retrieved from http://emedicine.medscape.com/article/155919-treatment#aw2aab6b6b2

CHAPTER

7

Epidemiology in Community Health Care

"Let me tell you the secret that has led me to my goal. My strength lies solely in my tenacity."

—Louis Pasteur

KEY TERMS

Causality
Endemic
Epidemic
Epidemiology
Global health patterns
Immunity
Incidence
Morbidity rate
Mortality rate
Natural history
Pandemic
Prevalence

LEARNING OBJECTIVES

Upon mastery of this chapter, you should be able to:

- Explore the historical roots of epidemiology.
- Explain the host, agent, and environment model.
- Describe theories of causality in health and illness.
- Explain a *web of causation* matrix that assists you with recognizing multicausal factors in disease or injury occurrences.
- Define immunity and compare passive immunity, active immunity, cross-immunity, and herd immunity.
- Explain how epidemiologists determine populations at risk.
- Identify the four stages of a disease or health condition.
- List the major sources of epidemiologic information.
- Distinguish between incidence and prevalence in health and illness states.
- Use epidemiologic methods to describe an aggregate's health.
- Discuss the types of epidemiologic studies that are useful for researching aggregate health.
- Use the seven-step research process when conducting an epidemiologic study.

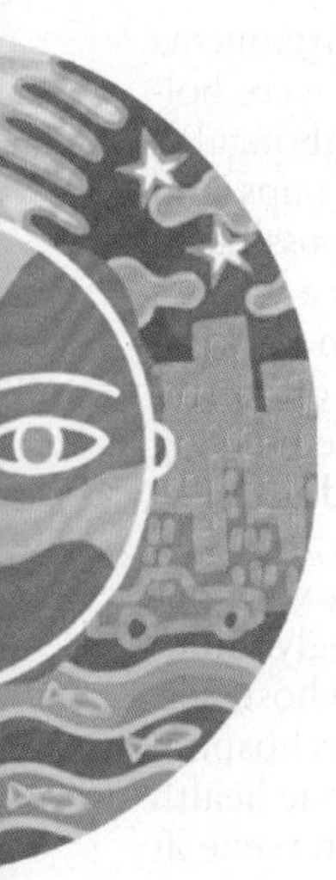

Epidemiology is "concerned with the distribution and determinants of health and diseases, morbidity, injuries, disability, and mortality in populations" (Friis & Sellers, 2009, p. 6). It is a specialized form of scientific research that can provide health care workers, including community health nurses, with a body of knowledge on which to base their practice and methods for studying new and existing problems. The term is derived from the Greek words *epi* (upon), *demos* (the people), and *logos* (knowledge): the knowledge or study of what happens to people. Epidemiologists ask such questions as the following:

- What is the occurrence of health and disease in a population?
- Has there been an increase or decrease in a health state over the years?
- Does one geographic area have a higher frequency of disease than another?
- What characteristics of people with a particular condition distinguish them from those without the condition?
- What factors need to be present to cause disease or injury?
- Is one treatment or program more effective than another in changing the health of affected people?
- Why do some people recover from a disease and others do not?

The ultimate goals of epidemiology are to "determine the extent of disease in a population, identify patterns and trends in disease occurrence, identify the causes of disease, and evaluate the effectiveness of prevention and treatment options" (Aschengrau & Seage, 2008, p. 33). With knowledge regarding the scale and nature of human health problems, solutions to prevent disease can be sought, thereby contributing to the improved health of the entire population.

Epidemiology offers community health nurses a specific methodology for assessing the health of aggregates. Furthermore, it provides a frame of reference for investigating and improving clinical practice in any setting. For example, if a community health nursing goal is to lower the incidence of sexually transmitted diseases (STDs) in a given community, such a prevention plan requires information about population groups. How many STD cases have been reported in this community in the past year? What is the expected number of STD cases (the morbidity rate)? Which members of the community are at highest risk of contracting STDs? To be effective, any program of screening, treatment, or health promotion regarding STDs must be based on this kind of information about population groups. Whether the community health nurse's goals are to improve a population's nutrition, control the spread of human immunodeficiency virus (HIV), deal with health problems created by a flood, protect and promote the health of battered women, or reduce the number of automobile crash injuries and fatalities at a specific intersection, epidemiologic data are essential.

HISTORICAL ROOTS OF EPIDEMIOLOGY

The roots of epidemiology can be traced to Hippocrates, a Greek physician who lived from about 460 to 375 BCE and who is sometimes referred to as the first epidemiologist. Hippocrates and other members of the Hippocratic School believed that disease not only affects individuals but also affects the masses. This was one of the earliest associations of the occurrence of disease with lifestyle and environmental factors, specifically geographic location (Lawson & Williams, 2001). Not until the late 19th century, however, did modern epidemiology come into existence.

An **epidemic** refers to a disease occurrence that clearly exceeds the normal or expected frequency in a community or region. In past centuries, epidemics of cholera, bubonic plague, and smallpox swept through community after community, killing thousands of people, changing the community structure, and altering the lifestyle of masses of people. When an epidemic, such as the bubonic plague (also called pneumonic plague or the Black Death) or acquired immunodeficiency syndrome (AIDS), is worldwide in distribution, it is called a **pandemic**.

Epidemic and pandemic diseases clearly prompted the development of epidemiology as a science. Epidemiology became a distinct branch of medical science through its concern with massive waves of infectious diseases. In 1348 and 1349, the Black Death (likely caused by the bacillus *Yersinia pestis*) swept through continental Europe and England, killing millions of people. In England alone, the epidemic resulted in the deaths of 30% to 60% of the population (Theilmann & Cate, 2007).

The plague continued in Europe, but with less force, for three centuries and then waned, only to reappear in an epidemic in Hong Kong in 1894. Discovery of the plague bacillus was first attributed to Shibasaburo Kitasato (1852–1931), a Japanese bacteriologist (Solomon, 1997). Procedural issues with Kitasato's work, however, eventually resulted in the attribution to Alexandre Yersin (1863–1943), who worked in Hong Kong at the same time (Solomon, 1997). Within 4 years, another scientist, Paul-Louis Simond, had traced the bacillus life cycle from rats to fleas to humans; he postulated that the bite of a *Yersinia*-infected flea caused plague in humans. Although viewed with skepticism, by 1906 the scientific community finally accepted the route of disease transmission described by Simond and others (Simond, Godley, & Mouriquand, 1998). With this combined knowledge, intervention was now possible, and public health officials declared war on rats, seeking to make ships and wharf buildings rat-proof.

One early example of a community-wide campaign against rats occurred after the outbreak of plague in

California in 1900 (Evans, 1939). The campaign proved successful and bolstered confidence in efforts to control disease outbreaks by attacking the likely source. Understanding the role that rats played in the transmission of the disease led to an effective approach for disease control. Unfortunately, plague has not been eradicated, and wild rodents, especially ground squirrels, as well as rabbits and domestic cats remain a natural reservoir of the plague bacillus (Heymann, 2009). Cases still occur occasionally in the western half of the United States, and the disease is an ongoing threat in major areas of Africa, Asia, and South America, especially in rural regions (World Health Organization [WHO], 2012). The continuing presence of a disease or infectious agent in a given geographic area, such as plague in Vietnam or malaria in the tropics of Brazil and Indonesia, means that the disease is **endemic** to that area.

As the threat of the great epidemic diseases declined, epidemiologists began to focus on other infectious diseases, such as diphtheria, infant diarrhea, typhoid, tuberculosis, and syphilis. They also studied diseases linked to occupations, such as scurvy among sailors and scrotal cancer among chimney sweeps. In recent years, epidemiologists turned to the study of major causes of death and disability, such as cancer, cardiovascular disorders, AIDS, violence, mental illness, accidents, arthritis, and congenital defects.

Florence Nightingale: Nurse Epidemiologist

Nursing's epidemiologic roots can be traced to Florence Nightingale (1820–1910). Her detailed records, morbidity (sickness) statistics, and careful description of the health conditions among the soldiers in the Crimean War represent one of the first systematic descriptive studies of the distribution and patterns of disease in a population. She used wedge-shaped graphs that were shaded and colored to illustrate preventable deaths of the hospitalized Crimean soldiers, compared with hospitalized soldiers in England at the time. The sophisticated level of detail in her studies heralded her as the first nurse researcher. Changes made according to her suggestions, which are common knowledge now—establishing a clean environment, providing edible foods, cleaning wounds and using new bandages, and separating infectious soldiers from injured soldiers—brought dramatic proof of the authenticity of her observations and knowledge. Forty-four of every hundred British troops were dying in the Crimea before Nightingale instituted environmental and nutritional changes in the hospital and field. When her work was finished, the mortality (death) rate was only 2% (Gabriel & Metz, 1992).

William Farr

Nightingale's epidemiologic approach grew from her decades-long collaboration with friend and colleague William Farr (Kudzma, 2006). Farr, a physician and self-taught mathematician, is considered one of the founders of modern epidemiology (Aschengrau & Seage, 2008). As head of the Office of the Registrar General for England and Wales (Kudzma, 2006), he developed a "more sophisticated system for coding medical conditions than was previously in use" (Friis & Sellers, 2009, p. 31). Arguments for the health care reforms Nightingale sought were bolstered by her collaboration with Farr. With Nightingale's data on the frequency of mortality among groups and Farr's broader population statistics, it was now possible to make "comparisons to the population at risk as a whole" (Kudzma, 2006, p. 63). The professional liaison between Nightingale and Farr is a wonderful example of collaborative practice in addressing public health; the merging of expertise from these two disciplines resulted in much more than either could accomplish individually.

Nightingale's use of statistical data, along with her commitment to environmental reform, strongly influenced nursing's evolution into a profession whose service addressed public health problems as well as hospital care (Kopf, 1978). As nursing has evolved, public health nurses have been increasingly challenged to intervene at the aggregate level, using epidemiologic approaches to address the needs of high-risk groups and populations.

Eras in the Evolution of Modern Epidemiology

Modern epidemiology can be described as having four distinct eras, each based on causal thinking, sanitary statistics, infectious disease epidemiology, and chronic disease epidemiology. In light of new research, the eco-epidemiology era is emerging.

Early causal thinking was dominated by the *miasma theory,* which had its origins in the work of the Hippocratic School and was formally developed in the early 1700s. This theory held that a substance called *miasma* was composed of malodorous and poisonous particles generated by the decomposition of organic matter and was the cause of disease. Prevention based on this theory attempted to eliminate the sources of the miasma or polluted vapors. Despite the faulty reasoning, this type of prevention had positive consequences because it made people aware that decaying organic matter can be a source of infectious diseases. This theory dominated until the first half of the 19th century. Nightingale herself never accepted the link between microorganisms and disease (Kudzma, 2006) and based her practice on this same approach. Her work in the Crimea, with its emphasis on sanitation, had positive results nonetheless.

Similarly, the pioneering work of John Snow in identifying the source of cholera in England in the mid-1800s was based on a faulty assumption that the climate was involved. Even so, he was able to trace the source of the infectious agent to the water supply and brought public attention to the link between sanitary conditions and disease. We owe much to these individuals; that they didn't understand the exact mechanisms in disease causation does not diminish their pioneering work in applied epidemiology (see Fig. 7-1).

The era of infectious disease epidemiology was dominated by the *contagion theory* of disease, which developed by the mid-18th century. Prompted by the development of increasingly sophisticated microscopes, this theory attempted to identify the microorganisms that cause diseases as a first step in prevention. It inspired various theories of immunity and even prompted

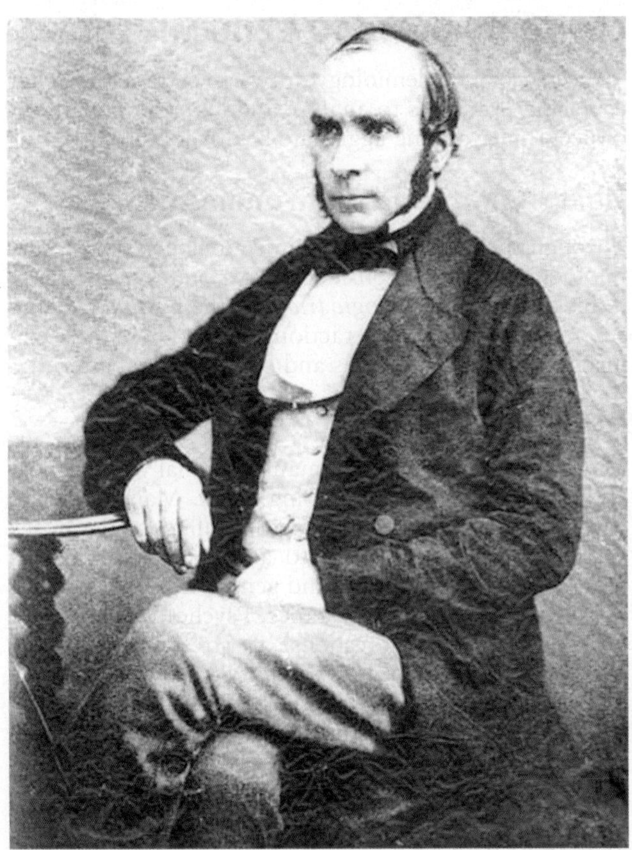

FIGURE 7-1. John Snow (National Library of Medicine—Images from the History of Medicine, 2012). Retrieved from http://ihm.nlm.nih.gov/luna/servlet/view/search?q=B08304

some initial attempts at vaccination against smallpox. Additionally, once an agent had been identified, measures were taken to contain its spread. Fumigating ships to kill rats, protecting wharf buildings and human habitations from rats, and removing rat food supplies from easy access were all measures taken to protect the public by further preventing the spread of plague bacilli. Based on the work of Louis Pasteur, Jakob Henle, and Robert Koch (see Koch's Postulates, Display 7.1), the contagion theory was refined and became best known as the *germ theory of disease* (Aschengrau & Seage, 2008), which was predominant from the late 19th century through the first half of the 20th century (Lawson & Williams, 2001).

In the era of infectious disease epidemiology, scientists viewed disease in terms of a simple cause-and-effect relationship. Finding a single cause (plague bacilli) and attacking it (eliminating rats) seemed to be the solution for preventing many diseases. In the case of bubonic plague, this approach appeared to be quite effective. However, scientific research eventually revealed that disease causation was much more complex than first suspected. For example, although most members of a group might be exposed to the plague, many did not contract it.

With bubonic plague, as with many other infectious diseases, the characteristics of the host can determine both the spread of the disease and its individual impact. Not everyone in a population is at equal risk; it is now known that untreated bubonic plague has a case fatality rate of 50% to 60%, meaning that about half of those who contract the disease and are not treated will eventually die (Heymann, 2009). Furthermore, the agent and course of transmission can be quite complex. Although a flea carries the bacilli from rats to humans in bubonic plague, many infectious diseases spread directly from one human being to another. Finally, the environment must be considered as part of the cause of disease. Evidence suggests that the plague originated in the high plains of Asia and spread to other parts of the world. However, questions remain as to whether the bacillus spread from rats to ground squirrels or had always been part of the squirrels' ecology.

After World War II, the causative agents of major infectious diseases were identified, methods of prevention were recognized, and antibiotics and chemotherapy were added to the arsenal to fight communicable diseases. The focus then became understanding and controlling the new chronic disease epidemics. Researchers completed case-control and cohort studies (discussed later) that linked the causative factors of cholesterol levels and smoking with coronary heart disease and associated smoking with lung cancer. Today, the major causes of mortality in the United States are noninfectious diseases. Chronic diseases of the heart and malignant neoplasms account for nearly 50% of all US deaths, with a near equal number of deaths attributed to chronic lower respiratory diseases (5%), cerebrovascular diseases (CVDs) (5%), and unintentional injuries (5%) (Murphy, Jiaquan, & Kochanek, 2012). These major health problems are not caused by infectious agents.

We are entering a new era of *ecoepidemiology*, distinguished by transforming global health patterns and technological advances. **Global health patterns**, the route,

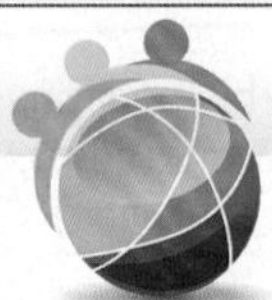

DISPLAY 7.1 KOCH'S POSTULATES

1. The microorganism must be observed in every case of the disease.
2. It must be isolated and grown in pure culture.
3. The pure culture must, when inoculated into a susceptible animal, reproduce the disease.
4. The microorganism must be observed in, and recovered from, the experimentally diseased animal.

King, L. S. (1952). Dr. Koch's postulates. *Journal of Historical Medicine*, 350–361. As cited in Friis, R. H., & Sellers, T. A. (2009). *Epidemiology for public health practice* (4th ed., p. 31). Sudbury, MA: Jones and Barlett Publishers.

form, and virulence in which diseases appear in countries around the world, with consideration of environmental, ecologic, human, technologic, and political factors, are in transformation. The West Nile virus, influenza A (H1N1), multidrug-resistant TB (MDR TB), and the HIV epidemic illustrate this transformation. In most cases, causative organisms and critical risk factors are known, yet diseases occur, spread, and suddenly appear in countries or regions previously free of them. We know which social behaviors need to change, but we are at a loss about how to create a climate of permanent change, even when entire populations are at stake. For example, we know how to prevent the transmission of HIV, yet thousands of new cases are reported each year. How can preventive practices be promoted in populations at risk for communicable diseases? The same is true for many current chronic diseases. How many nurses smoke? Do you exercise as you know you should? Do you know your cholesterol level and eat appropriate foods accordingly? Do you regularly use sunscreen? What are we missing to effectively change social behaviors?

Developments in technology drive research, primarily in biology and biomedical techniques and in information system capabilities. For example, the possibility now exists through DNA studies to recognize both viral and genetic components in insulin-dependent diabetes. HIV, tuberculosis, and other infections can be tracked from person to person through identifying the molecular specificity of the organisms, and a gene to track and mark one form of breast cancer has been identified. On a broader scale, using new technology, we are now able to track the geographic distribution of disease and correlate that data with other important health risks. For instance, using these geocoding systems, overweight and obesity in children can be correlated with other factors, such as after-school recreation opportunities, distribution of fast-food restaurants, farmer's markets, or socioeconomic status. The possibilities of learning through technology have just begun in this current epidemiologic era. Table 7-1 summarizes the four eras in the evolution of modern epidemiology.

CONCEPTS BASIC TO EPIDEMIOLOGY

The science of epidemiology draws on certain basic concepts and principles to analyze and understand patterns of occurrence among aggregate health conditions.

Host, Agent, and Environment Model

Through their early study of infectious diseases, epidemiologists began to consider disease states generally in terms of the *epidemiologic triad*, or the *host, agent, and environment model*. Interactions among these three elements explained infectious and other disease patterns.

Host

The **host** is a susceptible human or animal who harbors and nourishes a disease-causing agent. Many physical, psychological, and lifestyle factors influence the host's susceptibility and response to an agent. Physical factors include age, sex, race, and genetic influences on the host's vulnerability or resistance. Psychological factors, such as outlook and response to stress, can strongly influence host susceptibility. Lifestyle factors also play a major role. Diet, exercise, sleep patterns, and healthy or unhealthy habits all contribute to either increased or decreased vulnerability to the disease-causing agent.

The concept of resistance is important for public health nursing practice. People sometimes have an ability to resist pathogens. This is called *inherent resistance*. Typically, these people have inherited or acquired characteristics, such as the various factors mentioned earlier, that make them less vulnerable. People who maintain a healthful lifestyle may not contract influenza even if exposed to the flu virus. Resistance can be promoted through preventive interventions that support a healthful lifestyle. For example, one study found that regular use of a multivitamin in the periconceptual period reduced the risk of preeclampsia by 45% (n = 1,835) but only in those women who were not overweight (Bodnar et al.,

Table 7.1 Eras in the Evolution of Modern Epidemiology

Era	Paradigm	Analytic Approach	Prevention Approach
Sanitary statistics (1800–1850)	Miasma: poisoning from foul emanations	Clustering of morbidity and mortality	Drainage, sewage, sanitation
Infectious disease epidemiology (1850–1950)	Germ theory: single agent related to specific disease	Laboratory isolation and culture from disease sites and reproduce lesions	Interrupt transmission (vaccines, isolation, and antibiotics)
Chronic disease epidemiology (1950–2000)	Exposure related to outcome	Risk ratio of exposure to outcome at individual level in populations	Control risk factors by modifying lifestyle (diet), agent (guns), or environment (pollution)
Ecoepidemiology (emerging)	Relations within and between localized structures organized in a hierarchy of levels	Analysis of determinants and outcomes at different levels of organization using new information systems and biomedical techniques	Apply both information and biomedical technology to find leverage at efficacious levels

Adapted from Susser, M., & Susser, E. (1996a). Choosing a future for epidemiology: I. Eras and paradigms. *American Journal of Public Health, 86*(5), 668–673 and Susser, M., & Susser, E. (1996b). Choosing a future for epidemiology: II. From black box to Chinese boxes and eco-epidemiology. *American Journal of Public Health, 86*(5), 674–677.

2006). Adding to this body of evidence, Walker et al. (2011) demonstrated that participants (n = 7,867) taking multivitamins with folic acid during the early second trimester were 63% less likely to have preeclampsia. If confirmed by additional studies, multivitamin use with folic acid could be recommended as a preventive measure for preeclampsia. The American Academy of Pediatrics and the U.S. Public Health Service already recommend that women capable of becoming pregnant take 400 μg of folic acid each day to prevent neural tube defects such as spina bifida (AAP, 2011). Further study may reveal other benefits from the use of folic acid during pregnancy.

Agent

An *agent* is a factor that causes or contributes to a health problem or condition. Causative agents can be factors that are present (e.g., bacteria that cause tuberculosis, rocks on a mountain road that contribute to an automobile crash) or factors that are lacking (e.g., a low serum iron level that causes anemia or the lack of seat belt use that contributes to the extent of injury during an automobile crash).

Agents vary considerably and include five types: biologic, chemical, nutrient, physical, and psychological. Biologic agents include bacteria, viruses, fungi, protozoa, worms, and insects. Some biologic agents are infectious, such as influenza virus or HIV. Chemical agents may be in the form of liquids, solids, gases, dusts, or fumes. Examples are poisonous sprays used on garden pests and industrial chemical wastes. The degree of toxicity of the chemical agent influences its impact on health. Nutrient agents include essential dietary components that can produce illness conditions if they are deficient or are taken in excess. For example, a deficiency of niacin can cause pellagra, and too much vitamin A can be toxic. Physical agents include anything mechanical (e.g., chainsaw, automobile), material (rock slide), atmospheric (ultraviolet radiation), geologic (earthquake), or genetically transmitted that causes injury to humans. The shape, size, and force of physical agents influence the degree of harm to the host. Psychological agents are events that produce stress leading to health problems (war).

Agents may also be classified as infectious or noninfectious. Infectious agents cause communicable diseases, such as AIDS or tuberculosis—that is, the disease can be spread from one person to another. Certain characteristics of infectious agents are important for community health nurses to understand. Extent of *exposure* to the agent, the agent's *pathogenicity* (capacity to cause disease in the host), its *infectivity* (capacity to enter the host and multiply), its virulence (severity of disease), *toxigenicity* (capacity to produce a toxin or poison), *resistance* (ability of the agent to survive environmental conditions), *antigenicity* (ability to induce an antibody response in the host) (Friis & Sellers, 2009), and its structure and chemical composition all influence the effect of the agent on the host. (Chapter 8 examines the subject of communicable disease in greater depth.) Noninfectious agents have similar characteristics in that their relative abilities to harm the host vary with type of agent and intensity and duration of exposure.

Environment

The environment refers to all the external factors surrounding the host that might influence vulnerability or resistance. The physical environment includes factors such as geography, climate and weather, safety of buildings, water and food supply, and presence of animals, plants, insects, and microorganisms that have the capacity to serve as reservoirs (storage sites for disease-causing agents) or vectors (carriers) for transmitting disease. The psychosocial environment refers to social, cultural, economic, and psychological influences and conditions that affect health, such as access to health care, cultural health practices, poverty, and work stressors, which can all contribute to disease or health.

Host, agent, and environment interact to cause a disease or health condition. For example, the agent responsible for Lyme disease is the spirochete Borrelia burgdorferi; humans of all ages are susceptible hosts, along with dogs, cattle, and horses. Ticks that feed on wild rodents and deer transfer the spirochete to human hosts after feeding on them for several hours. Environmental factors, such as working or playing in tick-infested areas, influence host vulnerability. The host, agent, and environment model, shown in Figure 7-2, offered the epidemiologists who first studied Lyme disease in 1982 a plan for intervention. As soon as the agent was identified, measures could be taken to keep the spirochete from infecting human hosts, such as wearing protective clothing or tick repellent in tick-infested areas and promptly removing the attached ticks (Heymann, 2009).

In another example, the West Nile virus, which was widespread in Africa and the Middle East, arrived in the United States in 1999 and began to spread (Heymann, 2009). The first reported cases were in New York, where 45 people were infected. In that year, the region experienced a total of 59 hospitalized cases of West Nile disease, resulting in seven deaths. By 2006, West Nile virus had been reported in 43 states and the District of Columbia, with a total of 4,269 cases and 177 deaths. In 2011, there were 690 confirmed cases and 43 deaths in the United States. As of January 2012, only Alaska, Hawaii, and Oregon had no confirmed presence of the

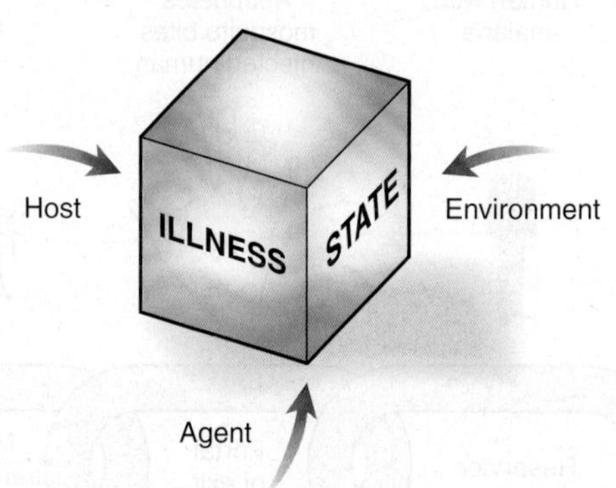

FIGURE 7-2. Epidemiologic triad. Epidemiologists study the causal agent, the susceptible host, and environmental factors that contribute to an illness, an injury, or a wellness state. Intervention may focus on any of these three to prevent the spread of illness or to improve health in a population.

virus in humans, birds, animals, or mosquitoes (Centers for Disease Control and Prevention [CDC], 2011b). The encephalitis-causing disease is transmitted by a mosquito bite. The virus survives winter in the body of the adult Culex mosquito (Heymann, 2009). The infected mosquito bites a bird and infects it. Other mosquitoes bite the bird and in turn become infected. The infected mosquitoes pass the virus on to birds, humans, or horses. Many dead birds in an area may mean that the virus is circulating between the bird and mosquito populations and should be reported. In humans and animals with intact immune systems, the virus is usually destroyed in the bloodstream. If the virus survives in the body, it can infect membranes around the spinal cord and brain and cause encephalitis. Those at highest risk are the elderly, children, and people with impaired immune systems.

Prevention of West Nile virus infection includes avoiding mosquito bites by applying insect repellent containing *N,N*-diethyl-meta-toluamide (DEET) when outdoors; wearing long-sleeved clothing and long pants treated with DEET-containing repellents; staying indoors at dawn, dusk, and in the early evening; eliminating standing water sources where mosquitoes lay their eggs; reporting dead birds; and ensuring that an organized mosquito control program exists in the area (CDC, 2011b). Using the model in Figure 7-2, can you categorize each of these six recommendations by their target (host, agent, or environment)?

Causality

Causality refers to the relationship between a cause and its effect. A purpose of epidemiologic study has been to discover causal relationships to understand why conditions develop and offer effective prevention and protection. As scientific knowledge of health and disease has expanded, epidemiology has changed its view of causality. The following section discusses some of those changes in thinking that began in the 1960s and are continually refined to this day.

Chain of Causation

As the scientific community's thinking about disease causation and the tripartite model (host–agent–environment) grew more complex, epidemiologists began to use the idea of a chain of causation (Fig. 7-3). The chain begins by identifying the reservoir (i.e., where the causal agent can live and multiply). With plague, that reservoir may be other humans, rats, squirrels, and a few other animals. With malaria, infected humans are the major reservoir for the parasitic agents, although certain nonhuman primates also act as reservoirs (Heymann, 2009). Next, the agent must have a portal of exit from the reservoir as well as some mode of transmission. For example, the bite of an *Anopheles* mosquito provides a portal of exit for the malaria parasites, which spend part of their life cycle in the mosquito's body; the mosquito in this case is the mode of transmission. The next link in the chain of causation is the agent itself. Malaria, for example, actually consists of four distinct diseases caused by four kinds of microscopic protozoa (Heymann, 2009). The next link is the portal of entry. In the case of malaria, the mosquito bite provides a portal of exit as well as a portal of entry into the human host.

The box surrounding the chain of causation in Figure 7-3 represents the environment, which can have a profound influence at almost any point along the chain. Consider the impact of environmental factors on the 1934 to 1935 malaria epidemic in Sri Lanka (an island country in the Indian Ocean off southern India, formerly known as Ceylon). Historically, malaria occurred frequently in the dry northern area, where sparse vegetation allowed pools of water to be exposed to the sun, providing excellent breeding grounds for the Anopheles

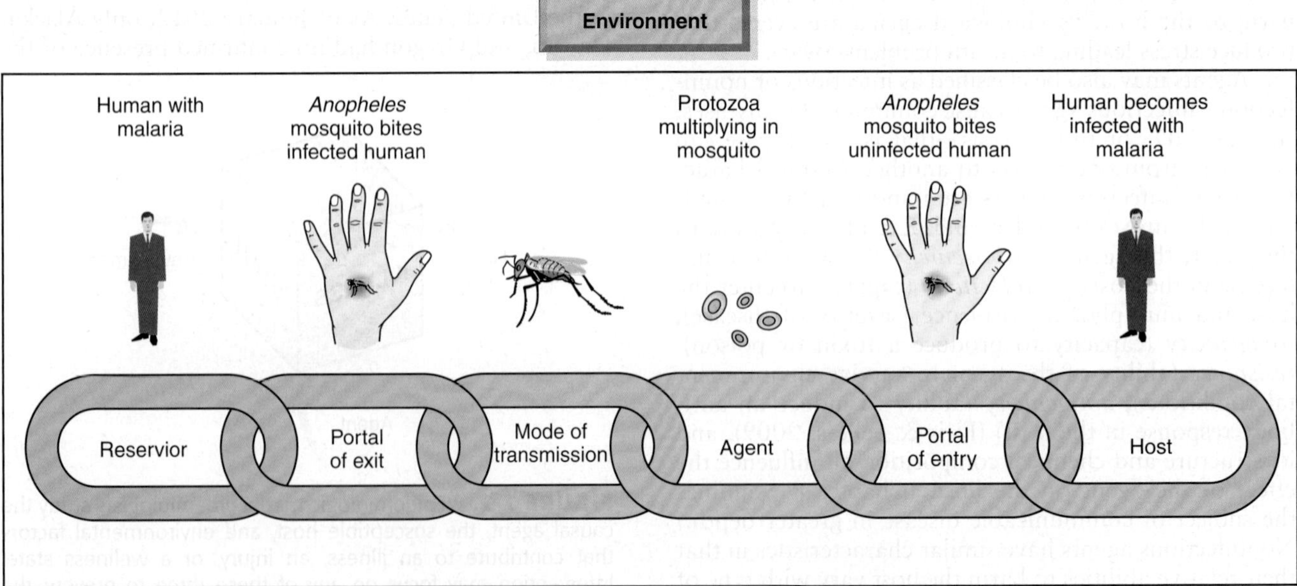

FIGURE 7-3. Chain of causation in infectious disease.

mosquito. In contrast, the more populous southwestern area usually had heavy monsoon rains and was relatively free from malaria. In 1934, however, a severe drought changed this environment drastically; throughout Sri Lanka, rivers almost dried up, leaving stagnant pools of water for mosquito breeding. Widespread crop failure caused the population to become badly undernourished, which added to conditions that would foster a malaria epidemic. The epidemic occurred in October 1934, affecting 2 to 3 million people and causing 80,000 deaths. The environment must certainly be seen as a major part of this causal chain (Burnet, 1962).

Another tragic example of the influence of environment on the causal chain occurred in the African country of Rwanda in July of 1994. Civil war caused a large percentage of the population to flee in the face of mass genocide of "unprecedented swiftness" that left up to 800,000 dead (U.S. Department of State, 2012). Hundreds of thousands of people filled refugee camps to overflowing. Conditions of squalor and poor sanitation led to contaminated water and resulted in a large-scale epidemic of cholera and the resulting severe watery diarrhea. The diarrhea typical of cholera is often referred to as "rice water" diarrhea due to the mucus that is present in the fluids. Relief workers had limited supplies of intravenous or oral rehydration solutions and could do little to help. Estimates were that over 12,000 refugees died during the epidemic (Siddique, 1994). The unstable political environment, unsanitary conditions, scarcity of clean water, and malnourishment were all part of the causal chain.

Causation in Noninfectious Disease

With the availability of vaccines and antibiotics in the United States and the developed world, attention shifted to the causes of noninfectious diseases such as cancer and diabetes. A new causal paradigm was clearly needed. The linear thinking embodied in models such as the *chain of causation* was insufficient in understanding the causes of these emerging health threats. Beginning in the 1950s, there was a growing interest in the role smoking played in the development of lung cancer. In 1964, the publication of *Smoking and Health: Report of the Advisory Committee to the Surgeon General of the Public Health Service* concluded that smoking caused lung and laryngeal cancer in men (U.S. Public Health Service [USPHS], 1964). The committee's conclusions were based on review of over 7,000 articles and utilized five criteria for judging the significance of the link between smoking and lung cancer (Friis & Sellers, 2009).

One year later, Sir Austin Bradford Hill proposed expanding those criteria to nine when evaluating the relationship between environmental exposure and potential health outcomes. Although these guidelines are often viewed as necessary for causal attribution, Hill stressed that they were a tool, not strict criteria (Legator & Morris, 2003). The elements added by Hill included biologic gradient, plausibility, experiment, and analogy. The criteria can be used with infectious disease, yet their significance lies with attributing cause in noninfectious disease. Each of the nine elements is summarized below (Aschengrau & Seage, 2008; Friis & Sellers, 2009):

1. *Strength of association:* This refers to the ratio of disease rates in those with and without the suspected causal factor. A strong association would be noted if disease rates are much higher in the group with the factor than in the group without it.
2. *Consistency:* An association is demonstrated in varying types of studies among diverse study groups (i.e., replication).
3. *Specificity:* A cause leads to one effect (not always the case in noninfectious diseases).
4. *Temporality:* Exposure to the suspected factor must precede the onset of disease (i.e., time order or time sequence).
5. *Biological gradient:* This relationship is demonstrated if, with increasing levels of exposure to the factor, there is a corresponding increase in occurrence of the disease (i.e., dose–response relationship).
6. *Plausibility:* The hypothesized cause makes sense based on current biologic or social models (i.e., it is possible).
7. *Coherence of explanation:* The hypothesized cause makes sense based on current knowledge about the natural history or biology of the disease (i.e., scientific knowledge).
8. *Experiment:* Experimental and nonexperimental studies support the association (e.g., reduced tobacco use in a population should lead to reduced lung cancer rates).
9. *Analogy:* Similarities between the association of interest and others (e.g., potential links to birth defects from new drugs is a concern since we already recognize this potential from the use of the drug thalidomide during the 1950s and early 1960s).

Based on the work of Hill and others, a basis was formed to critically assess causality in noninfectious diseases as well as in new and emerging infectious diseases. The elements described by Hill are still utilized by epidemiologists and provide the fundamental principles community health nurses can use to evaluate evidence of disease causation in all types of published reports, both scientific and lay. In health education, these principles can be utilized to teach disease causation risk, especially when the evidence is not yet complete. For instance, a pregnant teen asks a nurse if she should drink diet soda while she is pregnant. The nurse can share with her that the evidence to date supports the safety of artificial sweeteners for most adults (experiment) but that it is probably not wise to drink diet soda while pregnant. When she asks why (since there isn't any reported risk), the nurse can respond that any chemical has the potential to cause harm (plausibility and analogy), and the effects on a growing fetus (biologic gradient) are often unknown until decades later (temporality and experiment).

Multiple Causation

As health care professionals began to understand the complexity of many of the infectious and noninfectious disease threats, they came to realize that causation was never completely straightforward. Even with long-recognized contagious diseases like cholera, the organism was only part of the equation. Factors such as availability of clean water, the number of trained nurses and doctors, the overall nutrition of the population, and even political upheaval could influence the spread of disease and the number who ultimately died. Causation was beginning to be viewed as multifactorial. Fortunately, with recognition of the complexity of each health threat came multiple opportunities to find solutions. The following section discusses the complexity of causal factors on health outcomes and implications for reduced morbidity and mortality.

Web of Causation

In the 1960s, the concept of multiple causation emerged to explain the existence of health and illness states and to provide guiding principles for epidemiologic practice. A causal paradigm that gained attention was referred to as the web of causation. The implication was that intervention (or breaking of the web at any point nearest to the disease) could profoundly impact the development of that disease (Aschengrau & Seage, 2008). This was a significant shift in thinking about disease and health, positing that the combination of multiple factors was the deciding factor in the development of poor outcomes. This refinement in causal thinking also provided opportunities for health care interventions at a variety of levels. Another common term used for this approach is causal matrix.

Utilizing the multicausal approach, Figure 7-4 depicts a causal matrix for infant mortality. Data from birth and death certificates were used to identify the complex interactions among multiple causal factors that produce a negative health condition leading to infant mortality. Another example (Fig. 7-5) shows a web of causation for automobile crashes. All of the numerous factors involved must be considered when diagramming a web of causation. Speed, faulty equipment, heavy traffic, confusing traffic patterns, road construction, poor visibility, weather conditions, driver inexperience, and drinking or drug use, in any combination, can cause an automobile crash.

All health conditions can be diagramed to depict a matrix of causation. A communicable disease with one clearly identified organism as the agent has the ability to be diagramed based on factors such as availability of emergency services (treatment), diagnostic skill of health professionals (early diagnosis), availability of medications and vaccines to treat the disease (reduced morbidity), and community communication networks (public awareness). Any of these factors could greatly influence the progression of disease within the community.

Association is a concept that is helpful in determining multiple causality. Events are said to be associated if they appear together more often than would be the case by chance alone (see Perspectives Student Voice). Such events may include risk factors or other characteristics affecting disease or health states. Examples are the frequent association of cigarette smoking with lung cancer, obesity with heart disease, and severe prematurity with infant mortality. The study of associated factors suggests possible causality and points for intervention. Contemporary epidemiologists continue to explore new and more comprehensive ways of viewing health and illness. The associations among lifestyle, behavior, environment, and stress of all kinds and the ways in which they affect health states are gaining importance in epidemiology.

In the host, agent, and environment model, a shifting emphasis of investigation over time may be noted. Early epidemiologists worked to identify and manage the causative agent; the focus of concern was the disease state. The emphasis then shifted to the host: Who was susceptible? What characteristics led to susceptibility? Through immunization and health promotion, efforts were made to improve host resistance. Increasingly, however, public health workers came to realize the limitations imposed on individual control of

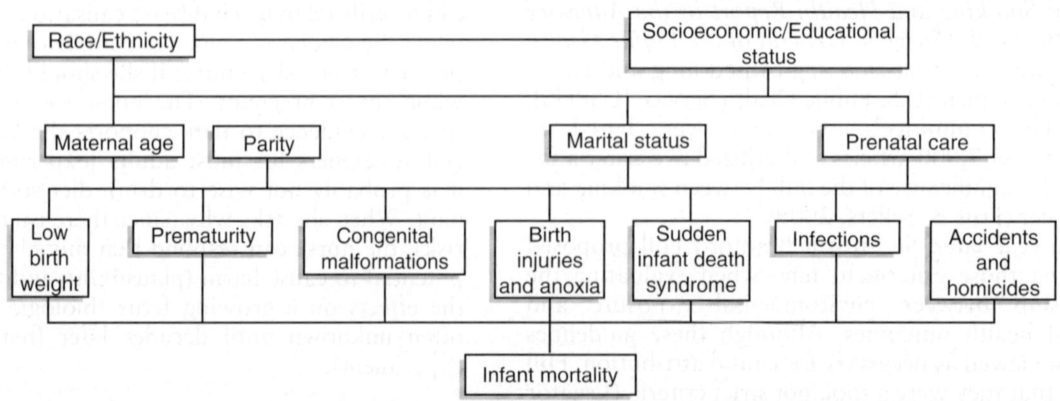

FIGURE 7-4. Web of causation for infant mortality based on information available from birth and death certificates. (From Anderson, E. T., & McFarlane, J. (2011). *Community as partner* (6th ed.). Philadelphia, PA: Wolters Kluwer/Lippincott Williams & Wilkins, with permission.)

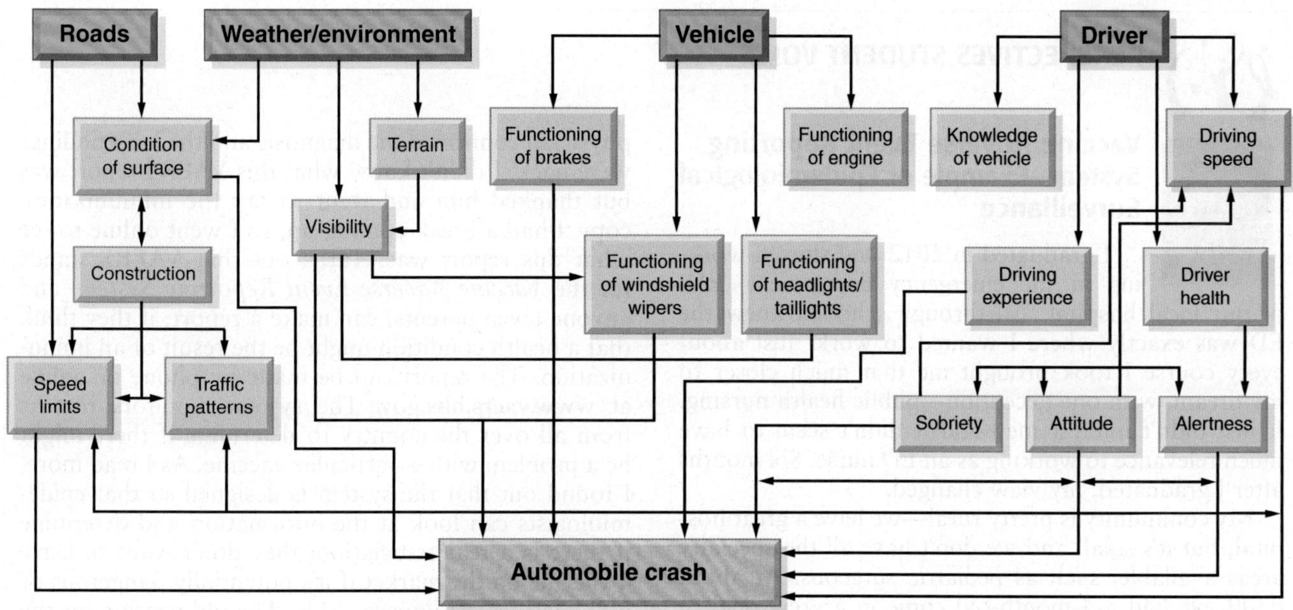

FIGURE 7-5. Web of causation for automobile crashes.

health. Even individuals who are in the best of health cannot withstand toxic agents in the workplace—for example, nuclear wastes in the atmosphere from power plant accidents—or other debilitating conditions created by modern society. More and more, public health professionals are studying the environment and looking for methods to change conditions that contribute to illness.

Immunity

Immunity refers to a host's ability to resist a particular infectious disease–causing agent. This occurs when the body forms antibodies and lymphocytes that react with the foreign antigenic molecules and render them harmless. For public health nursing, this concept has significance in determining which individuals and groups are protected against disease and which may be vulnerable. Four types of immunity are important in community health: passive immunity, active immunity, cross-immunity, and herd immunity.

Passive Immunity

Passive immunity refers to short-term resistance that is acquired either naturally or artificially. Newborns, through maternal antibody transfer, have natural passive immunity that lasts up to 1 year for certain diseases (CDC, 2011a). This maternally provided protection seems to work best with measles, rubella, and tetanus, and less well with other diseases (e.g., polio and pertussis). Artificial passive immunity is attained through inoculation with antibody products to provide temporary resistance. Examples of such products include immune globulin (hepatitis A and measles), hyperimmune globulins (hepatitis B, rabies, tetanus, and varicella), and hyperimmune serum (equine antitoxin for use with botulism and diphtheria). These products are used to boost a susceptible person's immunity, and administration must be repeated periodically to maintain immunity levels (CDC, 2011a).

Active Immunity

Active immunity is long-term and sometimes lifelong resistance that is acquired either naturally or artificially. Naturally acquired active immunity comes through host infection. That is, a person who contracts a disease often develops long-lasting antibodies that provide immunity against future exposures. Artificially acquired active immunity is attained through vaccine inoculation. Such vaccines are prepared from killed (inactivated) or live attenuated (weakened) organisms administered to artificially produce or increase immunity to a particular disease (CDC, 2011a). The concept of active immunity underlies public health immunization programs that have successfully kept polio, diphtheria, smallpox, and other major diseases under control worldwide.

Cross-Immunity

Cross-immunity refers to a situation in which a person's immunity to one agent provides immunity to a related agent as well. The immunity can be either passive or active. Sometimes, infection with one disease, such as cowpox, gives immunity to a related disease, such as smallpox. The concept of cross-immunity has also been useful in the development and administration of vaccines. Inoculation with a vaccine made from one disease-causing organism can provide immunity to a related disease-causing organism. Field trials in Uganda and Papua New Guinea and a study in India in the 1990s examined the administration of bacille Calmette-Guérin (BCG) vaccine, which is used to

PERSPECTIVES STUDENT VOICE

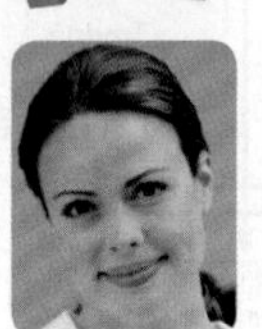

Vaccine Adverse Event Reporting System—Example of Epidemiological Surveillance

I graduated in 2012 and started working in the emergency department (ED) of our local hospital. All through school I knew the ED was exactly where I wanted to work. Just about every course I took brought me that much closer to my dream, with one exception—public health nursing. It just didn't interest me—and it didn't seem to have much relevance to working as an ED nurse. Six months after I graduated, my view changed.

My community is pretty rural—we have a great hospital, but it's small and we don't have all the specialty areas available, such as pediatric surgeons. At about 0300, we had a 4-month-old come in a great deal of distress, vomiting and crying inconsolably. While I was interviewing the mother, she said he had been a very healthy baby up until about 8 hours ago and had even been seen by his pediatrician a few days earlier for his regular checkup. She handed me his immunization record as proof. We ended up airlifting the baby to the nearest children's hospital when it seemed likely that he had intussusception, which is a folding of the bowel on itself and pretty serious. After the child and the mother were gone, I realized that I still had the child's immunization record and hadn't yet looked at it either. I called the other hospital to tell them I had the immunization record and that I could fax over a copy. The nurse I spoke with asked me which immunizations the child had recently received. Thinking he just wanted to see if the child was up-to-date, I told him he just had a well-child visit a few days ago. He persisted and told me he needed to know the exact dates and which vaccines were given. As I read through the list, I realized I wasn't familiar with one of the vaccines and asked him what it was. He explained that it was the rotavirus vaccine and had been licensed since 2006—adding that an earlier vaccine had been pulled off the market in 1999 due to an association with intussusception. He had my attention! The nurse wanted to know if the lot numbers for the vaccines were on the record—and they were. I asked if he thought the child's condition was due to the vaccine—he didn't believe so, but that he would be making a VAERS report on the case once the physician confirmed the diagnosis and the lab's findings were back. I didn't know what this VAERS report was but thanked him and went to fax the immunization copy. I had a break coming up, so I went online to see what this report was. Turns out that VAERS stands for the *Vaccine Adverse Event Reporting System,* and anyone (even parents) can make a report, if they think that a health condition might be the result of an immunization. The report can be made by phone or online at www.vaers.hhs.gov. The system monitors reports from all over the country to determine if there might be a problem with a particular vaccine. As I read more, I found out that the system is designed so that epidemiologists can look at the information and determine if there is a real association; they don't want to leave a vaccine on the market if it's potentially dangerous or pull vaccines off unnecessarily. The old vaccine for the rotavirus was pulled off the market after reports came in from VAERS and other sources. While I was sitting there taking this all in, I started recognizing that I had encountered two public health situations with just this one patient, and I had missed both of them. The first was assuming that because the child had a well-child checkup that he was up-to-date with his immunizations (I should have checked the record). The second was disease surveillance—if I had paid attention to the current recommendations for the rotavirus vaccine, I might have been alert to the potential connection with intussusception and been aware of the VAERS system. Since that night, I have done some research on the vaccine's safety, and so far, it looks like the association with intussusception is no more than would be expected in unvaccinated children—but I'll keep checking. I'm now the nurse that everyone comes to for information on vaccines, the need to make sure all the children we treat are up-to-date, and how to provide data to help monitor potential problems with vaccines. Who knew you could use public health nursing skills in an ED?

—Minerva G., RN/BSN (a.k.a. PHN)

For more information please see:

Centers for Disease Control and Prevention. (2010). *Vaccines and Preventable Diseases: Statement Regarding Rotarix® and RotaTeq® Rotavirus Vaccines and Intussusception.* Retrieved from http://www.cdc.gov/vaccines/vpd-vac/rotavirus/intussusception-studies-acip.htm

Centers for Disease Control and Prevention. (2011). *Vaccine Adverse Event Reporting System (VAERS).* Retrieved from http://www.cdc.gov/vaccinesafety/Activities/vaers.html

prevent tuberculosis, to people who had been exposed to Hansen disease (leprosy). The vaccine against Mycobacterium tuberculosis appeared to provide these individuals with a degree of cross-immunity to the related infectious agent, Mycobacterium leprae, and prevented their contracting disease (Heymann, 2009).

Herd Immunity

Herd immunity describes the immunity level that is present in a population group. A population with low herd immunity is one with few immune members; consequently, it is more susceptible to a particular disease.

Nonimmune people are more likely to contract the disease and spread it throughout the group, placing the entire population at greater risk. Conversely, a population with high herd immunity is one in which the immune people in the group outnumber the susceptible people; consequently, the incidence of a particular disease is reduced (Friis & Sellers, 2009). The level of herd immunity may vary with diseases. For instance, a level of community immunity of between 85% and 90% may be necessary for rubella, but for diphtheria a level of 70% may be effective (Friis & Sellers, 2009). Mandatory preschool immunizations and required travel vaccinations are applications of the herd immunity concept.

Risk

To determine the chances that a disease or health problem will occur, epidemiologists are concerned with risk, or the probability that a disease or other unfavorable health condition will develop. For any given group of people, the risk of developing a health problem is directly influenced by their biology, environment, lifestyle, and system of health care (Dever, 1984). A person's inherited health capacity, the environment lived in, the person's lifestyle choices, and the quality and accessibility of the health care system either negatively or positively affect health, thereby increasing or decreasing the likelihood that a health problem will occur. Negative influences are called risk factors. For example, low-birth-weight babies (biology, environment, and system of health care) tend to be at greater risk for health problems, as are people who smoke cigarettes, have diets high in cholesterol, and are sedentary (lifestyle). The degree of risk is directly linked to susceptibility or vulnerability to a given health problem.

Epidemiologists study populations at risk. A *population at risk* is a collection of people among whom a health problem has the possibility of developing because certain influencing factors are present (e.g., exposure to HIV) or absent (e.g., lack of childhood immunizations, lack of specific vitamins in the diet), or because there are modifiable risk factors present (e.g., CVD). A population at risk has a greater probability of developing a given health problem than other groups do. Epidemiologists measure this difference using the *relative risk ratio,* which statistically compares the disease occurrence in the population at risk with the occurrence of the same disease in people without that risk factor.

$$\text{Relative risk ratio} = \frac{\text{Incidence in exposed group}}{\text{Incidence rate in unexposed group}}$$

If the risk of acquiring the disease is the same regardless of exposure to the risk factor studied, the ratio will be 1:1, and the relative risk will be 1.0. A relative risk >1.0 indicates that those with the risk factor have a greater likelihood of acquiring the disease than do those without it, for instance, a relative risk of 2.54 means that the exposed group is 2.54 times more likely to acquire the disease than the unexposed group. This statistic may be used, for example, to compare the incidence of heart disease among smokers (smoking is a risk factor) with the incidence among nonsmokers, assuming that all other factors are the same. The relative risk ratio assists in determining the most effective points for community health intervention in regard to particular health problems. It also provides a more easily understood method for explaining the risk of certain behaviors in the development of illness or injury to the public.

Natural History of a Disease or Health Condition

Any disease or health condition follows a progression known as its **natural history**; this refers to events that occur before its development, during its course, and during its conclusion. This process involves the interactions among a susceptible host, the causative agent, and the environment. The natural progression of a disease occurs in four stages as they affect a population—susceptibility, preclinical (subclinical) disease, clinical disease, and resolution (Fig. 7-6). The last stage, resolution, includes recovery, disability, or death (Gerstman, 2003).

Susceptibility Stage

The first stage is susceptibility. During this state, the disease is not present and individuals have not been exposed. However, host and environmental factors could very likely influence people's susceptibility to a causative agent and lead to development of the disease. For example, college students with poor eating habits and fatigue from lack of sleep during final examinations present risk factors that promote the occurrence of the common cold. "If exposure to an agent occurs at this time, a response will take place. Initial responses reflect the normal adaptation response of the cell or functional system (e.g., the immune system). If these adaptation responses are successful, then no disease occurs and the process is arrested" (Valanis, 1999, p. 22). In 1994, the overcrowded conditions and poor sanitation of Rwandan refugee camps in Africa, described earlier, as well as refugees' stress, fatigue, and malnutrition, made them extremely vulnerable to contracting cholera and other diseases. However, in a later tragedy in Kosovo in 1999, the thousands of refugees fleeing for their lives from Yugoslavian Serbs were housed in refugee border camps with adequate supplies and services, and many found temporary or permanent refuge in other countries, including the United States. They endured a shorter period of stress and fatigue with better nutrition than the refugees in Rwanda; as a result, malnutrition was not as rampant. Because improved conditions in refugee camps eliminated major outbreaks of cholera and other diseases, susceptibility to disease in the group as a whole was reduced. Nevertheless, the psychological trauma from the attempts at "ethnic cleansing" of the people in Kosovo remained an existing health problem for years.

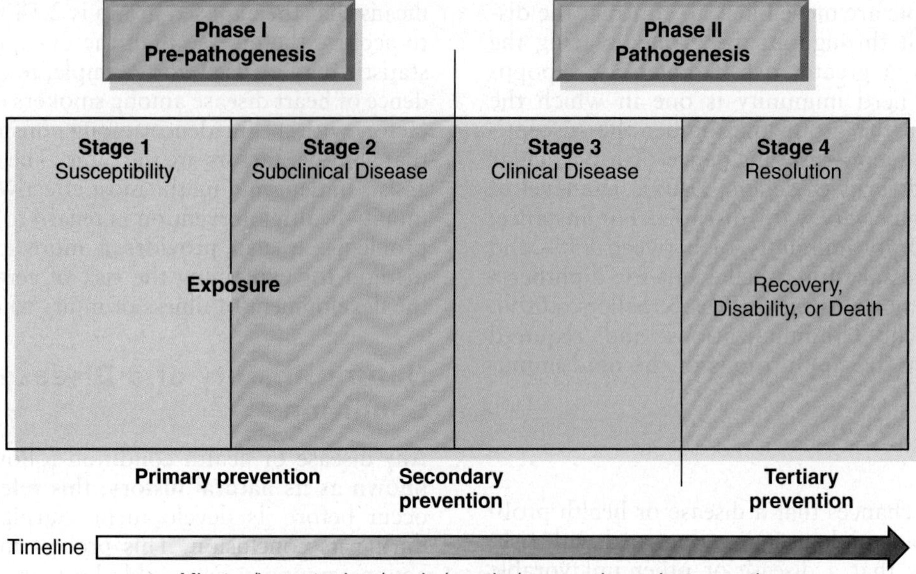

FIGURE 7-6. Natural history stages of a disease or health condition. (Adapted from Gerstman, B. B. (2003). *Epidemiology kept simple: An introduction to traditional and modern epidemiology* (2nd ed.). Hoboken, NJ: Wiley-Liss, Inc.)

Subclinical Disease Stage

The stage of subclinical disease begins when individuals have been exposed to a disease but are as yet asymptomatic. It is followed by an incubation period, during which the organism multiplies to sufficient numbers to produce a host reaction and clinical symptoms. Vulnerable children who have been exposed to chickenpox (varicella) but do not yet display signs of fever or lesions are in this stage. For diseases caused by infectious agents, the incubation period is relatively short, hours to months. One noteworthy exception to this is infection with HIV, which has an incubation period of 1 to 3 months, with progression to AIDS from 1 to 15 years or longer (Heymann, 2009). In other conditions caused by noninfectious agents, the time from exposure to onset of symptoms, known as the induction period or latency period, is often years to decades. For example, children exposed to radiation may have a 5-year latency period for leukemia. Lung cancer caused by exposure to asbestos may have a latency period of 40 years between exposure and detection of the disease.

Clinical Disease Stage

During the clinical disease stage, signs and symptoms of the disease or condition develop. In the early phase of this period, the signs may be evident only through laboratory test findings, such as tubercular lesions on radiographs or premalignant cervical changes evident on Papanicolaou (Pap) smears. Later in this stage, acute symptoms are clearly visible, as in the case of widespread enterocolitis in a salmonellosis (food poisoning) outbreak. In this early clinical stage or early discernible lesions stage, evidence of the disease or condition is present and diagnosis occurs.

Resolution Stage

In the resolution stage, the disease or health condition causes sufficient anatomic or functional changes to produce recognizable signs and symptoms. Disease severity may vary from mild to severe. The disease may conclude with a return to health, a residual or chronic form of the disease with some disabling limitations, or death. This can also be called the advanced disease stage because the disease or condition has completed its course.

Community health nurses can intervene at any point during these four stages to delay, arrest, or prevent the progression of the disease or condition. Primary, secondary, and tertiary prevention can be applied to each of the stages (see Levels of Prevention Pyramid).

Epidemiology of Wellness

The public health science of epidemiology has traditionally studied the occurrence of disease and health problems. Because of their devastating effect on the health of populations, infectious diseases such as plague, cholera, and AIDS, as well as chronic illnesses such as heart disease

LEVELS OF PREVENTION PYRAMID

SITUATION: Apply the levels of prevention during the four stages of the natural history of a disease to eradicate or reduce risk factors (examples of possible conditions provided)

GOAL: Using the three levels of prevention, negative health conditions are avoided, or promptly diagnosed and treated, and the fullest possible potential is restored.

<table>
<tr><th colspan="3">TERTIARY PREVENTION</th></tr>
<tr><th>Rehabilitation</th><th colspan="2">Primary Prevention</th></tr>
<tr><td rowspan="2">• Reduce the extent and severity of a health problem to minimize disability
• Restore or preserve function</td><td>Health Promotion & Education</td><td>Health Protection</td></tr>
<tr><td>• Training for employment —homeless population
• Group treatment and rehabilitation—adolescent drug users
• Food, shelter, rest/sleep, exercise</td><td>• Health services
• Immunizations as needed</td></tr>
<tr><th colspan="3">SECONDARY PREVENTION</th></tr>
<tr><th>Early Diagnosis</th><th colspan="2">Prompt Treatment</th></tr>
<tr><td>The third stage in the natural history of disease, the early pathogenesis or onset stage:
• Screening programs—breast and testicular cancer, vision and hearing loss, hypertension, tuberculosis, diabetes</td><td colspan="2">• Initiate prompt treatment
• Arrest progression
• Prevent associated disability</td></tr>
<tr><th colspan="3">PRIMARY PREVENTION</th></tr>
<tr><th>Health Promotion & Education</th><th colspan="2">Health Protection</th></tr>
<tr><td>May include:
• Nutrition counseling—diabetes
• Sex education—pregnancy
• Smoking cessation—lung cancer</td><td colspan="2">May include:
• Improved housing and sanitation—waterborne diseases
• Immunizations—communicable diseases
• Removal of environmental hazards—accidents</td></tr>
</table>

or cancer, and fatal or debilitating injuries all require a continued epidemiologic focus. Nonetheless, the need to examine the epidemiology of wellness grows increasingly urgent, for if we continually examine and uncover new health promotion practices and encourage them, we can focus on wellness at the ideal primary level of prevention.

Epidemiology has moved from concentrating only on illness to examining how host, agent, and environment are involved in wellness at various levels. In response to an escalating need for improved methods of health planning and health policy analysis, epidemiology has developed more holistic models of health (Dever, 1984, 1991). These evolving epidemiologic models are organized around four attributes that influence health: (1) the physical, social, and psychological environment; (2) lifestyle with its self-created risks; (3) human biology and genetic influences; and (4) the system of health care organization. In the United States, *Healthy People 2020* (USDHHS, 2010) and greater recognition of the importance and cost-effectiveness of illness prevention and health promotion are driving new efforts to develop policy and research initiatives to improve the public's health (see Display 7.2). There is also growing recognition of the collective impact of social determinants of health on health outcomes and conditions, not merely their individual role. Social determinants of health are "conditions in the environments in which people are born, live, play, worship, and age that affect a wide range of health, functioning, and quality of life outcomes and risks" (USDHHS, 2012). Population disparities result when these social determinants disproportionately impact individuals due to race/ethnicity, socioeconomic status, gender, age, disability status, sexual orientation, and geographic location (USDHHS, 2010).

Wellness models that at first focused on individual behavior now include approaches that encompass aggregates. A variety of wellness models can be found for groups of seniors (see Chapter 24), in occupational health

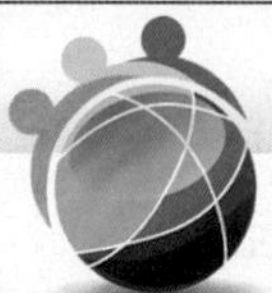

DISPLAY 7.2 *HEALTHY PEOPLE 2020*

Epidemiological Focus Objectives—Data and Information Systems

PHI-7—(Developmental) Increase the proportion of population-based *Healthy People 2020* objectives for which national data are available for all major population groups

PHI-8—Increase the proportion of *Healthy People 2020* objectives that are tracked regularly at the national level

PHI-9—(Developmental) Increase the proportion of *Healthy People 2020* objectives for which national data are released within 1 year of the end of data collection

PHI-10—Increase the number of states that record vital events using the latest US standard certificates and report (including birth, death, and fetal death)

Public Health Organizations

PHI-11—Increase the proportion of tribal and state public health agencies that provide or assure comprehensive laboratory services to support essential public health services (including integrated data management)

PHI-13—Increase the proportion of tribal, state, and local public health agencies that provide or assure comprehensive epidemiology services to support essential public health services (including state epidemiologists with formal training in epidemiology)

Source: U.S. Department of Health and Human Services. (2010). *Healthy People 2020: Public health infrastructure.* Retrieved from http:/www.healthypeople.gov/2020/topicsobjectives2020/objectiveslist.aspx?topicId=35

settings (see Chapter 31), at innovative schools where wellness programs for children and teens are initiated (see Chapter 22), and throughout the services provided for beginning and growing families (see Chapter 21). Programs designed for aggregates focus on a wellness approach to growth and development. Examples include programs for pregnant teens and for infant and child development (e.g., Healthy Start, Head Start) that are funded by state and federal monies. Societal changes such as the aging population, the communication revolution, the global economy, environmental threats, technology development, and the holism and wellness movements are driving these new approaches.

The four stages of the natural history of disease can apply to an understanding of any health condition, including wellness states. In stage one, *susceptibility*, people can become amenable to healthier practices and improved health system organization. In stage two, *subclinical*, a community can learn about these health-promoting behaviors. Stage three, *clinical disease stage*, could be a period of trying out the beneficial policies and activities, and stage four, *resolution*, could encompass full adoption and a higher level of wellbeing for the community. This approach has important implications for preventive and health promotion practices in community health nursing.

Community health nursing can play a primary role in the investigation and identification of factors that not only prevent illness but also promote health. This means sharpening skills in epidemiologic research to uncover the factors that contribute to a full measure of healthful living. The time for an epidemiology of wellness has come.

Causal Relationships

One of the main challenges to epidemiology is to identify causal relationships in disease and health conditions in populations. As was previously suggested, the assessment of causality in human health is difficult at best; no single study is adequate to establish causality. Causal inference is based on consistent results obtained from many studies. Frequently, the accumulation of evidence begins with a clinical observation or an educated guess that a certain factor may be causally related to a health problem.

A *cross-sectional study* (which explores a health condition's relation to other variables in a specified population at a specific point in time) can show that the factor and the problem coexist. For example, one study compared the incidence of gonorrhea in a 55-block area in urban New Orleans with a "broken window index," which measured housing quality, abandoned cars, graffiti, trash, and public school deterioration (Cohen et al., 2000). The broken window index predicted the variance for gonorrhea rates more accurately than did a poverty index measuring income, unemployment, and low education.

A *retrospective study* (which looks backward in time to find a causal relationship) allows a fairly quick assessment of whether an association exists. Looking back at the use of lead in interior paint in the United States, history shows that even though the particular dangers to children were documented in English language literature as early as 1904, the US lead industry did nothing to discourage the use of lead paint on interior walls and woodwork. In fact, some paint companies (e.g., Dutch Boy Paint) used children in their advertising through the 1920s (Markowitz & Rosner, 2000). Not until the 1950s did the industry adopt a voluntary standard limiting the amount of lead in interior paints and then only under increasing pressure. Not until 1978 was interior lead paint prohibited.

A *prospective study* (which looks forward in time to find a causal relationship) is crucial to ensure that the presumed causal factor actually precedes the onset of the health problem. The prospective approach is concerned with current information and provides a direct measure of the variables in question. For example, the U.S. Nurses' Health Study provided an opportunity for a prospective analysis of the association between night shift work and sleep deprivation and the risk of developing Parkinson's disease. In a sample of nearly 85,000 registered nurses, those with 15 or more years of night shift work had a 50% lower risk of developing the disease than those nurses who never worked the night shift. Increased sleep duration was positively associated with disease risk. The data suggested one of two options: that night shift work is protective against the development of Parkinson's disease or that low tolerance for night shift work is an indicator of the disease (Chen, Schernhammer, Schwarzschild, & Ascherio, 2006). Other U.S. Nurses' Health Study findings included 24% increase in risk of endometrial cancer in postmenopausal women who used perineal talcum powder at least once per week (Karageorgi, Gates, Hankinson, & De Vivo, 2010) and the association between greater physical activity and lower urinary albumin excretion in nondiabetic women (high levels of ACR are predictive of CVD, hypertension, and chronic kidney disease) (Robinson, Fisher, Forman, & Curhan, 2010). Studies such as these provide a mechanism to evaluate a variety of factors that precede the development of disease and then assess issues of association and ultimately causation.

Finally, if ethically possible, an *experimental study* (in which the investigator controls or changes factors suspected of causing the condition and observes results) is used to confirm the associations obtained from observational studies (in which the investigator merely observes data or people without controlling or changing any factors). It often requires many years to accumulate enough evidence to suggest a causal relationship.

Epidemiologically, a causal relationship may be said to exist if two major conditions are met: The factor of interest (causal agent) is shown to increase the probability of occurrence of the disease or condition as observed in many studies in different populations, and evidence suggests that a reduction in the factor decreases the frequency of the given disease. The synthesis of data begins by selecting as many of the various types of epidemiologic studies of the problem as possible. After those studies that are not methodologically sound are discarded, the studies are reviewed. The better the data meet the criteria outlined by Hill (discussed earlier), the more likely it is that the factor of interest is one of several causes of the disease (strength of association, consistency, specificity, time sequence, biologic gradient, plausibility, coherence, experiment, and analogy).

The goal of any epidemiologic investigation is to identify causal mechanisms that meet these nine criteria and to develop measures for preventing illness and promoting health. The community health nurse may need to gather new data for this type of investigation, but pertinent existing data should be thoroughly examined first. This type of information can be obtained by the community health nurse from a variety of sources, which are discussed in the next section.

SOURCES OF INFORMATION FOR EPIDEMIOLOGIC STUDY

Epidemiologic investigators may draw data from any of three major sources: existing data, informal investigations, and scientific studies. The public health nurse will find all three sources useful in efforts to improve the health of aggregates.

Existing Data

A variety of information is available nationally, by state, and by section, such as county, region, or urbanized area. This information includes vital statistics, census data, and morbidity statistics on certain communicable or infectious diseases. Local health departments often can provide these data on request. Public health nurses seeking information on communities may find local health system agencies helpful. These agencies collect health information for groups of counties within states and interact with health planning authorities at the state level. They have access to many types of information and can give advice on specific problems.

Vital Statistics

Vital statistics refers to the information gathered from ongoing registration of births, deaths, adoptions, divorces, and marriages. Certification of births, deaths, and fetal deaths are the most useful vital statistics in epidemiologic studies. The community health nurse can obtain blank copies of a state's birth and death certificates to become familiar with the information contained in each (Displays 7.3 and 7.4). Much more information is recorded than the fact and cause of death on the death certificate. Birth certificates also can provide helpful information (e.g., weight of the infant, amount of prenatal care received by the mother), which can be used to identify high-risk mothers and infants.

Sources for vital statistical information include state Web sites on the Internet, local and state health departments, city halls, and county halls of records (see list of Internet resources at the end of this chapter). Statistics regarding general morbidity and mortality for specific states are located in the aggregate from CDC at the national level (National Center for Health Statistics [NCHS]). State statistics are obtained from state health departments, and county information (specific cities or census tracts) can be obtained from either the state or the county health department.

Census Data

Data from population censuses taken every 10 years in many countries are the main source of population statistics. This information can be a valuable assessment tool for the community health nurse who is taking part in health planning for aggregates. Population statistics can be analyzed by age, sex, race, ethnic background, type of occupation, income gradient, marital status, educational level, or other standards, such as housing

DISPLAY 7.3 STANDARD BIRTH CERTIFICATE

U.S. STANDARD CERTIFICATE OF LIVE BIRTH

LOCAL FILE NO. BIRTH NUMBER:

CHILD

1. CHILD'S NAME (First, Middle, Last, Suffix)
2. TIME OF BIRTH (24 hr)
3. SEX
4. DATE OF BIRTH (Mo/Day/Yr)
5. FACILITY NAME (If not institution, give street and number)
6. CITY, TOWN, OR LOCATION OF BIRTH
7. COUNTY OF BIRTH

MOTHER

8a. MOTHER'S CURRENT LEGAL NAME (First, Middle, Last, Suffix)
8b. DATE OF BIRTH (Mo/Day/Yr)
8c. MOTHER'S NAME PRIOR TO FIRST MARRIAGE (First, Middle, Last, Suffix)
8d. BIRTHPLACE (State, Territory, or Foreign Country)
9a. RESIDENCE OF MOTHER-STATE
9b. COUNTY
9c. CITY, TOWN, OR LOCATION
9d. STREET AND NUMBER
9e. APT. NO.
9f. ZIP CODE
9g. INSIDE CITY LIMITS? □ Yes □ No

FATHER

10a. FATHER'S CURRENT LEGAL NAME (First, Middle, Last, Suffix)
10b. DATE OF BIRTH (Mo/Day/Yr)
10c. BIRTHPLACE (State, Territory, or Foreign Country)

CERTIFIER

11. CERTIFIER'S NAME:
TITLE: □ MD □ DO □ HOSPITAL ADMIN. □ CNM/CM □ OTHER MIDWIFE
□ OTHER (Specify)__________
12. DATE CERTIFIED ___/___/___ MM DD YYYY
13. DATE FILED BY REGISTRAR ___/___/___ MM DD YYYY

INFORMATION FOR ADMINISTRATIVE USE

MOTHER

14. MOTHER'S MAILING ADDRESS: 9 Same as residence, or: State: City, Town, or Location:
Street & Number: Apartment No.: Zip Code:
15. MOTHER MARRIED? (At birth, conception, or any time between) □ Yes □ No
IF NO, HAS PATERNITY ACKNOWLEDGEMENT BEEN SIGNED IN THE HOSPITAL? □ Yes □ No
16. SOCIAL SECURITY NUMBER REQUESTED FOR CHILD? □ Yes □ No
17. FACILITY ID. (NPI)
18. MOTHER'S SOCIAL SECURITY NUMBER:
19. FATHER'S SOCIAL SECURITY NUMBER:

INFORMATION FOR MEDICAL AND HEALTH PURPOSES ONLY

MOTHER

20. MOTHER'S EDUCATION (Check the box that best describes the highest degree or level of school completed at the time of delivery)
□ 8th grade or less
□ 9th - 12th grade, no diploma
□ High school graduate or GED completed
□ Some college credit but no degree
□ Associate degree (e.g., AA, AS)
□ Bachelor's degree (e.g., BA, AB, BS)
□ Master's degree (e.g., MA, MS, MEng, MEd, MSW, MBA)
□ Doctorate (e.g., PhD, EdD) or Professional degree (e.g., MD, DDS, DVM, LLB, JD)

21. MOTHER OF HISPANIC ORIGIN? (Check the box that best describes whether the mother is Spanish/Hispanic/Latina. Check the "No" box if mother is not Spanish/Hispanic/Latina)
□ No, not Spanish/Hispanic/Latina
□ Yes, Mexican, Mexican American, Chicana
□ Yes, Puerto Rican
□ Yes, Cuban
□ Yes, other Spanish/Hispanic/Latina
(Specify)__________

22. MOTHER'S RACE (Check one or more races to indicate what the mother considers herself to be)
□ White
□ Black or African American
□ American Indian or Alaska Native (Name of the enrolled or principal tribe)__________
□ Asian Indian
□ Chinese
□ Filipino
□ Japanese
□ Korean
□ Vietnamese
□ Other Asian (Specify)__________
□ Native Hawaiian
□ Guamanian or Chamorro
□ Samoan
□ Other Pacific Islander (Specify)__________
□ Other (Specify)__________

FATHER

23. FATHER'S EDUCATION (Check the box that best describes the highest degree or level of school completed at the time of delivery)
□ 8th grade or less
□ 9th - 12th grade, no diploma
□ High school graduate or GED completed
□ Some college credit but no degree
□ Associate degree (e.g., AA, AS)
□ Bachelor's degree (e.g., BA, AB, BS)
□ Master's degree (e.g., MA, MS, MEng, MEd, MSW, MBA)
□ Doctorate (e.g., PhD, EdD) or Professional degree (e.g., MD, DDS, DVM, LLB, JD)

24. FATHER OF HISPANIC ORIGIN? (Check the box that best describes whether the father is Spanish/Hispanic/Latino. Check the "No" box if father is not Spanish/Hispanic/Latino)
□ No, not Spanish/Hispanic/Latino
□ Yes, Mexican, Mexican American, Chicano
□ Yes, Puerto Rican
□ Yes, Cuban
□ Yes, other Spanish/Hispanic/Latino
(Specify)__________

25. FATHER'S RACE (Check one or more races to indicate what the father considers himself to be)
□ White
□ Black or African American
□ American Indian or Alaska Native (Name of the enrolled or principal tribe)__________
□ Asian Indian
□ Chinese
□ Filipino
□ Japanese
□ Korean
□ Vietnamese
□ Other Asian (Specify)__________
□ Native Hawaiian
□ Guamanian or Chamorro
□ Samoan
□ Other Pacific Islander (Specify)__________
□ Other (Specify)__________

Mother's Name __________

Mother's Medical Record No. __________

26. PLACE WHERE BIRTH OCCURRED (Check one)
□ Hospital
□ Freestanding birthing center
□ Home Birth: Planned to deliver at home? 9 Yes 9 No
□ Clinic/Doctor's office
□ Other (Specify)__________

27. ATTENDANT'S NAME, TITLE, AND NPI
NAME: __________ NPI: ______
TITLE: □ MD □ DO □ CNM/CM □ OTHER MIDWIFE
□ OTHER (Specify)__________

28. MOTHER TRANSFERRED FOR MATERNAL MEDICAL OR FETAL INDICATIONS FOR DELIVERY? □ Yes □ No
IF YES, ENTER NAME OF FACILITY MOTHER TRANSFERRED FROM:
____

REV. 11/2003

MOTHER

29a. DATE OF FIRST PRENATAL CARE VISIT ______/______/______ MM DD YYYY □ No Prenatal Care

29b. DATE OF LAST PRENATAL CARE VISIT ______/______/______ MM DD YYYY

30. TOTAL NUMBER OF PRENATAL VISITS FOR THIS PREGNANCY ______________ (If none, enter A0".)

31. MOTHER'S HEIGHT ______ (feet/inches)

32. MOTHER'S PREPREGNANCY WEIGHT ______ (pounds)

33. MOTHER'S WEIGHT AT DELIVERY ______ (pounds)

34. DID MOTHER GET WIC FOOD FOR HERSELF DURING THIS PREGNANCY? □ Yes □ No

35. NUMBER OF PREVIOUS LIVE BIRTHS (Do not include this child)

35a. Now Living Number _____ □ None

35b. Now Dead Number _____ □ None

36. NUMBER OF OTHER PREGNANCY OUTCOMES (spontaneous or induced losses or ectopic pregnancies)

36a. Other Outcomes Number _____ □ None

37. CIGARETTE SMOKING BEFORE AND DURING PREGNANCY For each time period, enter either the number of cigarettes or the number of packs of cigarettes smoked. IF NONE, ENTER A0".

Average number of cigarettes or packs of cigarettes smoked per day.

	# of cigarettes		# of packs
Three Months Before Pregnancy	______	OR	______
First Three Months of Pregnancy	______	OR	______
Second Three Months of Pregnancy	______	OR	______
Third Trimester of Pregnancy	______	OR	______

38. PRINCIPAL SOURCE OF PAYMENT FOR THIS DELIVERY
□ Private Insurance
□ Medicaid
□ Self-pay
□ Other (Specify) ____________

35c. DATE OF LAST LIVE BIRTH ______/______ MM YYYY

36b. DATE OF LAST OTHER PREGNANCY OUTCOME ______/______ MM YYYY

39. DATE LAST NORMAL MENSES BEGAN ______/______/______ MM DD YYYY

40. MOTHER'S MEDICAL RECORD NUMBER

MEDICAL AND HEALTH INFORMATION

41. RISK FACTORS IN THIS PREGNANCY (Check all that apply)

Diabetes
□ Prepregnancy (Diagnosis prior to this pregnancy)
□ Gestational (Diagnosis in this pregnancy)

Hypertension
□ Prepregnancy (Chronic)
□ Gestational (PIH, preeclampsia)
□ Eclampsia

□ Previous preterm birth

□ Other previous poor pregnancy outcome (Includes perinatal death, small-for-gestational age/intrauterine growth restricted birth)

□ Pregnancy resulted from infertility treatment-If yes, check all that apply:
□ Fertility-enhancing drugs, Artificial insemination or Intrauterine insemination
□ Assisted reproductive technology (e.g., in vitro fertilization (IVF), gamete intrafallopian transfer (GIFT))

□ Mother had a previous cesarean delivery If yes, how many ________

□ None of the above

42. INFECTIONS PRESENT AND/OR TREATED DURING THIS PREGNANCY (Check all that apply)
□ Gonorrhea
□ Syphilis
□ Chlamydia
□ Hepatitis B
□ Hepatitis C
□ None of the above

43. OBSTETRIC PROCEDURES (Check all that apply)
□ Cervical cerclage
□ Tocolysis

External cephalic version:
□ Successful
□ Failed

□ None of the above

44. ONSET OF LABOR (Check all that apply)
□ Premature Rupture of the Membranes (prolonged, ∃12 hrs.)
□ Precipitous Labor (<3 hrs.)
□ Prolonged Labor (∃ 20 hrs.)
□ None of the above

45. CHARACTERISTICS OF LABOR AND DELIVERY (Check all that apply)
□ Induction of labor
□ Augmentation of labor
□ Non-vertex presentation
□ Steroids (glucocorticoids) for fetal lung maturation received by the mother prior to delivery
□ Antibiotics received by the mother during labor
□ Clinical chorioamnionitis diagnosed during labor or maternal temperature ≥38°C (100.4°F)
□ Moderate/heavy meconium staining of the amniotic fluid
□ Fetal intolerance of labor such that one or more of the following actions was taken: in-utero resuscitative measures, further fetal assessment, or operative delivery
□ Epidural or spinal anesthesia during labor
□ None of the above

46. METHOD OF DELIVERY

A. Was delivery with forceps attempted but unsuccessful?
□ Yes □ No

B. Was delivery with vacuum extraction attempted but unsuccessful?
□ Yes □ No

C. Fetal presentation at birth
□ Cephalic
□ Breech
□ Other

D. Final route and method of delivery (Check one)
□ Vaginal/Spontaneous
□ Vaginal/Forceps
□ Vaginal/Vacuum
□ Cesarean
If cesarean, was a trial of labor attempted?
□ Yes
□ No

47. MATERNAL MORBIDITY (Check all that apply) (Complications associated with labor and delivery)
□ Maternal transfusion
□ Third or fourth degree perineal laceration
□ Ruptured uterus
□ Unplanned hysterectomy
□ Admission to intensive care unit
□ Unplanned operating room procedure following delivery
□ None of the above

NEWBORN INFORMATION

NEWBORN

48. NEWBORN MEDICAL RECORD NUMBER

49. BIRTHWEIGHT (grams preferred, specify unit)
____
9 grams 9 lb/oz

50. OBSTETRIC ESTIMATE OF GESTATION:
______________ (completed weeks)

51. APGAR SCORE:
Score at 5 minutes: ______________
If 5 minute score is less than 6,
Score at 10 minutes: ______________

52. PLURALITY - Single, Twin, Triplet, etc.
(Specify)______________

53. IF NOT SINGLE BIRTH - Born First, Second, Third, etc. (Specify) ______________

54. ABNORMAL CONDITIONS OF THE NEWBORN (Check all that apply)
□ Assisted ventilation required immediately following delivery
□ Assisted ventilation required for more than six hours
□ NICU admission
□ Newborn given surfactant replacement therapy
□ Antibiotics received by the newborn for suspected neonatal sepsis
□ Seizure or serious neurologic dysfunction
□ Significant birth injury (skeletal fracture(s), peripheral nerve injury, and/or soft tissue/solid organ hemorrhage which requires intervention)
9 None of the above

55. CONGENITAL ANOMALIES OF THE NEWBORN (Check all that apply)
□ Anencephaly
□ Meningomyelocele/Spina bifida
□ Cyanotic congenital heart disease
□ Congenital diaphragmatic hernia
□ Omphalocele
□ Gastroschisis
□ Limb reduction defect (excluding congenital amputation and dwarfing syndromes)
□ Cleft Lip with or without Cleft Palate
□ Cleft Palate alone
□ Down Syndrome
□ Karyotype confirmed
□ Karyotype pending
□ Suspected chromosomal disorder
□ Karyotype confirmed
□ Karyotype pending
□ Hypospadias
□ None of the anomalies listed above

56. WAS INFANT TRANSFERRED WITHIN 24 HOURS OF DELIVERY? 9 Yes 9 No
IF YES, NAME OF FACILITY INFANT TRANSFERRED TO:______________

57. IS INFANT LIVING AT TIME OF REPORT?
□ Yes □ No □ Infant transferred, status unknown

58. IS THE INFANT BEING BREASTFED AT DISCHARGE?
□ Yes □ No

Mother's Name ______________

Mother's Medical Record No. ______________

Rev. 11/2003

NOTE: This recommended standard birth certificate is the result of an extensive evaluation process. Information on the process and resulting recommendations as well as plans for future activities is available on the Internet at: http://www.cdc.gov/nchs/vital_certs_rev.htm.

DISPLAY 7.4 STANDARD DEATH CERTIFICATE

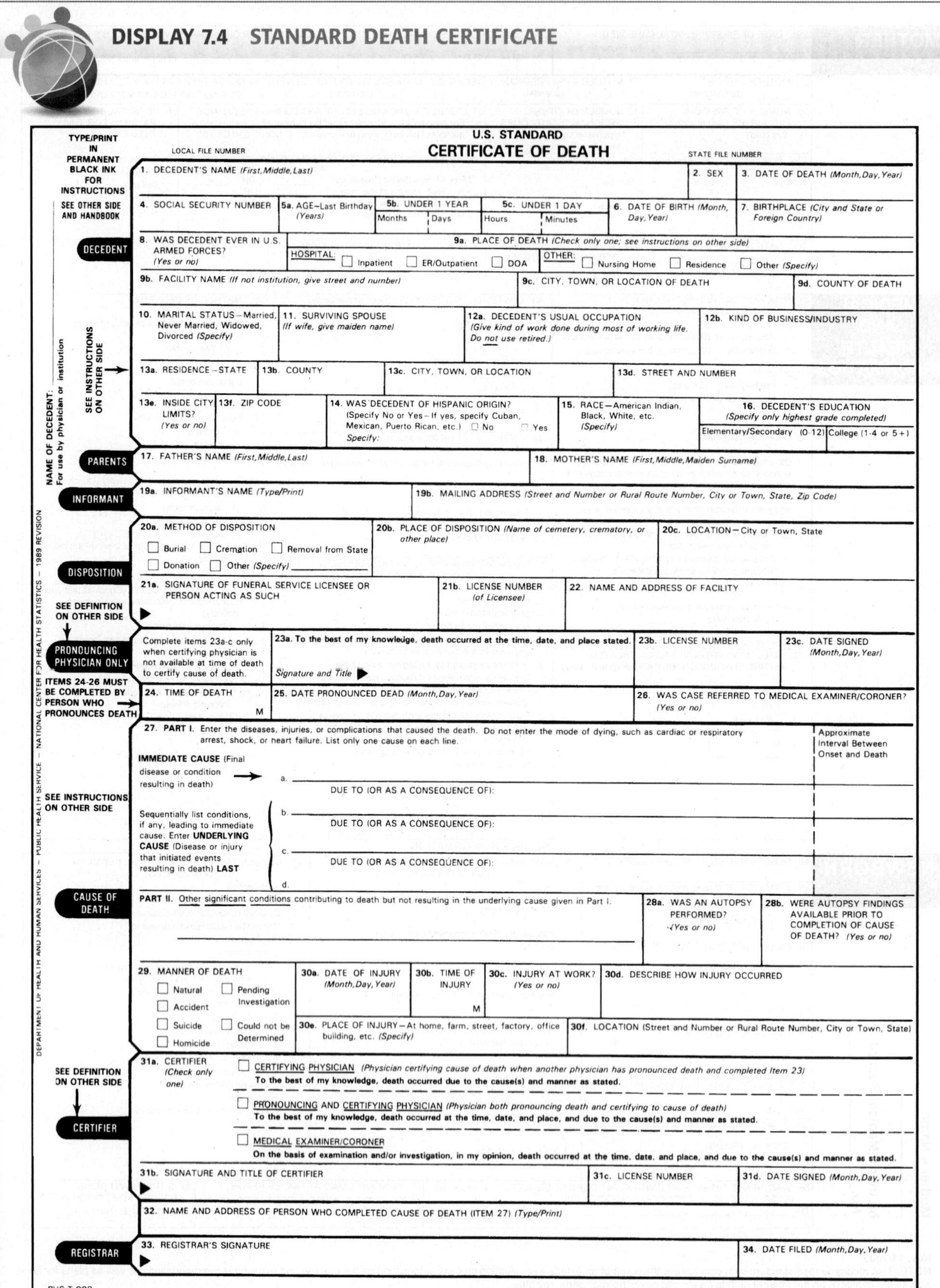

TYPE/PRINT IN PERMANENT BLACK INK FOR INSTRUCTIONS

SEE OTHER SIDE AND HANDBOOK

LOCAL FILE NUMBER

U.S. STANDARD

CERTIFICATE OF DEATH

STATE FILE NUMBER

DECEDENT

1. DECEDENT'S NAME *(First, Middle, Last)*
2. SEX
3. DATE OF DEATH *(Month, Day, Year)*
4. SOCIAL SECURITY NUMBER

5a. AGE—Last Birthday *(Years)*

5b. UNDER 1 YEAR: Months | Days

5c. UNDER 1 DAY: Hours | Minutes

6. DATE OF BIRTH *(Month, Day, Year)*
7. BIRTHPLACE *(City and State or Foreign Country)*
8. WAS DECEDENT EVER IN U.S. ARMED FORCES? *(Yes or no)*

9a. PLACE OF DEATH *(Check only one; see instructions on other side)*
HOSPITAL: ☐ Inpatient ☐ ER/Outpatient ☐ DOA
OTHER: ☐ Nursing Home ☐ Residence ☐ Other *(Specify)*

9b. FACILITY NAME *(If not institution, give street and number)*

9c. CITY, TOWN, OR LOCATION OF DEATH

9d. COUNTY OF DEATH

10. MARITAL STATUS—Married, Never Married, Widowed, Divorced *(Specify)*
11. SURVIVING SPOUSE *(If wife, give maiden name)*

12a. DECEDENT'S USUAL OCCUPATION *(Give kind of work done during most of working life. Do not use retired.)*

12b. KIND OF BUSINESS/INDUSTRY

SEE INSTRUCTIONS ON OTHER SIDE →

13a. RESIDENCE—STATE

13b. COUNTY

13c. CITY, TOWN, OR LOCATION

13d. STREET AND NUMBER

13e. INSIDE CITY LIMITS? *(Yes or no)*

13f. ZIP CODE

14. WAS DECEDENT OF HISPANIC ORIGIN? (Specify No or Yes—If yes, specify Cuban, Mexican, Puerto Rican, etc.) ☐ No ☐ Yes Specify:
15. RACE—American Indian, Black, White, etc. *(Specify)*
16. DECEDENT'S EDUCATION *(Specify only highest grade completed)* Elementary/Secondary (0-12) | College (1-4 or 5+)

NAME OF DECEDENT: ______ For use by physician or institution

PARENTS

17. FATHER'S NAME *(First, Middle, Last)*
18. MOTHER'S NAME *(First, Middle, Maiden Surname)*

INFORMANT

19a. INFORMANT'S NAME *(Type/Print)*

19b. MAILING ADDRESS *(Street and Number or Rural Route Number, City or Town, State, Zip Code)*

DISPOSITION

20a. METHOD OF DISPOSITION
☐ Burial ☐ Cremation ☐ Removal from State
☐ Donation ☐ Other *(Specify)* ______

20b. PLACE OF DISPOSITION *(Name of cemetery, crematory, or other place)*

20c. LOCATION—City or Town, State

21a. SIGNATURE OF FUNERAL SERVICE LICENSEE OR PERSON ACTING AS SUCH ▶

21b. LICENSE NUMBER *(of Licensee)*

22. NAME AND ADDRESS OF FACILITY

SEE DEFINITION ON OTHER SIDE

PRONOUNCING PHYSICIAN ONLY

Complete items 23a-c only when certifying physician is not available at time of death to certify cause of death.

23a. To the best of my knowledge, death occurred at the time, date, and place stated. Signature and Title ▶

23b. LICENSE NUMBER

23c. DATE SIGNED *(Month, Day, Year)*

ITEMS 24-26 MUST BE COMPLETED BY PERSON WHO PRONOUNCES DEATH →

24. TIME OF DEATH M
25. DATE PRONOUNCED DEAD *(Month, Day, Year)*
26. WAS CASE REFERRED TO MEDICAL EXAMINER/CORONER? *(Yes or no)*

CAUSE OF DEATH

SEE INSTRUCTIONS ON OTHER SIDE

27. **PART I.** Enter the diseases, injuries, or complications that caused the death. Do not enter the mode of dying, such as cardiac or respiratory arrest, shock, or heart failure. List only one cause on each line.

Approximate Interval Between Onset and Death

IMMEDIATE CAUSE (Final disease or condition resulting in death) → a. ______

DUE TO (OR AS A CONSEQUENCE OF):

Sequentially list conditions, if any, leading to immediate cause. Enter **UNDERLYING CAUSE** (Disease or injury that initiated events resulting in death) **LAST**

b. ______

DUE TO (OR AS A CONSEQUENCE OF):

c. ______

DUE TO (OR AS A CONSEQUENCE OF):

d. ______

PART II. Other significant conditions contributing to death but not resulting in the underlying cause given in Part I.

28a. WAS AN AUTOPSY PERFORMED? *(Yes or no)*

28b. WERE AUTOPSY FINDINGS AVAILABLE PRIOR TO COMPLETION OF CAUSE OF DEATH? *(Yes or no)*

29. MANNER OF DEATH
☐ Natural ☐ Pending Investigation
☐ Accident
☐ Suicide ☐ Could not be Determined
☐ Homicide

30a. DATE OF INJURY *(Month, Day, Year)*

30b. TIME OF INJURY M

30c. INJURY AT WORK? *(Yes or no)*

30d. DESCRIBE HOW INJURY OCCURRED

30e. PLACE OF INJURY—At home, farm, street, factory, office building, etc. *(Specify)*

30f. LOCATION (Street and Number or Rural Route Number, City or Town, State)

SEE DEFINITION ON OTHER SIDE

CERTIFIER

31a. CERTIFIER *(Check only one)*

☐ CERTIFYING PHYSICIAN *(Physician certifying cause of death when another physician has pronounced death and completed Item 23)*
To the best of my knowledge, death occurred due to the cause(s) and manner as stated.

☐ PRONOUNCING AND CERTIFYING PHYSICIAN *(Physician both pronouncing death and certifying to cause of death)*
To the best of my knowledge, death occurred at the time, date, and place, and due to the cause(s) and manner as stated.

☐ MEDICAL EXAMINER/CORONER
On the basis of examination and/or investigation, in my opinion, death occurred at the time, date, and place, and due to the cause(s) and manner as stated.

31b. SIGNATURE AND TITLE OF CERTIFIER ▶

31c. LICENSE NUMBER

31d. DATE SIGNED *(Month, Day, Year)*

32. NAME AND ADDRESS OF PERSON WHO COMPLETED CAUSE OF DEATH (ITEM 27) *(Type/Print)*

REGISTRAR

33. REGISTRAR'S SIGNATURE ▶
34. DATE FILED *(Month, Day, Year)*

DEPARTMENT OF HEALTH AND HUMAN SERVICES — PUBLIC HEALTH SERVICE — NATIONAL CENTER FOR HEALTH STATISTICS — 1989 REVISION

PHS-T-003

quality. Analysis of population statistics can provide the community health nurse with a better understanding of the community and help identify specific areas that may warrant further epidemiologic investigation. Data from the 2010 Census can be found on the U.S. Census Bureau Web site (see the Internet section at the end of this chapter) and is an easily accessed source of population-level data.

Reportable Diseases

Each state has developed laws or regulations that require health organizations and practitioners to report to their local health authority cases of certain communicable and infectious diseases that can be spread through the community (Heymann, 2009). This reporting enables the health department to take the most appropriate and efficient action. All states require that diseases subject to international quarantine regulations be reported immediately. However, many of these diseases (e.g., plague, cholera, yellow fever, and polio) are virtually unknown now in developed countries (WHO, 2007). Health care professionals have not had experience identifying another reportable disease, smallpox, because no cases have been reported since 1977 (CDC, 2007). In 1980, the WHO declared the global eradication of smallpox after more than 10 years of international effort. (Chapter 17 discusses the concern over the use of smallpox as a bioterrorism threat.) Numerous other diseases under surveillance by WHO (e.g., tuberculosis, malaria, and viral influenza) must also be reported [WHO, 2007]. Other reportable diseases (numbering between 20 and 40 in each state) are usually classified according to the speed with which the health department should be notified. Some should be reported by phone or e-mail, others weekly by regular mail. They vary in potential severity from varicella (chickenpox) to rabies and include AIDS, encephalitis, meningitis, syphilis, and toxic shock syndrome. Community health nurses should obtain the list of reportable diseases from their local or state health department office. Following-up on occurrences of these diseases is a task frequently assigned to public health nurses working for local health departments. Chapter 8 includes an example of a confidential morbidity report (CMR) used to report and track communicable diseases at the local, regional, and national level.

Disease Registries

Some areas or states have disease registries or rosters for conditions with major public health impact. Tuberculosis and rheumatic fever registries were more common when these diseases occurred more frequently. Cancer registries provide useful incidence, prevalence, and survival data and assist the community health nurse in monitoring cancer patterns within a community. Community health nurses can access these registries through state health department Web sites. At the federal level, the Agency for Toxic Substances and Disease Registry (ATSDR, 2011) maintains three registries of major public concern: the World Trade Center Health Registry (comprehensive and confidential health survey of those directly exposed to fallout and debris on September 11, 2001), the National Amyotrophic Lateral Sclerosis (ALS) Registry, and the National Toxic Substances Incidents Program (collects and combines information regarding spills and leaks of toxic substances).

Environmental Monitoring

State governments, through health departments or other agencies, now monitor health hazards found in the environment. Pesticides, industrial wastes, radioactive or nuclear materials, chemical additives in foods, and medicinal drugs have joined the list of pollutants (see Chapter 9 for a detailed discussion). Concerned community members and leaders view these as risk factors that affect health at both community and individual levels. Public health nurses can also obtain data from federal agencies such as the Food and Drug Administration (FDA), the Consumer Product Safety Commission, the Environmental Protection Agency (EPA), and as previously mentioned, the ATSDR.

National Center for Health Statistics Health Surveys

The NCHS furnishes valuable health prevalence data from surveys of Americans. Published data are also frequently available for regions. The National Health Interview Survey (formerly known as National Health Survey) was established by Congress in 1956 and provides a continual source of information about the health status and needs of the entire nation (NCHS, 2012a). The National Health Interview Survey includes interviews from approximately 43,000 households each year and provides information about the health status and needs of the entire country (NCHS, 2012a). The National Nursing Home Survey primarily samples institutional records of hospitals and nursing homes; it provides information on those who are using these services, along with diagnoses and other characteristics (NCHS, 2012b). The National Health and Nutrition Examination Survey (NHANES) reports physical measurements on smaller samples of the population and augments the information provided by interviews. It also provides prevalence information on injuries, diseases, and disabilities that appear frequently in the population. The National Survey of Family Growth (NSFG) focuses on fertility and family planning as well as other aspects of family health (NCHS, 2012b). Other studies investigate vital statistics events and characteristics of ambulatory patients in physicians' community practices.

Each of these nationally sponsored efforts suggests ways in which community health nurses can examine health problems or concerns affecting their communities (see From the Case Files). Interviews, physical examinations of subsets of community members, and surveillance of institutions, clinics, and private physicians' practices can be carried out locally after needs are identified and funds made available. Other sources may be found in data kept routinely but not centrally on the health problems of workers in local industries or the health problems of schoolchildren, a key issue for many community health nurses. Existing epidemiologic data can be used to plan parent education programs, health promotion among students, and almost any other type of service.

From the Case Files I

I am one of only four Public Health Nurses in our county—which is not many considering that our service area is very large, very rural, and very poor. Before I came, which was about 10 years ago, they had at least 10 nurses, and the population was maybe half of what it is now. We have growing numbers of residents with tuberculosis (TB), high teenage pregnancy, and too many low-birth-weight babies, and to top it off, many of our residents lack health insurance. The county is in a budget crisis (again), and public health is high on the list for further reductions. I have been asked to speak at the next county supervisors meeting about what public health nurses do and basically fight to keep us in the budget. I don't have much time to pull together information to give them and will only have about 15 minutes for the presentation. They are all business owners, so I know they will appreciate data. I know other counties have all their morbidity and mortality figures online, but not here. Where to even start?

In preparing for this presentation, what specific types of data would you recommend to this nurse? What would be the sources of this data? Are those sources from local, state, or national resources? How could *Healthy People 2020* help frame this presentation?

Another service of the CDC is its important publication, the *Mortality and Morbidity Weekly Report* (MMWR). This publication presents weekly summaries of disease and death data trends for the nation. It includes reports on outbreaks or occurrences of diseases in specific regions of the country and international trends in disease occurrences that may affect the US population. Most health departments subscribe to this publication, which provides important information both for epidemiologists and community health nurses. It is also available free online from the CDC.

Informal Observational Studies

A second information source in epidemiologic study is informal observation and description. Almost any client group encountered by the community health nurse can trigger such a study. If, for example, the nurse encounters an abused child at a clinic, a study of the clinic's records to screen for additional possible instances of child abuse and neglect could lead to more case findings. If several cases of diabetes come to the attention of a nurse serving on a Navajo reservation, a widespread problem might come to light through informal inquiries about the incidence and age at onset of the disease among this Native American population. Informal observational study often raises questions and suggests hypotheses that form the basis for designing larger-scale epidemiologic investigations.

Scientific Studies

The third source of information used in epidemiologic inquiry involves carefully designed scientific studies. The nursing profession has recognized the need to develop a systematic body of knowledge on which to base nursing practice. Already, systematic research is becoming an accepted part of the community health nurse's role. Findings from epidemiologic studies conducted by or involving nurses are appearing more frequently in the literature. For example, concern regarding negative birth outcomes prompted exploration on the association between maternal chronic disease and preterm birth (PTB), low birth weight (LBW), and infant mortality (Graham, Zhang, & Schwalberg, 2007). Working in collaboration with other health professionals, the nurse researchers examined birth and death certificates between 1999 and 2003 in a cohort of over 200,000 singleton infants born to African American and White mothers. The research showed that, irrespective of maternal race, chronic hypertension and diabetes were significantly associated with at least one negative birth outcome. Concerning too was the finding that, for African American mothers, cardiac disease was strongly associated with LBW and PTB (Graham et al. 2007). Another example was a study to determine landlord attitudes and behaviors regarding the impact of smoke-free policies. This descriptive, cross-sectional survey conducted both by telephone and by mail ($N = 392$) showed that the perception of landlords that smoke-free polices would increase vacancy rates and turnover was not supported by the findings. The results showed that the vacancy rate and turnover was actually much less in rentals with a smoke-free policy. When presented with these results, more than one-third of the landlords who allowed smoking expressed interest in learning more about implementing a smoke-free policy for their properties (Cramer, Roberts, & Stevens, 2010). Systematic studies as well as informal studies and existing epidemiologic data can provide the community health nurse with valuable information that can be used to positively affect aggregate health.

METHODS IN THE EPIDEMIOLOGIC INVESTIGATIVE PROCESS

The goals of epidemiologic investigation are to identify the causal mechanisms of health and illness states and to develop measures for preventing illness and promoting health. Epidemiologists employ an investigative process that involves a sequence of three approaches that build on one another: descriptive, analytic, and experimental studies. All three approaches have relevance for community health nursing (see Chapter 4 for a more detailed description).

Descriptive Epidemiology

Descriptive epidemiology includes investigations that seek to observe and describe patterns of health-related conditions that occur naturally in a population. For example, a community health nurse might seek to learn how many children in a school district have been immunized for measles, how many home births occur each year in the county, how many cases of STDs have occurred in the city in the past month, or how many automobile crashes have occurred near the community high school. At this stage in the epidemiologic investigation, the researcher seeks to establish the occurrence of a problem. Data from descriptive studies suggest hypotheses for further testing. Descriptive studies almost always involve some form of broad-based quantification and statistical analysis.

Counts

The simplest measure of description is a count. For example, an epidemiologic study to assess the impact of the varicella vaccine (licensed in 1995) on death due to the disease examined data from the NCHS (1990–2001) Multiple Cause-of-Death Mortality Data (Nguyen, Jumaan, & Seward, 2005). Data from the period prior to and following vaccine availability showed that varicella-related deaths dropped by more than 45%, from an average 145 per year between 1990 and 1994 to 66 per year during 1999 to 2001. The findings also showed that varicella-related deaths declined among children and adults (20 to 49 years) alike and for all racial and ethnic groups. As positive as these results were, reported deaths occurred among those who were eligible to receive the vaccine and not among those with high-risk conditions such as HIV, as might be expected. The most current figures from the CDC reflect an even more precipitous drop, with only two reported varicella-related deaths during 2008 (Hall-Baker et al., 2010).

Obtaining a count of this type always depends on the definition of what is being counted and when it was counted. This particular count, for example, utilizes a large database that takes time to be made public and therefore may not provide a current picture of actual deaths. Use of this type of data should always consider the time delay involved. If a community health nurse needs more current information within a specific community or state, hospital records or death certificates may be another source. However, before making use of any statistics, whether from official state offices, the Census Bureau, or a health agency, it is necessary to determine what the information represents.

Rates

Rates are statistical measures expressing the proportion of people with a given health problem among a population at risk. The total number of people in the group serves as the denominator for various types of rates. To express a count as a proportion, or rate, the population to be studied must first be identified. For instance, total West Nile virus fatalities in the United States for 2011 were 43 out of 690 confirmed infections (CDC, 2011b). If those deaths are considered in relation to the total number of cases in the country, there will be one rate; if, however, those fatalities are considered in relation to the total population, there will be a quite different rate. It is important when reviewing rates that you understand which measures are being compared.

In epidemiology, the population represents the universe of people defined as the objects of a study. Because it is often difficult, if not impossible, to study an entire population, most epidemiologic studies draw a sample to represent that group. Sometimes, it is important to seek a random sample (in which everyone in the population has an equal chance of selection for study and choice is made without bias). At other times, a sample of convenience (in which study subjects are selected because of their availability) is sufficient. In many small epidemiologic studies, it may be possible to study almost every person in the population, eliminating the need for a sample. Several rates have wide use in epidemiology. Those most important for the public health nurse to understand are the prevalence rate, the period prevalence rate, and the incidence rate.

Prevalence refers to all of the people with a particular health condition existing in a given population at a given point in time. The *prevalence rate* describes a situation at a specific point in time (Friis & Sellers, 2009). If a nurse discovers 50 cases of measles in an elementary school, that is a simple count. If that number is divided by the number of students in the school, the result is the prevalence of measles. For instance, if the school has 500 students, the prevalence of measles on that day would be 10% (50 measles/500 population).

$$\text{Prevalence rate} = \frac{\text{Number of persons with a characteristic}}{\text{Total number in population}}$$

In the study of varicella deaths, on the other hand, the investigators had a count for 1-year periods from 1991 to 2001 (Nguyen et al., 2005). Rather than portraying only 1 day, this number covered an extended period of time (1 year). The prevalence rate over a defined period of time is called a *period prevalence rate*:

$$\text{Period prevalence rate} = \frac{\text{Number of persons with a characteristic during a period of time}}{\text{Total number in population}}$$

Not everyone in a population is at risk for developing a disease, incurring an injury, or having some other health-related characteristic. The incidence rate recognizes this fact. **Incidence** refers to all new cases of a disease or health condition appearing during a given time. Incidence rate describes a proportion in which the numerator is all new cases appearing during a given period of time and the denominator is the population at risk during the same period. For example, some childhood diseases give lifelong immunity. The school children who have had such diseases would be removed from the total number of children at risk in the school population. Three weeks after the start of a measles epidemic in a school, the incidence rate describes the number of cases of measles appearing during that period in terms of the number of persons at risk:

$$\frac{200}{1{,}000} \text{ or } \frac{200 \text{ new cases}}{1{,}000 \text{ persons at risk}}$$

The health literature is not always consistent in the use of the term incidence; sometimes, this word is used synonymously with prevalence rates, and the reader must take this into consideration.

$$\text{Incidence rate} = \frac{\text{Number of persons developing a disease}}{\text{Total number at risk per unit of time}}$$

Another rate that describes incidence is the attack rate. An attack rate describes the proportion of a group or population that develops a disease among all those exposed to a particular risk. This term is used frequently in investigations of outbreaks of infectious diseases such as influenza. If the attack rate changes, it may suggest an alteration in the population's immune status or that the disease-causing organism is present in a more or less virulent strain.

Computing Rates

To make comparisons between populations, epidemiologists often use a common base population in computing rates. For example, instead of merely saying that the rate of an illness is 13% in one city and 25% in another, the comparison is made per 100,000 people in the population. This population base can vary for different purposes from 100 to 100,000. To describe the **morbidity rate**, which is the relative incidence of disease in

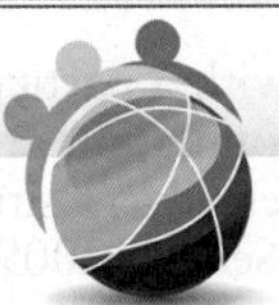

DISPLAY 7.5 COMMON EPIDEMIOLOGIC RATES

General Mortality Rates

Crude Mortality Rate =

$$\frac{\text{Number of Reported Deaths During 1 Year}}{\text{Estimated Population as of July 1 of Same Year}} \times 100{,}000$$

Case-Specific Mortality Rate =

$$\frac{\text{Number of Deaths From a Stated Cause During 1 Year}}{\text{Estimated Population as of July 1 of Same Year}} \times 100{,}000\text{M}$$

Case Fatality Rate =

$$\frac{\text{Number of Deaths From a Particular Disease}}{\text{Total Number With the Same Disease}} \times 100$$

Proportional Mortality Ratio =

$$\frac{\text{Number of Deaths From a Specific Cause Within a Given Time Period}}{\text{Total Deaths in the Same Time Period}} \times 100$$

Age-Specific Mortality Rate =

$$\frac{\text{Number of Persons in a Specific Age Group Dying During 1 Year}}{\text{Estimated Population of the Specific Age Group as of July 1 of Same Year}} \times 100{,}000$$

Specific Rates for Maternal and Infant Populations

Crude Birth Rate =

$$\frac{\text{Number of Live Births During 1 Year}}{\text{Estimated Population as of July 1 of Same Year}} \times 1{,}000$$

General Fertility Rate =

$$\frac{\text{Number of Live Births During 1 Year}}{\text{Number of Females Aged 15 - 44 as of July 1 of Same Year}} \times 1{,}000$$

Maternal Mortality Rate =

$$\frac{\text{Number of Deaths From Pueperal Causes During 1 Year}}{\text{Number of Live Births During Same Year}} \times 100{,}000$$

Infant Mortality Rate =

$$\frac{\text{Number of Deaths Under 1 Year of Age for Given Year}}{\text{Number of Live Births Reported for Same Year}} \times 1{,}000$$

Perinatal Mortality Rate =

$$\frac{\text{Number of Fetal Deaths Plus Infant Deaths Under 7 Days of Age During 1 Year}}{\text{Number of Live Births Plus Fetal Deaths During Same Year}} \times 1{,}000$$

a population, the ratio of the number of sick individuals to the total population is determined. The **mortality rate** refers to the relative death rate, or the sum of deaths in a given population at a given time. Display 7.5 includes formulas for computing rates commonly used in community health.

The goal of descriptive studies is to identify the patterns of occurrence of any health-related condition. They can be *retrospective* (identify cases and controls, then go back to review existing data) or *prospective* (identify groups and exposure factors and then follow them forward in time). In a descriptive study of child abuse, for example, the investigator would note the age, gender, race or ethnic group, and physical and emotional conditions of the children affected. In addition, data would be collected that described the economic status and occupation of parents, the location and setting of abusive behavior, and the time and season of the year when abuse occurred. In the retrospective study on reported varicella deaths, the investigators described the age, sex, ethnic background, and birthplace of victims and other information, such as whether varicella was an underlying or contributing cause of death (Nguyen et al., 2005). Describing facets of these deaths provides information for further study and suggests avenues for intervention or prevention.

Analytic Epidemiology

A second type of investigation, *analytic epidemiology*, goes beyond simple description or observation and seeks to identify associations between a particular human disease or health problem and its possible causes. Analytic studies tend to be more specific than descriptive studies in their focus. They test hypotheses or seek to answer specific questions and can be retrospective or prospective in design. Analytic studies fall into three types: prevalence studies, case–control studies, and cohort studies.

Prevalence Studies

When examining prevalence, it is helpful to remember that the health condition may be new or may have affected some people for many years. A *prevalence study* describes patterns of occurrence, as in the study of varicella-related deaths. It may examine causal factors, but a prevalence study always looks at factors from the same point in time and in the same population. Hypothesized causal factors are based on inferences from a single examination and most likely need further testing for validation.

Case–Control Studies

A *case–control study* compares people who have a health or illness condition (number of cases with the condition) with those who lack this condition (controls). These studies begin with the cases and look back over time (retrospectively) for presence or absence of the suspected causal factor in both cases and controls. In a case–control study to explore the risks of delivering a small-for-gestational-age (SGA) infant based on certain occupational patterns, women delivering single births between 1997 and 1999 were interviewed by telephone after delivery (Croteau, Marcoux, & Brisson, 2006). Comparisons between the cases and controls revealed that irregular and shift work increased the risk of a SGA birth but that changing those occupational patterns before 24 weeks could reduce the risk substantially. In a case–control study, the two groups should share as many characteristics as possible, to isolate possible causes. In the study by Croteau et al., the control group mothers were randomly selected from all singleton births during that same period and in the same region of the country. In this way, differences between the cases (SGA births) and those with a normal-weight infant are more easily identified.

Cohort Studies

A *cohort* is a group of people who share a common experience in a specific time period. Examples are a group of the elderly or the employees of an industry. In epidemiology, a cohort of people often becomes a focus of study. Cohort studies, rather than measuring the relationship of variables in existing conditions, study the development of a condition over time. A cohort study begins by selecting a group of people who display certain defined characteristics before the onset of the condition being investigated. In studying a disease, the cohort might include individuals who are initially free of the disease but are known to have been exposed to a particular factor. They would be observed over time to evaluate which variables were associated with the development or nondevelopment of the disease. These types of studies are often utilized with environmental hazard exposures, as with the World Trade Center Health Registry and the National Toxic Substance Incidents Program discussed earlier (ATSDR, 2011). These sources of data provide the capability to conduct a cohort study on postexposure disease development and enable those affected to access the most current information on their exposure risks.

In 1993, the Women's Health Study, a 10-year national longitudinal, experimental, cohort study involving nearly 40,000 female health professionals was initiated (National Institutes of Health, 2012). Sponsored by the National Heart, Lung, and Blood Institute and the National Cancer Institute, it consisted of a randomized trial evaluating the benefits and risks of low-dose aspirin and vitamin E in the prevention of cancer and CVD. Depending on the random assignment of the women, participants took 100 mg of aspirin or placebo and 600 IU of vitamin E or placebo every other day. This was a double-blind study: Neither the participants nor the researchers knew which subjects were taking the study drugs or placebos. The study was funded through 2009 to provide observational follow-up of study participants. The study findings were that women over age 65 may benefit from low-dose aspirin to prevent strokes. The aspirin regimen was not effective in preventing a first heart attack or death from cardiovascular causes. The research findings support adopting healthy lifestyle habits including "eating for heart health, getting regular physical activity, maintaining a healthy weight, not smoking, and controlling high cholesterol levels, high blood pressure, and diabetes" (Nabel, 2005). With respect to cardiovascular health and vitamin E, there was no demonstrated benefit or risk.

In practice, the various types of studies just discussed are frequently mixed. A case–control study may include description and analysis with a retrospective focus; a cohort study may be conducted prospectively or retrospectively. The Women's Health Study just discussed is an example of a case–control study, a cohort study, and an experimental study. Flexibility is essential to allow the investigator as much freedom as possible in choosing the most useful methodology.

Experimental Epidemiology

Experimental epidemiology follows and builds on information gathered from descriptive and analytic approaches. It is used to study epidemics, the etiology of human disease, the value of preventive and therapeutic measures, and the evaluation of health services (Valanis, 1999). In an experimental study, the investigator actually controls or changes the factors suspected of causing the health condition under study, then observes what happens to the health state. In human populations, experimental studies should focus on disease prevention or health promotion rather than testing the causes of disease, which is done primarily on animals.

Experimental studies are carried out under carefully controlled conditions. The investigator exposes an experimental group to some factor thought, improve health, prevent disease, or influence health in some way (as in the Women's Health Study). Simultaneously, the investigator observes a control group that is similar in characteristics to the experimental group but without the exposure factor.

The public health nurse should be alert for opportunities to conduct experimental studies in the course of working with groups. A study need not be elaborate to provide important data for future nursing practice. For example, a community health nurse can provide focused instruction to 20 new mothers encouraging them to breast-feed and then compare the health of their infants with infants of 20 mothers in the same service area who use formula.

A nurse can look at the number of automobile crashes at an intersection where there is a traffic light compared with a similar intersection that has stop signs. Based on the results of the investigation, the nurse may bring the information to the city council and petition for a stop light at the intersection. Study results can be used to bring about change in the community and are not limited to communicable or chronic diseases. Improving community safety is also an essential outcome.

An expanding area of experimental epidemiology involves the use of computers to simulate epidemics. With mathematical models, it is possible to determine the probabilities of various aspects of disease occurrence. This approach is making an increased contribution to epidemiologists' knowledge of etiology and prevention.

Occasionally, an experiment occurs naturally, thus affording the researcher the chance to make important discoveries. John Snow discovered such a "natural experiment" in London in 1854 (as discussed earlier in the chapter). In his seminal study of an epidemic of cholera, he observed one group that contracted the disease and another that did not. Closer inspection revealed that the major difference between these groups was their water supply. Eventually, the spread of cholera was traced to the water supply of the group with the high morbidity rate (Valanis, 1999).

A *community trial* is a type of experimental study done at the community level. Geographic communities are assigned to intervention (experimental) or nonintervention (control) groups and compared to determine whether the intervention produces a positive change in the community. Community trials can be extremely expensive and are not undertaken unless there is substantial evidence that the intervention will make a difference at the aggregate level. There are times when these community trials occur spontaneously, and it is important for the community health nurse to recognize these opportunities. For instance, one community public health department institutes an aggressive campaign to educate health care workers on the signs of elder abuse. Selecting a similar community where that level of training is not available, the community health nurse can then compare the rates of elder abuse reporting between these two communities. If you were conducting this research, what outcome would you expect in the community with the enhanced training? Where could you obtain this information? Think about what other measures you might be interested in comparing between these two communities.

CONDUCTING EPIDEMIOLOGIC RESEARCH

The community health nurse who engages in an epidemiologic investigation becomes a kind of detective. First, there is a problem to solve, a puzzle to unravel, or a question to answer. The nurse begins to search for basic information, for clues that might help answer the question. Information is never self-explanatory, and like a detective, the nurse must analyze and interpret every additional clue. Slowly, there is a narrowing of possible suspects until the causes of a disease, the consequences of a prevention plan, or the results of treatment are identified. On the basis of this investigation, the nurse can draw further conclusions and make new applications to improve health services.

As discussed previously, epidemiologic studies are a form of research. The steps outlined here are similar to those discussed in Chapter 4. Epidemiologic research involves seven steps. Everything from an informal study in the course of nursing practice to the most comprehensive epidemiologic research project can be undertaken with these steps:

1. Identify the problem.
2. Review the literature.
3. Design the study.
4. Collect the data.
5. Analyze the findings.
6. Develop conclusions and applications.
7. Disseminate the findings.

Each step is considered here in the context of a single nursing study that examined receipt of lead poisoning prevention information by parents of children enrolled in one state's Medicaid program (Polivka, 2006). Although research as a community health nursing role is covered in a separate chapter, the analysis of one epidemiologic study reinforces the integration of research in the nurse's role.

Identify the Problem

Community health nurses are constantly confronted with threats to the health and wellbeing of the community. Almost daily, questions are raised, puzzles presented, and problems identified. Pregnant women who smoke or use cocaine threaten the health of their unborn children: What can be done to reduce this behavior? Rape is increasing: What can be done to prevent such violence or to bring aid to victims? Children are injured and die from bicycle accidents: Why do these occur and how can they be prevented? Many farm workers have been killed or injured in farm equipment accidents: What can be done to prevent them? Any threat to the health of a group offers fertile ground for epidemiologic investigation.

One nurse researcher was concerned with lead poisoning prevention education among parents of young children. To explore this issue, the researcher sought to examine parental receipt of educational materials on lead poisoning prevention as well their preferred method of receiving that information (Polivka, 2006). Using a cross-sectional design, parents of 1- to 2-year-old children who were enrolled in the Medicaid program were mailed a survey developed by the researcher. From the nearly 90,000 children meeting the study criteria, a sample of 1,656 was selected, which allowed for a low but realistic 24% return rate. The response rate ($n = 532$) was actually higher than predicted, and the majority of the respondents reported receiving lead poisoning prevention information. Of concern, however, was that only 28% reported receipt of some type of reminder to have their child's blood drawn for a lead level assessment. The findings also indicated that most respondents preferred to receive lead poisoning prevention information from brochures/pamphlets (71%) or directly from health care providers (48%).

Review the Literature

All too often, after identifying a problem, health professionals rush to take immediate action without reviewing solutions that have been tried previously. Every epidemiologic investigation should begin with a review of the literature. Even discovering that little research has been done on the problem can be valuable information. Conversely, if many studies have already been conducted in the area, this information can help narrow the study to areas not previously investigated or allow researchers to replicate earlier studies to confirm findings in a different setting. One of the most valuable sources in the literature is the review article, which essentially summarizes all the research that has been conducted on a subject.

A review of the literature often suggests hypotheses from discoveries made in other studies. In the lead poisoning prevention education survey, a review of the literature provided helpful background information (Polivka, 2006). The literature review also revealed that other studies have found varied levels of receipt of lead poisoning prevention education among parents and caregivers, from as low as about 30% to as high as 60%.

Design the Study

The first step in designing a study is to formulate one or more specific questions to answer or hypotheses to test. Sometimes, the question or hypothesis emerges from the review of the literature; it also may be developed through the researcher's own analysis and hunches. It is a good idea to write out one or more hypotheses to test or questions to answer. In the lead poisoning education survey, the researcher did not explicitly state a hypothesis; however, in previous focus groups conducted by the researcher and a colleague, "parents revealed they had little knowledge regarding the sources of lead poisoning, and they preferred to receive information via videos and television ads" (Polivka & Gottesman, 2005). This piece of information helped inform the current study and the current research questions:

- Have parents received lead poisoning prevention information or reminders about lead testing?
- With whom have parents talked about lead poisoning?
- How would parents prefer to receive lead poisoning prevention education? (Polivka, 2006)

The next step is to plan what study type (descriptive, analytic, or experimental) or combination of study types best suits the goals of the research and how the study will be conducted. Will the data be collected retrospectively from existing records, or will new data be collected? Who will conduct interviews? What kinds of data will be needed to measure the outcomes of intervention? Polivka (2006) used a retrospective analytic approach in the design of this cross-sectional survey. A mailed survey was selected as an effective means to sample the population of interest.

Collect the Data

The survey tool used in the Polivka (2006) study was a researcher-developed instrument that was assessed for both face and content validity by a team of experts in the field. The next step was to pilot test the survey tool with individuals similar to the target population. In this case, the researcher used a small group of women who were enrolled in the WIC program (Special Supplemental Nutrition Program for Women, Infants, and Children, U.S. Department of Agriculture) and revised the survey based on their suggestions.

Following review by a human subjects committee, the survey was mailed to the identified parents along with a cover letter and stamped preaddressed envelope. To increase the return rate from the parents, a small incentive was included in the survey, and a thank you card and reminder to return the survey (for nonrespondents) was mailed out 1 week later. For those not returning surveys after 3 to 7 weeks, another survey was sent out in hope of increasing the rate of return. For those who completed the survey, a small thank you gift was mailed out. The steps taken by the researcher were all important to achieving a return rate of 32%, well over the expected rate of 24%.

As in the Polivka (2006) study, it is useful to perform a pilot study that pretests an interview guide, questionnaire, or treatment. If one wishes to interview women about battering during pregnancy, it might be useful to prepare a guide and interview one or two people, then revise the guide on the basis of the experience. If development of a questionnaire to assess the nutritional needs of elderly people living alone is part of the study design, it would be helpful to test the survey on some volunteers to determine its clarity and relevance. And if the study is to provide a specific treatment such as coaching, teaching, or demonstration, it is important to practice it on a small group of people with characteristics similar to those of the subjects. In community health nursing, data collection often can occur as part of ongoing practice. Unless the study has been carefully designed, however, data may be collected for months or years, only to discover that important questions have been omitted.

Analyze the Findings

In most epidemiologic studies, data analysis consists of summarizing the findings, computing rates and ratios, and displaying the findings in tables and graphs. At this stage, the data are used to address the original question or test the original hypothesis. Was the hypothesis supported or not supported by the data? Summarized data can also generate more questions or indicate areas that warrant further investigation. For example, in the Polivka (2006) study, 60% of the parents reporting receipt of some type of lead poisoning prevention information tended to be over age 25, unmarried, and with more than a high school education. These results certainly suggest that younger parents and those with less education should be a target of educational interventions to address lead poisoning prevention. Moreover, any educational materials developed should keep in mind the reading capability of those parents.

Develop Conclusions and Applications

Stating conclusions is an outcome of analysis and interpretation. The investigators summarize the results and their meaning for the purpose of making this information useful to other health services providers. Many times, research has direct practical application for improving health services, continuing or discontinuing services, or conducting future research. It is also important to describe mistakes made and lessons learned about study design and other aspects of the research, to assist future investigators.

In the Polivka study, the researcher suggests that "public health nurses need to collaborate with other health care providers in implementing individual, community, and system level lead-poisoning prevention educational interventions for parents of at-risk children" (2006, p. 55). Citing the continued need for efforts to reduce lead poisoning and the *Healthy People 2010* goal of eliminating lead poisoning in US children, the author also stated that "public health nurses can be pivotal in educational reminder efforts by determining specific targeted population segments and identifying appropriate educational methods for those segments at the individual, community, and system levels" (Polivka, 2006, p. 56). The author had clearly outlined the leadership role that community health nurses can and should take to reach this national goal.

Disseminate the Findings

Finally, research findings should be shared. Information gained from epidemiologic studies must be disseminated throughout the professional community to strengthen the knowledge base for improved practice and to promote future research. In the lead poisoning prevention education study, the author selected a well-known nursing journal, one that specifically focuses on public health nursing practice. Careful selection of this specialty venue helps assure that those practicing in community and public health nursing are more likely to read the article. The author's use of the term *lead poisoning* in the title of the article was also very important for dissemination. Nurses interested in lead poisoning are very likely to have this article selected in a database reference search, such as the Cumulative Index to Nursing & Allied Health Literature (CINAHL), based on the use of that term alone.

SUMMARY

Epidemiology is the study of the distribution and determinants of health, health conditions, and disease in human population groups. It shares with community health nursing the common focus of the health of populations. It is a specialized form of scientific research that can provide public health professionals with a body of knowledge on which to base their practice and methods for studying new and existing problems. To understand epidemiology, one must first understand some basic epidemiologic concepts: the host, agent, and environment model; causality; immunity; the natural history of disease or health conditions; risk; and prevention strategies.

Community health nurses can use three sources of information when conducting epidemiologic investigations: existing epidemiologic data, informal investigations, and carefully designed scientific studies.

Epidemiology employs three investigative approaches: descriptive studies, analytic studies, and experimental studies. Although studies can be either retrospective or prospective, some merely describe existing conditions (descriptive studies), whereas others seek to explain causes (analytic studies). Experimental studies seek to confirm causal relationships identified in descriptive and analytic studies. Analytic studies can be of three types: prevalence, case–control, or cohort. In practice, all these types of studies often become combined in various ways. They also make use of quantitative concepts such as count, prevalence rate, incidence rate, mortality rate, and various types of morbidity (sickness) rates.

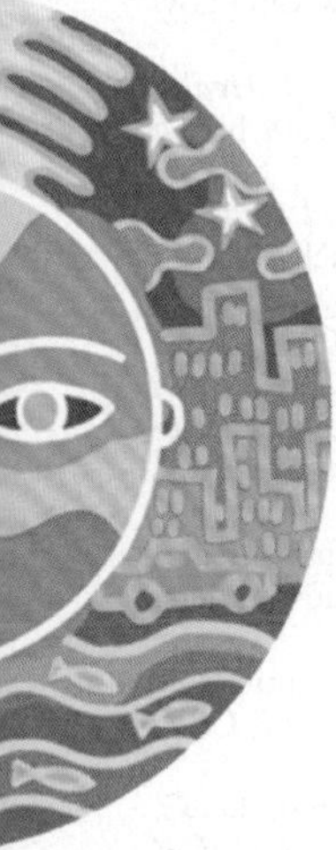

Epidemiologic research includes seven steps:

1. Identify the problem, which is usually a threat to the population's health.
2. Review the literature to determine what other studies have found.
3. Carefully design the study.
4. Collect the data.
5. Analyze the findings.
6. Develop conclusions and applications.
7. Disseminate the findings.

Thinking epidemiologically can significantly enhance community health nursing practice. Epidemiology provides both the body of knowledge—information on the distribution and determinants of health conditions—and methods for investigating health problems and evaluating services.

ACTIVITIES TO PROMOTE **CRITICAL THINKING**

1. Identify an aggregate-level health problem in your community. Using the host, agent, and environment model, explain who is the host, what are the causative agents, and what environmental factors have promoted or delayed the development of the problem.
2. Select an aggregate health (wellness) condition, such as preschoolers' normal growth and development or elders' healthy aging, and list all the causal factors that might contribute to this healthy state. Now, plot these schematically in a diagram to show the web of causation model for this condition.
3. Using the same health condition that you selected in the previous exercise, describe the natural history of this condition, outlining its four stages. Identify three preventive nursing interventions, one for each level of prevention that could apply to this condition.
4. Select an article that reports an epidemiologic study from a recent nursing or public health journal, and record your responses to the following questions:
   - What prompted the study, and what was its purpose?
   - Was it descriptive, analytic, or experimental research?
   - Was the study design retrospective or prospective?
   - Why did the investigators choose this design?
   - What existing sources of epidemiologic data did this study use? List all sources specifically, such as *Morbidity and Mortality Weekly Report* or incomes by household in census data.
   - What were the study findings? Identify the population group that will benefit from this research.
5. Interview one or more practicing public health nurses in your community, and identify an aggregate-level problem that needs epidemiologic investigation. Propose a rough draft study design to research this problem.

REFERENCES

Agency for Toxic Substances and Disease Registry. U.S. Department of Health and Human Services. (2011). *Data resources*. Retrieved from http://www.atsdr.cdc.gov/dataresources.html

American Academy of Pediatrics. (2011). *Where we stand: Folic acid*. Retrieved from http://www.healthychildren.org/English/ages-stages/prenatal/pages/Where-We-Stand-Folic-Acid.aspx

Aschengrau, A., & Seage, G. R. (2008). *Essentials of epidemiology in public health* (2nd ed.). Sudbury, MA: Jones and Bartlett Publishers.

Bodnar, L. M., Tang, G., Ness, R. B., Harger, G., & Roberts, J. M. (2006). Periconceptual multivitamin use reduces the risk of preeclampsia. *American Journal of Epidemiology, 164*, 470–477.

Burnet, M. (1962). *Natural history of infectious diseases* (3rd ed.). Cambridge, England: Cambridge University Press.

Centers for Disease Control and Prevention. (2007). *Smallpox fact sheet: Smallpox disease overview*. Retrieved from http://emergency.cdc.gov/agent/smallpox/overview/disease-facts.asp

Centers for Disease Control and Prevention. (2011a). *Epidemiology and prevention of vaccine preventable diseases: The Pink Book, course textbook* (12th ed.). Retrieved from http://www.cdc.gov/vaccines/pubs/pinkbook/index.html

Centers for Disease Control and Prevention, Division of Vector-borne Diseases. (2011b). *West Nile Virus: Statistics, surveillance, and control archive*. Retrieved from http://www.cdc.gov/ncidod/dvbid/westnile/surv&control.htm

Chen, H., Schernhammer, E., Schwarzschild, M. A., & Ascherio, A. (2006). A prospective study of night shift work, sleep duration, and risk of Parkinson's disease. *American Journal of Epidemiology, 163*, 726–730.

Cohen, D., Spear, S., Scribner, R., Kissinger, P., Mason, K., & Wildgen, J. (2000). "Broken Windows" and the risk of gonorrhea. *American Journal of Public Health, 90*, 230–236.

Cramer, M. E., Roberts, S., & Stevens, E. (2010). Landlord attitudes and behaviors regarding smoke-free policies: Implications for voluntary policy change. *Public Health Nursing, 28*, 3–12. doi: 10.1111/j.1525-1446.2010.00904.x.

Croteau, A., Marcoux, S., & Brisson, C. (2006). Work activity in pregnancy, preventive measures, and the risk of delivering a small-for-gestational-age infant. *American Journal of Public Health, 96*, 846–855.

Dever, G. E. A. (1984). *Epidemiology in health services management*. Rockville, MD: Aspen Systems Corporation.

Dever, G. E. A. (1991). *Community health analysis: Global awareness at the local level* (2nd ed.). Gaithersburg, MD: Aspen Publishers, Inc.

Evans, G. H. (1939). Bubonic plague outbreak in San Francisco: Year 1900. *California West Medicine, 50*(2), 121–123. Retrieved from http://www.pubmedcentral.nih.gov/articlerender.fcgi?artid=1659815

Friis, R. H., & Sellers, T. A. (2009). *Epidemiology for public health practice* (4th ed.). Sudbury, MA: Jones and Bartlett Publishers.

Gabriel, R. A., & Metz, K. S. (1992). *A history of military medicine: From the Renaissance through modern times*, Vol. II. New York: Greenwood Press.

Gerstman, B. B. (2003). *Epidemiology kept simple: An introduction to traditional and modern epidemiology* (2nd ed.). Hoboken, NJ: Wiley-Liss, Inc.

Graham, J., Zhang, L., & Schwalberg, R. (2007). Association of maternal chronic disease and negative birth outcomes in a non-Hispanic Black-White Mississippi birth cohort. *Public Health Nursing, 24*, 311–317.

Hall-Baker, P. A., Nieves, E., Jojosky, R. A., Adams, D. A., Sharp, P., Anderson, W. J., et al. (2010). Summary of notifiable diseases: United States, 2008. *Morbidity and Mortality Weekly Report, 57*(44), 1–94.

Heymann, D. L. (Ed.). (2009). *Control of communicable diseases manual* (19th ed.). Washington, DC: American Public Health Association.

Karageorgi, S., Gates, M. A., Hankinson, S. E., & De Vivo, I. (2010). Perineal use of talcum powder and endometrial cancer risk. *Cancer Epidemiology, Biomarkers & Prevention, 19*(5), 1269–1275.

Kopf, E. W. (1978). Florence Nightingale as statistician. *Research in Nursing and Health, 1*(3), 93–102.

Kudzma, E. C. (2006). Florence Nightingale and healthcare reform. *Nursing Science Quarterly, 19*, 61–64.

Lawson, A. B., & Williams, F. L. R. (2001). *An introductory guide to disease mapping*. Chichester, UK: John Wiley & Sons.

Legator, M. S., & Morris, D. L. (2003). What did Sir Bradford Hill really say? *Archives of Environmental Health, 58*, 718–720.

Markowitz, G., & Rosner, D. (2000). Public health then and now. "Cater to the children": The role of the lead industry in a public health tragedy, 1900–1955. *American Journal of Public Health, 90*, 36–46.

Murphy, S. L., Jisquan, X., & Kochanek, K. D. (2012). Deaths: Preliminary data for 2010. *National Vital Statistics Reports, 60*(4). Retrieved from http://www.cdc.gov/nchs/data/nvsr/nvsr60/nvsr60_04.pdf

Nabel, E. G. (2005). *Statement from Elizabeth G. Nabel, M.D., Director of the National Heart, Lung, and Blood Institute of the National Institutes of Health on the Finding of the Women's Health Study. NIH News*. Retrieved from http://www.nih.gov/news/pr/mar2005/nhlbi-07.htm.

National Center for Health Statistics. (2012a). *National Health Interview Survey (NHIS). About NHIS*. Retrieved from http://www.cdc.gov/nchs/nhis.htm

National Center for Health Statistics. (2012b). *Surveys and data collection systems*. Retrieved from http://www.cdc.gov/nchs/

National Institutes of Health. (2012). *Women's Health Study*. Retrieved from http://clinicaltrials.gov/ct2/show/record/NCT00000479

Nguyen, H. Q., Jumaan, A. O., & Seward, J. F. (2005). Decline in mortality due to Varicella after implementation of varicella vaccination in the United States. *New England Journal of Medicine, 352*, 450–458.

Polivka, B. J. (2006). Needs assessment and intervention strategies to reduce lead-poisoning risk among low-income Ohio toddlers. *Public Health Nursing, 23*, 52–58.

Polivka, B. J., & Gottesman, M. M. (2005). Parental perceptions of barriers to blood lead testing. *Journal of Pediatric Health Care, 19*(5), 276–284.

Robinson, E. S., Fisher, N. D., Forman, J. P., & Curhan, G. C. (2010). Physical activity and albuminuria. *American Journal of Epidemiology, 171*, 515–521.

Siddique, A. K. (1994). Cholera epidemic among Rwandan refugees: Experience of ICDDR,B in Goma, Ziaire. *Glimpse, 16*(5), 3–4.

Simond, M., Godley, M. L., & Mouriquand, P. D. E. (1998). Paul-Louis Simond and his discovery of plague transmission by rat fleas: A centenary. *Journal of the Royal Society of Medicine, 91*, 101–104

Solomon, T. (1997). Hong Kong, 1894: The role of James A. Lowson in the controversial discovery of the plague bacillus. *Lancet, 350*, 59–62.

Susser, M., & Susser, E. (1996a). Choosing a future for epidemiology: I. Eras and paradigms. *American Journal of Public Health, 86*, 668–673.

Susser, M., & Susser, E. (1996b). Choosing a future for epidemiology: II. From black box to Chinese boxes and eco-epidemiology. *American Journal of Public Health, 86*, 674–677.

Theilmann, J., & Cate, F. (2007). A plague of plagues: The problem of plague diagnosis in Medieval England. *Journal of Interdisciplinary History, 37*, 371–393.

U. S. Department of Health and Human Services (USDHHS). (2012). *Social determinants of health: Understanding social determinants of health*. Retrieved from http://www.healthypeople.gov/2020/topicsobjectives2020/overview.aspx?topicid=39

U.S. Department of Health and Human Services (USDHHS). (2010). *Healthy People 2020: Public health infrastructure*. Retrieved from http://www.healthypeople.gov/2020/topicsobjectives2020/objectiveslist.aspx?topicId=35

U. S. Department of State—Bureau of African Affairs. (2012). *Background note: Rwanda*. Retrieved from http://www.state.gov/r/pa/ei/bgn/2861.htm

U.S. Public Health Service. (1964). *Smoking and health: Report of the Advisory Committee to the Surgeon General of the Public Health Service*. Washington, DC: Author. Retrieved from http://profiles.nlm.nih.gov/ps/retrieve/Narrative/NN/p-nid/60/p-docs/true

Valanis, B. (1999). *Epidemiology in health care* (3rd ed.). Stamford, CT: Appleton & Lange.

Walker, M. C., Finkelstein, S. A., Rennicks White, R., Shachkina, S., Smith, G. N., Wen, S. W., et al. (2011). The Ottawa and Kingston (OaK) Birth Cohort: Development and achievements. *Journal of Obstetrics and Gynaecology Canada, 33*, 1124–1133.

World Health Organization. (2012). *Initiative for vaccine research (IVR): Zoonotic infections*. Retrieved from http://www.who.int/vaccine_research/diseases/zoonotic/en/index3.html

World Health Organization. (2007). *International health regulations 2005*. Retrieved from http://www.who.int/ihr/en/

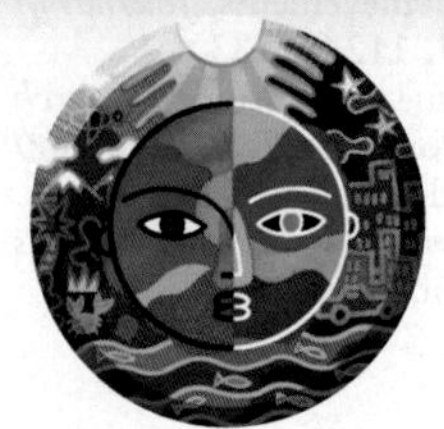

CHAPTER 8

Communicable Disease Control

"All interest in disease and death is only another expression of interest in life."

—***Thomas Mann*** (1875—1955)

KEY TERMS

Active immunity
Communicable disease
Direct transmission
Fomites
Herd immunity
Immunization
Incubation period
Indirect transmission
Infectious
Isolation
Novel
Passive immunity
Quarantine
Reservoir
Ring vaccination
Screening
Surveillance
Vaccine
Vector

LEARNING OBJECTIVES

Upon mastery of this chapter, you should be able to:

- Discuss the nurse's role in communicable disease control.
- Describe the three modes of transmission for communicable diseases.
- Explain the strategies used for the three levels of prevention in communicable disease control.
- Explain the significance of immunization as a communicable disease control measure.
- Describe major issues that affect the control and elimination of tuberculosis (TB).
- Discuss specific ways to prevent sexually transmitted diseases, including HIV/AIDS.
- Discuss the consequences of biologic terrorism with weapons such as anthrax and smallpox.
- Discuss ethical issues affecting communicable disease and infection control.

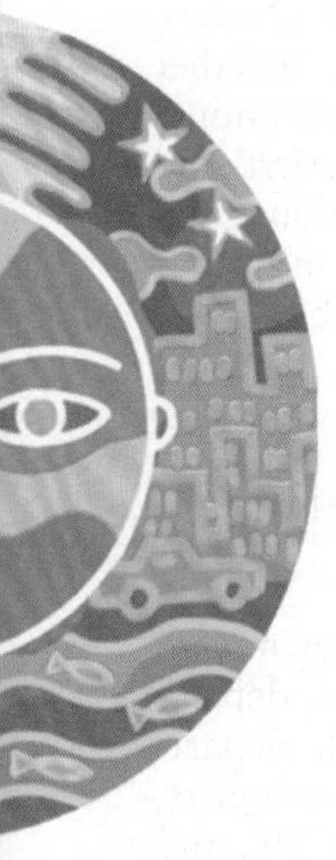

Communicable diseases pose a major threat to public health and are of significant concern to community/public health nurses. A **communicable disease** is one that can be transmitted from one person to another, is caused by an agent that is **infectious** (capable of producing infection), and is transmitted from a source, or **reservoir**, to a susceptible host (Heymann, 2008). The majority of communicable diseases that the public health nurse will encounter and investigate are considered infectious; other diseases are not infectious but are just as potentially problematic to a community. An example of a noninfectious disease is Lyme disease. The infections or diseases that are investigated are reportable through a process mandated by the individual state in which the nurse practices (Heymann, 2008).

Knowledge of communicable diseases is fundamental to the practice of community/public health nursing because these diseases typically spread through communities of people. Understanding the basic concepts of communicable disease control, as well as the numerous surrounding issues, helps a public health nurse work effectively to prevent and control communicable disease in populations and groups. It also helps nurses teach important and effective preventive measures to community members, advocate for those affected, and protect the wellbeing of uninfected persons (including nurses themselves).

In the last century, numerous changes occurred in the lives of people both nationally and globally related to issues of public health. Achievements in health, safety, longevity, and disease control improved the lives of many populations in developed nations, and with the work of many global organizations, will continue to improve for developing nations as well. With progress come challenges, and concerns necessitate ongoing work of the community/public health nurse in advocating for the health of individuals and communities through disease prevention and health promotion. Examples of ongoing issues include

- Higher morbidity among various age and population groups related to communicable diseases, rather than death
- Continuing disproportionate morbidity and mortality among lower socioeconomic populations
- Emergent, newly identified, or resurging diseases related to changing environments, global mobility, and need for space. Examples of these are Hanta virus, West Nile virus, malaria, and Avian and the novel H1N1 strains of influenza.
- Development of antibiotic resistant strains of bacteria that pose significant occupational health challenges as well as practice issues for health workers. Examples include multi- and/or extreme drug-resistant tuberculosis (MDRTB, XDRTB) and methicillin-resistant staphylococcus aureus.
- Potential terrorist attacks utilizing biologic agents
- Ongoing public empowerment through education regarding healthy life practices, and current health research associated with disease and cancer prevention through diet, immunization, and the environment (Centers for Disease Control and Prevention [CDC] 1999b, 2010e; Schlipköter & Flahault, 2010).

This chapter provides information to better understand communicable diseases in communities. It describes ways to plan and implement appropriate prevention interventions, including immunization of children and adults, environmental interventions, community education, screening programs, and disease investigation and case/contact finding. Ethical issues of communicable disease control are also discussed. A list of communicable disease information sources useful to you, the community/public health nurse, is provided on thePoint.

BASIC CONCEPTS REGARDING COMMUNICABLE DISEASES

Communicable diseases have challenged health care providers for centuries. They have led to the development of countless nursing and medical preventive measures, from simple procedures such as hand washing, sanitation, and proper ventilation to the research and development of vaccines and antibiotics (CDC, 1999b).

Evolution of Communicable Disease Control

Because preventive measures have greatly reduced the spread of communicable diseases, many people consider communicable diseases to be a threat of the past. Yet this is not the reality. Communicable diseases, particularly those of epidemic and pandemic probability, such as TB, influenza, or AIDS, continue to cost millions of lives and billions of dollars to the global human society every year (Schlipköter & Flahault, 2010).

As mentioned in Chapter 7, the first documented global threat from a communicable disease began in the 13th century in the form of bubonic plague. It was responsible for killing 25% of the population in some European countries over the years following the Crusades and during the years of exploration and trade by ship—in the 1400s to 1600s.

As commerce and industry continued to grow, people migrated from rural areas to towns and cities. However, health and hygiene practices that worked in remote areas did not transfer to the new urban settings. In tenements and overcrowded parts of towns, water for drinking easily became contaminated with human waste. Mounting garbage and trash, unable to be composted or buried as was done in farming communities, created a rich habitat for rodents and other animals and insects, encouraging them to breed and become vectors for many communicable diseases.

Not until the 1700s and 1800s were the causative organisms for various infectious diseases recognized through the assistance of increasingly sophisticated microscopes. With these discoveries came early attempts to create ways to prevent the spread of such organisms, either by decreasing their power or by eliminating them. Pasteurization of milk was invented, and efforts to eliminate rats from ships and food storage areas began. These measures commenced a global effort to eliminate communicable diseases (Schlipköter & Flahault, 2010).

As mentioned in Chapter 6, the World Health Organization (WHO) came into existence as an arm of the United Nations (UN) in 1948. It was established to tackle world health issues such as malaria, women's and children's health, TB, venereal diseases, nutrition, and environmental sanitation. The WHO continues to be a very active part of the UN. It has evolved into a multifaceted agency providing services such as ongoing health/illness research, education, medical response, and disease control response worldwide (WHO, 2007).

Also mentioned in Chapter 6 is the CDC, a branch of the U.S. Department of Health and Human Services (USDHHS). Originally tasked with the elimination of malaria in war areas, it has evolved over the years into a health promotion and disease prevention agency. It is recognized globally for its partnerships in disease surveillance, research, data collection, and analysis, as well as responding nationally and globally with peer agencies to disease outbreaks (CDC, 2012b). One disease, smallpox, is a classic example of a communicable disease control success story. For centuries, the infectious disease of smallpox killed millions of people and scarred survivors for life—in fact, it is thought that smallpox is responsible for more deaths than any other infectious disease (Children's Hospital of Philadelphia, 2010). Smallpox first responded to a crude vaccine that was developed in the 18th century. The vaccine was studied and perfected and used globally for decades. A major worldwide eradication campaign began in 1967. The last naturally acquired case of smallpox in the world occurred in October 1978; global eradication was certified 2 years later by the WHO and confirmed by the World Health Assembly in May 1980. Since then, no cases of naturally acquired smallpox have been identified in any country (Heymann, 2008).

Despite strides in controlling major disease outbreaks, the threat of biologic warfare using smallpox or other disease organisms raises concerns about how to prepare for the future. The CDC continues to strengthen the National Biosurveillance System, which searches for and is ready to respond to a national biological weapons attack. The Global Public Health Intelligence Network (GPHIN), developed by the Public Health Agency of Canada, provides a secure Internet-based multilingual early-warning tool that continuously searches global media sources such as news wires and web sites to identify information about disease outbreaks and other events of potential international public health concern (CDC, 2012b; Nuzzo, 2009; Public Health Agency of Canada, 2012). Together with data from the CDC, GPHIN, and other international public health programs, the WHO's Global Alert and Response Network (GAR) provides an international and integrated GAR system to address epidemics and other public health emergencies (WHO, 2012a, 2012b).

Community Health Nurse's Role: Process of Investigating Reportable Communicable Diseases

Each state has a State Health Department, but not all states have local level sites like a county health department. Some of the state and/or local health departments utilize a combination of nurses, epidemiologists, and communicable disease investigators. The CDC and WHO provide guidance documents that assist state public health agencies develop investigation policy and procedures for the local level investigator to use. The local investigations process must meet the requirements of the state and federal reporting laws that derive from state, federal, and global health regulations. Individual states utilize the national notifiable infectious disease list as the guidance for developing the state's reportable diseases and may add to this list as they choose, reflecting the types of conditions that are unique to a state or region of the United States (2012f). State health departments commonly specify two other circumstances that must be reported: any outbreak or unusually high incidence of *any* disease, and any occurrence of an unusual disease of public health importance (CDC, 2011h). The CDC is ready and willing to provide active guidance and recommendations to any state health department when a disease issue becomes too large for the local or state to provide response to (CDC, 2010j). The CDC is also available to each individual citizen via mail, phone, or the Internet (Centers for Disease Control and Prevention, 1600 Clifton Rd, Atlanta, Georgia 30333, United States; 800-CDC-INFO (800-232-4636); TTY: (888) 232-6348, 24 Hours/Every Day; cdcinfo@cdc.gov).

The local health department/agency is the initial point of notification of a communicable disease investigation. In most states, reporting known or suspected cases of a reportable disease is generally considered to be an obligation of

- Physicians, dentists, nurses, and other health professionals
- Medical examiners
- Administrators of hospitals, clinics, nursing homes, schools, and nurseries

Some states also require or request reporting from

- Laboratory directors
- Any individual who knows of or suspects the existence of a reportable disease

Each state has a disease report form; California uses a form titled "Confidential Morbidity Report" (Display 8.1 is an example of a reporting form). Each

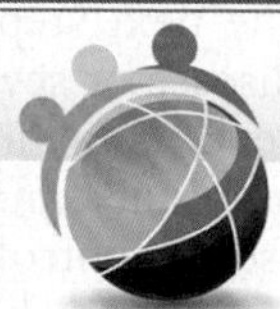

DISPLAY 8.1 CONFIDENTIAL MORBIDITY REPORT

CONFIDENTIAL MORBIDITY REPORT

NOTE: For STD, Hepatitis, or TB, complete appropriate section below. Special reporting requirements and reportable diseases on back.

DISEASE BEING REPORTED:

Patient's Last Name | **Social Security Number**

First Name/Middle Name (or initial) | **Birth Date** Month Day Year | **Age**

Address: Number, Street | **Apt./Unit Number**

City/Town | **State** | **ZIP Code**

Area Code | **Home Telephone** | **Gender** M F | **Pregnant?** Y N Unk | **Estimated Delivery Date** Month Day Year

Area Code | **Work Telephone** | **Patient's Occupation/Setting**
- ❒ Food service
- ❒ Day care
- ❒ Correctional facility
- ❒ Health care
- ❒ School
- ❒ Other

Ethnicity (✓ one)
- ❒ Hispanic/Latino
- ❒ Non-Hispanic/Non-Latino

Race (✓ one)
- ❒ African-American/Black
- ❒ Asian/Pacific Islander (✓ one):
  - ❒ Asian-Indian
  - ❒ Japanese
  - ❒ Cambodian
  - ❒ Korean
  - ❒ Chinese
  - ❒ Laotian
  - ❒ Filipino
  - ❒ Samoan
  - ❒ Guamanian
  - ❒ Vietnamese
  - ❒ Hawaiian
  - ❒ Other:
- ❒ Native American/Alaskan Native
- ❒ White:
- ❒ Other:

DATE OF ONSET Month Day Year

DATE DIAGNOSED Month Day Year

DATE OF DEATH Month Day Year

Reporting Health Care Provider

Reporting Health Care Facility

Address

City | **State** | **ZIP Code**

Telephone Number ( ) | **Fax** ( )

Submitted by | **Date Submitted** (Month/Day/Year)

REPORT TO

(Obtain additional forms from your local health department.)

SEXUALLY TRANSMITTED DISEASES (STD)

Syphilis
- ❒ Primary (lesion present)
- ❒ Secondary
- ❒ Early latent < 1 year
- ❒ Latent (unknown duration)
- ❒ Late latent > 1 year
- ❒ Late (tertiary)
- ❒ Congenital

❒ **Neurosyphilis**

Syphilis Test Results
- ❒ RPR Titer:
- ❒ VDRL Titer:
- ❒ FTA/MHA: ❒ Pos ❒ Neg
- ❒ CSF-VDRL: ❒ Pos ❒ Neg
- ❒ Other:

Gonorrhea
- ❒ Urethral/Cervical
- ❒ PID
- ❒ Other:

Chlamydia
- ❒ Urethral/Cervical
- ❒ PID
- ❒ Other:

- ❒ **PID (Unknown Etiology)**
- ❒ **Chancroid**
- ❒ **Non-Gonococcal Urethritis**

STD TREATMENT INFORMATION

❒ **Treated (Drugs, Dosage, Route):** | Date Treatment Initiated Month Day Year

❒ **Untreated**
- ❒ Will treat
- ❒ Unable to contact patient
- ❒ Refused treatment
- ❒ Referred to:

VIRAL HEPATITIS

		Pos	Neg	Pend	Not Done
❒ **Hep A**	anti-HAV IgM	❒	❒	❒	❒
❒ **Hep B**	HBsAg	❒	❒	❒	❒
❒ **Acute**	anti-HBc	❒	❒	❒	❒
❒ **Chronic**	anti-HBc IgM	❒	❒	❒	❒
	anti-HBs	❒	❒	❒	❒
❒ **Hep C**	anti-HCV	❒	❒	❒	❒
❒ **Acute**	PCR-HCV	❒	❒	❒	❒
❒ **Chronic**					
❒ **Hep D (Delta)**	anti-Delta	❒	❒	❒	❒
❒ **Other:**		❒	❒	❒	❒

Suspected Exposure Type
- ❒ Blood transfusion
- ❒ Other needle exposure
- ❒ Sexual contact
- ❒ Household contact
- ❒ Child care
- ❒ Other:

TUBERCULOSIS (TB)

Status
- ❒ **Active Disease**
  - ❒ Confirmed
  - ❒ Suspected
- ❒ **Infected, No Disease**
  - ❒ Convertor
  - ❒ Reactor

Site(s)
- ❒ Pulmonary
- ❒ Extra-Pulmonary
- ❒ Both

Mantoux TB Skin Test

Date Performed Month Day Year ❒ Pending

Results: ______ mm ❒ Not Done

Chest X-Ray

Date Performed Month Day Year

- ❒ Normal
- ❒ Pending
- ❒ Not done
- ❒ Cavitary
- ❒ Abnormal/Noncavitary

Bacteriology

Date Specimen Collected Month Day Year

Source

Smear: ❒ Pos ❒ Neg ❒ Pending ❒ Not done

Culture: ❒ Pos ❒ Neg ❒ Pending ❒ Not done

Other test(s)

TB TREATMENT INFORMATION

❒ **Current Treatment**
- ❒ INH
- ❒ RIF
- ❒ PZA
- ❒ EMB
- ❒ Other:

Date Treatment Initiated Month Day Year

❒ **Untreated**
- ❒ Will treat
- ❒ Unable to contact patient
- ❒ Refused treatment
- ❒ Referred to:

REMARKS

PM 110 (8/05) (Edited 9/05)

local health department/agency will investigate a specific disease using a protocol set by the local, state, or federal public health official (CDC, 2011h).

Disease investigation requires a systematic approach. Some diseases are terminal in the human host, not infectious to others, for example, Lyme disease (Heyman, 2008). Other diseases are passed from host to susceptible host, such as *Salmonella*. Whether it is a single case of illness in a small town, or a multijurisdictional outbreak, similar investigation steps are followed. These steps include interviewing individuals, contact and additional case finding, analyzing information gathered from surveillance, intervening to control the disease, and elimination and/or eradication (CDC, 2007).

Prior to contacting an individual for an interview:

- Review the information received from mandated reporters for completeness.
- Clarify that the disease is suspect or lab confirmed. Some infections can be reported if they meet a set of clinical criteria or are part of a larger outbreak and a case definition has been defined.
- Review the case definition. A case is the individual who either has a laboratory confirmed reportable disease or meets the clinical definition in an investigation.
- Review the disease information—reservoir, incubation period, infectious period, symptoms, and treatment.
- Many diseases have specific questionnaires that are useful when interviewing the client. Review the questionnaire prior to contacting the client, so you understand the intent. If no questionnaire exists, you may have to write a narrative report including the information related to onset of illness, symptoms, medical evaluation, treatment if received, recovery state, and individuals the person has been in contact with depending upon the nature of the disease. Display 8.2 provides one example of a generic disease investigation form (Directors of Public Health Nursing, 2008).

The Interview:

- Maintaining a neutral and nonjudgmental attitude during the interview process will elicit information more readily, especially when discussing an STD, for example.
- The interview may be by telephone or in person. The way an interview is pursued depends upon the department protocol and/or disease being addressed.
- Introduction of self and purpose of the confidential nature of the interview is essential.
- Eliciting what the individual knows about the disease may give the nurse an idea of the individual's knowledge base and what education or reeducation to provide.
- Gathering the information by using a disease-specific questionnaire may lead to a possible source of the disease, or to additional infected contacts.
- The nurse will contact individuals identified as possibly infected by the identified case. By pursuing contacts, the possibility of outbreak status may appear.

Surveillance of reportable diseases is the next step. The nurse may have individual cases of a disease or several cases that make up a cluster or outbreak. It is this awareness of the disease threat to the community and when to take prompt action that is key to disease control. Information is sent from the local investigation to the next higher level of government. If an outbreak is occurring, it may be from the next level of government that assistance is garnered (Heymann, 2008). Next is *disease control*. Control is determined by the disease. Prompt action is crucial to arresting a possible outbreak. Control actions may be achieved by offered testing, counseling, education, vaccination, treatment, or prophylaxis as appropriate, or environmental intervention like draining standing water (CDC, 2007; Heymann, 2008).

Effective surveillance and control can lead to *elimination and eradication* of a disease in many cases. Elimination is the stopping of a disease in a defined geographical region, whereas eradication is the extinction of naturally occurring disease (CDC, 1999a). An example of elimination is that in the United States, there are no natural cases of measles. By maintaining high levels of immunization, only imported cases of measles have occurred for years. An example of eradication of a disease is smallpox.

Modes of Transmission

As discussed in Chapter 7, the reservoir of infection can be a person, animal, insect, or inanimate material in which the infectious agent lives and multiplies and which serves as a source of infection to others. Transmission of a communicable disease can occur by direct, indirect, airborne, or vector methods.

Direct Transmission

Direct transmission occurs by immediate transfer of infectious agents from a reservoir to a new susceptible host. It requires direct contact with the source, through touching, biting, kissing, or sexual intercourse—that is, contact with oral secretions, blood, or other potentially infectious fluid, such as the drainage from a skin lesion. Coughing or sneezing secretions into the face of a susceptible individual can directly transmit respiratory infections, such as measles or pertussis. Close proximity is required, like sharing the space in a car, to transmit an organism from one person to another (Heymann, 2008) (see Fig. 8-1)

Indirect Transmission

Indirect transmission occurs when the infectious agent is transported within contaminated inanimate materials such as air, water, or food. It is also commonly referred to as *vehicle-borne transmission*. Chapter 9 describes both the government's role and the nurse's role in helping to prevent food and water contamination by infectious agents (Heymann, 2008).

Food- and Water-Related Illness

Food- or water-related illness can be caused by viruses, toxins, bacteria, or parasites, such as *Salmonella*,

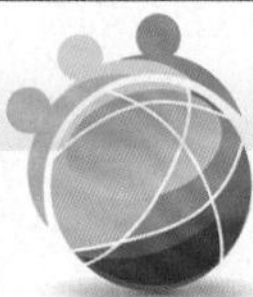

DISPLAY 8.2 SAMPLE GENERIC DISEASE INVESTIGATION FORM

SAMPLE GENERIC DISEASE INVESTIGATION FORM

Name: ______________________ DOB/age: __________

Address: ______________________

Telephone(s): ______________________

Race/ethnicity: __________ Occupation: __________ Gender: __________

Risk Factors

Recent travel outside US? __________ Outside of the County? __________

If yes, location(s) & date(s) ______________________

Was client born in US? __________

If no, country of birth __________ Year arrived in US __________

In 10 days prior to this illness, has individual participated in the following activities? If yes, please explain.

Attended a social gathering ______________________

Was food served? If yes, list foods consumed ______________________

Eaten at restaurants, including fast-food restaurants ______________________

____

Eaten rare/raw animal products, home-canned /unusual foods ______________________

____

Visited a day care or medical facility ______________________

Had visitors in his/her home? __________ Were any of them ill? __________

If yes, sex and dates of illness ______________________

Drunk water from/or swam/bathed in pools, lakes, hot tubs, etc. __________

If yes, where and when: ______________________

What is usual source of drinking water? ______________________

Does client have contact with domestic or wild animals? __________

Were any animals sick? If so, date of contact ______________________

I. Comments:

California Public Health Nursing Disaster Handbook IV-4
Second Edition 2008

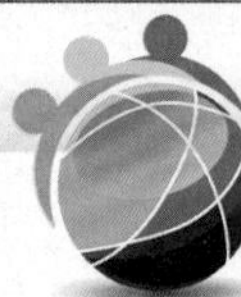

DISPLAY 8.2 SAMPLE GENERIC DISEASE INVESTIGATION FORM *(Continued)*

Clinical Information

Date/time of onset: ____________ Duration of symptoms: ____________

Symptoms: (check all that apply)

☐ Fever ____________

☐ Chills ☐ Nausea ☐ Vomiting ☐ Abdominal Cramps

☐ Diarrhea ☐ Headache ☐ Neck Stiffness ☐ Cough

☐ Runny Nose ☐ Shortness of Breath

Others: ____________

____

____

Did client see health care provider? ____________

If yes, name of provider, phone and date seen ____________

What was diagnosis? ____________

Was any lab work ordered? ____________

If yes: Test: ____________ Results ____________

Test: ____________ Results ____________

Test: ____________ Results ____________

Was any medication prescribed? ____________

Was client hospitalized? ____________ Where ____________

What was outcome? ____________

Does client have any chronic illnesses? List ____________

What medications does client normally take? ____________

Does client use any home remedies? ____________

Allergies to foods or medications ____________

Recent immunizations ____________

Is client aware of anyone else with similar symptoms? ____________

If yes, please give identifying information ____________

Females: Are you pregnant? ____________ If yes, EDC ____________

Is there any other information you think may be important for us to know regarding this Illness?

____

____

Initial telephone contact by ____________ Phone: ____________ Date: ____________

Person conducting the interview: ____________ Phone: ____________ Date: ____________

California Public Health Nursing Disaster Handbook
Second Edition 2008 IV-5

Source: Directors of Public Health Nursing. (2008). California public health nursing disaster handbook (2nd ed.). Retrieved from http://www.phncalifornia.org/pdf/phn-disaster-manual.pdf

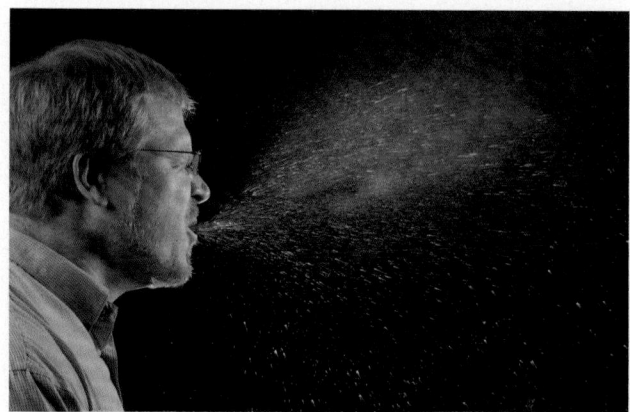

FIGURE 8-1. Sneeze in progress–Revealing the plume of droplets expelled in a large cone-shaped array. (From Centers for Disease Control and Prevention. Public Health Image Library. (2009). Photo Image ID #11161–James Gathany.)

Shigella, Escherichia coli 0157, and *Camplyobacter*; the protozoan agent *Giardia*; *Staphylococcus*, and the viral agent hepatitis A. These microorganisms cause intestinal illness, and sometimes even death. The contamination can occur at the source (e.g., contamination by animal into the food or water chain) or through unsanitary food handling or practices, which are referred to as the *fecal–oral route*. Improper food storage can also create an environment for microorganisms to grow. Ingestion of the pathogenic organism sets in motion the events of a food- or water-related illness (Heymann, 2008).

Most commonly, exposure to contaminated food or water results in symptoms related to gastrointestinal function, including diarrhea, nausea, vomiting, stomach cramps, and bloating. Fever may accompany these infections as well. Onset of symptoms may occur within a few hours after exposure or not until days or even weeks later, depending on the microorganism. This time interval between exposure and onset of symptoms is called the **incubation period**.

Microorganism contamination of food resulting in human illness occurs as a result of either infection or intoxication. Infection is related to a pathogen that occurs through ingestion of food contaminated with adequate doses of *Salmonella, Shigella, E. coli,* or other pathogens. The cycle begins when the infectious agent multiplies and grows in the food medium. The agent subsequently invades the host after ingestion of the food. Then infection occurs—which is the entry and development or multiplication of an infectious agent in the body. Infection is usually accompanied by an immune response, such as the production of antibodies with or without clinical manifestation. The infectious organism produces illness by direct irritation of the normal gastrointestinal mucosa. By contrast, intoxication is caused by the production of toxins as a by-product of the normal bacterial life cycle. This commonly occurs when cooked food is left standing at room temperature or is living on skin of a food preparer and inoculates the food. It is ingestion of the toxin, rather than the microbe itself, that produces the illness (Heymann, 2008). One well recognized example is the neurotoxin Botulinum which is produced by the bacteria *Clostridium botulinum*.

The distinction between infection and intoxication is relevant for a number of reasons. Toxins may be difficult to isolate and identify, particularly in the absence of the bacteria; some suspected food-borne illnesses go unidentified for this reason. Although the bacteria may be killed after heating of foodstuffs before consumption, some bacteria-produced toxins are stable at normal cooking temperatures, so that food cannot be rendered safe. Bacteria established in the human gastrointestinal system may require medical treatment to be eradicated. In contrast, individuals with food intoxication typically require supportive care while in the process of ridding themselves of the toxin (Heymann, 2008).

The most important aspects of food- or water-related diseases for nurses in community health is to recognize that outbreaks of illness affecting large numbers of people can occur, despite well-recognized standards for decontamination of water supplies and safe commercial food preparation. The public health nurse may receive similar reports of illness that requires looking for a common source and then may need a higher level of investigatory assistance, such as the state health department (CDC, 2011c). Outbreaks may not be detectable by local surveillance means alone because of the mobility of individuals or the routine transportation of foods from one state or country to the other. It may not be identified as an outbreak until the various reports of illness and laboratory reports from effected communities (or in one if it is a local outbreak) are processed and forwarded to a public health laboratory, and then onto the state public health laboratory. It is at this point that the sentinel surveillance system is triggered. Some states have local county public health laboratories that may make the identification of organism clusters. Unfortunately, many states or regions rely primarily on the state public health laboratory for organism identification, which has the potential for delays (CDC, 2011c).

The CDC has a system of surveillance called PulseNet; it is a network of public health and food regulatory agencies working together. This program uses laboratory testing to identify organisms that may come from the same source. This is determined by pulse-field gel electrophoresis or DNA fingerprinting of organisms. Once the common source is identified, the food regulatory agency will work with the source to clean up the problem or close the facility down. Several agencies may coordinate response when a food- or water-related contamination is identified: the CDC (2011j), the U.S. Food and Drug Administration (2009, 2010), or the U.S. Department of Agriculture Food Safety and Inspection Service (2010b).

For example, in one outbreak of *Salmonella enteritidis*, a common form of the bacteria, was traced to a large egg farm in the Midwest that sold to numerous local and national retailers. This illness outbreak was detected when multiple state laboratories identified identical bacterial fingerprints from specimens that were compared through PulseNet. The various state health

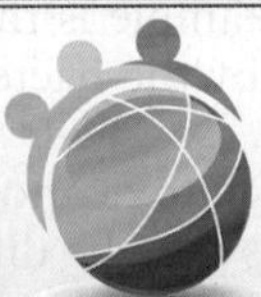

DISPLAY 8.3 CORRECT METHODS FOR PRESERVING THE SAFETY AND CLEANLINESS OF FOOD

Before handling food:

- Wash hands and all food preparation surfaces and utensils thoroughly with soap and water.

When preparing food:

- Wash foods that are to be eaten raw and uncooked thoroughly in clean water. This includes foods that are to be peeled that grow on the ground or come in contact with soil.
- Cook all meat products thoroughly.
- Do not allow cooked meats to come in contact with dishes, utensils, or containers used when the foods were raw and uncooked.

When storing leftover foods:

- Cool cooked foods quickly; store under refrigeration in clean, covered containers.

When reheating leftover foods:

- Heat foods thoroughly. Bacteria contaminating food grow and multiply in a temperature range between 39°F and 140°F.

departments were able to utilize this sentinel data from the surveillance network to identify contamination sources. Identification of the common source enabled the local regulators to guide the farmer in cleaning up the production process, in turn preventing further problems (CDC, 2010d).

Such outbreaks can serve to remind all community health practitioners of the continuing need to teach and observe the most basic methods for preventing food and water contamination. Display 8.3 summarizes correct methods for maintaining the safety and cleanliness of food.

Vector Transmission

When transmission occurs through a **vector** (a nonhuman carrier such as an animal or insect), it is known as vector-borne transmission. Rabies and Hantavirus are examples of illnesses passed from animals. Insects such as mosquitoes, fleas, and ticks are responsible for transmission of malaria, plague, and Lyme disease. Transmission can be through a bite of the insect or animal or exposure to the infected animal's body fluids, such as the urine from the Hantavirus-infected rodent (Heymann, 2008).

Control strategies directed toward vector-borne diseases typically involve community education and environmental measures to hinder the vector from reaching the host (U.S. Department of Agriculture, 2010a).

Control strategies may include the following:

- Reduce the population of insects.
- Eradicate rodents that carry diseases, such as rats.
- Use of mechanical or chemical barriers to protect from exposure to vectors, such as mosquitos or ticks—for example, sprays or mesh bed nets.
- Public education about preventive and protective measures, including avoiding vector habitats, and how to respond when exposed to a vector to prevent disease from developing.

Airborne Transmission

Airborne transmission occurs through droplet nuclei—the small residues that result from evaporation of fluid from droplets emitted by an infected host. Sneezing and coughing are common examples of airborne transmission. Because of the small size and weight of droplet nuclei, they can remain suspended in the air for long periods before they are inhaled into the respiratory system of a host. Small particles of dust from soil containing fungus spores may cling to clothing, bedding, or floors. The spores may become separated from dry soil by the wind and then be inhaled by the host (Heymann, 2008).

MAJOR COMMUNICABLE DISEASES IN THE UNITED STATES

Community health nurses encounter any number of communicable diseases in their practice. Many are reportable, but some are not—although they are just as transmittable to others as the reportable infections. As mentioned previously, each state department of health has the capacity to determine which diseases will be reportable based upon the federal reportable disease list. These diseases are frequently diagnosed and treated in the community care setting rather than the hospital. The following sections discuss some of the more common communicable diseases, but the list is not inclusive of all that are reportable. Diseases are presented in groups by similarity, rather than by virulence or prevalence.

Influenza (Seasonal or Novel) and Pandemic Preparedness

Influenza (flu) is identified as an acute communicable viral disease of the respiratory tract characterized by fever, headache, myalgia, prostration, coryza, sore throat, and cough. Influenza A virus causes the most severe and widespread disease (pandemics); influenza B causes milder disease outbreaks; and influenza C is connected with only sporadic cases of milder respiratory disease. Influenza is usually seasonal in nature, but may be found year round if testing is done. Seasonal flu preparedness is in the form of vaccine preparation, utilizing the previous year's flu strain information to calculate the next year's subtype through complex formulations done globally and nationally by public health authorities (CDC, 2010g).

Influenza derives its importance from the rapidity with which epidemics evolve, the widespread morbidity, and the seriousness of complications, namely pneumonias (Heymann, 2008). Influenza, an Italian word that means *influence of the cold*, has been recognized since 412 BCE and was first described by Hippocrates. It existed throughout the early centuries, and about 30 probable pandemics have been documented in the past 400 years. Three have occurred in the 20th century—in 1918, 1957, and 1968. The 1918 "Spanish flu" pandemic was the most devastating, with an estimated death toll of 50 to 100 million worldwide; in the United States, roughly 675,000 died (CDC, 2010f). This was a novel influenza strain (a new strain of the virus), which spread easily from person to person, devastating the world population.

Influenza infections occur primarily in the winter months, affecting individuals in all age groups and causing thousands of deaths and hospitalizations annually in the United States alone. Children have the highest rates of infection, but individuals age 65 years and older, children younger than 2 years of age, and those with medical conditions who are at risk for complications have the highest rates of hospitalizations, and of serious morbidity and mortality. Older adults account for more than 90% of the deaths attributed to influenza and pneumonia (CDC, 2010a).

Influenza immunization is available every flu season; vaccines are closely matched to the circulating strains of the virus. The CDC (2011a; 2011i) recommends key universal immunization of *all people 6 months of age and older*. Children younger than 6 months need to be protected by immunization of the individuals surrounding them. The most important message is to promote immunization of those that may suffer the poorest of outcomes and those caring for them:

- Health care workers and personal care providers
- Children younger than 5, but especially children younger than 2 years old
- Adults 65 years of age and older
- Pregnant women
- Individuals with asthma
- Those with chronic disease of any system of the body (neurologic, cardiac, pulmonary, hemologic, renal, hepatic, immune, or metabolic, endocrine, and anyone on long-term medication for an illness)

The injectable influenza vaccine is inactivated. The nasally inhaled version is a live attenuated vaccine (see Fig. 8-2). In the elderly, immunization may be less effective in preventing illness, but may reduce the severity of disease. With immunization, the incidence of complications and death among the elderly is reduced (CDC, 2010a; Heymann, 2008). The vaccine should be given every year *before* influenza is expected in the community. The season can begin as early as October, so vaccinating in September may be indicated, but usually it is the end of October in most of the United States. For those living or traveling outside the United States, timing of the immunization should be based on the seasonal patterns of influenza in the area to which they are traveling

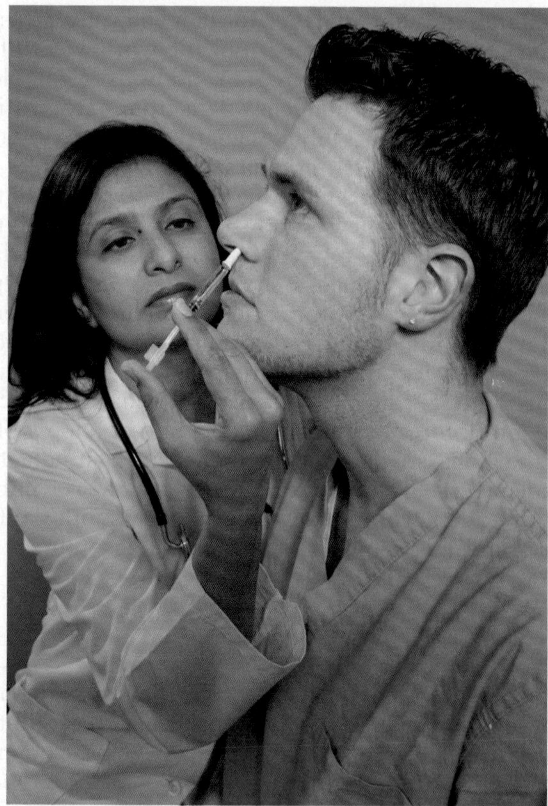

FIGURE 8-2. Administration of nasal-spray flu vaccine. (Centers for Disease Control and Prevention. Public Health Image Library. (2009). Photo Image ID #11864–James Gathany.)

(CDC, 2009e). Community/public health nurses play a major role in primary prevention. Influenza immunization clinics are frequently planned and organized by or with the local public health agency, with the injections usually administered by community/public health nurses.

Influenza pandemics occur when a flu subtype has not circulated previously (novel strain) or has reemerged in a population that has never been exposed (CDC, 2010f). The most recent **novel** or new strain of influenza was identified as H1N1, a strain that had not been experienced by the current world population. In the spring of 2009, two cases of this H1N1 strain were identified in the United States. There were ongoing cases of this new strain documented across the United States into the summer of 2010. The spread of this virus was occurring globally as well. There was a rapid response by the WHO and the CDC, in investigating, typing this strain, and initiating the production of a vaccine. Within 6 months, a monovalent (single strain) vaccine was available to the public. According to the CDC, 90 million doses of vaccine were made and 80 million doses were administered during that first season (CDC, 2010i).

The WHO's GAR is an integrated GAR system for epidemics and other public health emergencies with electronic support from the Network for Global Influenza Surveillance and FluNet. This program involves 116 national influenza centers worldwide and maintains constant vigilance for new influenza viruses. FluNet is an Internet-based tool for worldwide influenza surveillance. This program allows for the electronic submission of influenza data from participating global laboratories. Only designated users can submit data, but the results—graphics, maps, and tables of influenza activity on a global scale—are available to the general public. As new data arrive and are verified, the maps and tables are revised to give users an up-to-date overview of the influenza situation. FluNet has expedited the sharing of information on influenza patterns and virus strains, and is becoming an essential tool in preparing for and preventing influenza pandemics. Collaborating Influenza Surveillance Centers have created a task force of influenza experts to develop a plan for the global management and control of an influenza pandemic. These influenza experts and world public health leaders work diligently to prevent another influenza pandemic similar to the devastating outbreak of 1918 (WHO, 2012a).

Pneumonia

Pneumonia is a pulmonary infection that causes inflammation of the lobes of the lungs, bronchial tree, or interstitial space. In the United States, the most common bacterial cause of pneumonia is *Streptococcus pneumoniae* (pneumococcus) and the most common viral causes are influenza, parainfluenza, and respiratory syncytial viruses. Symptoms of pneumonia include sudden onset with a shaking chill, fever, pleural pain, dyspnea, a productive cough of "rusty" sputum, and tachypnea. The onset is less abrupt in elderly individuals, and the diagnosis may need to be confirmed by radiographic studies. In infants and young children, fever, vomiting, and convulsions may be the initial symptoms (CDC, 2012g).

Community-acquired pneumonia is a significant cause of morbidity and mortality. An increased incidence of pneumonia often accompanies epidemics of influenza. In 2007, 1.2 million people in the United States were hospitalized with pneumonia and more than 52,000 people died from the disease. Globally, pneumonia kills more than one and a half million children younger than 5 years of age each year. This is greater than the number of deaths from any other infectious disease, such as AIDS, malaria, or TB (CDC, 2012g). Hospital admissions and mortality related to pneumonia are far more common among people older than age 65; the mortality rate is approximately 50%. Although this is not a reportable infectious disease, it can nevertheless have a great impact upon the community (Heymann, 2008).

The incidence of pneumonia is highest in winter. Pneumonia is spread by droplets, by direct oral contact, and through **fomites**, which are any inanimate objects freshly soiled with respiratory discharges. People most susceptible to pneumonia are the elderly and people with a history of chronic diseases, a compromised immune system, or any condition affecting the anatomic or physiologic integrity of the lower respiratory tract (CDC, 2012g; Heymann, 2008).

Pneumococcal vaccine is available for high-risk groups, ages 2 years old and up. High-risk groups include those with chronic diseases, immune-suppressing health conditions, or those who are asplenic. Reimmunization is recommended only for high-risk children or adults over 65 years who had their first vaccination before age 65. The vaccine is not effective in children younger than 2 years of age and is not recommended for the healthy population between the ages of 2 and 65 years. For these people, education about preventing pneumonia is a major part of the community/public health nurse's role (CDC, 2012g).

Hepatitis

Of the five viral hepatitis infections that constitute serious liver disease, three commonly reported types are hepatitis A, B, and C. The number of people infected with hepatitis is a global epidemic. Substantial progress is being made in the elimination of hepatitis viruses through the primary prevention practices of education and immunization with hepatitis A and B vaccines.

Hepatitis A

Hepatitis A, caused by infection with the hepatitis A virus (HAV), occurs worldwide and is sporadic and epidemic, with cyclic recurrences affecting children and young adults most frequently. Case rates are high in Central and South America, the Caribbean, Mexico, Asia (except Japan), Africa, and southern and eastern Europe. Hepatitis A is identified by the presence of immunoglobulin M antibodies against HAV in the serum of acutely or recently ill individuals (Heymann, 2008). The disease is transmitted from person to person by the fecal–oral route and is characterized by the abrupt onset of symptoms including fever, malaise, anorexia, nausea, and abdominal discomfort, followed by jaundice in more severe cases. Mild illnesses last 1 to 2 weeks, but more severe cases last 1 month or longer. It is generally a self-limited disease that does not result in chronic infection or chronic liver disease. Recovery from HAV usually confers immunity to the individual (Heymann, 2008).

In areas of the world where environmental sanitation conditions are poor, endemic infection may exist and cause infection at an early age. In this setting, the majority of adults have immunity. In industrialized countries, cases will tend to occur in the older population rather than children, in households of the infected, and among travelers returning from countries where the disease is endemic. At times, common-source outbreaks are related to contaminated water, food contaminated by infected food handlers, raw or undercooked shellfish harvested from contaminated water, or contaminated produce (Heymann, 2008).

Hepatitis A vaccine has been available for use since 1995; it is an inactivated hepatitis A vaccine (CDC, 2012c). Administered in a two-dose series, these vaccines induce protective antibody levels in virtually all who are immunized. This has been a boon to eliminating this disease as a public health problem in the United States. The vaccine is recommended as a routine vaccine for children and, as of 2005, it was made available to children older than 12 months. Community/public health nurses play an important role in the prevention and control of this disease. Offering hepatitis A vaccine to travelers, case investigation, education, and identifying exposed contacts that need referral or assistance in obtaining postexposure prophylaxis and vaccination are vital to preventing and controlling this disease (CDC, 2012c).

Hepatitis B

Hepatitis B is a serious disease. The hepatitis B virus (HBV) is often a lifelong infection and may cause cirrhosis (scarring) of the liver, liver cancer, liver failure, and death. In a very few cases, the infection will resolve, conferring immunity (Heymann, 2008). This is a blood and body fluid pathogen; common transmission patterns are parenteral and sexual.

Hepatitis B is a global problem. Approximately 2 billion people have evidence of resolved or current HBV infection, and 350 million people are chronic carriers of the virus. In countries with high endemicity, the primary cause of infection is from mother to fetus (Heymann, 2008). The chance of a child developing a chronic HBV infection is 90% if infected at birth, 30% if infected between 1 and 5 years of age, and only 5% to 10% if infected after the age of 5 years (CDC, 2012c). Symptoms of HBV range from unnoticeable to fulminating, and include anorexia, vague abdominal discomfort, nausea and vomiting, and rash, often progressing to jaundice. The diagnosis is confirmed by the presence of specific antigens to HBV in serum (Heymann, 2008).

Immunization is the most effective way of preventing HBV transmission. Following WHO recommendations, 158 member states have integrated hepatitis B vaccine into their national immunization programs. The WHO and the United Nations Children's Fund (UNICEF) have sought means to help the poorest and neediest countries procure the vaccine (Rani, Yang, & Nesbit, 2008). In the United States, not every state has implemented universal newborn hepatitis B immunization, but it is recommended (CDC, 2011a). Community/public health nurses have an important role in the prevention and control of hepatitis B. Most importantly, this role includes teaching that encourages immunization compliance and consistent adherence to universal precautions, especially for people in high-risk lifestyles or occupations.

Hepatitis C

Hepatitis C (HCV) was first identified by a formal designation in 1989. Prior to this, the virus was referred to a non-A-non-B hepatitis. It causes a complex infection of the liver and is one of the leading known causes of liver disease in the United States. It is a common cause of cirrhosis and hepatocellular carcinoma, as well as liver transplantation. It is believed that at least 130 to 170 million people in the world are infected with HCV (Heymann, 2008).

HCV is more widespread than AIDS, and many infected people are unaware that they are infected. Symptoms are similar to those of hepatitis A and B, and may be unrecognizably mild to fulminating. Diagnosis depends on the demonstration of antibody to HCV and a screening test for blood donors was established in 1992. Before there was a specific test for HCV; this virus was the most common cause of posttransfusion hepatitis worldwide. The CDC (2010b) recommends that individuals at greater risk of developing HCV infection should consider testing

- People who inject drugs, including those who injected once or a few times in the past and do not consider themselves drug users
- Individuals who received transfusions or organ transplants before 1992 and recipients of blood from a positive donor
- People with selected medical conditions, including recipients of clotting factors before 1987, people undergoing chronic hemodialysis, and those with persistently elevated alanine aminotransferase levels
- Those exposed to HCV-positive sources, such as needlesticks, sharps, or mucosal exposures

There is currently no vaccine for HCV. The public health nurse's role is primarily supportive, encouraging testing for people who identified as having HCV infection risk factors, and referring individuals for care and treatment and to support/educational groups. As with HBV, teaching adherence to universal precautions in the home is important as well (Heymann, 2008).

HIV/AIDS

The *HIV* is a retrovirus that attacks the body's immune system. HIV is contracted through blood and body fluids from an infected person to a susceptible person. Transmission can occur during unprotected sex, sharing of contaminated needles, placental transmission from mother to fetus, and may also be transmitted through blood or blood components. Two types have been identified: type 1 (HIV-1) and type 2 (HIV-2). These viruses are relatively distinct serologically and geographically, but they have similar epidemiologic characteristics. The pathogenicity of HIV-2 appears to be less than that of HIV-1 (Heymann, 2008). More than 25 years have passed since the identification of this infection, and it is viewed by many to be a chronic, manageable disease process, especially in the developed world. In most parts of the world, HIV continues to devastate populations of people who do not have access to life-extending medical care and medications. An HIV-infected individual may remain symptom free for long periods, but viral replication is active during all stages of infection.

AIDS is a severe, life-threatening condition, representing the late clinical stage of infection with HIV, in which there is progressive damage to the immune and other organ systems—particularly the central nervous system. AIDS has been staved off in many individuals by the use of medications during the HIV stage of the spectrum (see "Selected Readings" at avert.org)

Tuberculosis

TB is a disease primarily of the lungs and larynx, caused by the mycobacterium tuberculosis (MTB) complex, *M. africanum*, *M. tuberculosis*, and *M. canettii*, all Gram-positive bacilli. TB can also infect other parts of the body; it is then referred to as *extrapulmonary TB* (outside of the lungs). TB has two stages: latent infection, which is noninfectious to others, and active disease, which is highly infectious to others. TB is airborne, and is spread by droplet nuclei, sprayed from the mouth by coughing, sneezing, laughing, yelling, singing, or any way in which air is expelled vigorously from the lungs through the mouth. Infection occurs after inhaling the bacilli exhaled by the person with active TB. The incubation time for TB is approximately 10 to 12 weeks (Heymann, 2008). Exposure to TB does not lead to actual disease in all cases. A latent period may persist for many years before the infected person develops disease and becomes infectious, if ever. The probability of becoming infected depends primarily on the amount of exposure to air contaminated with *M. tuberculosis*, the proximity to the infectious person, and the degree of ventilation.

Most individuals exposed to people with TB do not become infected. Of those who do, all but about 5% to 10% will remain disease free. The remaining 90% harbor the organism; although they are not infectious, they represent a persistent pool of potential cases in a population. The likelihood of being among the 10% who develop clinical infectious disease is variable, depending on the initial dose of infection and certain other risk factors. Groups at increased risk include children younger than 3 years of age, adolescents and young adults, the aged, the immunosuppressed, and those who are early in their infection (<2 years) (Heymann, 2008). Health factors can contribute to the development of active TB. Poor nutrition, health status, and chronic illness like diabetes can inhibit the immune system's ability to prevent TB activation from the dormant state. Figure 8-3 shows the geographic distribution of TB in the United States.

Once almost eradicated, TB has reemerged as a serious public health problem. There were a total of 10,521 new TB cases reported in the United States in 2011, or 3.4 cases per 100,000 population. This rate was 6.4% lower than in 2010 and represented the lowest recorded rate since 1953 (when national reporting was instituted). Although this is good news, there is evidence of sharply disparate rates among foreign-born and racial/ethnic minority populations—the TB case rates per 100,000 populations were 6.3 in African-Americans; 5.9 in Hispanic Americans; 21.4 in Asian-Americans; 5.4 in American Indians or Alaska Natives; 16.8 in Pacific Islanders and Native Hawaiians; and Whites had the lowest rate at 0.8 (CDC, 2012j). In 2011, over 50% of foreign-born persons with TB originated from five countries: Mexico, the Philippines, Vietnam, India, and China. The pattern of TB infections has changed dramatically over the past decade. Non-Hispanic Asians are now the largest population group among TB patients with a rate that is 25 times greater than non-Hispanic whites. These figures serve to emphasize the need for continued vigilance, especially in high-risk populations. The worldwide picture of TB has worsened over the past two decades, especially in Africa because of the HIV/AIDS epidemic (a fatal association exists between TB and HIV/AIDS). According to the WHO estimates, in 2008, 35% of the cases of TB occurred in Southeast Asian regions; however, twice as many cases occurred in sub-Saharan Africa. Deaths in Africa were estimated at 1.7 million in 2009 (WHO, 2010a, 2010b).

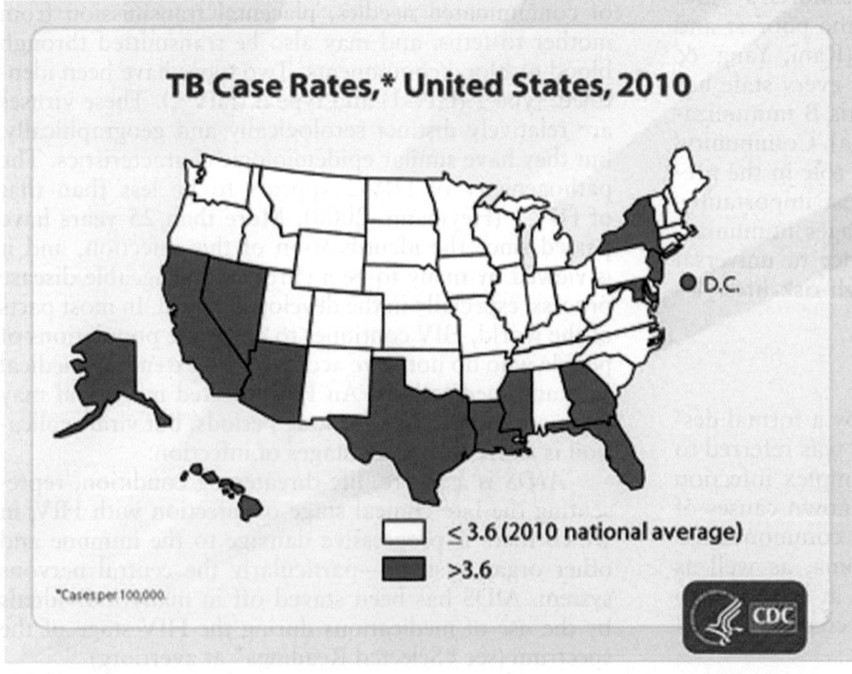

FIGURE 8-3. TB case rates by state. (From Centers for Disease Control and Prevention. (2012). *Tuberculosis in the United States National Tuberculosis Surveillance System highlights from 2010.* Retrieved from http://www.cdc.gov/tb/statistics/surv/surv2010/default.htm)

HIV infection contributes dramatically to the development of active TB. Immune-suppressed individuals can develop active TB within weeks after exposure to the mycobacterium, and the disease progresses much faster than in those with a normal, competent immune system. Consequently, a suspected case of TB in a person with HIV/AIDS is usually treated immediately, without waiting for the results of sputum tests or chest x-ray (CDC, 2012k).

Screening

Mantoux tuberculin skin testing is the standard method for evaluating TB infection. It is a simple skin test that measures—by visible reaction—whether the body has had immunologic experience with *M. tuberculosis* (Table 8-1). From there, evaluation procedures determine the classification status of the disease, ranging from 0 to 5. The two most used terms are *infected without current disease* (classification 2) and *with current TB disease* (classification 3) (Table 8-2). The skin test itself is not diagnostic of disease.

The Mantoux test delivers 0.1 mL of PPD (purified protein derivative) by intradermal injection. Because the dose is measured at the time of injection, the Mantoux test is considered to be reliable. Interpretation of the tuberculin test is critical to subsequent evaluation of the client's status. The interpretation of this screening method must be as sensitive as possible while maintaining specificity for exposure (Heymann, 2008). Recently, an interferon-gamma release assay (IGRA) or quantiferon TB test became available. It is a blood test that measures a person's immune reactivity to *M. tuberculosis*. This test has a high specificity and reliability. However, as noted by the CDC (2011d), there are advantages and disadvantages to this test:

Advantages of IGRAs:

- Necessitates only one visit to be tested
- Twenty-four-hour turnaround time on results
- Does not boost responses measured by subsequent tests
- No false-positive results from past immunization with BCG (Bacille Calmette-Guérin)

Disadvantages and limitations of IGRAs:

- Blood samples must be processed within 8 to 16 hours after collection.
- Collecting or transporting errors of the blood specimens or in running and interpreting the assay can decrease the accuracy of IGRAs.
- Limited data on the use of IGRAs to predict who will progress to TB disease in the future.
- Limited data on the use of IGRAs for
  - Children younger than 5 years of age
  - Persons who may be incubating *M. tuberculosis*
  - Immunocompromised persons
  - Serial testing
- Tests may be expensive.

The community health nurse may encounter an individual who, at the time of the TB skin test, discloses having had the BCG vaccine in their home country. The BCG

Table 8.1 Classification of the Tuberculin Skin Test Reaction

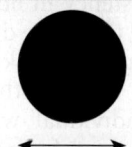

5 or More Millimeters	10 or More Millimeters	15 or More Millimeters
An induration of **5 or more millimeters** is considered positive for • human immunodeficiency virus-infected persons • Recent contacts of persons with infectious tuberculosis (TB) • People who have fibrotic changes on a chest radiograph • Patients with organ transplants and other immunosuppressed patients (including patients taking a prolonged course of oral or intravenous corticosteroids or TNF-α antagonists [tumor necrosis factor])	An induration of **10 or more millimeters** is considered positive for • People who have come to the United States within the last 5 yrs from the areas of the world where TB is common (e.g., Asia, Africa, Eastern Europe, Russia, or Latin America) • Injection drug users • Mycobacteriology lab workers • People who live or work in high-risk congregate settings • People with certain medical conditions that place them at high risk for TB (silicosis, diabetes mellitus, severe kidney disease, certain types of cancer, and certain intestinal conditions) • Children younger than 4 yrs • Infants, children, and adolescents exposed to adults in high-risk categories	An induration of **15 or more millimeters** is considered positive for • People with no known risk factors for TB

From Centers for Disease Control and Prevention. (2011). *Core curriculum on tuberculosis: What the clinician should know. Table 3.2 interpreting the TST reaction.* Retrieved from http://www.cdc.gov/tb/education/corecurr/pdf/chapter3.pdf

Table 8.2 Classification System for Tuberculosis (TB)

Class	Type	Description
0	No TB exposure *Not* infected	• No history of TB exposure and no evidence of *M. tuberculosis* infection or disease • Negative reaction to tuberculin skin test (TST) or interferon-gamma release assay (IGRA)
1	TB exposure No evidence of infection	• History of exposure to *M. tuberculosis* • Negative reaction to TST or IGRA (given at least 8 to 10 wk after exposure)
2	TB infection No TB disease	• Positive reaction to TST or IGRA • Negative bacteriological studies (smear and cultures) • No bacteriological or radiographic evidence of active TB disease
3	TB clinically active	• Positive culture for *M. tuberculosis OR* • Positive reaction to TST or IGRA, plus clinical, bacteriological, or radiographic evidence of current active TB
4	Previous TB disease (*not* clinically active)	• May have past medical history of TB disease • Abnormal but stable radiographic findings • Positive reaction to the TST or IGRA • Negative bacteriologic studies (smear and cultures) • No clinical or radiographic evidence of current active TB disease
5	TB suspected	• Signs and symptoms of active TB disease, but medical evaluation **not** complete

From Centers for Disease Control and Prevention. (2011). ***Core curriculum on tuberculosis: What the clinician should know. Table 2.8 TB classification system***. Retrieved from http://www.cdc.gov/tb/education/corecurr/pdf/chapter2.pdf

vaccine is an attenuated strain of *Mycobacterium bovis* (*M. bovis*) (bovine strain), which is not used in the United States, except in very rare incidences (CDC, 2011b). The efficacy of the BCG vaccine is questionable, as the protective value wanes over time and there is no consistency in how the vaccine is made. It is recommended the nurse disregard this immunization when interpreting the TB skin test because the test does not distinguish between the *M. bovis* strain and the MTB, and the individual who received the injection most likely emigrated from a TB endemic country and was most likely exposed to TB (California Tuberculosis Controllers Association, 2010). The BCG immunization has been demonstrated to have protective value to infants and children, even though it may not deflect infection. Infants and small children who develop TB can quickly succumb to meningitis, miliary, or extrapulmonary TB (CDC, 2011b).

Prevention and Intervention

According to the CDC Division of TB Elimination (DTBE) (CDC, 2009d), a well-functioning TB control program must focus resources on those at risk for TB exposure and treating latent TB and active TB. TB activation risk factors can be poor health (HIV/AIDS, chronic disease), lack of access to health care, poverty, malnutrition, and fear of deportation (nonresident status). Prevention and rapid treatment of infection can help prevent active TB and the possible emergence of drug-resistant TB. The functional aspect of the program should ideally strive for

- Standardized public health practices for investigating, case and contact finding, and care and treatment
- Case management of care and treatment of the individual with TB to ensure medication compliance and barriers to treatment completion are dealt with so treatment completion will occur
- Close monitoring for sputum conversion in people with active disease, in order to adjust medication as necessary
- A high completion-of-therapy rate within 1 year after diagnosis
- Assurance of adequate funding and a dedicated TB control infrastructure

One of the most effective ways to achieve a high completion-of-therapy rate is through directly observed treatment (DOT). In endemic countries, such as Africa, directly observed treatment short-course (DOTS) is used. This strategy assures treatment success because the client takes the medication in the presence of a health care worker. The DOT(S) strategy has been demonstrated to work, and it is supported by the CDC and in turn by state and local health departments. It is not mandatory, but health officers may use the laws surrounding TB prevention and public protection to institute policy and statute to mandate its use. By using DOT(S) with the client with active TB, there is a reduction in ongoing potential sources of infection in the community (CDC, 2011e; Moonan et al., 2011; WHO, 2010c).

The DOT approach is obviously labor-intensive, but according to the WHO, it has made a difference in fighting the spread of this disease. The more difficult clients are those who do not realize their personal or social responsibility for health and those who do not have the resources to focus on health when there are other stressors or diversions in their life. For these reasons, clients such as alcohol and drug abusers, transient homeless people, and people stressed by socioeconomic problems may become the source for new cases of TB. DOT therapy ensures that clients take a daily or intermittent dose of prescribed medication, locating them wherever they may be—in neighborhood bars, sleeping on the sidewalk, in a homeless shelter, or in a drug rehabilitation center. Most health departments and TB control programs have a percentage of their clients receiving DOT therapy, with licensed staff or community health workers assigned to administer the TB drug regimen. These outreach workers and sometimes public health nurses meet the people where they are, school, shelter, church, bar, or job, wherever it supports adherence to the mediation regimen. These ancillary staff members are often former program participants, trained and supervised by professional health workers. A program like DOTS needs sustained political commitment, with the governments of nations recognizing the long-term benefits of providing the resources and staff necessary to ensure its proper implementation (Moonan et al., 2011; WHO, 2010c).

Multidrug-Resistant Tuberculosis

Epidemiologists and communicable disease specialists cite a number of factors that contribute to the development and spread of TB strains resistant to one or more of the standard arsenal of TB drugs. Strains now exist that are resistant to almost all of the standard anti-TB drugs. According to the WHO, one in four persons contracting XDRTB dies rapidly, within months from the disease. Chief among the factors contributing to drug resistance seems to be the political and social response to declining rates of TB over past decades, which has resulted in funding cuts for surveillance, treatment, and research, and a premature sense that TB was defeated. Figure 8-4 demonstrates the disproportionate prevalence of MDRTB in foreign-born persons. On an individual case basis, the most common means by which resistant organisms are acquired is by noncompliance with therapy for the full, recommended period. As previously mentioned, the DOTS intervention can help those with TB successfully treat and cure the disease (Moonan et al., 2011; WHO, 2010c).

When candidates for drug therapy are identified, it is essential to provide program support to ensure that the maximum number of individuals comply with their medication regimen for the full duration of therapy. Isoniazid therapy for individuals who are infected with TB but have no evidence of active disease has been shown to be highly effective in preventing progression to infectiousness and clinical symptoms. Isoniazid (also known as INH) is a key component of the treatment for active disease (Heymann, 2008; Inge &Wilson, 2008).

Clients with HIV and TB

HIV infection is associated with an increased possibility of developing primary TB after exposure to a source. The person living with coinfection of latent TB infection and HIV infection has a 50% higher risk of developing active TB than the immune-competent individual (Heymann, 2008).

People with HIV infection and TB infection should be counseled thoroughly about the benefit of preventive treatment and possibility of TB activation without treatment. For HIV-infected people, preventive therapy usually consists of isoniazid daily for up to 1 year (the usual regimen for preventive therapy is 6 to 9 months). These clients must be monitored closely for effectiveness

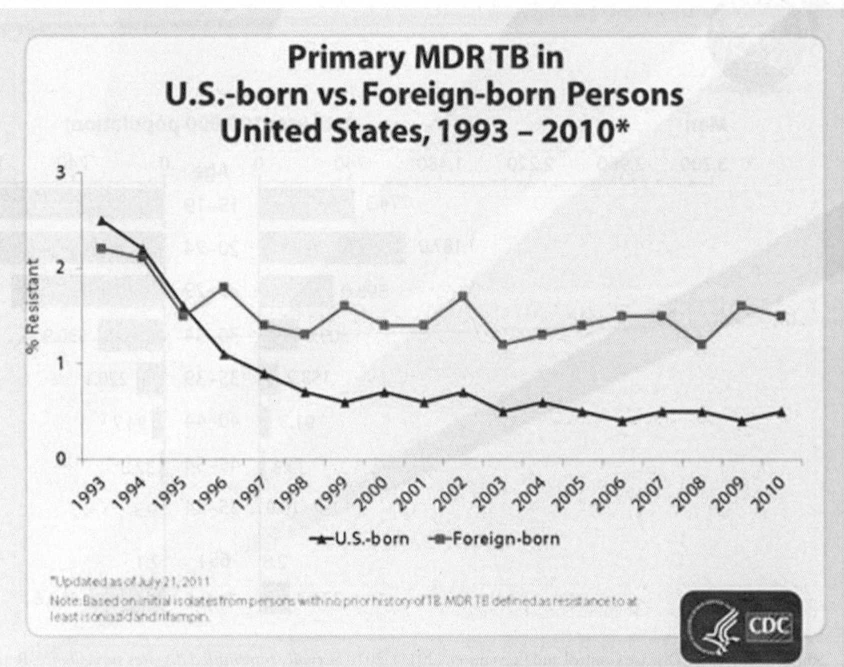

FIGURE 8-4. Multidrug-resistant TB patterns. (From Centers for Disease Control and Prevention. (2012). *Tuberculosis in the United States National Tuberculosis Surveillance System highlights from 2010.* Retrieved from http://www.cdc.gov/tb/statistics/surv/surv2010/default.htm)

of the preventive therapy and for tolerance to isoniazid. This drug has the capacity to develop adverse reactions or negative side effects. Isoniazid can cause hepatitis or damage the liver; close monitoring and regular follow-up are necessary to detect early symptoms such as nausea, vomiting, abdominal pain, fatigue, and dark urine signifying bleeding. Any combination of these symptoms is sufficient to initiate liver function tests (Heymann, 2008).

The HIV-positive client may not have the ability to react to a skin test for TB because of a weakened immune system. Therefore, other methods to determine TB status are employed. If it is determined that TB disease is present, HIV-infected clients should begin a regimen of drugs according to the accepted national and global medication schedule used in their country. The client should be closely monitored for response to treatment; if they do not seem to be responding, they should be reevaluated. Drug sensitivity is key to correct and successful treatment.

TB Case Management

Community health nurses have a responsibility to individuals who are HIV-infected and also infected with TB, to experience a successful TB treatment regimen. As previously mentioned, a component of a successful TB program is case management of care and treatment, which includes monitoring for adherence to treatment, administering medications (either directly through DOT or through DOT supervision by ancillary staff), interviewing the individual for signs and symptoms of adverse reactions, collecting lab specimens in a timely manner and monitoring for culture conversion, monitoring for overall health and wellbeing, educating, and making referrals (CDC, 2011p).

Sexually Transmitted Infections

Chlamydia

Chlamydia trachomatis (CT) infections are the most commonly reported notifiable STD in the United States. Since 1994, CT has made up the largest proportion of all STDs reported to the CDC. In women, Chlamydia infections, which are usually asymptomatic, may result in pelvic inflammatory disease (PID)—a major cause of infertility, ectopic pregnancy, and chronic pelvic pain. Chlamydia is a sexually transmitted bacterial infection of great concern. The CDCs 2010 report on CT infections was 1,307,893 cases or a case rate of 426 per 100,000 persons (CDC, 2011l).

Until recently, chlamydia was probably the least recognized of the STDs. People with uncomplicated infection are quite often symptom free until late and serious complications occur. Women can experience PID, ectopic pregnancy, and infertility. Infants born to infected women can be adversely affected by conjunctivitis with the possibility of blindness or severe pneumonia (Heymann, 2008).

Screening programs have been extremely effective in reducing the chlamydia burden. The use of the highly sensitive nucleic acid amplification urine tests is easy and more acceptable to most individuals who may be symptomatic or asymptomatic (CDC, 2011k). As a result of increased screening efforts in many settings outside of the medical office, reported rates of chlamydia continue to increase, especially in women aged 15 to 24 years (Display 8.4). The current CDC (2011k) guidelines for screening recommendations are as follows:

- Assess for risk factors at each medical contact with a sexually active person.
- Screen sexually active 24-year-olds and younger

DISPLAY 8.4 CHLAMYDIA—RATES BY AGE AND SEX, UNITED STATES, 2010

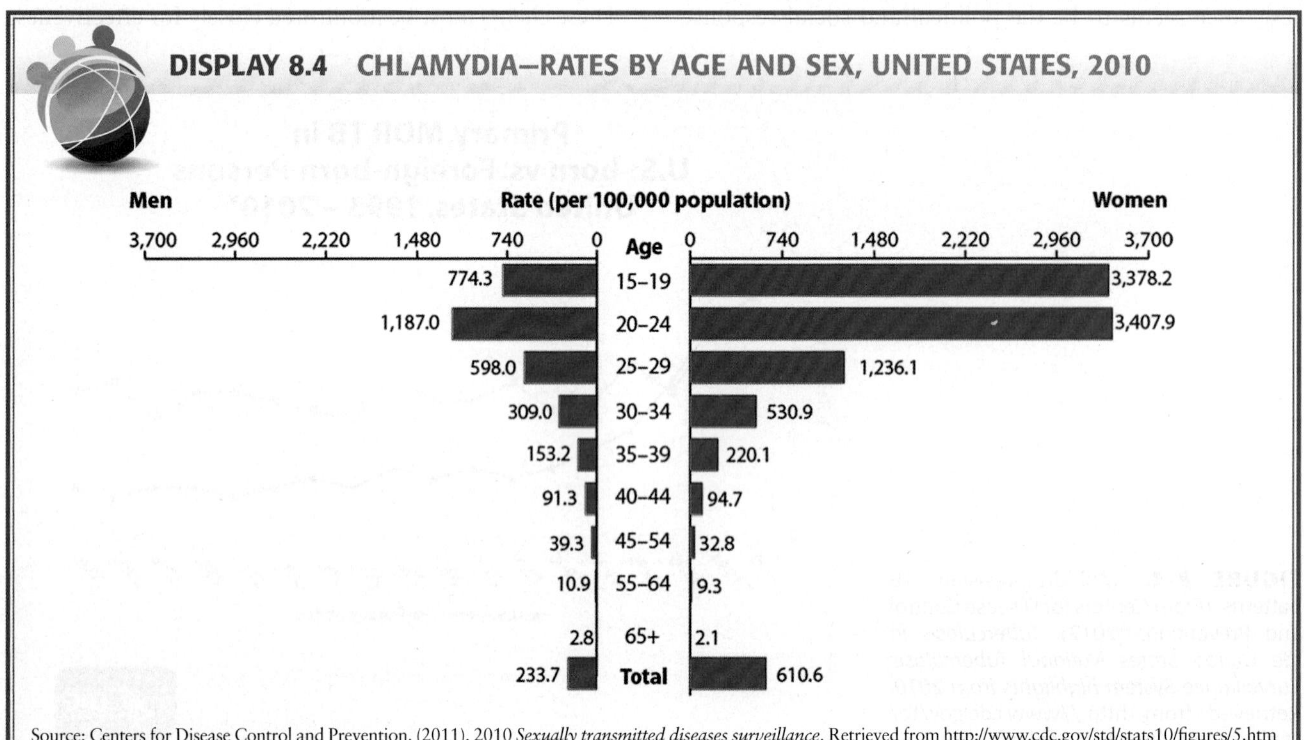

Source: Centers for Disease Control and Prevention. (2011). 2010 *Sexually transmitted diseases surveillance*. Retrieved from http://www.cdc.gov/std/stats10/figures/5.htm

- Screen those with multiple sexual partners
- Screen those with partners who have multiple sex partners within the last year
- Screen all pregnant women at least one time, no matter the age, and those who plan to terminate a pregnancy.
- Consider retesting any infected teens who may be at risk for reinfection.

Barriers exist to successful prevention, diagnosis, and treatment of chlamydia. Stigma surrounding seeking care, access to affordable care, and completion of extended antibiotic treatment may keep individuals from getting care and treatment. Using a one-dose treatment is far more acceptable than two to three times a day for 7 days treatment plan (CDC, 2011k).

"Patient-delivered partner treatment" or "expedited partner treatment" is the giving of either a prescription or medication to the infected patients to in turn give to their sex partner. This intervention has been shown to be more effective than encouraging the patient to notify their partner(s) to seek testing and treatment. Each state may have its own legal requirements related to this treatment option; the nurse needs to review and understand their states' law (CDC, 2012e). Another aspect to this method of treatment is to provide very specific written instructions that include self-administration of the medication, when to seek medical care, and how to prevent reinfection (CDC, 2012e; McBride, Goldsworthy, & Fortenberry, 2009). However, for men who have sex with men, this practice is not as customary, as there may be other coinfection issues that need evaluation and treatment as well (CDC, 2011k). To minimize the risk for reinfection, clients should be instructed to abstain from sexual intercourse until all of their sex partners have been treated and advised to use condoms as a continued STD prevention method. Testing for cure of infection depends upon the type of antibiotic used and if the person is pregnant or not (CDC, 2011k).

Gonorrhea

The overall rate of gonorrhea (GC) in the United States has decreased to 100.6 cases per 100,000 in 2010, compared with the 2008 case rate of 110.7 cases per 100,000; but slightly more than the 2009 rate of 98.1 (CDC, 2011l). The causative agent is gonococcus bacteria—*Neisseria gonorrhoeae*. Consistently, the highest rates have been among women age 15 to 19 years (570.9 cases per 100,000 females) and 20- to 24-year-old males (421 cases per 100,000 males) (CDC, 2011m).

Antimicrobial resistance continues to be a concern in treating gonorrhea. Overall, 27% of isolates collected in the United States in 2007 from the Gonnococcal Isolate Surveillance Project STD clinic sites were resistant to penicillin, tetracycline, or both. This antibiotic resistance is of great concern because this organism has an affinity to resistance. Since 2006, quinolones have been discontinued for use with GC within the United States and in many countries globally (Workowski, Berman, & Douglas, 2008).

Gonorrhea commonly manifests in men as a purulent drainage from the penis, accompanied by painful urination within 2 to 7 days after an infecting exposure. In women, the symptoms may be so mild as to go unnoticed. Progression of untreated gonorrhea in women can lead to serious reproductive system involvement causing PID and subsequent infertility. Screening criteria are similar to chlamydia; refer back to "Chlamydia" section.

Treatment for uncomplicated gonorrhea may include one of the following: ceftriaxone injectable, oral cefixime, or a combination of a single dose injectable cephalosporin plus either azithromycin or doxycycline. There are many complex situations that can exist with GC infection, for example, pregnancy or newborn exposure, and these take more medical intervention. (Please refer to the citation for the current STD guidelines in the reference section for further reading). Sex partners need to be referred to a medical provider for testing and treatment, but if this is not possible, expedited partner treatment can be used. This is not the preferred method with GC, but it has been used. Once again, refer to your state's regulations surrounding this method of treatment (CDC, 2011k). Because treatment failure with the combined ceftriaxone/doxycycline regimen is rare, a follow-up test of cure is not considered essential except for pregnant women, who should have a culture performed (CDC, 2011k).

Syphilis

Syphilis, a genital ulcerative disease, manifests in several forms during the life cycle of the disease. Approximately 3 weeks after exposure, a primary lesion called a *chancre* characteristically appears as a painless ulcer at the site of initial invasion of the causative organism *Treponema pallidum*, a spirochete. This first stage is considered primary syphilis. After 4 to 6 weeks, the chancre heals without treatment, to be replaced by the development of a more generalized secondary skin eruption, classically appearing on the soles of the feet and palms of the hands, often accompanied by fatigue. This stage is secondary syphilis. These secondary manifestations resolve spontaneously, and a latent period follows, which may last from weeks to years. These latent stages are referred to as latent, late latent, and tertiary or neurosyphilis. Unpredictably, severe systemic involvement with disability or even death may occur (Heymann, 2008). Sexual transmission of syphilis to partners is thought to occur only when mucocutaneous syphilitic lesions are present. Although such symptoms are unusual after the first year of infection, persons exposed sexually to a patient who has syphilis in any stage should be referred for clinical evaluation and lab tests (CDC, 2011k).

Syphilis is the first STD for which control measures were developed and tested. The incidence of primary and secondary syphilis cases in the United States increased between 2006 and 2010, from 9,756 to 13,774 reported cases (respective rates 3.3 and 4.5 per 100,000). This increase reflects outbreaks among men having sex with men (CDC, 2011l). Syphilis often contributes to HIV transmission. Elimination of syphilis would have far-reaching public health implications because it would remove two devastating consequences of the disease—increased likelihood of HIV transmission and compromised ability to have healthy babies due to spontaneous abortions, stillbirths, and multisystem disorders caused by congenital syphilis acquired from mothers with syphilis (CDC, 2011k). Treatment for syphilis is Penicillin G, injectable for all stages of syphilis. The preparation used (i.e., benzathine, aqueous procaine, or aqueous crystalline), the dosage, and the length of treatment depend on the stage and clinical manifestations of the disease. Clients should be reexamined serologically at 3 and 6 months after treatment to ensure cure; however, the single-dose treatment is considered effective therapy even if the client fails to return (CDC, 2011k).

Genital Herpes

Genital herpes is an STD caused by the herpes simplex viruses, type 1 (HSV-1) and type 2 (HSV-2). Most cases of genital herpes are caused by HSV-2. In women, sites of primary disease are the cervix and the vulva. Recurrent disease generally involves the vulva, perineal skin, legs, and buttocks. In men, lesions appear on the penis, and in the anus and rectum of those engaging in anal sex. Typically, another outbreak can appear weeks or months after the first, but it is almost always less severe and briefer than the first outbreak. The infection can remain in the body indefinitely, and the number of outbreaks will decrease over a period of years (Heymann, 2008).

Nationwide, at least 45 million people aged 12 and older, or 1 in 5 adolescents and adults, have had genital HSV infection. Genital HSV-2 infection is more common in women (approximately one of four women) than in men (almost one of five). This may be due to male-to-female transmissions being more likely than female-to-male transmission. Transmission can occur from an infected partner who does not have a visible sore and may not know that he or she is infected (CDC, 2011k).

Most people infected with HSV-2 are not aware of their infection. However, if signs and symptoms occur during the first outbreak, they can be quite pronounced. The first outbreak usually occurs within 2 weeks after the virus is transmitted. Other signs and symptoms during the primary episode may include a second crop of sores, and flu-like symptoms, including fever and swollen glands. Most individuals with HSV-2 infection may never have sores, or they may have very mild signs that they do not even notice or that they mistake for insect bites or another skin condition (CDC, 2011k).

Health care providers can diagnose genital herpes by visual inspection if the outbreak is typical, and by taking a sample from the sore(s) and testing it in a laboratory. HSV infections can be difficult to diagnose between outbreaks. Blood tests that detect HSV-1 or HSV-2 infection may be helpful, although the results are not always clear (Heymann, 2008).

Antiviral medications provide clinical benefit for genital herpes. Intravenous antiviral therapy is provided for clients who have severe disease or complications that necessitate hospitalization, such as disseminated infection, pneumonitis, hepatitis, or complications of the central nervous system (e.g., meningitis, encephalitis). Antiviral medications can shorten and prevent outbreaks during the period when the person takes the medication. In addition, daily suppressive therapy for symptomatic herpes can reduce transmission to partners (CDC, 2011k).

Viral Warts

Condyloma acuminata, verruca vulgaris, papilloma venereum, and the common wart are all forms of a viral disease manifested by a variety of mucous membrane and skin lesions (Heymann, 2008). All are transmitted by direct contact, but condyloma acuminata, or genital warts caused by HPV, are usually sexually transmitted.

Researchers have identified more than 100 types of papilloma viruses, and at least 30 of these types of the virus are sexually transmitted. Several of the subtypes of HPV are associated with cervical dysplasia and genital cancers, which can occur 5 to 30 years after the initial infection, accounting for more than 70% of cervical cancers and 90% of genital warts. The CDC estimates that about 50% of sexually active individuals will suffer infection of viral warts in their lifetime (CDC, 2011k).

Sexually active individuals are at risk for contracting any one or several of the types of genital warts that exist. Because few produce the actual bumpy, visual signs of warts, and some produce no notable symptoms, many cases go undiagnosed. This asymptomatic state leads to ongoing transmission between or among sexual partners (CDC, 2011k). Sexually active women can be diagnosed at the time of Papanicolaou (Pap) smear during the woman's health examination. This test can detect abnormal cytological changes, and viral tests can be performed on the sample to determine the presence of HPV. Biopsy of the site may also be needed to examine the tissue more thoroughly (CDC, 2011k).

Treatment depends on the size and location of the warts. Even though the warts may be removed, the viral infection cannot be cured, which is why the warts often return. Some of the medications used to treat genital warts cannot be used during pregnancy, so it is important for clients to tell their doctors if they could be pregnant. Small warts may be treated with medications applied to the skin. In some cases, applying liquid nitrogen (cryotherapy) to warts will freeze the tissue and make warts disappear. Some larger warts require laser treatment or surgical removal (CDC, 2011k).

Two vaccines are available for the prevention of Human papilloma virus (HPV), one of the types of viral warts infection. The vaccine, Gardasil, protects against four HPV types (6, 11, 16, and 18), which together cause 70% of cervical cancers and 90% of genital warts. The other vaccine is Cervarix that protects against HPV type 16 and 18. These vaccines are available to both female and males between the ages of 9 and 26 years. It is preferable the vaccine be given prior to onset of sexual activity (CDC, 2011k).

Sexually Transmitted Disease Prevention and Control

Human history has been shaped by disease, and all historical events played a part in creating the preconditions for epidemics. Of all the communicable diseases, perhaps none are as closely interrelated with human activities and attitudes as STDs. Many have occurred in epidemic proportions; most have existed for centuries.

The community/public health nurse needs to be concerned with the fact that women and children suffer an inordinate STD burden. Aside from the risk of AIDS and subsequent death, the most serious complications of STDs are PID, sterility, ectopic pregnancy, cancer associated with HPV, fetal and infant death, birth defects, blindness, and mental retardation, which has been discussed in previous sections of specific STDs. The medically underserved, particularly the poor and marginalized, as well as ethnic and racial minorities shoulder a disproportionate share of this problem—experiencing higher rates of disability and death from STDs than the population as a whole. Some notable disproportionately affected groups are sex workers, adolescents, adults in detention, and migrant workers (Hogben & Leichliter, 2008).

Changes in behavior require diverse and multidisciplinary interventions over an extended period. Such interventions must integrate the efforts of parents, families, schools, religious organizations, health departments, community agencies, and the media. Education programs that provide adolescents with the knowledge and skills to refrain the early onset of sexual intercourse, to make informed decisions related to sexual behavior and health, and to increase the use of condoms as well as other contraceptive measures among those unwilling to postpone onset of sexual activity are important to lifelong sexual health (Avert, 2009; CDC, 2009b).

Infectious Diseases of Bioterrorism

Information about anthrax and smallpox is presented here because of the threat that these diseases present to the community as weapons of terrorism (see Chapter 17 regarding disasters and terrorism). Because of the type of work public health nurses do in the community, they are in a position of responsibility to allay fears, to provide correct information, and to help people in the decision-making process regarding immunization in regard to possible terrorist attacks. Although other disease-causing organisms may be weaponized, anthrax and smallpox have a history of use as terrorist weapons and are discussed here (Putra, Petpichetchian, & Maneewat, 2011).

Anthrax

Shortly after the terrorist attacks of September 11, 2001, the U.S. population was further terrorized by anthrax. Several people who handled or delivered mail inhaled and touched anthrax spores concealed in envelopes. Many acquired anthrax, and deaths were reported. The pervasiveness of the fear this act created was felt nationwide.

In nature, anthrax is primarily a disease of herbivores, with humans and carnivores as incidental hosts. There are infrequent and sporadic human infections in most industrialized countries. It is an occupational hazard among workers who process animal hides, hair, bone and bone products, and wool in some countries. In fact, it has been called *woolsorter disease* and *ragpicker disease* (Heymann, 2008).

In humans, anthrax is an acute bacterial disease that affects mainly the skin or respiratory tract. The two main forms—cutaneous anthrax and inhalation anthrax—account for most human anthrax cases. The case-fatality rate for cutaneous anthrax is 5% to 20%. The skin becomes itchy where exposed, a lesion becomes papular and then vesicular, and in 2 to 6 days, a depressed black eschar, surrounded by extensive edema, develops. The infection may spread to the lymph system and cause septicemia. With inhalation anthrax, the initial symptoms are mild and nonspecific but progress to respiratory distress. Fever and shock follow in 3 to 5 days, and death is the expected outcome (Heymann, 2008).

The causative organism, *Bacillus anthracis* is a Gram-positive, encapsulated, spore-forming agent found in livestock and wildlife as the main reservoirs. The incubation period is short (hours to 1 week), and most cases occur within 48 hours after exposure. Transmission from person to person is rare, but articles and soil contaminated with spores may remain infective for decades (Heymann, 2008).

An anthrax vaccine exists, and all lots of this vaccine are owned by the Department of Defense. Troublesome side effects (fatigue, muscle or joint pains, and mental impairment) are experienced by 5% to 35% of recipients, and six doses are required over an 18-month period in addition to yearly booster doses. This vaccine is limited in its use, mainly for those laboratory scientists handling specimens and some veterinarians who may have work-related exposure risk (Heymann, 2008).

Smallpox

Smallpox is a disease from our history books. In fact, the last case of smallpox was reported in 1978, and in 1980, WHO declared the disease eliminated worldwide. However, as recently as 1966, the disease was widespread in 31 countries. Some 10 to 15 million people were contracting smallpox annually, 2 million people died each year, and millions more were permanently disfigured or blinded (Sibley, 2002). By the late 1970s, just over one decade later, the global eradication campaign had pushed smallpox to the brink of extinction. The last known naturally occurring case of smallpox was in Somalia in 1977. Smallpox was declared globally eradicated in May, 1980. Officially, the smallpox virus presently exists at only two places: the CDC in Atlanta and the State Research Centre of Virology and Biotechnology, Koltsovo, Novosibirsk Region, Russian Federation (Heymann, 2008).

In the United States, routine vaccination against smallpox ended in 1972, for health care workers in 1976, and for the military in 1990. Few health care practitioners today have seen cases of smallpox or have administered the vaccine. In 2002, as a result of presidential decision to promote emergency preparedness, public health nurses across the nation became involved in the primary prevention of smallpox and learned the intricate techniques of smallpox vaccination and treatment of vaccine side effects in preparation for large-scale population immunization (see Fig. 8-5). That year, voluntary smallpox vaccinations were resumed for the first time in three decades. Initially, key military units were inoculated, beginning in 2002, followed by "first responders" such as emergency health care providers and health department personnel. The general public is not currently targeted for immunization.

The response plan for smallpox exposure, disease, and investigation preparedness utilized the previously successful **ring vaccination** strategy—containing an outbreak by rapidly isolating and vaccinating people who have had close, face-to-face contact with the victim. This method refers to ring of people around the exposed or ill person. However, one bright spot with smallpox prevention is that people who come in contact with a victim can receive protection if they are vaccinated within 7 days after exposure. This is unlike other vaccine-preventable diseases (VPDs) and provides a window of time to reach exposed people (CDC, 2012c; Heymann, 2008).

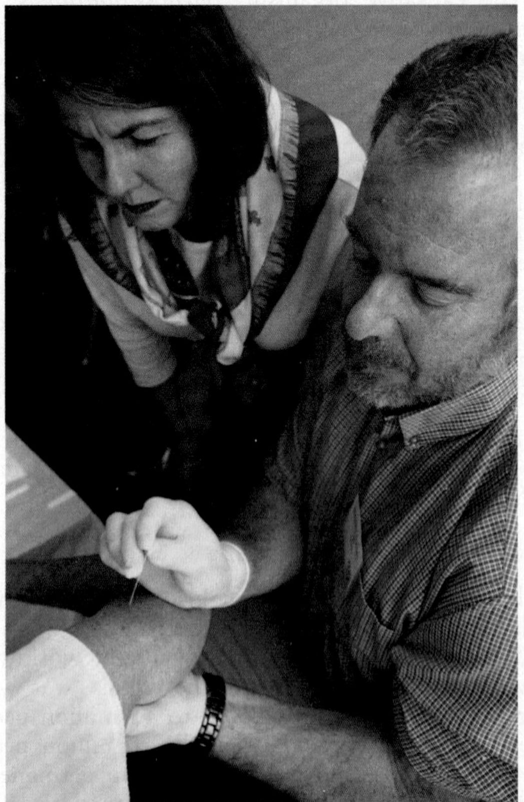

FIGURE 8-5. Smallpox inoculation of public health worker. (From Centers for Disease Control and Prevention. Public Health Image Library. (2002). Photo Image ID #2825–James Gathany.)

The smallpox vaccine does not contain variola (the smallpox organism) but is made from cowpox, a similar organism that confers protection to smallpox. Smallpox vaccination has risks. It is not a benign vaccine, and some experts allege that the morbidity associated with the vaccine has been understated. One to two deaths per 1 million recipients of the vaccine can be expected, in addition to hundreds of cases of generalized vaccinia, eczema vaccinatum, and postvaccinal encephalitis (CDC, 2012c; Heymann, 2008). Less severe but more common side effects include the formation of satellite lesions, regional lymphadenopathy, fever, headache, nausea, muscle aches, fatigue, and chills. In addition, the vaccine is contraindicated for the immunosuppressed, those with eczema, pregnant women, and infants younger than 1 year (CDC, 2012c).

The variola virus causes smallpox and is transmitted from person to person. Initial infection begins with a febrile prodromal period that occurs 1 to 4 days before the onset of the rash. Fever is 101°F or higher, and victims experience at least one of the following: prostration, headache, backache, chills, vomiting, and severe abdominal pain. These physical symptoms are followed by the classic smallpox lesions—characterized as deep-seated, firm/hard, round, well-circumscribed vesicles or pustules. The lesions are in the same stage of development, anywhere on the body. The smallpox lesion can be confused with other conditions, such as varicella (chicken pox), disseminated herpes zoster, impetigo, drug eruptions, contact dermatitis, scabies, or disseminated HSV (CDC, 2012c; Heymann, 2008). (Chapter 17 discusses the role of the community/public health nurse in emergency preparedness.)

PRIMARY PREVENTION

In the context of communicable disease control, two approaches are useful in achieving primary prevention: education using mass media with targeting health messages to aggregates and immunization.

Education

Health education in primary prevention is directed both at helping individuals understand their risk and at promoting healthy behaviors. Chapter 11 deals more extensively with the concepts of learning theory and the variety of health education approaches and materials available to community/public health nurses today. In planning and implementing an educational program, one very helpful document is *Simply Put: A Guide for Creating Easy-to-Understand Materials* available from the CDC (2009c)

Targeting Meaningful Health Messages to Aggregates

To effectively deliver a health promotion and disease prevention message, the message must reach the target (at-risk) population. This requires correct identification of the characteristics of the target audience in terms of educational level, salience of the issue, involvement of the target audience with the issue, and access of the target audience to the media channels used. Cultural issues affect people's interpretation of messages and must be considered in the presentation of a disease-prevention message to ethnic and racial minority groups (CDC, 2012c). Principles for adapting health messages to specific population subgroups include the following:

1. Develop educational materials from the community perspective, reflecting respect for community values and traditions, relevance to community needs and interests, and participation of the community in the preparation and use of the materials.
2. Materials must be related to the delivery of health services that are available, accessible, and acceptable to the target population.
3. All materials must be pretested and have demonstrated attractiveness, comprehension, acceptability, ownership, and persuasiveness.
4. Materials must have a readability level for the intended audience.

Ways to Communicate

Information technology is advancing at a fast pace. The use of traditional and new communication technologies can serve the global population. Radios, television, in person interactions, and print/signage have been used for years to promote health messages (e.g., signage in liquor stores, warning pregnant women of the dangers of alcohol, and the relation to fetal defects). The Internet has been used for some time now as a repository of information, some reliable and some not. The use of cell phones, Internet, texting, tweeting, and use of social networks like Facebook are examples of new ways to send messages and communicate to and with people. Many of the health sites on the Internet have ways to access information for phones and i-pods. Both the WHO and the CDC offer access to podcasts, Facebook, twitter, and Internet for reliable, factual, and current information (Hughes, 2010).

Immunization

Control of acute communicable diseases through immunization has been a common practice since the 19th century in the United States. **Immunization** is the process of introducing a form of a disease-causing organism into a person's system to promote the development of antibodies that will resist that disease. This process stimulates the individual's immune system to create antibodies to the particular infectious disease. Immunization and control of infectious diseases remains a national focus through *Healthy People 2020* (USDHHS, 2010c). Table 8-3 highlights select objectives related to immunization and infectious diseases.

The schedule for administration of vaccines for various populations and age groups is reviewed by the Advisory Committee on Immunization Practices (ACIP). The ACIP consists of 15 experts in the field of VPD. This group is chosen by the Secretary of the USDHHS; it functions to guide and advise on immunization practices (CDC, 2011a). In 1993, the CDC initiated the first National Immunization Survey, and in April of 1994, the first national data set obtained. This data set analyzed the immunization rates of children. Currently, there are data collection surveys for children, adolescents, and adult immunization rates.

As of 2010, 72.7% of children 19 to 35 months of age at the time of the survey had received all of the recommended immunizations (excluding Hib as there was a shortage of vaccine in 2007) (CDC, 2011g). The 2010 national data for adolescent immunization rates for four recommended vaccines were as follows: tetanus–diphtheria–acellular pertussis (Tdap) 68.7%; meningococcal conjugate vaccine 62.7%; hepatitis B vaccine series 91.6%; and female teens who had completed the three-dose series of HPV vaccine 69.6% (CDC, 2011f). Perceived barriers that may impact adolescent immunization levels may include lack of parental knowledge, inadequate access to medical care, and inadequate or no insurance coverage. The community/public health nurse can educate parents to the availability of federal programs that pay for vaccines for children (VFC) under the age of 19 (Birkhead, Orenstein, & Almquist, 2009; CDC, 2012l).

Adult vaccines include Tdap/Td, pneumococcal, zostavax (shingles prevention), influenza, hepatitis A and B, and for some young adults catch up on MMR. For many years, the emphasis has been on the adult receiving pneumococcal and influenza immunizations, but with recent evidence of pertussis spread from adults to vulnerable infants and young children, Tdap has been given greater emphasis. As of 2010, Tdap is now recommended for adults 19 to 64 years of age regardless of the interval since the last tetanus or diphtheria containing vaccine (CDC, 2011a, 2012h).

On the personal level, health care providers, public health nurses, and school nurses are in positions to review, educate, and provide opportunities for a child to obtain immunizations. Some children do not enter into the system for immunization review until entry into school, where they may or may not have been immunized (Omer, Salmon, Orenstein, deHart, & Halsey, 2009). Preschool-age children represent a major proportion of all cases of VPDs and are the group at highest risk for infection. Although childhood immunization rates historically have been lower in minority populations compared with the Caucasian population, rates for minority preschool children have been increasing at a more rapid pace, and the gap has significantly narrowed. Data for 2010 indicates that 73.5% of children 19 to 35 months

Table 8.3 ***Healthy People 2020***

Immunization and Infectious Diseases–Select Objectives	
IID-1	Reduce, eliminate, or maintain elimination of cases of vaccine-preventable diseases
IID-5	Reduce the number of courses of antibiotics for ear infections for young children
IID-6	Reduce the number of courses of antibiotics prescribed for the sole diagnosis of the common cold
IID-7	Achieve and maintain effective vaccination coverage levels for universally recommended vaccines among young children
IID-11	Increase routine vaccination coverage levels for adolescents
IID-14	Increase the percentage of adults who are vaccinated against zoster (shingles)
IID-16	(Developmental) Increase the scientific knowledge on vaccine safety and adverse events
IID-18	Increase the proportion of children under 6 yr of age whose immunization records are in fully operational, population-based immunization information systems
IID-22	Increase the number of public health laboratories monitoring influenza virus resistance to antiviral agents
IID-24	Reduce chronic hepatitis B virus (HBV) infections in infants and young children (perinatal infections)
IID-27	Increase the percentage of persons aware they have a hepatitis C infection
IID-28	(Developmental) Increase the percentage of persons who have been tested for HBV within minority communities experiencing health disparities

From U.S. Department of Health and Human Services. Office of Disease Prevention and Health Promotion. (2010c). *Healthy People 2020*: Improving the health of Americans. Immunization and infectious diseases objectives. Washington, DC. Retrieved from http://www.healthypeople.gov/2020/topicsobjectives2020/objectiveslist.aspx?topicId=23

living below poverty and 75.5% at or above poverty were fully immunized. Despite the minimal difference in rates, efforts to increase access to immunization programs need to be continued particularly for children living in poverty (Omer et al., 2009).

The majority of American society has accepted immunizations as a part of overall health care. However, there are some who challenge the notion of immunizing their children for many reasons. Some oppose government mandates, the sheer number of vaccinations, and others want to veer from the recommended spacing schedule for alternative immunization spacing and will eventually complete the childhood series. Although the ACIP may set the recommendations for immunizations, there are no laws mandating a child be immunized. Each state has set laws exempting immunizations for various reasons, religion, philosophy, or medical. Not all states accept all of these reasons. The public health nurse should look to their state's immunization agency for the accepted exemption criteria (Immunization Action Coalition, 2010). (This subject is further discussed under "Barriers to Immunization Coverage.")

It is important for health care providers working with any family with children to be aware of their own knowledge and beliefs regarding immunization and how to support a family in their decisions. Providing parents with opportunities to ask questions, feel supported, develop a trusting relationship, and offering science-based information about both the vaccine and the preventable disease is important to parents when making decisions about such an important health care matter (Gust, Darling, Kennedy, & Schwartz, 2008; Omer et al., 2009).

It is critical to discover the social and cultural characteristics affecting health status, attitudes about preventive measures, behaviors in seeking services, acceptability of interventions, and perceptions of health care providers that determine parental action in having a child immunized in a regular and timely fashion (see From the Case Files and Display 8.5). This is a unique area of health care delivery, one in which nurses must rely on parental initiative to obtain a form of care for the well child that may be perceived as producing pain and temporary illness for no observable benefit (Omer et al., 2009).

Vaccine-Preventable Diseases

VPDs, such as hepatitis A and B, *H. influenza* type b, measles, polio, diphtheria, pertussis, influenza, and chickenpox, are a few examples of diseases that can be prevented through immunization. Immunity may be either passive or active. **Passive immunity** is short-term

From the Case Files

Personal Belief Exemption and Immunization

A whooping cough (pertussis) outbreak occurred in a small rural community. Whooping cough is a vaccine-preventable disease. It is highly contagious, and can have devastating outcomes in the very young and very old. In this community, the population is not very ethnically diverse, but it is philosophically diverse. Many community members are against vaccinating their children. The outbreak of pertussis occurred in a small charter school, where the majority of the children were unvaccinated for reasons of parental personal belief objections. Personal belief exemption to vaccination is an option for a family. Unfortunately, with a large unvaccinated population, as in this school, the spark of a contagious, vaccine-preventable infection can spread rapidly. This is what happened in this school, with 22 cases of pertussis among children and family members. The school had to be closed a week early for winter break to help halt continued disease spread. Three waves of illness occurred in this school from November to April.

One might think the entire problem rests with the group of individuals who will not vaccinate their children, but this is not what was discovered upon investigation. The issue of personal belief exemption was discussed among public health nurses and school nurses in this community. The issue was discussed with parents and teachers at the charter school. The two highlights from our discussions were that parents signed the exemption either out of true conviction or out of frustration that the school was hounding them to get their child vaccinated. For whatever reason, some parents just cannot seem to make the time to get the necessary immunizations completed. These parents can be the high-risk families who keep a school nurse busy. It was discovered that in some of the schools with high-risk families, the personal belief exemption was signed in order to not be pestered.

So, which group do you extend your efforts to as a public health nurse? The answer is both. The parents who will not vaccinate their children will not be convinced otherwise. Parents who chose the easy way out may need more assistance. The county's immunization coordinator, the community's immunization coalition, and the school nurses determined that the school secretaries were the point of entrance to school registration. It was discovered that these individuals needed an in-service on how to properly offer the exemption to a family and what information parents would need to make an informed decision before signing the exemption.

The immunization coordinator developed an education tool that explained to the parents their responsibility to the community at large if their child were to become ill with a vaccine-preventable illness. The document covered points such as the family having a medical plan with their physician, learning how to care for and isolate the child, working with a public health nurse, and so on (see Display 8.5). The school secretaries were asked to give this document to parents who were interested in exempting and community resource information where to send families who may not have access to affordable immunizations.

The parents at the charter school were very accepting of the information on what to do for an ill child, and the school secretaries expressed relief regarding dealing with parents who may want to exempt out for convenience rather than conviction.

Karen, PHN

resistance to a specific disease-causing organism; it may be acquired naturally (as with newborns through maternal antibody transfer) or artificially through inoculation with pooled human antibody (e.g., immune globulin) that gives temporary protection. **Active immunity** is long-term (sometimes lifelong) resistance to a specific disease-causing organism; it also can be acquired naturally or artificially. Naturally acquired active immunity occurs when a person contracts a disease and develops long-lasting antibodies that provide immunity against future exposure. Artificially acquired active immunity occurs through inoculation with a vaccine, such as the diphtheria, pertussis, tetanus vaccination series given to children. A **vaccine** is a preparation made from a live organism or an inactivated form of the organism. Live attenuated vaccines are made from weakened wild virus organisms that are used to create an immune response in the recipient. It only takes a small amount to initiate an immune response, and the organisms must replicate to be effective. Inactivated vaccines are made from a viral organism that has been inactivated by heat or chemicals. These vaccines cannot replicate in the recipient (CDC, 2012c).

Because of the success of immunization strategies, few practicing nurses in the United States today have treated clients with tetanus or diphtheria, or even measles (although some have cared for clients with residual polio disabilities). However, VPDs still exist in force in the developing world, and outbreaks occur in the United States in groups of nonimmunized or

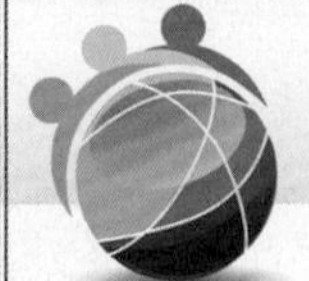

DISPLAY 8.5 WHAT PARENTS SHOULD KNOW WHEN SIGNING A PERSONAL BELIEFS AFFIDAVIT EXEMPTION OF IMMUNIZATION

1. Measles, mumps, rubella, chicken pox, pertussis, diphtheria, polio, *Haemophilus influenza* type b, hepatitis A, and hepatitis B are infectious to others and are avoidable through immunization.
2. Please educate yourself to the symptoms and possible complications that can arise from a vaccine-preventable disease (VPD). Information for parents about these diseases may be found at the National Immunization Program site http://www.cdc.gov/nip/ or by calling ***Insert Local County Public Health Department Name & Phone Number***.
3. These diseases have many symptoms that require close monitoring and care so that complications are minimized. It is essential to have a plan of care, coordinated with your health care provider, to act upon the mildest to most severe symptoms of the disease.
4. The school or school nurse is responsible for maintaining a list of the school children who have parent-signed exemption to immunization for medical, religious, or personal belief. This list allows the school nurse to quickly identify any child who is at risk of exposure to a VPD.
5. An unimmunized child will be excluded from school by the County Health Officer when a VPD is identified in the school. The ill child will also be excluded from school.
6. When a child is excluded from school, it is the responsibility of the parent or guardian to keep the child isolated* from the public at large to prevent spread of infection to the community.
7. VPDs are considered **reportable communicable diseases** under the Health and Safety Codes of California. If your child contracts one of these diseases, a Public Health Nurse will contact you. Be prepared to provide information about the illness to the investigator. **This information is confidential.**
8. The parent or guardian is also at risk of contracting any of these diseases when exposed to an ill child. If unimmunized, the parent or guardian may also be considered exposed and incubating the disease, since this may continue the cycle of infection to others. This in turn requires that the parent or guardian remain in isolation from the community through the incubation period.
9. The child who is exposed to the disease may be offered preventive medication or immunization to prevent the disease from occurring—either may keep the child from being excluded from school.

______________________ ________
Parent signature Date

*The isolation time frame is determined by the county health officer. Isolation means that the exposed or ill child cannot leave home except for medical care. No social gatherings!

susceptible populations. For example, certain people are medically exempt from immunization, and others decline immunization for religious or personal reasons. Even with global and national efforts at reducing and eliminating VPDs, some national goals have not been met. There is evidence that as the immunization rates fall, VPD rises that in turns strains a community's herd protection of its vulnerable individuals (Omer et al., 2009).

Schedule of Recommended Immunizations

A schedule for the administration of childhood vaccinations, based on recommendations by the ACIP, the American Academy of Pediatrics (AAP), the American Academy of Family Physicians, and the CDC, is published annually (Table 8-4). The CDC also provides "catch-up" schedules for children not receiving their first immunizations at birth, according to the standard schedule. Current recommendations call for a child to receive 10 different vaccines or toxoids (many in combination form and all requiring more than one dose) in 6 or 7 visits to a health care provider between birth and school entry, with boosters in the preteen to early teen years (CDC, 2011a, 2012c, 2012i).

Factors influencing the recommended age at which vaccines are administered include the age-specific risks of the disease, the age-specific risks of complications, the ability of persons of a given age to produce an adequate and lasting immune response, and the potential for interference with the immune response acquired from passively transferred maternal antibodies. In general, vaccines are recommended for the youngest age group at risk whose members are known to develop an acceptable antibody response to vaccination (CDC, 2012c).

Recommendations for vaccine administration may be revised in light of specific circumstances. For example, it is now recommended that infants receive hepatitis B

Table 8.4 Vaccines for Infants and School Entry

Recommended immunization schedule for persons aged 0 through 6 years—United States, 2012

Vaccine ▼ / Age ►	Birth	1 month	2 months	4 months	6 months	9 months	12 months	15 months	18 months	19–23 months	2–3 years	4–6 years
Hepatitis B[1]	**Hep B**	**HepB**					**HepB**					
Rotavirus[2]			**RV**	**RV**	**RV**[2]							
Diphtheria, tetanus, pertussis[3]			**DTaP**	**DTaP**	**DTaP**		*see footnote*[3]	**DTaP**				**DTaP**
Haemophilus influenzae type b[4]			**Hib**	**Hib**	**Hib**[4]		**Hib**					
Pneumococcal[5]			**PCV**	**PCV**	**PCV**		**PCV**				**PPSV**	
Inactivated poliovirus[6]			**IPV**	**IPV**			**IPV**					**IPV**
Influenza[7]								**Influenza (Yearly)**				
Measles, mumps, rubella[8]							**MMR**			*see footnote*[8]		**MMR**
Varicella[9]							**Varicella**			*see footnote*[9]		**Varicella**
Hepatitis A[10]								**Dose 1**[10]			**HepA Series**	
Meningococcal[11]								**MCV4 — see footnote**[11]				

Range of recommended ages for all children

Range of recommended ages for certain high-risk groups

Range of recommended ages for all children and certain high-risk groups

This schedule includes recommendations in effect as of December 23, 2011. Any dose not administered at the recommended age should be administered at a subsequent visit, when indicated and feasible. The use of a combination vaccine generally is preferred over separate injections of its equivalent component vaccines. Vaccination providers should consult the relevant Advisory Committee on Immunization Practices (ACIP) statement for detailed recommendations, available online at http://www.cdc.gov/vaccines/pubs/acip-list.htm. Clinically significant adverse events that follow vaccination should be reported to the Vaccine Adverse Event Reporting System (VAERS) online (http://www.vaers.hhs.gov) or by telephone (800-822-7967).

1. **Hepatitis B (HepB) vaccine.** (Minimum age: birth)
   At birth:
   - Administer monovalent HepB vaccine to all newborns before hospital discharge.
   - For infants born to hepatitis B surface antigen (HBsAg)–positive mothers, administer HepB vaccine and 0.5 mL of hepatitis B immune globulin (HBIG) within 12 hours of birth. These infants should be tested for HBsAg and antibody to HBsAg (anti-HBs) 1 to 2 months after completion of at least 3 doses of the HepB series, at age 9 through 18 months (generally at the next well-child visit).
   - If mother's HBsAg status is unknown, within 12 hours of birth administer HepB vaccine for infants weighing ≥2,000 grams, and HepB vaccine plus HBIG for infants weighing <2,000 grams. Determine mother's HBsAg status as soon as possible and, if she is HBsAg-positive, administer HBIG for infants weighing ≥2,000 grams (no later than age 1 week).

   Doses after the birth dose:
   - The second dose should be administered at age 1 to 2 months. Monovalent HepB vaccine should be used for doses administered before age 6 weeks.
   - Administration of a total of 4 doses of HepB vaccine is permissible when a combination vaccine containing HepB is administered after the birth dose.
   - Infants who did not receive a birth dose should receive 3 doses of a HepB-containing vaccine starting as soon as feasible (Figure 3).
   - The minimum interval between dose 1 and dose 2 is 4 weeks, and between dose 2 and 3 is 8 weeks. The final (third or fourth) dose in the HepB vaccine series should be administered no earlier than age 24 weeks and at least 16 weeks after the first dose.
2. **Rotavirus (RV) vaccines.** (Minimum age: 6 weeks for both RV-1 [Rotarix] and RV-5 [Rota Teq])
   - The maximum age for the first dose in the series is 14 weeks, 6 days; and 8 months, 0 days for the final dose in the series. Vaccination should not be initiated for infants aged 15 weeks, 0 days or older.
   - If RV-1 (Rotarix) is administered at ages 2 and 4 months, a dose at 6 months is not indicated.
3. **Diphtheria and tetanus toxoids and acellular pertussis (DTaP) vaccine.** (Minimum age: 6 weeks)
   - The fourth dose may be administered as early as age 12 months, provided at least 6 months have elapsed since the third dose.
4. ***Haemophilus influenzae* type b (Hib) conjugate vaccine.** (Minimum age: 6 weeks)
   - If PRP-OMP (PedvaxHIB or Comvax [HepB-Hib]) is administered at ages 2 and 4 months, a dose at age 6 months is not indicated.
   - Hiberix should only be used for the booster (final) dose in children aged 12 months through 4 years.
5. **Pneumococcal vaccines.** (Minimum age: 6 weeks for pneumococcal conjugate vaccine [PCV]; 2 years for pneumococcal polysaccharide vaccine [PPSV])
   - Administer 1 dose of PCV to all healthy children aged 24 through 59 months who are not completely vaccinated for their age.
   - For children who have received an age-appropriate series of 7-valent PCV (PCV7), a single supplemental dose of 13-valent PCV (PCV13) is recommended for:
     — All children aged 14 through 59 months
     — Children aged 60 through 71 months with underlying medical conditions.
   - Administer PPSV at least 8 weeks after last dose of PCV to children aged 2 years or older with certain underlying medical conditions, including a cochlear implant. See *MMWR* 2010:59(No. RR-11), available at http://www.cdc.gov/mmwr/pdf/rr/rr5911.pdf.
6. **Inactivated poliovirus vaccine (IPV).** (Minimum age: 6 weeks)
   - If 4 or more doses are administered before age 4 years, an additional dose should be administered at age 4 through 6 years.
   - The final dose in the series should be administered on or after the fourth birthday and at least 6 months after the previous dose.
7. **Influenza vaccines.** (Minimum age: 6 months for trivalent inactivated influenza vaccine [TIV]; 2 years for live, attenuated influenza vaccine [LAIV])
   - For most healthy children aged 2 years and older, either LAIV or TIV may be used. However, LAIV should not be administered to some children, including 1) children with asthma, 2) children 2 through 4 years who had wheezing in the past 12 months, or 3) children who have any other underlying medical conditions that predispose them to influenza complications. For all other contraindications to use of LAIV, see *MMWR* 2010;59(No. RR-8), available at http://www.cdc.gov/mmwr/pdf/rr/rr5908.pdf.
   - For children aged 6 months through 8 years:
     — For the 2011–12 season, administer 2 doses (separated by at least 4 weeks) to those who did not receive at least 1 dose of the 2010–11 vaccine. Those who received at least 1 dose of the 2010–11 vaccine require 1 dose for the 2011–12 season.
     — For the 2012–13 season, follow dosing guidelines in the 2012 ACIP influenza vaccine recommendations.
8. **Measles, mumps, and rubella (MMR) vaccine.** (Minimum age: 12 months)
   - The second dose may be administered before age 4 years, provided at least 4 weeks have elapsed since the first dose.
   - Administer MMR vaccine to infants aged 6 through 11 months who are traveling internationally. These children should be revaccinated with 2 doses of MMR vaccine, the first at ages 12 through 15 months and at least 4 weeks after the previous dose, and the second at ages 4 through 6 years.
9. **Varicella (VAR) vaccine.** (Minimum age: 12 months)
   - The second dose may be administered before age 4 years, provided at least 3 months have elapsed since the first dose.
   - For children aged 12 months through 12 years, the recommended minimum interval between doses is 3 months. However, if the second dose was administered at least 4 weeks after the first dose, it can be accepted as valid.
10. **Hepatitis A (HepA) vaccine.** (Minimum age: 12 months)
    - Administer the second (final) dose 6 to18 months after the first.
    - Unvaccinated children 24 months and older at high risk should be vaccinated. See *MMWR* 2006;55(No. RR-7), available at http://www.cdc.gov/mmwr/pdf/rr/rr5507.pdf.
    - A 2-dose HepA vaccine series is recommended for anyone aged 24 months and older, previously unvaccinated, for whom immunity against hepatitis A virus infection is desired.
11. **Meningococcal conjugate vaccines, quadrivalent (MCV4).** (Minimum age: 9 months for Menactra [MCV4-D], 2 years for Menveo [MCV4-CRM])
    - For children aged 9 through 23 months 1) with persistent complement component deficiency; 2) who are residents of or travelers to countries with hyperendemic or epidemic disease; or 3) who are present during outbreaks caused by a vaccine serogroup, administer 2 primary doses of MCV4-D, ideally at ages 9 months and 12 months or at least 8 weeks apart.
    - For children aged 24 months and older with 1) persistent complement component deficiency who have not been previously vaccinated; or 2) anatomic/functional asplenia, administer 2 primary doses of either MCV4 at least 8 weeks apart.
    - For children with anatomic/functional asplenia, if MCV4-D (Menactra) is used, administer at a minimum age of 2 years and at least 4 weeks after completion of all PCV doses.
    - See *MMWR* 2011;60:72–6, available at http://www.cdc.gov/mmwr/pdf/wk/mm6003. pdf, and Vaccines for Children Program resolution No. 6/11-1, available at http://www. cdc.gov/vaccines/programs/vfc/downloads/resolutions/06-11mening-mcv.pdf, and *MMWR* 2011;60:1391–2, available at http://www.cdc.gov/mmwr/pdf/wk/mm6040. pdf, for further guidance, including revaccination guidelines.

This schedule is approved by the Advisory Committee on Immunization Practices (http://www.cdc.gov/vaccines/recs/acip), the American Academy of Pediatrics (http://www.aap.org), and the American Academy of Family Physicians (http://www.aafp.org).
Department of Health and Human Services • Centers for Disease Control and Prevention

vaccine at birth, whether or not their mothers have a positive or negative response to the hepatitis B surface antigen. This approach will catch any infant born to mothers who lack prenatal testing, or who may live in households with individuals with unknown hepatitis B status (USDHHS, 2010a). Influenza vaccine is now recommended for all infants/children and adults over the age of 6 months; this is a newer recommendation in light of the introduction of the novel influenza strain H1N1 (CDC, 2011a, 2012i).

Herd Immunity

Herd immunity is central to understanding immunization as a means of protecting community health. As described in Chapter 7, herd immunity is the immunity level present in a particular population of people. If few immune persons exist within a community, herd immunity is low, and the spread of disease is more likely (see Fig. 8-6). Immunization of more individuals in the community contributes to a high proportion with acquired resistance to the infectious agent, playing a role in higher herd immunity. High herd immunity reduces the probability that the few unimmunized persons will come in contact with one another, making spread of the disease less likely (Heymann, 2008; USDHHS, 2010b). (See Evidence-Based Practice.)

Assessing Immunization Status of the Community

Determining the immunization status of children in a community can be a time-consuming but worthwhile task. Public health nurses can access the childcare and school entry immunization data through their state's immunization agency as well as state immunization registries. This data is of value when determining where to focus outreach energy in raising immunization rates or monitoring for potential disease activity (CDC, 2008a, 2012a).

Other community settings in which community/public health nurses may identify underimmunized children include homeless shelters and other public service settings or agencies used by families and children, including local religious centers. A family with one underimmunized child may have underimmunized children of other ages, as well as any number of other unmet preventive health care needs that the nurse can help address (AAP, 2010).

Barriers to Immunization Coverage

Improving immunization coverage requires examination of the reasons why children are not immunized. Many barriers exist. As mentioned earlier, each state may provide exemptions for parents who may not want to immunize their child. These exemptions may be religious, philosophical, or medical, and then there may be other barriers that are not exemption related but may be financial, social, cultural, or provider limitation issues. These are challenges the community health nurse may have to deal with when working with the community and working to effect adequate immunization coverage for the general public and protection from VPDs (Pickering et al., 2009)

Religious Barriers

The right to religious freedom gives individuals in the United States the constitutional right to exemption from immunization if they object to vaccination on religious grounds. Children from these families are identified at school entry. Such exemptions must be specifically enacted by law, and although it is not necessary to belong to a specific denomination, courts have required those seeking religious exemption to demonstrate that such belief against immunization is sincere and that no clear danger exists from the particular disease. Problems arise when members of exempted groups are found together in school or community settings, raising the risk of disease spread because of a lower herd immunity (McFall, 2008; Omer et al., 2009).

Financial Barriers

Access to affordable immunization programs may be a significant factor for immunization delays in families with limited incomes. Such families may have had more immediate priorities than vaccinations for an otherwise well child. In the late 1990s, two major initiatives significantly improved the financing of childhood immunizations. The VFC program and the Child Health Insurance Program (CHIP) cover children on Medicaid, uninsured children, and American Indian and Alaska Native children (CDC, 2012l). In addition, underinsured children who receive immunizations at federally qualified health centers and rural health clinics are covered. These initiatives should eliminate low income as a barrier (Birkhead, Orenstein, & Almquist, 2009).

Social and Cultural Barriers

Education levels, transportation problems, as well as access to health facilities can pose essential barriers to adequate immunization coverage for children and all family members. The paperwork involved in obtaining the informed consent of parents may be intellectually intimidating for some parents. Working parents may find it difficult, if not impossible, to reach an immunization clinic with their child during working hours. Requirements for appointments (instead of walk-in clinics) or for a physical examination before vaccination may present additional deterrents. Urban and rural areas may not be able to support clinics, which adds to the access problem. These pockets of need continue to exist adding substantially to the number of underimmunized children. The potential exists for disease outbreaks.

Meeting the immunization needs of minority groups involves understanding cultural concepts related to health care and preventive measures. Language barriers may lead parents to feel confused, overwhelmed,

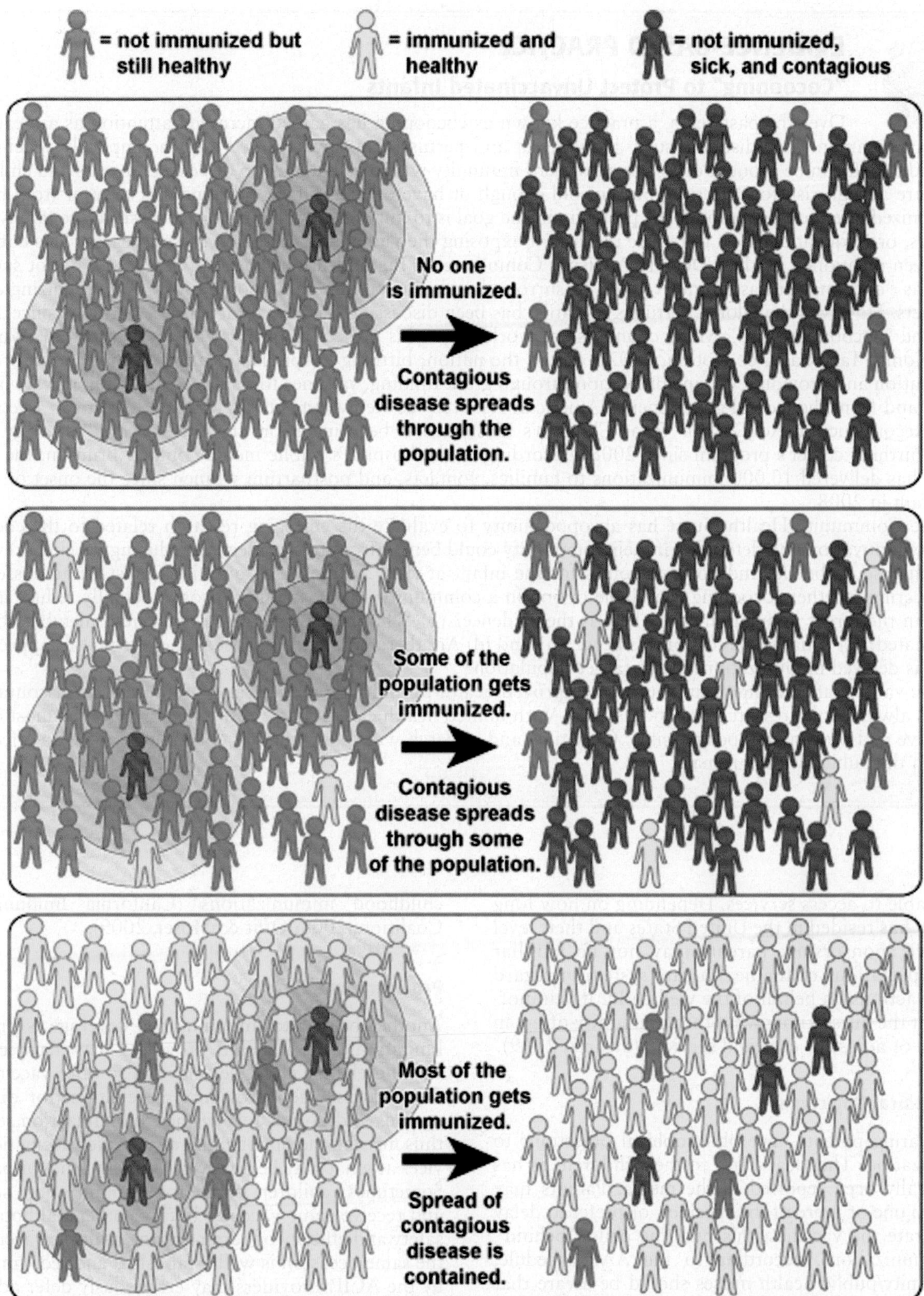

FIGURE 8-6. Community immunity/herd immunity. (From National Institute of Allergies and Infectious Diseases [NIAID].)

EVIDENCE-BASED PRACTICE

"Cocooning" to Protect Unvaccinated Infants

Over the past years, a practice known as cocooning has gained increased attention as a means to prevent communicable diseases, such as influenza and pertussis, in unvaccinated and incompletely vaccinated individuals. It can be thought of as a form of herd immunity within a small group of people. Infants and children who are at high risk for infection, but not old enough or have other health conditions that prevent from being immunized, are the target groups for protection. The goal is to immunize (influenza or pertussis) close family and friends, or frequent contacts to reduce the risk of exposing the vulnerable person to these diseases. This concept has been mentioned by the CDC and Advisory Committee on Immunization Practice (CDC, 2008b) not specifically as "cocoon," but as an intervention to surround and protect vulnerable populations by immunizing close contacts. However, the Global Pertussis Initiative has been discussing the global increase of pertussis since 2001 and the "cocoon strategy." Many countries are working on this project in birthing hospitals (Forsyth, Wirsing von Konig, Tan, Caro, & Plotkin, 2007). Across the nation, birthing hospitals are utilizing the cocoon project innovation and providing vaccine protection through grant funding, vaccines for children program, private insurance, and from the federal government's American Recovery & Reinvestment Act of 2009 (American Recovery and Reconstruction Act, 2010). Texas Children's Hospital has been incorporating the "cocoon" strategy into their birthing center's program since 2008. According to the hospital's public media contact, Brunton, the program has delivered 10,000 immunizations to families, contacts, and postpartum women since the onset of their program in 2008.

The Community Health Nurse has an opportunity to evaluate the emerging research related to the cocoon project innovation and determine if their community could benefit from this strategy in reducing vaccine preventable disease outbreaks and poor outcomes for the infant at risk. A number of questions must be addressed in considering whether cocooning is a viable option in a community: (a) Does this approach actually reduce infections in the target population and where is the evidence? (b) What is the risk to the household members being vaccinated? (c) What is the cost of this program? and (d) Are there unintended consequences from this approach, such as delayed immunizations in the target population?

Innovations are an important source of improved health-promoting practices and should not be discouraged, but as always, solid research evidence is vital. With limited health care dollars, efforts must target the most cost-effective and proven methods possible. Only time and research will show whether cocooning can be an effective tool in the public health arsenal.

and unable to access services. Depending on how long a family has resided in the United States and their level of active sponsorship, parents may not be familiar with expectations of the health care system in regard to their actions on behalf of the well child. It is important that the nurse know what the community offers in the way of access to care and services (Swartz, 2009).

Philosophical Objections

Many caring parents have philosophical objections to immunization. They fear harm to their children, as has periodically been reported in the media. Parents may object to one or more of the vaccines, or prefer to delay or separate the vaccines; this puts the child "behind" on immunizations, according to the AAP schedule. Community/public health nurses should be aware that caring parents are talking about these issues, reading about them, and trying to make informed decisions. When possible, it may be helpful to offer information or websites that address many myths surrounding childhood immunizations (California Immunization Coalition, 2008; Offit & Moser, 2009).

Provider Limitations

Another barrier to immunization coverage is provider limitations. Health care providers may have contact with an eligible child, yet may fail to offer vaccination. This occurs when providers see children for different reasons and do not review their immunization records, thus missing the opportunity to provide vaccination services at what may be a very convenient time for parents. Sometimes, children come for immunization services and receive some vaccines but not others, although the safety and efficacy of administering multiple vaccines on the same occasion is well established and recommended by the ACIP. Providers may erroneously defer administration of a vaccine based on a condition (e.g., symptom of illness) that is not a true contraindication to immunization. Another provider limitation or barrier to timely immunization coverage is that few providers have the initiative and resources to establish a uniform system for recall and notification when the next immunization is due. It is very important for the health care provider (physician or nurse) to establish a trusting relationship in order that the parents can share their concerns and fears and the provider can ally them (AAP, 2010).

Planning and Implementing an Immunization Campaign

Immunization campaigns targeting specific subgroups can be effective if they include the following: (a) community assessment for the target group(s) and (b) assessment of and planning for the needs of the target group(s), such as transportation, need for language interpreters, provision of child care, or dealing with high illiteracy rates. Successful outreach efforts are motivated by the desire to reach the target population, even if specific or unusual accommodations must be made. Clinics can be scheduled and held at times and places specifically intended to make the service more accessible and convenient to the target group. Materials in multilingual form can be obtained through the state's immunization agency or the CDC. The CDC and state immunization agencies have campaigns throughout the year for the public health nurse to participate in and provide to the public. Tool kits with the materials and tips for planning and implementing are available through the state immunization agency. Display 8.6 outlines an example of the necessary steps and considerations for administering an immunization campaign in a community setting.

Adult Immunization

Many people assume that vaccinations are for children only. Well-advertised influenza vaccination campaigns

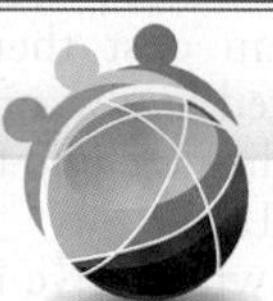

DISPLAY 8.6 ADMINISTRATIVE ASPECTS OF IMMUNIZATION CAMPAIGNS

Study the Target Community

- Assess disease incidence and level of immunization coverage.
- Identify the target group.
- Assess conditions in the community: Is the target group scattered or localized?
- Assess level of community involvement and awareness of the problem.
- Identify means of communicating with target group: Through the media or through leaders or other.
- Consider political and social structure of the community. Identify important leaders.
- Identify sites for immunization clinics that are appropriate, accessible, and available.

Plan the Immunization Campaign

- Review budget for immunization services.
- Determine goals for clinic performance or outcome measures.
- Communicate with target group to notify them of need and promote involvement and participation.
- Estimate needs for vaccines and supplies and obtain them. Plan care of vaccines before, during, and after clinic.
- Develop team coordination among staff.
- Plan clinic logistics: Available supply of needed materials, medical waste disposal, anaphylaxis supplies, records and means of clinic registration, staffing, floor plan for traffic control, and efficient management of crowds.
- Prepare staff with information regarding objectives for clinic, criteria for who shall not be immunized, and mechanisms for referral of clients with other health needs.

Publicity

- Inform target group of date, location, and times of immunization clinic.
- Provide information on reasons for and benefits of (and contraindications to) immunization.
- Encourage parents to bring existing immunization records to clinic.
- Provide contact information for those with questions or inquiries.

Immunization Clinic

- Registration system and records (for parent and clinic) ready.
- Registrar or assistant(s) ready to assist parents not familiar with language of paperwork.
- Parent education: informed consent, reporting of adverse reactions, date next vaccine due.
- System for call-back, follow-up.
- System for dealing with other health issues and/or adverse events.

Evaluation of Campaign

- Assess numbers of immunizations given in relation to goals.
- Assess suitability of approach in identification of target group, selection of sites, means of communication with group, availability of resources, and so forth.
- Invite parental as well as community and staff feedback.
- Evaluate results in relation to expenditures.

in recent years have, to some extent, helped to correct this notion. Adults are at as great a risk for a VPD as is a child if they are un- or underimmunized. Some of the immunizations that wane are tetanus, pertussis, influenza, and pneumococcal. The CDC (2012h) provides an adult immunization schedule of recommendations.

Pertussis is a disease that adults can acquire and pass onto vulnerable children and individuals, as well as can cause pneumonia as an outcome. It has recently been on the rise and is highly recommended that adults receive a dose of Tdap (CDC, 2011a). Shingles vaccine has been available to adults >60 years old since 2006 and is protective for shingles. Shingles is the latter version of dormant chickenpox. Shingles appear along the dermatomes, are painful, and can be debilitating (National Center for Biotechnology Information, 2011).

Adults may require immunizations to prevent occupational exposure to blood, blood products, or other potentially contaminated body fluids. The Occupational Safety and Health Administration (OSHA) has established the requirements for hepatitis B immunization for those whose profession may put them at risk (OSHA, 2010). All persons should receive tetanus vaccine every 10 years unless they experience sharp object injury. If such a wound is sustained, the individual should receive a booster of a tetanus toxoid-containing vaccine on the day of the injury if more than 5 years has elapsed since the last tetanus toxoid-containing dose.

Other reasons for promoting adult vaccination include history of high-risk conditions, such as heart disease, diabetes, and chronic respiratory diseases; international travel; and suspected failure of earlier vaccines to produce lasting immunity. Substantial numbers of VPDs still occur among adults despite the availability of safe and effective vaccines (USDHHS, 2009). Factors that may contribute to low vaccination levels among adults are as follows:

1. Limited comprehensive vaccine delivery systems are available in the public and private sectors for adults, similar to the VFC program for children.
2. Although statutory requirements exist for vaccination of children, no such requirements exist for all adults.
3. Health care providers may not be current with the adult-recommended immunizations and miss opportunities to vaccinate adults during contacts in offices, outpatient clinics, and hospitals.
5. Comprehensive vaccination programs have not been established in settings where healthy adults congregate (e.g., the workplace, senior centers).
6. Clients and providers may fear adverse effects after vaccination.

International Travelers, Immigrants, and Refugees

As Americans interact more and more with their neighbors in other parts of the world, the incidence of Americans with tropical or imported diseases also rises. Within about 36 hours of beginning a trip, any destination in the world can be reached by air flight. An average flight can equal an incubation period of infectious diseases, and microbial agents could be spread around the globe.

Information necessary for a potential traveler to travel to new and exotic places, remain healthy, and return healthy can be found at the CDC Travelers Health Internet site (CDC, 2011o). At a minimum, all international travelers should take steps to be adequately immunized as required by international health practices. These steps include being immunized with the recommended vaccines for the particular area of the world, having the necessary chemical prophylaxis on hand (i.e., antimalaria medications as prescribed), and being knowledgeable about food and water hygiene precautions as well as basic first aid for the care of simple injuries (CDC, 2011o). Every year, travelers who neglect to take the recommended travel vaccines or medications end up with generally preventable illnesses, which can cost them time, money, and their health. In the United States, one can find a tropical medicine or travel medicine clinic to prepare for international travel (CDC, 2011n).

Refugees and international travelers who arrive in the United States can be unfamiliar with U.S. health systems, health precautions, and practices. Refugees and immigrants must follow prescribed guidelines for their acculturation, including extensive health screening mandated by U.S. immigration laws (CDC, 2012d). More than ever before, community/public health nurses have professional contact with these new Americans, whether close to their time of arrival or later, in schools, immunization clinics, or other locations. Visitors from other countries may also require the assistance of other community health professionals. For this reason, public health nurses are encouraged to develop and maintain a global perspective on communicable diseases. (See Chapter 16 for more information on global health.)

SECONDARY PREVENTION

Two approaches to secondary prevention of communicable disease are possible: (a) screening and (b) disease case and contact investigation and notification (previously discussed).

Screening

The term **screening** is used in community health and disease prevention to describe programs that provide disease testing opportunities to detect disease in groups of asymptomatic, apparently healthy individuals. Common screening measures can include: (a) prenatal hepatitis B, (b) urine chlamydia and gonorrhea, and (c) Mantoux tuberculin skin tests for TB infection. For HIV, several screening tests are available—including oral fluids testing, rapid finger stick, or the more sensitive screening enzyme immunoassay. The HIV screening tests must be confirmed by a supplemental test such as the Western blot or an immunofluorescence assay when positive results arise (CDC, 2010c). Screening is a secondary prevention method because asymptomatic cases can be discovered and provided with prompt early treatment.

It is important to remember that the screening test itself is not diagnostic, but rather a method to identify those persons with positive or suspicious test findings who then require further medical evaluation or treatment. Public health nurse working with clients in a screening setting must be prepared to clearly and correctly explain to individuals that screening tests are not definitive and that positive findings require subsequent investigation before diagnostic conclusions can be drawn.

Criteria for Screening Tests

Some important criteria are used in deciding whether to carry out a screening intervention in a community. They include validity and reliability, and predictive value and yield.

Validity and Reliability

The screening test must be valid and reliable. *Validity* refers to the test's ability to accurately identify those with the disease. *Reliability* refers to the test's ability to give consistent results when administered on different occasions by different technicians.

Predictive Value and Yield

The *predictive value* of a screening test is important for determining whether the screening intervention is justified. *Yield* refers to the number of positive results found per number tested. The predictive value and the yield of screening tests become important in planning screening programs for communicable disease detection and prevention because they can help planners locate screening efforts in areas or within population groups that are known to be at high risk for the disease. The predictive value of screening tests increases as the prevalence of the disease increases. For example, a screening test for TB among refugees would have a greater predictive value and yield than TB screening in the population at large, due to a higher endemicity of TB in many countries outside of the United States.

Epidemiologic criteria for screening interventions for the detection of health problems include the following:

1. Is the disease an important public health problem?
2. Is there a valid and reliable test?
3. Is there an effective and tolerable treatment that favorably influences the early stages of the disease?
4. After a positive screening result, are facilities for diagnosis and treatment available and accessible?
5. Is there a recognizable early asymptomatic or latent stage in the disease?
6. Do clear guidelines for referral and treatment exist?
7. Is the total cost of the screening justifiable compared with the costs of treating the disease if left undiscovered?
8. Is the screening test itself acceptable?
9. Will screening be ongoing?

The ethics or values represented by these statements include a clear and unwavering respect for the dignity and worth of individuals across racial, gender, religious, sexual, tribal, ethnic, and geographic lines. They include a commitment to ensuring that resources are allocated to areas where they will have the most benefit in preventing disease and premature death. Socioeconomically disadvantaged persons are often at greatest risk for disease, yet they are the least likely to receive screening services because of financial barriers, including lack of health insurance coverage for preventive care (CDC, 2007).

Tertiary Prevention

The approaches to tertiary prevention of communicable disease include care and treatment of the infected person, isolation and quarantine of the infected person and safe handling and control of infectious wastes.

Care and Treatment

Communicable diseases have care and treatment specific to the disease. As mentioned previously, with respect to investigation, the nurse needs to understand the disease, the treatment and follow-up requirements, and the educational component to discuss with the infected person. There are many information resources for the community health nurse to utilize, such as the CDC and state agency resources. The public health agency may have policies and protocols for the community health nurse to utilize as well.

Isolation and Quarantine

Communicable disease control includes two methods for keeping infected persons and noninfected persons apart to prevent the spread of a disease. **Isolation** refers to separation of the infected persons (or animals) from others for the period of communicability to limit the transmission of the infectious agent to susceptible persons. **Quarantine** refers to restrictions placed on healthy contacts of an infectious case for the duration of the incubation period to prevent disease transmission if infection should develop (Heymann, 2008).

Safe Handling and Control of Infectious Wastes

The control of infection in community health also relies upon the proper disposal of contaminated wastes. The CDC supports and encourages *universal precautions* that stress that health care workers think of all blood and body fluids and materials that they may come in contact with as potentially infectious (CDC, 2009a). Although universal precaution observance is primarily considered while the nurse is giving hands-on treatment or care to a patient, keeping these principles in mind while making community health visits in the primary and secondary setting is paramount to the safety of both the client and the nurse (Heymann, 2008).

Universal precautions include the following:

- Hand washing after contact with the client or with potentially contaminated articles and before care of other clients
- Bagging and discarding articles contaminated with infectious material into an appropriate labeled container before it is sent for decontamination
- Use of proper personal protective equipment while dealing with an individual in isolation. This isolation is based on the mode of transmission of the specific disease, which may include strict isolation, contact isolation, respiratory isolation, TB isolation (acid-fast bacilli isolation), enteric precautions, or drainage/secretion precautions.

Infectious waste is waste capable of producing an infectious disease. The agency notes that for waste to be infectious, it must contain pathogens with sufficient virulence and quantity so that exposure to the waste by a susceptible host could result in an infectious disease. Requirements for medical waste disposal are for waste to be segregated into categories of (a) used and unused sharps, (b) cultures and stocks of infectious agents, (c) human blood and blood products, and (d) human pathologic, isolation, and animal waste. Although incineration has long been recognized as an efficient method for disposing safely of sharps and other contaminated medical waste, fewer incinerators are available now because of increasing regulation of emissions, and particularly those regulations related to burning chemical wastes (Heymann, 2008; OSHA 2010).

Four key elements of an infectious waste management program are applicable to community practice:

1. Health professionals must be able to correctly distinguish waste that poses a significant infection hazard from other biomedical waste that poses no greater risk than general municipal waste, and such infectious waste must be clearly defined.
2. The waste management program must have administrative support and authority to institute practice guidelines and provide the containers and other resources needed for safe disposal of infectious wastes.
3. Handling of the infectious wastes must be minimized. Containers should be rigid, leak resistant, and impervious to moisture; they should have sufficient strength to prevent rupture or tearing under normal conditions; and they should be sealed to prevent leakage. Containers for sharps must also be puncture resistant.
4. An enforcement or evaluation mechanism must be in place to ensure that the goal of reducing the potential for exposure to infectious waste in the community is met.

USING THE NURSING PROCESS FOR COMMUNICABLE DISEASE CONTROL

As mentioned in Chapters 4 and 7, the nursing process has steps similar to the research process and the epidemiologic process when approaching any health problem or condition. Therefore, using the nursing process to achieve communicable disease control should be an important and natural process for community health nurses.

Assessment

The first step of the nursing process, assessment, aligns itself with case-identification and case-finding in communicable disease control. The community health nurse must use all assessment skills and tools available during contact with clients, so as not to overlook the possibility of a communicable disease. Assessment must be comprehensive, producing physical, social, and environmental data. There is no place for assumption. At times, a nurse can become lulled into the usual patterns of inquiry, and this oversight may prove fatal to the client. An example follows:

> "Baby Josephine is irritable," says the mother. "Well, babies sometimes are," says the nurse. "How are you feeding her? Show me how you hold her. Does she sleep well? Try rocking her in the rocking chair before bedtime. And burp her more frequently. I'll check back with you in 2 weeks." Did the nurse record the baby's temperature, look at her for a rash, compare present weight with last weight, ask about bowel habits or vomiting, inquire about illnesses in the family, check on breast-feeding technique or watch while the mother demonstrated formula preparation, inspect the family's water source, ask about other foods the baby is eating, and so forth?

Broader inquiry into such a simple statement from the mother in this example may lead to the discovery of a life-threatening, undiagnosed communicable disease.

Assessment in the broader sense with respect to communicable disease control relates to the surveillance for disease. As mentioned previously, communicable diseases are reportable and the public health nurse may be the first to notice a trend in a rise in a particular disease rate.

Planning

The planning step in the nursing process involves different activities, depending on whether the intervention is for an individual, family, group, or entire community. At the individual level, the nurse may assist a client or family to obtain an immunization or definitive treatment. Or, the nurse may assist the client through education about self-care related to disease symptoms that provide relief and in reducing the chance of transmitting the disease to others in the family or community. With groups and communities, planning interventions includes the collaboration with community members and/or organizations. Whether a teen immunization campaign is proposed or a flu shot day is planned for senior citizens, there are location, staff, and supplies to prepare, which may include writing grants, establishing contracts, and training and orienting staff, before implementation can begin.

Implementation

During the implementation step, the nurse actually takes the action that was identified as necessary during assessment and planning. In the implementation step, the nurse may actually deliver the service or may supervise other staff or volunteers, as with a large immunization event. Implementing plans with small groups or families may involve arranging for transportation, so that several people can get to the immunization site or can be seen by a primary care provider. It may include gathering clinical specimens for laboratory analysis from a family recovering from a *Salmonella* infection. Education on primary prevention to prevent future infections is an essential part of the implementation phase. Agency record keeping, state-required contact investigation, and reports to the next level of government oversight of a communicable disease are essential in this phase.

Evaluation

Evaluation is an essential step in the nursing process with all services community health nurses provide. When dealing with communicable diseases, it is most important to determine whether actions have achieved the established goals. Have the outcomes been accomplished? Are all family members immunized? Are all family members free of the disease? Do families know how to prevent the diseases recurring? What needs to be done now to keep the community safe from communicable diseases? Are there funding issues, programs nearing completion that need support, or growth of services needed that can be addressed before a critical need occurs? These are examples of questions that need answers during evaluation. The community health nurse who is concerned with the health and safety of the community follows the steps of the nursing process to achieve healthy community goals.

LEGAL AND ETHICAL ISSUES IN COMMUNICABLE DISEASE CONTROL

Enforced Compliance

Legally, the responsibilities of public health officials in communicable disease control include the police power to enforce compliance with treatment or restrict the activity of infectious people to protect the welfare of others. Regulations that enforce compliance with disease prevention strategies are a justifiable restriction if the measures proposed are demonstrably effective and grounded in ethical principles (U.S. Food and Drug Administration, 2009).

Confidentiality, Privacy, and Discrimination

To carry out communicable disease interventions, client needs for confidentiality and privacy must be ensured. As agency and national data systems and programs continue to evolve, it is essential to make confidential data protection measures clear priorities (CDC, 2009d; USDHHS, 2010a).

Human society has a long-standing aversion to infectious diseases. Ostracism, which in the past included people with leprosy and other contagious conditions, has shifted to discrimination against people with TB or AIDS, for example. People are protected from discrimination under the Americans with Disability Act, but not with respect to posing a public health treat, such as with the contagious state of TB (Jones, 2008).

Confidentiality for individuals being interviewed about communicable disease is structured like any other health-related interview. It is important to assure the individual that the information will be maintained in a confidential manner, and the goal is care and treatment. It is also important to inform the individual that identified contacts will be notified in a confidential manner, without source identification. The CDC TB module on confidentiality related to the investigation offers techniques to use when conducting a confidential interview and maintain privacy (CDC, 2010h)

SUMMARY

Communicable diseases pose a major threat to the public's health and have done so since the beginning of humankind. In today's world, such diseases are transmitted globally as the result of mobile populations, increased urbanization, and international travel. Communicable diseases can be transmitted through direct contact from one person to another or indirectly through contaminated objects (air, water, food) or a vector (animal or insect). Communicable diseases affect all types of people and have worldwide significance.

Ideally, prevention of communicable diseases is accomplished through primary prevention methods such as utilizing mass media education campaigns, one-on-one education, and immunization. Knowledge of VPDs, the schedule of vaccinations, a community's immunization status, herd immunity, barriers to immunization coverage, planning and implementing immunization campaigns, adult immunizations, and the immunization needs of international travelers, immigrants, and refugees have been discussed. Health care workers need to practice universal precaution and the safe handling of infectious wastes to maintain worksite safety.

Secondary prevention activities of screening and disease investigation are steps taken when primary prevention activities have failed. Tertiary prevention is needed to ensure additional people are not infected and those who are ill receive care and treatment. Ongoing disease transmission can be interrupted through treatment, isolation, or quarantine.

Becoming familiar with the major communicable diseases affecting our nation is essential baseline information for community health nurses. TB, resurging since the 1980s, may be one of the biggest public health problems in the new millennium. Nurses must be aware of the populations at risk, how the disease is prevented, and the use of appropriate interventions during diagnosis and treatment. Issues compounding the control of TB are twofold: increasing infections with MDR strains, and the increasing number of people with TB and HIV/AIDS, making diagnosis and treatment more complicated.

A second major disease, HIV/AIDS, was first identified in the 1980s. With the success of antiviral drugs, HIV/AIDS is becoming a chronic disease for clients in industrialized nations, with an average life expectancy of 10 to 15 years after diagnosis. Africa is deeply affected by the massive numbers of women and children who are HIV positive, without access to the life-prolonging drugs available to people in developed nations.

STDs threaten the health and lives of millions of citizens. At greater risk are the sexually active, nonmonogamous. Control of STDs can be accomplished through effective screening, treatment, contact investigation, and aggressive public education. Several common STDs were discussed, including gonorrhea, syphilis, chlamydia, genital herpes, and viral warts.

Hepatitis is more common than HIV, and can lead to life-threatening events, such as cirrhosis and liver cancer. Yet, these diseases do not garner the attention they need. Most of the public is unaware of the types of hepatitis, prevention, transmission, and treatment. Vaccines for two of the forms (hepatitis A and hepatitis B) are available.

Influenza and pneumonia are "old" diseases that cause increased morbidity. These diseases cause the most morbidity and mortality in the frailest citizens—the immune compromised, very young, and the very old—although vaccines are available to prevent them.

Smallpox (an eradicated disease) and anthrax have been identified as potential bioterrorism weapons. The community/public health nurse has several areas of responsibility in regard to bioterrorism. First, the nurse must know the signs and symptoms of potential infectious diseases used as weapons. Also, the nurse has a responsibility to the community to allay fears about bioterrorism and to provide information about prevention.

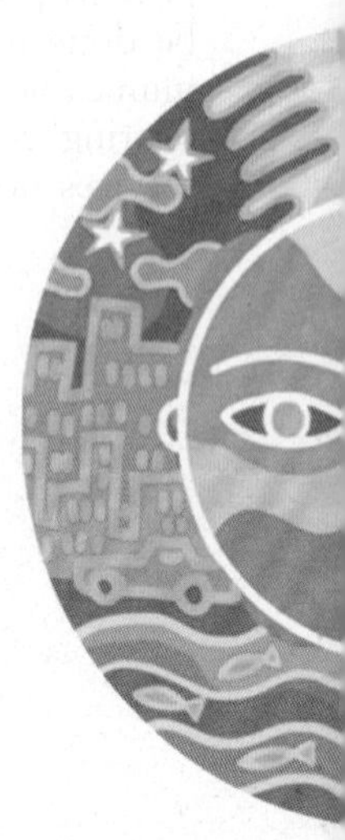

Community/public health nurses use the nursing process in their important role with regard to all populations at risk for communicable diseases. Nurses concerned with communicable disease control must recognize who is at risk, where the potential reservoirs and sources of infectious disease agents are located, what environmental factors promote their spread, and what are the characteristics and vulnerability of community members and groups. Community health nurses must work collaboratively with other public health professionals to establish immunization and education campaigns, work to improve community communicable disease control policies, and develop a broad range of services for at-risk community members.

Ethical issues in communicable disease control include enforced compliance, the justifiability of screening, preservation of confidentiality and privacy, and the avoidance of discrimination against infected people.

ACTIVITIES TO PROMOTE **CRITICAL THINKING**

1. Interview a professional in your local or state health department who works in communicable disease control. Determine (a) how she conducts communicable disease surveillance, (b) what diseases must be reported in your state, and (c) which communicable diseases are posing the greatest threat to the health of your state's citizens.
2. Compare a recent issue of *Mortality and Morbidity Weekly Report* with the same issue published a year earlier, in terms of cases of specific notifiable diseases in the United States. Which diseases appear to be increasing? Decreasing? Select one disease and read at least one recent publication on this subject to determine the reasons for its rise or decline.
3. Determine, through your local health department, what percentage of preschool children are immunized in your city or county. Is this a safe level of herd immunity? Propose some recommendations for preserving or raising this level.
4. Select one high-risk population discussed in this chapter and list the factors that make this group vulnerable to communicable disease. Use at least one other published source to enhance your understanding. Propose one nursing intervention (such as a specific screening or educational program) and outline how it might be accomplished.
5. Interview a professional who works in STD services or with the HIV-infected population. Determine what methods she uses for contact investigation. How does this health care worker preserve privacy and confidentiality? What measures have proved most effective in reaching contacts? What is your evaluation of their success?
6. Access the CDC through the Internet (***http://www.cdc.gov***) and browse the site to learn about its various services. Are there special travelers' warnings in certain countries at this time? What are some of the CDC's current concerns regarding communicable diseases? Select a communicable disease and identify the number of cases presently reported. Return to the same Web site 1 month later. Has the incidence of the disease increased or decreased?

REFERENCES

American Academy of Pediatrics. (2010). Policy statement increasing immunization coverage. *Pediatrics, 125*(6), 1295–1304.

American Recovery & Reinvestment Act. (2009). Retrieved from http://www.recovery.gov/About/Pages/The_Act.aspx

Avert. (2009). Sex *education that works*. Retrieved from http://www.avert.org/sex-education.htm

Birkhead, G. S., Orenstein, W. A., & Almquist, J. R. (2009). *Reducing financial barriers to vaccination in the United States*. Retrieved from http://pediatrics.aappublications.org/content/124/Supplement_5/S451.full.html

Brunton, C. (2010). *Nation's first "cocoon strategy" vaccination program delivers 10,000th immunization. Texas children's vaccine experts protect newborns from whooping cough*. Retrieved from http://www.texaschildrens.org/About-Us/News/Cocoon-Strategy-delivers-10,000th-immunization/

California Immunization Coalition. (2008). Vaccine *safety: Responding to parents' top 10 concerns*. Retrieved from http://www.cdph.ca.gov/programs/immunize/Documents/IMM-917.pdf

California Tuberculosis Controllers Association. (2010). CDHS/*CTCA joint guidelines for targeted testing and treatment of latent tuberculosis infection in adults and children*. Retrieved from http://ctca.org/index.cfm?fuseaction=page&page_id=5074

Centers for Disease Control and Prevention. (1999a). Achievements in public health, 1990–1999: Control of infectious diseases. *Morbidity and Mortality Weekly Report, 48*(29), 621–629.

Centers for Disease Control and Prevention. (1999b). Ten great public health achievements: United States 1900–1999. *Morbidity and Mortality Weekly Report, 48*(12), 241–243.

Centers for Disease Control and Prevention. (2007). *Principles of epidemiology in public health practice. An introduction to applied epidemiology and biostatistics* (3rd ed.). Atlanta, GA: Department of Health and Human Services, 1.15–1.17.

Centers for Disease Control and Prevention. (2008a). *2008 NCRID Annual Report*. Retrieved from http://www.cdc.gov/ncrid/annual-rpts/default.html

Centers for Disease Control and Prevention. (2008b). Prevention of pertussis, tetanus, and diphtheria among pregnant and postpartum women and their infants. *Morbidity and Mortality Weekly Report, 57*(RR-4), 1–56.

Centers for Disease Control and Prevention. (2009a). *Environmental health services. Biological and infectious waste*. Retrieved from http://www.cdc.gov/nceh/ehs/etp/biological.htm

Centers for Disease Control and Prevention. (2009b). School *connectedness: Strategies for increasing protective factors among youth*. Atlanta, GA: U.S. Department of Health and Human Services.

Centers for Disease Control and Prevention. (2009c). *Simply put. A guide for creating easy-to-understand materials* (3rd ed.). Atlanta,

GA: Centers for Disease Control and Prevention. Retrieved from http://www.cdc.gov/healthliteracy/pdf/Simply_Put.pdf

Centers for Disease Control and Prevention. (2009d). *Tuberculosis control laws and policies: A handbook for public health and legal practitioners*. The Centers for Law & the Public's Health. A collaborative at Johns Hopkins and Georgetown Universities. Retrieved from http://www.cdc.gov/tb/programs/TBlawPolicyHandbook.pdf

Centers for Disease Control and Prevention. (2009e). Use of northern hemisphere influenza vaccines by travelers to the southern hemisphere. *Morbidity Mortality Weekly Report, 58*(12), 312. Retrieved from http://www.cdc.gov/mmwrhtml/mm5812a4.htm

Centers for Disease Control and Prevention. (2010a). Estimates of deaths associated with seasonal influenza – United States, 1976–2007. *Morbidity and Mortality Weekly Report, 59*(33), 1057–1062.

Centers for Disease Control and Prevention. (2010b). *Hepatitis C general information*. Retrieved from http://www.cdc.gov/hepatitis/HCV/PDFs/HepCGeneralFactSheet.pdf

Centers for Disease Control and Prevention. (2010c). HIV *testing basics for consumers*. Retrieved from http://www.cdc.gov/hiv/topics/testing/resources/qa/index.htm

Centers for Disease Control and Prevention. (2010d). Investigation *update: Multistate outbreak of human salmonella enteritidis infections associated with shell eggs*. Retrieved from http://www.cdc.gov/salmonella/enteritidis/

Centers for Disease Control and Prevention. (2010e). *Our history – our story*. Retrieved from http://www.cdc.gov/about/history/ourstory.htm

Centers for Disease Control and Prevention. (2010f). *PanFlu storybook*. Retrieved from http://www.cdc.gov/about/panflu/default.htm

Centers for Disease Control and Prevention. (2010g). Seasonal *Influenza (Flu): Recommendations of the Advisory Committee on Immunization Practices (ACIP)*. Retrieved from http://www.cdc.gov/flu/professionals/acip/

Centers for Disease Control and Prevention. (2010h). *Self-study modules on tuberculosis. Module 7: Confidentiality in tuber culosis control reading materials. Measures to protect patient confidentiality*. Retrieved from http://www.cdc.gov/tb/education/ssmodules/module7/ss7reading4.htm

Centers for Disease Control and Prevention. (2010i). The *2009 H1N1 Pandemic: Summary highlights, April 2009–April 2010*. Retrieved from http://www.cdc.gov/h1n1flu/cdcresponse.htm

Centers for Disease Control and Prevention. (2010j). *Vision, mission, core values, and pledge*. Retrieved from http://www.cdc.gov/about/organization/mission.htm

Centers for Disease Control and Prevention. (2011a). *Advisory Committee on Immunization Practices (ACIP). General recommendations on immunization*. Retrieved from http://www.cdc.gov/vaccines/pubs/ACIP-list.htm

Centers for Disease Control and Prevention. (2011b). BCG *vaccine. Fact Sheet*. Retrieved from http://www.cdc.gov/tb/publications/factsheets/prevention/BCG.htm

Centers for Disease Control and Prevention. (2011c). *Detecting a possible outbreak*. Retrieved from http://www.cdc.gov/outbreaknet/investigations/detection.html

Centers for Disease Control and Prevention. (2011d). Interferon-*gamma release assays (IGRAs) – blood tests for TB infection*. Retrieved from http://www.cdc.gov/tb/publications/factsheets/testing/IGRA.htm

Centers for Disease Control and Prevention. (2011e). *Menu of suggested provisions for state tuberculosis prevention and control laws/ C. treatment/ 1. Case management, treatment guidelines, and required treatment*. Retrieved from http://www.cdc.gov/tb/programs/laws/menu/treatment.htm

Centers for Disease Control and Prevention. (2011f). National and state vaccination coverage among adolescents aged 13 through 17 Years—United States, 2010. *Morbidity Mortality Weekly Report, 60*(33), 1117–1123.

Centers for Disease Control and Prevention. (2011g). National and state vaccination coverage among children aged 19–35 months—United States, 2010. *Morbidity and Mortality Weekly Report, 60*(34), 1157–1163.

Centers for Disease Control and Prevention. (2011h). *Nationally notifiable infectious conditions, United States 2011*. Retrieved from http://www.cdc.gov/osels/ph_surveillance/nndss/phs/infdis2011.htm

Centers for Disease Control and Prevention. (2011i). Prevention and control of influenza with vaccines. Recommendations of the Advisory Committee on Immunization Practices (ACIP), 2011. *Morbidity and Mortality Weekly Report, 60*(33), 1128–1132.

Centers for Disease Control and Prevention. (2011j). *PulseNet*. Retrieved from http://www.cdc.gov/pulsenet/

Centers for Disease Control and Prevention. (2011k). *Sexually transmitted diseases (STDs): 2010 STD treatment guidelines*. Retrieved from http://www.cdc.gov/std/treatment/2010/default.htm

Centers for Disease Control and Prevention. (2011l). *2010 sexually transmitted diseases surveillance. Cases of sexually transmitted diseases reported by state health departments and rates per 100,000 population, United States, 1941–2010*. Retrieved from http://www.cdc.gov/std/stats10/tables/1.htm

Centers for Disease Control and Prevention. (2011m). *2010 sexually transmitted diseases Surveillance. STDs in adolescents and young adults*. Retrieved from http://www.cdc.gov/std/stats10/adol.htm

Centers for Disease Control and Prevention. (2011n). *Travelers' health. Find a clinic*. Retrieved from http://wwwnc.cdc.gov/travel/page/find-clinic.htm

Centers for Disease Control and Prevention. (2011o). *Travelers' health. Stay healthy and safe when you travel*. Retrieved from http://wwwnc.cdc.gov/travel/page/stay-healthy.htm

Centers for Disease Control and Prevention. (2011p). *TB guidelines: Tuberculosis infection control and prevention*. Retrieved from http:www.cdc/gov/tb/topic/infectioncontrol/default.htm.

Centers for Disease Control and Prevention. (2012a). *Centers for Disease Control and Prevention FY 2012 Online Performance Appendix*. Retrieved from http://www.cdc.gov/fmo/topic/Performance/performance_docs/FY2012_CDC_Online_Performance_Appendix.pdf

Centers for Disease Control and Prevention. (2012b). *CDC organization*. Retrieved from http://www.cdc.gov/about/organization/cio.htm

Centers for Disease Control and Prevention. (2012c). *Epidemiology and prevention of vaccine preventable diseases: the Pink Book* (12th ed.). Washington, DC: Public Health Foundation.

Centers for Disease Control and Prevention. (2012d). *Immigrant and refugee health*. Retrieved from http://www.cdc.gov/immigrantrefugeehealth/

Centers for Disease Control and Prevention. (2012e). *Legal status of expedited partner therapy (EPT)*. Retrieved from http://www.cdc.gov/std/ept/legal/default.htm

Centers for Disease Control and Prevention. (2012f). Notifiable disease and mortality tables. *Morbidity and Mortality Weekly Report, 61*(14), 184–198.

Centers for Disease Control and Prevention. (2012g). *Pneumonia can be prevented. Vaccines can help*. Retrieved from http://www.cdc.gov/Features/Pneumonia/

Centers for Disease Control and Prevention. (2012h). *Recommendations and guidelines: 2012 adult immunization schedule*. Retrieved from http://www.cdc.gov/vaccines/recs/schedules/adult-schedule.htm

Centers for Disease Control and Prevention. (2012i). *Recommended immunization schedule for persons aged 0 through 6 years—United States, 2012*. Retrieved from http://www.cdc.gov/vaccines/recs/schedules/downloads/child/0-6yrs-schedule-pr.pdf

Centers for Disease Control and Prevention. (2012j). Trends in Tuberculosis, 2011. *Morbidity and Mortality Weekly Report, 61*(11), 181–185.

CHAPTER 9

Environmental Health and Safety

"When we try to pick out anything by itself, we find it hitched to everything else in the Universe."

—*John Muir*, 1911

KEY TERMS

Bioaccumulation
Biomonitoring
Brownfield's
Built environment
Climate change
Ecology
Environmental epidemiology
Environmental justice
Epigenetics
Exposure pathway
Integrated Pest Management
Precautionary principle
Risk assessment
Risk management
Superfund
Sustainability
Toxicology

LEARNING OBJECTIVES

Upon mastery of this chapter, you should be able to:

- Apply the ecological perspective to human and environmental relationships.
- Discuss concepts of prevention and upstream approaches to health impact and environmental health.
- Discuss guiding documents for public health nursing.
- Discuss how the core functions of public health can be applied to public health nursing.
- Relate the effect of environmental hazards to human health.
- Describe how nurses can collaborate with other professionals, government agencies, and communities to reduce environmental threats to health.

The World Health Organization (WHO) defines environment, as it relates to health, as "all the physical, chemical, and biological factors external to a person, and all the related behaviors" WHO (1948/2011). The ability to live in a healthy environment not only increases the number of years of a healthy life but also one's quality of life. Increasingly, a number of environmental factors have been recognized as detrimental to health, including exposures to hazardous materials in air, water, food, and soil; the rise in development and use of synthetic chemicals not well tested for safety; the adverse effects of natural and man-made disasters; and, more recently, the built environment (U.S. Department of Health and Human Services [USDHHS], 2011a). In the most recent version of Healthy People, *Healthy People 2020*, the definition of environmental health "comprises those aspects of human health, disease, and injury that are determined or influenced by factors in the environment. This includes not only the study of the direct pathological effects of various chemical, physical, and biological agents, but also the effects on health of the broad physical and social environment, which includes housing, urban development, land-use and transportation, industry, and agriculture" (USDHHS, 2011b).

ENVIRONMENTAL HEALTH AND NURSING

Nurses are charged to incorporate knowledge of the environment into their nursing practice. Historically, public health and occupational health nurses (OHNs) have been leaders in this effort. Despite this history, the need for nursing knowledge, environmental health assessment, engagement with community members to address environmental health issues and policy, and advocacy efforts must be increased. During the past two decades in particular, several documents challenge nurses to advance their environmental health nursing knowledge and skills. In 1995, the Institute of Medicine report, *Nursing Health and the Environment* (Pope, Snyder, & Mood, 1995), addressed nursing education, practice, and research. The Agency for Toxic Substances and Disease Registry (ATSDR) launched their "Nursing and the Environment" initiative. Public health nursing led the profession with the publication of the *Environmental Health Principles for Public Health Nursing* in 2005 (see Table 9-1). The ANA produced the *ANA's Principles of Environmental Health for Nursing Practice with Implementation Strategies* in 2007 (see Table 9-2). And most recently, in 2010, the American Nurses Association(ANA) *Nursing: Scope and Standards of Practice* added a new standard, Standard 16 Environmental Health (see Display 9.1). These guiding documents and initiatives call for all nurses to incorporate environmental health into all areas of nursing practice.

Importance of Environmental Health for Nursing

Nurses are essential to improve environmental health through nursing education, research, and practice. More than a decade ago, the ATSDR developed the national Environmental Health Nursing Initiative to engage nurses to work collaboratively with federal agencies, nursing organizations, health departments, educational programs, and nongovernmental organizations. The agency selected nurses as important professionals because nurses "play key roles in protecting the health of all people; are in direct contact with patients, families, and communities from many cultural and socioeconomic backgrounds; and have the credibility and access that enables them to provide scientifically sound information about environmental issues and toxic exposures" (ATSDR, 2011).

The Alliance of Nurses for Healthy Environments offers reasons why nurses are important to environmental health that include the role of nurses in promoting healing and safe environments for people. Nurses work with diverse populations in homes, workplaces, and communities and are the largest population of health care providers in the United States with almost 3 million registered nurses. In addition, nurses are one of the most trusted professionals, are able to communicate complex information to their patients and communities, and interact with many other health care organizations and in policy setting roles (Smith, 2010).

CONCEPTS AND FRAMEWORKS FOR ENVIRONMENTAL HEALTH

Ecology

Ecology can be defined as the study of the interactions and relationships between living organisms and their environments. Ecosystems are dynamic communities of plant, animal, and microorganisms as well as the nonliving environments in which they live. No organism including humans can live removed from their ecosystem or other species. Ecosystems help regulate water, gases, waste recycling, nutrient cycling, pollination, infectious disease, climate, and biology as well as provide recreational and cultural opportunities for human use (Frumkin, 2010; Wright, 2008). The scientific study of ecosystems provides the science to understand the synergistic relationship between humans and the environment and why knowledge of environmental health is so important for nurses. The term ecomedicine refers to the adverse human impact upon the environment that in turn creates new patterns of disease and poverty (Science and Environmental Health Network, 2011). Specific threats to the environment for human health are discussed using a sustainability perspective.

Table 9-1 Guiding Documents—Environmental Principles for Public Health Nursing

Environmental Health Principles for Public Health Nursing

1. Safe and sustainable environments are essential conditions for the public's health.
2. Environmental health is integral to the role and responsibilities of all public health nurses.
3. All public health nurses should possess environmental health knowledge and skills.
4. Environmental health decisions should be grounded in sound science.
5. The precautionary principle is a fundamental tenet for all environmental health endeavors.
6. Environmental justice is a right of all populations.
7. Public awareness and community involvement are essential in environmental health decision making.
8. Communities have a right to relevant and timely information for decisions on environmental health.
9. Environmental health approaches should respect diverse values, beliefs, cultures, and circumstances.
10. Collaboration is essential to effectively protecting the health of all people from environmental harm.
11. Environmental health advocacy must be rooted in scientific integrity, honesty, respect for all persons, and social justice.
12. Environmental health research addressing the effectiveness and public health impact of nursing interventions should be conducted and disseminated.

Sustainability is "the ability to meet the needs of the present without compromising the ability of future generations to meet their own needs; an environmental protection strategy designed to protect the Earth's resources" (Hilgenkamp, 2006, p. 1). When the concept of sustainability is applied to human systems, the importance for the public to protect the environment and promote healthy characteristics in the population and community in which they live is evident. Currently, much of human–environment interactions are not sustainable

Table 9-2 ANA's Principles of Environmental Health for Nursing Practice

ANA Principles 2007

All nurses are to be aware of the principles of environmental health for nursing. We are to integrate these principles into our practice, education, and research.

ANA's Principles of Environmental Health for Nursing Practice

1. Knowledge of environmental health concepts is essential to nursing practice.
2. The precautionary principle guides nurses in their practice to use products and practices that do not harm human health or the environment and to take preventive action in the fact of uncertainty.
3. Nurses have a right to work in an environment that is safe and healthy.
4. Healthy environments are sustained through multidisciplinary collaboration.
5. Choice of materials, products, technology, and practices in the environment that impact nursing practice are based on the best available evidence.
6. Approaches to promoting a healthy environment reflect a respect for the diverse values, beliefs, cultures, and circumstances of patients and their families.
7. Nurses participate in assessing the quality of the environment in which they practice and live.
8. Nurses, other health care workers, patients, and communities have the right to know relevant and timely information about the potentially harmful products, chemicals, pollutants, and hazards to which they are exposed.
9. Nurses participate in research of best practices that promote a safe and healthy environment.
10. Nurses must be supported in advocating for and implementing environmental health principles in nursing practice.

Source: *ANA'S principles of environmental health for nursing practice with implementation strategies.* (2007). Silver Spring, MD: 2007 American Nurses Association.

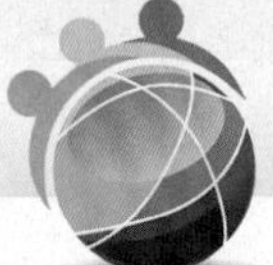

DISPLAY 9.1 AMERICAN NURSES ASSOCIATION NURSING: SCOPE AND STANDARDS OF PRACTICE

Standard 16. Environmental Health

The registered nurse practices in an environmentally safe and healthy manner.

Competencies:

The Registered Nurse:

Attains knowledge of environmental health concepts, such as implantation of environmental health strategies

Promotes a practice environment that reduces environmental health risks of workers and health care consumers

Assesses the practice environment for factors such as sound, odor, noise, and light that negatively affect health

Advocates for the judicious and appropriate use of products used in health care

Communicates environmental health risks and exposure reduction strategies to health care consumers, families, colleagues, and communities

Utilizes scientific evidence to determine if a product or treatment is a potential environmental threat

Participates in strategies to promote healthy communities

Additional Competencies for the Graduate-Level Prepared Specialty Nurse and the Advanced Practice Registered Nurse

Create partnerships that promote sustainable environmental health policies and conditions

Analyze the impact of social, political, and economic influences upon the environment and human health exposures

Critically evaluate the manner in which environmental health issues are presented by the popular media

Advocate for implementation of environmental principles for nursing practice

Support nurses in advocating for and implementing environmental principles in nursing practice

Source: American Nurses Association (ANA). (2010). *Nursing: Scope and Standards of Practice* (2nd ed.). Silver Spring, MD: Nursebooks.org). 2010 American Nurses Association. Reprinted with permission.

in that energy use exceeds supply, pollutants are changing the natural landscape of plant and animal life, and threatening both human life and ecosystems. Solutions to improve sustainability for humans and the environment include strategies that are socially desirable, economically feasible, and ecologically viable (Wright, 2008). One example of how increased human demands for energy impact sustainability is the increased use of fossil fuels for home heating and cooling. Increased use of coal, for example, increases air pollution from the toxic emissions released in coal-fired power plants that are often referred to as greenhouse gases and contribute to global warming. Current estimates indicate that the global need for oil has exceeded available resources that are not sustainable.

Public health nurses find that the science of ecology has been applied to social ecological perspectives that identify not only the physical environment but also the social and cultural factors that exist for populations. In public health, the ecological model of population health is used to illustrate that determinants of health (biological, behavioral, and environmental) interact to affect health (Friis, 2012) In addition, the *Healthy People 2020* approach emphasizes the need to include social, cultural, and environmental conditions into assessments for health determinants. Health behaviors occur within various levels of the ecological model and must be considered to clearly identify the most effective interventions for health promotion (USDHHS, 2011a) (see Figure 9-1).

Upstream Focus

Many public health nurses incorporate an "upstream" focus into their work with populations. That approach emerged from the seminal publication by John McKinley in 1979, "A Case for Focusing Upstream" that identifies root causes of disease and manufacturers of illness. It considers socioeconomic factors and also the environmental origins of disease and health problems. To illustrate this he uses examples in the food and tobacco industries (McKinley, 1979). Public health nurses work in prevention and health promotion areas, but an upstream approach moves our thinking to those factors that are at the institutional and system level rather than looking solely at healthy lifestyle issues. For example, a program to improve heart health in a community using a lifestyle approach would promote healthy diets, increased physical activity, and smoking cessation. An upstream focus looks at the social factors such as secondhand smoke in public places, unhealthy food choices available in schools and other public places, and how the built environment promotes or impedes safe outdoor physical activity. Butterfield (2002) claims that nursing has been focused upon the consequences of disease rather than the causes, particularly those that emerge from the physical, chemical, and biologic environmental influences upon health. She reminds us that nurses, particularly public health nurses, with our presence in worksites, homes, schools, and other community settings can serve to reduce

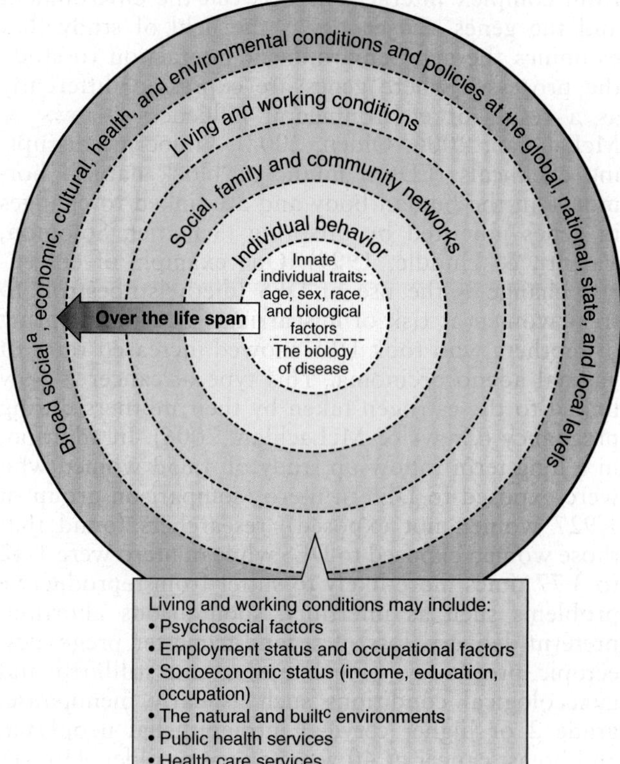

FIGURE 9-1. Ecological Model for Public Health. Institute of Medicine (2002). *The future of the public's health in the 21st century*. Washington, DC: National Academies Press. Adapted from Dahlgren, G. & Whitehead, M. (1991). *Policies and strategies to promote social equity in health*. Institute for Future Studies, Stockholm (Mimeo). Reprinted with permission from the National Academies Press, Copyright 2002, National Academy of Sciences.

risks. Public health nurses are often the "sentinels of surveillance" (Butterfield, 2002, p. 33) who detect unusual illness patterns and respond to environmental emergencies in work and community settings. With emphasis upon data estimates that as much as 33% of disease occurrence is attributable to environmental exposures and that the prevalence of environmentally linked health problems such as asthma, neurological problems, certain cancers, and birth defects are all on the rise, a case can be made for why nurses must use an upstream framework to assess, monitor, educate, advocate, and create policy to reduce environmental health risks. Butterfield identifies three specific opportunities for nurses to impact these health threats: (1) by nursing presence in hospitals, clinicians' worksites, schools, and home settings; (2) because nurses have skills to translate technical information into messages that nonhealth professionals can understand; and (3) nurses have skills to promote health at both the individual and community level. Strategic actions that can be considered as part of an upstream framework are to include:

- Using an environmental health history in nursing assessments in order to create better tracking of environmental exposures
- Embedding environmental health information into nursing practice settings
- Increasing educational efforts to inform individuals and families of environmental health hazards
- Knowing information
- Engaging in environmental health research to advance our understanding of etiology and prevention
- Advocating for individuals and groups who are at specific risks

By using an upstream approach, public health nurses can impact the prevalence of disease by intervening where the root causes exist (Butterfield, 2002).

Precautionary Principle

The **precautionary principle** states that in the absence of clear data that indicate the safety of an action, chemical, or material that poses a threat to human health, it should not be used. The origin of the precautionary principle is in Germany and was used as early as 1970 to restrict the impact of potentially toxic air emissions. In the United States, the adoption of this perspective that was used in Europe grew during the 1990s and culminated in 1998, when an interdisciplinary team met in Wisconsin at the Wingspread Center to address the environment and human health. The *Wingspread Statement on the Precautionary Principle* is rooted in precaution, scientific uncertainty, and human rights. The Wingspread Statement posits that based upon the release and use of toxic substances, the failure of environmental regulations to adequately protect human health and evidence that supports adverse human health effects from environmental exposures necessitate the implementation of the precautionary principle. The principle states, "When an activity raises threats of harm to human health or the environment, precautionary measures should be taken if some cause and effect relationships are not fully established scientifically. In this content the proponent of an activity, rather than the public, should bear the burden of proof" (Raffensperger & Tickner, 1999, pp. 353–354).

The precautionary principle has been applied to public health and the core functions. First, the core function of assessment includes two essential services: (1) monitoring health status and (2) the diagnosis and investigation of health hazards into the community. Environmental health surveillance is supported by the precaution principle. Most certainly the role of risk assessment that is central to environmental health meets the concern for evidence to determine the safety of activities that can pose environmental threats to health. Policy development addresses the guidance from the precautionary principle through the essential services that inform and educate the public, mobilize the community to address health issues, and develop policies to address those issues. The precautionary principle engages scientists to analyze and develop policies to ensure health based upon sound evidence. The core function of assurance requires that policies be enforced. The precautionary principle charges that instead of a focus upon remediation that those activities that could be harmful not be undertaken (Chaudry, 2008). The application of the precautionary principle to public health nursing can be noted in the *Environmental Health Principles and Recommendations for Public Health Nursing*, where Principle 5 states that the precautionary principle is a "fundamental tenet for all environmental health endeavors" (American Public Health Association, 2005). Chaudry (2008) reports that the precautionary principle is relevant for public health nursing interventions that include surveillance, community organizing, and advocacy and must be incorporated into nursing practice.

Specific Vulnerabilities

Various groups are at more risk at specific times of physical development, through comorbid health issues or from issues related to where they live, work, or attend school. Pregnant women's exposures create a number of risks to both mother and fetus and can produce lifelong or intergenerational adverse outcomes. Some of these effects include fetal loss, low birth weight infants, menstrual abnormalities, recurrent miscarriage, malformations of the reproductive system, reduced fertility, hormonal changes, intrauterine growth restriction, altered semen quality, and alterations in onset of puberty (Chalupka & Chalupka, 2010; Leffers, 2010).

Infants and children are at risk for a number of reasons related to their stage of physical development, behavioral factors, and specific environments such as NICUs, schools, and homes. Children's exposures begin in utero when many pollutants reach the developing fetus. Although breast-feeding is the best source of nutrition for infants, many chemicals such as polychlorinated biphenyls (PCBs), dichlorodiphenyltrichloroethane (DDT), dioxin, and benzene have been identified in breast milk. The stage of physical development of the respiratory, neurological, and excretory systems can all lead to increased risk of exposure and decreased ability to metabolize toxins. Childhood behaviors such as hand-to-mouth exploration, crawling and playing on or near the ground, and use of toys all contribute to specific vulnerability to hazards. Toxic materials on floors or in soil where children play and playthings, such as pressure-treated wood, toys, and paints, can all increase risk for childhood exposures. Lead, mercury, and PCB exposures increase the risk for developmental disabilities. Studies suggest that the rise in ADHD (attention deficit hyperactivity disorder) antisocial and aggressive behavior diagnoses can be attributed to the harmful effects of neurotoxicants in the environment (Stein, Schettler, Wallinga, & Valenti, 2002).

Prenatal Exposure to EDCs and Effect on Future Generations

Evidence indicates that many chronic diseases arise from complex interactions between the environment and the genes. **Epigenetics** is the field of study that examines the gene–environment interaction to study the processes where genes are expressed differently as a result of environmental influences (Crews & McLachlan, 2006; Olden, 2002). Endocrine disrupting chemicals (EDCs) mimic or block natural hormones in the human body and are linked to changes in genes inherited by offspring (Schettler, Solomon, Valenti, & Huddle, 1999). One example of epigenetic change is the use of DES (diethylstilbestrol) to treat women at risk of miscarriage. Female offspring of mothers who took DES showed increased rates of vaginal adenocarcinoma. This type of cancer is now linked to the estrogen taken by their mothers during pregnancy (Crews & McLachlan, 2006). In addition, in a long-term follow-up study of 4,653 women who were exposed to DES in utero (comparison group of 1,927 women not exposed), researchers found that those women exposed to DES while in utero were 1.42 to 3.77 times more likely to suffer from reproductive problems such as infertility, spontaneous abortion, preterm delivery, loss of second-trimester pregnancy, ectopic pregnancy, preeclampsia, and stillbirth and gynecological conditions such as early menopause, grade 2 or higher cervical intraepithelial neoplasia, and breast cancer at 40 years of age or older (Hoover et al., 2011). Experts argue that the genetic changes that result from epigenetic processes create negative effects on the health of future generations and contribute to rising rates of neurological conditions, alterations in reproductive organ development, and cancer (Schettler et al., 1999).

Brief History of Occupational/ Environmental Health Movement in Nursing

Environmental health assessment and nursing interventions have been part of nursing practice since Florence Nightingale and the early days of the profession. Nightingale emphasized the importance of the environment for health and recovery in her *Notes on nursing: What it is and what it is not* written in 1859. Nightingale cited the role of clean air, water, and overall sanitation for both health and recovery from illness (Nightingale, 1860/1969). Nurses who first worked with hazardous exposures in the workplace were often called industrial nurses. Now those who work in industry are called OHNs where they both assess worker's health status, and work to ensure worker safety and prevent adverse health effects from hazards in the workplace. With specific education and training in toxicology, epidemiology, workplace hazards, regulations, and prevention strategies, OHNs can be certified through the American Board of Occupational Health Nurses. Public health has included environmental health as a central aspect of health promotion and disease prevention. More recently, the nursing profession has responded to the call of nurses to establish environmental health competencies for nursing practice.

In 1995, the Institute of Medicine released the report of their meeting on *Nursing, Health and the Environment* (Pope et al., 1995) that called for nurses to become more knowledgeable about the scientific principles of the relationship between health and environment, to advance their assessment and referral skills for environmental hazards, to advocate for patients and communities to reduce adverse health effects, and to understand policy and legislation related to environmental health. More specifically, the report called for nurses to recognize pathways of exposure, prevention and control strategies, and the importance of research to develop sound and effective interventions. Interventions would include education and appropriate risk communication (Pope et al., 1995).

From 1995 until 2008 in response to this pivotal report, many schools and colleges increased their capacity to include environmental health into the nursing curriculum. In addition, nurses in practice incorporated environmental health into practice and were instrumental in making significant change in practice settings to reduce hazardous exposures to both health professionals and patients. Nursing research to address nursing interventions for environmental health increased, and nurses became involved in a number of policy and advocacy efforts.

In December 2008, 50 nurse leaders representing a range of nursing organizations including the American Public Health Association (APHA) Public Health Nursing Section, the Association of Community Health Nursing Educators, the Association of State and Territorial Directors of Nursing, and ANA met to develop an agenda for environmental health nursing. The organization, Alliance of Nurses for Healthy Environments (ANHE), was formed to advance nursing knowledge of environmental health and engage nurses in collaboration to advance environmental health nursing (ANHE, 2011). Four workgroups were formed: education, research, practice, and advocacy/policy. Since that time, a number of initiatives have placed environmental health at a forefront for nursing education and practice. The ANHE Education Workgroup developed competencies for nursing practice in 2009. Working collaboratively with the ANA, Standard 16 Environmental Health was included in the 2010 *Nursing: Scope and Standards of Practice* (ANA, 2010). With the publication of this document, all nurses must include environmental health in their nursing practice. In addition to the success with the development of competencies and standards, the nurses who work with ANHE have advanced their advocacy and policy voice, prepared research priorities for environmental health nursing, and held conferences and workshops for nursing practice, education, and advocacy efforts (ANHE, 2011). While public health nurses have been at the forefront of environmental health nursing, the new competencies provide guidance for all nursing practice and can be applied in community settings.

Guiding Documents

In addition to the previously mentioned Environmental Health Principles for Public Health Nursing (APHA, 2005), the ANA Principles of Environmental Health for Nursing Practice (ANA, 2007), and the Scope and Standards of Nursing Practice (ANA, 2010), nurses are guided by other public health documents. These include the federal guidelines from the Surgeon General report on healthy people and the core functions of public health developed by the Institute of Medicine.

Healthy People 2020 Initiatives

In 1979, the Surgeon General released a report, *Healthy People: The Surgeon General's Report on Health Promotion and Disease Prevention*, to set goals for improving health for the nation. In 1990, the Healthy People initiative set specific objectives to reduce disease, promote health, and improve healthy years of life. Revisions in 2000, 2010, and most recently for 2020 continue this focus upon targets for health improvement. This document provides guidance for nurses to identify targets for health and is used for many public health nursing interventions. The *Healthy People 2020* framework offers specific goals and objectives for environmental health. The overall goal is to "promote health for all through a healthy environment" (USDHHS, 2011b). The most recent release of the *Healthy People 2020* Environmental Health objectives focus on six areas that include outdoor air quality, surface and ground water quality, toxic substances and hazardous wastes, homes and communities, infrastructure and surveillance, and global environmental health. A number of health conditions are linked to poor air quality such as respiratory disease, cardiovascular disease, and cancer. Toxins found in water have been linked to neurological problems, endocrine disruption, and cancer. While not all mechanisms for disease from toxic exposures are fully understood or studied, various hazardous chemicals have been linked to birth defects, neurological problems, endocrine disruption, and cancer (USDHHS, 2011a). See Display 9.2 for a full listing of the *Healthy People 2020* Environmental Health objectives.

Core Functions of Public Health

In 1988, the Institute of Medicine convened to address what they called "the disarray of public health" and developed the mission, role of government in fulfilling this mission, and specific responsibilities for level of government. This resulted in the core functions of public health and the ten essential services. The core functions: assessment, policy development, and assurance will be applied to the important aspects of environmental health for public health nursing. Assessment includes the investigation of health hazards, surveillance

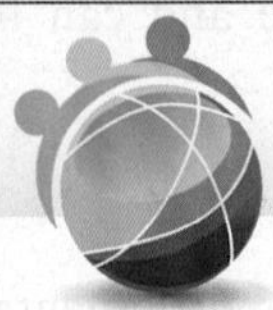

DISPLAY 9.2 *HEALTHY PEOPLE 2020* OBJECTIVES FOR ENVIRONMENTAL HEALTH TOPIC AREA

Goal: Promote health for all through a healthy environment.

Topic and Number Objective:

Outdoor Air Quality

EH-1 Air Quality Index (AQI) does not exceed 100
EH-2 Increase use of alternative modes of transportation for work
EH-3 Reduce air toxic emissions to decrease the risk of adverse health effects caused by airborne toxics

Water Quality

EH-4 Increase the proportion of persons served by community water systems who receive a supply of drinking water that meets the regulations of the Safe Drinking Water Act
EH-5 Reduce waterborne disease outbreaks arising from water intended for drinking among persons served by community water systems
EH-7 Increase the proportion of days that beaches are open and safe for swimming

Toxics and Waste

EH-8 Reduce blood lead levels in children
EH-9 Minimize the risks to human health and the environment posed by hazardous sites Minimize the risks to human health and the environment posed by hazardous sites
EH-10 Reduce pesticide exposures that result in visits to a health care facility Reduce pesticide exposures that result in visits to a health care facility
EH-11 Reduce the amount of toxic pollutants released into the environment
EH-12 Increase recycling of municipal solid waste

Healthy Homes and Healthy Communities

EH-13 Reduce indoor allergen levels
EH-14 Increase the number of homes with an operating radon mitigation system for persons living in homes at risk for radon exposure
EH-15 Increase the percentage of new single-family homes (SFHs) constructed with radon-reducing features, especially in high-radon-potential areas
EH-16 Increase the proportion of the nation's elementary, middle, and high schools that have official school policies and engage in practices that promote a healthy and safe physical school environment
EH-17 (Developmental) Increase the proportion of persons living in pre-1978 housing that has been tested for the presence of lead-based paint or related hazards
EH-18 Reduce the number of US homes that are found to have lead-based paint or related hazards
EH-19 Reduce the proportion of occupied housing units that have moderate or severe physical problems

Infrastructure and Surveillance

EH-20 Reduce exposure to selected environmental chemicals in the population, as measured by blood and urine concentrations of the substances or their metabolites
EH-21 Improve quality, utility, awareness, and use of existing information systems for environmental health
EH-22 Increase the number of states, territories, tribes, and the District of Columbia that monitor diseases or conditions that can be caused by exposure to environmental hazards
EH-23 Reduce the number of new schools sited within 500 feet of an interstate or Federal or State highway

Global Environmental Health

EH-24 Reduce the global burden of disease due to poor water quality, sanitation, and insufficient hygiene

of health issues such as disease or injury, examining causes, and assessing needs. Policy development relies upon science for decision making and educates people to create community involvement in order to develop polices. Assurance is a function that seeks innovative solutions to health issues, guarantees necessary services are provided, as well as provides oversight to policy implementation (Institute of Medicine, 1988).

Public health nurses fulfill these functions but extend them by their strong emphasis upon education for health promotion, disease prevention, as well as advocacy by integrating nursing knowledge and practice into these functions. In addition, public health nurses work collaboratively with others in the community to promote health for the people they serve. This chapter reviews essential environmental health information for public health nurses using the core functions as an organizational framework.

Some of the most commonly recognized areas of public health nursing practice where nurses address environmental impacts upon heath are in schools, homes, and broader community issues such as the built environment. School nurses have been leaders in addressing indoor air quality in schools particularly as rates of asthma in children rise. Many collaborate with the U.S. Environmental Protection Agency (EPA) and their IAQ Tools for Schools program (U.S. EPA, 2011j). More recently, in response to FIFRA (Federal Insecticide, Fungicide, and Rodenticide Act), school nurses are serving as advocates for IPM (**Integrated Pest Management**) programs for pest prevention without increasing exposure to harmful toxins. PHNs have been part of the Healthy Homes Initiative (HHI). OHNs have served to educate, enforce safety standards, monitor health, and advocate for workers' health. At the community level, nurses are involved with efforts to reduce pediatric obesity by participation in efforts to improve the built environment through safe walking paths, advocating for safe parks and recreational areas, and in reduction in exposure to pesticides in playgrounds (Gilden, 2011).

Assessment

The breadth of environmental health information available exceeds the scope of this chapter. Our discussion can be organized around the settings where people live, work, and go to school; the routes of exposure; the types of hazards; and the health effects of environmental toxins. In particular for nurses in the community, it is important to identify priority concerns for the locations where people spend the majority of their time (home, work, school) to better prepare health promotion and disease prevention interventions. To help the learner,

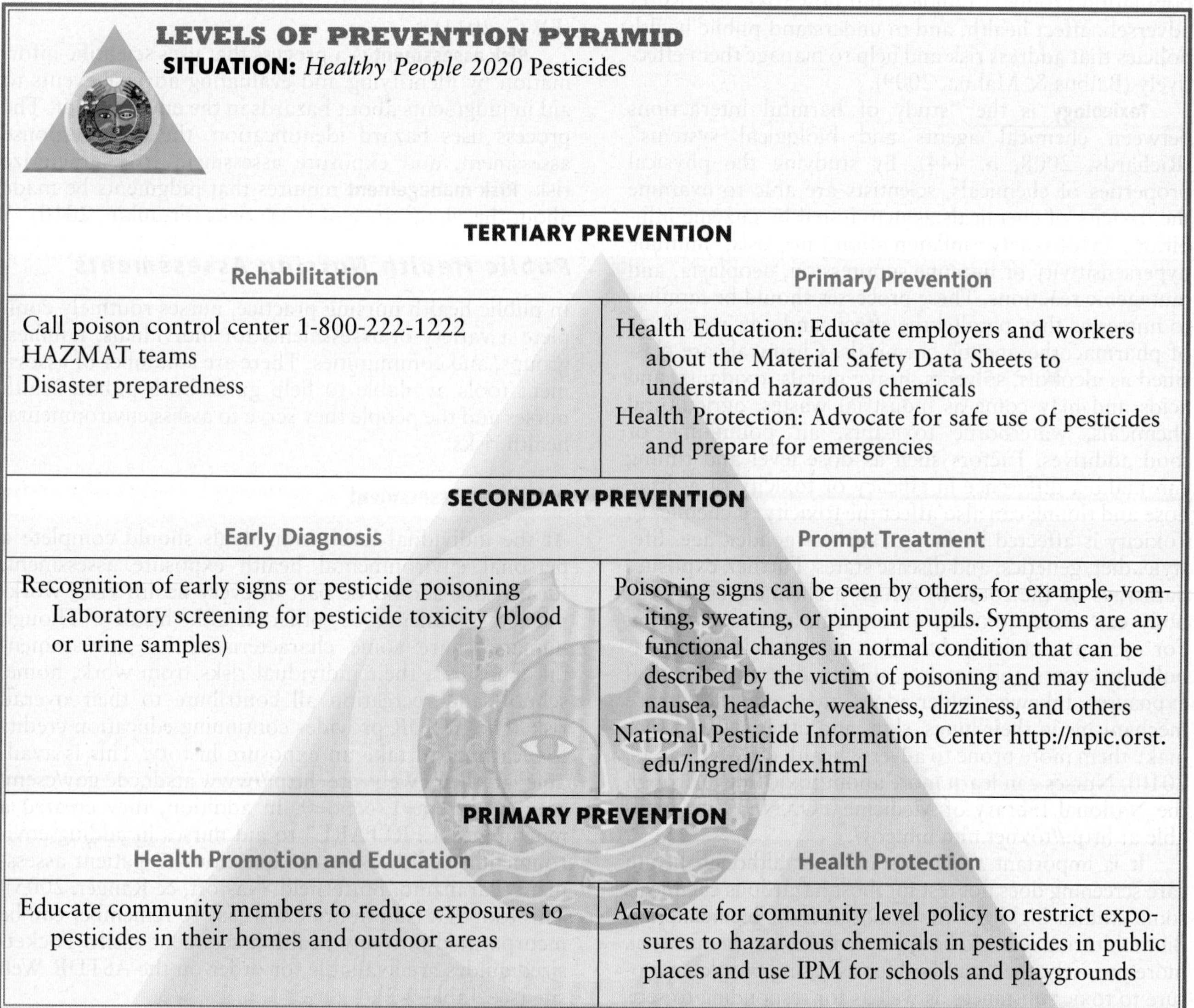

LEVELS OF PREVENTION PYRAMID

SITUATION: *Healthy People 2020* Pesticides

TERTIARY PREVENTION

Rehabilitation	Primary Prevention
Call poison control center 1-800-222-1222 HAZMAT teams Disaster preparedness	Health Education: Educate employers and workers about the Material Safety Data Sheets to understand hazardous chemicals Health Protection: Advocate for safe use of pesticides and prepare for emergencies

SECONDARY PREVENTION

Early Diagnosis	Prompt Treatment
Recognition of early signs or pesticide poisoning Laboratory screening for pesticide toxicity (blood or urine samples)	Poisoning signs can be seen by others, for example, vomiting, sweating, or pinpoint pupils. Symptoms are any functional changes in normal condition that can be described by the victim of poisoning and may include nausea, headache, weakness, dizziness, and others National Pesticide Information Center http://npic.orst.edu/ingred/index.html

PRIMARY PREVENTION

Health Promotion and Education	Health Protection
Educate community members to reduce exposures to pesticides in their homes and outdoor areas	Advocate for community level policy to restrict exposures to hazardous chemicals in pesticides in public places and use IPM for schools and playgrounds

we begin with some common types of exposures and the resultant adverse health effects. Later in the chapter, we will discuss the settings and common exposures there.

Assessment Role of PHN and Knowledge Base

While community assessment and epidemiology are essential skills for public health nursing, the ability to perform critical assessments for environmental health requires background in the environmental health sciences. Environmental health sciences include **environmental epidemiology**, toxicology, risk assessment, and risk management. Environmental epidemiology is a particular branch of epidemiology that focuses upon environmental exposures and the risks that contribute to adverse health effects such as cancer, developmental disabilities, neurological problems, reproductive health issues, or death. Environmental epidemiology seeks to better understand the specific vulnerabilities of population groups, to understand how toxic exposures adversely affect health, and to understand public health policies that address risk and help to manage them effectively (Balbus & Malina, 2009).

Toxicology is the "study of harmful interactions between chemical agents and biological systems" (Richards, 2008, p. 444). By studying the physical properties of chemicals, scientists are able to examine the toxicity of chemicals as manifested by enzyme inhibition, cytotoxicity, inflammation, necrosis, immune hypersensitivity or immune suppression, neoplasia, and mutagenic reactions. These processes should be familiar to nurses as they parallel the effects and adverse effects of pharmacotherapeutic chemicals. Chemicals are classified as alcohols, solvents, heavy metals, oxidants, and acids and may come as industrial wastes, agricultural chemicals, waterborne toxicants, air pollutants, or food additives. Factors such as dose level and timing can make a difference in efficacy or toxicity of a drug; dose and timing can also affect the toxicity of chemicals. Toxicity is affected by factors such as gender, age, lifestyle, diet, genetics, and disease states. Further, **exposure pathways** or the route by which a chemical enters the body can affect toxicity, absorption, and metabolism. For example, children have less well-developed metabolic processes and are less able to detoxify chemical exposures. Likewise, older adults have reduced defense mechanisms in their lungs, skin, and other systems that make them more prone to adverse health effects (Leffers, 2010). Nurses can learn more about toxicology through the National Library of Medicine TOXNET site available at http://toxnet.nlm.nih.gov/.

It is important to understand that although health care screening does not test for most hazardous chemicals some studies highlight the importance of **biomonitoring.** Biomonitoring refers to body burden of toxic chemicals or, more precisely, the "standard for assessing people's exposure to toxic substances as well as for responding to serious environmental public health problems" (U.S. Centers for Disease Control and Prevention [CDC], 2011b).

Nurses can learn more about the CDC National Biomonitoring Program on the CDC Web site (U.S. CDC, 2011c). Of particular interest to nurses is the study conducted by the Physicians for Social Responsibility (PSR) and titled "Hazardous Chemicals in Health Care: Snapshot of Chemicals in Doctors and Nurses." This study involved the testing of 20 doctors and nurses from a variety of practice settings around the United States for six chemicals or chemical groups totaling 62 chemicals. Each participant was found to have at least 24 hazardous chemicals in their bodies. This study is significant not only to health care workers but also their patients who are exposed to the same health care environments and chemicals (PSR, 2011). In addition, the Environmental Working Group video, "10 Americans," is a compelling argument for body burden and the importance of biomonitoring (EWG, 2011). A blood sample from a random sample of ten Americans showed that they had 287 chemicals in their blood representing exposures from waste products, commonly used chemicals in the home, as well as more than 200 chemicals and pesticides that were banned more than 30 years ago (EWG, 2011).

Risk assessment is a process that uses scientific information by identifying and evaluating adverse events to aid in judgments about hazards in the environment. The process uses hazard identification, the dose response assessment, and exposure assessment to characterize risk. **Risk management** requires that judgments be made about the significance of those risks (Frumkin, 2010).

Public Health Nursing Assessments

In public health nursing practice, nurses routinely complete a variety of assessments for individuals, families, groups, and communities. There are a number of assessment tools available to help guide both public health nurses and the people they serve to assess environmental health risks.

Individual Assessment

At the individual level, individuals should complete a personal environmental health exposure assessment. Ideally, this should be part of every health visit, workplace assessment, or other health history. Though humans share some characteristics for environmental exposures, their individual risks from work, home, school, and recreation all contribute to their overall risk. The ATSDR provides continuing education credits for learning to take an exposure history. This is available at their Web site http://www.atsdr.cdc.gov/csem/csem.asp?csem=17&po=0. In addition, they created a mnemonic "I PREPARE" to aid nurses in adding environmental health exposure questions to patient assessment (Paranzino, Butterfield, Nastoff, & Ranger, 2005). This tool that is both brief and easy to remember can be incorporated into any health assessment easily. Pocket-sized guides are available for order on the ASTDR Web site (see Table 9-3).

While completing an individual assessment, it is important to consider those exposures specific to the

Table 9.3 Environmental Health Assessment "I PREPARE"

Mnemonic Cue	Examples of Questions
I Investigate potential exposures	Do you have symptoms that occur in one setting? Have you had a sickness after coming in contact with a chemical?
P Present work	What chemicals are you exposed to in your work setting? Do you know where the MSDS safety sheets are kept?
R Residence	When was your residence built? What chemicals are stored on your property? What is your drinking water source?
E Environmental concerns	Are there environmental concerns in your neighborhood? Do you live near a hazardous waste site? Power plant? Farm? Industry?
P Past work	What work have you done in the past? Location?
A Activities	What are your hobbies? Use of pesticides?
R Referrals and resources	EPA, ASTDR, NLM, www.envirn.org
E Educate	Are materials available for education?

Source: Paranzino, G. K., Butterfield, P., Nastoff, T., & Ranger, C. (2005). I PREPARE: Development and clinical utility of an environmental exposure history mnemonic. *AAOHN Journal, 53*(1), 37–42.

workplace, school, or neighborhood. Workplace exposures are often addressed by OHNs, but include not only physical hazards such as injuries from machinery, burns, falls, and crushing injuries but also hazardous exposure to toxic chemicals, particulate matter in the form of dust, volatile organic compounds (VOCs) and aerosols, heavy metals, and components of "sick building syndrome." Sick building syndrome refers to exposures from buildings that cause adverse health effects that result from inadequate ventilation and chemical contaminants in the building. Symptoms include headaches; dizziness; nausea; irritation to the eyes, nose, or throat; coughs; and fatigue (U.S. EPA, 2011k).

School nurses often address children's and adult's exposures in school settings, but it is very important for public health nurses to identify potential risks in order to educate parents about environmental hazards in the school setting. Similar to the workplace, many schools have issues of "sick building syndrome" with the increased use of synthetics in building materials and reduced access to outdoor air. Neighborhood exposures affect individual health but are discussed in the community assessment section of this chapter. Specifically important to assess for hazards for school-aged children are the routes to school and playgrounds.

Home Assessment

Home assessments are generally completed by public health nurses who visit in a home for case-finding, follow-up, screening, or other public health services. Home assessments often look for safety hazards in the home but often do not include potential hazardous environmental toxic exposures. Families can be exposed to a number of serious environmental toxins in their own homes. Allison Del Bene Davis, PhD, RN, created a Home Environmental Health and Safety Assessment Tool at the University of Maryland Environmental Health Education Center in 2007 that is easy to use and addresses key exposure topics (Davis, 2007). These are grouped in areas such as the home itself, source of heat, gas appliances, source of water and lead pipes, fire safety, and carbon monoxide detector. This is available at www.envirn.org. In addition, public health nurses must assess the home for environmental tobacco smoke, possibility of asbestos in the home, lead paint, and other hazardous materials. Public health nurses should ensure that the family has their home tested for radon (U.S. EPA, 2011d). Likewise, family members should be reminded to safely dispose of their mercury thermometers and any other devices containing mercury. Cleaning products, paints, varnishes, strippers and other home remodeling materials, gardening fertilizers and pesticides, pest management insecticides and other materials, air fresheners, and presence of mold and moisture can all be sources of exposure in the home and land around the home. Pets can bring pesticides applied to lawns and gardens into the home, and adults and children can carry pesticides into the home on their shoes. Finally, a home assessment should address nearby environmental hazards or potential sources of hazards such as coal-fired power plants, farms, industries, Brownfield's, toxic waste sites, highways, and contaminated waterways. Frequently, these hazards are visible in the neighborhood, but often there are hidden routes of exposure from contaminated groundwater, ambient air, and contaminated soil. See Table 9-4 for common exposures in the home setting.

Community Assessment

A comprehensive community health assessment considers environmental factors in a number of ways. In Chapter 15 of this book, community health assessment

Table 9-4 Common Hazards in the Home Setting

Hazard	Source	Exposure Pathway	Risk Groups	Health Effects
Asbestos	Asbestos is a fiber that has been used for insulation and as a fire retardant. Used in shipbuilding and other occupational exposures to metal work	Inhalation	Children of metal workers Home residents	Lung cancer (mesothelioma) and lung disease
Arsenic	Used in pressure-treated wood, was formerly used in industrial sites, can be present in soil and water	Drinking water Inhalation from indoor or outdoor air	Children playing in playgrounds with pressure-treated wood, those with contaminated water supply	High levels are lethal Exposure can cause decreased red and white blood cells
Carbon monoxide	Colorless and odorless gas that is a by-product of combustion from home-heating sources as well as automobiles housed in attached garage	Inhalation	Persons with respiratory and cardiovascular disease	Unconsciousness and death due to hypoxia
Environmental tobacco smoke	Cigarette smoking	Inhalation	Those people in areas where smoking occurs in indoor space/home	Lung disease, lung cancer, cardiovascular problems
Formaldehyde	Carpeting, particle board, glues, adhesives used in home construction or decorating, also some personal care products	Inhalation		Cancer
Lead	Paint used prior to 1978; leaded gasoline prior to ban in 1970s; ceramics, pottery, pipes, soil; some alternative medical therapies	Ingestion from dust in home or soil	Children	Nervous system
Mold	Normal growth of fungi in and outside of home Can produce VOCs	Spores travel in the air Inhalation	Those people most sensitive to molds	Respiratory symptoms
Pests	Mites, cockroaches	Inhalation, physical contact with droppings	Children and those with asthma	Exacerbation of asthma
Pesticides	Used in homes and outside lawns and gardens to protect plants from pests, home from insects	Indoor or outdoor air inhalation Dermal absorption	Children All people exposed	Specific types of pesticides have been linked to neurological problems, others to cancer and many to endocrine disrupting chemicals (EDCs)
Radon	Naturally occurring radioactive gas	Seeps into homes through cracks in foundation of home	Residents of home	Lung damage particularly lung cancer
Solvents such as paint thinners, varnishes, and resins (ethers)	Dry cleaning, home improvements	Inhalation Percutaneous absorption	Home residents	Neurological problems; renal, liver, and reproductive effects
Personal care products	Shampoo, soaps, cosmetics	Percutaneous	Individuals using them, children, adolescents	Varied EDCs, cancer, and neurological effects
Volatile organic compounds (VOCs)	Alcohols, ketones, and esters that are present in thousands of products such as paint thinners, cleaning supplies, pesticides, building materials, office equipment, copiers, printers, glues, adhesives	Inhalation	Those exposed in indoor settings	Eye, nose, and throat irritation; headaches, kidney damage, and central nervous system

is introduced with a focus on aspects of the community that promote health or provide risks to health. Environment refers to more than the natural environment but also includes the **built environment,** that is, all structures (homes, schools, workplaces, and business areas), roadways, and parks and recreational areas. It includes waste disposal areas and changes in land use for agriculture and other purposes. The impact of the built environment is both indoor and outdoor physical environments, which in turn affect social environments where people live, work, and engage with others.

Community assessment is central to public health nursing practice and to the core functions of public health. For environmental health, it is imperative that nurses incorporate key assessment data into the overall assessment to identify community risks from environmental sources. Typically, a *windshield* or walking survey is very useful for observation of environmental hazards (see Chapter 15). By incorporating knowledge of likely hazards in the community, the public health nurse can identify many possible toxins simply by observation while traveling in the community. Various tools have been developed to assist nurses in their work. Though most community assessment tools address environment, it is important that public health nurses also consider specific threats for areas more broadly assessed. For air quality, nurses should look for visible sources of air pollution from smokestacks, identify exhaust from various vehicles, and learn of significant industries, power sources, and incinerators in the community. To better understand water quality, public health nurses must identify the source of drinking water as public or private, understand water treatment and quality, recognize evidence of pollution and whether there are fish alerts for local waterways, examine stagnant water and possible vectors, and identify issues related to sewer function and possible overflow and contamination and likelihood of floods and other water emergencies. Land use is another area for possible exposures. Nurses must assess not only the current land use but also how the land was formerly used. **Superfund** refers to funding made possible in 1980 by the Comprehensive Environmental Response, Compensation, and Liability Act of 1980 to address those contaminated areas of the United States that needed to be remediated. Well-known examples are Love Canal in New York State and Times Beach, Missouri. This funding is referred to as the Superfund and is administered by the EPA. Nurses must be aware of such sites in their communities that are listed on the National Priorities List. These sites can be located by searching on the EPA Web site (U.S. EPA, 2011w). **Brownfield's** sites "means real property, the expansion, redevelopment, or reuse of which may be complicated by the presence or potential presence of a hazardous substance, pollutant, or contaminant" (U.S. EPA, 2011b). These sites may remain undeveloped in communities but can also be redeveloped for public or private use. Playgrounds and schools that have been built upon former Brownfield's sites alarm community residents who often express concerns for the safety of their children. The EPA Brownfield's program seeks to ensure that the hazards are removed prior to redevelopment. EPA also promotes the successful redevelopment of sites such as the redevelopment of the Standard Times Field in New Bedford, Massachusetts, from a Brownfield's site of a former textile mill into a new industrial development in a harbor area that has brought industry and jobs to the community (U.S. EPA, 2011e). While this is a success story for the community, residents have been alarmed by the dumping of PCBs from manufacture of electrical transformers and capacitors in the city from 1935 until 1971. The PCBs were dumped on a site where the New Bedford High School, the new Keith Middle School, and the playing fields are now located. Citizens requested an environmental health assessment from the Massachusetts Department of Environmental Health as well as suing a major chemical company to recover some of the millions of dollars spent on the recovery (Evans, 2009). This example is not unique but one of thousands of examples of urban and rural communities nationwide that address the risks in their community and have a voice to advocate for the citizens of their localities.

Built Environment

The built environment refers to all aspects of our human environment that are not naturally occurring and includes not only the physical structures (dams, roadways, buildings) but also the features that contribute to social cohesiveness or disruption. Recently, environmental health experts have called for a shift from a focus upon disease causation as a result of lack of discipline and lifestyle choices and to a focus that examines how the built environment contributes to health (Jackson, 2003; Srinivasan, O'Fallon, & Dearry, 2003). Evidence suggests that many physical and mental health problems are related to the built environment such as asthma, cardiovascular disease, lung conditions, obesity, and cancer. Efforts to conduct research that demonstrates the positive effect of well-designed communities with safe walking and biking paths, environmentally safe public transportation, public spaces to encourage social interaction, and accessible green spaces for recreation will provide evidence to increase efforts to improve the built environment for health. Neighborhoods must be designed to encourage social interaction such as parks with shady areas that encourage people to congregate, ponds and trees that also help our ecological environment, and safe walkways and bikeways for access.

Public health nurses also must assess the quality of the housing stock. Buildings that were constructed prior to 1978 are likely to have lead-based paint. Homes or buildings constructed between 1930 and 1950 are likely to have asbestos in the insulation as well as in the hot water and steam pipes (U.S. Consumer Product Safety Commission, 2011). The overall condition of the community indicates sanitation factors, safe waste disposal, and contamination sources in the community. The location of schools, playgrounds, public transportation, and access to green spaces should be part of the community

PERSPECTIVES STUDENT VOICE

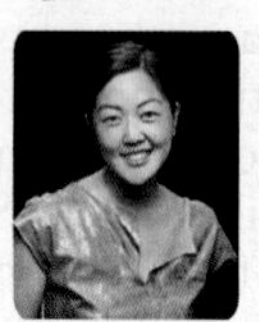

A Student's Viewpoint on Community Health Nursing: Environmental Health

Now that I am a senior nursing student, who is taking my community health nursing course and working part-time in a hospital as a collegiate aide, I am dismayed to see how much I did not know about the environment and health. What I have learned now astonishes me! I have taken steps to reduce the harmful chemicals that I am personally exposed to and have brought that information to my family and friends. After watching *The Story of Stuff* movie by Annie Leonard, I was determined to become more sustainable in my personal and professional life. I found it was not as difficult as I thought to change to less toxic products, to reduce consumption, and to recycle what I use. At work, I asked my supervisor if I might (though only a student and nurse aide) help to develop a "Green Team" to examine policies at our hospital that can be improved to reduce harmful exposures for staff and patients alike. For my community project in my clinical practicum in community health, I helped develop a carbon monoxide poisoning prevention program for the families at the federally qualified community health center where I spent the semester. We were able to disseminate the information to about 50% of the families (we serve about 15,000 city residents) and evaluations indicated that most planned to obtain carbon monoxide detectors and to take action to address specific risks in their homes. What was amazing about my project was that a fierce ice storm that came early in October forced many people to rely on generators while they were without power for more than 1 week. Many of them reported to us how grateful they were to learn about the risks of carbon monoxide poisoning while using a home generator. Wow, I never realized that I could save lives in the community too! I am now very interested in pursuing a career in public health nursing!

assessment. Examination of the overall community environment provides nurses who work in the community with essential information about how the residents can use the environment to maintain health or how the residents are more likely to be at risk for adverse health outcomes.

Sustainable Communities

Community assessments can provide evidence that a community is striving to be sustainable in practices to promote health for community members and to protect the natural environment. The President's Council in 1993 defined sustainable communities as "healthy communities where natural and historic resources are preserved, jobs are available, sprawl is contained, neighborhoods are secure, education is lifelong, transportation and health care are accessible, and all citizens have opportunities to improve the quality of their lives" (Clinton, 1993). This definition uses examples that are often considered causes of unsustainable practices such as urban sprawl that increases automobile use, use of highways, and the likelihood of agricultural practices that increasingly use pesticides and products to produce larger yields of food (Srinivasan et al., 2003). Many communities have made a commitment to become more sustainable in their city design and practices. One example is Oakland, California, where the city has established a "Sustainable Oakland" program in 1997 (City of Oakland, 2012). Oakland had suffered from poor land-use planning that created many sources for toxic exposures, noted by high rates of asthma and other environmentally related health problems (Jackson, 2012). Their goal is to provide city residents opportunities to live safe, happy, and healthy lives through sustainable development. They focus upon buildings, energy, climate, housing, land use, transportation, waste, natural resources, health, safety, education, and economic prosperity. The city has been recognized as a bicycle-friendly city, a Top Ten city by the National Resource Defense Council, and a Top Ten Sustainable City as well as recognition for solar efforts, storm management, and climate protection.

Climate issues are a great concern for health. In the community assessment, the nurse can note the presence of animal and insect vectors that can transmit disease. With **climate change**, there have been changes in the distribution of infection due to global warming. For example, locally transmitted malaria has been reported in Florida, Georgia, and Texas. Scientists track these changes and note that health professionals must be aware of the changing patterns of disease transmission from warming trends. In addition, there will likely be risks related to food and water quality and availability, heat stress for those most vulnerable, increased air pollution, and severe weather-related events. Vulnerable populations such as infants, children, and older adults must be protected from the impacts of climate change (U.S. Global Change Research Program, 2003). Severe weather events such as flooding, droughts, hurricanes, and tornados require emergency preparedness and disaster response from the public health sector (McMichael, Woodruff & Hales, 2006). Specially public health nurses must be prepared for surge events with skills such as ability to (1) be personally prepared, (2) comprehend state and local disaster plans, (3) conduct a rapid needs assessment, (4) investigate outbreaks, (5) perform public health triages, (6) communicate risk effectively,

(7) participate effectively in mass dispensing interventions, and (8) respond post event to the debriefing and public health impact of the event (Polivka et al., 2008).

Land Use

Topics that must be considered to address land use for a community health assessment include zoning regulations and enforcement; industries and their toxic releases; types of transportation with an emphasis upon sidewalks, bikeways, and public transportation; recreational space including green space; what fertilizers or pesticides are applied to the fields; safe play areas for children; and information regarding a tree ordinance to promote health environments. School locations should be examined for accessibility by foot or bicycle, surrounding area, and the use of pesticides on school fields. The community should be assessed for commercial lots, their safety and use, as well as vacant lots or unused property. Specific commercial businesses such as gas stations, auto repair shops, and dry cleaners are often sources of toxic exposures. If the community has agricultural areas, these must be assessed for irrigation practices, use of pesticides, runoff, and land-use practices. In addition, waste can be a source of environmental hazards, so public health nurses must assess the presence of landfills or municipal waste incinerators, medical waste incinerators, and municipal trash collection or presence of dumpsters throughout the community.

Leading researchers in environmental health report a research agenda that would examine the impact of community design and land use on the health of the public. Recent evidence suggests that land-use and transportation patterns and plans can influence the health of the community. The design of a city, community, or neighborhood affects physical activity, automobile dependence, ability of those of older age and physical disabilities to navigate the community, and opportunities for children to walk to school. Community design also highlights concerns for environmental justice when those who live in areas of low accessibility and high exposure to pollution are more likely to be living in poverty or of minority status. Areas they promote for further research include walking as an indicator of community health; measuring physical activity levels and contributory factors; examining the public health consequences of public safety design choices; determining the types and determinants of travel to school; examining the influence of community design on risk of injury; explaining the influence of community design on emissions of overall and specific pollutants; measuring physical activity, mobility, and social integration in persons with disabilities; characterizing social equity and health outcomes in relation to community design; and examining the influence of physical setting characteristics on mental health. For example, zoning codes that require minimum requirements for parking areas per housing unit but do not require sidewalks promote dependence upon automobile travel that increases air emissions and poor air quality, possible water contamination from auto exhaust, and risk of injury or death and reduce opportunities for safe areas for physical activity (Dannenberg et al., 2006).

Types of Toxic Exposures

Air

Air quality is a major variable in the health of populations. Those geographic areas that suffer poor air quality demonstrate higher rates of disease and adverse health effects. Ambient air, the air humans breathe, can be affected by a number of air pollutants. Air pollution is comprised of a number of materials such as aerosols, criteria air pollutants (carbon monoxide, lead, ground-level ozone, nitrogen dioxide, sulfur dioxide, particulate matter), VOCs, hydrofluorocarbons, radon, and other gases that contain toxins harmful to health. In response to the Clean Air Act of 1970, air quality is monitored by the EPA. The public is informed of air quality through the Air Quality Index (AQI) that is often reported in media sources on a daily basis. The AQI measures the criteria air pollutants in communities to see if they exceed the national air quality standard set by the EPA. The EPA publishes a *Plain English Guide to the Clean Air Act* available on their Web site for the public to learn about air quality (U.S. EPA, 2011p; 2011x).

Reports from the EPA monitoring of air pollution indicates that from 1990 to 2008 the overall levels of the six major pollutants measured by the federal government (carbon monoxide, ozone, sulfur dioxide, nitrogen dioxide, lead, and particulate matter) declined by a high of 78% for lead and a low of 14% for ozone. However, more than 127 million people in 2008 lived in areas that exceeded the national ambient air quality standard set by the U.S. EPA (2011m).

The outdoor and indoor air humans breathe can be affected by a variety of factors. Ambient air, or that air that is comprised of gases such as nitrogen, oxygen, argon, carbon dioxide, hydrogen, neon, helium, and other gases, is part of the atmosphere. It also contains moisture and particulate matter. The amount of hazardous matter that is contained in ambient air is the reason that the Clean Air Act of 1970 was created.

In an effort to inform citizens about the air quality in their own community, the EPA created the AQI, as seen in Table 9-5. The AQI is a tool to report daily air quality in communities. It is calculated for four of the six criteria air pollutants (ground-level ozone, particle pollution, carbon monoxide, and sulfur dioxide) with an emphasis upon how these affect health. On their Web site, they provide a guide for citizens to understand the importance of monitoring the ambient air, what the six criteria air pollutants are and how they affect health, and efforts to monitor air quality to provide public health advisories (U.S. EPA, 2011a).

Public health nurses must understand the adverse effects of ambient air pollution in order to assess, monitor, and advocate for those most vulnerable that include children, people with lung disease, older adults, and even healthy individuals who are active outdoors. Health

Table 9-5 Air Quality Index

AQI Value	Level of Health Concern	Color
When AQI is in this range ...	Air quality conditions are ...	As symbolized by this color
0–50	Good	Green
51–100	Moderate	Yellow
101–150	Unhealthy for sensitive groups	Orange
151–200	Unhealthy	Red
201–300	Very unhealthy	Purple
301–500	Hazardous	Maroon

AIRNow. Air Quality Index (AQI)—A Guide to Air Quality and Your Health http://www.epa.gov/airnow/aqi_brochure_08-09.pdf
Each category corresponds to a different level of health concern. The six levels of health concern and what they mean are:

- "Good" AQI is 0–50. Air quality is considered satisfactory, and air pollution poses little or no risk.
- "Moderate" AQI is 51–100. Air quality is acceptable; however, for some pollutants, there may be a moderate health concern for a very small number of people. For example, people who are unusually sensitive to ozone may experience respiratory symptoms.
- "Unhealthy for sensitive groups" AQI is 101–150. Although general public is not likely to be affected at this AQI range, people with lung disease, older adults, and children are at a greater risk from exposure to ozone, whereas persons with heart and lung disease, older adults, and children are at greater risk from the presence of particles in the air.
- "Unhealthy" AQI is 151–200. Everyone may begin to experience some adverse health effects, and members of the sensitive groups may experience more serious effects.
- "Very unhealthy" AQI is 201–300. This would trigger a health alert signifying that everyone may experience more serious health effects.
- "Hazardous" AQI >300. This would trigger a health warning of emergency conditions. The entire population is more likely to be affected.

effects include irritation of the respiratory system with inflammation of the cell lining. This makes the lungs more susceptible to infection. Air pollution can also exacerbate asthma, chronic lung disease, and reduced lung function and cause permanent lung damage. In addition, air pollution causes increased risk of cardiac disease, in particular, acute myocardial infarctions and arrhythmias (U.S. EPA, 2011a). Indoor air quality is particularly important for home, school, and workplace assessments. During advisories when the ambient AQI is high and people are asked to remain inside, humans are exposed to those pollutants that commonly affect indoor air. Air pollution in homes occurs from exposure to heating or combustion sources such as oil, coal, kerosene, or wood; radon gas; secondhand smoke from cigarettes; building materials and furniture that contains pressed wood products; carpeting and adhesives that emit VOCs; asbestos in insulation; cleaning products, paints, varnishes, and paint removers; personal care products; and sources used around the home such as pesticides. Mild health effects might be headaches and nausea; the more serious health effects include damage to the liver, kidneys, and central nervous system as well as cancer. In addition, molds, dust, and known asthma triggers in the home can exacerbate not only the asthma symptoms but also cause irritation to those with heart and lung conditions. Air quality in school buildings is very important for staff, teachers, and students. More than 53 million children and 6 million adults spend up to 6 to 8 hours in school each day. In particular, children are at increased risk for a variety of reasons. Young children are more likely to spend time on or near the floor where toxins are likely to settle and use more hand-to-mouth behavior, and they take in more air per size than adults. While exposures can be the same as in the home, those who attend or work in schools are in the same air environment for 6 to 8 hours or more where they are exposed to the toxins for long periods of time (U.S. EPA, 2011v). Nurses who work in the school setting can access information through the EPA Web site to aid in assessments and interventions to improve air quality in schools. The HealthySEAT tool (Healthy School Environments Assessment Tool) is available on their Web site (U.S. EPA, 2011i).

Water

Water is an element for human survival as the human body is composed of upwards of 50% to 60% water. So too, water is necessary for human survival. In public health, the concern is for safe water consumption, safe lakes, rivers, and streams for recreation, as well as safe waterways to support animal and plant life necessary for transport of nutrients and ecology of the environment. Globally, the availability of clean water is becoming a very serious threat to human survival. Estimates are that by 2025, 1.8 billion people will be living in countries or regions with severe water scarcity (United Nations, 2011). Reports identify the lack of safe drinking water as the leading cause of hunger, disease, and poverty worldwide (Global Water, 2011).

Water in the environment is available in two forms: surface water and ground water. Lakes, rivers, and streams are examples of surface water as is the surface runoff from rainfall. Groundwater is found in underground aquifers that run beneath the surface of the earth. Both are sources of contamination or pollution. Drinking water is available from both surface and groundwater. Surface water sources include lakes and streams and municipal reservoirs for water use. Underground sources include aquifers that run beneath the ground level and are reached via wells and springs. Many municipalities use reservoirs and other surface sources for their water supply, while in many areas people rely upon wells to provide their source of water. Safe drinking water is essential for human health. Public water systems provide water for community members through pipes for human consumption. More than 90% of Americans are served by public water systems. Public water systems are monitored and regulated through the EPA. These regulations require that public water suppliers protect consumers from microorganisms that harm health. The EPA does not regulate private sources of water from private wells and individual users must be responsible for monitoring their own wells. As a result, those using private wells are likely to have fecal contamination or microorganisms in their water as well as a number of toxic agents that are linked to bladder, kidney, and liver cancers (Friis, 2012).

Water can become contaminated from a number of sources both point and nonpoint sources. Point sources are those that can be traced to one source such as a wastewater facility release into municipal water or discharge from an industrial site. Nonpoint sources are runoff from agricultural areas, gasoline stations, and other contaminants carried by rain and waterways. Some common water contaminants are microbial (frequently Cryptosporidium and Giardia), and to rid public water systems of microorganisms, disinfection processes are used. These disinfects that are chlorine based produce disinfection by products that can also be hazardous to health. Additionally, other inorganic (such as nitrogen derivatives, arsenic, lead, fluoride, cadmium, and mercury) and organic chemicals (commonly organophosphates, phthalates) as well as radionuclides are frequent contaminants (U.S. EPA, 2011g). More recently, there is a global concern about pharmaceutical waste contaminants in water. In a study by the U.S. Geological Survey in 1999 to 2000, chemicals such as medications for humans and animals, natural and synthetic hormones, metabolites, pesticides, insecticides, plasticizers, and fire retardants were found in 80% of the streams sampled (Health Care Without Harm, 2011). Not only are pharmaceuticals used by humans, excreted in their urine, and discarded into locations where they can reach water supplies, but also animals are fed hormones and antibiotics in animal feeding operations that also leech into water supplies (Snyder, Westerhoff, Yoon, & Sedlak, 2003). Public health nurses must be aware of this source of water contamination that puts vulnerable population groups such as the growing fetus, infants and children, older adults, and those with compromised immunity at great risk. Organizations such as Health Care Without Harm seek to address the pharmaceutical waste issue though measures that address production, use, discharge and disposal, treatment in wastewater facilities, and collection of unused medications.

Food

Food quality and safety is essential to human health. Food quality refers to the relative nutritional value, cost, and variety of food available. The Centers for Disease Control and Prevention (CDC) estimates that each year more than 3,000 people die from foodborne illness and one in six Americans become ill from food consumption (U.S. CDC, 2011a). Public health nurses work closely with environmental sanitarians in state and local health departments who routinely monitor food establishments for their safety in order to prevent exposure to microbial agents that cause foodborne illness. Issues that affect food quality extend beyond the microbial exposures and include the availability of adequate nutritious food, chemical exposures through food additives and from agrichemicals and antibiotics, contaminated food from diseased animals, and improper food handling. Pesticides are ubiquitous in the environment and are transmitted to humans through foods. Fresh fruits and vegetables must be thoroughly washed to remove pesticide residue. In addition, antibiotics fed to animals in animal feeding operations are transmitted through food (U.S. EPA, 2011o).

Risks occur at all points from food production to food consumption. For example, agrichemicals such as chemical fertilizers and pesticides are applied in the production of fruits and vegetables while hormones and antibiotics are often fed to animals in animal feeding operations. Pesticides have been found in foods, particularly in strawberries, blueberries, and apples (Gilden, Huffing, & Sattler, 2010). After production, many foods are processed for market. Food additives such as dyes and flavors provide the color and often improve flavor of foods. Leavening and thickening agents improve consistency while preservatives keep food from spoiling on the shelf. Many of these additives can be harmful to health with examples being linked to cancer and endocrine disruption. Recently, there is a concern about genetically modified foods being marketed. These concerns address not only the safety of the food for human consumption but raise questions about the ecological impact and sustainability. While the U.S. Department of Agriculture sets policy for practices such as this, many organizations call for a more thorough examination of the consequences of this practice (Baker & Burnham, 2001; U.S. EPA, 2011t; Whitney, Maltby, & Carr, 2004). In addition, food is often irradiated to kill microorganisms. While many experts cite the safety of this process that can reduce the risk of microbial contamination, there can be concern for the use of radiation in any form to the workers and local community members (U.S. CDC, 2011b). After production, food is stored, transported, and prepared for sale in markets. At each phase of this food cycle, there are risks from improper food handling, refrigeration, or time in transit that affect the quality and safety of the food.

Microbial outbreaks are common from a variety of bacteria (*Shigella*, *Salmonella*, *Campylobacter*, *Escherichia coli*) and parasites (*Cryptosporidium parvum*, *amoeba*). While the public often hears about these outbreaks through the media, they may not be as aware of the risks from chemical contaminants. The U.S. Food and Drug Administration is charged with the responsibility to ensure the safety of food produced, shipped, imported, and sold in the United States. This includes not only the monitoring of microbial toxins but also chemicals such as lead and cadmium, pesticides, food additives, and packaging (U.S. FDA, 2011). While the FDA operates to insure that the genetically modified foods meet the same safety standards as other foods, the technology used to modify or engineer new food varieties from plant and animal breeding techniques is expanding rapidly (U.S. EPA, 2011t).

Vulnerable Groups

Public health nurses must also be aware of the increased vulnerability of certain groups. For example, pregnant women are likely to transmit their exposure to chemicals, pesticides, and toxins to the unborn fetus; children are more susceptible to hazards from food due to their immature gastrointestinal systems and increased food intake per size compared to adults; and those with altered immunity due to cancer, diabetes, and other health conditions are more likely to be affected by food exposures.

In addition, the effect of climate change upon weather extremes (droughts, foods, and storms) changes in rainfall and water supply for soil, and the ecology of microbial growth will have negative impacts upon the food supply. Globally, these changes can also affect human health (U.S. EPA, 2011f). Scientists report the risks for waterborne and foodborne pathogens in drinking water, seafood, and fresh produce from climate variability and the potential for ecological changes that can affect watershed and drainage (Rose et al., 2001)

Exposure to waterborne and foodborne pathogens can occur via drinking water (associated with fecal contamination), seafood (due to natural microbial hazards, toxins, or wastewater disposal), or fresh produce (irrigated or processed with contaminated water). Weather influences the transport and dissemination of these microbial agents via rainfall and runoff and the survival and/or growth through such factors as temperature. Federal and state laws and regulatory programs protect much of the US population from waterborne disease; however, if climate variability increases, current and future deficiencies in areas such as watershed protection, infrastructure, and storm drainage systems will probably increase the risk of contamination events. Knowledge about transport processes and the fate of microbial pollutants associated with rainfall and snowmelt is key to predicting risks from a change in weather variability. Although recent studies identified links between climate variability and occurrence of microbial agents in water, the relationships need further quantification in the context of other stresses. In the marine environment as well, there are few studies that adequately address the potential health effects of climate variability in combination with other stresses such as overfishing, introduced species, and rise in sea level. Advances in monitoring are necessary to enhance early-warning and prevention capabilities. Application of existing technologies, such as molecular fingerprinting to track contaminant sources or satellite remote sensing to detect coastal algal blooms, could be expanded. This assessment recommends incorporating a range of future scenarios of improvement plans for current deficiencies in the public health infrastructure to achieve more realistic risk assessments.

Toxic Waste

Waste Management

Individuals, families, schools, governmental agencies, health care facilities, and industries all create waste that must be managed to minimize environmental impact and to protect human health. The EPA reports that in 2009, Americans generated about 243 million tons of trash, a rate higher than all other countries. However, Americans also recycled and composted 82 million tons of these waste products. In response to efforts nationwide to reduce, reuse, and recycle, the average amount of waste per person sent to landfills has decreased during the last 50 years to a low of 2.36 pounds per person per day. This means that since 1990 the amount of municipal solid waste headed for landfills decreased from 145.3 million in 1990 to 131.9 million tons in 2009 (U.S. EPA, 2011l). As landfills enlarge, many municipalities have chosen to incinerate municipal waste. Waste incineration produces particulate air pollution and releases toxins into areas where they affect water and food sources.

More problematic for human health are the hazardous wastes that are produced. These wastes include solvent wastes, dioxins, and wastes from electroplating and other metal finishing operations, wastes from oil refineries, organic chemicals, pesticides, explosives, lead processing materials, and wood preservatives. Communities may be burdened with many Brownfield's sites as well as those listed on the National Priorities List of hazardous sites as Superfund sites (U.S. EPA, 2011w). Humans are exposed to these chemicals if they are aerosolized into the ambient air, leech into groundwater or wells, and reach the soil where children play or crops are produced. What is particularly dangerous for human exposure is the fact that most community members are unaware of the hazards in their communities. See from the case files.

Toxic Waste and Communities

Many nurses have become aware of communities affected by toxic waste through films such as "A Civil Action" and "Erin Brockovich." Both films highlighted real community stories where community residents were exposed to hazards through the water they drank from public water systems. In the first movie released in 1998, residents of Woburn, Massachusetts, were exposed to trichloroethylene (TCE) through contamination of the town's water supply. The hazardous chemical leeched from buried storage at the site of a former tannery, affected residents of the community, and was identified as the source of a leukemia cluster in the community. The latter film, released in 2000, depicted the true story of Erin Brockovich who worked for an attorney in Hinckley, California, and brought suit against Pacific

From the Case Files I

Scenario

Harbor City is a small coastal New England city of about 85,000 residents. Formerly, much of Harbor City's economy came from industries that supported manufacturing of textiles, electronic components, dyes, metals, and other industrial materials. Some still operate while others have closed. This has also had a negative impact upon the economy of the community, both public services and private incomes. Currently, there are many Brownfield's located in the community and one Superfund site. Recently, there have been increasing rates of various cancers, birth defects, and neurological disorders. As a public health nurse working in this community, you have been asked to help a local citizen's group to better understand what they perceive is an increase in illness in their community related to environmental causes. Community residents indicate that recent publicity surrounding this issue has caused concern about housing values, safety for children in city schools, and fears about what is not known about neighborhood exposures.

Questions:

1. Discuss how to obtain accurate assessment data about the morbidity rates of the various cancers, birth defects, and neurological disorders.
2. Describe the role of the public health nurse working with communities to improve their environmental health and safety.
3. Identify three interventions that you might employ. Be sure to consider collaboration with other groups or organizations.
4. Discuss how interventions that might address the following levels of prevention: primary, secondary, and tertiary.
5. How would you evaluate any nursing intervention?
6. Identify ethical concerns for the public health nurse working with this community.
7. How might you identify issues related to environmental justice in this situation?

Gas and Electric for the contamination of residential water supply with hexavalent chromium used to prevent rust in the machinery at the plant. Hexavalent chromium is a known carcinogen. The suit represented more than 1,000 people affected by the release of hexavalent chromium in their water.

Radiation

Humans are exposed to radiation in a variety of forms. Risks and forms of radiation are generally categorized as ionizing and nonionizing radiation. Ionization refers to the process where the atomic particle (ion) breaks away from the nucleus of the atom. Ionizing radiation occurs in natural forms as radon gas and cosmic radiation from the atmosphere. Radon is a leading cause of death from lung cancer. As an odorless gas, it can seep into the foundation of homes from the ground and expose home residents to the radiation effects. Nonionizing radiation refers to radiation from sources such as infrared, microwave, and radio wave radiation (U.S. EPA, 2011q, 2011r).

Policy Development

Community health nurses, once informed about the risks to health through environmental exposures, participate in the other core functions of public health for environmental health nursing. Policy development is the core function that addresses the need for legislation to protect human health but also the opportunities for nurses to engage communities to address their own health and create policy specific to their needs.

Nurses must be a catalyst for change in order to protect community members from hazards in the environment. To advocate for change, public health nurses must be informed about the hazards in the community, existing legislation that protects people in the community, and governmental and nongovernmental groups in communities that can be partners in the efforts to protect health (Gilden, 2003). To advance nursing knowledge in Michigan, The Nurse and the Environment: Tools for Action (NETFA) program was developed to increase nurse's knowledge of environmental risks and promote advocacy for change (Ortner, 2004).

Nurses can begin their advocacy work by writing letters to their legislators to support strengthening laws as TSCA (Toxic Substances Control Act) or FIFRA (Federal Insecticide, Fungicide, and Rodenticide Act). Recommendations to reform TSCA include roles for nurses to lobby their legislators but to also inform community members about the need for reform (Denison, 2009). Additionally, letters to local newspapers and periodicals can remind community members of safe practices in the home and personal use of chemicals. Nurses can present testimony at public forums or hearings. As knowledgeable and trusted members of the community, public health nurses help to educate and empower community members (Afzal, 2003).

Public health nurses can organize public educational programs in schools and agencies in their community to inform the public about local hazards in their homes, schools, and communities and to learn about resources to help reduce their exposures. In order to facilitate community involvement in environmental health issues, nurses can help build coalitions in the community to partner with other organizations to promote healthy communities. Public health nurses serve on local and national committees and boards to advocate for change. Examples of agencies where nurses play an advocacy role are the Children's Environmental Health Network,

EPA Children's Health Protection Advisory Committee, Just Green Partnership, local and country environmental groups, state nurses association environmental affairs committees, EPA Pesticide Committee, and Health Care Without Harm to name just a few. Nurses engaged in environmental health research can share the findings of successful environmental health nursing interventions to promote policy change.

In order for nurses to function effectively as advocates for safer environments, it is essential to be aware of important legislation for environmental health. To learn more about important legislation for environmental protection, see Display 9.3 for a list of laws enacted in the United States. Nurses can also use the EnviRN Web site to follow current advocacy efforts in nursing practice (EnviRN, 2011). An example where nurses participated in important advocacy was the National Day of Action on August 10, 2011, where nurses across the United States took action to promote healthier environments by calling attention the Safe

DISPLAY 9.3 IMPORTANT ENVIRONMENTAL PROTECTION LEGISLATION

Clean Air Act (CAA) 1970

The Clean Air Act was established in 1970 to exact controls on air quality through regulation of both stationary (industrial) sources and mobile sources. Through this act, the National Ambient Air Quality Standards were created, and the Environmental Protection Agency (EPA) was created and assumed the regulatory responsibility for monitoring these standards. While this legislation has been amended at various times since 1970, it continues to be the major source of control for air pollution.

Occupational Safety and Health Act (OSHA) 1970

In 1970, congress passed the Occupational and Safety Health Act to protect workers and promote workplace safety. This act served to protect workers in their place of employment from hazards to their safety and health. This act is regulated through the Occupational Safety and Health Administration and is supported by the work of the National Institute for Occupational Safety and Health. It is designed to protect workers from exposure to toxic chemicals, heat or cold stress, and mechanical dangers in the workplace, unsafe noise levels, or unsanitary conditions.

Federal Insecticide, Fungicide, and Rodenticide Act (FIFRA) 1972

Congress passed an early version of the Federal Insecticide, Fungicide, and Rodenticide Act (FIFRA) in 1947. Through this act, EPA regulates pesticides through the registration process of chemical manufacturing and enforcement of compliance with banned or unregistered pesticides.

Safe Drinking Water Act (SDWA) 1974

Congress passed the Safe Drinking Water Act (SDWA) in 1974 to protect health by ensuring that water quality of the public water supply would comply with water quality standards. This act is regulated by the EPA to oversee that state and local water supplies meet standards. This act has been amended since 1974, and threats to safe water are reviewed regularly. Primary contaminant sources include human and animal waste, pesticides, hazardous chemicals, and some naturally occurring hazards that get into the water supply.

Toxic Substances Control Act (TSCA) 1976

The Toxic Substances Control Act passed in 1976 addresses the production, use, and disposal of specific chemicals, but various materials such as food, drugs, pesticides, cosmetics, and personal care products are excluded.

Clean Water Act (CWA) 1977

The Clean Water Act (CWA) provides basic structure for regulating discharges of pollutants into the waters of the United States as well as regulating quality standards for surface waters. Wastewater standards are set and regulated to control hazardous contamination of water.

The Comprehensive Environmental Response, Compensation, and Liability Act (Superfund) 1980

Superfund is the name given to the environmental program established to address abandoned hazardous waste sites. It is also the name of the fund established by the Comprehensive Environmental Response, Compensation, and Liability Act (CERCLA) of 1980, commonly referred to as Superfund, created a program to fund remediation of hazardous waste sites. CERCLA was created in response to the discovery of toxic waste dumps in the 1970s. By taxing the petroleum and chemical industries, the funds were provided for the cleanup of the most damaging toxic waste sites.

Emergency Planning and Right to Know Act 1986

This act is often referred to as "Community Right to Know." This legislation helps communities to ensure environmental safety from hazardous chemicals. Through state and local planning, communities establish emergency planning committees. This act enables the pubic to gain access to information to increase their knowledge of chemicals in individual locations, their uses, and how they are released into the environment.

Chemicals Act of 2011 introduced on April 15, 2011, by Senator Frank Lautenberg (D—NJ). This legislation would improve the regulation of chemical toxins that are currently regulated under the Toxic Chemicals Safety Act (TSCA) of 1976. The limitations of TSCA are that more than 60,000 of the 80,000 chemicals in use today are not tested for safety due to the fact that their safety was "grandfathered" in 1976 (EnviRN, 2011).

Assurance

The regulatory function for policy ensures that appropriate services are provided. This public health function demands that public health nurses must incorporate environmental health principles into practice. For example, a nurse can educate families to reduce their risks from environmental hazards in the home, an OHN will ensure that safety regulations are followed in the work settings, or a school nurse can ensure that indoor air quality is monitored for the school setting. Assurance guarantees that policy and regulatory functions are followed through the provision of essential services. Nurses are vital to assuring that essential services are provided in the community. The following examples illustrate how community nurses fulfill the assurance function.

Home

People spend large amounts of time in their homes where environmental hazards contribute to serious adverse health effects and death. Nurses who work with families and in communities participate in research programs and collaborative projects that can impact home environments. The Healthy Children, Healthy Homes project implemented in Miami, Florida, provides educational programs for parents of children in elementary school on asthma triggers in the home and how to best reduce those exposures (Brooten et al., 2008). To address some of the health issues, particularly for children, the U.S. Department of Housing and Urban Development (HUD) (2001) created the Healthy Homes Initiative to protect children and their families from health and safety hazards in their homes. The program targets multiple childhood diseases and injuries in the home by using a comprehensive approach. Some of the environmental health concerns addressed by the Healthy Homes Initiative are lead, carbon monoxide, pesticides, radon, mold, home safety, and asthma. In Ohio, public health nurses collaborated with other professionals (program manager, health educator, sanitarians, community outreach worker) through a Healthy Homes Program grant to perform housing control assessments, education, and interventions in housing units. The interventions included home visits and education and were found to reduce asthma symptoms, schools days missed, work days missed, and number of emergency room visits for asthma events (Polivka, Chaudry, Crawford, Bouton, & Sweet, 2011). A Healthy Homes Program headed by public health nurses in Baltimore, MD, focused upon home assessments for environmental health risks (lead, asthma triggers, carbon monoxide, pesticide use, environmental tobacco smoke as well as source of heating in the home). Other components of the program were educational sessions to review home environmental health risks and a targeted hazard reduction intervention (U.S. Department of HUD, 2001; 2011b). In Lowell, Massachusetts, public health nurses were involved in a Healthy Homes grant to improve training and education among community and faith-based organizations to develop culturally appropriate home assessments and educational tools for a culturally diverse population in the community (U.S. Department of HUD, 2001; 2011a). Researchers have examined public awareness of risks of radon in the home and determined that knowledge of radon risk was low, and as a result, families did not use radon detectors to reduce their risks (Hill, Butterfield, & Larsson, 2006). In response to this finding, public health nurses should increase their efforts to educate community members about radon risks.

Severe Weather Events

A second area for nurses to assure that essential services are provided to community members is in response to severe weather events. In 2011, extreme weather events caused damage and destruction across the United States. Severe blizzards in the north began in early January, followed by more than 1,500 confirmed tornados during the spring and summer causing damage in many areas of the country and killing more than 500 people. Flooding of the Mississippi and Missouri Rivers caused serious damage from northern Montana to areas of the south, while Hurricane Irene caused widespread flooding in New England and the mid-Atlantic areas. Texas reported more than 100 days where the temperature was above 100 degrees and severe drought in Texas and Oklahoma caused wildfires that destroyed more than 3 million acres of land (Erdman, 2011). While the world's attention was focused upon the serous earthquake and tsunami in Honshu, Japan, in March 2011, the United States had notable earthquakes in Alaska, Arkansas, California, Colorado, Oklahoma, Oregon, and Virginia during that same year. While none were as serious as those reported in other parts of the world, the loss of power from earthquakes and hurricanes put many people at risk from natural disasters (U.S. Geological Survey, 2011).

While Chapter 17 discusses disasters and the role for public health, there are some specific issues related to environmental risks that occur after severe weather events. These include power outages, safe water and food supply, wastewater, mold, and toxic exposures. For example, when there is a power outage, many families depend upon generators to supply electricity. These can be a source of carbon monoxide poisoning if not effectively functioning or not well ventilated. During cold weather, families may use wood or kerosene for heat that can pose danger of fire, explosion, and asphyxiation from carbon monoxide, but kerosene heaters can also emit other pollutants including carbon dioxide, nitrogen dioxide, and sulfur dioxide. In particular, pregnant

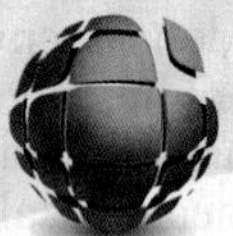

EVIDENCE-BASED PRACTICE

Public Health Nurses' Interventions to Address Environmental Health Risks in the Home Setting

In a study to test the effectiveness of a multirisk social cognitive intervention with low-income parents in the rural Northwest, researchers found that public health nursing interventions were effective in increasing self-efficacy and precaution adoption. Ten county public health nurses in Whatcom County, Washington, and in Gallatin County, Montana, delivered the intervention that included four home visits over a 4- to 6-week period. Biomarkers for lead and cotinine as well as household samples for water quality, radon, carbon monoxide, and evidence of moisture were collected from 235 families (including 399 adults and 441 children) to identify specific environmental risks in each single dwelling home. The intervention was developed using the CDC Healthy Homes Initiative (CDC). As part of the home visits, the public health nurses used an interactive book to review environmental health risks common in the home setting. These included carbon monoxide, radon, mold/mildew, lead, environmental tobacco smoke, and water quality. Public health nurses shared the results of the biomarker and household measures with the participants to share what were below or above threshold levels and to teach the parents about remediation for those risks above threshold levels using standard messages developed in consultation with technical experts. The results of the screening showed that 64% of the homes had at least one risk and 23% had more than one risk. In particular, the study examined parent's environmental self-efficacy and stage of environmental health precaution adoption using the Weinstein Precaution Adoption Process Model. The results indicated that the increase in self-efficacy scores pre- and postintervention time periods increased 1.5 (general effects) and three times greater (risk-specific effects) for those who received the public health nurse intervention than for the control group. Of all the specific risks, the only one that did not show significant change in precaution adoption was environmental tobacco smoke. This study demonstrates that public health nursing interventions to inform families about and to take appropriate precautions for environmental health risks are effective in increasing self-efficacy and precaution adoption.

Questions:

- This study was conducted in a rural region—would you expect to see similar results in a more urban setting; why or why not?
- What may have been contributing factors for the low demonstrated reduction in tobacco smoke?
- Do the study results have implications for other types of PHN interventions?

Reference: Butterfield, P. G., Hill, W., Postma, J., Butterfield, P. W., & Odom-Maryon, T. (2011). Effectiveness of a household environmental health intervention delivered by rural public health nurses. *American Journal of Public Health,* 101(S1), S262–S270.

women, asthmatics, individuals with cardiovascular disease, older adults, and young children are at particular risk from these toxic emissions. Nurses must inform community members of safety in the home when using alternate sources of heat or power. If a home is without power, there is a risk for food storage and safety. If the home has a well and water pump, there may not be access to water during the power outage. Community members should be informed of issues related to safe storage of food and the need to dispose of improperly refrigerated foods.

Homes that have septic systems may find that they have overflowed if there is any flooding from a severe storm. It is important to understand when it is safe to return to using a well or septic system after ground-level flooding. Floods also pose a problem to residents who have water enter their home. Standing water can cause mold and mildew, possibly harm home furnaces, pose a risk of fire, and release toxins into the water and air. Small children and older adults are at more risk of environmental exposures during and after a natural disaster and the public health nurse must address not only emergency planning but also safe remediation strategies to avoid toxic exposures among community members (U.S. EPA, 2011n).

Food Safety in the Community

Another area where nurses can assure health and safety for environmental health risks is for food safety. Public health nurses participate in efforts to ensure food safety through the prevention of foodborne illness. A great resource for families and community members is the Partnership for Food Safety Education (2011) that promotes safe food handling and education for both children and adults. However, as discussed earlier, food can also be a source of hazardous chemicals both from pesticides and fertilizers used but also from other chemicals found in soil, packaging, and cookware. Nurses can be a resource to ensure that community members learn about the specific risks, particularly in their own localities and identify ways to decrease their risk. The

EPA produces a booklet entitled *Citizen's Guide to Pesticides and Pesticide Safety* that is available from the EPA Web site (U.S. EPA, 2011c). The booklet is written to help nonprofessionals understand pesticides. While it is not directly focused upon pesticides in food, it helps community members understand the hazards present in pesticides and strategies to reduce their use and to ensure safety when using pesticides. The Pesticide Action Network (2011) uses data from the USDA Pesticide Program to identify commonly applied pesticides for many foods. Consumers can consult their Web site to be informed of foods that pose the most serious threats to health, particularly for the most vulnerable groups.

One specific area where nurses have been involved in education, advocacy, and policy efforts is with fish advisories. The EPA National Listing of Fish Advisories reports that 18.3 million lake acres and 1.5 million river miles are under advisory. This represents 44% of the nation's lake acreage and 41% of the nation's total river miles. Advisories warn consumers of contaminants (mercury, PCBs, chlordane, dioxins, and DDT). These contaminants persist in the environment, particularly in river and lake sediments where fish consume them from bottom-feeding organisms. **Bioaccumulation** refers to the process where toxins accumulate in greater concentration in an organism than the rate of elimination. Toxins can accumulate from direct exposure or from eating contaminated food products. Through biomagnifications, the toxins present at lower levels of the food chain are in greater concentration in those species further up the chain. Therefore, humans who eat contaminated fish are exposed to toxins at all levels across the food chain. Public health nurse and Georgetown University faculty member, Dr. Laura Anderko (2011) has been involved with fish advisories for many years. She prepared the educational set of four modules in collaboration with the EPA: *Fish Facts for Health Professionals: Methylmercury Exposure, Fish Consumption, and Health Risks/Benefits*. This is available through the Web site www.fish-facts.org.

Nurses who work with community agencies can use collaborative strategies to ensure that the population served is protected from environmental hazards, learns how to advocate for a safer community, and identifies appropriate sources of information. The Right to Know legislation and use of material Data Safety Sheets are ways that the public can be protected and learn how to protect themselves as well. Public health nurses can direct community members to consult the EPA Web site to learn about their right to know. One link connects to "your own community" and how to learn more about the risks for one's own community and how to address specific pollution and ensure safe drinking water (U.S. EPA, 2011s). Nurses can teach their community partners how to access a consumer confidence report. Every public water system is required to provide information to consumers that identify any detected contaminants or factors that affect the water quality for those customers that they serve. Common contamination is microbial or from chemicals in fertilizers and others such as lead and arsenic. This responsibility to provide the public with information about public water systems is mandated through the Safe Drinking Water Act enacted in 1974 that established standards for safe drinking water. Individuals can access information from their own water supplier or can visit the EPA Web site (U.S. EPA, 2011u). In addition, public health nurses can access for themselves and their community partners, the EPA resource, *Water on Tap: What you Need to Know* that is available in English, Chinese, and Spanish through the EPA Web site. This guide not only discusses the safety of public water systems but what individuals using well water can do to ensure the safety of their drinking water. Ways to conserve water use are addressed as well as the various types of treatment devices such as filters that can be used at the point of entry or point of use for the water in one's home (U.S. EPA, 2011y).

Environmental Justice

One final area where nurses must be informed to promote health in communities is the issue of environmental justice. The EPA defines **environmental justice** as "the fair treatment and meaningful involvement of all people regardless of race, color, national origin, or income with respect to the development, implementation, and enforcement of environmental laws, regulations, and policies" (U.S. EPA, 2011h). In communities across the United States, people of color, low-income, and tribal communities bear a higher burden of exposures to environmental risks where they live (Bullard, Johnson, & Torres, 2011). In a study of 368 communities in the Commonwealth of Massachusetts using U.S. Census Data, environmental data, income data, and geographic information on 17 different types of environmentally hazardous sites, researchers found that hazardous sites were disproportionately located in communities of color and where the population was low income (Faber & Krieg, 2002). Children are at particular risk in such disadvantaged communities where they have cumulative risk from exposures in homes, schools, and neighborhoods. Developmental and behavioral factors make children more vulnerable to environmental contaminants, and they have little control over where they live, what they eat, or the socioeconomic factors of their lives. Poor and minority children who are more likely to live in neighborhoods with incinerators, industrial plants, toxic waste sites, and poor quality housing show higher rates of asthma, learning disabilities, and elevated blood lead levels than nonminority children and those who come from more affluent families (Powell & Stewart, 2001). A variety of factors contribute to environmental health disparities; those living in affected areas experience challenges related to physical infrastructure, vulnerability/susceptibility, proximity to sources or environmental hazards, unique exposure pathways, multiple cumulative environmental burdens, chronic psychosocial stress, and diminished capacity to participate in decision making (Bullard, 2005; Nweke et al., 2011).

Findings such as these are noted in all areas of the United States. Strategies to address the inequalities and improve the safety of all communities include building capacity within affected communities to proactively leverage resources with government and other institutions, promoting dialogue to achieve environmental justice, and to identify successful models of collaboration (Lee, 2002). Communities are able to promote healthier environments through community development, community organizing, and community empowerment by working with advocacy groups, networking, and educational programming (Powell & Stewart, 2001).

Nurses who work in communities observe the impact of health disparities with those people living in poverty or of minority status bearing the greatest health burdens. Through community-based participatory research, partnering with local organizations, and collaborating with community members to identify risk maps of hazards (Postma, 2006), nurses can build relationships with community members that strengthen their voice to address the environmental risks they face. Public health nurses' skills in building relationships with community members, working collaboratively with community partners, and advocating for change through governmental programs make them important contributors to environmental justice work (Perry, 2005; Postma, 2006; Powell & Slade, 2002). (See Displays 9.4 and 9.5 for further sources of environmental health information.)

Global Environmental Health

Nurses must engage in strategies to protect human health in their communities through the core functions of public health: assessment, policy development, and assurance. To effectively do this, nurses must think globally in order to be effective locally. That means that considering global conditions of climate change and the effect upon human health is an important beginning (McMichael, Friel, Nyong, & Corvalen, 2008). However, broadening thinking to consider foods imported from countries around the world, toys made in other countries and used in the United States, and the manufacture of products in locations where the regulation for safety is not as stringent (or in some cases more stringent) as in the United States assists nursing in addressing environmental health knowledge and advocacy. Nurses who work for "green nursing" by promoting more ecological and environmentally safe practices in their workplace are making an impact upon global environmental health. While it is now illegal in most countries to dump waste into the ocean or to ship waste to less developed countries with less stringent laws to protect their citizens from toxins, large quantities of toxic industrial waste, medical waste, toxic ash from incinerators, as well as the growing issue of e-waste from computers and other electronic products has found its way to ocean waters and poorer countries. In order to fully promote the health of populations, nurses must take personal action to reduce their use of products (particularly those with toxic chemicals), reuse as much as possible, and recycle (in safe processes) to decrease their personal environmental footprint. Nurses must also incorporate the environmental health knowledge and skills mandated by the ANA *Scope and Standards of Nursing Practice* into their nursing practice.

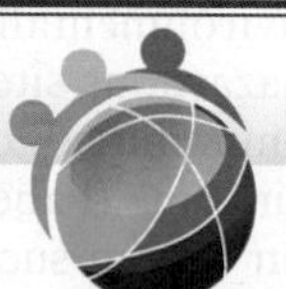

DISPLAY 9.4 ENVIRONMENTAL HEALTH REGULATORY AGENCIES

Environmental Protection Agency (EPA)

This federal agency was established in December 1970 for the purpose of standard setting, monitoring, and enforcement of environmental protection in order to work for a cleaner and healthier environment for America. The agency works to ensure that Americans are protected from risks to health in their homes, schools, and workplaces. The agency relies on the best scientific evidence to promote the development of policies to protect the environment and health and enforces federal laws to protect human health.
http://www.epa.gov/aboutepa/history/publications/print/origins.html

Food and Drug Administration (FDA)

The FDA or USFDA is an agency of the United States Department of Health and Human Services that regulates food safety, dietary supplements, prescription and over-the-counter pharmaceuticals, cosmetics, biopharmaceuticals, blood transfusions, and tobacco products.

Consumer Product Safety Commission (CPSC)

The U.S. CPSC was created in 1972 as an agency of the US Government to protect the public from risks of injury or death from consumer products. Commonly reported products are cribs, toys, household chemicals, and power tools but include any commercially traded product. As an independent agency, the CPSC does not report to any other agency of the US Government.
http://www.cpsc.gov/about/about.html

Occupational Safety and Health Administration (OSHA)

The OSHA was created in 1970 as a regulatory federal agency of the United States to assure safe working conditions. OSHA sets and enforces standards for health and safety in work environments.
http://www.osha.gov/

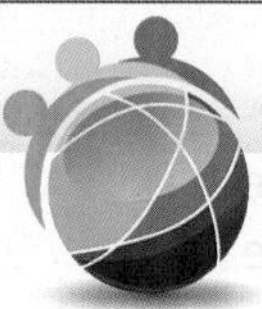

DISPLAY 9.5 ENVIRONMENTAL HEALTH RESOURCES

ASTDR: Agency for Toxic Substances and Disease Registry

ATSDR is a federal public health agency of the U.S. Department of Health and Human Services and division of the CDC. Using science, ATSDR serves the public to take responsive public health actions, by providing information to prevent harmful exposures and diseases. http://www.atsdr.cdc.gov/

ANHE: Alliance of Nurses for Healthy Environments

Alliance of Nurses for Healthy Environments (ANHE) is an organization for nurses and health care providers to promote health through knowledge, networking, and action. Their "EnviRN Knowledge Network" serves as an active learning environment for learning essential environmental health information from experts and connecting with others. Through workgroups that focus upon education, research, practice, and policy/advocacy, nurses can increase their capacity for environmental health nursing.
http://envirn.org/

CDC: Centers for Disease Control and Prevention

The overall mission of the CDC "is to collaborate to create the expertise, information, and tools that people and communities need to protect their health – through health promotion, prevention of disease, injury and disability, and preparedness for new health threats" (http://www.cdc.gov/about/organization/mission.htm). In the area of environmental health, they include topics related to air quality, air pollution, biomonitoring, children's health, climate and health, environmental health sciences, rodent control, sun protection, and water. Additionally they address specific risks such as asbestos, carbon monoxide, lead, mold, natural disasters, radiation, smoking and tobacco use, and wildfires.
http://www.cdc.gov/Environmental/

NLM: National Library of Medicine

The U.S. National Library of Medicine is the worlds' largest medical library. Their Web site offers a large number of resources useful for nurses to learn about environmental health.

TOXNET is a large set of databases on environmental health, toxicology, hazardous chemicals, and toxic releases. It also includes a household products database.

TOXMAP is an environmental Health e-Map that allows the user to explore toxic chemical releases and hazardous waste sites from the EPA's Toxics Release Inventory (TRI) and the Superfund National Priorities List (NPL).

TOX TOWN is an interactive site that includes a variety of settings from town, to city, to farm, to port to US border lands. In each setting, the user is able to view nontechnical descriptions of chemicals, how the environment affects human health, as well as other Internet resources on topics useful to the user. The color, graphics animation, and sounds make it an effective strategy to each adolescent, educator, and the general public about environmental exposures.

NIEHS: National Institute of Environmental Health Sciences

The National Institute of Environmental Health Sciences (NIEHS) is a part of the National Institutes of Health (NIH), which is an institute of the Department of Health and Human Services (DHHS). The mission is to understand how the environment influences health. To accomplish this, NIEHS focuses upon research, global health, and research training.
http://www.niehs.nih.gov/

NIOSH: National Institute for Occupational Safety and Health

The National Institute for Occupational Safety and Health (or NIOSH) is a US federal agency that is responsible for both conducting research and translating knowledge into recommendations for the prevention of work-related injury and illness. Created in 1970 in response to the Occupational Safety and Health Act, 1970, NIOSH was established to help ensure safe and healthful working conditions.
http://www.cdc.gov/NIOSH/

OSHA: Occupational Safety and Health Administration

The Occupational Safety and Health Administration was created in 1970 as a regulatory federal agency of the United States to assure safe working conditions. OSHA sets and enforces standards for health and safety in work environments.
http://www.osha.gov/

SUMMARY

Environmental health is a discipline encompassing all of the elements of the environment that influence the health and wellbeing of its inhabitants. Public health nurses need to monitor and determine causal links between people and their environment with a concern as to how they may promote the health and wellbeing of both. An ecologic perspective of environmental health is important to understand the human–environment relationship and how the health of one affects the health of the other. Prevention and strategic or long-range concerns are also important in considering environmental health, because what is done today may affect the health of many generations in the future. Examples such as DES use in pregnancy and the effects on the children of those women is a cautionary tale of the unintended consequences of toxic substances, even when used for beneficial purposes. The precautionary principle reminds us that absence of proof that an action, chemical, or material poses a threat to individuals and the environment is not proof of its safety.

Use of an "upstream" approach challenges the public health nurse to address factors that are at the institutional and system level rather than looking solely at healthy lifestyle issues. The disproportionate impact of environmental hazards on low income and people of color argue for the use of environmental justice to remedy those situations. The built environment can both negatively and positively influence the health of a community. Efforts made to promote sustainability, community cohesiveness, and healthy lifestyles can and are being successfully implemented across the country.

Both public and private sectors are involved in regulating, monitoring, and preventing environmental health problems. Health professionals, especially public health nurses, and the general public should be aware of reliable sources of information so that best evidence can inform decisions. Utilizing the core functions of public health, the public health nurse recognizes the key role of assessment, assurance, and policy development to influence change in the health of individuals, families, communities, and the environment. The public health nurse should be a leader of the team of health professionals who promote and protect the reciprocal relationship between the environment and the public's health.

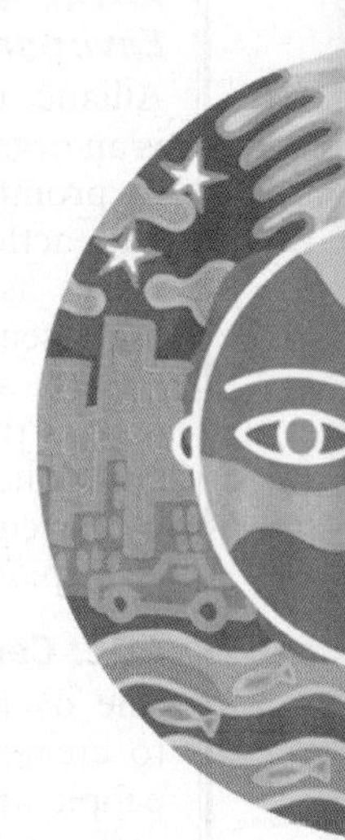

ACTIVITIES TO PROMOTE **CRITICAL THINKING**

Understanding Body Burden by Examining the Risks to Health From Personal Care Products

Many people lack awareness of their exposures to harmful chemicals in the environment. Children and adolescents are most vulnerable to exposures from personal care products due to their developmental stage. To gain a better understanding of common risks to health from commonly used personal care products, you will use the resources of the Environmental Working Group.

1. Begin by watching the Environmental Working Group video "10 Americans." There is an 8-minute version available on "YouTube." Then consider one specific area where humans are exposed to toxic chemicals: personal care products. This includes not only cosmetics but also soaps, toothpaste, and other products used several times a day for personal care.
2. Visit the EWG Web site http://www.ewg.org/. Select their "Skin Deep" database of commonly used products. Search for those you use frequently and identify the risks posed to your personal health.
3. Next, select a population group in the community that might be at risk (neonates, adolescents, etc.) and consider how you might educate that group about their body burden or exposures.

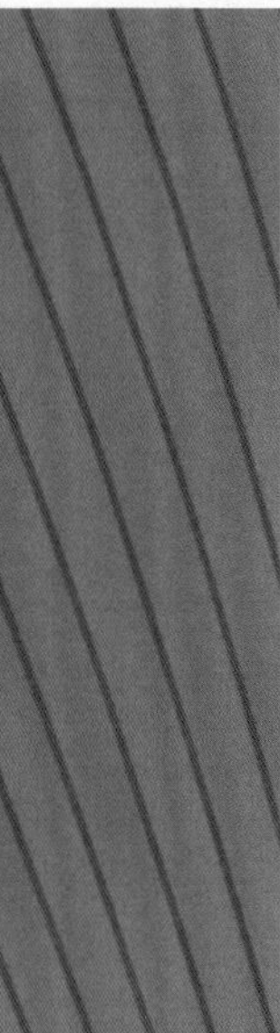

Environmental Protection Agency Activity

As a nursing student, it is important for you to know about common community hazards in order to educate the community members. Visit the EPA "My Environment" site and enter your home zip code or that of the community where you work. The link for this site is http://www.epa.gov/myenvironment/. There you will find headings for "MyAir," "MyWater," "MyHealth," "MyEnergy," "MyLand," "MyEnvironmentReports," and "MyCommunity."

1. Look through these headings to identify the hazards in your community. What is the air quality? Are there particular industries, power plants, or high areas for auto emissions that affect health? What about water quality? How might you advise community members to learn about their water quality? Are there significant toxic waste sites? What types of exposures are there in the community?
2. Can you identify possible risks from climate change and severe weather events? What might be ways to ensure emergency preparedness for those most at risk?
3. Using the framework of this chapter, the core public health functions, select a strategy for each area: assessment, policy development, and assurance that is most appropriate for your community.

REFERENCES

Afzal, B. M. (2003). Protecting the health of American communities: Access to information. *Policy Politics and Nursing Practice, 4*, 22–28. Doi:10.1177/1527154402239451

Agency for Toxic Substances and Disease Registry, Centers for Disease Control and Prevention. (2011). *Environmental health nursing initiative*. Retrieved from http://www.atsdr.cdc.gov/EHN/

Alliance of Nurses for Healthy Environments. (2011). *Alliance of nurses for healthy environments*. Retrieved from http://envirn.org/pg/groups/world/?tag=anhe

American Nurses Association. (2007). *ANA's principles of environmental health for nursing practice with implementation strategies*. Silver Spring, MD: Author.

American Nurses Association. (2010). *Nursing: Scope and standards of practice* (2nd ed.). Silver Spring, MD: Author.

American Public Health Association. (2005). *Environmental health principles for public health nursing*. Retrieved from http://www.apha.org/membergroups/newsletters/sectionnewsletters/public_nur/winter06/default.htm#{D58E85AF-5B7D-4549-A5B3-EC45B9B1216B}

Anderko, L. (2011). *Fish facts for health professionals: Methylmercury exposure, fish consumption and health risks/benefits*. Retrieved from www.dhs.wisconsin.gov/eh/fish/.../fishfactsworkbook2009.pdf

Baker, G. A., & Burnham, T. A. (2001). Consumer response to genetically modified foods: Market segment analysis and implications for producers and policy makers. *Journal of Agricultural and Resource Economics, 26*(2), 387–403.

Balbus, J. M., & Malina, C. (2009). Identifying vulnerable subpopulations for climate change health effects in the United States. *Journal of Occupational and Environmental Medicine, 51*, 33–37.

Brooten, D., Youngblut, J. M., Royal, S., Cohn, S., Lobar, S. L., & Hernandez, L. (2008). Outcomes of an asthma program: Healthy children, healthy homes. *Pediatric Nursing, 34*(6), 448–455.

Bullard, R. D. (2005). *The quest for environmental justice: Human rights and the politics of prevention*. San Francisco, CA: Sierra Club.

Bullard, R. D., Johnson, G. S., & Torres, A. O. (2011). *Environmental health and racial equity in the United States: Building environmentally just, sustainable and livable communities*. Washington, DC: American Public Health Association.

Butterfield, P. G. (2002). Upstream reflections on environmental health: An abbreviated history and framework for action. *Advances in Nursing Science, 25*(1), 32–49.

Butterfield, P. G., Hill, W., Postma, J., Butterfield, P. W., & Odom-Maryon, T. (2011). Effectiveness of a household environmental health intervention delivered by rural public health nurses. *American Journal of Public Health, 101*(S1), S262–S270.

Chalupka, S., & Chalupka, A. N. (2010). The impact of environmental and occupational exposures on reproductive health. *Journal of Obstetric, Gynecologic, and Neonatal Nursing, 39*, 84–102. Doi: 10.1111/j.1552-6909.2009.01091.x

Chaudry, R. V. (2008). The precautionary principle, public health, and public health nursing. *Public Health Nursing, 25*(3), 261–268.

City of Oakland, California. (2012). *Sustainable Oakland*. Retrieved from http://www2.oaklandnet.com/Government/o/PWA/o/FE/s/SO/a/ProgramOverview/index.htm

Clinton, W. J. (1993). Executive Order 12852. *President's Council on Sustainable Development*. Retrieved from http://clinton1.nara.gov/White_House/EOP/pcsd/info/executive-order.html

Crews, D., & McLachlan, J. A. (2006). Epigenetics, evolution, endocrine disruption, health and disease. *Endocrinology, 147*(6), (Suppl) S4–S10. Doi: 10.1210/en.2005-1122

Dahlgren, G. & Whitehead, M. (1991). *Policies and strategies to promote social equity in health*. Institute for Future Studies, Stockholm (Mimeo).

Dannenberg, A. L., Jackson, R. J., Frumkin, H., Schieber, R. A., Pratt, M., Kochtitzky, C., et al. (2003). The impact of community design and land-use choices on public health: A research agenda. *American Journal of Public Health, 93*(9), 1500–1508.

Davis, A. (2007). Home environmental health risks. *Online Journal of Issues in Nursing, 12*(4), Manuscript 4. Retrieved from http://www.nursingworld.org/MainMenuCategories/ANAMarketplace/ANAPeriodicals/OJIN/TableofContents/Volume122007/No2May07/HomeEnvironmentalHealthRisks.html

Denison, R. A. (2009). *Ten essential elements in TSCA reform*. Washington, DC: Environmental Law Institute. Retrieved from http://www.edf.org/sites/default/files/9279_Denison_10_Elements_TSCA_Reform_0.pdf

ENVIRN. (2011). *ENVIRN Knowledge Network*. Retrieved from http://envirn.org/pg/groups/all/

Environmental Working Group. (2011). *10 Americans*. Retrieved from http://www.ewg.org/10-americans

Erdman, J. (2011). *2011's incredible weather extremes*. Retrieved from http://www.weather.com/outlook/weather-news/news/articles/2011-extreme- weather_2011-09-28

Evans, B. W. (2009). New Bedford sues Monsanto, Cornel-Dubilier over buried toxic chemicals. *South Coast Today*. Retrieved from http://www.southcoasttoday.com/apps/pbcs.dll/article?AID=/20091213/NEWS/912130326

Faber, D. R., & Krieg, E. J. (2002). Unequal exposure to ecological hazards: Environmental injustices in the commonwealth of Massachusetts. *Environmental Health Perspectives, 110*(S2), 277–288.

Friis, R. H. (2012). *Essentials of environmental health* (2nd ed.). Sudbury, MA: Jones and Bartlett.

Frumkin, H. (2010). *Environmental health: From global to local.* San Francisco, CA: John Wiley.

Gilden, R. C. (2003). Community involvement at hazardous waste sites: A review of policies from a nursing perspective. *Policy, Politics, and Nursing Practice, 4*, 29–35. Doi:10.1177/1527154402239452

Gilden, R. (2011). *Potential health effects related to pesticide use on athletic fields.* Presented at the American Public Health Association Meeting, Washington, DC.

Gilden, R., Huffing, K., & Sattler, B. (2010). Pesticides and health risks. *Journal of Obstetrical, Gynecological, and Neonatal Nursing, 39*, 103–110.

Global Water. (2011). *Why water.* Retrieved from http://globalwater.org/whywater.htm

Health Care without Harm. (2011). *Pharmaceuticals.* Retrieved from http://www.noharm.org/us_canada/issues/pharmaceuticals/resources.php

Hilgenkamp, K. (2006). *Environmental health: Ecological perspectives.* Sudbury, MA: Jones and Bartlett.

Hill, W. G., Butterfield, P., & Larsson, L. S. (2006). Rural parent's perceptions of risks associated with their children's exposure to radon. *Public Health Nursing, 23*, 392–399.

Hoover R. N., Hyer, M., Pfeiffer, R. M., Adam, E., Bond, B., Cheville, A. L., et al. (2011). Adverse health outcomes in women exposed in utero to diethylstilbestrol. *New England Journal of Medicine, 365*(14), 1304–1314.

Institute of Medicine. (1988). *Future of public health.* Washington, DC: National Academy Press.

Institute of Medicine (2002). *The future of the public's health in the 21st century.* Washington, DC: National Academies Press

Jackson, R. L. (2003). The impact of the built environment on health: An emerging field. *American Journal of Public Health, 93*(9), 1382–1384.

Jackson, R. L. (2012). *Designing healthy communities.* San Francisco, CA: Jossey-Bass.

Lee, C. (2002). Environmental justice: Building a unified vision of health and the environment. *Environmental Health Perspectives, 110* (S2), 141–144.

Leffers, J. (2010). *Vulnerable populations. EnviRN essentials.* Retrieved from http://envirn.org/pg/groups/16/vulnerable-populations/

McKinley, J. (1979, June). A case for focusing upstream: The political economy of illness. *Proceedings of the American Heart Association Conference: Applying Behavioral Science to Cardiovascular Risk*, Seattle, WA.

McMichael, A. J., Friel, S, Nyong, A., & Corvalan, C. (2008). Global environmental change and health: Impacts, inequalities, and the health sector. *British Medical Journal, 336*, 191–194.

McMichael, A. J., Woodruff, R. E., & Hales, S. (2006). Climate change and human health: Present and future risks. *The Lancet, 387*(9513), 859–869.

National Library of Medicine. (2011). *TOXNET.* Retrieved from http://toxnet.nln.nih.gov/

Nightingale, F. (1860/1969). *Notes on nursing: What it is and what it is not.* New York: Dover Publications, Inc.

Nweke, O. C., Payne-Sturges, D., Garcia, L., Lee, C., Zenick, H., Grevatt, P., et al. (2011). Symposium on integrating the science of environmental justice into decision-making at the Environmental Protection Agency. *American Journal of Public Health, 101*(S1), S19–S26.

Olden, K. (2002). *Gene-environment interaction… the centerpiece for disease prevention.* Retrieved from http://www.help.senate.gov/imo/media/doc/Olden.pdf

Ortner, P.M. (2004). The nurse as change agent: An approach to environmental health advocacy training. *Policy Politics and Nursing Practice, 5*(2), 125–130. Doi:10.1177/1527154404263890.

Paranzino, G. K., Butterfield, P., Nastoff, T., & Ranger, C. (2005). I PREPARE: Development and clinical utility of an environmental exposure history mnemonic. *AAOHN Journal, 53*(1), 37–42.

Partnership for Food Safety Education. (2011). *Food safety.* Retrieved from http://www.fightbac.org/

Perry D. (2005). Transcendent pluralism and the influence of nursing testimony on environmental justice legislation. *Policy Politics and Nursing Practice, 6*(1), 60–71.

Pesticide Action Network. (2011). *What's on my food?* Retrieved from http://whatsinmyfood.org/index.jsp

Physicians for Social Responsibility. (2011). *Hazardous chemicals in health care: Snapshot of chemicals in doctors and nurses.* Retrieved from http://www.psr.org/resources/hazardous-chemicals-in-health.html

Polivka, B. J., Chaudry, R. V., Crawford, J., Bouton, P., & Sweet, L. (2011). Impact of an urban Healthy Homes Intervention. *Journal of Environmental Health, 73*(9), 16–20.

Polivka, B. J., Stanley, S. A., Gordon, D., Taulbee, K., Kieffer, G., & McCorkle, S. M. (2008). Public health nursing competencies for public health surge events. *Public Health Nursing, 25*(2), 159–165.

Postma, J. (2006). Environmental justice: Implications for occupational health nurses. *AAOHN Journal, 54*(11), 489–498.

Pope, A. M., Snyder, M. A., & Mood, L. H. (1995). *Nursing, health and the environment: Strengthening the relationship to improve the public's health.* Washington, DC: National Academy Press.

Powell, D., & Slade, D. (2002). Advocating for environmental justice: Protecting vulnerable communities from pollution. In B. Sattler, & J. Lipscomb (Eds.), *Environmental health and nursing practice* (pp. 321–338). New York: Springer Publishing.

Powell, D. L., & Stewart, V. (2001). Children. The unwitting target of environmental injustices. *Pediatric Clinics of North America, 48*(5), 1291–1305.

Raffensperger, C., & Tickner, J. (1999). *Protecting public health and the environment: Implementing the precautionary principle.* Washington, DC: Island Press.

Richards, I. S. (2008). *Principles and practice of toxicology in public health.* Sudbury, MA: Jones and Bartlett.

Rose, J. B., Epstein, P. R., Lipp, E. K., Sherman, B. H., Bernard, S. M., & Patz, J. A. (2001). Climate variability and change in the United States: Potential impacts on water- and food borne diseases caused by microbiologic agents. *Environmental Health Perspectives, 109*(S2), 211–221.

Schettler, T., Solomon, G., Valenti, M., & Huddle, A. (1999). *Generations at risk: Reproductive health and the environment.* Cambridge, MA: MIT Press.

Science and Environmental Health Network. (2011). *Ecological medicine.* Retrieved from http://www.sehn.org/emandeh.html

Snyder, S. A., Westerhoff, P., Yoon, Y., & Sedlak, D. L. (2003). Pharmaceuticals, personal care products, and endocrine disruptors in water: Implications for the water industry. *Environmental Engineering Science, 20*(5), 449–469. Doi: 10.1089/109287503768335931.

Srinivasan, S., O'Fallon, L. R., & Dearry, A. (2003). Creating healthy communities, healthy homes, healthy people: Initiating a research agenda on the built environment and public health. *American Journal of Public Health, 93*(9), 1446–1450.

Smith, C. (2010). *Why nursing and environmental health.* Retrieved from http://envirn.org/pg/pages/view/1785/why-nursing-and-environmental-health

Stein, J., Schettler, T., Wallinga, D., & Valenti, M. (2002). In harm's way: Toxic threats to child development. *Developmental and Behavioral Pediatrics, 23*, S13–S22.

United Nations. (2011). *UN water.* Retrieved from http://www.unwater.org/downloads/WWD2012_water_scarcity.pdf

U.S. Centers for Disease Control and Prevention. (2011a). *CDC and Food Safety.* Retrieved from http://www.cdc.gov/foodsafety/cdc-and-food-safety.html

U.S. Centers for Disease Control and Prevention. (2011b). *Food irradiation.* Retrieved from http://www.cdc.gov/ncidsd/dbmd/diseaseinfo/foodirradiation.htm

U.S. Centers for Disease Control and Prevention. (2011c). *National biomonitoring program.* Retrieved from http://www.cdc.gov/biomonitoring/about.html

U.S. Consumer Product Safety Commission. (2011). *Asbestos in the home.* Retrieved from http://www.cpsc.gov/cpscpub/pubs/453.html

U.S. Department of Health and Human Services. (2011a). *Healthy People 2020.* Retrieved from http://www.healthypeople.gov/2020/about/default.aspx

U.S. Department of Health and Human Services. (2011b). *Healthy People 2020 Environmental Health Objectives*. Retrieved from http://www.healthypeople.gov/2020/topicsobjectives2020/overview.aspx?topicid=12

U.S. Department of Housing and Urban Development. (2011a). *Healthy Homes Program. Abstracts by Region. Region 1 New England*. Retrieved from http://portal.hud.gov/hudportal/HUD?src=/program_offices/healthy_homes/hhi/hhabstracts

U.S. Department of Housing and Urban Development. (2011b). *Healthy Homes Program. Abstracts by Region. Region 3 Mid-Atlantic*. Retrieved from http://portal.hud.gov/hudportal/HUD?src=/program_offices/healthy_homes/hhi/hhabstracts

U.S. Department of Housing and Urban Development. (2001). *Healthy Homes Demonstration Grant Program*. Retrieved from http://portal.hud.gov/hudportal/HUD?src=/program_offices/healthy_homes/hhi/hhd

U.S. Environmental Protection Agency. (2011a). *Air quality*. Retrieved from http://www.epa.gov/airquality/peg_caa/

U.S. Environmental Protection Agency. (2011b). *Brownfield's*. Retrieved from http://epa.gov/brownfields/overview/glossary.htm

U.S. Environmental Protection Agency. (2011c). *Citizen's guide to pesticides and pesticide safety*. Retrieved from http://www.epa.gov/oppfead1/Publications/Cit_Guide/

U.S. Environmental Protection Agency. (2011d). *Citizen's guide to radon*. Retrieved from http://www.epa.gov/radon/pubs/citguide.html

U.S. Environmental Protection Agency. (2011e). *City of New Bedford, MA*. Retrieved from http://www.epa.gov/region1/brownfields/success/newbedford1.html

U.S. Environmental Protection Agency. (2011f). *Climate change and agriculture*. Retrieved from http://www.epa.gov/climatechange/effects/agriculture.html

U.S. Environmental Protection Agency. (2011g). *Drinking water contaminants*. Retrieved from http://water.epa.gov/drink/contaminants/index.cfm

U.S. Environmental Protection Agency. (2011h). *Environmental justice*. Retrieved from http://www.epa.gov/environmentaljustice/

U.S. Environmental Protection Agency. (2011i). *Healthy Schools Environments Assessment Tool: Healthy Seat*. Retrieved from http://www.epa.gov/schools/healthyseat/

U.S. Environmental Protection Agency. (2011j). *IAQ Tools for Schools*. Retrieved from http://epa.gov/iaq/schools/

U.S. Environmental Protection Agency. (2011k). *Indoor air quality: Sick Building Syndrome*. Retrieved from http://www.epa.gov/iaq/pubs/sbs.html

U.S. Environmental Protection Agency. (2011l). *Municipal solid waste (MSW) in the United States: Facts and figures*. Retrieved from http://www.epa.gov/osw/nonhaz/municipal/msw99.htm

U.S. Environmental Protection Agency. (2011m). *National air quality standards*. Retrieved from http://www.epa.gov/airtrends/2010/report/highlights.pdf

U.S. Environmental Protection Agency. (2011n). *Natural disasters and weather emergencies*. Retrieved from http://www.epa.gov/naturaldisasters/general.html

U.S. Environmental Protection Agency. (2011o). *Pesticides and food: What you and your family need to know*. Retrieved from http://www.epa.gov/pesticides/food/

U.S. Environmental Protection Agency. (2011p). *Plain English guide to the Clean Air Act*. Retrieved from www.epa.gov/air/peg/peg.pdf

U.S. Environmental Protection Agency. (2011q). *Radiation protection*. Retrieved from http://epa.gov/radiation/understand/ionize_nonionize.html#nonionizing

U.S. Environmental Protection Agency. (2011r). *Radon health risks*. Retrieved from http://www.epa.gov/radon/healthrisks.html

U.S. Environmental Protection Agency. (2011s). *Resources in your community*. Retrieved from http://epa.gov/epahome/community.htm

U.S. Environmental Protection Agency. (2011t). *Risk management research: Genetically modified foods*. Retrieved from http://www.epa.gov/nrmrl/news/052010/news052010.html

U.S. Environmental Protection Agency. (2011u). *Safe Drink Water Act*. Retrieved from http://water.epa.gov/lawsregs/rulesregs/sdwa/

U.S. Environmental Protection Agency. (2011v). *Schools*. Retrieved from http://www.epa.gov/schools/

U.S. Environmental Protection Agency. (2011w). *Superfund*. Retrieved from http://www.epa.gov/superfund/about.htm

U.S. Environmental Protection Agency. (2011x). *Urban air*. Retrieved from http://www.epa.gov/airquality/urbanair/

U.S. Environmental Protection Agency. (2011y). *Water on tap*. Retrieved from http://water.epa.gov/drink/guide/

U.S. Food and Drug Administration. (2011). *Food safety*. Retrieved from http://www.fda.gov/

U.S. Global Change Research Program. (2003). *Climate change impacts the U.S. Southeast*. Retrieved from http://www.usgcrp.gov/usgcrp/nacc/education/southeast/se-edu-6.htm

U.S. Geological Survey. (2011). *Significant earthquakes*. Retrieved from http://earthquake.usgs.gov/earthquakes/eqinthenews/

Whitney, S. L., Maltby, H. J., & Carr, J. M. (2004). "This food may contain…" What Nurses need to know about genetically engineered foods. *Nursing Outlook, 52*, 262–266.

World Health Organization. (1948/2011). *WHO definition of health*. New York: World Health Organization. Retrieved from https://apps.who.int/aboutwho/en/definition.html

Wright, R. T. (2008). *Environmental science: Toward a sustainable future* (10th ed.). Upper Saddle River, NJ. Prentice Hall.

thePoint: Everything You Need to Make the Grade!

thePoint Visit http://thePoint.lww.com/Allender8e
for selected readings, study aids for all learning styles, and more!

UNIT 3

COMMUNITY HEALTH NURSING TOOLBOX

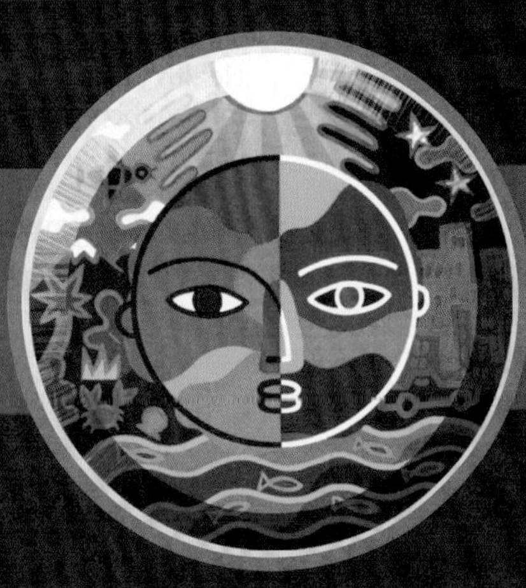

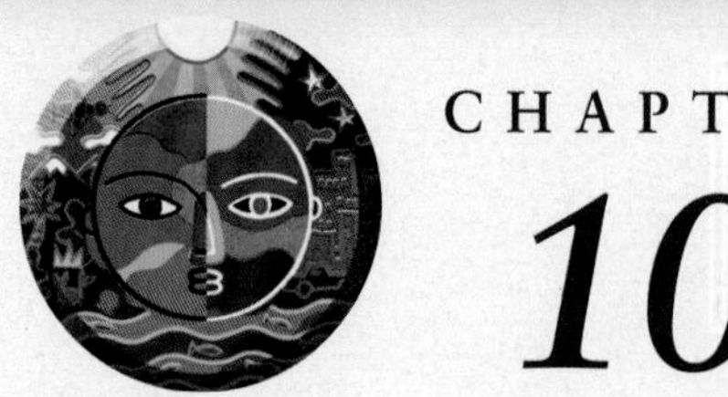

CHAPTER 10

Communication, Collaboration, and Contracting

"Think like a wise man but communicate in the language of the people."

—***William Butler Yeats*** (1865–1939)

KEY TERMS

Active listening
Asset-based community development
Brainstorming
Carefronting
Channel
Collaboration
Communication
Community-based participatory research
Contracting
Critical pathway
Decoding
Electronic meetings
Empathy
Encoding
Feedback loop
Formal contracting
Group process
Health literacy
Informal contracting
Message
Multivoting
Nominal group technique
Nonverbal messages
Nursing informatics
Paraphrasing
Receiver
Sender
Verbal messages

LEARNING OBJECTIVES

Upon mastery of this chapter, you should be able to:

- Identify the seven basic parts of the communication process.
- Describe five barriers to effective communication in community health nursing and how to deal with them.
- Explain three sets of skills necessary for effective communication in community health nursing.
- Summarize the key issues related to health literacy.
- Explain the stages of group process.
- Differentiate between task roles and maintenance roles.
- Describe five characteristics of collaboration in community health.
- Compare the three phases common to the collaboration process.
- Identify four features of contracting in community health nursing.
- Discuss the value of contracting to both clients and community health nurses.
- Design a contract useful in community health nursing.

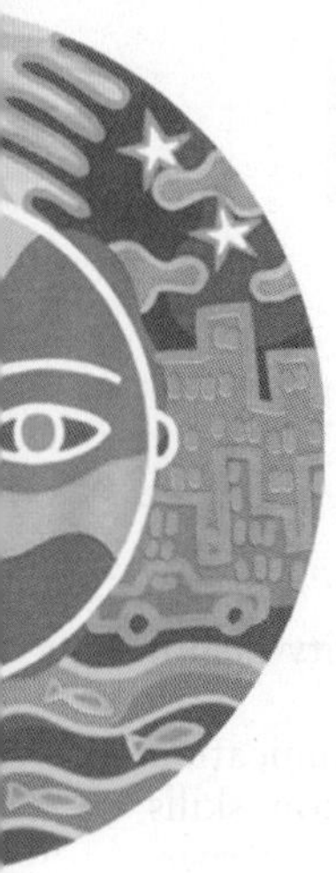

Communication, collaboration, and contracting are primary tools for community health nurses. They form the basis for effective relationships that contribute both to the prevention of illness and to the protection and promotion of population health. To use these concepts skillfully in community health practice, it is important to understand their meaning and value. Because of its relationship to health promotion and disease prevention and management, **health literacy** is a concept that is becoming more important to health care providers, especially those in public settings. For the nurse accustomed to communicating one-on-one with clients, communicating with community groups, along with a wide range of professionals and lay community workers, requires new skills. Group work is a key component of community health nursing and effective application of group process skills will facilitate work with both task and support groups. Advances in technology bring opportunities to develop innovative ways to deliver community-based health services to individual clients, their families, populations, and communities. The computer, with its teleconferencing, telehealth, Internet, and e-mail capabilities, as well as ever-changing smartphone technology, global positioning, and information systems, enriches communication and virtually brings the world into home and work settings.

Unlike ordinary social relationships, collaborative relationships are based on a team approach with shared responsibilities and mutual participation in establishing and carrying out goals. Effective professional collaboration can improve health outcomes and foster organizational commitment. The concept of contracting can further assist the collaborative process. Clients and health care professionals enter into a working agreement, or contract, tailored to address specific client needs. This chapter examines these tools and discusses their integration into community health nursing practice.

COMMUNICATION IN COMMUNITY HEALTH NURSING

The importance of communication is often taken for granted since people spend most of their waking hours communicating; speaking, listening, reading, or writing. Yet, the quality of people's communication has far-reaching effects. In nursing, lack of effective communication can lead to misunderstanding, poor performance, interpersonal conflict, ineffective program development, medical mistakes, and many other undesirable outcomes. Therefore, for effective communication "nurses must be as proficient in communication as they are in clinical skills" (Zavertnik, Huff, & Munro, 2010, p. 65).

Effective communication is vital to all areas of nursing but is considered to be a fundamental core competency needed in community health nursing practice (Education Committee of the Association of Community Health Nurse Educators [ACHNE], 2010). The Quad Council PHN Competencies (2003) includes communication skills as one of the eight essential core competencies. Communicating effectively, soliciting input from others, and listening to others in a nonjudgmental way are a few of the necessary skills highlighted in that document. Nurses working in community health must be skilled in effective communication to be able to maintain relationships with individual clients, family members and aggregate populations, members of the health care team, and community partners. Good communication skills will enable community health nurses to provide quality health care and health education; advocate effectively for clients, families, and populations; initiate public health policy; and implement programs designed to meet the needs of the clients (Young, 2009). In community health nursing, effective individual and group communication will improve patient outcomes, enhance professional collaboration, and foster organizational commitment (Propp, Apker, Zabava-Ford, Wallace, Serbenski, & Hofmeister, 2010).

Communication provides a two-way flow of information that nourishes professional–client and professional–professional relationships. It also establishes the base of information on which health planning decisions are made and programs developed. For communication to take place, clients and professionals need to send and receive messages. As participants in the communication process, community health nurses play both roles: sender and receiver. The nurse working with a group of abused women must learn to "read" the messages these women send. Similarly, as a member of a health planning team, the nurse must be able to elicit ideas as well as contribute to the planning process by speaking and acting in ways that promote information sharing.

Communication serves several functions in community health nursing. It provides information for decision making at all levels of community health. From the choice of goals for a small client support group to health policy affecting a population at risk, decisions are enhanced through effective communication. Communication functions as a motivator by clarifying information, so that consensus is reached and the people involved can move forward with commitment to shared goals. Effective communication facilitates the expression of feelings and promotes closer working relationships. It also controls behavior by providing clear expectations and boundaries for group-member actions.

The Communication Process

Communication in its simplest form is the sending and receiving of a **message**; a process by which one assigns and conveys meaning in an attempt to create shared understanding. This process incorporates the conventional aspects of communication—sender, receiver,

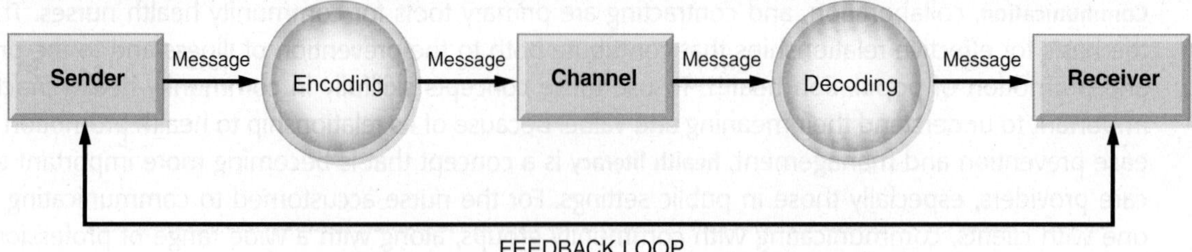

FIGURE 10-1. The communication process (the feedback loop).

message, channel, feedback, the **encoding**, and the **decoding** of the messages (Tonn, 2009). This seven-step process is described in Figure 10-1.

It is often suggested that the message is the most important aspect of communication because without the message, there can be no communication. However, for effective communication to occur, we must take a closer look at the seven steps of the communication process. First, the **sender** must effectively encode the message for the receiver. To transmit the message, the sender must decide which specific signals or codes, such as language, words, gestures, and body language, to use. The degree of the sender's success in encoding a message is influenced by the sender's communication skills, knowledge about the topic, attitudes, and feelings related to the message.

The **channel** is the medium through which the sender conveys the message. The channel may be a written, spoken, or nonverbal expression; and communication channels may be formal, such as a written grant proposal, or informal, such as a face-to-face verbal statement. Other examples include e-mail messages, a written report to provide information, a written care plan, or a facial expression indicating confusion. Once the sender has conveyed a message through a channel, the **receiver** must translate (decode) the message into an understandable form. The receiver's ability to decode the message is influenced by knowledge of the topic, skills in reading and listening, and attitudes, beliefs, and sociocultural values.

Although communication has been exchanged, this does not mean that the exchange is meaningful. All communication involves perception and expectation. We interpret messages based upon prior experiences with either the sender/receiver or with others who have influenced our lives. The final part of the communication process, the **feedback loop**, allows both the sender and the receiver to check on the success of the transference of meaning and to renegotiate the message to allow for clarity and better understanding. Effective communication is seen only when the message sent is received and interpreted by the receiver as intended (Borkowski, 2011).

Communication Barriers and Strategies to Overcome Them

Community health nurses should be aware of the barriers that block effective communication. Display 10.1 lists barriers that nurses working in community health may encounter.

Overcoming barriers to effective communication requires development of sound communication skills that include sending skills, receiving skills, and interpersonal skills.

Sending Skills

Sending skills enable nurses to transmit messages effectively. Through these skills, nurses convey information to clients and other persons. Two important considerations influence the clarity and effectiveness of message sending. First, the extent of the nurse's self-awareness affects communication. Does the nurse feel anxious, angry, tired, impatient, or concerned? Does the nurse find certain individuals irritating or offensive? What motives and interests prompt the communication? Second, the nurse's awareness of the receiver influences the sending of messages. What do clients or the professionals with whom the nurse is interacting want or need? Is the message suited to their cultural background and level of understanding? Does the message have significance for them? How are receivers responding as the nurse sends the message?

Two main channels are used to send messages: nonverbal and verbal. **Nonverbal messages**, those conveyed without words, constitute a large portion of the messages transmitted in normal communication. Nonverbal statements may enhance or discredit what someone says verbally, and thus, are even more important than the spoken words (Rollnick, Miller, & Butler, 2008). People send messages nonverbally in many ways. Nonverbal messages can be sent through personal appearance, dress, posture, facial expression, gestures, and physical distance between sender and receiver. Body language often speaks louder than words. Facial expressions can convey acceptance or rejection, interest or boredom, anger or patience, and fear or confidence. Gestures and bodily movements, such as clenched hands, crossed arms, tapping fingers, hands on hips, or a turned shoulder, can negatively affect communication. Eye contact or lack of it, tone of voice, and use of silence also send important nonverbal messages. A nurse's awareness that nonverbal messages may have different cultural meanings or social interpretations can save considerable misunderstanding (Spector, 2009).

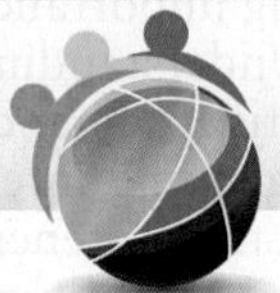

DISPLAY 10.1 BARRIERS TO EFFECTIVE COMMUNICATION IN COMMUNITY HEALTH NURSING

Selective Perception

Receivers in the communication process interpret a message through their own perceptions, which are influenced by their own experience, interests, values, motivations, and expectations. They project this perceptual screen onto the communication process as they decode a message; leading to possible distortion or misinterpretation of the meaning from the sender's original intent. Nurses can overcome this barrier by using the feedback loop to ask clients or others involved to voice their understanding of the message. This provides an opportunity for clarification and correction of misunderstandings, which is an essential step in the communication process and helps to prevent miscommunication that can lead to mistakes.

Filtering

Filtering is described as the manipulation of information by the sender in order to make it seem more favorable to the receiver. To gain favor with receivers, senders sometimes say what they believe receivers want to hear rather than the whole truth (CBS Interactive, 2010).

Clients sometimes use filtering during a needs assessment process, giving only partial or distorted information because they think this is what health professionals want to hear. Filtering can also affect PHNs. Cole (1990), in a classic work, notes that we have "filters" through which we view others—often influenced by culture, ethnicity, and socioeconomic class or even gender—and these can lead to miscommunication. Cole's premise is that dissimilar people actually view the world differently, thus confounding communication and leading to prejudice and stereotyping. Community health nurses should consider the communication style and preferences of the people whom they come in contact with and avoid stereotyping (Berman, Snyder, Kozier, & Erb, 2008). Another intent of filtering is to slant information. Prepared minutes from a meeting or a department's quarterly report can emphasize some points and omit or de-emphasize others, giving (sometimes unintentionally) false impressions that influence decision-making.

Emotional Influence

How a person feels at the time a message is sent or received influences its meaning. Senders can distort messages and receivers can interpret messages incorrectly when emotions cloud their perception. Emotions can interfere with rational and objective reasoning, thus blocking communication. Nurses need to be aware of their own emotions as they send messages. To avoid misunderstandings, they also need to ascertain the emotional status of clients or health professionals with whom they are communicating. For example, it is important for community health nurses to remain calm and unruffled when dealing with families in crisis. Family communication may be angry, blaming, and confrontational because of a serious health crisis with a child, for instance. A community health nurse who responds with frustration, defensiveness, or anger only heightens the family's emotional reactions. A calm, firm, reassuring presence can go far in diffusing the situation and promoting clearer and more constructive communication. It is always helpful to be aware of the receiver's emotional status and help the receiver to identify it. You may say, "I sense that you are feeling upset about Joey's diagnosis. Are there any questions I can answer for you? How can I be helpful?"

Language Barriers

People interpret the meaning of words differently, depending on many variables, such as age, education, cultural background, and primary spoken language. An adolescent understands the terms sweet and tight to mean that something is fashionable or desirable, whereas an 80-year-old woman might understand the terms to mean sugary and confining, respectively. In community health, nurses work with a wide range of clients and professionals whose disparate ages, education levels, and cultural backgrounds lead to different communication patterns.

Language of Nursing

The context of health care provides nurses with a unique vocabulary that may not be understood by clients, family, and community members. The use of scientific terminology or jargon by some health professionals can be confusing. For example, the terms critical pathways or case-management approach may have little meaning to a community group. Community health nurses should be able to adjust their communication styles as appropriate; that is, communication techniques would be different when educating a new mother on proper breast-feeding techniques than when discussing community health needs with the director of a community health department (Hearnden, 2008).

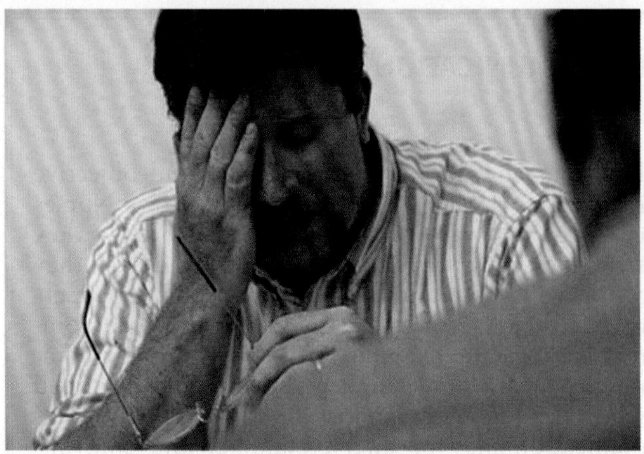

Verbal messages are communicated ideas, attitudes, and feelings transmitted by speaking or writing. Effective sending skills depend on asking for feedback to make certain that receivers have understood the verbal message's intent. Nurses cannot always assume clients or other professionals completely understand the exact intent of their words. Communication is more effective if speakers avoid using jargon that is unfamiliar to clients. Like all occupations, nursing has its own vocabulary, or jargon, which may not be understood by clients and that may make them feel ignorant or inferior. Nurses must make a special effort to avoid using jargon that is part of nursing's everyday language.

The basic rules for effective sending can be summarized in this manner:

1. Keep the message honest and uncomplicated.
2. Use as few words as possible to state it.
3. Ask for reactions (feedback) to make certain that the message is understood.

Receiving Skills

Receiving skills are as important to communication as sending skills. They involve not only listening to what people say but also observing their behavior and nonverbal cues. They enable nurses to receive accurate and complete messages. Effective receiving skills require attending to nonverbal as well as verbal messages and seeking feedback to understand their meaning.

If members of a seniors' exercise class agree to certain exercises but do not participate in them, they are sending a message. What message is their behavior sending? Were the proposed exercises too difficult? Did they misunderstand the nurse's instructions about how to perform the exercises? Are they resisting in other areas of the program? The nurse's role is to clarify the intent of the message through effective communication skills.

An essential skill needed for receiving messages is **active listening** or reflective listening, which is considered to be the most useful and important listening skill. Active listening is the skill of assuming responsibility for and striving to understand the feelings and thoughts in a sender's message, thus giving importance to the person speaking (Nadig, 2010). Understanding the message from the sender's perspective demands careful attention, which arises from a genuine interest in what the speaker has to say. Active listeners demonstrate their interest, perhaps by remaining quiet when appropriate, sitting forward with arms relaxed, sustaining eye contact, nodding the head, and asking occasional questions for clarification (Active Listening, 2010; Scheingold, 2010). The content and feeling of the sender's message may be overwhelming at times, and you can become preoccupied with formulating a response rather than listening actively so it is important to tune out distractions. Let the speaker's words "ring" in your ears; mentally repeating key words as your client speaks will help reinforce your understanding and keep you from straying from the conversation (University of Kentucky, 2009). At times, **paraphrasing**, or repeating back to the sender what the receiver heard, is helpful in clarifying the sender's meaning. Summarizing your perceptions at the end of a home visit, for instance, helps to ensure that the client's communication has been accurately interpreted.

Active listening helps to communicate acceptance and increase trust, especially when the listener is emphatic and nonjudgmental. However, often we listen to our own personal beliefs and values when clients are speaking, and we make judgments about their messages. A critical response to the client's message by the nurse cuts off communication. Many nurses note that "a curtain drops"—a visible change of expression takes place—when the client *disengages* in response to a nurse's judgmental response. Refraining from making any negative judgments of the message or the way it is delivered will allow clients to be heard and acknowledged, which ultimately increases acceptance of suggestions (Nadig, 2010).

Nurses also can listen actively by asking reflective questions that restate what clients or others have said to clarify the received meaning. Reflective questions have a twofold purpose: to show a sincere attempt to understand the sender's message and to demonstrate the importance of the message. An example of a reflective question follows:

> *Client states*: "Quitting smoking is impossible."
> *The nurse asks*: "Do you feel you can't quit smoking?"

By asking reflective questions, the nurse continues to clarify the messages clients send. You can reflect back to clients their:

- Account of the facts
- Thoughts and beliefs
- Feelings and emotions
- Wants, needs, and motivations
- Hopes and expectations (Nadig, 2010).

Active listening allows us to more accurately understand another person's viewpoint and helps to bring issues and concerns into the open where they can be more easily resolved. And if a misunderstanding has occurred, active listening will allow community health nurses to address any misunderstanding immediately (Nadig, 2010).

Interpersonal Skills

Effective communication in community health nursing also requires interpersonal skills. Three types of interpersonal skills build on sending and receiving skills, but go beyond the mere exchange of messages. They are showing respect, empathizing, and developing trust and rapport.

Showing Respect

Showing respect means conveying the attitude that clients and others have importance, dignity, and worth—a concept basic to nursing practice (International Council of Nurses (ICN), 2010). Community health nurses can express respect by treating clients' ideas and comments as valuable and worthy of attention. You can demonstrate an interest in wanting to understand the situation from the other person's point of view. We show respect by the manner in which we address people—for instance, by using the courtesy titles of "Mr." or "Mrs." until it is determined how the client wants to be addressed. On a more subtle level, the tone of voice the nurse uses can show respect or make people feel inferior and insignificant. Nonverbal cues and active listening can indicate to clients that you are fully engaged and interested in their issues. Clients, community members, and other professionals all need to feel respected if they are to enter fully into the mutual exchange necessary for effective communication and optimal health care (Boutain, 2008).

Empathizing

Empathy is a critical component of the communication process as it "involves not only understanding a client's feelings, it involves a level of self-awareness that allows (the PHN) to accurately demonstrate this understanding to the client" (Webster, 2010, p. 87). The capacity to empathize communicates a sensitive awareness of another person's feelings, emotional state, and point of view. We show empathy by striving to put ourselves in our client's shoes—by reflecting their feelings and expressing the message in the receiver's language. This action allows us to convey the message, "This is the way it seems to me. Is that correct?" The nurse should keep validating the speaker's true feelings to be certain that the message is being interpreted correctly. The nurse should use the same terms and, if possible, the same tone of voice as the other person did. For example, you should assume a serious manner if the speaker seems serious. Effective empathetic responses facilitate the development of mutual trust and a sense of shared understanding (Williams & Stickley, 2010).

Developing Trust and Rapport

Building trust and rapport with clients is usually the first goal for community health nurses, and the strongest tool a community health nurse can use in order to develop a trusting relationship is communication. Effective communication can aid in establishing a trusting relationship that is open, genuine and demonstrates true concern for their clients (Current Nursing, 2010). Clients note that a trusting relationship is developed when the community health nurse shows respect and enhances their dignity by being open, accepting, nonjudgmental, and showing empathy (Browne, Doane, Reimer, MacLeod, & McLellan, 2010). Clients appreciate nurses using a transparent process of communication; this includes being reliable, honest, and admitting when they don't have all of the answers (Browne et al., 2010). However, power differences that may exist between the nurse and client may present difficulties in creating a trusting relationship. This is important to understand as clients and others will not express their true feelings if they do not fully trust the nurse (Eriksson & Nilsson, 2008). Many times, clients may say what they think the nurse wants to hear. They may agree to a plan of action simply because they do not want to displease the nurse, or they may hide their true feelings because they think that the nurse is eager for a decision. Also, agreeing with others, especially with people who are in powerful positions and from more dominant cultures, is the polite and respectful thing to do in some cultures (Spector, 2009). The nurse who is unaware of this fact may mistakenly interpret the client's agreement as understanding, thus a "teachable moment" is lost.

Building a trusting relationship is a dynamic process essential in community health nursing. A trusting relationship can enable our clients to have the necessary strength needed to accomplish important lifestyle changes (see Evidence-Based Practice 10.1). Therefore, we need to promote trust in all relationships by:

- Committing to have knowledge and experience of the patient and situation (Eriksson & Nilsson, 2008).
- Clarifying expectations, anticipated behaviors, and boundaries of the nurse–client relationship.
- Demonstrating consistency.
- Being aware of attitudes and behaviors that do not promote trust (Browne et al., 2010).

Factors Influencing Communication

In a helping relationship, it is important for the public health nurse to demonstrate effective communication. Display 10.2 lists key components that assist in promoting a helping relationship.

Effective communication is also strongly influenced by previous experiences and culture of the nurse and the client. Previous experiences of both sender and receiver influence their perceptions and the meanings they attach to messages. For example, adolescents who are having

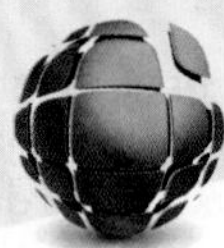

Evidence-Based Practice

Community Health Nurse–Client Communication

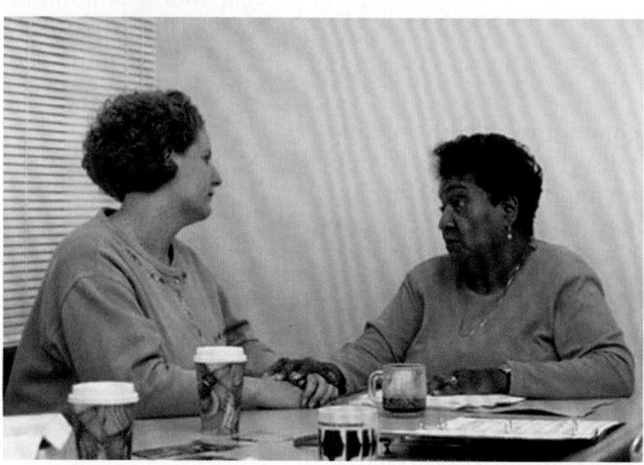

Early research on community health nurse–client communication revealed that this relationship supported self-confidence through the verbal communication patterns of information sharing/advising, negotiating, encouraging, calming, confirming, joking, listening, and silence (Vehvilamen-Julkunen, 1992, p. 900). Newer research has verified the importance of establishing rapport and trust, understanding our clients, and the complex communication skills used by community health nurses with their clients (Philibin et al., 2010; Porr, 2005; Winters et al., 2007).

One study examined the preconditions needed for establishment of a trusting relationship during health counseling, a common PHN activity (Eriksson & Nilsson, 2008). This small qualitative study using open-ended interviews of district nurses in Sweden revealed two main themes: nurse competence and the nurse–client meeting. Nurses were aware of the importance of communication (both verbal and nonverbal) in the development of a trusting relationship with their clients. They noted that they needed to master their reactions to client discouragement or negative emotions, as well as their own situations of stress or workload constraints, because a calm environment where the client feels "welcome and important during the meeting" (p. 2355) was a prerequisite to the development of a trust-based relationship. The appropriate use of touch, the balance of information giving and receiving, and the imperative to be seen by the client as uncritical and nonjudgmental further engendered trust. The ability to meet clients "at their own level" (p. 2355), taking into account their capacity for lifestyle change, and to understand their "everyday life and identify the motives for change" (p. 2355) was found to help create a climate that ensures participation and closeness. Professional credibility was also important, and all health teaching should be evidence-based and up-to-date. During the first meeting with the client, the importance of reserving a sufficient amount of time to "build the base for a trusting relationship" (p. 2356), and sufficient time at follow-up visits were common themes. Continuity was another important precondition for a trusting relationship, as the nurse responds to the client's needs during subsequent visits and helps them "understand that they are important and that the district nurse is there for them" (p. 2356). Respectful communication was described as best demonstrated by using active listening, as well as displaying sensitivity and humility. The nurses noted that it is helpful to listen to the client's concerns, even when not related to the purpose of the visit, as striving to see the whole picture is important to trust building. A "fair and effective conversation" was described as the nurse listening, asking open questions, explaining health terms or teaching concepts, and assuming a "manner of negotiation and power sharing" with clients (p. 2357).

While no systematic review exists on this topic, themes remain fairly consistent. Discuss these research findings with your PHN preceptor or instructor and see if he or she concur with the results.

Eriksson, I., & Nilsson, K. (2008). Preconditions needed for establishing a trusting relationship during health counseling—an interview study. *Journal of Clinical Nursing, 17*(17), 2352–2359.

difficulty with parents' authority may hear the nurse's suggestion to "learn more about sexually transmitted diseases" as an authoritarian command or effort to exert control. Requests for clarification help to verify that messages are being received as intended.

The respective cultures of sender and receiver influence both understanding and acceptance of messages. Communication between health care providers and clients who share the same culture and language background is often complex, but differences in culture,

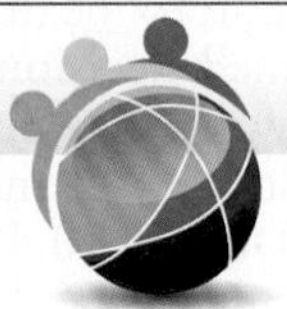

DISPLAY 10.2 CHARACTERISTICS OF A HELPING RELATIONSHIP

In a helping relationship, it is important to promote:

- Openness, genuineness, trustworthiness, and self-awareness (ability to reflect on one's strengths and weaknesses)
- Sensitivity, acceptance, and concern for the client
- Respect for the client as an individual, which includes:
  - Encouraging client to take an active role in health care and to be included in all decisions and choices
  - Considering ethnic and cultural backgrounds
  - Considering family background, beliefs, and values (Department of Health: Australia, 2010)
- Knowledge, self-confidence, creativity, compassion, and empathy
- Ability to problem-solve and to confront or direct when necessary (Rollnick et al., 2008).

ethnicity, and linguistics pose even greater challenges in establishing a helping relationship (see From the Case Files 10.1).

In community health nursing, nurses often find themselves communicating cross-culturally (sometimes through an interpreter), which requires patience and constant effort to ensure accurate and inoffensive messages. For example, a nervous laugh, appropriate as an outlet in one culture, may appear rude and disrespectful to someone from another culture. Silence, which in Native American cultures indicates patience and thoughtfulness, may be interpreted as weakness or indifference to someone not familiar with these cultural practices. As culture is dynamic, community health nurses can never assume they know what is typical of another's culture; however, it has been shown that knowledge of someone's cultural background can aid in providing quality care within the cultural context of the client (Hearnden, 2008; Spector, 2009).

Health Literacy and Health Outcomes

"Health literacy is the degree to which individuals have the capacity to obtain, process, and understand basic health information and services" (United States Department of Health and Human Services [USDHHS], 2010e, p. 1.) Health literacy includes the ability to understand information on prescription drug bottles, doctor's directions, health information educational materials, and the ability to navigate complex health care systems (National Network of Libraries of Medicine, 2010). Comprehension of health information, either verbal or written, is important for clients in maintaining their health and the health of their families. However, many people lack the ability to read, understand, and act on health information presented to them on a regular basis. Research has shown that limited health literacy affects people of all races, incomes, ages, and educational levels, with the impact of limited health literacy disproportionately affecting minority and lower socioeconomic groups, and nearly 9 out of 10 adults have difficulty with using the health information that is routinely presented to them (USDHHS, 2010e). (See Display 10.3 for further explanation).

Low health literacy has a negative impact on a patient's health status and health outcomes. Research studies show that patients with limited reading skills are:

- Less likely to engage in health screenings and preventive action
- Less likely to have chronic disease under control
- More likely to be hospitalized
- More likely to report being in poor health
- More likely to die (Rudd, 2010)

Poor health literacy skills have been associated with poorer health status and increased health care costs as patients with a low health literacy level are less knowledgeable about their health conditions and are less likely to seek preventative care (DeMarco & Nystrom, 2010). A systematic review of 31 articles assessed health literacy rates for patients seeking care through hospital emergency departments (EDs). Findings showed evidence that a substantial portion of patients seen in EDs have limited health literacy and that adults at age 65 or over with lower health literacy were more likely to use the ED as a primary source for care, thus increasing health care costs (Herndon, Chaney, & Carden, 2011). For children, low literacy skills in both the children and their caregivers led to poor health outcomes. A systematic review of 13 studies found that children with low literacy skills had worse health behaviors. Parents with lower health literacy had less knowledge about their child's condition and were less likely to produce behaviors that would help improve their child's condition, thus leading to worse health outcomes for their children (DeWalt & Hink, 2009).

Health literacy is characterized as critical to health promotion and disease prevention; therefore it is important to recognize that health literacy goes beyond the basic definitions of literacy and can include such things as cultural literacy and computer literacy, as well as scientific, media, and technological literacy (USDHHS, 2010e). Recognizing the factors that affect health literacy is important as we strive to improve health literacy as "basic health literacy is fundamental to the success of each interaction between health care professionals and patient" (USDHHS, 2010e, p. iii).

The USDHHS developed the National Action Plan to Improve Health Literacy based on the vision and

From the Case Files

Mr. Sanchez Needs an Interpreter

I am a student in community health nursing now, but I work as an extern at our small, local county hospital helping out in the ED. A man came in one Saturday a month or so ago with a bad cut to his right hand from a push lawnmower—you know, the kind without a motor. Mr. Sanchez was trying to clean the grass from the blades and cut himself pretty badly. The ED doc asked him if he had received a tetanus shot recently, and he quickly nodded "yes." He spoke a little English, but I could tell that he was having some trouble understanding some of our questions. His friend, who brought him to the ED, did not speak English at all. We couldn't find an interpreter—they are always stretched so thin. None of us spoke Spanish. Anyway, we didn't give him a tetanus booster—just cleaned his wound, closed it with stitches, bandaged it, and told him to keep it clean. He was given a prescription for an antibiotic medication. It was a busy night, and I didn't think about it much. A few weeks later, Mr. Sanchez was back in the hospital because his wound had gotten infected and he had used a needle to drain some pus from his hand (he hadn't gotten the prescription filled because he had no insurance and no money because he was off work now). Unfortunately, by poking around with the needle, he had provided a perfect, anaerobic place for tetanus to flourish. He now was in the ICU with full-blown tetanus. I have never seen anything like this! He was on a ventilator and had to be "paralyzed," so that we could get air into him. I had only read about opisthotonos—in which the body arches with only feet and head touching the bed because of a tetanic spasm—but now I was seeing it firsthand. This poor man was completely rigid, and we were trying to give him meds to relax him and permit the ventilator to work, but at the same time we were working to keep his blood pressure from dropping too low from the meds. Mr. Sanchez spent 30 agonizing days in ICU—all because he nodded "yes" to the doc's question about the tetanus booster. With hindsight I think he probably just wanted to get out of the ED and didn't truly understand the question. A $5 tetanus booster could have prevented all of this misery and expense. (He had no insurance and was an illegal alien, so the county paid the bill.) We should have used an interpreter; should have insisted on it; should have waited until one was available. They are always in short supply—but I truly understand the importance of a translator now. I have some Spanish-speaking clients in my community health nursing rotation. I do my best to speak with them, but when I need to be sure that something is fully understood, I request that an interpreter accompany me on my home visits. I remember Mr. Sanchez and what happens when you don't use an interpreter.

Amy, age 24

principles that "(1) everyone has the right to health information that helps them make informed decisions and (2) health services are delivered in ways that are understandable and beneficial to health, longevity, and quality of life" (USDHHS, 2010e, p. 16) (Display 10.4).

To be sure that these goals are being met, the improvement of health literacy and health communication for our population continues to be a priority in the *Healthy People 2020* goals (Display 10.5).

Health communication encompasses the concept of health literacy, but also incorporates health messages and campaigns, along with mass media and consumer health issues that are targeted to populations. Population health promotion is best achieved by health communication that uses multiple communication channels to reach individuals, families, and community members. Those sources may include TV, radio, newspapers, Web sites, social media sites, educational pamphlets, health care providers, nutrition, and medication labels. To manage disease and promote health, we must make sure our patients can understand the health information they see, hear, and read from multiple sources (USDHHS, 2010e). More information on these topics can be found in Chapter 11.

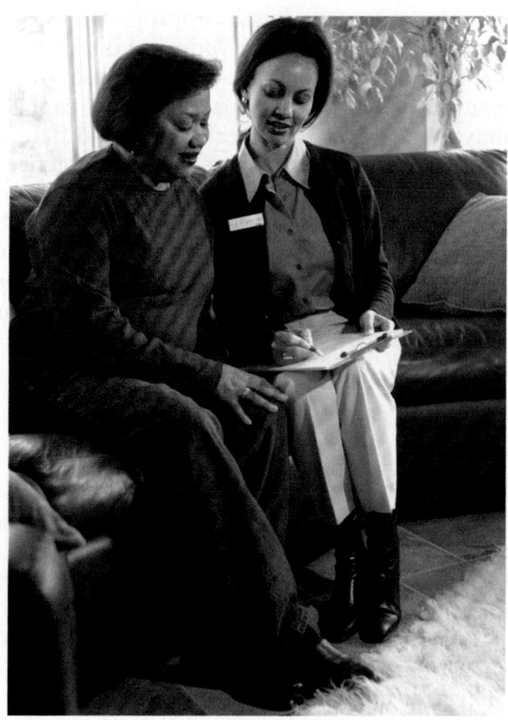

Communicating with Groups

An important aspect of communication in community health nursing involves working with groups of people. Community health nurses are regularly involved in committees, task forces, and other work-related groups; they also work with aggregates in small groups—often teaching and facilitating support groups. Group communication patterns can be complex, and interaction requires skill on the nurse's part to elicit feedback from all members and to generate a common understanding among the group's members. Since the relationships among

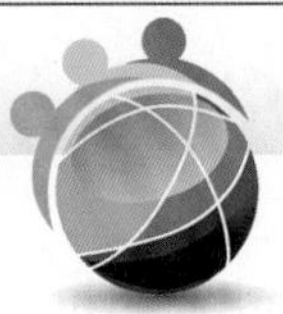

DISPLAY 10.3 HEALTH COMMUNICATION—ONE DISPARITY: LOW-LITERACY CLIENTS

Most poorly educated populations, those with the lowest literacy levels, have the highest mortality and morbidity. Changing demographics suggest that low literacy is an increasing problem among adults over age 65, certain racial and ethnic groups, recent refugee and immigrant populations, low-income populations, people with less than a high school degree or GED, nonnative speakers of English, and those living with chronic mental and/or physical health conditions (National Network of Libraries of Medicine [NNLM], 2010; USDHSS, 2010e). Yet it has been well documented that most health information pamphlets, brochures, and other materials cannot be read or comprehended by low-literacy adults. Communication with these high-risk groups should be simplified and should include easy-to-read materials. At the same time, there is the danger of making the communication so simple that the reader feels insulted. Low literacy does not necessarily mean low intelligence. How does the nurse find the right balance?

The goal of communication is to achieve understanding. If clients are to understand health communication—whether the messages are spoken or written—they must be given ample opportunity to provide feedback. Before final printing and distribution, pamphlets and other written health information should be reviewed by their intended audiences. Proposed users should comment on the readability and acceptability of both text and graphics. With spoken communication, nurses should regularly solicit feedback to make certain that messages are understood.

group members can significantly influence the effectiveness of communication, community health nurses need to understand how to organize groups and how groups function and develop over time, as well as techniques for facilitating group support and decision making.

Group Development

Think about the first time you walked into a nursing classroom—you didn't know the teacher or any of the other students in your group. What were your feelings? What did you expect or need the teacher to do? How did your feelings and expectations about the students and teacher change by the end of the term? Changes in "group dynamics" over time are termed **group process.**

In 1977, Tuckman and Jenson were credited with identifying the five most commonly used stages of group development (Display 10.6). The first stage of their model is termed *forming*. This stage is characterized by members feeling awkward and hesitant, needing to be reassured and accepted. Members depend on the group leader or facilitator to help them develop

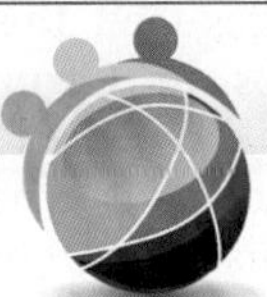

DISPLAY 10.4 THE NATIONAL ACTION PLAN TO IMPROVE HEALTH LITERACY

Vision for the Future

- An engaged and informed public that values health promotion, protection and preparedness

The vision informing this plan is of a society that:

- Provides everyone with access to accurate and accountable health information
- Delivers person-centered health information and services
- Supports lifelong learning and skills to promote good health

This vision depends on achieving the following seven goals:

1. Develop and disseminate health and safety information that is accurate, accessible, and actionable.
2. Promote changes in the health care system that improves health information, communication, informed decision-making, and access to health services.
3. Incorporate accurate, standards-based, and developmentally appropriate health and science information and curricula in child care and education through the university level.
4. Support and expand local efforts to provide adult education, English language instruction, and culturally and linguistically appropriate health information services in the community.
5. Build partnerships, develop guidance, and change policies.
6. Increase basic research and the development, implementation, and evaluation of practices and interventions to improve health literacy.
7. Increase the dissemination and use of evidenced-based health literacy practices and interventions.

From: U. S. Department of Health and Human Services: Office of Disease Prevention and Health Promotion. (2010) *National action plan to improve health literacy*. Retrieved from http://www.health.gov/communication/HLActionPlan/pdf/Health_Literacy_Action_Plan.pdf

DISPLAY 10.5 HEALTH COMMUNICATION, HEALTH INFORMATION TECHNOLOGY, AND HEALTH LITERACY

Selected *Healthy People 2020* objectives related to health literacy or health communication are listed below:

Health Communication (HC) and Health Information Technology (HIT)

HC/HIT-1: Improve the health literacy of the population.

HC/HIT-2: Increase the proportion of persons who report that their health care providers have satisfactory communication skills.

HC/HIT–3: Increase the proportion of persons who report that their health care providers always involved them in decisions about their health care as much as they wanted.

HC/HIT-4: Increase the proportion of patients whose doctor recommends personalized health information resources to help them manage their health.

HC/HIT-5: Increase the proportion of persons who use electronic personal health management tools.

HC/HIT-6: Increase individuals' access to the Internet.

HC/HIT-7: Increase the proportion of adults who report having friends or family members whom they talk with about their health.

HC/HIT–8: Increase the proportion of quality, health-related Web sites.

HC/HIT–9: Increase the proportion of online health information seekers who report easily accessing health information.

HC/HIT–10: Increase the proportion of medical practices that use electronic health records.

HC/HIT–11: Increase the proportion of meaningful users of HIT.

HC/HIT-12: Increase the proportion of crisis and emergency risk messages intended to protect the public's health that demonstrate the use of best practices.

HC/HIT-13: Increase social marketing in health promotion and disease prevention.

United States Department of Health and Human Services: *Healthy People 2020. (2010d). Health communication and health information technology.* Retrieved from http://www.healthypeople.gov/2010/topicsobjectives2020/overview.aspx?topicid=18

mutual trust and give them structure and guidance (Gilley, Morris, Waite, Coates, & Veliquette, 2010). At this stage, the group leader's task is to help the members become oriented to each other and to the work or purpose at hand.

"Ice-breaker" activities, to introduce members to each other and move past the awkwardness and hesitancy, are often used at the first group meeting. Conflict and sensitive topics, or too much self-disclosure by leaders or group members, are to be avoided at this stage. Rather, it is important to set ground rules (e.g., no sharing personal information outside of support group) and define the scope of work and timeline for completion. As group interaction is established in the first stage, task roles are the major focus with maintenance roles emerging in later stages (see Task, Maintenance, and Nonfunctional Roles in Group, Display 10.7).

The next stage is called *storming*, which is when the group begins to work together. In this stage, conflict and competition become more common as different agendas, ideas, and approaches begin to compete

DISPLAY 10.6 STAGES OF GROUP DEVELOPMENT

Forming—Group dependent on facilitator; anxiety high, need safe environment, structure, and avoid too much self-disclosure; agree on guidelines for group work/behavior; orient to task or purpose of group

Storming—Competition and conflict; need for structure; problem-solving; need to draw out quiet members; continue to clarify group task or purpose

Norming—Group now more cohesive and creative; acknowledge others' contributions; shared leadership; trust increases; work moves along more quickly

Performing—Not reached by all groups; true interdependence—can work as group, or as individuals, and in subgroups; most productive; least reliant on facilitator

Adjourning—The termination phase; conclusion of activities and resolution of relationships; formal acknowledgment of group work

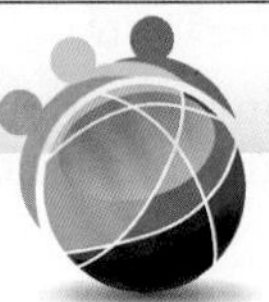

DISPLAY 10.7 TASK, MAINTENANCE, AND NONFUNCTIONAL ROLES IN GROUPS

Task Roles: Required in selecting and carrying out group tasks.

Maintenance Roles: Required in strengthening and maintaining group relationships and activities.

Nonfunctional Roles: Roles that harm the group and its work—often self-oriented behavior.

Task Role Behaviors

Initiating Activity: Proposing solutions; suggesting new ideas, new definitions of the problem, and new approaches to the problem or new organization of material.

Seeking Information: Asking for clarification of suggestions; requesting additional information or facts.

Seeking Opinions: Looking for an expression of feeling about something from members; seeking clarification of values, suggestions, or ideas.

Giving Information: Offering facts or generalizations; relating one's own experiences to the group problem to illustrate a point.

Giving Opinions: Stating an opinion or belief concerning a suggestion or suggestions; particularly concerning its value rather than its factual basis.

Elaborating: Clarifying, giving examples or developing meanings, trying to envision how a proposal might work if adopted.

Coordinating: Showing relationships among various ideas or suggestions, trying to pull ideas and suggestions together, trying to draw together activities of various subgroups or members.

Summarizing: Pulling together related ideas or suggestions; restating suggestions after the group has discussed them.

Maintenance Role Behaviors

Encouraging: Being friendly, warm, and responsive to others, praising others and their ideas, agreeing with and accepting contributions of others.

Gatekeeping: Trying to make it possible for another member to make a contribution to the group by saying "We haven't heard anything from Jim yet," or suggesting limited talking time for everyone, so that all will have a chance to be heard.

Standard Setting: Expressing standards for the group to use in choosing its content or procedures or in evaluating its decisions; reminding the group to avoid decisions that conflict with group standards.

Following: Going along with decisions of the group; thoughtfully accepting ideas of others; serving as audience during group discussion.

Expressing Group Feelings: Summarizing what group feeling is sensed to be; describing reactions of the group to ideas or solutions.

Both Task and Maintenance Role Behaviors

Evaluating: Submitting group decisions or accomplishments to compare with group standards; measuring accomplishments against goals.

Diagnosing: Determining sources of difficulties; appropriate steps to take next; analyzing the main block to progress.

Testing for Consensus: Tentatively asking for group opinions in order to find out whether the group is nearing consensus on a decision; sending up trial balloons to test group opinions.

Mediating: Harmonizing, conciliating differences in points of view, suggesting compromise solutions.

Relieving Tension: Draining off negative feelings by jesting or pouring oil on troubled waters; putting a tense situation in a wider context.

Types of Nonfunctional Behaviors

Being Aggressive: Working for status by criticizing or blaming others; showing hostility toward the group or some individual; deflating egos or status of others.

Blocking: Interfering with the progress of the group by going off on a tangent; citing personal experiences unrelated to the problem; arguing too much on a point; rejecting ideas without consideration.

Self-confessing: Using the group as a sounding board; expressing personal, nongroup-oriented feelings or points of view.

Competing: Vying with others to produce the best idea, talk the most, play the most roles, gain favor with the leader.

Seeking Sympathy: Trying to induce other group members to be sympathetic to one's problems or misfortunes; deploring one's own situation, or disparaging one's own ideas to gain support.

Special Pleading: Introducing or supporting suggestions related to one's own pet concerns or philosophies, lobbying.

Horsing Around: Clowning, joking, mimicking, disrupting the work of the group.

Seeking Recognition: Attempting to call attention to one's self by loud or excessive talking, extreme ideas, unusual behavior.

Withdrawal: Acting indifferent or passive, using excessive formality, daydreaming, doodling, whispering to others, wandering off the subject.

Adapted from: Kirst-Ashman, K., & Hull, G. (2011). *Understanding generalist practice* (6th ed.). Belmont, CA: Brooks-Cole; Boyd, M., & Foley, M. (2009). *Psychiatric nursing: Contemporary practice.* (4th ed.) Philadelphia, PA: Lippincott, Williams & Wilkins.

for attention. However, this period of role ambiguity is necessary to allow group members to identify roles and expectations and get a feel of how the group will work together. The storming stage can be difficult, but an effective group leader can guide group members in problem solving and setting goals. Modeling maintenance roles such as encouraging all group members to participate, asking for a quiet member to share an idea with the group, and summarizing group feelings, is helpful in moving group members along in maintenance as well as task roles.

By the time group members begin to show signs of cohesiveness, they have moved on to the *norming* stage, and work begins to progress. Trust and openness are much more apparent, and there is a shared sense of "belonging" to the group. Creativity and shared ideas and opinions characterize this stage. Until this time, most groups function at the task level, but by this stage, maintenance activities are more apparent as members draw others in and constructively share feelings. The leader should continue to role model good maintenance behaviors to move the group along in its work.

The *performing* stage may not occur with all groups; it is characterized by the ability to work as a total group, in subgroups or independently. This is considered the most productive stage as group members are motivated and able to handle the decision-making process in a competent and autonomous manner. A high level of team satisfaction is seen in this stage as members are now able to work together more smoothly and do not need a lot of direction from the facilitator.

When either work or support groups end, the final stage of development is termed *adjourning*. In adjourning the emphasis is on wrapping up the project, and this results in a withdrawal from both task and relationship or maintenance activities. Group members often feel happy that they have accomplished their goal, but are sad about the loss or disbandment of the group. Therefore, group leaders may plan a small party or ceremony—something to formally commemorate the group's time together and help members successfully disengage (Gilley et al., 2010).

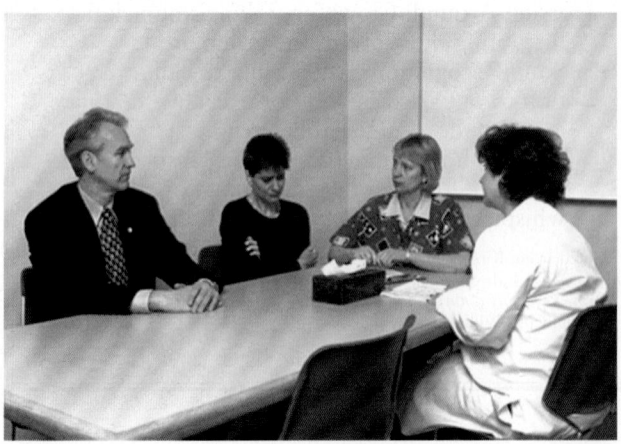

Group Functions in Decision Making

Groups, regardless of size, perform many functions. Four functions of particular relevance to group decision making include:

1. *Group members share information.* In community health nursing, groups often include clients, health professionals, and community members who share their experience and expertise to arrive at solutions and decisions. Something one member says may spur others to think of more creative solutions or share similar problems allowing group members to gain insight and develop trust (Gilley et al., 2010).
2. *Groups are heterogeneous and present diverse views* that enrich the number and types of alternatives in the problem-solving process. Group decisions are often better than individual ones because of the diversity of experiences and perspectives. However, group facilitators should promote open, prejudiced-free attitudes within the group to increase the positive benefits of diversity (van Dick, van Knippenberg, Hagele, Guillaume, & Brodbeck, 2008).
3. *Groups influence their members, thinking* by broadening their perspectives and presenting new ways of thinking about the issues. This allows group members to gain more insight in understanding the issue at hand (Hare, 2010). This influencing function can improve the quality of group decision making and increase the likelihood of decisions that support positive outcomes (Gilley et al., 2010).
4. *Groups progress toward consensus* or resolution by planning tasks that allow members to discuss a set of alternatives and arrive at solutions to meet established goals. Time pressures and desire for completion help to move this process along (Gilley et al., 2010).

Techniques for Enhancing Group Decision Making

As a member of many decision-making groups in the community, the community health nurse can facilitate the process through certain techniques. Three strategies commonly used in community health settings include brainstorming, multivoting technique, and **nominal group technique**.

Brainstorming

Brainstorming is an idea-generating process that encourages group members to freely offer suggestions. When brainstorming, group members are asked to present ideas. They are encouraged to be creative and "think out of the box"; no idea is too bizarre or wild. Furthermore, no criticism or discussion is allowed until all ideas have been exhausted and recorded. This technique is helpful for generating creative possibilities and is most useful in the early stages of decision making. Research has shown that brainstorming is considered to be the most widely used method of generating creative ideas, but is often less effective than nominal group techniques (Heslin, 2009).

Multivoting

Multivoting is a decision-making tool that enables members to prioritize a long list of ideas with minimal discussion and difficulty. Multivoting often follows brainstorming to narrow the list to a few items worthy of immediate attention. All of the ideas are listed on a flip chart and members are allowed to vote on one-third of the total number of items. For example, if there are 60 items, members are given 20 stickers to place their "vote" beside their top priorities on the flip chart. Once everyone has voted, the stickers are tallied to arrive at a shorter list of priorities (Bens, 2005).

Nominal Group Technique

Nominal group technique is a group decision-making method in which group members are asked to not speak to each other but instead are asked to write down their ideas, along with the advantages and disadvantages of the issue being addressed. After everyone has completed the task, the members' ideas are presented to the group and discussion takes place so that the information can be categorized and prioritized (Ohio State University, 2009). This technique was used in a study of 44 African American men and women to "determine what foods African Americans most associate with their culture and if they consider these foods healthy or unhealthy" (Jefferson et al., 2010, p. 344). Based on results of this study, researchers can develop culturally appropriate dietary interventions to reduce blood pressure in African American populations (Jefferson et al., 2010). Nominal group technique affords researchers a means of collecting data that are inclusive and respectful of participants' opinions, while allowing both shy and talkative members to join in the discussion.

Other Group Communication Techniques

Not all community health nursing work with groups involves group process and group decision making. Sometimes, community health nurses are asked to speak to groups of concerned citizens at public meetings to raise awareness of an issue (e.g., preparing for disasters), or provide information to parent-teacher groups (e.g., immunization compliance). Often, they are called upon to incorporate group-teaching methods to change behaviors (see Chapter 11 for more on health teaching). One example of an effective group-teaching intervention is a randomized controlled trial to increase parent–adolescent sexual risk communication conducted in Mexico by community health nursing professors (Villarruel, Cherry, Cabriales, Ronis, & Zhou, 2008). After randomly assigning 791 parents to either an intervention (HIV risk reduction) or control (health promotion) group, testing was done at baseline, posttest, and 6- and 12-month postintervention. Six 60-minute teaching modules (using similar principles, activities, and homework) were used for both intervention and control groups—with one focusing on pregnancy and HIV-prevention, support of sexual-specific communication, overcoming discomfort with sexual topics, and general adolescent–parent communication; and the control group focusing on general health behaviors (e.g., diabetes, heart disease, cancer prevention), behavior changes (e.g., diet, exercise, not smoking), and parental roles in health promotion. Adolescents received similar information from trained facilitators (nurses, others). Results showed "significantly more general communication ($p < 0.005$), more sexual risk communication ($p < 0.001$), and more comfort with communication ($p < 0.001$) among parents and teens in the intervention group than in the control intervention" (p. 371).

Group or public education and communication occur routinely in public health nursing. However, it is even more critical during disasters and other public health emergencies. Consistent public messages, interagency communication, and providing education and guidance on disaster preparedness were found to be lacking in a study of public health professionals who participated in focus groups on the topic of previous emergency responses (Rebmann, Carrico, & English, 2008). Researchers also noted "effective communication is necessary to maintain public trust" (p. 344).

Health Information Technology

The use of health information technology (HIT) is essential to the communication process in all areas of nursing practice. Since the 1970s nurses have partnered with multidisciplinary team members in the delivery of health care and in the design and implementation of HIT systems within many health care settings. Since that time nurses have continued to embrace the potential that HIT has to transform health care, with nurses guiding and developing nursing informatics (NIs) into a well-established specialty within nursing.

Nursing Informatics

Nursing informatics (NI) integrates information and communication technology (ICT) with the practice of nursing, thus enhancing individual and group decision making while also providing a framework for interdisciplinary study and research. Currently, there are more than 5,000 nursing informaticists and 25 distinct NIs organizations in the United States. NIs will continue to grow as a specialty as nurses continue to find innovative ways to use HIT to increase patient safety and improve quality outcomes (Murphy, 2010).

Nurses must be competent in using 21st century technology advances that have the potential to improve patient care and safety. The application of ICTs will allow community health nurses to deliver innovative health care strategies that promote the health of individuals, families, and communities (Jette, Tribble, Gagnon, & Mathieu, 2010; Murphy, 2010). For example, utilizing technology, such as telehealth, nurses working in underserved areas will deliver health care that overcomes barriers such as lack of transportation and limited access to care (Luptak, Daily, Juretic, Rupper, Hill, Hicken, et al., 2010).

Effective use of communication and technology by community health nurses has the potential to:

- Improve health care quality and safety (e.g., in-home patient monitoring systems)
- Support care in the community and home (e.g., provision of specialty care through telehealth)
- Build health care skills and knowledge (e.g., use of simulation for teaching clinical skills)
- Facilitate clinical and consumer decision making (e.g., quality, health-related websites) (USDHHS, 2010e)

Computerized Systems

The first computer systems were installed in hospitals in the late 1960s and since that time, the computer has changed all aspects of health care (Murphy, 2010). Currently, various practitioners use computers to access Internet databases in order to research diseases, treatment methodologies, clinical trials, and educational resources for clients. In many community health settings, computer databases aid in the documentation of assessment data and practice activities. Examples include statewide immunization tracking systems and identification of epidemiological health problems in the community through health and disease data systems (ACHNE, 2010). Computers also allow the use of shared workplaces for groups to utilize group decision-making techniques for recording ideas and research findings, tabulating rankings, voting and election of officers in professional organizations, and conducting simulations for disaster planning.

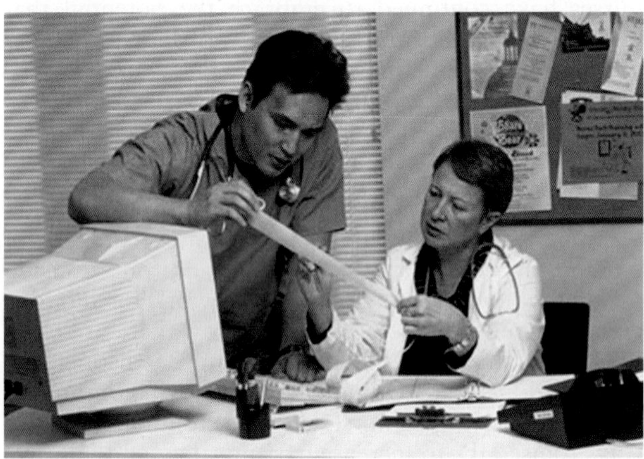

Computers allow community health nurses to access educational opportunities that include online journals, workshops, courses, and conferences for professionals. With advancing computer technology, online educational opportunities are increasing rapidly with the quality of the programs improving every day. To assist in maintaining a quality work force in community health nursing, health care organizations and nursing programs are designing computerized programs that address specific topics. For example, the threat of a terrorist attack is a concern for national security. To educate and train nurses how to respond to an attack that utilizes biological agents, faculty at the University of California have designed a computerized program that is able to present nurses with six case scenarios that allow them to develop and utilize critical thinking skills to diagnose infectious agents rapidly in an effort to prevent mass destruction (Nyamathi, Casillas, Gresham, Pierce, Farb, & Weichmann, 2010).

Patient self-management, utilizing information technology, is becoming an important factor in the way health care is delivered. Patients now have a vast amount of consumer-oriented health information available to them through the web and many consumers are now visiting Web sites for their health care information. Consumers can conduct their own research by surfing the web; however, because of quality control issues many health care professionals are now referring their clients to specific Internet to obtain disease-related information. These websites include WebMD, MedlinePlus, Centers for Disease Control and Prevention (CDC) or disease-specific sites such as the American Cancer Society.

For particular diseases, health care practitioners are beginning to use information technology to support clinical services. Currently researchers are studying how computer technology can be used effectively and efficiently in the treatment of diabetes. Soon patients with diabetes will input data related to blood sugar results, insulin dosage, physical activity, weight, and mood into an interactive program that analyzes the information and formulates a tailored message back to them based on their needs at that point in time. Also, interactive links will allow patients with diabetes to link directly to other family and friends for needed support and link to others with diabetes so they can learn how to integrate diabetes into their everyday life (Kaufman, 2010).

Electronic Health Records

Historically, the documentation process has increasingly involved the computer, with paperless charting becoming commonplace. With the passage of the Patient Protection and Affordable Care Act of 2010, technology will continue to be involved in all aspects of health care. One aspect will be an increased emphasis on the use of HIT to implement electronic health records (EHRs). EHRs, an electronic version of a client's medical history, will allow for the documentation of structured, electronic clinical information (Hertelendy, Fenton, & Griffin, 2010) that will provide "meaningful use" to accurate and complete information. Meaningful use involves the use of a certified EHR "in a meaningful manner, such as e-prescribing....electronic exchange of health information to improve quality of care" and the use of "EHR technology to submit clinical quality and other measures" (USDHHS, 2010b, para. 3). The EHR automates access to a client's medical information, and this ready access to accurate and timely information will allow better coordination of care to:

- Diagnose health problems earlier
- Reduce medical errors, duplication of tests and delays in treatment and

- Allow clients to become well informed of their health status and partner in the decision making process thus facilitating better client-focused decisions (USDHHS, 2010c).

In the future, the use of the EHR will expand beyond the use in medical home and acute care settings. Soon community health nurses may be able to swipe a card and access a patient's health history and current health data (e.g., laboratory and x-ray results) in community clinics and home health settings.

Portable Technology Devices

Other information technology advances such as the smartphone, iPad, and tablet personal computers (PCs) have become popular because of their wireless connectivity and portability features. Recent advances in low-power computing and advances in battery life have allowed a plethora of handheld devices to stay powered longer and have greater computing power. Their computer processing capabilities and wireless Internet connection allow nurses to access the Internet in seconds. This instant access allows community health nurses to immediately retrieve large amounts of health and educational materials that can be effectively utilized in mobile outreach programs and disaster responses to promote and protect the health of communities. For example, in 2008 extreme flooding in Iowa caused widespread devastation and the displacement of thousands of families. In response to the flooding, public health officials capitalized on accessibility of the Internet and cellular telephone networks to educate affected community members on important issues, such as contaminated well water, mold and mold removal, and beneficial vaccinations (Murphy, Iqbal, Sanchez, & Quinlisk, 2010).

Organizations and coalitions across the country are utilizing the widespread availability of smartphones and wireless connectivity to provide health prevention messages to community members utilizing free mobile information services. The National Healthy Mothers, Healthy Babies Coalition has launched a campaign that provides pregnant women and new mothers with three free text messages each week during the pregnancy up until the child's first birthday. These messages focus on a variety of topics related to maternal and child health including prevention of birth defects, prenatal care, breast-feeding, nutrition, car seat safety, oral health, safe sleep, and immunizations. The goal of these messages is to help participants care for their own health and give their babies the best possible start in life, which ultimately will have a positive impact on maternal and child health on a national level (National Healthy Mothers, Healthy Babics Coalition, 2009). Short message service (SMS), or text messaging, was also employed in a study of parents of 124 adolescent girls needing follow up on human papillomavirus (HPV) vaccine doses 2 and 3 (Kharbanda et al., 2011). On-time subsequent vaccines among the texting group were greater (51.6%) than for the group not receiving text message reminders (35%). And in diabetes treatment, researchers have found that providing supportive care through smartphone text messaging improves health care outcomes by increasing knowledge and improving self-efficacy (Kaufman, 2010).

Although there are several disadvantages to smartphones, such as limited screen size making some information difficult to read, it is expected that the use of this type of technology will continue to increase in all health care settings (Putzer & Park, 2010). Demonstration projects in medically underserved areas, such as the Mobile Health Information System in South Africa, are using wireless technology that allows health care practitioners to access relevant and accurate clinical information while in the field thus improving health service delivery (QualComm, 2010).

Geographic Information System

To effectively plan and implement public health programs, up-to-date and relevant information must be communicated to public health officials and community leaders. One communication method utilizes computerized geographic information systems (GIS) to visually display, analyze, and manipulate spatial data.

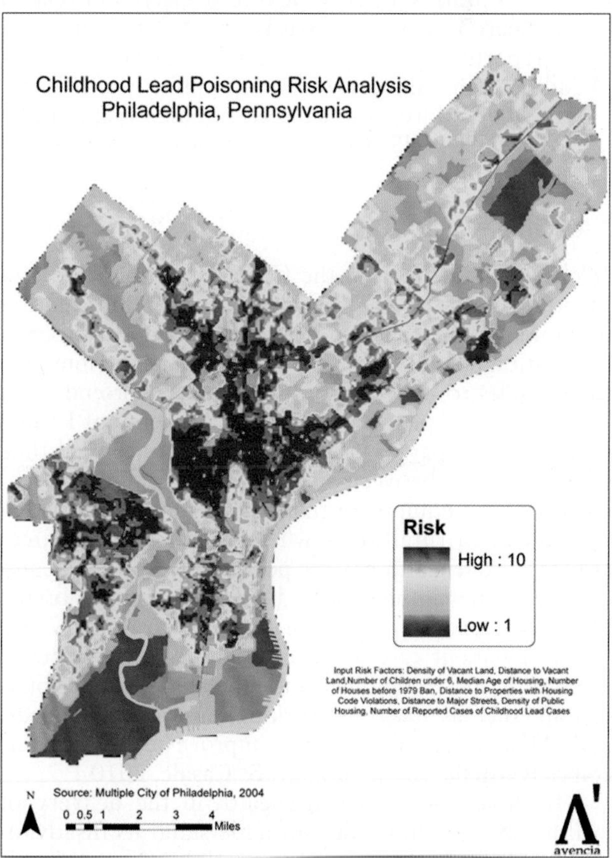

Example of GIS use in a lead poisoning project. (Photo courtesy of USA.gov.) Retrieved from: http://www.cdc.gov/gis/images/maps/LeadPoisoiningRisk.png

This technology allows community health and safety organizations to use three-dimensional graphics to locate and track diseases, toxic waste sites, ground water sources, and vehicle crashes on roads in a region, county, or census tract, and so on. With such information, community health and safety can be enhanced and traffic patterns can be altered to make roads safer; health care personnel resources can be redistributed based on disease distribution; and dumps and waste sites can be relocated to protect valuable ground water sources. Real life examples of the use of GIS in community health include:

- Assisting public health officials in Rhode Island to identify children under age 6 years who have an increased risk of lead poisoning. GIS mapping has assisted public health officials to focus cleanup efforts in areas where lead poisoning is the worst (Brown University, 2010).
- Motor vehicle-related injuries are the leading cause of death for people aged 1 to 34 in the United States and are considered a significant public health issue. To assist communities in addressing this issue, the National Highway Traffic Safety Administration (NHTSA) utilizes GIS mapping to document fatality data on all vehicle crashes in the United States that occur on a public roadways (NHTSA, n.d.).
- The Center for Disease Control and Prevention (CDC) utilizes a GIS system to display data related to heart disease and stroke mortality. This data is reported by geography, gender, and ethnicity. It allows communities to develop public health initiatives that address these diseases in high-risk populations (USDHHS: Centers for Disease Control and Prevention [CDC], n.d.).

Telehealth

Telehealth is defined by the Centers for Medicare and Medicaid Services as "the integration of information technologies, medical and health technologies, telecommunication technologies, and human–machine interface technologies to deliver health care and to promote the health status of people" (American Academy of Family Practice, 2011, para. 1). This exchange involves real-time communication between a patient and a health care provider utilizing equipment that includes audio and video equipment. In rural areas where health care resources are scarce, telehealth has the potential to address health care disparities in underserved populations by allowing health care providers to increase access to primary and specialty patient care, education, and support systems. Telehealth can be combined with other technologic applications, such as social networking, on-line chat boards, and SMSs for text messaging to improve health care outcomes (Castelli, 2010; Gibbons & Casale, 2010).

To effectively utilize telehealth in the delivery of health care, it is important to understand its disadvantages and barriers to use. One possible consequence is the breakdown in the relationship between the patient and health care provider. Communication breakdowns could occur from poor interpersonal skills and cultural and linguistic differences among health care professionals and patients, as well as poor mastery of the telehealth technology. Other barriers include costs of services, equipment malfunctions, network failures, malpractice concerns related to licensing issues, lack of adequate reimbursement, and lack of evidence about cost-effectiveness and efficiency of telehealth applications (Sarhan, 2009).

Despite its current limitations, telehealth holds great potential to deliver quality health care and increase access to care in many communities. Telehealth programs are already showing evidence of decreased hospital admissions by 46% in patients diagnosed with chronic heart failure (Berkley, Bauer, & Rowland, 2010), and telehealth is being explored as an option to keep the high costs of chronic illness lower in diseases, such as diabetes and hypertension (Schlachta-Fairchild, Varghese, Deickman, & Castelli, 2010).

Electronic Groups and Social Networking

Electronic meetings are similar to telehealth, as electronic meeting systems involve using video and audio equipment to allow conferences and meetings to be held with participants scattered across a building, counties, the state, or even the globe. Electronic group meetings are considered an effective form of group-decision support as facilitators can encourage, organize, and prioritize ideas from all participants. Participants do not have to spend travel time and money away from their normal location, allowing electronic meetings to promote more efficient use of time and effective decision making by groups (Electronic Meeting Systems, 2011).

Information technology now allows community health nurses to utilize shared online workspaces to collaborate with professional colleagues and community partners to share resources, negotiate ideas, and coordinate collaborative efforts regardless of their geographic location. Examples of shared online workspaces that allow groups to share information and receive feedback include many sites that utilize Wiki software, such as Google Groups and PBworks (http://pbworks.com/). Many other online collaborative management tools exist and will continue to be developed allowing groups

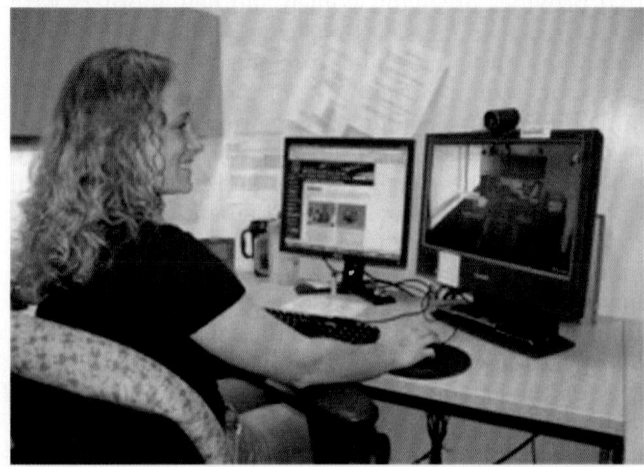

Telehealth gives the community health nurse an opportunity to see and speak with clients located at remote sites. (Photo courtesy of USA.gov.) Retrieved from: http://www.albuquerque.va.gov/images/Feature/Telenutrition1.jpg

to share minutes of meetings and real-time information, conduct surveys, and schedule meetings. Shared online workspaces can increase communication in collaborative relationships. Educational institutions are now using shared online workspaces to educate students in various areas and the potential exists for using shared online resources for education and support of clients in community health nursing (Wang, 2010).

Nurses also communicate with clients and communities through online social networking that connects people with colleagues, family, and friends. Social networking sites, such as Facebook, allow you to upload videos, create a blog, post events, join groups, and send messages. There are many social network sites available on the Internet, many of which are tailored to specific health-related topics. For example, social networks related to HIV infection aim to:

- Reach people with HIV prevention, testing, and treatment information
- Form support groups for those living with or affected by HIV or AIDS
- Inform people about HIV-related events and activities

Examples of social networking sites for HIV-related information include AIDS.gov's MySpace page, AIDS.gov's Daily Strength group page and CDC's Facebook page (AIDS.gov, 2011).

HIT is now considered an essential tool for improving health communication for clients, families, and communities. As technology-assisted decision making becomes increasingly useful and available, community health nurses should strive to understand and be trained in all forms of computer and telecommunication technologies. However, it is also important to understand that not all population groups have the resources or capability to access these technologies. In brief, the term *digital divide* refers to the gap between people who have access to digital or Internet information and those who have not.

For example, older adults with lower incomes or from rural areas might not own a computer or have Internet access. And, even if they have Internet access, many older adults may have unique physical challenges, impaired vision, cognitive impairment, and low health literacy that can affect their ability to access health information digitally. Also, cultural and linguistic diversity may be a barrier to an individual's ability to access information using digital technology. For example, it has been found that older Italian and Greek migrants in South Australia are minimal users of computer technology and cell phones; many express no interest in learning about new technologies (Goodall, Ward, & Newman, 2010). In community health nursing, it is important to assess a client's ability to access and use information technology. For many clients, such as older adults, migrants, those living in low socioeconomic communities and those with lower literacy levels, a nondigital means of communication might be the most appropriate way to meet their needs (Chu, Huber, Mastel-Smith, & Cesario, 2009; Goodall et al., 2010).

COLLABORATION AND PARTNERSHIPS IN COMMUNITY HEALTH NURSING

Effective interdisciplinary and interprofessional collaboration is essential in the health care system to achieve quality health care and assure successful outcomes (Boon, Mior, Barnsley, Ashbury, & Haig, 2009). The definition of collaboration implies working together for the greater good; however, a more detailed definition will help facilitate the development of collaboration into practice for community health nurses. When working in community health, **collaboration** means a purposeful interaction among nurses, clients, other professionals, and community members to develop strategies for improving the health of individuals, families, and communities (Petri, 2010).

Although collaboration is a complex dynamic process there are really only two basic features of collaboration: (1) it has a goal, and (2) it involves several parties assisting one another to achieve that goal. The overriding purpose or goal of collaboration in community health practice is to benefit the health of the public. Therefore, many players must work together (e.g., agencies, professionals, clients, lay health workers) to effectively achieve that goal. Partners will be able to meet their goals more effectively if the collaborative process promotes an atmosphere of mutual trust and respect, maintains open and honest communication, and accepts the roles and skills of the participating partners (Petri, 2010).

Asset-based community development (ABCD) is a methodology that starts with community assets and strengths including local persons, community associations and networks, natural resources, and institutions as a means of working with residents to create sustainable communities. Rather than a needs-focused approach, ABCD starts with identifying the types of skills and resources in the community and then consults with the community members on improvements they would like to make (Asset-based Community Development Institute, 2009). Similarly **community-based participatory research** (CBPR) involves community members in the entire research process from identifying a topic of importance to the community through implementation and dissemination (Community-Campus Partnerships for Health, 2011; Pavlish, & Pharris, 2012). See more on CPBR in Chapter 4. Involving stakeholders in planning and implementing programs and research increases their buy-in and the likelihood of success.

Key principles for establishing partnerships and collaboration with communities and interprofessional team members include:

- Think "outside the box" when looking for partners or collaborators.
- Plans are guides toward a goal; stay flexible.
- Partners must be part of the planning; continuously widen the circle of participants.
- When adding new partners, be prepared to replan.

- Maintain different levels of collaboration (different team members have more resources, come in later to the project, or leave the project earlier).
- Use consensus-building techniques that are creative and visual.
- Establish a shared vision; then share the plans and leadership (USDHHS 2010a; Petri, 2010; Asset Based Community Development, 2009).

To meet the needs of aggregate populations, community health nursing practice draws on the expertise and assistance of numerous individuals. The list of team members can include health planners, policy makers, epidemiologists, biostatisticians, community citizens, demographers, environmentalists, educators, politicians, housing experts, safety professionals, and industrial hygienists in addition to nurses, physicians, social workers, psychologists, physical therapists, dentists, and other professionals involved in health services. All partners should be encouraged and allowed to utilize their skills and knowledge to optimize outcomes (Kilgore & Langford, 2009).

Depending on the need to be addressed, community health nurses may work with many people on a single project or on multiple endeavors and it is important to remember to involve the most important team players. Therefore, representatives from the identified client population should always be included as key members of the collaborative process. For example, to address the increasing prevalence of childhood obesity, research has provided evidence that family-based interventions are the most successful. Therefore, overweight and obese children and their parents should be included in the process of designing and implementing childhood obesity programs. By including members of the identified population, potential barriers, such as inconvenient appointment times, lack of transportation, and excessive length of the program, can be identified and addressed (Grimes-Robison & Evans, 2008). Another example is when developing a culturally based intervention program to address HIV/AIDS among Latino youth, the collaborative process should include members of the targeted population while also including HIV prevention and treatment providers, HIV case management agencies, funding partners, and community members. By involving the appropriate interdisciplinary members, effective community health programs can be designed and implemented (Villarruel, Gal, Eakin, Wilkes, & Herbst, 2010). A case study illustrating the concept of community collaboration is described in Display 10.8.

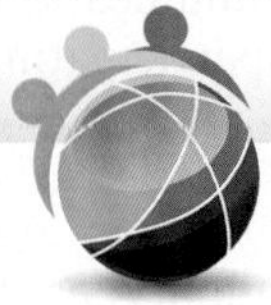

DISPLAY 10.8 COMMUNITY COLLABORATION

Case Study: Community Health Improvement Partnership: the Health Provocateur Project in Sarasota County, Florida

The proportion of people who are uninsured in the United States has steadily increased over the last 25 years. In the state of Florida, new data from the Census Bureau indicates that one in four Floridians under the age of 65 lack health insurance that puts Florida third on the list of states with the highest percentage of uninsured. This high percentage of uninsured residents in Florida affects all Floridians through higher medical costs, insurance premiums, and taxes.

The health insurance crisis in Florida puts all communities at risk. Floridians without health insurance are more likely to be sicker as access to care is late or not at all, thus impacting quality of life greatly. In Sarasota County, Florida, 38% of uninsured residents report that they delayed or did not get needed medical care when sick, with 12% reporting their health care status as fair or poor.

What can a community do to address the growing number of uninsured in their neighborhoods? In Sarasota County, community leaders believe a community is only as strong as its weakest member and that finding ways to expand coverage and increase access to affordable care for the uninsured is vital to the health of their entire county.

The responsibility for solving the problem of the uninsured must be shared among federal, state, and local government, private and public organizations, insurers, hospitals, and individuals. The Community Health Improvement Partnership (CHIP) in Sarasota County brings together a dynamic collaboration of individuals, community leaders, not-for-profit organizations, and hospitals that are dedicated to improving the physical, mental, social, and environmental health of all citizens in Sarasota County. Community Health Action Teams (CHAT), comprising community volunteers and organizational partners, were formed in several areas of the county to focus on improving the health of a specific community. CHATs identify and study health issues, and then take action to tackle priority issues. For example, the North Port CHAT helped bring additional health care and transportation services to its community, and also promoted youth activities and efforts to reduce substance abuse.

The Health Provocateur Project is another example of CHIP's initiatives. This initiative convenes major stakeholders of the local health care system, including hospital chief executive officers (CEOs) and health department administrators on a quarterly basis to

(continued)

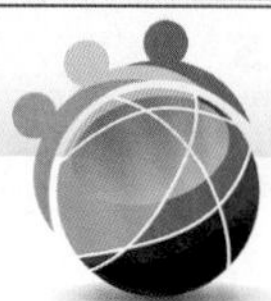

DISPLAY 10.8 COMMUNITY COLLABORATION *(Continued)*

discuss and act on local issues. In 2006, a team of collaborators from 12 hospitals and health departments created Sarasota Healthcare Access, a model system of care to improve services to the uninsured. Using a large-scale systems approach, the goals of this initiative include:

- Creating a formal system of the exchange of patient health information, data and information on program/providers services
- Developing a universal referral system
- Utilizing existing capacity of providers to increase the number of residents who are enrolled in primary care and oral health service programs
- Providing case management services for uninsured clients with identified medical conditions to reduce unnecessary emergency room visits and hospital readmissions
- Enhancing access to low cost medication
- Increasing community awareness of available health care resources for the uninsured.

Effective collaboration in Sarasota County has led to the creation of a coordinated system of care that will move Sarasota County one step closer to improving the quality of life for all its residents. (Ellingstad, K., & Clarke, L. L. (2007). *Uncovered: Health and the uninsured in Sarasota county. Community Health Improvement Partnership 2007.* Sarasota, FL: Sarasota County Health Department; Sarasota County Health Department. (2011). *Community health improvement partnership.* Retrieved from http://www.sarasotahealth.org/communityprograms/chip.htm)

Case Study Analysis Questions

Directions: Explore the CHIP website (http://www.chip4health.org) to learn more about this initiative and help answer the following questions:

1. What characteristics of collaborative partnerships are evident in this case study? Provide examples
2. How are community members engaged in the CHIP initiatives? What is the role of CHAT teams?
3. What barriers to communication would you anticipate in working with CHIP teams?
4. Provide examples of three task and maintenance roles that the community health nurse can use to facilitate effective communication during for CHIP and Health Provocateur Project meetings.
5. Discuss the stages of group development that you would expect the CHAT team to experience. What interventions can the community health nurse employ to help the CHAT move to the performing stage.
6. The hospitals and health departments in the Health Provocateur Project are a mix of government, for-profit, and not-for-profit organizations. What are the benefits and challenges of them working together?
7. What barriers to collaboration would you expect in the Health Provocateur Project? What communication interventions could the community health nurse use to address the barriers?

In the Levels of Prevention display, the levels of prevention pyramid are utilized to provide a framework of the collaborative process in community health nursing. One of the objectives seen in *Healthy People 2020* is Environmental Health objective HP2020-13: Eliminate elevated blood lead levels in children (*Healthy People 2020, 2011*). To achieve this objective, community health nurses need to be able to collaborate effectively with community partners in the design and implementation of health programs that address this very significant issue. However, the same nurses may work directly with individuals and families to educate them on the importance of having their children tested for elevated lead blood levels and once a child is identified with an elevated lead blood level, the nurse may collaborate with individual clients to understand the importance of medical treatment for their child.

Culture and Collaborative Services

Culture is a set of shared understandings related to knowledge, attitudes, and behaviors that give meaning to an experience. In community health nursing, clients and providers are often separated by their own distinct set of understandings or culture. Therefore, clients' cultural background, experience in collaboration and partnership building, perspectives, and expressions of need provide important information for the planning and delivery of services (Display 10.9). Community health nurses, by being aware of one's own culture and the difference between their culture and their clients', will be able to participate in cultural exchanges with clients that will promote stronger alliances, allowing them to develop greater understanding, acceptance, and commitment to more fully use the health programs designed for their benefit (Palinkas, 2010). See Chapter 5 for more on culture in community health nursing.

Characteristics of Collaborative Partnerships in Community Health Nursing

To explore the meaning of collaboration in the context of community health nursing, this section examines five

LEVELS OF PREVENTION PYRAMID APPLIED TO CHILDREN'S HEALTH AND THE ENVIRONMENT: COLLABORATIVE OPPORTUNITIES FOR COMMUNITY HEALTH NURSES AT ALL THREE LEVELS OF PREVENTION

SITUATION: High lead blood levels were identified in a community

GOAL: Using the three levels of prevention:

- Programs and policies will be developed to prevent childhood lead poisoning.
- Children will be screened for elevated blood levels.
- Lead-poisoned infants and children will receive appropriate medical care and environmental follow-up.

TERTIARY PREVENTION (REDUCE THE MORBIDITY RELATED TO LEAD EXPOSURE OR POISONING)	
Prevent Death and Further Disability	**Interventions**
• Restore child to healthful state. • Restore the environment to a healthful state	• Medical treatment as indicated; may include chelation therapy. • Removal of child from environment • Aggressive environmental remediation
SECONDARY PREVENTION (MINIMIZE ABSORPTION OF LEAD AND ELIMINATE CHRONIC EXPOSURE)	
Early Diagnosis	**Prompt Treatment**
Surveillance and screening activities for early detection, treatment and referral for management of environmental lead exposure	Identification of children with elevated blood lead levels. Routine maintenance and repair of homes in high-risk communities
PRIMARY PREVENTION (REMOVE LEAD FROM THE ENVIRONMENT SO THAT EXPOSURE CANNOT OCCUR)	
Health Promotion and Education	**Health Protection**
• Identify high-risk areas, populations and activities associated with housing-based lead exposure. • Use local data and expertise to expand resources and motivate action for primary prevention • Develop strategies and ensure the creation of lead-safe housing • Collaborative partnerships in communities to provide educational programs to increase knowledge of lead safety in at-risk populations • Evaluate and redesign current prevention programs to achieve primary prevention while ensuring adequate secondary interventions.	• Use surveillance, demographic and housing data to identify high-risk geographic areas • Identify high risk families who could benefit from immediate assessment and services to reduce lead exposure • Educate community partners on the cost of inaction to the community and affected families; highlight risk disparities • Incorporate lead hazard screening into home visits by community health nurses • Assure current programs are meeting the community's needs or readjust priorities.

Adapted from Centers for Disease Control and Prevention: CDC's Childhood Lead Poisoning Prevention Program, 2011.

characteristics that distinguish collaboration from other types of interaction: shared goals, mutual participation, maximized resources, clear responsibilities, and set boundaries.

Shared Goals

First, collaboration in community health nursing is goal-directed. The nurse, clients, and others involved in the collaborative effort or partnership recognize specific reasons for entering into the relationship. For example, a lumber company with 150 employees seeks to develop a wellness program. The community health nurse, company employee representatives, a safety expert, an industrial hygienist, a health educator, an exercise therapist, a nutritionist, and a psychologist might work together to develop specific physical and mental health goals. The team enters into the collaborative relationship with broad needs or purposes to be met and specific objectives to accomplish.

Mutual Participation

Second, in community health nursing, collaboration involves mutual participation; all team members contribute and are mutually benefited (Petri, 2010). Collaboration involves a reciprocal exchange, in which

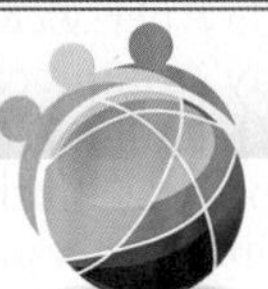

DISPLAY 10.9 CROSS-CULTURAL GUIDELINES

1. Community health nurses should strive to ensure all population members receive care and services that are respectful and sensitive to their client's cultural beliefs and practices.
2. Be aware of your own belief system and values; understand and acknowledge that cultural differences may exist.
3. Develop a basic understanding and knowledge of other cultures, but do not use generalizations about other cultures to stereotype or oversimplify your ideas to another person or group. Remember there are differences within each cultural group that are influenced by individual characteristics and geographical location; therefore never assume you understand what a person from another culture thinks or feels.
4. Demonstrate a genuine interest in the client's personal circumstances and seek to establish trust. Suspend judgments and respect the opinion of others.
5. Be aware of power imbalances and the effect on communication. Identify members who are accorded higher status and authority in family or group and respect the status hierarchy. Respect gender and age differences.
6. Do not assume that there is only one way (yours) to communicate. Keep working on ways to improve your cross-cultural communication skills. For example, avoid using jargon or slang that may not be understood cross-culturally. Use very clear and simple English.
7. Unspoken communication can be powerful; be aware and use appropriate body language.
8. Practice active listening. Try to put yourself in the other person's shoes, especially when another person's ideas or perceptions are different from your own. Be willing to step outside your comfort zone.
9. Do not assume that just because clients say they understand the information that they really do. Clarify questions and statements. Seek feedback by reframing the question in a different form to ensure understanding.
10. Apologize for cultural mistakes. Admit your own limitations and state willingness to learn from others. Show appreciation for the opportunity to learn from others.
11. Easily understood information and services should be delivered in the preferred language of the population served. Whenever possible, utilize interpreters who are trained in culturally competent care, and if possible, avoid using family members or friends to interpret. Look directly at the client, not the interpreter, when speaking.
12. Practice—we get better at cross-cultural collaboration when we practice it.

Adapted from Eubanks, R. L., McFarland, M. R., Mixer, S. J., Munoz, C., Pacquiao, D. F., & Wenger, A. F. (2010). Chapter 4: Cross-cultural communication. *Journal of Transcultural Nursing, 22*(Suppl 1), 137S–150S; Rowe, J., & Paterson, J. (2010). Culturally competent communication with refugees. *Home Health Care Management Practice, 22*(5), 334–338.

individual team players discuss their intended involvement and contribution, and it is important for all members of a team to feel equally valued—no hierarchies should exist (Miller & Hafner, 2008). The lumber company representatives may outline assessed areas of need, such as back-strengthening exercises to facilitate lifting and reduce strain. The professionals, including the nurse involved in the collaboration, will offer their own specific ideas and expertise to design the wellness program. In interdisciplinary teams, physicians, nurses, lay community health workers, clients, outside agency personnel, and others must be able to effectively share ideas and frustrations on an equal, reciprocal basis.

Maximized Use of Resources

A third characteristic of collaboration is that it maximizes the use of community assets (Hamner, Pattillo, Faulk, Lazenby, & Wilder, 2008). That is, the collaborative partnership is designed to draw on the expertise of those who are most knowledgeable and in the best positions to influence a favorable outcome. If the lumber company team has identified a need for health education materials, the nurse and other members of the collaborating team may explore health education resources through the local health department and within their own professions. In this age of dwindling resources, it is now common for community health agencies to seek additional funding assistance from other agencies to support new community health programs or to provide educational information or interventions. Acute care hospitals and public health agencies may align over common interests (e.g., influenza, diabetes, and other lifestyle diseases). Outside funding agencies, both government and nonprofit, are increasingly looking for proof of effective collaboration and coalition building before approving grant or government funding. Being able to demonstrate fiscal responsibility and evidence-based outcomes will assist community health nurses in sustaining health promotion efforts on a long-term basis, and this may be facilitated by collaborative partnerships.

Clear Responsibilities

Fourth, the collaborating team members work in partnership and assume clearly defined responsibilities. As in a football team, each member in the partnership plays a specific role with related tasks. The nurse may play a case-management or group-leadership role, whereas others assume roles appropriate to their areas of expertise. Effective collaboration clearly designates what each member will do to accomplish the identified goals. The nurse, for example, might coordinate the planning effort for the lumber company wellness program and work with the health educator to develop classes on various topics. The psychologist might advise on a chemical dependency program, and the industrial hygienist would provide assistance with safety measures. Each member of the team develops an understanding of individual responsibilities based on realistic and honest expectations. This understanding comes through effective communication. The collaborating partners explore necessary resources, assess their capabilities, and determine their willingness to assume tasks.

Boundaries

Fifth, collaboration in community health practice has set boundaries, with a beginning and an end, that fall within the goals of the partnership. An important part of defining collaboration is determining the conditions under which it occurs and when it will be terminated. The temporal boundaries sometimes are determined by progress toward the goal, sometimes by the number of team member contacts and often by setting a time limit. The collaborating group might target 6 months as a completion date for the lumber company wellness program and establish a timeline with designated activities to reach the goal. Once the purpose for the collaboration has been accomplished, the group as a formal entity can be terminated.

In some settings, the partnership may desire to continue to work on other, mutually agreed upon activities. If so, the process begins again with different goals. Some partnerships are ongoing. For example, a university with a department of nursing might use a neighborhood community center for clinical experiences for their students. The community center has needs that may include health assessments and in-home health teaching among community members, flu shots given at the center for elders without transportation, or health education classes for the adults in an English-as-a-Second-Language (ESL) class or for preschoolers in a Head Start program. The center and the university work in partnership so that, each semester, ongoing services are provided by the nursing students and coordinated by a faculty member or graduate nursing student in collaboration with the community center staff. Each partner wins. The students receive a rich educational experience, and the neighborhood center gets services they would otherwise do without. Within such a model, there are opportunities for students and volunteers. Students from other educational disciplines—social work, theater arts, physical therapy, early elementary education, and other areas—can be integrated into a center that serves people of all ages. Professionals (e.g., dentists, pediatricians) who are willing to volunteer (e.g., one-half or 1 day per week) enhance the services provided, as can lay volunteers, who can read to the children, answer the telephone, or participate in fund raising. Any number of possibilities exist when people collaborate and work in partnership together.

Fostering Client Participation

This chapter has stressed that communication and collaboration are based on mutual participation. The extent of clients' involvement in that participation varies, however, depending on their readiness and ability to participate (Estes, 2008). The client's level of wellness at the time of the initial professional–client encounter directly influences participation. Some people are not physically or emotionally well enough to assume an active role in the relationship. Women recently discharged from the hospital after a mastectomy, for example, have many physical and emotional adjustments with which to cope. Their families, too, must expend additional energies to provide needed support and to cope with the temporary loss of the woman's usual role in the family. They may find it difficult to engage actively in identifying their needs and goals at the start of the collaborative process. The nurse may have to take a stronger initial leadership role; however, the goals of collaboration are not abandoned. Gradually, as the client's wellness level improves or the client's family becomes more involved, the nurse can encourage more active participation. Developmentally disabled clients, or others who are cognitively impaired, may not have the full capacity for true collaboration, but a collaborative team can work together with them in designing an effective plan.

Engaging clients in a collaborative process may be difficult at times. Clients with lower literacy skills or from low-income levels, or minority or different cultural backgrounds may need extensive encouragement to actively participate in a collaborative relationship. Sometimes a client's previous experience with health personnel limits participation in collaboration; clients who were not previously encouraged to participate in decision making by physicians, nurses, or other professionals may follow the pattern of a passive role and not truly collaborate. Unless the nurse persists in efforts to reduce the dependence of clients, the relationship can fall short of therapeutic goals.

The nurse's own view of collaboration also influences the degree of client participation. Nurses who are accustomed to relating to clients in an adult-to-child manner restrict client involvement. If nurses see their position as more informed, and the client's position as one of complete ignorance and need, a paternalistic relationship may develop. All clients have resources on which to build, and the community health nurse should help clients to discover these resources and use them to enhance collaboration and attain health goals.

DISPLAY 10.10 STAGES OF COLLABORATION

Competition: Competing backgrounds, ideas, and motivations, and a search to find shared values, goals, and ethical principles.

Networking/Communication: Sharing information promotes development of trust and role clarity, and reduces miscommunication caused by stereotypical views of other disciplines, professions, or entities.

Cooperation/Coordination: More sharing of resources, less duplication, and formal communication through structure and agreements; more mutual respect.

Coordination/Partnership: Becoming more invested in the success of all partners, better able to manage and share resources, and full support of agencies involved.

Coalition: Shared leadership and decision-making; resources benefit all members; sufficient power and authority to work collectively.

Collaboration: Shared mission and vision, open and trusting communication, strong relationships, sense of belonging, and shared accomplishments and goals.

TA&D Network. (2010). *Stages of collaboration*. Retrieved from http://www.tadnet.org/; United States Department of Health and Human Services: Office of Public Health and Science. (n.d.). What is collaboration? *Office of population affairs*. Retrieved from http://www.hhs.gov/opa/familylife/tech_assistance/etraining/collaboration/sustainabilty/whatiscollaboration.

Structure of Collaborative Relationships

Like group process, collaboration among agencies or groups of people may occur in stages (Display 10.10). During this process, the work of identifying and meeting the client's needs takes place. Because most collaborative and partner relationships are bound by time, the structure involves several phases: (1) a beginning phase when the team relationship is just being established; (2) a middle, working phase; and (3) a termination phase when the relationship or project ends.

The first phase is a period of establishing and defining the team relationship. All of the team members, including clients, are getting to know each other; they seek to establish communication patterns and develop trust. In this phase, they identify the clients'/projects' needs and determine the goals toward which they will work.

The second phase occurs when team members start working together to accomplish desired goals. Their work may include assessment and planning as well as implementation and evaluation. The cycle of the nursing process is repeated as needed during this working phase until goals are satisfactorily accomplished.

The third or termination phase occurs when the need for team members to work together has ended. When team members have grown close in the relationship, termination can be difficult. Termination should never occur abruptly or without participation. It often requires careful advance preparation to make certain that all parties understand when and why it is taking place. Termination helps to ensure a clear-cut end to the collaborative relationship. For example, a nurse, physician, social worker, psychologist, and nutritionist collaborated with a refugee group for almost 1 year. As the group's multiple needs declined, the professionals began to taper off their assistance. Two months before the relationship was ended, termination of the group was discussed. At first, client group members were frightened at the loss of group support, but slowly they took ownership and control, and with their newly acquired skills, they assumed more responsibility for their health needs.

Barriers to Effective Collaboration

Communication barriers and miscommunication can inhibit effective collaboration. This is sometimes caused by misconceptions on the part of team members regarding the professional knowledge and motives of other team members. Stereotypes and the perception of unequal power and authority granted to certain disciplines can sabotage the effectiveness of communication and true collaboration. Apprehension about sharing information with the team, inflexibility and uneasiness with the more fluid boundaries required in collaboration, and a failure to develop a common purpose and goals are all barriers for effective teamwork and collaboration. It is essential that team members share information about their respective disciplines and backgrounds, as well as personal expectations related to collaborative efforts that includes their perspective on what they see as the goal of the process (Goldsmith, Wittenberg-Lyles, Rodriguez, & Sanchez-Reilly, 2010). Organizational or structural factors, such as inadequate time, lack of resources, and lack of agency support are also cited as barriers to effective collaboration (Petri, 2010).

Conflict is inevitable when dealing with groups of diverse individuals, but how potential anger, resentment and mistrust are handled is the key (Sluzki, 2010). Open, honest communication must prevail. One strategy to handle conflict is to introduce "**carefronting**"—described as a method of addressing and resolving conflict by confronting others in a caring, responsible, yet self-asserting manner. This method involves honest communication that sends the message that both parties in the situation should be treated with respect. Using "I" messages ensures that all parties in the conflict matter and that you care enough to negotiate differences so that common goals can be met. It is more fruitful to focus on the issue or problem at hand in a safe environment where all members can voice their opinions openly, and not on personal determinations of who is right or wrong (Kupperschmidt, 2008; Thomas, 2010).

CONTRACTING IN COMMUNITY HEALTH NURSING

Contracting means negotiating a working agreement between two or more parties in which they come to a shared understanding and mutually consent to the purposes and terms of the transaction. Some kinds of contracts are familiar, such as when a buyer signs a contract agreeing to pay a certain amount over a certain period of time to purchase an automobile. Paying tuition for an education involves a form of contracting. Although no formal document is signed, students agree with an educational institution on a purpose (to obtain a degree), with the terms of the contract being regular tuition payments and regular learning opportunities over a specified period of time. For students in individual university courses, the syllabus is an informal contract. It spells out what is offered, what is expected, and what the outcomes may include. Sometimes, learning contracts are utilized within a course to further clarify roles and responsibilities, and students may "contract" for a grade—agree to do a specific number of assignments in exchange for a predetermined grade.

In contrast to legal contracts, which are written and legally binding, contracts in community health nursing can be either a verbal or written agreement that clients make with themselves, with family members, or with health care practitioners. This agreement commits clients to a set of behaviors, with the goal to improve adherence to a health promotion program or plan (Bosch-Capblanch, Abba, Prictor, & Garner, 2009). Display 10.11 shows a contract used by community health nurses when counseling clients who desire to stop smoking. Contracts in a collaborative relationship or a nurse–client alliance are flexible and changing, and are based on mutual understanding and trust. The flexibility built into nurse–client contracting makes it a valuable tool for community health nurses.

The same format is followed with clients who are receiving home health care services. The contract that develops from the partnership between client and home health care nurse often is referred to as a **critical pathway.** It consists of the written plans for client care with a timetable. This represents a more formal type of contracting: it is typically a fiscally driven and agency-required tool designed to document standards and quality of care while reducing costs (see Chapters 12 and 32).

Characteristics of Contracting

The concept of contracting, as used in the collaborative relationship, incorporates four distinctive characteristics: partnership and mutuality, commitment, format, and negotiation.

Partnership and Mutuality

All aspects of contracting involve shared participation and agreement between team members; they become partners in the relationship. There is also mutuality to the nurse–client relationship: If we were to document nurse–client collaboration on a continuum, paternalism would be at one extreme and autonomy at the other. Mutuality becomes the midpoint balance, or ideal of these two extreme positions. For example, a parenting group of 15 couples requested community health nursing involvement. The group entered into a mutual partnership with the nurse and came to an agreement on what they needed and what the nurse could provide. Together, they developed goals, outlined methods to meet those goals, explored resources to help achieve them, defined the time limits for the contract, and outlined their separate responsibilities. The contract involved reciprocal negotiation and shared evaluation. A partnership with mutuality means that all parties are responsible for setting up and carrying out the terms of the agreement within a dynamic balance.

Commitment

Second, every contract implies a commitment. The involved parties make a decision that binds them to fulfilling the purpose of the contract. In community health collaboration, contracting does not mean making a binding agreement in the legal sense, rather, it is a pledge of trust and dedication. Accompanying that sense of dedication is a strong motivation to see the contract through to completion. All parties feel responsible for keeping promises; all want to achieve the intended outcomes. When the nurse and the parenting group identified their separate tasks, they committed themselves: "Yes, we will do thus and so."

Format

Format, the third distinctive feature of contracting, involves outlining the specific terms of the relationship. Clients and professionals gain a clear idea of the purpose of the relationship, their respective responsibilities, and the specific limits within which they will work. Expectations are clarified for all parties involved. The format of contracting provides the framework for collaboration. Once the terms of the contract have been spelled out, there is no question about what has to be done, who is to do it, or within what timeframe it is to be accomplished. This format helps to avoid the difficulty of terminating long-term relationships and shifts health care responsibilities from the professionals to the individual or group. At times, having something

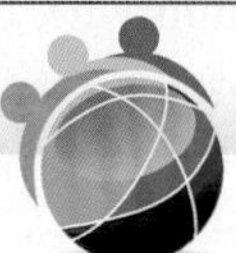

DISPLAY 10.11 CLIENT SERVICE PLAN WITH CONTRACT

Madera County Public Health Department
Public Health Nursing: Client Individual Service Plan

Client Name: Angelica Luz-Smith   Client's Signature: ______________

RN Case Manager: J. Allender, PHN   Start Date: 3//1/2011

Date: 3/1/2011	Client Goal:	Case Manager: Teaching/ Counseling/ Referral Case Manager will:	Follow-up/Reassessment Date: 5/2011
Strengths Identified: Angelica desires to improve the length and quality of life; to be healthier to spend time with grand-children **Problems/Risks:** Has smoked 1–2 packs per day for 20 years	ANGELICA will decrease to fewer than 10 cigarettes per day within the next 2 months. Contract agreement: Angelica will avoid temptations or situations associated with pleasurable aspects of smoking by: • Instead of smoking after meals, brush teeth or take a walk • Limit social activities to where smoking is prohibited • Find new activities that make smoking difficult such as swimming or bicycle riding • Identify new activity to spend time on during work breaks (reading, crosswords, etc.). • Avoid alcoholic drinks • Keep oral substitutes such as carrots, pickles, sugarless gum handy. • Take a yoga class to learn relaxation techniques Angelica will explore community resources: • American Lung Association Program: Freedom from Smoking • California Smokers' Helpline: 1-800-NO-BUTTS	• Promote positive expectations for success, encourage self-efficacy. • Prepare Angelica for relapse. • Assist in developing timeframe with goal ultimately to be that Angelica will stop smoking completely • Partner with Angelica for evaluation, feedback, and revision of health plan as needed • Provide resources for Freedom from Smoking and California Smoker's Helpline	**Outcome/Evaluation** Angelica will be smoking fewer than 10 cigarettes (1/2 pack) per day by 5/2011.

Adapted from Gulanik, M., & Myers, J. (2010). Nursing Care Plans: Nursing Diagnosis and Intervention. (7th ed.). St. Louis, MO: Elsevier/Mosby.

in writing helps the client "legitimize" the nurse–client interaction.

Negotiation

Finally, contracting always involves negotiation. The nurse and other team members propose to accept certain responsibilities and then ask whether the clients agree. The nurse might ask, "What do you feel you can do to achieve this goal?" A period of give-and-take then occurs in which ideas are discussed and conclusions and consensus are reached—no coercion should be involved. Team members may find over time that terms or goals on which they had agreed need modification. Perhaps clients have assumed more responsibility than they can realistically handle at this time and need to redefine their specific responsibilities. Perhaps the nurse feels a need to involve another professional in the collaborative process. The importance of effective interpersonal communication between clients and professionals to keep contracts updated is emphasized. Negotiation during contracting allows for changes that facilitate the ultimate achievement of goals. It provides built-in flexibility and encourages ongoing communication among all team members. Negotiation gives contracting a dynamic quality. Also, we need to remember that, although we may be experts in community health nursing and feel that we know best what is needed for our clients, they know more about their life circumstances and how health and illness impact them (Eriksson & Nilsson, 2008; Pavlish & Pharris, 2012). Mutual respect and regard are necessary before effective contracting can take place.

Value of Contracting

The value of contracting has been demonstrated in many settings and disciplines. Contracts have been used for many years in psychiatric and other nursing settings to promote client self-respect, problem-solving skills, autonomy, and motivation. Other disciplines, such as social work, have long used contracting as a tool in helping to enhance realistic planning and emphasize partnership. For example, both nurses and social workers can utilize contracting to help a frustrated young mother develop a child safety plan. If a young mother feels that she may hit her child out of anger or frustration, a plan can be developed to identify a family member or friend who can be called in a time of crisis. This process identifies the potential problem and allows the mother to identify a resource that can help her in a time of need—ultimately keeping her baby safe (Hepworth, Ronney, Rooney, Gottfried, & Larsen, 2010). Educational contracts between students and instructors have proven valuable for facilitating learning. Negotiating with students to develop contracts gives them the opportunity to realize that what they want does matter, and it allows them to become more responsible for their own work and more enthusiastic about their education (International Reading Association, 2011).

Community health nursing has used the concept of contracting for many years; developing partnerships with clients to address issues such as weight loss, exercise, and substance abuse. Without always labeling it contracting, community health nurses have used these techniques with clients who, for example, want to lose weight. In this case, the contract involves mutual agreement on certain exercise and eating patterns for clients and teaching and support responsibilities for the nurse. Often, it has a set time limit, such as 6 months, within which to achieve the intended weight loss. For chronically ill older adults, community health nurses can help take a complex behavior and break it into manageable steps. For example, the idea of exercise may seem overwhelming to an older adult struggling with chronic health issues, however, contracting to walk at a moderate pace for 30 minutes three times a week may seem feasible. And, success in meeting the contract may aid in stimulating future efforts to increase exercise activities (Ruppar & Conn, 2010). In each case, a partnership is developed, with agreement about the partnership and the conditions under which it will be carried out. Nurses and clients are, in effect, contracting even though they may see it simply as setting goals with clients, and no written documentation is developed.

As more nurses seek to promote client autonomy and self-care, the wide applicability of contracting within nursing practice is being increasingly recognized. Community health nurses are, and will continue to use, contracting when implementing health promotion programs. Examples of community health interventions that have utilized the concept of contracting are stopping or reducing substance abuse, changing eating habits, increasing physical activity, diabetes care, and addressing depression and medication compliance (Bosch-Capblanch et al., 2009). Display 10.12 is a simple contract that can be used by community health nurses and other providers when working with families to combat childhood obesity.

The advantages of contracting in community health nursing can be summarized as follows: It

1. Involves clients in promoting their own health
2. Motivates clients to perform necessary tasks
3. Focuses on clients' unique needs, regardless of aggregate size
4. Increases the possibility of achieving the health goals identified by collaborating team members
5. Enhances all team members' problem-solving skills
6. Fosters client participation in the decision-making process
7. Promotes clients' autonomy and self-esteem as they learn self-care
8. Makes nursing service more efficient and cost-effective

Contracting can also be done with groups or aggregates, and also with agencies (e.g., schools, businesses). For instance, a school district may want to contract with a public health agency to provide community health nurses and health educators to address pregnancy prevention. The nurse working with the adolescents in the pregnancy prevention program may want to informally contract with them about sharing information gleaned in the small-group teaching exercises with their parents to encourage adolescent–parent communication.

Potential Problems with Contracting

Emphasis on contracting as a method rather than a concept can create problems. If a client has experienced contracts only in a business setting, it is possible to carry the stereotype of a cold, formal arrangement into the nursing practice setting. Some nurses fear that asking clients to negotiate a contract will place clients under stress, impede the development of trust, and negatively influence the relationship. Others have found that some clients prefer to have the nurse make decisions for them and are not ready to enter into any kind of negotiation. These problems in contracting can be overcome by understanding the true concept of contracting. Contracting is not a panacea. Some clients cannot fully participate in a collaborative relationship. Developmentally delayed clients and those with serious mental or cognitive impairments (e.g., mental illness, dementia) may be unable to fully participate in the nurse–client contract. Also, the use of contracting should not be used in place of developing a therapeutic relationship with clients. For example, when working with clients with suicidal ideations practitioners may use contracting to address suicide prevention—developing a written agreement between the health care provider and the client stating that the client will refrain from suicidal behavior for a specified time period. However, it has been found that formal contracting in suicide prevention is often used in place of a therapeutic alliance and also can weaken an existing therapeutic relationship. Suicide prevention contracting should be done very carefully as it has the potential to produce negative outcomes when used in high-risk patients who are unlikely to be able to give informed consent (Edwards & Sachman, 2010).

Problems can arise when contracting with aggregates or agencies, as well. In the earlier example of contracting with a school district on pregnancy prevention, the

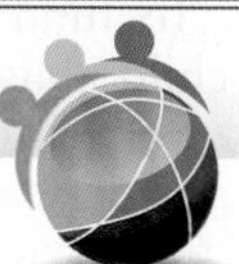

DISPLAY 10.12 Rx FOR HEALTHIER LIVING

IDEAS FOR HEALTHIER LIVING

5 Eat at least 5 fruits and vegetables every day.
2 Limit screen time (for example, TV, video games, computer) to 2 hours or less per day.
1 Get 1 hour or more of physical activity everyday
0 Drink fewer sugar-sweetened drinks. Try water and low-fat milk instead.

MY HEALTHY LIFE STYLE

- Eat____ fruits and vegetables each day.
- Reduce screen time to ____ minutes per day.
- Get _____ minutes of physical activity each day
- Reduce number of sugared drinks to ___ per day.

__________________________ Client's name/signature

__________________________ Parent's/Caregiver Signature

__________________________ Provider's signature

___________ Date

Adapted from Let's Move: America's Move to Raise a Healthier Generation of Kids. (2010). Retrieved from http://www.letsmove.gov/prescribe-activity-and-healthy-habits

community health nurse may need to take into account the culture of the school, as well as the community in general. If the school is concerned about teen pregnancy, but the community is against "sex education" it may be an untenable alliance. The community or agency culture may prevent real progress on this issue.

Principles of Contracting

Contracting applies the basic principles of adult education: self-direction, mutual negotiation, and mutual evaluation. It need not be a formal, written, or complex negotiation; it may be formal or informal, written or verbal, simple or detailed, and signed or unsigned by client and nurse. It should be adapted to the particular client's abilities to assess, plan, implement, and evaluate, which may vary greatly from situation to situation (Berman, Snyder, Kozier, & Erb, 2008; McKenzie, Neiger, & Thackeray, 2009). The tool shown in Display 10.12 seeks input from the client. The client's goals are mutually set, and the goals are spelled out. Initial interventions are dated, as are follow-up and reassessment visits. In addition, there is a place for a continuing assessment of outcomes and for evaluation on future dates. Like all nursing tools, contracting enhances a client's health only if it is adapted to each particular set of client needs and abilities.

Contracting in Steps

Contracting follows a sequence of steps. As a working agreement, it depends on knowing what clients want, agreeing on goals, identifying methods to achieve these goals, knowing the resources that collaborating members bring to the relationship, using appropriate outside resources, setting limits, deciding on responsibilities, and providing for periodic reviews. Each of these tasks requires discussion among members of the contractual group. The tasks are incorporated into the contracting process and can be described in eight phases that follow the nursing process.

Assessment

1. *Explore needs*: Assess clients' health and needs: done by clients, nurse, and other relevant persons

Nursing Diagnosis/Goal Setting

2. *Establish goals*: Discussion followed by agreement among contracting members on goals and objectives

Plan/Intervention

3. *Explore resources*: Define what each member has to offer and can expect from the others; identify appropriate resources and agencies
4. *Develop a plan*: Identify methods, activities, and a timeline for achieving the stated goals
5. *Divide responsibilities*: Negotiate the activities for which each member will be responsible
6. *Agree on time frame*: Setting limits for the contract in terms of length of time or number of meetings

Evaluation

7. *Evaluation*: Formative and summative assessments of progress toward goals occur at agreed-on intervals
8. *Renegotiation or termination*: Agree to modify, renegotiate, or terminate the contract

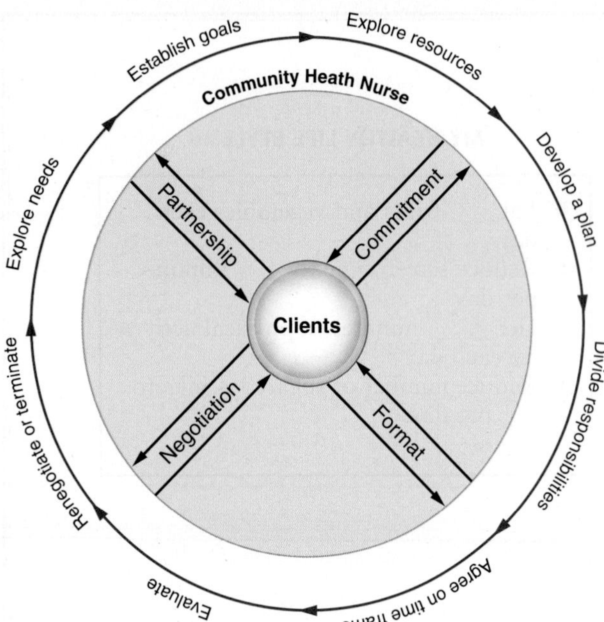

FIGURE 10-2. The concept and process of contracting. Contracting is based on four distinctive features, shown here as spokes that support a wheel. These features form the basis for a reciprocal relationship among clients, nurse, and other persons. This relationship is not static; it is a dynamic process that moves through phases, represented here as the outer rim of the wheel. The process moves forward, focused on meeting clients' needs, and enables the collaborating group to facilitate ultimate achievement of clients' goals.

As community health nurses use this process to negotiate a contract, they must adapt it to each situation. The sequence of phases may change, and some steps may overlap. Nevertheless, the basic elements remain important considerations for successful contracting (Fig. 10.2).

Levels of Contracting

Community health nurses use contracts at levels ranging from formal to informal. The degree of formality depends on the demands of the situation. To fund a community health program for preventing child abuse, for example, a formal contract in the form of a written grant proposal may be needed. To conduct a wide-scale needs assessment of a homeless population, the services of an epidemiologist and statistician may require a formal contract to clarify roles and expectations, as well as fees. **Formal contracting** involves all parties' negotiating a written contract by mutual agreement, signing the agreement, and sometimes having it witnessed or notarized. This level of contract has been used with mental health or substance-abusing clients, where the seriousness of the working agreement and the need to actively involve the client are important aspects of therapy.

Some situations best lend themselves to a modified and less formal use of contracting, in which the nursing plan becomes the written contract. For example, a school nurse forms a support group for pregnant adolescents. The nurse uses modified contracting by discussing with the girls the purpose of the group and the number of sessions needed and obtaining their agreement to attend all sessions.

Informal contracting involves some form of verbal agreement about relatively clear-cut purposes and tasks. A client group may agree to prioritize their list of needs, the nurse may agree to conduct health teaching sessions, the social worker may agree to obtain informational materials, and so on. Sometimes, nurses use contracting informally without realizing it. They conclude a session with clients by agreeing with them about the purpose and time of the next meeting. Conscious use of contracting, however, is a more effective way to provide structure for the relationship and foster client involvement, regardless of the level at which it is applied.

The level of contracting also may change during the development of communication and collaboration. Clients often need education about their options. Initially, they may have difficulty in identifying needs and making choices. The professional team can work to promote clients' self-confidence and help them assume increasing responsibility for their own health. Through these efforts, contracting becomes a consciously recognized part of the relationship, and clients become fully participating partners.

SUMMARY

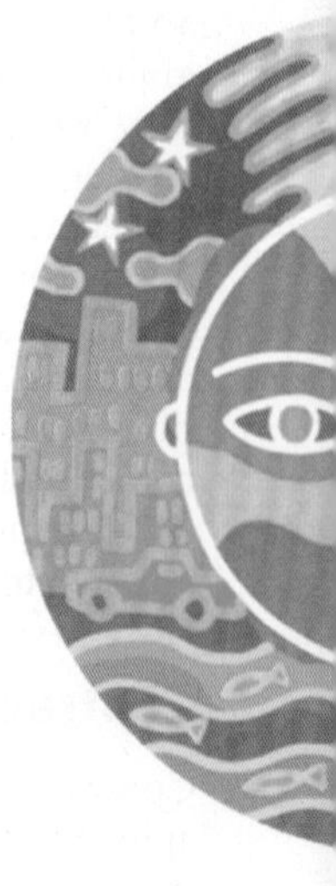

Communication and collaboration are important tools for community health nurses to promote aggregate health. Communication involves the transfer and understanding of meaning between individuals (see Display 10.13).

The communication process comprises seven parts: a message, a sender, a receiver, encoding, a channel, decoding, and a feedback loop. Barriers to effective communication include selective perception, language barriers, clients filtering out parts of the message, and emotional influence. Core skills essential to effective communication in community health nursing include sending skills, which allow the nurse to transmit messages effectively; receiving skills, which allow the nurse to receive accurate and complete messages; and interpersonal skills, which allow the nurse to interact and respond to the messages from clients. These skills include special techniques of active listening, the ability to

DISPLAY 10.13 EXPERIMENT IN COMMUNICATION

Purpose

The experiment will demonstrate the differences between one-way and two-way communication and demonstrate the advantages of the latter.

Setting

The experiment can be conducted in the classroom with any size group. Each person will need paper and pencil.

Procedure

Have the group members select one person who everyone believes can communicate clearly and effectively to be the "sender." Place this person so that he or she is out of sight but can be clearly heard by the rest of the group (the "receivers"). The sender is to describe a diagram, and the receivers are to draw it. The sender should explain the diagram with the intention that the receivers will be able to recreate it exactly, without any further communication with the sender or with other group members. Time the exercise. When the receivers are finished, rank the accuracy of their drawings by placing them on a Likert scale (a 10-point scale, with 1 as least accurate to 10 as most accurate). Ask receivers how they felt and how the sender probably felt. Ask the sender how she or he felt.

Next, begin the two-way communication demonstration by allowing the sender to remain in sight of the group as he or she explains a second diagram and the receivers draw it. Allow the receivers to ask questions. The sender may reply, but may not use gestures. Record the time required and rank the drawings for accuracy. Discuss how the receivers felt and how the sender probably felt. Ask the sender how she or he felt this time.

Analysis

Compare your findings with the following statements:

1. Two-way communication takes longer.
2. Two-way communication results in greater accuracy among the drawings.
3. In one-way communication, the sender often feels relatively confident; the receiver, uncertain or frustrated.
4. In two-way communication, the sender may feel frustrated or angry; the receiver relatively confident.

show respect regardless of the message (whether positive or negative), the ability to empathize with clients' thoughts and feelings, and the ability to develop trust. Many factors can influence the quality of communication, such as negative previous experience, cultural influence, and relationships among the people involved. The community health nurse must consider all of these factors when trying to foster good communication.

In community health, nurses frequently need to promote communication in groups and in-group decision-making. Decisions made by groups have many advantages, including sharing of members' experience and expertise, diversity of opinions, potential for broadening members' perspectives, and a focus on arriving at consensus solutions. Several methods of enhancing group decision-making are available, including brainstorming, nominal group technique, and multivoting technique. NIs, encompassing all of the computer-generated tools created to enhance communication, is changing the form of communication in community health nursing, as it has in the acute care setting.

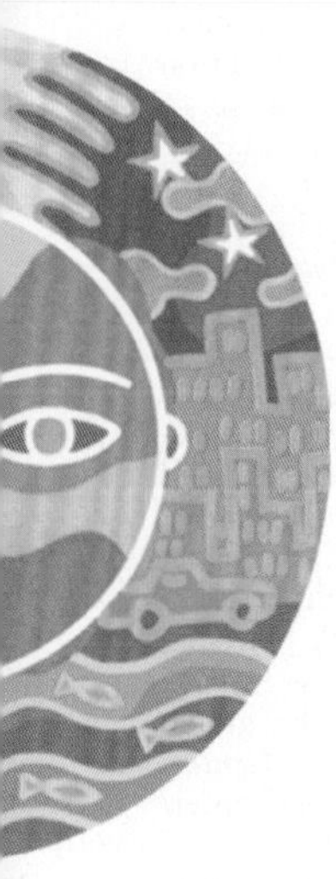

Collaboration and partnership building is a purposeful interaction among the nurse, clients, community members, and other professionals based on mutual participation and joint effort. It is characterized by shared goals, mutual participation, maximized use of resources, clear responsibilities, and set boundaries. Clients play an important role in the collaborative relationship.

Contracting is a helpful tool in promoting clients' participation, independence, and motivation. It is used at all levels in community health nursing to promote partnership in the collaborative process, to encourage commitment to health goals, and to ensure a format and a means for negotiation among the collaborating group. Contracts can be formal or informal, written or verbal, simple or complex. The nurse must know the needs and abilities of clients and must tailor the type of contracting to best suit the client's particular situation.

ACTIVITIES TO PROMOTE **CRITICAL THINKING**

Discuss how you would handle the communication barrier of selective perception with a group of clients.

1. Practice active listening with a colleague and subsequently analyze the factors that interfered with your total concentration. Identify three actions to take to improve your active listening and apply them during the next week, keeping a log of your progress.
2. Think of a patient you have worked with who may have low health literacy. What kinds of things can you do to help them better communicate with their physician and other health professionals? Why is good health literacy important not only for the patient as an individual, but for the community and society as a whole?
3. Use nominal group technique with a group of classmates to arrive at a rank ordering of barriers to cross-cultural communication. What did you learn about arriving at a quality decision in the process?
4. Attend an open meeting (e.g., student body council, school board, city council) and watch for task and maintenance roles among the members. Are any members displaying nonfunctional role behaviors? Can you recognize task, maintenance, and nonfunctional role behaviors in some of the student groups in which you participate?
5. Organize a group of classmates to represent a group of clients, professionals, and community members who are collaborating to address the needs of an inner-city homeless population. Analyze how well you integrated the five characteristics of collaboration into your activity.
6. Explain the concept of contracting as it applies to aggregates. Discuss its four distinctive characteristics and the advantages that contracting offers to the community health nurse.
7. Develop a hypothetical contract with a group of elderly widows who need support and outlets to alleviate their loneliness. What other community members and professionals might be helpful as part of a collaborative team to address the widows' needs?
8. Become a good listener. This exercise asks you to list your closest friends, relatives, school peers, and work associates. Rank them on a scale of 1 to 10, with 1 meaning always fascinating and 10 meaning boring. If you find that you've labeled most as boring, you probably have one of two problems: you are either socializing or working with the wrong people, or you are a poor listener. The likelihood is the latter. To improve listening skills, compliment people and encourage them; this increases the chance that they will continue conversing with you, and it is a valuable skill in both your personal and professional life.
9. Experiment in communication. The activity described in Display 10.14 can be used with your peers or as part of a group-teaching project on communication with elementary or high school students.

REFERENCES

Active Listening. (2010). *Care notes*. Retrieved from http://www.galenet.com.lp.hscl.ufl.edu/servlet/HWRC/hits?r=d&origSearch=true7bucket

AIDS.gov. (2011). *Social network sites*. Retrieved from http://aids.gov/using-new-media/tools/social-network-sites/

American Academy of Family Practice. (2011). *Telehealth discussion paper*. Retrieved from http://www.aafp.org/online/en/home/membership/ruralcommunity/governmentandnongovernmentresources/telemedicine/telehealth.html

Asset-Based Community Development Institute. (2009). *Welcome to ABCD*. Retrieved from http://www.abcdinstitue.org/

Association of Community Health Nursing Educators [ACHNE]. (2010). Essentials of baccalaureate nursing education for entry-level community/public health nursing. *Education Committee of the Association of Community Health Nurse Educators, 27*(4), 371–382.

Bens, Ingrid. (2005). *Advanced facilitation strategies: tools and techniques to master difficult situations*. San Francisco, CA: Jossey-Bass.

Berkley, R., Bauer, S. A., & Rowland, C. (2010). How telehealth can increase the effectiveness of chronic heart failure management. *Nursing Times, 106*(26). Retrieved from http://www.lexisnexis.com.lp.hscl.ufl.edu

Berman, A., Snyder, S. J., Kozier, B., & Erb, G. (2008). *Fundamentals of nursing: concepts, process and practice* (8th ed.). Upper Saddle River, NJ: Pearson Education.

Boon, H. S., Mior, S. A., Barnsley, J., Ashbury, F. D., & Haig, R. (2009). The difference between integration and collaboration in patient care: results from key informant interviews working in multiprofessional health care teams, *Journal of Manipulative and Physiological Therapeutics, 32*(9), 715–722.

Borkowski, N. (2011). *Organizational behavior in health care*. Sudbury, MA: Jones and Bartlett.

Bosch-Capblanch, X., Abba, K., Prictor, M., & Garner, P. (2009). Contracts between patients and healthcare practitioners for improving patients' adherence to treatment, prevention and health promotion activities. *The Cochrane Database of Systematic Reviews, 3*. Retrieved from http://ovidsp.tx.ovid.com.lp.hscl.ufl.edu/sp-3/2/4b/ovidweb

Boutain, D. M. (2008). Social justice as a framework for undergraduate community health clinical experiences in the United States. *International Journal of Nursing Education Scholarship, 5*(1), Article 35.

Boyd, M., & Foley, M. (2009). *Psychiatric nursing: Contemporary practice*. (4th ed.) Philadelphia, PA: Lippincott, Williams & Wilkins.

Brown University. (2010). *Lead poisoning maps in R.I. reveal huge disparities, guide cleanup*. Brown University Press Release. Retrieved from http://news.brown.edu/pressreleases/2010/11/lead?printable

Browne, A. J., Doane, G. H., Reimer, J., MacLeod, M., & McLellan, E. (2010). Public health nursing practice with 'high priority' families: the significance of contextualizing 'risk'. *Nursing Inquiry, 17*(1), 27–38.

Castelli, D. (2010). Telehealth technologies addressing the global impending nursing shortage. *Lippincott's Nursing Center*. Retrieved from http://www.nursingcenter.com/CareerCenter/static.aps?eid=880469

CBS Interactive. (2010). *Interpersonal Communication*. Retrieved from http://www.search.com/reference/Interpersonal-Communication

Centers for Disease Control and Prevention. (2011). *CDC's childhood lead poisoning prevention program*. Retrieved from http://www.cdc.gov/nceh/lead/about/program.html

Chu, A., Huber, J., Mastel-Smith, B., & Cesario, S. (2009). "Partnering with seniors for better health": Computer use and Internet information retrieval among older adults in a low socioeconomic community. *Journal of the Medical Library Association, 97*(1), 11–19.

Cole, J. (1990). *Filtering people: Understanding and confronting our prejudices*. Philadelphia, PA: New Society Publishers.

Community-Campus Partnerships for Health. (2011). *Community-based participatory research*. Retrieved from http://depts.washington.edu/ccph/commbas.html

Current Nursing. (2010). *Nursing theories: Jean Watson's philosophy of nursing*. Retrieved from http://currentnursing.com/nursing_theory/Watson.html

DeMarco, J., & Nystrom, M. (2010). Health literacy: the importance of health literacy in patient education. *Journal of Consumer Health on the Internet, 14*(3), 294–301.

Department of Health: Australia. (2010). Enhancing communication and clinical practice to help realise healthcare rights. *Australian Charter of Healthcare Rights in Victoria*. Retrieved from http://www.health.vic.gov/au/[patientcharter/services/clinical/htm

DeWalt, D. A., & Hink, A. (2009). Health literacy and child health outcomes: a systematic review of the literature. *Pediatrics, 124*(S3), S265–274.

Edwards, S. J., & Sachmann, M. D. (2010). No-suicide contracts, no-suicide agreements, and no-suicide assurances: A study of their nature, utilization, perceived effectiveness, and potential to cause harm. *Crisis: The Journal of Crisis Intervention and Suicide Prevention, 31*(6), 290–302.

Electronic Meeting Systems. (2011). *Tips on using computer aided meeting systems to improve conference efficiency*. Retrieved from http://www.articlesbase.com/business-articles/tips-on-using-computer-aided-meeting-systems-to-improve-conference-efficiency-4639657.html

Ellingstad, K., & Clarke, L. L. (2007). *Uncovered: Health and the uninsured in Sarasota county. Community Health Improvement Partnership 2007*. Sarasota, FL: Sarasota County Health Department.

Eriksson, I., & Nilsson, K. (2008). Preconditions needed for establishing a trusting relationship during health counseling—an interview study. *Journal of Clinical Nursing, 17*(17), 2352–2359.

Estes, T. S. (2008). Assessing collaborative management in asthma: a pilot study. *The Journal of Theory Construction and Testing, 12*(2), 63–67.

Eubanks, R. L., McFarland, M. R., Mixer, S. J., Munoz, C., Pacquiao, D. F., & Wenger, A. F. (2010). Chapter 4: Cross-cultural communication. *Journal of Transcultural Nursing, 22*(Suppl 1), 137S–150S.

Gibbons, M. C., & Casale, C. R. (2010). Reducing disparities in health care quality: The role of health IT in undersourced set tings. *Medical Care and Research Review, 67*(5), 155S–162S.

Gilley, J. W., Morris, M. L., Waite, A. M., Coates, T., & Veliquette, A. (2010). Integrated theoretical model for building effective teams. *Advances in Developing Human Resources, 12*(1), 7–28.

Goldsmith, J., Wittenberg-Berg, E., Rodriguez, D., & Sanchez-Reilly, S. (2010). Interdisciplinary geriatric and palliative care team narratives: collaboration practices and barriers. *Qualitative Health Research, 20*(1), 93–104.

Goodall, K., Ward, P., & Newman, L. (2010). Use of information and communication technology to provide health information: what do older migrants know, and what do they need to know? *Quality in Primary Care, 18*(1), 27–32.

Grimes-Robinson, C., & Evans, R. R. (2008). Benefits and barriers to medically supervised pediatric weight-management programs. *Journal of Child Health, 12*(4), 329–343.

Hamner, J., Pattillo, R., Faulk, D., Lazenby, R., & Wilder, B. (2008). Collaborative change: An interdependent model of nursing education. *Southern Online Journal of Nursing Research, 8*(1), Article 6.

Hare, A. P. (2010). Theories of group development and categories for interaction analysis. *Small Group Research, 41(1)*, 106–140.

Healthy People 2020. (2011). *2020 Topics and objectives*. Retrieved from http://www.healthypeople.gov/2020/topicsobjectives2020/default.aspx

Herndon, J. B., Chaney, M., & Carden, D. (2011). Health literacy and emergency department outcomes: A systematic review. *Annals of Emergency Medicine*, *57*(4), 334–345.

Hearnden, M. (2008). Coping with differences in culture and communication in health care. *Nursing Standard, 23*(11), 49–59.

Hepworth, D. H., Rooney, R. H., Rooney, G. D., Strom-Gottfried, K., & Larsen, J. (2010). *Direct social work: Theory and skills* (8th ed.). Belmont, CA: Brooks/Cole.

Hertelendy, A., Fenton, S. H., & Griffin, D. (2010). The implications of health reform for health information and electronic health record implementation efforts. *Perspectives in Health Information Management* (Summer 2010), 1–2.

Heslin, P. A. (2009). Better than brainstorming? Potential contextual boundary conditions to brainwriting for idea generation in organizations. *Journal of Occupational and Organization Psychology, 82*, 129–145.

International Council of Nurses. (2010). *Code of ethics for nurses*. Retrieved from http://www.ich.sh/about-icn/code-of-ethics-for-nurses/

International Reading Association: ReadWriteThink (2011). *Student contracting*. Retrieved from http:///www.readwrite.think.org/classroom-resources

Jefferson, W. K., Zunker, C., Feucht, J. C., Fitzpatrick, S. L., Greene, L. F., Shewchuk, R. M., et al. (2010). Use of the nominal group technique (NGT) to understand the perceptions of the healthiness of foods associated with African Americans. *Evaluation and Program Planning, 33*(4), 343–348.

Jette, S., Tribble, D. S., Gagnon, J., & Mathieu, L. (2010). Nursing student's perceptions of their resources toward the development of competencies in nursing informatics. *Nurse Education Today, 30*(2010), 742–746.

Kaufman, N. (2010). Internet and information technology use in the treatment of diabetes. *The International Journal of Clinical Practice, 64*(Suppl 166), 41–46.

Kharbanda, E. O., Stockwell, M., Fox, H., Andres, R., Lara, M., & Rickert, V. (2011). Text message reminders to promote HPV vaccination. *Vaccine, 29*(14), 2509–2648.

Kilgore, R. V., & Langford, R. W. (2009). Reducing the failure risk of interdisciplinary teams. *Critical Care Nursing Quarterly/April-June 2009, 32*(2), 81–88.

Kirst-Ashman, K., & Hull, G. (2011). *Understanding generalist practice* (6th ed.). Belmont, CA: Brooks-Cole.

Kupperschmidt, B. R. (2008). Conflicts at work? Try care fronting. *Journal of Christian Nursing, 25*(1), 10–17.

Let's Move: America's Move to Raise a Healthier Generation of Kids. (2010). *Rx for healthier living*. Retrieved from http://letsmove.gov

Luptak, M., Dailey, N., Juretic, M., Rupper, R., Hill, R. D., Hicken, B. L., et al. (2010). The care coordination home telehealth (CCHT) rural demonstration project: A symptom-based approach for serving older veterans in remote geographic settings. *Rural and Remote Health, 10*(2). Retrieved from http://www.rrh.org.au/articles/subviewnew.asp?ArticleID=1375

McKenzie, J. F., Nieger, B. L., & Thackeray, R. (2009). *Planning, implementing, and evaluating: Health promotion programs* (5th ed.). San Francisco, CA: Pearson Education.

Miller, P., & Hafner, M. (2008). Moving toward dialogical collaboration: A critical examination of a university-school-community partnership. *Educational Administration Quarterly, 44*(1), 66–110.

Murphy, J. (2010). Nursing informatics: The intersection of nursing, computer and information sciences. *Nursing Economics, 28*(3), 204–207.

Murphy, M. W., Iqbal, S., Sanchez, C. A., & Quinlisk, M. P. (2010). Post-disaster health communication and information sources: The Iowa flood scenario. *Disaster Medicine and Public Health Preparedness, 4*(2), 129–134.

Nadig, L. A. (2010). *Tips on effective listening*. Retrieved November 5, 2010 from http://www.drnadig.com/listening.htm.

National Healthy Mothers, Healthy Babies Coalition. (2009). *Welcome to HMHB: text4baby announces plan to reach one million moms*. Retrieved from http://www.hmhb.org/

National Highway Traffic Safety Administration (NHTSA). (n.d.). *Fatality analysis reporting system (FARS)*. Retrieved from http://www.nhtsa.gov/FARS

National Network of Libraries of Medicine. (2010). *Health literacy*. Retrieved from http://nnlm.gov/outreach/consumer/hlthlit.html

Nursing Care Plans: Nursing Diagnosis and Intervention. (2010). Nursing Diagnosis: health-seeking behaviors. Retrieved from http://www1.us.elsevierhealth.com/MERLIN/Gulanick/Constructor

Nyamathi, A. M., Casillas, A., King, M. L., Gresham, L., Pierce, E., Farb, D., et al. (2010). Computerized bioterrorism education and training for nurses on bioterrorism attack agents. *The Journal of Continuing Education in Nursing, 41*(8), 375–384.

Ohio State University. (2009). Building dynamic groups: Nominal group technique; *Ohio State University Extension*. Retrieved from http://www.ag.ohio-state.edu/~bdg/pdf_docs/d/F06.pdf

Palinkas, L. A. (2010). Commentary: Cultural adaptation, collaboration and exchange. *Research on Social Work Practice, 20*(5), 544–546.

Pavlish, C. P., & Pharris, M. D. (2012). *Community-based collaborative action research: A nursing approach*. Sudbury, MA: Jones & Bartlett Learning.

Petri, L. (2010). Concept analysis of interdisciplinary collaboration. *Nursing Forum, 45*(2), 73–82.

Philibin, C., Griffiths, C., Byrne, G., Horan, B., Brady, A. M., & Begley, C. (2010). The role of the public health nurse in a changing society. *Journal of Advanced Nursing 66*(4), 743–752.

Porr, C. (2005). Shifting from preconceptions to pure wonderment. *Nursing Philosophy, 6*, 189–195.

Propp, K. M., Apker, J., Zabava-Ford, W. S., Wallace, N., Serbenski, M., & Hofmeister, N. (2010). Meeting the complex needs of the health care team: Identification of nurse-team communication practices perceived to enhance patient outcomes. *Qualitative Health Research, 20*(1), 15–28.

Putzer, G. J., & Park, Y. (2010). The effects of innovation factors on smartphone adoption among nurses in community hospitals, *Perspectives in Health Information Management, 7*(Winter), 1–20.

Quad Council. (2003). *Quad Council PHN Competencies*. Retrieved from http://www.resourcenter.net/images/ACHNE/Files/Final_PHN_Competencies.pdf

QualComm. (2010). 3G wireless technology provides clinical information to public health care workers through mobile health information system project. Retrieved from http://multivu.prnewswire.com/mnr/qualcomm/47225/

Rebmann, T., Carrico, R., & English, J. (2008). Lessons public health professionals learned from past disasters. *Public Health Nursing, 25*(4), 344–352.

Rollnick, S., Miller, W. R., & Butler, C. C. (2008). *Motivational interviewing in health care: Helping patients change behavior*. New York: The Guilford Press.

Rowe, J., & Paterson, J. (2010). Culturally competent communication with refugees. *Home Health Care Management Practice, 22*(5), 334–338.

Rudd, R. E. (2010). *Literacy and health*. Retrieved from Harvard University, Harvard School of Public Health website: http://www.hsph.harvard.edu/healthliteracy/files/overview_slides.pdf

Ruppar, T. M., & Conn, V. S. (2010). Interventions to promote physical activity in chronically ill adults. *American Journal of Nursing, 110*(7), 31–37.

Sarasota County Health Department. (2011). *Community health improvement partnership*. Retrieved from http://www.sarasota-health.org/communityprograms/chip.htm

Sarhan, F. (2009). Telemedicine in healthcare 1: Exploring its uses, benefits and disadvantages. *Nursing Times, 105*, 10–13. Retrieved from http://www.lexisnexis.com.lp.hscl.ufl.edu/lnacui2api/frame.do?reloadEntirePage=true

Scheingold, L. (2010). Active listening. *Clinical References Systems, 2010* (1). http://smexchange.ogilvypr.com/wp-content/uploads/2010/11/OW_SM_WhitePaper.pdf

Schlachta-Fairchild, L., Varghese, S. B., Deickman, A., & Castelli, D. (2010). Telehealth and telenursing are live: APN policy and practice implications. *The Journal for Nurse Practitioners, 6*(2), 98–106.

Sluzki, C. E. (2010). The pathway between conflict and reconciliation: Coexistence as an evolutionary process. *Transcultural Psychiatry, 47*(2010), 55–69.

Spector, R. E. (2009). *Cultural diversity in health and illness* (7th ed.). Upper Saddle River, NJ: Prentice-Hall Allied Health.

TA&D Network. (2010). Stages of collaboration. Retrieved from http://www.tadnet.org/

Thomas, C. M. (2010). Teaching nursing students and newly registered nurses strategies to deal with violent behaviors in the professional practice environment. *The Journal of Continuing Education in Nursing, 41*(7), 299–328.

Tonn, V. L. (2009). A systemic world of communication. *China Media Research, 5*(3), 45–58.

United States Department of Health and Human Services: Administration of Children and Families. (2010a). *Establishing partnerships*. Office of Community Services. Retrieved from http://www.acf.hhs.gov/programs/ocs/ccf/about_ccf/gbk_ep/ep_gbk_toc.html

United States Department of Health and Human Services: Centers for Disease Control and Prevention. (n.d.). *Geographic Information Systems (GIS) at CDC*. Retrieved from http://apps.nccd.cdc.gov/GISCVH2/Selection.aspx

United States Department of Health and Human Services: Centers for Medicare and Medicaid Services. (2010b). EHR *incentive programs: meaningful use*. Retrieved from https://www.cms.gov/EHRIncentivePrograms/30_Meaningful_Use.asp

United States Department of Health and Human Services: Centers for Medicare and Medicaid Services. (2010c). *Electronic health records: overview*. Retrieved from https://www.cms.gov/EhealthRecords/

United States Department of Health and Human Services: Healthy People 2020. (2010d). *Health communication and health information technology*. Retrieved from http://www.healthypeople.gov/2010/topicsobjectives2020/overview.aspx?topicid=18

United States Department of Health and Human Services: Office of Disease Prevention and Promotion. (2010e). *National action plan to improve health literacy*. Retrieved from http://www.health.gov/communication/HLActionPlan/pdf/Health_Literacy_Action_Plan.pdf

United States Department of Health and Human Services: Office of Public Health and Science. (n.d.). What is collaboration? *Office of population affairs*. Retrieved from http://www.hhs.gov/opa/familylife/tech_assistance/etraining/collaboration/sustainabilty/whatiscollaboration

University of Kentucky. (2009). Active leadership. *Leadership development: office of student involvement*. Retrieved from http://getinvolved.uky.edu/leadership/resources.html

van Dick, R., van Knippenberg, D., Hagele, S., Guillaume, Y. R. F., & Brodbeck, F. C. (2008). Group diversity and group identification: The moderating role of diversity beliefs. *Human Relations, 61*(10), 1463–1492.

Vehvilamen-Julkunen, K. (1992). Client-public health nurse relationships in child health care: A grounded theory study. *Journal of Advanced Nursing, 17*, 896–904.

Villarruel, A. M., Cherry, C., Cabriales, E. G., Ronis, D., & Zhou, Y. (2008). A parent-adolescent intervention to increase sexual risk communication: Results of a randomized controlled trial. *AIDS Education and Prevention, 20*(5), 371–383.

Villarruel, A. M., Gal, T. L., Eakin, B. L., Wilkes, A., & Herbst, J. H. (2010). From research to practice: The importance of community collaboration in the translation process. *Research and Theory for Nursing Practice: An International Journal, 24*(1), 25–34.

Wang, Q. (2010). Using online shared workspaces to support group collaborative learning. *Computers and Education, 55*(2010), 1270–1276.

Webster, D. (2010). Promoting empathy through a creative reflective teaching strategy: A mixed-method study. *Journal of Nursing Education, 49*(2), 87–94.

Williams, J., & Stickley, T. (2010). Empathy and nurse education. *Nurse Education Today, 30*(8), 752–755.

Winters, L., Gordon, U., Atherton, J., & Scott-Samuel, A. (2007). Developing public health nursing: Barriers perceived by community nurses. Public Health, 121(8), 623–633.

Young, S. (2009). Professional relationships and power dynamics between urban community-based nurses and social work case managers: Advocacy in action. *Professional Case Management, 14*(6), 312–320.

Zavertnnik, J. E., Huff, T. A., & Munro, C. L. (2010). Innovative approach to teaching communication skills to nursing students. *Journal of Nursing Education, 49*(2), 65–71.

thePoint: Everything You Need to Make the Grade!

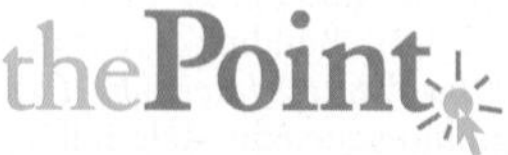

Visit http://thePoint.lww.com/Allender8e for selected readings, study aids for all learning styles, and more!

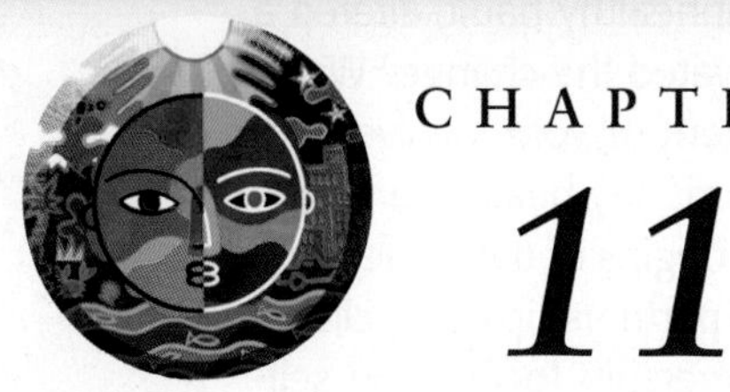

CHAPTER

11

Health Promotion: Achieving Change Through Education

"As I see it, every day you do one of two things: build health or produce disease in yourself."

—*Adelle Davis*

KEY TERMS

Adult learning
Affective domain
Anticipatory guidance
Cognitive domain
Empiric–rational change strategy
Health promotion
Normative–reeducative change strategy
Planned change
Power–coercive change strategy
Psychomotor domain
Social determinants of health
Stages of change

LEARNING OBJECTIVES

Upon mastery of this chapter, you should be able to:

- Explain the three stages of change.
- Identify three planned-change strategies.
- Summarize six principles for effecting change in community health.
- Describe the community health nurse's role as educator in promoting health and preventing or postponing morbidity.
- Identify educational activities for the nurse to use that are appropriate for each of the three domains of learning.
- Identify health-teaching models for use when planning health education activities.
- Develop teaching plans focusing on primary, secondary, and tertiary levels of prevention for clients of all ages.
- Identify teaching strategies for the community health nurse to use when encountering clients with special learning needs.
- Describe social determinants of health and how each relate to health inequities domestically and internationally.

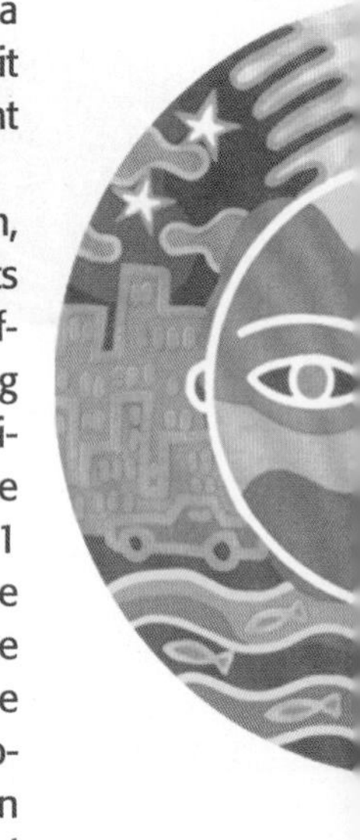

Think of a time when you were so influenced by a teacher that you stopped an unhealthy habit, altered a long-held belief, or embarked on a new endeavor. What precisely was it that motivated the change? Was it simply the content of the teaching, or was it how the teacher presented the content or your involvement in the learning process? What is good teaching, and why is it so important to community health nursing?

Teaching has been a critical part of the community health nurse's role since the origins of the profession, and it frequently is the primary role or function. Community health nurses develop partnerships with clients to achieve behavior changes that promote, maintain, or restore health. This partnership focuses on self-care—the ability to effectively advocate and manage a person's own health. The rationale for health teaching is to equip people with the knowledge, attitudes, and practices that will allow them to live the fullest possible life for the greatest length of time. The vision of *Healthy People 2020* is for "a society in which all people live long, healthy lives" (U.S. Department of Health and Human Services [USDHHS], 2010a). Figure 11-1 depicts a graphic model of *Healthy People 2020*, including overarching goals. This model demonstrates the influence of social determinants of health to the positive health outcomes envisioned in the Healthy People initiative. *Healthy People 2020* objectives for educational, community-based programs, which address the goal of increasing the "quality, availability and effectiveness of educational and community-based programs designed to prevent disease and injury, improve health and enhance the quality of life," are listed in Table 11-1 (USDHHS, 2010b). These objectives when viewed in the broader context depicted in the model can be used to identify client needs and align educational efforts that will advance this national initiative.

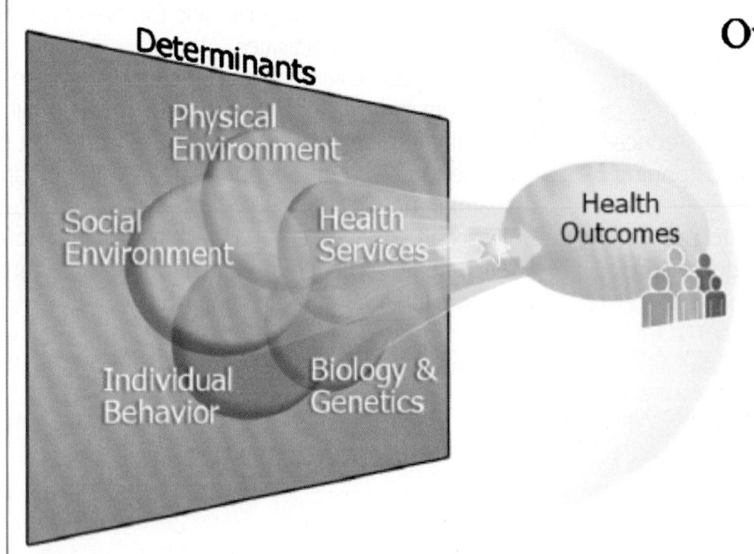

FIGURE 11-1. Health people 2020 framework. (From USDHHS, Office of Disease Prevention and Health Promotion. (*Healthy People 2020*). *Healthy People 2020 Framework: The vision, mission, and goals of Healthy People 2020*. Retrieved from http://healthypeople.gov/2020/consortium/HP2020Framework.pdf)

Table 11.1 ***Healthy People 2020*** **Objectives for Education and Community-Based Programs**

	Objective	2020 Goal
ECBP–1	Preschool health education	Increase the proportion of preschool Early Head Start and Head Start programs that provide health education to prevent health problems in the following areas: unintentional injury; violence; tobacco use and addiction; alcohol and drug use, unhealthy dietary patterns; and inadequate physical activity, dental health, and safety
ECBP–2	School health education	Increase the proportion of elementary, middle, and senior high schools that provide comprehensive school health education to prevent health problems in the following areas: unintentional injury; violence; suicide; tobacco use and addiction; alcohol or other drug use; unintended pregnancy, HIV/AIDS, and STD infection; unhealthy dietary patterns; and inadequate physical activity.
ECBP–3	School health education standards	Increase the proportion of elementary, middle, and senior high schools that have health education goals or objectives that address the knowledge and skills articulated in the National Health Education Standards
ECBP–4	School health education on personal growth and wellness	Increase the proportion of elementary, middle, and senior high schools that provide school health education to promote personal health and wellness in the following areas: hand washing or hand hygiene; oral health; growth and development; sun safety and skin cancer prevention; benefits of rest and sleep; ways to prevent vision and hearing loss; and the importance of health screenings and checkups
ECBP–5	School nurse-to-student ratio	Increase the proportion of the Nation's elementary, middle, and senior high schools that have a full-time registered school nurse-to-student ratio of at least 1:750
ECBP–6	High school completion activities	Increase the proportion of the population that completes high school education
ECBP–7	Health-risk behavior information in higher education	Increase the proportion of college and university students who receive information from their institution on each of the priority health risk behavior areas (all priority areas; unintentional injury; violence; suicide; tobacco use and addiction; alcohol and other drug use; unintended pregnancy, HIV/AIDS, and STD infection; unhealthy dietary patterns; and inadequate physical activity)
ECBP–8	Worksite health promotion programs	Increase the proportion of worksites that offer an employee health promotion program to their employees
ECBP–9	Participation in employer-sponsored health promotion	Increase the proportion of employees who participate in employer-sponsored health promotion activities
ECBP–10	Community-based primary prevention services	Increase the number of community-based organizations (including local health departments, tribal health services, nongovernmental organizations, and State agencies) providing population-based primary prevention services in the following areas: injury, violence, mental illness, tobacco use, substance abuse, unintended pregnancy, chronic disease programs, nutrition, physical activity
ECBP–11	Culturally appropriate community health programs	Increase the proportion of local health departments that have established culturally appropriate and linguistically competent community health promotion and disease prevention programs
ECBP–12	Clinical prevention and population health training—M.D.–granting medical schools	Increase the inclusion of core clinical prevention and population health content in M.D.–granting medical schools

(Continued)

Table 11.1 ***Healthy People 2020*** **Objectives for Education and Community-Based Programs** ***(continued)***

	Objective	2020 Goal
ECBP–13	Clinical prevention and population health training—D.O.–granting medical schools	Increase the inclusion of core clinical prevention and population health content in D.O.–granting medical schools
ECBP–14	Clinical prevention and population health training —undergraduate nursing	Increase the inclusion of core clinical prevention and population health content in undergraduate nursing
ECBP–15	Clinical prevention and population health training—nurse practitioner	Increase the inclusion of core clinical prevention and population health content in nurse practitioner training
ECBP–16	Clinical prevention and population health training —physician assistant	Increase the inclusion of core clinical prevention and population health content in physician assistant training

ECBP, education and community-based program.

When the community health nurse identifies a need that is best met through health education, the nurse is faced with a series of questions: What is the overall goal? How can I teach effectively? What content should I cover? What method of presentation will communicate most effectively? What resources can I use as teaching tools? How do I know when the client has grasped the information or mastered the skills? How do I involve the client in the learning process? How do I help clients with special learning needs? The nurse must understand what makes teaching effective, how teaching skills are acquired, and how mastery is measured. The nurse might also need to consider why some individuals adopt new health practices and others do not and how social determinants influence health outcomes. This chapter addresses these questions and discusses teaching as a basic intervention tool in community health nursing practice. For health education to be effective, awareness of the underlying principles of behavior change is vital. The community health nurse should consider what motivates people to adopt new behaviors and what factors may inhibit or prevent that change. By understanding the principles of teaching and behavior change, the community health nurse can work toward the ultimate goal of health promotion for individuals, families, groups, and communities.

HEALTH PROMOTION THROUGH CHANGE

Health promotion has been defined as "behavior motivated by the desire to increase wellbeing and actualize human health potential" (Pender, Murdaugh, & Parsons, 2011). Another term often confused with health promotion is *disease prevention* (or *health protection*), which is "behavior motivated by a desire to actively avoid illness, detect it early, or maintain functioning within the constraints of illness" (Pender et al., 2011). These two terms, so often used interchangeably, are clearly both important aspects of health education efforts, yet they imply a decidedly different motivation. For the community health nurse, both terms are aligned to practice at the primary level of prevention. The Levels of Prevention Pyramid at the end of this chapter describes educational activities within both of these approaches in relation to primary prevention. For instance, a community health nurse may plan an educational program for community-dwelling older adults to learn about the need for a balanced diet, rich in fruits and vegetables. This would be an example of a health promotion focus, since there is no clear disease or condition at issue. As the nurse continues to work with these individuals, the nurse learns that several clients have had recent falls. Fortunately, none of the falls was serious, yet the nurse recognizes the need to discuss foods that will help reduce bone loss and promote healthy bone growth. To protect the clients' health, the nurse provides information on a variety of foods rich in calcium and explains the need for adequate vitamin D. This effort would be still primary prevention, but with the purpose of health protection.

For the community health nurse, teaching is the primary means to influence health at all levels, primary, secondary, and tertiary. But consider the community health nurse's educational program just described: He or she has provided a well-developed educational program that was well received by the participants. They listened attentively, took the nurse's well-prepared handouts home, and even promised to add more fruits, vegetables, and calcium-rich foods to their diet. A few weeks later, in another educational program, the nurse learns from the participants that they have not altered their dietary patterns in the slightest. This is an example of how understanding the principles of behavior change may have provided guidance to this nurse in planning a more effective program, with greater prospects for success.

The Nature of Change

To be a community health nurse is to be a health educator with the goal of effecting change in people's behaviors. When nurses suggest that families adopt

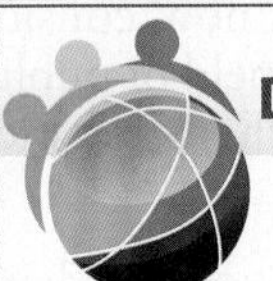

DISPLAY 11.1 CHANGING BEHAVIOR

- People decide to change for lots of different reasons.`
- People try and fail several times before they successfully change habits.
- Working at some changes can be lifelong.
- Most people change on their own; they don't need special programs.
- What works for one person may not help another.

Adapted from Center for the Advancement of Health. (2006). *What we know about changing behavior*. Retrieved from http://www.cfah.org/about/whatweknow.cfm

healthier communication patterns, they are asking them to change. Teaching parenting skills to teenagers is introducing a change. Promoting a community's self-determination in choosing a safer environment requires that the individuals involved must change. Therefore, it becomes imperative for community health nurses to understand the nature of change, how people respond to it, and how to effect change for improved community health (see Display 11.1).

Definitions and Types of Change

Change is "any planned or unplanned alteration of the status quo in an organism, situation, or process" (Lippitt, 1973, p. 37). This classic definition explains that change may occur either by design or by default. Over the years, various theorists have contributed to understanding the nature of change. From a systems perspective, change means that things are out of balance or the system's equilibrium is upset (Roussel, 2013; Rowitz, 2006). For instance, when a community is devastated by a flood, its normal functioning is thrown off balance. Adjustments are required; new patterns of behavior become necessary.

Other classic theorists have explained change as the process of adopting an innovation (Spradley & McCurdy, 1994). Something different, such as an organization-wide smoke-free policy, is introduced; change occurs when the innovation is accepted, tried, and integrated into daily practice. Some have explained change in terms of its effect on behavior—change requires adjustment in thinking and behavior, and people's responses to change vary according to their perceptions of it. Change threatens the security that people feel when following established and familiar patterns. It generally requires adopting new roles. Change is disruptive. The way people respond to change depends partly on the type of change. The change process can be described as sudden or drastic (revolutionary) or gradual over time (evolutionary).

Evolutionary change is change that is gradual and requires adjustment on an incremental basis. It modifies rather than replaces a current way of operating. Some examples of evolutionary change include becoming parents, gradually cutting back on the number of cigarettes smoked each day, and losing weight by eliminating desserts and snacks. Because it is gradual, this kind of change does not require radical shifts in goals or values. For the most part, people resist discarding their own ideas. Accepting another's idea can reduce their self-esteem and is resisted. Gradual change may "ease the pain" that change brings to some individuals. Sometimes this type of change may be viewed as *reform*.

Revolutionary change, in contrast, is a more rapid, drastic, and threatening type of change that may completely upset the balance of a system. It involves different goals and perhaps radically new patterns of behavior. Sudden unemployment, stopping smoking overnight, losing the town's football team in a plane accident, removing children from abusive parents, or rapidly replacing human workers with computers are examples of revolutionary changes. In each instance, the people affected have little or no advance warning and little or no time to prepare. High levels of emotional, mental, and sometimes physical energy and rapid behavior change are required to adapt to revolutionary change. If the demands are too great, some may experience defense mechanisms such as incapacitation, resistance, or denial of the new situation.

The impact of a proposed change on a system clearly depends on the degree of the change's evolutionary or revolutionary qualities, a factor to be considered in planning for change. Some situations lend themselves better to one kind of change than another. A community in need of improved facilities for the handicapped (e.g., ramps, wider doors) can introduce this change on an evolutionary, incremental basis, whereas a community that is involved in an unsafe, intolerable, or life-threatening situation, such as a flood or serious influenza epidemic, may require revolutionary change.

Stages of Change

The phrase **stages of change** refers to the three sequential steps leading to change: unfreezing (when desire for change develops), changing (when new ideas are accepted and tried out), and refreezing (when the change is integrated and stabilized in practice). These stages were first described by Kurt Lewin in the 1940s and early 1950s, and they have become a cornerstone for understanding the change process in more recent years (Lewin, 1947, 1951; Lippitt, Watson, & Westley, 1958).

Unfreezing

The first stage, unfreezing, occurs when a developing need for change causes disequilibrium in the system. A system in disequilibrium is more vulnerable to change. People are motivated to change either intrinsically or by some external force. People have a sense of dissatisfaction; they feel a void that they would like to fill. The unfreezing stage involves initiating the change. Unfreezing may occur spontaneously: A family requests help in solving a problem with alcoholism, a group seeks assistance in adjusting to retirement, and a community desires a solution to noise pollution. However, the nurse as change agent may need to initiate the unfreezing stage by attempting to motivate clients, through education or other strategies, to see the need for change. What we do know is that people have a tendency to be reactive rather than proactive when it comes to managing their health behaviors (Center for Advancing Health, 2010). This has been termed as "just-in-time" involvement, when clients are motivated to change once illness seems imminent. This concept is discussed further in Chapter 17 in relation to emergency preparedness.

Changing/Moving

The second stage of the change process, changing or moving, occurs when people examine, accept, and try the innovation. For instance, this is the period when participants in a prenatal class are learning exercises or when elderly clients in a senior citizens' center are discussing and trying ways to make their apartments safe from accidents. During the changing stage, people experience a series of attitude transformations, ranging from early questioning of the innovation's worth, to full acceptance and commitment, to accomplishing the change. The change agent's role during this moving stage is to help clients see the value of the change, encourage them to try it out, and assist them in adopting it.

Refreezing

The third and final stage in the change process, refreezing, occurs when change is established as an accepted and permanent part of the system. The rest of the system has adapted to it. Because it is no longer viewed as disruptive, threatening, or new, people no longer feel resistant to it. As the change is integrated, the system becomes refrozen and stabilized. It is evident that refreezing has occurred when weight-loss clients, for example, are routinely following their diets and losing weight, or when senior citizens are using grab bars in their bathrooms and have removed scatter rugs from their homes, or when a community has erected stop signs and established crosswalks at dangerous intersections.

Refreezing involves integrating or internalizing the change into the system and then maintaining it. Because a change has been accepted and tried does not guarantee that it will last. Often, there is a tendency for old patterns and habits to return. Consequently, the change agent must take special measures to ensure maintenance of the new behavior. A later section discusses ways to stabilize change.

Planned/Managed Change

Leaders in community health nursing have been change agents for decades. They have planned and managed change in a variety of systems. **Planned change** is a purposeful, designed effort to effect improvement in a system with the assistance of a change agent (Spradley, 1980). Planned change, also known as managed change (Roussel, 2013) is crucial to the development of successful community health nursing programs. In fact, the ability to manage and influence change is now considered to be an important competency in the field of public health (Thompson, 2010). The following characteristics of planned change are key to its success:

The change is purposeful and intentional: There are specific reasons or goals prompting the change. These goals give the change effort a unifying focus and a specific target. Unplanned change occurs haphazardly, and its outcomes are unpredictable.

The change is by design, not by default: Thorough, systematic planning provides structure for the change process and a map to follow toward a planned destination.

Planned change in community health aims at improvement: That is, it seeks to better the current situation, to promote a higher level of efficiency, safety, or health enhancement. Planned change aims to facilitate growth and positive improvements. Plans to provide shelter and health care for a homeless population, for example, are designed to improve this group's wellbeing.

Planned change is accomplished through an influencing agent: The change agent is a catalyst in developing and carrying out the design; the change agent's role is a leadership role; often as an educator.

Planned-Change Process

The planned-change process involves a systematic sequence of activities that follows the nursing process. Following its eight basic steps leads to the successful management of change: (1) recognize symptoms, (2) diagnose need, (3) analyze alternative solutions, (4) select a change, (5) plan the change, (6) implement the change, (7) evaluate the change, and (8) stabilize the change (Spradley, 1980). Figure 11-2 shows how forces acting on a system create a need for change using the planned-change model.

Step 1: Recognize (Assess) Symptoms

The first step in managing change is to recognize and assess the symptoms that indicate a need for change. This step requires gathering and examining the presenting evidence, not diagnosing or jumping ahead to treatment. For instance, assume that a group of clients shows interest in receiving help with parenting skills. The nurse cannot assume that these clients feel inadequate in the parent role, nor can the nurse assume that they lack information about parenting or are having difficulty with their children. The nurse must assess the specific needs to discover that some of the parents have trouble talking to their teenagers, others wonder whether their children's behavior is normal, a few question how strictly they should set limits, and still others are not certain about how to handle punishment. These symptoms are pieces of evidence that will assist diagnosis in the next step. This first step is an assessment phase. Before

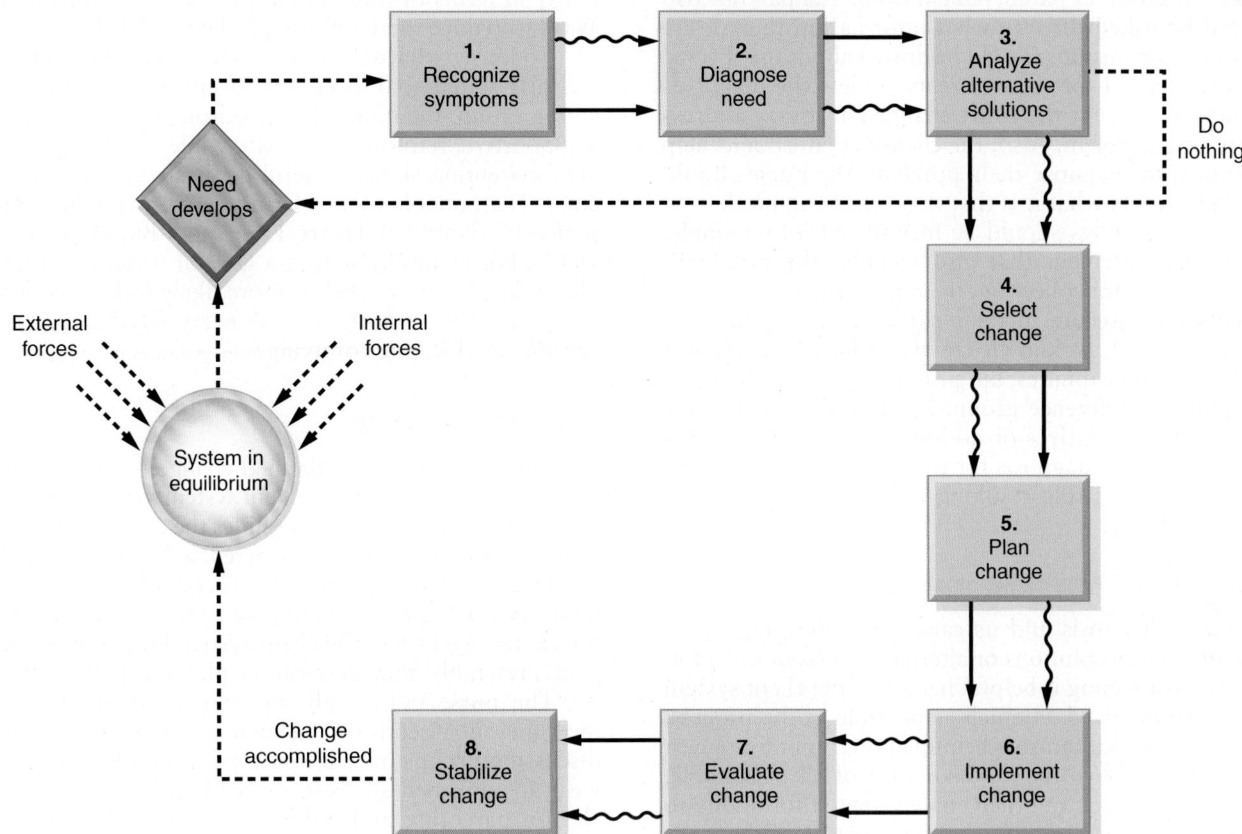

FIGURE 11-2. Planned-change model. The planned-change process begins when one recognizes a need. When the change agent fails to respond to a need for change, the need continues and may escalate. Client system (those involved and affected by the change) and change agent must work together throughout the entire planned-change process. Their respective roles vary depending on the situation and the players' abilities, but no planned change is truly effective without utilization of this collaborative relationship. The client system (*wavy arrow*), which may be an entire community, will fluctuate in its involvement with the change process. The change agent (*straight arrow*), as a good leader, analyzes the situation thoroughly, plans carefully, and sets a steady course for effecting the change.

moving on, however, change agents need to ask themselves what their motives are for pursuing this change. Inappropriate motives on the change agent's part, such as wanting to feel needed, can cloud judgment and interfere with effective management of change.

Step 2: Diagnose Need

Diagnosis involves analyzing the symptoms and reaching a conclusion about what needs changing. First, describe the situation as it is now (the real) and compare it with the way it should be (the ideal). For example, loud arguing and conflict may be normal and functional behavior for an adolescent support group. There is no discrepancy between the real and the ideal and, therefore, no need for change within the group. If, however, a discrepancy exists between the real and the ideal, then a need exists and a change effort is justified (Hersey, Blanchard, & Johnson, 2008). For example, the community health nurse, in talking with a group of parents, hears the following comment: "I'm not sure how much freedom to allow Karen. She came in late twice last week and I'm not sure how to punish her." Clearly, the nurse notices a discrepancy between this family's present and ideal situations; hence, a need exists.

The next step is to determine the nature and cause of the need. Gathering data by questioning clients, checking the literature, or seeking consultation is important for making a more accurate diagnosis. The parents should be questioned in more detail about the difficulties that they are having with their children. The nurse asks questions such as the following: How do they feel about being parents? What are the most difficult aspects of parenting for them? Have they read any books or used any other resources to help them in their parenting activities? To whom do they talk about parenting problems? When they have a problem raising their children, how do they usually solve it? Secondary data should be obtained by checking the literature to determine the most effective approaches to solving parenting problems or by consulting an expert on family life to get ideas about what this group of parents might need. The parents also should be asked directly what information they desire or need. Conclusions should be drawn about the specific changes needed for these parents. Unless the diagnosis is made accurately, the entire change effort may address the wrong problem. Also, the client system should help the nurse to diagnose their problem; the nurse should ask the parents what it is that they want and need.

These findings should be formulated into a single, diagnostic statement that also includes the problem's cause. After data collection, the nurse discovers that the parents are insecure in their parenting roles, partially because of lack of knowledge about how to carry out parental responsibilities, but primarily because they lack a supportive reference group. Most of them live some distance from relatives or no longer maintain close ties with them. The diagnosis for these parents is insecurity in the parenting role resulting from a lack of support and knowledge.

Step 3: Analyze Alternative Solutions

Once the diagnosis and its cause are determined, it is time to identify solutions or alternative directions to follow. Brainstorming is helpful here, and the client system should be involved as much as possible in the process. Reviewing the literature is helpful at this point to suggest solutions tried by others. Make a list of all reasonable, broad alternatives and then analyze them thoroughly to determine the advantages, disadvantages, possible consequences, and risks involved in each. For the parents, general alternatives might be considered, such as family counseling, a support group, or education in family life. Each of these alternatives includes some advantages and disadvantages toward meeting the parents' need for confidence in their roles.

Next, each alternative should be analyzed. For example, the counseling solution could provide insight and awareness into family behavior. It would give family members opportunities to express feelings and gain understanding of how other family members feel. However, it would not provide a frame of reference that the clients could use to compare their own parenting behaviors with other acceptable ones, nor would it provide adult peer support for the parents. The consequences of this alternative most likely would be to promote parents' self-understanding and better family communication. Risks would include the possibility that children, especially teenagers, might not be willing to participate and that parents might not gain self-confidence in their roles. Each alternative should be examined to determine its usefulness and feasibility; again literature and other resources (e.g., consultants) can be used to learn the best ways to meet the parents' need for change.

Step 4: Select a Change

After all alternatives have been carefully analyzed, the best solution must be selected. The parents favor the idea that the best solution is a parenting support group. The risks involved in the choice of change should be reexamined, such as whether this action might be too costly in terms of time, money, or potential for failure. Ways to reduce these risks might be explored.

To know what the change is aiming to accomplish, a clearly stated goal should be formulated. For this parenting group, the mutually agreed-on goal is to provide a supportive, reinforcing climate while increasing members' parenting skills. "Useful goals should be (1) specific; (2) attainable (doable); and (3) forgiving [less than perfect]" (National Heart Lung and Blood Institute, 2012). For example, setting a goal of walking 30 minutes a day, 5 days a week is more likely to be successful than a goal of walking 5 miles every day because it is specific, doable, and forgiving.

Step 5: Plan the Change

Step 5 is at the heart of planned change, because at this stage, the change agent and client system together prepare the design, or blueprint, that guides the change action. In steps 1 through 4, data are gathered, a diagnosis is made, resources are assessed, and a goal is established—all preparatory actions for planning the change. The plan tells the change agent and the client system how to meet that goal. Preferably, they develop the plan together.

The nurse talks with the parents about ways to meet their goal, considering such possibilities as weekly discussion groups on selected topics, monthly meetings with an informed speaker, or reading books and articles on parenting and holding regular sessions to discuss their application. After analysis and discussion, the group decides to meet one evening a month, rotating the location among members' homes. Group sessions will include a variety of approaches: a speaker will be invited every 4 months, a book or article discussion will be held quarterly, and the remaining meetings will be spent on topics of the group's choice. All sessions will provide opportunities for parents to discuss their concerns or problems. The nurse and the group design this plan around a set of objectives.

The most important activity in planning is to have clear, specific objectives. These should be measurable and, preferably, stated as outcomes. For example, the following objective is measurable and describes an outcome: "By the end of the second session, each parent in the group will have participated in the discussion at least once." It is helpful to prepare a list of activities to help accomplish each objective and to develop a time plan. It also is important to assess the potential costs in terms of time, money, materials, and the number of people needed and to determine the resources available. Then the evaluation plan is designed, and a list of ways to stabilize (refreeze) the change is made.

During planning, it is useful to perform a *force field analysis* (Hersey et al., 2008), a technique developed by Kurt Lewin for examining all positive (driving) and negative (restraining) forces that are influencing a change situation. *Force field theory* describes driving forces, which favor change, and restraining forces, which decrease or discourage change. Examples of driving forces include clients' desire to be healthier, to be more productive, or to

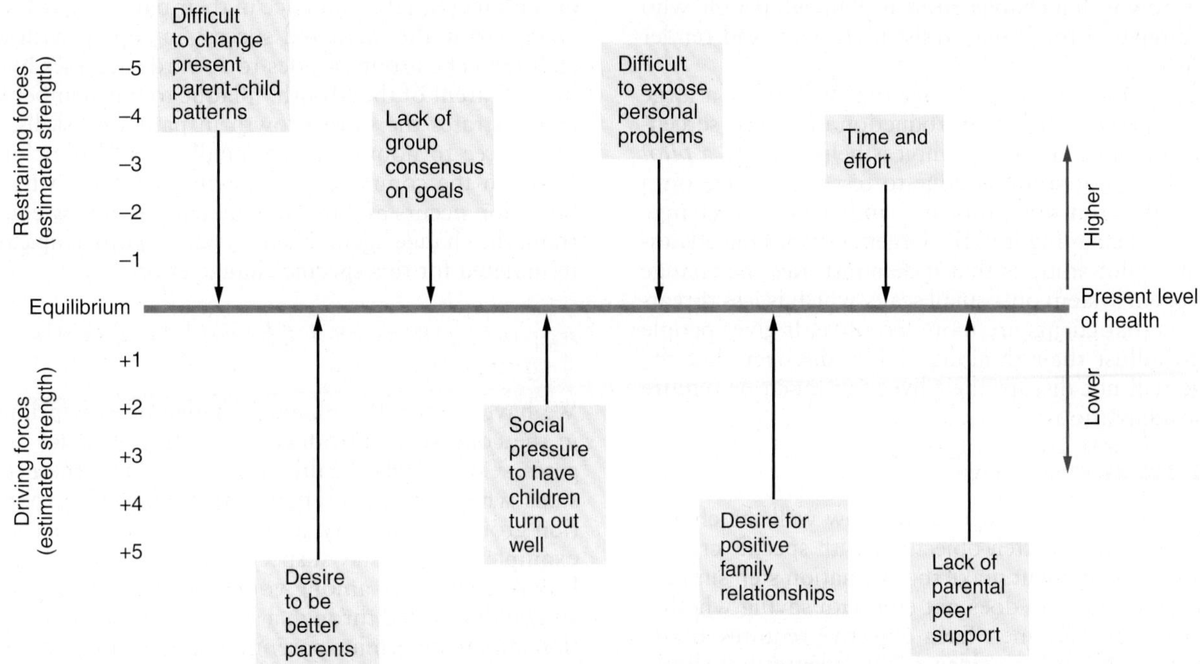

FIGURE 11-3. Analysis of restraining and driving forces.

have a safer environment. Examples of restraining forces include apathy, habits, fear of something new, perceived loss of power, low self-esteem, insecurity, and hostility (Roussel, 2013). When the strength of the driving forces is equal to the strength of the restraining forces, equilibrium exists. To introduce a change and move the client system to a higher level of health, that balance must be altered. The change agent either increases the driving forces, decreases the restraining forces, or both. The change agent uses force field analysis to study both sets of forces and to develop strategies to influence the forces in favor of the change (Fig. 11-3).

The procedure for conducting a force field analysis follows a few simple steps. The change agent may perform the analysis alone but preferably consults with clients and a change-planning resource group such as community health colleagues. The steps for conducting force field analysis are as follows:

1. Brainstorm to produce a list of all driving and restraining forces. (For the parenting group, one driving force is the parents' desire to be more successful parents; a restraining force might be lack of group agreement on discussion topics.)
2. Estimate the strength of each force.
3. Plot the forces on a chart such as the one shown in Figure 11-3.
4. Note the most important forces, then research and analyze them.
5. List and document possible responses or actions that might strengthen each important driving force or weaken each important restraining force.

Finally, as a consideration in planning the change and in analyzing the driving and restraining forces, the change agent studies the social network and interactions within the system involved in the change. The change agent needs to be aware of formal and informal leaders, cliques within larger groups, influential persons, and all other social network influences on the change process. For instance, one nurse attempting to improve the infant-feeding practices among a group of young Southeast Asian mothers failed to consider the strong cultural influence of the infants' grandmothers living nearby. The older women had strong opinions based on long-held cultural traditions about what infants were to eat and how they were to be fed. To ignore their influence could cause the proposed change to fail; involving the grandmothers could be a way of turning their influence into a driving force for the change.

Step 6: Implement the Change

The implementation step involves enacting the change plan. Because the objectives and activities have been clearly defined in previous steps, the change agent and client system know what needs to be done and how to begin the process. For example, the parenting group and their nurse/change agent begin group discussions meeting every Tuesday evening at a local school.

At the start of implementation, be certain that all persons concerned clearly understand and are prepared for the change. When working with an aggregate, for example, the nurse may do most of the planning with a few key members. The nurse must be sure that each member who will be affected by the proposed change understands (a) what to expect, (b) the meaning of the change, and (c) what will be required of them in adapting to it. An unprepared client system, especially in a large group or organization, may bring disaster. No matter how well a change effort is planned, people who are unprepared for it may resist it strongly and render it useless.

When implementing change that will affect a large group of people, such as introduction of a mass screening or immunization program, it is helpful to do a *pilot study*. The pilot study is done to test the change on a small scale, iron out problems, and revise the change before implementing it in the larger system. One advantage of a pilot study is that it demonstrates the change to the client system on a small scale, which is less threatening, so that clients are more receptive. It gives people time to adjust their thinking and to discover that the change will not disrupt their lives too much or require drastic adaptations.

Step 7: Evaluate the Change

The success of step 7 depends on how well the change is planned. Well-written objectives with specific criteria for their measurement make the evaluation step simpler. However, evaluation does not end with saying whether the objectives were met. Each objective requires analysis: Was it met? What evidence (documentation) shows that it was met? Was it accomplished using the best means possible, or would another method have been better? The objective for the parenting group stated that each member should enter into the discussion by the end of the second session. Although this objective could easily be evaluated by the nurse leader, the objective could have been improved by a more specific description of how this participation would occur. A better method to achieve this objective would have been to suggest that more active group members solicit ideas from those who did not have an opportunity to speak. This would facilitate more group participation, rather than having the nurse educator call on nontalkers to speak. Finally, considering the evaluation, the change agent makes needed modifications in the change before stabilization.

Step 8: Stabilize the Change

The final step in the planned-change process requires taking measures to reinforce and maintain the change. A well-developed change plan includes a design for stabilization. The change agent actively encourages continued use of the innovation by establishing two-way communication. In this way, future resistance can be overcome, and the client's full commitment to the change can be maintained. Stabilization occurs by soliciting reactions from the client system. Do the clients perceive any potential problems? Do they have doubts? Reinforcing the desired behavior and following up on the change as long as necessary will help to ensure its permanence.

Alcoholics Anonymous, for example, stabilizes the change to nondrinking by providing a regular support group that reinforces the nondrinking pattern. The group rewards compliance with praise and replaces drinking with other satisfying experiences, such as social acceptance, to keep the alcoholic from returning to the old behavior. In the example of the parenting group, the nurse stabilizes changed behaviors by focusing on the group's increased confidence in their parenting roles and emphasizing the increased success in coping with their children. The group decides to reward successes by giving a "Parent of the Month" plaque to the member who demonstrates the most growth in parenting skills, and they agree to nominate one member as "Parent of the Year" in the community newspaper contest. After stabilization occurs and the system achieves a new equilibrium, the change agent–client system relationship can be terminated for this specific change effort.

Applying Planned Change to Larger Aggregates

We have viewed the planned-change process primarily in the context of introducing change to smaller aggregates. Community health nurses also use these eight steps when managing change at organization, population group, community, and larger aggregate levels. For example, a nurse may suspect that there is a widespread lack of confidence among young parents. This hypothesis could be tested through a survey using a mailed questionnaire to determine parenting needs among the entire community's population of young parents. If symptoms are present (step 1), the nurse, in collaboration with health department personnel or other appropriate professionals, could analyze the symptoms and reach a diagnosis (step 2), perhaps that many young parents in the community are lacking in confidence and knowledge of parenting skills. Several approaches to meeting this need could be considered, such as instituting a parenting center in the community with satellite clinics, organizing churches or clubs to sponsor parenting support groups, or working through the community college system to hold workshops and classes on parenting skills (step 3). The most feasible and useful alternative could be selected (step 4), and a parenting program for the community could be planned (step 5) and implemented (step 6). The nurse, with parents and other professionals involved, would then evaluate the outcomes (step 7) and make necessary adjustments in the parenting program before finally stabilizing it (step 8), making certain that this change, undertaken to meet a population group need, remains an established and effectively functioning service.

Planned-Change Strategies

Here we focus on the three major change strategies: (1) empiric–rational, (2) normative–reeducative, and (3) power–coercive. In a given situation, the change agent may use one or a combination of these strategies to effect a change.

Empiric–Rational Change Strategies

Empiric–rational change strategies are used to effect change based on the assumption that people are rational and, when presented with empiric information, will adopt new practices that appear to be in their best interest. To use this approach, which is common in community health, new information is offered to people. For instance, most family planning programs use empiric–rational strategies. Clients are given basic information (communication-related strategy) on reproductive anatomy and physiology, and they are told about the benefits of contraception with an explanation of a variety of family planning methods. Health workers hope that once clients have this information, they will adopt some method of family planning. Some clients respond well to this approach, and others do not. The difference lies in client ability and interest in self-help. The nurse/change agent uses empiric–rational strategies with clients who can assume a relatively high degree of responsibility for their own health.

Normative–Reeducative Change Strategies

Normative–reeducative change strategies are used to influence change that not only presents new information but also directly influences people's attitudes and behaviors through persuasion. It is a sociocultural reeducation. This approach assumes that people's attitudes and practices are determined by sociocultural norms and that they need more than presentation of information to change behavior. This approach strengthens client self-understanding, self-control, and commitment to new patterns through direct urging and influence. For example, a health education program that aims to increase safety practices in an industrial setting not only provides safety information, such as posters and warning signs, but also uses persuasive tactics, such as individual rewards for safe practices, division recognition for minimum number of accidents, or discipline for noncompliance. Nurses use normative–reeducative strategies with clients who have a measure of self-care skill but at the same time need external assistance to effect lasting behavioral change. This type of client is found in teaching, counseling, and therapy situations.

Power–Coercive Change Strategies

Power–coercive change strategies use coercion based on fear to effect change. Change agents may derive power from the law (health regulations, administrative policies), from position (political, social, or managerial), from a group (social, work, or professional), or from personal power (personal charisma, competence, respect of followers). They use this power to coerce change; the result is forced compliance on the part of the client system. Some situations, particularly those that are life-threatening, may require power–coercive strategies. In community health practice, power–coercive strategies may be used with people who cannot help themselves or in situations that threaten individuals' safety or the public's health. An example is the stringent enforcement of infection control policies regarding the treatment of contaminated objects such as used needles and the safe disposal of infectious wastes. In another example, if officials find a restaurant to be in violation of health codes, they will either force compliance with the code or close the restaurant. Occasionally, clients cannot exercise responsibility because of temporary or permanent physical or psychological incapacitation; examples may include mentally ill individuals, abusive parents, or developmentally disabled persons. In such cases, the nurse may need to use the power of the law to effect changes that are in clients' best interests. Although power–coercive strategies are appropriate in some situations, they should be used with caution because they can rob people of opportunities to grow in autonomy and capacity for self-care.

Planned-change strategies may be combined; for instance, a normative–reeducative approach might have a power–coercive backup. This combination is evident in programs that educate and persuade groups of people to be immunized against an impending epidemic or to keep their garbage contained to avoid insect and rodent infestation. Behind this normative–reeducative strategy is an implied coercive threat of official disapproval, or worse, if the clients are noncompliant.

The effectiveness of a change strategy varies with each situation and particularly with the degree of client capacity for self-care. The community health nurse as a change agent must adapt strategies to fit each change situation. It is important to remember that "the central issue in change is not just strategy, structure, culture, or systems change, but how people see the proposed change and how it affects their feelings about the changes proposed" (Rowitz, 2006, p. 437).

Principles for Effecting Positive Change

Community health nurses introduce change every day that they practice. Every effort to solve a problem, prevent another problem from occurring, meet a potential community need, or promote people's optimal health requires changes. For these changes to be truly successful, so that desired outcomes are reached, they must be managed well. The following six principles provide guidelines for effecting positive change: (1) principle of participation, (2) principle of resistance to change, (3) principle of proper timing, (4) principle of interdependence, (5) principle of flexibility, and (6) principle of self-understanding.

Principle of Participation

Persons affected by a proposed change should participate as much as possible in every step of the planned-change process. This involvement is important for several reasons. Collaboration with those who have a vested interest in the change can produce a wealth of ideas and insights that can greatly improve the change plan. Furthermore, such participation can help remove obstacles and reduce resistance. Participation ensures a greater likelihood that the change will be accepted and maintained. One nurse, for instance, when planning with a school's parent–teacher association for a drug education program, involved students as well as teachers and parents. As a result, the nurse secured this group's support and cooperation, gained many helpful suggestions that had not been previously considered, and discovered that students were more responsive to the program because the change plan was specifically tailored to their needs. In cross-cultural or international arenas, community participation is paramount to effective change. For example, a project targeting improved sanitation and hygiene practices in Bangladesh involved community members throughout the project cycle, resulting in sustainable behavior change and true community ownership (Kausar, 2012).

Principle of Resistance to Change

Because all systems instinctively preserve the status quo, the change agent can expect people to resist change. The homeostatic mechanism operating in any system seeks to maintain equilibrium; change poses a threat to that stability and security. Furthermore, all systems experience inertia, that is, they resist beginning movement. People do not undertake a change until they are convinced of its worth. Resistance may also come from a conflict over goals and methods or from misunderstanding about what the change will mean and require. Involving people in the planned-change process, as discussed in the previous section, is one way to overcome resistance. Another way is establishing and maintaining open lines of communication to make ideas clearly understood and to resolve disagreements quickly. The nurse must prepare clients thoroughly for the change, provide support and patience during the change process, and encourage response and expression of feelings.

Principle of Proper Timing

Sometimes a change, even a well-designed and much-needed one, should be postponed because it is not the right time to introduce it. For example, perhaps the client system is experiencing too many other changes to handle the stress of this one. Other projects or activities in which the client system is currently engaged may compete for energy and other resources, depleting the energy and resources needed to make the proposed change successful. For example, in November, some middle-aged women, eager to start a book club that focused on preparing for midlife changes (including menopause, "empty-nest" syndrome, and planning for retirement), had to postpone the project because the holidays were approaching. Shopping, entertaining, and vacations made it impossible to give the kind of time and energy needed to make the book club effective.

Proper timing is as important to a planned change as well-timed seed planting is to a good harvest. The change idea must be appropriate, the change recipient prepared, the climate right, and the resources available before the change can be fostered to grow into full maturity and usefulness.

Principle of Interdependence

Every system has many subsystems that are intricately related to and interdependent on one another. A change in one part of a system affects its other parts, and a change in one system may affect other systems. For example, a county community nursing agency made a change in its use of home health aides. Because many homebound clients needed more care than the agency staff could provide, the agency contracted with a private home-care service for extra home health aides. These paraprofessionals worked in the homes of agency clients, supplementing the care given by agency staff. The private company preferred to supervise its own aides, whereas the county agency had a policy of using community health nurses to supervise aides. The county agency was legally responsible and professionally accountable for the quality of care given to clients. The private company wanted to retain control of its workers. The matter was resolved by contracting with a different private service that would accept the county agency's supervision. The change, however, had affected the roles of nurses and aides within the system, as well as the relationships between the two systems.

This principle of interdependence reminds the nurse that change does not take place in a vacuum. When workers learn new health and safety practices associated with their jobs, their relationships with one another, and their bosses, their overall productivity in the organization may easily be affected. One must anticipate and prepare for the impact of the proposed change on the clients involved, other persons, departments, organizations, or even geographic areas.

Principle of Flexibility

Unexpected events can occur in every situation. This fifth principle—flexibility—emphasizes two points. First, the nurse needs to be able to adapt to unexpected events and make the most of them. Perseverance and flexibility are the marks of a creative change manager (Clampitt & DeKoch, 2001; Roussel, 2013). One community health nurse had tried unsuccessfully to contact a young mother who was reportedly abusing her 2-year-old son. After several phone calls and visits to an empty house, the nurse finally found the mother and son at home with a neighbor who insisted on staying for the entire visit. At first, the nurse was irritated by the neighbor's presence and viewed it as interfering with the goal of getting to know the mother and child. When the nurse realized that the neighbor's presence offered an opportunity to learn more about the situation through the neighbor's input, the nurse viewed it as an opportunity to influence another client as well. She asked whether the neighbor had children, and began to include both women in the discussion, explaining what could be offered in terms of health teaching and support. This nurse was flexible in her approach to this situation.

The second point to remember about flexibility is that a good change planner anticipates possible blocks or problems by preparing strategies and alternative plans. During step 3 of the planned-change process, it is helpful to rank the alternative solutions considered. Then, if the first choice does not work out for some reason, an alternative is ready to be put into action. Flexibility involves a willingness to consider a variety of options and suggestions from many sources (Clampitt & DeKoch, 2001).

Principle of Self-Understanding

Self-understanding is essential for an effective change agent (Hersey et al., 2008). The community nurse (as change agent) should be able to clearly define his or her role and learn how others define it. It is important to understand one's values and motives in relation to each change that one might ask people to make. Nurses should also understand their own personality traits, so that they can capitalize on or alter them to be more effective change agents. Understanding oneself is crucial to learning to make use of one's best qualities and skills to effect change.

Change is inevitable. It can be seen as the "process of moving from what has become an obsolete present into a revitalized present with an eye on the future ... the old rules do not seem to be working anymore, and new rules and procedures need to be developed for the changing context in which we live today" (Rowitz, 2006, p. 431). Understanding the principles of planned change can assist the community health nurse in guiding individuals, families, and communities toward achieving the highest level of health.

SOCIAL DETERMINANTS OF HEALTH

Social justice has long been a tenant of our society, dating back to the industrial revolution (Hofrichter & Bhatia, 2010). Social justice, as it relates to health, is an increasing concern primarily because of the growing inequity in the distribution of disease, illness and wellness across our society. **Social determinants of health** are "conditions in the environments in which people are born, live, learn, work, play, worship, and age that affect a wide range of health, functioning, and quality-of-life outcomes and risks" (USDHHS, 2010c). *Healthy People 2020* addresses social determinants of health as a new topic, with the goal of "creating social and physical environments that promote good health for all" (USDHHS, 2010c).

Understanding social determinants of health requires examination of numerous factors, beyond individual behavior, that contribute to our state of health. Factors that influence an individual's ability to maintain good health include social, economic, and physical factors such as access to social and economic opportunities; safe housing; quality education; clean water, food, and air; safe workplaces; equitable social interactions (class, race, and gender); and adequate community resources (USDHHS, 2010c, 2010e). Addressing these factors in a manner that has a positive impact on social, economic, and physical conditions and supports positive health behavior change can improve the health of our communities over time.

"Nursing has a clear mandate to ensure access to health and health-care by providing sensitive empowering care to those experiencing inequities and working to change underlying social conditions that result in and perpetuate health inequities" (Reutter & Kushner, 2012, p. 269). The community health nurse can play a significant role in addressing social determinants of health by first being aware and educated about factors that influence health beyond an individual's choices, looking at root causes of disease.

Secondly, the community health nurse can incorporate social determinant factors when assessing individuals, families, and communities. One resource for this is the Health Impact Project, found at: http://www.healthimpactproject.org/. This project seeks to advance policies for healthier communities by examining social, economic, and environmental influences; building consensus across community members and other stakeholders; and advocating for health considerations in all policies (Health Impact Project, 2011).

Finally, community health nurses can educate their client base on the social determinants of health, facilitate community action that supports positive change, and advocate for policies that address the root causes of disease and health inequities (USDHHS, 2010c, 2010e).

The Robert Wood Johnson Foundation conducted research to determine the most effective messages on social determinants of health that are meaningful and understandable to Americans (Robert Wood Johnson Foundation, 2010). The community health nurse educator can use these messages to communicate concepts about social determinants of health to clients and communities (see Display 11.2).

Facilitating community action is most effective when using participatory action research approaches (Hofrichter & Bahatai, 2010). One such approach is known as the Community Action Model (Fig. 11-4) that seeks to identify actions that are achievable, sustainable, and compels change for the wellbeing of all. This model builds on concepts presented in the planned-change process earlier in this chapter. The cyclical five-step process

DISPLAY 11.2 SIX WAYS TO TALK ABOUT SOCIAL DETERMINANTS OF HEALTH

1. Health starts—long before illness—in our homes, schools, and jobs.
2. All Americans should have the opportunity to make the choices that allow them to live a long, healthy life, regardless of their income, education, or ethnic background.
3. Your neighborhood or job shouldn't be hazardous to your health.
4. Your opportunity for health starts long before you need medical care.
5. Health begins where we live, learn, work, and play.
6. The opportunity for health begins in our families, neighborhoods, schools, and jobs. (Robert Wood Johnson Foundation, 2010, p. 7)

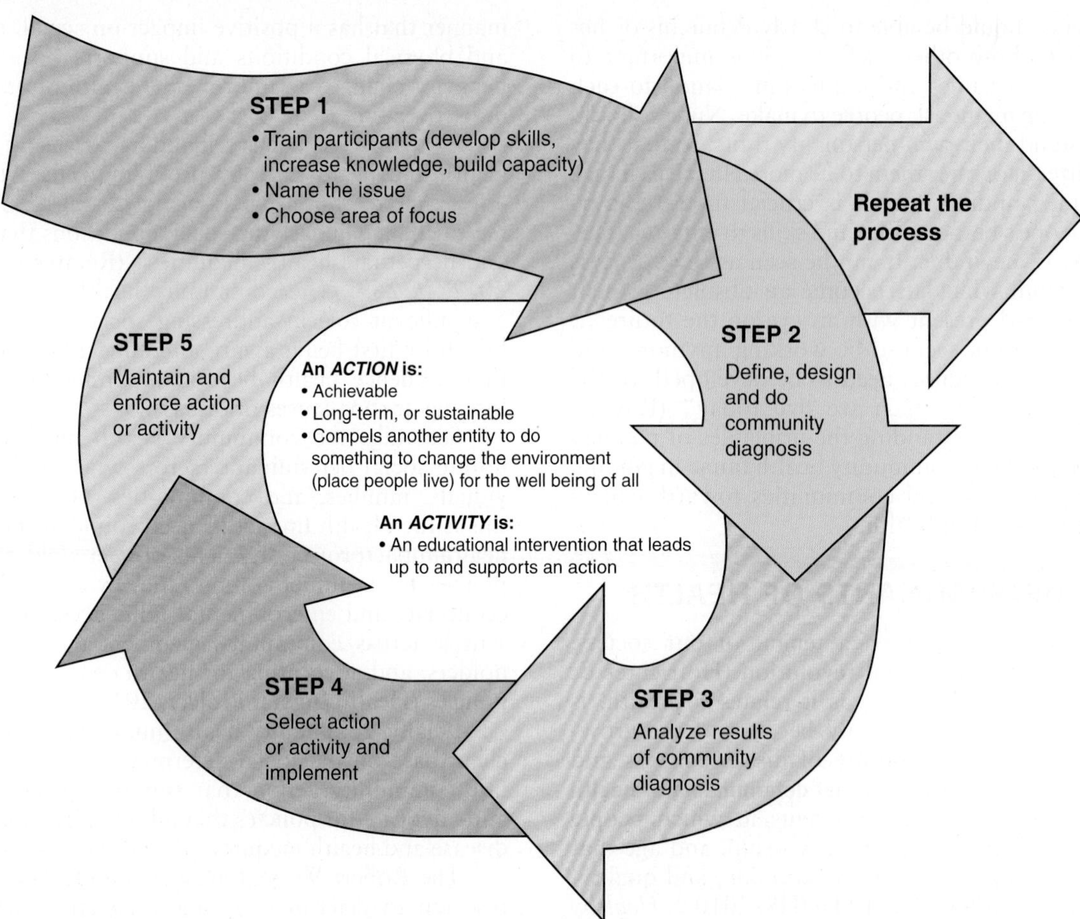

FIGURE 11-4. Community action model—creating change by building community capacity. (From Community Health Education Section, San Francisco Department of Public Health. (2002). *Community Action Training.* Retrieved from http://www.sfdph.org/dph/files/CAMdocs/intro_and_overview/CAMCreatingChangebyBuildingCommunityCapacity.pdf)

is outlined in Display 11.3. The community health nurse educator can use this model to facilitate community participation and ownership of change that has a positive impact on the community's health. An example of a successful application of the Community Action Model involved tobacco divestment on college campuses, which was carried out as a part of the San Francisco Tobacco Free Project (Hofrichter & Bahatai, 2010). Further information and curriculum on the Community Action Model can be found at: http://sftfc.globalink.org/AdaptCAM-En.pdf and http://www.sfdph.org/dph/comupg/oprograms/CHPP/CAM/default.asp

Policy advocacy is most successful when approached through intersectoral collaboration involving key stakeholders as well as beneficiaries of the policies (Reutter & Kushner, 2012). This requires that the community health

DISPLAY 11.3 FIVE-STEP COMMUNITY ACTION MODEL

Step 1 Skills-based trainings where advocates choose an area of focus

Step 2 Action research where advocates define, design, and do a community diagnosis (action research)

Step 3 Analysis where advocates analyze the result of the diagnosis and prepare findings

Step 4 Organizing where advocates select, plan, and implement an action for change and education to support it

Step 5 Implementing where advocates ensure that the policy outcome is enforced and maintained. (Hofrichter & Bahati, 2010, p. 360)

educator think beyond health and engage with sectors to tackle inequities through policy analysis and advocacy. Advocating for "Health in All Policies" (HiAP) is one approach to addressing multisector policy change as it relates to social determinants of health (World Health Organization [WHO], 2010). Since many factors outside of health impact health outcomes, it is vital that all policies, regardless of the sector, be viewed from a health lens. Examples of sectors that often have a direct impact on health include agriculture, education, energy, environment, global warming, housing, trade, and transportation, among others (The Aspen Institute, 2012).

CHANGE THROUGH HEALTH EDUCATION

Early in this chapter, you were introduced to one definition of health promotion, with a clear focus on individual and aggregate behavior (Pender et al., 2011). Consider another definition: "any combination of educational, organizational, environmental, and economic supports for behavior and conditions of living that are conducive to health" (Ottoson & Green, 2008, p. 614). This definition points out the need for a system-wide approach to promoting healthy behaviors, one that includes education. For the community health nurse, health education is a foundation of practice. Whether the nurse is providing one-on-one education to a new mother about the benefits of breast-feeding or briefing county officials on the need to maintain breast-feeding support centers, educational techniques are being used to promote health in the community. Knowledge of educational theories and teaching methods can assist the nurse to frame these "health messages" for the greatest impact and chance of success.

Teaching is a specialized communication process in which desired behavior changes are achieved. The goal of all teaching is learning. Learning is thought to mean gaining knowledge, comprehension, or mastery. These are nebulous terms, and a more acceptable definition suggests that *learning* is a process of assimilating new information that promotes a permanent change in behavior. All people have been presented with information that was not interesting, relevant to their needs, or comprehensible. In such situations, learning is difficult, if not impossible. The nurse as teacher seeks to transmit information in such a way that the client demonstrates a relatively permanent change in behavior. After learning, clients are capable of doing something that they could not do before learning took place. Effective teaching is a cause; learning becomes the effect. To teach effectively, especially in the community where teaching is the focus of care, nurses need to understand the various domains of learning and related learning theories.

DOMAINS OF LEARNING

Learning occurs in several realms or domains: cognitive, affective, and psychomotor. Understanding of the differences among the domains and of the related roles of the nurse provides the background necessary to teach effectively.

Cognitive Domain

The cognitive domain of learning involves the mind and thinking processes. When the meaning and relationship of a series of facts is grasped, cognitive learning is experienced. The **cognitive domain** deals with the recall or recognition of knowledge and the development of intellectual abilities and skills (Bloom, 1956). There are six major levels in the cognitive domain (Gronlund, 1970; Miller, Linn, & Gronlund, 2009): knowledge, comprehension, application, analysis, synthesis, and evaluation. To *operationalize* these levels (i.e., put these ideas or concepts into words that can be used), verbs are used. As the goal of the learning or behavioral objective changes, so do the verbs, indicating the learning to be accomplished within that particular level of the cognitive domain. Notice that the objectives at the beginning of each chapter in this text follow this format, using a variety of verbs to indicate the expected level of learning. A representative sample of behavioral objectives focusing on nutrition and appropriate cognitive-level verbs is included in the discussion of each level.

Knowledge

Knowledge, the lowest level of learning according to Bloom's taxonomy (1956), involves recall. If students remember material previously learned, they have acquired knowledge. This level may be used with clients who are unable to understand underlying reasons or rationales, such as young children or people who have had strokes. Stroke clients may need to remember that medication should be taken daily, that regular exercise restores function, and that drinking alcohol should be avoided, although they may not grasp the reasons behind these measures. Five-year-olds may need to identify healthful foods rather than understand why they are nutritious.

A knowledge-level behavioral objective might be "The client can *recall* the names of six fruits to eat as nutritious snacks." Other knowledge-level verbs include *define*, *repeat*, *list*, and *name*.

Comprehension

The second level of cognitive learning, comprehension, combines remembering with understanding. Teaching aims at instilling at least a minimal understanding. Nurses want clients to grasp the meaning and to recognize the importance of suggested health behaviors.

An example of a comprehension-level behavioral objective might be, "The pregnant client will *describe* a well-balanced diet during pregnancy." Other appropriate verbs at the comprehension level include *discuss*, *explain*, *identify*, *tell*, and *report*.

Application

Application is the third level of cognitive learning, in which the learner cannot only understand material but also apply it to new situations. Application approaches the possibility of self-care when clients use their knowledge to improve their own health. The test of application is a transfer of understanding into practice. Therefore, to encourage application, the nurse can design teaching plans that provide clients with knowledge that can be put into practice. In the home setting, a nurse may suggest that a diabetic client write down glucometer readings to show the nurse at the next visit. A school nurse could ask adolescents in a weight-loss group to keep a diet record for a week, draw up a diet plan, and share this plan with the group at the next meeting. In contrast, the construction worker who understands on-the-job hazards but seldom wears a protective hat in the work area has yet to transfer knowledge and comprehension into practice or application.

An example of an application-level behavioral objective might be, "The client will *practice* eating well-balanced meals at least two times a day." Other verbs at this level include *apply*, *use*, *demonstrate*, and *illustrate*.

Analysis

The fourth level of cognitive learning is analysis; at this level, the learner breaks down material into parts, distinguishes between elements, and understands the relationships among the parts. This level of learning becomes a preliminary step toward problem-solving. The learner carefully scrutinizes all of the variables or elements and their relationships to each other to explain the situation. A family that studies its own communication patterns to identify sources of conflict is using analysis. A mother analyzes when she seeks to determine the cause of an infant's crying. After viewing the total situation, she breaks it down into variables such as hunger, pain, overstimulation, loneliness, type of crying, and intensity of crying. She examines these parts and draws conclusions about their relationships. In health teaching, community health nurses foster clients' analytic skills by (a) demonstrating how to isolate the parts in a situation and (b) encouraging the clients to consider the relationships among the parts and to draw conclusions from their thinking.

An analysis-level behavioral objective for senior citizens trying to learn more about low-fat foods might be, "The seniors should be able to *compare* the fat content in a variety of packaged foods." Other verbs at the analysis level include *differentiate*, *contrast*, *debate*, *question*, and *examine*.

Synthesis

Synthesis, the fifth level of cognitive learning, is the ability not only to break down and understand the elements of a situation but also to form elements into a new whole. Synthesis combines all of the earlier levels of cognitive learning to culminate in the production of a unique plan or solution. Clients who achieve learning at this level not only analyze their problems but also find solutions for them. For example, a nurse may assist mental health clients in a therapy group to examine their frequent depression and then to generate their own plan for alleviating it. A young couple who want to toilet train their 2-year-old child may learn the physiologic and psychological dimensions of toilet training, analyze their own situation, and then develop strategies (their own plan) for training the child. Nurses facilitate synthesis by assisting and encouraging clients to develop their own solutions with specific plans. After a problem is identified, the client should be asked, "What are some possible causes? Do you see anything that has been overlooked about the problem?" If the client asks for a solution, the nurse should encourage synthesis by asking, "What are some possible solutions to this problem that you might carry out?"

An example of a synthesis-level behavioral objective for a client on a sodium-restricted diet might be, "The client will be able to *prepare* an enjoyable meal using low-sodium foods." Other verbs at this level include *compose*, *design*, *formulate*, *create*, and *organize*.

Evaluation

The highest level of cognitive learning is evaluation: at this level, the learner judges the usefulness of new material compared with a stated purpose or specific criteria (Miller et al., 2009). Clients can learn to judge their own health behavior by comparing it with standards established by others—such as complete abstinence from smoking, maintenance of normal weight, or exercising three times a week. Alternatively, clients may establish their own criteria. For example, a parent support group might design activities to enhance parent–child communication, and then judge their performance by using their desired outcomes as evaluation criteria. When nurses aim for this level of client learning, they have made self-care a concrete objective. Evaluation, because it goes beyond attempts at problem-solving, enables the client to judge the adequacy of solutions, to critique lifestyle and health-related behaviors, and to anticipate needed improvements.

An example of a behavioral objective at the evaluation level might be, "The clients in a nutrition class will be able to *measure* the cholesterol content in one portion of the low-cholesterol dish they brought to share." Other verbs at this level include *judge*, *rate*, *choose*, and *estimate*.

How to Measure Cognitive Learning

Cognitive learning at any of the levels described can be measured easily in terms of learner behaviors. Nurses know, for instance, that clients have achieved teaching objectives for the application of knowledge if their behavior demonstrates actual use of the information taught. Client roles in cognitive learning range from relatively passive (at the knowledge level) to active (at the evaluation level). Conversely, as clients become more active, the nurse's role becomes less directive. Notice that not all clients need to be brought through all levels of cognitive learning, nor does every client need to reach the evaluation level for each aspect of care. For some clients and situations, comprehension is an adequate and effective level; for others, the nurse should focus on the application level as the level of achievement. Table 11-2 illustrates client and nurse behaviors for each cognitive level.

Table 11.2 Cognitive Learning: Case Study in Controlling Diabetes

Level	Illustrative Client Behavior	Illustrative Nurse Behavior
Knowledge (recalls, knows)	States that insulin, if taken, will control own diabetes	Provides information
Comprehension (understands)	Describes insulin action and purpose	Explains information
Application (uses learning)	Adjusts insulin dosage daily to maintain proper blood sugar level	Suggests how to use learning
Analysis (examines, explains)	Discusses relationships between insulin, diet, activity, and diabetic control	Demonstrates and encourages analysis
Synthesis (integrates with other learning, generates new ideas)	Develops a plan, incorporating above learning, for controlling own diabetes	Promotes client formulation of own plan
Evaluation (judges according to a standard)	Compares degree of diabetic control (outcomes) with desired control (objectives)	Facilitates evaluation

Affective Domain

The **affective domain** in which learning occurs involves emotion, feeling, or *affect*. This kind of learning deals with changes in interest, attitudes, and values (Bloom, 1956). Here, nurses face the task of trying to influence what clients value and feel. Nurses want clients to develop an ability to accept ideas that promote healthier behavior patterns, even if those ideas conflict with the clients' own values.

Attitudes and values are learned. They develop gradually, as the way an individual feels and responds is molded by family, peers, experiences, and cultural influences (Hollinger, 2005). These feelings and responses are the result of imitation and conditioning. In this way, clients acquire their health-related beliefs and practices. Because attitudes and values become part of the person, they are difficult to change unless the nurse is aware of how they develop.

Affective learning occurs on several levels as learners respond with varying degrees of involvement and commitment. At the first level, learners are simply receptive; they are willing to listen, to show awareness, and to be attentive. The nurse aims at acquiring and focusing learners' attention (Miller et al., 2009). This limited goal may be all that clients are ready for during the early stages of the nurse–client relationship.

At the second level, learners become active participants by responding to the information in some way. Examples are a willingness to read educational material, to participate in discussions, to complete assignments (e.g., keeping a diet record), or to voluntarily seek out more information.

At the third level, learners attach value to the information. Valuing ranges from simple acceptance through appreciation to commitment. For example, a nurse taught members of a therapy group several principles concerning group effectiveness. An explanation of the importance of a democratic group process and ways to improve group skills was given. Members showed acceptance when they acknowledged the importance of these ideas. They showed appreciation of the ideas by starting to practice them. Commitment came when they assumed responsibility for having their group function well.

The final level of affective learning occurs when learners internalize an idea or value. The value system now controls learner behavior. Consistent practice is a crucial test at this level. Clients who know and respect the value of exercise but only occasionally play tennis or go for a walk have not internalized the value. Even several weeks of enthusiastic jogging is not evidence of an internalized value. If the jogging continues for 6 months, 12 months, or longer, learning may have been internalized.

Affective learning often is difficult to measure (Rankin, Stallings, & London, 2005). This elusiveness may influence community health nurses to concentrate their efforts on cognitive learning goals instead. Yet, client attitudes and values have a major effect on the outcome of cognitive learning—desired behavioral changes. Therefore, both cognitive and affective domains must remain linked in teaching, otherwise, results quickly fade.

Attitudes and values can change in the same way that they were first learned, that is, through imitation and conditioning. Role models, particularly individuals from the client's peer group who practice the desired health behaviors, can be a strong influence. Support groups, such as mastectomy or chemical dependency support groups, can have a powerful role-model effect. Frequently, the nurse is viewed as a role model by clients; for this reason, nurses should be careful to demonstrate healthy behaviors.

Attitudes often change when the nurse provides clients with a satisfying experience during the learning process. The nurse who recognizes clients' participation in a group, praises them for completing assignments, or commends them for sticking to diet plans will have more success than the nurse who only criticizes failures.

Table 11.3 Affective Learning: Case Study in Family Planning

Level	Illustrative Client Behavior	Illustrative Nurse Behavior
Receptive (listens, pays attention)	Attentive to family planning instruction	Directs client's attention
Responsive (participates, reacts)	Discusses pros and cons of various methods	Encourages client involvement
Valuing (accepts, appreciates, commits)	Selects a method for use	Respects client's right to decide
Internal consistency (organizes values to fit together)	Understands and accepts responsibility for planning for desired number of children	Brings client into contact with role models
Adoption (incorporates new values into lifestyle)	Consistently practices birth control	Positively reinforces healthy behaviors

Another point to remember is that clients can develop a close relationship with the nurse during the teaching–learning process. When this occurs, some limited sharing of the nurse's experiences in managing personal health issues may be appropriate to let clients know that the nurse, too, is human. This can be an effective addition to teaching strategies if it feels comfortable and is used wisely. Table 11-3 shows client and nurse behaviors for each level of affective learning.

To influence affective learning requires patience. Values and attitudes seldom change overnight. Remember that other forces continue to reinforce former values. For example, a middle-aged housewife may want to pursue a career for self-fulfillment, but she might not do so because she has children in high school and feels that their needs come first. A young man who can verbalize to the nurse the importance of safe sex may be uncomfortable discussing the subject with his partner, thus jeopardizing his compliance with the nurse's instruction.

Psychomotor Domain

The **psychomotor domain** includes visible, demonstrable performance skills that require some kind of neuromuscular coordination. Clients in the community need to learn skills such as infant bathing, temperature taking, breast or testicular self-examination, prenatal breathing exercises, range-of-motion exercises, catheter irrigation, walking with crutches, and how to change dressings.

For psychomotor learning to take place, three conditions must be met: (1) learners must be capable of the skill, (2) learners must have a sensory image of how to perform the skill, and (3) learners must practice the skill.

The nurse must be certain that the client is physically, intellectually, and emotionally capable of performing the skill. An elderly diabetic man with tremulous hands and fading vision should not be expected to give his own insulin injections; it could frustrate and harm him. An accessible person who is more physically capable should be enlisted and taught the skill. Clients' intellectual and emotional capabilities also influence their capacity to learn motor skills. It may be inappropriate to expect persons of limited intelligence to learn complex skills. The degree of complexity should match the learners' level of functioning. However, educational level should not be equated with intelligence. Many clients have had limited formal schooling but are able to learn complex skills for themselves or as caregivers after thorough instruction. Developmental stage is another point to consider in determining whether it is appropriate to teach a particular skill. For example, most children can put on some article of clothing at 2 years of age but are not ready to learn to fasten buttons until well past their third birthday.

Learners also must have a sensory image of how to perform the skill through sight, hearing, touch, and sometimes taste or smell. This sensory image is gained by demonstration. To teach clients motor skills effectively, the nurse has to provide them with an adequate sensory image. The nurse must demonstrate and explain slowly, one point at a time, and sometimes repeatedly, until clients understand the proper sequence or combination of actions necessary to carry out the skill.

The third necessary condition for psychomotor learning is practice. After acquiring a sensory image, clients can start to perform the skill. Mastery comes over time as clients repeat the task until it is smooth, coordinated, and unhesitating. During this process, the nurse should be available to provide guidance and encouragement. In the early stages of practice, the nurse may need to use hands-on guidance to give clients a sense of how the performance should feel. When clients give return demonstrations, the nurse can make suggestions, give encouragement, and thereby maximize the learning. For example, a nurse demonstrates passive range-of-motion exercises on a client's wife to show her how the exercises should feel (giving her a sensory image). The wife then learns to perform the exercises on her husband. During practice, feedback from the nurse enables the wife to know whether the skill is being performed correctly.

The psychomotor domain, like the cognitive and affective domains, ranges from simple to complex levels of functioning. It is necessary to exercise judgment in assessing a client's ability to perform a skill. Even clients with limited ability often can move to higher levels once

Table 11.4 Nurse Behaviors in Psychomotor Learning

The Nurse	Provides Sensory Image	Encourages Practice
Determines capability: Assesses client's physical, intellectual, and emotional ability	Demonstrates and explains	Uses guidance and positive reinforcement

they have mastered simple skills. Nurse behavior that influences psychomotor learning is shown in Table 11-4.

LEARNING THEORIES

A *learning theory* is a systematic and integrated look into the nature of the process whereby people relate to their surroundings in such ways as to enhance their ability to use both themselves and their surroundings more effectively. Each nurse has and uses a particular theory of learning, whether consciously or unconsciously, and that theory, in turn, dictates the way of teaching of the nurse. It is useful to discover what each nurse's learning theory is and how it affects the nurse's role as health educator.

Some of the learning theories developed by educational psychologists in the 20th century remain influential. They are grouped into four categories: behavioral, cognitive, social, and humanistic. Additionally, the adult learning theory of Malcolm Knowles (1980, 1984, 1989, 1990) has influenced client teaching. A brief examination of these categories and the specific theories of each follows.

Behavioral Learning Theories

Behavioral theory (also known as stimulus-response or conditioning theory) approaches the study of learning by focusing on behaviors that can be observed, measured, and changed. Developed early in the 20th century, behavioral theory work is associated primarily with three famous names: Ivan Pavlov (1957), Edward Thorndike (1932, 1969), and B. F. Skinner (1974, 1987). To a behaviorist, learning is a behavioral change—a response to certain stimuli. Therefore, the behavioristic teacher seeks to significantly change learners' behaviors through a series of selected stimuli.

The stimulus–response "bond" theory proposes that, with conditioning, certain causes (stimuli) evoke certain effects (responses). The teacher promotes acquisition of the desired stimulus–response connections so that transfer of learning can occur in another situation having the same stimulus–response elements. Pavlov's early work with stimulus–response and involuntary reflex actions is the best-known application of this theory. Pavlov conditioned a dog to anticipate food by ringing a bell at feeding time. Initially, the dog would salivate as the food was brought to the cage. However, after time, the dog would salivate at hearing the bell, before seeing or smelling the food.

Two other behavioral theories are conditioning with no reinforcement (Thorndike) and conditioning through reinforcement (Skinner). No-reinforcement theorists focus on the learner's innate reflexive drives to accomplish the desired response after conditioning, such as when the nurse repeatedly emphasizes to a group of pregnant women that their prenatal classes promote a positive delivery experience and healthy newborns. In contrast, the reinforcement theorists use successive, systematic changes in the learner's environment to enhance the probability of desired responses. For example, a school nurse might give rewards (balloons, coloring books, crayons) to children who attend each class on safety.

Cognitive Learning Theories

Jean Piaget is the most widely known cognitive theorist. His theory of cognitive development contributed to the theories of Kohlberg (moral development) and Fowler (development of faith). Piaget (1966, 1970) believed that cognitive development is an orderly, sequential, and interactive process in which a variety of new experiences must exist before intellectual abilities can develop. His work with children led him to develop five phases of cognitive development, from birth to 15 years of age (Table 11-5).

Table 11.5 Piaget's Five Phases of Cognitive Development

Age	Stage	Behavior
Birth to 2 y	Sensorimotor stage	The child moves focus from self to the environment (rituals are important)
2–4 y	Preconceptual stage	Language development is rapid and everything is related to "me"
4–7 y	Intuitive thought stage	Egocentric thinking diminishes, and words are used to express thoughts
7–11 y	Concrete operations stage	Child can solve concrete problems and recognize others' viewpoints
11–15 y	Formal operations stage	Child uses rational thinking and can develop ideas from general principles (deductive reasoning) and apply them to future situations

Each stage signifies a transformation from the previous one, and a child must move through each stage sequentially. The three abilities of *assimilation* (reacting to new situations by using skills already possessed), *accommodation* (being sufficiently mature so that previously unsolved problems can now be solved), and *adaptation* (the ability to cope with the demands of the environment) are used to make the transformation. Nurses must understand their audience's learning stage to ascertain how to approach teaching for that developmental stage. The nurse can see how the use of puppets with 3-year-olds may be a beneficial addition to a presentation on safety, whereas a group of young teens with diabetes may respond to information on the consequences of taking or not taking their insulin.

The Gestalt-field family of cognitive theories assumes that people are neither good nor bad—they simply interact with their environment, and their learning is related to perception (Wertheimer, 1945/1959, 1980). A principal assumption of this approach is that "each person perceives, interprets, and responds to any situation in his or her own way" (Braungart & Braungart, 2008, p. 61).

The first Gestalt-field theory, called *insight theory*, regards learning as a process in which the learner develops new insights or changes old ones. Learners sense their way intuitively and intelligently through problems. However, the "insight" is useful only if the learner understands its significance. For example, Lana dropped out of high school after the birth of her daughter; after attending a career planning class offered by a community health nurse, she realizes that she has limited job skills and that if she knew how to use a computer, she could get a better job. This learner understood the significance of her insight.

The second theory, *goal–insight*, is similar to the insight theory but goes beyond intuitive hunches to tested insights. Teachers subscribing to this theory promote insightful learning but assist learners in developing higher-quality insights. For example, Lana takes a beginning and then an advanced computer class and is offered a higher-paying job. The community health nurse discusses Lana's successes with her, asks Lana whether she ever thought about going to college, and mentions the added benefits of college-level course work. Lana reflects on this for a while and begins to think about completing the requirements to go to community college, because if she had an associate degree she could be promoted to supervisor.

In the third theory, *cognitive-field theory*, the learner is seen as purposive and problem-centered. Teachers seek to help learners gain new insights and restructure their lives accordingly. For example, Lana confers with the community health nurse about her choices and has changed her thinking about herself so much that she is planning to get an apartment in a neighborhood that is better for her child, and she may continue taking classes "for the fun of it" after she completes her degree in a few months.

Social Learning Theories

The aim of social learning theory is to explain behavior and facilitate learning. An important social theorist, Bandura (1977, 1986), pointed out that apparent but not real relationships often are dysfunctional, producing undesirable or inappropriate behavior. He described three ways that dysfunctional beliefs develop:

1. In *coincidental association*, outcomes typically are preceded by numerous events, and the client selects the wrong events as predictors of an outcome. For example, Juanita had a negative experience with a man who wore a hearing aid. Afterward, all of her experiences with men who wore hearing aids were negative. She reached the conclusion that all men who wear hearing aids were undesirable. This client's beliefs became a self-fulfilling prophecy.
2. In *inappropriate generalization*, one negative experience provokes negative feelings for future experiences. For example, Shauna had a purse snatched by a teenager and generalized that all teenagers are bad. Three-year-old Ryan accidentally drank some spoiled milk. He generalized that milk tastes bad and now refuses to drink it.
3. In *perceived self-inefficacy*, "Persons who judge themselves as lacking coping capabilities, whether the self-appraisal is objectively warranted or not, will perceive all kinds of dangers in situations and exaggerate their potential harmfulness" (Bandura, 1986, p. 220). For example, an older client, William, tells the community health nurse about two missing Social Security checks, but he refuses to take a bus to the post office. He states that he does not know what to say to the postal clerk and has read about senior citizens getting mugged on buses. He refused to follow up on his lost income.

Social learning theory focuses on the learners. They are benefitted by role models, building self-confidence, persuasion, and personal mastery. Self-efficacy can lead to the desired behaviors and outcomes. Juanita may begin to separate her negative experiences with men from their hearing disabilities after attending a class on building self-esteem suggested by the nurse. Through some positive experiences with teenagers organized by the nurse, Shauna may learn that not all teenagers are bad. The nurse can suggest to Ryan's mother that he may be persuaded to drink chocolate milk. She then can slowly reintroduce plain milk. William might find the courage and self-confidence to solve future problems after the nurse introduces him to another gentleman in the apartment complex who feels confident in the neighborhood.

Humanistic Learning Theories

Humanistic theories assume that people possess a natural tendency to learn and that learning flourishes in an encouraging environment. Two of the best-known humanists are Abraham Maslow and Carl Rogers. Abraham Maslow developed the classic hierarchy of human needs in the 1940s. It suggests that a person's first needs are physiologic (air, food, water). Once these needs are met, people work to fulfill safety and security needs. Next is the need for love and a sense of belonging; then come self-esteem needs (positive feelings of self-worth). Only after these needs are met do people work toward self-actualization or "becoming all that we can be" (Maslow, 1970).

In community health nursing, the clients' needs must be considered when planning health education programs. For example, it would be difficult for a group of young mothers to concentrate on learning about proper infant nutrition if they are worried about their babies crying in the next room or about an abusive partner who doesn't want them out of the house. Their need to care for their children (need for love and belonging) or for their personal wellbeing (security and safety) would be greater than the need to learn about future health considerations (self-esteem and self-actualization). Likewise, it is impossible for learning to take place if a room is so warm that the participants are falling asleep (i.e., physiologic needs are not being met).

Carl Rogers developed the client-centered counseling approach that has long been important in psychotherapy. He believed the role of the therapist should be nondirective and accepting, and proposed approaching clients in a warm, positive, and empathetic manner to get in touch with their feelings and thoughts. Rogers (1969, 1989) soon applied his beliefs to education, suggesting that the learning environment be learner-centered. The outcome of a learner-centered educational environment is that students become more self-directed and guide their own learning. Rogers believed that the learner is the person most capable of deciding how to find the solutions to problems. The client identifies the problem and, given time and space, can find a way through the problem to a solution. The nurse acts as a facilitator in this learning process, as for example, when a 55-year-old man wants to quit smoking after a prolonged upper respiratory tract infection, aggravated by his habit, and comes to a stop-smoking class conducted by a nurse in the county health department.

Knowles' Adult Learning Theory

In the last 20 to 30 years, a variety of techniques have been developed to help adults learn. One of the main discoveries is that adults as learners are different from children. They do not learn differently, but rather are a different kind of learner. Knowles (1984) suggested that there are four characteristics of adult learners, and these characteristics have implications for **adult learning**. Adults are self-directed in their learning; they have a lifetime of experience to draw on when learning; their readiness to learn is focused on requirements for their personal and occupational roles; and adults have a problem-centered time perspective, in that the learners have a need to learn so that it can be applied and tried out quickly. Display 11.4 describes the characteristics of adult learners and implications for nurses working with adults in more detail.

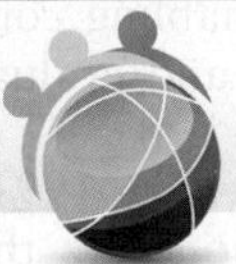

DISPLAY 11.4 CHARACTERISTICS AND IMPLICATIONS FOR KNOWLES' ADULT LEARNING THEORY

Characteristics	*Learning Implications*
Self-Concept	
Adult learners are self-directed.	Openness and respect between teacher and learner. The learner plans and carries out own learning activities. Learner evaluates own progress toward self-chosen goals.
Experience	
Adults have a lifetime of experience and define self in terms of this experience.	Teaching methods focus on experiential activities. Discovering how to learn from experience is key to self-actualization. Mistakes are opportunities for learning.
Readiness to Learn	
Learning is focused on social and occupational roles.	Experiential learning opportunities focus on requirements for occupational and social roles. Learning peaks when there is a need to know. Adults can best assess own readiness to learn and teachable moments.
Need to Learn	
Adults have a problem-centered time perspective.	Teaching needs to be problem-centered rather than theoretically oriented. Teacher needs to teach what the learners need to learn. Learners need to apply and try out learning quickly.

HEALTH-TEACHING MODELS

Theories on learning provide a general understanding of how people learn. In addition, various health-teaching models specifically focus on explaining individual health experiences, behaviors, and actions. These models fit with the learning theories to give nurses a more accurate picture of the client and the clients' learning needs. Three useful models are described here: the Health Belief Model (HBM), Pender's Health Promotion Model (revised) (HPM), and the PRECEDE and PROCEED models.

The Health Belief Model

This section and the next describe two closely associated health models. The HBM, which was developed by social psychologists and brought to the attention of health care professionals by Rosenstock (1966), has undergone much empiric testing. The HBM is useful for explaining the behaviors and actions taken by people to prevent illness and injury. It postulates that readiness to act on behalf of a person's own health is predicated on the following (Strecher & Rosenstock, 1997):

- Perceived susceptibility to the condition in question
- Perceived seriousness of the condition in question
- Perceived benefits to taking action
- Barriers to taking action
- Cues to action, such as knowledge that someone else has the condition or attention from the media
- Self-efficacy—the ability to take action to achieve the desired outcome

For example, researchers in Turkey developed a 33-item Health Belief Model Scale for use with diabetic patients in their country (Kartal & Ozsoy, 2007). Building on similar studies with other cultural groups, they studied the validity and reliability of the tool with 352 patients with type 2 diabetes mellitus. Their findings supported the use of this tool with this population and noted that it could provide a means to test the effectiveness of intervention strategies. Community health nurses may find the use of the HBM (and variations) to be helpful in assessing the health behaviors and beliefs of culturally diverse populations.

Pender's Health Promotion Model

First published by Pender in the early 1980s, the HPM was envisioned as a framework for exploring health-related behaviors within a nursing and behavioral science context (Pender, 1996). Reflecting the growing body of literature relevant to the HPM, Pender revised the model to reflect a number of major theoretical changes. Consistent with the original, the revised model is derived from social cognitive theory and expectancy-value theory. The revised HPM includes three general areas of concern to health-promoting behavior: *Individual characteristics and experiences* are seen to interact with *behavior-specific cognitions and affect* to influence specific *behavioral outcomes* (Pender et al., 2011). The revised HPM modifies the HBM and focuses on predicting behaviors that influence health promotion. In addition, the HPM includes the variable of interpersonal influence of others, including family and health professionals.

Being able to predict health promotion behaviors enhances the community health nurse's ability to work with clients. Awareness of their characteristics, experiences, comprehension of their health-related issues, perceived barriers, self-efficacy, support (or lack of it) from significant others, and commitment provides the nurse with a picture that clarifies the client–nurse role and gives direction for action taking. The HPM (Fig. 11-5) is based on the theoretical propositions found in Display 11.5.

Using these propositions, researchers explored clients' health behaviors in many studies conducted in the 1980s, 1990s, and into the 21st century. Examples of research using the model include surveying health-promoting behavior among low-income elderly Korean women (Shin, Kang, Park, Cho, & Heitkemper, 2008), surveying health promotion in adolescents (Srof & Velsor-Friedrich, 2006), in older Iranian adults (Morowatisharifabad, Ghofranipour, Heidarnia, Ruchi, & Ehrampoush, 2006), and low-income pregnant minority women (Esperat, Feng, Zhang, & Owen, 2007).

The PRECEDE and PROCEED Models

First published by Green in 1974, the PRECEDE model was developed for educational diagnosis. The acronym PRECEDE has been slightly revised from the original to stand for *p*redisposing, *r*einforcing, and *e*nabling *c*onstructs in *e*ducational/ecological *d*iagnosis and *e*valuation (Green & Kreuter, 2005).

The PROCEED model (Green & Kreuter, 1991) works in tandem with the PRECEDE model as the community health nurse proceeds to plan, implement, and evaluate health education programs. This acronym stands for *p*olicy, *r*egulatory, and *o*rganizational *c*onstructs for *e*ducational and *e*nvironmental *d*evelopment. The entire PRECEDE–PROCEED model includes eight phases in the formulation and evaluation of health educational programs. The first five of these phases are included in the PRECEDE portion of the model and include: (1) social, (2) epidemiologic, and (3) education/ecological assessments, followed by (4) administrative and policy assessment and intervention alignment, and (5) implementation. The PROCEED model is emphasized in the last three phases: (1) process evaluation, (2) impact evaluation, and (3) outcome evaluation.

A hallmark of the PRECEDE–PROCEED model is the emphasis on the desired outcome. The model both begins and ends with *quality of life*, which includes "subjectively defined problems and priorities of individuals and communities" (Green & Kreuter, 2005, p. 11). The emphasis on what the individual or community perceives as the problem, not what the professional believes it to be, is crucial. Outcome evaluation is logically linked back to that same individual or community in assessing achievement of the desired change.

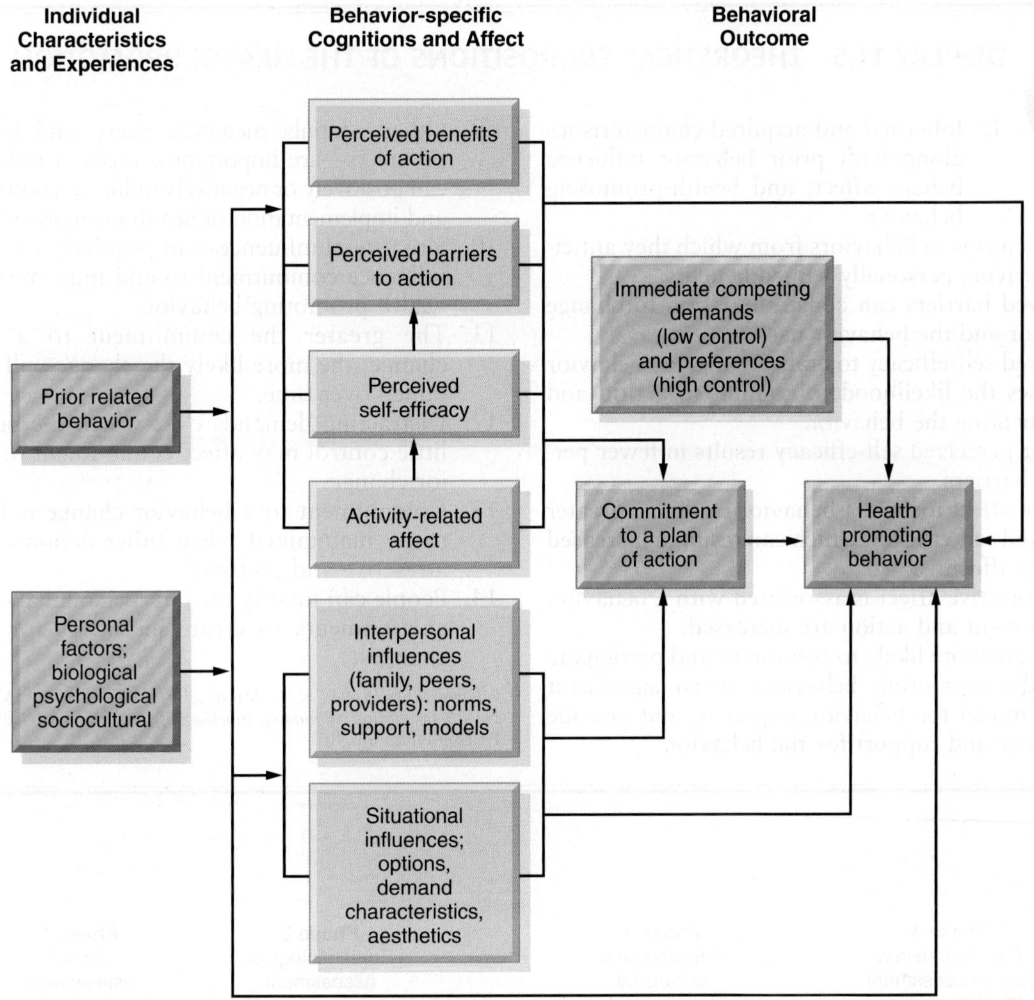

FIGURE 11-5. Health promotion model. (From Pender, N. J., Murdaugh, C. L., & Parsons, M. A. (2011). *Health promotion in nursing practice* (6th ed.). Upper Saddle River, NJ: Pearson Education, Inc., with permission.)

The steps in this model are similar to those of the nursing process. Because of this familiarity, the model has become a useful tool for nurses teaching in the community. The nurse builds on the assessment formulated from the PRECEDE model, determines the best interventions, and then proceeds to evaluate the outcome of those interventions. The emphasis on the perceived needs of the individual or community as the starting point for all community efforts is consistent with community health nursing practice. The model reminds us of the importance of an organized approach to health educational programs, one that begins and ends with the "experts"—the individuals, families, and communities we hope to help through our efforts. The PRECEDE–PROCEED model can be seen in Figure 11-6.

TEACHING AT THREE LEVELS OF PREVENTION

Nurses should develop teaching programs that coincide with the level of prevention needed by the client. The three levels of primary, secondary, and tertiary prevention are demonstrated in the Levels of Prevention Pyramid for nurses who teach clients, families, aggregates, or populations.

Ideally, the community health nurse focuses teaching at the primary level. If nurses were able to reach more people at this level, it would help to diminish years of morbidity and limit subsequent infirmity. Many people experience disabilities that could have been prevented if primary prevention behaviors had been incorporated into their daily activities.

Because the primary level of prevention is not possible in all cases, a significant share of the nurse's time is spent teaching at the secondary or tertiary level. An example is an 88-year-old woman with a fractured hip who has returned home after 3 weeks of physical therapy at a skilled nursing facility. The nurse assesses the client's environment, gait, functional limitations, safety, and adherence to medication, and initiates needed referrals. The teaching focuses on rehabilitation and prevention of a secondary problem that may affect the healing process and the client's health and safety in general.

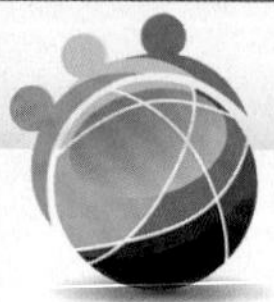

DISPLAY 11.5 THEORETICAL PROPOSITIONS OF THE HEALTH PROMOTION MODEL

1. Inherited and acquired characteristics along with prior behavior influence beliefs, affect, and health-promoting behavior.
2. People engage in behaviors from which they anticipate deriving personally valued benefits.
3. Perceived barriers can constrain action to change behavior and the behavior itself.
4. Perceived self-efficacy to embrace a given behavior increases the likelihood to commit to action and implementing the behavior.
5. Greater perceived self-efficacy results in fewer perceived barriers.
6. Positive affect toward a behavior results in greater perceived self-efficacy, which can result in increased positive affect.
7. When positive affect is associated with a behavior, commitment and action are increased.
8. People are more likely to commit to and participate in health-promoting behaviors when significant others model the behavior, expect it, and provide assistance and support for the behavior.
9. Others—family members, peers, and health care providers—are important sources of influence that can positively or negatively influence commitment to and implementation of health-promoting behavior.
10. Situational influences can positively or negatively influence commitment to and implementation of health-promoting behavior.
11. The greater the commitment to a behavior change, the more likely the change will be maintained over time.
12. Distracting demands over which the person has little control may affect commitment to a behavior change.
13. Commitment to a behavior change is less likely to be maintained when other actions are more attractive and preferred.
14. People can modify the interpersonal and physical environments to create incentives for behavior changes.

Adapted from Pender, N. J., Murdaugh, C. L., & Parsons, M. A. (2011). *Health promotion in nursing practice* (6th ed.). Upper Saddle River, NJ: Pearson Education, Inc.

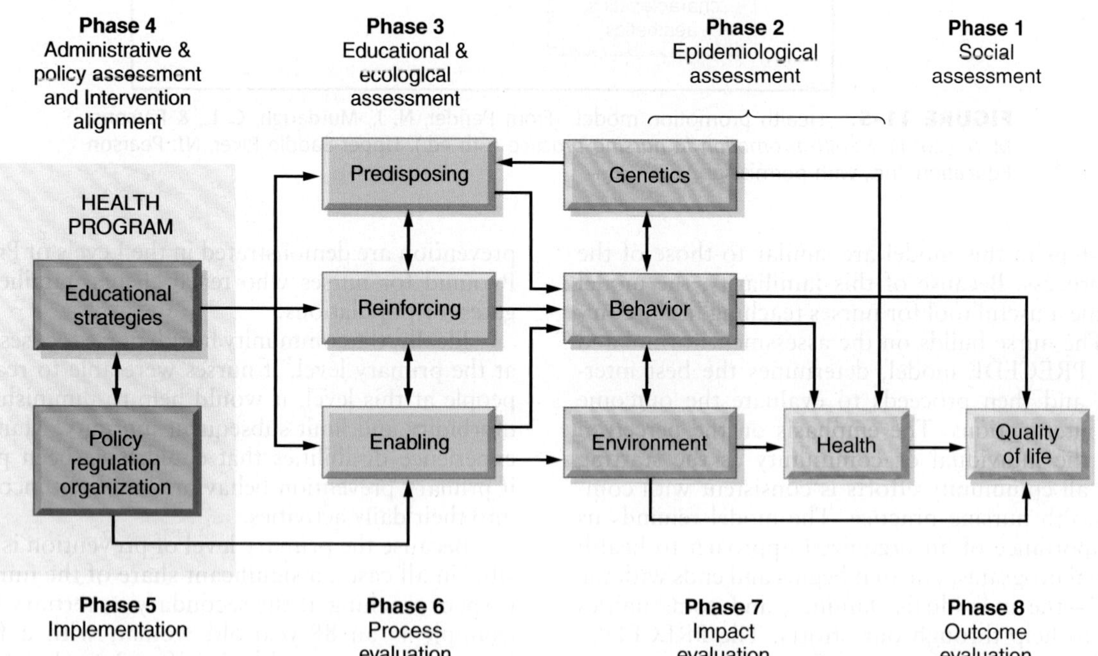

FIGURE 11-6. The PRECEDE–PROCEED model. (From Green, L. W., & Kreuter, M. W. (2005). *Health program planning: An educational and ecological approach* (4th ed., p. 10). New York: McGraw-Hill, with permission.)

LEVELS OF PREVENTION PYRAMID

SITUATION: Several examples of teaching at three levels of prevention.

GOAL: Using the three levels of prevention, negative health conditions are avoided, or promptly diagnosed and treated, and the fullest possible potential is restored.

TERTIARY PREVENTION		
Rehabilitation	**Primary Prevention**	
	Health Promotion & Education	*Health Protection*
• Restore function: a nurse teaches a stroke survivor about home safety, alternative housing options, physical therapy, and retraining opportunities	• Health teaching: a nurse teaches about the importance of diet, rest, and exercise to prevent a secondary health problem	• Maintenance: a nurse observes clients with tuberculosis where they live while taking their oral medication on a daily basis (DOT - Directly Observed Therapy)

SECONDARY PREVENTION	
Early Diagnosis	**Prompt Treatment**
• Screening and case finding: a nurse takes blood pressure measurements from all family members at each home visit and teaches them the importance of maintaining a healthy blood pressure reading	• Treatment: a nurse teaches clients how to navigate through the complexities of the health care delivery system to receive prompt treatment

PRIMARY PREVENTION	
Health Promotion & Education	**Health Protection**
• Health education: a nurse teaches a class on sensible weight control for teenagers	• Immunizations: a nurse teaches about the importance of pneumonia and flu vaccines for seniors, followed by an immunization clinic

EFFECTIVE TEACHING

Teaching is an art. It was described in the classic book *The Educational Imagination* by E.W. Eisner (1985). Teaching can be performed with such skill and grace that the client becomes part of a well-orchestrated event, with learning as the natural outcome. Instead of relying on prescribed teaching methods, the skillful nurse can make judgments based largely on client qualities, situations, and needs that guide the experience to fruition. The desired changes emerge in the course of the interaction rather than at a level conceived before the teaching. Before the community health nurse can reach this level of artistry, there is much to learn about being an effective teacher.

Teaching–Learning Principles

Teaching lies at one end of a continuum. At the other end is learning. Without learning, teaching becomes useless in the same way that communication does not occur unless a message is both sent and received. Both the teacher and the learner have responsibilities on that continuum. Learners must take responsibility for their own learning (Braungart & Braungart, 2008). Teachers obstruct that process if they assume complete responsibility for bringing about changed behavior. Clients can be directed toward health knowledge, but they will not learn unless they have the desire to learn. Teaching, then, becomes a matter of facilitating both the desire and the best conditions for satisfying it. Teaching in community health nursing means to influence, motivate, and act as a catalyst in the learning process. Nurses bring information and learners together and stimulate a reaction that leads to a change (Rankin et al., 2005). Nurses facilitate learning when they make it as easy as possible for clients to change. To do this, the nurse needs to understand the basic principles underlying the art and science of the teaching–learning process and the use of appropriate materials to influence learning (Table 11-6).

Client Readiness

Clients' readiness to learn influences teaching effectiveness. Four facets of client readiness have been identified (Kitchie, 2008) and must be assessed by the nurse: (1)

Table 11.6 Seven Principles for Maximizing the Teaching–Learning Process

Teaching Principles	Learning Principles
1. Adapt teaching to clients' level of readiness	1. The learning process makes use of clients' experience and is geared to their level of understanding
2. Determine clients' perceptions about the subject matter before and during teaching	2. Clients are given the opportunity to provide frequent feedback on their understanding of the material taught
3. Create an environment that is conducive to learning	3. The environment for learning is physically comfortable; offers an atmosphere of mutual helpfulness, trust, respect, and acceptance; and allows for free expression of ideas
4. Involve clients throughout the learning process	4. Clients actively participate. They assess needs, establish goals, and evaluate their learning progress
5. Make subject matter relevant to clients' interest and use	5. Clients feel motivated to interest and learn
6. Ensure client satisfaction during the teaching–learning process	6. Clients sense progress toward their goals
7. Provide opportunities for clients to apply material taught	7. Clients integrate the learning through application

Adapted from Knowles, M. (1980). *The modern practice of adult education: Andragogy versus pedagogy* (2nd ed.). Chicago, IL: Follett.

physical readiness, which deals with ability, complexity of the task, environment, health status, and gender; (2) emotional readiness, which deals with the state of receptivity to learning; (3) experiential readiness, which reflects the learner's past experiences with learning; and (4) knowledge readiness, which encompasses the learner's knowledge and understanding. For instance, one community health nurse found that a young primipara was not ready for prenatal teaching on fetal growth and development. She had strong fears, the nurse discovered, that "losing her figure" would make her sexually unattractive to her partner. Until these anxieties had subsided, the teaching would remain ineffective. Clients' needs, interests, motivation, stress, and concerns determine their readiness for learning.

Another factor that influences readiness is educational background. If a group of women who never completed grade school meet to learn how to care for a sick person in the home, material should be presented simply, factually, and in terms that they understand. To discuss complex concepts of health, illness, and scientific research would be above their level of readiness. However, increasingly complex concepts can be introduced as the nurse works with the women and assesses their readiness to assimilate advanced concepts.

Maturational level also affects readiness. An adolescent mother who is still working on the normal developmental tasks of her age group, such as seeking independence or selecting a career path, may not be ready to learn parenting skills. Readiness of the client determines the amount of material presented in each teaching session. The pace or speed with which information is presented must be manageable. A moderate amount of anxiety often increases client receptivity to learning; however, high or low levels of anxiety can have the opposite effect.

Client Perceptions

Clients' perceptions also affect their learning, serving as a screening device through which all new information must pass. Individual perceptions help people interpret and attach meaning to things. A wide range of variables affects human perception. These variables include values, past experiences, culture, religion, personality, developmental stage, educational and economic level, surrounding social forces, and the physical environment. One client may view the experience of parenting as a positive, growth-producing relationship; another may see it as a conflict-ridden, unhappy experience to avoid. Each kind of perception has a different consequence for teaching and learning. In another example, the nurse working with adolescents to educate them about the dangers of substance abuse should understand that adolescents seeking independence need to feel that they have options and choices and do not want to be told what to do.

Frequently, clients use selective perception. They screen out some statements and pay attention to those that fit their values or personal desires. For example, a nurse is teaching a client about the various risk factors in coronary disease; the individual screens out the need to quit smoking and lose weight, paying attention only to factors that would not require a drastic change in lifestyle. Nurses must know their clients, understand their backgrounds and values, and learn about their perceptions before health teaching can influence their behavior.

Educational Environment

The setting in which the educational endeavor takes place has a significant impact on learning (Kitchie, 2008). Students probably have had the experience of sitting in a cold room and trying to concentrate during a lecture or of being distracted by noise, heat, or uncomfortable seating. Physical conditions such as ventilation, lighting, decor, room temperature, view of the speaker, and whispering must be controlled to provide the environment most conducive to learning.

Equally important for learning is an atmosphere of mutual respect and trust. The nurse needs to convey this attitude both verbally and nonverbally. The way the nurse addresses clients, shows courtesies, and gives recognition makes a considerable difference in establishing clients' respect and trust. Both nurse and clients need to be mutually helpful and considerate of one another's needs and interests. All participants in the educational experience should feel free to express ideas, should know that their views will be heard, and should feel accepted despite differences of opinion and perspective. According to Knowles, this requires that the nurse refrain from seeming judgmental or inducing competitiveness among learners. Knowles (1980, p. 58) adds that the teachers should share their own feelings and knowledge "as a co-learner in the spirit of inquiry."

Client Participation

The degree of participation in the educational process directly influences the amount of learning. One nurse discovered this principle while working with a group of clients who were nearing retirement. After talking to them about the changes they would face and receiving little response, the nurse shifted to a different method of teaching. Pamphlets on Social Security benefits were distributed, and everyone was asked to read them during the week and come the next week with questions generated by the pamphlets. This strategy prompted the group to slowly begin to participate in their own learning.

When the nurse works with clients in a learning context, one of the first questions to discuss is, What does the client want to learn? As Carl Rogers (1969, p. 159) stated:

> Learning is facilitated when the student participates responsibly in the learning process. When he chooses his own directions, helps to discover his own learning resources, formulates his own problems, decides his own course of action, lives with consequences of each of these choices, then significant learning is maximized.

The amount of learning is directly proportional to the learners' involvement. In another example, a group of senior citizens attended a class on nutrition and aging, yet made few changes in eating patterns. It was not until the members became actively involved in the class, encouraged by the nurse to present problems and solutions for food purchasing and preparation on limited budgets that any significant behavioral changes occurred.

Contracting, in which the client participates in the process as a partner to determine goals, content, and time for learning, can contribute to client learning (see Chapter 10). Contracting in the context of teaching assists clients to develop a sense of accountability for their own learning (Rankin et al., 2005).

Subject Relevance

Subject matter that is relevant to the client is learned more readily and retained longer than information that is not meaningful. Learners gain the most from subject matter that is immediately useful to their own purposes. This is particularly true for adult learners, who have more life experiences that can be related to learning and who tend to see the immediate relevance of the material taught (Knowles, 1980).

Consider two middle-management men taking a physical fitness course offered by their employer. One, the father of a Boy Scout, has agreed to co-lead his son's troop on a 2-week backpacking trip in the mountains. He wants to get in shape. The second man is taking the course because it is required by the company. Its only relevance to his own purposes is that it prevents incurring the disfavor of his boss. There is little question about which man will learn and retain the most. The course has considerable relevance and meaning to the first man and little to the second.

Relevance also influences the speed of learning. Diabetic clients, who must give themselves daily injections of insulin to live, learn that skill quickly. When clients see considerable relevance in the learning, they accomplish it with speed. According to Rogers (1969), 65% to 85% of the time allotted for learning various subjects could be deleted if learners perceived the material to be related to their own purposes. When the subject matter is relevant to the learner, more knowledge is retained. On seeing the usefulness of the material, the learner develops a strong motivation to acquire and use it, and he is less likely to forget it. Even in instances when a previously learned motor skill has not been used for years, it often is quickly recaptured when it is needed.

Client Satisfaction

To maintain motivation and increase self-direction, clients must derive satisfaction from learning. Learners need to feel a sense of steady progress in the learning process. Obstacles, frustrations, and failures along the way discourage and impede learning. Many clients who have had strokes and have potential for rehabilitation often give up trying to regain speech or move paralyzed limbs because they become frustrated, discouraged, and dissatisfied. On the other hand, clients who experience satisfaction and progress in their speech and muscle retraining maintain their motivation and may work on exercises without prompting. Nurses can promote client satisfaction through support and encouragement.

Realistic goals contribute to learner satisfaction. Objectives should be set within the learner's ability, thereby avoiding the frustration resulting from a task that is too difficult and the loss of interest resulting from one that is too easy. Setting objectives requires agreement on goals, periodic reviews, and revision of goals if they become too easy or too difficult. Nurses further promote clients' learning satisfaction by designing tasks with rewards. One school nurse led a class for obese adolescents, and together they set the goal of a weekly 2-pound weight loss. The nurse helped the group to design a plan that included counting calories, reducing fat in their diets, increasing physical activity, and a buddy system to bring about behavior change. As members in the group achieved monthly goals, they were encouraged to reward themselves with a pair of earrings, new nail polish, or a special outing as a group. These students found this learning experience satisfying because goals were attainable, and their progress was rewarded. Instead of competing with one another, the group members set out to help each member achieve the goal. As a result, most kept the weight off after the class finished.

Client Application

Learning is reinforced through application. Learners need as many opportunities as possible to apply the learning in daily life. If such opportunities arise during the teaching–learning process, clients can try out new knowledge and skills under supervision. Learners are given an opportunity to begin integrating the learning into their daily lives at a time when the teacher is there to help reinforce that pattern. Take a prenatal class as an example. The learning begins with explanations of proper diet, exercise, breathing techniques, hygiene, and avoidance of alcohol and tobacco. More learning occurs as the group members discuss these issues and apply them intellectually, exploring ways to practice them at home. Additional reinforcement comes by demonstrating how to do these activities. Sample diets, demonstrations of exercises, posters, pamphlets, or models may be used. The group can begin application in the classroom by making diet plans, exercising, role-playing parenting behavior, or engaging in group problem solving. The members then can be encouraged to apply these activities on a daily basis at home and to share their results with the group at future sessions.

Frequent use of newly acquired information fosters transfer of learning to other situations. The major goal of illness prevention and health promotion depends on such a transfer. For instance, mothers who learn and practice a well-balanced diet that is free of nonnutritious snacks can be encouraged to offer more nourishing foods to other family members. A family that practices asepsis and good hand-washing techniques when caring for a family member's postsurgical wound can learn to transfer this same principle to prevention of infection in daily living.

Teaching Process

The process of teaching in community health nursing follows steps similar to those of the nursing process:

1. *Interaction:* Establish basic communication patterns between clients and nurse.
2. *Assessment and diagnosis*: Determine clients' present status and identify clients' need for teaching (keeping in mind that clients should determine their own needs).
3. *Setting goals and objectives*: Analyze needed changes and prepare objectives that describe the desired learning outcomes.
4. *Planning:* Design a plan for the learning experience that meets the mutually developed objectives; include content to be covered, sequence of topics, best conditions for learning (place, type of environment), methods, and materials (e.g., visual aids, exercises). A written plan is best; it may be part of the written nursing care plan.
5. *Teaching*: Implement the learning experience by carrying out the planned activities.
6. *Evaluation:* Determine whether learning objectives were met and if not, why not. Evaluation measures progress toward goals, effectiveness of chosen teaching methods, or future learning needs.

Interaction

Reciprocal communication must occur between nurse and client. It is essential in the nurse–client relationship and requisite to effective use of the nursing process. Community health nurses need to develop good questioning techniques and listening skills to determine clients' learning needs and levels of readiness.

Assessment and Diagnosis

Identifying clients' learning needs presents a challenge to the nurse. Too often, teaching occurs based on the nurse's assumption of what the learner needs to know. In client education, nurses have a responsibility to tailor their teaching to clients' real and perceived needs. Knowles (1980, 1984, 1989) described educational needs as gaps between what people know and what they need to know to function effectively. He related that the potential learners, the sponsoring organization, and the community all help to determine the needs to be addressed in the teaching–learning situation.

Assessing educational needs may be accomplished in several ways. The nurse can use surveys, interviews, open forums, or task forces that include representative clients as members. The principle to remember is that clients should be involved in identifying what they want to learn. When a "need" to learn something, such as the importance of immunizing children, is identified by the nurse rather than by clients, the nurse may need to "sell" clients on the importance of the topic. Nurses need to use approaches that assist clients toward their own awareness of the need.

Setting Goals and Objectives

Once a need has been clearly identified, the nurse and clients can establish mutually agreed-on goals and objectives. *Goals* are broad statements of intent, and *objectives* are more specific descriptions of intended outcome (Mager, 1975). Sometimes, in a teaching situation, an objective may be broken down into short- and long-term goals. For example, the nurse may have identified a group's desire to stop smoking. The need and teaching goals might be stated as follows:

Need: A group of smokers wish to end their addiction to nicotine.

Short-term goal: All members of the group will stop smoking within 1 month.

Long-term goal: Ninety percent of group members will remain tobacco-free for 6 months.

Objectives should be stated in measurable behavioral terms, using a grammatical structure that contains a subject, verb, condition/criterion, and time frame. That is, each objective should include a single idea that describes an outcome that can be measured within a certain time frame. To accomplish the short- and long-term goals of smoking cessation, educational objectives are developed from the levels of cognitive learning covered earlier in this chapter. Each behavioral objective is stated in measurable terms and includes a verb that coincides with one of the six levels within the cognitive domain (Display 11.4). Objectives might appear as follows:

At the end of the program all clients should be able to

1. *List* three reasons why smoking is unhealthy.
2. *Identify* at least two factors that influenced their smoking habit.
3. *Apply* a series of action steps leading to smoking cessation within 1 month.
4. *Examine* the steps as they contribute to living tobacco-free in the first 3 months.
5. *Design* a way to live a fulfilled, tobacco-free life.
6. *Evaluate* successful strategies to remain tobacco-free for 6 months.

Each of these objectives (a) refers to a subject; (b) can be readily measured, because each describes a specific outcome, condition, criterion, or expected behavior; (c) uses a verb for stating cognitive outcomes; and (d) includes a specific time frame (see Display 11.6). Well-written objectives meet these four criteria and enhance evaluation of the success of the educational effort.

Planning

Teaching preparation and the planning of it are all-important (Bastable & Doody, 2008). Although nurses teach individuals and families informally, it is generally best to have a written plan when teaching. The formalization of creating a written plan provides a framework within which the nurse can function securely, knowing that the topic is well thought out and presented and individualized for a specific client group. This plan should include the following eight items: (1) purpose, (2) statement of the overall goal, (3) list of objectives, (4) outline of the related content, (5) instructional methods, (6) time allotted for the teaching of each objective, (7) instructional resources, and (8) evaluation methods and criteria (Bastable & Doody, 2008).

Teaching

The class, seminar, workshop, or small-group teaching should be conducted according to the plan described earlier. Even with one-on-one teaching, these eight steps should be planned in advance, because each client has a different cultural background, education, intellectual level, and learning need. Use of a variety of teaching

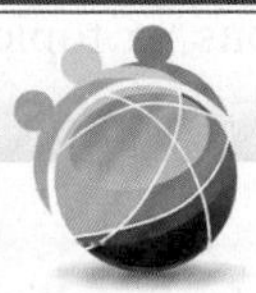

DISPLAY 11.6 SAMPLE VERBS FOR STATING COGNITIVE OUTCOMES

Knowledge	*Comprehension*	*Application*	*Analysis*	*Synthesis*	*Evaluation*
Define	Translate	Interpret	Analyze	Compose	Judge
Repeat	Restate	Apply	Distinguish	Plan	Appraise
Record	Describe	Employ	Appraise	Propose	Evaluate
List	Discuss	Use	Calculate	Design	Rate
Recall	Recognize	Practice	Experiment	Formulate	Value
Name	Explain	Operate	Differentiate	Arrange	Revise
Relate	Express	Schedule	Test	Assemble	Score
Underline	Identify	Sketch	Compare	Collect	Select
	Locate	Shop	Contrast	Construct	Choose
	Report	Practice	Criticize	Create	Assess
	Review	Demonstrate	Diagram	Set up	Estimate
	Tell		Inspect	Organize	Measure
			Debate	Manage	
			Inventory	Prepare	
			Question		
			Relate		
			Categorize		
			Examine		

methods addresses the unique needs of learners and makes the teaching interesting. Include and combine such methods as lectures, discussions, role playing, demonstrations, and videos (see "Teaching Methods and Materials").

If necessary, assignments can be made, such as readings, presentations, journaling, practice experiences, or return demonstrations can be designed to reinforce and synthesize the learning. The teaching methods used and activities selected are important parts of the teaching plan. The teacher will find that a well-designed plan enhances the smoothness and effectiveness of the teaching situation. Problems in teaching often can be related to a poorly developed plan.

Evaluation

The final step of evaluation is critical in the teaching–learning process. According to Tyler (1949, p. 106), "evaluation is the process for determining the degree to which changes in behavior are actually taking place." At this point, the nurse determines whether the goals and objectives for the educational experience have been met and, if not, why not. Clear, measurable objectives facilitate evaluation.

If objectives have not been met or have been met only partially, this too requires attention. The nurse should explore this outcome with clients to determine what factors hindered their success and what actions might be helpful. Partially met objectives give the nurse a place to begin with the group at follow-up sessions and should not be considered a failure.

Teaching Methods and Materials

Teaching occurs on many levels and incorporates various types of activities. It can be formal or informal, planned or unplanned. Formal presentations, such as group lectures, usually are planned and fairly structured. Some teaching is less formal but still planned and relatively structured, as in group discussions in which questions stimulate the exploration of ideas and guide thinking. Informal levels of teaching, such as counseling or **anticipatory guidance** (in which the client is assisted in preparing for a future role or developmental stage), require the teacher to be prepared, but there is no defined plan of presentation. Perhaps the nurse uses a pamphlet or agency protocol steps as a guide. All nurses use one or a combination of methods and a variety of materials to facilitate the teaching–learning process. However, nurses need to expand their repertoire of teaching methods and avoid relying on only one or two methods. Generating a variety of teaching methods stimulates creative thinking. Nurses use knowledge from physiology, pathology, sociology, and psychology in their practice, and, when teaching, nurses can benefit from using concepts, principles, and teaching methods derived from education, especially adult education. This chapter closes by discussing four commonly used teaching methods (lecture, discussion, demonstration, and role playing), teaching materials for enhanced learning, and how to effectively teach the client with special learning needs.

Lecture

The community health nurse sometimes presents information to a large group, such as a local parent–teacher association, a women's club, or a county board of commissioners. Under such circumstances, the lecture method, a formal kind of presentation, may be the most efficient way to communicate general health information. However, lecturers tend to create a passive learning environment for the audience unless strategies are devised to involve the learners. Many individuals are visual rather than auditory learners. To capture their attention, slides, overhead projections, computer-generated slide presentations, or videotapes can supplement the lecture. Allowing time for questions and discussion after a lecture also actively involves learners. This method is best used with adults, but even they have a limited attention span, and a break at least midway through a presentation of 1 hour or longer will be appreciated. Distributing printed material that highlights and summarizes the content shared, or supplements it, also reinforces important points.

Discussion

Two-way communication is an important feature of the learning process. Learners need an opportunity to raise questions, make comments, reason out loud, and receive feedback to develop understanding. When discussion is used in conjunction with other teaching methods, such as demonstration, lecture, and role playing, it improves their effectiveness. In group teaching, discussion enables clients to learn from one another as well as from the nurse. The nurse must exercise leadership in controlling and guiding the discussion so that learning opportunities are maximized and objectives are met. Discussions that are organized around specific questions or topics are most fruitful.

Demonstration

The demonstration method often is used for teaching psychomotor skills and is best accompanied by explanation and discussion, with time set aside for return demonstration by the client or caregiver. It gives clients a clear sensory image of how to perform the skill. Because a demonstration should be within easy visual and auditory range of learners, it is best to demonstrate in front of small groups or a single client. Use the same kind of equipment that clients will use, show exactly how the skill should be performed, and provide learners with ample opportunity to practice until the skill is perfected.

This is an ideal method to use in a client's home as well as in groups. The materials and supplies that the client will use when unaided by the nurse should be used in the demonstration. This might be the time when the nurse uses improvising skills. Helping families figure out ways to accomplish goals with materials found at home often becomes the hallmark of an experienced community health nurse. The new mother learns how to bathe her baby safely in the kitchen sink. The nurse assists several low-income parents in using household items to make inexpensive toys (e.g., mobiles from plastic coat hangers, string, and pictures from a magazine; bean bags using dry beans and scraps of fabric). The husband learns how to change dressings over his wife's central venous line site using sterile technique while conserving supplies purchased on their fixed income. Each activity takes a different type of psychomotor skill and ingenuity on the part of the nurse.

Role Playing

At times, having clients assume and act out roles maximizes learning. A parenting group, for example, found it helpful to place themselves in the role of their children; their feelings about various ways to respond became more apparent. Reversing roles can effectively teach spouses in conflict better ways to communicate. To prevent role playing from becoming a game with little learning, plan the proposed drama with clear objectives in mind. What behavioral outcomes should be achieved? Define the context (the "stage") clearly, so that everyone shares in the situation. Then define each role ahead of time, making sure that participants understand their performance roles. Emphasize that no wrong or right performance exists, and that participants should behave the way people behave in everyday life. Avoid having people play themselves, because it can embarrass them and make it difficult for them to achieve objectivity. After the drama has concluded, elicit discussion with carefully prepared questions. This technique can be used with staff, coworkers, young children, teenagers, and adults. However, it can be a risk-taking experience for some people, and they may be reluctant to participate. The nurse should use judgment, begin with volunteers, and avoid pushing this technique on unwilling or nonreceptive people. Build up to full participation.

Teaching Materials

Many different kinds of teaching materials are available to the nurse. They often are used in combination and are useful during the teaching process. Visual images—such as PowerPoint presentations, pictures, slides, posters, chalkboards, flannel boards, DVDs, bulletin boards, flash cards, pamphlets, flyers, charts, and gestures—can enhance most learning. Some tools, such as tapes and compact disks, provide an auditory stimulus as well. Americans readily learn from television and the Internet; appeals to vision and hearing senses and more or less grabs attention. Learning of both positive and negative health behaviors through television or the Internet can be more effective and efficient than traditional teaching methods. Other tools, such as anatomic models and improvised or purchased equipment, provide clients with both visual and tactile learning experiences. Still others, such as interactive computer games or instruction, actively involve the learners.

The choice of teaching materials varies with the clients' interests and abilities and the resources available. Teaching often occurs in casual conversations, spontaneously in situations in which clients raise unexpected questions, or when a crisis arises. In these instances, nurses draw on their background of knowledge and exercise professional judgment in their selection of content, methods, and materials.

Several different types of printed educational support materials are available, such as pamphlets, brochures, booklets, flyers, and informational sheets. Each should be evaluated for its appropriateness and effectiveness with particular individuals, families, or groups. Many come from state and local official sources. Nurses can create their own handouts by using the Internet and a computer, customizing them to the needs of individual clients. The Internet has vast health resources that can be combined with the desktop publishing capabilities of the nurse's computer to create one-of-a-kind materials for clients. The nurse can get educational information from state, federal, and international health agencies such as state health departments, the U.S. Food and Drug Administration (FDA), the Centers for Disease Control and Prevention (CDC), the National Institutes of Health (NIH), and the WHO. Other materials come from nonprofit national agencies such as the American Diabetes Association (ADA), the March of Dimes, the American Association for Retired Persons (AARP), and the American Heart Association (AHA). Materials from these sources can be acquired in large quantity for free or at a nominal cost to the nurse or agency. Major manufacturers of infant formulas, foods, diapers, and toys are good sources for literature on growth and development, safety, and caring for infants and children. Pharmaceutical companies develop educational materials for the public, as do the manufacturers of in-home supplies and equipment. Usually, these are excellent sources of information for families or groups; however, the nurse needs to assess the material for appropriateness. Also, be sure that the commercial message in the literature does not outweigh the educational impact, thus making it misleading or confusing to the client.

Factors to be considered with all educational literature include the material's content, complexity, and reading level. There are several ways to assess the readability of the printed word. One easy way is to use the Fog Index. It is a rough way of determining the years of schooling needed to understand printed material. It works by analyzing words and sentence length. The higher the Fog Index, the more difficult the reading level. A Fog Index of 6 is a sixth-grade reading level, and 11 is the junior year in high school (Bastable, 2008). Fortunately, most word processing programs now include a feature to allow assessment of the reading level in text. Another very common tool is the Fleish Reading Ease program, which evaluates the material on a 100-point scale, with 90 to 100 being rated as very easy to read, and 60 to 70 as the standard; a rating of under 59 indicates a more difficult level (Bastable, 2008). Similar to the Fog Index, the Flesch-Kincaid Grade Level readability score rates the material in terms of typical grade level; a score of 8 would indicate that an eighth grade student should be able to read and understand the material. For most health promotion materials, a reading level of sixth grade is normally sufficient (Doak, Doak, & Root, 1996). The nurse should always consider the population when selecting a reading level, as many individuals cannot understand materials at that high a grade level.

Culturally appropriate health education materials must be acquired or developed for the predominant cultural and linguistic minority populations taught by the nurse. Developing printed materials is an important first step, but the development of video, audio, and public service announcements in community-appropriate languages is also necessary. When translating printed materials from English into another language, it is strongly suggested that a separate translator, "back-translate" the materials. This added step helps assure that the meaning from the original has not been distorted or lost in the translation. Essentially one person or group translates the material and another individual or group translates it back into English. This can add time and cost to the project, but it may prevent inaccuracies in the final material.

Finally, nurses teach by example. Actions speak louder than words. If a nurse teaches the importance of washing hands to reduce disease transmission and then begins a newborn assessment without hand-washing, the message of observed actions carries more impact than the words. Nurses who exhibit healthy practices use themselves as teaching tools and serve as role models as well as health teachers.

Clients with Special Learning Needs

At times, the nurse experiences a challenging teaching situation with an individual, family, or group. These challenges may involve clients who have cultural or language differences, hearing impairments, developmental delays, memory losses, visual perception distortions, and problems with fine or gross motor skills, distracting personality characteristics, or demonstrations of stress or emotions. Regardless of the situation, the nurse will feel most comfortable and confident if he or she is prepared to deal with these situations before they are experienced.

Before beginning to teach a client, family, or aggregate, thorough preparation is important for successful learning to occur. This includes finding out whether it is possible to teach in English or whether other modifications are needed as the teaching plan is being developed. Nurses should never assume anything, including the primary language spoken by clients, their visual or hearing ability, or their capacity to understand. When teaching unfamiliar groups, the nurse can obtain information regarding the interests and abilities of the members from a center manager, caretaker, or program director. These human resources are invaluable in planning any teaching when English may be a second language or when other barriers exist that may impede success if they are not known by the nurse. The phases of the nursing process continue to guide the nurse as a teacher.

Another difficulty that can arise is unexpected behavior from a client who disrupts the group process. The client may monopolize the discussion, answer questions asked of others, burst out with personal experiences that have no relevance to the topic, become irate at the comments of others, or sit silently and never speak. This can be unnerving to even the most experienced nurse. Any behavior that has the potential to distract the other learners must be diffused by the nurse. This is accomplished by caringly giving the recognition sought by the person while also setting limits.

SUMMARY

The purpose of health education is to effect change, which alters the equilibrium in a system. Change may occur gradually, with time for people involved to adjust, or it may occur in a drastic fashion, such as in a crisis or natural disaster. Change occurs in three stages: *unfreezing* when the system is ready for change, *changing* when the innovation is implemented, and *refreezing* when the change is stabilized.

Planned or managed change is a purposeful, designed effort to effect improvement in a system with the help of a change agent. It involves a process of eight steps, similar to the nursing process, which nurses can use to create change. These steps include assessing symptoms, diagnosing need, analyzing alternative solutions, selecting a change, planning the change, implementing the change, evaluating the change, and stabilizing the change. During planned change, the nurse can use one or a combination of several change strategies. However, the three major change strategies—a rational approach of providing information to influence people to change, an educative approach of combining new information with persuasion to effect change, and a coercive approach of enforcing compliance—are encompassing strategies. Several important principles serve as guidelines for community health nurses to effect change. They include involving all persons affected by the change, introducing change in a timely fashion, considering the impact of the change on other systems, being flexible, and understanding oneself and one's own qualities, which can be groomed to provide the most effective leadership.

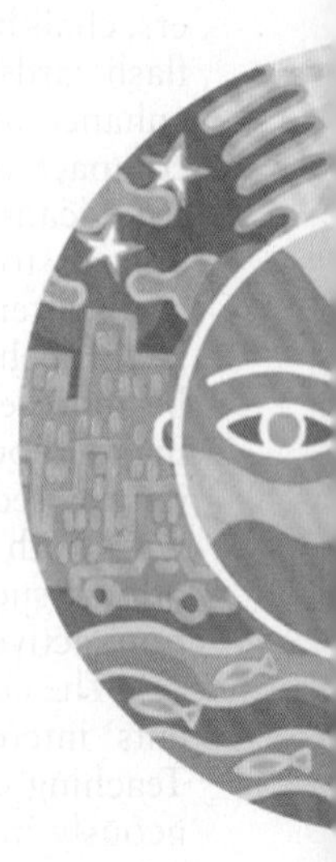

Much of community health nursing practice involves teaching. More than simply giving health information to clients, the purpose of teaching is to change client behavior to healthier practices. If these practices are internalized and implemented regularly, years of morbidity and premature mortality can be avoided, thus contributing to the quality and length of the human lifespan. Recognition that social determinants of health must be factored into any educational or health promotion efforts is a focus of *Healthy People 2020*.

Understanding the nature of learning contributes to the effectiveness of teaching in community health. Learning occurs in three domains: cognitive, affective, and psychomotor. The cognitive domain refers to learning that takes place intellectually. It ranges in levels of learner functioning from simple recall to complex evaluation. As learners move up the scale of cognitive learning, they become more self-directed; the nurse then assumes a more facilitative role.

Affective learning involves the changing of attitudes and values. Learners may experience several levels of affective involvement, from simple listening to adopting the new value. Again, as the client increases involvement, the nurse becomes less directive.

Psychomotor learning involves the acquisition of motor skills. Clients who learn psychomotor skills must meet three conditions: they must be capable of the skill, they must develop a sensory image of the skill, and they must practice the skill.

Learning theories can be grouped into four broad categories: (1) behaviorist theories, which view learning as a behavioral change accomplished through stimulus–response or conditioning; (2) cognitive learning theories, which seek to influence learners' understanding of problems and situations through promoting their insights; (3) social learning theories, which explain dysfunctional behavior and facilitate learning; and (4) humanistic theories, which assume that people have a natural tendency to learn and that learning flourishes in an encouraging environment. Knowles' adult learning theory provides a framework for understanding adult characteristics and appropriate teaching interventions.

Health-teaching models work together with the learning theories to give nurses a more accurate picture of the client and the client's learning needs. Three models were explored in this chapter. The HBM is useful in explaining the behaviors that are triggered by people with an interest in preventing diseases, and the revised HPM modifies the HBM and focuses on predicting behaviors that influence health promotion. The PRECEDE–PROCEED model is designed to guide health educational program development. The model has a strong focus on the perceived problems and priorities of a particular individual or group as they impact quality of life. Educational interventions are developed following a thorough assessment, which includes administrative and policy issues, and evaluation is conducted at three levels: process, impact, and outcome.

Teaching in community health nursing is the facilitation of learning that leads to behavioral change in the client. Ideally, this is done at the primary level of prevention. However, much of the nurse's work is done at the secondary and tertiary levels. The nurse uses several teaching–learning principles to facilitate the learning process, such as clients' readiness for learning, clients' perceptions, learners' physical and emotional comfort within an educational setting, degree of client participation, relevant subject matter, allowing clients to derive satisfaction from learning, and reinforcing learning through application.

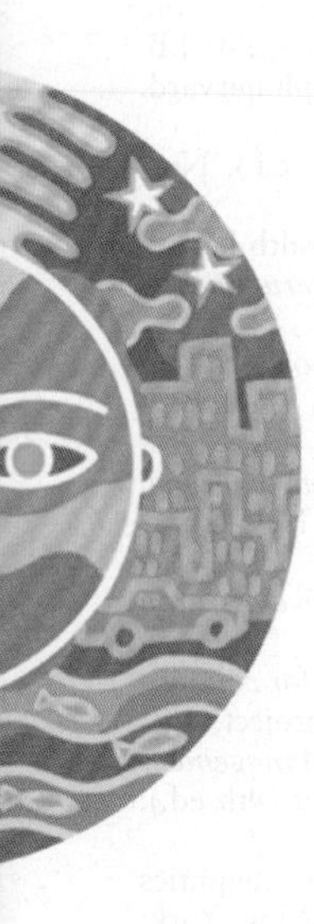

The teaching process in community health nursing is similar to the nursing process, including steps of interaction, assessment and diagnosis, goal setting, planning, teaching, and evaluation. The teaching may be formal or informal, planned or unplanned, and methods may range from structured lecture presentations and discussions to demonstration and role playing.

Selection of teaching materials depends on how well they suit learners and help to meet the desired objectives. Sources of teaching materials that are free or inexpensive can enhance the nurses' teaching efforts, but need to be evaluated for effectiveness and appropriateness. The nurse needs to know how to help learners with special needs, those with physical or mental disabilities, those who are from a different culture or who speak a different language, and those who monopolize the discussion, become emotional, or are hostile. The nurse must be prepared for each situation to effectively teach the individual, family, or group.

ACTIVITIES TO PROMOTE **CRITICAL THINKING**

1. As a staff community health nurse, you have been asked to chair an ad hoc committee in your health department made up of interdisciplinary colleagues and community members. The committee's task is to plan a health fair for the local community.
   a. Outline the specific planned-change steps that your committee needs to ensure a successful health fair with outcomes that promote improved levels of community health.
   b. Select one specific objective of your health fair (e.g., cholesterol screening of an at-risk aggregate with the goal of reduced cholesterol levels in a year). Does the proposed objective require an evolutionary or revolutionary change in citizens' health-related behaviors? Justify your choice of the type of change.
   c. Explain the strategies that you would use to effect the change.
   d. Six principles for effecting positive change are presented in this chapter. Briefly discuss how you would use each one as you and your committee develop the health fair.
2. What learning theories discussed in this chapter most closely reflect your own position? How can they be applied in your practice?
3. Your city governmental officials often make decisions that appear to reflect a lack of knowledge regarding health and health care. How might you "educate" them using the concepts and principles described in this chapter?
4. Using behavioral objectives that match the learning level desired, develop a flyer or program for an educational presentation for clients.
5. Select one of the health-teaching models. Use the model to plan an educational program for a group of teenagers. How did the use of the model enhance your teaching?
6. You are teaching an aggregate of middle-aged women about menopause. One woman monopolizes the class by telling stories and talking negatively about her husband. The other women are getting upset with her. How do you resolve the situation?
7. Using the list of Internet resources at the end of this chapter, review the type and quality of free or low-cost educational materials that they offer. Try to locate additional resources from other companies, public service agencies, and voluntary health agencies. Either request useful material to be used with clients now or bookmark a selection of sites to refer to later as needed, developing a resource file.

REFERENCES

Bandura, A. (1977). *Social learning theory*. Englewood Cliffs, NJ: Prentice-Hall.

Bandura, A. (1986). *Social foundations of thought and action: A social cognitive theory*. Englewood Cliffs, NJ: Prentice-Hall.

Bastable, S. B. (2008). Literacy in the adult client population. In S.B. Bastable (Ed.), *Nurse as educator: Principles of teaching and learning for nursing practice* (3rd ed., pp. 229–283). Boston: Jones & Bartlett.

Bastable, S. B., & Doody, J. A. (2008). Behavioral objectives. In S.B. Bastable (Ed.), *Nurse as educator: Principles of teaching and learning for nursing practice* (3rd ed., pp. 383–427). Boston: Jones & Bartlett.

Bloom, B. (Ed.). (1956). *Taxonomy of educational objectives: The classification of educational goals. Handbook I: Cognitive domain*. New York: Longman.

Braungart, M. M., & Braungart, R. G. (2008). Applying learning theories to healthcare practice. In S. B. Bastable (Ed.), *Nurse as educator: Principles of teaching and learning for nursing practice* (3rd ed., pp. 51–89). Sudbury, MA: Jones & Bartlett.

Center for Advancing Health. (2010). *Snapshot of people's engagement in their health care*. Retrieved from http://www.cfah.org/pdfs/CFAH_Snapshot_Summary_2010.pdf

Clampitt, P. G., & DeKoch, R. J. (2001). *Embracing uncertainty: The essence of leadership*. Armonk, NY: M.E. Sharpe.

Doak, C. C., Doak, L. G., & Root, J. H. (1996). *Teaching patients with low literacy skills* (2nd ed.). Philadelphia, PA: J.B. Lippincott Company. Retrieved from http://www.hsph.harvard.edu/healthliteracy/resources/doak-book/

Eisner, E. W. (1985). *The educational imagination* (2nd ed.). New York: Macmillan.

Esperat, C., Feng, D., Zhang, Y., & Owen, D. (2007). Health behaviors of low-income pregnant minority women. *Western Journal of Nursing Research, 29*, 284–300.

Green, L. W., & Kreuter, M. W. (1991). *Health promotion planning: An educational and environmental approach* (2nd ed.). Mountain View, CA: Mayfield.

Green, L. W., & Kreuter, M. W. (2005). *Health program planning: An educational and ecological approach* (4th ed.). New York: McGraw Hill.

Gronlund, N. E. (1970). *Stating behavioral objectives for classroom instruction*. New York: Macmillan.

Health Impact Project. (2011). *Advancing smarter policies for community health*. Retrieved from http://www.healthimpactproject.org/

Hersey, P., Blanchard, K., & Johnson, D. E. (2008). *Management of organizational behavior: Leading human resources* (9th ed.). Upper Saddle River, NJ: Prentice-Hall.

Hofrichter, R., & Bhatia, R. (2010). Tackling health inequities through public health practice, theory to action. New York: Oxford University Press.

Hollinger, B. (2005). Integration of cultural systems and beliefs. In S. H. Rankin, K. D. Stallings, & F. London (Eds.), *Patient education in health and illness* (5th ed., pp. 47–71). Philadelphia, PA: Lippincott Williams & Wilkins.

Kartal, A., & Ozsoy, S. A. (2007). Validity and reliability study of the Turkish version of Health Belief Model Scale in diabetic patients. *International Journal of Nursing Studies, 44,* 1447–1458.

Kausar, R. (2012). *Sustaining behavior change through participatory approaches in project cycle.* Presented at the Asia Regional Sanitation and Hygiene Practitioners Workshop. Retrieved from http://www.irc.nl/page/68130

Kitchie, S. (2008). Determinants of learning. In S. B. Bastable (Ed.), *Nurse as educator: Principles of teaching and learning for nursing practice* (3rd ed., pp. 93–145). Boston, MA: Jones & Bartlett.

Knowles, M. (1980). *The modern practice of adult education: Andragogy versus pedagogy* (2nd ed.). Chicago, IL: Follett.

Knowles, M. (1984). *The adult learner: A neglected species* (3rd ed.). Houston, TX: Gulf.

Knowles, M. (1989). *The making of an adult educator: An autobiographical journey.* San Francisco, CA: Jossey-Bass.

Knowles, M. (1990). *The adult learner: A neglected species* (4th ed.). Houston, TX: Gulf Publishing.

Lewin, K. (1947). Frontiers in group dynamics: Concept, method, and reality in social science; social equilibria and social change. *Human Relations, 1*(1), 5–41.

Lewin, K. (1951). *Field theory in social science: Selected theoretical papers.* New York: Harper & Row.

Lippitt, G. L. (1973). *Visualizing change: Model building and the change process.* La Jolla, CA: University Associates.

Lippitt, R., Watson, J., & Westley, B. (1958). *The dynamics of planned change.* New York: Harcourt.

Mager, R. F. (1975). *Preparing instructional objectives* (2nd ed.). Belmont, CA: Pitman Learning.

Maslow, A. H. (1970). *Motivation and personality* (2nd ed.). New York: Harper and Row.

Miller, D. M., Linn, R., & Gronlund, N. E. (2009). *Measurement and assessment in teaching* (10th ed.). Upper Saddle River, NJ: Pearson.

Morowatisharifabad, M. A., Ghofranipour, F., Heidarnia, A., Ruchi, G. B., & Ehrampoush, M. H. (2006). Self-efficacy and health promotion behaviors of older adults in Iran. *Social Behavior and Personality, 34,* 759–768.

National Heart Lung and Blood Institute. (2012). Guide *to behavior change.* Retrieved from http://www.nhlbi.nih.gov/health/public/heart/obesity/lose_wt/behavior.htm

Ottoson, J. M., & Green, L. W. (2008). Public health education and health promotion. In L. F. Novik, C. B. Morrow, & G. P. Mays (Eds.), *Public health administration: Principles for population-based management* (2nd ed., pp. 589–619). Sudbury, MA: Jones & Bartlett.

Pavlov, I. P. (1957). *Experimental psychology and other essays.* New York: Philosophical Library.

Pender, N. J. (1996). *Health promotion in nursing practice* (3rd ed.). Stamford, CT: Appleton & Lange.

Pender, N. J., Murdaugh, C. L., & Parsons, M. A. (2011). *Health promotion in nursing practice* (6th ed.). Upper Saddle River, NJ: Pearson Education, Inc.

Piaget, J. (1966). *The origin of intelligence in children.* New York: Norton.

Piaget, J. (1970). Piaget's theory. In P. H. Mussen (Ed.), *Charmichael's manual of child psychology* (Vol. 1). New York: Wiley.

Rankin, S. H., Stallings, K. D., & London, F. (2005). *Patient education in health and illness* (5th ed.). Philadelphia, PA: Lippincott Williams & Wilkins.

Reutter, L., & Kushner, K. E. (2012). Health equity through action on the social determinants of health: Taking up the challenge in nursing. *Nursing Inquiry,* 17(3), 269–280.

Robert Wood Johnson Foundation. (2010). A new way to talk about social determinants of health. Retrieved from http://www.rwjf.org/files/research/vpmessageguide20101029.pdf

Rogers, C. (1969). *Freedom to learn.* Columbus, OH: Merrill.

Rogers, C. (1989). *Freedom to learn for the eighties.* Columbus, OH: Merrill.

Rosenstock, I. M. (1966). Why people use health services. *Milbank Memorial Fund Quarterly, 44,* 94–127.

Roussel, L. A. (2013). *Management and leadership for nurse administrators* (6th ed.). Sudbury, MA: Jones & Bartlett.

Rowitz, L. (2006). *Public health for the 21st century: The prepared leader.* Sudbury, MA: Jones & Bartlett.

Shin, K. R., Kang, Y., Park, H. J., Cho, M. O., & Heitkemper, M. (2008). Testing and developing the health promotion model in low-income, Korean elderly women. *Nursing Science Quarterly,* 21, 173–178.

Skinner, B. F. (1974). *About behaviorism.* New York: Knopf.

Skinner, B. F. (1987). *Upon further reflection.* Englewood Cliffs, NJ: Prentice-Hall.

Spradley, B. W. (1980). Managing change creatively. *Journal of Nursing Administration, 10*(5), 32–37.

Spradley, J., & McCurdy, D. (1994). *Conformity and conflict: Readings in cultural anthropology* (8th ed.). New York: Harper Collins.

Srof, B. J., & Velsor-Friedrich, B. (2006). Health promotion in adolescents: A review of Pender's health promotion model. *Nursing Science Quarterly, 19,* 366–373.

Strecher, U. J., & Rosenstock, I. M. (1997). The health belief model. In K. Glanz, F. M. Lewis, & B. K. Rimer (Eds.), *Health behavior and health education: Theory, research and practice* (2nd ed., pp. 41–59). San Francisco, CA: Jossey-Bass.

The Aspen Institute. (2012). *Health in all policies.* Retrieved from http://www.aspeninstitute.org/policy-work/health-biomedical-science-society/health-stewardship-project/principles/health-all

Thompson, J. M. (2010). Understanding and managing organizational change: Implications for public health management. *Journal of Public Health Management & Practice, 16*(2), 167–173.

Thorndike, E. L. (1932). *The fundamentals of learning.* New York: Teachers College Press.

Thorndike, E. L. (1969). *Educational psychology.* New York: Arno Press.

Tyler, R. W. (1949). *Basic principles of curriculum and instruction.* Chicago, IL: University of Chicago Press.

U. S. Department of Health and Human Services. (2010a). *Healthy People 2020: About Healthy People.* Retrieved from http://www.healthypeople.gov/2020/about/default.aspx

U. S. Department of Health and Human Services. (2010b). *Healthy People 2020: Education and community based programs.* Retrieved from http://www.healthypeople.gov/2020/topicsobjectives2020/objectiveslist.aspx?topicId=11

U. S. Department of Health and Human Services. (2010c). *Healthy People 2020: Social determinants of health.* Retrieved from http://www.healthypeople.gov/2020/topicsobjectives2020/overview.aspx?topicid=39

U. S. Department of Health and Human Services. (2010d). *Healthy People 2020 Framework: The vision, mission, and goals of Healthy People 2020.* Retrieved from http://healthypeople.gov/2020/consortium/HP2020Framework.pdf

U. S. Department of Health and Human Services. (2010e). *Secretary's advisory committee on health promotion and disease prevention objectives for 2020.* Retrieved from http://www.healthypeople.gov/2010/hp2020/advisory/societaldeterminantshealth.htm

Wertheimer, M. (Ed.). (1945/1959). *Productive thinking.* New York: Harper & Row.

Wertheimer, M. (1980). Gestalt theory of learning. In G. M. Gazda, & R. H. Corsini (Eds.), *Theories of learning: A comparative approach.* Itasca, IL: Peacock.

World Health Organization, Government of South Australia. (2010). *Adelaide statement on health in all policies.* Retrieved from http://www.who.int/social_determinants/hiap_statement_who_sa_final.pdf

thePoint: Everything You Need to Make the Grade!

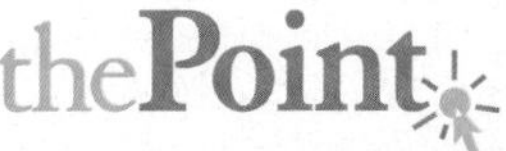

Visit http://thePoint.lww.com/Allender8e
for selected readings, study aids for all learning styles, and more!

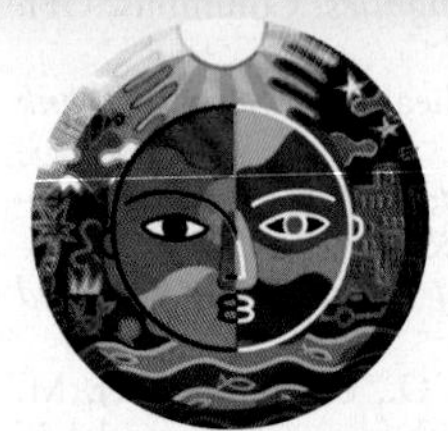

CHAPTER

12

Planning and Developing Community Programs and Services

"True genius resides in the capacity for evaluation of uncertain, hazardous, and conflicting information."

***—Winston Churchill (1874–1965)**, British Prime Minister during World War II*

KEY TERMS

Advisory group
Authoritative knowledge
Benchmarking
Enabling factors
Geographic information system (GIS)
Grant
Letter of inquiry
Predisposing factors
Reinforcing factors
Request for proposal (RFP)
Social marketing

LEARNING OBJECTIVES

Upon mastery of this chapter, you should be able to:

- List sources of information that can be used to identify group and community health problems.
- Identify change strategies that maximize cooperation of target populations.
- Identify methods to gain input from target populations to define the scope of a health problem.
- Identify and evaluate the effectiveness of intervention methods targeting health problems.
- Classify health problems based on their changeability.
- Identify barriers to solving health problems.
- Discuss the role of the nurse within quality measurement and improvement programs in community/public health nursing.
- Recognize the role of social marketing in health promotion programs.
- Locate appropriate grant funding sources for select health promotion programs.

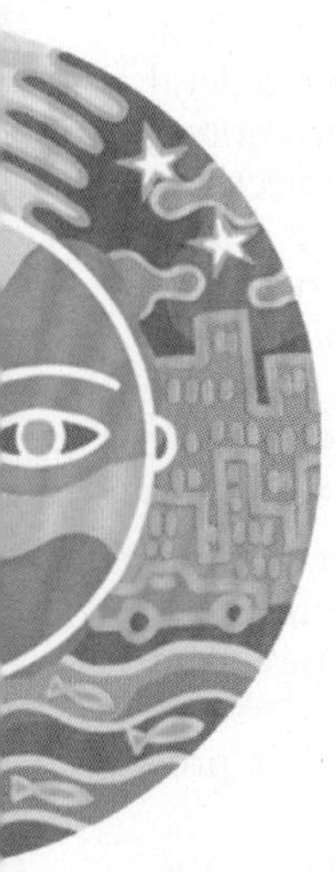

A public health nurse collaborates with the county housing authority to implement a comprehensive fall-prevention program for community-dwelling seniors; another nurse works into the night to complete a multimillion-dollar grant to fund comprehensive human immunodeficiency virus (HIV) educational programs in Kenya; community health nursing students volunteer to do a weekly radio program on health issues. The efforts described may seem very different, but each represents a health promotion program targeting populations, not just individuals. A fall-prevention program could potentially reduce the number of hospitalizations in the community resulting from serious falls, the HIV program may ultimately save tens of thousands from contracting this dreaded disease, and the radio program may reach thousands in the community, prompting them to think about their own health habits. Each of these examples represents the emerging role of the public health nurse and argues for the acquisition of a new set of skills. The skills of grant writing, radio programming, and collaborating with county officials all require new abilities that may require additional training or working with a mentor. These roles may seem foreign to you now, as you begin your career, but they may be the very skills needed to help bring vital health promotion programs to fruition.

In many communities across the country, local health departments struggle to recruit nurses to provide much-needed services. With shrinking budgets, many communities are forced to change long-held views on the scope and nature of services provided by public health nurses. The home visiting model, once a mainstay of public health nursing, has been eliminated in many communities. Increasingly, public health nurses find themselves providing health promotion and educational programs to larger and larger audiences. To meet this need, public health nurses must become skilled at planning and implementing health promotion programs. As with any activity, the need for the program must be justified, and with limited resources, the benefit to the community must be demonstrated. Additionally, communities are rarely in a position to fund the entire realm of needed health programs and must turn to outside agencies for funding, either through grants or contracts. The responsibility for locating, securing, and maintaining grant funding is often assumed by the public health nurse.

Whether the program is funded by the county or an outside agency, results must be assessed. Evaluation of programs is vital for their continuation and is a requirement of most funders, whether public or private. A nurse who receives $500 to start an emergency preparedness program with low-income families may not be expected to provide the level of evaluation data that a million-dollar effort to address methamphetamine use in the community would likely require. However, some level of evidence showing the impact of the program will be needed. Even the populations served want to know whether the programs were successful and why. For instance, a mother agrees to have her daughter enrolled in an after-school program to increase self-esteem. At the end of the first 6-week session, the mother is asked to give permission for her daughter to attend the second session. Her daughter says she enjoys the sessions but would also like to go to a dance class that is held at the same time. With competing demands on the daughter's time, the mother may ask for details on what was accomplished in the first session and what expectations the providers have for this second session. With this information, she can discuss various options with her daughter. The funders, consumers, and the nurse all need to be aware of the demonstrated outcomes of programs.

In Chapter 11, you were introduced to the concept of change—how it influences the adoption of health behaviors and what factors impede change in individuals. Educational methods are often used to influence change in behaviors and play a vital role in those efforts. In this chapter, we build on the concepts of change and appropriate educational techniques and apply them to larger groups and populations. The discussion of the PRECEDE–PROCEED model (Green & Kreuter, 1999, 2005; Ottoson & Green, 2008) will be expanded upon as you are introduced to the basics of health program planning, intervention, and evaluation to maximize successful results. Meeting the Institute of Medicine (IOM, 2003) call for enhanced quality and safety in nursing education and the impact this has on performance and outcome assessment of community health programs and services will be addressed, as well as the Quality and Safety Education for Nurses (QSEN, 2012) project that evolved from this call for action. Within this overall context, the subsequent IOM reports, the *Future of Nursing* (2010) and *For the Public's Health* (2012) will build on the challenges specific to public health and public health nursing. *Social marketing*, a relatively new tool for reaching large audiences with health information will be presented. Several well-known models familiar to nurses will be explored in terms of facilitating the evaluation of programs and services. Finally, as the need for grant funding becomes increasingly important, information on the various types of available funding will be provided.

PROGRAM PLANNING: THE BASICS

Ottoson and Green (2008, p. 590) define public health education programs as interventions "designed to inform, elicit, facilitate, and maintain positive health practices in large numbers of people." Even the American Nurses Association (ANA), *Public Health Nursing: Scope and Standards of Practice* (2007), is centered on the role of the nurse in planning, implementing, and evaluating population-focused health promotion/health education programs. Specifically, Standard 5B calls on the public health nurse to "employ multiple strategies to promote health, prevent disease, and ensure a safe environment for populations" (p. 23), through programs and services that include appropriate teaching–learning methods, that are culturally and age-appropriate, and that include an evaluation component.

With so much emphasis on planning and developing health education/health promotion programs, the process can seem overwhelming to the new public health nurse, or even to the acute care nurse who may be involved in some aspect of health initiative development within an agency. The first part of this chapter is designed to take some of the mystery out of the process. You will be guided through the complex problem of obesity in school-aged children. This particular issue is of great importance to the health of our children, and the principles applicable to this example can be utilized in other situations and other programs, even those that are very broad in scope and involve many practice partners. In your nursing program, you may even have been tasked with developing a health program, working on an existing community program, or simulating the process in a written assignment. Whatever your experience level, the essential elements are the same. As you begin this next section, think about past experiences you have had, such as taking blood pressures at a local health fair or developing a pamphlet on the need for prostate screening in non–English speaking residents. Did these actions have the impact you hoped for? Successful health promotion programs do not occur by accident; they take skill, time, patience, and most of all listening to and understanding the needs and opinions of the individuals who are the focus of your program (the target population).

IDENTIFYING GROUP OR COMMUNITY HEALTH PROBLEMS

Nursing education emphasizes practice with a focus on individuals, families, and communities, yet nurses often practice at the individual and family level. When is it appropriate for a nurse to expand her practice to the community level? Perhaps the most natural time is when a nurse identifies an ongoing issue that does not change with traditional interventions. Examples might include overuse of the emergency room for urgent care; recurrent hospitalization of the elderly from several nursing homes for dehydration, sepsis, and malnutrition; or hospitalization of 6- to 8-year-olds for injuries caused by insufficient car seat restraint. These types of recurrent problems might lead the nurse to investigate the feasibility of a community-based intervention.

Individually or in a group, identify a possible issue to explore—one that you believe is leading to poor health outcomes in your community. How do you know if this problem is widespread or if others also find it to be a problem? Several methods can be used to validate the importance of the issue. One method would be to consider *Healthy People 2020* objectives for the nation (U.S. Department of Health and Human Services [USDHHS], 2010). What are the major issues that are of concern to improving health outcomes for the United States? What are the priorities of the state in which you live? You might take some time to review Web sites for federal agencies to identify the programs they are promoting to meet the *Healthy People 2020* goals and objectives. Your state department of health may also have a Web site with information on achievement of *Healthy People 2020* objectives, including those objectives that remain challenging. Local communities also establish priorities that reflect the *Healthy People 2020* objectives for the nation. These overarching national goals are as follows:

- Attain high-quality, longer lives free of preventable disease, disability, injury, and premature death.
- Achieve health equity, eliminate disparities, and improve the health of all groups.
- Create social and physical environments that promote good health for all.
- Promote quality of life, healthy development, and healthy behaviors across all life stages.

Community agencies and organizations frequently network to establish community-wide goals. This work is often spearheaded by the local health department. It may also be organized by community-based health agencies and volunteer organizations. Improved outcomes for individuals who have diabetes or asthma are issues a local community might want to address. Another topic of concern is childhood obesity. Nurses can work collaboratively with these types of special interest groups to find solutions for individuals and families with identified problems.

As a specific problem is identified, it is crucial to analyze the extent to which individuals and families are affected by the problem. It is a poor use of resources to set up a program if there is a very small incidence of the condition or situation. For example, it would be a waste of resources to establish a program on diabetes and pregnancy for a local homeless shelter that only serves 35 women a year. Of those 35 women, none may be pregnant, and since 2% to 10% of the population of pregnant women develops gestational diabetes (USDHHS, 2011), it may be a number of years before an eligible client is found. A better use of resources would be to target a community with a higher proportion of individuals at risk for diabetes during pregnancy. An example might be a program targeting a community with a large population of young Asian Indian families, as the incidence of gestational diabetes is higher in this population (11%) versus non-Hispanic Whites (4%). Yet another target group may be foreign-born Hispanic or Filipina women who are also at increased risk (Hedderson, Darbinian, & Ferrara, 2010). There are many ways a nurse can decide if a problem has affected a sufficient percentage of the population to warrant intervention. The best way to start is by reviewing the local, state, and national data available through government repositories. This can be done through the Internet, by going to a university library for assistance, and by asking for sources of specific data from your local health and social service agencies, police and judicial departments, and local school districts. Hospital discharge data are also reported to state agencies, and this information is sometimes available at the local level. As nurses and other community groups narrow their focus, they can often map data by zip codes and neighborhoods, which helps to identify the best places to target groups and communities. Currently, many organizations have this ability and are able to identify target groups by race, age, and family status. This type of data, known as **geographic information system (GIS)** information, is widely available. At the federal level, the National Center for Health Statistics (NCHS) Web site maintains GIS maps on the major causes of mortality in the country. Additional GIS data can be found through a variety of federal sources, including the CDC, the National Cancer Institute, the Center for Mental Health Services, the National Library of Medicine, and the Environmental Protection Agency (Public Health Partners, 2012). Another effective approach is to talk to other nurses and other health care professionals within and outside of your organization. Get their ideas about the problem and ideas about what should be done to alleviate the problem. In addition, find out what has been tried in the past and get their input on why past interventions failed. One very helpful source of information is the *Guide to Community Preventive Services: What Works to Promote Health?* (2012), a federally sponsored initiative that provides recommendations regarding population-based interventions, including which are recommended, which need more evidence to determine effectiveness, and which are not recommended. The interventions with limited evidence may actually be very effective but need to be demonstrated by more studies; perhaps your idea is among those listed. Publication of program results is not only professionally gratifying but adds to the body of evidence on which health promotion programs can be evaluated. For example, in Chapter 6 of the guide, recommendations to increase community demand for vaccinations include client reminder and recall systems, yet there is not enough evidence to support client or family incentives, or the use of patient-held medical records (pp. 223–224).

The next step of intervention is the most important of all, as it will determine whether your interventions succeed or fail. A nurse may think, "I know what the problem is—now I will think up an intervention to alleviate it!" This approach may be well intentioned, but will lead the nurse down the path of failure. At this point, only part of the assessment is completed; the most important part of the assessment is to find out the views of the target population about the identified problem. What do they think causes it? What ideas do they have about solving it? Which approaches do they think will work, and which are doomed to failure? These are all important questions the nurse needs to ask. It is crucial that the views of the target population be heard and respected. Anthropologists talk about a concept called **authoritative knowledge**. This is "whose knowledge is respected," not "whose knowledge is right" (Sargent & Davis-Floyd, 1997). Nurses may think that they know more about a topic, such as diabetes, than their target population does, and therefore their solutions are better than the target population's solutions. Members of a target population hold just as strongly to their own belief systems. If nurses don't learn about the target population's beliefs and only consider their own, they will not be able to work out an acceptable and appropriate solution with the target population. Interventions that fail to engage the target population will likely be unsuccessful because of this. It is crucial that interventions utilize health resources effectively and that positive working relationships be established with high-risk target communities.

Getting Started

When working with target groups, it's important to get as much information about the population as possible. Start by asking those whom you know, as colleagues and as patients/clients, about their local community. What do they see as issues regarding the problem about which you are concerned? What do they think about the quality of services currently available? What do they see as barriers to services? What about barriers to adherence to treatment and other health care recommendations?

Additional issues to explore include: Who else do they think you should speak with to gain insight about the issues relevant to this problem? Who are key people with whom you should build relationships? What are their customs in regard to health care? Who are the leaders within a family? If you want to establish linkages with this population, what is the best method? Who are their *formal* and *informal leaders*? What types of events bring them together? What are the roles of family, church, and health care providers within their community? Should you go through church groups, school groups, or other organizations? What radio stations do they listen to, and what television stations are they most likely to watch? What are the most common Web sites used by this population when accessing health topics? This information will not only help you gain insight into factors influencing the health problem, it will also give you information about how most effectively to reach out to the target population.

As you start to gain insight into the environmental and social factors that influence the problems about which you are concerned, you are also building interest in the issue. As you participate in discussions with others, be open to their input. It may be that the ideas you start out with need to change in response to feedback from members of the target and service communities. For example, an experienced public health nurse was involved in a project developed to serve Hispanic women with gestational diabetes. When interviewed, the monolingual Spanish-speaking women expressed concern that they were told to go on a diabetic "diet" and were then chastised for not eating enough. To these women, going on a "diet" meant they should eat less. They were also told that if they followed the diabetic diet they wouldn't have such "big babies." They thought a "big" baby was a healthy baby and couldn't understand why they were being told to avoid having a larger baby. These were simple issues to fix, but required knowledge of how the "diabetic teaching plan" was interpreted by the target audience. Another key factor was that the clinic was a family event; thus, all of the children were brought along. The clinic staff had been consistently irritated by the presence of large groups of children, but learned that they needed to alter the clinic setup and resources to accommodate the expectations of their clients. Modifications were made based on dialogue with members of the target population that positively influenced the eventual success of the clinic's program.

This example demonstrates how use of *local knowledge* can increase the effectiveness of a community-based intervention. The participation of members of the target population also builds greater community capacity for resolution of health problems within target communities. Working with community partners, including members of target populations, is a technique that has been used in providing services within developing countries. This type of approach ensures community *buy-in* for an intervention. It also builds networks that can continue to increase the capacity of communities to resolve other health care issues, both current and emerging (Butaet al., 2011; Lavery et al., 2005; Zlotnick, Wright, Sanchez, Kusnir, & Te'o-Bennett, 2010).

It is essential to review literature regarding health problems, factors influencing the outcomes of interventions, and the role of families and communities in adherence to interventions. The literature review can offer the opportunity to develop additional insights that may shape interviews with members of the target and service communities. How does this target group compare to other target groups? What else should be addressed that wasn't found in the literature? Another public health nurse conducted a study that addressed use of the emergency room for after-hours urgent care. The literature focused heavily on "misuse" of emergency rooms by parents to treat urgent ambulatory care health problems, such as otitis media. Based on input from an emergency room nurse, families were asked what their doctors had told them to do if their child became ill at night. The families indicated that they were told to take their children to the emergency room! None of the literature addressed what the families had been told to do for after-hours care. This is an example of how being open to information from a variety of sources (in this case the emergency room nurse) enhanced the researcher's understanding of the problem beyond what could be learned by solely relying on the literature.

As nurses work with community members to identify factors contributing to a health problem, individuals will begin to stand out because of their knowledge, their network capabilities, and their interest in the subject. A key factor for ensuring the success of any intervention is to appoint an **advisory group** that includes representatives from the target and service communities. Findings from interviews, literature reviews, and data analyses need to be reviewed with this advisory group. To ensure success of the advisory group, all meetings should be carefully planned, so that they are well organized, punctual, and efficient. Strategies to encourage input from the advisory group should be employed; meetings should focus on getting the advisory group to interpret findings and community feedback and to develop possible solutions. Contributions from each member should be sought and valued equally. Depending on the size of the group, it may be most effective to have some breakout sessions as well as larger group sessions. An evaluation should be done by each member after each meeting, so that any problems can be addressed before the next meeting. Maintaining a record of these meetings—either in the form of minutes or a brief written overview—is also very helpful. Be certain to also keep a record of attendees. Maintaining a *paper trail* is always important.

Delineating the Problem to Be Addressed

With the help of the advisory group, it's important to delineate the problem or problems to be addressed. The following is a case example. A group of nurses identified childhood obesity as a problem. Input from community members, as well as a review of data, demonstrated a higher rate of childhood obesity in a local elementary school, where a high proportion of the children were African American. Although the original plan made by the nurses was to establish a special educational program for overweight children, ages 10 to 12, input from members of the service and target community indicated major problems with this approach:

1. It would be embarrassing for any child identified as needing the program.
2. Children this age usually don't pick the menu for their home or school.
3. Diet is culturally dependent, and the nurses knew very little about the dietary practices of African American families within the targeted community.

The use of an advisory group helped the nurses first identify what behavioral factors contributed to childhood obesity in the target population. These behavioral factors included the following:

- School breakfasts and lunches served were high in fat and salt, with limited fresh vegetable and fruit choices.
- Physical education classes were conducted for 45 minutes, once a week.
- No sports equipment was available for use during school recess and lunch periods.
- Participation in after-school sports cost $150 per student for uniforms and fees.
- The students aged 10 to 12 preferred to drink sodas and eat French fries for lunch.
- Most parents were working and often bought "fast food" for their children for dinner.
- Local parks were unsafe for children to play in, and there were no outdoor recreational activities that were free (no cost).
- Children in the target group described feeling very stressed due to high homework demands and expectations to score well on national tests.
- Children in the target group indicated that they went home after school and watched TV or played video games because their parents wouldn't allow them to play outside while they were at work.

- When asked what they did when stressed, children in the target group indicated they watched TV, listened to music, played video games, and had snacks.
- The favorite after-school snacks eaten by children in the target group were macaroni and cheese from a box or packaged noodles—both of which are high in fat, carbohydrates, and salt.

Rating the Importance and Changeability of Identified Behavioral Factors

To achieve success, programs must narrow their focus to a limited number of health behaviors that can be addressed successfully within a specific time frame (Green & Kreuter, 1999, 2005). To prioritize which behaviors to address, Green and Kreuter (2005) suggest that they be rated in terms of importance and changeability. The final list should include problems that are both important and easy to change.

Importance is determined by rating how frequently the identified behavior occurs and how strongly it is linked to a health problem. The advisory group for childhood obesity ranked the importance of the identified behaviors; their ranking and rationale (basis) for the ranking can be seen in Table 12-1. For instance, the lack of available sports equipment was not rated very highly since the advisory group observed that children can be physically active without sports equipment. A highly rated item was the poor quality of the school-provided breakfasts and lunches; as a primary source of nutrition for many of the school's children, it could contribute to obesity in this population.

Table 12.1 Importance of Behaviors Contributing to Childhood Obesity at Stevens Place Elementary School

Important	Basis for Rating
• School breakfasts and lunches were served that were high in fat and carbohydrate, with limited fresh vegetable and fruit choices.	A number of children ate their main meals at school, and studies have shown that high-fat, high-carbohydrate diets contribute to childhood obesity.
• Physical education classes were conducted for 45 min once a week.	Increasing exercise frequency will increase muscle mass as well as metabolic rates.
• The students aged 10–12 preferred to drink sodas and eat French fries for lunch.	Peer pressure can adversely influence food choices.
• Most parents were working and often bought "fast food" for their children for dinner.	Fast foods are high in carbohydrates and fat.
• Children in the target group described feeling very stressed due to high homework demands and expectations to score well on national tests.	High stress levels in adults contribute to obesity by increasing cortisol levels.
• Children in the target group indicated they went home after school and watched TV or played video games because their parents wouldn't allow them to play outside while they were at work.	Sedentary activities contribute to childhood obesity.
• When asked what they did when stressed, children in the target group indicated they watched TV, listened to music, played video games, and had snacks.	Sedentary activities contribute to childhood obesity.
• The favorite after-school snacks eaten by children in the target group were macaroni and cheese from a box or packaged noodles–both of which are high fat, high carbohydrate, and high salt.	These foods are high in fat and carbohydrates.
Less Important	
• There was no sports equipment available for use during school recess and lunch periods.	Children can be physically active without sports equipment.
• Participation in after-school sports cost $150 per student for uniforms and fees.	High costs for participation in sports are a deterrent for low-income children.
• Local parks were unsafe for children to play in and there were no outdoor recreational activities that were free.	Although important, there isn't a direct linkage between the lack of safe parks and free recreation and childhood obesity.

The advisory group was then asked to rate the changeability of the behaviors. Green and Kreuter (1999, p. 138) indicate that those that are easiest to change:

- Are still in the developmental stages
- Have only recently been established
- Are not deeply rooted in cultural patterns or lifestyle
- Have been found to change in previous attempts

The advisory group's changeability ratings for the behaviors can be seen in Table 12-2. In this round of assessments, the advisory group found that the lack of sports equipment, although not as important, could be potentially changed. This rating was based on the fact that the underfunding of the play equipment was a relatively new occurrence, and funding might be redirected if attention was brought to the problem. The poor nutritional quality of the breakfasts and lunches was seen as less changeable due to existing contracts with outside businesses to provide the meals.

After rating the identified problems based on changeability and importance, the nurses and advisory group sought to narrow their focus to specific goals. Green and Kreuter (1999) suggest ranking the behaviors in a simple table, as seen in Table 12-3. This effort yielded a table with the problems categorized in four groups: more important/more changeable, less important/more changeable, more important/less changeable, and less important/less changeable. The issues seen as most important and changeable included fifth and sixth grade students choosing high-fat, high-sugar foods for lunch and breakfast; children feeling stressed by homework demands; and children engaging in sedentary activities.

Table 12.2 Changeability Ratings of Behaviors Contributing to Childhood Obesity at Stevens Place Elementary School

More Changeable	Basis for Rating Behavior
There was no sports equipment available for use during school recess and lunch periods.	Trends in underfunding school play equipment are relatively recent.
The students aged 10–12 preferred to drink sodas and eat French fries for lunch.	Peer pressure often changed student behavior and could be used to encourage healthy choices.
Children in the target group described feeling very stressed due to high homework demands and expectations to score well on national tests.	Pressure for children to perform well on standardized tests is a recent phenomenon of questionable value.
When asked what they did when stressed, children in the target group indicated they watched TV, listened to music, played video games, and had snacks.	This was rated as easier to change due to the newer interactive video games that include movement.
Less Changeable	
Physical education (PE) classes were conducted for 45 min once a week.	Trends to decrease PE time per week are relatively recent —limited funding creates barriers to PE.
School breakfasts and lunches were served that were high in fat and salt, with limited fresh vegetable and fruit choices.	For a number of years, schools have contracted out for lunch services from businesses based on bids.
Participation in after-school sports cost $150 per student for uniforms and fees.	Sports have been privately funded for a number of years.
Most parents were working and often bought "fast food" for their children for dinner.	Most parents are working, and fast food restaurants have become part of the American culture.
Local parks were unsafe for children to play in, and there were no outdoor recreational activities that were free.	Funding for parks and recreation has steadily declined for a number of years.
Children in the target group indicated they went home after school and watched TV or played video games because their parents wouldn't allow them to play outside while they were at work.	This has become commonplace in the modern culture.
The favorite after-school snacks eaten by children in the target group were macaroni and cheese from a box or packaged noodles—both of which are high fat, high carbohydrate, and high salt.	These are cheap and easy foods to fix.

Table 12.3 Rankings of Behaviors Contributing to Childhood Obesity at Stevens Place Elementary School by Importance and Changeability

	More Important	Less Important
More Changeable	Fifth and sixth grade students chose high-fat, high-sugar foods for lunch and breakfast. Children stressed by homework demands Children engaged in sedentary activities (watch TV, play video games) after school.	Limited sports equipment
Less Changeable	High-fat and high-carbohydrate school food Limited physical education classes Favorite after-school snacks high fat, high carbohydrate, and high salt	Participation in after-school sports cost $150 per student Parents often bought "fast food" for dinner Local parks unsafe; lack of free recreational activities

The use of this grid enabled the advisory group to focus on more changeable and important issues. They wrote behavioral objectives for each identified factor they hoped to change. These objectives identified *who* was targeted, *what* they hoped would change or what action would be taken, *how* the change would be measured, and what the *time frame* was for achieving the expected outcome. The following are their behavioral objectives:

1. By the end of the fall semester, 75% of the fifth and sixth grade students will choose a breakfast and lunch diet that includes fruit, vegetables, protein, dairy, and starch (bread, potatoes) at each meal.
2. By the end of the school year, the teachers will schedule homework that can easily be done by a low-average student within a half hour.
3. By the end of the fall semester, all fifth and sixth grade students will be provided physically interactive games free of charge.

Factors that Influence Behavior Change: Predisposing, Reinforcing, and Enabling Factors

Green and Kreuter (1999, 2005) suggest that three categories of factors affecting individual behavior be addressed, as they can break down factors that contribute to successful behavioral change and create barriers to behavioral change. These factors are:

> **Predisposing factors** are antecedents to behavior that provide the rationale or *motivation* for the behavior.
> **Reinforcing factors** are factors following a behavior that provide the continuing reward or incentive for the persistence or repetition of the behavior.
> **Enabling factors** are antecedents to behavior that allow a motivation to be realized (1999, p. 153).

Predisposing factors include the knowledge, beliefs, values, attitudes, and confidence of the target population that influence their behavioral choices. **Reinforcing factors** include the knowledge, values, beliefs, and attitudes of the family and friends of the target population. It also includes authority figures such as teachers or managers, as well as agency and community decision makers, as these individuals also influence the target population. Finally, **enabling factors** include the availability of resources; the accessibility of resources, laws, and government support for the health behaviors or for the health program; as well as skills (Green & Kreuter, 2005).

The advisory group, following the Green and Kreuter model, identified the predisposing, enabling, and reinforcing factors that affected each behavioral objective. Table 12-4 shows the grid they developed for the first behavior objective—"By the end of the fall semester, 75% of the fifth and sixth grade students will choose a breakfast and lunch diet that includes fruit, vegetables, protein, dairy and starch (bread, potatoes) at each meal." For example, one enabling factor that supported the change was the identification of a community group that agreed to provide incentives to students making positive food choices. On the other hand, the lack of school funding for educational intervention programs for obese children was seen as inhibiting change.

The advisory group decided to establish a peer mentoring program, in which student leaders would work with the advisory group and model food choices from all food groups. The advisory group had teachers nominate students for this intervention. The principal allowed the nominated students to attend special educational classes conducted by the nurses to increase their knowledge about the food groups. The nurses worked collaboratively with the students to ensure their teaching approaches were effective. Students suggested rewards that the students could work for that would encourage them to eat more balanced meals. One of the rewards students felt should be offered is sports equipment for student use during recess and lunch periods. One local community-based organization offered to sponsor a fund raising event that would allow them to purchase sports equipment for the school.

Grids similar to that shown in Table 12-4 were developed for the remaining two objectives. This process allowed the nurses and the advisory group to develop program intervention strategies that maximized their potential to achieve desired outcomes. Working

Table 12.4 Predisposing, Enabling, and Reinforcing Factors That Influence Meal Choices of Fifth and Sixth Grade Students Attending Stevens Place Elementary School

Factors That Support the Change	Factors That Inhibit the Change
Predisposing	
Fifth and sixth grade students tend to believe what they are taught by teachers, thus educating them on food choices could positively affect their choices. Fifth and sixth grade students like to be similar to other children their age.	Fifth and sixth grade students are beginning to feel some independence from adults and may like to eat what they want vs. what adults tell them they should do. Students like the taste of sodas and French fries more than balanced food choices.
Reinforcing	
Students emulate behavior of popular students. Teachers and parents are concerned about poor food choices being made by fifth and sixth grade students. Local community leaders expressed outrage about the obesity rates of African American children at Stevens Place Elementary School.	Media shows teens eating French fries and drinking sodas.
Enabling	
A local community-based organization has offered to provide incentives to students who model positive food choices. The principal has offered to allow time for the nurses to work with an identified group of student leaders to educate them about modeling better food choices. The local Parent Teacher Association has offered to help monitor student behavioral changes.	The school has no funding for educational intervention programs for obese children.

with the advisory group, the nurses developed a program plan map outlining activities for each objective, as well as who was responsible for the activity, date by which the activities were to be accomplished, and how outcomes would be documented. Display 12.1 shows the program plan that was developed for the first objective. This type of mapping allows the group to stay focused, share responsibilities, and monitor outcomes. For instance, student leaders were tasked with modeling balanced food choices at breakfast and lunch and completing a checklist of their food choices each day. The nurses were tasked with meeting each week with the student leaders to provide peer mentoring training sessions.

Working with the advisory group allowed the nurses to contextualize the problem about which they were concerned within the target community. The advisory group ensured that the nurses identified solutions that were culturally acceptable, appropriate, and ultimately effective. This process also helped them to develop outcome measures that were consistent with the concerns of the community. As data were gathered, findings could be interpreted with input from the advisory group. This approach grounded the findings and ensured that interpretations were culturally consistent with the target population. Evaluation was facilitated by clearly defined goals that could be measured against actual results.

This particular case study is an example of the program development needed in schools to address obesity and overweight. The *Guide to Community Preventive Services* (2012) systematic review of published school-based programs indicated that more evidence was needed to determine the effectiveness of these types of programs. Although they noted some positive effects in the studies reviewed, the results were too varied to make any conclusions. Their review supports continued efforts to demonstrate program effectiveness in school-based programs. Clear and verifiable outcome measures are needed.

EVALUATION OF OUTCOMES

The IOM report, *The Future of the Public's Health in the 21st Century* (2002), called for examining the benefits of accrediting governmental public health departments (Benjamin, Fallon, Jarris, & Libbey, 2006; IOM, 2002). Responding to this challenge, the Exploring Accreditation Steering Committee published *Final Recommendations for a Voluntary National Accreditation Program for State and Local Public Health Departments* in 2006, outlining this first-ever accreditation program for health departments (Benjamin et al., 2006). The benefits of this program were described as:

- Promoting high performance and continuous quality improvement
- Recognizing high performers that meet nationally accepted standards of quality

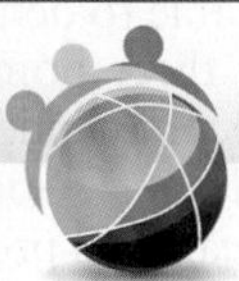

DISPLAY 12.1 SAMPLE PROJECT PLAN MAP

Goal: Fifth and sixth grade students attending Stevens Place Elementary School will engage in behaviors designed to decrease their obesity levels.

Objective	*Activity*	*Who Is Responsible*	*Due Date*	*Evaluation*
1. By the end of the Fall semester, 75% of the fifth and sixth grade students will choose a breakfast and lunch diet that includes fruit, vegetables, protein, dairy, and starch (bread, potatoes) at each meal	1a. Teachers will identify student leaders from the fifth and sixth grade classes who can participate in leadership training for peer mentoring.	1a. J. Jamison, school principal	September 20, 2012	1a. A list of student leaders will be available for review.
	1b. Students will be approached to participate in the program.	1b. J. Jamison, school principal	September 25, 2012	1b. Student response will be documented.
	1c. Permission slips for student leaders to participate will be sent home to parents.	1c. J. Jamison, school principal	September 27, 2012	1c. Copies of permission slips will be maintained by the principal.
	1d. Nurses will meet with the student leaders weekly during the designated time period to provide them training for their peer mentoring.	1d. Nurses	September 28–October 31, 2012	1d. Copies of the meeting notes and educational plans will be maintained by the nurses.
	1e. Student leaders will model balanced food choices during breakfast and lunch meals.	1e. Student leaders	November 1–December 22, 2012	1e. Student leaders will provide a check list of their food choices to the principal at the end of each day.
	1f. A check list of possible food choices for students' breakfast and lunch meals using the school menus will be developed.	1f. Nurses	December 1, 2012	
	1g. PTA volunteers will monitor student food choices during breakfast and lunch meals 1 day each week for 3 weeks.	1g. PTA volunteers	December 3, 12, 17, 2012	1g. Results of checklists will be tabulated and available for review.

- Clarifying the public's expectations of state and local health departments
- Increasing the visibility and public awareness of governmental public health, leading to greater public trust, increased health department credibility and accountability, and ultimately a stronger constituency for public health funding and infrastructure (p. 4)

In 2008, 16 states were selected to "lead a national initiative to advance accreditation efforts and quality improvement strategies in public health departments" (National Network of Public Health Institutes, 2010, p. 1). Areas explored by these states in the initiative included culturally appropriate services, use of health data, and integration of customer service into health programs. Made clear in the IOM report and by the Public Health Accreditation Board (PHAB; incorporated in 2007 to implement and oversee accreditation), this voluntary accreditation program is an effort to assure quality through measurable outcomes and standards of practice in the programs and services provided by both state and local health departments (PHAB, 2012a). With the 2011 publication of the *Guide to National Health Department Accreditation*, health departments are now able to apply for accreditation (PHAB, 2011a). Per the PHAB, accreditation if open to a "governmental entity that has the primary statutory or legal responsibility for public health in a Tribe, state, territory, or at the local level" (2012b, para. 1). Of the 12 standards for accreditation, three are particularly applicable to program development and outcome measurement (PHAB, 2011b):

Domain 4: Engage with the community to identify and address health problems.
Domain 9: Evaluate and continually improve processes, programs, and interventions.
Domain 10: Contribute to and apply the evidence base of public health.

As more agencies seek accreditation, there will likely be increased pressure to achieve this status at all levels (local, county or state) to demonstrate excellence. Public health nurses can work with state and local health departments to achieve accreditation. Accreditation serves not only to promote high-quality services to the public and demonstrate a commitment to meeting the specific needs in these communities but also supports the need for public health nursing services to meet those challenges.

The previous section of this chapter discussed the issues of program planning, implementation, and evaluation as they related to a small health program. This section focuses on the programs and services provided by the agencies. Although the scope of the effort to address outcome evaluation is understandably broader, the concepts are essentially the same. The accreditation initiative has raised the issue of demonstrating in real and objective terms the outcomes resulting from health promotion programs provided through public health agencies. The principles discussed have relevance in many community settings and should be considered whenever health promotion programs and services are provided. Public health nurses are instrumental to many of the health promotion programs and services offered through health departments; their expertise with and understanding of the communities served are invaluable to assuring ongoing quality assurance and outcome evaluation.

Setting Measurable Goals and Objectives

Planned programs should have specific goals to help identify who the program is supposed to serve, what services are provided, the length of time the services are to be provided, and the resources that are needed. Then, measurable objectives are developed that describe the expected outcomes. Use of selected verbs indicates the expected level of achievement, such as "clients will be able to demonstrate safe administration of insulin after three home visits," or "parents will have their infants' recommended immunizations up to date by 24 months of age." Goal setting is imperative when developing an educational program (see Chapter 11) for an entire health program or service. These statements of measurable goals are then examined during the program evaluation. Without such statements, accurate evaluations cannot be conducted.

One helpful acronym, SMART has been attributed to a number of authors since the 1960s including a 1981 publication by G.T. Doran (Morrison, 2010). Regardless of the original source the acronym is frequently used in developing outcome measures. The general consensus is that SMART stands for *S*pecific, *M*easureable, *A*ttainable, *R*elevant, and *T*imely, and often, *E*valuate and *R*eevaluate are added (SMARTER). Display 12.2 describes specific questions that must be asked and answered at each step of the SMART process.

In evaluating programs and care, outcomes must be measured against certain standards. *Standards* are generic guidelines of expected functioning. They can focus on the client, the caregiver, or the organization (finances). All care and services must also be measured against these guidelines. The core standards of care, practice, and finance must be integrated and compatible if they are to ensure quality care.

Evaluating Outcomes

The outcomes or results of care (having the right things happen) are the desired effect of the structure (having the right things) and the processes (doing the right things). The focus on client outcomes demands continued analysis of structure and process, because these two components produce the desirable or undesirable outcomes. With the focus on outcomes, there has been an impetus to include positive outcome terms such as improved health status, functional ability, perceived quality of life, and client satisfaction. Client satisfaction is measured by how closely a client's expectations of nursing care match the perception of the nursing care actually received (Gordon, 1998). Client satisfaction, as one outcome measurement, can be determined by a telephone survey or a mailed questionnaire (Donabedian, 1969) as well as confidential online surveys.

If the responses indicate that a program is meeting its goals, maintaining set standards, and having positive client outcomes and satisfied clients, the program is providing quality care. However, the accuracy of using outcomes as a primary measure of quality care is limited, because some clients have unsatisfactory outcomes despite receiving good care. Factors other than specific health interventions influence outcomes. These factors include a client's adherence to medically prescribed treatments; the progress of chronic or terminal disease beyond the capabilities of medicine, nursing care, or client behaviors; and the client's ability to respond to care as a result of such situations as a compromised immune system. Public health nurses need to keep such factors in mind when evaluating care.

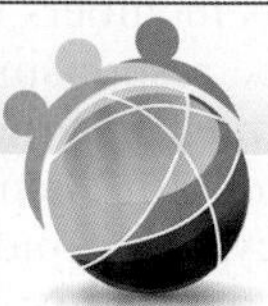

DISPLAY 12.2 DEVELOPING SMART OBJECTIVES

Specific
- What: What do we want to accomplish?
- Why: Specific reasons, purpose, or benefits of accomplishing the goal.
- Who: Who is involved?
- Where: Identify a location.
- Which: Identify requirements and constraints.

Measurable
- How much?
- How many?
- How will we know when it is accomplished?

Attainable
- How can the goal be accomplished?

Relevant
- Does this seem worthwhile?
- Is this the right time?
- Does this match our other efforts/needs?
- Are we the right group or agency?

Time-Bound or Timely
- When?
- What can we do 6 months from now?
- What can we do 6 weeks from now?
- What can we do today?

Sources: Doran, G. T. (1981). There's a S.M.A.R.T. way to write management's goals and objectives. *Management Review (American Management Association Forum), 70*(11) 35–36; Meyer, P. J. (2003). What would you do if you knew you couldn't fail? Creating S.M.A.R.T. Goals. *Attitude is everything: If you want to succeed above and beyond.* Meyer Resource Group, Incorporated; Wikipedia. (2012). *SMART criteria.* Retrieved from ttp://en.wikipedia.org/wiki/SMART_criteria

Quality indicators of client outcomes are the quantitative measures of a client's response to care (Gordon, 1998). Defining and quantifying client outcomes from these indicators are worthwhile processes that enable the nursing staff to evaluate the results of the care they provide. The goal of care in the community is successful client outcomes. By starting with measurable indicators, successful outcomes can be demonstrated in quantifiable terms. When client care meets the standards set, client satisfaction—another quality outcome indicator—is greater.

Quality indicators are part of the broader quality management program and are used to determine goal achievement. A chart audit is a useful method by which to measure the frequency of quality indicator occurrence. For example, an agency may have a quality indicator such as, "all infants younger than 6 months of age are weighed on each home visit." Every fifth chart of infants visited in March, June, September, and December during a designated year is audited for documentation of the number of home visits and the number of infant weights recorded. A sampling of charts is sufficient to measure goal achievement and specific quality indicators. It is generally accepted that a sample of 20 randomly selected cases will provide useful information. If the population to be sampled numbers more than 200, some sources recommend that the sample include more than 20 cases.

Quantifying the indicators also can be accomplished through a rate or ratio of events for a defined population and time frame. Such indicators can be tailored to express almost any patient outcome (Williams, 1991). For example, in Display 12.3, the nursing staff sets a standard for the number of urinary tract infections (UTIs) the agency will tolerate in clients with indwelling urinary catheters (perhaps 5% to 7%, depending

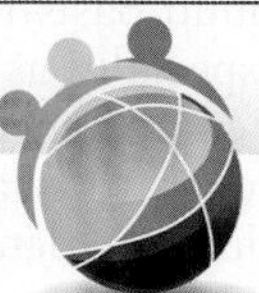

DISPLAY 12.3 QUANTIFYING OUTCOME INDICATORS

$$\text{Outcome indicators} = \frac{\text{Number of patient care events}}{\text{Total number of clients of total number of times at risk for event during a given period}}$$

Example:

$$\begin{array}{l}\text{Occurrence of urinary tract infections in}\\ \text{clients with indwelling urinary catheters}\end{array} = \frac{\begin{array}{c}\text{Number of clients experiencing urinary tract infections related}\\ \text{to long - term use of indwelling urinary catheters from}\\ \text{January 1 to March 1, 2012}\end{array}}{\begin{array}{c}\text{Number of clients with long - term indwelling urinary catheters}\\ \text{from January 1 to March 1, 2012}\end{array}}$$

on client age, diagnosis, family support, and home environment). In another situation, a community/public health nursing service has a standard to make home visits within 5 days of delivery to first-time mothers and babies born at one hospital 95% of the time. To evaluate this goal, the dates of initial home visits to first-time mothers and the birth dates of the infants are measured from a sample of client records during several measurement periods. These are both examples of assessing quality outcome indicators.

It is necessary to have indicators when setting standards in order to measure the success and quality of programs at home or in the community. The same types of indicators are used in acute care settings, with the focus appropriate to that population. If the standards are being met, but client outcomes are unacceptable, the process indicators are explored for possible areas of weakness. Such areas may need further study to identify the cause of the poor client outcomes. For example, a process indicator such as the catheter-care protocol used by an agency or the communication system between hospital and health department nurses may be examined to determine, respectively, the cause of infections or the reason why initial home visits are delayed. In addition, Medicaid and Medicare regulations in some states mandate that a percentage of records be audited each year.

While striving for excellence and best practices, agencies use the benchmarking process. **Benchmarking** uses continuous, collaborative, and systematic processes for measuring and examining internal programs' strengths and weaknesses; benchmarking includes studying another's processes in order to improve one's own (Lewis & Latney, 2002). Internal benchmarking occurs within the organization, between departments or programs. External benchmarking occurs between similar agencies providing like services. For example, a home care agency may have developed a clinical pathway that has proved useful with clients with congestive heart failure; another agency could benefit by using the same clinical pathway. In another example, an agency may use clinical practice guidelines obtained from a specialty organization along with information from a national database; another agency could benefit from this knowledge. In this way, an agency identifies what is achievable while comparing and contrasting how others provide quality services. One example of benchmarking is a descriptive, comparative study of benchmark attainment by maternal and child health clients using the Omaha System (discussed later). This study supported the use of benchmarking to compare both individual progress toward benchmark standards and to assess overall attainment of standards between programs offering similar services (Monsen, Radosevich et al., 2011).

Role of the Nurse in Quality Measurement and Improvement

Although nurses who deliver care directly to clients are not managers, as such, improving quality is a "management" activity, not only of administration personnel, but of the practicing nurses, as members of the team. Public health nurses may not be responsible for a staff or agency budget and functioning, but they may be responsible for managing a caseload of clients with needs of varying degrees of urgency. With judicious use of the resources available, they must provide priority services that promote the highest possible level of personal and group functioning and health. Any activities the public health nurse engages in to realize these goals contribute to the quality management program.

Some quality improvement activities for public health nurses include daily prioritizing of care needs for a caseload of clients, seeking supervision or skills development for a difficult case, systematizing charting so that needed documentation is efficiently completed (e.g., using flow sheets to chart maternal–child health visits), proposing better ways to organize care of chronically ill clients, and establishing new agency procedures. All of these actions demonstrate that nurses are evaluating their work and looking for ways to improve care. Staff meetings, peer review, and case conferences are common settings for nurses to bring the lessons of their practices to the larger group for examination and potential adoption.

It is the role of nursing administration to develop a formalized quality management program that includes a three-pronged focus, based on a classic approach to quality management: (1) review organizational structure, personnel, and environment; (2) focus on standards of nursing care and methods of delivering nursing care (process); and (3) focus on the outcomes of that care (Donabedian, 1985). These formal evaluations include peer review audits (documented care delivered by peers), client satisfaction assessments, review of agency policies and procedures, analysis of demographic information, and the like (ANA, 2007; Issel, 2009; Stubbs & Achat, 2011). The issue of quality and safety has more recently been addressed through the QSEN project (QSEN, 2012). Building on the IOM reports *To Err is Human: Building a Safer Health System* (1999) and *Keeping Patients Safe: Transforming the Work Environment for Nurses* (2004), the project provides a framework for nursing education but also forms a sound basis for community health program evaluation, especially as it relates to professional quality. The QSEN competencies are consistent with the Donabedian approach to quality improvement. The project is discussed in more detail later in this chapter.

Nurses who are new to formal quality improvement activities in the work setting need to recognize the value of these efforts and their part in ensuring that quality care is being delivered. Direct service providers are the best judges of care problems and their potential solutions. For this reason, it is critical that quality assurance reviews and other quality improvement activities focus on issues relevant to staff and client concerns and be structured so that they can be accomplished quickly and with minimal effort. When these activities are clear, concise, and well-integrated into daily routines, they become less time-consuming, and staff members can see the positive client outcomes as rewards for their contributions to the process. Moreover, when health care providers have the opportunity to systematically examine the care they provide, they can generate useful ideas for improving that care and can identify care issues sooner.

Whether small or large, health care agencies are complex organizations with interrelated components. The nursing staff has input into or some control over the quality of care delivered to clients who use the services of the agency. The following paragraphs review the nurse's role in each of the three areas of structure, process, and outcomes.

Structure

The organizational structure and financial stability of the agency should allow the mission statement or philosophy to be realized. The agency should be client-focused, with sufficient resources to maintain present services and introduce additional services as needed. Public agencies need to operate within budget and also have a well-developed system of acquiring additional funding for new services through grants and contract expansion. Private agencies should operate efficiently enough to realize a profit that encourages the owners and boards of directors to continue to support the services. They should look for additional ways to solicit clients, in addition to employing highly motivated and qualified staff.

Process

The agency should maintain standards set by the professional staff that comply with or surpass those recommended by the relevant accrediting bodies. The staff is encouraged to contribute to the evaluation of the standards and to revise them as needed. Staff members need to keep themselves current by attending in-service training sessions and acquiring additional education appropriate to their job requirements. The staff members work collaboratively with others across disciplines to improve the quality of care given in the community by using a variety of participative management tools (e.g., audit instruments, peer review). The agency is supportive of its staff and the needs of individuals. Staff turnover is minimal because employee values are compatible with the goals of the agency. Administration and staff have a compatible working relationship. A system of quality review is in place, and each staff member contributes to this process as a member of a peer review committee or quality improvement or assurance committee. Staff members also listen to clients and provide an outlet to evaluate the care received (e.g., questionnaires, surveys, interviews), and the agency acts on client suggestions and comments.

Outcomes

All services an agency provides should be reviewed periodically to determine whether standards are meeting the present needs of the population and whether the nursing staff are implementing these standards. The nursing services used most frequently, such as well-child care, self-care education with chronically ill adults, and various screening programs, are excellent places to begin the review. Usually, these services involve the entire nursing staff and consume a significant amount of nursing care time.

The focus on commonly served high-risk groups presents an opportunity to optimize care delivery as well as to benefit high-risk clients. Children living in neighborhoods that are known to have high lead toxicity rates from leaded paint in older homes stand to benefit tremendously from a consistently implemented lead screening, treatment, and advocacy program. Without review, such a program may not achieve its goals of decreasing toxic levels of lead in the area's children.

Incidents of poor client outcomes are important areas for further study. Through clinic or home visit records, community nurses can routinely review documentation of deceased or hospitalized clients to assess whether any aspect of the clinic's care or home visit activities might have prevented these occurrences. For instance, the case of a child with repeated high serum lead levels who requires hospitalization for chelation might stimulate a clinic's examination of the adequacy of parent education regarding environmental sources of lead. The clinic could also explore the effectiveness of its advocacy with the area's lead-abatement staff to ensure needed repairs in leaded homes and the removal of families to safe housing while repairs are being made.

As another example, a review of the charts of hospitalized clients who take multiple medications can be conducted to ascertain whether teaching or compliance issues regarding medication contributed to each client's hospitalization. The results may prompt a change in home visit teaching techniques, an increase in the frequency of visits, or a change in vital sign parameters for notifying a physician. Persistence of problems and deficiencies could be a clue that the public health nurse needs additional education in this area or that the nurse's caseload is too heavy and therefore exceeds the ability of the nurse to provide minimally expected care. Once the cause is determined, implementation of appropriate changes can commence, after allowing adequate time for the staff to address critical issues. Should additional education be needed, it is the responsibility of the coordinating, in-service, or staff education nurse to provide or arrange for the needed education.

Given adequate resources, including sufficient time, information, and support, good care is the norm. Occasionally, quality-of-care problems result from an individual provider's performance. Recommendations are made for counseling or another type of intervention by that person's supervisor, and appropriate corrective action should be taken to resolve the problem and preserve the employee's potential contributions as a successful team member.

Identification of quality health care characteristics and "checkpoints" for quality helps the community/public health care practitioner recognize the quality indicators of best practice. These also give public health nurses direction for their role in quality measurement and improvement. This role is grounded in the structure, process, and outcomes of caregiving and services provided.

MODELS USEFUL IN PROGRAM EVALUATION

Models of client caregiving are based on structure, process, and outcome; ideally, they provide *structure* to guide nurses through the *nursing process* to reach desired *client outcomes*. Each of the following models has all three components; some work more effectively than others, depending on the agency and its philosophy.

Donabedian Model

Donabedian (1966, 1969, 1981, 1985, 2002), the country's premier researcher on health care quality, proposed a model for the structure, process, and outcome of quality that has been widely used as the framework for more elaborate models. The care environment structure—from philosophy, to facility resources, to personnel—is the first component. Next are the processes responsible for improving or stabilizing the client's health status, such as standards, attitudes, and effectiveness of tools used in caregiving (e.g., nursing care plans). Finally, the resultant outcomes are causally linked indicators of quality, such as client health care goals and effectiveness of service. The Donabedian model is recognized as a simplistic and basic method of measuring quality. Structure, process, and outcome can be depicted in a box-shaped model (see Fig. 12-1).

Quality Health Outcomes Model

Mitchell, Ferketich, and Jennings (1998) took the time-tested Donabedian model a step further. The Quality Health Outcomes Model includes the client in the model and proposes a two-dimensional relationship among components. Interventions always act through the system and the client, creating a dynamic model. The uniqueness of this model is the postulate that there are "dynamic relationships with indicators that not only act upon, but reciprocally affect the various components" (Mitchell et al., 1998, p. 43). A major criticism of other models is that they do not lend themselves to the population focus of community/public health nursing. However, this model includes community as a client. Figure 12-2 depicts the Quality Health Outcomes Model.

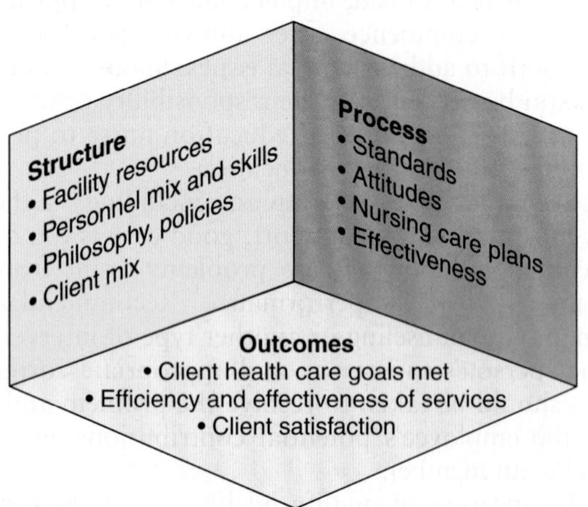

FIGURE 12-1. Structure, process, and outcome of quality model.

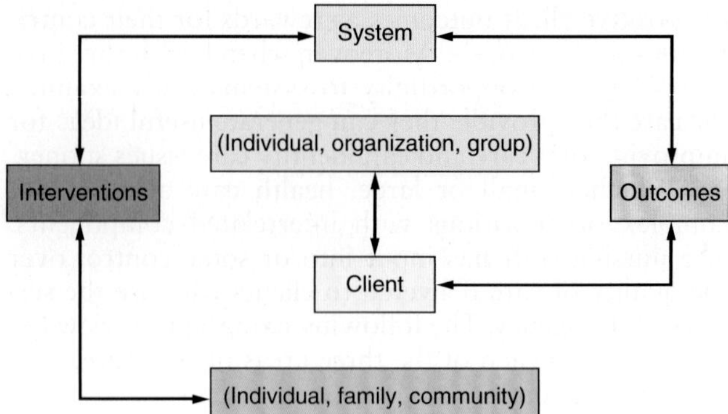

FIGURE 12-2. Quality Health Outcomes Model.

Omaha System

Also discussed in Chapter 14, the Omaha System has measurement approaches that make it a useful model for determining the quality of nursing care provided to individuals, families, and communities. Evaluation focuses on process indicators, client outcome measures, and satisfaction with care (Martin, Leak, & Aden, 1997). With the use of this multifocal approach, measurement of nursing practice becomes comprehensive. Although originally designed to evaluate care to individuals and families, the model has been modified to include the community (Martin, 2005). This revision was prompted by the wider use of the model to document population-based and community-level interventions. The inclusion of community as a modifier is seen as a work in progress, awaiting further research and testing.

Community is defined as "groups, schools, clinics, neighborhoods, or other larger geographic areas that share a common physical environment and ownership of a health-related problem" (Martin, 2005, p. 464). In this model, outcomes are rated in terms of knowledge (what the client knows), behavior (what the client does), and status (how the client is). This approach allows for quantifying a range of severity, as well as progress toward or away from optimal health. Ongoing monitoring of these aspects as they relate to individual, family, or community problems allows for evaluation of nursing interventions—a necessary component of both quality assurance and outcome assessment. For instance, individuals enrolled in a 6-week health promotion program on weight management can be assessed initially for their knowledge of healthy eating and exercise, their current behaviors relative to both, and their current health status (e.g., body mass index [BMI]). The outcome of the program can be assessed by measuring those same indicators and then comparing the initially obtained individual and aggregated data with data collected after the program is concluded. Whereas individual positive changes, such as decreased BMI, are a positive indicator, the impact on the entire group is of even more importance in terms of community-level health status.

The following is a case study exemplifying another use of the Omaha System. A group of county health department public health nurses conducted an assessment of a community's need for a satellite health clinic in a rural part of the county. The nurses gathered data on population needs, age, health status, and accessibility to health care by surveying clients who lived in rural zip code areas and used the main health department. They also conducted a survey by mail of additional residents who were not presently using the health department clinic system for immunizations, screening for tuberculosis or sexually transmitted diseases, or well-baby visits, to see whether these people had unmet needs. After carefully analyzing the data, they began operating three 4-hour clinics during the first week of each month in an empty storeroom of the community pharmacy.

After funding the clinics for 6 months, the health department evaluated the effectiveness of this nursing service. The number of emergency room visits for infants in the area was compared with the number of visits during a similar period before the satellite clinic was established, as was the number of cases of influenza and pneumonia among residents older than 65 years of age. Finally, clients were surveyed in regard to their satisfaction with nursing care and services and were asked if there were any additional services they needed. Survey outcomes were supportive of continuing the clinics and adding an additional well-baby clinic, a dental clinic, and a prenatal clinic. Clients liked the convenience—older residents did not have to drive the 35 miles to the main clinic, parents were able to keep more closely to the recommended schedule for their children's immunizations, and they liked the shorter wait. Follow-up after HIV screening included the formation of an HIV/AIDS support group for clients and families in the rural area, meeting a need that no one had previously identified. The nurses combined clinic responsibilities with home visits in the area on clinic days and were able to do case finding, thus improving the overall health of this rural area.

The nurses were evaluated, and their charts were audited with the use of traditional tools, and clients received the same periodic surveys. Case conferences continued to be held among the nurses serving the rural area, and at times, cases were presented among the larger group of nurses. By utilizing the comprehensive Visiting Nurse Association of Omaha measurement approaches, they met the quality measurement needs of a population. The Omaha System provides an organized method to assess individual-, family-, and community-level health. With ongoing research efforts, the utility of the model with respect to program evaluation will be enhanced. Program evaluation studies such as verifying interrater reliability (Monsen, Lytton et al., 2011), exploring the models utility in nondirect patient interventions by nurse managers (Monsen & Newsom, 2011), and the body of evidence created from this standardized data (Bowles, 2011) continue to support the broader use of the Omaha System to assess programmatic effectiveness.

The Quality Practice Setting Attributes Model

This model, developed by the College of Nurses of Ontario in Canada, provides the foundational framework for a unique quality improvement approach to creating quality practice environments. The College of Nurses of Ontario is the regulatory body for registered nurses and registered practical nurses in the Province of Ontario, Canada; it has functions similar to those of the Board of Registered Nursing in each state in the United States. The Quality Practice Setting Attributes Model is used as a tool to assist in ensuring the quality of nursing practice and the nursing profession by promoting continuing competence among nurses in Canada (MacKay & Risk, 2001). The model provided the framework of the Practice Setting Consultation Program (MacKay & Risk, 2001); later known as the Quality Practice Environment Consultation Program (MacKay, 2007) of the College & Association of Registered Nurses of Alberta (CARNA), The program was developed to "help nurses and agencies identify and cultivate characteristics in their workplace that support quality professional practice" (Brookes & Tansey, 2003).

This nurse-centered model of quality improvement is designed to contribute to the best possible health outcomes for the client, regardless of health care setting. The components of this quality assurance program include reflective nursing practice, practice review, and practice setting consultation. The first two components focus on nurses' individual responsibility for maintaining competence throughout their career; the practice setting consultation focuses on the practice environment in which nursing care is delivered. The governing body for nurses in Ontario, Canada, has relied on the Quality Practice Setting Attributes Model to improve nursing care quality in their province. As mentioned earlier, it also serves as a framework in Alberta (CARNA) in their nursing quality practice program. The model identifies seven key systems attributes in the work environment that create a quality practice setting. Figure 12-3 portrays this model and its components.

Quality and Safety Education For Nurses

As was mentioned earlier, the issue of quality and safety in health care was brought to the public's attention with

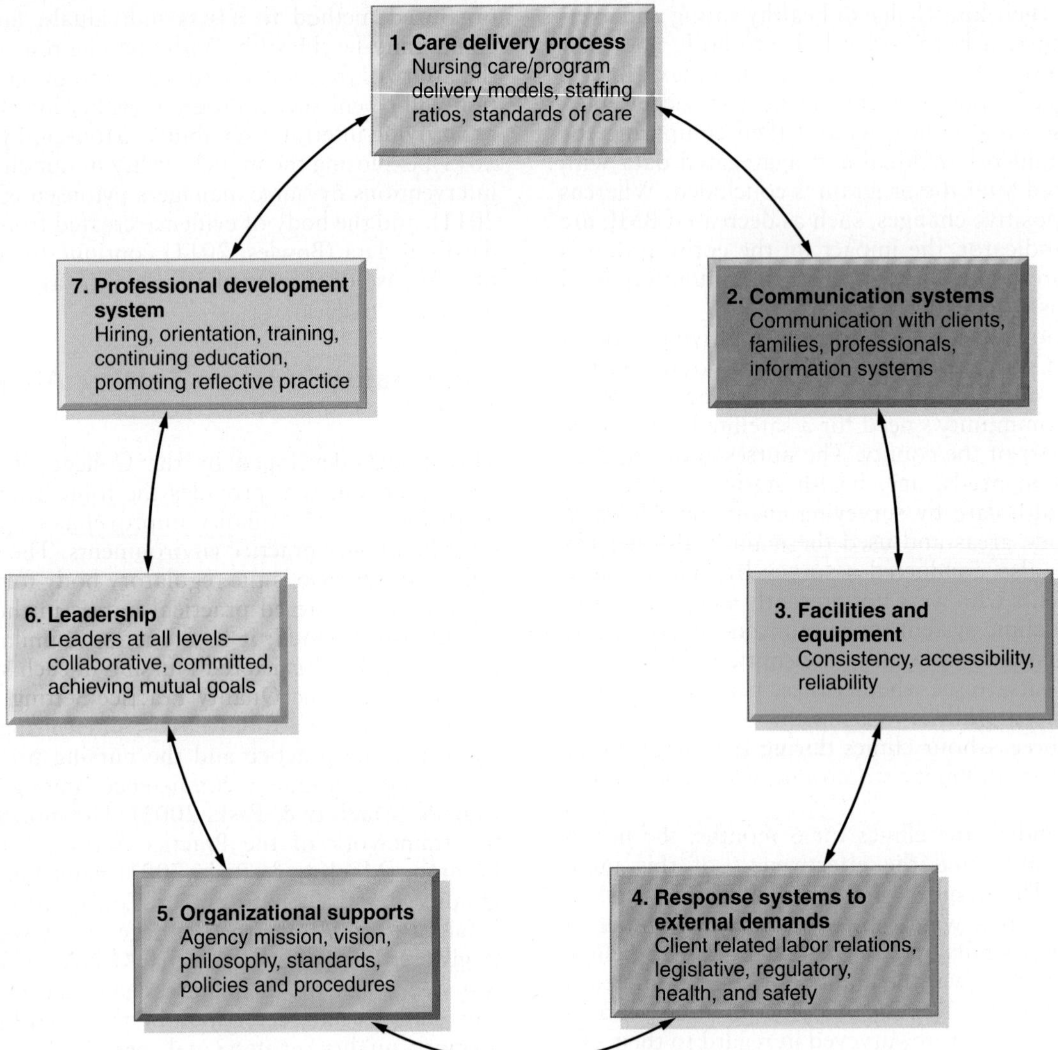

FIGURE 12-3. The Quality Practice Setting Attributes Model.

the groundbreaking 1999 IOM report on medical errors and the subsequent 2004 report that focused on nursing quality and safety. This recognition promoted the funding by the Robert Wood Johnson Foundation of what has become known as the QSEN project. The purpose of the project is "the challenge of preparing future nurses who will have the knowledge, skills and attitudes (KSAs) necessary to continuously improve the quality and safety of the health care systems within which they work" (QSEN, 2012). Although QSEN is not presented in a diagrammatic form, it is nevertheless a model of quality improvement. Consistent with the taxonomy of educational objectives (Bloom, 1956; Krathwohl, 1964; Simpson, 1972) as discussed in Chapter 11, the foundational competencies delineated by KSAs can also be described as falling within the cognitive, psychomotor, and affective domains. The KSAs are also similar to the Omaha System outcome measures of knowledge (what the client knows), behavior (what the client does), and status (how the client is). Specific to QSEN, the prelicensure KSAs include:

- Patient-centered care
- Teamwork and collaboration
- Evidence-based practice
- Quality improvement
- Safety
- Informatics

Of most relevance to community/public health program assessment is quality improvement which is defined as: "use data to monitor the outcomes of care processes and use improvement methods to design and test changes to continuously improve the quality and safety of health care systems" (Cronenwett et al., 2007). The significance to community/public health nursing practice is that the QSEN competencies provide a method of both evaluating individual nurse performance but to use aggregated data to assess programmatic outcomes. The KSAs can be used in all settings that a nurse works, whether hospital, outpatient center, home care, hospice or community/public health nursing services.

SOCIAL MARKETING

Each of the five program evaluation models presented provides a mechanism to plan, implement, and evaluate community-based programs and services. Emphasizing the importance of demonstrating quality through measurable outcomes is a crucial aspect of community health. Health promotion and health education programs must demonstrate achievement of stated goals to justify continuation. Likewise, the overall program, be it a health department or a community-based health center staffed by volunteers, is challenged to demonstrate quality outcomes through ongoing evaluation efforts. Community health services are also challenged to provide programs in ways that reach and engage their target populations. In this section, the role of social marketing is explored as an additional tool for community health care professionals to influence health behaviors and lifestyle choices. These methods must be selected carefully and evaluated against the same standards as previously presented, perhaps more so, due to the potentially higher costs of this type of intervention.

Are you of an age that when you hear the words *"Smoky the Bear,"* your mind finishes the phrase with *"only you can prevent forest fires!"*? Or, perhaps, when you see two golden arches you start craving a hamburger and fries? The ideas that are imbedded in your psyche are all due to marketing. Businesses have long recognized that providing "catchy" advertisements in a way that is memorable to the potential customer is vital to their success. Marketing can literally make or break their business. If the message is effective, they often have more business; if not, they may lose customers. The military has even begun to recognize the effectiveness of these advertising methods, using those same techniques in television and print advertising to increase recruitment. Children as young as 2 years have been found to be "branded" with current fast food items and beverages, meaning they recognize and prefer one particular brand or logo over another. The techniques used by some of these businesses and corporations have in many ways contributed to health issues we currently face as a nation (i.e., obesity in children, teenage smoking).

The public health care sector has only recently begun to recognize the power of marketing health messages. Although used in some capacity since the 1960s, not until the 1990s—when federal agencies, such as the Centers for Disease Control and Prevention (CDC) spearheaded efforts—did it gain the attention it now has in addressing health issues (Andreasen, 2006). The term **social marketing** refers to "influencing the behavior of target audiences" (Andreasen, p. vii). Lotenberg and Siegel go on to explain that in "the public health context, marketing efforts are undertaken to improve societal health, either through influencing changes in health behaviors of individuals, in policies that impact health behaviors, or in perceptions of and support for public health as an institution" (2008, pp. 621–622). The integration of marketing with public health practice is seen as a useful method to increase the effectiveness of public health practitioners (Lotenberg & Siegel, 2008).

Concepts that are important in marketing are applicable to social marketing as well. The following concepts are outlined by Lotenberg and Siegel (2008):

- Exchange: An individual gives something to get something; the person weighs the cost and the perceived benefits.
- Self-interest: People act in their own interests in most cases.
- Behavior change: Change in behavior is the focus; thoughts and ideas may also need to change but are not the ultimate goal.
- Competition: Selecting one option (or action) inherently involves giving up another option (or action).
- Consumer orientation: Problem-solving process is directed at the target—the consumer (could be an individual, group, or organization).
- Product, price, place, and promotion: Also called the marketing mix; each can be altered to increase market share.
- Partners and policy: Other organizations that share similar interests and could provide opportunities to work together; identification of policy changes necessary for behavioral change, those supportive of the change, and those that the organization could help influence.

These principles seem rather straightforward, yet public health practitioners are often at a disadvantage when attempting to implement social marketing campaigns (Lotenberg & Siegel, 2008). They often lack training in the necessary skills, may be outspent by the competition (e.g., the fast food industry), or have limited access for the distribution of their message (e.g., public service announcements). One example of a very successful social marketing campaign is the *Go Red for Women* initiative begun in 2004 by the American Heart Association (2012). Using a red dress as the symbol of the program, the initiative seeks to raise awareness of heart disease among women. Another less well-known campaign was the American Cancer Society's *Polyp Man* campaign, designed to bring awareness to the need for colon cancer screening. The 2002 campaign featured the funny little polyp-shaped man with the line: "Get the test, get the polyp, get the cure" (Cohen & Falco, 2002). These health issues are equally important, but one has a more broadly recognized campaign; the other was humorous but not necessarily well received. Ultimately, the issue is whether or not behaviors have been changed and health outcomes improved as a result of these social marketing campaigns. Time will be the judge of all these efforts.

One international example of social marketing was an effort to increase consumption of iron-fortified soy sauce among women in China (Sun, Guo, Wang, & Sun, 2007). Nearly 400 women living in both urban and rural areas of Guizhou province participated in this study. Using the marketing techniques of product, price, place, promotion, policy, and partnership, they demonstrated that mass media campaigns can be effective. In the study, availability of the iron-fortified soy sauce increased in all areas, and purchases were increased by nearly 30% more in the intervention groups as compared to the control groups. The researchers point to the feasibility of the campaign and the impact it had on knowledge, intention to purchase, and actual consumption as justification for use of other mass media campaigns. For health care providers, use of mass media is an option, but for cost reasons, it is not always practical.

Cates, Otiz, Shafer, Romocki, and Coyne-Beasley (2012) reported on a qualitative study to explore messaging that was most effective in promoting vaccination for human papillomavirus (HPV) of preteen age boys. Focus groups of parents were conducted and transcripts coded using a constant comparison method to interpret themes. While the parents knew little about HPV and the vaccine, they supported vaccination of their children, yet did express concern about safety and cost. From a social marketing perspective, the messages that were most motivating focused on infection risk and those that included images of the parents with their sons, providing a visual and more personal link to the parental role (Cates et al., 2012). This study exemplifies the importance of framing health-related messages in a manner that is appealing, relevant to the situation, and acceptable to the audience.

How can social marketing principles be utilized when you have a limited budget, limited time, and limited creativity? University campuses hold a wealth of oft-untapped expertise. For nursing students working on a health promotion program, the substance of the effort (the health issue) is often pretty straightforward, but the presentation is more challenging. Many schools of nursing are providing collaborative experiences for students, supporting partnering with nonnursing students and faculty in addressing health education needs. The following is one example of how collaboration can be effective: Two nursing students recognized that off-campus housing lacked sufficient smoke detectors due to a "loophole" in state and local building codes. This meant that students living in the most high-risk housing for fires (older buildings) might only have one smoke detector in the entire apartment; this was clearly inadequate. After discussing the issue with their faculty member, they sought input from several student organizations. From those discussions, they identified a low level of knowledge about the issue and modest concern by the students present. Recognizing that college students are not prone to worrying about how many smoke detectors they have, the nursing students sought help from the university housing department. The staff of housing agreed that this was an important issue, and they were willing to post information on the housing Web site regarding the need to install additional smoke detectors. The students didn't know how to develop online materials, but based on input from the student groups, they knew that it had to be eye-catching and quickly present a message. In conjunction with their faculty advisor, they contacted the graphic arts department and found an instructor who was willing to include the development of an online smoke detector campaign as part of a class assignment. The nursing students provided the educational information that needed to be included, and the graphic arts students proceeded to develop a campaign within those parameters. In the end, several outstanding examples were submitted, and one was selected and posted on the housing Web site. The campaign was particularly effective with parents who saw the campaign on the Web site as they helped in apartment searches. Many messages were sent to the Web site by the parents regarding the campaign, and the responses were handled by the nursing students. The campaign was not expensive, identified the most skilled individuals for each task (health information: nursing students; Web-based campaign: graphic arts students), and provided much-needed health and safety information to the university students and their parents. Even though they had targeted the college students, the nursing students found that the parents were much more interested in the campaign. The results of this initial effort provided vital information for future campaigns that might target parents, students, apartment management, and the local building code enforcement office.

When planning for and beginning development of a social marketing approach, there are many resources available to the public health nurse and other public health professionals. The CDC offers an excellent Web site that includes links to a wide variety of resources as well as the *Social Marketing for Nutrition and Physical Activity Web Course* available through the Division of Nutrition, Physical Activity, and Obesity (CDC, 2011). Another very helpful publication is *Using Social Media Platforms to Amplify Public Health Messages* (Oglivy Public Relations Worldwide & the Center for Social Impact Communication, 2010).

Social marketing is not a panacea, but it does provide techniques that can support health education and health promotion programs. The method can be very expensive and very elaborate, or it can provide simple, straightforward messages. The point is that well-presented marketing can be the difference in whether behavior changes are made or not. Media messages are not a replacement for a sound health promotion program; they are just one tool that can be used for great impact.

GRANTS

Grants are a reality in public health efforts. They are not easy to locate, easy to secure, or easy to manage once you have one, but they are vital to providing a wide range of programs and services in the community. Many local and county health departments see them as an integral part of their service delivery, even hiring grant writers and grant managers in some cases. For most health departments, community agencies, and volunteer service providers, the task of locating grant funds, writing the grant application, and doing the work stipulated by the grant all falls on the nurses and other professionals within those agencies. On the positive side, it provides an opportunity for community health nurses to explain to others what they can provide to the community in terms of services and programs targeting the community's health. Some basic knowledge about grants can demystify the topic.

Even if you aren't ever required to write a grant, you will likely be involved in some part of a programmatic grant at some point in your career, either in the delivery of services stipulated by the grant (product) or in evaluating the outcomes of the services provided (i.e., satisfaction surveys). You may even be asked to provide ideas for specific services to be included in the grant application; take advantage of these opportunities. The experience you gain will enhance your knowledge of the process and may prove instrumental in future efforts you may be involved with. The grant process, although arduous, provides the opportunity to focus clearly on what you intend to accomplish, why it is needed, and what part you will play in the successful outcome of the project. This is similar to a job interview, in which your prospective employer asks you *"Why should we hire you? What will you contribute to this organization?"* You have a limited amount of time to express your worth. You have to be very specific and concise about what you and your organization or group will be doing to address a specific need. You are making the case that providing you with support is the best choice.

What exactly is a grant? A **grant** is, very simply, one individual or group providing another individual or group the support (i.e., money) for a specified purpose. In health promotion and education, it generally means funding for program development or project support. These types of grants fall into the following common categories: planning grants (i.e., initial project development), start-up grants (i.e., seed money), management or technical assistance grants (e.g., for fund raising or marketing), and facilities or equipment grants (e.g., money for a building, computer, or van) (Minnesota Council on Foundations, 2010). This money doesn't typically need to be paid back; however, it is a contractual agreement, and the terms and conditions are usually clearly delineated. For federal grants, the following definition applies: "award of financial assistance from a federal agency to a recipient to carry out a public purpose of support or stimulation authorized by a law of the United States" (Grants.gov, 2012). Federal grants are available from 26 grant-making agencies. The funding categories most applicable to community health include community development, disaster preparation and relief, food and nutrition, and health. Federal grants are available to a wide variety of groups, but typically, health-related grants are available to state or local governments, which include public health departments, public housing organizations, educational organizations, and nonprofit organizations.

What is a *nonprofit organization*? Nonprofit means that the organization was not established to earn a profit. This does not mean that it doesn't generate income, only that there are restrictions on how those funds can be used. Of particular importance to the discussion of grants is the term *501c3*. This is a designation that refers to the Internal Revenue Service (IRS) tax-exempt status granted to certain nonprofit organizations. To be granted this designation, an organization must be organized and operated exclusively for specific purposes, which include charity, science, education, or the prevention of cruelty to children or animals (IRS—Department of the Treasury, 2011). Some grants are only available to 501c3 organizations, and the funders will request proof of this in the grant application. Only corporations, community chests, funds, or foundations can receive this designation; individuals or partnerships do not qualify (IRS, 2011). Essentially, the 501c3 organization can be the provider of the grant funding or the organization seeking the funding.

Grants are available from government sources, private philanthropic sources, and corporations. Federal grants can be found on the Web site www.grants.gov or on individual federal agency Web sites. Private organizations often have sections on their Web sites with information on available grant funding. This is likewise the case with corporations. This broad search approach is not a terribly effective way to find grants; to improve search efficiency, a number of proprietary grant-locating programs are available. These programs are very expensive and, because of cost considerations, often are licensed only to large organizations, such as universities and medical centers. They allow the user the ability to limit the search (e.g., type of funder, health issue, age group, program or research grant, funding limits, and time frame for submission). For the small nonprofit organization seeking funding, one effective approach is to partner with a local university, which allows for more access to grant-locating programs, as well as the expertise offered on the campuses (e.g., content area experts, experienced researchers, statisticians, business plan experts). In a discussion of academic/community partnerships, Chorpita and Mueller (2008) caution that these relationships can be complicated and "projects should be based on a win-win-win proposition, in which consumers, researchers, and service agencies all stand to benefit" (pp. 144–145). Sieber (2008) notes that "productive collaboration requires long-term commitment by the academic researcher despite all the conditions that make this difficult" (p. 137). The community organization and the academic institution both stand to gain from these types of arrangements as do, of course, the target populations.

Some grant funders allow letters of inquiry to be submitted prior to an actual full grant application. The letter of inquiry may be by invitation-only or be part of the original advertisement of the grant funding. In any case, this letter is normally only two or three pages in length and includes a concise overview of the project. For example, a **letter of inquiry** would likely include an overview of your organization and its purpose, the reason for the funding request, clearly stated need or problem to be addressed, overview of the proposed project or program, and other funding sources for your project or program (prospective and committed) (National Service-Learning Clearinghouse, 2012). This letter is brief, yet clearly lays out your plan. Your goal is to be invited to submit a full proposal for consideration. If this approach is successful, you will be asked to complete the organization's application process (the proposal), which can vary in length and complexity depending on the organization.

Crucial to either the letter of inquiry or the full proposal is that you have selected a funder that is a good match for your organization and your program/project. For instance, applying to a faith-based organization that supports abstinence-only educational programs would not be a good fit for your program to provide contraceptive information in an after-school program for teens. Before you spend valuable time and energy writing a letter of inquiry or a grant application, be sure to do your homework. The Internet provides a quick method for reviewing potential funders, their vision, mission, and types of previous funding. You may even be able to find out the monetary range of grants funded by the organization. Perhaps you have a small grant request and find that the organization you are reviewing only funds large multimillion-dollar projects; it might be best to look for other options. The Web site will likely have contact information; making a phone call can assure you that this organization is a good match for your project and can give you an opportunity to start building a relationship with their staff.

Grants are most often competitive—which means you can expect to have competition from other deserving groups—so be prepared. A well-prepared grant—one that carefully follows the application guidelines specified in the request for proposals (RFPs) and very clearly describes the program you are seeking support for—is more likely to be funded. The **request for proposals (RFPs)** outlines the specific requirements of the application, the information to include and in what order, and what supplemental forms to include, if any. Submitting a grant after the deadline and not including all required items will mean that your grant application is not likely to be reviewed. If your grant is not selected, make certain to contact the funder to see if they will provide you with a review of your submission; this is common with government-sponsored grants. With knowledge of what hampered your selection, you will be in a much better position to resubmit to this funding source again, or to be more prepared for other grant opportunities. Another suggestion for new grant writers is to seek the help of an experienced mentor—someone who has been successful in grant writing—as they can critique your proposal prior to submission and offer suggestions.

The following tips may be helpful as you begin the process of seeking grant funding (Corporation for Public Broadcasting, 2012):

1. Define your project:
   - Clarify the purpose of your project and write a concise mission statement.
   - Define the scope of work to focus your funding search.
   - Determine the broad project goals, then identify the specific objectives that define how you will focus the work to accomplish those goals.
2. Identify the right funding sources.
3. Contact the funders; think of the funder as a resource.
4. Acquire proposal guidelines.
5. Know the submission deadline.
6. Determine personnel needs.
7. Update your timeline.

One reality of grant funding is that experience counts. If you have a proven record in securing grants and completing the requirements specified in those grants, you or your organization will have an easier time securing additional funding. For the new grant seeker, this can be a bit discouraging. So, where to begin? Don't start with the most complicated grants available. Look for small local grants with a proven track record in grant management, and build your reputation. Work with partners. A school of nursing could partner with a home health agency to write a grant to provide worksite wellness programs for uninsured agricultural workers. Or, several faith-community groups could partner in a grant application to provide free health screenings for uninsured adults in their area. Finally, be certain that the grant will allow you to meet the mission and goals of your program. The grant funder will also be looking to see if their support will enable you to provide a service that you have both the skill and expertise to accomplish. With limited funds available, funders are looking for proof of the sustainability of your program after their support ends. For instance, a breastfeeding support program sought funding in a high-risk area where there was a clear need. Although the need was demonstrated, the agency had no plan for continuing the program after the funding ended; they did not receive funding. Grant support is often seen as funding to get programs started—not to provide for long-term operations.

Many courses are available to assist you in understanding how to locate grants, write them, and be successful in your attempts. Your local library is another source of information, and a wide variety of information is available on the Internet. Some examples of helpful Web sites are included in the Internet Resources found on thePoint.

SUMMARY

Successful community health programs require that the nurse listen to the target population and not determine the problem and solution without their assistance. Awareness of predisposing, reinforcing, and enabling factors facilitates the assessment of health-related behaviors. Importance and changeability are important considerations when determining priorities among competing behavioral targets. An advisory group, with representation from the target and service communities, is an effective tool in helping to identify the problem, select appropriate interventions to address the problem, and evaluate the outcomes of the interventions chosen. Outcome measures should be consistent with the concerns of the community. Evaluation can be facilitated by clearly defined goals that can be measured against actual results.

The multiple models or frameworks on which quality management systems are based include a classic way of looking at programs through organizational structure, process, and outcomes, along with the interrelatedness of each component. The five models presented in this chapter are structured in unique ways that enable them to meet the differing needs of community agencies. Whether quality measurement and improvement techniques are formally or informally practiced, whenever nurses monitor, assess, and judge the quality and appropriateness of care as measured against professional standards, the interests of clients are being served.

Social marketing is one tool that can enhance health promotion efforts in the community. Media messages are particularly helpful in reaching large audiences. The basis of social marketing is similar to product marketing to consumers. The goal of consumer marketing is not necessarily to change the way people think, but the way they behave. Social marketing seeks to first change behavior and then to influence how people think about health, lifestyle, and the choices they make every day that influence their health. One example of social marketing is the American Heart Association *Go Red for Women* campaign, which seeks to bring attention to heart disease risk among women. Social marketing, like any consumer-focused marketing, must consider the target population in the design, implementation, and evaluation of the effort. Successful outcomes are imperative for continuation of this type of program, as with any other health promotion campaign.

Grants are increasingly vital to providing health promotion programs and services in the community. Community health nurses frequently are involved in some aspect of a grant program, whether in the writing, implementation of the program or services stipulated in the grant, or in the evaluation of the outcomes for the grant. Grants are available from government sources, private philanthropic sources, and corporations. Successful grant proposals comply with the instructions provided in the RFPs. Community agencies and academic programs can collaborate in providing community services and evaluation research that seeks to improve the lives of the target population. Mastering the grant process, from formulating the goal to defining the evaluation methods, is a skill that can benefit all manner of health promotion programs, whether funded or not.

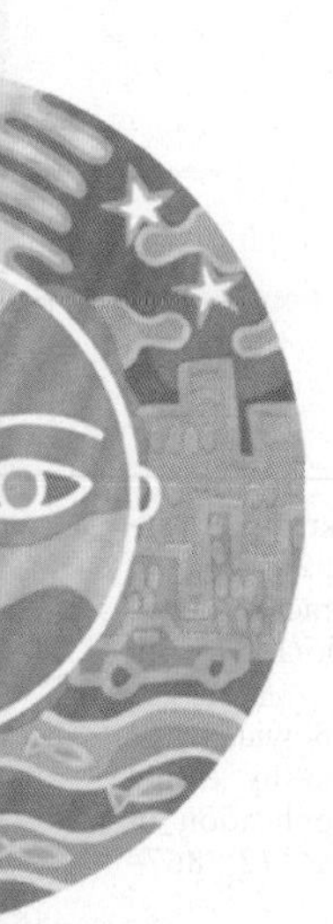

Community/public health nurses are in a key position to plan, implement, and evaluate all types of health promotion/health education programs. Knowledge of the target population and engaging the target population in determining the problem and solutions is vital to successful outcomes. Ongoing use of quality measurement techniques and application of recognized professional standards helps assure effective and appropriate service delivery. Social marketing is a tool that can be effective in reaching large audiences with valuable health messages. Finally, the skills gained in working on any portion of a grant effort can be utilized in future programmatic efforts, whether supported through funding or not.

ACTIVITIES TO PROMOTE **CRITICAL THINKING**

1. A group of student PHNs are approached by a faculty member who teaches acute care nursing. She informs them that there is a high incidence of chlamydia infection in a local community among Spanish-speaking people. The hospital where she has students wants to do something to reduce the incidence of chlamydia. The faculty member has found a pamphlet online that describes chlamydia infection, how it's diagnosed, and how it's treated. She thinks it would be a wonderful idea for the student PHNs to translate the pamphlet into Spanish.
   - **a.** Is this the appropriate intervention?
   - **b.** What data should be gathered? What literature should be reviewed?
   - **c.** What agencies, organizations, and groups should the students contact?
   - **d.** Who is the target population?
   - **e.** What outreach should be done with this population? What information should be gathered from the population prior to developing any educational materials?
   - **f.** What steps should the students take to ensure that the target population finds the educational materials they develop to be appropriate, acceptable, and understandable?
2. A school nurse works in a rural agricultural community. The main crop is rice. Every year after harvesting the rice, the local farmers burn their rice fields. The school nurse notes a significant increase in absences during this period for respiratory problems, especially asthma. She notes that even the teachers have increasing respiratory problems. She believes that the respiratory problems are aggravated by the burning rice fields. She mentions her concerns about the relationship between the fields burning and increased respiratory-related illnesses to the school principal. He responds that while it may be true, the local farmers control the local community—without them, the community would collapse. He states that kids and adults will just have to adjust.
   - **a.** What can the nurse do to find out if the burning rice fields are a threat to the health of children and adults in the local area? (What data should be gathered, what literature should be reviewed, to whom should she talk?)
   - **b.** What steps should she take to increase interest in addressing this problem?
   - **c.** What agencies, organizations, and groups should she contact?
3. Identify a health-related social marketing campaign that you viewed recently on the television or in a store or billboard advertisement. Has this campaign effectively reached out to the target audience?

REFERENCES

American Heart Association. (2012). *Go Red for Women: About the movement*. Retrieved from http://www.goredforwomen.org/about_the_movement.aspx

American Nurses Association. (2007). *Public health nursing: Scope and standards of practice*. Silver Spring, MD: Nursesbooks.org.

Andreasen (2006). *Social marketing in the 21st century*. Thousand Oaks, CA: Sage.

Benjamin, G., Fallon, M., Jarris, P. E., & Libbey, P. M. (2006). *Final recommendations for a voluntary national accreditation program for state and local public health departments*. Retrieved from http://www.rwjf.org/pr/product.jsp?id=23495

Bloom, B. S. (1956). *Taxonomy of educational objectives: Handbook I. Cognitive domain*. New York, NY: D. McKay.

Bowles, K. H. (2011). Achieving meaningful use with standardized data. *Online Journal of Nursing Informatics, 15*(2). Retrieved from http://ojni.org/issues/?p=574

Brookes, N. L., & Tansey, M. R. (2003). Visionary leadership in psychiatric and mental health nursing. Presented at the *2003 Sigma Theta Tau International Biennial Convention*. Abstract retrieved from http://www.nursinglibrary.org/vhl/handle/10755/148157?mode=full&submit_simple=Show+full+item+record

Buta, B., Brewer, L., Hamlin, D. L., Palmer, M. W., Bowie, J., & Gielen, A. (2011). An innovative faith-based healthy eating program: From class assignment to real-world application of PRECEDE/PROCEED. *Health Promotion Practice, 12*, 867–875. doi: 0.1177/1524839910370424

Cates, J. R., Ortiz, R., Shafer, A., Romocki, L. S., & Coyne-Beasley, T. (2012). Designing messages to motivate parents to get their preteenage sons vaccinated against human papillomavirus. *Perspectives on Sexual and Reproductive Health, 44*(1), 39–47. doi: 10.1363/4403912

Centers for Disease Control and Health Promotion. (2011). *Social marketing resources*. Retrieved from http://www.cdc.gov/nccdphp/DNPAO/socialmarketing/index.html

Chorpita, B. F., & Mueller, C. W. (2008). Toward new models for research, community, and consumer partnerships: Some guiding principles and an illustration. *Clinical Psychology: Science & Practice, 15*, 144–148.

Cohen, E., & Faleo, M. (2002, January 30). American Cancer Society: Ad campaign uses humor to fight colon cancer. *CNN Health. Turner Broadcasting System, Inc*. Retrieved from http://articles.cnn.com/2002-01-30/health/polyp.man.ad_1_colon-cancer-american-cancer-society-ads?_s=PM:HEALTH

Corporation for Public Broadcasting. (2012). *Grant proposal writing tips*. Retrieved from *http://www.cpb.org/grants/grantwriting.html*

Cronenwett, L., Sherwood, G., Barnsteiner, J., Disch, J., Johnson, J., Mitchell, P., et al. (2007). Quality and safety education for nurses. *Nursing Outlook, 55*(3), 122–131. doi: 10.1016/j.outlook.2007.02.006

Donabedian, A. (1966). Evaluating the quality of medical care. *Milbank Memorial Fund Quarterly, 44*, 166–206.

Donabedian, A. (1969). Medical care appraisal: Quality and utilization. In *Guide to medical care administration*. New York, NY: American Public Health Association.

Donabedian, A. (1981). *The criteria and standards of quality*. Ann Arbor, MI: Health Administration Press.

Donabedian, A. (1985). *Explorations in quality assessment and monitoring* (Vol. 3). Ann Arbor, MI: Health Administration Press.

Donabedian, A. (2002). *An introduction to quality assurance in health care*. New York: Oxford University Press.

Doran, G.T. (1981). There's a S.M.A.R.T. way to write management's goals and objectives. *Management Review (American Management Association Forum), 70*(11), 35–36.

Gordon, M. (1998, September 30). Nursing nomenclature and classification system development. *Online Journal of Issues in Nursing, 3*(2). Retrieved from http://www.nursingworld.org/MainMenuCategories/ANAMarketplace/ANAPeriodicals/OJIN/TableofContents/Vol31998/No2Sept1998/NomenclatureandClassification.html

Grants.gov. (2012). *Who is eligible for a grant?* Retrieved from http://www.grants.gov/aboutgrants/eligibility.jsp

Green, L. W., & Kreuter, M. W. (1999). *Health program planning: An educational and environmental approach* (3rd ed.). Mountain View, CA: Mayfield Publishing Company.

Green, L. W., & Kreuter, M. W. (2005). *Health program planning: An educational and ecological approach* (4th ed.). New York, NY: McGraw-Hill.

Guide to Community Preventive Services. (2012). *The community guide: What works to promote health*. Retrieved from http://www.thecommunityguide.org/index.html

Hedderson, M. M., Darbinian, J. A., & Ferrara, A. (2010). Disparities in the risk of gestational diabetes by race-ethnicity and country of birth. *Paediatric and Perinatal Epidemiology, 25*(5), 441–448. doi: 10.1111/j.1365-3016.2010.01140.x

Institute of Medicine. (1999). *To err is human: Building a safer health system*. Washington, DC: National Academies Press.

Institute of Medicine. (2002). *The future of the public's health in the 21st century*. Washington, DC: National Academies Press.

Institute of Medicine. (2003). *Health professions education: A bridge to quality*. Washington, DC: National Academies Press.

Institute of Medicine. (2004). *Keep patients safe: Transforming the work environment of nurses*. Washington, DC: National Academies Press.

Institute of Medicine. (2010). *The future of nursing: Leading change, advancing health*. Washington, DC: National Academies Press.

Institute of Medicine. (2012). *For the public's health: Investing in a healthier future*. Washington, DC: National Academies Press.

Internal Revenue Service—Department of the Treasury. (2011). *Tax-exempt status for your organization*. Retrieved from http://www.irs.gov/publications/p557/index.html

Issel, L. M. (2009). *Health program planning and evaluation: A practical, systematic approach for community health* (2nd ed.). Burlington, MA: Jones and Bartlett.

Krathwohl, D. R. (1964). *Taxonomy of educational objectives: Handbook II. Affective domain*. New York, NY: D. McKay.

Lavery, S. H., Smith, M. L., Esparza, A. A., Hrushow, A., Moore, M., & Reed, D. F. (2005). The community action model: A community-driven model designed to address disparities in health. *American Journal of Public Health, 95*, 611–616. doi:10.2105/AJPH.2004.047704

Lewis, P. S., & Latney, C. (2002). Achieve best practice with an evidence-based approach. *Nursing Management, 33*(12), 24–30.

Lotenberg, L. D., & Siegel, M. (2008). Using marketing in public health. In L. F. Novick, C. B. Morrow, & G. P. Mays (Eds.). *Public health administration: Principles for population-based management* (2nd ed., pp. 621–656). Sudbury, MA: Jones & Bartlett Publishers.

MacKay, S. A. (2007). *President's update*. Alberta RN, 63(1). Retrieved from http://nurses.ab.ca/carna-admin/Uploads/AB_RN_jan_07_web.pdf

MacKay, G., & Risk, M. (2001). Building quality practice settings: An attributes model. *Canadian Journal of Nursing Leadership, 14*(3), 19–27.

Martin, K. S. (2005). *The Omaha System: A key to practice, documentation, and information management* (Reprinted 2nd ed.). Omaha, NE: Health Connections Press.

Martin, K., Leak, G., & Aden, C. (1997). The Omaha system: A research-based model for decision making. In B. W. Spradley, & J. A. Allender (Eds.). *Readings in community health nursing* (5th ed., pp. 316–324). Philadelphia, PA: Lippincott-Raven.

Minnesota Council on Foundations. (2010). *Common types of grants*. Retrieved from http://www.mcf.org/nonprofits/common-types-of-grants

Mitchell, P. H., Ferketich, S., & Jennings, B. M. (1998). Quality health care outcomes model. *Image: Journal of Nursing Scholarship, 30*, 43–46.

Monsen, K. A., Lytton, A. B., Ferrari, S., Halder, K. M., Radosevich, D. M., Kerr, M. J., et al. (2011). Evaluating reliability of assessments in nursing documentation. *Online Journal of Nursing Informatics, 15*(3). Retrieved from http://ojni.org/issues/?p=899

Monsen, K. A., & Newsom, E. T. (2011). Feasibility of using the Omaha System to represent public health nurse manager interventions. *Public Health Nursing, 28*, 421–428. doi: 10.1111/j.1525-1446.2010.00926.x

Monsen, K. A., Radosevich, D. M., Johnson, S. C., Farri, O., Kerr, M. J., & Geppert, J. S. (2011). Benchmark attainment by maternal and child health clients across public health nursing agencies. *Public Health Nursing, 29*, 11–18. doi: 10.1111/j.1525-1446.2011.00967.x

Morrison, M. (2010). *History of SMART objectives. Introduction to SMART objectives and SMART goals*. Retrieved from http://rapidbi.com/history-of-smart-objectives/

National Network of Public Health Institutes. (2010). *Multi-state Learning Collaborative: Lead states in public health quality improvement*. Retrieved from http://www.nnphi.org/program-areas/accreditation-and-performance-improvement/multi-state-learning-collaborative

National Service-Learning Clearinghouse. (2012). *Grant-writing tools for non-profit organizations*. Retrieved from http://www.servicelearning.org/funding_source/non-profit-guides-grant-writing-tools-non-profit-organizations

Oglivy Public Relations Worldwide & the Center for Social Impact Communication. (2010). *Using social media platforms to amplify public health messages: An examination of tenets and best practices for communicating with key audiences*. Retrieved from http://csic.georgetown.edu/involved/fellowships/188086.html

Ottoson, J. M., & Green, L. W. (2008). Public health education and health promotion. In L.F. Novick, C. B. Morrow, & G. P. Mays (Eds.). *Public health administration: Principles for population-based management* (2nd ed., pp. 589–619). Sudbury, MA: Jones & Bartlett Publishers.

Public Health Accreditation Board. (2011a). *Guide to national public health department accreditation*. Retrieved from http://www.phaboard.org/accreditation-process/guide-to-national-public-health-accreditation/

Public Health Accreditation Board. (2011b). *Standards: An overview.* Retrieved from http://www.phaboard.org/wp-content/uploads/PHAB-Standards-Overview-Version-1.0.pdf

Public Health Accreditation Board. (2012a). *Public health department accreditation background.* Retrieved from http://www.phaboard.org/about-phab/public-health-accreditation-background/

Public Health Accreditation Board. (2012b). *Who is eligible?* Retrieved from *http://www.phaboard.org/accreditation-overview/who-is-eligible/*

Public Health Partners. (2012). *Statistical Information by Subject. Geographic Information Systems (GIS).* Retrieved from http://phpartners.org/tutorial/03-hs/3-sources/3.3.6.html

Quality and Safety Education for Nurses. (2012). *Competency KSAs (pre-licensure).* Retrieved from http://www.qsen.org/

Sargent, C. F., & Davis-Floyd, R. E. (1997). *Childbirth and authoritative knowledge: Cross cultural perspectives.* Berkeley, CA: University of California Press.

Sieber, J. E. (2008). When academicians collaborate with community agencies in effectiveness research. *Clinical Psychology: Science & Practice, 15*, 137–143.

Simpson, E. J. (1972). *The classification of educational objectives in the psychomotor domain.* Washington, DC: Gryphon House.

Stubbs, J. M., & Achat, H. M. (2011). Monitoring and evaluation of a large-scale community-based program: Recommendations for overcoming barriers to structured implementation. *Contemporary Nurse, 37*(2), 188–196.

Sun, X., Guo, Y., Wang, S., & Sun, J. (2007). Social marketing improved the consumption of iron-fortified soy sauce among women in China. *Journal of Nutrition Education & Behavior*, 39, 302–310.

U.S. Department of Health and Human Services. (2010). *Healthy People 2020: Improving the health of Americans.* Retrieved from http://www.healthypeople.gov/2020/default.aspx

U.S. Department of Health and Human Services. National Diabetes Information Clearinghouse. (2011). *National diabetes Statistics, 2011. Gestational diabetes in the United States.* Retrieved from *http://diabetes.niddk.nih.gov/dm/pubs/statistics/#Gestational.*

Williams, A. D. (1991). Development and application of clinical indicators for nursing. *Journal of Nursing Care Quality, 6*(1), 1–5.

Zlotnick, C., Wright, M., Sanchez, R. M., Kusnir, R. M., & Te'o-Bennett, I. (2010). Adaptation of a community-based participatory research model to gain community input on identifying indicators of successful parenting. *Child Welfare, 89*(4), 9–27.

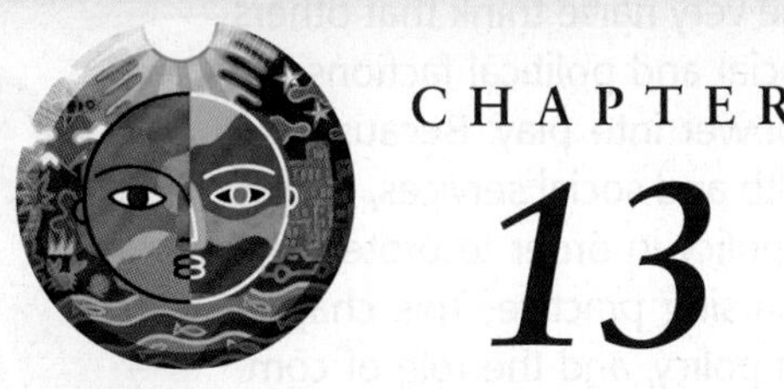

CHAPTER 13

Policy Making and Community Health Advocacy

"Never doubt that a small group of thoughtful citizens can change the world. Indeed, it is the only thing that ever has."

—Margaret Mead

KEY TERMS

Advocacy
Community health advocacy
Distributive health policy
Empowerment
Grassroots
Health center
Health policy
Lobbying
Lobbyists
Polarization
Policy
Policy analysis
Political action
Political action committee (PAC)
Politics
Power
Public policy
Redistributive health policy
Regulatory health policy
Social justice
Special interest groups

LEARNING OBJECTIVES

Upon mastery of this chapter, you should be able to:

- Define health policy and explain how it is established.
- Analyze the influence of health policy on community health and nursing practice.
- Explain the role of special interest groups in health care reform and policy making.
- Explain the role that professional organizations play in public policy.
- Define power and empowerment and the roles these concepts play in policy development.
- Identify the four stages in the policy process and briefly explain what each entails.
- Explain the processes of policy analysis and strategy development.
- Explain the role of community health nurses in determining a community's health policy needs.
- Discuss the difference between advocacy and lobbying and the influence of both on policy.
- Identify the 10 steps of mobilizing a community for political action.
- Describe the steps involved in how a bill becomes law.
- Discuss several methods of communicating with legislators on policy issues.

Behind all legislation and health care regulation lie power struggles. Only the very naive think that others will be persuaded by facts alone. In all legislative activities and reforms, social and political factions are at work—special interest groups, business, and industry each bring their power into play. Because the outcomes of these struggles determine the availability and quality of all health and social services, nurses need to develop a working knowledge of the political process and health policy in order to protect the individuals, families, and communities they serve, as well as their own nursing practice. This chapter examines health policy, the political process involved in determining health policy, and the role of community health nursing in the process. Community health nurses should provide not only input to policy circles through advocacy but also leadership at decision-making tables. Community health nurses must understand and emphasize their powerful role in providing an essential influence and unique perspective in health care.

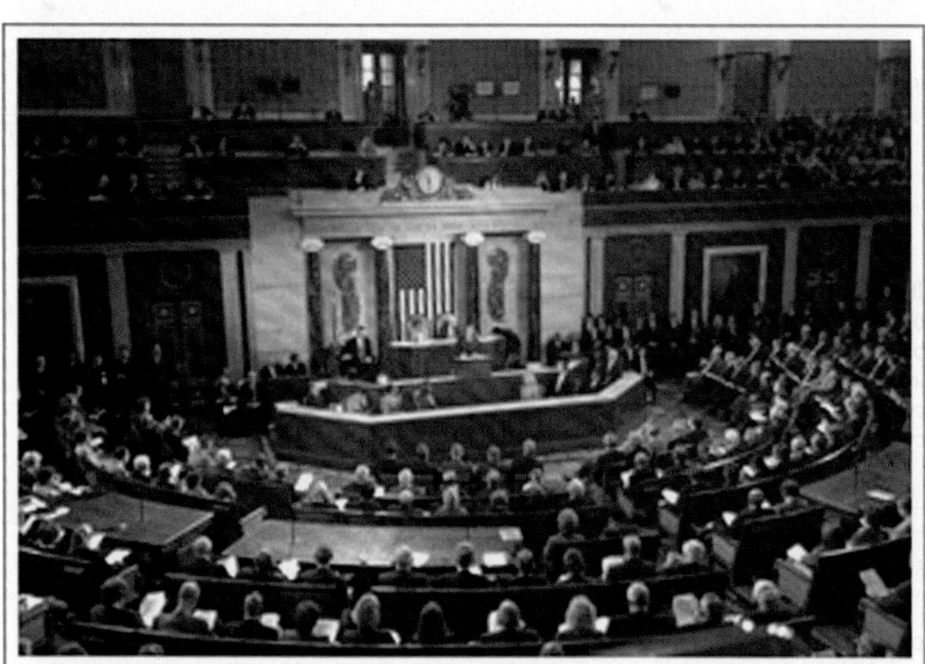

U.S. Congress in session. (Photo courtesy of USA.gov.)

EVOLUTION AND EFFECTS OF CURRENT U.S. HEALTH POLICIES

The United States is often touted as having the best health care system in the world. It is recognized worldwide for achievements in the medical and auxiliary sciences that have contributed to the mapping of the genome, advances in biomedical technologies, and increasing numbers of pharmaceuticals that hold promise for addressing the myriad chronic and acute illnesses that affect the world's populations. People often come from other countries to the United States to access our high-quality medical care.

Uninsured and Underinsured

As discussed in Chapter 6, while we claim to have the best health care available, the U.S. Census Bureau (2010) reports that 50.7 million people (16.7% of the population) were uninsured in 2009. This was the 1st year to show an actual drop in the number of people with health insurance since tracking of these data first occurred in 1987. A shift has also occurred between the numbers of those insured privately (e.g., insurance provided by employers and individuals) and publicly (e.g., paid by government through Medicaid or Medicare). A large-scale study examined public records of bankruptcy filers, following up with questionnaires and telephone interviews, and found that over 60% of bankruptcy filings were linked to medical expenses (Himmelstein, Thorne, Warren, & Woolhandler, 2009). Three fourths of the medical debtors had health insurance, and most were educated middle-class people. This is further proof that the underinsured, along with those individuals without health insurance, are at risk of financial disaster when confronted with a serious medical emergency or long-term illness. Additionally, millions of citizens suffer death and disease because of ethnic disparities (Gehlert & Colditz, 2011; Smedley, 2008; Smedley, Stith, & Nelson, 2003), and there continues to be an imbalance in the ethnic makeup of our professional health care providers—nurses, physicians, dentists, and others (Gilliss,

Powell, & Carter, 2010; Grumbach & Mendoza, 2008; Johansson, Jones, Watkins, Haisfield-Wolfe, & Gaston-Johansson, 2011; Sullivan Commission, 2004). Our medical care system is the most expensive in the world, but our longevity is lower than in countries that spend much less than we do for health care while still providing care for their entire populations (Preston & Ho, 2009; Squires, 2011). In the United States, infant mortality rates—a marker for quality of health care—are near the bottom of industrialized nations, with a rate of 6.71 per 1,000 births (MacDorman & Matthews, 2008). The maternal mortality rate is 1 in 4,800—"one of the highest in the developed world" (Save the Children, 2010, p. 34). Our publicly financed health system—Medicaid and Medicare—is constantly under siege, and increasing numbers of medical errors are harming 1.5 million patients per year (Goodman, Villareal, & Jones, 2011; Institute of Medicine [IOM], 2000, 2002a, 2003, 2006; Van Den Bos et al., 2011). The changing demographics and social indicators of our society, along with other issues, such as immigration, shortages of professional health care providers, increased use of alternative and complementary medicine, and most importantly, the shift from a non-profit to a for-profit health care system, affects our society in innumerable ways (Pauly, 2011; Werner, Kolstad, Stuart, & Polsky, 2011). (See What Do You Think?)

What do *you* think?

Martin Luther King Jr. Memorial. (Photo courtesy of NPS. org.)

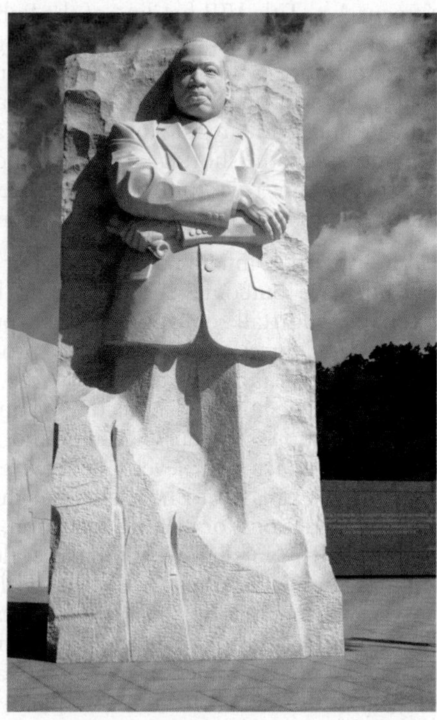

Of all the shocking and inhumane in society; the lack of access to health care is the most inhumane.

—Dr. Martin Luther King

In the decade or so leading up to President Clinton's attempt at health care reform, the debate about access to health care centered on whether health care was a *right* or a *privilege*. What do you think? Given that so many Americans are now without any access to insurance or health care, should there be some basic rights to access to services as found in most other developed nations (e.g., a safety net)? Or is this a privilege that should be earned? What are your thoughts on President Obama's health care reform law?

Economic Effects

The 1990s ushered in an era of health care reform, and with it came downsizing—registered nurses (RNs) in the acute care setting were thought to be dispensable and were replaced by less-prepared staff (Pringle, 2009). In the first half of the following decade, hiring of nurses increased along with signing bonuses and competition for new graduates. This has slowed in most areas in the latter half of the decade as a result of economic downturn and fewer nurses retiring, along with uncertainty about health care reform (Bureau of Labor Statistics, 2011).

The core functions of public health—assessment, assurance, and policy development—became underfunded and underappreciated by local and state governments. As this chapter was being written, health departments continued to be in crisis as a result of economic downturns that necessitated nursing staff layoffs. In addition, the normal attrition of licensed staff led to a substantial reduction in programs and services (National Association of County & City Health Officials [NACCHO], 2009). The average age of public health nurses (PHNs) is 49.5, and the rate of public health workers dropped from 219 to 158 per 100,000 people (Robert Wood Johnson Foundation, 2008). The pipeline for future nurses has also diminished, as schools of nursing have had to slash programs and reduce admissions due to budget problems (University Bound News, 2011). We have yet to recover from the earlier downsizing of nursing schools, and it is now exacerbated by the continuing nursing shortage despite the economic downturn beginning in 2008. The cyclical changes in health workforce patterns are accentuated by the graying of our workforce. RNs over the age of 50 will soon become the largest age group within the profession of nursing. By 2025, a shortage of more than 260,000 nurses is projected. This is twice the size of the largest previous nursing shortage (Buerhaus, Auerbach, & Staiger, 2009). Additionally, the shortages of nursing faculty also hinder our nursing schools from accommodating students interested in entering the profession. The American Association of Colleges of Nursing (AACN) reported that "U.S. nursing schools turned away 67,563 qualified applicants from baccalaureate and graduate nursing programs in 2010 due to an insufficient number of faculty, clinical sites, classroom space, clinical preceptors, and budget constraints. Almost two-thirds of the nursing schools responding to the survey pointed to faculty shortages as a reason for not accepting all qualified applicants into baccalaureate programs" (AACN, 2011a, para. 3).

Federal nursing programs, including the Nurse Reinvestment Act, Title VIII funding of the Public Health Service Act, and various state funding programs are attempting to address these issues. Linda Aiken et al. (2009) called for adapting Title VIII and Medicare to fund baccalaureate and graduate nursing education as a mechanism for addressing the shortage of faculty and nurses to serve in primary care roles and other advanced practice roles. According to National League for Nursing (NLN):

> Health disparities, inflated costs, and poor quality of health care outcomes are deepening because of today's shortfall of appropriately prepared (workforce). Nurses are the primary professionals of quality health care delivery in the nation. Yet, the nursing shortage is affecting communities across the nation. The nurse faculty and nursing shortage is outpacing the level of federal resources allocated by Congress to help alleviate the situation. Appropriations for nursing education, such as the Title VIII—Nursing Workforce Development Programs, are inconsistent with the health care reality facing our nation. Insufficient investments will diminish human resource development, a shortsighted course of action that potentially further jeopardizes access to and the quality of the nation's delivery of health care (2011a, para. 2).

As an example, California and Florida have loan forgiveness programs in return for a commitment to work in designated areas (e.g., state facilities or underserved areas) for a specified period of time. Additionally, California is offering loan forgiveness for graduate students to become nursing instructors for 3 to 5 years, with the impetus being that these graduates will remain as nursing instructors after the term of the agreement expires. Many other states are offering various incentives to attract and retain their public health personnel (AACN, 2011a; NLN, 2011a).

The health care system is evolving. What was originally a retrospective payment system has now moved through managed care to pay-for-performance—and subsequently nonpayment for preventable conditions (see Chapter 6). Health care coverage and access are ongoing policy discussions in the United States, with the cost of care high and growing each year. Health care insurance coverage is often provided through employers, and as costs rise, employers are passing on more costs to the worker. Co-pays and deductibles have increased. With the recession, more people lost jobs and subsequently were also without employer-sponsored insurance. The costs of insurance are increasing, with the annual premium for an individual (not a group insurance member) between the ages of 55 and 64 rising to $5,349 in 2008 (America's Health Insurance Plans, 2009). As the numbers of elderly Americans increase, costs to provide health coverage for them are growing exponentially. However, despite the recessionary period, the major health insurance companies posted record profits (30% higher than projected) while Americans were either forgoing or postponing needed medical care. And many of these health insurers have requested higher premiums (Abelson, 2011).

In 2010, President Barack Obama signed into law the Patient Protection and Affordable Care Act (see Chapter 6) providing greater access to health care coverage for Americans.

Some changes that were immediately instituted included establishing a temporary national high-risk pool for individuals with preexisting conditions, prohibiting health plans from placing lifetime limits on coverage or rescinding coverage (except for fraud) as well as excluding children for preexisting conditions, and extending dependent coverage for children to age 26. Later, Medicaid and Medicare expansion to individuals under age 65 for those with an income 133% of the federal poverty level will be added, as will establishment of state-based Health Benefit Exchanges so that individuals and businesses can purchase health insurance at reasonable rates (Kaiser Family Foundation, 2011). See more on health care reform in Chapter 6.

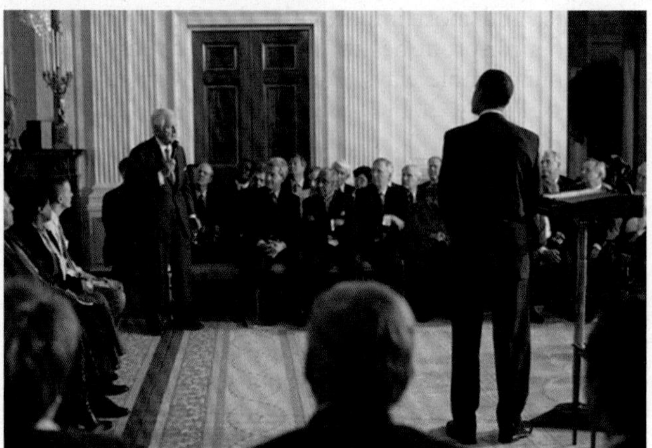

White House Forum on Health Reform. (Photo courtesy of USA.gov.)

Need for Action to Change

This health reform legislation represents a marked change in health policy. Most people agree that health care policy in the United States must change, but there is little agreement among policy makers and citizens about how this should occur (Cillizza, 2010). Some believe market forces should be allowed to work this problem out; others believe the government should assume responsibility—as in other countries—and ensure that all have access to health care coverage. Public health activists believe that if every person adhered to a healthful lifestyle, the need for medical care would lessen.

Policy discussions at the state and local level determine access to care for their residents; other issues, such as high rates of unemployment, health care allotments in state and local budgets, and increasingly heated discussions on the role that undocumented residents play in the costs of health care affect how health care is delivered. The latter issue is a discussion that occurs more frequently in those states with significant numbers of undocumented workers (see Chapter 29). Nonetheless, the numbers of uninsured or underinsured result in patients who lack access to primary care, or who delay care, resulting in higher morbidity, mortality, and costs. This ultimately increases the burden on the health care system and the taxpayers. Disadvantaged populations are more likely to be uninsured because of unemployment or underemployment, resulting in low or no income, health disparities, poor housing, and neighborhoods that may be unsafe (see Chapter 25). Recent studies document that uninsured or underinsured patients have difficulty maintaining economic and social stability (Himmelstein et al., 2009; Kogan et al., 2010; Nance-Nash, 2011; Schoen, Collins, Kriss, & Doty, 2008; Schoen, Doty, Robertson, & Collins, 2011). This has further impact within our economic systems—housing, banking, automobile sales, and the credit industry, as well as state and local governments (Families USA, 2009). Larger employers complain that they are subsidizing those firms that don't provide coverage, and this also drives up the cost of the premiums they have to pay. Loss of insurance coverage leads to increases in charity care that, in turn, impacts health care facilities' ability to continue to provide care. People with health insurance pay higher deductibles and co-pays as a result of the lack of universal health coverage. Disproportionate-share hospitals are closing, while others are implementing diversion policies to ensure greater equity in the care of patients without sufficient health care insurance. The economic downturn and the increasing numbers of uninsured, along with funding cuts in federal, state, and local health programs, have also had a huge affect on community-based health clinics. These are the safety net providers (venues where those with limited resources receive care). The Health Resources and Services Administration (HRSA) defines **health centers** as:

> Community-based and patient-directed organizations that serve populations withlimited access to health care. These include low-income populations, theuninsured, those with limited English proficiency, migrant and seasonal farm workers, individuals and families experiencing homelessness, and those living in public housing (n.d., para. 2).

Without a safety net and adequate resources, people are more vulnerable to illness. Despite advances in caring for and addressing infectious diseases, one of the scourges of an earlier time, tuberculosis (TB), has resurfaced. Although the increased incidence of AIDS accounts for some of this resurgence, drug resistance to the TB bacillus and the influx of immigrants from endemic areas, coupled with budget cuts, have impeded the labor-intensive measures of tracking patients, directly observing therapy, and providing continuous follow-up for these patients (see Chapter 8).

Despite the availability of vaccines against childhood diseases, the number of children fully vaccinated has dropped—only about 73% of 2-year-olds are completely immunized (Centers for Disease Control and Prevention [CDC], 2009). Because of a complicated vaccination schedule coupled with access issues, many youngsters are not fully immunized; consequently, periodic outbreaks of childhood diseases (e.g., measles, pertussis, and meningitis) occur. At the same time, with the increased emphasis on terrorism, public health departments are being called on to address critical disaster preparedness plans that each state and local jurisdiction will need in the event of a major disaster (Inglesby, 2011).

In a classic article, Peters (2002, p. 2) puts forth the premise that the "valuing of physician primacy has led to an undervaluing of nursing and their contribution to health care." Physicians have historically been the dominant group in shaping health policy because of their perceived expertise, not their numbers (Aries, 2011). Hospitals and academic medical centers have also greatly influenced health policy and funding for technology. "White, male physicians and administrators achieved control of the health care industry and its workers, including nurses, at the start of the 20th century" (Ballou & Landreneau, 2010, p. 71). This gender-biased, authoritarian system has been difficult to change. Nurses, however, are the largest group of health care professionals, and nursing has long promoted health maintenance with a broader definition than just the absence of disease. A lack of understanding at the highest levels of policy making has led to systems of care that focus on physician-oriented cure and has disproportionately affected nursing, resulting in a lack of emphasis on prevention and early intervention. Additionally, by concentrating on nursing tasks, rather than nursing knowledge, the displacement of nursing adds to poor patient outcomes, exacerbates the nursing shortage, and is detrimental to overall system effectiveness. While Milstead (2008) noted that nursing's link to public policy may have begun in the 1960s with a push for federally funded nursing research, it has greatly intensified as advanced practice nurses have utilized the policy arena to "fight battles for recognition as professionals" and reimbursement for services (p. 7). The need for nurses to become even more involved in **policy analysis** and development is obvious (Hewison, 2007). As Catherine Dodd, a nurse and former Regional Director for the U.S. Department of Health & Human Services, reminds us "those who fail to participate in the political process are allowing the decisions to be made by people who may seek to control resources for their own personal or political gain" (2011, p. 15).

With the health care arena in flux, nurses are beginning to take on more of a role in health policy. It is instructive to discuss policy, power, and how the community health nurse can be a catalyst for change in the health policy arena. In the 111th Congress (2009–2010), there were three former nurses: Lois Capps, (D-CA), a former school nurse; Eddie Bernice Johnson (D-TX), a former chief psychiatric nurse at the Dallas Veteran's Administration and the first nurse to be elected to the U.S. Congress; and Carolyn McCarthy, (D-NY), a former licensed practical nurse who was elected to serve vowing to fight for more stringent gun laws after her son and husband were shot on the New York subway (Dodd, 2008). These representatives carry on the legacy of nurses involved in influencing health policy in the United States. They have proved, as others before them, to be instrumental in the introduction and passage of policies that affect the health of us all. The 112th Congress brought three more nurses whose stories differ somewhat from their colleagues who have served in Congress for some time. First, Renee Ellmers is a Republican representing North Carolina's second district. After passage of the *Patient Protection and Affordable Care Act*, which she opposed, she became involved in local Republican politics. She is a former surgical intensive care nurse and worked with her husband, a physician, as Clinical Director of Trinity Wound Care Center in Dunn, NC. Congresswoman Diane Black is the Representative for Tennessee's sixth Congressional District. She is a former emergency room nurse, as well as a former Tennessee state representative and senator, having served in the State Senate Republican Caucus. The other nurse most recently elected to the 112th Congress is Ann Marie Buerkle, a Republican representative from New York's 25th Congressional District. She worked as a substitute school nurse before going to law school at Syracuse University. She served as the Assistant Attorney General of New York beginning in 1997 and, upon being elected to the Congress, voted in 2011 to repeal the *Patient Protection and Affordable Care Act* (Rutgers Center for American Women & Politics, 2010).

Other nurses in the public eye include Dr. Mary Wakefield, Jennie Chin Hansen, and Dr. Catherine Dodd. Mary Wakefield was appointed by President Obama in 2009 to head the HRSA. She was a nursing educator and advocate for rural health issues before her appointment.

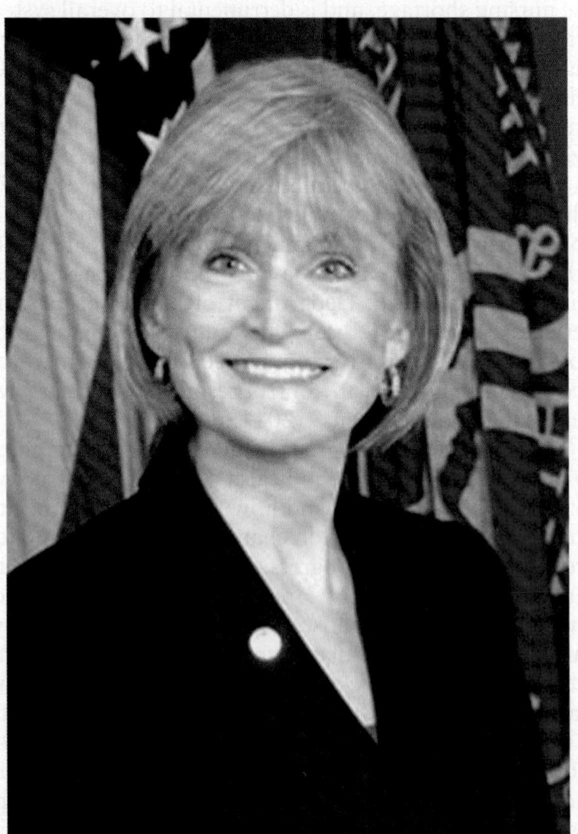

Mary Wakefield, PhD, RN, Administrator, HRSA. (Photo courtesy USA.gov.)

Jennie Chin Hansen was elected president of the American Association of Retired Persons for 2008–2010. She has taught nursing for the past few years at San Francisco State University and before that served for 25 years as the executive director of a nonprofit organization providing primary, long-term care and community-based services. Catherine Dodd is the Director of the San Francisco Health Services System and was formerly Deputy Chief of Staff to San Francisco Mayor Gavin Newsom and District Chief of Staff to Speaker of the House Nancy Pelosi. She previously served as Region IX Director of U.S. Health & Human Services and has been actively engaged in health policy for many years, some of them in association with the American Nurses Association (ANA). In her nursing career, she provided physical examinations to farm workers and served as a perinatal nurse for high-risk families (Mason, Leavitt, & Chaffee, 2012; U.S. Department of Health & Human Services Archive, 1999).

FOUNDATIONS OF POLITICAL ACTION AND ADVOCACY

The basic concepts of public health have evolved over the last 150 years. From an emphasis on the individual to a population focus, this is evidenced through policy development that has a broader effect through "healthy policies—education, adequate and affordable housing, living wage, and environmental concerns" (IOM, 2002b, p. 46, 2006; Hansen & Jones, 2011).

Public Health

The concept of social justice is seen as the very foundation of public health nursing (deChesnay & Anderson, 2012; Perez & Martinez, 2008). The AACN (2011b) emphasizes that the guiding values of nursing include social justice, and the ANA *Code of Ethics with Interpretative Statements* (2001, preface) states that "nurses should act to change those aspects of society that detract from health and wellbeing." The ANA's *Public Health Nursing: Scope and Standards of Practice* document also highlights the basic value of social justice in community health nursing (2007). The many definitions of social justice depend on the discipline involved; for purposes of this chapter, **social justice** is "a fair allocation of the costs and rewards of group membership," focusing on the processes, perceptions, and roles (Barusch, 2009, p. 6). Boutain (2008) further clarifies this as "the equalizing of the balance of societal burdens ad benefits" (p. 2). However, it has been noted that nurses "lack a multidisciplinary vocabulary to discuss, critique and strategize about injustice" (Boutain, 2005, p. 10).

We often want things to be fair, but do not clearly define what that means, or sufficiently promote specific actions needed to ensure it. We may feel frustration about situations we see everyday, but need to be better equipped to address them (Boutain, 2008; Paquin, 2011). You may be caught in a "Catch-22" situation, working within a market-based system that is inherently unfair and often leads to health and social disparities for ethnic and other disadvantaged groups while having pledged to alleviate suffering within the groups you serve (Logsdon & Davis, 2010; Manthey, 2008).

As a community health nurse, you are expected to give voice to the disparities found in the communities you serve (e.g., substandard housing, high rates of unemployment, death and disability)—disparities that often could be prevented or alleviated at early stages. Your efforts through nursing interventions can address not only health issues but also the educational, social, and economic issues that give rise to these disparities (deChesnay & Anderson, 2012; Perez & Martinez, 2008). The Minnesota Department of Public Health Nursing Section has developed a public health interventions model that gives a broad overview of public health nursing. The model is based on the type of intervention and practice levels that allows a range of activities, such as advocacy, community organizing, coalition building, case management, and policy development, which you as a public health practitioner can activate (see Chapter 14). The nexus between social justice, advocacy, and policy is interrelated, complex, and one that will affect every aspect of your community health nursing career.

History of Public Health Nursing Advocacy

Nurses have a long history of action in social justice and **advocacy**, which can be defined as pleading the case of another or championing a cause (see Chapter 2). It is a "fundamental nursing role—whether on behalf of patients, communities, or the profession, and in crafting policy solutions" (Mason, Leavitt, & Chaffee, 2012, p. 37). To advocate is to try to influence outcomes that affect people, communities, and systems. Additionally, advocacy is a process, not an outcome, one that includes identifying an issue, collecting information, identifying who can be influenced/who can make the decision sought, building support, and taking action. Advocacy can present itself in a variety of ways—self-advocacy, which is advocating for oneself; individual advocacy, which is pleading the case of others; and legislative advocacy, which is changing or modifying state or federal laws (MacDonnell, 2009). Advocacy also includes litigation and public education campaigns. Finally, advocacy is also the process of empowering those less able to present their views or needs, with the goal of giving them a voice and/or achieving their objectives. Nurses have long been advocates for their patients, and advocacy can and does affect the larger systems of care (deChesnay & Anderson, 2012; Paquin, 2011; Perez & Martinez, 2008). **Community health advocacy** refers to efforts aimed at creating awareness of and generating support for meeting the community's health needs. Both nurses and communities have a common goal—the best possible health services for all.

The term and concept of *public health nursing* was coined in 1893 by Lillian Wald, who described PHNs as "those nurses working outside the hospital in poor and middle-class communities" (Jewish Women's Archive, 2011, para. 2). These nurses specialized "in both preventative care and the preservation of health, these nurses responded to referrals from physicians and patients, and received fees based on the patient's ability to pay" (para. 2). In 1893, Lillian Wald and Mary Brewster established the Visiting Nurses Service, and a year later the famed Henry Street Settlement House was established (see Chapter 2).

Public health as a concept grew out of Wald's exposure to the plight of newly arrived immigrants to the lower east side of Manhattan and their appalling living conditions. She was determined that these immigrants and other poor people, regardless of ethnicity or religious affiliation, would have access to health care and adequate housing. Remarkably, in the 21st century, the Henry Street Settlement (n.d.) still provides many of the services established by Wald and her associates—currently, the organization advocates for the homeless, builds AIDS awareness, fights illiteracy and domestic violence, and provides youth and senior programs. Understanding the critical concepts of primary care, prevention, and early intervention, and the role they played in assuring a healthy childhood, Lillian Wald advocated for the hiring of public school nurses. In 1902, Lina Rogers became the first school nurse in New York City "as a one- month experiment," and within a year's time New York City had hired an additional 12 school nurses (Haninck, 2011; Schumacher, 2002; Woodfill & Beyrer, 1991, p. 5). Wald also went on to encourage the establishment of the Department of Nursing and Health at Columbia University's Teachers College through a series of lectures she presented starting in 1910. She also was instrumental in creating the U.S. Children's Bureau in 1912, an agency that oversaw fair child labor laws.

The importance of these nurses—Lillian Wald and her compatriots, Sojourner Truth, Margaret Sanger, Clara Barton, Mary Seacole, Susie King Taylor, Mary Mahoney, and others—is that they wielded influence at a time when women were not even allowed to vote. In fact, many women in the 1800s, regardless of socioeconomic status, did not attend school. African American women in the early 20th century were legally forbidden to learn to read and write (Foreman, 2009; Nickitas, Middaugh, & Aries, 2011). Historically, women—both Black and White—volunteered their services during crises although nursing, as a profession, didn't exist (University of Medicine & Dentistry of New Jersey, 2011). For these women to be successful and influential during the 19th century is a tribute to their ability to take on the system in which they lived and to triumph over it. Women during these times rarely, if ever, voiced their opinions about issues affecting their lives, the lives of their children, their families, or their communities; it was neither expected nor accepted. These early pioneers also are seen as feminists, and the entrance of these women into the political arena opened the way for others. In the 110th Congress, we had the first-ever female Speaker of the House, Nancy Pelosi of California. There are currently three female Supreme Court justices. Additionally, in the 112th Congress (2011–2013), there were 90 women serving—17 in the Senate and 73 in the House of Representatives (Rutgers Center for American Women & Politics, 2010).

Professional Advocacy

One of the chief ways in which nurses have been successful in advocating is through membership in their professional organizations. The late 19th century may be seen as the beginning of nurse activism. The Nurses Associated Alumnae of the U.S. and Canada and the American Society of Superintendents of Training Schools of the U.S. and Canada were formed in 1890s (ANA, 2011a; NLN, 2011b). Out of these groups came the ANA and the NLN. However, in the 1980s, with the stratification of nursing into various specialties and organizations, representing an assortment of specialty groups, came the realization that the many nursing groups needed to coordinate efforts in order to be more successful (Cohen et al., 1996). Throughout the next few decades, the nursing organizations realized, regardless of internal differences and competition, that to be politically successful they must join together to work toward their common political goals. The formation of the following coalitions occurred:

Tri-Council for Nursing—comprising ANA, AACN, NLN, and the American Organization of Nurse Executives

American College of Nurse Practitioners (NPs)—state and national NP groups initially met for a national forum and eventually to influence health policy

Nursing Organizations Alliance (The Alliance)—an alliance of National Federation of Specialty Nursing Organizations and Nursing Organizations Liaison Forum

Nurses Coalition for Legislative Action—National Association of Pediatric Nurse Practitioners, American College of Nurse Midwives, Association of Women's Health, Obstetric, and Neonatal Nurses, American Nephrology Nurses Association, and the National Association of Orthopedic Nurses.

These and other coalitions permitted the organizations to lobby for common nursing issues (e.g., maintenance of federal funding for nursing education and research) and ultimately the establishment of the National Institute of Nursing Research within the National Institutes of Health (Milstead, 2008). Many of the current state nurse practice acts and expanded responsibilities for NPs are the result of these new coalitions. But more significantly, nursing now has a better understanding that there is a difference between "self-interest" and "selfishness" (Cohen et al., 1996; Fyffe, 2009; Wilson, 2002). One of the most significant outcomes of this time was the development of *Nursing's Agenda for Health Care Reform* (ANA, 1994), this document exemplified the maturing of nursing as a special interest group, but more importantly demonstrated consensus building and collaboration among the more than 60 nursing and various health care provider organizations. Despite nursing's early history of political activism and the fact that nurses are the largest group of health care providers in the United States, widespread political involvement has yet to be fully realized (Nickitas et al., 2011). Nursing is still not consistently regarded as a major player in Washington when discussing health care policy (Harrington & Estes, 2008). For a more recent example of successful professional advocacy, see *From the Case Files—Nurse Practitioners Part of the Prescription for Pennsylvania.*

Large professional organizations have the resources, relationships with policy makers, success at coalition building, and reputation for the ability to compromise needs to assure viable outcomes. Being a part of your professional organization demonstrates your professionalism, promotes your organization's viability, and demonstrates your social responsibility to advocate for the needs of your patients. Nurses must take advantage of how the public views the profession. For more than a decade, nurses have ranked highest in a Gallup poll for honesty and ethical standards (Jones, 2010). Clearly, there is favorable impression of nursing as a profession among the general public. Despite criticism about special interest and professional organizations "protecting their turf," professional nursing organizations demonstrate how a critical mass can be influential and successful in moving the discussion forward on health care and the public's perception of nursing. It is the professional nursing organizations that have elevated nursing professionalism, given voice to the inequities that affect our society, and developed the paradigms that influence and affect public health at the institutional, state, and national level in the 21st century. A united voice on public policy is more powerful than individual nurses pleading with their legislators.

The pursuit of personal agendas over the common good results in a piecemeal approach to problems and promotes polarization. **Polarization** is the process by which a group is severely split into two or more factions over a political issue. Polarization can be so intense that people perceive one another as good or wicked, depending on their ideological opinions. One of the primary goals of a professional nursing association is to build a collective voice for nurses. A strong professional association limits polarization by developing the political skills of its members and ensures that its structure and processes equitably meet the needs of its constituencies. This is the essence of politics: people must listen to each other, learn from others' viewpoints, and compromise to ensure the most positive outcomes from their endeavors.

Nursing's Role in Health Care Reform

Since the 1950s, the ANA has advocated for reforms in health care that will benefit both nurses and their patients. Their involvement in federal health care reform began in the 1960s with the passage of Medicaid and Medicare. In the 1970s, ANA formed a **political action committee (PAC)**. PACs are organizations that raise money to contribute to political parties or candidates, with the understanding that those receiving financial and political support will be sympathetic toward issues of interest to members of the PAC.

In 1991, ANA released *Nursing's Agenda for Health Care Reform: A Call to Action—a* plan so ambitious and forward looking that Senator Kennedy referenced this document when introducing his legislation on health care reform. Even though this legislation failed to pass, ANA and other nursing organizations gained wide recognition

From the Case Files

Nurse Practitioners Part of the Prescription for Pennsylvania

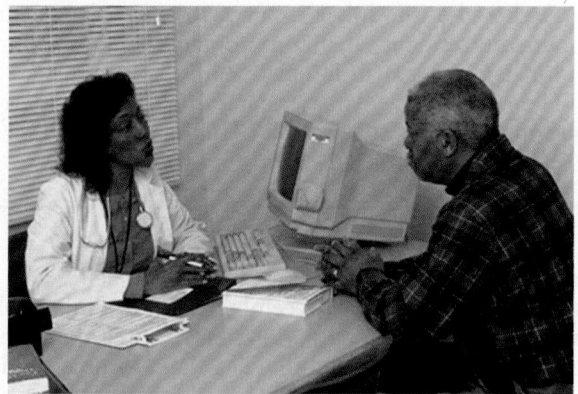

In their article, "How Advanced Practice Nurses Became Part of the Prescription for Pennsylvania," Hansen-Turton, Ritter, & Valdez (2009) describe how advanced practice nurses in that state successfully advocated for "nursing-related legislative reforms" as part of the "Prescription for Pennsylvania" health care reform legislation, sponsored by Governor Edward Rendell (p. 7). The Pennsylvania Coalition of Nurse Practitioners began in the 1980s with only three nurse practitioners (NPs) and by 2005 was composed of 17 regional groups throughout the state. Some of their accomplishments since the year 2000 include gaining prescriptive authority, signatory authority for disability placards and license plates, and permission for oral and written orders in hospitals. The many years of lobbying, coalition building, and hard work led to nursing-related bills heard in the Pennsylvania Assembly in 2007 regarding expanded scope of NP practice—for instance, prescriptive authority for controlled substances, home visits for chronically ill patients, the ability to order wheelchairs and other medical devices, and referral power to other professionals, such as occupational and physical therapists. This has paved the way for a large health care provider, Highmark Inc., to seek out independent NPs as "primary care practitioners" to meet the anticipated demand when 32 additional Americans will gain health insurance coverage in the next few years. Medicare payments for NPs are currently at 85% of payments for physicians, and nurse-managed clinics may become more prevalent as health care reform moves into high gear (Johnson, 2010; Toland, 2011). We must seize this opportunity and "learn to speak with a unified voice and build strong relationships with a broad range of bipartisan policy makers, funders, civic leaders, business leaders, and legislative advocates" as the Pennsylvania nurse practitioners did (Hansen-Turton et al., 2009, p. 7).

Hansen-Turton, T., Ritter, A., & Valdez, B. (2009). Developing alliances: How advanced practice nurses became part of the prescription for Pennsylvania. *Policy, Politics, & Nursing, 10*(1), 7–15.

Johnson, C. K. (2010, April 16). 28 states consider expanding nurses' roles. Associated Press. Retrieved from http://www.usatoday.com/news/health/2010-04-16-nurse-doctors_N.htm

Toland, B. (2011, January 20). Nurse practitioners' role expanding? *Pittsburgh-Post Gazette*. Retrieved from http://www.post-gazette.com/pg/11020/1119222-28.stm

for their policy acumen and leadership abilities. During the Clinton-era health care debate, ANA continued to play a key role in the policy and political discussions on health care reform. As research and experience continued to show the need for health care reform, ANA remained steadfast in its advocacy and updated the policy agenda on health care reform. In 2005, the revised 1991 document *ANA's Health Care Agenda 2005* was released, moving forward the discussion on the shortages of health care providers, particularly nurses, and its effect on the health of the nation. *ANA's Health System Reform Agenda* is the 2008 revision of the 2005 document, and the newer document called for a "movement away from the overuse of expensive, technology-driven, acute, hospital-based services in the model we now have" and progress toward a more balanced approach incorporating primary care, community-based care, and preventive services (2008, p. 3). This policy statement also supported the development of a single-payer system. With this document guiding them, the critical issues for discussion were quality, cost, access, and the nursing workforce (ANA, 2008; Kaiser Family Foundation, 2009).

Understanding the time was ripe for health care reform, the ANA-PAC identified those legislators supportive of ANA's legislative and regulatory agenda. They provided financial and political support and increased their grassroots organizing. RNs nationwide responded and through multiple activities (e.g., contacting members of Congress, testifying at hearings, sharing personal stories, participating in high-profile press conferences, attending rallies and events) lobbied for action (see Display 13.1). The frontline nurses also joined ANA's health care reform team, and through these concentrated efforts and collaborations, health care reform became a reality in March 2010 (ANA, 2010). With the successful passage of HR 3590 (Public Law 111-148), *The Patient Protection and Affordable Care Act*, on March 23 and the March 25 passage of HR 4872 (PL 111-152), *Health Care and Education Affordability Reconciliation Act of 2010*, amending HR 3590, the long quest for health care system reform occurred. Both pieces of legislation are referred to as the *Affordable Care Act* (ACA). See Chapter 6 for more on health care reform.

DISPLAY 13.1 AMERICAN NURSES ASSOCIATION (ANA) LOBBYING EFFORTS TOWARD HEALTH CARE REFORM

ANA and its members played a critical role in advocating for health reform. Below is a list of their activities, over a 15-month period:

- Participated in hundreds of media interviews
- Participated in dozens of local media events
- Testified before three Congressional Committees
- Met with White House and Congressional health care reform staff
- Participated in two presidential press conferences at the White House: ANA was one of only 150 representatives invited to participate in the White House Health Care Summit on March 5, 2009
- Participated in the June 25, 2009 rally—*Health Care for America Now*
- Gathered at the July 15, 2009, Rose Garden event where President Obama personally thanked ANA for its involvement in health care reform efforts
- Helped organize America's national-call-in day to Congress in October 2009 (ANA, 2011b).

The importance of nurses being politically active is gathering steam and in December 2009, a new nursing organization, the 160,000 member National Nurses United (NNU), a national advocacy association was formed with the purpose of influencing national health policy and assisting nurses across the country to introduce and pass a patient ratio law, similar to California's 1999 law. Three existing unions came together to form NNU—the California Nurses Association (CNA—not affiliated with the ANA), operating in California and four other states; the Massachusetts Nurses Union, organizing nurses in the northeast; and the United American Nurses, organizing nurses in the Midwest (NNU, 2011).

Nurses are increasingly becoming shapers of policy on both the local and federal level; this is occurring because of our experience, perspective, and expertise in health care. The realization that improving conditions for nursing also improves conditions for the communities we serve, and the larger society in which we live and work has enhanced our ability to organize. This increases our visibility, access to policy makers, and, more importantly, our capacity to influence the political process.

Nurses who represent the largest number of health care practitioners in America—more than 3 million—are poised at the frontline in patient care to play a major role in implementing of health care reform. Being fully involved in the regulatory framework development (e.g., how the law will be implemented) will further demonstrate the advocacy of nurses as they work to improve the health care delivery system and remove barriers that prevent nurses from providing high-quality, competent, appropriate care. However, to change the existing system, the barriers to competent, quality care (e.g., nursing shortages, faculty shortages, a lack of proper education and training) that prevent nursing from taking its rightful place among the cadre of providers must be addressed. To that end, in 2008, the Robert Wood Johnson Foundation in collaboration with the IOM began the activities necessary to "assess and transform" nursing. The document resulting from this evaluation is *The Future of Nursing: Leading Change, Advancing Health* (IOM, 2011). To encourage and assure public participation, three forums were held around the country. Beginning in October 2009, the first forum addressing acute care was held in Los Angeles, CA; the second forum, held in December 2009 in Philadelphia, addressed primary care, long-term care, community health, and public health. The last forum, held in Houston, TX, in February 2010, addressed nursing education (Robert Wood Johnson Foundation, 2009).

The Future of Nursing is a seminal document that addresses the need to reform the health care and public health system of the 21st century and outlines nursing's pivotal role in this. This is the first time *nurses* are seen as key to "meeting current and future health care needs" (Schultz, 2010, p. 345). In the development of this document, the process was open to all. This allowed nursing to address challenges to the profession, while simultaneously putting forth solutions that result in a rationale and a comprehensive approach to the delivery of high-quality health care for all. It also encourages system responsiveness to the needs of those accessing care.

As expected, the nursing organizations were active in the process of developing this document and participated in the National Summit on Advancing Health through Nursing held in late 2010 to discuss the implications of the recommendations for the future of health care and the future role of nurses in America (Robert Wood Johnson Foundation, 2010). Four key messages from *The Future of Nursing: Leading Change, Advancing Health* (IOM, 2011, p. 4) include the following:

1. Nurses should practice to the full extent of their education and training.
2. Nurses should achieve higher levels of education and training through an improved education system that promotes seamless academic progression.
3. Nurses should be full partners, with physicians and other health professionals, in redesigning health care in the United States.
4. Effective workforce planning and policy making require better data collection and an improved information infrastructure.

The resulting eight recommendations are

Recommendation1—*Remove scope of practice barriers*. Advanced practice RNs should be able to practice to the full extent of their education and training (p. 9).

Recommendation 2—*Expand opportunities for nurses to lead and diffuse collaborative improvement efforts.* Private and public funders, health care organizations, nursing education programs, and nursing associations should expand opportunities for nurses to lead and manage collaborative efforts with physicians and other members of the health care team to conduct research and to redesign and improve practice environments and health systems. These entities should also provide opportunities for nurses to diffuse successful practices (p. 11).

Recommendation 3—*Implement nurse residency programs.* State boards of nursing, accrediting bodies, the federal government, and health care organizations should take actions to support nurses' completion of a transition-to-practice program (nurse residency) after they have completed a prelicensure or advanced practice degree program or when they are transitioning into new clinical practice areas (p. 11).

Recommendation 4—*Increase the proportion of nurses with a baccalaureate degree to 80% by 2020.* Academic nurse leaders across all schools of nursing should work together to increase the proportion of nurses with a baccalaureate degree from 50% to 80% by 2020. These leaders should partner with education accrediting bodies, private and public funders, and employers to ensure funding, monitor progress, and increase the diversity of students to create a workforce prepared to meet the demands of diverse populations across the lifespan (p. 12).

Recommendation 5—*Double the number of nurses with a doctorate by 2020.* Schools of nursing, with support from private and public funders, academic administrators and university trustees, and accrediting bodies, should double the number of nurses with a doctorate by 2020 to add to the cadre of nurse faculty and researchers, with attention to increasing diversity (p. 13).

Recommendation 6—*Ensure that nurses engage in lifelong learning.* Accreditingbodies, schools of nursing, health care organizations, and continuing competencyeducators from multiple health professions should collaborate to ensure that nurses and nursing students and faculty continue their education and engage in lifelong learning to gain the competencies needed to provide care for diverse populations across the lifespan (p. 13).

Recommendation 7—*Prepare and enable nurses to lead change to advance health.* Nurses, nursing education programs, and nursing associations should prepare the nursing workforce to assume leadership positions across all levels, while public, private, and governmental health care decision makers should ensure that leadership positions are available to and filled by nurses (p. 14).

Recommendation 8—*Build an infrastructure for the collection and analysis of interprofessional health care workforce data.* The National Health Care Workforce Commission, with oversight from the Government Accountability Office and the HRSA, should lead a collaborative effort to improve research and the collection and analysis of data on health care workforce requirements. The Workforce Commission and the HRSA should collaborate with state licensing boards, state nursing workforce centers, and the Department of Labor in this effort to ensure that the data are timely and publicly accessible (p. 14).

Nurses are realizing that they are an important force in health care and should be at the table with other stakeholders when important decisions are being made. The IOM report on nursing is a clear hallmark of our growth in the area of health policy and health reform. The recently passed health care reform legislation has the potential to transform the current system to be more responsive to the least among us, is more focused on primary care and prevention, and encourages wellness and disease prevention. The resulting system change will be based on research and data collection that fosters better patient outcomes and high quality care, but more importantly, without the anticipated transformation of nursing it cannot occur. "Nurses' regular, close proximity to patients and scientific understanding of care processes across the continuum of care give them a unique ability to act as partners with other health professionals and to lead in the improvement and redesign of the health care system and its many practice environments, including hospitals, schools, homes, retail health clinics, long-term care facilities, battlefields, and community and public health centers" (IOM, 2011, p. S-3). This is a mandate for community health nurses to be actively involved in advocacy and influencing the future development of our health care system.

CURRENT PUBLIC HEALTH NURSING ADVOCACY

Lois Capps, Eddie Bernice Johnson, and Carolyn McCarthy, three of the nurses currently serving in Congress, all ran for office because of their commitment to improving the lives of their communities. The stories of how they came to serve in Congress are indicative of dedicated people wanting to make a difference for their communities. For example, when Carolyn McCarthy's husband was killed and her son badly injured during an attack by a lone gunman, she began to work on promoting legislation for an assault weapons ban. When her Congressman voted against it, she was so outraged she decided to run for office. With strong **grassroots** (political movement driven by community members, a bottom-up rather than a top-down process) support, she won this seat representing the citizens of New York in 1996. Eddie Bernice Johnson ran for office because she believed her work as a volunteer in a low-income immunization program could be augmented. Again, with a grassroots movement behind her, she won in 1992 and is now serving her ninth term in the House of Representatives on behalf of the people of Texas. Lois Capps' story is somewhat similar. Her husband, the Representative for

California's 23rd Congressional District, died suddenly in 1998, and she was drafted to run in his place. Capps, a former school nurse, founded the House Nursing Caucus, and subsequently sponsored HR 4903, the National Nurse Act of 2006. This legislation was also supported by the 91 members of the House Nursing Caucus and would have amended the Public Health Service Act to establish the Office of National Nurse. At the time, Capps stated "the National Nurse would be an advocate for nursing issues when the profession faces growing demands for its skills and an increasing shortage of qualified personnel to meet current challenges" (Orlovsky, 2006, para. 10). However, this legislation was never heard during the 109th Congress, and bills that have not passed prior to the end of each 2-year legislative session are cleared from the books. In February 2010 (111th Congress), Representative Earl Blumenauer of Oregon introduced HR 4601, legislation similar to HR 4903. Through the leadership of Lois Capps and Congressman Steven LaTourette (Republican, Ohio), we now have the bipartisan Congressional Nursing Caucus, and it is anticipated nursing issues will have a greater voice and advocacy.

Theresa Polick and Teri Mills, both RNs, were the impetus behind both HR 4903 and HR 4601. They stated they wanted to do something about the health care crisis and in an op-ed piece for the *New York Times*. Teri Mills called for an Office of the National Nurse. Polick joined with her to form the National Nurse Team and headed to Capitol Hill (Polick, 2006). To further the work of having a National Nurse, the National Nursing Network Organization has been formed as a 501(c) 4 to:

- Establish an Office of a National Nurse to complement the work of the U.S. Surgeon General, filling this position from among the ranks of the existing United States Public Health Service nurse leaders.
- Build a network of volunteer teams of nurses and other health professionals who will promote, encourage, and support nationwide efforts that focus on wellness and disease prevention (2011, para. 5).

What Teri and Theresa engaged in is known as **lobbying**, which is the process of influencing legislators or other policy makers to make decisions on policy issues. Professional organizations or other **special interest groups** (individuals who share a common interest and work politically to make their goals a reality) may retain paid lobbyists. **Lobbyists** are professionals who know the rules governing the state or federal political process, have or develop relationships with policy makers, provide guidance for members of the organizations employing them on how to impact public policy decisions, and work behind the scenes to influence policy discussions and outcomes. States and the federal government have laws and regulations that determine the legal actions of lobbyists as well as the organizations that employ them (Mason et al., 2012; Milstead, 2008).

Universal health and social issues affecting communities include health care access, affordable housing, safe neighborhoods, domestic and youth violence, safe schools, gun control, and many others. Dr. Deborah Prothrow-Stith, a young physician in the mid-1980s, was weary of seeing young victims of violence in the emergency rooms of inner city Boston, so she started a movement that swept across the country. She changed the way youth violence was viewed by recognizing that youth violence was a public health issue, not merely a criminal issue. She believed that applying public health principles of prevention could decrease the incidence of violence. She wrote about this in her groundbreaking book *Deadly Consequences: How Violence Is Destroying Our Teenage Population and a Plan to Begin Solving the Problem*. Because of her belief in prevention and early intervention, she developed a discipline that is now recognized and taught throughout the country and the world—*violence prevention*. Dr. Prothrow-Stith also developed the precursor to violence prevention curricula for schools and communities: *The Violence Prevention Curriculum for Adolescents* is still in use today (Harvard School of Public Health, 2011).

POLICY

Community health nursing, as it has evolved, puts nurses where the people are—in schools, homes, neighborhood centers, health clinics, and churches. Community health nurses are in a position to see and understand the issues affecting people at an individual and group level. With this access to information and the issues affecting the communities they serve, who better than nurses to advocate for policy changes in the health care system? **Policy** is defined as a plan of action or an agenda that outlines steps or actions to implement a stated goal or objective. Policies are laws, regulations, or administrative rulings; when issued by national, state, or local governments they are called **public policy**. **Health policy** refers to specific policies involving health care. The legislative and regulatory process may start with lofty goals, but the final product is usually the result of compromise often encouraged by special interest groups, coalition groups, political realities, or the current economic environment. Although the study of politics has a long history, the systematic study of public policy, on the other hand, can be said to be a 20th-century creation. According to Daniel McCool, in his classic treatise on policy (1995), the study of public policy dates to 1922, when political scientist Charles Merriam sought to "connect the theory and practices of politics to understanding the actual activities of government, which is public policy" (p. 4).

Health policies can be distributive or regulatory. A **distributive health policy** promotes nongovernmental activities that are thought to be beneficial to society as a whole. An example of a distributive policy is the Nurse Training Act, Title VIII of the Public Health Service Act, which was established in 1965 and provided federal subsidies for nursing education in an effort to address the need for more nurses. A **redistributive health policy** changes the allocation of resources from one group to another, usually to a broader or different group. Medicare is an example of redistributive policy, in that provisions under Medicare were expanded to provide a broader range of benefits and coverage to needy groups—such as those older than age 65 and the permanently disabled of any age (McGrath, 2009).

A **regulatory health policy** is one that attempts to control the allocation of resources by directing those agencies or persons who offer resources or provide public services. For example, certain government regulations set standards for the licensure of health care organizations (e.g., hospitals) and health care providers (e.g., nurses). Regulatory public health policy is often used to protect the health of the community (Kovner & Knickman, 2011). In the United States, one example is the mandatory reporting of certain communicable diseases. On the international level, regulatory health policy has a broad scope, including areas such as international communicable disease control, trade, human rights, armed conflict and arms control, and the environment (Beaglehole & Bonita, 2009; also see Chapter 16).

Regulatory policy can be further categorized as either competitive or protective. *Competitive regulation* limits, or structures, the provision of health services by designating exactly who is permitted to deliver them. A case in point is the ruling by the Centers for Medicare and Medicaid Services (CMS) regarding Certified Registered Nurse Anesthetists (CRNAs). Until 2001, federal supervision requirements were in place for CRNAs; they were required to work under the direction of a physician. States can now opt out of that requirement, and 16 have done so (American Association of Nurse Anesthetists, 2010). A large retrospective analysis of Medicare data from 1999 to 2005 found that opting out of the requirement for physician oversight did not increase inpatient complications or deaths, and the researchers called for CMS to remove restrictions on CRNAs (Dulisse & Cromwell, 2010). *Protective regulations* set conditions under which various private activities can be undertaken. Although professional licensure is most commonly identified as having the primary purpose of protecting the public, such policy is really competitive regulation in terms of its social impact. Protective regulation is more clearly evident in utilization review organizations, regulatory bodies that critically examine health agency utilization patterns, or certificates of need, the legal requirement that a potential provider agency demonstrate the need for its services before a license to practice is granted (see Chapter 6).

As the medical system slowly moves from an emphasis on diagnosis and treatment to prevention and health promotion, nurses are uniquely situated to provide guidance in developing health policy. The aforementioned activities are fundamentally nursing functions, and we must realize that public policy affects nursing practice regardless of venue (Taft & Nanna, 2008). Nurses must have a clear and present voice in the development of policy (O'Byrne & Holmes, 2009). As noted earlier, nursing tasks have been assigned to lesser-prepared staff, and this is most prevalent in the school setting. California gives us an example of how policy changes occur when school funding cuts, school nurse shortages, and a lack of understanding of disease processes converge to influence schools to permit unlicensed, nonmedical school personnel to provide vital health services to school children. The ANA, its California affiliate (ANA-CNA), and the California School Nurses Organization united to oppose a 2007 agreement between the California Department of Education and the American Diabetes Association (ADA) authorizing unlicensed school personnel (e.g., secretaries, health aides, and teachers) to administer insulin to diabetic children in the school setting. This agreement was developed in response to a 2005 lawsuit brought by the ADA and four school-aged children claiming that student rights were being violated according to two federal laws—Section 504 of the Rehabilitation Act and the Individuals with Disabilities Education Act. In June 2010, the court upheld nursing's position that only licensed nurses can administer insulin in the schools, and that this agreement to authorize unlicensed school personnel to administer insulin was a violation of the California Nurse Practice Act (Neiberg, 2010). Setting policy does not only occur in the halls of the capitol, but in the courts when an interpretation of existing law is required.

Policy can also be viewed as the key interests of professional organizations (e.g., *Nursing's Agenda for Healthcare Reform*, ANA, 1994); government agencies (e.g., *Healthy People 2020*); think tanks, such as the Heritage Foundation (e.g., *A Recipe for Reform: Success of Consumer-Driven Principles In Medicare Programs*, Nix, 2011); or advocacy groups, such as the Children's Defense Fund—the originators of the *Leave No Child Behind* movement that advocates for legislation and policies that ensure every child a "healthy start, a head start, a fair start, a safe start, and a moral start" (2011, para. 3). These disparate groups reflect various political persuasions that influence which policies are debated at the national and state levels (Taft & Nanna, 2008). How effective these groups are in influencing policy development and implementing change is also tied to the political environment, or more specifically, to who is in power. Each major political party has differing political agendas that impact the policies that eventually become law.

Workplaces also implement policy, such as workplace rules and regulations that affect how the workplace functions and what is required of an employee (e.g., dress code, policy and procedure manuals, hours of work, who has access to e-mail, what is acceptable behavior in the workplace, and so forth). The roles and responsibilities of unlicensed versus licensed personnel, as mentioned earlier, are also health care workplace issues that generate policy development, as do rulings related to collective bargaining (see Display 13.2). It should be noted that all licensed health care personnel operate under the licensure acts of each state. Laws regulate nursing and are enforced by a state agency. For nurses, it is usually the Board of Registered Nursing that defines and interprets the functions and responsibilities of their licensees. Changes cannot occur unless the practice acts are revised or the courts interpret the existing laws. There are frequently issues that arise in the workplace relating to turf battles; many times, the issues

DISPLAY 13.2 AN INCONSISTENT RULING AFFECTING NURSING

An October 2006 ruling by the National Labor Relations Board (NLRB) determines which employees are seen as "supervisors" or staff employees. One nursing union has interpreted this as a policy that will severely impact who can belong to a union, based on their job classification. This decision grew out of a 2001 Supreme Court case stating that an NLRB ruling in a Kentucky nursing facility case was flawed. The board at that time, composed mainly of Democrats, ruled that the registered nurses (RNs) at the nursing home were not supervisors because they did not "exercise independent judgment." The Supreme Court, in reviewing the case, sent it back to the board, stating that the role and duties of a supervisor should be more carefully reviewed. The board members at that time were mainly Republicans. A later decision by the NLRB found that Oakwood Healthcare failed to prove that an RN, acting as a relief clinical coordinator (10% to 15% of time), exercised "independent judgment in assigning nursing staff" and was, therefore, a supervisor (NLRB, 2009, p. 19). However, they also ruled that permanent charge nurses did fall into that category. The current board consists of two members, one Democrat and one Republican (Matthews, 2010).

From Matthews, J. (2010). When does delegating make you a supervisor? *Online Journal of Issues in Nursing, 15*(2), manuscript 3; *NLRB Annual Report*, 2009.

relate to reimbursement or a disagreement on what a licensed group can legally do.

Policies affect our daily lives, regardless of whether they are health or work related. So, community health nurses must have an understanding of health policy to better understand the issues affecting the communities they serve. It must be recognized that nurses have differing opinions on health policy, even down to the basic premise of whether nurses should become involved in political issues and the political process. According to Plato, "One of the penalties for refusing to participate in politics is that you end up being governed by your inferiors."

Process of Public Policy

The development of public policy is rarely easy, straightforward, or even rational. Myriad concerns determine whether one is successful with any attempt to make policy. Increasingly, the complexity of public–private interactions plays a strong role in how policy is developed, because of both the privatization of health care and the increased consolidation of health care providers and insurers. As noted earlier, managed care that is regulated by federal and state policies has a direct effect on how health care is delivered at the local level. Many states have applied for waivers that allow them to demonstrate how they can better provide access, save money, and increase the numbers of people covered if they don't have to follow the existing federal regulations. This has, in some cases, created unforeseen problems. For example, during the 1990s, 27 states under the federal state children's health insurance program established new non-Medicaid programs and, as a result, the states were unable to collect Vaccines for Children funds (VCF) for those in managed care because the CMS interpreted the new laws to mean that these children were in private health plans. The providers of vaccines for children, who obtained their care through Medicaid's Early Periodic Screening Diagnosis and Treatment, were eligible to acquire vaccines through the VCF program, as were providers of care to Native Americans, the uninsured, and rural or federally qualified health clinics. The states were not eligible to capture VCF and bore the costs for immunizing those children enrolled in the non-Medicaid plans. This demonstrates the unintended consequences of regulatory and legislative changes if all aspects are not known or adequately investigated or if disagreement arises regarding interpretation.

The public policy process is similar to advocacy or **political action** and involves a number of steps that are synonymous with the nursing process. The policy/advocacy process may appear linear, but it involves overlap, reordering of priorities, mobilization of resources, and development of stakeholders. The overarching issues in advocacy or public policy development are timing, funding, and politics. Each year, thousands of measures at the state and federal level are introduced, but only a fraction of them complete the legislative process (Figs. 13-1 and 13-2). This falloff can be attributed to a number of reasons: conflicting sides of the issue with the strongest side winning out, timing of bill introduction or an unwillingness to put it on the agenda based on other influences or competing issues, or the inability to identify a funding source.

How and Where to Start

It can be very tricky to come into a community and determine that an existing problem can be addressed politically. If you are aware of the problems, there are, no doubt, others who are also aware. It would be incumbent upon you to identify the leaders or elders of the community and determine if they have previously addressed the issue and, if so, what the outcome was. It is helpful to ask if they feel that the issue is something that should be reopened if they were not successful, or if they were satisfied with the previous outcome. It helps to know how these problems relate to the priorities of the city or county, and if there are stakeholders

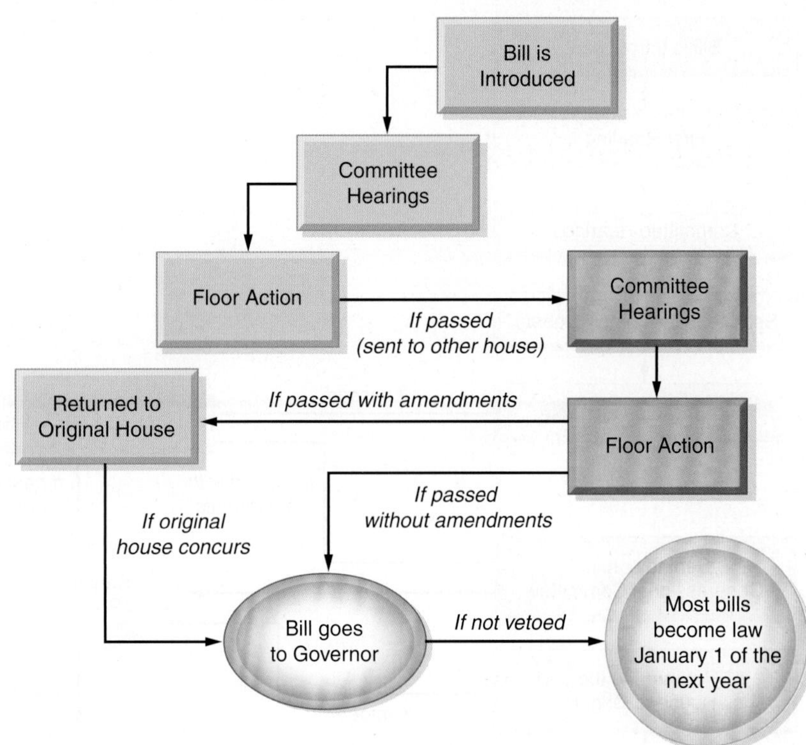

FIGURE 13-1. How a bill becomes a law—state process. The process may vary by state, but generally the schematic shows how the process unfolds. Source: California Legislative Counsel.

who are willing to become engaged in the issue. Costs or possible effects of addressing these issues must be considered. These are by no means exhaustive questions, but should be considered prior to assuming leadership in addressing the issues or problems affecting a community.

If you determine you are on safe ground and others are willing to be involved, various steps can be used to put forth the agenda of issues or problems the community will be addressing and may agree to take forward to their political representatives. Nurses can take several approaches when analyzing a policy that affects the health of a community or target population (Milstead, 2008). They can look at the reasons for policy formulation, the groups of people affected by the policy, or the policy's possible long-range consequences. When doing a **policy analysis**, nurses need to answer two general questions: Who benefits from this policy? Who loses from this policy? Whether the community, as a whole, should advocate for the policy depends on the degree to which the policy benefits the community without being detrimental to individuals or the country.

Figure 13-3 provides a simple model for studying health policy. If nurses know something about the forces shaping health policy and the policy process, they are in a better position to influence policy outcomes. The model identifies four major stages in the policy process: formulation, adoption, implementation, and evaluation.

- *Policy formulation* involves identifying goals, problems, and potential solutions.
- *Policy adoption* involves the authorized selection and specification of means to achieve goals, resolve problems, or both.
- *Policy implementation* follows adoption and occurs when the policy is put to use.
- *Policy evaluation* compares policy outcomes or effects with the intended or desired effects.

Stages 1 and 2: Policy Formulation and Adoption

Health policy formulation is the stage at which a policy is conceptualized and ultimately defined. It is approached in at least two ways. Most commonly, a health problem is identified, such as the increased infant mortality rate associated with teenage pregnancy, and health policy is developed to correct that particular problem. Another approach to policy formulation emphasizes health planning more than corrective actions, at least initially (Milstead, 2008). This is a goal-oriented approach. Health goals and strategies for achieving the goals are identified. In this more proactive approach, resources may be created as well as allocated for health services. Although either approach to policy formulation may lead to the solution of a health problem, the goal-oriented approach is less reactive in that it does not require problem identification before creating health policy.

The social and political conditions that affect policy formulation are limitless, but public need and public demand *should* be the strongest influences (Kovner & Knickman, 2011). Health care providers can stimulate a community to identify its health needs and demand health policies to fulfill its needs. During this process, the community health nurse should recognize that each community is unique, with its own mix of health services and public expectations.

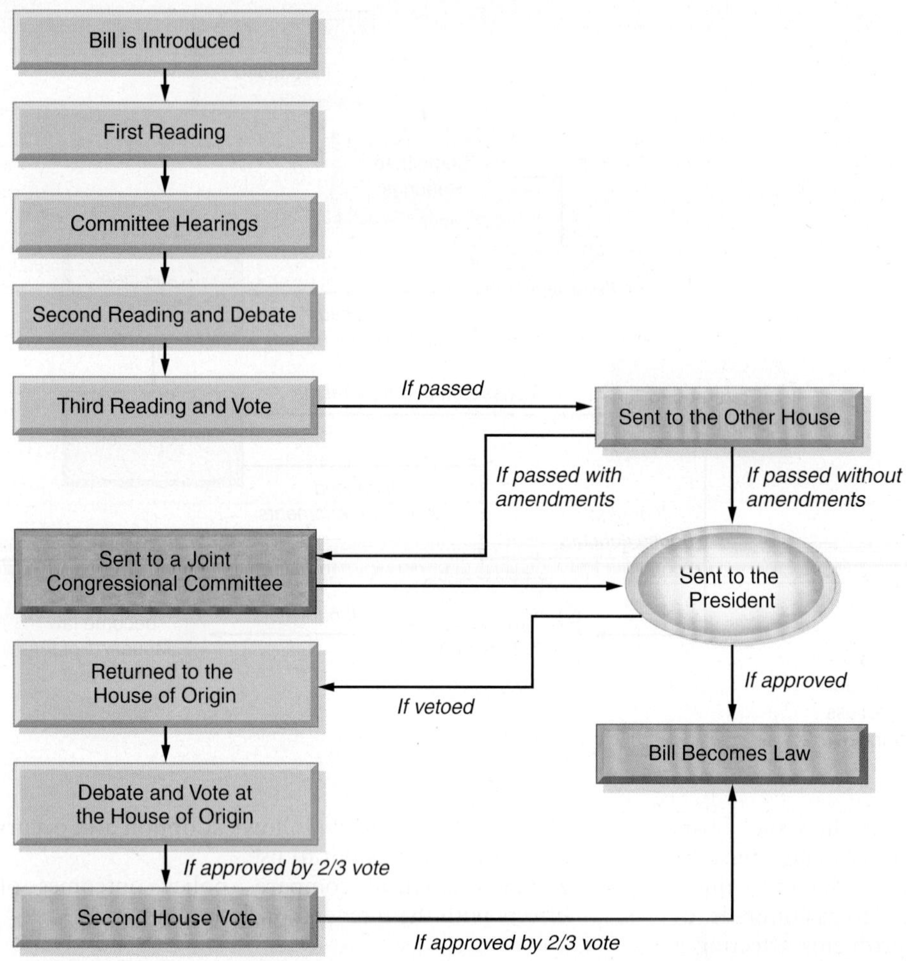

1. **Bill is Introduced**. Ideas for laws can come from a legislator, constituent, staff member, or organization.
2. **First Reading**. A legislator introduces the bill, and sends it to the clerk of his or her corresponding body (Senate or House), who gives it a number and title. This is the *first reading*, and the bill is referred to the proper committee.
3. **Committee Hearings**. The committee may decide the bill is unwise or unnecessary and *table* it, thus killing it at once. Or it may decide the bill is worthwhile and hold hearings to listen to facts and opinions presented by experts and other interested persons. After members of the committee have debated the bill and perhaps offered amendments, a vote is taken; if the vote is favorable, the bill is sent back to the floor of the house.
4. **Second Reading and Debate**. The clerk reads the bill sentence by sentence to the house; this is known as the *second reading*. Members may then debate the bill and offer amendments.
5. **Third Reading and Vote**. The *third reading* is by title only, and the bill is put to a vote, which may be by voice or roll call, depending on circumstances and parliamentary rules.
6. **Sent to the Other House**. The bill then goes to the other house of Congress, where it may be defeated or passed, with or without amendments.
7. **Sent to a Joint Congressional Committee**. If the bill is passed with amendments, a joint congressional committee must be appointed by both houses to resolve the differences.
8. **Sent to the President**. After its passage by both houses, the bill is sent to the president.
9. **Returned to the House of Origin**. If the president *vetoes* the bill, it is sent back to the house of origin with his reasons for the veto.
10. **Debate and Vote at the House of Origin**. The president's objections are read and debated, and a roll-call vote is taken.
11. **Second House Vote**. If the bill receives a two-thirds vote or greater in the house of origin, it is sent to the other house for a vote.
12. **Bill Becomes Law**. If the president approves the bill, or if his veto is overridden by a 2/3 vote in both houses, the bill becomes a law.

Note: Should the president desire neither to sign nor to veto the bill, he may retain it for ten days (Sundays excepted) after which time it automatically becomes a law without signature. However, if Congress has adjourned within those ten days, the bill is automatically killed, that process of indirect rejection being known as a *pocket veto*.

FIGURE 13-2. How a bill becomes a law—federal process.

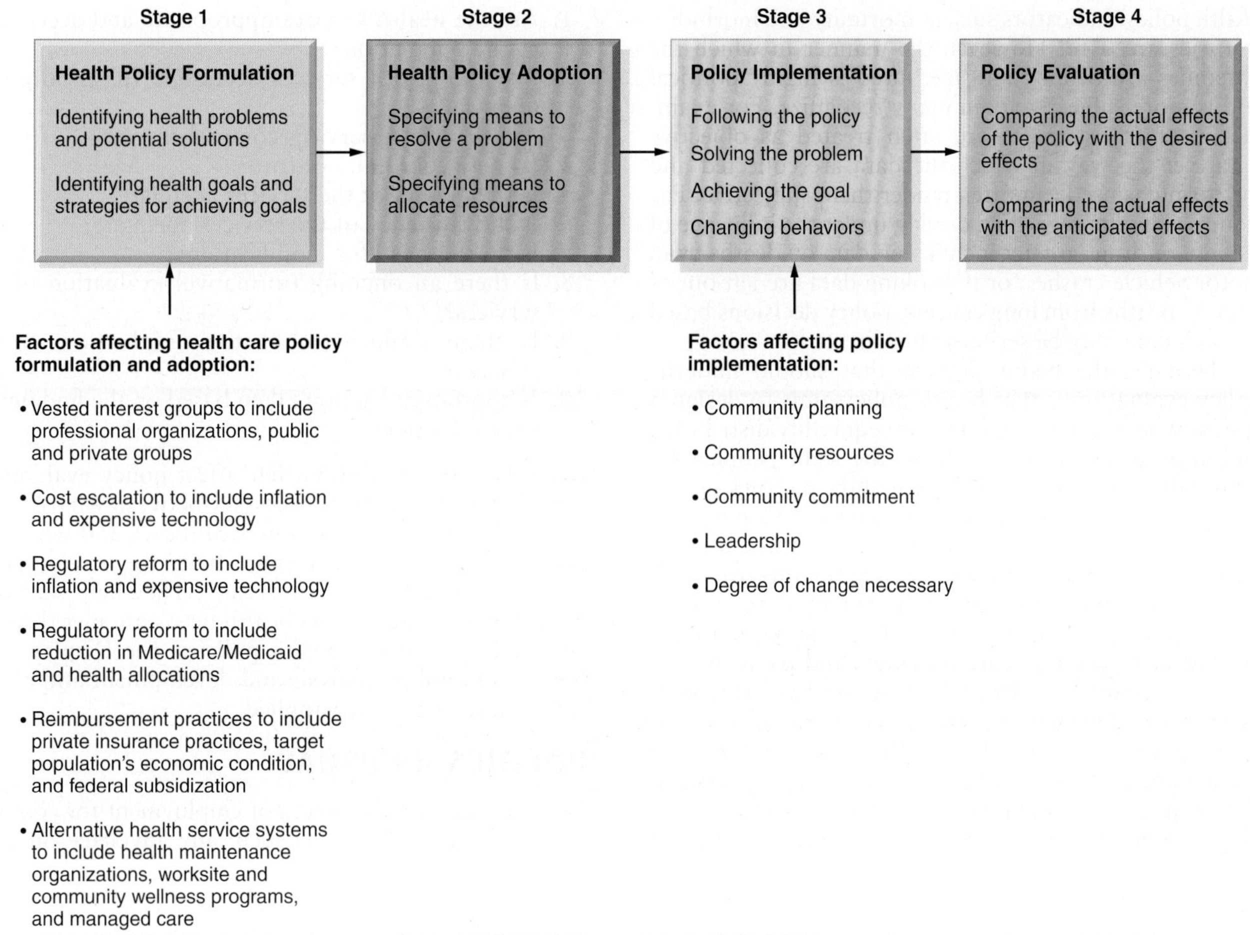

FIGURE 13-3. Policy analysis model.

Stage 3: Policy Implementation

Implementation of health policy occurs when an individual, group, or community puts the policy into use. It involves overt behavior changes as the policy is put into nursing practice. The extent of compliance with a policy is the most direct measure of the policy's implementation (Harrington & Estes, 2011). *Noncompliance* refers to conscious or unconscious refusal to follow the policy directives. Community health nurses have always been health policy implementers and, recently, evaluators, regardless of whether these roles were consciously chosen.

Implementation of health policy is an essential part of effective, comprehensive client care for many documentable reasons. It should now be apparent that policies come in many forms and can have statutory or nonstatutory origins. Nurses are most cognizant of the latter, in the form of procedure manuals and institutional guidelines. Communities are most aware of policies that limit or restructure their activities and growth, such as curfews and zoning regulations.

Once a health policy is written and adopted, its successful implementation depends heavily on the manipulation of many variables. For example, the implementation of day care standards depends, in part, on how they are interpreted and what resources are available to enforce them. As an implementer, the community health nurse assesses the capacity of the community to formulate and define strategies that will enhance the community's compliance with the policy. This phase of policy analysis does not focus on the merits or shortcomings of the policy, in contrast to policy formulation, adoption, and evaluation.

Stage 4: Policy Evaluation

Comparing what a policy does with what it is supposed to do is *evaluation*. Evaluation of a policy should result in continuation of the policy in its original form, revision or modification of the policy, or termination of the policy. Laws and policies are created to express the collective and powerful interests of the political system that generated them (Kovner & Knickman, 2011; Milstead, 2008). The need for a particular health policy may be temporary, but a policy may be difficult to change once it is adopted and implemented. Once a policy system is in operation, vested interests evolve as a result and become political influences. These vested interests, under the guise of jobs, positions, titles, and wealth, are perceptibly jeopardized by any change in the health policy that helped create them. Hence, tradition, in the form of old policies, tends to prevail (as in the case of CRNAs supervised by physicians, noted previously).

One form of policy evaluation examines the health outcomes that are believed to be attributable to the health policy. Indicators such as mortality and morbidity statistics are used. However, the manner in which the outcomes are defined and measured is highly political and is more subjective than many recognize. For example, mortality statistics are often treated as objective data, yet the way in which the data are collected and the formulas used can often render them subjective. For example, if data regarding driving under the influence of alcohol or drugs are not included in data on deaths from motor vehicle crashes, or if smoking data are left out of data on deaths from lung cancers, policy decisions based on such data may be seriously misdirected.

Perhaps, the major premise that should underlie policy evaluation is that health policy aims to design a system wherein health services are equitably distributed and appropriate care is given to the right people at a reasonable cost. Representing one of the nation's safety-net providers, the National Association of Community Health Centers noted that health care reform policies should make "significant and meaningful improvements in the accessibility and quality of primary care" (2009, p. ii). They would like to see investment in developing a workforce of primary care providers and payment systems that reward results and quality of care, as well as assurance of a primary health care home and investment in the primary care safety net. This is a shift from the fragmented system we have had that rewards specialization. When evaluating policy and programs, one should keep in mind the following basic criteria for evaluation:

1. Are the health services appropriate and acceptable to the population?
2. Are the health services accessible (physically and financially)?
3. Are the health services comprehensive?
4. Is there continuity of care?
5. Is the quality of the services adequate?
6. Is the efficiency of the services adequate?
7. Is there a need for modifications?
8. Is there an ongoing (formative) evaluation of the services?
9. Is there a final (summative) evaluation of the services?
10. Is appropriate action taken based on the findings of the evaluations?

Regardless of the factors that affect policy evaluation, continual comparison is necessary between what a community believes and wants in health care and what it is getting. Nurses have a responsibility to increase community awareness of health issues. They help the community make sure that its health needs are met through productive, desirable health policies. See Display 13.3 for steps in policy analysis and development and places where influence can be applied.

POLITICS AS USUAL

Communities are the places of employment for community health nurses and, as such, any advocacy on your

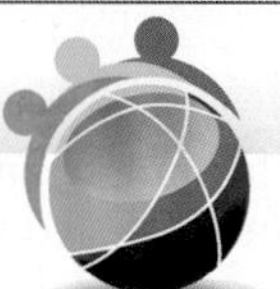

DISPLAY 13.3 STEPS IN POLICY ANALYSIS AND DEVELOPMENT

A number of models can be used to address these issues; the following steps are an amalgamation of models available for policy/advocacy development:

Policy Analysis

Looking at public problems and determining the appropriate solution—may consist of the following steps:

1. **Define the problem.** What is the problem and how will you solve it? It should be succinctly worded, so that those not familiar with the issue can understand it. A concept or issue paper may assist in clarifying the ideas and thoughts of the group.
2. **Gather information.** Be sure that information is accurate. Can you identify trends—increase or decrease over time, demographics? There must be agreement on the analysis of the facts and data.
3. **Find alternatives to your approach.** Don't reinvent the wheel. Have other communities solved this problem? How did they address it? Will their approach work in this community? If not, what is necessary to make it workable in your situation? There should be multiple alternatives, but the fewer the better to make it more manageable. There should also be agreement on consequence.
4. **Choose the most appropriate approach.** Which objectives will work, either long- or short-term? What is the cost of your approach and where will you get the funding? Can you determine the consequences of your actions? The approach must be strong and the message clear and understandable.

Strategy Development

Strategy development will tell you where you are, where you want to go, and how to get there. It is best to determine:

1. **Objective.** Clear and concise goals and objectives as determined by the policy analysis process. Objectives must be measurable.
2. **Audience.** Who is the audience that you must influence? Is this an issue addressed by local authorities—city (city council) or county (board of supervisors)—or by state (legislature, state agencies) or federal (Congress, federal agencies) authorities? Is this an issue that warrants people's attention?
3. **Message.** Frame the discussion. The message should be accurate and reflect the self-interest of

DISPLAY 13.3 STEPS IN POLICY ANALYSIS AND DEVELOPMENT *(Continued)*

the receiver. Receptivity also depends on whether the people are ready to hear the message. Messages should be tailored to each audience. Get the message out in various ways, for example, press conferences, letter writing, public presentations, and the like. Timing is critical in getting the message out.

4. **Messenger.** The messenger must be creditable—a member of the community or someone with ties to the community. Messengers can be seen as "experts" or speaking from experience. How does the group assist the messenger?
5. **Resources.** What do you already have, and what do you need to be successful? Build on the resources you currently have and determine what gaps exist. How can resources be increased if necessary? Are your coalitions reflective of the groups within the community and if not, how can others be brought aboard? Maintain open communication with all involved.
6. **Evaluation.** Is this working? Is your message meeting with success, and how is the audience responding? Review the goals and objectives and change if necessary. Ask what isn't working? Are we getting support on these issues?

How to Influence Public Policy

Several arenas exist in which one can influence public policy:

1. **Legislative.** Influence in this arena is done through bills or measures introduced by our representatives but may be the result of issues brought to them by individuals, professional organizations, or state/federal agencies. If these measures can complete the legislative process and be signed by the governor or president, these measures become law. This is a process for the development and passage of the majority of our laws or statutes. The process whereby this occurs is called the *legislative process*, and the public must be involved to ensure that the needs of various communities are met. Laws/policies determine how the society functions, how services and programs are distributed, and who can access them. Public comment and involvement allow for the development of sound public policy, hopefully with few unintended consequences. Each state has a nurse practice act that determines the roles and responsibilities of registered nurses and how they can legally function. One approach to addressing the nursing shortage was initiated by the National Council of Boards of Nursing–Nurse Licensure Compacts. By changing the laws and regulations of each state, it allows nurses licensed and in good standing to practice in another state if both are "compact states." These nurses have "multistate licenses." Currently, more than 20 states have changed their laws to allow nurses to move from one state to another while licensed in only one state.
2. **Judicial.** In the judicial arena, disputes relating to laws and/or regulations are brought before the court for affirmation or invalidation. Scope of practice and licensing laws, many times, are played out judicially. Professional organizations, employers, and unions may be more likely than individuals to use the courts for rulings on licensing, scope of practice, and workplace rules. However, there have been rulings on controversial health and social issues, such as minors' access to abortions and same-sex marriages, as well as findings relating to medical malpractice.
3. **Regulatory.** The regulatory arena involves implementation of existing laws. Codes of Regulations are issued by the agency that has oversight of the laws passed by the legislature. Regulations provide the specificity of the statute; for example, regulations accompanying a state nurse practice act provide the detail of how the act is to be implemented. The process allows for public comment prior to implementation; it is critical for nurses to be involved in the regulatory process, as many have a direct effect on individual nursing practice. For example, a California regulation—California Standards of Competence, Title 16, Section 1443.5 (6)—states that nurses must be patient advocates.
4. **Executive Order.** This order can be issued only by presidents or governors. President Obama in March 2009 issued an executive order that established the White House Office of Health Reform.
5. **Initiative.** An initiative is also called a *referendum* or *proposition*. It is a local process in which groups can qualify an issue for the ballot by collecting a percentage of names of voters, usually based on the numbers of voters in the last election. This is an example of direct democracy by voters bypassing our representative process. As an example, in the 2010 elections, four states had initiatives to determine if mandatory participation in federal health care should be prohibited.
6. **Budgetary.** The budgetary arena involves federal or state plan/legislation for funding services and programs. The federal or state budgets are reflective of what policy makers or those who are influential deem important. Being involved in the budget process is important for the implementation of various policies, as *most* policies require funding to be effective. The state–federal health programs of Medicaid and Medicare are affected by the funding appropriated in the state budgets. The state children's health insurance program is a children's health program instituted to cover those children who qualify based on certain criteria. This is a state–federal program; the amount of money coming from the federal government is based on the amount of money allocated by the state, this is called a "match."

part and/or policy changes will affect those within the communities you serve (Manthey, 2008). Your role is to be responsive to the needs of the community you serve and its attendant politics. **Politics** is defined as the art or science of government, or governing of a political entity. It can be and is often defined as the art of using influence to bring about change. However, you may already be aware that politics can represent the machinations in which groups or individuals engage to influence, gain power, or get their way. Politics can also be labeled as the relationships between elected officials and their constituents; it can also be seen as the interplay between staff nurses and their head nurse or nursing supervisor. Politics can be described as the practice of public ethics. A clear example of this is the conflict between individual needs and the needs of a community—such as the debate around assisted suicide or the continuing debate regarding universal health care. Within communities, it may be the debate on whether to have and/or where to locate a family planning clinic, or the most appropriate and effective methods to address teen pregnancy issues. As stated by the late Massachusetts congressman and former Speaker of the House, Tip O'Neill, "*All politics is local.*"

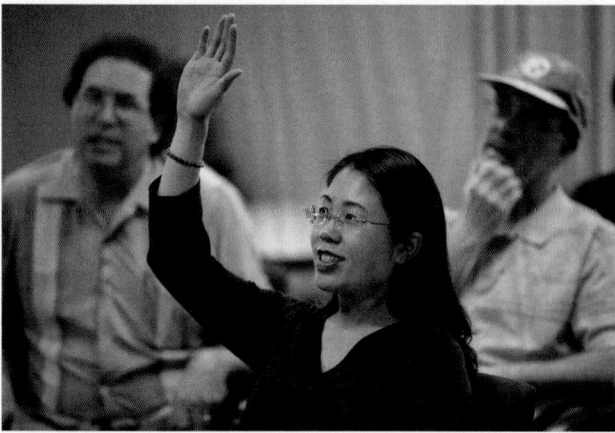

Town hall meetings promote community participation. (Photo courtesy of CDC Photo Image Library.)

Public health practice is inherently political because it involves the differing values and worldviews that exist in communities based on ethnicity, language, and culture. It is the primacy of these perspectives that influence which needs are addressed and the ultimate direction of public policy issues. Be aware that issues change over time; for example, chronic disease management and safety and quality issues take front stage currently, but in the 1970s substance abuse was a high priority and in the 1990s, it was violence prevention. These shifts reflect the dynamic nature of public health policy and how differing policies attract public attention and funding. The funding issues for public health have also changed over time, with private funding (e.g., managed care) now providing much of the care for low-income populations. This funding shift has also encouraged a swing back to the primary mission of public health—assurance, assessment, and policy development (see Chapter 1). It is imperative to understand that policy and politics go hand in hand; neither exists without the other (Milstead, 2008).

POWER AND EMPOWERMENT

Eliciting services and programs for unserved or underserved populations is a never-ending issue. Citizen participation is never particularly easy in communities that are excluded from political or economic resources. Sherry Arnstein, in her classic 1969 treatise *A Ladder of Citizen Participation*, stated that "citizen participation is citizen power," and without access to information about how the system functions, these populations cannot obtain the resources they need to make their communities livable and nurturing (p. 217). Arnstein goes on to point out that those in power prevent those in need from accessing the process:

> The idea of citizen participation is a little like eating spinach: no one is against it in principle because it is good for you. Participation of the governed in their government is, in theory, the cornerstone of democracy—a revered idea that is vigorously applauded by virtually everyone. The applause is reduced to polite handclaps, however, when this principle is advocated by the have-not Blacks, Mexican Americans, Puerto Ricans, Indians, Eskimos, and Whites. When the have-nots define participation as redistribution of power, the American consensus on the fundamental principle explodes into many shades of outright racial, ethnic, ideological, and political opposition (p. 216).

Although Arnstein writes about the anger that disenfranchised populations feel, she does offer possible solutions that allow each party to "share power through partnership," as outlined by engaging in the process discussed in her treatise (p. 217). (See more on this in Chapter 15.) **Power** can be defined as the ability to act or produce an effect, possession of control, or authority or influence over others. As public health professionals, nurses have a commitment to social justice and working with disadvantaged communities. This means that nurses have a responsibility to ensure community participation in issues affecting them, and they must continually examine the relationship and position they hold within these communities. The term **empowerment** has been used to explain a process of assisting communities to come together to express their values and ideas to those outside the community (Cawley & McNamara, 2011). Generally, the issue of empowerment comes up when outside forces are behaving in a way that the community considers detrimental to its well-being. The various definitions of empowerment and the expansion of the definition of health, which now includes the social, political, and economic determinants of health, have changed our thinking on how best to interact with the communities we serve. Theorists have suggested that if power is the ability to control, predict, and participate in one's environment, then empowerment is the process whereby individuals and communities take power and transform their lives (Laverack, 2006; Yoo, Butler, Elias, & Goodman, 2008) (see *Perspectives—Student Voices*).

PERSPECTIVES STUDENT VOICE

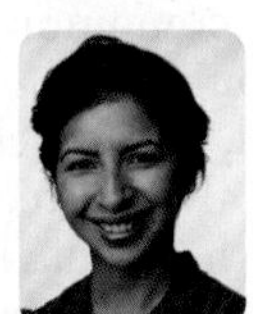

Advocacy for the Ages

I remember being told in nursing school that we needed to become "politically active" and should be prepared to "legislatively advocate for our clients." I always thought that it would be up to someone else—someone older, more experienced, more eloquent, and knowledgeable. I didn't really think they were talking about me. Well, I realize now that anyone can be a political advocate! I read about Bria Brown, a 13-year-old girl from Florida, who was diagnosed with osteosarcoma at age 6. She was an inpatient at Miami Children's Hospital for a year and now describes herself as a cancer survivor. While at Miami Children's she met 18 other children who succumbed to their cancers—one of them her best friend, Chendarlyn Williams. But despite all of this, she has raised over $120,000 for the American Cancer Society (ACS) and is now an ACS Ambassador. She has spoken to her state legislature in Florida, urging them to provide help for children with cancer. And, she and her family have gone to Washington, D.C., and met with local congressional leaders in order to promote increased funding for cancer research. She advocates on the local, state, and national levels. What an inspiring story! She now wants to study to be a pediatrician, to help children who are also fighting cancer (Nestle, 2010). If a young girl can be a political advocate and can lobby for health issues, I certainly need to rethink my priorities and get to work! After all, I have a wealth of knowledge and experiences I can share to help persuade my legislator to vote for issues and policies I believe are important.

Cara, Age 24, Oncology Nurse

This also suggests a change in the relationship between professionals and communities—a change from the customary hierarchical patient–provider relationship to one of a partnership (Baxamusa, 2008). However, one must be mindful that professionals hold the power and authority by virtue of their place in the bureaucracy. They have access to information, are better connected politically, and are more cognizant of how to make the system positively respond to the issues they bring forth.

How does one make sure that preconceived ideas about certain communities are not forced on the community in order to meet the goals and objectives of the public health agency? In the past, community health promotion practice often only met the bottom rung of Arnstein's ladder by using the rhetoric of community participation while the professionals working with the community actually set the agenda. Health promotion may best be facilitated by the use of empowerment, and assisting individuals and communities in articulating their problems and solutions. Discovering what is most important to the community and providing access to that information, while supporting leadership from within the community, and by encouraging them to overcome bureaucratic hurdles to action are important parts of community empowerment. This helps to improve problem-solving skills and abilities (Wong, Zimmerman, & Parker, 2010). This is a concept also enforced in the IOM (2002b) report *The Future of the Public's Health in the 21st Century*.

INFLUENCING POLICY

So, how can PHNs influence policies that affect the communities they serve? We have discussed how you, as a professional, can empower your communities, based on your knowledge of how to influence others and your ability to encourage those within your communities to join with you in advocating policies that positively impact their lives. Health care policies are usually the result of legislative action at the state and federal levels, and the regulations that are implemented as a result of this legislation provide the specifics of how each law is to be carried out. So, how do we influence policy makers to hear our concerns and act on them?

Seasoned advocates have developed skills in influencing policy decisions; ground rules also exist by which to play the game. Some call them the "ten commandments of lobbying." However these steps are described, advocates adhere to the basic ideas inherent in the following:

1. **Honesty is the best policy**. Being known as someone who has integrity is a lasting virtue. Never mislead a legislator or someone who is likely to support your interests, as it is difficult to regain credibility once you lose it. Speaking beyond your level of expertise gets advocates into trouble. If you don't know the answer, say so; but if you promise to get the answer, then do so. Do not promise what you can't deliver.
2. **Start early**. Planning always takes longer than you think it will. Your interests are not everyone's interests and convincing others they should be involved always involves time. If you are planning policy change at the state or federal level, it is vital to know the legislative process and the critical time lines.
3. **Know what you want.** Be aware of all sides of the issue prior to approaching a policy maker, know the pros and cons, and be prepared to answer questions and provide data on both sides of the issue. Understand the role politics plays in getting what you want and how policy makers may respond to your issue. Targeting your story to the goals, emotions, and interests of the legislator is important and may result in a positive outcome. Be *clear* about what you are asking the legislator for—to carry legislation, or to vote no or yes on specific legislation. Asking your legislator to vote a certain way is perfectly legitimate, and if you don't ask, the opposition will.
4. **KISS** (Keep it simple, stupid). Be able to articulate your issues in a clear and concise manner. Do not confuse possible supporters with complicated arguments. Key issues should be concise and clear and

on one page, no more than two. Leave behind an informational packet with pertinent information about the community and/or services and programs.

5. **No permanent enemies, no permanent friends.** Political affiliation doesn't always determine what interests a person has or whether they are likely to support your interests. It behooves you to speak with everyone on your issue; if nothing else, you may find out who they are and why they may oppose your concerns. Remember, in politics, there are only permanent interests.
6. **Know your opponents.** Visit with all possible supporters—just because someone opposed you in the past doesn't mean they won't support you on a current issue. Respectful disagreement keeps the door open for future agreement and compromise.
7. **Compromise.** Ask for much more than you think you can get. When negotiating, you can give up something without hurting your priorities or your bottom line. In politics, rarely does anyone get all they want, but priority setting is key: What do we expect to accomplish with this activity?
8. **There is strength in numbers.** The more groups involved, the more likely you are to be successful. Any opportunity for networking is an opportunity to enlarge your coalition. Including disparate groups means you may have accessed conflicting political persuasions. Additionally, having groups who can speak with those who are not seen as "friends" is useful. Cross-fertilization of groups is politically expedient, but understand that next time you or they may be in opposition.
9. **Work at the local level.** Legislators are interested in their constituents—these are the people who elected them to office and who will keep them in office. To be noticed by policy makers, sharing information with them about their constituents is the surest way to capture their attention. Information sharing should occur on issues both in the community where you live and in the one where you work.
10. **Thank you.** Everyone loves to be told, "Job well done." To maintain your coalitions, always recognize the work of others. Spreading the credit is like sowing seeds: the wider the spread, the more bountiful the crop.

Finally, it is important for those new to advocacy to understand that the thing with the most critical influence on policy is *money*. Nurses, even with the passage of the recent health care reform legislation, must become even more actively involved in the process of influencing policy. How many nurses understand that the nurse practice acts, or portions thereof, under which they work are developed by legislators or special interest groups who don't have a background in health care? How many nurses know who their legislators are at either the state or federal level? How many nurses have written their legislators about pending health care legislation or legislation that affects nursing? (see Display 13.4).

The 2010 federal midterm election was the most expensive midterm election in history, with $4.2 billion spent on television campaign ads (Gardner, 2010). Money—who has it and who gives it—is increasingly becoming an issue in state and federal elections. Sadly, money is important in assuring that your legislator or candidate can maintain or win a seat whether at the state or federal level. Campaign financing is important because TV ads, direct mailers, campaign staff, not

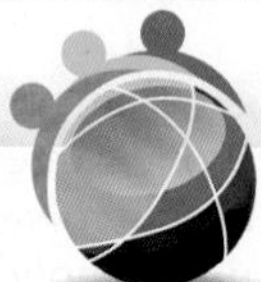

DISPLAY 13.4 HOW TO HELP YOUR LEGISLATOR KNOW THE COMMUNITY

1. **Know who your legislators are—local, state, and federal:**
   - Include their contact information on your e-mail and regular mailing lists.
   - Develop a relationship with them or their staff.
2. **Assign a constituent to the legislator:**
   - Keep all critical information on legislators up to date.
   - What are the key committees they sit on?
3. **Keep legislators and staff informed:**
   - Keep them aware of any actions occurring in the community.
   - Share any printed materials.
   - Provide them with updated, current promotional information.
   - Send copies of news articles, radio interviews, and alerts.
   - If you have a website, blog, podcasts, etc., send URL.
   - Invite legislators to your facility or community tour for "show and tell."
4. **When passing out awards, think of your legislators:**
   - Recognize any actions by legislators that benefit the community in which you serve.
   - Invite legislators to award ceremonies and/or community events.
5. **Communicate with your policy maker:**
   - Write your policy maker about issues important to the communities in which you serve or issues important to your profession.
   - Provide real stories or examples of the issue.
   - Use personal letters; postcards, phone calls, form letters, and e-mail are not always the most effective way to deliver your message.

withstanding volunteers, and political consultants all require adequate funding. Anyone running for a political position knows that in order to compete, money is required; those with the most financing can get their message out and encourage potential voters to vote for them. While spending the most money doesn't always guarantee success, without sufficient financing you can be assured your message will *not* be heard. As stated by Jesse Unruh, the Speaker of the California Assembly in the 1960s, "*money is the mother's milk of politics.*"

Political Action Committees

One reason why nurses are less politically active can be tied to a lack of money. Nurses don't earn as much money or appear not to have access to as much money as other health care interests (e.g., hospitals, physicians, insurance companies, and health care plans), and as such there is much less money for nursing organizations to use for lobbyists or to assist chosen candidates. As mentioned earlier, the ANA has a political action committee (PAC) that supports federal candidates on a nonpartisan basis; candidates must demonstrate an interest in and willingness to vote for nursing issues or issues that nurses support. To participate in the PAC, you must be a member of ANA (this also allows your family to contribute to the PAC). By giving to the ANA-PAC, one maximizes their contribution by joining with other nurses—this power in numbers increases our influence with those candidates we choose to endorse. ANA-PAC has instituted the "Race for the Million" campaign to raise money in support of candidates and legislators who back nurses' issues (Song, n.d.). However, giving to your personal legislator can keep you on their mailing list, and it may get you invited to local legislative activities. It also lets your legislator know you are interested in whether she remains in office. Being in regular contact with your legislators provides an avenue for introducing legislation that impacts nursing or other health-related issues, and when you call to ask for a vote "for" or "against" an issue, the legislator is more likely to entertain your request. Aren't you more likely to respond to someone you know, rather than someone who comes to you out of the blue to ask for a favor?

Volunteering

Money is *not* the only way to build a relationship with your legislator. Volunteering your time can be just as important (see *Perspectives—Voices from the Community*). Candidates for office need bodies to get things done (e.g., phone banking, stuffing mailers, answering phones, putting up flyers and campaign posters, walking door to door to spread the message, and assisting in the development of issue papers). Candidates develop issue papers to tell their constituents where they stand on key campaign concerns. Nurses have the expertise to assist legislators in developing an agenda on health care policy, or at the least to review and comment on issue papers.

PERSPECTIVES
VOICES FROM THE COMMUNITY

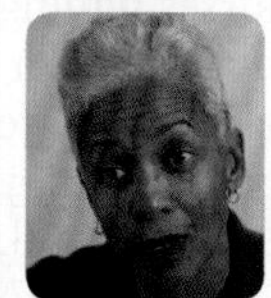

Volunteer Service for the Long Term

A registered nurse (RN) who had been through what I called the women's legislative career ladder—School Board, City Council, County Board of Supervisors—was now posed to run for the state legislature. Because we had had numerous contacts and I believed she would make a good state legislator and a voice for nursing and health care, I volunteered to work in her campaign office. I primarily answered the phones on the evenings I worked, but I met the office staff—many of them were much younger than me. And, even once, she came in while I was there. I talked with the staff about some of my experiences as a lobbyist, and they shared their experiences; many of them were fresh out of college.

She was successful in her run for office, and whenever I needed to meet with her or her staff, I was shown right in. I was also asked my opinion about the hiring of certain staff. Her staff knew me by name—many of them did not work on her campaign, but they were told about me by those campaign staff who were still around. After 3 years in office, she was appointed chairperson of a key committee, and I maintained access to her committee consultants and to her when necessary. We were able to work together quite successfully and, although we didn't always agree on every policy issue, I think the weeks I put in volunteering 3 years earlier really paid off for the clients and the issues I was representing.

L.B., Professional Lobbyist

Relationships are critical in policy development and in affecting public policy. As demonstrated earlier, being a friend can reap huge benefits when health care policy is on the line. Being involved in local and state elections can take many forms. Voting, for instance, is vital—RNs represent a substantial block of potential voters (Nickitas et al., 2011). Joining your local and state professional organizations is vital to having the voice of nursing heard at all levels. You can become more actively involved by writing legislators about the health care issues that impact the communities, both where you live and work. It is also vital to understand the importance of critically timing those communications. Effective communications with legislators should be tied to times when the issues are being heard in policy committee—thus, you must know when your issue is scheduled to be discussed in committee. For example, it is prudent to send letters on your issue—via fax or regular mail—close to the time of the committee hearing. Holding a press conference or getting other media coverage when the bill is introduced, or on the day it will be heard in committee, is quite effective in drawing attention to your issue. Writing letters to the editor of your local newspaper on health issues and writing articles for various publications are also effective methods of persuading others to back your issue. Other methods for influencing health policy or nursing issues include applying for positions on boards and commissions; each local area has advisory committees for their locally elected officials at the city and county level. The state board of RNs needs nurses willing to sit on their board or to serve on various advisory committees and task forces. At your state capitols, there are usually vacancies on policy committees, or legislators may be looking for new staff—either personal or policy. And, who better to serve in this capacity than a nurse! Who else has more knowledge about health issues than nurses? When all else fails, *run for office*.

A Call to Action

The need for health care reform has become critical as the costs of health care continue to rise. The United States spends a disproportionate percentage of the national budget on health care, yet major segments of the population still do not have adequate access to quality health services. Because of these economic concerns, health care reform and policy making have become politically charged issues involving many groups and factions that include not only health care providers and health care professionals but also government, third-party payers, insurance companies, and others with vested interests.

Many people are just beginning to realize that health care is a business. It has always been a business—we are just more aware of it now because of the scarcity of resources. Many believe that business interests and efforts to curb rising costs may divert public services away from community health issues, such as preventive and primary care. Because community health nurses know community needs and the value of such services, they need to be a major force in the political arenas where health policy decisions are being made. Community health nurses need to become politically aware and active to ensure quality health services by working as community health advocates. They must collaborate with community constituents and with nurses and other professionals to ensure the safety and wellbeing of groups and populations at risk.

Health care is the talk of the nation, and nurses must be involved in the process of setting policy for themselves and their communities. Although nursing's influence has been limited in the recent past, we are making progress and must continue to learn how to empower ourselves as professionals, individuals, and the communities with whom we work by becoming politically active and aware. If we are to fulfill our mission of promoting, protecting, and preserving the health of aggregates, we must become policy makers as well as policy implementers. We must learn to use policy systems and the political process, so that our voice is heard and we have influence in policy decision making. We must learn to formulate, implement, and evaluate health policies. We must understand the legislative process and how to influence that process. The politically involved nurse should aim to accomplish three primary goals: (1) generate support for one's views by communicating ideas effectively and getting to know and influence representatives at local, state, and national levels; (2) create professional legitimacy by keeping abreast of current issues in health care and nursing and becoming involved in professional nursing organizations, community boards or committees, or political office at the local, state, or national level; and (3) resolve conflict and effectively negotiate and compromise.

We have a rich history of advocacy, of using data and statistics to influence public policy, of speaking out about the injustices in our society, and of providing leadership in the development of services and programs that uplift and enrich the lives of the least among us. The inequities in our system, both socially and politically, add to the existing health disparities (National Association of Community Health Centers, 2009).

Chapters 5 and 10 of this text highlighted the need for cultural and linguistic competency, and it is clear that our institutions of higher learning must become more actively involved in developing and implementing curricula that educates and trains our health care providers with an understanding of, appreciation for, respect for, and competency in dealing with diverse cultures and languages. These programs must also challenge our individual values relating to other cultures and their worldviews. After all, these are the populations with whom you will work, and they will look to you for advice and leadership.

We also must do a better job of encouraging people of color to enter and complete courses of study in the health professions, for it is only when we have a critical mass of diverse providers and educators that we can we hope to alleviate some of the health inequities that challenge us today. *It is not enough to be clinically competent; one must be culturally competent.*

Nurses, despite their numbers and past history of public health nursing advocacy, have not really challenged the society in which they function. This duality has also hindered nurses' development as policy developers and advocates. Because of pressing health care concerns and the nursing shortage, many of us have become politically active and will remain so as the development of the regulatory framework implements ACA. With our successful participation in the passage of health care reform, many realize the importance of political advocacy and the effect it can have on nursing and the issues we represent. We are still gaining knowledge and experience in empowering the communities we serve by working with them to identify their strengths, examining the system rather than blaming the individual, and engaging with them in the development and implementation of preventive and health promotional behaviors that allow communities to grow and to become independent and self-reliant. When we "work with" communities, and do not "direct" them, we achieve personal growth as well.

Finally, community health nursing is a proud discipline with a rich foundation of helping the less fortunate and addressing issues that impact poorer communities. We are continually working toward empowering ourselves and our profession, as well as the larger communities that often suffer because of societal inequities. Community health nurses must honor this mandate to become policy advocates, to influence policy, and to learn how the policy process works, so that their voices and the voices of their communities are heard.

SUMMARY

This chapter has reviewed the political processes inherent in the development of health policies and the community health nurse's policy and advocacy roles within those processes. The foundations of political action and advocacy stem from a rich history of PHNs, like Lillian Wald, who strived to provide a voice for vulnerable and disenfranchised populations. Social justice remains a pillar of our current practice.

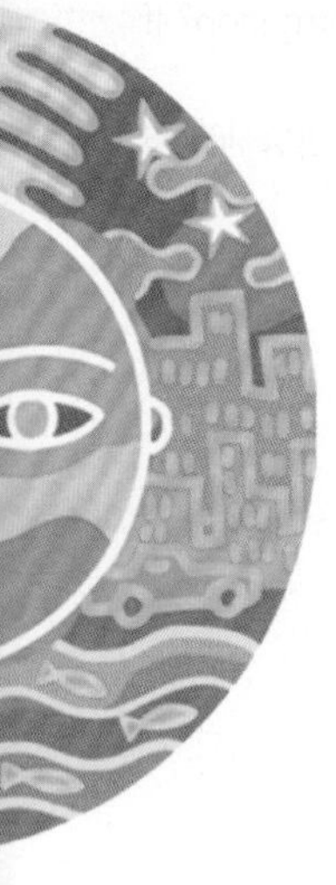

Advocacy for our clients is always important, but professional advocacy through affiliation and activity in our professional nursing organizations is also vital so that we, as PHNs, may have a "collective voice." This chapter highlighted examples of nurses who are serving as elected officials—many of whom came to power through grassroots efforts. Politics may be uncomfortable and foreign to many of us, yet it provides the methods for needed change through lobbying or influencing legislators. Nurses and special interests groups can gain access to legislators individually or through the services of a professional lobbyist or PACs.

Policies are actions or agendas that can be used to implement important goals and objectives, such as the health objectives found in *Healthy People 2020*. Distributive, redistributive, and regulatory health policies were defined and discussed, along with the processes that can be used by PHNs to impact policy formulation, adoption, implementation, and evaluation. Tips on how to influence policy makers were outlined, and nurses may consider volunteering time to a candidate of their choice as a means of gaining greater access to the political process. Nurses' role in health care reform was discussed, along with IOM's *The Future of Nursing*, and lobbying efforts by the ANA.

Community health nursing is by nature political because we deal with many issues that affect the health and wellbeing of the diverse populations we serve. Power and empowerment are important concepts to both public health nursing and politics, and political action and advocacy skills should be honed by every community health nurse.

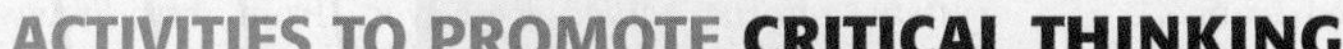

ACTIVITIES TO PROMOTE **CRITICAL THINKING**

1. Investigate a major health policy system in your community or state, discover how it works, and determine whether community health nurses are represented in this system. Areas to investigate include the boundaries of the system, the authority by which the system generates health policy, how the system receives input (formally and informally), resources the policy system uses and allocates to others, and the system's output over the past few years.
2. Describe a legislative bill related to community health at either the state or federal level and the issues involved in it. Identify who is sponsoring the bill, who is opposing it, and why. Determine who will be affected by the bill if it passes and in what ways they will be affected. Discuss what you, as a community health nurse, could do to be involved in this bill and then develop a political action plan to support or oppose the bill. Write a letter to your legislator regarding your position.
3. Carefully review your own health care insurance plan and determine whether you believe it is an adequate and equitable plan. Describe the plan and the issues involved in it. Include what health services are covered and who is authorized to provide services and receive direct reimbursement. Also determine who qualifies for the plan, who is excluded, and what conditions can disqualify a person or a family once they have been covered by the plan. Survey your class and determine the percentage of students not covered by some type of health insurance and who is for or against the Obama health reforms (anonymous ballot).
4. Attend a meeting of a professional organization, board of directors, government agency, or council when a health policy or health care issue is on the agenda. Analyze the positions of the major interest groups involved and describe to what extent economics comes into the discussion. Describe who controls the discussion and how this is done.
5. Interview a health care administrator in your local area and determine this person's position on health care reform and the rationale for his position. Determine at what levels this administrator is politically active and involved in influencing policy.

ACTIVITIES TO PROMOTE **CRITICAL THINKING** *(Continued)*

6. Several websites for government agencies and organizations are shared in this chapter. Contact two or three of them. What resources can you get from these sites? How can you use the political advocacy information as a community health nurse? Did these sites lead you to other sites? If they did, contact these additional sites and write down the additional website addresses in the margin of the chapter for future reference.
7. What issues or events occurred in the United States that reduced the willingness of nurses to speak out about health care issues? Examine the years starting with the 1930s. What events or issues changed, if any, to reinvigorate nurses serving as political activists?
8. Are nurses the most qualified group to articulate national health care issues? If so, why? If not, why not?
9. Do you consider it an ethical or human rights issue to provide appropriate and accurate health information? If yes, why? If not, why not?
10. Who are your state legislators? What are the critical health issues in your state, and how have your legislators responded to the issues? If there has been health care-related legislation introduced
    - What is the issue?
    - What party introduced the bill?
    - Where is the bill in the legislative process?
    - What groups support or oppose the legislation?
    - What is the reasoning for the groups' support or opposition?
11. How active is your state professional nursing organization in policy issues?
    Are you a member of the organization? If not, why not?
    What are the public policy issues the organization is involved in?
    How successful have they been?
    Does the group have a paid lobbyist or does it rely on volunteer lobbyists?

REFERENCES

Abelson, R. (2011, May 13). Health insurers making record profits as many postpone care. *The New York Times*. Retrieved from http://www.nytimes.com/2011/05/14/business/14health.html

Aiken, L. H., Cheung, R. B., & Olds, D. M. (2009). Education policy initiatives to address the nurse shortage in the United States *Health Affairs, 28*(4), w646–w656.

American Association of Colleges of Nursing (AACN). (2011a, April). *Nursing faculty shortage: Fact sheet*. Retrieved from http://www.aacn.nche.edu/Media/Factsheets/facultyshortage.htm

American Association of Colleges of Nursing (AACN). (2011b, May). *Clinical nurse leader*. Commission on Nurse Certification. Retrieved from http://www.aacn.nche.edu/CNC/pdf/SOC.pdf

American Association of Nurse Anesthetists. (2010). *Fact sheet concerning state opt-outs and November 13, 2001 CMS rule*. Retrieved from http://www.aana.com/Advocacy.aspx?id=2573

American Nurses Association (ANA). (1994). *Nursing's agenda for healthcare reform*. Washington, DC: Author.

American Nurses Association (ANA). (2001). *Code of ethics for nurses with interpretive statements*. Retrieved from http://www.nursingworld.org/ethics/code/protected _nwcoe303.htm

American Nurses Association (ANA). (February, 2008). *ANA's health system reform agenda*. Silver Springs, MD: Author.

America's Health Insurance Plans. (2009, October). *Individual health insurance 2009: Comprehensive survey of premiums, availability, and benefits*. Retrieved from http://www.ahipresearch.oprg/pdfs/2009IndividualMarketSurveyFinalReport.pdf

American Nurses Association (ANA). (2010, March 30). *ANA's nurses' efforts pay off in historic health care bill signing*. Press Release. Retrievedfromhttp://www.nursingworld.org/MainMenuCategories/HealthcareandPolicyIssues/HealthSystemReform/What-ANA-is-Doing/Health-Care-Bill-Signing.aspx

American Nurses Association (ANA). (2010, December 20). *Capitol update: Four new nurses to join 112th Congress in January*. Retrieved from http://www.capitolupdate.org/index.php/2010/12/four-new-nurses-to-join-112th-congress-in-january/

American Nurses Association (ANA). (2011a). *ANA history*. Retrieved from http://www.nursingworld.org/history

American Nurses Association (ANA). (2011b). *At the health system reform table*. Retrieved from http://www.nursingworld.org/MainMenuCategories/HealthcareandPolicyIssues/HealthSystemReform/What-ANA-is-Doing/At-the-Table.aspx

Aries, N. (2011). To engage or not engage: Choices confronting nurses and other health professionals. In D. Nickitas, D. Middaugh, & N. Aries (Eds.). *Policy and politics for nurses and other health professionals: Advocacy and action* (pp. 3–24). Sudbury, MA: Jones and Bartlett Publishers.

Arnstein, S. (1969). A ladder of citizen participation. *Journal of American Planning Association, 35*(4), 216–224.

Ballou, K. A., & Landreneau, K. J. (2010). The authoritarian reign in American health care. *Policy, Politics, & Nursing, 11*(1), 71–79.

Barusch, A. S. (2009). *Foundations of social justice in human perspective* (3rd ed.). Belmont, CA: Brooks/Cole.

Baxamusa, M. H. (2008). Empowering communities through deliberation: The model of community benefits agreements. *Journal of Planning, Education, & Research, 27*(3), 261–276.

Beaglehole, R., & Bonita, R. (Eds.). (2009). *Global public health: A new era* (2nd ed.). New York: Oxford University Press.

Boutain, D. M. (2005). Social justice as a framework for professional nursing. *Journal of Nursing Education, 44*(9), 404–408.

Boutain, D. M. (2008). Social justice as a framework for undergraduate community health clinical experiences in the United States. *International Journal of Nursing Education Scholarship, 5*(1), 1–12.

Buerhaus, P., Auerbach, D., & Staiger, D. (2009). The recent surge in nurse employment: Causes and implications. *Health Affairs, 28*(4), 657–668.

Bureau of Labor Statistics. (2011). *Occupational outlook handbook 2010-11 edition*. U. S. Department of Labor. Retrieved from http://www.bls.gov/oco/ocos083.htm

Cawley, T., & McNamara, P. (2011). Public health nurse perceptions of empowerment and advocacy in child health surveillance in West Ireland. *Public Health Nursing, 28*(2), 150–158.

Centers for Disease Control and Prevention (CDC). National Immunization Program (2009). *NIS data, tables, Jan-Dec 09*. Retrieved from http://www.cdc.gov/vaccines/stats-surv/nis/data/tables_2009.htm

Children's Defense Fund (CDF). (2011). *CDF mission statement*. Retrieved from http://www.childrensdefense.org/about-us/

Cillizza, C. (2010, March 21). Five myths about the politics of health-care reform. *The Washington Post*, B03. Retrieved from http://www.washingtonpost.com/wp-dyn/content/article/2010/03/18/AR2010031801518.html

Cohen, S. S., Mason, D. J., Kovner, C., Leavitt, J. K., Pulcine, J. & Sochalshi, J. (1996). Stages of nursing's political development: Where we've been and where we ought to go. *Nursing Outlook, 44*(6), 259–66.

deChesnay, M., & Anderson, B. A. (2012). *Caring for the vulnerable: Perspectives in nursing theory, practice, and research* (3rd ed.). Burlington, MA: Jones & Bartlett Learning.

Dodd, C. (2008). Play to win: Know the rules. In C. Harrington & C. Estes (Eds.). *Health policy: Crisis and reform in the U.S. health care delivery system* (5th ed.) (pp. 15–26). Sudbury, MA: Jones & Bartlett Publishers.

Dulisse, B., & Cromwell, J. (2010). No harm found when nurse anesthetists work without supervision by physicians. *Health Affairs, 29*(8), 1469–1475.

Families USA. (2009, October). *Fact sheet: Medicaid and the Children's Health Insurance Program (CHIP) soften the blow during tough economic times. Retrieved from* http://www.familiesusa.org/assets/pdfs/medicaid-chip-soften-blow.pdf

Foreman, P. G. (2009). *Activist sentiments: Reading Black women in the 19th century*. Chicago, IL: University of Illinois Press.

Fyffe, T. (2009). Nursing shaping and influencing health and social care policy. *Journal of Nursing Management, 17*(6), 698–706.

Gardner, D. (2010, November 9). The real cost of the midterms: How politicians spent $4 billion on ads—more than any other election in U.S. history. *Mail Online*. Retrieved from http://www.dailymail.co.uk/news/article-1327814/Mid-term-Elections-2010-Politicians-spent-4-2bn-adverts.html

Gehlert, S., & Colditz, G. (2011). Cancer disparities: Unmet challenges in the elimination of disparities. *Cancer Epidemiology Biomarkers and Prevention, 20*(9), 1809–1814.

Gilliss, C., Powell, D., & Carter, B. (2010). Recruiting and retaining a diverse workforce in nursing: From evidence to best practices to policy. *Policy, Politics, & Nursing Practice, 11*(4), 294–301.

Goodman, J., Villarreal, P., & Jones, B. (2011). The social cost of adverse medical events, and what we can do about it. *Health Affairs, 30*(4), 590–595.

Grumbach, K., & Mendoza, R. (2008). Disparities in human resources: Addressing the lack of diversity in the health professions. *Health Affairs, 27*(2), 413–422.

Haninck, E. (2011). Linda Rogers, the first school nurse: Spearheading an intervention to keep kids in school. *Working Nurse*. Retrieved from http://www.workingnurse.com/articles/Lina-Rogers-the-First-School-Nurse

Hansen, M. M., & Jones, M. (2011). Public health policy: Promotion, prevention, and protection. In D. M. Nickitas, D. J. Middaugh, & N. Aries (Eds.). *Policy and politics for nurses and other health professionals: Advocacy in action* (pp. 181–208). Sudbury, MA: Jones & Bartlett Publishers.

Harrington, C., & Estes, C. L. (2008). *Health policy & nursing: Crisis & reform in the US healthcare delivery system* (5th ed.). Sudbury, MA: Jones & Bartlett Publishers.

Harvard School of Public Health. (2011). *Deborah Prothrow-Stith*. Retrieved from http://www.hsph.harvard.edu/faculty/deborah-prothrowstith/

Health Resources & Services Administration (HRSA). (n.d.). *What is a health center?* Retrieved from http://bphc.hrsa.gov/about/

Henry Street Settlement. (n.d.). *About us*. Retrieved September 19, 2011 from http://www.henrystreet.org/about/

Hewison, A. (2007). Policy analysis: A framework for nurse managers. *Journal of Nursing Management, 15*(7), 693–699.

Himmelstein, D. A., Thorne, D., Warren, E., & Woolhandler, S. (2009). Bankruptcy in the US, 2007: Results of a national study. *American Journal of Medicine, 122*(8), 741–746.

Inglesby, T. V. (2011). Progress in disaster planning and preparedness since 2001. *Journal of the American Medical Association (JAMA), 306*(12), 1372–1373.

Institute of Medicine (IOM). (2000). *To err is human: Building a safer health system*. Washington, DC: The National Academies Press.

Institute of Medicine (IOM). (2002a). *Health insurance is a family matter*. Washington, DC: The National Academies Press.

Institute of Medicine (IOM). (2002b). *The future of the public's health in the 21st century*. Washington, DC: The National Academies Press.

Institute of Medicine (IOM). (2003). *A shared destiny: Community effects of uninsurance*. Washington, DC: The National Academies Press.

Institute of Medicine (IOM). (2006). *Preventing medication errors: Quality chasm series*. Washington, DC: The National Academies Press.

Institute of Medicine (IOM). (2011). *The future of nursing: Leading change, advancing health*. Washington, DC: National Academies Press.

Jewish Women's Archive. (2011). *Public health nursing: Lillian Wald, 1867–1940*. Retrieved from http://jwa.org/historymakers/wald/public-health-nursing

Johansson, P., Jones, D., Watkins, C., Haisfield-Wolfe, M., & Gaston-Johansson, F. (2011). Physicians' and nurses' experiences of the influence of race and ethnicity on the quality of healthcare provided to minority patients, and on their own professional careers. *Journal of the National Black Nurses Association, 22*(1), 43–58.

Jones, J. (2010, December 3). *Nurses top honesty and ethics list for 11th year*. Gallup Poll. Retrieved from http://www.gallup.com/poll/145043/nurses-top-honesty-ethics-list-11-year.aspx

Kaiser Family Foundation. (2009, March). National health insurance: A brief history of reform efforts in the U.S. Retrieved from http://www.kff.org/healthreform/upload/7871.pdf

Kaiser Family Foundation. (2011, April 15). Focus on health reform: Summary of new health reform law. Retrieved from http://www.kff.org/healthreform/upload/8061.pdf

Kogan, M., Newacheck, P., Blumberg, S, Ghandour, R., Singh, G., et al. (2010). Underinsurance among children in the United States. *New England Journal of Medicine, 363*, 841–851.

Kovner, A. R., & Knickman, J. R. (Eds.). (2011). *Jonas & Kovner's health care delivery in the United States* (10th ed.). New York: Springer Publishing Company.

Laverack, G. (2006). Improving health outcomes through community empowerment: A review of the literature. *Journal of Health, Population, and Nutrition, 24*(1), 113–120.

Logsdon, C., & Davis, D. W. (2010). Social justice as a wider lens of support for childbearing women. *Journal of Obstetric, Gynecologic & Neonatal Nursing, 39*(3), 339–348.

MacDonnell, J. A. (2009). Fostering nurses' political knowledge and practices: Education and political activation in relation to lesbian health. *Advances in Nursing Science, 32*(2), 158–172.

MacDorman, M. F., & Matthews, M. S. (2008, October). *Recent trends in infant mortality in the United States*. National Center for Health Statistics Data Brief No. 9. Retrieved from http://www.cdc.gov/nchs/data/databriefs/db09.pdf

Manthey, M. (2008). Social justice and nursing: The key is respect. *Creative Nursing, 14*(2), 62–65.

Mason, J., Leavitt, J., & Chaffee, M. (2012). *Policy and politics in nursing and healthcare* (6th ed.). St. Louis, MO: Elsevier Saunders.

McCool, D. (1995). *Public policy theories, models and concepts: An anthology*. Old Tappan, NJ: Prentice Hall.

McGrath, R. J. (2009). Implementation theory revisited....again: Lessons from the State Children's Health Insurance Program. *Politics and Policy, 37*(2), 309–336.

Milstead, J. A. (2008). *Health policy and politics: A nurse's guide (3rd ed.)*. Sudbury, MA: Jones & Bartlett Publishers.

Nance-Nash, S. (2011, September 9). *Number of underinsured adults rises by 80%*. Daily Finance. Retrieved from http://www.dailyfinance.com/2011/09/09/number-of-underinsured-adults-rises-by-80/

National Association of Community Health Centers. (2009, March). *Primary care access: An essential building block of health reform*. Bethesda, MD: Author.

National Association of County & City Health Officials (NACCHO). (2009, January). *NACCHO survey of local health departments' budget cuts and workforce reductions*. Retrieved from http://www.naccho.org/advocacy/upload/2008-LHD-budget-cut-report.pdf

National League for Nursing (NLN). (2011a). *Public policy: Nursing shortage/nurse workforce development*. Retrieved from http://www.nln.org/publicpolicy/hcreform_shortage_info.htm

National League for Nursing (NLN). (2011b). *About the NLN.* Retrieved from http://dev.nln.org/aboutnln/info-history.htm

National Nurses United (NNU). (2011). *About the NNU.* Retrieved from http://www.nationalnursesunited.org/pages/about

Neiberg, B. (2010, September 14). *California law affects insulin administration in schools.* Retrieved from http://gcrlegal.com/news/in-the-news/california-law-affects-insulin-administration-in-schools.php

Nestle. (2010). *Nestle very best in youth: 2007 winner Bria Brown.* Retrieved from http://verybestinyouth.nestleusa.com/alumni/AlumniDetail.aspx?Winner=dc681634-0bf7-4787-a1a0-7be376d41c81&year=0&search=&state=All&page=5

Nickitas, D. M., Middaugh, D. J., & Aries, N. (Eds.). (2011). *Policy and politics for nurses and other health professionals: Advocacy and action.* Sudbury, MA: Jones & Bartlett Publishers.

Nix, K. (2011, August, 10). A recipe for reform: Success of consumer-driven principles in Medicare programs. *The Heritage Foundation.* Retrieved from http://www.heritage.org/Research/Reports/2011/08/Consumer-Driven-Medicare-Reform-Models-for-Success

O'Byrne, P., & Holmes, D. (2009). The politics of nursing care: Correcting deviance in accordance with the social contract. *Policy, Politics, and Nursing Practice, 10*(2), 153–162.

Orlovsky, C. (2006). *National Nurse Act introduced in House of Representatives.* AMN Healthcare Education Services. Retrieved from http://w3.rn.com/News/headlines_details.aspx?Id=8334

Paquin, S. O. (2011). Social justice advocacy in nursing: What is it? How do we get it? *Creative Nursing, 17*(2), 63–67.

Pauly, M. V. (2011). The trade-off among quality, quantity, and cost: How to make it—if we must. *Health Affairs, 30*(4), 574–580.

Perez, L. M., & Martinez, J. (2008). Community health workers: Social justice and policy advocates for community health and wellbeing. *American Journal of Public Health, 98*(1), 11–14.

Peters, R. M. (2002). Nurse administrator's role in health policy: Teaching the elephant to dance. *Nursing Administration Quarter, 26*(4), 1–8.

Polick, T. (2006, October 13). Grassroots nursing. *Advance for Nurses.* Retrieved from http://nursing.advanceweb.com/Article/Grassroots-Nursing-2.aspx

Preston, S. H., & Ho, J. Y. (2009, August). *Low life expectancy in the United States: Is the health care system at fault?* The National Bureau of Economic Research (NBER) Working Paper No. 15213.

Pringle, D. (2009). Alert: Return of 1990s healthcare reform. *Nursing Leadership, 22*(3), 14–15.

Robert Wood Johnson Foundation. (2008, September). *Strengthening public health nursing: Part I.* Charting Nursing's Future. Washington, DC: Author.

Robert Wood Johnson Foundation. (2009, September 17). *Forum on the future of nursing: Acute care.* Retrieved from http://www.rwjf.org/pr/product.jsp?id=48528

Robert Wood Johnson Foundation. (2010, November 30). *Robert Wood Johnson Foundation launches national campaign to advance health through nursing.* Retrieved from http://www.rwjf.org/pr/product.jsp?id=71510

Rutgers Center for American Women and Politics. (2010). *Women serving in the 112th Congress (2011–2013).* Retrieved from http://www.cawp.rutgers.edu/fast_facts/levels_of_office/Congress-Current.php

Save the Children. (2010). *Women on the front lines of health care: State of the world's mothers 2010.* Retrieved from http://www.savethechildren.org/atf/cf/%7B9def2ebe-10ae-432c-9bd0-df91d2eba74a%7D/SOWM-2010-Women-on-the-Front-Lines-of-Health-Care.pdf

Schoen, C., Collins, S., Kriss, J., & Doty, M. (2008). How many are underinsured? Trends among U.S. adults, 2003 and 2007. *Health Affairs, 27*(4), w298–w309.

Schoen, C., Doty, M., Robertson, R., & Collins, S, (2011). Affordable Care Act reforms could reduce the number of underinsured US adults by 70 percent. *Health Affairs, 30*(9), 1762–1771.

Schumacher, C. (2002). Lina Rogers: A pioneer in school nursing. *The Journal of School Nursing, 18*(5), 247–249.

Schultz, C. (2010). Transformation: The Institute of Medicine report on The Future of Nursing. *Nursing Education Perspectives, 31*(6), 345.

Smedley, B. D. (2008). Moving beyond access: Achieving equity in state health care reform. *Health Affairs, 27*(2), 447–455.

Smedley, B., Stith, A., & Nelson, A. (Eds). (2003). *Unequal treatment: Confronting racial and ethnic disparities in health care.* Washington, DC: The National Academies Press.

Song, A. (n.d.). *ANA-PAC wraps up first half of the "Race for the Million" campaign.* ANA Capitol Update. Retrieved from http://www.rnaction.org/site/PageServer?pagename=CUP_Arch_022908_en1_racemillion&ct=1

Squires, D. A. (2011, July). *Issues in international health policy: The US health system in perspective—a comparison of twelve industrialized nations.* The Commonwealth Fund Publication 1532.

Sullivan Commission. (2004). *Missing persons: Minorities in the health professions* (Vol. 16). Washington, DC: Institute of Medicine.

Taft, S., & Nanna, K. (2008). What are the sources of health policy that influence nursing practice? *Policy, Politics, and Nursing Practice, 9*(4), 274–287.

The National Nursing Network Organization. (2011). *The national nurse for public health: About us.* Retrieved from http://nationalnurse.org/aboutUs.shtml

University Bound News. (2011, February 24). *Nursing schools forced to cut enrollment.* Retrieved from http://news.university-bound.com/2011/02/24/nursing-schools-forced-to-cut-enrollment/

University of Medicine & Dentistry of New Jersey. (2011). *Black nurses in history: A bibliography and guide to web resources.* Camden Campus Library. Retrieved from http://www.umdnj.edu/camlbweb/blacknurses.html

U.S. Census Bureau. (2010, September 16). *Income, poverty and health insurance coverage in the United States: Summary of key findings.* Retrieved from http://www.census.gov/newsroom/releases/archives/income_wealth/cb10-144.html

U.S. Department of Health & Human Services Archive. (1999). *Catherine Dodd appointed HHS region IX director.* Retrieved September 21, 2011 from http://archive.hhs.gov/news/press/1999pres/990507.html

U.S. Department of Health & Human Services. (2011). *About Healthy People.* Retrieved from http://www.healthypeople.gov/2020/about/default.aspx

Van Den Bos, J., Rustagi, K., Gray, T., Halford, M., Ziemkiewicz, E., & Shreve, J. (2011). The $17.1 billion problem: The annual cost of measurable medical errors. *Health Affairs, 30*(4), 596–603.

Yoo, S., Butler, J., Elias, T., & Goodman, R. (2009). The 6-step model for community empowerment: Revisited in public housing communities for low-income senior citizens. *Health Promotion Practice, 10*(2), 262–275.

Werner, R., Kolstad, J., Stuart, E., & Polsky, D. (2011). The effect of pay-for-performance in hospitals: Lessons for quality improvement. *Health Affairs, 30*(4), 690–698.

Wilson, D. M. (2002). Testing a theory of political development by comparing the political action of nurses and non-nurses. *Nursing Outlook, 50*(1), 30–34.

Wong, N. T., Zimmerman, M. T., & Parker, E. A. (2010). A typology of youth participation and empowerment for child and adolescent health promotion. *American Journal of Community Psychology, 46*(1–2), 100–114.

Woodfill, M. M., & Beyrer, M. K. (1991). *The role of the nurse in the school setting: A historical perspective.* Kent, OH: American School Health Association.

thePoint: Everything You Need to Make the Grade!

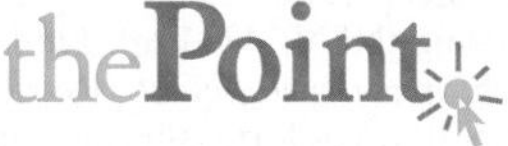

Visit http://thePoint.lww.com/Allender8e for selected readings, study aids for all learning styles, and more!

UNIT 4

THE COMMUNITY AS CLIENT

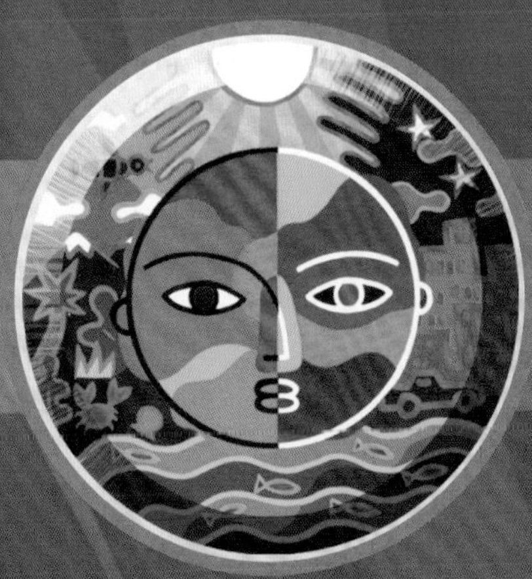

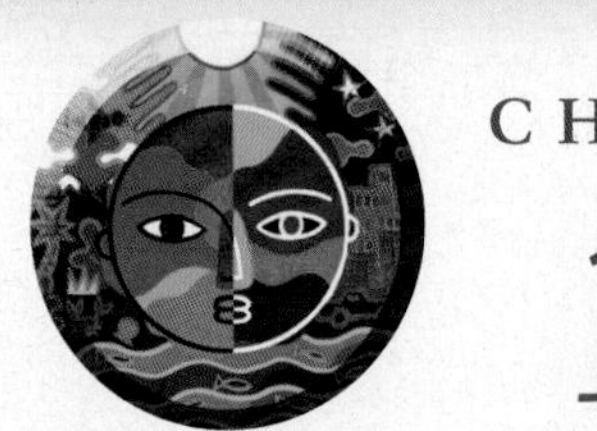

CHAPTER

14

Theoretical Basis of Community/Public Health Nursing

"We know a great deal more about the causes of physical disease than we do about the causes of physical health."

—*M. Scott Peck,* The Road Less Traveled

KEY TERMS

Bioterrorism
Community-oriented, population-focused care
Conceptual model
Genetics
Genomics
Genetic engineering
Global economy
Migration
Model
Nursing theory
Principle
Relationship-based care
Technology
Theory

LEARNING OBJECTIVES

Upon mastery of this chapter, you should be able to:

- Discuss three essential characteristics of nursing service when a community is the client: community-oriented, population-focused care, and relationship-based care.
- Describe the contributions of at least five models of nursing practice to community/public health nursing practice.
- Explain the benefits of applying the eight principles of public health nursing to community/public health nursing.
- Identify at least five social issues that influence contemporary community/public health nursing care.

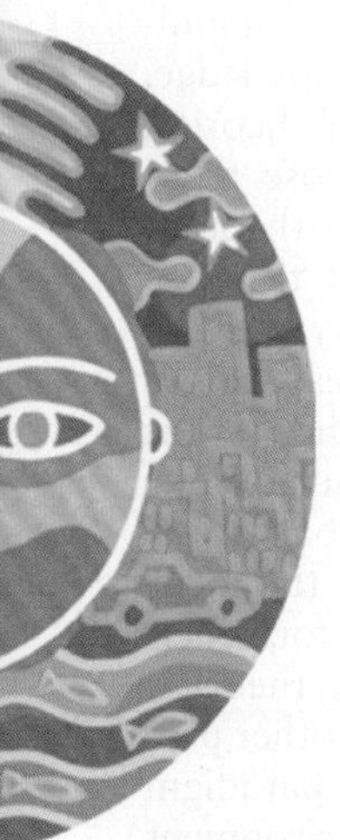

When you open the door of a senior center where you will be promoting cardiovascular fitness, advocating for exercise equipment, and suggesting changes in the on-site meal program, how might theories of public health nursing contribute to your success? When you approach your city council about the need to increase staffing of public health services, what models of public health nursing practice might support your argument? What is meant by *theories, models*, and *principles*, and what is their relevance to day-to-day public health nursing practice? These are the key issues explored in this chapter. First, however, we revisit some of the fundamental characteristics of community/public health nursing that we began to explore in Unit 1.

WHEN THE CLIENT IS A COMMUNITY: CHARACTERISTICS OF COMMUNITY/ PUBLIC HEALTH NURSING PRACTICE

Nursing exists to address people's health care needs, and nurses fulfill this purpose through their work in various specialty areas. Specialties are characterized by the unit of care for which the specialty is responsible and by the goal of the specialty. Each specialty requires a particular area of knowledge and a set of skills for excellence in practice.

Public health nursing is a specialty in which the unit of care is a specific community or aggregate, and the nurse has responsibility to promote group health. The goal of this specialty is health improvement of the community. Some of the skills required for excellence in public health nursing practice include epidemiology, research, teaching, community organizing, and interpersonal relational care.

In summary, community/public health nursing is characterized by community-oriented, population-focused care and is based on interpersonal relationships. In the following sections, each of these characteristics is examined in more depth.

Community-Oriented, Population-Focused Care

As was discussed in Chapter 1, a *community* is a group of people who have some characteristics in common, are bounded by time, interact with one another, and feel a connection to one another. For example, members of an Internet-based support group for people with colitis are a community. They share similar experiences and concerns, and they often influence one another's behavior. For instance, they may recommend food choices or complementary therapies to one another. Members of a class of community/public health nursing students are also a community. Because they begin and end their studies in a particular month and year, they are bonded by time, and they most likely share certain values and feel a sense of connection to one another.

Community orientation is a process that is actively shaped by the unique experiences, knowledge, concerns, values, beliefs, and culture of a given community. For example, when an outbreak of hepatitis occurs, the public health nurse does more than simply treat infection in individuals. The nurse also

- Uses disease-investigation skills to locate possible sources of infection.
- Determines how the community's knowledge, values, beliefs, and prior experiences with infectious disease may influence its interpretation of the disease, response to the outbreak, and treatment preferences.
- Uses knowledge and suggestions gathered from the community to develop, in collaboration with other health professionals, a community-specific program to prevent future outbreaks.

A community-oriented nurse who provides education about sexually transmitted diseases to a group of students at a Catholic university includes consideration of community values regarding sexual behavior. Similarly, a community-oriented nurse who provides nutritional counseling to a community of Hispanic seniors considers the meaning of food in this culture, the types of food most commonly consumed, and the cooking methods most commonly used.

A *population* is any group of people who share at least one characteristic, such as age, gender, race, a particular risk factor, or disease. Smokers and breast cancer survivors are two populations. The concept of population may also include delineation by time (e.g., all children born in the year 2012). The nurse's place of employment commonly limits the population that the nurse serves. For example, a nurse who works for a county health department is limited professionally to caring for the population of that county.

A *population focus* implies that a nurse uses population-based skills such as epidemiology, research in community assessment, and community organizing as the basis for interventions. For example, a population-focused nurse employed by an autoworkers' union may study all cases of repetitive-use injury occurring in the auto industry in the United States in the past 5 years, develop a program for reducing repetitive-use injury, and lobby industry executives for adoption of the program.

Community-oriented, population-focused care employs population-based skills and is shaped by the characteristics and needs of a given community. Public health nurses provide community-oriented, population-focused care when they count and interview homeless people sleeping in a park and, based on these data, help develop a program to provide food, clothing, shelter, health care, and job training for this population.

Relationship-Based Care

Relationship-based care incorporates the value of establishing and maintaining a reciprocal, caring relationship with the community. It is a necessary and feasible aspect of public health nursing practice and is foundational to caring effectively for the community's health. A reciprocal, caring relationship with the community involves listening, participatory dialogue, and critical reflection, and it may also involve sociopolitical elements of practice such as advocacy, community empowerment, and movement to action (Shields & Lindsey, 1998).

Public health nurses provide relationship-based care when they meet regularly with groups of female inmates to learn about their physical and psychosocial health care needs and the needs of their families, and then use the information gathered to advocate for this population with prison officials and other professionals in the community. A public health nurse also provides relationship-based care when working with parents of children with cancer, a psychologist, and a hospital chaplain to determine the needs of each family and to facilitate formation of a self-help group. In both these examples, public health nurses are working to establish and maintain ongoing relationships with other professionals in the community and with their communities of clients.

THEORIES AND MODELS FOR COMMUNITY/PUBLIC HEALTH NURSING PRACTICE

A **theory** is a set of systematically interrelated concepts or hypotheses that seek to explain or predict phenomena. For example, the "big bang theory" seeks to explain the series of events that occurred during the earliest moments in the history of our universe. A theory is based either explicitly or philosophically on a conceptual model (also referred to as a conceptual framework, a conceptual system or a paradigm). A **conceptual model** as defined by Fawcett (2005, p. 16) "is a set of relatively abstract and general concepts that address the [things that are] of central interest to a discipline, the propositions that broadly describe those concepts, and the propositions that state relatively abstract and general [associations] between two or more of the concepts."

The evolution of conceptual model and theory development in nursing dominated the last half of the 20th century. The scholarly and creative efforts of those nurse leaders and researchers sought to explain what nursing is and how it influences individuals, families, or communities, providing a basis for building nursing knowledge. From those early efforts came more testable theories, many from those same nurse researchers; those theories are typically referred to as middle-range theories. Although less abstract than conceptual models, the need for an even more practical approach to theory use and testing led ultimately to practice-based theories. Walker and Avant note that "the essence of practice theory was a desired goal and prescriptions for action to achieve the goal" (2005, p. 14), clearly emphasizing the goal directedness of nursing practice. Most significantly, the focus on practice has opened up new opportunities for generalist nurses to both understand and use nursing theories.

One feature separating **nursing theory** from other professional theories is the use of the nursing metaparadigm concepts: nursing, client/patient, health, and environment (Fawcett, 1989; Walker & Avant, 2005). A metaparadigm is defined as "a global statement that identifies the subject matter of each discipline or field of study" (Fawcett & Gerity, 2009, p. 5). As you read through the descriptions of the theories and conceptual models, see if you can determine which ones conform to the nursing metaparadigm and which ones can be used by nurses as well as other health care professionals (see Activities to Promote Critical Thinking at the end of this chapter).

To more fully understand the elements inherent in a nursing theory and the underlying conceptual model, a pictorial representation, or graphic model, is often used. These models provide a visual means to understand the relationships between, for instance, the nurse and the environment, the nurse and the client, or the client and stressors. However complex these models, comprehension of the entire work can only be derived from reading the theorist's descriptions of the conceptual model, the theory(ies), and the subsequent research testing those theory(ies). Both theories and conceptual models have been developed to describe, clarify, and guide nursing practice. Theories and conceptual models that have particular relevance to the practice of community/public health nursing are described here.

Nightingale's Theory of Environment

Florence Nightingale's environmental theory has great significance to nursing in general and to public health nursing specifically, because it focuses on preventive care for populations. While organizing and supervising a nursing service for soldiers in the Crimean War, Nightingale kept meticulous records. Her observations suggested that disease was more prevalent in poor environments, and that health could be promoted by providing adequate ventilation, pure water, quiet, warmth, light, and cleanliness. The crux of her theory was that poor environmental conditions were bad for health and that good environmental conditions reduced disease (Nightingale, 1859/1992).

There is no consensus of opinion on specific conditions that ensure people's health. Some people believe that, in addition to a clean environment, social services such as public transportation, education, and health care are necessary. This more expansive approach can best be described as social determinants of health and is included in the *Healthy People 2020* objectives. Examples of social and physical determinants of health can be seen in greater detail in Displays 14.1 and 14.2 (U.S. Department of Health and Human Services [U.S. DHHS], 2010). As you think about services included in Display 14.1, it is useful to consider

- Why these services were created.
- Who benefits from the services.
- Who pays for the services.
- The cost to the people using the services.
- The public's perception of the services.

For example, if ventilation in a city's homeless shelter is inadequate, the public health nurse who plans to advocate for capital improvements to the shelter needs to consider who pays for the shelter as well as the public's perception of the shelter.

One contemporary example of the utility of Nightingale's theory is the work of Shaner-McRae, McRae, and Jas (2007), who sought to bring attention to the need for nurses to optimize environments for healing. Although they specifically focused on the health care setting, describing ways to manage both "upstream and downstream waste (solid, biohazard, and hazardous chemical wastes)" (p. 1), their premise can be easily applied to the home, community, or even the public health department. Controlling environmental contaminants and protecting the environment are important goals in a wide variety of settings. Nightingale's influence on the way nurses approach health issues impacting communities today remains a powerful force.

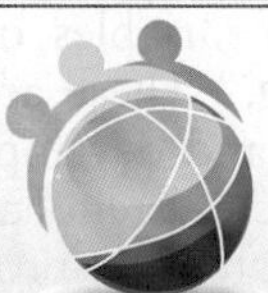

DISPLAY 14.1 EXAMPLES OF SOCIAL DETERMINANTS OF HEALTH

- Availability of resources to meet daily needs (e.g., safe housing and local food markets)
- Access to educational, economic, and job opportunities
- Access to health care services
- Quality of education and job training
- Availability of community-based resources in support of community living and opportunities for recreational and leisure-time activities
- Transportation options
- Public safety
- Social support
- Social norms and attitudes (e.g., discrimination, racism, and distrust of government)
- Exposure to crime, violence, and social disorder (e.g., presence of trash and lack of cooperation in a community)
- Socioeconomic conditions (e.g., concentrated poverty and the stressful conditions that accompany it)
- Residential segregation
- Language/literacy
- Access to mass media and emerging technologies (e.g., cell phones, the Internet, and social media)
- Culture

U.S. Department of Health and Human Services. (2010). *Healthy People 2020: Social determinants of health*. Retrieved from http://www.healthypeople.gov/2020/topicsobjectives2020/overview.aspx?topicid=39

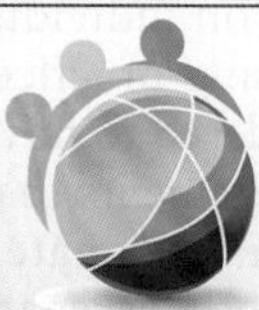

DISPLAY 14.2 EXAMPLES OF PHYSICAL DETERMINANTS OF HEALTH

- Natural environment, such as green space (e.g., trees and grass) or weather (e.g., climate change)
- Built environment, such as buildings, sidewalks, bike lanes, and roads
- Worksites, schools, and recreational settings
- Housing and community design
- Exposure to toxic substances and other physical hazards
- Physical barriers, especially for people with disabilities
- Aesthetic elements (e.g., good lighting, trees, and benches)

U.S. Department of Health and Human Services. (2010). *Healthy People 2020: Social determinants of health*. Retrieved from http://www.healthypeople.gov/2020/topicsobjectives2020/overview.aspx?topicid=39

Orem's Self-Care Model

Dorothy Orem (1914–2007), a nurse administrator and educator, focused on the concept of *self-care*—learned, goal-oriented actions to preserve and promote life, health, and wellbeing. She described people who need nursing care as those who lack ability in self-care (Orem, 2001). If a demand for self-care exceeds the client's ability, the client experiences a self-care deficit, and nursing intervention becomes appropriate. The goal of nursing action is to help people recognize their self-care demands and limitations and increase their self-care ability. Nursing care also functions to meet clients' self-care needs until they are able to care for themselves.

Orem further described three types of requirements that influence people's self-care abilities:

- Universal requirements are activities common to all human beings, which are essential to meet physiologic and psychosocial needs.
- Developmental requirements are activities necessary to help people progress developmentally.
- Health-deviation requirements are activities needed to help people deal with a diminished level of wellness.

Although Orem's model focused primarily on individuals, it can be applied to public health nursing practice. Populations and communities can be considered to have a collective set of self-care actions and requirements that affect the wellbeing of the total group. If an aggregate's demands for self-care exceed its ability, the aggregate experiences a self-care deficit, and public health nursing intervention is indicated. According to this interpretation, the goal of nursing is to promote a community's collective independence and self-care ability. Kagan expanded on Orem's interpretation of self to reflect a more unitary link between humans and their environment; considering human–environment as one entity. With this worldview, she emphasized that nurses "can learn new information, make ethical and political decisions, and act to take care of the environment including regulation of human interaction with, and impact on, the environment" (Kagan, 2011, p. 73)

For example, a riverside community that ingests large quantities of fish contaminated with heavy metals might have self-care deficits related to the lack of awareness that eating local fish is dangerous and that some subpopulations, such as pregnant women and young children, are especially vulnerable. The public health nurse should help the community become aware of the risk and identify other food sources. The nurse should also help the community lobby government and industry to reduce pollution and clean up the river.

Three specific theories have been derived from the original model: the Self-Care Deficit theory, the Theory of Self-Care, and the Theory of Nursing System (Gast & Montgomery, 2005). The applicability of the Self-Care Deficit theory to public health nursing was demonstrated in a study of adherence to latent tuberculosis therapy among Latino immigrants (Ailinger, Moore, Nguyen, & Lasus, 2006), and in a pilot study of mother's knowledge of childhood immunizations (Wilson, Baker, Nordstrom, & Legwand, 2008). The theory of self-care was also utilized to identify self-care behaviors of school-aged children with heart disease (Fan, 2008) and to improve glycemic control and blood sugar stability in adult women with type 2 diabetes mellitus (Evans, 2010). Clearly the model and the derived theories have shown applicability to public health practice directed at improving health outcomes for a variety of populations in the community setting.

Neuman's Health Care Systems Model

Betty Neuman, a leader in mental health nursing and nursing education, proposed a systems model (Neuman, 1982; Neuman & Fawcett, 2002) that can be adapted to view clients as aggregates. In this model, people are seen as open systems that constantly and reciprocally interact with their environments. Each system is greater than the sum of its parts, and wellness exists when the parts of the system interact in harmony with each other and with the system's environment. Four sets of variables, or influences, make up each system's "whole." These are physiologic, psychological, sociocultural, and developmental variables. Given these variables, each system has a unique response to stressors and to those tension-producing stimuli that may cause disequilibrium or illness.

A system's response to stressors may be envisioned as a series of concentric circles (Fig. 14-1). In the center is a core of basic survival abilities, such as a community's

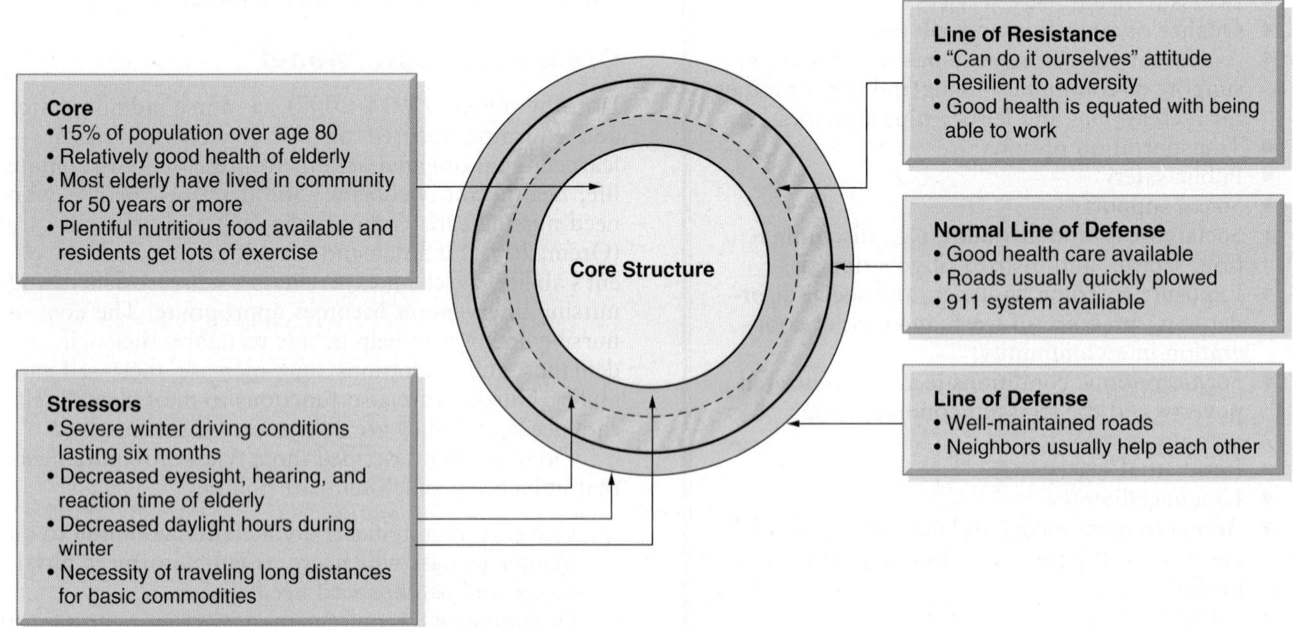
Core
• 15% of population over age 80
• Relatively good health of elderly
• Most elderly have lived in community for 50 years or more
• Plentiful nutritious food available and residents get lots of exercise
Stressors
• Severe winter driving conditions lasting six months
• Decreased eyesight, hearing, and reaction time of elderly
• Decreased daylight hours during winter
• Necessity of traveling long distances for basic commodities
Core Structure
Line of Resistance
• "Can do it ourselves" attitude
• Resilient to adversity
• Good health is equated with being able to work
Normal Line of Defense
• Good health care available
• Roads usually quickly plowed
• 911 system availiable
Line of Defense
• Well-maintained roads
• Neighbors usually help each other

FIGURE 14-1. Neuman's health care systems model applied to a rural county regarding traffic safety issues concerning the elderly by D. Block, from Allender, J., & Spradley, B. (2001). *Community health nursing: Concepts and practice* (5th ed.). Philadelphia, PA: Lippincott, with permission.

ability to make the best use of its natural resources. Surrounding this core are three boundaries. The innermost boundary is a flexible line of resistance that encompasses internal defenses, such as a community's collective sense of responsibility for raising healthy children. The second boundary is the system's normal line of defense, such as a community's police force or voluntary fire brigade. The third boundary is a dynamic, flexible line of defense, a buffer that prevents stressors from invading the system's normal line of defense. An example is regular maintenance of a community's roads and bridges.

In Neuman's model, stressors can originate from the internal environment or the external environment. Examples of internal stressors include a high proportion of low-income residents or an inadequate system of water purification. External stressors might include natural disasters, war, or a downturn in the global economy. The role of public health nursing, then, is to assist communities in remaining stable within their environments. The applicability of the Neuman model to public health nursing was clearly demonstrated in a comprehensive literature review of published studies between 1983 and 2005 (Skalski, DiGerolamo, & Gigliotti, 2006). This review yielded 13 studies dealing with stressors in client populations with the vast majority pertinent to public health nursing practice (i.e., spousal alcoholism, long-term cancer survivors, informal caregivers of head-injured adults, and telephone counseling). In a more recent example, Greenawalt and Wacheter (2011) applied the model to health care workplace safety, further demonstrating the utility to both occupational health nursing and nursing education. In this example the authors identified the stressors (hazards or risk) as intrapersonal (poor body mechanics, lack of adherence to safety and health rules), interpersonal (violence, intimidation, or untimely dissemination of information on hazards to workers), and extrapersonal (blood-borne pathogen exposure, natural and other disasters).

In 2007, Neuman and Reed (p. 111) noted that "the language of the model concepts is understandable to those in other cultures, enabling them to make inference to healthcare situations specific to them." The international and cross-cultural relevance can be demonstrated in the increasing number of non-English publications of nursing research utilizing the Neuman model. One international example was the research done by Kaur and Kaur (2012) regarding cervical cancer awareness of Indian women. In this descriptive study, 62.3% of the sample had inadequate awareness of cervical cancer despite the fact that this type of cancer is the easiest female cancer to prevent through screening and early intervention. Factors such as educational status, age at marriage, occupation, and monthly family income were associated with awareness.

Rogers' Model of the Science of Unitary Human Beings

Not typically linked with community/public health nursing practice, this model can be useful for the public health nurse in promoting holistic and healthful community–environment interactions. Martha Rogers (1915–1994) established the first visiting nursing service in Arizona in the mid-1940s; it was one of the first in the nation (Tomasson, 1994). A nursing administrator and long-time nurse educator, Rogers is responsible for modern nursing's emphasis on the whole person (Hemphill & Muth Quillin, 2005). In 1970, she developed a nursing conceptual model based on systems theory. Her model emphasized that the whole is greater than the sum of its parts; that is, focusing on the parts of a community, such as its health care or housing, does not provide an adequate picture of its totality.

Rogers also incorporated developmental theory into her model by describing the development of "unitary" persons or systems according to three principles: (1) life proceeds in one direction along a rhythmic spiral, (2) energy fields follow a certain wave pattern and organization, and (3) human and environmental energy fields interact simultaneously and mutually, leading to completeness and unity (Rogers, 1990). Using this model, the public health nurse can focus on community–environment interaction; the community functions interdependently with others and with the environment.

Even after her death, Rogers continues to garner a strong following. Talley, Rushing, and Gee (2005) utilized Rogers' model as a framework to create a profile of a small rural community in a southern state. This profile was used to exemplify the link between the model and community assessment, providing a comprehensive and thoughtful view of community needs and a clear basis for nursing interventions. A number of nurse researchers have expanded on Rogers' work from a theoretical perspective. Reed (2010) applied Rogers' conceptual model and elements of caring science to develop a unitary-caring conceptual model for use in palliative care. These two world views were seen to create "an opportunity for human healing during the journey of health, illness, death, and dying" (p. 26). In yet another example, Barrett (2010) derived a theory of power (both individual and group) from the science of unitary human beings. Although noting that Rogers never wrote specifically about power in the model, knowingly participating in change as a form of power was not seen as inconsistent with Rogers' views. In a final example, Zahourek and Larkin (2009) sought to link the concepts of conscience, intentionality and community within a unitary framework. Exploration of this relationship offers nurses the "potential to utilize their capacity to focus consciousness in community with expanded intentions for health and healing" (p. 15).

King

Imogene King (1923–2007), nursing scholar and educator, was one of the early nurse theorists to provide a conceptual model of nursing (Messmer & Palmer, 2008). Her groundbreaking work *Toward a Theory for Nursing* (1970) and the subsequent *A Theory for Nursing: Systems, Concepts, Process* (1981) were both designed to "promote conceptual learning in undergraduate and graduate nursing programs" (1981, p. vii) and can be utilized by the public health nurse to define the nurse–client relationship. From the original general systems model which demonstrated the interrelationship between social, interpersonal, and personal systems (Killeen & King, 2007), King formulated the *Theory of Goal Attainment*. The theory focuses on the personal and interpersonal systems of the conceptual model. The basis of the theory is that, in any nurse–client encounter, both the nurse and the client come to the situation with their own goals and expectations. Optimal success at goal achievement is only possible when the nurse and the client work together to set goals, thus recognizing the expectations of both parties rather than the preeminence of one over the other. For instance, a public health nurse may have planned to speak to a teen mother about birth control on a home visit. The teen, however, has nearly run out of formula and has exhausted all her cash. In this instance, the teen's priorities are to locate formula or the resources to obtain formula, while the nurse may be concerned that the teen has resumed sexual activity and may become pregnant again. The immediate priority would clearly be the formula, but the nurse can also provide birth control information within that context after the teen is aware that a solution to the formula issue can be found. King's theory is a reminder of the importance of the reciprocal relationship between the nurse and the client. Negotiation is a skill inherent in the theory; only through recognition of the perceived needs and goals of the client can the public health nurse help maintain or improve the client's health and wellbeing. The principles of public health nursing discussed later in this chapter (American Nurses Association [ANA], 2007) also emphasize the need to treat the client as an equal partner—a strong reminder of King's legacy to nursing practice.

The conceptual model and the Theory of Goal Attainment remain relevant to nursing practice. In discussing the role of the nurse in palliative care, Whelton (2008) notes that the emphasis on the relationship, and on mutual goal setting, is especially important. The progress of terminal illness leaves patients especially vulnerable, fearful, and helpless. Care providers reach beyond this potential for despair to be present with, and provide personal affirmation and hope to, the patient and their loved ones (p. 85).

Alligood (2010) emphasized the application of the conceptual system and theory of goal attainment to a "theory-driven program of research for practice" in family health care (p. 99). Exemplars include family health care with a mentally ill child (Doornbos, 1995, 2007) or a child with type 1 diabetes or asthma (Frey, 1995; Frey, Ellis, & Naar-King, 2007), and when a family member has chronic obstructive pulmonary disease (Wicks, 1995; Wicks, Rice, & Tally, 2007). These and many other examples demonstrate the utility of King's work to current practice in public health.

Parse's Theory of Human Becoming

Rosemarie Rizzo Parse developed her theory, initially called the "man-living-health" theory, in 1981. In 1992, she changed the name to "Human Becoming Theory" to better reflect all people. The theory posits quality of life from each person's own perspective as the goal of nursing practice. The theory is structured around three themes (Parse, 1981, 1998):

Meaning. People coparticipate in creating what is real for them through self-expression by living their values in their own chosen way.

Rhythmicity. The unity of life encompasses apparent opposites in rhythmic patterns of relating. While living moment to moment, one shows and does not show the self, creating both opportunities and limitations that emerge as moving with and moving apart from others.

Transcendence. Moving beyond the moment and forging a unique personal path for oneself in the midst of ambiguity and continuous change.

These three themes apply effectively to the community. The nurse must know what the community means to its inhabitants, identify and be aware of the rhythmicity of the people as attempts are made to create positive health changes in the community, and realize the transcendence that occurs when people work in the presence of ambiguity and continuous change, characteristics inherent in a community. Use of this theory as a guide enhances the ability of community members to work together to accomplish identified goals. Examples of the use of the theory most applicable to public health nursing practice include nursing's engagement in health policy (Poirier, 2012), the act of being "present" in professional practice (Zyblock, 2010), and supporting caring–healing–sustainable nursing practices (Clark, 2012).

Building on her research, Parse has developed what she terms a Human Becoming Community Model (Parse, 2012). The model emphasizes the change concepts of moving–initiating, anchoring–shifting, and pondering–shaping. She clarifies the significance of community such that "when people come together as a group, the individual communities bring their histories to the emerging now, and this creates an entity of coevolving histories, which confirms individual as community and group as community" (pp. 44–45). The work of Parse and others brings a unique and holistic perspective to community/public health nursing practice.

Pender's Health Promotion Model

As we have noted throughout this text, health promotion is a priority in community/public health nursing practice. Pender defined health promotion as actions that are directed toward increasing the level of wellbeing and self-actualization in individuals or groups (Pender, Murdaugh, & Parsons, 2011). It is a proactive set of behaviors in which people act on their environment rather than react to stressors arising from the environment.

Pender's *Health Promotion Model* seeks to explain this proactive behavior. The model, based on social learning theory, stresses cognitive processes that help regulate behavior such as perceptions people have that directly influence their motivation to begin or continue health-promoting behaviors. These include, for example, perceptions of control of health, health status, benefits of health-promoting behaviors, and barriers to engaging in health-promoting behaviors.

Five types of modifying factors influence people's perceptions about pursuing health-promoting behaviors:

- Demographic factors, such as age and race
- Biologic characteristics, such as height and weight
- Interpersonal influences, such as the expectations of others
- Situational factors, such as availability of healthful foods
- Behavioral factors, such as stress-coping patterns

Using Pender's model, a public health nurse might interview the residents of a low-income housing project to determine their perceptions about improving health and safety. Research of demographic, situational, and other factors that might influence the residents' motivation and ability to change their circumstances could then be conducted. Pender's model is being increasingly used as a framework in studies of health promotion in diverse populations: preventing farm accidents in children (Conway, McClune, & Nosel, 2007), self-efficacy and health-promoting behaviors in older adults in Iran (Morowatisharifabad, Ghofranipour, Heidarnia, Ruchi, & Ehrampoush, 2006), adolescent health-promoting behavior (Srof & Velsor-Friedrich, 2006), and health-promoting behaviors of low-income elderly Korean women (Shin, Kang, Park, Cho, & Heitkemper, 2008). More recently, Espositio and Fitzpatrick (2011) conducted a study of nurses' beliefs about the benefits of exercise and their own exercise behavior, in relation to their recommendation of exercise for health promotion or treatment. The findings showed positive correlations between exercise benefits, physical activity, and the recommendation of exercise to patients. This study supports the role modeling aspect of nursing practice on patient teaching.

Although pertinent to public health nursing practice, the model is not strictly speaking of a conceptual model of nursing, as was discussed earlier in this chapter. The metaparadigm concepts of patient/client, health, and environment are present, but the model does not stipulate that the provider of health educational services be a nurse—and can in fact be from other disciplines. Pender's model is further discussed in relation to client education in Chapter 11.

Roy's Adaptation Model

Sister Callista Roy's model describes people as open and adaptive systems that experience stimuli, develop coping mechanisms, and produce responses. These responses, which may be adaptive or maladaptive, provide feedback that influences the amount and type of stimuli that can be handled in the future (Andrews & Roy, 1991; Roy, 2009; Roy & Andrews, 1999). This model helps the public health nurse understand how a community's ability to adapt to stressors will affect the health of the community.

Roy describes two response processes. In the *regulator* process, stimuli from the internal and external environments are received, and this combination of information is then processed to produce a response. In the *cognator* process, perceptions, learning, judgment, and emotion are considered in formulating a response to stimuli. An example of the regulator process might begin with a community's desire to keep adolescents from smoking (internal stimulus) and new state regulations prohibiting the sale of tobacco products to minors (external stimulus). These combined stimuli lead to a city ordinance that prevents the sale of cigarettes to minors (coping mechanism), resulting in reduced levels of smoking (response) among this population. A cognator process might begin with the stimulus of heavy rainfall in a riverside community. Residents' perceptions of the amount of rainfall, memories of past floods, insights about preventing or managing floods, and the level of anxiety all contribute to their plans for evacuation, sandbagging, and soliciting county or state assistance.

In applying Roy's conceptual model to public health nursing, it is important to remember that communities are made up of many parts and are influenced by many variables. The community's collective adaptation level is constantly changing. The public health nurse must assess a community's coping mechanisms and help its members use these collective abilities in adapting to challenges. For example, if a community is doing nothing to respond to the increased number of teen pregnancies, nursing actions can be designed to encourage more healthful coping patterns and adaptive responses.

Roy's model has been utilized in a number of studies with direct applicability to community health: bulimia nervosa (Hannon-Engel, 2008), self-concept of children with HIV/AIDS in the United States and Kenya (Waweru, Reynolds, & Buckner, 2008), and as the basis for developing an antenatal assessment instrument (Lee, Tsang, Wong, & Lee, 2011). This particular instrument focuses on assessment of behaviors in the four adaptive modes in Roy's model: physiologic, self-concept, role functioning, and interdependence. Further instrument development and psychometric testing are needed, but the tool can serve to focus client education in the community setting by identifying clients' ineffective and effective behaviors.

Salmon's Construct for Public Health Nursing

Marla Salmon, a leader in public health nursing administration, nursing education, and public health policy in the United States, proposed a model to specifically guide community health nursing practice. In *Construct for Public Health Nursing*, Salmon (1982) described public health as an organized societal effort to protect, promote, and restore the health of people, and public health nursing as focused on achieving and maintaining public health.

The model describes three practice priorities. These priorities are prevention of disease and poor health, protection against disease and external agents, and promotion of health. There are three general categories of nursing intervention:

- Education that is directed toward voluntary change in the attitudes and behavior of the subjects
- Engineering which is directed at managing risk-related variables
- Enforcement that is directed at mandatory regulation to achieve better health

The scope of practice spans individual, family, community, and global care. Interventions target determinants in four categories: human/biologic, environmental, medical/technologic/organizational, and social. Using Salmon's approach, a public health nurse attempting to reduce the transmission of tuberculosis would use education, engineering, and enforcement in working with the population of affected individuals and families. The nurse would also collaborate with the client community on a variety of interventions, from medications to teaching to social support, to prevent further disease in the community and to promote global health.

Salmon's editorial entitled *Public Health Nursing: The Opportunity of a Century* again stressed the importance of the central functions of public health nursing practice: "assessment, surveillance, policy, and health promotion and disease and injury prevention activities" (1993, p. 1674). In *Public Health Nursing: Scope and Standards of Practice* (ANA, 2007) the Salmon model is cited as an exemplar of an ecological approach to public health nursing interventions.

PUBLIC HEALTH PRACTICE MODELS

Minnesota Wheel—The Public Health Interventions Model

The Minnesota Department of Health, Division of Community Health Services, Public Health Nursing Section, devised a **model** that depicts public health interventions and applications for public health practice. In the form of a wheel, the model presents 17 different interventions within three levels of public health practice: population-based community-focused practice, systems-focused practice, and individual-focused practice. The "Minnesota Wheel" (2001) is depicted in Figure 14-2.

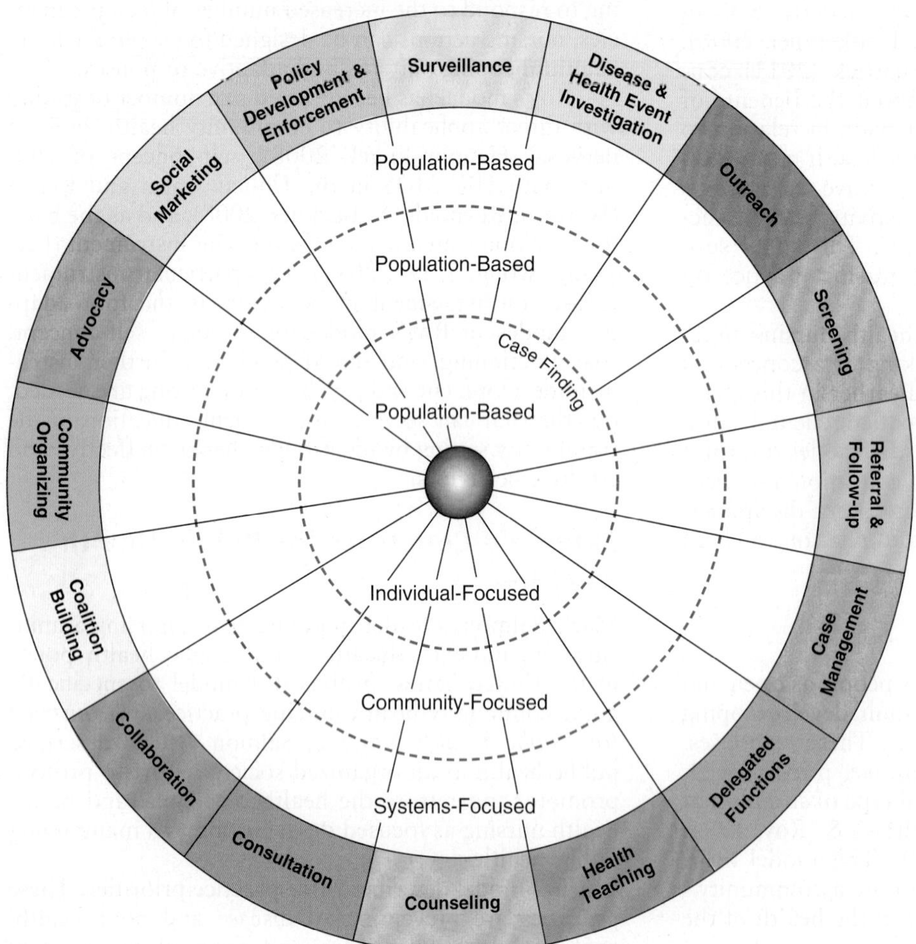

FIGURE 14-2. The Minnesota Wheel. (*Source*: Minnesota Department of Health, Division of Community Health Services, Public Health Nursing Section.)

The intervention wheel was first proposed in 1998 (Keller, Strohschein, Lia-Hoagberg, & Schaffer, 1998) as a practice model for population-based public health nursing. It can be applied in a variety of venues including public health practice, nursing education, and management. Keller and colleagues emphasized that "use of the Wheel has empowered nurses to explain in a better way how their practice contributes to the improvement of population health" (Keller, Strohschein, Lia-Hoagberg, & Schaffer, 2004, p. 454). The wheel is useful for public health nurses because it visually depicts the comprehensive list of interventions nurses must consider in the scope of practice. Saewyc, Solsvig, and Edinburgh (2007) utilized the Minnesota Wheel in an evaluation of "a coalition formed to address a growing issue of young Hmong girls in a Midwest state running away from home, being truant from school, and experiencing subsequent sexual exploitation" (p. 69). The outcomes of the task force were assessed relative to best practices identified in the model. This example shows just one of the many ways the model can assist the novice nurse, the expert practitioner, as well as other public health disciplines.

Public Health Nursing Practice Model

The need for a model that could blend public health nursing practice and the principles of public health, and could be applicable to both the generalist nurse and nurses working in specific programs, was the impetus for development of the Public Health Nursing Practice Model (Smith & Bazini-Barakat, 2003). The model was created by Los Angeles County, Department of Health Services (LAC-DHS), Public Health Nursing, with input from the California Conference of Local Health Department Nursing Directors (CCLHNDN) Southern Region and other public health nurse leaders. Referred to as the LAC PHN Practice Model (2007), it is described as integrating the Public Health Nursing Standards of Practice, the 10 Essential Public Health Services, the 10 Leading Health Indicators from *Healthy People 2010*, and the Minnesota Public Health Nursing Interventions Model. "The LAC PHN Practice Model provides a conceptual framework that assists in clarifying the role of the public health nurse and presents a guide for public health practice applicable to all public health disciplines" (Smith & Bazini-Barakat, 2003, p. 42).

As described by Smith and Bazini-Barakat (2003), the principles of population-based practice are included in the LAC PHN Practice Model. Public health nurses integrate assessment, policy development, and assurance into their work. The three levels of population-based practice—individuals and families, community, and systems—are addressed, with the nursing process applied throughout the model. Seventeen interventions, as first presented in the Minnesota Public Health Nursing Model, are also incorporated into the LAC PHN Practice Model. The LAC PHN Practice Model promotes the concepts of an interdisciplinary public health team working together, with an emphasis on primary prevention. It also recognizes the importance of active participation of the individual, family, and community (Smith & Bazini-Barakat, 2003). See Figure 14-3 for a depiction of the LAC PHN Model.

Omaha System

The Omaha System was developed and refined during four research projects conducted between 1975 and 1992 in the Omaha Visiting Nursing Association. It was designed to increase the effectiveness and efficiency of nursing practice in the agency (Bowles & Naylor, 1996; Martin, Leak, & Aden, 1997). The system is now finding increasing utility in facilitating evidence-based practice, documentation, and information management (Martin, 2005), all of which are critical to contemporary public health care systems. It is a comprehensive system, including the following components (Martin, 2005):

- Problem classification scheme. Offers nurses a holistic, comprehensive method for identifying clients' health-related concerns. It includes domains, problems, modifiers, and signs/symptoms. Problems can be identified at the individual, family, or community level.
- Intervention scheme. Provides a framework for documenting plans and interventions in the client record in the areas of health teaching, guidance, and counseling; treatments and procedures; case management; and surveillance
- Problem rating scale for outcomes. Consists of a Likert-type scale that is a systematic and recurring method used to document the progress of clients in the record and in case conferences during their time of service in the agency. It is used in conjunction with any problem in the Problem Classification Scheme. Central to problem rating is quantifying outcomes in three dimensions: knowledge (what the client knows), behavior (what the client does), and status (how the client is).

The Omaha System is based on universal principles of nursing practice. The model was judged to be consistent with the Nightingale model of environmental health (Zurakowski, 2005). Citing some variations in language use, Gast and Montgomery (2005) found that Orem's model of self-care was also consistent with the premises of the Omaha System. The *Omaha System Model of the Problem Solving Process* (Fig. 14-4) shows the interrelationship between the practitioner and the client in addressing health problems. The model guides the nurse through the six steps in the process: (1) collecting and assessing data, (2) stating the problem, (3) identifying the problem rating on admission, (4) planning and actual interventions, (5) identification of interim or dismissal problem rating, and finally, and (6) evaluating the problem outcome. The model is applicable to individuals, families, and communities, and provides a mechanism to evaluate both individual and group change over time. With ongoing pressure for public health program funding, outcome data is vital and can be achieved through the application of the Omaha System.

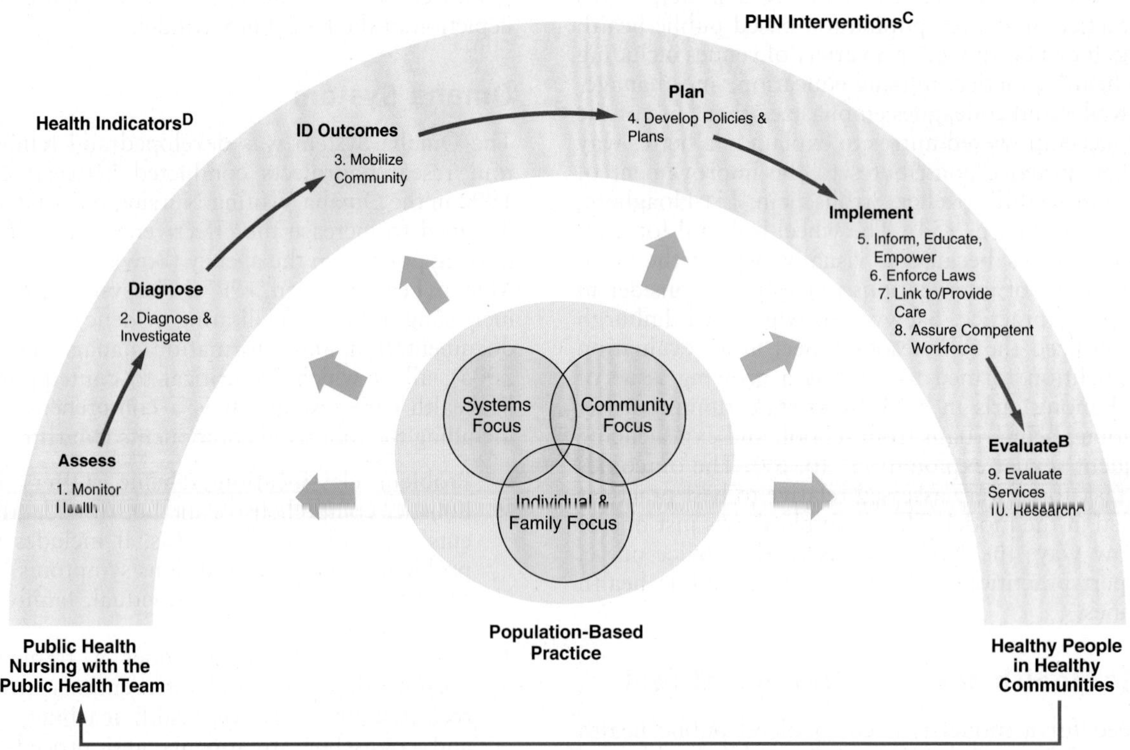

FIGURE 14-3. Public health nursing practice model, used with permission of Los Angeles County Department of Public Health, Public Health Nursing.

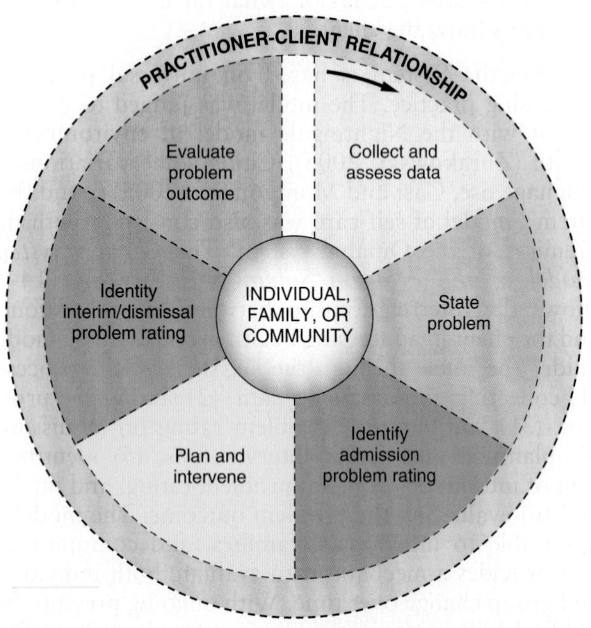

FIGURE 14-4. Omaha System Model of the Problem Solving Process. From Martin, K. S. (2005). *The Omaha System: A key to practice, documentation, and information management* (2nd ed. reprinted). Omaha, NE: Health Connections Press with permission.

Research regarding the contribution of the Omaha System to program evaluation has included assessment of interrater reliability of nursing documentation (Monsen, Lytton et al., 2011), measuring public health manager interventions (Monsen & Newsom, 2011), and benchmarking of population health status and home visiting program outcomes (Monsen, Radosevich et al., 2011). In a practice-related approach, health promotion lifestyle profiles and quality of life in Turkish women was explored using the Omaha System (Erci, 2012). The findings of this study demonstrated that application of system interventions improved measurements of self-actualization, health responsibility, interpersonal support, and stress management. These are but a few of the examples of research adding to the body of knowledge regarding the role of the Omaha System in affecting individual and group change and providing a reliable measure of programmatic effectiveness.

PRINCIPLES OF COMMUNITY/PUBLIC HEALTH NURSING

The word **principle** can be defined variably as a rule or code of conduct, or an underlying aptitude or ability (Merriam-Webster, 2012). Whatever the definition,

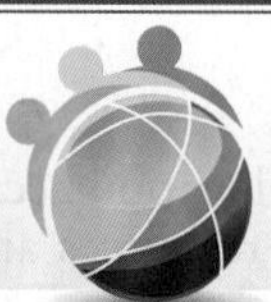

DISPLAY 14.3 PRINCIPLES OF PUBLIC HEALTH NURSING

1. **Focus on the Community.** The client or unit of care is the population
2. **Give Priority to Community Needs.** The primary obligation is to achieve the greatest good for the greatest number of people or the population as a whole
3. **Work in Partnership With the People.** The processes used by public health nurses include working with the client as an equal partner
4. **Focus on Primary Prevention.** Primary prevention is the priority in selecting appropriate activities
5. **Promote a Healthful Environment.** Public health nursing focuses on strategies that create healthy environmental, social, and economic conditions in which populations may thrive
6. **Target All Who Might Benefit.** A public health nurse is obligated to actively identify and reach out to all who might benefit from a specific activity or service
7. **Promote Optimum Allocation of Resources.** Optimal use of available resources to ensure the best overall improvement in the health of the population is a key element of the practice
8. **Collaborate with Others in the Community.** Collaboration with a variety of other professions, populations, organizations, and other stakeholder groups is the most effective way to promote and protect the health of the people

Adapted from American Nurses Association. (2007). *Public health nursing: Scope and standards of practice* (pp. 7–9). Silver Spring, MD: Nursesbooks.org.

there are universals in practice that can guide public health nursing practice in a way that can help achieve the most beneficial outcomes. The goals of public health nursing, to promote and protect the health of communities, are facilitated by adhering to eight principles identified by the ANA (2007) for public health nursing practice. These principles are summarized in Display 14.3 (ANA, 2007).

Principle 1: Focus on the Community

The first principle reminds us that the ultimate responsibility of public health nursing is to direct services to the population as a whole. Even though public health nurses may intervene to address individual, family, or group needs, the entire community is the client.

Principle 2: Give Priority to Community Needs

The second principle deals with the ethical obligation of the public health nurse to give priority to the needs and preferences of the whole community over those of one individual. This means that the nurse must consider interventions that will lead to the greatest good for the most people. For example, programs that make mammograms for early detection of breast cancer available to all women regardless of income level are given priority over those that provide bone marrow transplantation for women with advanced metastatic breast cancer.

Principle 3: Work in Partnership with the People

The third principle requires the public health nurse to work in partnership with the community. The nurse and the community members (or groups) each bring their own values, beliefs, and expertise to the partnership. Policy development and assurance are more likely to be accepted and applied if there is mutual consideration of and respect for these elements. Developed policies need to be communicated in language that reflects an understanding of the community. For these reasons, an essential part of establishing a partnership with a community is getting to know the members and groups within that community.

Principle 4: Focus on Primary Prevention

The fourth principle of public health nursing underscores the importance of primary prevention in promoting the health of people. Most fields of medicine, including acute care nursing, are primarily concerned with illness, and with efforts to prevent complications from and reoccurrence of the illness. In contrast, public health nursing has an obligation to prevent health problems and to promote a higher level of wellness. Public health nurses take the initiative to seek out high-risk groups, potential health problems, and situations that contribute to health problems. They then institute preventive programs. For example, if community assessment revealed a large number of new mothers with postpartum depression, public health nurses would address secondary prevention by establishing mental health programs. Equally as important, they would attend to primary prevention by working to change the conditions in the community that increase the risk for postpartum depression.

Principle 5: Promote a Healthful Environment

The fifth principle recognizes the importance of ensuring that people live in conditions conducive to health. Therefore, it is aligned with Nightingale's Environmental Theory of Health. People are less likely to be healthy if they live in a community with high unemployment, crowded housing, and dirty air, or where it is difficult to obtain inexpensive, healthful food. They are also less likely to be healthy if the community's norms include acceptance or even encouragement of activities such as smoking, binge drinking, drug use, or unsafe sex. To change these conditions requires commitment, perseverance, patience, resourcefulness, and a long-range view.

Principle 6: Target All Who Might Benefit

The sixth principle involves outreach strategies to meet the obligation to serve all people who might benefit from an intervention. This tenet requires that the nurse examine policies or programs to determine whether they are accessible and acceptable to the entire population in need and advocate for change if necessary.

In one community, families with young children had a high (80%) rate of compliance with regulations requiring the use of infant and toddler car seats, but assessment revealed that more than 90% of the seats were being used incorrectly. For example, the harness straps were too loose, the seats were not properly installed, or the model used had been recalled because of safety problems. A coalition of public health nurses and law-enforcement officials implemented a summer-long, monthly car seat checkup service in the parking lot of a local mall and advertised the service in a media campaign. In evaluating the program, the coalition acknowledged that the campaign had not affected the transport of children born after the intervention period had expired or residents who were out of town for the summer, nor had it increased the knowledge of car seat safety among expectant parents or the community in general.

The questions in Display 14.4 can help the nurse evaluate a planned program's success in reaching people who might benefit. These questions should guide the design, implementation, and evaluation of outreach strategies.

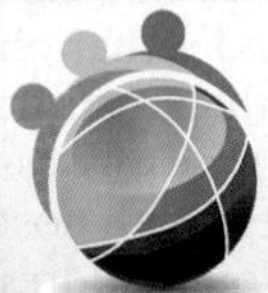

DISPLAY 14.4 DETERMINING WHETHER PROGRAMS SERVE INTENDED POPULATIONS

- Is the service offered in a manner that encourages utilization?
    - Are the services located conveniently?
    - Do the hours of the service fit with the work or school life of the people?
    - Are the services offered in a manner that is respectful of the values, beliefs, mores, and traditions of the people?
    - What kind of marketing strategies have been used to inform the people of the service?
- What is the satisfaction level of users of the service?
- Why are some people not using services?

Principle 7: Promote Optimum Allocation of Resources

The seventh principle addresses resource-allocation decisions. In most communities, the available resources are not sufficient to meet all the needs of all the people. The nurse must ensure that the community is using limited resources in ways that lead to the greatest improvement in health. To promote optimum allocation of resources, the nurse must

- Know the latest research on the effectiveness of various programs in addressing needs
- Collect information about the short- and long-term costs of programs
- Evaluate existing programs and policies for ways to improve or discontinue them
- Communicate this information to community decision makers, so that they can make resource allocation decisions that are most likely to improve the community's health

Principle 8: Collaborate with Others in the Community

The eighth principle underscores the importance of collaboration with other nurses, health care providers, social workers, educators, spiritual leaders, business leaders, and government officials within the community. This interdisciplinary collaboration is essential to establish and maintain effective programs. Programs that are planned and implemented in isolation can lead to fragmentation, gaps, and overlaps in health services. For instance, without collaboration, a well-child clinic may be started in a community that already has a strong developmental screening program but does not have community prenatal services. Without collaboration, programs may also fail to be effective. Another example, a Saturday-morning cardiovascular fitness program designed without consultation with spiritual leaders may be totally ineffective in a devout Jewish community, where members devote Saturdays to religious observances.

SOCIETAL INFLUENCES ON COMMUNITY-ORIENTED, POPULATION-FOCUSED NURSING

Society is constantly changing and these changes influence a community's health, either positively or negatively. For this reason, public health nurses need to continually adapt their strategies to respond to these changing conditions. An example is international air travel, which increases risk for communicable disease in a small city with a new international airport. Public health nurses in this city must be proactive in developing strategies to control the spread of communicable disease. Social changes may also affect the availability of resources necessary to ensure that effective intervention strategies are available. For example, a downturn in the stock market may prompt closure of a community business that once generously supported local community services.

Contemporary public health nurses must be especially aware of the mutual interaction between nursing and technology. The term **technology** refers to the application of science to change processes of production or industry; or simply the practical application of knowledge (Merriam-Webster, 2012). Ideally, technologic innovations lead to improvements in processes for creating products or services. The 20th century was filled with technologic innovations that simultaneously disrupted old patterns of production and created new opportunities to increase production, but new technology also presents new challenges. Two technologic changes that are highly relevant to contemporary public health nursing are communication technology and genetic engineering.

Communication Technology

Changes in communication technology present new opportunities and challenges for community-oriented, population-focused care. Because of advances in satellite and telecommunications technology, communication is possible anywhere in the world where resources are available to purchase equipment and services. This means that a public health nurse, whether working in the Australian outback or at a public health clinic in Anchorage, Alaska, can contact clients, consultants, and agencies worldwide, if resources are available to take advantage of the technologies.

In addition, Internet technology has made it possible to access local, state, national, and international data for community assessment, planning, and evaluation. Nurses who require data for a new intervention strategy, for example, can search the Internet for information from consumer groups, researchers, and other experts worldwide. To keep apprised of emerging issues and trends in public health, the nurse can join numerous Internet-based electronic discussion groups or listservs (electronic discussions distributed by way of e-mail). The challenge to the nurse is to manage the volume of information and to weigh its worth.

Health care consumers face similar opportunities and challenges. Most diseases and disabilities can be researched online; information is available on the Internet, and consumers are increasingly searching the Net for health-related data. Certainly, the validity and reliability of information on the Internet can vary widely. Research is needed to understand how people decide what information to use from the Internet, how they use it, and how its use affects their health. As health educators, public health nurses can provide guidelines to help people decide how to use health information found on the Internet (Display 14.5). At the same time, public health nurses need to be actively involved in creating technology resources, such as Internet sites, to provide health information specific to their targeted communities.

The Internet is a superb vehicle for rapidly tracing the international spread of infectious diseases. For example, the World Health Organization has an Internet site for countries to report epidemiologic and laboratory data on influenza. The Centers for Disease Control and Prevention (CDC) offers current data on communicable diseases through the online publication *Morbidity and Mortality Weekly Report*. In addition, many local health departments and health agencies have their own Web sites that can provide information and resources specific to the needs of the local communities.

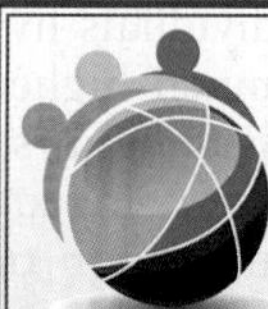

DISPLAY 14.5 DETERMINING WORTH OF HEALTH INFORMATION ON THE INTERNET

- What are the credentials and affiliation of the author?
- Is it easy to determine who is the publisher or sponsor of the Web site? Evaluate how the publisher or sponsor might gain economically through your use of the information
- Is the date of publication of the Web site included? Is the information current?
- Are both sides of an issue described? Does the author discuss pros and cons of information presented?
- What references are included to substantiate the information in the article?

New forms of technology continue to be introduced. Today, forms of communication can range from cell phones and text messages to instant messaging and social networking. This new technology provides innovative ways to enhance health communication and social marketing. Nurses can utilize social media such as Web blogs, Facebook, and Twitter to disseminate health messages to specific target populations (CDC, 2011). Health messages distributed through a variety of modalities including mass media such as television and radio, small media such as brochures, social media such as computer networking, and interpersonal communication such as face-to-face interactions increase the exposure of the message to a wider swath of the population (CDC, 2011). Internet-enabled mobile devices and social networking have even been used to promote an exercise program among 15- to 24-year-olds receiving mental health treatment (Killackey et al., 2011). In yet another example, authors Huang, Chan, and Hyder propose the creation of an Internet social networking emergency response system. Citing the effectiveness of Internet social networking and mobile technology used by community residents during the 2009 typhoon disaster in Taiwan, this technology holds promise for establishing "a reliable and accessible tunnel for proximal and distal users in disaster preparedness and management (Huang et al., 2010, p. 1)

With so much technology at our finger tips, nurses must remember that not everyone has access to or regularly uses the Internet. A study by Rains (2008) supported the notion that younger, more educated individuals living in urban areas utilize the Internet at much higher rates than do other groups. The public health nurse must be vigilant, so that access issues do not impede access to health information for the many poor or elderly clients who might be less likely to have access to computers. Supporting the need for increased access for older adults are the findings of Hogeboom, McDermott, Perrin, Osman, and Bell-Ellison (2010) suggesting that Internet use can strengthen social networks in adults over 50 years of age. Examining the results of the 2004 Health and Retirement Survey (n = 2,284), a significant positive association was found between Internet use and frequency of contact with friends and family and attendance at organized meetings (not religious services).

Genetics, Genomics, and Genetic Engineering

Genetics, the science of heredity and **genomics**, the study of the entire genome, are terms that have gained increased attention from nurses over the past decade. An outgrowth of this knowledge is **genetic engineering**, which can be defined as "the group of applied techniques of genetics and biotechnology used to cut up and join together genetic material and especially DNA from one or more species of organism and to introduce the result into an organism in order to change one or more of its characteristics" (Merriam-Webster, 2012). The development of the field was made possible by the discovery of certain enzymes that can "cut" DNA from two or more different sources into pieces that can be recombined in a test tube. Gene manipulation also required the development of methods for inserting these recombinant DNA molecules into cells by the use of so-called *vectors* such as viruses.

Genetic engineering allows scientists to alter the herbicide, pest, and stress resistance of crops and to increase the nutrition and attractiveness of the foods we eat. Genetic engineering also allows scientists to develop new kinds of medicines and to cure diseases by replacing absent or faulty genes. Mapping of the DNA sequence that makes up the "genetic blueprint" of human beings has provided new opportunities for protecting human health (Ellsworth & Manolio, 1999; Jenkins & Calzone, 2007). In addition to increasing understanding of the contribution of genetic material to health and disease, genetic research has created new opportunities for early identification, prevention, and treatment of people at risk for disease. For example, techniques for DNA screening of newborns allow early detection of risk for certain diseases and disabilities, thereby permitting early intervention. Genetic counseling, previously only available to a limited population, is being used increasingly by women in the preconception and prenatal periods (Dolan, Biermann, & Damus, 2007). Now, genome studies help in the diagnosis of diseases, identification of individual health needs based on genetic makeup, and with providing insight and guidance for treatment of specific health conditions (National Human Genome Research Institute, 2011).

Despite the enthusiasm of many groups, especially commercial concerns, genetic engineering has generated much controversy (Biotech Opponents, 2011; Cahill, Morley, & Powell, 2010). The controversy emerges from a number of different concerns. One concern is the inability to know for certain the long-term consequences of genetic alteration of foods or organisms such as bacteria, insects, or human beings. For example, the release of a genetically altered weed or insect could be catastrophic if that weed or insect reproduces prolifically and damages the ecosystem. Fears of negative effects of engineered gene transfers between species in genetically engineered food include allergic reactions, spread of diseases across crop species, and emergence of new diseases because of unpredictable mutations in the genetic code.

The Human Genome Project has opened dramatic possibilities for health and wellbeing, as well as created ethical challenges in the near future. The potential scientific capacity to alter methods of human reproduction raises concerns about creating unintended consequences for the human race. Another source of concern is that science is "playing God." For some people, the possibility of being able to select the gender, intelligence, or eye color of a child raises concerns about interfering with nature and creates conflict with religious or ethical views. In addition, genetic screening could be used to deny rights and opportunities to people. For example, someone who is found to carry a gene that increases the risk for heart disease might be denied health insurance coverage. Another source of concern is the distrust many people have of government, large commercial enterprises, and the scientific community. Some people believe that they are not being told the truth about scientific or other issues. Because genetic alteration of food or humans can affect the survival of individuals, groups, or society as a whole, this distrust results in some strong opposition to any type of genetic engineering (Biotech Opponents, 2011; Cahill et al., 2010).

In dealing with these concerns, it is the public health nurse's responsibility to be aware of the latest scientific information when educating communities, so that the decisions made best fit the community's value system. Advocating for the highest scientific rigor in genetic engineering research is another important role of public health nurses. Public health nurses need to advocate for research that not only maps DNA but also identifies interventions that can change the outcome for people at risk for genetic disorders. Nurses need to balance what is good for the community as a whole against potential costs to people at risk, advocating for policies and regulations that ensure such a balance. Despite growing evidence of the need to establish essential nursing competencies in this area, Jenkins and Calzone (2007) note that "the relevance of genetics and genomics to nursing practice is not fully appreciated and many nurses still consider it a subspecialty that is not relevant to the entire profession" (p. 11). Nevertheless, *Essentials of Baccalaureate Education for Professional Nursing Practice* (American Association of Colleges of Nursing, 2008) emphasized the impact of advances in genetics and genomics. Specifically, Essential VII: Clinical Prevention and Population Health stresses that the graduate be prepared to: (1) "Assess protective and predictive factors, including genetics, which influence the health of individuals, families, groups, communities, and populations" and (2) "Conduct a health history, including environmental exposure and a family history that recognizes genetic risks, to identify current and future health problems" (p. 24).

Global Economy

Hundreds of years ago, the economies of communities were largely local. If drought led to a reduction in crop yield in one region, only that region and perhaps its closest neighbors would be affected. Since World War II, however, there has been a consistent trend toward international trade, investment, travel, and ownership of information and ideas (Moller, 1999), yet disparities in economic prosperity and health have widened over that same period (Benatar, Gill, & Baker, 2011). This increasingly **global economy** is evidenced by the creation of the European Economic Community and the passage of the North American Free Trade Agreement. This globalization has contributed to a strong economy for many developed nations, including the United States, but has also led to increased instability of all economies as problems in markets in distant countries affect markets worldwide.

This interrelationship was made clear after the terrorist attacks in the United States on September 11, 2001. Key markets in the world experienced downturns, as did the economies of the United States and other nations. The United States and other countries are still experiencing the effects of that day, which were only compounded by the severe global economic downturn that became evident in 2008. Entire countries are having to reassess national priorities in light of high unemployment and stressed economies. Added to this pressure on world economic health is the rising cost of fuels, predominately oil. As world economies grow, so too does their need for oil. With increasing global demand (despite economic challenges) and limited growth in production capacity, the price of a barrel of oil is no longer a discussion only on Wall Street, but on Main Street as well.

A global economy also permits rich countries in need of skilled workers to recruit them from developing countries, causing a shortage of skilled labor in those countries that need it most. In countries able to recruit labor, the presence of new immigrant groups may be seen as a threat to the local culture or economy, causing an increase in ethnic, racial, and religious tensions. Even people with jobs that pay well may react negatively because they see their world changing and their own future as more uncertain. At the same time, when citizens in developing nations perceive their country or its citizens as suffering unjustly because of unfair economic changes, there may be an increase in nationalism and even international terrorism.

Medical tourism is another response to the current economic challenges in accessing health care resources. Patients from industrial countries seek out health care in foreign countries for a variety of reasons including affordability, access to prompt treatment, availability of procedures not available in their home country, or privacy reasons (Johnson, Crooks, Adams, Snyder, & Kingsbury, 2011). Central and South America, Asia, India, Thailand, and Singapore are popular destinations for foreign health care (Hopkins, Labonte, Runnels, & Packer, 2010; Mechinda, Serirat, Anuwichanont, & Gulid, 2010). Health care in these countries is more affordable to the medical tourist since "the lower cost of health care is appropriate for the economic environment in which the care is provided" (Horowitz & Rosensweig, 2007, p. 26). A specific form of medical tourism, reproductive tourism is a growing concern in many less developed countries and within poorer communities. This practice typically targets low-income females who serve as surrogates or candidates for egg donation, either of which may result in poor health outcomes for these women, both short and long term (Donchin, 2010). This industry raises ethical and social justice issues that are only just beginning to be explored.

More recently, the national economy has been impacted by a major decline in U.S. home values, precipitated by imprudent and possibly illegal lending practices by some residential mortgage lenders. The result has been thousands of home mortgage foreclosures, as families found they were unable to afford the escalating costs of mortgages with adjustable interest rates. With rising foreclosures, others who were continuing to pay their mortgages on time found their homes' values decreasing at an alarming rate, due in part to the large inventory of foreclosed houses in their neighborhoods. Fear that the housing market could decline further kept many prospective buyers out of the market. The resulting impact on available and affordable rental properties is felt most by those with limited incomes. As more and more people compete for limited rental housing options, rental costs rose accordingly. The impact on the international community of the U.S. housing decline continues to take a toll on American residents.

Finally, the economic trends of the late 20th century and into the new millennium have contributed to greater worldwide disparities in wealth, health, and *relative poverty*, a measurement of an individual's income against the average for the society in which that individual lives. In the United States, economic disparity has been fueled by increased demand for skilled workers and decreased demand for unskilled laborers. When the demand for skilled workers (e.g., software engineers) exceeds the supply, these workers can demand increased wages, resulting ultimately in increased costs for housing, health care, products, and services, even for those unskilled laborers whose wages have decreased proportionately. The number of people living in poverty in the United States today is the highest it has been in 52 years (U.S. Census Bureau, 2011).

The World Bank was founded in 1946 and has become a source of financial and technical support for underdeveloped countries (Ruger, 2005). Its purpose at the time of its inception was to support the redevelopment of Europe after World War II. Since then, the focus of the World Bank efforts has turned to promoting health in underdeveloped countries (Ruger, 2005). Using a collaborative approach, the World Bank is able to mobilize funds to support improved nutrition, health education, and systems change to promote health in impoverished regions (Ruger, 2005). As a result of the recent global economic crisis, financial instability among developed countries has impacted access to funding resources. The World Bank has continued to support developing countries by funding schools and health clinics, and providing microloans for women (World Bank, 2012).

Reducing income disparity and its numerous effects is a challenge for all people who work in service to humanity. Public health nurses have an obligation to read the latest research, so that they can better understand the relationship of poverty to health. At the same time, they need to advocate for policies that will reduce adverse effects of poverty and income disparities. As mentioned earlier, it is imperative for nurses to ensure that limited resources are utilized in ways that lead to the greatest improvement in health.

Migration

Migration is the act of moving from one region or country to another, temporarily, seasonally, or permanently. Throughout history, people have migrated from place to place to seek improved opportunities or to escape intolerable conditions in their home countries. In the late 20th century and the early years of the 21st century, a dramatic increase occurred in the number of *refugees* who migrated from their homes to escape invasion, oppression, or persecution (World Health Organization, 2012). We also saw an increased reliance on migrant farm workers, people who move from one region to another seasonally, following the crops.

The health care needs of migrants and migrant refugees are enormous. Environmental factors are a primary reason for compromised health, and include inadequate waste disposal, crowded and often unsanitary living conditions, lack of access to healthful foods, and air pollution from an increased concentration of vehicles used for moving refugees. Compounding these problems are language and cultural barriers, as well as distrust and fear that may interfere with meeting the needs of these vulnerable populations. The potential detriments to health associated with migration require that public health nurses ensure that surveillance systems able to detect emerging health problems are in place; programs to prevent health problems and treat existing conditions also need to be developed.

Terrorism and Bioterrorism

Terrorism is one way in which a small number of people who perceive that they have been unfairly treated can exert influence on a larger group or nation. Groups wishing to harm other countries need sophisticated skills and coordination for most conventional weapons. Terrorists may also use unconventional weapons when highly motivated, such as flying planes into buildings, strapping bombs to their bodies, or even allowing bombs to be implanted in their bodies.

Some methods of bioterrorism may be even cheaper and easier to use. **Bioterrorism** is the use of living organisms, such as bacteria, viruses, or other organic materials, to harm or intimidate others, in order to achieve political ends. Some of the possible biologic agents used include *Bacillus anthracis*, smallpox virus, *Brucella*, and botulinum toxin (see Chapter 17). An increasingly proactive approach has been adopted by the federal government to reduce the risk of both natural occurring and deliberate outbreaks of disease. This approach requires a melding of biodefense needs with an increased emphasis on biosecurity, balancing both public health and national security interests (Koblentz, 2012).

Because of escalating concerns about bioterrorism, public health workers increasingly recognize the need for skills in dealing with a bioterrorist attack. They need to do the following (CDC, 2008):

- Ensure that adequate surveillance systems are in place for early detection.
- Educate emergency and other health personnel about symptoms, treatment, and prevention of further spread.
- Establish coordinated response plans with health and law-enforcement officials.

Perhaps more importantly, public health nurses need to be involved in primary prevention of bioterrorism through advocating for the elimination of biologic weapons and addressing the root causes of terrorism, such as poverty, hunger, poor housing, limited educational opportunities, lack of clean water, and inadequate or no health care.

Climate Changes

Climate changes can be considered societal changes because they may be influenced by economics. Since the Industrial Revolution, increased amounts of carbon dioxide, methane, and nitrous oxide created by manufacturing industries, automobile emissions, and consumer products have been introduced into the earth's atmosphere. These increases have contributed to climate changes that are expected to affect sea level; the production of food, fiber, and medicines; and the spread of infectious diseases. Conversely, significant increases in fuel efficiency and efforts to reduce pollution could avoid millions of deaths around the world. Population-focused nurses need to educate the public about the potential dangers of continuing to contaminate the environment and to advocate for changes in public policy that reduce air and water contaminants. In 2008, the American Nurses Association's House of Delegates passed a Global Climate Change initiative that encourages nurses to "advocate for change on both individual and policy levels; to support local public policies that endorse sustainable energy sources and reduce greenhouse gas emissions; and ... to support initiatives to decrease the contribution to global warming by the healthcare industry" (ANA, 2012). This built on elements of the 2007 Public Health Nursing: Scope and Standards of Practice most notably in terms of ethics in practice, challenging nurses to contribute to "resolving social and environmental issues and barriers to healthy living conditions" (p. 34). Chapter 9 explores health-related environmental issues in detail.

SUMMARY

Public health nursing is a community-oriented, population-focused nursing specialty that is based on interpersonal relationships. The unit of care is the community or population rather than the individual, and the goal is to promote healthy communities.

Theories and models of community/public health nursing practice aid the nurse in understanding the rationale behind community-oriented care. Florence Nightingale's environmental theory emphasizes the importance of improving environmental conditions to promote health. Orem's self-care model provides a framework, within which the public health nurse can promote a community's collective independence and self-care ability. Neuman's health care systems model describes the nurse's role as one of assisting clients to remain stable within their environment, whereas Rogers' model of the science of unitary man focuses on client–environment interaction and holistic health. King's Theory of Goal Attainment reminds nurses to work in partnership with clients to achieve the best health outcomes. Parse's Human Becoming Theory posits quality of life from each person's own perspective as the goal of nursing practice. Pender's model focuses on the promotion of health behaviors in people; the goal of nursing is to enhance the likelihood that people will engage in health-promoting behaviors by assessing and influencing perceptual and modifying factors. Roy's adaptation model describes the nurse's goal as one that promotes healthful coping mechanisms and adaptive responses to stressors. Salmon's construct for public health nursing prescribes education, engineering, and enforcement with individuals, families, communities, and nations. Finally, the models used in public health nursing practice, the Minnesota Intervention "Wheel," the Los Angeles County–Public Health Nursing Practice Model, and the Omaha System Model of the Problem Solving Process provide a mechanism for public health nurses to assess, plan, intervene, and evaluate the care they provide in their communities.

The eight principles of public health nursing applied to community/public health nursing practice provide a framework within which the nurse works to promote and protect the health of populations. They emphasize the primacy of prevention, the need for outreach, and the importance of working in collaboration for the greatest good of the greatest number of people.

Nurses must anticipate and adapt to societal changes in order to fulfill their mission of promoting the health of all people. Contemporary societal influences on public health nursing include communication technology, genetic engineering, the global economy, migration, terrorism, and climate changes?

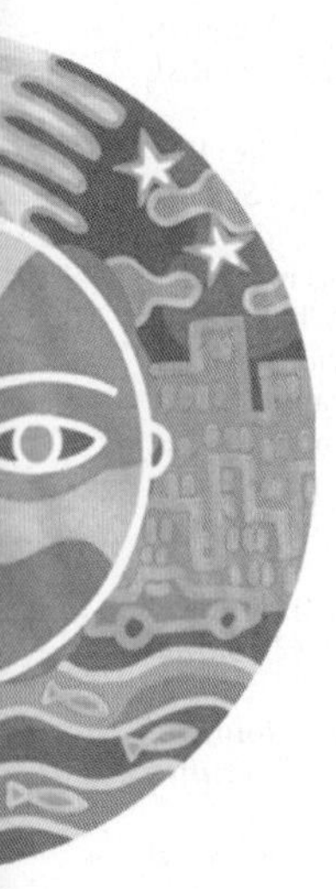

ACTIVITIES TO PROMOTE **CRITICAL THINKING**

1. Interview a public health nursing director to determine what population-focused programs are offered in your locality. Explore nursing's role in the assessment, development, implementation, and evaluation of these programs. Discuss with the director how public health nurses might expand their population-focused interventions
2. Describe a situation in community/public health nursing practice in which the use of an educational intervention would be most appropriate. Do the same with engineering and enforcement interventions. Discuss what made you match each situation with that intervention
3. Assume you have been asked to make a home visit to a 75-year-old man, living alone, whose wife recently died. In addition to assessing his individual needs, what factors should you consider for assessment and intervention that would indicate an aggregate- or community-focused approach?
4. Select one of the societal influences on a community or population. How would the theories or models for community/public health nursing practice that were discussed in this chapter guide your practice concerning that societal issue? Choose three models or theories to discuss.
5. Explore one of the societal influences on community or population using the Internet. Using the information in Display 14.3, try to determine the worth of the information available on several Internet sites
6. Select five or six conceptual models used in nursing research with a community/public health focus. Make a chart that shows how each model defines the nursing metaparadigm concepts: nurse, client/patient, health, and environment. Which of these conceptual models include all these concepts? Where the provider of services is defined, can public health nurse be substituted for another provider of services?

REFERENCES

Ailinger, R. L., Moore, J. B., Nguyen, N., & Lasus, H. (2006). Adherence to latent tuberculosis infection therapy among Latino immigrants. *Public Health Nursing, 23*, 307–313.

Alligood, M. R. (2010). Family healthcare with King's Theory of Goal Attainment. *Nursing Science Quarterly, 23(2)*, 99–104, doi: 10.1177/0894318410362553

American Association of Colleges of Nursing. (2008). *The essentials of baccalaureate education for professional nursing practice*. Washington, DC: Author.

American Nurses Association. (2012). *Climate change*. Retrieved from http://nursingworld.org/MainMenuCategories/WorkplaceSafety/Environmental-Health/Issues/Climate

American Nurses Association. (2007). *Public health nursing: Scope and standards of practice*. Silver Spring, MD: Nursesbooks.org.

Andrews, H. A., & Roy, C. (1991). *The Roy adaptation model: The definitive statement*. Norwalk, CT: Appleton-Lange.

Barrett, E. A. (2010). Power as knowing participation in change: What's new and what's next. *Nursing Science Quarterly, 23*(1), 47–54, doi: 10.1177/0894318409353797

Benatar, S. R., Gill, S., & Bakker, I. (2011). Global health and the global economic crisis. *American Journal of Public Health, 101*, 646–653, doi:10.2105/AJPH.2009.188458

Biotech Opponents. (2011, October 12). U.S.: Biotech opponents demand genetically engineered labeling. *European Environment & Packaging Law Weekly, 269*, 30–31.

Bowles, K. H., & Naylor, M.D. (1996). Nursing intervention classification systems. *Journal of Nursing Scholarship, 28*(4), 303–308.

Cahill, S., Morley, K., & Powell, D. A. (2010). Coverage of organic agriculture in North American newspapers. Media; Linking food safety, the environment, human health and organic agriculture. *British Food Journal, 112*, 710–722, doi: 10.1108/00070701011058244

Centers for Disease Control and Prevention. (2008). *CDC Emergency Preparedness and Response*. Retrieved from http://www.bt.cdc.gov/.

Centers for Disease Control and Prevention (2011). *The community guide*. Retrieved from http://www.thecommunityguide.org/healthcommunication/campaigns.html.

Clark, C. S. (2012). Beyond holism: Incorporating an integral approach to support caring-healing-sustainable nursing practices. *Holist Nursing Practice*, 26(2), 92–102, doi: 10.1097/HNP.0b013e3182462197

Conway, A. E., McClune, A. J., & Nosel, P. (2007). Down on the farm: Preventing farm accidents in children. *Pediatric Nursing, 33*(1), 45–48.

Dolan, S., Biermann, J., & Damus, K. (2007). Genomics for health in preconception and prenatal periods. *Journal of Nursing Scholarship, 39*, 4–9.

Donchin, A. (2010). Reproductive tourism and the quest for global gender justice. *Bioethics, 24*(7), 323–332.

Doornbos, M. M. (1995). Using King's systems framework to explore family health in the families of the young chronically mentally ill. In M. A. Frey & C. L. Sieloff (Eds.), *Advancing King's systems framework and theory of nursing* (pp. 192–205). Thousand Oaks, CA: Sage.

Doornbos, M. M. (2007). King's conceptual system and family health theory in the families of adults with persistent mental illnesses—an evolving conceptualization. In C. L. Sieloff & M. A. Frey (Eds.), *Middle-range theory development using King's conceptual system* (pp. 31–49). New York: Springer.

Ellsworth, D. L., & Manolio, T. A. (1999). The emerging importance of genetics in epidemiologic research. I. Basic concepts in human genetics and laboratory technology. *Annals of Epidemiology, 9*(1), 1–16.

Erci, B. (2012). The effectiveness of the Omaha System intervention on the women's health promotion lifestyle profile and quality of life. *Journal of Advanced Nursing, 68*, 898–907, doi: 10.1111/j.1365-2648.2011.05794.x.

Esposito, E. M., & Fitzpatrick, J. J. (2011). Registered nurses' beliefs of the benefits of exercise, their exercise behavior and their patient teaching regarding exercise. *International Journal of Nursing Practice, 17*, 351–356, doi:10.1111/j.1440-172X.2011.01951.x

Evans, M. M. (2010). Evidence-based practice protocol to improve glucose control in individuals with type 2 diabetes mellitus. *MEDSURG Nursing, 19*(6), 317–322

Fan, L. (2008). Self-care behaviors of school-age children with heart disease. *Pediatric Nursing, 34*, 131–138.

Fawcett, J. (1989). *Analysis and evaluation of conceptual models of nursing* (2nd ed.). Philadelphia, PA: F.A. Davis.

Fawcett, J. (2005). *Contemporary nursing knowledge: Analysis and evaluation of nursing models and theories* (2nd ed.). Philadelphia. PA: F. A. Davis.

Fawcett, J., & Gerity, J. (2009). *Evaluating research for evidence-based nursing*. Philadelphia, PA: FA Davis.

Frey, M. A. (1995). Toward a theory of families, children, and chronic illness. In M. A. Frey & C. L. Sieloff (Eds.), *Advancing King's systems framework and theory of nursing* (pp. 109–125). Thousand Oaks, CA: Sage.

Frey, M. A., Ellis, D. A., & Naar-King, S. (2007). Testing theory with intervention research. In C. L. Sieloff, & M. A. Frey (Eds.), *Middle-range theory development using King's conceptual system* (pp. 273–286). New York: Springer.

Gast, H. L., & Montgomery, K. S. (2005). Orem's model of self-care. In J. J. Fitzpatrick, & A. L. Whall (Eds.). *Conceptual models of nursing: Analysis and application* (4th ed. pp. 101 115). Upper Saddle River, NJ: Pearson Education, Inc.

Greenawalt, J., & Wachter, J. K. (2011). Applying the Neuman Stressor Model for workplace safety. *Journal of Healthcare Risk Management, 30*(3), 16–22, doi: 10.1002/jhrm.20056

Hannon-Engel, S. L. (2008). Knowledge development: The Roy Adaptation Model and bulimia nervosa. *Nursing Science Quarterly, 21*, 126–132.

Hemphill, J. C., & Muth Quillin, S. I. (2005). Martha Rogers' model: Science of unitary beings. In J. J. Fitzpatrick, & A. L. Whall (Eds.). *Conceptual models of nursing: Analysis and application* (4th ed. pp. 247–272). Upper Saddle River, NJ: Pearson Education, Inc.

Hogeboom, D. L., McDermott, R. J., Perrin, K. M., Osman, H., & Bell-Ellison, B. A. (2010). Internet use and social networking among middle aged and older adults. *Educational Gerontology, 36*, 93–111, doi: 10.1080/03601270903058507.

Hopkins, L., Labonte, R., Runnels, V., & Packer, C. (2010). Medical tourism today: What is the state of existing knowledge? *Journal of Public Health Policy, 31*(2), 185–198.

Horowitz, M. D., & Rosensweig, J. A. (2007). *Medical tourism-Health care in the global economy. The Physician Executive* (November–December), 24–30.

Huang, C., Chan, E., & Hyder, A. (2010). Web 2.0 and Internet social networking: A new tool for disaster management?—Lessons from Taiwan. *BMC Medical Informatics and Decision Making, 10*(57), 1–5. Retrieved from http://www.biomedcentral.com/1472-6947/10/57

Jenkins, J., & Calzone, K. A. (2007). Establishing the essential nursing competencies for genetics and genomics. *Journal of Nursing Scholarship, 39*, 10–16.

Johnson, R., Crooks, V. A., Adams, K., Snyder, J., & Kingbury, P. (2011). An industry perspective on Canadian patients' involvement in medical tourism: Implications for public health. *BMC Public Health, 11*, 1–8. Available at http://www.biomedcentral.com/1471-2458/11/416

Kagan, P. N. (2011). Catastrophe and response: Expanding the notion of 'self' to mobilize nurses' attention to policy and activism. *Nursing Science Quarterly, 24*(1), 71–78, doi: 10.1177/0894318410389076.

Kaur, S., & Kaur, B. (2012). A descriptive study to assess the awareness of the women regarding cervical cancer. *International Journal of Nursing Education, 4*(1), 66–68.

Keller, L. O., Strohschein, S., Lia-Hoagberg, B., & Schaffer, M. A. (1998). Population-based public health interventions: A model from practice. *Public Health Nursing, 15*, 207–215.

Keller, L. O., Strohschein, S., Lia-Hoagberg, B., & Schaffer, M. A. (2004). Population-based public health interventions: Practice-based and evidenced-supported. Part I. *Public Health Nursing, 21*, 453–468.

Killackey, E., Anda, A. L., Gibbs, M., Alvarez-Jimenez, M., Thompson, A., Sun, P., et al. (2011). Using internet enabled mobile devices and social networking technologies to promote exercise as an intervention for young first episode psychosis patients. *BMC Psychiatry, 11*, 1–6. Retrieved from http://www.biomedcentral.com/1471-244X/11/80

Killeen, M. B., & King, I. M. (2007). Viewpoint: Use of King's conceptual system, nursing informatics, and nursing classification systems for global communication. *International Journal of Nursing Terminologies and Classifications, 18*(2), 51–57.

King, I. M. (1970). *Toward a theory for nursing*. New York: John Wiley & Sons.

King, I. M. (1981). *A theory for nursing: Systems, concepts, process*. Albany, NY: Delmar Publishers, Inc.

Koblentz, G. D. (2012). From biodefence to biosecurity: The Obama administration's strategy for countering biological threats. *International Affairs, 88*(1), 131–148.

Lee, L. Y., Tsang, A. Y., Wong, K. F., & Lee, J. K. (2011). Using the Roy Adaptation Model to develop an antenatal assessment instrument. *Nursing Science Quarterly, 24*(4), 363–369, doi: 10.1177/0894318411419209.

Los Angeles County, Department of Public Health. (2007). *Public health nursing practice model*. Retrieved from http://admin.publichealth.lacounty.gov/PHN/docs/NarrativePHNModela2007.pdf.

Martin, K. S. (2005). *The Omaha System: A key to practice, documentation, and information management* (2nd ed. reprinted). Omaha, NE: Health Connections Press. St. Louis, MO: Elsevier.

Martin, K., Leak, G., & Aden, C. (1997). The Omaha System: A research-based model for decision making. In B. W. Spradley, & J. A. Allender (Eds.). *Readings in community health nursing* (5th ed. pp. 316–324). Philadelphia, PA: Lippincott-Raven.

Mechinda, P., Serirat, S., Anuwichanont, J., & Gulid, N. (2010). An examination of tourist's loyalty towards medical tourism in Pattaya, Thailand. *International Business & Economics Research Journal, 9*(1), 55–70.

Merriam-Webster. (2012). *Merriam-Webster online dictionary*. Retrieved from http://www.merriam-webster.com/netdict.htm

Messmer, P., & Palmer, J. (2008, First Quarter). *In honor of Imogene M. King. Reflections on Nursing Leadership*. Retrieved from http://nursingsociety.org/RNL/Current/ in_touch/tribute_king.html.

Minnesota Wheel. (2001). *Public health interventions*. Minneapolis, MN: Minnesota Department of Health, Division of Community Health Services, Public Health Nursing Section.

Moller, J. O. (1999). The growing challenge to internationalism. *The Futurist, 33*(3), 22–27.

Monsen, K. A., Lytton, A. B., Ferrari, S., Halder, K. M., Radosevich, D. M., Kerr, M. J., et al. (2011). Evaluating reliability of assessments in nursing documentation. *Online Journal of Nursing Informatics, 15*(3). Retrieved from http://ojni.org/issues/?p=899.

Monsen, K. A., & Newsom, E. T. (2011). Feasibility of using the Omaha System to represent public health nurse manager interventions. *Public Health Nursing, 28*, 421–428, doi: 10.1111/j.1525-1446.2010.00926.x

Monsen, K. A., Radosevich, D. M., Johnson, S. C., Farri, O., Kerr, M. J., & Geppert, J. S. (2011). Benchmark attainment by maternal and child health clients across public health nursing agencies. *Public Health Nursing, 29*, 11–18. Doi: 10.1111/j.1525-1446.2011.00967.x.

Morowatisharifabad, M. A., Ghofranipour, F., Heidarnia, A., Ruchi, G. B., & Ehrampoush, M. H. (2006). Self-efficacy and health promotion behaviors of older adults in Iran. *Social Behavior and Personality, 34*, 759–768.

National Human Genome Research Institute (2011). *A brief guide to genomics*. Retrieved from http://www.genome.gov/18016863

Neuman, B. (1982). *The Neuman systems model: Application to nursing education and practice*. Norwalk, CT: Appleton-Lange.

Neuman, B., & Fawcett, J. (2002). *The Neuman systems model* (4th ed.). Upper Saddle River, NJ: Prentice Hall.

Neuman, B., & Reed, K. S. (2007). A Neuman System Model perspective on nursing in 2050. *Nursing Science Quarterly*, 20, 111–113, doi: 10.1177/0894318407299847.

Nightingale, F. (1859/1992). *Florence Nightingale's notes on nursing* [Edited with an introduction, notes, and guide to identification by V. Skretkowicz]. London, England: Scutari Press.

Orem, D. E. (2001). *Nursing: Concepts of practice* (6th ed.). St Louis, MO: Mosby.

Parse, R. R. (1981). *Man-living-health: A theory of nursing*. New York, NY: Wiley & Sons.

Parse, R. R. (1998). *The human becoming school of thought: A perspective for nurses and other health professionals*. Thousand Oaks, CA: Sage.

Parse, R. R. (2012). New humanbecoming conceptualizations and the humanbecoming community model: Expansions with sciencing and living the art. *Nursing Science Quarterly, 25*(1), 44–52, doi: 10.1177/0894318411429068

Pender, N. J., Murdaugh, C. L., & Parsons, M. A. (2011). *Health promotion in nursing practice* (6th ed.). Upper Saddle River, NJ: Pearson Education, Inc.

Poirier, P. A. (2012). Humanbecoming: Transcending the now to explore the possibles in health policy. *Nursing Science Quarterly, 25*(1), 104–110, doi: 10.1177/0894318411429036.

Rains, S. A. (2008). Health at high speed: Broadband internet access, health communication, and the digital divide. *Communication Research, 35*, 283–297.

Reed, S. M. (2010) A Unitary-caring conceptual model for advanced practice nursing in palliative care. *Holistic Nursing Practice, 24*(1), 23–34.

Rogers, M. (1990). Nursing: Science of unitary, irreducible human beings: Update 1990. In E. A. M. Barrett (Ed.). *Visions of Rogers' science-based nursing*. (pp. 5–11). New York, NY: National League for Nursing.

Roy, C. (2009). *The Roy adaptation model* (3rd ed.). Upper Saddle River, NJ: Pearson

Roy, C., & Andrews, H. A. (1999). *The Roy adaptation model*. Stamford, CT: Appleton-Lange.

Ruger, J. P. (2005). The changing role of the World Bank in global health. *American Journal of Public Health, 95*, 60–70.

Saewyc, E. M., Solsvig, W., & Edinburgh, L. (2007). The Hmong youth task force: Evaluation of a coalition to address the sexual exploitation of young runaways. *Public Health Nursing, 25*, 69–76.

Salmon, M. E. (1982). Construct for public health: Where is it practiced, in whose behalf, and with what desired outcome. *Nursing Outlook, 30*(9), 527–530. (Originally published under the author name Marla Salmon White.)

Salmon, M. E. (1993). Public health nursing: The opportunity of a century. *American Journal of Public Health, 83*(12), 1674–1675.

Shaner-McRae, H., McRae, G., & Jas, V. (2007). Environmentally safe health care agencies: Nursing's responsibility, Nightingale's legacy. *Online Journal of Nursing Issues, 12*(2), 1.

Shields, L. E., & Lindsey, A. E. (1998). Community health promotion nursing practice. *Advances in Nursing Science, 20*, 23–36.

Shin, K. R., Kang, Y., Park, H. J., Cho, M. O., & Heitkemper, M. (2008). Testing and developing the health promotion model in low-income, Korean elderly women. *Nursing Science Quarterly, 21*, 173–178.

Skalski, C. A., DiGerolamo, L., & Gigliotti, E. (2006). Stressors in five client populations: Neuman systems model-based literature review. *Journal of Advanced Nursing, 56*, 69–78.

Smith, K., & Bazini-Barakat, N. (2003). A public health nursing practice model: Melding public health principles with the nursing process. *Public Health Nursing, 20*, 42–48.

Srof, B. J., & Velsor-Friedrich, B. (2006). Health promotion in adolescents: A review of Pender's health promotion model. *Nursing Science Quarterly, 19*, 366–373.

Talley, B., Rushing, A., & Gee, R. M. (2005). Community assessment using Cowling's Unitary appreciative inquiry: A beginning exploration. *Visions: The Journal of Rogerian Nursing Science, 13*(1), 27–40. Retrieved from http://drtcbear.servebbs.net:81/Visions/.

Tomasson, R. E. (1994, May 24). *Martha Rogers, 79, an author of books on nursing theory*. The New York Times. Retrieved from http://www.nytimes.com/.

U.S. Census Bureau (2011). *Poverty*. Retrieved from http://www.census.gov/hhes/www/poverty/index.html

U.S. Department of Health and Human Services. (2010). *Healthy People 2020: Social determinants of health*. Retrieved from http://www.healthypeople.gov/2020/topicsobjectives2020/overview.aspx?topicid=39

Walker, L. O., & Avant, K. C. (2005). *Strategies for theory construction in nursing* (4th ed.). Upper Saddle River, NJ: Pearson Education, Inc.

Waweru, S. M., Reynolds, A., & Buckner, E. B. (2008). Perceptions of children with HIV/AIDS from the USA and Kenya: Self-concept and emotional indicators. *Pediatric Nursing, 34*(2), 117–124.

Whelton, B. J. (2008). Human nature: A foundation for palliative care. *Nursing Philosophy, 9*, 77–88.

Wicks, M. N. (1995). Family health as derived from King's framework. In M. A. Frey & C. L. Sieloff (Eds.), *Advancing King's systems framework and theory of nursing* (pp. 97–108). Thousand Oaks, CA: Sage.

Wicks, M. N., Rice, M. C., & Talley, C. H. (2007). Further explorations of family health within the context of chronic obstructive pulmonary disease. In C. L. Sieloff & M. A. Frey (Eds.), *Middle-range theory development using King's conceptual system* (pp. 215–236). New York: Springer.

Wilson, F. L, Baker, L. M., Nordstrom, C. K., & Legwand, C. (2008). Using the teach-back and Orem's self-care deficit nursing theory to increase childhood immunization communication among low-income mothers. *Issues in Comprehensive Pediatric Nursing, 31*, 7–22.

World Bank (2012). *Financial crisis*. Retrieved from http://www.worldbank.org/financialcrisis/

World Health Organization. (2012). *Humanitarian health action*. Retrieved from http://www.who.int/hac/en/

Zahourek, R. P., & Larkin, D. M. (2009). Conscience, intentiality, and community: Unitary perspectives and research. *Nursing Science Quarterly, 22*(1), 15–22, doi: 10.1177/0894318408329244

Zurakowski, T. L. (2005). In J. J. Fitzpatrick, & A. L. Whall (Eds.). *Conceptual models of nursing: Analysis and application* (4th ed. pp. 21–45). Upper Saddle River, NJ: Pearson Education, Inc.

Zyblock, D. M. (2010). Nursing presence in contemporary nursing practice. *Nursing Forum, 45*(2), 120–124.

thePoint: Everything You Need to Make the Grade!

thePoint Visit http://thePoint.lww.com/Allender8e for selected readings, study aids for all learning styles, and more!

CHAPTER 15

Community as Client: Applying the Nursing Process

A community needs a soul if it is to become a true home for human beings. You, the people, must get it this soul.

—*Pope John Paul II* (1920–2005)

KEY TERMS

Assets assessment
Coalition
Community as client
Community development
Community diagnoses
Community needs assessment
Community subsystem assessment
Comprehensive assessment
Descriptive epidemiologic study
Evaluation
Familiarization assessment
Goals
Implementation
Interaction
Key informants
Location variables
Objectives
Outcome criteria
Partnerships
Planning
Population variables
Priority setting
Problem-oriented assessment
Social class
Social determinants of health
Social system variables
Survey
Windshield survey

LEARNING OBJECTIVES

Upon mastery of this chapter, you should be able to:

- Describe the characteristics of a healthy community.
- Describe the meaning of community as client.
- Articulate three specific considerations of each of the three dimensions of the community as client.
- Explain methods the community health nurse might use to interact with the community.
- Discuss methods of community needs assessment.
- Compare and contrast five types of community needs assessment.
- Delineate five sources of community data.
- Describe the role of the community health nurse as a catalyst for community development.

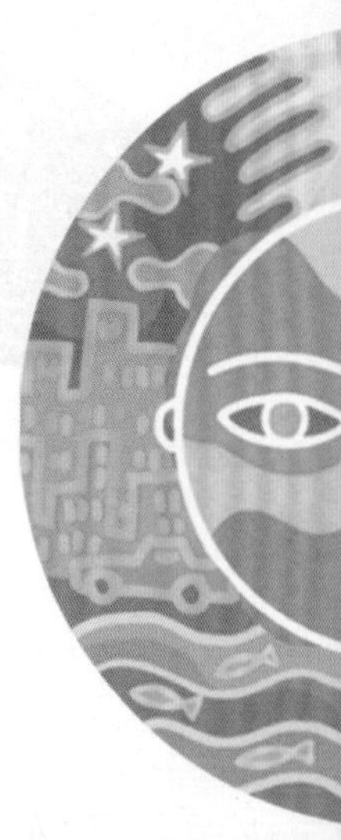

By this point in your nursing education, you are familiar with the use of the nursing process in caring for individuals in the acute care setting. It is a new experience to think of an entire community as your focus of care, but similar principles apply. Although community health nursing practice involves the care of individuals, families, and groups, the care of communities is vital to promoting health and preventing disease. The term community has been well defined in the nursing literature. A community is a collection of people interacting with one another because of geography, common interests, characteristics, or goals. These interactions include social institutions, such as schools, government agencies, and social services. The concept of **community as client** refers to a group or population of people as the focus of nursing service (Anderson & McFarlane, 2010). As described in Chapter 1, understanding the concept of the community as client is a prerequisite for effective service at every level of community nursing practice. Population health and epidemiology are core competencies for the Doctor of Nursing Practice (DNP) degree (Curley & Vitale, 2011). It is this population-focused practice that distinguishes community health nursing from other nursing specialties (American Nurses Association [ANA], 2007; American Public Health Association [APHA], 2012; Baisch, 2009; Issel et al., 2011; Radzyminski, 2007). The Quad Council of Public Health Nursing (PHN) Organizations, building on the work of the Council on Linkages Between Academia and Public Health Practice (COL) developed a list of "Core Competencies for Public Health Nurses." These competencies help clarify the role of the community health nurse within the context of community as client (Quad Council, 2011). See Display 15.1.

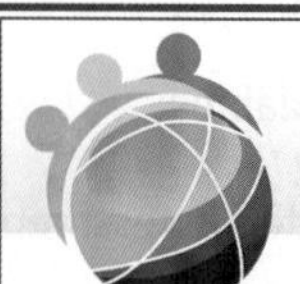

DISPLAY 15.1 QUAD COUNCIL CORE COMPETENCIES OF PUBLIC HEALTH NURSING (2011)

Tier 2 Community Based, Population Focused

1. **Analytic and Assessment Skills**
    - Assesses health status of populations and related determinants of health and illness.
    - Develops public health nursing (PHN) diagnoses for individuals, families, communities, and populations (identifies assests/needs, values/beliefs, resources and relevant environmental data).
    - Utilizes variety of relevant variables for health conditions measurement of a community or population.
    - Develops a data collection plan using epidemiology, demography, biostatistics, etc. to collect quantitative/qualitative data on community or population.
    - Uses multiple methods/sources when collecting/analyzing data for a comprehensive community/population assessment.
    - Critiques validity, reliability, and comparability of data collected for communities/populations.
    - Identifies gaps/redundancies in data sources; examines effect of data gaps on PH practice/program planning.
    - Ensures application of ethical, legal, and policy principles in collection, maintenance, use and dissemination of data/information.
    - Synthesizes qualitative/quantitative data during analysis for comprehensive assessment; uses various data collection methods/sources to conduct a comprehensive assessment.
    - Incorporates an ecological perspective in data analysis; partners with groups, communities, health professionals, and stakeholders to review/evaluate collected data.
    - Utilizes information technology effectively in collection/analysis/storage/retrieval of data.
    - Practices EBP PHN to promote health of communities/populations.
    - Collects data related to social determinants of health (SDH) and community resources to plan for community-oriented and population-level programs; analyzes data; incorporates results.
2. **Policy Development/Program Planning Skills**
    - Identifies valid/reliable data; conducts/uses policy analysis to address specific PH issues.
    - Plans population-level interventions guided by research and relevant models.
    - Conducts/uses policy analysis to address PH issues; incorporates a wide range of policy options into planning/delivery of services.
    - Plans population-level interventions; uses planning models, epidemiology, etc. in evaluating population-level interventions; critiques evidence; conducts/uses policy analysis to address PH issues.
    - Selects an appropriate method of decision analysis for an issue relevant to an identified group/community/population; uses planning models, epidemiology, etc. in development/implementation of population-level interventions.
    - Manages delivery of community/population-based health services; evaluates/ensures compliance with PH laws/regulations.
    - Develops plans to implement programs/policies; works as member of interdisciplinary team.

DISPLAY 15.1 QUAD COUNCIL CORE COMPETENCIES OF PUBLIC HEALTH NURSING (2011) *(Continued)*

- Manages implementation of organizational policies/programs for areas of responsibility.
- Designs evaluation plans that address multiple variables, both process/outcome measures, and uses multiple data collection methods.
- Identifies variety of sources/methods to access PH information; utilizes technology to collect data to monitor/evaluate quality/effectiveness of programs for populations.
- Develops QI indicators/core measures as part of the process to improve PH programs/services; utilizes these as part of process to improve PH programs/services.

3. **Communication Skills**
   - Assesses the health literacy of communities/populations served.
   - Communicates effectively in writing, orally, and electronically; communication characterized by critical thinking/complex decision making.
   - Solicits input from community/population members/stakeholders when planning health care programs.
   - Utilizes a variety of methods to disseminate PH information/EBP outcomes to multiple audiences, including community/professional groups.
   - Communicates effectively with community groups/partners/and interprofessional teams.
   - Articulates role of PHN within the overall health system to internal/external audiences.
4. **Cultural Competency Skills**
   - Utilizes social/ecological determinants of health to develop culturally responsive interventions with communities/populations.
   - Uses epidemiological data/concepts, other evidence to analyze SDH when developing/tailoring population-level health services; applies multiple methods/sources of information technology to better understand impact of SDH on communities/populations.
   - Plans health services to meet cultural needs of diverse communities/populations.
   - Explains interplay of multiple forces contributing to cultural diversity.
   - Serves as an advocate to build a diverse PH workforce.
   - Uses evidence/awareness of cultural models to tailor interventions to diverse populations; evaluates current population health programs for evidence of cultural tailoring; evaluates staff development needs related to cultural competency.
   - Uses evidence/cultural models to tailor program-level interventions.
5. **Community Dimensions of Practice Skills**
   - Utilizes an ecological perspective in health assessment/planning/interventions with communities/populations.
   - Provides population health expertise for community-based participatory research teams.
   - Identifies need for community involvement/partners to create community groups/coalitions.
   - Identifies mechanisms for enhancing collaboration among stakeholders in population-focused health interventions; develops partnerships with key stakeholders/groups.
   - Partners effectively with key stakeholders/groups in care delivery to communities/populations.
   - Identifies areas for community involvement in agency programs/initiatives; critiques evidence on approaches to fostering community partnerships/involvement; uses EBP guidelines and effective group processes to partner with community members/groups.
   - Explains to community groups/partners the role of government and the private/nonprofit sectors in delivery of community health services.
   - Utilizes community assets/resources to promote/deliver care to communities/populations.
   - Uses input from a variety of community/aggregate stakeholders in development of PH programs/services.
   - Advocates for PH policies/programs/resources that better serve populations.
6. **Basic Public Health Sciences Skills**
   - Utilizes PH/nursing science in practice at population/community level.
   - Describes influence of sentinel events on current PHN practice.
   - Uses EBP to assure population level programs contribute to meeting core PH functions and the 10 essential services.
   - Uses descriptive/analytical methods and PH sciences to design/implement/evaluate interventions at community/population level.
   - Synthesizes research across disciplines related to PH concerns/population-level interventions.
   - Identifies gaps in scientific evidence related to PH issues/concerns/population-level interventions.
   - Identifies a wide variety of sources/methods to access PH information (e.g., geographic information system (GIS) mapping); identifies gaps/inconsistencies in research evidence for practice.
   - Incorporates the requirements of patient confidentiality, human subjects protection, and research ethics into data collection/processing.

(continued)

DISPLAY 15.1 QUAD COUNCIL CORE COMPETENCIES OF PUBLIC HEALTH NURSING (2011) *(Continued)*

- Disseminates theory-guided and/or EBP outcomes in peer-reviewed journals/national level meetings; facilitates research projects with organizations.

7. **Financial Management and Planning Skills**
   - Collaborates with relevant public and/or private systems for managing program in PH.
   - Supervises operations of health programs within federal/state/tribal/local PH agencies.
   - Develops partnerships with communities/agencies within federal/state/tribal/local levels of government that have authority over PH situations (e.g., emergency preparedness).
   - Implements judicial/operational procedures of governing body and/or administrative unit designated with oversight of PH organizational operations.
   - Develops a programmatic budget.
   - Manages care delivery to communities/populations within current/forecasted budget constraints.
   - Develops strategies for determining budget priorities based on financial input from federal/state/tribal/local sources.
   - Assesses impact of organizational budget priorities on PHN programs/practice; establishes organization PHN resource priorities that assure effective PHN practice.
   - Designs evaluation plans for population-focused programs; implements plans.
   - Leads revisions to population-focused programs based on formative/summative evaluation results.
   - Develops proposals for funding from external sources.
   - Applies basic human relations/conflict management skills in interactions with direct reports/other professionals/health care team members.
   - Identifies opportunities to use health care technologies/informatics to improve PH program/business operations; incorporates health care technology/informatics to improve PH program/business operations.
   - Assists in development of contracts/other agreements for provision of services.
   - Describes how cost-effectiveness/cost-benefit/cost-utility analyses affect programmatic prioritization/decision making; employs these measures.
   - Participates in implementation/evaluation of performance management systems.
8. **Leadership and Systems Thinking Skills**
   - Addresses ethical issues related to the PHN care of communities/populations.
   - Applies system theory to PHN practice with communities/populations.
   - Leads team/community partners in identifying vision/values/principles for community action.
   - Analyzes internal/external factors that may impact the delivery of essential PH services; implements strategies to assure quality/collaboration/coordination in delivery of PHN services.
   - Leads interprofessional team/organizational learning opportunities; provides leadership in staff development.
   - Implements opportunities to mentor/advise/coach/develop peers/direct reports, and other members of PH workforce.
   - Uses EBP models to design/implement quality initiatives; establishes indicators to monitor organizational performance.
   - Adapts program delivery to communities/populations in consideration of changes in PH system, and larger social/political/economic environment; assesses outcomes of current health policy relevant to PH/PHN practice.

Note: Tier 1 competencies cover generalist PHNs, Tier 2 competencies cover PHNs with program implementation, supervisory/management duties that may include clinical services, home visiting, community-based/population-focused programs. Tier 3 competencies refer to senior management or executive level PHNs in administrative/leadership roles at public health agencies or organizations. Refer to complete document for complete list of competencies at all three levels.

Adapted from Quad Council (2011, Summer). *Quad Council PHN Competencies for Public Health Nurses*. Retrieved from http://www.resourcenter.net/images/ACHNE/Files/QuadCouncilCompetenciesForPublicHealthNurses_Summer2011.pdf

WHAT IS A HEALTHY COMMUNITY?

What is a healthy community? Just as health for an individual is relative and will change, all communities exist in a relative state of health. A community's health can be viewed within the context of health being more than just the absence of disease, and including things that promote the maintenance of a high quality of life and productivity. A key vision for healthy communities is presented in *Healthy People 2020*, the national health promotion and disease prevention agenda published by the U.S. Department of Health & Human Services (USDHHS). Its four overarching goals for the health of the nation are:

- To attain high quality, longer lives free of preventable disease, disability, injury, and premature death.
- To achieve health equity, eliminate disparities, and improve the health of all groups.
- To create social and physical environments that promote good health for all.
- To promote quality of life, healthy development, and healthy behaviors across all life stages (USDHHS, 2012, para. 5).

The 42 topic areas and 1,200 objectives are discussed in more detail elsewhere (see Chapter 1 describing *Healthy People 2020*) These objectives and targets provide guidelines for communities to follow in order to promote the health of their members. By encouraging collaboration across communities, empowering individuals to make better choices, and measuring progress toward set benchmarks, *Healthy People 2020* provides a road map for achieving longer and healthier lives for all Americans.

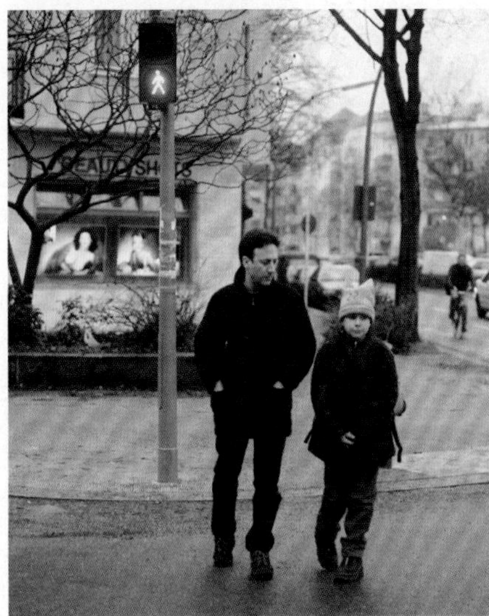

Healthy communities promote productivity and a good quality of life for their residents.

DIMENSIONS OF THE COMMUNITY AS CLIENT

The health of a community can be characterized through a number of perspectives. One such view is by examining three dimensions: status/people, structure, and process (LeBan, 2011).

Status/People is the most common measure of the health of a community. It typically comprises morbidity and mortality data identifying the physical, emotional, and social determinants of health (SDH). Physical and social indices include vital statistics, leading causes of death and illness, suicide rates, and rates of drug and alcohol addiction. Social determinants can be identified by crime rates and functional ability level, or by high school dropout rates or average income levels. Other demographic characteristics, such as single, female-headed households, are also helpful status measures. Informal leaders and resource persons can impact the health of communities outside the formal health care system.

Structure of a community refers to its services and resources. Community associations, groups, and organizations provide a means for accessing needed services. Adequacy and appropriateness of health services can be determined by examining patterns of use, number and types of health and social services, and quality measures. Classification as a medically underserved area is indicative of a lack of sufficient health care providers (e.g., nurses, physicians, dentists). Demographic data, such as socioeconomic and racial distribution, age, gender, and educational level, are also important indicators of community structure. These measures provide key information and correlate to health status.

Process reflects the community's ability to function effectively. It includes processes within the community (collaboration between subsystems of education and health, for instance) and between the community and the state or national levels. In a classic work, Cottrell (1976) describes *community competency* as a key component to the process dimension. Just as nurses assess the strengths and limitations of clients when working with individuals, the community health nurse must assess the strengths and limitations of the community when working with the community as client. Strengths must be enhanced and limitations addressed to achieve agreed-upon goals. Characteristics of a competent community follow. A competent community can

- Collaborate effectively in identifying community needs and problems
- Achieve a working consensus on goals and priorities
- Agree on ways and means to implement the agreed-upon goals
- Collaborate effectively to take the required actions.

These characteristics are discussed in more detail later in the discussion on "Planning to Meet the Health Needs of the Community." See Chapter 1 for more information on healthy communities.

Addressing community health by examining the process in addition to the structure and status dimensions provides a broader view into the complexities of community health and community actions for change. It is key to examine not only the individual components of the community but also the sum of all the parts—*the whole*—including interactions among all the constituents (Hawe, Shiell, & Riley, 2009).

Another perspective identifies the community as having three features: a location, a population, and a social system. Figure 15-1 presents a visual interpretation of

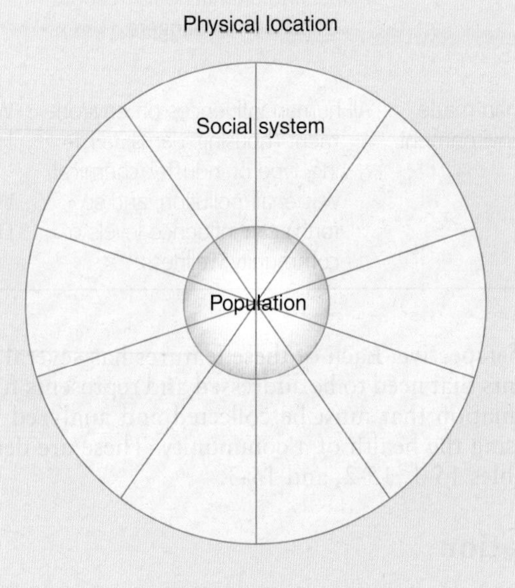

FIGURE 15-1. Three features of a community. The community has (1) a physical location, represented here by the square boundary, (2) a population, shown here by the central circle, and (3) a social system, divided here into subsystems.

Table 15.1 Community Profile Inventory: Location Perspective

Location Variables	Community Health Implications	Community Assessment Questions	Information Sources (For All–Various Internet Sites)
Boundary of community	Community boundaries serve as basis for measuring incidence of wellness and illness, and for determining spread of disease.	Where is the community located? What is its boundary? Is it a part of a larger community? What smaller communities does it include?	Atlas State maps County maps City maps Telephone book City directory Public library
Location of health services	Use of health services depends on availability and accessibility.	Where are the major health institutions located? What necessary health institutions are outside the community? Where are they?	Telephone book Chamber of commerce State health department County or local health departments Maps Public library
Geographic features	Injury, death, and destruction may be caused by floods, earthquakes, volcanoes, tornadoes, or hurricanes. Recreational opportunities at lakes, seashore, mountains promote health and fitness.	What major landforms are in or near the community? What geographic features pose possible threats? What geographic features offer opportunities for healthful activities?	Atlas Chamber of commerce Maps State health department Public library
Climate	Extremes of heat and cold affect health and illness. Extremes of temperature and precipitation may tax community's coping ability.	What are the average temperature and precipitation? What are the extremes? What climatic features affect health and fitness? Is the community prepared to cope with emergencies?	Weather atlas Chamber of commerce State health department Maps Local government Weather bureau Public library
Flora and fauna	Poisonous plants and disease-carrying animals can affect community health. Plants and animals offer resources as well as dangers.	What plants and animals pose possible threats to health?	State health department Poison control center Police department Emergency rooms Encyclopedia Public library
Human-made environment	All human influences on environment (housing, dams, farming, type of industry, chemical waste, air pollution, and so forth) can influence levels of community wellness.	What are the major industries? How have air, land, and water been affected by humans? What is the quality of housing? Do highways allow access to health institutions?	Chamber of commerce Local government City directory State health department University research reports Public library

this perspective. Each of these features has several components that need to be addressed and represents further information that must be collected and analyzed when assessing the health of a community. These are detailed in Tables 15-1, 15-2, and 15-3.

Location

Every physical community carries out its daily existence in a specific geographic location. The health of a community is affected by location, because placement of health services, geographic features, climate, plants, animals, and the human-made environment are intrinsic to geographic location. The location of a community places it in an environment that offers resources and also poses threats (Mitchell & Popham, 2008; Nykiforuk et al., 2012). The healthy community is one that makes wise use of its resources and is prepared to meet threats and dangers. In assessing the health of any community, it is necessary to collect information not only about variables specific to location but also about relationships between the community and its location. Do groups cooperate to identify threats? Do health agencies cooperate to prepare for an emergency such as a flood or earthquake?

Does the community make certain that its members are given available information about resources and dangers? Table 15-1 describes the location perspective of the Community Profile Inventory, including the six **location variables:** community boundaries, location of health services, geographic features, climate, flora and fauna, and the human-made environment.

Community Boundaries

To talk about the community in any sense, one must first describe its boundaries (Theiss-Morse, 2009). Measurements of wellness and illness within a community depend on defining the outer geographic limits of the unit under consideration, and also the more informal boundaries that are present (Swarts, 2011). Nurses need to be clear, for example, that a target community of the elderly includes a description of age and location (e.g., all persons age 65 and older in a given city or county). Some communities are distinctly separate, such as an isolated rural town, whereas others are closely situated to one another, such as the suburbs of a large metropolis. Therefore, it is important for the nurse to know the nature of each location and explicitly define its boundaries.

Location of Health Services

If the members of a town must travel 200 miles to the nearest clinic or dental office, the health of the community will be affected. When assessing a community, the community health nurse needs to identify the major health centers and know where they are located (Hawe, Shiell, & Riley, 2009). For example, an alcoholism treatment center for indigent alcoholics was located 30 miles outside one city. This location presented transportation problems and profoundly affected the willingness of clients to voluntarily seek treatment and the length of time they remained at the center. If a well-baby clinic is located on the edge of a high-crime district, parents may be deterred from using it. It is often enlightening to plot the major health institutions, both inside and outside the community, on a map that shows their proximity and relationship to the community as a whole.

Geographic Features

Communities have been constructed in every conceivable physical environment, and environment certainly can affect the health of a community (see Chapter 9). A healthy community is one that takes into consideration the geography of its location, identifies possible problems and likely resources, and responds in an adaptive fashion (Ory, Liles, & Lawlor, 2010). For example, Anchorage, Alaska and San Francisco, California, are both located on a geologic fault line and subject to major earthquakes. In such places, the health of the community is determined, in part, by its preparedness for an earthquake and its ability to cope and respond quickly when such a crisis occurs. In Ontario, Canada, a series of lakes called the Lac la Croix is a valuable food resource for Ojibway Indian communities because they depend on fish from the lakes for their livelihood. Over the years, acid rain generated from coal-burning power plants in the United States and Canada has begun to affect the lakes and the fish, thus contaminating a major food supply of the Ojibway communities. In another example, high levels of arsenic are found in the ground and surface water and are linked to various health problems in several locations in India (Das et al., 2009). These conditions must be addressed in order to prevent disease and injury.

Climate

The climate also has a direct influence on the health of a community (Eby & Semenza, 2008; Knowlton et al., 2007). When Buffalo, New York, is blanketed with deep winter snows, members of the community sometimes are immobilized for days. Deaths from coronary occlusion increase as people attempt to shovel their sidewalks and uncover their cars. Falls in the elderly have been associated with colder climate (Stevens, Thomas, & Sogolow, 2007). The intense summer heat of a location such as Phoenix, Arizona, can create many health problems (e.g., heat stroke, heat exhaustion). Asthma and other lung diseases are exacerbated in the Central San Joaquin Valley of California because mountains surround this area, and create an air inversion, trapping vehicle and agricultural by-products in what can be described as a "large bowl" and causing smog during many months of the year. In Minnesota, one study reported higher rates of asthma among children living in housing tracts facing intersections with major highways and railroads (Juhn et al., 2010). Skin cancer incidence is associated with unprotected sun exposure, which increases the risk for people who live in warm, sunny regions (Townsend et al., 2011). Climate can also affect infectious disease rates (Lafferty, 2009; Ebi. & Semenza, 2008).

A healthy community encourages physical activity among its members, but the climate affects this activity. Although long, cold winters can restrict activity, one community, St. Paul, Minnesota, holds an annual Winter Carnival. Sporting events, parades, ice sailing, dog sledding, a treasure hunt, and hot air balloon races bring thousands of Minnesotans outdoors at a time when they might otherwise be confined by the weather.

Flora and Fauna

Plant and animal populations in a community are often determined by location. The way a community responds to these populations, whether wild or domesticated, can affect the health of the community. Exposure of inner-city children to cockroaches has been associated with higher levels of hospitalization for asthma (Rabito et al., 2011). Poison oak, ivy, and sumac can be found across the United States, and these plants produce an allergic contact dermatitis in many people who come in contact with it (Petersen, 2011). In the Sierra foothill communities of central California, black widow and tarantula spiders, scorpions, and rattlesnakes are resident populations that pose potential health threats. The poison from a single snakebite may cause serious injury or death (Seifert et al., 2009). In the south–central Midwest, the bite of the brown recluse spider injects a toxin that can lead to necrotic skin ulcers as well as systemic symptoms (Rhoads, 2007). In the Northeast and Mid-Atlantic states, increased deer populations—and consequently deer ticks—bring with them an increased incidence of Lyme disease.

The community health nurse needs to know about the major sources of danger from plants and animals affecting the community under study. Are there community agencies that provide educational information about these dangers? Does the populace understand their significance? Are emergency services, such as a poison control center, available to community members?

Human-Made Environment

Every community is located in the midst of an environment created and transformed by human ingenuity. People build houses and factories, dump wastes into streams or vacant lots, fill the air with gases, and build dams to control streams. All of these human alterations of the environment have important implications for community health (Aboelata, 2010). A community health nurse might improve the health of a community by working for legislation to prevent disposal of waste chemicals into water or landfills. Such legislation might have prevented the disaster at Love Canal in the state of New York, where groundwater contaminated with toxic wastes continued to seep into residential areas for many years, severely affecting the community's health and spurring community activism that led to the creation of the federal Superfund program to clean up areas with hazardous wastes. Early research revealed somewhat higher rates of birth defects and cancer from the 1978 event, but a mortality study examining data from 1979 to 1996 found no clear association between the exposure and mortality when compared to a comparison population (Gensberg et al., 2009). However, the true pattern may not yet be apparent and further studies are planned.

Population Characteristics

When one considers the community as the client, examining the health status of the total population in a given community is a critical component. Population consists not of a specialized aggregate, but of all the diverse people who live within the boundaries of the community.

The health of any community is greatly influenced by the attributes of its population. Various features of the population suggest health needs and provide a basis for health planning (Lantz, Golberstein, House, & Morenoff, 2010; Schoenbaum, Schoen, Nicholson, & Cantor, 2011). A healthy community has leaders who are aware of the population's characteristics, know its various needs, and respond to those needs. Community health nurses can better understand any community by knowing about its **population variables**: size, density, composition or demography, rate of growth or decline, cultural characteristics, social class structure, and mobility. Table 15-2 presents the population perspective section of the Community Profile Inventory.

Table 15.2 Community Profile Inventory: Population Perspective

Population Variables	Community Health Implications	Community Assessment Questions	Information Sources (For All–Various Internet Sites)
Size	The number of people influences number and size of health care institutions. Size affects homogeneity of the population and its needs.	What is the population of the community? Is it an urban, suburban, or rural community?	State health department Census data Maps City or town officials Chamber of commerce
Density	Increased density may increase stress. High and low density often affects the availability of health services.	What is the density of the population per square mile?	Census data State health department
Composition	Composition of the population often determines types of health needs.	What is the age composition of the community? What is the sex composition of the community? What is the marital status of community members? What occupations are represented and in what percentages?	Census data State health department Chamber of Commerce U.S. Department of Labor Statistics
Rate of growth or decline	Rapidly growing communities may place excessive demands on health services. Marked decline in population may signal a poorly functioning community.	How has population size changed over the past two decades? What are the health implications of this change?	Census data State health department

Table 15.2 Community Profile Inventory: Population Perspective *(Continued)*

Cultural differences	Health needs vary among subcultural and ethnic populations. Utilization of health services varies with culture. Health practices and extent of knowledge are affected by culture.	What is the ethnic breakdown of population? What racial groups are represented? What subcultural populations exist in the community? Do any of the subcultural groups have unique health needs and practices? Are different ethnic and cultural groups included in health planning?	Census data State health department Social and cultural research reports Human rights commission City government Health planning boards
Social class	Class differences influence the utilization of health services. Class composition influences cost of public health services.	What percentage of the population falls into each social class? What do class differences suggest for health needs and services?	State health department Census data Sociological reports
Mobility	Mobility of the population affects continuity of care. Mobility affects availability of service to highly mobile populations.	How frequently do members move into and out of the community? How frequently do members move within the community? Are there any specific populations, such as migrant workers, that are highly mobile? How does the pattern of mobility affect the health of the community? Is the community organized to meet the health needs of mobile groups?	State health department Census data Health agencies serving migrant workers Farm labor offices Program serving transients and the homeless
Poverty Level	Economic disparities may lead to health disparities.	What percentage of the population is below federal poverty levels? How many children qualify for free or reduced cost school lunch?	Census data State data Local data (schools)
Education level	Education disparities may lead to health disparities.	What percentage of the population has less than high school education? What is the literacy rate?	State data Local data (schools)
Unemployment rate	Health insurance is often tied to employment. Lack of regular income can be a family stressor. Both can lead to health disparities.	What is the rate of unemployment? How variable is this rate?	U.S. Department of Labor State data Local data
Population by age	A high proportion of children and elderly can overburden health care and social systems.	What is the dependency ratio? Has this rate changed dramatically? What is the trend?	Census data State data Local data
Health status	Community members' status relative to the 10 Leading Health Indicators can impact overall community health.	What is the rate of obesity/overweight? What are the rates of tobacco use and substance abuse? What is the immunization rate? What are rates of injury and violence? What are the STD and HIV/AIDS rates?	State data Local data Centers for Disease Control and Prevention (CDC) data Vital statistics—Numbers of births, deaths, marriages, and infant mortality rate. (Compare local to state data; state to national data.)
Environmental health status	Poor environmental health (e.g. presence of coliform bacteria in well water, toxic chemicals, or poor air quality) can lead to increased incidence of communicable or chronic diseases.	What are rates of communicable or chronic diseases (e.g., *E. coli* infections, asthma)? What is the Toxic Release Inventory?	CDC data State data Local data

Size

Dover, Delaware (with ~35,000 people) and the city of Los Angeles, California (with around 4 million people) have radically different health problems. If a single case of *Salmonella* poisoning occurred in Dover, health officials would probably quickly learn of it. It would be relatively easy to trace the course, check the few restaurants in town, and interview people about sanitation practices. However, many cases might occur in Los Angeles without the health department's knowledge. Moreover, once the cases were discovered, tracing the source of contamination might involve a long and complicated search. This is only one small way in which population size can affect the health of a community. The size of a community also influences the presence of inadequate housing, the heterogeneity of the population, and almost every conceivable aspect of health needs and services. Knowing a community's size provides community health nurses with important information for planning. See Chapter 29 for issues related to rural and urban health of populations.

Density

In some communities, thousands of people are crowded into high-rise apartment buildings. In others, such as farm communities, people live at great distances from one another. The full impact of living in high-density communities is being researched, and some research has already shown that crowding affects individual and community health. Motor vehicle exhaust from highways has been shown to be associated with higher risk of asthma and reduced lung function in children, as well as higher pulmonary and cardiac mortality in adults (Brugge, Durant, & Rioux, 2007). When compared with rural populations, urban populations in Ireland have a higher incidence of lung cancer and respiratory disease, thought to be associated with higher air pollution levels (O'Reilly, O'Reilly, Rosato, & Connolly, 2007).

A low-density community, however, may have problems. When people are spread out, health care provision can become difficult. There may not be enough resources in the form of taxes to support public health services. Rural communities often suffer from inadequate distribution of health care personnel, including private physicians and community health nurses. An Oregon study of families receiving food stamps found that rural children, despite access to health insurance, had more problems accessing dental care and had greater unmet health needs than urban children (DeVoe, Krois, & Stenger, 2009). Artnak, McGraw, and Stanley (2011) note that "quality health care services in rural communities for the chronically ill and dying remain problematic" (p. 140). In some cases, higher rates of hospitalization have been found (Laditka, Laditka, & Probst, 2009). One large study found that populations using critical access rural hospitals had higher mortality rates for acute myocardial infarction, congestive heart failure, and pneumonia when compared with patients at nonrural hospitals (Joynt, Harris, Ora, & Jha, 2011). Other rural health risks include greater rates of injuries from traffic accidents (Tiesman, Zwerling, Peek-Asa, Sprince, & Cavanaugh, 2007) and illnesses related to agricultural pesticide exposure. One or more high pesticide exposures can lead to central nervous system problems, and almost one fourth of 693 participants in one study reported ever having an exposure (Starks et al., 2011).

A healthy community takes into consideration the density of its population. It organizes to meet the differing needs created by its density levels (e.g., it recognizes differences in density between the inner city and the suburbs and allocates services accordingly). See Chapter 29 for more on health risks specific to rural and urban areas.

Composition/Demographics

Communities differ in the types of people who live within their boundaries. A retirement community in Florida whose members are mostly older than age 65 has one set of interests and concerns, whereas a city with a large number of women in their childbearing years will have another set of concerns. A healthy community is one that takes full account of its constituents and provides for their differences. Age, sex, educational level, occupation, and many other demographic variables affect health concerns (Lantz, Golberstein, House, & Morenoff, 2010). In communities with a high proportion of low-income families, considerations must be made to accommodate the needs of the poor (Lee et al., 2011). Occupation can also affect health. For example, in a town where 75% of the workers are employed in a textile mill, the community lives with the threat of brown lung disease, which is caused by cotton dust. In areas where tobacco is the main source of income and a large proportion of the population is engaged in its production, green tobacco sickness—or acute nicotine poisoning—is a concern because workers can absorb nicotine through the skin, and precautions must be taken to prevent this from happening (Arcury et al., 2008). Understanding a community's composition is an important early step in determining its level of health.

Rate of Growth or Decline

Community populations change over time. Some grow rapidly. The unparalleled recent growth of Las Vegas, Nevada, as a popular place to live has placed extreme demands on the environment, along with the provision of health care and other services. Other populations may experience a decline because of economic change, for example, those areas of the United States where steel manufacturing has declined. Any significant fluctuation in population size can affect the health of the community. As people leave to find new employment or better living conditions, consumption of goods and services drops. Community morale may suffer, and community leadership may decline. Even a stable community can have problems (e.g., members may resist needed change because they notice little fluctuation in their population; commercial and residential properties may be abandoned or left vacant).

Cultural Characteristics

A community may be composed of a single cultural group, such as Ojibway Indians on their reservation in Wisconsin, or it may be made up of many cultures or subcultures. For instance, if a city has a large Hispanic population, along with a group of Native Americans living in the inner city and a cluster of Vietnamese refugees, the cultural differences among these members will influence the health of the community. These differences can create conflicting or competing demands for resources and services or create intergroup hostility. A healthy community is aware of such cultural differences and acts to promote understanding among cultural subgroups (Spector, 2009).

Social Class and Educational Level

Social class refers to the ranking of groups within society by income, education, occupation, prestige, or a combination of these factors. There is no absolute agreement on income levels or other criteria to designate social class categories (upper, middle, lower), other than the government formula used to compute poverty level (USDHHS, 2007). Although class distinctions are not clearly defined, class rankings based on occupation, education, and wealth (income plus assets) seem to correlate with many different social patterns and are used frequently in research (Cargan, 2007). Occupational level, in particular, has historically and consistently proven to be a reliable measure, with surprisingly similar rankings among all societies for which data exist (Adcock & Brown, 1957). This classic research has shown that people with higher occupational levels generally have higher incomes and education, exert greater political influence, and are more highly esteemed by others. Newer research, linking educational attainment with mortality, indicates that income (linked to education and occupation) is often the best predictor for mortality (Lantz et al., 2010). *Healthy People 2020* identified the relationship between these factors and others by defining **social determinants of health:**

> Social determinants of health reflect social factors and the physical conditions in the environment in which people are born, live, learn, play, work, and age.... Social and physical determinants of health....impact a wide range of health, functioning, and quality of life outcomes (USDHHS, 2012, para. 10).

For example, socioeconomic conditions (e.g., poverty), resources to meet daily needs (opportunities for quality education and employment; access to healthy food), social norms and attitudes (e.g., segregation, discrimination), public safety and transportation (e.g., crime, violence, sanitation, mass transit), and social support/interactions (e.g., cell phones, Internet, mass media, families/friends) are part of the larger construct of SDH. Physical determinants of health include things like the natural environment (e.g., climate, plants), the built environment (e.g., transportation, buildings), housing and neighborhoods (e.g., density, condition), exposure to hazards (e.g., physical, toxic), barriers (e.g., disabled), and aesthetic elements (e.g., green belts, lighting). Health promotion and preventive health services are often most needed by low-income groups and people with fewer years of education, although the community, as a whole, will benefit from effective community health efforts. Frieden's (2010) Health Impact Pyramid has as its base socioeconomic factors (or social determinants of health), as these can have the greatest impact on populations, followed by changing context to make default decisions more healthy (e.g., when most people don't smoke, it is easier to be a nonsmoker), then protective interventions that are long lasting (e.g., immunizations, colonoscopies), and finally clinical interventions (e.g., ongoing monitoring for chronic conditions like heart disease) and counseling/education (e.g., health education to improve diet/exercise).

It is generally known that different social classes have different health problems, as well as a variety of resources for coping with illness and diverse ways of using health services. A healthy community recognizes these differences and creates health care services to meet these varied needs.

Mobility

Americans are a mobile population. Between 2010 and 2011, 11.6% moved, however, that is a record low compared to 20.2% in 1985, and this is most likely due to tenuous housing and job markets (U.S. Census Bureau, 2011). People move to go to college, take a new job, join other family members or friends, or seek a new climate after retirement. This mobility has a direct effect on the health of communities (Gushulak & MacPherson, 2006, 2011). If the population turnover is extensive, continuity of services may suffer. Leadership for improving the health of the community may change so frequently that concerted action becomes difficult. High turnover may necessitate special attention to health education about local conditions.

Population groups may arrive and depart in seasonal swings; fluctuations in the number of migrant farm workers, tourists, or college students can affect a community. Border health issues are of special concern, as people continually move across borders, bringing with them health issues such as communicable diseases (Ramos et al., 2009). Immigrants and refugees may represent a significant population subgroup in many areas of a country, and public health officials must meet their unique needs. The community health nurse also needs to identify those populations that are seasonally mobile. These subgroups present special health needs and place an added burden on a community (e.g., migrant workers). If a town of 3,000 people has an annual influx of 10,000 students who disappear in the summer, residents must prepare to meet this population instability. The small towns of the San Juan Islands in Puget Sound, Washington, can command such high prices for accommodations in the summer that some low-income, year-round residents camp in tents during those months because they are unable to pay the high rents. Thus, the lives of many families are disrupted each year. A healthy community neither ignores nor overreacts to this kind of mobility. Rather, it identifies the nature of the population change, determines the needs created by such change, and organizes to meet those needs.

Social System

In addition to location and population, every community has a third feature—a social system. The various parts of a community's social system that interact and influence the health of a community are called **social system variables**. These variables include health, family, economic, educational, religious, welfare, political, recreational, legal, and communication. Whether assessing a community's health, developing new services for the mentally ill within the community, or promoting the health of the elderly, the community health nurse needs to understand the community as a social system. A community health nurse working in a tiny village in Alaska needs to understand and work with the social system of that village no less than a nurse practicing in New York City. Table 15-3 guides the nurse in assessing a community's social system variables.

The Concept of a Social System

A social system is an abstract concept and can be more readily understood by first considering the people who make up the community's population. Each person enacts multiple roles, such as parent, spouse, employee, citizen, church member, and political volunteer. People in certain roles tend to interact more closely with others in related roles, such as a nursing supervisor with a staff nurse or a customer with a sales clerk. The patterns and communication that emerge from these interactions form the basis of organizations. Some organizations are informal (e.g., an extended family group). Other organizations, such as a city police department or a software business, are more formal. However, all organizations are constructed from roles that are enacted by individual citizens. Organizations, in turn, interact with one another, forming linkages. For example, a medical equipment company and a laboratory establish contracts (linkages) with a home care agency. When a group of organizations are linked and have similar functions, such as all those providing social services, they form a community system or subsystem (Fig. 15-2). The various community systems have a profound influence on one another. Because this interaction among parts determines the health of the whole, it is the total social system that concerns community health nurses.

The Health Care Delivery System as Part of the Social System

Although community health nurses must examine all the systems in a community and must understand how they interact, the health system is of particular importance. The major function of the health system is to promote the health of the community. Community assessment asks not only whether, but also how well, the system is functioning. What is the level of health promotion carried out by the health system of a community? To answer this question, one that can be applied to any system, the PHN needs a clear notion about the subsystems,

Table 15.3 Community Profile Inventory: Social System Perspective

Social System Variables	Community Health Implications	Community Assessment Questions	Information Sources. (For All–Various Internet Sites)
Health system Family system Economic system Educational system Religious system Welfare system Political system Recreational system Legal system Communication system	Each system must fulfill its functions for a healthy community. Collaboration among the systems to identify goals and problems affects health of community. Undue influence of one system on another may lower the health of the community. Agreement on the means to achieve community goals affects community health. Communication among organizations in each system affects community health.	What are the functions of each major system? What are the major subsystems of each system? What are the major organizations in each subsystem? How well do the various organizations function? Are the subsystems in each major system in conflict? Is there adequate communication among the major systems? Is there agreement on community goals? Are there mechanisms for resolving conflict? Do any parts of the total system dominate the others? What community needs are not being met?	Chamber of Commerce Telephone book City directory Organizational literature Officials in organizations Community self-study Community survey Local library Key informants

Community Systems
Health
Family
Economic
Education
Religious
Welfare
Political
Recreation
Legal
Communication
Subsystems
Organizations
Roles
Population

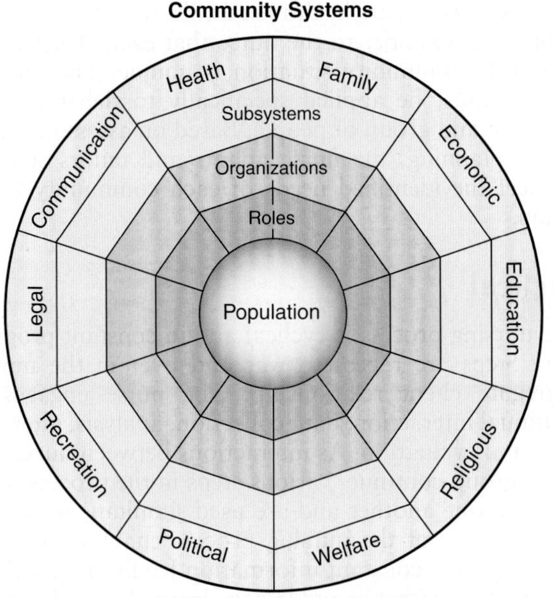

FIGURE 15-2. The community as a social system. Each of the 10 major systems of a community includes a number of subsystems that are made up of organizations. Members of the community occupy roles in these organizations.

organizations, and roles that make up the system. Any evidence of inadequate functioning becomes a warning signal for more careful assessment. For example, a high rate of teenage pregnancies in a city may signal inadequate functioning of several systems (e.g., family, educational, religious, health), so a closer look is in order. What community values influence sexual behavior among adolescents? What sex education programs are available to this population? Does the health system provide information and counseling?

The components of the health system, described in Figure 15-3, include eight major subsystems—each with one or more organizations. Although the community health nurse must be aware of all the systems in a community, the health system is of central importance.

THE NURSING PROCESS APPLIED TO THE COMMUNITY AS CLIENT

Consisting of a systematic, purposeful set of interpersonal actions, the nursing process provides a structure for change that remains a viable tool employed by the community health nurse. This chapter examines the use of the nursing process as applied at the aggregate or

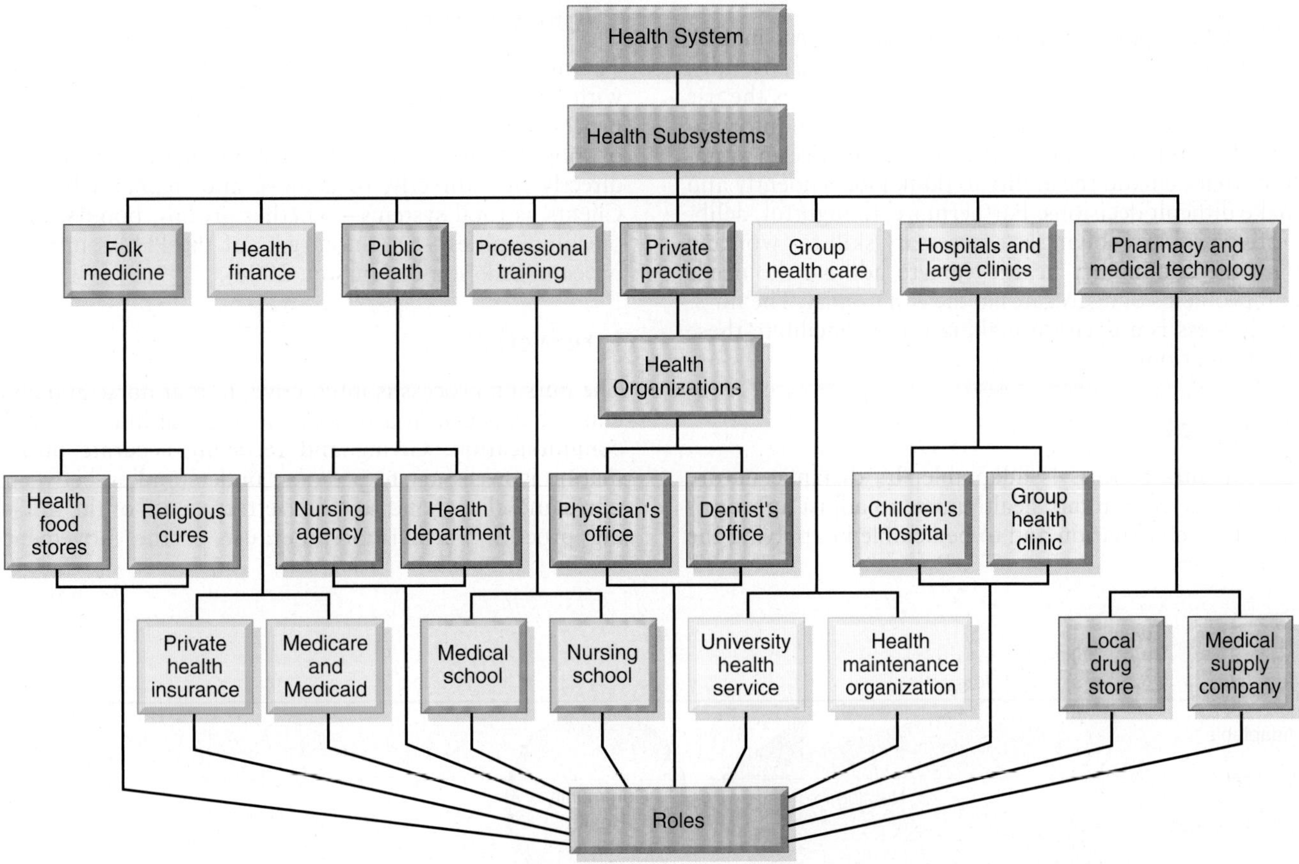

Health System
Health Subsystems
Folk medicine
Health finance
Public health
Professional training
Private practice
Group health care
Hospitals and large clinics
Pharmacy and medical technology
Health Organizations
Health food stores
Religious cures
Nursing agency
Health department
Physician's office
Dentist's office
Children's hospital
Group health clinic
Private health insurance
Medicare and Medicaid
Medical school
Nursing school
University health service
Health maintenance organization
Local drug store
Medical supply company
Roles

FIGURE 15-3. Components of the health system. This figure shows some representative types of organizations for each of the major subsystems. In turn, each of these organizations also has members with many different roles, and the health of the entire system depends, in part, on how well these roles are carried out.

community level. Five components—assessment, diagnosis, planning, implementation, and evaluation—give direction to the dynamics for solving problems, managing nursing actions, and improving the health of communities and community health nursing practice.

Three characteristics support the use of the nursing process in community health nursing. First, the nursing process is a problem-solving process that addresses community health problems at every aggregate level with the goals of preventing illness and promoting public health. Second, it is a management process that requires situational analysis, decision making, planning, organization, direction, and control of services, as well as outcome evaluation. As a management tool, the nursing process addresses all aggregate levels. Third, it is a process for implementing changes that improve the function of various health-related systems and the ways that people behave within those systems.

The nursing process provides a framework or structure on which community health nursing actions are based. Application of the process varies with each situation, but the nature of the process remains the same. Certain characteristics of that process are important for community health nurses to emphasize in their practices (Fig. 15-4).

Deliberative

The nursing process, like the research process in EBP (evidence-based practice), is deliberative—purposefully, rationally, and carefully thought out. It requires the use of sound judgment that is based on adequate information. Community health nurses often practice in situations that demand the ability to think independently and make difficult decisions. Furthermore, thoughtful, deliberative problem solving is a necessary skill for working with the community health team to address the needs and problems of aggregates in the community. The nursing process is a decision-making tool to facilitate these determinations.

Adaptable

The nursing process is adaptable. Its dynamic nature enables the community health nurse to adjust appropriately to each situation and to be flexible in applying the process to aggregate health needs. Furthermore, its flexibility is a reminder to the nurse that each client group and each community situation is unique. The nursing process must be applied specifically to the individual situation and group of people. Based on assessment and sound planning, the nurse adapts and tailors services to meet the identified needs of each community client group.

Cyclical

The nursing process is cyclical and in constant progression. Steps are repeated over and over in the nurse–aggregate client relationship. The nurse engages in continual interaction, data collection, analysis, intervention, and evaluation. As interactions between nurse and client group continue, various steps in the process overlap with one another and are used simultaneously. The cyclic nature of the nursing process enables the nurse to engage in a constant information feedback loop: The information gathered and lessons learned at each step of the process promote greater understanding of the group being served, the most effective way to provide quality services, and the best methods of raising this group's level of health.

Client Focused

The nursing process is client focused; it is used for and with clients. Community health nurses use the nursing process for the express purpose of addressing the health of populations. They are helping aggregate clients, directly or indirectly, to achieve and maintain health. Clients as total systems—whether groups, populations, or communities—are the targets of the PHN's nursing process (Eriksson & Nilsson, 2008).

Interactive

The nursing process is interactive, in that nurse and clients are engaged in a process of ongoing interpersonal communication. Giving and receiving accurate information is necessary to promote understanding between nurse and clients and to foster effective use of the nursing process. Furthermore, because of the movement

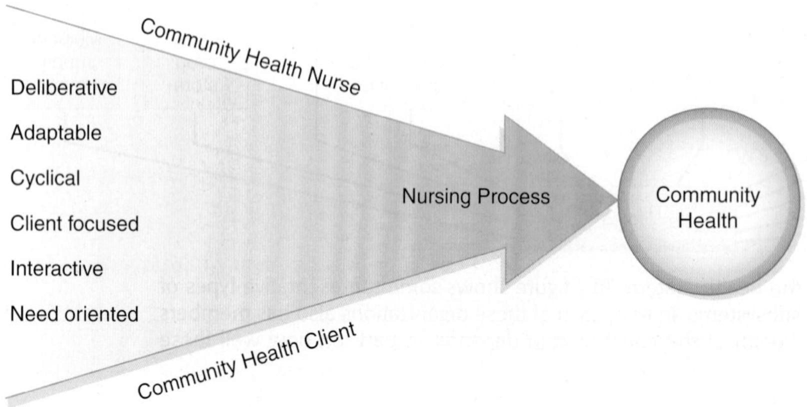

FIGURE 15-4. Nursing process characteristics emphasized in community health.

toward informed use of medical care, demands for clients' rights and the concept of self-care have gained emphasis. Client groups and community health nurses have increasingly joined forces to assume responsibility for promoting community health. The nurse–aggregate client relationship can and should be a partnership, a shared experience by professionals (nurses and others) and client groups (Chrisman, 2007).

Need Oriented

The nursing process is need oriented. A long association with problem solving has tended to limit the focus of the nursing process to the correction of existing problems. Although problem solving is certainly an appropriate use of the nursing process, the community health nurse can also use the nursing process to anticipate client needs and prevent problems. The nurse should think of nursing diagnoses as ranging from health problem identification to primary prevention and health promotion opportunities. This focus is needed if the goals of community health—to protect, promote, and restore the people's health—are to be realized.

Interacting With the Community

All steps of the nursing process depend on **interaction**, reciprocal exchange and influence among people. Although nurse–client interaction is often an implied or assumed element in the process, it is an essential first consideration for community health nursing (see Chapter 10 for more details). Listening to a group of elderly people, teaching a class of expectant mothers, lobbying in the legislature for the poor, working with parents to set up a dental screening program for children—all these involve relationships, and relationships require interaction. Mutual give and take between nurse and clients—whether a family, a group of mothers on a Native American reservation, or a population of school children—is an expected and much needed skill that should be integrated throughout the nursing process (Fig. 15-5).

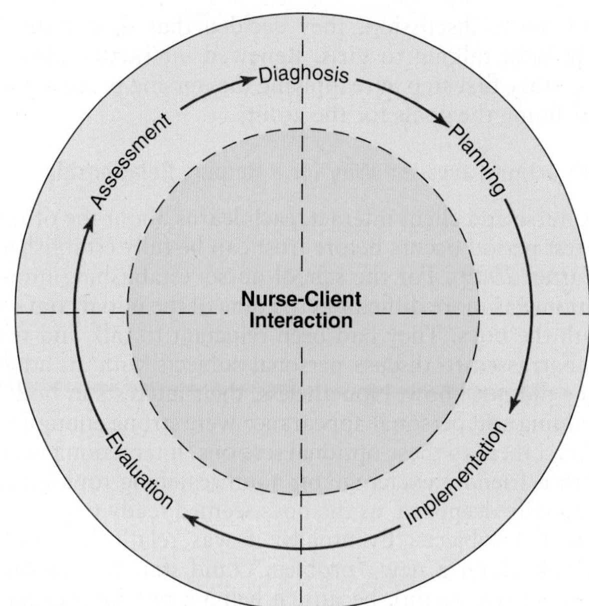

FIGURE 15-5. Nursing process components. Nurse–client interaction, a preamble structure, forms the core of the process. As a nurse and client maintain a reciprocal exchange of information and trust through interaction, they can effectively assess client needs, diagnose needs, and plan, implement, and evaluate care.

Need for Communication

When a community health nurse initially contacts a group of community leaders, for example, any information the nurse may have in advance can give only partial clues to that group's needs and wants. Unless everyone involved talks and listens, the steps of the nursing process will go awry (LeBan, 2011).

Interaction and Effective Communication

Through open, honest sharing, the nurse (and others on the health team) will begin to develop trust and establish lines of effective communication. For instance, the nurse explains who he is and why he is there. The nurse encourages the group members to talk about themselves. Nurse and group members together discuss their relationship and clarify the desired nature of that alliance (Pavlish & Pharris, 2012). Does the group want help to identify and work on its health needs? Would its members like this nurse to continue regular contacts? What will their respective roles be? Effective communication, as a part of interaction, is essential to develop understanding and facilitate a free exchange of information between nurse and client.

Interaction Is Reciprocal

Sharing of information, ideas, feelings, concerns, and self goes both ways. Nurses must avoid the temptation either to do all the talking or merely to listen while a few group members monopolize the conversation (Active Listening, 2010). A dynamic exchange must exist between two systems. The community health nurse (and other collaborating health professionals) represents one system and the client group represents the other. Health care professionals tend to prioritize based on their own perspective and many times neglect to take the clients' wishes into account. Whether the client is a parent group, a homeless population, or an entire community, this exchange involves a two-way sharing between the nurse and client group. The key elements of interaction are mutuality and cooperation.

Consider the following example: A dozen junior high school boys, most of whom were on the football team, met for several weeks with the school nurse to discuss physical fitness, nutrition, and other health topics. After their agreed-upon goals had been accomplished, the nurse wondered whether further meetings were needed. The nurse raised the question and offered several topics for possible future sessions, such as the use of steroids and other drugs and injury prevention. The boys were not interested in these suggestions, but, after more discussion, they decided that they wanted help with talking to girls. Renewed interaction was a necessary first step in reapplying the nursing process and redefining the goals for the group.

Interaction Paves the Way for a Helping Relationship

As nurse and client interact, each learns about the other. A test period occurs before trust can be fully established (Carter, 2009). For the school nurse, establishing interaction was more difficult at the time of the initial contact with the boys. They had been reluctant to talk and felt embarrassed to discuss personal subjects with an adult they did not know. Nonetheless, their interests in bodybuilding and personal appearance were strong enough to attract them to these optional sessions. Interaction began with a friendly exchange on nonthreatening topics and gradually deepened, as the boys seemed ready to discuss personal subjects. Eventually, it was relatively simple to talk about a new "problem" (and start the nursing process over again), because a helping relationship had already been developed. The nurse had a track record. The boys trusted, respected, and liked the nurse, so they were happy to interact around a newly stated need.

Aggregate Application

As noted in earlier chapters, community health practice focuses largely on the health of population groups; therefore, interaction goes beyond the one-on-one with individual patients. The challenge that the community health nurse faces is a one-to-aggregate approach. A group of parents concerned about teenage alcoholism, handicapped people needing access ramps, and a neighborhood's elderly population frightened by muggings and thefts are all aggregates or clients with different concerns and opinions. As defined in Chapter 1, an aggregate refers to a mass or grouping of distinct individuals who are considered as a whole and who are loosely associated with one another. Each person in an aggregate is influenced by the thoughts and behavior of other group members. Nursing interaction with an aggregate client demands an understanding of group behavior, group dynamics, and group-level decision making. It requires interpersonal communication at the group level. Interaction is more complex with an aggregate than with an individual, but it also can be challenging and rewarding. Once community health nurses acquire an understanding of aggregate behavior, they can capitalize on the potential of group influence to make a far-reaching impact on the health of the total community (see Perspectives for an example of a public health nurse partnering with law enforcement to provide preventive heath care to gang youth). Chapter 10 examines communication and interaction with groups more closely.

Forming Partnerships and Building Coalitions

Another important consideration in community-level nursing practice requires teamwork. The job of planning for the health of an entire community or a community subsystem requires that the nurse collaborate with other professionals. Usually, the nurse is part of an organized team, separate from the agency that employs the nurse. The team is brought together with the goal of improving the health of the community. Each group member brings expertise and a particular view of the problem. These interprofessional work groups are often formed as either partnerships or coalitions (Kaiser, Barry, Lopez, & Raymond, 2010).

Partnerships are agreements between people (and agencies) that support a joint purpose (Zahner, Kaiser, & Kapelke-Dale, 2005). A partnership can be large (e.g., a multinational corporation and several high schools; a city government and the county jail system), or it can be a more modest endeavor (e.g., a group of senior citizens and a preschool program; a Girl Scout troop and a community recycling program). Community wide partnerships require more planning and coordination than do small partnerships. For example, because of increased student enrollment, a college may need two additional temporary and part-time faculty members who can teach the community health nursing course. The county public health department is interested in more new graduate nurses coming to work in the agency. The nursing program and the health department form a partnership and design a plan to solve both problems. The health department selects two staff nurses who have master's degrees and are qualified to teach undergraduate clinical laboratories in community health nursing 1 day a week for two semesters. The benefits for everyone are numerous. The nursing program solves a temporary staffing problem; the nurses from the health department share their expertise with students, enhancing their practice and the students' learning experience; and the health department successfully introduces a pool of students who may be potential staff members to the agency and the services that it provides for the community.

A **coalition** is an alliance of individuals or groups that work together to influence the outcomes of a specific problem (Clark et al., 2011; Trinh-Shevrin et al., 2011). Coalitions are an effective means to achieve a collaborative and coordinated approach to solving community problems (Chrisman, 2007). Steps to coalition building include defining goals and objectives, conducting a community assessment, identifying key players or leaders, and identifying potential coalition members. Once these steps have been accomplished, the leader needs to keep the coalition active. This is best done by knowing and staying in touch with the coalition members, running effective meetings, and keeping every participant involved. An example of a successful coalition is an Asian American hepatitis B program using community-based participatory research (CBPR) as a means of community assessment and providing pooled resources for this community in New York City (Trinh-Shevrin et al., 2011).

Sound public health practice depends on pooling resources—including people—in ways that will best serve the public. Whether health service is aimed at families, groups, subpopulations, populations, or communities, the consumers of that service are equally important

PERSPECTIVES
VOICES FROM THE COMMUNITY

Public Health Nurse

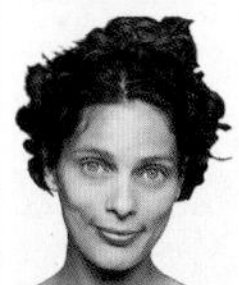

I am a public health nurse, married to a Los Angeles-area police officer. His job with a juvenile diversion program for 13- to 18-year old offenders (gang youth or those at risk of gang involvement) includes organizing a semester-long course to build confidence and self-esteem, as well as physical training and education in a classroom setting. Various officers teach the course, and they invite guest speakers. I ended up being a guest speaker for three 3-hour sessions and loved it! In order to prepare, I examined statistics and other assessment information about gangs as an aggregate. I noted that they have been found to have higher drug and alcohol use, earlier sexual initiation, and unsafe sexual practices with attendant higher rates of STIs (sexually transmitted infections). Higher rates of mental disorders, drug-related crime, and violent victimization are also hallmarks of gang membership. Basically, they are more likely to engage in high-risk behaviors, and I wanted to try to reach this aggregate that often has little access to health care. I thought this was a great opportunity to reach a vulnerable population and generate a discussion with them on health-related issues. I wanted it to be interactive and used examples they could identify with; I also spoke with some of their slang terms. The first session addressed major causes of morbidity and mortality among their age group. I showed them a photograph of a car involved in a crash due to driver texting, and discussed the dangers of racing cars, driving drunk, and driving while distracted (as this driver had done). I started a discussion with them about homicide statistics and asked how this has personally affected them. I also gave them information about suicide and hotline numbers. At the second session, I wanted to focus on major health issues (e.g., obesity, drug use, mental and sexual health), and addressed each by highlighting the health consequences, behaviors that needed to change, and how they could prevent problems and access care when needed. We discussed obesity, and I brought examples of food nutrition labels, especially from fast food restaurants they frequented. They were amazed at the calories and fat levels, so we discussed healthier alternatives. At the last session, I focused on health promotion and risk prevention. I emphasized testicular and breast self-exams (yes, there were girls) and encouraged medical screening for STIs, with information on free clinics in their areas.

While no formal evaluation of the program was done, I got great feedback from parents of the youth involved, who reported that their child's attitudes improved. Also, a good number of graduates of the program came back to work as student volunteers with subsequent cohorts. I felt a sense of accomplishment, having reached this difficult yet vulnerable population. I think that my openness and frankness in answering their questions and comfortable use of their slang terms developed rapport with them, and permitted me to reach them with health information that they really needed to hear. I would encourage you to look for opportunities to do the same!

Alisha, BSN

Adapted from: Sanders, B., Schneiderman, J., Loken, A., Lankenau, S., & Bloom, J. (2009). Gang youth as a vulnerable population for nursing intervention. Public Health Nursing, 26(4), 346–352.

members of the team. In planning for a community's health, the community (represented by appropriate individuals and agencies) must be involved. Community health nurses cannot lose sight of the need for client involvement at all levels and in all stages of community health practice.

Types of Community Needs Assessment

After considering the importance of community partnerships and coalitions, the community health nurse is ready to determine the community's needs. Assessment is the key initial step of the nursing process. Assessment for nurses means collecting and evaluating information about a community's health status to discover existing or potential needs and assets as a basis for planning future action (Anderson & McFarlane, 2010).

Several models or frameworks can be used for assessment. Three such models are Assessment Protocol for Excellence in Public Health (APEXPH), Protocol for Assessing Community Excellence in Environmental Health (PACE EH), and Mobilizing for Action through Planning and Partnerships (MAPP). All three of these models have been developed through partnership with the Centers for Disease Control & Prevention (CDC) to improve community assessment in relation to *Healthy People* goals (National Association of County & City Health Officials [NACCHO], 2007). An earlier tool, the Planned Approach to Community Health (PATCH) was developed to assist communities in assessing health promotion and chronic disease prevention programs (NACCHO, 2012). The *Healthy People 2020* Web site also provides planning tools and toolkits to assist local communities (see Internet Resources at end of chapter). These are all valuable resources that provide specific guidelines focusing on local-level strategies to improve the health of communities.

Assessment involves two major activities. The first is collection of pertinent data, and the second is analysis and interpretation of data. These actions overlap and are repeated constantly throughout the assessment phase of the nursing process. While assessing a community's ability to enhance its health, the nurse may simultaneously collect data on community lifestyle behaviors and interpret previously collected data on morbidity and mortality.

Community needs assessment is the process of determining the real or perceived needs of a defined community. In some situations, an extensive community study may be the first priority; in others, all that is needed is a study of one system or even one organization. At other times, community health nurses may need to perform a cursory examination or "windshield survey" to familiarize themselves with an entire community without going into any depth (Anderson & McFarlane, 2010).

Familiarization or Windshield Survey

A familiarization assessment is a common starting place in evaluation of a community. **Familiarization assessment** involves studying data already available on a community, then gathering a certain amount of first-hand data in order to gain a working knowledge of the community. Such an approach may utilize a **windshield survey**—an activity often used by nursing students in community health courses and by new staff members in community health agencies. Nurses drive (or walk) around the community of interest; find health, social, and governmental services; obtain literature; introduce themselves and explain that they are working in the area; and generally become familiar with the community and its residents. This type of assessment is needed whenever the community health nurse works with families, groups, organizations, or populations. The windshield survey provides knowledge of the context in which these aggregates live and may enable the nurse to better connect clients with community resources (Table 15-4). See an example in From the Case Files I.

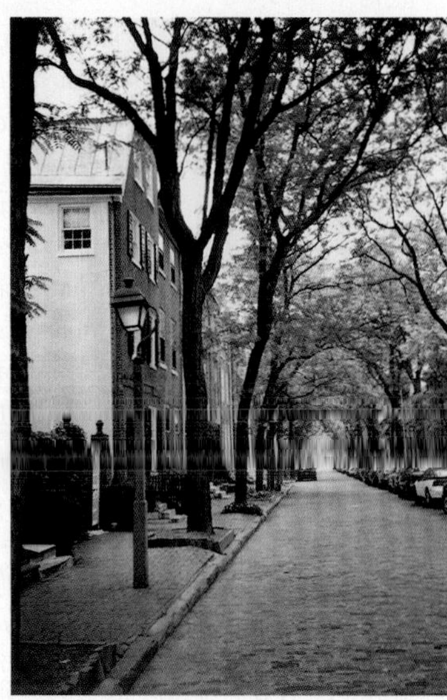

Windshield surveys are a quick way to become familiar with a new community and its residents.

Table 15.4 Community Familiarization (Windshield) Survey

This is often done to help you become familiar with a new community or public health service area. Walking/driving around neighborhoods and interacting with community members can provide a context for further community assessment. You might begin at the local Chamber of Commerce or government building to determine history, current statistics, and demographics, and to access maps and further resources for data you might use for a more formal community health assessment.

Physical

- Look at the age and conditions of the buildings, the density (apartments, houses on large lots) and materials used (bricks, plywood), and the zoning and maintenance of yards/empty lots. What clues does that give you about the community as a whole?
- How similar are the houses (are some neighborhoods very rich, others very poor)? Are there abandoned vehicles, piles of excess trash, large numbers of stray animals/for sale signs, or vacant houses?
- Are there open spaces (parks, agricultural areas, public/private areas like golf courses) and are they being used; by whom?
- Are there boundaries separating the community (e.g., natural boundaries like rivers, economic boundaries, commercial/residential boundaries)?
- What about air/water quality, signs of pollution?

Economic

- Does the area look like it is a thriving community?
- Are there areas where homeless gather? Soup kitchens, etc.?
- Is there adequate shopping (e.g., grocery stores, shopping centers)?
- Does it appear that food stamps are accepted/welcomed?
- Are there businesses, industries, manufacturing, and adequate places for employment? What is the unemployment rate?

Services

- Are there schools (how many, in what condition)? School nurses? What are the main concerns or problems with the educational system here (e.g., dropout rates)?
- Are there libraries? Do they provide additional services (e.g., Internet)? Are they well used?
- Are there recreational facilities (e.g., gyms, playgrounds, soccer fields, baseball diamonds); are these being used and by whom?
- How many churches do you see; what denominations?

Table 15.4 Community Familiarization (Windshield) Survey *(Continued)*

Services *(continued)*

- Is there adequate health care? Does the community have a hospital? Are there adequate health care services (e.g., physicians, clinics, nurses, mental health/substance abuse facilities, PH department services, nursing homes, traditional health care providers)? Is it a medically underserved area, a health professions shortage area?
- What types of social services are available (e.g., welfare/social workers, shelters, mental health counseling)? Do you see one main location for social services (e.g., government center) or are they dispersed around the community?
- What types of public/private transportation is available? Are highways and roads crowded with traffic? Accident rate? Are there bike paths/trails and adequate sidewalks? How is transportation access for the disabled?
- Does the community "feel" safe to you? Is there adequate fire and police protection? What is the crime rate, most common types of crimes?
- Are there signs of political activity (e.g., posters, notices of meetings, predominant party affiliations)? Do people feel that they can be involved in decisions made by their local government?

Social

- Are there common 'hangouts' (e.g., teen gathering spots, chess playing for older adults)? What about local newspapers, radio, TV (e.g., satellite dishes)?
- Who do you see on the streets? Indications of homogeneity or diversity of ethnicities, languages spoken, SES (socioeconmic status), occupations; how are people dressed?
- How do people feel about living in this community? What problems or concerns do they express? What strengths do they note? How "healthy" is their community?
- What are your impressions of this community?

Adapted from Anderson, E. T., & McFarlane, J. (2011). ***Community as partner: Theory and practice in nursing***. Philadelphia: Lippincott Williams & Wilkins.

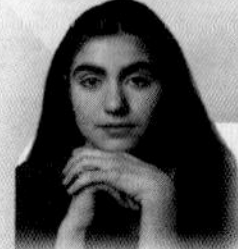

From the Case Files

The Angelo Family and a Familiarization Assessment

A community health nurse named Jean visited the Angelo family on the outskirts of Philadelphia. During the initial visit, she gathered information, learning that the family was Italian American and that there were four children, ranging in age from 15 to 3. The father had been out of work for 6 months; the mother worked on weekends as a maid in a motel; the oldest boy had been in trouble with the juvenile authorities; the 13-year old girl was deaf; and their house appeared rundown. Jean assessed this family, trying to determine its coping ability and its level of health. Furthermore, because community health nursing is population focused, her concern was not only for the Angelo family but also for the population of families with similar problems that this family represented.

However, the nurse's assessment was almost impossible without further knowledge of the community. Was theirs an Italian American neighborhood with specific cultural influences? What was the extent of unemployment in this city? What were the services for the deaf? Were all the houses in this part of town old and in need of repair? Once the nurse began working with the family, familiarity with the community became even more imperative. She discovered that, as a result of the Angelo's low income, family conflicts were intense. The family members seldom got out; they made almost no use of the community's recreational system. Before she could help them make use of it, however, the nurse had to find out what resources were available. As she familiarized herself with the community, she discovered Friends of the Deaf, which sponsored a group for parents of deaf children. The nurse could now help Mr. and Mrs. Angelo become part of that group. A quick survey of the religious system in the community revealed two job-transition support groups, one of which would welcome Mr. Angelo. In the meantime, the nurse chose to find out about the welfare system and how this family and other similar families could benefit from its services. Even her own attitude changed as she studied the community. For instance, she discovered that a strike had closed down the plant where Mr. Angelo worked for 20 years, and so could view his and others' unemployment from a broader perspective. Using a familiarization assessment helped this nurse to enhance her practice.

Whatever role nurses play in community health promotion, they will want to be making a continuous study, an ongoing assessment. Whether nurses become client advocates, work with the local government, or operate from a nursing agency serving the elderly, a familiarization assessment is prerequisite for their work.

Problem-Oriented Assessment

A second type of community assessment, **problem-oriented assessment**, begins with a single problem and assesses the community in terms of that problem. Suppose that Jean, the nurse who explored services available for the Angelo family's deaf child in From the Case Files I, had discovered that there were none. Confronted with this problem—one family with one deaf child—she could make a problem-oriented community assessment. Her first step would be to discover the incidence of childhood deafness, both in the community and in the state. Second, she might begin interviewing officials in the schools and health institutions to find out what had been done in the past to assist deaf children. She could check the local library or the Internet to locate available resources on the subject of deafness. Are there interpreters available for people who use sign language? How do hospitals and courts approach deafness? Are there any clubs or other organizations for deaf people? Are there school programs for the deaf, and, if so, where are they located?

The problem-oriented assessment is commonly used when familiarization is not sufficient and a comprehensive assessment is too expensive. This type of assessment is responsive to a particular need. The data collected will be useful in any kind of planning for a community response to the specific problem. Data should address the magnitude of the problem to be studied (e.g., prevalence, incidence), the precursors of the problem, information about population characteristics, along with the attitudes and behaviors of the population being studied (Issel, 2009).

Community Subsystem Assessment

In **community subsystem assessment**, the community health nurse focuses on a single dimension of community life. For example, the nurse might decide to survey churches and religious organizations to discover their roles in the community. What kinds of needs do the leaders in these organizations believe exist? What services do these organizations offer? To what extent are services coordinated within the religious system and between it and other systems in the community?

Community subsystem assessment can be a useful way for a team to conduct a more thorough community assessment. If five members of a nursing agency divide up the ten systems in the community and each person does an assessment of two systems, they could then share their findings to create a more comprehensive picture of the community and its needs.

Comprehensive Assessment

Comprehensive assessment seeks to discover all relevant community health information. It begins with a review of existing studies and all the data presently available on the community. A survey compiles all the demographic information on the population, such as its size, density, and composition. **Key informants** are interviewed in every major system—education, health, religious, economic, and others. Key informants are experts in one particular area of the community or they may know the community as a whole. Examples of key informants would be a school nurse, a religious leader, key cultural leaders, the local police chief or fire captain, a mail carrier, or a local city council person. Then, more detailed surveys and intensive interviews are performed to yield information on organizations and the various roles in each organization. A comprehensive assessment describes the systems of a community, and also how power is distributed throughout the system, how decisions are made, and how change occurs (Anderson & McFarlane, 2010; LeBan, 2011).

Because comprehensive assessment is an expensive, time-consuming process, it is not often undertaken. Performing a more focused study, based on prior knowledge of needs, is often a better and less costly strategy. Nevertheless, knowing how to conduct a comprehensive assessment is an important skill when designing smaller, more focused assessments. See Perspectives: Public Health Nursing Instructor.

Community Assets Assessment

The final form of assessment presented here is **assets assessment**, which focuses on the strengths and capacities of a community rather than its problems (Williams, Bray, Shapiro, Reisz, & Peranteau, 2009). The type of assessment depends on variables such as the needs that exist, the goals to be achieved, and the resources available for carrying out the study. Although it is difficult to determine the type of assessment needed in advance, understanding the various types of community assessment in advance helps to facilitate your decision. Based on a classic model developed by McKnight and Kretzmann in the 1980s (Kretzman & McKnight, 1993), the assets assessment provides a framework with which to conduct a complete functional community assessment and serves as a guide to the community for the nurse, as well as the foundation for community development. The previously mentioned methods are needs oriented and deficit based—in other words, they are *pathology* models, in which the assessment is performed in response to needs, barriers, weaknesses, problems, or perceived scarcity in the community. This may result in a fragmented approach to solutions for the community's problems rather than an approach focused on the community's possibilities, strengths, and assets. The assets assessment also provides the community the ability to "identify a variety and richness of skills, talents, knowledge, and experience of people" and "provides a base upon which to build new approaches and enterprises" (p. 4).

Assets assessment begins with what is present in the community (Kramer, Seedat, Lazarus, & Suffla, 2011). The capacities and skills of community members are identified, with a focus on creating or rebuilding relationships among local residents, associations, and institutions to multiply power and effectiveness. This approach requires that the assessor look for the positive or see the glass as half full. The nurse can then become a partner in community intervention efforts, rather than merely a provider of services. Assets assessment has three levels:

1. Specific skills, talents, interests, and experiences of individual community members such as individual businesses, cultural groups, and professionals living in the community.

PERSPECTIVES
PUBLIC HEALTH NURSING INSTRUCTOR

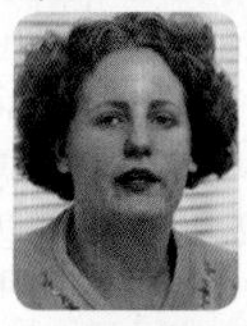

I have worked for many years in community and public health settings. I had been teaching community health nursing at a state university for 5 or 6 years when I decided to break from the "usual procedure" of having students do a comprehensive type of community assessment (all subsystems, vital statistics, etc.). This information did not change dramatically from the previous semester, or the prior 2 to 3 years for that matter. Students hate busy work and I do, too! They had complained to instructors about this repetitive assignment (a classic learning activity in public health nursing [PHN] coursework) for many years, and some were tempted to just repackage previous groups' assessments. I felt it would be more meaningful, but still have a population focus, if we could actually gather data and information for the small country health department where we were assigned. I asked several department heads to come up with ideas of aggregate or population assessment data that they needed (often related to grants they were writing or state-directed program evaluations). Several of them "pitched" these ideas and projects to our student group. The students then voted on the one they found most interesting or viable and we set about creating our own community assessment template, usually drawing from standardized assessment tools. Each semester it was different, depending upon the need. They would gather data, analyze it, and present it to the department head. From that assessment, they would create a project (often an educational intervention) that could be completed and evaluated within their timeframe. They were excited to gather this information; it was like a bunch of detectives chasing down leads! They problem-solved and worked together to achieve their goals. They worked with other agencies and NGOs; they spoke with local health care providers and members of the community. Once, the program director for a teen pregnancy program asked them to help with getting questionnaires distributed to local teens to gather information on sexual activity and attitudes. At that time, the county had the highest rate of teen pregnancy in the state, and one of the large universities in a metropolitan area was developing a survey to gather data on teen pregnancy and sexual activity in the state. This was a conservative county and many parents opposed *Sex Ed*. However, students were able to gather information and statistics on teen pregnancy in this county and compared it with state and national data. They investigated best practices for teen pregnancy prevention programs. Forming into smaller work groups, some met with school officials, high school students, teachers, and parents in order to educate them about this project. Others worked with the program director and local school nurses and counselors. They were able to convince one school superintendant to distribute this survey to high school students in his district. Students strategized about the best methods for distributing and collecting the surveys. The day came for the survey, and it was a rousing success, with no major roadblocks. They felt that their community assessment and project were worthwhile and very meaningful to this community. The health department and the university heartily agreed! I never went back to the "usual procedure," and I always encourage other instructors to try this approach.

Debbie, PHN Instructor

2. Local citizen associations, organizations, and institutions controlled largely by the community such as libraries, social service agencies, voluntary agencies, schools, and police.
3. Local institutions originating outside the community controlled largely outside the community such as welfare and public capital expenditures (p. 14).

The key, however, is linking these assets together to enhance the community from within. The community health nurse's role is to assist with those linkages.

COMMUNITY ASSESSMENT METHODS

Community health needs may be assessed using a variety of methods. Regardless of the assessment method used, data must be collected. Data collection in community health requires the exercise of sound professional judgment, effective communication techniques, and special investigative skills. Four important methods are discussed here: surveys, descriptive epidemiologic studies, community forums or town meetings, and focus groups.

Surveys

A **survey** is an assessment method in which a series of questions is used to collect data for analysis of a specific group or area. Surveys are commonly used to provide a broad range of data that will be helpful when used with other sources or if other sources are not available. To plan and conduct community health surveys, the goal should be to determine the variables (selected environmental, socioeconomic, and behavioral conditions or needs) that affect a community's ability to control disease and promote wellness. The nurse may choose to conduct a survey to determine such things as health care use patterns and needs, immunization levels, demographic characteristics, or health beliefs and practices.

The survey method involves self-report, or response to predetermined questions, and can include questionnaires, telephone or in person interviews (Polit & Beck, 2010). It can also be combined with other measures. In one study, the metric properties of the Neighborhood Inventory for Environmental Typology (NifETy) tool were examined by comparing NifETy data with self-reported youth alcohol/other drug exposure and violence with crime statistics. The data correlated with the crime statistics and self-reported use of alcohol and drugs (Furr-Holden et al., 2010).

Descriptive Epidemiologic Studies

A second assessment method is a **descriptive epidemiologic study**, which examines the amount and distribution of a disease or health condition in a population by person (Who is affected?), by place (Where does the condition occur?), and by time (When do the cases occur?). In addition to their value in assessing the health status of a population, descriptive epidemiologic studies are useful for suggesting which individuals are at greatest risk and where and when the condition might occur. They are also useful for health planning purposes and for suggesting hypotheses concerning disease etiology (Issel, 2009). Their design and use are detailed in Chapter 7.

Geographic Information System Analysis

In Chapter 10, the concept of geographic information systems (GIS) was introduced as a health information technology. Graves (2009) notes that GIS "mapping and visualization of health disparities and their relationship to the geographical location of health care services can allow for better resource allocations to disparate and underserved populations" (p. 52). It is now commonly used in community health assessment, in general, and for specific populations and problems. A review of current literature on GIS use in public health found four common themes: (1) disease surveillance, (2) risk analysis, (3) health access and planning, and (4) community health profiling (Nykiforuk & Flaman, 2011). A survey of the National Coalition of STD Directors found that 58% of those responding used GIS for data visualization and analysis, as well as for program intervention targeting; the remainder of respondents cited barriers (e.g., staffing, training) to using GIS (Bissette et al., 2009). Statewide use of GIS has identified poor access to food (or *food deserts*), overlapping with high poverty neighborhoods, in Vermont (McEntee & Agyeman, 2010). It has also been useful in identifying air pollutant risk exposure (Hammond et al., 2011), planning for rapid public health response during a natural disaster (Holt et al., 2008), and identification of colorectal screening resources for medically underserved communities (Gwede et al., 2010). GIS data are often combined with field observation (Neckerman et al., 2009) or census data and other survey results (Kazda et al., 2009) to provide powerful visualizations of data for analysis and intervention.

Community Forums or Town Hall Meetings

The community forum or town hall meeting is a qualitative assessment method designed to obtain community opinions. It takes place in the neighborhood of the people involved, perhaps in a school gymnasium or an auditorium. The participants are selected to participate by invitation from the group organizing the forum. Members come from within the community and represent all segments of the community that are involved with the issue. For instance, if a community is contemplating building a swimming pool, the people invited to the community forum might include potential users of the pool (residents of the community who do not have pools and special groups such as the Girl Scouts, elders, and disabled citizens), community planners, health and safety personnel, and other key people with vested interests. They are asked to give their views on the pool: Where should it be located? Who will use it? How will the cost of building and maintaining it be assumed? What are the drawbacks to having the pool? Any other pertinent issues the participants may raise are included. This method is relatively inexpensive, and results are quickly obtained. A drawback of this method is that only the most vocal community members, or those with the greatest vested interests in the issue, may be heard. This format does not provide a representative voice to others in the community who also may be affected by the proposed decision.

This method is used to elicit public opinion on a variety of issues, including health care concerns, political views, and feelings about issues in the public eye, such as gangs. Frequently, local cable television channels air important city government or school board meetings. Local news programs may hold town meetings, soliciting public opinion on regional issues. Other methods of opinion gathering include e-mailing (e.g., to a television news program) to support a particular view, Web-based survey sites (e.g., Survey Monkey), and using a toll-free phone number setup especially for text messaging a Yes or No vote on an issue. Now commonplace, chat rooms are available for a host of topics and interests. Electronic town meetings are designed to elicit grassroots opinions from local community members, and have been utilized by many entities, including those in favor of health care reform (Oberlander, 2010). Presidential debates are available over the Internet, with citizens sending in e-mail or Twitter questions for candidate responses in real time (Gough, 2007; Kavanaugh et al., 2010).

Focus Groups

This fourth assessment method, focus groups, is similar to the community forum or town hall meeting in that it is designed to obtain grassroots opinion. However, it has some differences. First, only a small group of participants, usually 5 to 15 people, is present (Polit & Beck, 2010). The members chosen for the group are homogeneous with respect to specific demographic variables. For example, a focus group may consist of female community health nurses, young women in their first pregnancy, or retired businessmen. Leadership skills are used in conjunction with the small group process to promote a supportive atmosphere and to accomplish set goals. The interviewer guides the discussion according to a predetermined set of questions or topics. The best use of focus group data includes not only analysis of individual communications, but of the interactions between participants (Willis, Green, Daly, Williamson, & Bandyopadhyay, 2009).

Major advantages of focus groups are their efficiency and low cost, similar to the community forum or town hall meeting format. A focus group can be organized to be representative of an aggregate, to capture community interest groups, or to sample for diversity among different population groups. One example is a research study involving Hmong youths and adults. Eight focus groups were held to determine perceptions of healthy diet and exercise among parents and children (Pham, Harrison, & Kagawa-Singer, 2007). Whatever the purpose, however, some people may be uncomfortable expressing their views in a group situation (Polit & Beck, 2010).

The choice of assessment method varies depending on the reasons for data collection, the goals and objectives of the study, and the available resources. It also varies according to the theoretical framework or philosophical approach through which the nurse views the community. In other words, the community health nurse's theoretical basis for approaching community assessment influences the purposes for conducting the assessment and the selection of methodology. For example, Neuman's health care systems model forms the basis for the "community-as-partner" assessment model developed by Anderson and McFarlane (2010). Additional resources on methodologies for assessing community health are available in the list of Internet Resources and Selected Readings at the end of this chapter.

SOURCES OF COMMUNITY DATA

The community health nurse can look in many places for data to enhance and complete a community assessment. Data sources can be primary or secondary, and they can be from international, national, state, or local sources. Web sites for many primary and secondary data sources are included at the end of this chapter.

Primary and Secondary Sources

Community health nurses make use of many sources in data collection. Community members, including formal leaders, informal leaders, and community members, can frequently offer the most accurate insights and comprehensive information. Information gathered by talking to people provides primary data, because the data are obtained directly from the community. Secondary sources of data include people who know the community well and the records such people create in the performance of their jobs. Specific examples are health team members, client records, community health (vital) statistics, census bureau data, reference books, research reports, and community health nurses. Because secondary data may not totally describe the community and do not necessarily reflect community self-perceptions, they may need augmentation or further validation through focus groups, surveys, and other primary data collection methods.

International Sources

International data are collected by several agencies, including the World Health Organization (WHO) and its six regional offices and health organizations, such as the Pan-American Health Organization. In addition, the United Nations and global specialty organizations that focus on certain populations or health problems, such as the United Nations Children's Fund, are major sources of international health-related data (WHO, 2008a). The WHO publishes an annual report of their activity, and international statistics for diseases and illness trends can be found on the Internet (WHO, 2008b). Information from these official sources can give the nurse in the local community information about immigrant and refugee populations he serves. More information on international health agencies can be found in Chapter 16.

National Sources

Community health nurses can access a wealth of official and nonofficial sources of national data (see Chapter 6 for more information). Official sources develop documents based on data compiled by the government. The following are the major official agencies:

- **USDHHS.** This is the main agency from which data can be retrieved, and its agency, the National Center for Health Statistics (NCHS) at the **Centers for Disease Control & Prevention** (CDC) was specifically established for the collection and dissemination of health-related data. This agency is the nation's principal health statistics agency, compiling data from many sources. These data provide information for many functions, including health status for various populations and subgroups, identification of disparities, monitoring trends, identifying health problems, and supporting research.
  - USDHHS also developed *Healthy People 2020* (USDHHS, 2012), which was designed to focus America's attention on the major national health problems, including realistic goals for national, state, and local agencies to work toward over one decade. Data from *Healthy People 2010* is available for analysis. Other data sources available through the CDC include Health Indicators Warehouse, Health Data Interactive, Surveillance Resource Center, and VitalStats (CDC, 2011).
- **U.S. Bureau of the Census.** This agency undertakes a major survey of American families every 10 years, gathering data on health, socioeconomic,

and environmental conditions. This information is available on the Web or on a CD-ROM, allowing numerous variables to be viewed in combination, for easier development of a community profile.

- **National Institutes of Health (NIH).** This system of 27 Institutes and Centers, a part of the USDHHS, focuses on improving the health of the nation. An emphasis is placed on discovery of new cures or treatments and preventing disease. Employees of these agencies prevent, diagnose, and treat diseases and conduct research and disseminate research findings (NIH, 2011).

Nonofficial agencies have data sources generated from research they conduct that focuses on the population, disease, or condition they were developed to serve. Each agency collects data at the national level; however, the more accessible arm for services function at state and local levels. Examples of these agencies are the American Cancer Society (ACS), the American Association of Retired Persons (AARP), Mothers Against Drunk Drivers (MADD), and Students Against Drunk Drivers (SADD). The Kaiser Family Foundation and the RAND Corporation have a variety of fact sheets and compilations of data from various sources. The Gallup Poll provides national survey information on various topics, including health. Information from such national sources allows community health assessment teams to compare local data with national and state statistics and trends—a very valuable function. Proprietary data sources include the American Hospital Association, the American Medical Association, or various health insurance companies. See Chapter 6 for a list of data collection systems.

State and Local Sources

For nurses, the most significant state source of assessment data comes from the state health department. This official agency is responsible for collecting state vital statistics and morbidity data. The Behavioral Health Surveillance System (BRFSS) is the world's largest telephone health survey that monitors health risk at the state level (CDC, 2012). Supported by the CDC, the information is used at various levels to identify risk and prevent disease. As a resource to local health departments, the state health department provides invaluable support services and it is the main source of health-related data on the state level. Nonofficial agencies have state chapters or headquarters and compile their information at the state level. Local nonofficial agency chapters have documents of compiled state and national data on the population, disease, or condition they address.

The U.S. Chamber of Commerce (2012) publishes the County and City Data Book, and state and county budgets or public health agency Web sites may also provide helpful information. All states collect vital statistics (e.g., births, deaths), and many collect information on hospitalization and morbidities related to infectious diseases, cancer, or cardiovascular disease. State departments of education may have school-based data on immunizations and overall school health. Information on traffic accidents, mental health, and environmental hazards are often available at the state level. States may also organize their statistics by county level, making it easier to compare your county's data with others.

Many sources of information may be obtained at the local level. Some key sources are the local visitor's bureau, city Chamber of Commerce, city planner's office, health department, hospitals, social service agencies, county extension office, school districts, universities or colleges, libraries, clergy, business and service organizations, and community leaders and key informants. Some of these sources compile their own statistics, but all have views of the community particular to their discipline, interest, or knowledge base. Some agencies at the local level develop city or county directories. These are updated periodically and are valuable resources for community health assessment teams and community health nurses. More detailed information on national, state, and local health agencies, and information available from them, can be found in Chapter 6.

DATA ANALYSIS AND DIAGNOSIS

This stage of assessment requires analysis of the information gathered, so that inferences or conclusions may be made about its meaning. Such inferences must be validated to determine their accuracy, after which a nursing diagnosis can be formed.

The Analysis Process

First, the data must be validated: Are they accurate, complete, representative of the population, and current (Northwest Center for Public Health Practice, n.d.)? Several validation procedures may be used:

1. Data can be rechecked by the community assessment team.
2. Data can be rechecked by others.
3. Subjective and objective data can be compared.
4. Community members can consider the findings and verify them.

Validated data are then separated into categories such as physical, social, and environmental data. In many instances, data spreadsheets are used to provide a structure for data organization. Next, each category is examined to determine its significance. At this point, there may be a need to search for additional information to clarify the meaning of the data. Only then can inferences be made and a tentative conclusion about the meaning of the data be reached (Anderson & McFarlane, 2010).

Some computer programs are designed to analyze community assessment data. For large, complex, or ongoing community assessment plans, this may be the best method. For smaller, one-time assessments, the paper-and-pencil method may be sufficient and less unwieldy. Some communities may hire an outside professional assessment service. These teams often use the latest technology when analyzing data. Not all communities can afford such a service, and if key leaders become familiar with assessment, analysis, and diagnostic processes, an investment in a computer program may be worthwhile. GIS technology, as noted earlier, is proving very useful in community assessment. These tools are becoming more user friendly and cost effective, and have been used to pinpoint incidences of various diseases, display environmental risks, note the location of health care facilities, and determine accurate community boundaries (Nykiforuk & Flaman, 2011). Regardless of the analysis method used, data interpretation remains a critical phase of the process.

In data interpretation, the ever-present danger exists of making inaccurate assumptions and diagnoses. The importance of validation cannot be overemphasized. Before making a diagnosis, all assumptions must be validated: Are they sound? Community members should participate actively in validation efforts by clarifying perceptions, explaining the circumstances surrounding the situation, and acting as sounding boards for testing assumptions. Other resources, such as the health team members and community leaders, are used to explore and confirm inferences. Data collection, data interpretation, and nursing diagnosis are sequential activities, with validation serving as the bridges between them (Table 15-5). When performed thoroughly, these steps lead to accurate diagnoses.

Community Diagnosis Formation

The next step of the nursing process, after analysis, is the development of the community diagnosis. Community diagnoses stems from analysis of assessment data. The diagnosis "describes a situation" and "implies a reason" or etiology focusing on a specific community (Anderson & McFarlane, 2011, p. 236). Various taxonomies and classification systems are used in nursing to describe specific nursing problems and each one has its limitations when dealing with community-level diagnoses. The North American Nursing Diagnosis Association (NANDA) is much more oriented to nursing diagnoses of individuals and families than to community-level problems. Nursing Outcomes Classification (NOC) is also generally individual oriented. The Omaha System, originally designed by the Omaha Visiting Nurse Association, is again primarily used in nursing diagnoses of individuals, families, and small groups, although some community health applications have been developed (Omaha System, 2011).

This chapter discusses nursing diagnosis as characterized by Neufeld and Harrison (1996), based on the classic work of Mundinger and Jauron (1975). These authors proposed the use of nursing diagnoses in the community by substituting the term *client, family, group*, or *aggregate* for the word *patient*. Their definition of a nursing diagnosis is (Neufeld & Harrison, 1996, p. 221):

> The statement of a [client's] response which is actually or potentially unhealthful and which nursing intervention can help to change in the direction of health. It should also identify essential factors related to the unhealthful response.

Neufeld and Harrison built on this work to form a wellness diagnosis by using the phrase *healthful response* instead of *unhealthful response*. Their definition of a wellness diagnosis is (p. 221):

> The statement of a client's [community's] healthful response which nursing intervention can support or strengthen. It should also identify the essential factors related to the healthful response.

In 1996, Stolte developed a manual dedicated solely to nursing wellness diagnosis. Carpenito (2008) incorporated both community diagnosis and wellness diagnosis into her well-known handbook on applying nursing diagnosis to clinical practice. By substituting the term *community* for client, family, group, or aggregate, the nursing or wellness diagnosis can be applied to the

Table 15.5 Assessment and Diagnosis Phases of the Nursing Process

Interpretation of data leads to diagnosis of a community's needs, the community responses, and expected outcomes.

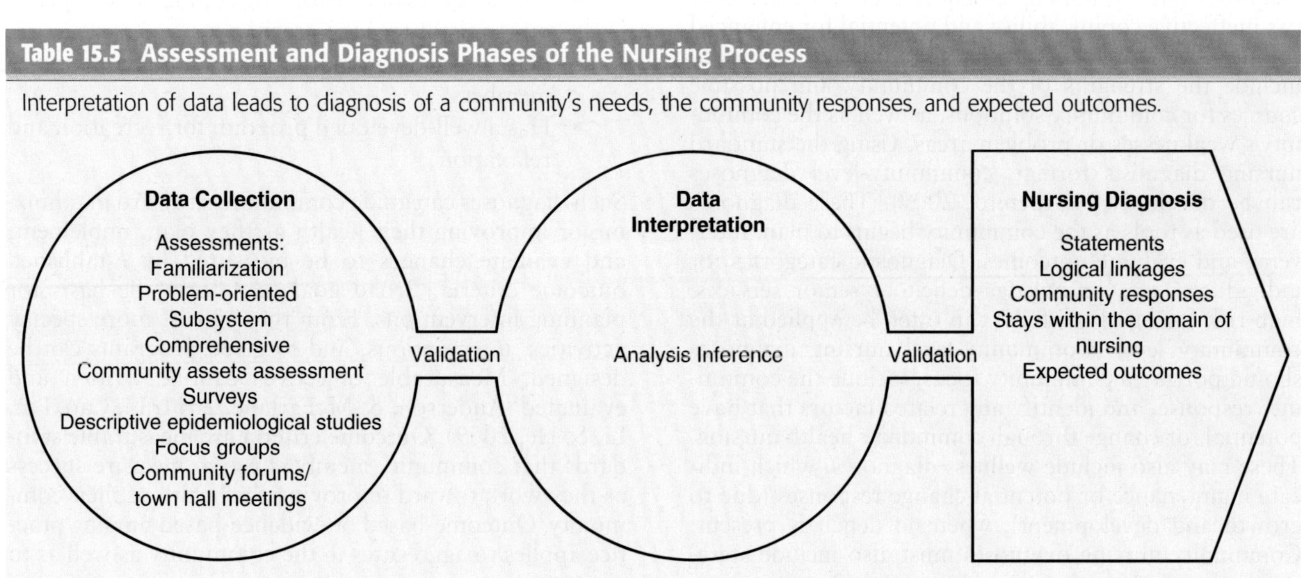

community as a whole. These diagnoses identify the conclusion the nurse draws from interpretation of collected data and describe a community's healthy or unhealthy responses that can be influenced or changed by nursing interventions. Change comes about through collaboration with other community and health team members.

In community health, nurses do not limit their focus to problems; they consider the community as a total system and look for evidence of all kinds of responses that may influence the community's level of wellness (as shown in Fig. 15-5). Responses encompass the whole health–illness continuum, from specific deficits, such as a lack of senior centers or day care programs, to opportunities for maximizing a community's health, such as promoting improvement of police protection or the safety of the roadways. The statement of community response—the diagnosis—can focus on a wide range of topics.

Community Diagnoses

Data have been gathered from a variety of sources and have been validated by several means. The data have been recorded, tabulated, analyzed, and synthesized, so that patterns and trends can be seen. The use of charts, graphs, and tables assists in visualizing the synthesized data. The community assessment team should present their findings to peers and colleagues, and use their expertise to assist in the formulation of the community diagnoses. Inferences are drawn from the data, and these statements refer to *actual* or *potential* problems. Additional statements involve *etiology*, by stating that this condition is *related to* certain conditions or problems. There may be a number of these statements, involving several subsystems, for every one diagnosis. Signs and symptoms of the diagnosis relate to the *magnitude* or *duration* of the problem, usually documented "as manifested by" (Anderson & McFarlane, 2011, p. 237).

Continuing with the nursing process format, nursing diagnoses for the community are developed. **Community diagnoses** refer to nursing diagnoses about a community's ineffective coping ability and potential for enhanced coping. The statements about the community should include the strengths of the community and possible sources for community solutions, as well as the community's weaknesses or problem areas. Using the standard nursing diagnosis format, community-level diagnoses can be developed (Carpenito, 2009). These diagnoses are used as tools as the community begins to plan, intervene, and evaluate outcomes. Diagnostic categories for individuals (e.g., knowledge deficit of senior services, high risk for injury or falls) can often be applied at the community level. Community-level nursing diagnoses should portray a community focus, include the community response, and identify any related factors that have potential for change through community health nursing. These may also include wellness diagnoses, which indicate maintenance or potential change responses (due to growth and development), when no deficit is present. Community nursing diagnoses must also include statements that are narrow enough to guide interventions, have logical linkages between community responses and related factors, and include factors within the domain of community health nursing intervention.

Examples of wellness and deficit community nursing diagnoses and several diagnoses for a specific community follow:

1. *Wellness nursing diagnosis for an assisted living community of elders.* The senior residents of an assisted living center (*community focus*) have the potential for achieving optimal functioning related to (*host factors*) their expressed interest in exercise, diet, and meaningful activities and to (*environmental factors*) their access to exercise opportunities, nutritional information, and social outlets.
2. *Deficit community nursing diagnosis for a rural farm-worker community.* The inhabitants of (*name of the town*) in (*name of the state*) are at risk for illness and injury related to (*host factors*) exposure to pesticides, lack of motivation to add or use safety devices on farm machinery, lack of safety knowledge, choice to take unnecessary risks (*environmental factors*), lack of family income to purchase newer equipment, and long hours of work that lead to stress and exhaustion.
3. *Community diagnoses for Anytown, Kansas.* Anytown, Kansas, is experiencing an increase in crime, a problem compounded by the small size of the police force and an influx of many new community members. The community has worked together constructively in the past, communicates well, and has strong recreational outlets for community members. The community:
   - Has expressed vulnerability and feels overwhelmed related to threats to community safety
   - Has failed to meet its own expectations related to inadequate law enforcement services
   - Has expressed difficulty in meeting the demands of change related to an influx of new community members
   - Has a successful history of coping with a previous crisis of teenage pregnancy
   - Has positive communication among community members
   - Has a well-developed program for recreation and relaxation

Such diagnoses can guide communities toward maximizing or improving their health as they plan, implement, and evaluate changes to be measured by established outcome criteria. Broad goals can form the basis for planning interventions. From these goals, more specific activities, interventions, and targeted programs can be designed. Measurable objectives can be written and evaluated (Anderson, & McFarlane, 2011; Li, Cao, Lin, Li, & He, 2009). **Outcome criteria** are measurable standards that community members use to measure success as they work toward improving the health of their community. Outcome-based or evidence-based nursing practice applies to aggregates in the community as well as to patients in acute-care settings.

Nursing diagnoses change over time because they reflect changes in the health status of the community; therefore, diagnoses need to be periodically reevaluated and redefined. The changing diagnosis can be a useful means of moving a community toward improved health because it gives community members a clear standard against which to measure progress.

PLANNING TO MEET THE HEALTH NEEDS OF THE COMMUNITY

Planning is the logical decision-making process used to design an orderly, detailed series of actions for accomplishing specific goals and objectives. Planning for community health is based on assessment of the community and the nursing diagnoses formulated, but assessment and diagnosis alone do not prescribe the specific actions necessary to meet clients' needs (Anderson, & McFarlane, 2011; Minnesota Department of Health, 2011). Knowing that a group of mothers at the well-child clinic need emotional support does not tell the nurse what further action is indicated. A diagnosis of culture shock (adjustment deficit to a contrasting culture) for a family newly arrived from Cuba does not reveal what action to take. The nurse must systematically develop an appropriate plan (see Levels of Prevention Pyramid).

Tools to Assist with Planning

Various tools may enhance planning for community health care provision and programs; these may include operational definitions of objectives and activities, conceptual frameworks, and models (Minnesota Department of Health, 2011). Such tools help to identify target population characteristics, clarify program goals, specify nursing interventions, and anticipate client outcomes. Tools that assist with planning also enable the nurse to test ideas and adjust solutions before actual implementation. Finally, the use of standardized tools enhances the planning process and promotes effectiveness of services, as well as professional standards of practice.

In addition to using tools, a systematic approach to planning guides the community health nurse to list

LEVELS OF PREVENTION PYRAMID

THE PROBLEM OF CHILD ABUSE

SITUATION: Desire to reduce the incidence of child abuse in a given community by 50% within 2 years.

GOAL: Using the three levels of prevention, negative health conditions are avoided, or promptly diagnosed and treated, and the fullest possible potential is restored.

TERTIARY PREVENTION

Rehabilitation	Primary Prevention	
	Health Promotion & Education	*Health Protection*
• Establish rehabilitation programs for abused children, including safe home placement, physical and emotional treatment, and self-esteem building • Rebuild the family unit if appropriate or possible	• Provide family life education programs for families • Develop resources to support health promotion programs	• If unable or inappropriate to rehabilitate the abuser or family, keep abuser away from victim through incarceration or court order

SECONDARY PREVENTION

Early Diagnosis	Prompt Treatment
• Develop early detection programs through schools, clinics, and physicians' offices • Promote enforcement of child protection laws	• Establish programs to provide prompt treatment for abused children and abusing parents

PRIMARY PREVENTION

Health Promotion and Education	Health Protection
• Assess factors contributing to child abuse • Institute family life education programs through schools and community groups • Develop community resources to support health protection programs	• Identify families in the community who are at greatest risk (e.g., parents with history of child abuse, families under great stress) • Develop community resources to support health promotion programs

needs in order of priority, establish goals and objectives, and record the plan. As they do in the rest of the nursing process, community health nurses collaborate with clients and other appropriate professionals throughout each of these planning activities.

The Health Planning Process

The health planning process is a four-stage system used to design new health-related programs or services in the community. The process is often used by health educators when designing educational programs, or by administrators in community health agencies when initiating new services. The nursing process is similar to the health planning process (Table 15-6). Each model helps to promote service effectiveness in addition to maintaining standards of practice. Community health nurses familiar with both the health planning process and the nursing process should be able to work collaboratively with community health professionals using either model.

Setting Priorities

Priority setting involves assigning rank or importance to the identified needs to determine the order in which goals should be addressed. There are numerous ways to set priorities in the planning process (Platonova, Studnicki, Fisher, & Bridger, 2010). Many have identified useful criteria that can guide ranking problems for order of action (CDC, n.d.; Office of the Assistant Secretary for Planning & Evaluation, n.d.; Rudan, Kapiriri, Tomlinson, Balliet, 2010; Sibbald, Singer, Upshur, & Martin, 2009). They are presented here as a combination of criteria:

1. Significance of the problem or the number of people affected in the community
2. Level of community awareness of the problem
3. Community motivation to act on the problem (or, Is this important to the community?)
4. Nurse and partnership's ability to reduce risk and/or influence the solution
5. Cost of risk reduction in terms of financial, social, and ethical capital
6. Ability to identify a specific target population for an intervention
7. Availability of expertise to solve the problem within the partnership, coalition, or community
8. Severity of the outcome if left unresolved or the consequences of inaction
9. Speed with which the problem can be resolved

For example, a community assessment revealed that a group of elderly residents living within a specific zip code were fearful of crime, but also identified the lack of public transportation as issues to be addressed. Using the above criteria, the community health nurse working in this community identified that 85% of residents of the community had fears about crime but did not see transportation as an issue. The residents saw crime as an important concern and were also motivated to act on the crime issue, but were not willing to explore the transportation issue at the current time. The nurse, along with the community coalition partners, would be better able to influence the crime problem by helping to form Town Watch groups and getting the local police district to provide increased patrols during evening hours when robberies were more likely to occur. However, the partners had little influence

Table 15.6 Comparison Between the Health Planning Process and the Nursing Process

Health Planning Process	Nursing Process
1. ASSESSMENT STAGE	**1. ASSESSMENT**
Determine data needed and collect data. Interpret data and identity needs. Set goals based on needs.	Determine data needed and collect data. Interpret data and identity needs. Set goals based on needs.
2. ANALYSIS AND DESIGN	**2. DIAGNOSIS**
Analyze findings and set specific objectives. Design alternative interventions. Analyze and compare pros and cons of various solutions.	Analyze findings and set specific objectives. Design alternative interventions. Analyze and compare pros and cons of various solutions. Formulate nursing diagnoses.
	3. PLANNING
Create a plan.	List needs in order of priority. Establish goals and objectives. Write an action plan.
3. IMPLEMENTATION STAGE	**4. IMPLEMENTATION**
Describe how to operationalize the plan. Design a method for monitoring progress.	Describe how to operationalize the plan. Design a method for monitoring progress.
4. EVALUATION STAGE	**5. EVALUATION**
Examine costs and benefits of proposed solution. Judge the potential outputs, outcomes, and impact of plan. Modify to achieve the best plan. Present plan to sponsoring group or agency. Obtain acceptance (and funding).	Examine costs and benefits of proposed solution. Judge the potential outputs, outcomes, and impact of plan. Modify to achieve the best plan. Present plan to sponsoring group or agency. Obtain acceptance (and funding).

to extend the hours of operation on buses or influence the creation of new bus routes. Members of the coalition included the local police chief and chamber of commerce director. If the crime problem was left unchecked, more people could be adversely affected, including businesses, because people would not be willing to leave their homes to shop or might even be forced to move away. Finally, these initiatives could be put in place rather quickly and inexpensively after the formation and training of volunteer Town Watch groups. There certainly are no adverse social, economic, or ethical consequences attached to addressing this problem. Therefore, it would seem that the crime issue would take priority over the transportation issue. It is important to remember that each community diagnosis is examined separately and then compared. Priorities for action are discussed, ranked, and then prioritized for action. Criteria for prioritizing health problems in the community include:

- Numbers of community members affected by the problem
- Community awareness of the problem
- Ability of team to reduce risk or influence the problem
- Cost of risk reduction (social, economic, and ethical)
- Ability to clearly identify a target or risk population
- Availability of expertise
- Consequences of inaction
- Speed of resolution (CDC, n.d.; Issel, 2009; NACCHO, n.d.)

Establishing Goals and Objectives

Goals and objectives are crucial to planning and should be feasible and specific (Anderson & McFarlane, 2011; USDHHS, 2012). The diagnosis that identifies needs must be translated into goals to give focus and meaning to the nursing plan. **Goals** are broad statements of desired outcomes. **Objectives** are specific statements of desired outcomes, phrased in behavioral terms that can be measured. Target dates for expected completion of each objective are also stated. Objectives are the stepping-stones to help one reach the end results of the larger goal. For the elderly group concerned about crime in the neighborhood, the need, the goal, and the objectives were defined as follows:

- *Need*: The group of elderly people has altered coping ability related to their fear of crime.
- *Goal*: Within 6 months, this group of elderly people will feel comfortable to walk the streets of their neighborhood without experiencing any incidents of criminal assault.
- *Objectives:*
  1. By the end of the first month, a safety committee (composed of senior citizens, nurses, police, and other appropriate community members) will be established to study the crime patterns in the neighborhood.
  2. The safety committee will develop strategies for crime reduction and elder protection, which will be presented to the city council for approval by the end of the third month.
  3. Safety strategies, such as increased police surveillance, Town Watch patrols, and escort services, will be implemented by the end of the fifth month.
  4. By the end of the sixth month, nursing assessment will determine that senior citizens feel free to walk about the neighborhood.
  5. By the sixth month, there will be no reported incidents of criminal assault.

Development of objectives depends on a careful analysis of all the ways in which one could accomplish the larger goal. One should first select the course of action that is best suited to meet the goal and then build objectives. For the group of elderly people, other alternatives, such as staying indoors or always walking in pairs, were considered and rejected. The ultimate choice was to find a way to make their environment safe and enjoyable.

Some rules of thumb are helpful when writing objectives. First, each objective should state a single idea. When more than one idea is expressed—as in an objective to both obtain equipment and learn procedures—it is more difficult to measure the completion of the objective. Second, each objective should describe *one* specific behavior that can be measured. For instance, the fourth objective from the list states that the seniors will report feeling free to walk outdoors within 6 months. It describes a behavior that can be measured at some point in time. One can more readily evaluate objectives that include specifics—such as what will be done, who will do it, and when it will be accomplished. Then it is clear to everyone involved exactly what has to be done and within what time frame. Writing measurable objectives makes a tremendous difference in the success of planning. (See Chapter 11 for more information on writing behavioral objectives.)

Planning means thinking ahead. The nurse looks ahead toward the desired end and then decides what intermediate actions are necessary to meet that goal. Sometimes, an objective itself describes the intermediate actions. At other times, an objective may be further broken down into several activities. For example, the second objective states that the safety committee will be charged with developing strategies, presenting them to the city council, and gaining their approval. Good planning requires this kind of detail.

Making decisions is an important part of planning. Decisions must be made during the process of establishing priorities. Decisions are necessary for selecting goals and for choosing the best course of action from many possible courses. Further decision making is involved in selecting objectives and taking action to accomplish the objectives.

To facilitate planning and decision making, the community health nurse involves other people. Clients must be included at every step because they are the ones for whom the planning is being done. Without their insight and cooperation, the plan may not succeed. Additionally, the involvement of other nurses may be important. Team meetings, nurse–supervisor conferences, and nurse–expert consultant sessions are all useful resources for planning. In addition, you may wish to confer with members of other health and professional disciplines (e.g., teachers, social workers, mental health professionals, city planners). Interdisciplinary team conferences are valuable for gaining a broader perspective and enlisting wider support for the evolving plan.

IMPLEMENTING PLANS FOR PROMOTING THE HEALTH OF THE COMMUNITY

Implementation is putting the plan into action. The nurse, other professionals, or clients carry out the activities of the plan. Implementation is often referred to as the action phase of the nursing process. In community health nursing, implementation includes not just nursing action or nursing intervention, but collaboration with clients and perhaps other professionals. When bringing about change in a community organization, implementation involves the greatest commitment of time and planning. This often includes an implementation timetable, as well as funding or organizing physical/informational/staff/management resources, collaboration with outside agencies, training staff and working with community volunteers as needed for program implementation, as well as actually putting into action those interventions created during the planning phase (Issel, 2009). Certainly, the nurse's professional expertise and judgment provide a necessary resource to the client group. The nurse is also a catalyst and facilitator in planning and activating the action plan. However, a primary goal in community health is to help people learn to help themselves in achieving their optimal level of health. To realize this goal, the nurse must constantly involve clients in the deliberative process and encourage their sense of responsibility and autonomy. Other health team members may also participate in carrying out the plan. All are partners in implementation.

Preparation

The actual course of implementation, outlined in the plan, should be fairly easy to follow if goals, expected outcomes, and planned actions have been designed carefully. Professionals and clients should have a clear idea of *who*, *what*, *why*, *when*, *where*, and *how*. Who will be involved in carrying out the plan? What are each person's responsibilities? Do all understand why and how to do their parts? Do they know when and where activities will occur? As implementation begins, nurses should review these questions for themselves, as well as for clients. This is the time to clarify any doubtful areas, thereby facilitating a smooth implementation phase. An operations manual may be needed, as well as organizational charts, clear budgets, and social marketing plans (Anderson & McFarlane, 2011; Issel, 2009).

Even the best planning may require adjustments. For example, some nurses who planned a health fair for seniors discovered that the target group would not have transportation to the site because the volunteering bus company had withdrawn its offer. To smoothly implement the plan, the nurses arranged for volunteers from local churches to pick up the seniors, bring them to the health fair, and deliver them afterward to their homes. Implementation requires flexibility and adaptation to unanticipated events.

Activities or Actions

The process of implementation requires a series of nursing actions or activities:

1. The nurse applies appropriate theories, such as systems theory or change theory, to the actions being performed.
2. The nurse helps to facilitate an environment that is conducive to carrying out the plan (e.g., a quiet room in which to hold a group teaching session or solicitation of support from local officials for an environmental cleanup project).
3. The nurse and other health team members prepare clients to receive services by assessing their knowledge, understanding, and attitudes and by carefully interpreting the plan to clients. This interaction nurtures open communication and trust between nurse and clients. Professionals and clients (or representatives if the aggregate is large) form a contractual agreement about the content of the plan and how it is to be carried out.
4. The plan is carried out, or modified and then carried out, by professionals and clients. Modification requires constant observation and interchange during implementation, because these actions determine the success of the plan and the nature of needed changes.
5. The nurse and the team monitor and document the progress of the implementation phase by process evaluation, which measures the ongoing achievement of planned actions.

EVALUATING IMPLEMENTED COMMUNITY HEALTH PLAN

Evaluation is usually seen as the final step, but since the nursing process is cyclic in nature, the nurse is constantly evaluating throughout the entire process. For instance, in the assessment phase, the nurse must evaluate whether the collected data are sufficient and appropriate to beginning planning. Evaluation methods must be addressed during the planning phase as goals and objectives, as well as interventions are identified (Anderson & McFarlane, 2011; Council on Education for Public Health [CEPH], 2011; Issel, 2009). **Evaluation** refers to measuring and judging the effectiveness of goal or outcome attainment. Too often, emphasis is placed primarily on assessing client needs and on planning and implementing service. The nursing process is really not complete until evaluation takes place. Actually, if you look at the nursing process as cyclical instead of linear, then the evaluation guides the next assessment (CEPH, 2011; Issel, 2009). How effective was the service? Were client needs truly met? How has health status changed? Professional practitioners owe it to their clients, themselves, and other health service providers to fully and effectively evaluate a program (see From the Case Files II).

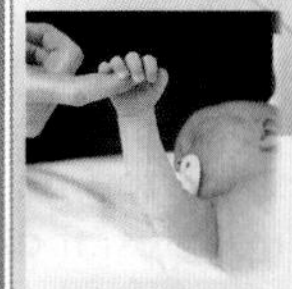

From the **Case Files**

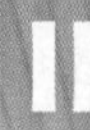

Evaluating Outcomes of a Home Care Postpartum Program

Scenario

As a nurse working as the liaison between Capitol City Hospital and its home health agency, you are given the job of reviewing your early postpartum discharge program. Your program has been in effect for 18 months. Client satisfaction is high. The program has increased revenue for the hospital as many clients choose to deliver at Capitol City Hospital because of the early discharge program.

The protocol for your early discharge program includes a postpartum home visit by an RN from the home health agency. These visits are provided as a service to the client. In some cases, visits are billable to insurance companies. Medicaid authorizes payment for one postpartum visit.

You have gathered the following information about the early discharge program:

I. Protocol: Standard is one visit within 48 hours after discharge which includes
   A. Education
      1. Newborn care
      2. Breast-feeding
      3. Warning signs warranting follow-up (mother and baby)
         —Infection
         —Hemorrhage
      4. Comfort
      5. Parenting
      6. Sexuality
         —Resumption of sexual activity
         —Contraception
      7. Community resources
      8. Nutrition
      9. Well and sick baby care
   B. Assessment
      1. Infant: Jaundice (heel stick performed if necessary)
         Mother: Hemorrhage, perineal lacerations, hematomas
         Both: Nutrition
         —Weight
         —Hydration
         —Breast-feeding
      2. Elimination

II. Cost:
   A. Fully reimbursed by some insurance companies
   B. All mother/baby dyads receive postpartum visits, regardless of insurance coverage
   C. Optional or additional methods of reimbursement have not been explored by the agency
   D. Agency makes money on reimbursed visits, loses money on nonreimbursed, but additional revenue generated by clients choosing the hospital because of the positive public perception. The program is thought to balance out cost of nonreimbursed visits.

Outcomes. Outcomes of postpartum early discharge with accompanying home visit (as compared to traditional length of postpartum stay)

I. Positive
   A. Higher percentage of successful (at least 2 months) breast-feeding
   B. Higher rate of immunization compliance
   C. Fewer inappropriate emergency room visits
   D. High client satisfaction
   E. Lower levels of maternal stress reported to pediatricians
II. Negative
   A. Higher incidence in jaundice in babies whose mothers participated in the early discharge program

Questions

1. What, if any, additional information do you need to make a recommendation regarding the program?
   • How will you obtain this information?
2. As the nurse making a recommendation for the continuation or termination of the postpartum early discharge program, what are your recommendations?
   • Should the program be abandoned?
   • Should the program be maintained?
3. What, if any, alterations would you make in the following areas:
   • Funding
   • Protocol
   —Client education
   —Assessment
   —Timing of visit
4. Outcome measurements are critical to demonstrate the efficacy of this program.
   • What will you evaluate?
   • How often?
   • Why?

As stated earlier, evaluation is an act of appraisal in which one judges value in relation to a standard and a set of criteria. Evaluation requires a stated purpose, specific standards and criteria by which to judge, and judgment skills.

Types of Evaluations

To determine the success of their planning and intervention, community health nurses use two main types of evaluation: formative and summative evaluation. The focus of *formative* evaluation is on process during the actual interventions. *Summative* evaluation focuses on the outcome of the interventions: Did you meet your goals? In formative evaluation, performance standards are developed and used to determine what is and is not working throughout the process (CEPH, 2011). They could include the physical and organizational structure of the agency, as well as resources that provide a foundation for any interventions. Formative evaluation essentially looks at the step-by-step process of program implementation. Could I do anything better or differently to increase my desired outcome? An example would occur when looking at the poor attendance at two sessions of an evening health-promotion class for senior citizens. The nurse identifies the reason for poor attendance as being seniors' reluctance to attend an evening class because they either don't drive at night or fear coming out in the dark. The class is rescheduled for midmorning, and the attendance dramatically increases.

Summative evaluation examines outcomes of the interventions. The *effect*, or degree to which an outcome objective has been met, informs the agency or program leader of the program's impact on clients' health. As an example, one manufacturing company had an 80% adherence rate for employees who were supposed to wear proper protective devices (goggles, safety shoes, and hard hats) in the plant. Noncompliance on the part of some workers was a concern to union representatives, the health and safety team, and the company management. They were concerned that 20% of their employees were at risk for injury that would cause pain, suffering, loss of work time, disruption to the manufacturing process, and reduced profitability. The occupational health nurse along with the safety officer began a month-long safety campaign that included safety miniclasses, posters, and incentives for departments with 100% safety equipment adherence. Three months after the program, 95% of the employees were adhering to the safety regulations. This 15% increase was attributed to the effect of the safety program. See Chapter 12 for more on program evaluation.

The *impact* of a program determines how close it comes to attaining its goals. In the earlier example, the objective of the safety campaign was to increase safety equipment use, and use was significantly increased as a result of the program. However, if the goal of the program had been to decrease accidents and save the company money, the result could be determined only with additional information. Were there fewer injuries caused by accidents? Were there fewer days lost to injuries? Did the company save money as the direct result of employee safety adherence? Depending on the answers to these questions, the overall goal of the program may or may not have been met, even though the objective of the program was met. The full impact of the program cannot be determined without additional data. See Chapter 12 for more on program evaluation.

Community Development Theory

An outcome of effective community-level nursing practice is community development. **Community development** is the process of collaborating with community members to assess their collective needs and desires for positive change and to address these needs through problem solving, the use of community experts, and resource development (Blakely & Leigh, 2010). A community development perspective assumes that community members participate in all aspects of change—assessment, planning, development, delivery of services, and evaluation. With this approach, the focus is on healthful community changes generated from within the community, as a partnership between health care providers and inhabitants, rather than a commodity dispensed by health care providers. The community as partner model exemplifies this approach (Anderson & McFarlane, 2011). Chapter 11 details community change theory.

The outcomes are more positive when community members have a sense of ownership in the health programs and services that address their needs. This enhances empowerment among members of the community and enables them to more effectively control and participate in transforming their environment and their personal circumstances. This implies that health care agency infrastructures are appropriate additions to services that are planned and delivered in an acceptable manner to the community (see Fig. 15-6, Arnstein's Ladder). This empowerment leads to greater resilience and ultimately, wellness (Norris, Stevens, Pfefferbaum, Wyche, & Pfefferbaum, 2008). See Chapter 13.

When applying community development theory, the agent of change (often the community health nurse) is considered a partner rather than an authority figure responsible for the community's health. To achieve acceptance as a partner, the nurse must listen and learn from the community members, because they are the experts with respect to their health care needs, culture, and values (Nadig, 2010; Timmons et al., 2007). They have mastered adaptation to the community, and they have firsthand knowledge of prevention methods and interventions that are appropriate to their lifestyles. For example, a randomized controlled trial with 285

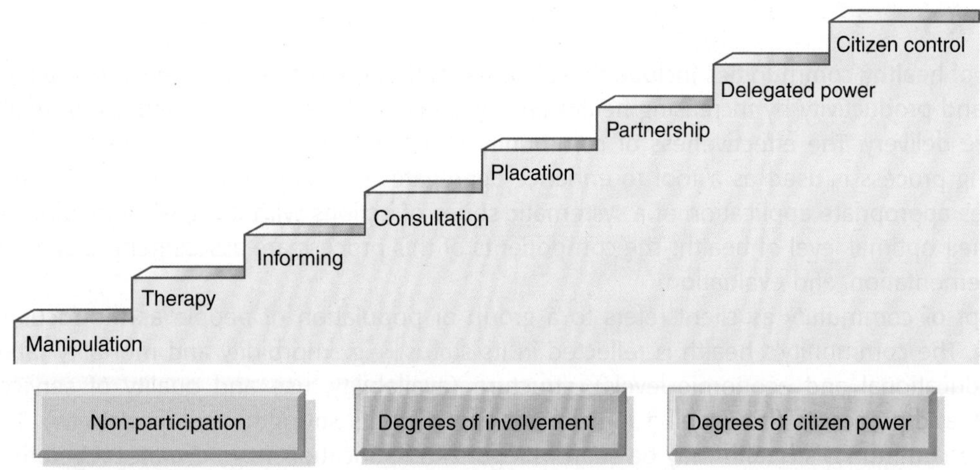

FIGURE 15-6. Arnstein's Ladder—Eight steps of citizen participation. (Adapted from Arnstein, S. R. (1969, July). A ladder of citizen participation. *Journal of the American Institute of Planners, 35*(4), 217–224.)

women having chronic health conditions and receiving Temporary Aid for Needy Families (TANF), and utilizing a CBPR approach, found that 9 months of PHN case management improved health outcomes for those in the intervention group (Kneipp et al., 2011). Medicaid knowledge and skills improved for both the intervention and control groups, but those in the intervention group had improved depression and functional status; they were also more likely to have a new mental health visit (Kneipp et al., 2011). The PHNs developed rapport with their clients and formed a partnership with them. The principles of CBPR involve this type of partnership (see Chapters 4, 13, and 25 for more information on this subject). Members of the community are engaged as coresearchers, and time is spent building trust and developing collaborative relationships with community members, stakeholders, and neighborhood health care providers. The expertise of community members is valued and can be useful in designing recruitment strategies, as well as in data analysis (Perry & Hoffman, 2010). This experience can enrich the community as a whole, as well as the actual participants.

The outcomes of the services provided by any organization can be benchmarked against those of other groups. *Benchmarking* involves comparing an organization's outcomes against those of a similar organization or an organization that is known for its excellence in a particular area of client care (Haustein et al., 2011). Information from this comparison can be used to identify an organization's areas of weakness and to focus attention on specific outcomes. The establishment of *best practice* activities entails constant comparisons between high- and low-performance programs and interventions (Glanz & Bishop, 2010; Hughes, Seymour, Campbell, Whitelaw, & Bazzarre, 2009).

From a global perspective, the Conference on Primary Health Care held at Alma-Ata in 1978 concluded that people have little control over their own health care services and that the emphasis should be on health problems identified by the members of the community in their attempts to attain a state of wellness (WHO, 1998). Since that time, the WHO, along with other agencies and groups, has been providing leadership in the use of community development methods to improve global health, based on the following concepts (Community Development Society, 2007):

- Promote active, representative participation to influence decisions affecting community members' daily lives
- Engage community members in economic, social, political, environmental, psychological, and other issues that impact them
- Interest them in learning more about alternative courses of action
- Incorporate diverse cultures, ethnic and racial groups, and varied interests in the process of community development
- Refrain from supporting efforts that are likely to adversely affect disadvantaged members of the community
- Actively work to build leadership capacity of community leaders and groups, and individuals
- Work toward long-term sustainability and community wellbeing

SUMMARY

Characteristics of healthy communities include those elements that enable people to maintain a high quality of life and productivity by increasing health and decreasing disease and disparities in health and health care delivery. The effectiveness of community health nursing practice depends on how well the nursing process is used as a tool to enhance aggregate or population health. The nursing process involves appropriate application of a systematic series of actions with the goal of helping clients achieve their optimal level of health. The components of this process are assessment, diagnosis, planning, implementation, and evaluation.

The concept of community as client refers to a group or population of people as the focus of nursing service. The community's health is reflected in its status (e.g., morbidity and mortality rates, crime rates, educational and economic levels), structure (availability, use and quality of services and resources), and processes (how well it functions in regard to its strengths and limitations). The dimensions of a community's health may be seen in regard to its location (e.g., climate, vegetation, boundaries), population (e.g., diversity or homogeneity, old, young, pregnant, addicted, or academic members), and social systems (e.g., schools, businesses, communications, health care, and religious organizations, among others).

Interaction is deeply integrated in the nursing process. Because nurse and clients must first establish a relationship of reciprocal influence and exchange before any change can take place, interaction could be considered the most essential step in the process. Effective communication is inherent in assessing needs and establishing trust between nurse and clients as partners in the nursing process. The first steps in interacting involve understanding group behaviors and dynamics, followed by interpersonal communication at the group level in the form of listening, teaching, building trust, seeking client involvement, sharing, and collaborating to build partnerships and teams.

Assessment for community health nurses means collecting and evaluating information about a community's health status to discover existing or potential needs and assets as a basis for planning future action. Assessment involves two major activities. The first is collection of pertinent data, and the second is analysis and interpretation of that data.

Community health nurses may use various assessment methods to determine a community's needs. They include *familiarization assessments*, such as windshield surveys, which involves studying data already available on a community; *problem-oriented assessment*, which focuses on a single problem and looks at the community in terms of that problem; *community subsystem assessment*, by which the community health nurse focuses on a single dimension of community life; a complicated and often time-consuming *comprehensive assessment*, to discover *all* relevant community health information; or an *assets assessment* that focuses on the strengths of a community as opposed to its deficits. Combinations may also prove useful (e.g., problem oriented and assets assessments).

Community data may be provided by surveys, descriptive epidemiologic studies, community forums or town meetings, focus groups, and primary and secondary sources, such people who are familiar with the community and its character and history, Web sites, government departments and agencies that compile statistics, such as the Bureau of the Census, the county health department, and others. Sources can include national international, state, county, and local agencies, as well as business and social organizations.

Using the nursing process in the community would not be complete without looking at the role of the community health nurse as a catalyst for community development. Community development theory is the foundation that supports citizen empowerment and use of key players in the community to plan for the health and safety of that community.

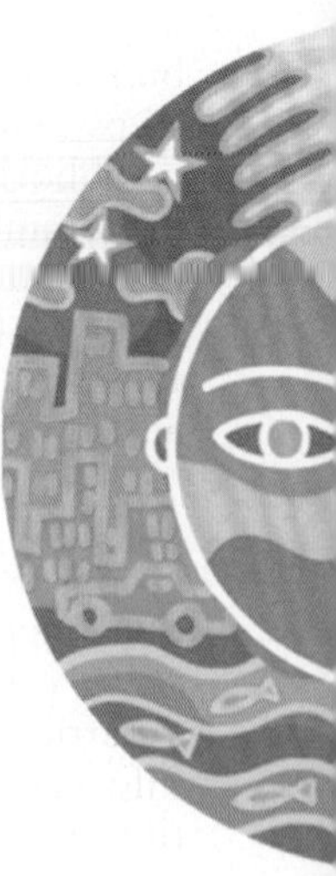

ACTIVITIES TO PROMOTE CRITICAL THINKING

1. Explain to a nonnursing friend why it is important to understand and work with the community as a total entity.
2. How does defining the community as the client change the community health nurse's practice? List some specific examples of how this concept can be applied.
3. If you were part of a health planning team concerned about the health needs of senior citizens in your community, what are some location, population, and social system variables you would want to assess? Name some of the sources from which you might collect the data.
4. Discuss under what circumstances you might choose to conduct a problem-oriented community health assessment. What method would you consider using to conduct this assessment, and how would you carry it out?
5. If possible, interview someone from your state or local health department who has recently conducted a community needs assessment survey. Or, access one on a state website. Analyze the process used, and compare it with the steps for conducting a survey described in this chapter. How are they similar? Different?
6. Use the Internet to contribute your ideas in response to a health-related survey taken by a television show, newspaper, or magazine, or share your opinions in a health-related chat room.

REFERENCES

Aboelata, M. J. (2010). The built environment and health: 11 profiles of neighborhood transformation. *Annals of the Rheumatic Diseases, 69*(12), 2062–2066.

Active Listening. (2010). *Care notes*. Retrieved from http://www.galenet.com.lp.hscl.ufl.edu/servlet/HWRC/hits?r=d&origSearch=true7bucket

Adcock, C., & Brown, L. (1957). Social class and the ranking of occupations. *The British Journal of Sociology, 8*(1), 26–32.

American Nurses Association (ANA). *Public health nursing: Scope and standards of practice*. Silver Springs, MD: Author.

American Public Health Association (APHA). Public Health Nursing Section. (2012). *The role of public health nurses*. Retrieved from http://www.apha.org/membergroups/sections/aphasections/phn/about/phnroles.htm

Anderson, E. T., & McFarlane, J. (2010). *Community as partner: Theory and practice* (6th ed.). Philadelphia, PA: Lippincott Williams & Wilkins.

Arcury, T. A., Vallejos, Q., Schultz, M., Feldman, S., Fleischer, A. B., Verma, A., & Quandt, S. A. (2008). Green tobacco sickness and skin integrity among migrant Latino farmworkers. *American Journal of Industrial Medicine, 51*(3), 195–203.

Artnak, K. E., McGraw, R. M., & Stanley, V. (2011). Health care accessibility for chronic illness management and end-of-life care: A view from rural America. *The Journal of Law, Medicine, and Ethics, 39*(2), 140–155.

Baisch, M. J. (2009). Community health: An evolutionary concept analysis. *Journal of Advanced Nursing, 65*(11), 2464–2476.

Bissette, J., Stover, J., Newman, L., Delcher, P., Bernstein, K. T., & Matthews L. (2009). Assessment of geographic information systems and data confidentiality guidelines in STD programs. *Public Health Reports, 124*(Suppl. 2), 58–64.

Blakely, E. J., & Leigh, N. G. (2010). *Planning local economic development: Theory and practice* (4th ed.). Thousand Oaks, CA: Sage Publications, Inc.

Brugge, D., Durant, J., & Rious, C. (2007). Near-highway pollutants in motor vehicle exhaust: A review of epidemiologic evidence of cardiac and pulmonary health risks. *Environmental Health, 6*, 23.

Cargan, L. (2007). *Doing social research*. Lanham, MD: Rowman & Littlefield.

Carpenito, L. J. (2008). *Nursing diagnosis: Application to clinical practice* (12th ed.). Philadelphia, PA: Lippincott Williams & Wilkins.

Carpenito, L. J. (2009). *Handbook of nursing diagnosis* (13th ed.). Philadelphia, PA: Lippincott Williams & Wilkins.

Carter, M. A. (2009). Trust, power, and vulnerability: A discourse on helping in nursing. *Nursing Clinics of North America, 44*(4), 393–405.

Centers for Disease Control & Prevention (CDC). (n.d.). *Prioritization*. Retrieved from http://www.cdc.gov/od/ocphp/nphpsp/documents/Prioritization.pdf

Centers for Disease Control & Prevention (CDC). (2011). *Data & statistics*. Retrieved from http://www.cdc.gov/datastatistics/

Centers for Disease Control & Prevention (CDC). (2012). *Behavioral Risk Factor Surveillance System*. Office of Surveillance, Epidemiology, and Laboratory Services. Retrieved from http://www.cdc.gov/brfss/

Chrisman, N. J. (2007). Extending cultural competence through systems change: Academic, hospital, land community partnerships. *Journal of Transcultural Nursing, 18*(Suppl. 1), S68–S76, discussion S77–S85.

Clark, C. R., Baril, N., Hall, A., Kunicki, M., Johnson, N., Soukup, J. et al. (2011). Case management intervention in cervical cancer prevention: the Boston REACH coalition women's health demonstration project. Progress in Community Health Partnerships, 5(3), 235–247.

Community Development Society. (2007). Principles of good practice. Retrieved from http://www.comm-dev.org

Cottrell, L. S., Jr. (1976). *The competent community*. In B.H. Kaplan, R.N. Wilson, & A.H. Leighton (Eds.). *Further explorations in social psychiatry* (pp. 195–209). New York: Basic Books.

Council on Education for Public Health (CEPH). (2011). *Outcomes assessment for school and program effectiveness: Linking planning and evaluation to mission, goals, and objectives*. Retrieved from http://www.ceph.org/pdf/LinkingProgramEvaluationtoMission.pdf

Curley, A. L., & Vitale, P. A. (Eds.). (2011). *Population-based nursing: Concepts and competencies for advanced practice*. New York: Springer Publishing Company.

Das, B., Rachman, M., Nayak, B., Pal, A., et al. (2009). Groundwater arsenic contamination, its health effects and approach for mitigation in West Bengal, India and Bangladesh. *Water Quality, Exposure and Health, 1*(1), 5–21.

DeVoe, J. E., Krois, L., & Stenger, R. (2009). Do children in rural areas still have different access to health care? Results from a statewide survey of Oregon's food stamp population. *The Journal of Rural Health, 25*(1), 1–7.

Ebi, K. L., & Semenza, J. C. (2008). Community-based adaptation to the health impacts of climate change. *American Journal of Preventive Medicine, 35*(5), 501–507.

Eriksson, I. & Nilsson, K. (2008). Preconditions needed for establishing a trusting relationship during health counseling—an interview study. *Journal of Clinical Nursing, 17*(17), 2352–2359.

Frieden, T. R. (2010). A framework for public health action: The health impact pyramid. *American Journal of Public Health, 100*(4), 590–595.

Furr-Holden, C., Campbell, K., Milam, A., Smart, M., Ialongo, N.A., & Leaf, P.J. (2010). Metric properties of the Neighborhood Inventory for Environmental Typology (NIfETy): An environmental assessment tool for measuring indicators of violence, alcohol, tobacco, and other drug exposures. *Evaluation Review, 34*(3), 159–184.

Gensberg, L. J., Pantea, C., Fitzgerald, E., Stark, A., Hwang, S. A., Kim, N. et al. (2009). Mortality among former Love Canal residents. *Environmental Health Perspectives, 117*(2), 209–216.

Glanz, K., & Bishop, D. (2010). The role of behavioral science theory in development and implementation of public health interventions. *Annual Review of Public Health, 31*, 399–418.

Gough, P. J. (2007). *Presidential candidates to debate over Internet*. The Hollywood Reporter. Retrieved from http://www.hollywoodreporter.com/hr/content_display/news/e3iaf82321e51c9ae093c3c40caeeba91eo0

Graves, A. (2009). A model for assessment of potential geographical accessibility: A case for GIS. *Online Journal of Rural Nursing and Health Care, 9*(1), 46–56.

Gushulak, B. D., & MacPherson, D. W. (2006). The basic principles of migration health: Population mobility and gaps in disease prevalence. *Emerging Themes in Epidemiology, 3*(3), 1–11. doi: 10.1186/1742-7622-3-3.

Gushulak, B. D., & MacPherson, D. W. (2011). Health aspects of the pre-departure phase of migration. *PLoS Medicine, 8*(5), e1001035. doi. 10.1371/journal.pmed.1001035.

Gwede, C., Ward, B., Luque, J., Vadaparampil, S., Rivers, D., Martinez-Tyson, D. et al. (2010). Application of geographic information systems and asset mapping to facilitate identification of colorectal cancer screening resources. *Online Journal of Public Health Informatics, 2*(1), 2893.

Hammond, D., Conlon, K., Barzyk, T., Chahine, T., Zartarian, V., & Schultz, B. (2011). Assessment and application of national environmental databases and mapping tools at the local level to two community case studies. *Risk Analysis, 21*(3), 475–487.

Haustein, T., Gastmeier, P., Holmes, A., Lucet, J., Shannon, R. P., Pittet, D., & Harbarth, S. (2011). Use of benchmarking and public reporting for infection control in four high-income countries. *The Lancet Infectious Diseases, 11*(6), 471–481.

Hawe, P., Shiell, A., & Riley, T. (2009). Theorising interventions as events in systems. *American Journal of Community Psychology, 43*, 267–276.

Holt, J., Mokdad, A., Ford, E., Simoes, E., Mensah, G., & Bartoli, W. (2008). Use of BRFSS data and GIS technology for rapid public health response during natural disasters. *Preventing Chronic Disease, 5*(3), A97.

Hughes, S. L., Seymour, R. B., Campbell, R. T., Whitelaw, N., & Bazzarre, T. (2009). Best-practice physician activity programs for older adults: Findings from the National Impact Study. *American Journal of Public Health, 99*(2), 362–368.

Issel, L. M. (2009). *Health program planning and evaluation: A practical, systematic approach for community health* (2nd ed.). Sudbury, MA: Jones & Bartlett Publishers.

Issel, L. M., & Bekemeier, B. (2010). Safe practice of population-focused nursing care: Development of a public health nursing concept. *Nursing Outlook, 58*(5), 226–232.

Issel, L. M., Berkemeier, B., & Baldwin, K. A. (2011). Three population-patient care outcome indicators for public health nursing: Results of a consensus project. *Public Health Nursing, 28*(1), 24–34.

Joynt, K. E., Harris, Y., Orav, J., & Jha, A. (2011). Quality of care and patient outcomes in critical access rural hospitals. *The Journal of the American Medical Association, 306*(1), 45–52.

Juhn, Y. J., Qin, R., Urm, S., Katusic, S., & Vargas-Chanes, D. (2010). The influence of neighborhood environment on the incidence of childhood asthma: A propensity score approach. *The Journal of Allergy and Clinical Immunology, 125*(4), 838–843.

Kaiser, K., Barry, T., Lopez, P., & Raymond, R. (2010). Improving access and managing population health through multidisciplinary partnerships. *Journal of Public Health Management and Practice, 16*(6), 544–552.

Kavanaugh, A., Perez-Quinones, M., Tedesco, J., & Sanders, W. (2010). Toward a virtual town square in the era of Web 2.0. In J. Hunsinger, L. Klastrup, & M. Allen (Eds.) *International Handbook of Internet Research* (pp. 279–294). New York: Springer.

Kazda, M., Beel, E., Villegas, D., Martinez, J., Patel, N., & Migala, W. (2009). Methodological complexities and the use of GIS in conducting a community needs assessment of a large U.S. municipality. *Journal of Community Health, 34*(3), 210–215.

Kneipp, S. M., Kairalia, J., Lutz, B., Pereira, D., Hall, A. G., Flocks, J. et al. (2011). Public health nursing case management for women receiving Temporary Assistance for Needy Families: A randomized controlled trial using community-based participatory research. *American Journal of Public Health, 101*(9), 1759–1768.

Knowlton, K., Lynn, B., Goldberg, R., Rosenzweig, C., Hogrefe, C., Rosenthal, J. K., & Kinney, P. L. (2007). Projecting heat-related mortality impacts under a changing climate in the New York City region. *American Journal of Public Health, 97*(11), 2028–2031.

Kramer, S., Seedat, M., Lazarus, S., & Suffla, S. (2011). A critical review of instruments assessing characteristics of community. *South African Journal of Psychology, 41*(4), 503–516.

Kretzman, J., & McKnight, J. (1993). *Building communities from the inside out: A path toward finding and mobilizing a community's assets*. Chicago, IL: ACTA Publications.

Laditka, J. N., Laditka, S. B., & Probst, J. C. (2009). Health care access in rural areas: Evidence that hospitalization for ambulatory care-sensitive conditions in the United States may increase with the level of rurality. *Health and Place, 15*(3), 761–770.

Lafferty, K. D. (2009). The ecology of climate change and infectious diseases. *Ecology, 90*, 888–900.

Lantz, P. M., Golberstein, E., House, J., & Morenoff, J. (2010). Socioeconomic and behavioral risk factors for mortality in a national 19-year prospective study of U.S. adults. *Social Sciences and Medicine, 70*(10), 1558–1566.

LeBan, K. (2011). *How social capital in community systems strengthens health systems: People, structure, processes*. Core Group. Retrieved from http://www.coregroup.org/storage/Program_Learning/Community_Health_Workers/Components_of_a_Community_Health_System_final10-12-2011.pdf

Lee, B. Y., Brown, S. T., Bailey, R. R., Zimmerman, R. K., Potter, M. A., McGlone, S. M. (2011). The benefits to all of ensuring equal and timely access to influenza vaccines in poor communities. *Health Affairs, 30*(6), 1141–1150.

Li, Y., Cao, J., Lin, H., Li, D., & He, J. (2009). Community health needs assessment with PRECEDE-PROCEED model: A mixed methods study. *BMC Health Services Research, 9*(10), 181. Retrieved from http://www.biomedcentral.com/1472-6963/9/181

McEntee, J., & Agyeman, J. (2010). Towards the development of a GIS method for identifying rural food deserts: Geographic access in Vermont, USA. *Applied Geography, 30*(1), 165–176.

Minnesota Department of Health. (2011). *Minnesota local public health assessment and planning*. Retrieved from http://www.health.state.mn.us/divs/cfh/ophp/system/planning/

Mitchell, R., & Popham, F. (2008). Effect of exposure to natural environment on health inequalities: An observational population study. *Lancet, 372*(9650), 1655–1660.

Mundinger, M. O., & Jauron, G. D. (1975). Developing a nursing diagnosis. *Nursing Outlook, 23*(2), 94–k98.

Nadig, L. A. (2010). *Tips on effective listening*. Retrieved from http://www.drnadig.com/listening.htm

National Association of County & City Health Officials (NACCHO). (n.d.). *First things first: Prioritizing health problems*. Retrieved from http://chfs.ky.gov/NR/rdonlyres/B070C722-31C1-4225-95D527622C16CBEE/0/PrioritizationSummariesandExamples.pdf

National Association of County & City Health Officials (NACCHO). (2007, November). *APEXPH, PACE EH, and MAPP: Local public health planning and assessment at a glance*. Retrieved from http://www.naccho.org/topics/infrastructure/mapp/upload/MappPaceApex.pdf

National Association of County & City Health Officials (NACCHO). (2012). *Integrating MAPP with other national initiatives: Questions and answers*. Retrieved from http://www.naccho.org/topics/infrastructure/mapp/QAnationalinitiatives.cfm

National Institutes of Health (NIH). (2011). *About NIH*. Retrieved from http://www.nih.gov/about/

Neckerman, K., Lovasi, G., Davies, S., Purciel, M., Quinn, J., Feder, E. (2009). Disparities in urban neighborhood conditions: Evidence from GIS measures and field observation in New York City. *Journal of Public Health Policy, 30*, s264–s285.

Neufeld, A., & Harrison, M. J. (1996). Educational issues in preparing community health nurses to use nursing diagnosis with population groups. *Nurse Education Today, 16*, 221–226.

Norris, F., Stevens, S., Pfefferbaum, B., Wyche, K., & Pfefferbaum, R. (2008). Community resilience as a metaphor, theory, set of capacities, and strategy for disaster readiness. *American Journal of Community Psychology, 41*(1–2), 127–150.

Northwest Center for Public Health Practice. (n.d.). *Module one: An overview of public health data*. Retrieved from http://www.nwcphp.org/docs/bcda_series/data_analysis_mod1_transcript.pdf

Nykiforuk, C., Flaman, L., Raine, K. D., Plotnikoff, R. C. et al. (2011). Geographic information systems (GIS) for health promotion and public health: A review. *Health Promotion Practice, 12*(1), 63–73.

Nykiforuk, C., Schopflocher, D., Vallianatos, H., Spence, J., et al. (2012). Community health and the built environment: Examining place in a Canadian chronic disease prevention project. *Health Promotion International*. doi: 10.1093/heapro/dar093.

Oberlander, J. (2010). Long time coming: Why health reform finally passed. *Health Affairs, 29*(6), 1112–1116.

Office of the Assistant Secretary for Planning & Evaluation. (n.d.). *Setting priorities and objectives*. USDHHS. Retrieved from http://aspe.hhs.gov/ezec/planning/setting.htm

Omaha System. (2011). *The Omaha System: Solving the clinical data-information puzzle*. Retrieved from http://www.omahasystem.org/overview.html

O'Reilly, G., O'Reilly, D., Rosato, M., & Connolly, S. (2007). Urban and rural variations in morbidity and mortality in Northern Ireland. *BMC Public Health, 7*, 123.

Ory, M., Liles, C., & Lawler, K. (2010). Building healthy communities for active aging: A national recognition program. *Generations, 33*(4), 82–84.

Pavlish, C. P., & Pharris, M. D. (2012). *Community-based collaborative action research: A nursing approach*. Sudbury, MA: Jones & Bartlett Learning.

Perry, C., & Hoffman, B. (2010). Assessing tribal youth physical activity and programming using a community-based participatory research approach. *Public Health Nursing, 27*(2), 104–114.

Petersen, D. D. (2011). Common plant toxicology: A comparison of national and Southwest Ohio data trends on plant poisonings in the 21st century. *Toxicology and Applied Pharmacology, 254*(2), 148–153.

Pham, K., Harrison, G., & Kagawa-Singer, M. (2007). Perceptions of diet and physical activity among California Hmong adults and youths. *Prevention of Chronic Disease, 4*(4), A93.

Platonova, E., Studnicki, J., Fisher, J., & Bridger, C. (2010). Local health department priority setting: An exploratory study. *Journal of Public Health Management and Practice, 16*(2), 140–147.

Polit, D., & Beck, C. T. (2010). *Essentials of nursing research: Appraising evidence for nursing pratice* (7th ed.). Philadelphia, PA: Lippincott Williams & Wilkins.

Quad Council. (2011, Summer). *Quad Council PHN Competencies for Public Health Nurses*. Retrieved from http://www.resourcenter.net/images/ACHNE/Files/QuadCouncilCompetenciesForPublicHealthNurses_Summer2011.pdf

Rabito, F. A., Carlson, J., Holt, E., Iqbal, S., & James, M. A. (2011). Cockroach exposure independent of sensitization status and association with hospitalizations for asthma in inner-city children. *Annals of Allergy, Asthma and Immunology, 106*(2), 103–109.

Radzyminski, S. (2007). The concept of population health within the nursing profession. *Journal of Professional Nursing, 23*(1), 37–46.

Ramos, R., Ferreira-Pinto, J., Brouwer, K., Ramos, M., Lozada, R. M., Firestone-Cruz, M., & Strathdee, S. A. (2009). A tale of two cities: Social and environmental influences shaping risk factors and protective behaviors in two Mexico-US border cities. *Health and Place, 15*(4), 999–1005.

Rhoads, J. (2007). Epidemiology of the brown recluse spider bite. *Journal of the American Academy of Nurse Practitioners, 19*(2), 79–85.

Rudan, I., Kapiriri, L., Tomlinson, M., Balliet, M., Cohen, B., & Chopra, M. (2010). Evidence-based priority setting for health care and research: Tools to support policy in maternal, neonatal, and child health in Africa. *PLoS Medicine, 7*(7), e10000308. doi: 10.1371/journal.pmed.10000308.

Sanders, B., Schneiderman, J., Loken, A., Lankenau, S., & Bloom, J. (2009). Gang youth as a vulnerable population for nursing intervention. *Public Health Nursing, 26*(4), 346–352.

Schoenbaum, S., Schoen, C., Nicholson, J., & Cantor, J. (2011). Mortality amenable to health care in the United States: The roles of demographics and health systems performance. *Journal of Public Health Policy, 32*, 407–429.

Seifert, S., Boyer, L., Benson, B., & Rogers, J. (2009). AAPCC database characterization of native U.S. venomous snake exposure, 2001–2005. *Clinical Toxicology, 4*, 327–335.

Sibbald, S. L., Singer, P. A., Upshur, R., & Martin, D. K. (2009). Priority setting: What constitutes success? A conceptual framework for successful priority setting. *BMC Health Services Research, 9*, 43. doi: 10.1186/1472-6963-9-43.

Spector, R. E. (2009). *Cultural diversity in health and illness* (7th ed.). Upper Saddle River, NJ: Prentice-Hall Allied Health.

Starks, S. E., Gerr, F., Kamel, F., Lynch, C. F., Alavanja, M. C., Sandler, D. P., & Hoppin, J. A. et al. (2011). High pesticide exposure events and central nervous system function among pesticide applicators in the Agricultural Health Study. *International Archives of Occupational and Environmental Health*. doi: 10.1007/s00420-011-0694-8.

Stevens, J., Thomas, K., & Sogolow, E. (2007). Seasonal patterns of fatal and nonfatal falls among older adults in the U.S. *Accidents: Annals of Prevention, 39*(6), 1239–1244.

Stolte, K. M. (1996). *Wellness: Nursing diagnosis for health promotion*. Philadelphia, PA: Lippincott Williams & Wilkins.

Swarts, H. (2011). Drawing new symbolic boundaries over old social boundaries: Forging social movement unity in congregation-based community organizing. *Sociological Perspectives, 54*(3), 453–477.

Theiss-Morse, E. (2009). *Who counts as an American? The boundaries of national identity*. Cambridge, UK: Cambridge University Press.

Tiesman, H., Zwerling, C., Peek-Asa, C., Sprince N., Cavanaugh J. E. (2007). Non-fatal injuries among urban and rural residents: The National Health Interview Survey, 1997–2001. *Injury Prevention, 13*(2), 115–119.

Timmons, V., Critchley, K., Campbell, B., McAuley, A., Taylor, J. P., & Walton, F. et al. (2007). Knowledge translation case study: A rural community collaborates with researchers to investigate health issues. *Journal of Continuing Education in the Health Professions, 27*(3), 183–187.

Townsend, J. S., Pinkerton, B., McKenna, S., Higgins, S., Tai, E., Steele, C. B. et al. (2011). Targeting children through school-based education and policy strategies: Comprehensive cancer control activities in melanoma prevention. *Journal of the American Academy of Dermatology, 65*(5, Suppl. 1), s104–s113.

Trinh-Shevrin, C., Pollack, H., Tsang, T., Park, J., Ramos, M. R., Islam, N. et al. (2011). The Asian American hepatitis B program: Building a coalition to address hepatitis B health disparities. *Progress in Community Health Partnerships, 5*(3), 261–271.

U.S. Census Bureau. (2011, November 15). *Mover rate reaches record low, Census Bureau reports*. Newsroom. Retrieved from http://www.census.gov/newsroom/releases/archives/mobility_of_the_population/cb11-193.html

U.S. Chamber of Commerce. (2012). *The marketing environment*. Retrieved from http://www.uschambersmallbusinessnation.com/toolkits/guide/P03_2046

U.S. Department of Health & Human Services. (2007). *The 2005 HHS poverty guidelines*. Retrieved July 25, 2008, from http://aspe.hhs.gov/poverty/05poverty.shtml

Williams, K., Bray, P., Shapiro, C., Reisz, I., & Peranteau, J. (2009). Modeling the principles of community-based participatory research in a community health assessment conducted by a health foundation. *Health Promotion Practice, 10*(1), 67–75.

Willis, K., Green, J., Daly, J., Williamson, L., & Bandyopadhyay, M. (2009). Perils and possibilities: Achieving best evidence from focus groups in public health research. *Australian and New Zealand Journal of Public Health, 33*(2), 131–136.

World Health Organization. (1998). *Primary health care in the 21st century is everybody's business*. Geneva, Switzerland: Author.

World Health Organization (WHO). (2008a). *Data and statistics*. Retrieved from http://www.who.int/research/en/

World Health Organization (WHO). (2008b). *The world health report*. Retrieved from http://www.who.int/whr/en/

Zahner, S., Kaiser, B., & Kapelke-Dale, J. (2005). Local partnerships for community assessment and planning. *Journal of Public Health Management Practice, 11*(5), 460–464.

CHAPTER

16

Global Health and International Community Health Nursing

"Our country is the world—our countrymen are mankind."

—***William Lloyd Garrison,*** American abolitionist (1805–1879)

KEY TERMS

Community health worker (CHW)
Control
Disability-adjusted life year (DALY)
Elimination
Era of Chronic, Long-Term Health Conditions
Era of Infectious Diseases
Era of Social Health Conditions
Eradication
Global burden of disease (GBD)
Global nursing
Health for All
Integrated management of childhood illness (IMCI)
Jakarta Declaration
Multilateral agencies
Oral rehydration therapy (ORT)
Ottawa Charter for Health Promotion
Pluralistic health care systems
Primary health care (PHC)
Universal imperatives of care
World Bank (WB)
World Health Assembly (WHA)
World Health Organization (WHO)
World Health Organization Collaborating Centers

LEARNING OBJECTIVES

Upon mastery of this chapter, you should be able to:

- Describe a context and framework for delivering community-based nursing within the context of international community health nursing.
- Describe the major health care conditions currently affecting the world's populations and the types and preparation of health care workers addressing them.
- Describe the community health nursing interventions and strategies commonly used within an international context.
- Recognize the factors that influence populations' perceptions of health and health status and their receptivity to community health nursing programs.
- Describe the personal and professional perceptions and biases you bring to providing community health nursing interventions within an international context.
- Identify the major international, national, regional, and local organizational structures and organizations that affect the ways in which community health nursing is practiced.
- Locate relevant resources as a basis for planning the assessment, implementation, and evaluation of community health nursing within an international context.

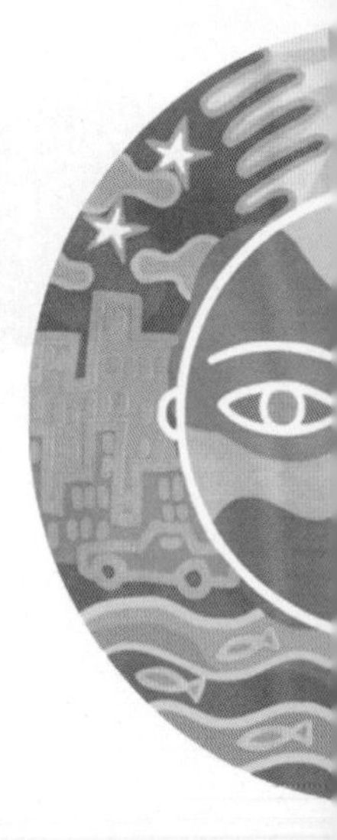

Let us suppose that you have completed your schooling and are ready to embark on a career in global community health nursing. **Global nursing** can range from providing clinical services to policy making at an international level. Perhaps you engaged in several years of successful clinical practice and are interested in pursuing an international opportunity to practice nursing in another country. You undertake a search of the World Wide Web, you talk to professional colleagues, and you read articles in nursing and other professional and popular journals.

You quickly realize that researching health care is a rather awesome undertaking, and the search for health care opportunities within a global context yields a plethora of Web sites, universities, and organizations going global. "By looking through a computer window, (students of your generation) are able, instantaneously, to see almost any place, to connect to almost any person, and to access information about almost any concept that has existed since people began to write down their ideas in the fourth millennium BCE" (Kanter, 2008, p. 115).

You also learn that community health care is complex and that it affects and is affected by multiple factors that have to do with geography, history, politics, culture, religion, and a nation's wealth. Your searches will be informative. You will notice that some countries' data are difficult to access, and you realize this may be because a country has been involved in a long, protracted civil war or has experienced continuous cycles of disasters or financial collapse.

In your search, you also find that people's conception of health, wellness, and illness varies from culture to culture and that the ways in which they view nurses and other health care providers is affected by their attitudes toward women, their culture, and belief systems. You will also notice patterns of privilege across countries and regions regarding who lives, who dies, the way people function on a day-to-day basis, the health care decisions they make, and the cost of the care they receive.

In your search, you also will learn a great deal about the health care providers that countries look to for nursing care and medical treatment. You will notice a disparity between the health status and health conditions of people in a country, as well as the kind of health care providers who are educated practicing in that country. For example, if you were to travel to mountainous areas, such as Nepal, you would see medications and treatments being administered without questions asked about the provider's credentials. The closest primary health care (PHC) station might be 20 miles away, and any relief from pain is welcome.

You may become sensitized to the difference between your kind of nursing education and that of the nurses in countries different from your own. The ways in which one is recruited and educated varies from country to country, as does legislation regarding licensure and entry to practice. For example, midwifery in the United States is based on a baccalaureate degree in nursing, while in Denmark, students have been admitted directly into a midwifery program without a nursing background and foundation. Yet in France, midwives are aligned with the field of medicine and see their practice from that standpoint rather than from a nursing perspective.

You will come across hundreds of references to international, national, and regional agencies that work in health care internationally. These references will be organized according to international agencies, national governments, universities, churches, and nongovernmental organizations (NGOs), including those with religious affiliations and those that are nondenominational.

Most importantly, you will become aware of your own approach to community health nursing. The ways in which practice takes place in an international context are influenced by all these factors and by your own personal background, your religious beliefs and attitudes, your orientation toward the theory of community health nursing practice, as well as your values and cultural beliefs. These factors and issues constitute a global framework for community health nursing, and they are the foci of this chapter. The question arises: How to put all of this in perspective, to apply a way of thinking to assist you in achieving your goal of an international nursing experience?

This chapter begins with a framework you can use to organize your thinking and around which you can structure your search as you expand your repertoire of knowledge and understanding. Those of us who work abroad need a framework in which to place our searches, professional dialogues, and readings. We need a compass to guide us as we conduct these searches for a match between us and the people we hope to serve. We also need a way of thinking about the communities, regions, or countries of the world and about the kinds of community health nursing interventions a country may need, given the elements described here.

A FRAMEWORK FOR GLOBAL COMMUNITY HEALTH NURSING

The Three P's

To guide your thinking, consider a global framework bounded by a context that includes three parts, the three "P's," and occurs over time through three generations of health care conditions. We begin with the three "P's"; these are the population, the provider, and the procedure. In community health nursing, our focus is on populations rather than individual patients. The provider refers to the health care team, which may include a community health nurse, a physician, a midwife, an "injector" (someone who is trained to only give injections), or a community health worker (CHW). The procedure refers to the interventions health care providers implement for or with populations.

In this global framework, alongside the three P's, think about three *eras* of health and health conditions. During our ancestors' time, populations of people died from the plague, tuberculosis (TB), puerperal fever, and other infectious diseases. Entire populations were sometimes eliminated through these infections. During this first era, families had many children, as they knew that most children would die before adulthood, and without any form of social security, children were their parents' only source of livelihood. Sons were preferred over daughters as sons ensured the family's livelihood and were capable of defending the community from enemies. This is referred to as the **Era of Infectious Diseases**. With the advent of antibiotics, people survived common infections. The lifespan of children was longer than that of their parents, but often, they suffered from chronic, long-term illnesses such as heart disease, cancer, and debilitating arthritis (King & Guralnik, 2010). This is referred to as the **Era of Chronic, Long-Term Health Conditions**. Despite changes and advances in health care, people continued to produce large families because of the cost or absence of birth control measures, persistent religious beliefs that influenced families regarding birth, and the intent of countries—such as Romania (before 1989)—to increase their populations for financial reasons. More recently, a new array of health conditions is affecting world populations, including addictions and obesity, and social conditions such as prostitution, sexual abuse, and deviant behavior. These are examples from the **Era of Social Health Conditions**. The popular press has exposed many of these conditions through documentaries on the effects of methamphetamine on entire communities, the obesity epidemic sweeping countries throughout the world, and the slave trade of young children (Skinner, 2010).

Continuing Emerging Health Conditions

Today, the communities of the world are experiencing all three eras of health conditions simultaneously. In one community, a population may be dealing with avian (bird) influenza, heart disease, cancer, adolescent prostitution, and mental illness. Most of these health conditions have been present for many years, some for thousands of years. Twenty-five years ago, public health specialists believed that infectious diseases would soon play a minor role in health. However, they are still the world's leading cause of death. Further, Davenport (2007), an expert in infection research, indicates that this era is experiencing what he calls a rebirth; some rates of infectious diseases have fallen but some have indeed risen. This trend is attributed, in part, to the increase in travel, the massive migration of populations occurring due to wars and civil uprising, and the economic situation forcing people to leave their home countries for employment. This chapter examines the context in which these conditions occur, the health care providers who work with them, and the ways in which interventions are applied through the work of many sponsoring global health organizations.

Universal Imperatives of Care

In addition to the three P's and the three eras of health conditions, community health nurses need to consider the current status of health in the community of interest. The **universal imperatives of care** is one useful paradigm. When we ask the question, how many nurses do a community need, part of answer have to do with these imperatives. These imperatives include mortality, morbidity, daily functioning, decision making, and cost of and access to health care. This paradigm underscores the notion of *first things first*. That is, one must be alive and well before interventions can focus on functioning or decision making (Fig. 16-1, Framework for Global Community Health Nursing).

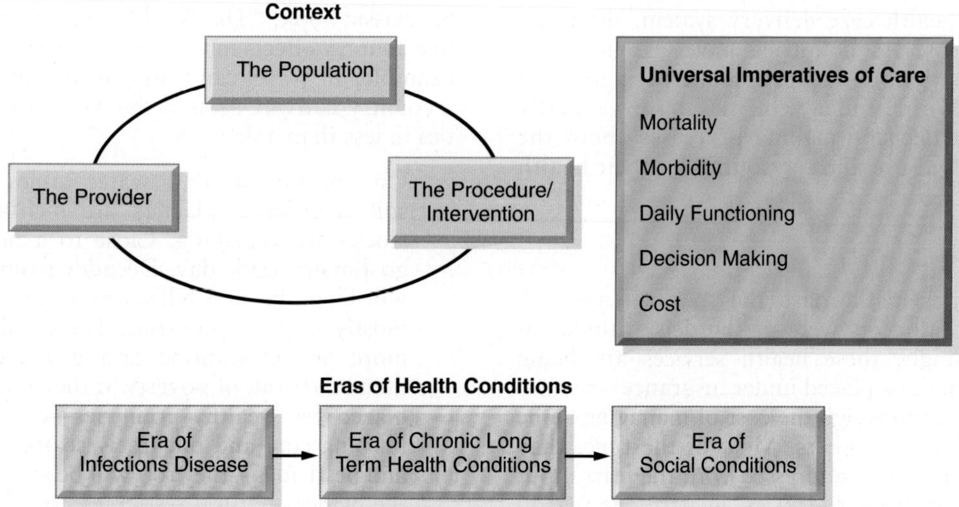

FIGURE 16-1. Framework for global community health nursing. (M. Farrell, 2012.)

Mortality

A government's first priority is to keep its population alive and free from illness. This is critical if a country is to survive, protect itself, and feed its population. In this regard, community health nurses may be frustrated that the disabled are going without community resources, programs are not created to help couples make informed decisions about abortion and birth control, or the mentally ill have no possibilities for therapy. However, when countries are poor, they will focus on preventing mortality and the evidence-based interventions that will ensure the survival of the people (Farrell, 2009). The health care team member required when mortality is a priority is the physician.

Morbidity

When people are not dying, a country can focus on its population's morbidity—the conditions that make people sick—and will look to physicians and nurses for assistance. Sickness derives from infectious diseases, long-term chronic health conditions, and the social conditions introduced above and will be discussed in more detail in upcoming sections.

Daily Functioning

In many countries, the ability to care for oneself—to bathe, secure food, and carry out other activities of daily living for fragile elderly or the disabled—is the purview of nurses, physical therapists, social services and social workers. However, in some countries, certain health care team members that nurses in the United States take for granted do not exist. Caring for an autistic child or a severely disabled parent is left entirely to the family. This is not because the government is negligent. It is because the universal imperatives in a country with constrained resources must focus on the necessities first.

Decision Making

In order to choose, one needs options. In countries with only one health care delivery system, there are no other options. As countries have expanded to include privatization, and as people increasingly have access to the World Wide Web, they have generally evolved in their decision-making processes about the providers they will use and the sources of their health information.

Cost

In many countries in the past, the state provided all health care, and all costs were the burden of the community. Increasingly, these health services are being rationed, restricted, or placed under insurance schemes. Nations are forced to weigh the cost of managing some health conditions over others. Most of the time, they opt for those that can be addressed with the least input and the maximum benefit. This is, in part, the reason that the Era of Social Conditions is not being addressed in many countries. The interventions that will reduce the incidence of these conditions are largely unknown, and the knowledge and research needed to access them are well beyond many countries' resources, thus encouraging these countries to work increasingly with the international community. Many countries do not have the resources to support the necessary research and programming to address the issues that may involve them and their border nations. In some countries with national health services that purport to provide all of a family's needs, a strong underground of health products and services is available to those who can afford to pay for them.

Access

Increasingly, a major concern is not only having the health services available to populations but the access to health services to the people. Access to health care refers to the ease with which an individual can obtain needed (health care) services. Several factors influence access worldwide. For example, people who speak the language, people who have insurance, and those who are part of the military establishment may have priority in some countries. Most often, the particular groups who go wanting include the poor, illiterate, those living in rural or remote areas, and in some places, women (due to religious taboos).

THE CONTEXT

A Context of Interdependency

The context of community health nursing suggests considering one planet of interdependent nations. This interdependence relates to virtually all areas of life, including health. By the end of 2011, the earth will be the home of seven billion people, with an estimated 10.5 billion by 2050. This number might be less, at 8 billion, if each woman has one child (Kunzig, 2011). As systems theory suggests and Friedman (2005) reiterates in his classic book, "The World is Flat," what happens in one country affects many others in important ways. For example, air travel can transport health problems from a country halfway around the world to new communities in less than a day.

> On our one Earth, "water tables are falling, soil is eroding, glaciers are melting, and fish stocks are vanishing. Close to a billion people go hungry each day. Decades from now, there will likely be two billion more mouths to feed, mostly in poor countries. There will be billions more people wanting and deserving to boost themselves out of poverty. If they follow the path blazed by wealthy countries—clearing forests, burning coal and oil, freely scattering fertilizers and pesticides—they too will be stepping hard on the planet's natural resources" (p. 43).

In addition to the number of people, the location and movement of populations is a major consideration. The number of migrants internationally has doubled over the past 25 years to 200 million people, and this migration trend Goldin, Cameron, and Balarajan (2011) predict will define the future more than environmental or weather patterns affecting the globe. These migrants sometimes settle in the country to which they have moved, others return to their native homeland. It is expected that the next wave will be people from Africa and will provide services that are needed in the recipient countries.

One example of a deadly migration involves the international spread of a virus. In New York, in the fall of 1999, 61 severe cases and 7 deaths were reported from a mysterious viral illness later identified as the West Nile virus (WNV), which had not previously been reported in the United States. Researchers now speculate that the virus may have traveled to the United States in smuggled exotic birds. The virus was closely related genetically to strains found in the Middle East. At its peak in 2003, a reported 9,862 cases related to WNV and 264 deaths had occurred in 46 states (Centers for Disease Control and Prevention [CDC], 2011a, 2011b).

The globalization of food commodities and food safety also affects health. For example, researchers suggest that a causal relationship exists between ongoing outbreaks in Europe of bovine spongiform encephalopathy, or *mad cow disease*, and the human disease called new variant Creutzfeldt–Jakob disease (vCJD). Of the worldwide total of 153 vCJD cases, 143 have occurred in the United Kingdom. Cattle are considered the only source of the disease (CDC, 2011c). Global health issues become everyone's concerns when they spread within or beyond one's borders, when we commit resources to a country in need, when we make a personal commitment to improve the health of a population beyond our shores, and when we import or export food.

These trends and examples underscore both the ways in which people are being exposed to the health conditions, food, and environmental effects that may originate in one part of the world and to the uniqueness of local communities with their own geography and environment, history, cultural traditions, religion, and ideas about health, wellness, disease, and death. The notion to think globally and act locally captures the essence of this seeming dichotomy. Each of these elements constitutes entire disciplines of study and requires years of interacting with people to understand the ways in which they affect health care in a particular country.

Geography and Environment

The environment in which people live includes air, climate, soil, and water, and each of these may undergo changes that turn natural elements into hazardous ones. Humans are exposed to pollutants in two basic ways: by exposure to the source or by release of the pollutant into air or water.

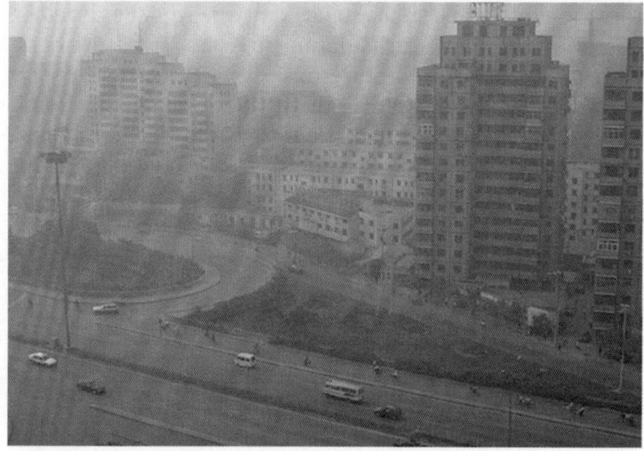

Air pollution in China. (Photo courtesy of CDC Photo Image Library.)

When people use streams and rivers to dispose of body wastes and then use the same body of water for cleaning and washing their clothes, they expose themselves to infections from those waters. For example, countries such as India, Indonesia, and Bangladesh—countries with large populations—have no choice as sewerage and clean water sources are not available in some parts of these countries. When people in villages build their homes around sources of water, they also invite mosquitoes that carry malaria, for instance. In this environment, community health nurses' interventions might include teaching people the steps to preventing malaria, such as placing netting around a bed during the night, cleaning pools of stagnant water around the home, covering the body with light cotton clothes (Heymann, 2008), and advising on the placement and maintenance of latrines.

People throughout the world are affected by the impact of major developments that may occur in their communities over which they have no control. Governmental authorities may build a dam, create a waterway, or move populations to clear land for crops (Reuters News Service, 2009). For example, populations in Ethiopia were moved from one part of the country to another as colonial rulers developed crops for their own use. In the process, they displaced farmers to other areas to grow crops about which they knew little and which were not appropriate for the soil and weather conditions. In the aftermath of a 6.9 magnitude earthquake in Armenian Soviet Socialist Republic (SSR), Union of Soviet Socialist Republics (USSR), the Italian Cooperation built temporary housing in the available surrounding areas. The government provided basic metal enclosures for housing that later were destroyed to provide long-term structures and roads, along with many other donations of goods and services from countries around the world (ReliefWeb, 2011).

Environmental experts have focused on these and other issues, such as the effects on communities when climate changes occur or when weather conditions affect entire regions. The volcano eruption in Iceland, the tsunami and subsequent damage to the nuclear reactors in Japan, the tsunami in Asia, and Hurricane Katrina in the United States are examples where entire communities were swept away (National Geographic Daily News, 2011). Over the past 5 years, the international meeting on the environment held in Copenhagen, Denmark, brought these issues to the forefront as did former United States Vice President and Nobel Prize winner, Al Gore, in his focus on global warming through his provocative and moving film, *An Inconvenient Truth*. In that film, Gore examined the ways in which our current habits and beliefs are affecting the world's temperature and environmental conditions (Bender, David, Chilcott, & Burns, 2006; Climate Crisis, n.d.).

Sometimes, change is intentional and is made in the interests of survival and daily functioning. For example, when governments address energy concerns for transportation and industry, they may move to nuclear sources of that energy—clearly as an effort to secure a local resource but also with some risk. The people in New Orleans experienced the aftermath of an oil rig disaster in the Gulf of Mexico as did the people of Chernobyl who found their homes a wasteland when the nuclear plant disaster polluted the region with cesium and iodine (Boston Globe, 2011). In a follow-up meeting to the Chernobyl accident, held a few years later in the Netherlands, representatives spoke of the population's fears and actions, including possessing machines that would measure the radioactivity near their homes. This accident prompted the discussion of disaster-preparedness strategies to evacuate entire cities of people after a nuclear environmental accident.

Classification of Environmental Hazards

The Organisation for Economic Co-operation and Development (OECD, 2010), World Health Organization (WHO, 2009b), and others have classified the environmental hazards affecting communities that include the impact of local climate changes on weather patterns and agriculture. The Blumenthal Classification lists classes of environmental hazards. They include infectious agents (e.g., bacteria and viruses), respiratory fibrotic agents (e.g., coal dust), asphyxiates (e.g., carbon monoxide), poison (e.g., pesticides), physical agents (e.g., noise), psychological agents (e.g., stressful synergisms such as crowding combined with noise), mutagens (e.g., dioxin), teratogens (e.g., cadmium), and carcinogens (e.g., cigarette smoke).

Contamination of Water Sources

Nearly 1 billion people lack access to safe water and 2.5 billion do not have improved sanitation; the implications for health are considered "staggering" (Water.org, 2011). More than 90% of waste water in developing countries is discharged untreated, polluting rivers, lakes, and coastal areas (Corcoran et al., 2010). In places such as Peru, Egypt, Bangladesh, India, Indonesia, and Thailand, raw sewage is released into rivers that are used for drinking and bathing. In Western Africa, parts of the ocean are contaminated with raw sewage. Such practices often result in diarrheal diseases, including cholera. The International Centre for Diarrhoeal Diseases Control Research (ICDDR) in Bangladesh specializes in those illnesses, including cholera that results from these practices, for which residents know of no alternative.

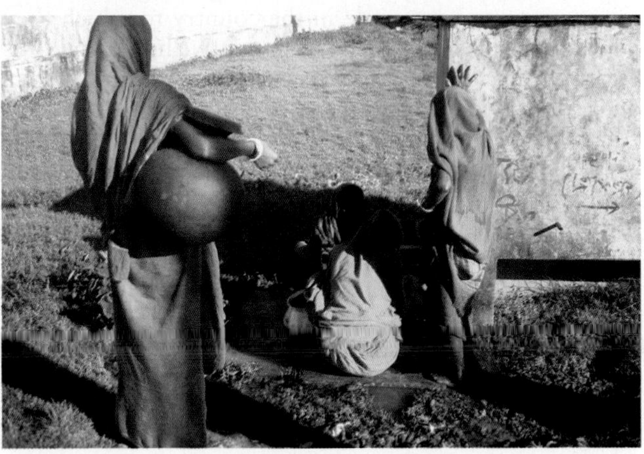

Women in a Bangladeshi village getting water from a communal well. (Photo courtesy of CDC Photo Image Library.)

Five million people die annually from illnesses linked to unsafe drinking water, poor household hygiene, and improper human and animal waste disposal. Ninety percent of all deaths caused by diarrheal diseases are children under 5 years of age, mostly in developing countries (United Nations-Water, 2008) (see Display 16.1, Major

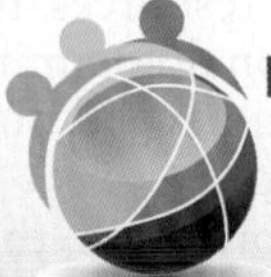

DISPLAY 16.1 ENVIRONMENTAL-RELATED KILLERS IN CHILDREN UNDER AGE 5

- Diarrhea kills 1.6 million children each year (mainly due to unsafe water and poor sanitation).
- Indoor air pollution kills 1 million children each year as a result of acute respiratory infections (due to use of biomass fuels for indoor cooking and heating).
- Malaria kills around 1 million children, mostly in Africa (exacerbated by poor management and storage of water, deforestation, and inadequate housing).
- Unintentional physical injuries account for 300,000 annual deaths due to drowning, fires, falls, poisoning, traffic accidents, and other causes (often related to community or household hazards).

From World Health Organization (WHO). (2012). *The environment and health for children and their mothers*. Retrieved from: http://www.who.int/ceh/publications/factsheets/fs284/en/

Environmental Killers in Children Under Age 5). Half of the population in the poor countries of the world suffers from one or more of the five main diseases associated with water and sanitation—diarrhea, ascariasis, hookworm, schistosomiasis, and trachoma—and one fourth of the world's population is without proper access to water and sanitation (WHO, 2009).

Water-related diseases arise from the ingestion of pathogens in contaminated water or food and from insects or other water-associated vectors. However, according to a classic text on developing countries, overall progress in reaching people deprived of adequate water and sanitation services has been poor since 1990 (Jamison et al., 2006).

The Ozone Layer

As the challenge of a depleted ozone layer is addressed, the incidence of cataracts and cancer (especially melanoma and basal cell carcinoma) is reduced. It is believed that human activities are contributing to the depletion of the ozone layer; these activities include the use of chlorofluorocarbons (CFCs) (used in the manufacture of air conditioners, refrigerators, aerosol propellants, and other products) and methyl bromides (found in pesticides and herbicides). Efforts are underway to phase out CFCs in 13 countries, including the United States (The Ozone Hole, n.d.).

History

If you have tea with a group of health care providers in Moscow, the conversation inevitably turns to the devastating effects of the major historical event that faced that country—World War II, or the Great Patriotic War. Despite the fact that this war occurred over 60 years ago, it remains in the collective memory of the Soviet people, their leaders, and many others in Eastern Europe, as 20 million Russians died along with thousands of people in other countries. That war, and the war that involved Bosnia–Herzegovina and Serbia, will affect people for decades to come and will influence the ways in which the health care systems of these countries will partner and collaborate with each other in the future.

The ways in which mental health was viewed historically was strongly influenced by its replacement in England of leprosy as a reminder of death and the need to rid the community of madness. Here, the response was to rid the community by sending the insane, first outside the gates of the cities, then on ships out to sea, in the famous Ships of Fools, only later to be turned over to doctors and housed in buildings referred to as "madhouses," through a process of incarceration enforced by the law. In this way, the mentally ill became inextricably linked to law enforcement (as described in the classic book by Foucault, 1965), and this link persists today. This form of power was expressed through laws that controlled not only the mentally ill but the poor and the unemployed.

Throughout the past century, other forms of power and control occurred throughout the world as countries were colonized and sometimes purged of their wealth. The relationship between those colonized and their colonizers persists today. These political relationships also affect the ways in which community health nurses might be recruited and practice. For example, given a country's history, health care providers with particular nationalities or religious backgrounds might not be acceptable to a country. While people in one country might consider these biases unacceptable, they remain as policy in other places, determining whether or not care providers of a particular nationality are allowed to enter and work in a country. These biases are often unexpected and may be puzzling. At first glance, one may wonder why Italy might want to support a disaster preparedness program in Ethiopia. But a review of the historical relationship between Italy and Ethiopia reveals a relationship that preceded the program initiative. In a similar way, for example, Chad has a past relationship with France, Mozambique with Portugal, the Congo with Belgium, Albania with Italy, and Indonesia with the Netherlands, to name just a few. This is further explained by Hochschild (1999) in his classic book. In addition to past relationships with other countries, communities also develop within the context of other relationships as well.

Community health nurses are involved in designing and implementing projects in collaboration with international governmental organizations and NGOs. In summary, the historical context of a country is paramount as people are selected for international positions and projects, for interventions that a community is willing to adopt, and organizations are chosen to intervene in a region.

Language

Often, a language connection exists between countries, and this linkage prompts health officials to seek nurses who speak the same language. For example, common history and language often connect Mozambique, Portugal, and Brazil, which are all Portuguese-speaking countries. Many people from Mozambique immigrated to Portugal during the 1970s, and the shared historical past affects current perceptions about the two countries' relationship with each other. Knowing that a shared language exists among countries may suggest ways of learning about cultural practices and about gathering existing health-related teaching and learning materials and can reduce the costs of production and language validation.

Political, Cultural, Religious Practices, and Context

A country's political orientation and practices affect the ways in which community health nurses are educated and function daily. For example, in some countries, nurses and midwives were not exposed to the emerging knowledge and practices concerning the HIV/acquired Immunodeficiency Syndrome (AIDS) epidemic. This happened, in part, because countries whose economies depended on tourism were fearful that high numbers of HIV-infected people would frighten away tourists. In other countries with closed borders and totalitarian regimes, health authorities were left out of the latest information on the epidemiology of diseases. In some countries, tribal practices took precedence over protection from the virus, and in other countries, the custom of visiting brothels resulted in epidemic rates of the virus. Consequently, national health policies and announcements denied the presence of the virus, people by the hundreds were infected, and nurses and midwives were not protected as they collected blood samples, administered injections, and delivered babies.

The culture and religion of a community represent the frame within which people understand who they are, why they are on the earth, and what their purposes are in life (Spector, 2008). Culture and religion influence the knowledge, attitudes, and practices of people about what they think will kill them or make them sick, will help them function or make decisions, or will affect their financial status. People in different cultures manage these in ways that may seem peculiar, ill-advised, immoral, or even criminal to someone outside the society. For example, Illyes (1979), in the classic book *People of the Puszta*, discussed the cultural practice of suicide in a part of Hungary, the Puszta, where people are characterized as "dirt poor." Yet, suicide is not a socially accepted option for people in other cultures. In the Philippines, some prostitutes see their activities as their daily work, not as a moral act. Efforts to dismantle the country's prostitution business have met with negative reactions from the prostitutes themselves, as this is their way of feeding their children and caring for their families.

Community health nurses will face their own beliefs when confronting female circumcision, the use of nonlicensed personnel to carry out medical treatments, and the use of Western interventions used simultaneously with local treatments. For example, in Chad, clients in a Chadian hospital received Western style medical treatment and nursing care through the interventions of French physicians and nurses while lines wound around the grounds of the hospital to the offices of the two Chinese acupuncturists. In rural villages in India, untrained midwives, or *dais*, may fail to treat a fever in women during the postpartum period regardless of its etiology.

Cultural issues are of concern when individuals and groups of a particular background from one country are often fiercely committed to "helping" their homeland. Here, both donors and recipients need to understand each other and their reasons for entering collaborative relationships. When this is thought through, the results can be most positive. In this regard, Armenian communities benefited enormously from the fund-raising efforts of U.S. community health nurses and physicians who knew well the Armenian communities in Boston, parts of Canada, and Los Angeles, and the American Albanian community was mobilized after the economic collapse of Albania in 1991. The same thing occurred after the "Arab Spring" uprisings in Egypt, with calls for wealthy Egyptian Americans to help support post-revolution Egypt (Eishinnawi, 2011).

Women and Culture

Women in most societies are viewed in ways that require close scrutiny. Historically, women in Western society during the Middle Ages and the Renaissance had an incentive to marry early as they had no legal status before the courts and had to generally be represented by a male proctor (DeMoor & Van Zanden, 2010). These practices persist today in some European countries and in other parts of the world where women, for example, must be accompanied by a male family member for health care (e.g., Saudi Arabia). Historically and today, poor women were and are particularly marginalized because of few opportunities for work. They were raised to produce children and were kept relatively secluded until marriage. If their spouses died, they entered a nunnery or prostituted themselves.

Women are seen as Madonnas, superheroes, warriors, nurturers, slaves, income producers, objects of sexual desire, concubines, negotiators, angels of mercy, and assistants. Although these characterizations may be repulsive to some, to others women in their communities have played these roles for so long that they are considered immutable and acceptable. In many countries, nurses are exclusively women and experience these projections as they carry out their daily work. In some places, women have no or little voice and are viewed as weak or ineffectual, despite their physiological hardiness and ability to survive above their male counterparts (Amanatullah & Morris, 2010). Kirk and Okazawa-Rey (2009) have documented the harmful economic, social, and military policies that they suggest have been imposed on the South and have wreaked havoc on U.S. working class and poor people of color as well as immigrant communities.

Community health nurses may perceive themselves as excellent practitioners with excellent theoretical and clinical backgrounds and expect to be respected for these qualities. Yet, in another country, their nursing notes may be torn up (who will read them?), their projects taken over by others (a nurse can't possibly lead a project), and their research may be published under someone else's name (anyone can write hypotheses, so what makes these so special?). In some countries, women (and nurses) are not expected to argue with authority, assume a team leadership role, or attend important meetings at high levels (Amanatullah & Morris, 2010).

These are challenging situations, some of which become teachable moments. Some may be events that alter the duration of one's assignment, or provide an opportunity to reframe interactions with others of differing persuasions, beliefs, and practices. Community health nurses need to determine their own position on these issues and come to terms with being placed in subservient positions or in roles that detract from their level of academic preparation, expectations for learning and developing, and ultimately, their sense of self. Yet, as noted below, women have played critical activist roles in the situations of crisis, conflict, and genocide.

Women carry the culture of a society, and they are inextricably linked with a country's history, conflicts, and their solutions. Here, women's issues intersect with issues of armed conflict, militarism, and their activism. In this section of this chapter, as in their lives, women provide a link between a society's culture and the wars in which the society engages. For example, Gallimore (2008) indicates that "women all over the African region have not only participated in, survived and resisted violent conflict, but played key roles in facilitating negotiations and peace-brokering efforts" (p. 6).

Armed Conflict, Uprisings, Wars, and Humanitarian Emergencies

An armed conflict is defined as major if the number of deaths has reached 1,000. Increasingly, conflicts are internal rather than between states. In their quest for economic and political power, the combatants target the lives and livelihoods of civilians associated with opposing factions. Typically, armed conflicts and uprisings initially cause governments and agencies to place a high priority on health care, but their ability to sustain health care is reduced as time goes on. Countries engaged in armed conflict form internal factions, including those supporting the government and those in conflict against them. Most conflicts occur between states for economic and political power. Currently, the world is experiencing another sea change as rebel forces in Egypt, Libya, Yemen, Syria, and other countries reject the existing regimes in power. Sometimes, outside nations support a country's factions, and fighting escalates and continues until the supporting powers win, lose interest, change their political orientation, or exhaust their financial sources. In this regard, community health nurses need to be aware of those involved in the immediate situation and of those who are influencing the situation from abroad. In turn, funding and sustaining nursing projects may depend ultimately on a variety of factors, not the least of which is being able to participate in situations that may be a threat to the nurse's safety and survival.

Countries that have long-standing conflicts suffer as current health care needs are unaddressed, and the long-term health status of an entire country may be affected—sometimes for decades. For example, Mozambique had endured a national conflict for over two decades. Two generations of young people had no formal education and were prepared only to fight. Countries in conflict deflect resources to the battlefield, and those fighting, identified as the males in the society, receive whatever resources are available despite the fact that women and children experience extreme devastation during these times. These conflicts are extremely complex social phenomena, for which the most rooted causes are inequity, cultural and religious intolerance, and ethnic discrimination (Sidel & Levy, 2008). The health infrastructure during conflicts and uprisings becomes vulnerable because of the instability. Often, opposing factions raid hospitals and clinics. For example, during the 1989 Romanian uprising, health providers told of instances in which the underground secret police feigned injury, transported themselves in rigged ambulances, and entered the emergency room areas of the capitol's major hospitals, all in an effort to kill or wound the hospitals' health care providers.

Between the end of World War II and the end of the Cold War, most conflicts occurred in developing countries in Africa, the Middle East, Asia, and Latin America. After the dissolution of the Soviet Union, major conflicts occurred in the emerging European states and subsequently in Yugoslavia (Brunner & Johnson, 2007). Wars in other areas of the world also were reignited, such as that between Eritrea and Ethiopia (Global Security, 2011). We have recently seen a similar situation in Iraq (Fearon, 2007).

The community interventions that nurses develop are informed by the situation and the layers of conflict that have occurred in the past and those that may be continuing (see From the Case Files I). During national conflicts, health services become disorganized and experience decreased resources. Outside help is needed in these instances, and international help is often available. For example, during the Romanian uprising, members of WHO/EURO international disaster preparedness team, along with the country's health officials, established an Interim Ministry of Health and identified key areas that required attention. Members of the team, including the Regional Nursing Advisor, met with NATO and COMECON ambassadors in the capitol and communicated the health needs of the population. They remained in Romania and established a WHO office, participating with groups, universities, and organizations to assist the country during this difficult period.

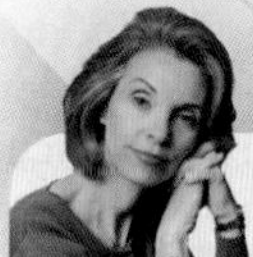

From the Case Files I

During the war in Yugoslavia, Bosnians and Serbs worked with the European Regional Office of the World Health Organization (WHO/EURO) in Copenhagen, Denmark, to develop interventions for women and children's health. WHO/EURO developed the training program to be held in Denmark but was not certain that the roads between Sarajevo and the coast would be open and safe for travel, as snipers continued to operate out of the mountains surrounding Sarajevo and along the roads to the country's borders. The workshop the nurses, physicians, and midwives attended in Copenhagen included both Bosnians and Serbs in the breakout sessions, but the facilitator had to ensure separate dining spaces, as the workshops occurred during the latter part of the war—a time during which communications were difficult and awkward.

Marie, WHO Regional Advisor

During wars and other man-made disasters, epidemics are almost inevitable. As conflict goes on, the health care needs of the combatants often take priority over those of civilians; consequently, thousands of children may be injured, orphaned, and at risk for disease. Additionally, conflict disrupts food cultivation, harvest, and distribution, leaving populations at risk for malnutrition and setting the stage for disease. Refugees from such events have special health and social needs. Often, refugee camps are developed by international organizations on the fringe of such conflicts to temporarily assist refugees with shelter, food, and the rudiments of health care. Such camps place a strain on the resources of neighboring countries, as illustrated during the recent war in Sudan (Warburg, 2010).

All of these factors can lead to complex humanitarian emergencies. The CDC describes complex humanitarian emergencies as situations that involve large civilian populations and factors related to war or civil strife, shortage of necessities such as food, and the dislocation of local populations. These situations and these factors result in mortality beyond that expected under normal circumstances (United Nations High Commissioner for Refugees [UNHCR], 2010).

Recovery after war is a long-term project. Any postwar recovery effort must deal with the disabled, the mentally ill, prisoners, widows, orphans, abandoned children, homeless and displaced persons, refugees, and the unemployed (Sidel & Levy, 2008; Siegel & Watson, 2006). In addition, livestock and domestic animals must be cared for or their carcasses buried or incinerated. These issues are complex; for example, in some African countries, if a family loses its land and its members cannot plant and harvest crops, the family dies. During the long conflict in that region, many women lost their husbands and their land. They required care from others who had very little to offer them. Currently, the rebel forces in the countries in conflict are poorly equipped, have experienced severe injuries, and require interventions from a population also under siege.

In these environments, populations are displaced and people find themselves living in war zones that are strewn with the remnants of the war (Sidel & Levy, 2008; UNHCR, 2010). Land mines have continued to injure or kill long after hostilities have ceased. This issue received international attention from Princess Diana of Wales, who made their removal one of her major projects before her untimely death and continues with her sons (The Halo Trust, 2011).

Health Promotion

It is not enough to strive to protect individuals from disease or adverse events, but as the title of this book states, health promotion is also vital. This paradigm shift was exemplified in the **Ottawa Charter for Health Promotion.** The first international conference on health promotion took place there in 1986, and prerequisites were outlined: peace, shelter, food, income, education, a stable ecosystem, sustainable resources, and social justice/equity (WHO, 2012i). The participants acknowledged that health is created by individuals each day as they care for themselves and others. The conference ended with this pledge:

- to move into the arena of healthy public policy and to advocate a clear political commitment to health and equity in all sectors
- to counteract the pressures toward harmful products, resource depletion, unhealthy living conditions and environments, and bad nutrition and to focus attention on public health issues such as pollution, occupational hazards, housing and settlements
- to respond to the health gap within and between societies; to tackle the inequities in health produced by the rules and practices of these societies; to acknowledge people as the main health resource; to support and enable them to keep themselves, their families, and friends healthy through financial and other means; and to accept the community as the essential voice in matters of its health, living conditions, and wellbeing
- to reorient health services and their resources toward the promotion of health and to share power with other sectors, other disciplines and, most importantly, with people themselves
- to recognize health and its maintenance as a major social investment and challenge and to address the overall ecological issue of our ways of living (WHO, 2012d, p. 3)

At the fourth international conference on health promotion in 1997, the **Jakarta Declaration** on Leading Health Promotion Into the 21st Century was developed (WHO, 2012e). This was the first health promotion conference held in a developing country (Jakarta, Indonesia). Participants acknowledged that "health is a basic right and is essential for social and economic development" (p. 1). They noted that comprehensive approaches are most effective, specific settings (e.g., workplaces, schools, cities, health care facilities) are best for implementation of these strategies, and that individual participation is critical and can be facilitated by proper information and education. Priorities for 21st century health promotion include the following:

- Promote social responsibility for health
- Increase investments for health development
- Consolidate and expand partnerships for health
- Increase community and empower the individual
- Secure an infrastructure for health promotion (p. 3)

Governments were called on to promote health within their own countries and work together to create alliances, and this was again emphasized at the sixth international conference in Bangkok, which produced the *Bangkok Charter for Health Promotion in a Globalized World* (WHO Media Centre, 2005). This document called for "policy coherence, investment and partnering across governments, international organizations, civil society and the private sector to work toward four key commitments": (1) keeping health promotion as a central focus of global development; (2) ensuring that all governments recognize health promotion as a core responsibility (legislation, regulation, policy development, investment); (3) promoting health as a factor of good corporate practice; and (4) advocating for health as a vital right of civil society (para 3).

Many countries have agencies that promote health within their boundaries and assist in health and development in other countries (e.g., Canadian International Development Agency [CIDA], National Primary Healthcare Development Agency [NPHCDA] in Nigeria, U.S. CDC). Nongovernmental organizations (NGOs) from many countries also work together to promote health and assist in community development (Aga Khan Development Network, Oxfam, Project HOPE).

Health Care Systems

Countries throughout the world have developed health care systems that they organize and structure in particular ways. When community health nurses find themselves in locations different from their own, they notice differences immediately, and their ability to practice within the context of these different ways of delivering health care services is critical to their success. The capacity to reflect on one's consciousness is an essential skill as one considers the ways in which people expect to govern others, provide people with what they need, determine who gets served and who does not, establish lines of authority and communication, and establish payment systems for health care services.

Important questions arise as one delivers community health nursing services within a country's health care system. For example, if a client has to wait 6 months for elective surgery, what does he or she do in the meantime? If a government provides all prenatal and obstetrical services but will not instruct couples on birth control, how do couples manage, and how do health authorities deal with prevalent practices that result in an abortion rate that is three times the birth rate (as documented in a classic article by Farrell et al., 1994) or that allow *under the table* reimbursement for these services? If a ministry of health is administered through a centrally governed model of decision making, how do decisions get made that require local—rather than district or national answers? If a local nursing group is interested in developing community health nursing standards of practice, and yet all nursing actions are reviewed by only a medical board of physicians, on what are the nursing standards based?

Pluralistic health care systems are found in many countries. They often consist of traditional healing systems, lay practices, household remedies, transitional health workers, and practitioners of Western medicine (Ginsburg, Doherty, Ralston, & Senkeeto, 2008). Traditional healing may be all that is available to populations in some rural areas and in some cities.

Western medicine was introduced to some countries during colonial times, and systems were operated either by colonial administrations or by missions. After independence, health systems tended to vary in their development. Some continue their colonial practices; others followed tax-financed government insurance or socialist health care systems (Crisp, 2010).

During the second half of the 20th century, curative health care expanded rapidly in urban areas, and the level of health care was raised in those areas. In the late 1970s, many countries adopted the PHC approach and the WHO regions of the world developed their own set of targets. For example, in the United States, *Healthy People 2000* and *Healthy People 2010* were developed (we now have *Healthy People 2020*); the European Region of WHO developed its *38 Regional Targets for Health*, and within these targets, nursing's program was elaborated. Throughout the world, countries used this approach to serve their urban and rural populations. Four major types of health care systems are currently operational throughout the world. These systems are entrepreneurial, welfare-oriented, comprehensive, and socialist systems.

- *Entrepreneurial health care systems.* A country's health care system is based, in part, on its political economy. An entrepreneurial health system is typically found in industrialized countries with free-market economies, abundant resources, large amounts of money allocated to health care, and decentralized governments. These countries operate from a highly individualistic perspective. For example, the health care system in the United States is typical of the entrepreneurial system (Ginsburg et al., 2008).
- *Welfare-oriented health care systems.* Statutory programs drive these systems that support the cost of health care for all, or almost all, of the population through their "national health insurance." In these, half of the health-related expenditures are covered by government sources, but most physicians and dentists remain in private practice. Western Europe, Japan, and Australia subscribe to welfare-oriented health care systems.
- *Comprehensive health care systems.* These systems are a step away from the welfare-oriented types in that substantial modifications exist in delivery and financing that result in universal entitlements. These systems abandon the separate and complex sources of financing found in the previous two systems. The Scandinavian countries, Great Britain, and New Zealand use a comprehensive health care delivery system.
- *Socialist health care systems.* These systems came about through social revolutions that abolished free-market economies and replaced them with socialism, in which the health care system is also socialized. The first overthrow of capitalism was in Russia in 1917, followed by Eastern Europe, Albania, Bulgaria, Czechoslovakia, Hungary, Poland, Romania, and later China. In these systems, health services were viewed as a social entitlement and a government responsibility. They emphasized prevention and engaged in central planning for health resources and services with one central health authority. They also prioritized special groups, such as industrial workers and children, and based health care work on scientific principles. Nonscientific and cultist practices were not permitted. Many of these countries are now in the process of democratization and are attempting to redesign their health care systems.

The four health systems described above apply to industrialized countries. The renowned health system researcher Roemer (1993) used the same typology for transitional and very poor countries. (Countries that are in the process of development are referred to as "transitional.") Such countries and their health care systems are moving effectively toward economic and social development. The global median gross national product (GNP) of these countries is $1,500 per capita. (It should be noted that some might object to this classification system that considers being financially poor synonymous with being socially underdeveloped. This suggests a bias in thinking and a Western perspective that determines what is "developed" and what "needs developing.")

Very poor countries are even less economically developed and have lower per capita GNPs than do the industrialized or transitional countries. Countries classified as "very poor" have historically included Ethiopia, Kenya, Ghana, Myanmar, Sri Lanka, and Mozambique. China's economic rise has moved it out of that classification. Other countries that do not easily fit into the health care system matrix are the oil-rich developing countries. In just a few years, the wealth in such countries exploded upward, from low levels typical of Africa and some Asian countries to levels equal to or greater than those of highly industrialized countries. Examples are Gabon, Libya, Saudi Arabia, and Kuwait. The governments of these countries have, to some degree, used their income to extend and improve health services for the general population. Entrepreneurial or socialist systems are not found in these countries. Gabon and Libya are classified as welfare-oriented because they have different schemes of social insurance for health services for a large percentage of the population. Saudi Arabia and Kuwait have been classified as universal and comprehensive systems that use government funding to provide complete health services to everyone. How some of these countries will be classified in the future, however, is a question, given the civil strife currently underway.

Trends Affecting Health Care Systems

Health care systems are affected by major social factors such as urbanization, industrialization, education, government structure, international trade, and demographic changes. Many national health systems have undergone major changes during the 1980s, 1990s, and 2000s. Specifically, these health care systems have changed the way they organize and are managed. For example, in England, health services were traditionally led by health care professionals. In the mid-1980s, the emerging view was that one did not have to be a health provider to manage the health services of the country. Increasingly, health care administrators who were not from the health service ranks assumed these positions, and the composition of health leadership changed. Health care systems that were totally funded by national health services are moving to privatization of their services, while the United States is heading toward health care reform.

Health care systems also expanded their resources and added personnel, facilities, and equipment. Meanwhile, populations grew, migrated, and became more educated. They demanded more and better health care services. Over the past decade, hospitals worldwide have shifted to outpatient services and home care, expanding the roles and positions of community health nurses. Currently, in the United States, this trend has resulted in the closing of community hospitals, to the consternation of many in the community (Tribble, 2011).

Hospitals in Denmark benefited from a surgical procedure for hip replacement that would allow a patient to be discharged from hospital to home in a much shorter time period than previously experienced. This meant that home care had to be ready to accept the patient within an abbreviated time frame, thus requiring innovations in discharge planning and teaching protocols. In addition to these advances, the PHC movement supported efforts to reduce the number of hospital buildings and to increase community-based nursing services (Husted et al., 2011).

Technological advances occurred to support this move, and ways of thinking about health promotion emerged with a variety of quality measures and, more recently, evidence-based practices that support nursing interventions on an outpatient basis and at lowered costs. The depopulation of some communities and the increasing number of empty beds have also been related to these closings.

Most importantly, people have begun to educate themselves through the Internet and World Wide Web. Ministries of health are training community care workers in communication, observation, and technical skills for telemedicine systems that link remote areas to academic health centers. For example, a health center in Almaty, Kazakhstan, is now connected through the Internet, even though it began as a relatively isolated center in what was referred to as Alma-Ata. Now, groups with relatively rare health care conditions can receive support and information from others in parts of the world formerly unknown to them.

THE POPULATION

The populations that community health nurses serve are complex and include clients' concerns, values, beliefs, physical symptoms, and health history. As described earlier, the framework that provides some boundaries for considering these issues focuses on context, the three eras of health conditions, and the universal imperatives of care.

Era of Infectious Diseases

Infectious diseases and conditions have killed people, made them sick, altered their daily functioning, influenced their decision making, and affected the costs of care. Thus, these infections and infectious processes involve all the universal imperatives of care but do so differently, depending on a variety of factors (Davies,

2008). These factors include the climate, geography, and other conditions infectious organisms need to survive and thrive and the populations the infectious agents invade–often infants and children. Thus, it is not surprising that 98% of all deaths in children younger than 15 years of age are in those countries in which infectious diseases are rampant. Eighty-three percent of deaths of those aged 15 to 59 years are in these countries as well. The probability of death before age 15 ranges from 22% in sub-Saharan Africa to only 1.1% in countries with established market economies. Five of the ten leading causes of death are communicable, perinatal, and nutritional maladies that largely affect children. Most of these are preventable. The major preventive measure, immunization, is described here, followed by brief descriptions of some of the major infectious diseases. (See Display 16.2 for a ranked listing of the leading causes of death worldwide.)

Immunization

The WHO estimates that 3 million more lives could be saved each year with immunizations. One of the most cost-effective interventions available has been developed through the WHO Expanded Program on Immunization (Reingold & Phares, 2006). Vaccines are one of the most cost-effective interventions found in public health. Today, almost three fourths of the world's children are being reached with essential vaccines, but many barriers make it difficult to maintain high levels of immunization in low- and middle-income countries. Measles deaths worldwide fell by 74% between 2000 and 2007 (Kiem, 2009), but in the United States, 2009 figures note that 10% of toddlers had not received any measles, mumps, and rubella (MMR) vaccinations (Goodman, 2011).

Barriers persist and include limited finances, lack of trained health care workers, physical obstacles to reaching remote areas, and civil wars; these factors have prompted the development of an interagency vaccine initiative entitled the Global Alliance for Vaccine and Immunizations. This initiative seeks to protect every child against vaccine-preventable diseases (Reingold & Phares, 2006). Strategies include funding, research, development, distribution of vaccines, and program sustainability. These approaches are expected to result in more immunized children and to move newer vaccines into developing countries more quickly.

Measles

Measles is a vaccine-preventable communicable disease. In 2008, the number of measles deaths was 164,000. The largest number of deaths—95%—occurred in low-income countries with inadequate health infrastructures (WHO Media Centre, 2011c). The intervention considered to have the greatest impact in reducing measles is the **integrated management of childhood illness (IMCI)**. This intervention promotes wide immunization coverage, rapid referral of serious cases, prompt recognition of secondary conditions, improved nutrition including breast-feeding, and vitamin A supplementation. Three main foci include improving health systems and case management skills, along with community and family health practice improvement (WHO, 2011). A WHO/UNICEF Measles Mortality Reduction and Regional Elimination Strategic Plan sought a 50% reduction in measles mortality worldwide by 2005—hoping eventually to eradicate the disease. Measles deaths actually fell worldwide by 74% between 2000 and 2007 (Kiem, 2009).

Poliomyelitis

In 1988, there were 35,000 annual cases of poliomyelitis (polio) in the world. By 1991, polio was eliminated from the Western hemisphere. Polio is now

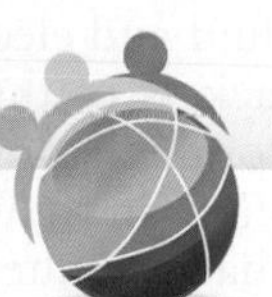

DISPLAY 16.2 RANKED DEATHS BY RISK FACTOR GROUP, WORLDWIDE

Child/Maternal Undernutrition

Child underweight
Suboptimal breastfeeding
Vitamin A deficiency
Zinc deficiency
Iron deficiency
Iodine deficiency

Diet/Physical Inactivity

High blood pressure
High blood glucose
Physical inactivity
Overweight/obesity
High cholesterol
Low fruit/vegetable intake

Environmental

Indoor smoke from solid fuels
Unsafe water/sanitation/hygiene
Urban outdoor air pollution
Global climate change
Lead exposure

Alcohol, Tobacco, Illicit Drug Use

Alcohol use
Illicit drugs
Tobacco use

Source: World Health Organization (WHO). (2009a). *Global health risks: Mortality and burden of disease attributable to selected major risks*. Geneva: Author.

almost eliminated worldwide, even in densely populated and war-torn countries. Yet this author witnessed parents in Chad, Africa, exercising their polio-handicapped child through daily exercises. Since the inception of the Global Polio Eradication Initiative, cases have fallen by over 99% and the number of polio-infected countries dropped from 125 to 10. Fifteen previously polio-free African countries were reinfected in 2009, and by late 2010, 10 of them were able to stop their outbreaks. Two endemic states in India—Uttar Pradesh and Bihar—had not reported any wild polios virus cases for over 6 months. Since 1985, over 1,000 children in 125 countries were paralyzed each day from polio. Rotary International contributed over $900 million dollars between 1985 and 2010 to help eradicate this disease. The CDC, WHO, UNICEF, and many national governments support the Global Polio Eradication Initiative. Only Afghanistan, India, Pakistan, and Nigeria remain endemic for polio (WHO Media Centre, 2011d).

Pandemic Influenza

The WHO, in cooperation with many other organizations and agencies, prepared for the H1N1 influenza pandemic of 2009 to 2010. The United States has a pandemic influenza plan (see *http://www.hhs.gov/pandemicflu/plan/*) that outlines public health and medical support, guidance for state and local health departments, and an operational plan for the U.S. Department of Health and Human Services. The response to this novel virus may have seemed to many to be an overreaction—this was simply "the flu." But an H1N1 virus was responsible for the 1918 influenza pandemic that killed over 50 million people worldwide (much more than the 16 million lost in World War I), and it appeared without warning in late spring. It surfaced again in fall and was much more virulent, with some victims dying "within hours of their first symptoms" (para 3). Young adults, along with children and the elderly, were most susceptible to complications and U.S. life expectancy "dropped by 12 years" during 1918 (National Archives & Records Administration, n.d., para 4).

Because of this earlier pandemic experience with H1N1, WHO issued worldwide cautions and preparations, and scientists raced to produce enough specific vaccine for global demand (Khazeni, Hutton, Garber, Hupert, & Owens, 2009). Researchers ran statistical models to predict transmissibility and control measures (Yang et al., 2009). Even though more recent reexaminations of preserved lung tissue samples from soldiers who died of influenza in 1918 found a majority of deaths due to bacterial pneumonia secondary to the flu, it was deemed important to take precautionary measures. This bacteria is commonly found in the nose and throat, but as H1N1 obliterated cells lining the bronchial tubes and lungs, it invaded the lungs causing pneumonia (National Institute of Allergy and Infectious Disease [NIAID], 2008). While we now have antibiotics to combat influenza complications, an influenza pandemic can still wreak havoc on economies and societies. And with medication-resistant bacteria now commonplace, our theoretical protection from previous flu pandemics in 1958 and 1967 may no longer hold (NIAID, 2008).

In August 2010, WHO announced that the world was no longer "in phase 6 of influenza pandemic alert" and that the virus had "largely run its course" and was now behaving more as a seasonal influenza (para 1). WHO cautioned that vigilance is still needed in this postpandemic period as the virus will continue to cause serious cases among the younger age groups, and pandemics are unpredictable (WHO, 2010).

Diarrheal Diseases

Diarrhea is defined as the passage of more than three stools during a 24-hour period for individuals older than 3 months of age. The incidence of diarrheal diseases is somewhat elusive because it depends on the definition of diarrhea used, the frequency of surveillance, and the population. Sometimes, public health professionals use the term *diarrhea* to mean dysentery, although the latter is usually characterized by the presence of blood in the stool, with or without looseness or specified frequency.

Among other causes, a host of enteric pathogens can result in diarrhea; these pathogens are most significant in countries where there is poverty, poor personal and domestic hygiene, infected water, low maternal education, and lower occupational status. These factors have been associated with diarrheal morbidity and mortality (Heymann, 2008; Zwane & Kremer, 2007).

The risk is highest among infants who are not breast-fed. Each year, an estimated 2.2 million children die from diarrhea and related illnesses (Rehydration Project, 2010).

Reductions in mortality rates have occurred; in some areas, as many as 90% fewer deaths have been reported. This was largely the result of the promotion of **oral rehydration therapy (ORT)**, a simple treatment available since the 1970s that mothers may administer to their children in order to replace lost fluid and electrolytes (PATH, 2008) (Display 16.3). Packets of this powder are added to clean water to make oral rehydration solution (ORS), and new lower sodium and glucose formulations (low-osmolarity ORS) have resulted in 25% reductions in stool output, 30% less vomiting, and one-third fewer unscheduled IV therapies (PATH, 2008). Actions need to prevent diarrheal disease include community programs that promote personal and domestic hygiene, water supply and sanitation facility improvements, promotion of breast-feeding and improved weaning practices, zinc treatment, and immunizations for cholera, measles, and rotavirus (Rehydration Project, 2010).

Wide implementation of seven preventive interventions (improved water sources, sanitation, and household water treatments; breast-feeding; hand washing with soap; vitamin A supplementation; rotavirus vaccination) and three treatment interventions (ORS, zinc supplementation, and use of antibiotics for dysentery)

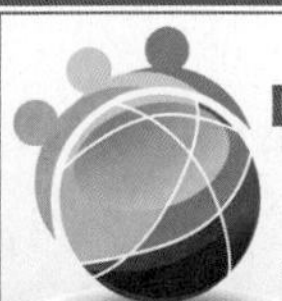

DISPLAY 16.3 HOW TO PREPARE HOMEMADE ORAL REHYDRATION SOLUTION (ORS)

- If ORS sachets are available: dilute one OR sachet in 1 L of safe water.
- Otherwise, make your own:

Use 1 L of safe water (clean or boiled and then cooled)—about 5 cups—and add:

Salt—1/2 level teaspoon
Sugar—6 level teaspoons

- Home remedy for watery diarrhea:

½ to 1 cup precooked rice baby cereal
(or 1½ tablespoon granulated sugar)
2 cups water
½ teaspoon salt

Note: Solutions should not taste saltier than human tears. Extra liquids are needed until diarrhea ceases.
From Rehydration Project. (2012). *Oral rehydration solutions made at home*. Retrieved from: http://rehydrate.org/solutions/homemade.htm#recipe

could drop the rate of child diarrheal deaths by 92% (Walker et al., 2011). No single type of intervention has greater overall impact on national development and public health than does the provision of safe drinking water and proper disposal of human excreta. Promising research in this area includes improvement of zinc treatments, vitamin A supplementation, and increased access to ORS packets, as well as increasing measles and rotavirus vaccination rates (Kosek et al., 2009).

Acute Respiratory Tract Infections

The most common illness in the world and a leading cause of mortality is acute respiratory tract infection (ARI). Three million deaths annually are attributed to ARI among children younger than 5 years of age, usually from pneumonia. Risk factors include low birth weight, poverty, crowding, lower educational levels, poor nutrition, inadequate child care practices, and a lack of health education about ARI. Additional risk factors include smoking and indoor and outdoor air pollution. Indoor air pollution is 20 times higher in villages in poor areas than in homes in those countries of the world where people smoke two packs of cigarettes (Schlein, 2007). The source of pollution is largely indoor cook stoves that use organic fuel. Indoor cooking stoves kill 2 million people annually more than malaria (Sheridan, 2011). A threat to the reduction of pneumonia, however, is the increase in drug-resistant organisms. Measures to better control ARI include immunizations, birth spacing, and improvement in nutrition and living conditions (including use of smokeless cooking stoves). A global commitment to reduce ARI was realized by a resolution at the World Summit for Children in 1990 that called for a one-third reduction in deaths from the condition. This goal has been difficult to achieve because of the varying clinical symptoms and causative organisms of pneumonia (see Levels of Prevention Pyramid).

Human Immunodeficiency Virus Infection and Acquired Immunodeficiency Syndrome

An estimated 33.2 million people worldwide are living with HIV infection, but true figures are difficult to reach. Human immunodeficiency virus (HIV) prevalence worldwide is thought to be 0.5% of the world's population, and prevalence rates for Africa are substantially higher than for Asia and North America (Brookmeyer, 2010). Recent research has led to the current practice in developing countries of early treatment for anyone with HIV. This has been due to the relatively recent success in the combination of antiretroviral treatment. This practice is tempered by the incidence of toxicity due to the treatment; nevertheless, delays are reportedly related to heightened illness and death. Experts expect policy shifts will focus on pregnant women and infants, antiretroviral interventions will become less costly, and strengthened delivery systems will be developed. Some also predict that "early interventions may have an impact on transition of the HIV virus" (Hobbs & Essajee, 2009, p. 222). Asia and Eastern Europe are experiencing epidemic rates of HIV/AIDS cases. Russia reported increases, and HIV is beginning to spread among high-risk populations in some Middle Eastern countries (Abu-Raddad et al., 2010). It is predicted that life expectancy in African countries is likely to decline by as much as 27%.

The virus attacks young adults in productive age groups, requiring older people to care for and support their terminally ill adult children and, later, their orphaned grandchildren. Often, these elders are themselves impoverished and in poor health and are left without caregivers when they require assistance in their later years. The HIV/AIDS epidemic threatens to upset and destabilize entire societies in Africa. Reduced productivity of adult workers and early death are counterproductive to economic and social development.

An expanded global response to the pandemic offered 12 essential interventions to reduce HIV transmission: mass media campaigns, public sector condom promotion and distribution, condom social marketing, voluntary counseling and testing programs, prevention of mother-to-child transmission, school-based programs, programs for out-of-school youth, workplace programs, treatment of sexually transmitted infections, peer counseling for sex workers, outreach to men who have sex with men, and harm reduction programs for injection drug users (Abu-Raddad et al., 2010). If this "window of opportunity" is missed, the economic burden on this reason will be great (p. S5).

There is also hope regarding treatment. Other research has demonstrated the effectiveness of circumcision for adult males in decreasing the spread of HIV (Abu-Raddad et al., 2010) and the importance of protecting HIV-positive

LEVELS OF PREVENTION PYRAMID

SITUATION: Prevent acute respiratory tract infections (ARIs) in children in developing countries

GOAL: Using the three levels of prevention, negative health conditions are avoided or promptly diagnosed and treated, and the fullest possible potential is restored.

TERTIARY PREVENTION		
Rehabilitation	**Primary Prevention**	
	Health Promotion & Education	*Health Protection*
• Restore child to optimal level of functioning through the recovery period.	• Continue to promote educational programs and individual teaching regarding practices that promote health and prevent diseases among family members.	• Educate on the prevention of recurrence and spread of disease.

SECONDARY PREVENTION	
Early Diagnosis	**Prompt Treatment**
• Get a prompt diagnosis of an acute ARI.	• Collaborate with families to combine the best of folk and home remedies with established Western medical practices. • Treat early with antibiotics (if indicated and available). • Provide culturally appropriate symptomatic care. • Teach caregiver signs and symptoms of complications.

PRIMARY PREVENTION	
Health Promotion & Education	**Health Protection**
• Promote general health education among community members. • Good prenatal care • Advocate breast-feeding, child spacing, and adequate nutrition. • Teach good hygiene and child care practices. • Teach when to seek medical attention. • Eliminate poverty and household crowding.	• Administer appropriate immunizations. • Eliminate indoor contaminants such as smoke from cook stoves without chimneys and cigarette, cigar, or pipe smoking. • Ventilate rooms to eliminate indoor smoke and allow fresh air in.

patients from malaria, as they become "supercontagious" and are more likely to spread HIV after contracting malaria (*The New York Times*, 2006, para. 2).

Tuberculosis

TB is an infectious disease caused by the tubercle bacillus. The disease has been known for hundreds of years and was commonly referred to as *consumption*. The causative organism has become resistant to the medications used to treat it, and currently, a worldwide TB epidemic is underway. One third of the world's population is thought to be currently infected by this bacteria, but only 5% to 10% of those become ill or can spread this to others within their lifetime. In 2009, it is estimated that 1.7 million people died from TB, with the highest number of deaths in Africa (50 per 100,000). TB is one of the illnesses that disproportionately affects poor people around the world, and it is estimated that the largest number of new cases of TB in 2008 were in Southeast Asia (WHO Media Centre, 2010d). Drug-resistant TB is a problem around the world. WHO began the Stop TB Strategy in 2006, and 41 million people have been treated using drug-observed therapy (DOTS). By 2015, the goal is to begin to reverse the TB incidence rate and to eliminate TB as a public health problem by 2050. It is believed that TB reached its peak in 2004, so the goals may be attainable (WHO Media Centre, 2010d).

Tuberculosis and Human Immunodeficiency Virus

TB alone is a pernicious illness. When TB and HIV occur in one individual, the combination is lethal, with each speeding the other's progress. TB is the leading cause of death among people who are HIV-positive (WHO Media Centre, 2010d). One study found that almost one quarter of all TB cases in the United States are among foreign-born individuals living here longer than 5 years for a rate of 21.5/100,000 compared to 2.7/100,000 for U.S.-born individuals. Many of the cases among the foreign-born are due to activation of latent TB infections (Cain et al., 2007).

Malaria

Malaria is a disease caused by the presence of the protozoan parasite *Plasmodium* in human red blood cells; the parasite is usually transmitted to humans by the bite of an infected female mosquito. "Humans are the only important reservoir of human malaria" (Heymann, 2008, p. 325). Fifty percent of the world population lives in malaria endemic areas. About 1 million deaths occur per year due to malaria, most are among African children (Heymann, 2008; WHO Media Centre, 2011e). In 2011, 216 million cases of malaria were estimated, but mortality rates have dropped by one fourth since 2000 (WHO Media Centre, 2011e).

The global disease burden from malaria is estimated to be >300 million acute illnesses and 1 million deaths per year. Ninety percent of the world's malaria cases occur in Africa, south of the Sahara. Malaria and the deaths it causes mainly affect two vulnerable groups—young children and pregnant women.

Malaria is resistant to multidrug therapy (MDT), and the mosquito, its tenacious vector, persists. Malaria is highly endemic in some areas, and its eradication depends on pesticides such as DDT. In addition, human and economic resources are not available to fully implement a malaria program. Perhaps the major contributors to lack of success have been failure to integrate the malaria eradication effort into basic health services, inadequate efforts to exploit the effective involvement of communities, and the absence of political will.

Currently, one part of the health strategy focuses on control and includes the following elements (Heymann, 2008; WHO Media Centre, 2011e):

1. Early case finding and treatment
2. Reduction of contact with mosquitoes (insecticide-treated mosquito nets)
3. Destruction of adult mosquitoes and larvae (vector control)
4. Source detection
5. Destruction of malaria parasites
6. Community education programs

The WHO Global Malaria Programme seeks to

- Form evidence-based policy and strategies
- Keep independent score of global progress
- Develop approaches for capacity building, strengthening systems, and surveillance
- Identify threats to malaria control and elimination, along with new areas for action (WHO Media Centre, 2011).

Over 500 partners, along with WHO, launched an initiative entitled the Roll Back Malaria (RBM) Program, which coordinates a worldwide action plan against malaria.

There is currently no licensed malaria vaccine, but one research vaccine is being evaluated in seven African countries. As with TB, malaria disproportionately affects the poor, and it has damaging effects on the economies of many poor countries. Up to 40% of public health expenditures and 30% to 50% of hospital admissions, as well as 60% of outpatient visits, are noted in disease-heavy countries (WHO Media Centre, 2011e).

West Nile Virus

WNV (*Flavivirus: Flaviviridae*) is considered the most widespread arbovirus worldwide and is most often transmitted to humans through the bite of an infected mosquito (Kramer, Styer, & Ebel, 2008). This virus may cause a fatal neurological disease, but 80% of those individuals infected do not demonstrate any symptoms. In those that develop West Nile fever, symptoms often are comprised of fever, body aches, nausea and vomiting, headache, fatigue, and sometimes a skin rash and enlarged lymph nodes. The sever disease, often termed West Nile encephalitis, is characterized by symptoms of headache, stiff neck, stupor, high fever, disorientation, coma, tremors, paralysis, and seizures. WNV can cause severe illness and death in horses, and contact with infected animals, their tissue or blood, can also be a source of transmission. It was first identified in the West Nile area of Uganda in 1937 and is commonly found in Africa, the Middle East, Europe, West Asia, and now North America. Birds are natural hosts, and mosquitoes most often transmit the infection from birds to humans. Sites for outbreaks are usually on major migratory routes for birds. However, the United States had a large outbreak between 1999 and 2010, thought to be imported from Israel or Tunisia. The virus has now spread to Venezuela and Canada.

No vaccine is available for humans, but there is one for horses. Treatment is most often supportive in nature (e.g., IV fluids, hospitalization). Active animal surveillance and early warning from veterinarians and public health officials are being used to prevent transmission. Education and reducing mosquito transmission (e.g., use of nets, spraying, eliminating mosquito breeding sources) are also being used (WHO Media Centre, 2011b).

Leprosy

Leprosy is a chronic granulomatous infection caused by *Mycobacterium leprae* (Hansen's bacillus). It affects various parts of the body including the skin of the face (*Medline Plus Merriam-Webster Medical Dictionary,* 2012). In 2011, the prevalence of leprosy was 192,246 cases. Most countries have eliminated this disease, but highly endemic countries include Central African Republic, Brazil, Nepal, Mozambique, United Republic of Tanzania, Democratic Republic of Congo, India, Madagascar, and Angola. Early diagnosis and treatment is the best course of action, and MDT is a key to elimination of the disease. WHO provides this free of charge to all individuals around the world (WHO, 2012f). People with leprosy have had access to this free effective drug treatment since 1995. Communities can help eradicate this disease through proper diagnosis and treatment and provision of care without stigma or isolation. A change in the image of leprosy, so that people with the condition will more readily present themselves for treatment, is essential.

Guinea Worm Disease (Dracunculiasis)

Dracunculiasis, or guinea worm disease, is a parasitic disease that is transmitted to humans when a person drinks water containing a worm's intermediate host, a water flea that can ingest and harbor guinea worm larvae. Once in a human body, the larvae migrate through the tissue and the mature adult worm attempts to emerge, usually from the lower leg. Farmers are the most commonly affected. Although there is no cure, once the larvae are ingested, the eradication strategy includes interruption of transmission, surveillance, health education, and certification.

Guinea worm disease is "on the verge of eradication with fewer than 1100 cases reported in 2011" (WHO Media Centre, 2012, para 1). In 2000, over 75,000 cases were reported by WHO (2012). In 2011, the incidence dropped by over 99%, and only Chad, Ethiopia, Mali, and South Sudan have reported cases. Most cases are in remote, often inaccessible areas (WHO Media Centre, 2012).

Era of Infectious Disease and the Universal Imperatives of Care

The infectious diseases and processes carry the potential for death, illness, and compromised functioning but when addressed promptly can be prevented. When left unmanaged, they can result in sickness and lifelong consequences to daily functioning. Some of these conditions involve decision making. For example, when national governments do not provide clear national policies or funding for immunization programs, entire populations are at risk for the consequences of diphtheria, pertussis, typhoid, measles, and polio. When families and communities are living in areas with infectious agents, or do not clear their land as needed, their members are exposed to malaria. When community health programs do not include sanitation and the building of latrines, the result is diarrheal diseases that affect an entire community (Zwane & Kremer, 2007).

Eradication, Elimination, and Control of Communicable Diseases

The primary global health goals related to communicable disease are eradication, elimination, and worldwide control. **Eradication** means interruption of person-to-person transmission and limitation of the reservoir of infection so that no further preventive efforts are required; it indicates a status whereby no further cases of a disease occur anywhere. At times, the term **elimination** is used when a disease has been interrupted in a defined geographic area. In 1991, WHO defined elimination as a reduction of prevalence to <1 case per 1 million population in a given area. In contrast, the term **control** indicates that a specific disease has ceased to be a public health threat. Control programs are aimed at reducing the incidence and prevalence of communicable and some noncommunicable conditions.

Although eradication is always the desired effect, extensive funding and much international cooperation are usually required to achieve such a goal (see What Do You Think?). The successful eradication of smallpox from the world came about because of the leadership of the WHO, and it was a tremendous accomplishment in public health. In 1959, several countries proposed the global eradication of smallpox, but progress was slow. The Intensified Smallpox Eradication Programme began in 1967, when smallpox was endemic in 31 countries, with 10 to 15 million individuals infected. Through enhanced surveillance and *ring vaccination* to prevent transmission between humans and control epidemics, progress improved. New cases were quickly identified and quarantined, and their close contacts were vaccinated and quarantined. Remarkably, by 1980, there were no cases in the world (Global Alert and Response, 2010). Clearly, if global eradication programs are to be successful, collaboration and partnerships are essential. Control of river blindness (onchocerciasis—the chief cause of blindness in many African countries) joined the growing list of global public health accomplishments (WHO, 2012g). These programs are dependent on comwmitment from involved governments, international bodies, NGOs, and the affected communities themselves. Global eradication and elimination programs that are close to meeting the goal include poliomyelitis and guinea worm disease. Eradication programs for leprosy and measles are continuing. Additional major efforts have increased to reduce, control, and prevent malaria, TB, HIV/AIDS, diarrheal diseases, and respiratory infections. Unfortunately, international terrorism threatens to reintroduce smallpox through acts of bioterrorism; smallpox vaccination programs have had to be reestablished to protect health workers and the populations at risk (Pease, 2010).

> **What do *you* think?**
>
> Imagine today's world without any international cooperation related to communicable disease knowledge or control. What would be some of the health, social, and economic consequences of such inaction?

New and Emerging Infectious Diseases and Conditions

Despite the advances made, new and emerging diseases, conditions, and syndromes have appeared in parts of the world. Health authorities thought that some of these were under control. Over the past 20 years, a number of previously unknown diseases have emerged, among them Ebola, Hantavirus pulmonary syndrome, Lyme disease, and severe acute respiratory syndrome (see Table 16-1) (WHO, 2012k).

The development of antimicrobial-resistant organisms, mainly as a result of the overuse and misuse of antibiotics, has fueled a resurgence of some diseases that were under control, such as TB. Medication-resistant TB is now estimated to comprise almost 15% of new TB cases in some parts of the world (Zagar & McNerney, 2008). Antimalarial medicines have become ineffective in some countries (Artzy-Randrup, Alonzo, & Pascual, 2010). The easy availability of global air travel and subsequent rapid transmission of microbes pose real health threats.

Another factor related to emergence of new and recycling conditions is migration (as discussed earlier in this chapter) and urbanization, which serves to concentrate large numbers of people in small geographic areas. With urbanization, deforestation continues, and the two phenomena may permit the infestation of microbes into human populations, as humans who move into the cleared forests may encounter previously unknown pathogens. Changes in agricultural practices, such as new dams and irrigation schemes, also present potential transmission scenarios. The ability of microbes to change and adapt rapidly is a persistent threat as well. Davenport (2007) reminds us that:

> In 1967, the United States Surgeon General proclaimed the end of infectious disease. But epidemiology, medicine, and basic biology have revealed that infectious diseases have not disappeared. Instead, the threat is a constantly changing one, and a concerted research effort from multiple fields is necessary to keep up with the challenge. (p. 1)

Table 16.1 Examples of Emerging Pathogens Identified Since 1973

Agent	Microbe	Disease
V	Rotavirus	Major cause of infantile diarrhea globally
V	*Cryptosporidium parvum*	Acute and chronic diarrhea
V	Ebola virus	Ebola hemorrhagic fever (Africa)
B	*Legionella pneumophila*	Legionnaires' disease/pneumonia
V	Hantaan virus (Sin Nombre virus)	Hemorrhagic fever with renal syndrome
B	*Campylobacter jejuni*	GI infections (infants/children) globally
V	Human T-lymphotropic virus 1 (HTLV-1)	T-cell lymphoma, leukemia globally
B	Toxin producing strains of *Staphylococcus aureus*	Toxic shock syndrome
B	*Escherichia coli 0157:H7*	Mild to severe diarrhea, hemorrhagic colitis, hemolytic uremic syndrome (beef)
V	HTLV-II	Hairy cell leukemia, paraparesis globally
S	*Borrelia burgdorferi*	Lyme disease
V	Human immunodeficiency virus (I and II)	Acquired immunodeficiency syndrome (AIDS) worldwide
B	*Helicobacter pylori*	Peptic ulcer disease
V	Hepatitis C	Hepatitis, cirrhosis, carcinoma globally
V	Guanarito virus	Venezuelan hemorrhagic fever
V	Junin virus	Argentine hemorrhagic fever
B	*Vibrio cholerae 0139*	New strain associated with epidemic cholera
B	*Bartonella henselae*	Catscratch disease, bacillary angiomatosis

(Continued)

Table 16.1 Examples of Emerging Pathogens Identified Since 1973 *(Continued)*

Agent	Microbe	Disease
V	Sabia virus	Brazilian hemorrhagic fever
V	Machupo virus	Bolivian hemorrhagic fever
V	Human herpesvirus-6, 7, 8	Roseola infantum/mononucleosis in adults, febrile childhood illness, Kaposi's sarcoma in AIDS patients
V	Norovirus	Acute vomiting, cramps, diarrhea
V	Parvovirus B19	Fifth disease, arthropathy, anemia worldwide
V	Nipah virus	Encephalitis
V	Hendra virus	Severe pneumonitis/meningitis
V	Marburg virus	Microvascular leakage/hemorrhages (Africa)
B	*Clostridium difficile*	Severe infections—toxic megacolon, sepsis, death (asymptomatic in healthy neonates, nosocomial adults)
V	Severe acute respiratory syndrome coronavirus (SARS-CoV)	SARS

From Dong, J., Olano, J., McBride, J., & Walker, D. (2008). Emerging pathogens: Challenges and successes of molecular diagnostics. *Journal of Molecular Diagnostics, 10*(3), 185–197; World Health Organization. (1998d). Examples of pathogens recognized since 1973. *WHO Fact Sheet No. 97, 4*. Geneva: Author; World Health Organization. (2001). *Nipah virus. WHO Fact Sheet, 262, 1–2*. Geneva, Author; World Health Organization (2003, 12 March). *WHO issues a global alert about cases of atypical pneumonia. Press Release WHO/22*. Geneva: Author.

Era of Chronic Long-Term Health Conditions

Despite the programs of control, many infectious diseases persist, but people survive and live on to experience chronic, long-term conditions. These conditions, while averting mortality, persist through their ongoing etiology and affect people's daily functioning, decision-making, and cost. Adding to the burden is the escalating sale of tobacco and the use of cigarettes by young populations in developing countries. The long-term effects of these practices for people in these countries will undoubtedly follow a similar trajectory as has occurred in developed countries with increases in lung cancer, heart disease, and other illnesses related to tobacco use. Thus, the longevity that has resulted from meeting the challenges of the Era of Infectious Diseases compounds the more recent emergence of chronic diseases in the many countries. Here, a transition occurs. As infectious diseases decrease, life expectancy lengthens and the population experiences the degenerative diseases seen in developed countries. The concept of epidemiologic transition explains the replacement of infectious disease morbidity and mortality with that of chronic disease. The ways in which people in remote areas will manage their heart disease or cope with the long-term effects of diabetes and cancer are yet to be understood. Formerly, those with mental illness, inborn genetic disorders, disabilities, or compromised activities of daily living were cared for by the family and were often hidden from the community. This was often due to religious and cultural beliefs, lack of knowledge, the availability of health providers with specialized expertise, and dedicated health care facilities or services for those chronic illness.

As families change their composition, members of families migrate to seek employment; the care of those who require daily assistance will also have to change. It will require a change in the response of the health care system in terms of provision of care, planning, and allocation of resources. Addressing these concerns is considered a cost-effective investment in a nation's human capital (Yach, Mensah, Hawkes, Epping-Jordan, & Steyn, 2011).

Era of Social Health Conditions

The WHO researchers suggest that overall, dramatic changes in health-related needs will occur within the next 20 years. There is evidence that noncommunicable diseases are rapidly replacing infectious diseases as the major causes of disability and premature death. Noncommunicable diseases are expected to account for seven of every 10 deaths in developing countries, compared with fewer than 5 of every 10 today. See Display 16.4 for Deaths Attributed to Leading Risk Factors.

Maternal and Perinatal Morbidity and Mortality

The WHO estimates that almost 400,000 women die yearly from complications of pregnancy and childbirth. Ninety-nine percent of these deaths are in economically poor countries. Pregnant women living in rural areas

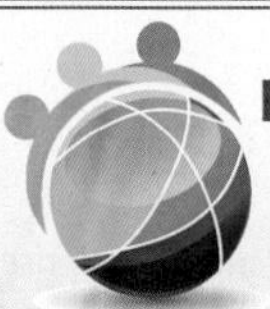

DISPLAY 16.4 DEATHS ATTRIBUTED TO 19 LEADING RISK FACTORS

1. High blood pressure	7.5 million deaths worldwide
2. Tobacco use	5.1
3. High blood glucose	3.4
4. Physical inactivity	3.2
5. Overweight/obesity	2.8
6. High cholesterol	2.6
7. Unsafe sex	2.4
8. Alcohol use	2.3
9. Underweight	2.2
10. Indoor smoke from solid fuels	2.0
11. Unsafe water, sanitation, and hygiene	Factors 11 through 15 below 2 million
12. Low fruit and vegetable consumption	
13. Suboptimal breast-feeding	
14. Urban outdoor air pollution	
15. Occupational risks	
16. Vitamin A deficiency	Remainder below 1 million
17. Zinc deficiency	
18. Unsafe health care injections	
19. Iron deficiency	

From World Health Organization (WHO). (2009a). *Global health risks: Mortality and burden of disease attributable to selected major risks.* Geneva. Author.

and adolescent mothers face higher mortality rates. The death of a mother profoundly affects the wellbeing of the entire family. Between 1990 and 2008, global rates of maternal mortality dropped by one third (WHO Media Centre, 2010c).

Early pregnancy, high fertility, and close child spacing are common in developing countries and are known to be major determinants of poor health for mothers and children. Poverty, illiteracy, poor nutrition, low weight gain, maternal age (highest when younger than 15), infections, smoke in the home, smoking, and poor health care are some of the major determinants associated with high health risks to mothers and children in the poorest nations of the world (WHO Media Centre, 2010c). As noted above, the added burden of long protracted civil wars has exacerbated these conditions as have the factors associated with migration. As men leave home to seek employment abroad, women remain behind to care for children, often managing heavy workloads and their pregnancies.

Prevention strategies include better general health for women through poverty alleviation, education, family planning guidance, prenatal care including food supplementation, immunization, local and regional care with referrals for complications, training of traditional birth attendants (TBAs), and effective postpartum care (Rosato et al., 2008).

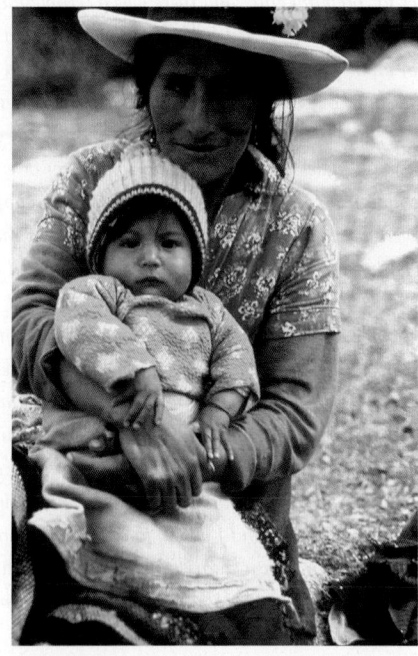

Maternal and perinatal morbidity and mortality are important global issues addressed by the World Health Organization. (Photo courtesy of CDC Photo Image Library.)

Mental Health Conditions

Mental illness has been thought of in a variety of ways over the centuries through drastic measures including exclusion from society, ridicule, and incarceration, as outlined in the classic book by Foucault (1965). Some suggest that it accounts for almost 14% of disease burden worldwide (Thomas & Lewis, 2009). The recent civil wars and popular uprisings and the major wars in Iraq and Afghanistan have taken their toll on members of the armed forces resulting in posttraumatic stress among soldiers as well as the inhabitants who have experienced war. These events and the recent financial downturn in the economies of the world have affected the mental health of people as they struggle to manage the multiple social, financial, and cultural issues facing them, not the least of which are the effects of unemployment and financial ruin for families throughout many parts of the world.

Tobacco

Over 100 million deaths were attributed to tobacco in the 20th century. Tobacco accounts for 1 death every 6 seconds in the world, or about 6 million people annually. Without some form of intervention, this trend will continue ultimately resulting in over 8 million annual deaths by 2030 and over one billion deaths within the

PERSPECTIVES
A NURSE MIDWIFE IN SUDAN

I am a nurse midwife in South Sudan. My husband, who works with local pastors, and I are Seventh-Day Adventist missionaries based out of Uganda. One evening I got a call about a lady in labor. I had not seen her for prenatal care, and there was a terrible rainstorm that night. I was told this was a first baby for the young woman, and she had been in labor for more than 24 hours. They wanted to take her to a hospital but could not get a vehicle to transport her there. The dirt roads are slippery and awful in this area, and the girl was 11 miles away from me (5 miles were dirt roads). I rode my bike in the rain, watching children on the sides of the road trying to capture ants to eat. They were beating on tin cans to lure them out of the ant holes, in order to gather the fat, winged ants that are considered tasty treats. As my assistant and I got close to the girl's thatched hut, we noticed groups of people gathered nearby. Villagers were often concerned about mothers and babies, but we were quickly told that the baby had just been born and was dead. I went into the hut and noticed a limp baby girl. I began to examine the baby and felt a faint heartbeat on the umbilical cord (still connected to the mother). I grabbed my bag and mask and began resuscitating the baby. The baby was on the mat covering the dirt floor, and I finally found an oral airway to keep the baby's mouth open, as the air did not seem to be getting through. Air finally began going into the lungs, and I checked the heartbeat (normal). I kept bagging the baby and watched the tiny chest rise and fall. The tiny hut was filled with concerned neighborhood women who had been wailing because they thought the baby had died. Now, they sat quietly, speaking softly to one another as they watched me intently. Other women were crowded around the doorway to the hut and still more sat outside. I looked over at the mother, who seemed to be alright, not bleeding too much. I asked the women for hot water so I could keep the baby warm, and I kept bagging the baby. Then, I tried shocking the baby with colder water, so that she would begin to breathe on her own. We went back and forth like this a few times, and the baby would take an occasional breath on her own. I inserted a nasogastric tube to remove any excess air that may have accumulated, and her color improved and muscle tone increased. After awhile, the baby began to breathe on her own. I checked the mother for any tearing (none apparent) and stayed with them for several hours to make sure there were no further signs of respiratory distress or other problems. Because the next day was market day, word of the baby's condition spread very fast. I don't know what will happen tomorrow, but I am grateful for the blessings of today!

Kristina, Nurse Midwife

Adapted from Reaching out to South Sudan: Meet the Muehlhausers. Retrieved February 1, 2012 from http://www.adventistmission.org/article.php?id=101

21st century. Most of the world's one billion smokers live in low-income or mid-income countries where premature death and the burden of disease prevent economic growth (WHO Media Centre, 2011a). The statistics are startling when one considers the lifelong smoker who is as likely to die from tobacco as he/she is from all other causes of death combined (Schaffer Library of Drug Policy, 2011). Yet, it is difficult for smokers to stop smoking. With medication and counseling, however, the chances of success in quitting smoking are doubled (WHO Media Centre, 2011a).

The WHO Framework Convention on Tobacco Control took effect in 2005. The treaty's signatory parties (over 170 representing 87% of the world population) agreed to implement comprehensive tobacco control programs and strategies. WHO introduced a tobacco control package, MPOWER, to help implement the provisions of the treaty. The six components are as follows:

- Monitor tobacco use and prevention policies
- Protect people from tobacco use
- Offer help to quit tobacco use
- Warn about the dangers of tobacco
- Enforce bans on tobacco advertising, promotion, and sponsorship
- Raise taxes on tobacco (WHO Media Centre, 2011, para 46)

This legally binding treaty and international effort represents an important step in global public health and is expected to reduce the impact of tobacco use in the decades to come.

Given that tobacco eventually kills about half of its users, this important global public health initiative should help save lives, improve standards of living and world economies, as well as improve global health.

Global Burden of Disease

If a member of your family dies, what does it cost? What does it cost if you miss a month of work or school due to an illness? What does it cost a country when the majority of adults smoke a package of cigarettes a day or when adults eat beetle nut several times a day? These questions are often irritating and are sometimes considered in poor taste. Yet insurance companies, governments, and community members do ask these questions—as they must carry the financial burden for them. But how does one go about putting a value on a life? Or a value on the cost of a disability? To capture these concerns, WHO coined the term: the ***global burden of disease*** **(GBD)**.

WHO's GBD studies numerically verified numerous long-held assumptions about disparities in the burden of disease worldwide, especially in regard to children, through landmark studies by Murray and colleagues that revealed startling statistics:

- 98% of all deaths of infants and children under 15 years occur in the developing world.
- 83% of deaths between ages 15 and 19 are in the developing world (Murray & Lopez, 1997).

In addition to causes of mortality, the GBD study quantified the burden of disease with a measure that is used for cost-effectiveness analysis. To compare across conditions and risk factors, researchers developed a measure called the **disability-adjusted life year (DALY)**, which are the combination of years of life lost due to premature mortality and years of life lived with disability adjusted for the severity of disability (WHO, 2012c). The 2004 GBD study ranked the leading risk factor causes of DALYs overall and by income group (see Table 16-2). Childhood underweight, unsafe sex, alcohol use, unsafe water/sanitation/hygiene, high blood pressure, tobacco use, suboptimal breast-feeding, high blood glucose, indoor smoke from solid fuels, and overweight/obesity were the top ten risk factors worldwide (WHO, 2009a).

Table 16.2 Ranking of 10 Leading Risk Factor Causes of DALYs: Worldwide and High-Income Countries

Risk Factor	Worldwide	High-Income Countries
Childhood underweight	1	n/a
Unsafe sex	2	n/a
Alcohol use	3	2
Unsafe water, sanitation, hygiene	4	n/a
High blood pressure	5	4
Tobacco use	6	1
Suboptimal breast-feeding	7	n/a
High blood glucose	8	5
Indoor smoke from solid fuels	9	n/a
Overweight and obesity	10	3
Physical inactivity	n/a	6
High cholesterol	n/a	7
Illicit drugs	n/a	8
Occupational risks	n/a	9
Low fruit and vegetable intake	n/a	10

From World Health Organization (WHO). (2009a). *Global health risks: Mortality and burden of disease attributable to selected major risks*. Geneva: Author. Adapted from Table 2, p. 12.

Eight risk factors are responsible for 61% of cardiovascular-related deaths: alcohol use, tobacco use, high body mass index, high cholesterol, high blood pressure, high blood glucose, low fruit and vegetable consumption, and physical inactivity (WHO, 2009). These same risk factors account for more than 75% of ischemic heart disease, the world's leading cause of death. These risk factors are present in countries with high, middle, and low incomes. If exposure to these risk factors could be reduced, life expectancy worldwide would increase by 5 years (WHO, 2009).

An estimated 39% of childhood deaths worldwide were attributable to preventable environmental risks, micronutrient deficiencies, underweight, and suboptimal breast-feeding. Environmental and behavioral risks, along with infectious causes, were the cause of 45% of global cancer deaths (WHO, 2009). See Table 16-3 for more on deaths attributable to specific risk factors.

The information obtained from the GBD and its analysis guides current decisions related to investments in health, research, human resource development, and physical infrastructure. Reassessment of global and regional information on diseases and injuries is expected to occur periodically, with the 2010 study currently underway.

PROVIDERS OF HEALTH CARE

The implications for community health nursing concerning the three eras of health conditions are many. The health provider most appropriate when death is a common occurrence, as it was during the Era of Infectious Diseases, is a physician. This category of health worker is best suited for saving lives and for delivering the medical interventions that keep people alive. Nursing and nursing personnel are health care providers who have traditionally served populations that experience long-term chronic illnesses. Nursing personnel worldwide serve populations in nursing homes, long-term care facilities, and in community-based programs for the elderly and disabled. The nursing services in Slovenia and Germany are excellent examples of the latter practice in Europe.

The caregiver needed for the Era of Social Conditions is evolving. For example, community health nurses and primary care physicians are developing new competencies for HIV/AIDS prevention among adolescent prostitutes, but also needed is a host of other interventions that require collaboration with other social service. In addition, some communities, because of their former political persuasion and cultural beliefs, have viewed the state as the provider of all health care services. For example, during the earthquake in Armenia, international workers recognized the need for social supports for those whose homes and community had been destroyed. At that time, these social structures, as they existed in North America, were not available to that population. While alcoholism has been rampant in parts of Eastern Europe, organizations such as Alcoholic Anonymous were not available. In other areas, such as South America, close-knit

Table 16.3 Percent of Deaths by Attributable Risk Factors, Low/Middle-Income Countries, High-Income Countries, World

Risk Factor	Low/Middle (%)	High (%)	World (%)
Childhood underweight	7.5	0	6.5
Hypertension	12.9	17.6	13.5
High cholesterol	6.3	10.7	6.9
Overweight/obesity[a]	3.6	7.8	4.2
Low fruit/vegetable intake[b]	4.8	4.2	4.7
Inadequate physical activity	3.2	4.8	3.4
Smoking[a,b]	6.9	18.5	8.5
Alcohol consumption[a,b]	3.9	0.3	3.4
Unsafe sex	5.8	0.4	5.1
Urban air pollution	1.5	1.0	1.4
Indoor air pollution (fuels)	3.7	0	3.2
Contaminated injections (health care settings)	0.8	<0.1	0.7

[a]Smoking, alcohol, and overweight/obesity are the most significant risk factors for 12 most common cancers in high-income countries.
[b]Smoking, alcohol, and low fruit/vegetable intake are the most significant factors for 12 most common cancers in low/middle-income countries.
Adapted from Lopez, A., Mathers, C., Ezzati, M., Jamison, D., & Murray, C. (Eds.). (2006). *Global burden of disease and risk factors*. Washington, DC: The World Bank. Danaei, G., Vander Hoorn, S., Lopez, A., Murray, C., Ezzati, M.; Comparative Risk Assessment Collaborating Group (Cancers). (2005). Causes of cancer in the world: Comparative risk assessment of nine behavioural and environmental risk factors. *Lancet, 366*(9499), 1784–1793.

family structures are vital. Yet few if any services are available to families living between the era of the close-knit family structure and one that requires outside help for emerging third era conditions.

In the future, community health care will be increasingly collaborative, and experienced as participatory partnerships with clear shifts in ownership and leadership. Formerly, international workers and consultants went to a country as outsiders and delivered their ideas, programs, and projects. The philosophy, beliefs, practices, and values of this dominant group of outsiders prevailed, and the recipient groups were considered a success to the extent that they adopted the dominant group's ways of being, living, and caring for their health.

In the future, partnerships that are sensitive to the dynamics of power and oppression, and which honor the need for local groups to be in control of their own projects and the resources that are used to implement them, will prevail. Freire's (1970) well-known advocacy for using *generative themes* that support education and critical consciousness has been adopted as collaborative projects demonstrate innovative ways of learning and conducting research. For example, in many countries, local experts and community members are forming partnerships with outside consultants and are insisting on striking changes in responsibility, authority, and ownership of data and innovations. In these emerging models, action research projects are being adopted over positivist, empirical studies with the community becomes the initiator of action.

Health Providers at District Levels

In earlier forms of PHC, the locus of decision-making was at the village level. However, after many years of effort, the WHO and other organizations realized that the power to sustain change required more than village-level involvement. Thus, the move to the district level of implementation is currently being practiced in many places.

Regardless of level, however, the essential point is the adage: think globally, act locally. Specifically, this means that expertise is needed from those at international, national, regional, and district levels, but the ways in which communities interpret the issues and actually decides to use the solutions belong to them. In local areas, communities adopt the health centers or organizations created to address community concerns. For example, in one Greek community, a local mayor sat through a week of deliberations on ways to bring PHC to his island. He heard the comments of members of the local community, its health workers, and an international WHO PHC team. Ultimately, the mayor realized that rooms for health providers would be needed, and he declared the community's full support to provide these rooms to further the work of the health center. In this way, his community was fully active and responsible for its own health status.

Community Health Workers

In some countries, particularly those in which professional health providers are scarce, the community identifies a local, respected, responsible person most often called the **community health worker (CHW)**. This person is selected from the village and is approved by the committee to serve the village people in health matters. CHWs usually provide 1 to 2 hours of health service per day, for which they may or may not be compensated by the community. In Ethiopia, refugees in camps erected after disasters identify responsible adults to serve as their kind of CHWs; these adults are known to and are trusted by newly established communities (described in a classic article by Farrell, 1986).

The CHW is trained in the fundamentals of promoting health and preventing and treating the most common health care conditions. This includes basic first aid, advice and assistance on simple treatments, and health teaching on personal hygiene, safe water supplies, safe disposal of human waste and refuse, and nutrition. Community health nurses often serve as consultants to the CHW and, in some places, are expected to supervise their work and provide ongoing education. These CHWs, as noted above, have demonstrated their effectiveness in controlling communicable diseases (e.g., malaria treatment) and promoting health (e.g., cervical cancer/mammography screenings) in this country and around the world (Viswanathan et al., 2009).

Village Midwife

The village midwife receives training in obstetrics and child care. This person provides basic antenatal, intrapartum, and postnatal care and makes referrals as required (Ensor, Quayyum, Nadjib, & Sucahya, 2009). In India, the village midwife is referred to as a trained *dai*. These are most often older women who may have had training from professional nurses and who are expected to call on professionals when needed. However, they often make their own decisions even though they have a referral source to professionals. Many times, adverse effects occur because cultural practices take precedence over knowledge-based practices that require collaborative decision-making.

In some countries, traditional health practitioners receive formal training and return to their villages to continue their services with new knowledge and skills to enhance their effectiveness. Countries such as Bangladesh implemented programs to train workers who would practice in ways similar to the "barefoot doctors" of China (Ho & Gostin, 2009; Valentine, 2005). This author (with Drs. Howard Barnum and Dr. Pierre Glacin) examined the work of these barefoot doctors as the Ministry of Health in Bangladesh was challenged in its efforts during the 1980s to provide health care to rural population. Because of cultural taboos, women were not allowed to leave their homes for training and, if they did, would rarely allow themselves to be posted in a village other than their own. This was because women were viewed as wayward if they were not with their families in their home environments. This issue also occurred in Indonesia, when community health nurses were placed in villages away from home. They did not have the respect of the local community, were not seen as experts, and were considered to be of dubious moral standing. This cultural barrier presents challenges to nursing education programs that focus on community rather than hospital-based experiences. A recent study of nurse midwives in Indonesia found that they can earn "a substantial private income" even in areas that are remote and rural, but they were often unwilling to move to remote areas for other (nonfinancial) reasons (Ensor et al., 2009, p. 26).

Community Health Nurses

Background and Age at Entry to Nursing Education

When community health nurses join their colleagues in a country other than their own, they often assume that "a nurse is a nurse, is a nurse." Nothing could be further from the truth. The ways in which women and men are socialized, recruited into, advanced through, and graduated from nursing programs vary considerable from country to country. So does the age at entry, the exposure that nursing students have to the social and behavioral sciences, the theoretical and clinical applications studied, and the kind and extent of supervision they receive. For example, in some countries, young people begin their study of nursing at age 15, studying nursing in programs designed, sequenced, and financed by the government. These graduates are expected to practice as fully experienced community health nurses by age 18. In some countries, the extent of responsibilities placed on these relatively young practitioners is beyond their ability or maturity levels; however, the expectations persist because the number of prepared health care personnel is often at a premium.

Curricula of Nursing Programs

In the United States, curricula in nursing are designed to serve the community in which the nursing program is based. Thus, a community prone to hurricanes, for example, would provide enhanced curricula for delivering nursing care in this kind of natural disaster. However, in some countries, nursing education curricula are conceived and designed at national levels and in this way, are not responsive to local situations. The opportunity this model provides is consistency of teaching and learning and the possibility to produce teaching–learning materials in a uniform way and in the language of the country. The risks are that local conditions are not included, and care practices essential for a region of a country may not be addressed. For example, during an earthquake in Armenia, this author, as WHO European Regional Advisor, requested that content related to earthquakes and disaster preparedness be added to the curriculum. Authorities decline, showing the consulting team and local nurse leaders the detailed content and hours developed for the curriculum designed in Moscow. No opportunities, at that time, were possible for this content to be added, despite the fact that 25,000 people had lost their lives in this natural disaster.

Nursing educational programs may still be based in hospitals, technical schools, or university. Specialty areas may be introduced as part of the basic curriculum, as is the practice in Denmark where midwifery is a basic program offered and is seen as a discipline different from nursing and in France where midwifery is aligned with medicine. This design differs from other countries in which nursing is the basic preparation upon which mental health, midwifery, and other areas are built and considered as advanced practice. In some countries, mental health is not included as part of the basic curriculum. For the graduates of these programs, moving to and working in countries that require mental health theory and practice requires additional schooling before the candidate is allowed to sit for the licensing examination.

International Migration of Nurses

While this chapter often focuses on U.S. nurses working in other countries, another, sometimes ominous component of global nursing is the migration of nurses from less-developed nations to more industrialized countries offering higher wages. Conditions in sub-Saharan Africa are very problematic. Having an already weak and poorly developed health system, countries in this region are now facing a serious crisis due to nursing shortages and migration of nurses to South Africa or other countries within the region where a better standard of living exists. Zambia, for instance, has a nurse to population ratio of 0.22 to 1,000 (about 40 times less than the U.S. ratio), and many African governments feel that their nurses are being enticed away by wealthier nations (Pittman, Aiken, & Buchan, 2007). They are asking that foreign aid be directed toward assisting them to provide better nursing education and salaries so that nurses remain in their own countries. Filipino nurses often immigrate to the United States, and this has caused changes to their nursing education system that the Philippine government feels is problematic. Canada and the United Kingdom often recruit nurses from outside their countries while at the same time losing Canadian nurses to the United States. The United States, with its history of nursing shortages and a large health care system, has often relied on foreign graduates of nursing schools to meet its demands. This has caused concern among other nations (Pittman et al., 2007).

Forces That Support Nursing Development

In many places, nursing has yet to distinguish itself with its own body of research, knowledge, managerial practices, standards of practice, and ethical tenets. However, it appears that nursing has thrived as a respected discipline in countries where, overall, women are respected and where those in leadership positions understand the value of the caring process and are willing to champion nursing at all levels, including at the national level. For example, Turkey stands out as a country with a cadre of doctor ally prepared nurses who were able to secure their education abroad thanks to Dr. Ihsan Dogramaci, an international figure, pediatrician, and child health specialist (Rose, 2008). Dr. Dogramaci sponsored nurses in Turkey, so that they were able to pursue higher education through the doctoral level of preparation. Nursing has developed in unusual ways in other countries as well. For example, conversations with Portuguese nurses reveal that many of the leaders of nursing in that country came from wealthy families and were committed to a contemporary view of nursing practice. In Denmark, an unusually strong nursing association and union of nursing and nursing personnel has fostered a strong presence for the discipline in that country and in the European Region.

In Indonesia, many types of nursing personnel had proliferated, and 25 categories of nursing personnel practiced in the country until the mid-1980s. The WHO worked diligently with the Ministry of Health to introduce PHC nursing, a transformation that was clearly a challenge in a country peppered with hundreds of islands, where providing community learning experiences requires time and financial resources to travel to clinical sites. This situation is exacerbated by the limited availability of qualified faculty and the nature of the clinical experiences available in remote locations.

A major challenge to community health nurses who have undergone theory and clinical experiences as learners is working with nurses who have not had community health experience. As is well understood, functioning well in a fully equipped hospital is different from working in a community or village where resources are not easily available. Exploring these differences is an essential part of one's own needs assessment as one embarks on an experience with a team from locations other than one's own.

THE PROCEDURES/INTERVENTIONS

Community health nurses consider the population as their patient or client. A population might refer to all those living in a catchment area, in a neighborhood, village, a district, or city. Countries might refer to their populations at national, regional, or international levels. Regardless of location or level, community health nurses practice within the context of some kind of health care system or organization.

Nurses and midwives constitute a majority of the qualified work force in many national health care systems, and they represent a powerful force for bringing health care to all populations. Nurses provide the spectrum of PHC services and conduct health research, and as the global population ages, average age of nurses is increasing; this further intensifies nursing shortages (International Centre for Human Resources in Nursing [ICHRN], 2008).

The interventions that community health nurses provide depend on the context in which they are working and on the population, its health status, and the health conditions it presents. These interventions also depend on the ways in which nursing is practiced in a country and on the organizations in which community health nurses are employed or with which they are collaborating. A key issue here is that community health nurses need to know the mission of the agencies with which they are working and the kinds of services and resources their employing organizations provide. This section describes selected organizations that provide interventions to address community health care issues and the ways in which community health nurses work within them.

Providing an intervention that "works" constitutes an achievement. Providing an intervention in community health constitutes a remarkable achievement. This is because interventions are complex, often costly, and involve considerable knowledge, planning, and expert execution and evaluation skills. This section also focuses on the interventions community health nurses provide in a context different from their own within the context of a sponsoring organization.

As noted, the first step is to understand what the community's health needs are, who is involved in addressing them, the roles they play, and the contributions they are able to bring to the issue. Again, knowing the context in which one is working and understanding the population and their health status and health conditions are also critical elements (and have been addressed earlier). A second but often overlooked step is to understand the reasons the interventions are being delivered and one's reasons for being involved. Specifically, what does the sponsoring agency believe is its mission and why now, why here? What does the community have to say? Does the community see itself as a recipient of donations or as partners and collaborators? How do they see the intervention? Did they identify the need and ask for assistance? Have the recipients been involved in identifying the issue, in planning strategies for the intervention? Are they committed to the issue and to the outcome? What is their level of involvement in the issue?

These are complex questions. In some countries, the number and seriousness of challenges may be overwhelming, and despite outsiders' authoritative view of what should be tackled first, the community's perspective will often determine the intervention's effectiveness. For example in Chad, of all the health information that the country could collect, Harvard University international consultants worked with the Ministry of Health and established an essential list that its people would find the most useful. At times, one's own interests may not be the ones the community needs to tackle.

Questions you need to ask yourself are the following: why are you there? What motivates you and what is your commitment? How does this fit with the scope of the work you will be undertaking, and will your time commitment see the project through, and if not, what effect will your leaving have on its success? In some places, a custom has been established of exchanges where the international project staff is accommodated and where the local staff expects the same when they join the international staff in their home country. This commitment may represent a time and financial commitment you are not prepared to make. You will want to examine this issue before you commit to a project and its sometimes unwritten expectations.

Criteria for Support of Interventions

Sustainability. One of the most important criterions for donor support is sustainability: Can the recipient unit, a village health center, a district hospital, and a regional health office manage the projects after external funds are no longer available? For example, in one project slated for an African country, this author was instructed to avoid any project under $5 million, as the donor agency did not want to manage what they considered "small projects."

Absorptive capacity. While many communities need support for their interventions, they often lack the personnel, structures, or processes to actually use the support. For example, in the project described above, the country's department requesting funding, although in dire need of help, was staffed at the national level with one full-time and one half-time person, with virtually no computer capability and no delivery system. In many countries, particularly after national disasters, well-intentioned donors flood a country with clothing, supplies, and equipment that go into warehouses as the infrastructure to receive, sort, transport, and deliver the goods are simply not functional.

Transferability. Many donor organizations and countries support pilot projects to assess their use in other places in the region, country, or throughout the world. For example, one country committed to its history of medicine requested funds from an international donor agency. The request was denied as this agency saw itself as promoting creative ideas and projects that might be applied to other places in the world.

When considering a project's funding, these questions need to be asked. Other questions need to be asked as well—about gender, political, and cultural issues. For example, if an organization plans to support the elimination of the practice of female circumcision, how will that be seen by the population? If a donor agency insists on a democratic process of decision-making, how do leaders implement this process when they have no background or skills in the democratic process and their positions are tied to their ability to make decisions without team input? How do CHWs implement sanitation programs that place farm animals in places segregated from humans when villagers see their cows as sacred and want to have them in the family compound? How does the community health nurse reduce the malaria fever of a newly delivered woman when the village midwife, the untrained *dais*, insists "you sponge her only on day three"? How do you provide international education for a country's highly intelligent practicing nurses when local physicians view the nurses as their assistants?

These and many other questions challenge the underlying assumptions about the process of change and the unplanned effects a well-intentioned intervention is designed to deliver. Yet another question relates to the way community health services are organized.

The most commonly involved organizations that provide health-related interventions and support are described here. An overall umbrella agency is the United Nations (UN). Most people know of the UN's work in peacekeeping. This body also focuses on working conditions through the International Labor Organization (ILO), educational issues through the United Nations Educational Scientific and Cultural Organization (UNESCO), and health issues, specifically, through WHO and UNICEF.

The World Health Organization

The leading global agency that focuses specifically on health is the **World Health Organization (WHO)**. The organization has regional offices in six parts of the world with its headquarters in Geneva, Switzerland. The six regional offices include WHO Regional Office for Americas (PAHO), WHO Regional Office for the Eastern Mediterranean (EMRO), WHO Regional Office for Europe (EURO), WHO Regional Office for Southeast Asia (SEARO), WHO Regional Office for Africa (AFRO), and WHO Regional Office for the Western Pacific (WPRO). The WHO established special offices in Addis Ababa, Ethiopia, to work with the new African Union (formerly the Organization of African Unity) and in Moscow to work with Eastern European countries and the newly independent states of Central Asia. These regional offices recruit and place community health nurses in their many projects throughout their regions.

The WHO, Its History and Its Work

The UN began in 1945, and discussions about the need for a global health organization began. The WHO developed its own constitution which went into effect on April 7, 1948, although it has been closely associated with the UN since its inception. It is responsible for its own programs, funded by regular and extra budgetary funds, and also for health-related initiatives sponsored and funded by UN agencies and other international bodies. The WHO carries out its work through the policies it creates with its member states throughout the world. It does this initially at its annual May meeting, the World Health Assembly (WHA). World Health Day is celebrated annually on the anniversary of WHO's inception (WHO, 2012d).

The World Health Assembly

The World Health Assembly (WHA) is the highest governing body within the WHO and includes 193 member countries. Representatives from each of the world's regions attend this assembly and bring the policies and recommendations to their respective regional offices for implementation and expression at regional and local levels. Staff members at the regional offices then work with their member countries through their annual September Regional Committee Meeting held each year after the WHA.

The WHO provides technical support and advises member states on strategies to meet their health care needs. The WHO serves as a catalyst to mobilize the resources of national governments, financial institutions and endowments, and bilateral partners for health development. Its six-point agenda includes promoting development, fostering health security, strengthening health systems, harnessing information/evidence/research, enhancing partnerships, and improving performance through its ongoing reforms (WHO, 2012h, 2012i). The WHO is not the organization of choice when vehicles, equipment, and medicines are required; the WHO can help a member state determine the drugs that are essential and will assist in developing health policy, project plans, and programs.

The WHO employs many types of professionals, including nurses. However, the organization does not focus on professional issues to support the development of particular health-related practitioners, such as nurses, midwives, social workers, or physicians. Nurses interested in these types of issues should explore opportunities with the International Council of Nurses (ICN) or nursing organizations at national or state levels. In the United States, these would include the American Association of Colleges of Nursing, the American Nurses Association, or National Council of State Boards of Nursing.

The WHO does focus on providing technical support related to the interventions these health professionals deliver, and for these, considerable effort is expended on developing nursing, midwifery, social work, and physician-related knowledge and skills that are basic to these interventions. However, the WHO works closely with the ICN and with national nursing organizations on policies and programming issues.

WHO Collaborating Centers

The WHO generally uses a 5-year planning cycle that is divided into 2-year cycles of projects, documentation, publications, and the development of information systems. Community health nurses are employed at the international level in Geneva, and they hold regional level positions as Regional Nursing Advisors. However, one or two Regional Nursing Advisors cannot possibly carry out the work of a region that might be the home to thousands of nursing personnel. To address this issue, WHO developed a network of **World Health Organization Collaborating Centers** in nursing and other fields. These centers focus on specific areas of expertise and carry out the work of the member countries in these areas. For example, the collaborating center network in nursing of the European Region has focused on PHC and information systems. The European Regional also developed a collaborating center network on disaster preparedness that included a 30-member international team of experts, including the Regional Advisor for Nursing, Midwifery, and Social Work. The network in the United

States has worked through universities in their respective areas of excellence. In the United States, early pioneer universities included the University of Illinois, the University of Pennsylvania, the University of Texas, the University of Alabama, and the University of California. Student nurses in these universities have the opportunity to participate in the research, nursing projects, and other international activities their universities sponsor, both in the United States and in their partnering countries. Sometimes, these collaborating centers represent the WHO and their countries at national and international meetings. They provide critical services that are recognized by but cannot be funded or staffed by the WHO. They also bring credibility to projects, as they come from the communities they represent, and they know the issues and interventions that have the greatest chances of succeeding (WHO, 2012a).

WHO and Its Collaborators

The WHO works closely with national governments, its collaborating center network, its universities, research centers, and NGOs. Experts from member countries are recruited throughout the year to deliberate on global health and health-related issues. For example, during the Chernobyl disaster, WHO/EURO called five internationally recognized nuclear experts to an emergency meeting to examine the issues and assist the member countries with next-step actions to protect their populations, livestock, and agricultural industries. Historically, the WHO has collaborated with centers of excellence throughout the world, including the CDC in the United States.

WHO as a Multilateral Agency

The WHO and other UN agencies are sometimes referred to as *multinational* or **multilateral agencies**. They support development efforts of governments, organizations, and universities in countries throughout the world. The WHO regional offices also collaborate with each other to address issues on which they can partner and provide resources. For example, during the civil wars in Africa, Chad, Angola, and Mozambique, WHO/AFRO and WHO/EURO collaborated to develop projects on rehabilitation for the countries with few nursing programs, no medical schools, and no comprehensive programs for the disabled. The WHO intervenes through its own staff's efforts and through those of its partnerships. In another example, the WHO's health promoting schools is a collaborative effort with UNESCO and UNICEF. Still, another example is the Human Reproduction Program, a global research program on reproductive health. It collaborates with two programs of the UN as well as the World Bank (WB). Similarly, the WHO has joined with several other organizations to fight hunger and improve food standards and has collaborated with UNICEF, the WB, and other agencies on *Deliver Now for Women + Children*, a program launched in 2007 to promote advocacy for women and children in South America, India, and other areas of the world (WHO, 2012b).

Health for All: A Primary Health Care Initiative

In its earlier years, the WHO personnel watched as hospitals and costly health establishments were built throughout the world. One of the world's leading economists, Dr. Brian Abel Smith, noted that countries could not afford to erect costly buildings, nor could they add large numbers of health professional to their cadres of personnel. Rather, he suggested that the health personnel available work with the population to manage their health care needs. His major assertion is that health care needs and wants may expand infinitely, but resources do not, and all must manage with the resources currently available. Many health leaders throughout the world recognized the trends emerging and believed that a major change in thinking and practice was needed. They met together in Alma-Ata, Kazakhstan, in the former Soviet Union and created a sweeping set of declarations that became the *Declaration of Alma-Ata* (see Chapter 1) or **Health for All**. The world body of 134 countries called on all members to reframe their expectations and implement PHC. In Europe, the 32-member countries developed its 38 regional targets for health. In the United States, health care professionals launched *Healthy People 2000*. After the year 2000, *Healthy People 2010* became the blueprint, and now *Healthy People 2020* outlines our goals and objectives for the future (U.S. Department of Health and Human Services, 2012).

Primary health care (PHC) is sometimes called a philosophy, a movement, a way of thinking, a way of working, a setting for health services, or a set of principles. Making it operational at the national level, however, meant that communities would focus on health care services at the local level rather than building large, tertiary hospitals that cater exclusively to urban, financially secure populations. This also meant that the education of health care providers would be located at this level with a de-emphasis on high-cost medical interventions and technology available only to relatively few in the population.

Health for All emphasizes PHC that is affordable, culturally acceptable, appropriate, accessible, and delivered through partnerships between national health services system and local communities. The communities take the leading responsibility for identifying their own priority health concerns and planning and implementing their own PHC service. These PHC services include prevention, health promotion, and curative and rehabilitative care provided by the people themselves (WHO, 2008). (See Figure 16-2 for an illustration of the organizational pattern of community-based PHC.)

Functions of Primary Health Care

Article VII of the *Declaration of Alma-Ata* (now Almaty) lists the eight basic elements of PHC (WHO, 1978):

1. Education concerning prevailing health problems and the methods of preventing and controlling them
2. Promotion of food supply and proper nutrition
3. An adequate supply of safe water and basic sanitation

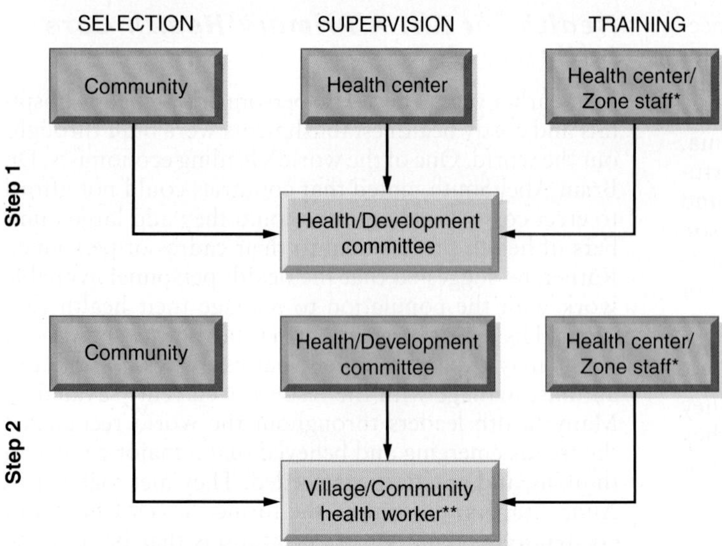

FIGURE 16-2. Community-based primary care.

4. Maternal and child health, including family planning
5. Immunization against major infectious diseases
6. Prevention and control of locally endemic diseases
7. Appropriate treatment of common diseases and injuries
8. Provision of essential drugs

Public health care also involves related sectors concerned with national and community development, including agriculture, animal husbandry, food, industry, education, housing, public works, and communication (Article VI, Section 4). Health for All by the year 2000 was the goal, but around 98% of global deaths occur in developing countries. Much assistance is needed there. Sachs (2008) has called for wealthy countries to devote 0.1% of the gross domestic product (GDP) to assist poor countries with their health issues. Further, he called on low-income countries to pledge 15% of their own budgets to health, and for a comprehensive, global plan for malaria control. HIV and TB should also be addressed by wealthy countries and assistance given to lower-income countries. He also encouraged ready access to sexual and reproductive health services worldwide and an even greater emphasis on PHC.

Deterrents to Primary Health Care

Fostering a PHC approach is one thing, implementing it is another. Initially, political reactions from professional groups feared their incomes would plummet as health services would be delivered not at the level of the tertiary hospital or office of the specialist but at the local level in the cubicle of the primary care provider. Universities and teaching institutions lacked the experience of working in communities and did not know how to educate professionals for PHC. Textbooks were based on education for treating diseases and assumed the backup of well-equipped and in some places, technically advanced hospital environments. Nursing faculty in developing countries adopted community health nursing textbooks from North America but did not understand the problems of placing student nurses in remote clinical areas with no faculty. Faculty was virtually nonexistent in rural areas and, if they were available, clients were not. Stationing young women in villages without supervision was seen in some countries as ill-advised, and clients refused to appear at these health centers. In addition, populations in some rural areas were used to traditional methods and indigenous practitioners, and even when available, professional nurses or midwives were not consulted. Inadequate supervision and follow-up led to misapplication of theory learned, and those in rural areas were not prepared for the situations they faced daily. Health care workers did not understand their responsibilities for maintaining, restocking, and securing medical supplies on a regular basis, and many had no knowledge of community-based principles of case finding, record keeping, community monitoring of immunizations, prenatal care, disease prevention, health promotion, and basic measures to ensure community sanitation. For example, in one rural health center in Southeast Asia, this author observed barrels of antibiotics, medicated creams, lotions, and other medications spoiled from running solutions that had not been sorted, shelved, or refrigerated.

In many places, referral systems to nearby hospitals were not effective, and health care workers were reluctant to place themselves in responsible positions without backup and accessible secondary and tertiary facilities. In one rural community in Spain, a nurse–physician pair who worked closely together confided that they worried that the distance between them and the nearest tertiary facility would threaten their success in securing help for those during periods of emergencies.

Natural environmental phenomena such as rain, floods, and poor or absent communication facilities periodically isolated areas and prevented transport of patients to nearby facilities. Other problems arose when expensive drugs were dispensed in place of less-expensive generic brands (or in some cases were given first to the family and friends of the health care workers) and when health centers failed to refer patients back to the referring CHW. (See Evidence-Based Practice for comparison of physician-led and nurse-led patient care.)

Achievements of Primary Health Care

In the 30 plus years since the 1978 proclamation of *Health for All* by WHO, there have been acknowledged significant global accomplishments. Childhood immunization rates have improved, as has the provision of safe water and sanitation. But the access to essential health care is still not available worldwide. Economic barriers, the shortage of health care personnel, and the worldwide HIV/AIDS epidemic have made it more difficult to achieve this worthwhile goal. One example of expansion of comprehensive services to their full population is Portugal (Waddington, 2008). Portugal organized Family Health Units (FHU), where groups of physicians, nurses, and staff work to provide care to patients and families and make decisions together with them about health needs. Since the 1970s, Portugal's infant mortality rate has dropped by 50% every 8 years; the 2006 rate was 3 per 1,000. Life expectancy jumped 9.2 years in one generation. Patients register for government-sponsored health services through a family physician, and MD/RN salaries are based on productivity and performance (Waddington, 2008). While Portugal has achieved provision of health care to most of its population and improved vital statistics, it still has a high out-of-pocket expenditure (about 22%). High-risk groups (e.g., pregnant women, children, people with diabetes) are exempt from these copayments.

Many other nations need to achieve *Health for All* by making health care a right for all citizens and expanding services to meet the needs of rural populations and high-risk groups. Future action regarding PHC calls for strengthened collaboration among governmental agencies and NGOs in both the public and private sectors. Only then will the world have a realistic chance of achieving all the goals set out in the *Declaration of Alma-Ata* (WHO, 1978).

The Way Forward

One of the greatest achievements of WHO has been the eradication of smallpox. In 1967, this disease threatened 60% of the world's population. It is projected that 20 million people would have died in the next two decades if smallpox had not been eradicated. In 2010, a statute was erected to commemorate the 30th anniversary of smallpox eradication (WHO Media Centre, 2010b). The WHO's other accomplishments include reduction of malaria, standardization of data collection systems, adoption of international standards for the control and reporting of morbidity and mortality, and publication of classic works for the prevention and management of disease. They have also partnered with Rotary International and UNICEF to provide measles, polio, and DPT immunizations to the world's children. In 1990, they reached the 80% mark. In addition, the WHO has been credited with preventing hundreds of millions of cases of tropical diseases. As the 21st century begins, new eradication/elimination programs are under way for polio, leprosy, guinea worm disease, and measles. Other initiatives include:

1. Reducing transmission and incidence of HIV/AIDS
2. Launching the *RBM* program
3. Stopping the transmission of TB

EVIDENCE-BASED PRACTICE

Physician Versus Nurse Interventions

A Cochrane Collaboration systematic review of 4,253 articles netting 16 studies between 1966 and 2002 found that "appropriately trained nurses can produce as high quality care as primary care doctors and achieve as good health outcomes for patients" (para. 9). Nurses in these studies included staff nurses, nurse practitioners, clinical nurse specialists, and advanced practice nurses.

Many lower-income countries rely on nurses to provide some or most primary care, as physicians are scarce. Nurses usually provide care at a lower cost. Quality of care, in this systematic review, was found to be similar. However, cost benefits were not determined. Nurses generally gave more health advice and teaching and achieved higher patient satisfaction than physicians.

Source: Laurant, M., Reeves, D., Hermens, R., Braspenning, J., Groi, R., & Sibbald, B. (2004). *Substitution of doctors by nurses in primary care*. The Cochrane Library. Retrieved from http://onlinelibrary.wiley.com/doi/10.1002/14651858.CD001271.pub2/abstract

4. Increasing access to essential pharmaceuticals
5. Improving the poor quality of some pharmaceuticals
6. Preventing and treating iron deficiency
7. Reducing maternal morbidity and mortality
8. Promoting healthful lifestyles for all age groups, including elders (WHO, 2012h)

Dr. Gro Harlem Brundtland, former Director General of WHO, characterized the 20th century as one encompassing the biggest social transformations of history. Living conditions, she noted, have dramatically improved for the large majority of human beings, and she identified health as the key to improving the productivity of people and nations. She noted the persistence of excess mortality and morbidity that disproportionately affect poor people and underscored the need to focus on those interventions that can achieve the greatest health gains possible using available resources.

International Governmental Organizations with National Governments

Sometimes, the WHO is the first to describe a health-related situation requiring international support. It then contacts other groups or organizations with the requisite expertise, assembling members of its international disaster preparedness teams from governmental organizations that represent various nations. Organizations such as church-related groups, universities, researchers, and governments provide international assistance.

Countries throughout the world are structured to fund within-country health issues and to contribute to the international agenda. The United States contributes internationally through its United States Agency for International Development (USAID). Some other countries' international arms include Denmark's DANIDA and Italy's Italian Cooperation. The European Union (EU) is an organization that provides funding for many health-related projects.

United States Agency for International Development

The USAID is an independent, bilateral agency of the executive branch that is under the guidance of the Secretary of State. It works to enhance long-term and equitable economic growth and to advance U.S. foreign policy by supporting countries in their efforts to recover from disaster, escape poverty, and engage in democratic reforms. The agency provides support to developing countries for economic development, agriculture and trade, global health, democracy, conflict prevention, and humanitarian assistance and does this through its collaboration with many governmental and private agencies to implement its programs (Nichols, 2011). This agency also hires nurses and other health care providers and often provides workshops to brief grant writers on the interventions currently under exploration.

American International Health Alliance

The USAID often collaborates with other organizations to implement its programs. The American International Health Alliance (AIHA) is one of these and operates under a cooperative agreement with USAID. It establishes and manages hospital partnerships between health care institutions in the United States and their counterparts in central and Eastern Europe and in the newly independent states of Central Asia. The AIHA is reportedly the U.S. hospital sector's most coordinated response to health care issues in those areas. AIHA manages programs and research in partnerships with countries in Eurasia (Central and Eastern Europe, Central Asia), Africa, Asia, and the Caribbean (AIHA, 2012).

World Bank

The **World Bank (WB)** is an agency that focuses on economic development, and it includes a health component. It partners with countries, the WHO, and other organizations to address poverty, build capacity, transfer knowledge, provide resources, and forge partnerships in the public and private sectors (The World Bank Group, 2011) (see Display 16.5).

Nongovernmental Organizations

Countries throughout the world provide interventions through formal governmental organizations and through NGOs. These organizations are not under government sponsorship or control. In the United States, they are designated as private voluntary organizations (PVOs) that focus on humanitarian and professional issues related to global health. Examples of PVOs are the Global Health Council (GHC), the Center for International Health and Cooperation, CARE, the Carter Center, and the ICN.

These organizations contribute in their particular areas of expertise and work with other international organizations, research centers, and universities. Some focus on children, such as Save the Children and the International Society of Prevention of Child Abuse and Neglect (SPCAN); some on medically focused interventions, such as Doctors without Borders; and some on logistics and supplies, such as Direct Relief International (DRI).

DISPLAY 16.5 WORLD BANK

The fight against poverty is not a fight for glory. It is about equity and social justice, about the environment and resources we all share, and about peace and security. It is a fight for a better life for all of us and for our children who will live in this very interconnected world.

From Wolfensohn, J. D., & Kircher, A. (2005). *Voice for the world's poor: Selected speeches and writings of World Bank President James D. Wolfensohn, 1995–2005* (quote excerpted from p. 167). Washington, DC: The World Bank.

Global Health Council

The GHC (formerly known as the National Council for International Health) is the world's largest membership alliance dedicated to saving lives by improving health throughout the world. The GHC advocates for needed policies and resources, builds networks and alliances among those working to improve health, and shares innovative ideas, knowledge, and best practices in health (GHC, 2012).

The GHC's membership includes hundreds of private and public organizations around the world, as well as several thousand professionals involved in global health. It is staffed by a multidisciplinary, cross-cultural board of directors, health professionals, student interns, volunteers, and members and serves as a "neutral convener of and information source for the global health community" (GHC, 2012, para 2).

Center for International Humanitarian Cooperation

The Center for International Humanitarian Cooperation (CIHC), founded in 1992, promotes peace and healing in countries shattered by war, regional conflicts, and ethnic violence, as well as natural disasters. Its belief is that health and other basic humanitarian actions often provide the only common ground for initiating dialogue and cooperation among warring parties. The center provides training in mental health issues, disaster management, and negotiation, as well as books on topics ranging from civil strife to epidemics (CIHC, n.d.).

CARE

The Cooperative for American Remittances to Europe (CARE) was founded in 1945, when 22 American organizations joined together to rush lifesaving *care packages* from individual American citizens, churches, clubs, and businesses to survivors of World War II. Millions of CARE packages followed in the next two decades. In the 1950s, CARE expanded its program to developing nations, using surplus American food to feed the hungry. In the 1960s, it pioneered PHC. Now renamed the Cooperative for Assistance and Relief Everywhere, CARE is affiliated with foundations and other organizations, as well as the UN and the EU. CARE intervenes by responding to famines and disasters worldwide with emergency food, supplies, and rehabilitative efforts. It delivers programs in education, health, population, water and sanitation, agriculture, environmental preservation, economic development, and community building (CARE, n.d.).

The Carter Center

Former United States President, Jimmy Carter, and his wife Roselyn, founded the Carter Center in 1986. The Carter Center intervenes in disease prevention and agriculture throughout the world and cites its fundamental mission as "human rights and alleviation of human suffering" (The Carter Center, 2012, para 2). The particularly successful interventions include the guinea worm disease eradication program and the program to eradicate river blindness, as well as trachoma and schistosomiasis control. Lymphatic filariasis elimination, malaria control, and mental health issues, along with an international task force on disease eradication, are also components of its health program.

International Council of Nurses

As noted earlier, the ICN represents the global interests and concerns of the nursing profession. ICN's mission is to maintain the role of nursing in health care through its global voice. Its current membership includes nursing organizations from 130 countries representing 13 million nurses (ICN, 2011).

National Governments Working Alone

Individual nations have considerable experience working across agencies and organizations, and they have traditions that they honor as they intervene. For example, the Federal Republic of Germany has one of the largest voluntary sectors in the world and is known for its work with the International Red Cross. The Finnish Nursing Organization has an outstanding international reputation for its work during the Armenian earthquake and in other international efforts throughout Europe. The Danish Nurses Organization has provided funds, leadership, and expertise to numerous projects in collaboration with the WHO and with the ICN.

At times, however, governments facing a crisis or disaster prefer to operate alone, without international assistance. This position must be respected, and because of this expectation, international organizations will not appear in a country until a formal request is received from representatives of the country in crisis. Furthermore, some countries are more receptive to certain kinds of assistance than others. Some countries do not welcome foreign professionals, as they believe they have enough of their own. They may prefer help in the form of equipment, transport, medications, or vital supplies, such as water and food. Those in disaster preparedness are well aware of what some refer to as the "second disaster," when well-intentioned groups send in truckloads of used clothing and articles that are useless in some environments. The recent disasters in Haiti lead to an outbreak of cholera that was brought into the country by international workers. This experience has added another layer of concern for those involved in relief work. Further, these disasters have also spurred the removal of children from affected countries; some of these are characterized as rescue missions, some are reported to arise out of groups dedicated to religious objectives, and some have been shown to occur out of financial interests (receiving payment for couples wishing to adopt children). At times, governments would prefer to work alone but do not have the resources to do so, nor can their authorities provide the personnel to sort the kinds of contributions donors provide during emergencies.

Organizations with Religious Affiliations

Many organizations are sponsored by religious groups, some of which include a religiously oriented agenda along with their interventions. Some, however, do not. Often, the work of these groups is similar to those with a non-religious focus, and the source of funding for a particular project may be the only overt connection to any religious group. Catholic Charities and other Christian organizations provide critical interventions, as do Muslim, Jewish, and other religiously oriented organizations. These organizations often recruit community health nurses and other health care providers for short- and long-term assignments. See Perspectives: One Nurse's Experience Overseas.

COMMUNITY HEALTH NURSING OPPORTUNITIES

Let us suppose that, after reading this chapter and some of its references, you have decided to work in a location other than your own. You are not alone.

> Global health programs are becoming increasingly prevalent at academic health centers. These programs range in scope from comprehensive, multidisciplinary, multi-professional initiatives—with patient care, research, and education components—to individual courses. The larger initiatives may involve collaborative efforts among schools of medicine, public health, nursing, and dentistry, and may have alliances with schools outside the health professions. This growth in the number of programs is accompanied by a surge of interest in every facet of global health among health science students and trainees. (Kanter, 2008, p. 115)

If you decided to pursue work abroad, you might begin your work at a local level, at a local health center in a village. You would be aware of your own issues and reasons for wanting this experience, and you would have selected the location because of some factors that draw you to it. How then might you go about preparing for the experience? In what kind of activities might you be involved? What might be the expectations and commitments you would make regarding the assignment?

Community health nurses, as shown in this chapter, carry major responsibility for managing health services in health centers, clinics, schools, workplaces, and community settings that range in population density and complexity from remote areas to major centers in large metropolitan areas. This work includes providing education, guidance, and professional supervision to other cadres of health care providers.

Before you travel, conduct your own preliminary needs assessment. You can use the logic of the thinking process developed in this chapter and move through the framework as a guide. Begin, as this chapter suggests, with a review of the context. Here, you would examine the location, climate, temperatures, weather conditions, travel routes, living arrangements, languages spoken,

PERSPECTIVES
ONE NURSE'S EXPERIENCE OVERSEAS

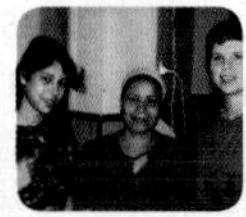

I had always wanted to be a nurse and work in a foreign country, so when I heard of an organization that sent health workers overseas, I got involved while I was in college. The experiential cross-cultural training that my husband and I received before we left made all the difference in preparing us to have a positive transition. We learned that our goal would be to become "servant learners," serving the local population and learning from them rather than coming in to solve their problems with our superior ways of doing things. This was a hard lesson to learn and we kept coming back to it in our 18 years abroad as we searched for the rationales behind customs that puzzled us. I also had to find a balance between "going native" in each new culture and keeping the parts of my own identity which were valuable.

When we first arrived, it was like nothing I expected. No one met us at the airport as planned, we did not speak the language, a luggage cart hit me from behind and cut my leg, and it was hot, crowded, and dirty. This was not a complete surprise as I had been prepared for the actual experience to differ from my expectations, but adjusting took conscious effort. I expected to go to a delta town and work in an established hospital. We were asked to go to a major seaport city and teach English! We did find an opportunity to work in community health with the goal of "working ourselves out of a job" by training national workers who would be far more effective in their country than we could ever be.

Flexibility, comfort with ambiguity, being able to laugh at ourselves, and patience when results seemed few and far between were essential skills. I learned much about myself and grew in my ability to cross cultures. I learned to actually prefer other ways of doing and being. My faith deepened and I learned to depend upon it like I never had before. We were accepted by people who brought us into their culture and treated us like family, which I consider the most valuable part of the whole experience as I look back upon our time there. Our children were born overseas and grew up feeling at ease in many settings and with a particular sensitivity to differing perspectives. I know what it is to live with war, to celebrate life in impossibly difficult circumstances, and to stand truly in another's shoes—experiences I would never have had at home but which expanded my life. Although I had no idea when I first got off that airplane that I would spend most of my adult life in foreign countries, I am so grateful for the opportunity I have had to live my dreams.

Karin Urso, RN, PHN
Missionary Nurse

cultural patterns, religious beliefs, and religious holidays. Locate novels and literature from the country, as this source of data is often more revealing than many of the statistical charts and information available from official sources. Interacting with people from the country often provides valuable insights not available from reading materials. In all probability, you will find enclaves of people living in the United States from the country in which you plan to work. For example, Armenian communities are located in Watertown, Massachusetts, and Los Angeles, California. There are many Ethiopian communities in Atlanta, Georgia; New York City, New York; and Los Angeles, California. There are groups and organizations of Albanian Americans, Polish Americans, Hungarian Americans, Romanian Americans, Indian Americans, Ethiopian Americans, and Mexican Americans. These groups maintain close contact with their mother country and receive and give support to their family members and organizations in those countries.

Next, examine the population's health status, at the regional levels (e.g., Europe, Asia, Africa), the country level (Chad, Nepal, India), and at the local level (Tete Provinces and villages in Tete Provinces, Mozambique). Here, you would review the data to identify the universals of care, that is, the causes of mortality and morbidity, the level of functioning in the community, decision making (if available), and cost of health care.

Then, move on to review evidence of the three eras of health conditions in the country and determine the age of the population and the health conditions they experience, given their history, location, and experiences with natural or man-made disasters. Look at birth rates, death rates, infant mortality rates, and maternal mortality rates, asking the following: how many infants are born? How many of these die at birth, during the first month of life, during the first year of life? How long do people live? What kills them? What makes them sick? How do people function everyday? What kinds of decisions do they have to make and how do they make them? What community supports exist to help people with these processes? What is the average income per capita? What do people buy with their money?

Review the conditions that account for the three eras of health conditions as described in this chapter and determine the prevailing health conditions that you will encounter. Review the kinds of health conditions that are reported both in the professional literature and in the popular literature and media.

Next, it's helpful to review the organization with which you will be associated. Examine its philosophy, its mission, its ways of working, its relationship to the community of interest, and the ways in which community health nurses are considered, placed, and function. Query the nature of the health care team of which you would become a member, those to whom you report, and those who would report to you. Review their scope of practice, the interventions they provide, and their ways of delivering health services.

It is helpful to identify the international governmental and NGOs working in the area and obtain their publications for review and their addresses and contact numbers (when you arrive in the area, visit these organizations and request a briefing). Review the projects currently under way, and examine their track record for the factors that suggest ill-conceived outcomes and evidence of those that produced successful outcomes.

If you are considering further education, you will find many opportunities available to you. Universities throughout North America have developed partnerships with universities, governments, and agencies in

PERSPECTIVES
VOICES FROM THE COMMUNITY

You cannot build a strong country on the backs of sick people.

Dr. Mohammad Akhter, Executive Director, American Public Health Association

Nurses and midwives play a crucial and cost-effective role in reducing excess mortality, morbidity, and disability and in promotion of healthy lifestyles.

Dr. Gro Harlem Brundtland, Director-General, World Health Organization

Global health nurses always receive far more than they give.

Cydne, former Peace Corps nurse

The developing world may be poor materially, but it is rich in hope and spirit.

Edith, missionary nurse

Nurses working in foreign lands make a big difference through their training and support of local nurses and others. Their professional dedication to quality health care and promotion of healthful living among their patients, families, and communities serves as an effective role model and has a profound impact on the wellbeing of the people they work with.

Tom, physician

Living overseas for many years was a challenging and rewarding experience. Raising a family was not always easy, but our six children, now adults, value the exposure they had to other cultures and the many interesting friendships they made.

Inez, spouse of a global health administrator

Nurses play an important role ministering to the health care needs of not only the indigenous population, but also the sometimes-sizable population of expatriates and their families.

Jennifer, teacher

There is nothing so powerful as seeing a community that has changed through individuals taking responsibility for them and their own community.

Lydia, volunteer PHN with Medical Ambassadors

other countries. The major universities and colleges that specialize in community health most often include schools of public health and graduate programs in nursing. Harvard's School of Public Health, Johns Hopkins University, Wayne State University, Duke University, the University of Illinois, the University of Pennsylvania, to name just a few, provide scholar practitioner education to those wishing to work toward providing access to health care, develop community partnerships to ensure health care for the uninsured, and serve as researchers, teachers, practitioners, community health administrators, or health information specialists. A world of challenges and a world of opportunity and self-learning are waiting—when you are ready.

Following this review, identify and remediate gaps in your knowledge of theory and practice. Most importantly, take the time to plan, to take care of yourself and your health, as your own health status is critical to your functioning in what may be a very different context from your own.

To explore specific opportunities, contact the organization of interest (see the listing of selected organizations at the end of the chapter). Some of the larger organizations, such as the WHO, require graduate education and at least 5 years of experience, but many organizations do not. Nurses can participate in numerous smaller organizations that are involved in health programs. Among such groups seeking nurses are the U.S. Peace Corps, religious and lay organizations, and private and governmental agencies, societies, and foundations. Health Volunteers Overseas (HVO) is an example of a private, nonprofit organization that seeks to improve health care quality and access in developing countries through education. Twelve professional organizations sponsor HVO, including the American Association of Colleges of Nursing (HVO, 2011). The GHC provides information on career opportunities in global health for community health nurses and others. It also offers career seminars and provides suggestions from global health experts for nurses interested in entering the field (GHC, 2008). University student nurses can also contact their campus office of global affairs for opportunities available overseas (see Perspectives: Voices from the Community).

SUMMARY

Community health nursing is practiced throughout the world and can be considered within a useful, worldwide framework. This framework considers first the context within which the population, the provider, and the procedures interact.

The context reflects a location's geography, history, weather, culture, religious patterns, and belief systems. This context is a critical element that community health nurses appreciate for its influences on the populations, the providers, and the interventions they are able to deliver.

Community health nurses work with populations that vary from country to country, and to serve them appropriately requires an understanding of the ways in which the context in which they are located interacts with their health status and health histories. In this regard, an examination is required to assess the universal imperatives of care, to identify the population's current health status, and to determine the focus of nursing interventions. That is, when a population is experiencing high mortality, the interventions must be targeted to that level and not, say, at the level of functioning.

Community health nurses also examine the population to assess the kinds of health conditions they experience, and the three eras are helpful guides in this assessment. These are the Era of Infectious Diseases, the Era of Chronic Long-Term Health Conditions, and the Era of Social Conditions. The three P's (population, providers, and procedures) relate to the interventions community health nurses deliver as they serve populations and are informed by the organization with which the community health nurse works. A number of international, national, and local organizations intervene in communities. Some of these agencies are intergovernmental and multilateral, such as the UN and WHO; others are bilateral, such as the USAID and the Peace Corps. Many NGOs (or PVOs) also assist with global health.

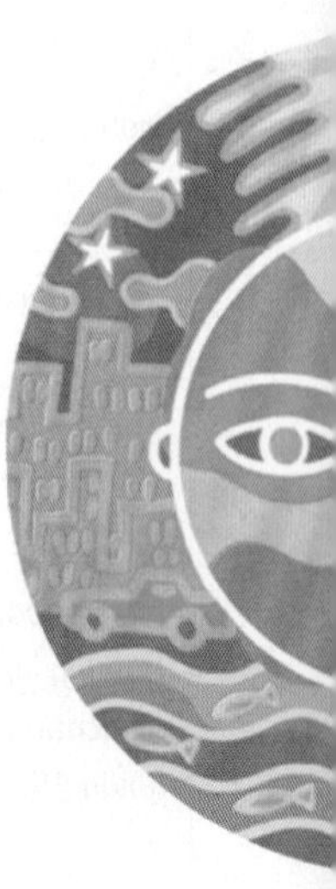

The focus remains on delivering PHC to populations throughout the world. The world's communities deliver health care in different ways, depending on their political economies. The entrepreneurial, welfare-oriented, comprehensive, and socialist systems provide for the health of their citizens in unique ways.

Variations of these systems exist, depending on whether the country is considered industrialized, transitional, or very poor. The GBD study has provided important quantifiable information about morbidity and mortality in the world, as well as disability measurements. Primary global health concerns include the eradication, elimination, or control of communicable disease, as well as immunization,

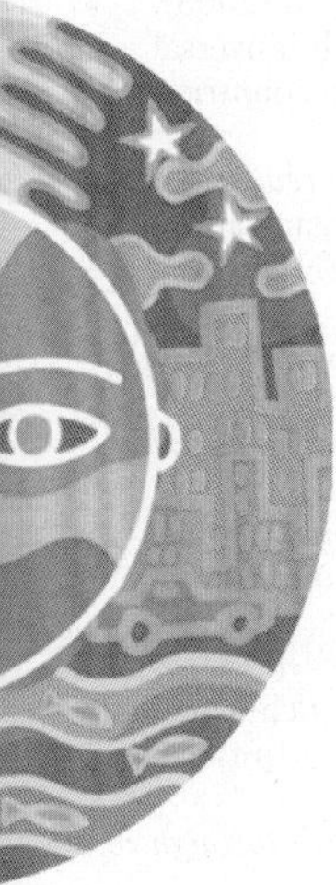

maternal and perinatal morbidity and mortality, tobacco-related diseases, chronic disease, environmental illness, and malnutrition. In addition to these age-old health problems, there are new, emerging, and reemerging diseases. Armed conflicts and political upheavals also adversely affect health; this is an important consideration because of the number of major armed conflicts occurring at any given time.

Community health nursing services are critical to the ultimate health of a community. They provide important primary, secondary, and tertiary levels of care and prevention throughout the world. In the future, community health nurses will continue as major contributors to global health.

ACTIVITIES TO PROMOTE **CRITICAL THINKING**

1. What infectious diseases are most commonplace around the world? What is being done to combat them?
2. Which of the worldwide leading risk factors also impact the United States? Why? What can you, as a public health nurse, do to address these risk factors?
3. Identify a country or community in which you would like to practice community health nursing. Before you begin a review of this community, write down your own knowledge, attitudes, and beliefs about the country, the people, and the culture. Examine your own reasons for wanting this experience. Identify the way you might feel if you were the recipient rather than the donor of the services you plan to provide.
4. Conduct your own needs assessment using the framework provided in this chapter. Given what you have found, what would you prioritize as the major focus of a community nursing intervention for that community? Provide your rationale for your choices.
5. Given what you have found, what organizations, groups, or references would you access before you left on your assignment?
6. Based on your examination, what questions would you want to ask of the employing agency before you left on your assignment? What additional actions would you take to protect yourself and your health, given the review you conducted?
7. What sources of information appear to be most informative? What data are you seeking that are not reported? Why do you think this is the case?
8. Identify a person or a group from the community in which you plan to work. Develop an interview protocol that includes questions that address the framework developed in this chapter. What are the most appropriate questions these individuals or groups can answer?

REFERENCES

Abu-Raddad, L., Hilmi, N., Mumtaz, G., Benkirane, M., Akala, F., Ayodeji, R., et al. (2010). Epidemiology for HIV infection in the Middle East and North Africa. *AIDS, 24,* S5–S23.

Amanatullah, E., & Morris, M. (2010). Negotiating gender roles: Gender differences in assertive negotiating are mediated by women's fear of backlash and attenuated when negotiating on behalf of others. *Journal of Personality & Social Psychology, 98*(2), 256–267.

American International Health Alliance. (2012). *What we do.* Retrieved from http://www.aiha.com/en/WhatWeDo/

Artzy-Randrup, Y., Alonso, D., & Pascual, M. (2010). Transmission intensity and drug resistance in malaria population dynamics: Implications for climate change. *PLoS ONE, 5*(10), e13588. doi: 10.1371/journal.pone.0013588. Retrieved from http://www.plosone.org/article/info%3Adoi%2F10.1371%2Fjournal.pone.0013588

Bender, L., David, L., Chilcott, L., & Burns, S. Z. (Producers) & Guggenheim, D. (Director) (2006). *An Inconvenient Truth* [Film]. United States: Paramount Home Entertainment.

Brookmeyer, R. (2010). Measuring the HIV/AIDS epidemic: Approaches and challenges. *Epidemiologic Reviews, 32*, 26–37.

Brunner, B., & Johnson, D. (2007). *Timeline: The former Yugoslavia*. Retrieved from http://www.infoplease.com/spot/yugotimeline1.html

Cain, K., Haley, C., Armstrong, L., Garman, K., Wells, C., Iademarco, M., et al. (2007). Tuberculosis among foreign-born persons in the United States: Achieving tuberculosis elimination. *American Journal of Respiratory Critical Care Medicine, 175*(1), 75–79.

CARE. (n.d.). *Frequently asked questions*. Retrieved January 31, 2012 from http://www.care.org/about/faqs.asp

Center for International Humanitarian Cooperation. (n.d.). *Promoting healing and peace*. Retrieved January 31, 2012 from http://www.cihc.org/

Centers for Disease Control and Prevention (CDC). (2011a). West Nile Virus: Virus history and distribution. Retrieved from http://www.cdc.gov/ncidod/dvbid/westnile/background.htm

Centers for Disease Control and Prevention (CDC). (2011b). *2003 West Nile Virus activity in the United States*. Retrieved from http://www.cdc.gov/ncidod/dvbid/westnile/surv&control CaseCount03_detailed.htm

Centers for Disease Control and Prevention (CDC). (2011c). *Preliminary investigation suggests BSE-infected cow in Washington State was likely imported from Canada*. Retrieved from http://www.cdc.gov/ncidod/dvrd/bse/bse_washington_2003.htm

Climate Crisis. (n.d.). *An inconvenient truth: The film*. Retrieved from http://www.climatecrisis.net/an_inconvenient_truth/about_the_film.php

Corcoran, E., Nellemann, C., Baker, E., Bos, D., Osborn, D., & Savelli, H. (Eds.). (2010). *Sick water? The central role of wastewater management in sustainable development*. United Nations Environmental Programme. Retrieved from http://www.unep.org/pdf/SickWater_screen.pdf

Crisp, N. (2010). *Turning the world upside down: The search for global health in the 21st century*. London: Royal Society of Medicine.

Davenport, R. J. (2007). A new century of new challenges: Infection research faces new threats. *Infection Research*. Retrieved from http://www.infection-research.de/perspectives/detail/pressrelease/infection_research_in_the_21th_century_old_enemies_new_threats/

Davies, S. E. (2008). Securitizing infectious disease. *International Affairs, 84*(2), 295–313.

DeMoor, T., & Van Zanden, J. (2010). Girl power: The European marriage pattern and labour markets in the North Sea region in the late medieval and early modern period. *The Economic History Review, 63*, 1–33.

Eishinnawi, M. (2011, June 7). *Egyptian Americans help post-revolution Egypt*. Voice of America: North Africa. Retrieved from http://www.voanews.com/english/news/africa/north/How-do-Egyptian-Americans-help-post-revolution-Egypt–123369318.html

Ensor, T., Quayyum, Z., Nadjib, M., & Sucahya, P. (2009). Level and determinants of incentives for village midwives in Indonesia. *Health Policy and Planning, 24*(1), 26–35.

Farrell, M. (1986). *Development of a WHO Centre in Addis Ababa, Africa for disaster preparedness and relief*. Ethiopia/Italian Ministries of Health and Foreign Affairs/WHO Regional Office for Europe.

Farrell, M. (2009). Living evidence: Translating research into practice. In T. Porter-O-Grady, & K. Malloch (Eds.). *Evidence-based practice: A professional resource* (2 nd ed.), (pp. 99–118). Sudbury, MA: Jones and Bartlett Publishers.

Farrell, M., Harkless, G., Orzack, L. H., Houd, S., Oakley, A., & Socenyi, C. (1994). Hungarian midwives and their practice: A national survey. *Midwifery, 10*, 67–72.

Fearon, J. D. (2007, March/April). Iraq's civil war. *Foreign Affairs*. Retrieved from http://www.foreignaffairs.com/articles/62443/james-d-fearon/iraqs-civil-war

Foucault, M. (1965). *Madness and civilization: A history of insanity in the age of reason*. New York: Vintage.

Freire, P. (1970). *Pedagogy of the oppressed*. New York: Continuum Publishing Company.

Friedman, T. L. (2005). *The world is flat: A brief history of the 21st century*. New York: Farrar, Straus & Giroux.

Gallimore, R. B. (2008). Militarism, ethnicity, and sexual violence in the Rwandan genocide. *Feminist Africa, 10*, 9–25.

Ginsburg, J. A., Doherty, R. B., Ralston, J. F, & Senkeeto, N. (2008). Achieving a high-performance health care system with universal access: What the United States can learn from other countries. *Annals of Internal Medicine, 148*(1), 55–75.

Global Alert and Response (GAR). (2010). *Scientific review of variola virus research, 1999–2010*. World Health Organization. Retrieved from http://whqlibdoc.who.int/hq/2010/WHO_HSE_GAR_BDP_2010.3_eng.pdf

Global Health Council. (2008). *Career network*. Retrieved from http://careers.globalhealth.org/

Global Security. (2011). *Ethiopia/Eritrea war*. Retrieved from http://www.globalsecurity.org/military/world/war/eritrea.htm

Goldin, I., Cameron, G., Balarajan, M. (2011). *Exceptional people: How migration shaped our world and will define our future*. Princeton, NJ: University Press.

Goodman, B. (2011, September 1). CDC: *Vaccination rates for toddlers rising*. WebMD. Retrieved from http://children.webmd.com/vaccines/news/20110901/cdc-vaccination-rates-for-toddlers-rising

Health Volunteer Overseas. (2011). *Improving global health through education*. Retrieved from http://www.hvousa.org/

Heymann, D. L. (Ed.). (2008). *Control of communicable diseases manual* (19th ed.) Washington, DC: American Public Health Association.

Ho, C. S., & Gostin, L. O. (2009). The social face of economic growth: China's health system in transition. *JAMA, 301*(17), 1809–1811.

Hobbs, C. V. & Essajee, S. M. (2009). Early treatment of HIV: Implications for resource-limited settings. *Current Opinion in HIV & AIDS, 4*(3), 222–231.

Hochschild, A. (1999). *King Leopold's ghost*. New York: Houghton Mifflin Co.

Husted, H., Lunn, T., Troelsen, A., Gaarn-Larsen, L., Kristensen, B., & Kehlet, H. (2011). Why still in hospital after fast-track hip and knee arthroplasty? *Acta Orthopaedica, 82*(6), 679–684.

Illyes, G. (1979). *People of the Puszta*. Budapest, Hungary: Franklin Printing House.

International Centre for Human Resources in Nursing (ICHRN). (2008). *An ageing nursing workforce*. Retrieved from http://www.icn.ch/images/stories/documents/publications/fact_sheets/2a_FS-Ageing_Workforce.pdf

International Council of Nurses (ICN). (2011). *About ICN*. Retrieved from http://www.icn.ch/about-icn/about-icn/

Jamison, D. T., Bremen, J. G., Measham, A. R., Allelyne, G., Claeson, M., Evans, D. B. et al. (Eds.). (2006). *Disease control priorities in developing countries* (2nd ed.). New York: Oxford University Press.

Kanter, S. (2008). Global health is more important in a smaller world. *Academic Medicine, 83*(2), 115–116.

Khazeni, N., Hutton, D., Garber, A., Hupert, N., & Owens, D. (2009). Effectiveness and cost-effectiveness of vaccination against pandemic influenza (H1N1) 2009. *Annals of Internal Medicine*. Retrieved from http://www.annals.org/content/early/2009/10/05/0003-4819-151-12-200912150-00157.full

Kiem, E. (2009, October 21). *State of the world's vaccines: Childhood immunization at record high*. UNICEF. Retrieved from http://www.unicef.org/immunization/index_51482.html

King, A. C., & Guralnik, J. M. (2010). Maximizing the potential of an aging population. *JAMA, 304*(17), 1944–1945.

Kirk, G., & Okazawa-Rey, M. (2009). *Women's lives: Multicultural perspectives* (5th ed.). New York: McGraw-Hill.

Kosek, M., Lanata, C., Black R. Walker, D., Snyder, J., Abdus, M. et al. (2009). Directing diarrhoeal disease research towards disease-burden reduction. *Journal of Health, Population and Nutrition, 27*(3), 319–331.

Kramer, L., Stuyer, L., & Ebel, G. (2008). A global perspective on the epidemiology of West Nile Virus. *Annual Review of Entomology, 53*, 61–81.

Kunzig, R. (2011). Population seven billion. *National Geographic, 219*(1), 32–69.

Medline Plus Merriam-Webster Medical Dictionary. (2012). *Leprosy*. Retrieved from http://www.merriam-webster.com/medlineplus/leprosy

Murray, C. J., & Lopez, A. D. (1997). Mortality by cause for eight regions of the world: Global Burden of Disease Study. *Lancet, 349*, 1269–1347.

National Archives and Records Administration. (n.d.). *The deadly virus: The influenza epidemic of 1918*. Retrieved from http://www.archives.gov/exhibits/influenza-epidemic/

National Geographic Daily News. (2011, March 15). *Japan tsunami: 20 unforgettable pictures*. Retrieved from http://news.nationalgeographic.com/news/2011/03/pictures/110315-nuclear-reactor-japan-tsunami-earthquake-world-photos-meltdown/

National Institute of Allergy and Infectious Diseases (NIAID). (2008, August 19). *Bacterial pneumonia caused most deaths in 1918 influenza pandemic: Implications for future pandemic planning*. News Release. Retrieved from http://www.nih.gov/news/health/aug2008/niaid-19.htm

Nichols, R. W. (2011). Moving USAID forward. *Science, 9*, 1381. doi: 10.1126/science.333.6048.1381-a

Organisation for Economic Cooperation and Development (OECD). (2010). *Joint meeting of the chemicals committee and the working party on chemicals, pesticides and biotechnology*. Retrieved from http://search.oecd.org/officialdocuments/displaydocumentpdf/?cote=env/jm/mono(2010)7&doclanguage=en

PATH. (2008). *Oral rehydration therapy/oral rehydration solution*. Retrieved from http://www.path.org/files/IMM_EDD-ort_fs.pdf

Pease, A. (2010). Smallpox bioterrorism. How big a threat? *Yale Journal of Medicine and Law, 6*(2). Retrieved from http://www.yalemedlaw.com/2010/02/smallpox-bioterrorism-how-big-a-threat/

Pittman, P., Aiken, L., & Buchan, J. (2007). International migration of nurses: Introduction. *Health Services Research, 42*(3 Pt 2), 1275–1280.

Rehydration Project. (2010). *Focus on diarrhea, dehydration, and rehydration*. Retrieved from http://rehydrate.org/diarrhoea/#65

Reingold, A. L., & Phares, C. R. (2006). Infectious diseases. In M. H. Merson, R. E. Black, & A. J. Mills (Eds.). *International public health diseases, program, system, and policies* (2nd ed.) (pp. 710–711). Gaithersburg, MD: Aspen.

ReliefWeb. (2011). *Armenia, USSR earthquake. December 1988 UNDRO situation reports 1-14*. Retrieved from http://reliefweb.int/node/34437

Reuters News Service. (2009). Brazil approves *Amazon hydro-power dam*. Environmental News Network. Retrieved from http://www.enn.com/top_stories/article/40015

Roemer, M. I. (1993). *National health systems of the world* (Vols. I & II). New York: Oxford University Press.

Rosato, M., Laverack, G., Grabman, L. H., Tripathy, P., Nair, N., Mwansambo, C. et al. (2008). Community participation: Lessons for maternal, newborn, and child health. *The Lancet, 372*(9642), 962–971.

Rose, K. W. (2008). *The Rockefeller Foundation's fellowship program in Turkey, 1925–1983*. Retrieved from http://www.rockarch.org/publications/resrep/pdf/roseturkey.pdf

Sachs, J. D. (2008, January). Primary health for all (extended version). *Scientific American*. Retrieved from http://www.scientificamerican.com/article.cfm?id=primary-health-for-all-extended

Schaffer Library of Drug Policy. (2011). *Worldwide trends in tobacco consumption and mortality*. Retrieved from http://druglibrary.net/schaffer/tobacco/who-tobacco.htm

Schlein, L. (2007, July 28). WHO says environmental hazards kill millions of children. *Voice of America News*. Retrieved October 1, 2008 from http://www.voanews.com/english/archive/2007-07/2007-07-28-voa27.cfm?CFID=48545824&CFTOKEN=37283846.

Sheridan, K. (2011, October 13). *Indoor cooking stoves kill 2 million yearly: Study*. AFP. Retrieved from http://www.google.com/hostednews/afp/article/ALeqM5ie2kolKAgQ65-FeWVnnWa9xNsr6A?docId=CNG.a3ab38cb5db8b5323b644de0172e361a.2b1

Sidel, V. W., & Levy, B. S. (2008). The health impact of war. *International Journal of Injury Control and Safety Promotion, 15*(4), 189–195.

Siegel, R., & Watson, I. (2006). *Lebanon begins post-war recovery effort*. National Public Radio broadcast. Retrieved December 12, 2011 from http://www.npr.org/templates/story/story.php?storyId=5671702&storyid=5671702

Skinner, E. B. (2010, January 18). South Africa's new slave trade and the campaign to stop it. *Time Magazine*. Retrieved from http://www.time.com/time/magazine/article/0,9171,1952335,00.html

Spector, R. E. (2008). *Cultural diversity in health and illness* (7th ed.). Upper Saddle River, NJ: Pearson.

The Boston Globe. (2011, April 25). *Chernobyl disaster 25th anniversary*. Retrieved from http://www.boston.com/bigpicture/2011/04/chernobyl_disaster_25th_annive.html

The Carter Center. (2012). *About us: Our mission*. Retrieved from http://www.cartercenter.org/about/index.html

The Halo Trust. (2011). *Prince Harry visits Halo Mozambique*. Retrieved from http://www.halotrust.org/media/news/prince_harry.aspx

The New York Times. (2006, December 18). *The AIDS-malaria connection*. Retrieved from http://www.nytimes.com/2006/12/18/opinion/18mon2.html

The Ozone Hole. (n.d.). *Montreal Protocol on ozone-depleting substances effective, but work still unfinished says Secretary General in message for International Day*. Retrieved December 12, 2011 from http://www.theozonehole.com/ozoneday2006.htm

The World Bank Group. (2011). *About us*. Retrieved from http://web.worldbank.org/WBSITE/EXTERNAL/EXTABOUTUS/0,pagePK:50004410~piPK:36602~theSitePK:29708,00.html

Thomas, L., & Lewis, G. (2009). The epidemiology of mental illness. In L. Gask, H. Lester, T. Kendrick, & R. Peveler (Eds.), *Primary care mental health* (pp. 3–15). London: Royal College of Psychiatrists.

Tribble, S. J. (2011, June 13). *East Cleveland's Huron Hospital closing despite best efforts of its longtime advocate*. Retrieved December 12, 2011 from http://www.cleveland.com/medical/index.ssf/2011/06/huron_hospital_closing_despite.html

United Nations High Commissioner for Refugees (UNHCR). (2010). *Public health equity in refugee and other displaced persons settings*. Retrieved from http://www.unhcr.org/cgi-bin/texis/vtx/home/opendocPDFViewer.html?docid=4bdfe1699&query=refugee%20health

United Nations-Water. (2008). *Tackling a global crisis: International Year of Sanitation*. Retrieved from http://esa.un.org/iys/docs/IYS_flagship_web_small.pdf

U.S. Department of Health and Human Services (USDHHS). (2012). *Healthy People 2020*. Retrieved from http://www.healthypeople.gov/2020/default.aspx

Viswanathan, M., Kraschnewski, J., Nishikawa, B., Morgan, L., Thieda, P., Honneycutt, A., et al. (2009, June). *Outcomes of community health worker interventions*. Rockville, MD: Agency for Healthcare Research and Quality (AHRQ); (Evidence Reports/Technology Assessments, No. 181.) Available from: http://www.ncbi.nlm.nih.gov/books/NBK44601/

Waddington, R. (2008). Portugal's rapid progress through primary health care. *Bulletin of the World Health Organization (WHO), 86*(11), 817–908.

Walker, C., Friberg, I., Binkin, N., Young, M., Walker, N., Fontaine, O. et al. (2011). Scaling up diarrhea prevention and treatment interventions: A lives saved tool analysis. *PLoS Medicine, 8*(3), e1000428. doi: 10.1371/journal.pmed.1000428

Warburg, G. (2010). A history of modern Sudan and war and survival in Sudan's frontierlands: Voices from the Blue Nile. *Middle Eastern Studies, 46*(2), 307–312.

Water.org. (2011). *Billions daily affected by water crisis*. Retrieved from http://water.org/water-crisis/one-billion-affected/

World Health Organization (WHO). (1978). *Primary health care: Alma Ata conference*. Geneva: Author. Retrieved from http://whqlibdoc.who.int/publications/9241800011.pdf

World Health Organization (WHO). (2008). *World health report 2008: Primary health care (now more than ever)*. Retrieved from http://www.who.int/whr/2008/en/index.html

World Health Organization (WHO). (2009a). *Global health risks: Mortality and burden of disease attributable to selected major risks*. Geneva: Author.

World Health Organization (WHO). (2009b, June 10). *Child deaths from preventable environmental hazards "can and must be stopped"*. News release. Western Pacific Region: Author. Retrieved from http://www.wpro.who.int/media_centre/press_releases/pr_20091006.htm

World Health Organization (WHO) Media Centre. (2010, August). *H1N1 in post-pandemic period*. Retrieved from http://www.who.int/mediacentre/news/statements/2010/h1n1_vpc_20100810/en/index.html

World Health Organization (WHO). (2011). *Integrated management of childhood illness (IMCI)*. Retrieved from http://www.who.int/child_adolescent_health/topics/prevention_care/child/imci/en/

World Health Organization (WHO). (2012a). *Collaborating centres: More on the collaborating centres*. Retrieved from http://www.who.int/collaboratingcentres/cc_historical/en/index.html

World Health Organization (WHO). (2012b). *Deliver Now for Women + Children: The initiative*. Retrieved from http://www.who.int/pmnch/activities/delivernow/en/index.html

World Health Organization (WHO). (2012c). *Health topics: Global burden of disease*. Retrieved from http://www.who.int/topics/global_burden_of_disease/en/

World Health Organization (WHO). (2012d). *History of WHO*. Retrieved from http://www.who.int/about/history/en/index.html

World Health Organization (WHO). (2012e). *Jakarta Declaration on Leading Health Promotion into the 21st Century*. Retrieved from http://www.who.int/healthpromotion/conferences/previous/jakarta/declaration/en/

World Health Organization (WHO). (2012f). *Leprosy elimination: Leprosy today*. Retrieved from http://www.who.int/lep/en/

World Health Organization (WHO). (2012g). *Priority eye diseases: Onchocerciasis (river blindness)*. Retrieved from http://www.who.int/blindness/causes/priority/en/index3.html

World Health Organization (WHO). (2012h). *Programmes and projects*. Retrieved from http://www.who.int/entity/en/

World Health Organization (WHO). (2012i). *The Ottawa Charter for Health Promotion*. Retrieved from http://www.who.int/healthpromotion/conferences/previous/ottawa/en/index.html

World Health Organization (WHO). (2012j). *The WHO agenda*. Retrieved from http://www.who.int/about/agenda/en/index.html

World Health Organization (WHO). (2012k). *Trade, foreign policy, diplomacy and health: Emerging diseases*. Retrieved from http://www.who.int/trade/glossary/story022/en/index.html

World Health Organization (WHO) Media Centre. (2005). *New Bangkok Charter for health promotion adopted to address rapidly changing health issues*. Retrieved February 1, 2012 from http://www.who.int/mediacentre/news/releases/2005/pr34/en/

World Health Organization (WHO) Media Centre. (2010a, June 18). *Anniversary of smallpox eradication*. Retrieved from http://www.who.int/mediacentre/multimedia/podcasts/2010/smallpox_20100618/en/

World Health Organization (WHO) Media Centre. (2010b, August). *H1N1 in post-pandemic period*. Retrieved from http://www.who.int/mediacentre/news/statements/2010/h1n1_vpc_20100810/en/index.html

World Health Organization (WHO) Media Centre. (2010c, November). *Maternal mortality*. Retrieved from http://www.who.int/mediacentre/factsheets/fs348/en/index.html

World Health Organization (WHO) Media Centre. (2010d, November). *Tuberculosis: Fact sheet No. 104*. Retrieved from http://www.who.int/mediacentre/factsheets/fs104/en/

World Health Organization (WHO) Media Centre. (2011a, July). *Tobacco: Fact sheet No. 39*. Retrieved from http://www.who.int/mediacentre/factsheets/fs339/en/index.html

World Health Organization (WHO) Media Centre. (2011b, July). *West Nile virus: Fact sheet No. 354*. Retrieved from http://www.who.int/mediacentre/factsheets/fs354/en/

World Health Organization (WHO) Media Centre. (2011c, October). *Measles: Fact sheet No. 286*. Retrieved from http://www.who.int/mediacentre/factsheets/fs286/en/

World Health Organization (WHO) Media Centre. (2011d, October). *Poliomyelitis: Fact sheet No. 114*. Retrieved from http://www.who.int/mediacentre/factsheets/fs114/en/

World Health Organization (WHO) Media Centre. (2011e, December). *Malaria: Fact sheet No. 94*. Retrieved from http://www.who.int/mediacentre/factsheets/fs094/en/

World Health Organization (WHO) Media Centre. (2012, January). *Dracunculiasis (guinea-worm disease): Fact sheet No. 359*. Retrieved from http://www.who.int/mediacentre/factsheets/fs359/en/

Yach, D., Mensah, G., Hawkes, C., Epping-Jordan, J., & Steyn, K. (2011). Chronic diseases and risks. In M. H. Merson, R. E. Black, & A. J. Mills (Eds.), *Global health: Diseases, programs, systems, and policies* (3rd ed.). Sudbury, MA: Jones & Bartlett Learning.

Yang, Y., Sugimoto, J., Halloran, E., Basta, N., Chao, D., Matrajt, L., et al. (2009). The transmissibility and control of pandemic influenza A (H1N1) virus. *Science, 326*(5953), 729–733.

Zagar, E. M., & McNerney, R. (2008). Multidrug-resistant tuberculosis. *BMC Infectious Diseases, 8*(10). doi:10.1186/1471-2334-8-10. Retrieved from http://www.biomedcentral.com/1471-2334/8/10

Zwane, A. P., & Kremer, M. (2007). What works in fighting diarrheal diseases in developing countries? A critical review. *The World Bank Research Observer, 22*(1), 1–24.

thePoint: Everything You Need to Make the Grade!

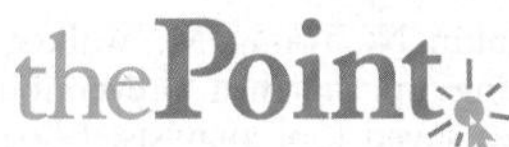

Visit http://thePoint.lww.com/Allender8e for selected readings, study aids for all learning styles, and more!

CHAPTER

17

Being Prepared: Impact of Disaster, Terrorism, and War

"I have an almost complete disregard of precedent, and a faith in the possibility of something better. It irritates me to be told how things have always been done. I defy the tyranny of precedent. I go for anything new that might improve the past."

—*Clara Barton*

KEY TERMS

Biologic warfare
Casualty
Chemical warfare
Complex emergency
Critical Incident Stress Debriefing (CISD)
Directly impacted by disaster
Disaster
Disaster planning
Displaced persons
Incident Command System
Indirectly impacted by disaster
Intensity
Man-made disaster
Mass-casualty incident
Moulage
Natural disaster
Nuclear warfare
Posttraumatic stress disorder (PTSD)
Refugee
Resilience
Scope
Terrorism
Triage

LEARNING OBJECTIVES

Upon mastery of this chapter, you should be able to:

- Describe a variety of characteristics of disasters, including causation, number of casualties, scope, and intensity.
- Discuss a variety of factors contributing to a community's potential for experiencing a disaster.
- Identify the four phases of disaster management.
- Describe factors involved in disaster planning.
- Describe the role of the community health nurse in preventing, preparing for, responding to, and supporting recovery from disasters.
- Use the levels of prevention to describe the role of the community health nurse in relation to acts of chemical, biologic, or nuclear terrorism.

What would you do if your local news station broadcasts an announcement that your community was directly in the path of a hurricane that earlier in the day had caused extensive damage and loss of life in a neighboring state? What would you do if you were shopping at a local mall, suddenly heard an explosive noise followed by shouts and cries for help, then noticed that a pungent odor was filling the air? What *did* you do on the morning of September 11, 2001, when the world of each American, especially those in New York City, in Washington, DC, and on a plane over rural Pennsylvania, changed forever? In March of 2011, were you glued to your television watching live coverage of the earthquake and tsunami in Japan? When you hear news of riots and violence in the Middle East and bombings of cities, do you think of it as a disaster? Even today, the impact of the 2005 hurricanes Katrina and Rita on the Gulf Coast continues to affect the lives of the residents of those communities devastated by the storms. As distant as some of these scenarios might seem from your own life, natural disasters and terrorism are ever-present possibilities, and nurses and other health care professionals have an obligation to respond appropriately. This chapter increases your understanding of the community health nurse's role in preparing for, responding to, and recovering from natural disasters and terrorism.

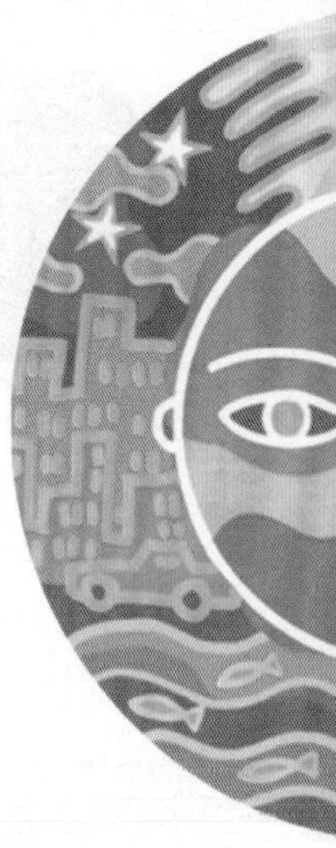

DISASTERS

A **disaster** is any natural or man-made event that causes a level of destruction or emotional trauma exceeding the abilities of those affected to respond without community assistance. The crash of a private plane over the Pacific Ocean in which no bodies are recovered and no environmental impact is felt is not a disaster by this definition, because no specific community-based response is required or even possible. Such a tragedy may, however, be felt for a lifetime by family members and friends who need emotional support and possibly long-term financial assistance. If a plane with 150 passengers crashes over land, destroying several homes in its path, the community affected is unable to cope with the resulting injuries, deaths, and property destruction without assistance; by the definition used here, this constitutes a disaster.

The geographic distribution of disasters varies because certain types of disasters are more common in some parts of the world. For example, California, Alaska, and Tennessee are associated with earthquakes and the Gulf Coast with hurricanes. Similarly, it is not surprising to hear of drought in Ethiopia, floods in India during the monsoon season, or bombings in Afghanistan. When certain types of disasters are anticipated, communities are usually better prepared for them. For instance, California has strict building codes to prevent destruction of structures in the event of earthquakes, but most California homes lack the basements and insulation that characterize homes in Iowa and Oklahoma often visited by tornados or winter storms. Similarly, residents of Germany, Austria, and Russia are better prepared for blizzards than for heavy rain, which explains in part the devastation caused in some communities by floods there in 2002.

Because the local media in the United States do not typically report on disasters unless there are mass casualties, one may be unaware of the frequency and variety of both natural and technologic disasters worldwide. Here is a brief sampling of major disasters that occurred in 2007 to 2011 (Infoplease, 2008, 2009; International Charter, 2008; Littleton, Axsom, & Grills-Taquechel, 2009; Press Information Bureau, 2008):

May 2007
- *Russia*: Explosion killed 38 coal miners in Yubileinaya, 2 months after a similar explosion in a nearby town killed 110.

April 2007
- *Virginia*: Worst mass shooting in US history at Virginia Tech University ended with 33 dead and 17 seriously wounded.

October 2007
- *California*: Wildfires burned more than 516,000 acres in Southern California. Seven died, and nearly ninety people were injured. Over 500,000 people were forced to evacuate their homes; 2,000 homes were destroyed.

November 2007
- *Bangladesh*: Cyclone killed nearly 3,500 people in southern Bangladesh; millions of people were left homeless.

January 2008
- *Kenya*: After an election, violent riots between tribes killed 300 people, and thousands of houses, farms, and businesses were burned.

February 2008
- *U.S. South*: Violent tornados struck Kentucky, Tennessee, Alabama, Mississippi, and Arkansas with little warning, resulting in 54 deaths and hundreds of injured, with widespread damage reported.

May 2008
- *China*: Earthquake struck eastern Sichuan, northwest of Chengdu. The tremor was felt throughout the region, with the death toll exceeding 65,000.

November 2008
- *India*: Terrorists attacked Mumbai with 10 coordinated bombings and attacks across the city. Terrorists killed 164 people and wounded over 300.

January 2010

- *Haiti*: Earthquake struck Port-au-Prince, Haiti. The tremor was felt throughout the region, with the death toll exceeding 222,570.

March 2011

- *Japan*: Earthquake and tsunami struck Pacific coastal areas of northeastern Japan. Estimates of over 9,000 dead and 18,000 missing.

Characteristics of Disasters

Disasters are often characterized by their cause. A **natural disaster** is caused by natural events, such as the earthquake and tsunami in Japan in 2011. A **man-made disaster** is caused by human activity, such as the 2008 shootings at Virginia Tech, the bombing of the World Trade Center in New York City in 2001, the displacement of thousands of Kosovars during their war with Serbia in 1999, or the riots in Kenya in 2008. Other man-made disasters include nuclear reactor meltdowns; industrial accidents; oil spills; construction accidents; and air, train, bus, and subway crashes. In fact, man-made disasters can and frequently do follow natural disasters, as occurred with the nuclear reactors in Japan following the earthquake and tsunami in 2011. A **complex emergency** is a "multifaceted crisis in a country, region or society where there is a total or considerable breakdown of authority resulting from internal or external conflict and which requires a multi-sectorial, international response" (UN Inter-Agency Standing Committee, 2008). Complex humanitarian emergencies disproportionately impact women and children.

A **casualty** is a human being who is injured or killed by or as a direct result of an accident. Although major disasters sometimes occur without any injury or loss of life, disasters are commonly characterized by the number of casualties involved. If casualties number more than two people but fewer than 100, the disaster is characterized as a *multiple-casualty incident*. Although multiple-casualty incidents may strain the health care systems of small or midsized communities, a **mass-casualty incident**—involving 100 or more casualties—often completely overwhelms the resources of even large cities. Preparedness for mass-casualty incidents is essential for all communities.

The possibility of being prepared is another characteristic that varies with different types of disasters. For instance, the path and time of landfall of a hurricane can be tracked, so that residents in the storm's path can be evacuated and families and businesses can be protected. Communities can also minimize devastation from flooding by building reservoirs or refusing to grant building permits in flood-prone areas and by reinforcing areas around waterways with sandbags during rainy weather. In fire-prone areas, communities can post notices to heighten awareness of fire danger and enforce regulations to cut back vegetation near structures in forested areas.

On the other hand, some disasters strike without warning. For example, the terrorist attacks in New York City caught thousands of civilians by surprise. They were trapped in buildings with limited escape routes and very little time to retreat to safety. For employees in the Pentagon on 9/11, survival depended on being in the right place at the right time. The number of fires in southern California in 2007 was unanticipated and uncharacteristically large, and control was hindered by heat and high winds. Residents were barred from reentering their communities for weeks, without any knowledge of whether they would have homes when they were allowed to return. The shootings at Virginia Tech in 2007 and in Tucson in 2011 that resulted in 6 deaths and seriously wounded Rep. Gabrielle Giffords occurred without warning and were both the result of a mentally unstable individual acting alone.

The **scope** of a disaster is the range of its effect, either geographically or in terms of the number of people impacted. The collapse of a 500-unit high-rise apartment building has a greater scope than the collapse of a bridge that occurs while only two cars are crossing.

The **intensity** of a disaster is the level of destruction and devastation it causes. For instance, an earthquake centered in a large metropolitan area and one centered in a desert may have the same numeric rating on the Richter scale, yet have very different intensities in terms of the destruction they cause.

Persons Impacted by Disasters

Because disasters are so variable, there is no typical person impacted in a disaster. Nor can anyone predict whether he or she will ever become impacted by a disaster. However, once disaster strikes, persons impacted may be characterized by their level of involvement. **Directly impacted by disaster** are the people who experience the event, whether fire, volcanic eruption, war, or bomb. They are the dead and the survivors, and even if they are without physical injuries, they are likely to have health effects from their experience. Some may be without shelter or food, and many experience serious psychological stress long after the event is over (Display 17.1).

Depending on the cause and characteristics of the disaster, some direct survivors may become displaced persons or refugees. **Displaced persons** are forced to leave their homes to escape the effects of a disaster. Usually, displacement is a temporary condition and involves movement within the person's own country. A common example is relocation of residents of flooded areas to schools, churches, and other shelters on higher ground. Typically, the term **refugee** is reserved for people who are forced to leave their homeland because of war or persecution. For example, over 2.5 million displaced people lived in camps in Darfur after fleeing ethnic cleansing by Sudanese government forces and militia. The United Nations (UN) estimates that an additional 2 million have been impacted by the conflict, resulting from the damage to local economies and trade (Human Rights Watch, 2008). Returning

DISPLAY 17.1 DIRECTLY AND INDIRECTLY IMPACTED PEOPLE OF A DISASTER

On September 11, 2001, almost 3,000 people died in the terrorist attacks on the World Trade Center in New York City. Although all of the employees and visitors in the two buildings were directly impacted by this disaster, the entire population of Manhattan can be considered indirectly impacted. Hotels, businesses, and apartments for blocks surrounding the Twin Towers suffered structural damage, blown-out windows, and interiors covered with inches of powdered cement and other debris. A year after this disaster, many residents in the surrounding areas still were unable to return home.

Many rescue workers who were survivors have lasting psychological effects from their own survival experiences and from losing close friends and colleagues. In addition, many rescuers inhaled the dust in the air for days and now suffer respiratory damage, which changes their status from indirectly to directly impacted by the disaster.

All people working or visiting in Manhattan that day were affected by the closing of the bridges and tunnels and were stranded in New York City until transportation routes opened again, thus becoming indirectly impacted. Other indirectly impacted persons included children attending school and living within sight of the Twin Towers. They received counseling in school for months, and in some cases years, after the disaster.

For 1 year after the attack, volunteer construction workers and rescue workers who lost fellow police officers, paramedics, or firefighters worked 24 hours a day. First, the efforts were geared to find survivors. Shortly after, workers knew that they were looking for the bodies or body parts of victims while removing thousands of tons of building pieces. Thousands of people involved in the recovery efforts can still be considered indirectly impacted.

Family members of the 2,980 deceased victims, who have been affected for a lifetime, also are indirectly impacted. Thousands of children lost a parent, some parents lost multiple children, and, in some cases, both spouses were lost because husband and wife worked in the World Trade Center. The ripples of tragedy extended beyond the borders of the United States, because there were hundreds of people working in the Twin Towers from many different countries whose family members remain indirectly impacted.

refugees can also place economic and social strains on the county of origin. One significant example is the return of almost 5 million refugees to Afghanistan over the past decade, increasing the total population by more than 20%. Along with needs for employment and shelter, this influx also raises concerns in the areas of early or forced marriages, child labor, and human trafficking (United Nations Refugee Agency, 2008). Whether the displacement of refugees is permanent or not, the lasting impact to both the country of origin and the host country is significant.

Indirectly impacted by disaster are the relatives and friends of persons directly impacted by disasters. Although these people do not experience the stress of the event itself, they often undergo extreme anguish from trying to locate loved ones or accommodate their emergency needs. If bodies cannot be found or are unidentifiable, indirectly impacted persons experience even greater anguish and may not be able to accept that their loved one has died. Family members of those killed on 9/11 in New York City have worked with architects to develop a complex of buildings and a memorial that meets the expectations of most of those indirectly impacted by the attack and honors their loved ones. This effort, along with the Flight 93 National Memorial (Shanksville, PA) and the Pentagon Memorial, will help with the long healing process. They also serve as a reminder of the impact that day had on each of our lives.

Factors Contributing to Disasters

It is useful to apply the host, agent, and environment model (epidemiological triad) to understand the factors contributing to disasters, because manipulation of these factors can be instrumental in planning strategies to prevent or prepare for disasters.

Host Factors

The *host* is the human being who experiences the disaster. Host factors that contribute to the likelihood of experiencing a disaster include age, general health, mobility, psychological factors, and even socioeconomic factors. For instance, elderly residents of a mobile home community may be unable to evacuate independently in response to a tornado warning if they can no longer drive. Impoverished residents of a low-income apartment complex in a large city may notice that their building is not compliant with city fire codes, but may avoid alerting authorities for fear of being forced to move to more expensive housing.

Agent Factors

The *agent* is the natural or technologic element that causes the disaster. For example, the high winds of a hurricane and the lava of an erupting volcano are agents, as are radiation, industrial chemicals, biologic agents, and bombs. The Station nightclub fire and the apartment deck collapse in Chicago (both in 2003) demonstrated that the irresponsibility of contractors and inspectors and failure to adhere to safety policies can act as agents of disaster, resulting in death and destruction.

Environmental Factors

Environmental factors are those that could potentially contribute to or mitigate a disaster. Some of the most common environmental factors are a community's level of preparedness; the presence of industries that produce harmful chemicals or radiation; the presence of flood-prone rivers, lakes, or streams; average amount of rainfall or snowfall; average high and low temperatures; proximity to fault lines, coastal waters, or volcanoes; level of compliance with local building codes; and presence or absence of political unrest.

Agencies and Organizations for Disaster Management

In 1803, just 10 years after the Treaty of Paris, the United States first recognized the need to prepare for emergencies through law and dedicated organizations. The first law was written as a direct response to a major disaster, the Portsmouth, New Hampshire, fire of 1803. The majority of subsequent legislation was also in response to specific crises and created many different agencies to respond to those disasters. The George Washington University (GWU) Institute for Crisis, Disaster and Risk Management (2011) found that from 1803 until the passage of the Disaster Relief Act of 1950 there were 125 pieces of legislation related to disaster assistance and many of these pieces of legislation changed the roles and responsibilities of government agencies. The one constant was that the "federal response to disasters was ad hoc and reactive" and only became coordinated with the establishment of the Federal Emergency Management Agency (FEMA) in 1979 and the passage of the Robert T. Stafford Disaster Relief and Emergency Assistance Act of 1988 (GWU Institute for Crisis, Disaster and Risk Management, 2011).

In response to World War II and the specter of all-out nuclear war with the Soviet Union, the United States created Civil Defense, a series of programs and agencies designed to protect the population from "counter-value" nuclear strikes and increase the survivability of a nuclear war. The earliest phases of the National Civil Defense Plan (NCDP) on record at the National Archives were started in 1952 and continued until the Federal Civil Defense Administration completed the first NCDP in 1956 (Carbine, 1961). The early goal was to make the plans as simple as a Boy Scout Manual.

The Department of Health, Education, and Welfare (USDHEW) created the *Handbook for Civil Defense Emergency Planning in Welfare Institutions*, which was a guide to protect individuals and help staff prepare for fallout from a nuclear event (USDHEW, 1961). Significant in this handbook was the attention given to family responsibilities and the likelihood that staff, including nurses, would choose family responsibilities over professional responsibilities. To help alleviate the problems associated with absenteeism as a result of the nurses' conflicting responsibilities, the handbook recommended (1) reminding staff of their responsibility as public servants, (2) providing shelter for families within the institution, (3) planning for getting families to the shelter, and (4) planning for families to assist the staff during a crisis (USDHEW, 1961).

Under the 1950 version for the United States Civil Defense Plan, health services were to remain under the control of existing health agencies to avoid unnecessary duplication of services, but would now also be subject to the rules and regulations of civil defense. The U.S. Public Health Service was responsible for providing staffing for civil defense offices and would work for the state health officer who would have the lead. The roles have been in continual transition since that time, but the basic principles remain the same.

Among disaster-relief organizations, perhaps none is as famous as the Red Cross, which is referred to as the American Red Cross in the United States and the Red Crescent Societies in Islamic countries. The American Red Cross was founded in 1881 by Clara Barton and was chartered by the U.S. Congress in 1905. It is authorized to provide disaster assistance free of charge across the country through its more than half a million volunteers and staff. The duties assumed by the Red Cross in the event of a disaster are to provide shelter, food, basic health and mental health services, and distribution of emergency supplies (American Red Cross, 2011). Even the role of this historic disaster response organization changed after September 11, 2001.

President George W. Bush sought to consolidate the roles and responsibilities of agencies and organizations involved in disaster response and to align them with the Emergency Support Functions (ESFs) (see Table 17-1). The Department of Homeland Security (DHS) was organized in 2002 and incorporates many of the nation's security, protection, and emergency response activities into a single federal department. In 2003, the Federal Emergency Management Agency (FEMA), along with parts of twenty-three agencies, became part of the DHS. The FEMA, established in 1979, is the federal agency responsible for assessing and responding to disaster events in the United States. It also provides training and guidance in all phases of disaster management. The DHS includes other widely known agencies including the Transportation Security Administration (TSA), U.S. Customs and Border Protection, U.S. Immigration and Customs Enforcement (ICE), U.S. Citizenship and Immigration Services (USCIS), U.S. Coast Guard, and U.S. Secret Service (DHS, 2006, 2011).

Under the oversight of FEMA is the National Incident Management System (NIMS), which was developed to allow responders from different jurisdictions and disciplines to work more cohesively in response to natural disasters, emergencies, and terrorist acts. "NIMS benefits included a unified approach to incident management; standard command and management structures; and emphasis on preparedness, mutual aid and resource management" (FEMA, 2008). Among the elements that

Table 17.1 ESF Responsibilities

ESF	Scope	Coordinating Agency
1. Transportation	Aviation/airspace management and control Transportation safety Restoration/recovery of transportation infrastructure Movement restrictions Damage and impact assessment	Department of Transportation
2. Communications	Coordination with telecommunications and information technology industries Restoration and repair of telecommunications infrastructure Protection, restoration, and sustainment of national cyber and information technology resources Oversight of communications within the federal incident management and response structures	Department of Homeland Security—National Communications System
3. Public works and engineering	Infrastructure protection and emergency repair Infrastructure restoration Engineering services and construction management Emergency contracting support for lifesaving and life-sustaining services	Department of Defense—U.S. Army Corps of Engineers
4. Firefighting	Coordination of federal firefighting activities Support to wildland, rural, and urban firefighting operations	United States Department of Agriculture—Forest Service
5. Emergency management	Coordination of incident management and response efforts Issuance of mission assignments Resource and human capital Incident action planning Financial management	Department of Homeland Security—Federal Emergency Management Agency
6. Mass care, housing, and human services	Mass care Emergency assistance Disaster housing Human services	Department of Homeland Security—Federal Emergency Management Agency
7. Resource support	Comprehensive, national incident logistics planning, management, and sustainment capability Resource support (facility space, office equipment and supplies, contracting services, etc.)	Department of Homeland Security—Federal Emergency Management Agency
8. Public health and medical services	Public health Medical Mental health services Mass fatality management	Department of Health and Human Services
9. Urban search and rescue	Lifesaving assistance Search and rescue operations	Department of Homeland Security—Federal Emergency Management Agency
10. Oil and hazardous materials response	Oil and hazardous materials (chemical, biological, radiological, etc.) response Environmental short- and long-term cleanup	Environmental Protection Agency
12. Energy	Energy infrastructure assessment, repair, and restoration Energy industry utilities coordination Energy forecast	Department of Energy

(Continued)

Table 17.1 ESF Responsibilities *(Continued)*

ESF	Scope	Coordinating Agency
13. Public safety and security	Facility and resource security Security planning and technical resource assistance Public safety and security support Support to access, traffic, and crowd control	Department of Justice
14. Long-term community recovery	Social and economic community impact assessment Long-term community recovery assistance to states, local governments, and the private sector Analysis and review of mitigation program implementation	Department of Homeland Security —Federal Emergency Management Agency
15. External affairs	Emergency public information and protective action guidance Media and community relations Congressional and international affairs Tribal and insular affairs	Department of Homeland Security

Department of Homeland Security. (2008). *National Response Framework*. Retrieved from http://www.fema.gov/pdf/emergency/nrf/nrf-core.pdf

nurses must understand is the **Incident Command System** (ICS) that was created in the 1970s after catastrophic wildfires in California resulted in many deaths (see Fig. 17-1). Nurses and other health care professionals must understand this system and are encouraged to take courses dealing with the ICS; these courses are available free online from FEMA Emergency Management Institute at http://www.training.fema.gov/EMI/. The most important courses for a nurse are (1) IS-100. HCb Introduction to the Incident Command System

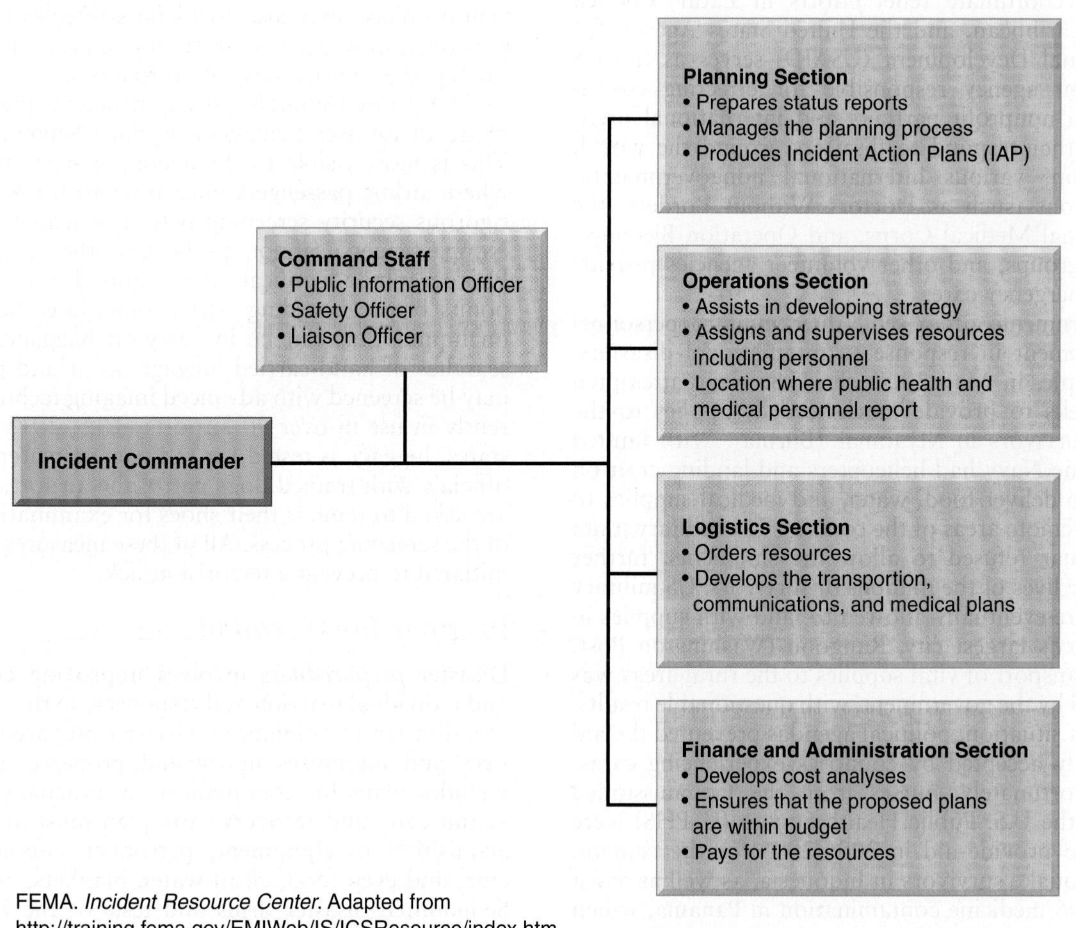
Planning Section
• Prepares status reports
• Manages the planning process
• Produces Incident Action Plans (IAP)
Command Staff
• Public Information Officer
• Safety Officer
• Liaison Officer
Operations Section
• Assists in developing strategy
• Assigns and supervises resources including personnel
• Location where public health and medical personnel report
Incident Commander
Logistics Section
• Orders resources
• Develops the transportion, communications, and medical plans
Finance and Administration Section
• Develops cost analyses
• Ensures that the proposed plans are within budget
• Pays for the resources

FEMA. *Incident Resource Center*. Adapted from http://training.fema.gov/EMIWeb/IS/ICSResource/index.htm

FIGURE 17-1. Incident command system

for Healthcare/Hospitals, (2) IS-700.a Introduction to the NIMS, and (3) IS-800.b Introduction to the Nation Response Framework.

The USDHHS is the lead federal agency for public health and medical services during a public health or medical disaster. Supplemental services are provided to state, local, and territorial governments. The services may include Disaster Medical Assistance Teams, U.S. Public Health Service officers, epidemiological personnel from the CDC, and veterinary support to name a few. The USDHHS preparedness and response efforts for public health and medical emergencies are led by the Assistant Secretary for Preparedness and Response, and recovery efforts are led by the Office of the Assistant Secretary for Public Health and Science. The USDHHS efforts to support human services needs, including disaster case management, are led by the Administration for Children and Families. When natural or man-made disasters within the United States are accompanied by civil disturbance, looting, or violent crime, the resources of local police departments may be overwhelmed. In such cases, the National Guard is often called in to restore order. This action is typically accomplished within each individual state, under the jurisdiction of the governor.

The World Health Organization's (WHO) Emergency Relief Operations provide disaster assistance internationally, the Pan American Health Organization works to coordinate relief efforts in Latin America and the Caribbean, and the United States Agency for International Development (USAID) serves as the US government agency responsible for directing contributions to nonprofit partners and international organizations that respond to disasters around the world. In addition, various international nongovernmental organizations (such as Doctors Without Borders, the International Medical Corps, and Operation Blessing), religious groups, and other volunteer agencies provide needed emergency care.

Governments often send their military personnel and equipment in response to international disasters. For example, in May 2008, the U.S. Navy attempted for 3 weeks to provide much-needed supplies to the cyclone survivors in Myanmar (Burma). With limited options, the Navy had helicopters and landing craft on standby to deliver food, water, and medical supplies to the most remote areas of the country. The military junta in Myanmar refused to allow the shipments, further risking the lives of the millions of survivors. US military planes were eventually allowed to land with supplies in the country's largest city, Rangoon (Washington Post, 2008). Transport of vital supplies to the rural areas was conducted by the government, with questionable results.

In this situation, political agendas prevented the aid so typically accepted by countries experiencing catastrophe. Fortunately, nurses from the Commissioned Corps of the U.S. Public Health Service (USPHS) were allowed to provide aid in 2004/2005 for the tsunami and earthquake survivors in Indonesia, as well as assist in the 2006 medicine contamination in Panama, which ultimately claimed the lives of over 100 people (USPHS, 2008). The USPHS has worked collaboratively with the U.S. Navy to provide nursing and other medical care on combined humanitarian missions to South America over the last 5 years. Chapter 30 contains additional information about the role of the USPHS Commissioned Corps Nurses and their role in emergency preparedness.

Phases of Disaster Management

In developing strategies to address the problem of disasters, it is helpful for the community health nurse to consider each of the four phases of disaster management: prevention, preparedness, response, and recovery. Additionally, some knowledge of the language typically used in disaster preparedness may be helpful and is included in Display 17.2.

Prevention Phase

During the *prevention phase*, no disaster is expected or anticipated. The tasks during this phase are to identify community risk factors, to develop and implement programs to prevent disasters from occurring or mitigate their impact, and to train personnel and educate citizens. Task forces typically include representatives from the community's local government, health care providers, social services providers, police and fire departments, major industries, local media, schools, and citizens' groups. Programs developed during the prevention phase may also focus on strategies to mitigate the effects of disasters that cannot be prevented, such as earthquakes, hurricanes, and tornadoes.

The United States has strengthened the preparedness phase of disaster management since September 2001. This is most visible to the average citizen at airports, where airline passengers must now go through a more rigorous security screening before boarding the plane. Nonpassengers cannot go beyond the security area. Photographic identification is required at two or more points before boarding. Strict limits have been placed on liquids that can be in carry-on baggage. Random searches of hand-carried luggage occur and passengers may be screened with advanced imaging technology currently in use in over 90 airports (TSA, 2011). In some states, luggage is tested for radioactive material, police officials with trained dogs patrol the airport, or people are asked to remove their shoes for examination as part of the screening process. All of these measures have been initiated to prevent a terrorist attack.

Preparedness Phase

Disaster *preparedness* involves improving community and individual reaction and responses, so that the effects of a disaster are minimized. Disaster preparedness saves lives and minimizes injury and property damage. It includes plans for communication, evacuation, rescue, victim care, and recovery. Any plan must also address acquisition of equipment, personnel, supplies, medicine, and even food, clean water, blankets, and shelter. Semiannual disaster drills and tests of the Emergency Broadcast System are examples of appropriate activities during the preparedness phase.

DISPLAY 17.2 COMMON TERMS USED IN EMERGENCY PREPAREDNESS AND RESPONSE

All-hazards preparation: Preparedness for domestic terrorist attacks, major disasters, and other emergencies

Chain of command: A series of command, control, executive, or management positions in hierarchical order of authority

Credential: A health volunteer's qualifications. Credentials are used to determine a health volunteer's emergency credentialing level (i.e., nursing license).

Designated equivalent source: Selected agencies that have been determined to maintain a specific item or items of credential information that is identical to the information at the primary source

Disaster, major (federal): Any natural catastrophe, or, regardless of cause, any fire, flood, or explosion, in any part of the United States, which in the determination of the President causes damage of sufficient severity and magnitude to warrant major disaster assistance to supplement the efforts and available resources of states, local governments, and disaster relief organizations

Emergency declaration: Refers to the state (or local) government's capacity to declare a general emergency or public health emergency, or state of disaster

Emergency Management Assistance Compact (EMAC): An interstate mutual aid agreement that allows states to assist one another in responding to all types of natural and man-made disasters

***Just-in-time* training**: Concise, targeted training, normally provided on-site after a disaster or emergency has occurred. It provides a minimum level of exposure for volunteers to select issues in disaster response. Examples could be use of self-protection equipment, documentation, mental health triage, or registration of casualties.

Hospital Emergency Incident Command System (HEICS): An emergency management system that employs a logical management structure, defined responsibilities, clear reporting channels, and a common nomenclature to help unify hospitals with other emergency responders

Incident Command System (ICS): The combination of facilities, equipment, personnel, procedures, and communications operating within a common organizational structure, designed to aid in the management of resources during incidents

National Electronic Disease Surveillance System (NEDSS): A CDC initiative promoting the use of data and information systems standards to improve disease surveillance systems at federal, state, and local levels

National Incident Management System (NIMS): The single all-hazards incident management system required by Homeland Security Presidential Directive 5 that governs the management of the National Response Plan

Public Health Information Network (PHIN): A framework providing the basis for information technology projects for CDC-funded programs including NEDSS, Health Alert Network (HAN), and others

Strategic National Stockpile: A national cache of drugs, vaccines, and supplies that can be deployed to areas struck by disasters, including bioterrorism

Surge capacity: The accommodation by the health system to a transient sudden rise in demand for health care following an incident with real or perceived adverse health effects

Adapted from U.S. Department of Health and Human Services–HRSA. (2005). ESAR–VHP interim technical and policy guidelines, standards, and definitions (Ver. 2) (Appendix 8: ESAR–VHP Guidelines glossary of terms). Washington, DC: U.S. Government Printing Office.

Disaster preparedness activities occur locally, regionally, and nationally. A town keeps its warning system working and tests it each month. Sections of the country coordinate larger warning systems to notify communities in the path of a tornado or hurricane, and the country has a plan to stockpile vital pharmaceuticals such as smallpox vaccine for mass immunization. The Centers for Disease Control and Prevention (CDC) reports that the Strategic National Stockpile (SNS) contains enough doses of smallpox vaccine to vaccinate every person in the United States should biological warfare become a threat (CDC, 2009). The last case of smallpox in the United States occurred in 1949, and routine immunization was halted in 1972 (CDC, 2009). In 1979, the global commission on smallpox agreed that smallpox had been eradicated from the world (Henderson, 2010). With a largely unvaccinated population, most people in the nation would need the vaccine. Having the vaccine ready is a demonstration of disaster preparedness, but also an admission that smallpox can be used as a terrorist weapon.

Community health nurses will be called upon during a terrorist attack involving biologic weapons like smallpox or anthrax to provide vaccines, prophylactic antibiotics, and screen suspected cases. The Department of Health and Human Services proposed programs for distribution of vaccinations and prophylactic medication to emergency personnel, including nurses. However, vaccines have side effects and the smallpox vaccine carries more serious risks than other vaccines. The smallpox vaccination program proposed by the Bush administration ended with fewer than 40,000 people vaccinated after it was found that there were no smallpox stores in Iraq and the state public health directors quit supporting the program (Henderson, 2010).

Response Phase

The *response phase* begins immediately after the onset of the disastrous event. Preparedness plans take effect immediately, with the goals of saving lives and preventing further injury or damage to property. Activities during the response phase include rescue, triage, on-site stabilization, transportation of injured, and treatment at local hospitals and clinics. Response also requires recovery, identification, and refrigeration of bodies, so that notification of family members is possible and correct, even weeks after a disaster. This care of the dead is demanding and time-consuming work that is often overlooked by people unfamiliar with disaster response. Persons trained in mortuary services are an essential part of any emergency planning efforts. The mortuary teams always have pastoral personnel with them to ensure that remains are always treated with respect and in accordance with religious traditions. Supportive care, including food, water, and shelter for survivors and relief workers, is also an essential element of the total disaster response. The extent of care provided for animals is an additional area of concern that should be addressed in the overall plan. Many shelters will not accept pets; those that do need to be identified as soon as possible to avoid unnecessary confusion and delays in sheltering.

Recovery Phase

During the *recovery phase*, the community takes actions to repair, rebuild, or relocate damaged homes and businesses and restore health, social, and economic vitality to the community. Psychological recovery must also be addressed. The emotional scars from witnessing a traumatic event may last a lifetime. Both survivors and relief workers should be offered mental health services to support their recovery (see Perspectives: Voices From the Community).

During the recovery phase, special attention should be given to the needs of children who are approximately

PERSPECTIVES
VOICES FROM THE COMMUNITY

It was 5:00 PM on October 17, 1989, in Santa Cruz, CA, a day that would change my view of life forever. I had just fed my newborn son and was rocking him in a soft, comfortable chair when the house began to shake. Without even thinking or being aware of what I was doing, I jumped up with my baby in my arms and headed for the nearest doorway, as I had done so many times before in an earthquake. I stood there holding my son in one arm and braced myself against the door jamb with the other one as the house continued to shake all around us. It was not until the shaking stopped that I began to feel fear and worry as I surveyed the damage to my house.

In my kitchen, all of the cupboard doors were flung open and their contents spilled onto the floor, which was now a mess of spilled food, sticky sauces, dented tin cans, and broken glass. Tears came to my eyes as I saw my son's infant seat, where he had been seated only moments before the quake, covered with glass shards and fallen tin cans. I realized he could have been killed, and I had no control over it. I became afraid for the safety of my 10-year-old daughter, who was at dancing lessons across town. Fortunately, when I got to her, she was safe.

The next few days continued to be very stressful. We had no gas or electricity and no running water that was safe to drink. I went to the drug store in a panic to buy premixed formula to feed my son, since I could not boil the water to mix with the powdered formula. Both the drug store and the grocery store were "trashed," all of the items were thrown off of the shelves and laying on the debris-strewn floors. The grocery store was giving away the ice cream because they had no power to keep it frozen. But who could eat ice cream?

There was something about seeing my favorite grocery store in such a disastrous condition that made me realize how little control I had over the consequences of what insurance companies call "acts of God." I couldn't just run to the grocery store for what I needed; it wouldn't be there for me. My family and I felt very unsafe as we all huddled together in the master bedroom at night. My son was in his bassinet at the foot of the bed and my daughter slept with me until she felt safe enough to return to her own room. I was attempting to regain control of my life as I cleaned up my house and waited for the water and electricity to be restored. Of all the losses, the greatest loss was the illusion of safety and the illusion that I had control over my life.

Over the next week, I experienced the loss of many services and products that made up my comfortable and safe lifestyle: homes were damaged, with their chimneys strewn across front lawns, there was no phone service for days, and a normal 10-minute drive took an hour and a half on clogged highways provided as an alternative route to highways and bridges damaged by the quake. As a community mental health nurse, I wanted to volunteer to help others who were experiencing the same feelings as I was, but I was told that they were not taking mental health volunteers from the immediate area because we, too, were victims of the disaster and needed to care for ourselves first. I think they were right, since I had many feelings that took a long while to heal and I have lost the illusion of control forever.

25% of the population in the United States and even higher in many countries. The National Commission on Children and Disasters recommended that the needs of children be comprehensively integrated into all phases of disasters. The NCCD specifically identified the needs for child care and schools to be supported to ensure that children return to a learning environment as soon as possible (NCCD, 2010).

Role of the Community Health Nurse

The community health nurse has a pivotal role in preventing, preparing for, responding to, and supporting recovery from a disaster. After a thorough community assessment for risk factors, the community health nurse may initiate the formation of a multidisciplinary task force to address disaster prevention and preparedness in the community.

Preventing Disasters

Disaster prevention may be considered on three levels: primary, secondary, and tertiary. These are applied to a natural disaster in the Levels of Prevention Pyramid.

Primary Prevention

Primary prevention of a disaster means keeping the disaster from ever happening by taking actions that

LEVELS OF PREVENTION PYRAMID

SITUATION: A natural disaster—tornado

GOAL: By using the three levels of prevention, negative health conditions are avoided, promptly diagnosed, and treated, and/or the fullest possible potential is restored.

TERTIARY PREVENTION

Rehabilitation	Primary Prevention: Health Promotion & Education	Primary Prevention: Health Protection
• Remain safe during the immediate recovery period • Accept help from others—friends, family, and community services • Rebuild family lives through counseling and other services to reestablish stable life physically, emotionally, spiritually, and financially	• Educate community members about the need to enhance planning against damage from future natural disasters, based on experiences with the current disaster	• Keep recommended immunizations current • Community physical structures need rebuilding, with infrastructure planning and supports that improve ability to withstand natural disasters

SECONDARY PREVENTION

Early Diagnosis	Prompt Treatment
• Remain in your position of safety until a community all-clear warning signal is sounded or until rescued • Leave a damaged building cautiously, if able and not seriously injured, and do not return until it is declared safe	• Rescue individuals promptly and get appropriate care for those injured as soon as possible • The infrastructure of the community becomes/remains intact, keeping community members safe from hazards such as live wires, broken gas lines, and fallen debris

PRIMARY PREVENTION

Health Promotion and Education	Health Protection
• Increase community awareness • Increase community preparation through education • Each person is as prepared as possible both physically and emotionally	• Community members know what to do and where to go, whether at home, work, school, or elsewhere in the community • Get to safety before the impact—southwest corner of a home's basement or an interior room away from windows and under heavy furniture

completely eliminate its occurrence. This is the first aspect of primary disaster prevention. Although it is obviously the most effective level of intervention, both in terms of promoting clients' health and containing costs, it is not always possible. Tornadoes, earthquakes, terrorist attacks, and other disasters often strike without warning, despite the use of every available technologic device for prediction and tracking.

If possible, primary prevention of disasters can be practiced in all settings: in the workplace and home with programs to reduce safety hazards and in the community with programs to monitor risk factors, reduce pollution, and encourage nonviolent conflict resolution. Primary disaster prevention efforts should take into account a community's physical, psychosocial, cultural, economic, and spiritual needs. The community health nurse has a role in each of these areas. As a teacher, the community health nurse educates people at home, at work, at school, or in a faith community about safety and security focused on preventing a disaster. The community health nurse can teach community members how to protect themselves from the effects of a natural disaster. The nurse can be a part of a safety team, if working as a school nurse or occupational health nurse. If working for a health department, the nurse can determine during home visits whether a family has a personal disaster plan and help them develop one if none exists. Nursing students can work with low-income community–dwelling elders to ensure that they have enough food, water, and medical supplies to "shelter in place" for at least 72 hours. There are many actions the nurse can initiate.

The second aspect of primary disaster prevention is anticipatory guidance. Disaster drills and other anticipatory exercises help relief workers experience some of the feelings of chaos and stress associated with a disaster before one occurs. It is much easier to do this when energy and intellectual processes are at a high level of functioning. Anticipatory work can dissipate the impact of a disastrous event. The community health nurse has a role in these disaster drills through committee membership, organization of drills at the place of employment, or activism at the grassroots level to assist in holding community-wide disaster drills on a regular basis (see Evidence-Based Practice).

Secondary Prevention

Secondary disaster prevention focuses on the earliest possible detection and treatment. For example, a mobile home community is devastated by a tornado. After the disaster the local health department's community health nurses work with the American Red Cross to provide emergency assistance. Secondary prevention corresponds to immediate and effective response. In a post Katrina study of the emergency planning and response by home health providers serving the poor in New Orleans during the emergency (Kirkpatrick & Bryan, 2007), the successes and challenges of these providers were identified. Agencies that provided early evacuation, identified shelters for special-needs patients outside the high-risk area, implemented volunteer cascading communication systems, conducted pre-event mock evacuation plans, and those that included volunteers in their disaster plan were most successful. Recommendations to improve response include identification of patients who may be reluctant to evacuate, the provision of adequate security at special-needs shelters, and, most importantly, practice drills (Kirkpatrick & Bryan, 2007). With appropriate planning, sound and easily understood emergency response can provide optimal care and services to those impacted by the disaster.

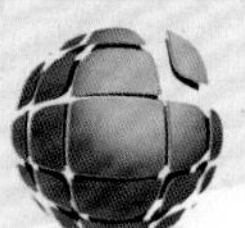

EVIDENCE-BASED PRACTICE

Effectiveness of an Unfolding Emergency Preparedness Training Exercise at Increasing Nursing Student Competence with Emergency Preparedness

Study: Public health emergency simulated exercise with undergraduate senior nursing students using an unfolding infectious disease outbreak scenario.

Findings: Quantitative (verbal) and qualitative (Likert-type scale) evaluations were conducted with the 79 undergraduate nursing students participating in the exercise. Examples of questions included in the quantitative evaluations were clarity of the simulation's purpose, the importance of delivering safe care during the exercise, and pre- and postsimulation debriefing effectiveness and participation. Of the seven questions posed, the responses ranged from 77% to 92% for ratings of strongly agreed/agreed. The qualitative portion of the evaluation included a group debriefing and a written reflection by each student. Overall, the findings of all the evaluation methods were positive and reflected satisfaction with the simulated exercise.

Nursing Implications: Simulated emergency preparedness training is a useful adjunct to a public health nursing clinical course for senior level students. The exercise supports the Quality and Safety Education for Nurses (QSEN) competencies. Students are able to "...practice assessment, treatment, delegation, organizational and leadership skills" and apply nursing skills and knowledge from previous course work.

Source: Morrison, A. M., & Catanzaro, A. M. (2010). High-fidelity simulation and emergency preparedness. *Public Health Nursing, 27*, 164–173. doi:10.1111/j.1525–1446.2010.00838.x

Tertiary Prevention

Tertiary disaster prevention involves reducing the amount and degree of disability or damage resulting from the disaster. Although it involves rehabilitative work, it can help a community recover and reduce the risk of further disasters. In this sense, it becomes a preventive measure.

An example from September 11, 2001, comes from a nurse living in the Boston area who, after that date, began to lose a sense of hope for her future. She often found it difficult to assist her patients with their needs because of her own insecurities and fears. She and a peer responded to a request from the Logan Airport Employee Assistance Program (EAP) asking for help with crisis counseling for United Airlines survivors of 9/11. The planes used in the attacks were from American and United Airlines, and the community of employees felt like survivors because they lived while fellow employees were lost in the disaster. Employees were in turmoil and their ability to function was affected. "The terrorists had taken away their colleagues, friends and sense of security" (DiVitto, 2002, p. 21). The most important interventions the nurses provided were a listening ear and validation that what the employees were feeling and experiencing was normal, and often essential, for healthy grieving. Some employees needed to talk about good times, others were quiet and sad, and others expressed a fear of flying again but did so with the support of family and friends. All demonstrated courage and an ability to continue their lives with a sense of strength and hope. Working with these employees enabled the nurse to recapture the essence and true meaning of her life (DiVitto, 2002).

Preparing for Disasters

Disaster planning is essential for a community, business, or hospital. It involves thinking about details of preparation and management by all involved, including community leaders, health and safety professionals, and lay people. A disaster plan need not be lengthy. Two weeks after the April 1995 Oklahoma City bombing of the Murrah Federal Building by two American citizens, one hospital distilled its 44-page manual into a 5-page disaster response guide. Such a concise plan should still contain information on the elements discussed in this and the following section. See Display 17.3 for a summary of these elements.

Personal Preparation

The preparation of a disaster plan for a community should be preceded by the need for all nurses to address their own personal preparedness to respond in a disaster. Display 17.4 describes the tragic outcome of one nurse's lack of preparation when she attempted to provide nursing care at the scene of the Oklahoma City bombing.

Personal preparedness means that the nurse has read and understood workplace and community disaster plans and has developed a disaster plan for his or her own family. The prepared nurse also has participated in disaster drills and knows cardiopulmonary resuscitation and first aid. Finally, nurses preparing to work in disaster areas should bring copies of their nursing license and driver's license, durable clothing, and basic equipment,

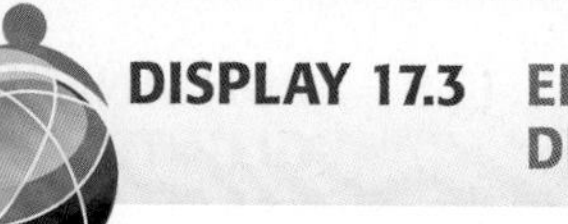

DISPLAY 17.3 ELEMENTS OF A DISASTER PLAN

A disaster plan should address all of the following:

Chain of authority
Lines of communication
Routes and modes of transport
Mobilization
Warning
Evacuation
Rescue and recovery
Triage
Treatment
Support of survivors and families
Care of dead bodies
Disaster worker rehabilitation

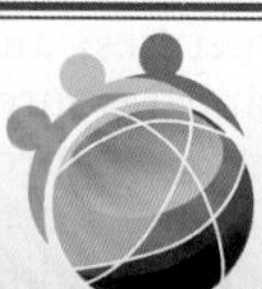

DISPLAY 17.4 NURSES AT DISASTER SITES: HELP OR HINDRANCE?

On April 19, 1995, 37-year-old Rebecca Anderson, a registered nurse working in Oklahoma City, after hearing a televised report of the bombing of the Federal Building, went to the site wearing jeans and a sweatshirt. Along with firefighters and other rescue workers in hardhats and other protective gear, she was allowed to enter the scene. Within a short time, Rebecca was struck on the back of the head by a concrete slab that fell from the building's wreckage. She died 5 days later of massive cerebral edema. Nurses can learn the following lessons from this tragedy:

- Never enter a disaster scene unless you are directed to do so by an emergency medical technician, firefighter, or law enforcement official.
- Contact local hospitals and clinics to offer your help; your medical expertise is more useful in the clinical environment.
- Take courses in first aid and emergency care. Contact your local Red Cross for a list of courses.
- Contact your local health department to learn more about your community's disaster plan and how you can contribute in the event of a disaster in your area.

DISPLAY 17.5 SPONTANEOUS VOLUNTEERS

Volunteers represent a potential resource to a community affected by a disaster, whether of natural or man-made origin. However, individuals who respond spontaneously and without appropriate training and verifiable qualifications can easily overwhelm the capabilities of local government and other agencies.

From Warner, K., & Hanna, B. (2007). *Disasters happen: Do you know your role?* Presented at 21st Century Nursing Challenges, Chico, CA: Kappa Omicron Chapter STTI.

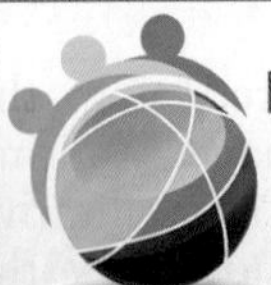

DISPLAY 17.6 FREE ONLINE EMERGENCY PREPAREDNESS TRAINING

CDC Emergency Preparedness and Response Training and Education: http://www.bt.cdc.gov/training/
Federal Emergency Management Agency (FEMA): http://www.fema.gov/about/training/emergency.shtm
Public Health Foundation—Train.org: https://www.train.org
National Nurse Emergency Preparedness Initiative (NNEPI): http://www.nnepi.org/
National Institutes of Health—Radiation Emergency Medical Management: http://www.remm.nlm.gov/training.htm
University of Minnesota, Center for Public Health Preparedness: http://www.sph.umn.edu/ce/umncphp/
Uniformed Services University of the Health Sciences Online Preparedness Education Program: http://opep.usuhs.edu/

such as stethoscopes, flashlights, and cellular phones. In the event of an emergency, many who are unprepared or untrained often present at the site of a disaster or at local hospitals to volunteer. These "spontaneous volunteers" can be an additional burden to those in charge (Display 17.5).

To increase understanding of and the ability to work within an emergency situation, every nurse should become familiar with the NIMS. The NIMS offers a "unified approach to incident management; standard command and management structures; and emphasis on preparedness, mutual aid, and resource management" (FEMA, 2008). In essence, it provides a common language for disaster response, to reduce confusion as much as possible. Free online courses are offered through FEMA (see Display 17.6). Additionally, every nurse should have up-to-date vaccinations; many biologic threats have the same initial presentations, and reducing susceptibility to common illnesses such as influenza can help with initial identification.

Assessment for Risk Factors and Disaster History

As noted earlier in the chapter, the community health nurse is uniquely qualified to perform a community assessment for risk factors that may contribute to disasters. In addition, the nurse should review the *disaster history* of the community. Have earthquakes, tornadoes, hurricanes, floods, blizzards, riots, or other disasters occurred in the past? If so, what (if any) were the warning signs? Were they heeded? Were people warned in time? Did evacuation efforts remove all people in danger? What were the community's on-site responses, and how effective were they? What programs were put in place to rehabilitate the community?

Establishing Authority, Communication, and Transportation

In addition to assessing for preparedness, the effective disaster plan establishes a clear chain of authority, develops lines of communication, and delineates routes of transport. Establishing a clear and flexible chain of authority is critical for successful implementation of a disaster plan. Usually, the chain is hierarchical, with, for example, the community's governmental head (e.g., mayor) initiating the plan, alerting the media to broadcast warnings, authorizing the police to begin evacuations, and so on. Within each level of the organization, the hierarchy continues. For example, at the local hospital, the hospital administrator may be responsible for alerting nurse managers to call in additional personnel. Flexibility is essential, because key authority figures may themselves be survivors of the disaster. If the home of the chief of police is destroyed in an earthquake, his second-in-command must have equal knowledge of the community's disaster plan and be able to step in without delay.

Effective communication is often a point of breakdown for communities attempting to cope with major disasters. After the terrorist attacks in Oklahoma City and New York City, phone lines were damaged and cellular sites were overwhelmed, making communication difficult. Communication was possible only through handheld radios or by way of couriers on foot. At times of heightened chaos and stress, as well as after physical damage to communication facilities and equipment, misinformation and misinterpretation can flourish, leading to delayed treatment and increased loss of life.

Again, clarity and flexibility are the watchwords for establishing lines of communication. How will warnings be communicated? What backups are available if the normal communication systems are destroyed in the disaster? How will communication between relief workers at the disaster site, hospital personnel, police, and governmental authorities be maintained? What role will local media play, both in keeping information flowing to the outside world and in broadcasting needs for assistance and supplies? Finally, how will friends and family members be informed of the whereabouts or health status of their loved ones? The characteristics of effective communication during disasters are summarized in Display 17.7.

Closed or inefficient routes of transportation can also increase injury and loss of life. For example, if a single, narrow mountainous road is the only means of transporting firefighters to or evacuating residents from the scene of a forest fire, then disaster planners should propose widening the road or clearing a second road. Disaster planners must also consider what routes emergency vehicles will take when transporting disaster survivors to local and outlying hospitals or health care workers to the disaster site. What if the chosen routes are inaccessible because of floodwaters, advancing fires, mountain slides, or building rubble? Are alternative routes designated?

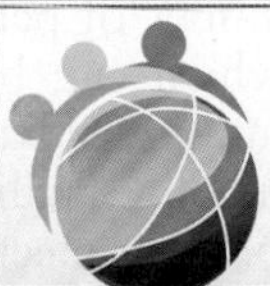

DISPLAY 17.7 EFFECTIVE COMMUNICATION DURING DISASTERS

To be effective, communication during disasters must elicit action. Communication that elicits action provides information that is

- Believable
- Current
- Unambiguous
- Authoritative
- Predictive of the probability of future events (what is going to happen next?)

Effective communication is

- Interactive—it allows for and addresses questions.
- Conclusive—it eliminates room for speculation and *catastrophizing*.
- Urgent—conveys seriousness without resorting to fear tactics
- Clear, simple, and repetitive
- Characterized by solutions and suggestions for success
- Personal—it uses people's names if possible and addresses their real and perceived needs.

Finally, because rumors can hinder effective action or provoke premature action, effective communication includes rumor control. It provides suggestions for constructive activity, reducing time and energy spent on rumor generation and perpetuation.

Mobilizing, Warning, and Evacuating

In many natural disasters, local weather service personnel, public works officials, police officers, or firefighters have the earliest information indicating an increasing potential for a disaster. These officials typically have a plan in place for providing community authorities with specific data indicating increased risk. They may also advise the mayor's office or other community leaders of their recommendations for warning or evacuating the public. Additionally, they may recommend actions the community can take to mitigate damage, such as spraying rooftops in the path of fires, sandbagging the banks of rising rivers, or imposing a curfew in times of civil unrest.

Disaster plans must specify the means of communicating warnings to the public, as well as the precise information that should be included in warnings. Planners should never assume that all citizens can be reached by radio or television or that broadcast systems will be unaffected by the disaster. Broadcast media may indeed be a primary means of communicating warnings, but alternative strategies, such as police or volunteers canvassing neighborhoods with loudspeakers, should also be in place. In multilingual communities, messages should be broadcast in multiple languages. Not only homes but also businesses must be informed. Information that should be communicated includes the nature of the disaster; the exact geographic region affected, including street names if appropriate; and the actions citizens should take to protect themselves and their property.

An evacuation plan is an essential component of the total disaster plan. The plan should cover notification of the police, local military personnel, or voluntary citizens' groups of the need to evacuate people, as well as methods of notifying and transporting the evacuees. A plan should also be made for responding to citizens who refuse to evacuate. For example, will police authorities forcibly remove an elderly citizen from his home to a shelter? Will evacuation plans include household pets? If farms or ranches are in the path of fires or floods, will animals be evacuated?

Responding to Disasters

At the disaster site, police, firefighters, nurses, and other relief workers develop a coordinated response to rescue, triage, and treat disaster survivors. One of the first obligations of relief workers is to remove survivors from danger.

Rescue

The job of rescue typically belongs to firefighters and Urban Search and Rescue teams that have personnel

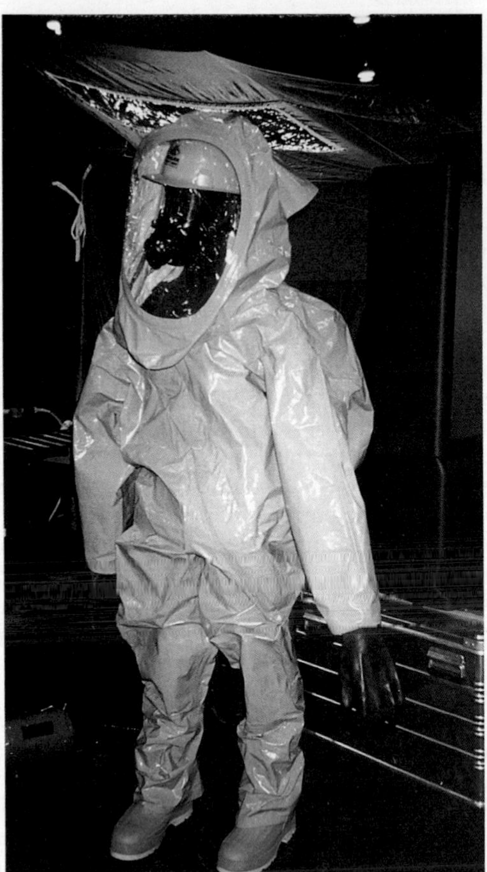

FIGURE 17-2. Hazardous materials suit used by the military and most fire departments. (Photo by Cynthia Tait.)

with special training in search and rescue. Depending on the disaster agent, protective gear, heavy equipment, and special vehicles may be needed, and dogs trained to locate dead bodies may be brought in (Fig. 17-2). Usually, the immediate disaster site is not the best place for the disaster nurse, who can be far more effective in triage and treatment of survivors. One of the lessons of the World Trade Center bombing was that the greatest need for medical professionals was at the local hospitals, not at the disaster site.

Rescue workers face the logistically and psychologically difficult task of determining when to cease rescue efforts. Some factors to consider include increasing danger to rescue workers, diminishing numbers of survivors, and diminishing possibilities for survival. For example, after a plane crash on a snowy mountain, rescue efforts may cease if it is deemed that anyone who might have survived the crash would subsequently have died of exposure.

Triage

Whereas emergency nurses daily determine which clients require priority care, the community health nurse may be at a loss as to where to start when faced with multiple persons impacted by a disaster. Knowing the principles and practice of triage allows the nurse to offer nursing skills most effectively. **Triage** is the process of sorting multiple casualties in the event of a war or major disaster. It is required when the number of casualties exceeds immediate treatment resources. The goal of triage is to affect the greatest amount of good for the greatest number of people. Figure 17-3 shows the four basic categories of the international triage system, as well as a triage tag. The most common method of triage used by first responders at a mass-casualty incident in the United States is the Simple Triage and Rapid Treatment (START) for adults and JumpSTART for pediatric patients. START and JumpSTART is the form of triage that is consistent with Figure 17-3.

Prioritization of treatment may be very different in a mass-casualty event as opposed to an average day in a hospital emergency department. Under normal circumstances, a person presenting to a hospital emergency department with a myocardial infarction and showing no pulse or respirations would receive immediate treatment and have a chance of recovery. At a disaster site, a person without a pulse or respirations would most likely be placed in the nonsalvageable category.

The term *mass casualty* refers to a number of persons impacted that is greater than that which can be managed safely with the resources the community has to offer (such as rescue vehicles and emergency facilities available to serve disaster survivors while also meeting the needs of the rest of the community). Frequently, in mass-casualty occurrences, the broader community needs to become involved, which necessitates calling in rescue vehicles, firefighters, and police officers from neighboring towns, or the use of neighboring hospitals. This adds another layer of disaster management coordination that must be considered.

Immediate Treatment and Support

Disaster nurses provide treatment on-site at emergency treatment stations, at mobile field hospitals, in shelters, and at local hospitals and clinics (see Display 17.8). In addition to direct nursing care, on-site interventions might include arranging for transport once survivors are stabilized and managing the procurement, distribution, and replenishment of all supplies. Disposable items might be in short supply, requiring resterilization procedures that may be unfamiliar to a nurse not accustomed to field work. These procedures may pose a challenge even to an experienced nurse because of the field environment. The nurse may also manage provision or distribution of food and beverages, including infant formulas and rehydration fluids, and arrange for adequate, accessible, and safe sanitation facilities, either on-site or in a shelter. Finally, the nurse often must also arrange for psychological and spiritual care of survivors of disasters.

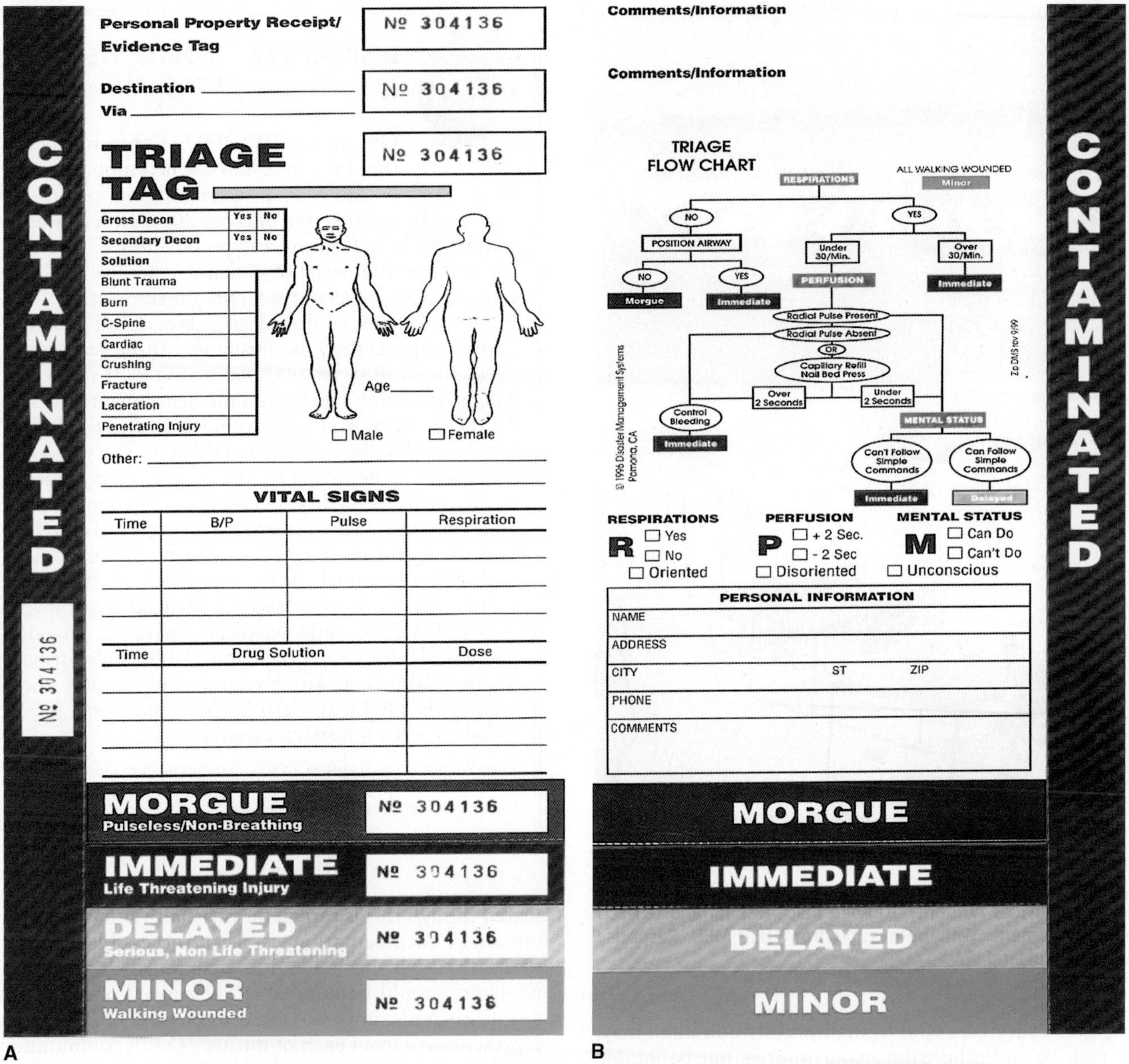

CONTAMINATED

Personal Property Receipt/ Evidence Tag № 304136

Destination ______ № 304136
Via ______

TRIAGE TAG № 304136

Gross Decon	Yes	No
Secondary Decon	Yes	No
Solution		

Blunt Trauma
Burn
C-Spine
Cardiac
Crushing
Fracture
Laceration
Penetrating Injury

Age____
☐ Male ☐ Female

Other: ______

VITAL SIGNS

Time	B/P	Pulse	Respiration

Time	Drug Solution	Dose

№ 304136

MORGUE Pulseless/Non-Breathing № 304136
IMMEDIATE Life Threatening Injury № 304136
DELAYED Serious, Non Life Threatening № 304136
MINOR Walking Wounded № 304136

A

Comments/Information

Comments/Information

TRIAGE FLOW CHART

RESPIRATIONS — ALL WALKING WOUNDED — Minor
NO — POSITION AIRWAY — NO — Morgue; YES — Immediate
YES — Under 30/Min. — PERFUSION; Over 30/Min. — Immediate
Radial Pulse Present / Radial Pulse Absent OR Capillary Refill Nail Bed Press
Over 2 Seconds — Control Bleeding — Immediate
Under 2 Seconds — MENTAL STATUS
Can't Follow Simple Commands — Immediate
Can Follow Simple Commands — Delayed

© 1996 Disaster Management Systems Pomona, CA

RESPIRATIONS R ☐ Yes ☐ No ☐ Oriented
PERFUSION P ☐ + 2 Sec. ☐ - 2 Sec ☐ Disoriented
MENTAL STATUS M ☐ Can Do ☐ Can't Do ☐ Unconscious

PERSONAL INFORMATION
NAME
ADDRESS
CITY ST ZIP
PHONE
COMMENTS

MORGUE
IMMEDIATE
DELAYED
MINOR

CONTAMINATED

B

FIGURE 17-3. Example of victim triage tag. Four basic categories are all applied when a medical system is overwhelmed with person impacted by the incident. (1) *Red*: Urgent/Critical. Victims in this category have injuries or medical problems that will likely lead to death if not treated immediately (e.g., an unconscious victim with signs of internal bleeding). (2) *Yellow*: Delayed. Victims in this category have injuries that will require medical attention; however, time to medical treatment is not yet critical (e.g., a conscious victim with a fractured femur). (3) *Green*: Minor/Walking Wounded. Victims in this category have sustained minor injury or are presenting with minimal signs of illness. Prolonged delay in care most likely will not adversely affect their long-term outcome (e.g., a conscious victim with superficial cuts, scrapes, and bruises). (4) *Black*: Dead/Nonsalvageable. Victims in this category are obviously dead or have suffered mortal wounds because of which death is imminent (e.g., an unconscious victim with an open skull fracture with brain matter showing). Lifesaving heroics on this group of victims will only delay medical care on more viable victims.

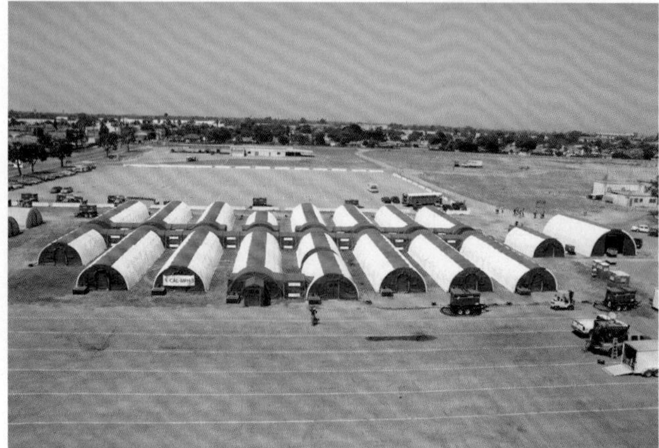

A

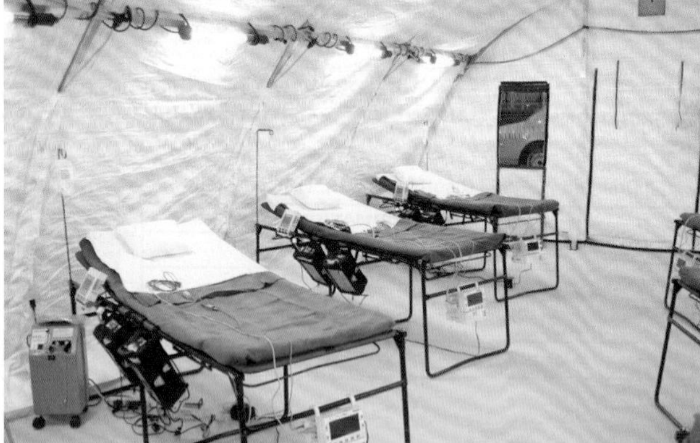

B

Mobile field hospital, interior and exterior. (A) CA Emergency Medical Services Authority 200-bed field hospital and (B) ICU with equipment. With permission from BLU-MED Response Systems, Kirkland WA

Some survivors who seem physically uninjured may, in fact, be suffering from major injuries but be unable to relate their symptoms to a relief worker because of shock or anxiety. For instance, a father pulling debris away from his collapsed house after a tornado may be so worried about a missing child that he does not realize that he has a broken arm.

Other survivors may be so emotionally traumatized by a disaster that they act out, disrupting efforts to assist them and other survivors and even engaging in dangerous activities. This may cause relief workers to focus on emotional care; however, such survivors must be assessed for head trauma and internal injuries, because their behavior may have a physical cause. If they are physically able, such survivors may be given a simple, repetitive task to perform, which serves as both a distraction and a means to restore, to a small extent, their sense of control over their environment.

Care of Bodies and Notification of Families

Identification and transport of the dead to a morgue or holding facility are crucial, especially if contagion is feared though this is rare in masscasualty situations. Toe tags make documentation visible and accessible. Records of deaths must be made and maintained, and family members should be notified of their loved ones' deaths as quickly and compassionately as possible. If feasible, a representative from each of the area's faith communities should be available to assist families awaiting news of missing loved ones. As stated earlier, a family's recovery from loss is often delayed when notification of relatives (indirectly impacted) is not possible because the persons' bodies are badly damaged or not found.

> **DISPLAY 17.8 MOBILE FIELD HOSPITAL**
>
> On August 25, 2007, California featured the first state-owned mobile field hospital in a statewide disaster-training exercise. The tent hospital is one of three 200-bed hospitals purchased by California and prepositioned around the state in the event of a major emergency. The hospital can be deployed and on-site within 72 hours and comes equipped for 7 days of full patient care. Used together, the hospitals can be reconfigured into a 400- or 600-bed hospital, if needed. This is the same type of mobile field hospital used by the military, and it was modeled after the hospitals used by the Air Force and Navy. The various units within the hospital mirror services provided in any modern facility including emergency room, surgical suite, laboratory, x-ray, surgical intensive care, and even a pediatric unit. The exercise included personnel from the Medical Reserve Corps (MRC), federal Disaster Medical Assistance Team (DMAT), state Medical Assistance Team, Mental Health Response Team, Ambulance Strike Team, California Air National Guard, and the California Highway Patrol. "Victims" were provided by a local nursing program.
>
> From Warner, K., & Hanna, B. (2007). *Disasters happen: Do you know your role?* Presented at 21st Century Nursing Challenges, Chico, CA: Kappa Omicron Chapter STTI.

Supporting Recovery from Disasters

Disasters do not suddenly end when the rubble is cleared and the survivors' wounds are healed. Rather, recovery is a long, complex process. It often includes long-term medical treatment, physical rehabilitation, financial restitution, case management, and psychological and spiritual support.

Long-Term Treatment

Long-term treatment may be required for many survivors of disasters, straining the local rehabilitative-care facilities and resources. Children who are survivors may have to deal with lifelong disabilities or scars from their ordeal, and families may be without adequate financial support for their child's medical care. Elderly citizens who had been in excellent health but who sustained serious injuries in the disaster might suddenly find that they can no longer live independently and must move to a long-term care facility. After floods, landslides, fires, or earthquakes, extensive property damage may cause some residents or businesses to relocate rather than rebuild on land they now deem to be disaster prone. A disaster that creates numerous persons impacted in a small community may alter the entire social fabric of that community permanently.

Long-Term Support

Disaster survivors may need funding to repair or rebuild their homes or to reopen businesses, such as stores, restaurants, child care facilities, and other services needed by the community. Insurance settlements, FEMA funding, and private donations may assist in financing community rehabilitation. Health care workers may be required to provide case management and assist survivors with necessary paperwork. Immediately after a disaster, some survivors may be unable to concentrate on anything beyond fulfilling their immediate needs and those of their family.

Psychological support is often required after a disaster, both for survivors and for relief workers. Some individuals may experience posttraumatic stress disorder (PTSD) (discussed later). Many survivors, especially elderly persons displaced from their homes, may quietly lose their will to live and drift into apathy and malaise. Individuals whose belief in God was unshakable before the incident may now question their faith, wondering how a loving God could have let this happen, especially if they lost a loved one. These survivors often require not only empathetic listening but also long-term skilled spiritual counseling. In assessing a community's citizens for counseling needs after a disaster, the nurse should not forget to include children. Often, children do not have words to express their feelings or fears and may act out in ways adults find difficult to understand, unless age-appropriate psychological intervention is provided.

Need for Self-Care

Self-care, including stress education for all relief workers after a disaster, is a common practice and actively encouraged in many communities. Proponents report that stress education helps to reduce anxiety and put the situation into proper perspective. **Critical Incident Stress Debriefing (CISD)** provides relief workers with professional debriefing in small groups or individually and becomes a mechanism for emotional reconciliation. CISD is generally provided between 24 and 72 hours after the disaster event. Proponents of CISD claim that it typically produces positive effects by

- Accelerating the healing process
- Equipping participants with positive coping mechanisms
- Clearing up misconceptions and misunderstandings
- Restoring or reinforcing group cohesiveness
- Promoting a healthy, supportive work atmosphere
- Identifying individuals who require more extensive psychological assistance

A CISD addresses all components of the human response to trauma, including physiologic effects, emotions, and cognition. Some studies show that CISD allows individuals to regain a sense of equilibrium much sooner than those not involved in CISD if participation is voluntary. However, the studies that have shown the effectiveness of CISD were not randomized clinical trials. The large randomized studies that have been done found that emotional debriefing had adverse effects on the participants and that at 4 months and 3 years the individuals that had forms of CISD suffered greater PTSD than individuals than those that did not have CISD (Mayou, Ehlers, Hobbs, 2003; Sijbrandij, Oiff, Reitsma, Carlier, & Gersons, 2006). Based on the conflicting research studies, nurses should be cautious about CISD, but should also be knowledgeable of it because it is so prevalent following a disaster. It can take years to end a popular practice even when it has been shown to be ineffective.

Self-care comes in many forms and is part of a prescription for emotional healing after a traumatic event. Self-care is not just for rescue workers but for everyone touched by trauma. Keep in mind the following self-care points (Peeke, 2002):

- *Give yourself time to heal.* You need time to adjust. Even though you want the pain to be over immediately, it is healthier to realize that this is a long-term recovery process.
- *Ask for emotional support.* Talk with family and friends around the country. It feels good to be connected with others. You listen and support one another as you share your feelings.
- *Take care of yourself;* it will improve your ability to deal with stress. Eat regularly, avoid alcohol, maintain sleep patterns, follow your exercise routine, and embrace each day as a gift.
- *Reestablish daily routines.* Getting back to your regular routine is important and gives you a sense of security and normalcy.
- *Use your time wisely.* A significant traumatic event gives you an opportunity to reprioritize how you spend your time each day. Are you living your dreams and passions? Traumatic events remind us of our fragile nature and that each moment should be savored and enjoyed.
- *Give something back.* Your life goes on. Demonstrate your gratefulness by becoming part of a global healing process. Donate to charities and give time to causes you have ignored. Seek ways to reach out to those who are in need of help.

Psychological Consequences of Disasters

In addition to physical injury, potential loss of life, and destruction of property that can occur from a disaster, people affected by the disaster can also suffer from psychological consequences, such as acute stress disorder, depression, and PTSD. The community health and community mental health nurses, through education, screening, assessment, and referral, have an important role in the primary, secondary, and tertiary prevention of psychological disturbances due to a disaster.

Primary Prevention

Although a disaster, by its very nature, is often unforeseen, people's ability to cope with the disaster can be determined in part by their previous level of coping and the resources available to help them. Stuart and Laraia (2005) explain that primary prevention in behavioral health care has two basic objectives:

- To help people avoid stressors or cope with them more adaptively
- To change the resources, policies, or agents of the environment so that they no longer cause stress but rather enhance people's functioning (pp. 208–209)

A community health nurse can engage in many activities to promote mental health and strengthen adaptive coping skills in individuals and the community. She or he can teach health education classes in positive stress adaptation, positive ways of coping, self-efficacy, and **resilience**, an important quality that enables people to cope with disaster. A definition of resilience is offered by the President's New Freedom Commission on Mental Health in their 2003 report *Achieving the Promise: Transforming Mental Health Care in America*.

> Resilience means the personal and community qualities that enable us to rebound from adversity, trauma, tragedy, threats, or other stresses—and to go on with life with a sense of mastery, competence, and hope. We now understand from research that resilience is fostered by positive individual traits, such as optimism, good problem-solving skills, and treatments. Closely knit communities and neighborhoods are also resilient, providing supports for their members (p. 5).

According to Stuart and Laraia (2005), the building of competency or resilience may be the most important primary prevention strategy, since a competent person or community can make informed decisions based on availability of resources and problem-solving skills. In a phone survey of more than 2,700 New York City residents (after September 11, 2001), Bonanno, Galea, Bucciarelli, and Vlahov (2007) found that the strongest variables associated with resilience pertained to the absence of additional life stressors, pointing to the need for more research on the role of resilience in recovery from extreme incidents.

In addition to working with individuals within the community to enhance their resilience, community health nurses can contribute to primary prevention in the face of disaster by being active advocates for improving the social structure of the community, including housing, work, schools, child care, and economic conditions for community members. At a time when governments are reducing spending and services, it is important for the community health nurse to advocate for the resources necessary for the community to meet both the physical and psychological challenges of a disaster.

Secondary Prevention

Despite community education and intervention, people involved in a disaster often feel anxious and overwhelmed. They are in a *mental health crisis*, defined as a state when people's usual coping mechanisms no longer are effective in the face of the overwhelming disaster (Stuart & Laraia, 2005). A crisis or disaster, an event that is out of the ordinary in magnitude and personal experience, is called an *adventitious crisis*. Examples of adventitious crises are natural disasters, such as floods, earthquakes, and fires, and national disasters such as terrorist attacks, war, riots, and airplane crashes (Varcarolis & Halter, 2009). When the stress of these disasters causes overwhelming anxiety, *crisis intervention* is a secondary prevention intervention that the trained community health or community mental health nurse can employ to minimize the psychological consequences of the disaster.

Crisis intervention is a short-term intervention, no longer than 6 weeks, designed to return an individual or community to its predisaster level of functioning and solve immediate psychological problems. Interventions are provided on several levels: environmental manipulation, general support, generic approach, and the individual approach (Stuart & Laraia, 2005). *Environmental manipulation* results in the change of a person's physical or interpersonal situation, providing situational support to relieve stress. An example of environmental manipulation is when a community health nurse coordinates the reunification of family members separated by the disaster. *General support* is defined as the caring, warmth, and concern the community health nurse conveys to the client as he or she delivers services (Stuart & Laraia, 2005).

The *generic approach* is an aspect of crisis intervention that is particularly well suited to the community health nurse. This approach is designed to reach high-risk individuals and large groups who have experienced the same disaster, teaching them about the expected emotional reactions to the type of disaster they have experienced and promoting adaptive responses. Grief reactions follow a known pattern, and large groups can be taught what to expect in the face of severe loss while giving individual members of the group an opportunity to express their feelings of loss. This generic approach is sometimes called *debriefing*. Individual crisis intervention is reserved for high-risk individuals who need special treatment because of the severity of their symptoms and is best provided by nurses trained in mental health treatment and crisis intervention (Stuart & Laraia, 2005).

Tertiary Prevention

People who have experienced or witnessed a disaster and have been unable to adequately cope with its consequences can develop long-term effects, such as *acute stress disorder* or **posttraumatic stress disorder (PTSD)**. According to the fourth edition of *Diagnostic and Statistical Manual of Mental Disorders*, text revision (DSM-IV-TR) (American Psychiatric Association [APA], 2000), both acute stress disorder and PTSD can occur after any traumatic event in which a person responds with intense fear, helplessness, or horror to an actual or threatened death or serious injury to oneself or others. Both natural and man-made disasters fit into this definition (see Evidence-Based Practice).

The DSM-IV-TR (APA, 2000) defines acute stress disorder as occurring within 1 month of the disaster and resolving within 4 weeks. A person experiencing acute distress disorder must have three symptoms of dissociation during or after the disaster:

- A subjective sense of numbing, or absence of emotional responsiveness
- A reduction of awareness of his or her surroundings (e.g., "being in a daze")
- Derealization (a sense of unreality regarding one's environment)
- Depersonalization (sense of unreality or self-estrangement)
- Dissociative amnesia (i.e., inability to recall an important aspect of the trauma) (p. 432)

If an acute reaction to the disaster lasts longer than 4 weeks, it can develop into the more chronic disorder of PTSD. According to the DSM-IV-TR (APA, 2000), the symptoms for both acute stress disorder and PTSD include the following:

- The traumatic event is persistently reexperienced in one (or more) of the following ways:
  1. Recurrent and intrusive distressing recollections of the event, including images, thoughts, or perceptions
  2. Recurrent distressing dreams of the event
  3. Acting or feeling as if the traumatic event were recurring (includes a sense of reliving the experience, illusions, hallucinations, and dissociative flashback episodes, including those which occur on awakening or while intoxicated)
  4. Intense psychological distress at exposure to internal or external cues that symbolize or resemble an aspect of the traumatic event
  5. Physiological reactivity on exposure to internal or external cues that symbolize or resemble an aspect of the traumatic event
- Persistent avoidance of stimuli associated with the trauma and numbing of general responsiveness (not present before trauma) as indicated by three (or more) of the following:
  1. Efforts to avoid thoughts, feelings, or conversations associated with the trauma
  2. Efforts to avoid activities, places, or people that arouse recollections of the trauma
  3. Inability to recall an important aspect of the trauma
  4. Markedly diminished interest or participation in significant activities
  5. Feelings of detachment or estrangement from others
  6. Restricted range of affect (e.g., unable to have loving feelings)
  7. Sense of a foreshortened future (e.g., does not expect to have a career, marriage, children, or normal life span)
- Persistent symptoms of increased arousal (not present before the trauma), as indicated by two (or more) of the following:
  1. Difficulty in falling or staying asleep
  2. Irritability or outburst of anger
  3. Difficulty concentrating
  4. Hypervigilance
  5. Exaggerated startle response (p. 428)

It is important for the community health nurse to be aware of the symptoms of these disorders so that she or he can refer the client for treatment, which should be left to the advanced practice mental health nurse and other mental health professionals.

TERRORISM

At the start of the 21st century, the world is a global community. This is particularly evident in the increased incidence and sophistication of terrorist threats and acts around the world. Incidents occurring on US soil, such as the bombing of the World Trade Center in 1993 and its destruction on September 11, 2001, alerted us to our vulnerability and dramatically emphasized the need for increased preparedness within our communities.

The July 2005 bombings in London that struck multiple transportation system sites, which killed 56 and injured over 700; the February 2008 bombings in Baghdad by remotely controlled bombs carried by two mentally disabled women, which killed 98 and wounded 200; and the 2007 bombings in Karachi, Pakistan, which killed 136 and injured 387, all confirm that our vulnerability exists in many areas. Biologic, chemical, and nuclear terror are tragically possible.

The U.S. Federal Bureau of Investigation (FBI) defines **terrorism** as "the unlawful use of force and violence against persons or property to intimidate or coerce a government, the civilian population, or any segment thereof, in furtherance of political or social objectives" (U.S. Department of Justice, 2006). A terrorist is over zealous and obsessed with an idea. Terrorism and terrorist acts are not new. The term *terrorism* can be traced to 1798, and the use of terrorist tactics precedes this date. A highly organized religious sect called the *Sicarii* attacked crowds of people with knives during holiday celebrations in Palestine at about the time of Christ. During the French and Indian War of 1763, British forces gave smallpox-contaminated blankets to Native Americans. During World War I, the German bioweapons program developed anthrax, glanders, cholera, and wheat fungus as weapons targeting cavalry animals. In World War II, the Japanese tested biologic weapons on Chinese prisoners.

Three major countries operated offensive bioweapons programs in recent years: the United Kingdom until 1957, the United States until 1969, and the former Soviet Union until 1990. Iraq started its bioweapons program in 1985 and continued to develop weapons until 2003. At least 17 other nations are currently suspected of operating offensive bioweapons programs (Evans, Crutcher, Shadel, et al., 2002). Bioweapons include mustard gas, sarin and VX gas, and anthrax. Terrorists typically use biologic or chemical agents, explosives, or incendiary devices to deliver the agents to their targets.

Nuclear warfare involves the use of nuclear devices as weapons and can take several forms. Terrorists who gain access to nuclear power plants could cause a chain of events that lead to a meltdown of the nuclear core, thereby releasing radioactive particles for hundreds of miles around the site. Nuclear accidents have occurred, but no known terrorist attacks have yet involved the use of nuclear power plants as weapons. A terrorist attack using nuclear weapons or destruction of a nuclear plant would cause multiple and prolonged deaths with extensive damage and negative effects for decades.

Chemical warfare involves the use of chemicals such as explosives, nerve agents, blister agents, choking agents, and incapacitating or riot-control agents to cause confusion, debilitation, death, and destruction (Yergler, 2002). Terrorists in the Middle East, willing to murder others and knowing they will be committing suicide, strap bombs to themselves and detonate the explosives in or near targets. Others crash vehicles loaded with explosives into crowds of people or into a building.

The aircraft used on September 11, 2001, were incendiary devices because they were carrying thousands of tons of jet fuel. The success of the mission depended on the surprise of the attack, severe damage to recognizable buildings, and the deaths of many people. Disaster responders and government officials did not expect the collapse of the buildings. If the planes had been low on fuel, the damage would have been less severe. The liquid fuel burned at such a high temperature that the internal structures of the buildings were weakened (National Institute of Standards and Technology, 2008).

Biologic warfare involves using biologic agents to cause multiple illnesses and deaths. Biological agents are graded as Category A, B, or C by the CDC (see Table 17-2). Typical biologic agents are anthrax, botulinum, bubonic plague, Ebola, and smallpox. These agents could be used to contaminate food, water, or air. Deliberate food and water contamination remains the easiest way to distribute biologic agents for the purpose of terrorism (Khan, Swerdlow, & Juranek, 2001).

Table 17.2 Categories of Biologic Agents

Category	Definition	Agents/Diseases
Category A	• High-priority agents pose a risk to national security. • Can be easily disseminated or transmitted from person to person • Result in high mortality rates and have the potential for major public health impact • Might cause public panic and social disruption • Require special action for public health preparedness	• Anthrax (*Bacillus anthracis*) • Botulism (*Clostridium botulinum* toxin) • Plague (*Yersinia pestis*) • Smallpox (variola major) • Tularemia (*Francisella tularensis*) • Viral hemorrhagic fevers (filoviruses [e.g., Ebola, Marburg] and arenaviruses [e.g., Lassa, Machupo])
Category B	• Second highest risk to national security • Are moderately easy to disseminate • Result in moderate morbidity rates and low mortality rates • Require specific enhancements of CDC's diagnostic capacity and enhanced disease surveillance	• Brucellosis (*Brucella* species) • Epsilon toxin of *Clostridium perfringens* • Food safety threats (e.g., *Salmonella* species, *Escherichia coli* O157:H7, *Shigella*) • Glanders (*Burkholderia mallei*) • Melioidosis (*Burkholderia pseudomallei*) • Psittacosis (*Chlamydia psittaci*) • Q fever (*Coxiella burnetii*) • Ricin toxin from Ricinus communis (castor beans) • Staphylococcal enterotoxin B • Typhus fever (*Rickettsia prowazekii*) • Viral encephalitis (alphaviruses [e.g., Venezuelan equine encephalitis, eastern equine encephalitis, western equine encephalitis]) • Water safety threats (e.g., *Vibrio cholerae*, *Cryptosporidium parvum*)
Category C	• Third highest priority agents include emerging pathogens that could be engineered for mass dissemination in the future because of: • Availability • Ease of production and dissemination • Potential for high morbidity and mortality rates and major health impact	• Emerging infectious diseases • Nipah virus • Hantavirus

From: CDC. Emergency Preparedness and Response. Retrieved from http://www.bt.cdc.gov/agent/agentlist-category.asp

The U.S. Office of Technology Assessment has speculated that the release of 220 pounds of anthrax spores from a crop-duster over the Washington, DC, area on a calm, clear night could kill between 1 and 3 million people (U.S. Army Chemical and Biological Defense Command, 1998).

The United States is very concerned about the possibility of biologic warfare or bioterrorism, as nations should be. The anthrax infections and deaths that occurred after September 11, 2001, added to these concerns. It was years before the government confirmed to the public that these incidents were committed by a domestic terrorist who was a single disturbed citizen. In 2008, the investigation led to a scientist at Ft. Detrick as the cause of this terroristic act. Although charges were never filed due to the individual's suicide, the FBI believes that he was solely responsible for this act of domestic terrorism (FBI, 2008). Regardless of the source of terrorism, the outcomes are the same: fear, death, and destruction.

Factors Contributing to Terrorism

Political factors are the most common contributors to terrorism. Anti-American sentiment runs high in many foreign countries, especially those that perceive the United States as a threat to their military, economic, social, or religious self-determination. Terrorist acts against American military installations abroad, in airports, in airplanes, at American embassies, and even on American soil targeting civilian populations have occurred frequently in the last decade as an expression of political unrest. The war in Iraq in 2003 was based on information about suspected bioterrorism weapons and reports that Iraq was harboring anti-Western terrorists; these two pieces of information resulted in the toppling of the Saddam Hussein political regime. However, hundreds of military lives were lost and thousands of civilians were killed, and no weapons of mass destruction were found. As of January 2011, more than 4,421 US military and civilian personnel have lost their lives, and some 1,935 are dealing with injuries in the ongoing military campaign (Operation Iraqi Freedom [OIF] U.S. Casualty Status, 2011). There have been 1,439 killed and 9,971 wounded in action in Afghanistan (OIF U.S. Casualty Status, 2011). Additionally, there have been approximately 109,422 Iraqi civilian deaths due to violence since the beginning of Operation Iraqi Freedom (Iraqi Body Count, 2011).

Within the United States, violence-prone members of militia movements, violent antiabortion activists, racial desegregation advocates, and other radical groups have performed terrorist acts, such as the bombing of health clinics offering abortions. In 1984, members of a religious cult, the Rajneeshees, lived in Wasco County, Oregon, and followed a self-proclaimed guru exiled from India. In an attempt to reduce voter turnout in an upcoming county election, they sprinkled *Salmonella* bacteria over items on salad bars in local restaurants and in the produce sections of grocery stores. They hoped that, with a reduced voter turnout, representatives friendlier to their group would win the election. Their attack failed to affect the election and killed no one; however, 751 people became sick (Bernett, 2006; McDade & Franze, 1998). The media underreported this event because domestic terrorism was not a topic of concern at that time in US history.

Role of the Community Health Nurse

Community health nurses need to be prepared for the possibility of terrorist activity. They have a role in primary, secondary, and tertiary prevention.

Primary Prevention

Community health nurses are in ideal situations within communities to participate in surveillance. They must look and listen within their communities for antigroup sentiments, for example, antireligion, antigay, or antiethnic feelings. The nurse should report any untoward activities accordingly.

Nurses should be alert to signs of possible terrorist activity. Specific indicators of possible chemical or biologic terrorism include unusual numbers of dead or dying animals; unexplained serious illnesses or deaths; an unusual liquid, spray, vapor, or odor; and low-lying clouds or fog unrelated to weather. Unusual swarms of insects might also indicate the use of biologic agents for terrorism. "Although not all nurses will want to become 'disaster' nurses, it is imperative that each nurse acquire a knowledge base and minimum set of skills to enable them to plan for and respond to a disaster in a timely manner" (Veenema, 2007, p. 17). Additionally, Secor-Turner and O'Boyle (2006) noted a lack of studies of nurses' responses to bioterrorism events in a literature review of studies between 2002 and 2004. They emphasized the need for bioterrorism plans that "incorporate strategies to support nurses and address their physical, psychological, and emotional issues" (p. 414). Less subtle forms of terrorism include bombings, mass shootings, and hijackings, which are more difficult to uncover in time to prevent injury or death.

Secondary and Tertiary Prevention

Although prevention of terrorist incidents is primarily the responsibility of the Department of Defense, the DHS, and public health and law enforcement agencies, community health nurses must be ready to handle the secondary and tertiary effects of such attacks. Knowing the lethal and incapacitating chemical, biological, and radiological weapons that may be used by terrorists is important. Many of the communicable disease organisms that could be used by terrorists were discussed in Chapter 8.

Realizing that terrorist attacks may result in large numbers of casualties, the community health nurse must be prepared to act safely, access information rapidly, and use resources effectively. Specifically, the community health nurse may be called on to provide direct care to survivors, to volunteer as a hospital–community liaison, to set up and administer mass immunizations, to support shelters, to make home visits to affected families, to establish a case management system for survivors, or to serve on committees responding to terrorist acts. Formulating, updating, and following a disaster plan is one of the most effective community-based strategies to minimize injury and mortality from terrorism.

Most community health nurses will not be on the front line of uncovering or immediately responding to terrorist activities, but their skills will be needed with groups, families, or individuals who experience a terrorist-related event. Some of the activities listed earlier in this chapter to help people deal with the aftermath of a disaster would also be appropriate if terrorism is the cause of the disaster. In addition, community health nurses may work with people who need help coping or who want to do something to help. After experiencing a traumatic event such as a terrorist attack, people do not know how to cope. We are warned to expect more attacks. We are told to be vigilant. The terror we are fighting is often our own. This is a new experience for most people, and assistance from the community health nurse can help them cope effectively. The following 10 tips were gathered from experts in many fields by Foley (2002) and are commonsense approaches to fighting anxiety:

- *Be a little afraid.* A certain level of fear is healthy if you learn to use it as positive energy. Use your pinch of anxiety to be more vigilant about your safety and that of your family, especially when you travel, and in taking care of your health.
- *Keep a courage journal.* Fear immobilizes, and courage takes action. Every time you take action, you are getting past fear. Even small steps are an opportunity to build more courage. Every time you take a courageous step—getting on a plane, opening your mail—write it down.
- *Reassure your children.* In the act of reassuring your children, you will reassure yourself.
- *Hang out with children.* Do things with your children—most young people carry a charge of positive energy that is infectious. If you do not have young children, volunteer at a school or read to children at a nearby day care center.
- *Cook something hearty, healthy, and large, and invite lots of people in to eat it.* The process of cooking is good for the soul. The aromas are good for the soul. And the chopping and dicing make you feel that you are doing something useful and concrete.
- *Give kindness to others.* We all need each other. Make a point of chatting with the woman at the checkout counter or letting a pedestrian cross the street when you are driving. Wave hello to strangers. You will be amazed how much it is true that in giving, we receive.
- *Get spiritual.* Reach out and participate in your faith community or get involved in one, if so inclined. Believing in a power greater than yourself can be comforting.
- *Laugh.* Laughter is the best medicine for fear. Spend evenings in good company—group laughter is better than laughing alone.
- *Get back to nature.* Spending interactive time with nature is a remedy for just about any soul sickness. Go to the park, take a walk, or work in your garden.
- *Find reasons to believe the sky is not falling.* All the unpleasant facts and figures get our "anxiety juices" flowing. Seek out positive people, and read literature that encourages positive thinking. Do not feed the "dark side." Turn off the news and opt for a funny movie or an inspirational story.

Community health nurses can make major differences in grassroots efforts to bring about change, but on a day-to-day basis, the little things they say and do with peers and clients can make just as big a difference.

Current and Future Opportunities

There are many ways in which nurses, especially nursing students, can prepare themselves both personally and professionally for emergency events in their own communities. Various governmental and educational programs have been developed to provide free online training covering a broad range of topics. A summary of some of those training opportunities is provided in Display 17.6. For the novice nurse, or nursing student, an important issue is your role, if any, in your local response plan. Many schools of nursing have now begun to formal ize their emergency preparedness plans in coordination with local hospitals, public health departments, or faith institutions. Take some time to discuss with your faculty what role you have in the event of a local emergency. If no organized plan exists, then perhaps you can work with the nursing faculty or your local student nurses association to prepare one. Knowing your role in an emergency will give you the peace of mind of knowing where you should go and what you are expected to do. Doing a little extra work by completing some of the online courses listed will help you to feel more involved and less fearful if the unimaginable were to happen. FEMA offers four particular courses within the Incident Command System (ICS 100, ICS 200, IS 700, & IS 800B); these are recommended for all health care personnel. Students who are also employed at local hospitals as interns or salaried employees should find out what role they have in the hospital's emergency plan. Finally, make sure you have a family plan to reconnect with and care for children, spouses, and parents.

Increasingly, communities are conducting emergency preparedness exercises (e.g., mass-casualty exercises and tabletop exercises; see Display 17.9) in response to the need to prepare local resources to coordinate emergency response efforts for maximum effectiveness (Center for Public Health Preparedness, 2007). As a student, you may be asked to participate in one of these exercises as a "victim." Take the opportunity. The knowledge you gain from this experience will enhance your understanding of the process, and you may be able to help identify

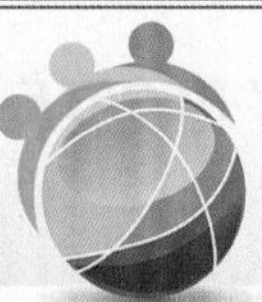

DISPLAY 17.9 WHAT IS A TABLETOP EXERCISE?

A tabletop exercise is a drill typically used by emergency planners and responders. It is designed to allow personnel to gather in a semiformal setting, so that they can participate in open discussions regarding their role in the event of an emergency situation. Participants typically assume their own role, but may be required to assume other key positions. A simulated disaster/emergency event is provided, called the *scenario*. This type of drill

- Does not require complete plans and procedures
- Allows for practice in coordinated emergency problem solving
- Permits discussion of the decisions reached
- Prepares personnel for larger, more costly exercises (i.e., mass-casualty exercises)

Adapted from Placer County Department of Health and Human Services (2005). *Table Top Exercises: What are they? Why do we have them?* Auburn, CA.

gaps in services or areas in need of improvement. With your expertise in nursing, you are a much greater asset to the exercise than untrained individuals. You may be asked to have **moulage** applied to simulate injuries, and you will likely be given a brief description of your trauma (see Display 17.10). Your assigned health problem may be emotional and not physical, allowing you

DISPLAY 17.10 WHAT IS MOULAGE?

Pronounced *mü-läzh*, the term *moulage* comes from the French word *mouler*, which means "to mold." In emergency preparedness training, moulage refers to the art of applying mock injuries for use in mass-casualty exercises. These injuries can be very simple or more complex, depending on available resources and the skills of the person applying the moulage. The use of moulage typically provides a more realistic experience for personnel participating in mass-casualty exercises.

Of the many online resources for information regarding equipment needed and how-to advice, one such Web site is Community Emergency Response Team (CERT) Los Angeles–*Moulage Information* at http://www.cert-la.com/education/moulage.htm.

to utilize your understanding of behavioral health issues and crisis intervention. Whatever your capacity, the experience will provide as close to a realistic event as possible. Just as immunizations help fight against infections, participating in an emergency preparedness drill can build your tolerance for responding appropriately in a real event.

Many organizations, both private and governmental, are seeking volunteers. As a student, you have more limited options; however, two major opportunities are available to you. Both require initial and ongoing training, but if you wish to become more active in emergency preparedness volunteer efforts, the American Red Cross and your local Medical Reserve Corps are two options. You can continue your relationship with these organizations after you receive your nursing license, and your role with them will likely evolve.

With your registered nurse license in hand, many more options are open to you. Each state is developing plans for a database of licensed health care providers who may be willing to volunteer in the event of local, state, or national emergencies. The exact criteria being developed for registration by each state may vary slightly, but as a licensed health care professional you may add your name to the registry along with your specialty training and contact information. Registration does not obligate you to any service; you agree only to be contacted if the need arises. The guidelines for these state-run databases were generated by the U.S. Department of Health and Human Services and can be reviewed in the document *Emergency Systems for Advance Registration of Volunteer Health Professionals* (ESAR-VHP) (USDHHS, 2011). The professional volunteer registry in Wisconsin is named WEAVR (*Wisconsin Emergency Assistance Volunteer Registry*). Using similar guidelines, California launched its version of the registry (*Disaster Healthcare Volunteers*). Mississippi has the *Volunteers in Preparedness Registry* (VIPR), and Arkansas nurses can register with the *Arkansas Volunteer Registry*. Check with your state's office of emergency preparedness and response for the link to your particular registry or information on availability.

As you progress in your career, many other high-intensity efforts are available for your involvement. At both the national and state level are Disaster Medical Assistance Teams (DMAT), groups of highly trained health professionals who can rapidly respond to emergencies within a state or nationally. The DMATs operate as part of the National Disaster Medical System (NDMS). Each DMAT has a sponsoring organization (i.e., major medical center, public health agency, non-profit organization). Check to see if your organization has sponsored a DMAT; if so, you might want to interview one of the members to learn more about his training and experiences.

For those assuming roles in public health nursing, competencies formulated by Gebbie and Qureshi (2002, 2006) provide a sound basis for practice. The work of Gebbie and Qureshi was included in the 2007 position paper *The Role of Public Health Nurses in Emergency Preparedness and Response* (Jakeway, LaRosa, Cary,

& Schoenfisch, 2008). The specific competencies can serve as an emergency preparedness guide for students and practicing public health nurses. They include the following:

1. Describe the public health role in responding to a range of likely emergencies
2. Describe the agency's chain of command in emergency response
3. Identify and locate the agency's emergency response plan
4. Describe one's functional roles and responsibilities in emergency response and demonstrate those roles in regular drills
5. Demonstrate the correct use of equipment (including personal protective equipment) and the skills required in emergency response during regular drills
6. Demonstrate the correct use of all equipment used for emergency communication
7. Describe communication role(s) in emergency response
8. Identify the limits of one's own knowledge, skills, and authority, and identify key system resources for matters that exceed these limits
9. Apply creative problem-solving skills and flexible thinking to unusual challenges within one's functional responsibilities, and evaluate the effectiveness of all actions taken
10. Recognize deviations from the norm that might indicate an emergency and describe appropriate action
11. Participate in continuing education to maintain up-to-date knowledge in areas relevant to emergency response
12. Participate in planning, exercising, and evaluating drills

Many options are available to you as both a student and a practicing nurse. What is important is that you are prepared. Assuring that you understand the role you may assume in the event of a local disaster or emergency situation is critical to your own welfare as well as to your community. You decide your level of participation, but resources are available for you to become as prepared as possible.

Healthy People 2020

The past decade of *Healthy People* has been devoted to increasing quality and years of healthy life and to eliminating health disparities (USDHHS, 2000). Formulated in the years before January 2000, many disasters, both natural and man-made, had yet to occur. The United States had not yet faced the national failures in the response to the hurricanes Katrina and Rita. We would also learn 18 months after the publication of *Healthy People 2010* that our nation was not immune from acts of terrorism. The objectives of *Healthy People 2020* directly address issues of emergency preparedness and response under the new topic of *Preparedness*. Additional topics also include preparedness activities, such as the objectives for Public Health Infrastructure. In the ensuing years, many of these objectives will help focus public's attention on health care during a disaster. The goal of the new topics and objectives are to improve the "Nation's ability to prevent, prepare for, respond to, and recover from a major health incident" (see Display 17.11). Those specific objectives provide the support needed to enhance public health surveillance activities, laboratories, training, development of professional competencies, and performance standards for public health organizations (USDHHS, 2010).

DISPLAY 17.11 *HEALTHY PEOPLE 2020*

PREP-1 (Developmental) Reduce the time necessary to issue official information to the public about a public health emergency

No current data are available, but CDC is listed as a potential data source.

PREP-2 Reduce the time necessary to activate designated personnel in response to a public health emergency

Baseline indicates that 66 minutes were needed for personnel to report to duty in 2009.

PREP-3 Increase the proportion of Laboratory Response Network (LRN) laboratories that meet proficiency standards

PREP 3.1 (Developmental) Proportion of LRN biological laboratories that meet proficiency standards for Category A and B threat agents

PREP 3.2 Proportion of LRN chemical laboratories that meet proficiency standards for chemical threat agents

PREP-4 Reduce the time for state public health agencies to establish after action reports and improvement plans following responses to public health emergencies and exercises

Baseline indicates that it took state public health agencies 46 days to establish after action improvement plans in response to a public health emergency in 2009.

PHI-11 Increase the proportion of tribal and state public health agencies that provide or assure comprehensive laboratory services to support essential public health service

PHI-11.8 response—only 66% of public health agencies provided comprehensive services for emergency response in 2008.

SUMMARY

A disaster is any event that causes a level of destruction that exceeds the abilities of the affected community to respond without assistance. Disasters may be caused by natural or man-made/technologic events and may be classified as multiple-casualty incidents or mass-casualty incidents.

The scope of a disaster is its range of effect, and its intensity is the level of destruction it causes. Persons impacted by disasters include those directly impacted (those injured or killed) and indirectly impacted (the loved ones of directly impacted). Displaced persons are those who are forced to flee their homes because of the disaster, and refugees are those who are forced to leave their homelands, usually in response to war or political persecution.

Host factors that contribute to the likelihood of experiencing a disaster include age, general health, mobility, psychological factors, and socioeconomic factors. The disaster agent is the fire, flood, bomb, or other cause. Environmental factors are those that could potentially contribute to or mitigate a disaster.

In developing strategies to address the problem of disasters, it is helpful for the community health nurse to consider each of the four phases of disaster management: prevention, preparedness, response, and recovery.

Primary prevention of disasters means keeping the disaster from ever happening by taking actions to eliminate the possibility of its occurrence. Secondary prevention focuses on earliest possible detection and treatment. Tertiary prevention involves reducing the amount and degree of disability or damage resulting from the disaster.

In addition to assessing for preparedness, an effective disaster plan establishes a clear chain of authority, develops lines of communication, and delineates routes and modes of transport. Plans for mobilizing, warning, and evacuating people are also critical elements of the disaster plan. At the disaster site, police, firefighters, nurses, and other relief workers develop a coordinated response to rescue survivors from further injury, triage survivors by seriousness of injury, and treat survivors on-site and in local hospitals. Care and transport of dead bodies must also be managed, as well as support for the loved ones of the injured, dead, or missing. Long-term support includes both financial assistance and physical and emotional rehabilitation.

In addition to the physical injuries resulting from disasters, people also suffer psychological trauma that can affect them for life. The importance of prevention, early crisis intervention, and ongoing treatment for those in need is evident. The community health nurse plays a key role in assessing individuals for symptoms of psychological trauma and intervening to prevent long-term consequences. Self-care, including stress education for all relief workers after a disaster, helps to lower anxiety and put the situation into perspective. CISD provides relief workers with a mechanism for emotional reconciliation and healing.

Terrorism is the unlawful use of force or violence against persons or property to intimidate or coerce a government or civilian population in the furtherance of political or social objectives. Terrorism may be nuclear, biologic, or chemical and may involve the use of nerve agents and explosive devices. The community health nurse should be alert to signs of possible terrorist activity and prepared to address the secondary or tertiary effects of such attacks. Preparation includes knowledge of the effects of specific biologic or chemical agents and how to help people cope with the terror they personally feel.

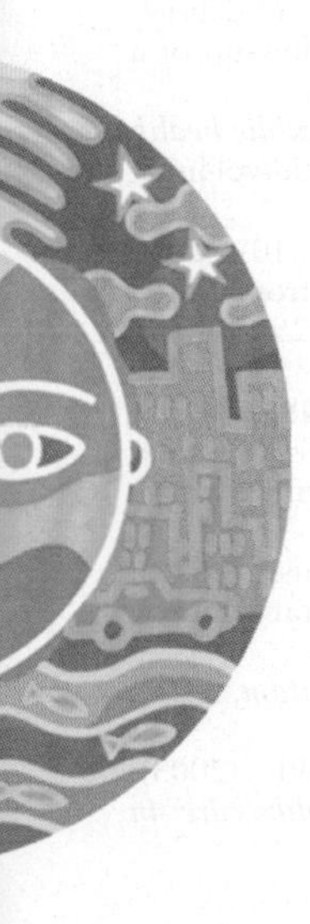

Many opportunities are available for both student nurses and experienced community health nurses to become involved in emergency preparedness and response efforts. Agencies such as the American Red Cross and the Medical Reserve Corps are options available to students and at a higher level of involvement, once licensed. Natural and man-made disasters are a too frequent occurrence. It is the obligation of all nurses to be involved in emergency preparedness and to seek training that will enable them to provide the best possible service if the unthinkable happens. With the development of *Healthy People 2020*, ongoing efforts to help communities prepare for disasters and emergencies will require more nurses willing and able to respond to a call for action.

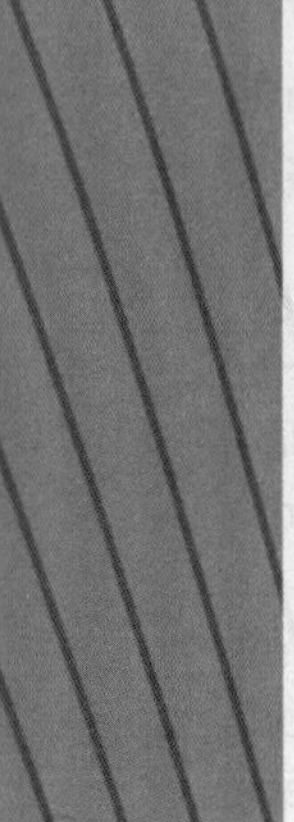

ACTIVITIES TO PROMOTE **CRITICAL THINKING**

1. Think about your own community and its residents. What are some host factors that might increase its risk of experiencing a disaster? What environmental factors might be significant? In each case, identify the likely agent. What interventions could be included in a disaster plan to reduce these risk factors?
2. The nightly news on TV shows that at least 200 people have been injured in an explosion in a neighboring community. At the disaster site, survivors are still being recovered from the wreckage, and local hospitals are overwhelmed with patients who have fractures, lacerations, and burns. You want to offer your assistance as a registered nurse. How should you go about volunteering your services?
3. Access one or more of the Internet sites listed in this chapter. Report on the change in statistics for disasters or terrorism since the year 2008. Have rates increased or decreased? What factors might be involved in this change?

REFERENCES

American Psychiatric Association. (2000). *Diagnostic and statistical manual of mental disorders*, 4th ed. [Text revision]. Washington, DC: Author.

American Red Cross. (2011). *American Red Cross guide to services*. Retrieved from http://www.redcross.org/www-files/Documents/GovernmentRelations/GuideToServices.pdf

Bernett, B. C. (2006). *U.S. biodefense and homeland security: Toward detection and attribution*. Unpublished master's thesis. Naval Postgraduate School, Monterey, California.

Bonanno, G. A., Galea, S., Bucciarelli, A., Vlahov, D., et al. (2007). What predicts psychological resilience after disaster? The role of demographics, resources, and life stress. *Journal of Consulting and Clinical Psychology, 75*, 671–682. Doi: 10.103710022 006X.75.5.671

Carbine, D. J. (1961). *Personal notes*. National Archives.

Center for Public Health Preparedness. (2007). *Conducting a BT-Table Top: A "how-to" guide. Decatur, GA: DeKalb County Board of Health*. Available from NACCHO (toolbox) website, http://www.naccho.org/toolbox/

Centers for Disease Control and Prevention. (2009). *What you should know about a smallpox outbreak*. Retrieved from http://www.bt.cdc.gov/agent/smallpox/basics/outbreak.asp

Department of Homeland Security. (2006). *Department of Homeland Security. Freedom of Information Act. Operational review and improvement plan*. Retrieved from http://www.dhs.gov/xlibrary/assets/foia/privacy_foia_improvement-plan_r.pdf

Department of Homeland Security. (2008). *National Response Framework*. Retrieved from http://www.fema.gov/pdf/emergency/nrf/nrf-core.pdf

Department of Homeland Security. (2011). *Creation of the Department of Homeland Security*. Retrieved from http://www.dhs.gov/xabout/history/gc_1297963906741.shtm

DiVitto, S. (2002). Giving hope, she found hope. *Reflections on Nursing Leadership, 28*(3), 21.

Evans, R. G., Crutcher, J. M., Shadel, B., et al. (2002). Terrorism from a public health perspective. *American Journal of the Medical Sciences, 323*, 291–298.

Federal Bureau of Investigation. (2008). *Anthrax investigation: Closing a chapter*. Retrieved from http://www.fbi.gov/page2/august08/amerithrax080608a.html

Federal Emergency Management Agency. (2008). *National incident management system*. Retrieved from http://www.fema.gov/emergency/nims/

Foley, D. (2002). Fight terror: Your own. *Prevention, 54*(2), 126–133, 174–176.

Gebbie, K. M., & Qureshi, K. (2002). Emergency and disaster preparedness: Core competencies for nurses. *American Journal of Nursing, 102*(1), 46–52.

Gebbie, K. M., & Qureshi, K. (2006). A historical challenge: Nurses and emergencies. *Online Journal of Issues in Nursing, 11*(3), 6.

George Washington University Institute for Crisis, Disaster, and Risk Management. (2011). *Disaster management in the 21st century*. Retrieved from http://www.seas.gwu.edu/~emse232/emse232book3

Henderson, D. A. (2010). *Smallpox: The death of a disease*. Amherst, NY: Prometheus Books.

Human Rights Watch. (2008). *Q & A: Crisis in Darfur*. Retrieved from http://hrw.org/english/docs/2004/05/05/darfur8536.htm

Infoplease. (2008). *2007 disasters*. Boston, MA: Pearson Education. Retrieved from http://www.infoplease.com/ipa/A0934966.html

Infoplease. (2009). *2008 disasters*. Boston, MA: Pearson Education. Retrieved from http://www.infoplease.com/ipa/A0001437.html.

International Charter. (2008). *Charter activations*. Retrieved from http://www.disasterscharter.org/

Iraqi Body Count. (2011). Retrieved from http://www.iraqbodycount.org/database/

Jakeway, C. C., LaRosa, G., Cary, A., Schoenfisch, S., et al. (2008). The role of public health nurses in emergency preparedness and response: A position paper of the Association of State and Territorial Directors of Nursing. *Public Health Nursing, 25*, 353–361. Doi: 10.1111/j.1525-1446.2008.00716.x

Khan, A. S., Swerdlow, D. L., & Juranek, D. D. (2001). Precautions against biological and chemical terrorism directed at food and water supplies. *Public Health Reports, 116*, 3–14.

Kirkpatrick, D. V., & Bryan, M. (2007). Hurricane emergency planning by home health providers serving the poor. *Journal of Health Care for the Poor and Underserved, 18*, 299–314.

Littleton, H., Axsom, D., & Grills-Taquechel, A. E. (2009). Adjustment following the mass shooting at Virginia Tech: The roles of resource loss and gain. *Psychological Trauma: Theory, Research, Practice, and Policy, 1*, 206–219.

Mayou, R., Ehlers, A., & Hobbs, M. (2003). Psychological debriefing for road traffic accident victims: Three-year follow-up of a randomized controlled trial. *FOCUS, 1*(3), 307–312.

McDade, J. E., & Franze, D. (1998). *Bioterrorism as a public health threat*. Retrieved from http://www.cdc.gov/ncidod/eid/vol4no3/mcdade.htm

National Commission on Children and Disasters. (2010). *2010 Report to the President and Congress*. Retrieved from http://cybercemetery.unt.edu/archive/nccd/20110427002908/http:/www.childrenanddisasters.acf.hhs.gov/index.html

National Institute of Standards and Technology. (2008). *Federal building and fire safety investigation of the World Trade Center disaster: Answers to frequently asked questions*. Retrieved from http://wtc.nist.gov/pubs/factsheets/faqs_8_2006.htm

Operation Iraq Freedom (OIF) U.S. Casualty Status. (2011). Retrieved from http://www.globalsecurity.org/military/library/news/2011/01/110104-casualty.pdf

Peeke, P. M. (2002). Reclaim your peace of mind. *Prevention, 54*(1), 92–97.

President's New Freedom Commission on Mental Health. (2003). *Achieving the promise: Transforming mental health care in*

America. Final report. Retrieved from http://store.samhsa.gov/product/SMA03-3831

Press Information Bureau, Government of India. (2008). *HM announces measures to enhance security*. Retrieved from http://pib.nic.in/release/release.asp?relid=45446

Secor-Turner, M., & O'Boyle, C. (2006). Nurses and emergency disasters: What is known. *American Journal of Infection Control, 34*, 414–420.

Sijbrandij, M., Oiff, M., Reitsma, J., Carlier, I. V., Gersons, B. P., et al. (2006). Emotional and educational debriefing after psychological trauma: Randomized controlled trial. *The British Journal of Psychiatry*, 189, 150–155.

Stuart, G., & Laraia, M. (2005). *Principles and practice of psychiatric nursing* (8th ed.). St. Louis, MO: Elsevier-Mosby.

Transportation and Safety Administration. (2011). *Advanced imaging technology*. Retrieved from http://www.tsa.gov/approach/tech/ait/index.shtm

United Nations Inter-Agency Standing Committee. (2008). *Civil-military guidelines and references for complex emergencies*. Retrieved from http://ochaonline.un.org/cmcs/guidelines

United Nations Refugee Agency. (2008). *Iraqi crisis fuels rise in asylum seekers in industrialized world*. Retrieved from http://www.unhcr.org/news/NEWS/47de99982.html

U.S. Army Chemical and Biological Defense Command. (1998). *Domestic preparedness program: Hospital provider course*. McLean, VA: Booz-Allen & Hamilton, Inc. and SAIC, Inc.

U.S. Department of Health, Education, and Welfare. (1961). *Handbook for Civil Defense Emergency Planning in Welfare Institutions (Draft)*. Unpublished. National Archives.

U.S. Department of Health and Human Services, Assistant Secretary for Preparedness and Response. (2011). *Emergency systems for advance registration of volunteer health professionals (ESAR-VHP)*. Retrieved from http://www.phe.gov/esarvhp/pages/default.aspx

U.S. Department of Health and Human Services. (2000). *Healthy People 2010: Understanding and improving health* (2nd ed.). Washington, DC: U.S. Government Printing Office.

U.S. Department of Health and Human Services. (2010). *Healthy People 2020: Preparedness*. Retrieved from http://www.healthypeople.gov/hp2020/

U.S. Department of Justice. (2006). *Terrorism 2002–2005*. Retrieved from http://www.fbi.gov/stats-services/publications/terrorism-2002–2005

U.S. Public Health Service, Commissioned Corps. (2008). *About the Commissioned Corps. Disaster response*. Retrieved from http://www.usphs.gov/AboutUs/emergencyResponse.aspx

Varcarolis, E., & Halter, M. J. (2009). *Foundations of psychiatric mental health nursing: A clinical approach* (6th ed.). St. Louis, MO: Elsevier-Mosby.

Veenema, T. G. (2007). *Disaster nursing and emergency preparedness for chemical, biological, and radiological terrorism and other hazards* (2nd ed.). New York, NY: Springer Publishing Company.

Washington Post. (2008). *U.S. Navy ends bid to ferry storm relief into Burma*. Retrieved from http://www.washingtonpost.com/wp-dyn/content/article/2008/06/04/AR2008060400978.html

Yergler, M. (2002). Nerve gas attack. *The American Journal of Nursing, 102*(7), 57–60.

UNIT 5

THE FAMILY AS CLIENT

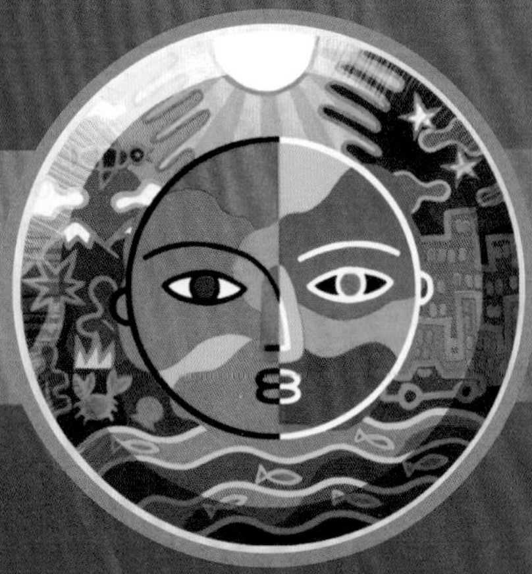

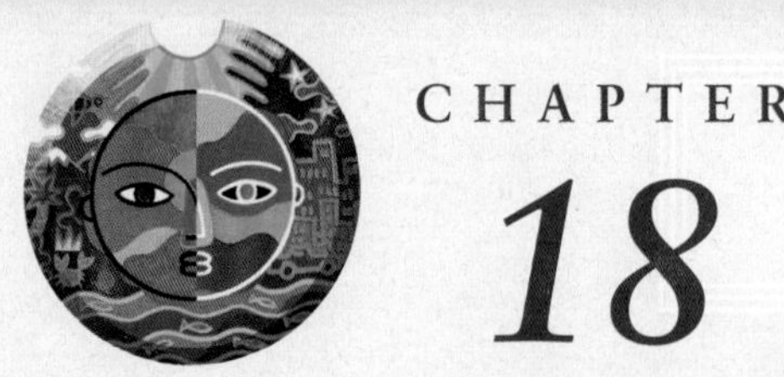

CHAPTER

18

Theoretical Basis for Promoting Family Health

"Call it a clan, call it a network, call it a tribe, call it a family. Whatever you call it, whoever you are, you need one."

—Jane Howard, 'Families'

KEY TERMS

Energy exchange
Family
Family culture
Family functions
Family health
Family life cycle
Family structures
Family system boundaries
Foster families
Gay and lesbian families
Homeless families
Kin-network
Roles

LEARNING OBJECTIVES

Upon mastery of this chapter, you should be able to:

- Define family health nursing.
- Analyze definitions of family.
- Discuss characteristics all families have in common.
- Identify the stages of the family life cycle and the developmental tasks of a family.
- Discuss how a family's culture influences its values, behaviors, and roles.
- Describe the functions of a family.
- Analyze the role of the community health nurse in promoting the health of the family.

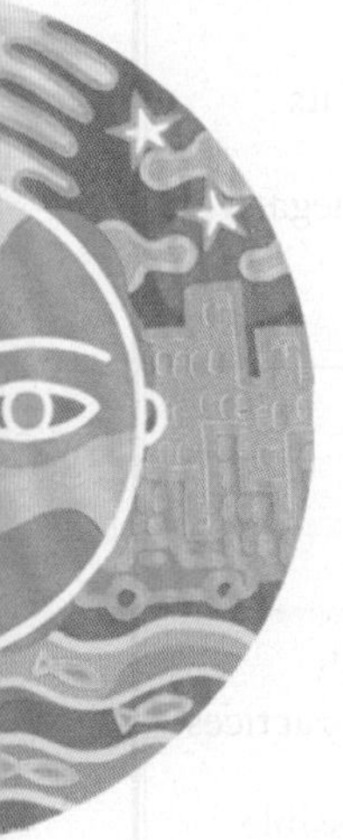

Community health nurses are intimately involved with families. The family plays a critical role in the health of its members. Health habits such as preventative care, diet, exercise, and physical activity are developed in the context of family (Campbell, 2006). Health beliefs, genetic influences, and care of the ill family member all take place within the family environment. The community health nurse is in a unique position to influence and promote family health.

The definition of a family varies by organization, discipline, and individual. The World Health Organization (1976) characterized the family as "the primary social agent in the promotion of health and wellbeing" (p. 17). Many family theorists suggest that a family consists of two or more individuals who share a residence or live near one another; possess some common emotional bond; engage in interrelated social positions, roles, and tasks; and share cultural ties and a sense of affection and belonging (Friedman, Bowden, & Jones, 2003; Kaakinen, Gedaly-Duff, Coehlo, & Hanson, 2010). There are many definitions of family. One definition that seems the most inclusive and yet the simplest is "family is whoever they say it is" (Wright & Bell, 2009, p. 50).

Today's community health nurse needs to understand and work with many types of families, each of which has unique health needs. For example, a young, single mother who is homeless seeks help in caring for her sick infant. A 55-year-old grandfather provides care for his elderly mother, who was recently discharged from the hospital after a stroke. A family from El Salvador needs instruction on the purchase and preparation of food. Why is it important for the community health nurse to understand and respect the unique characteristics, cultures, structures, and functions of each of these families? Do families have characteristics that affect the type of community health nursing intervention? The answer is an unqualified yes. The effectiveness of the community health nurse depends on knowing how to work with all kinds of families.

This chapter explores the nature of families and family health. It draws from various theories to strengthen the student's understanding and appreciation of families as clients. This information will promote the effectiveness of interventions with families at the primary, secondary, and tertiary levels of prevention. See Level of Prevention Pyramid.

FAMILY HEALTH

Kaakinen et al. (2010) define **family health** as a "dynamic changing relative state of wellbeing which includes the biological, psychological, spiritual, sociological, and culture factors of the family systems" (p. 5). Family health is concerned with how well the family functions together as a unit. It involves not only the health of the members and how they relate to other members but also how well they relate to and cope with the community, outside the family. In fact, family health, like individual health, ranges along a continuum from wellness to illness. A family may be at one point on that continuum now and at a much different point 6 months from now. Family health refers to the health status of a given family at a given point in time (Kaakinen et al., 2010).

WHAT IS FAMILY HEALTH NURSING?

There are multiple ways that community health nurses can approach families. Nurses can provide care to individuals within the family or to the family as the client (family as context) or to the family as a system. Some nurses view family nursing as part of other specialties such as community health nursing, maternal child nursing, or mental health nursing. However, some nurses view family nursing as its own distinct specialty, rich with its own body of literature and research. Each of these approaches with families has their own distinct set of beliefs.

Nurses work with individuals within families every day. Most often, the individual is the recipient of care. While assessing the needs of the individual, the nurse needs to include the family in the assessment, as the family is the pivotal provider of care. This may represent family as context. How does the family assist the individual family member? What are their available resources (physically, emotionally, and spiritually)? This approach is frequently used in the care of infants and children (Kaakinen et al., 2010).

Nurses working with families as a system view the family as part of a larger suprasystem that includes many subsystems. The family becomes greater than the sum of all of its parts. A change within the family system not only affects just the individual member but all of the family members (Wright & Leahey, 2009). When visualizing a family as a system, it may help to compare it to a mobile. Think of all the pieces suspended freely by a string. If you pull lightly on one piece, all the pieces move.

Examples of Level of Care

How can this make more sense to us? A nurse receives a referral to visit a new adolescent mother in her home. The baby girl (Rose) is currently 2 weeks old. Her mother (April) is 15 years old. April lives with her mother and three other children (13, 11, and 9 years of age).

LEVELS OF PREVENTION PYRAMID

SITUATION: The family will provide the emotional and material resources necessary for its members' growth and wellbeing.

GOAL: Using the three levels of prevention, negative health conditions are avoided, negative health conditions are promptly diagnosed and treated, and/or the fullest possible potential is restored.

TERTIARY PREVENTION		
Rehabilitation	**Primary Prevention**	
	Health Promotion & Education	*Health Protection*
• After the family suffers a crisis, the members recognize the need for help and accept that help • Families draw on personal resources to rebuild relationships and heal the family unit	• The family continues using resources that enhance the growth and wellbeing of individuals and the family as a unit	• Engage in family strengthening practices to protect the family from possible inhibitors to growth and wellbeing

SECONDARY PREVENTION	
Early Diagnosis	**Prompt Treatment**
• Identification of a family member's personal problems that affect the family as a whole • Early recognition that problems exist in the relationship among or between family members	• The family seeks out the appropriate resources that brings the family to the highest level of wellness possible

PRIMARY PREVENTION	
Health Promotion & Education	**Health Protection**
• Adults are well prepared for the responsibilities of their union • Adults enter the relationship with the personal resources necessary to promote the growth and development of their family unit	• Adults are able to provide for basic needs (housing, nutrition, safety)

On the referral, Rose is listed as the client and the recipient of care. The nurse assesses Rose's feeding, sleeping, and her interaction with her mother. The focus is clearly on the needs of the infant and intervening with any information that may be needed to meet the needs of Rose.

The nurse on the same visit includes information about the family on the assessment from the perspective of the family as context. How would this change the initial approach with the family? Who assists in the care of Rose? Will April remain in school? Who takes care of Rose while she attends school?

The nurse includes information on the assessment looking at the family as a system of care. The nurse would observe Rose and April as members of a family. How are they adjusting to their new roles within the family? How has the birth of Rose changed the family? What is different in the family with the birth of Rose?

DEFINITIONS OF FAMILY

Throughout history, the **family** has been the most basic unit. One of the first steps of the nurse is to define the family. How nurses define a family influences the care that they provide and how they interact with the family. What comes to mind when you hear the word family? How would you define your own family? Is your grandmother a member of your family? Your niece? Your neighbor? A friend? A family pet?

Most of us were raised in families and spent a good portion of our lives within families. Our first experiences with others are from our families. So we come to our nursing practice with ideas about families based on our own experiences. As the nurse begins working with families, it is important to first reflect on our own definition of a family.

The United Nations (UN) defines family "as the basic unit of society" (2011). They recognize that there have

DISPLAY 18.1 DEFINITION OF FAMILY

How do you define family? How would you define your own family? Who do you include as family members? What are your first memories of family?

been many changes in families in the last 50 years due to societal forces such as delayed marriage and childbearing, smaller family size, increases in divorce rates, and migration (UN, 2011). The U.S. Census Bureau (2011) views family as "a householder and one or more other persons living in the same household who are related to the householder by birth, marriage, or adoption. All persons in a household who are related to the householder are regarded as members of his or her family." Kaakinen et al. (2010) defines family as "two or more individuals who depend on one another for emotional, physical, and economical support. The members of the family are self-defined" (p. 6). See Display 18.1 for some questions to ask yourself about your own family.

UNIVERSAL CHARACTERISTICS OF FAMILIES

Several observations can be made about families in general. First, each family is unique, with its own distinct set of strengths. When you approach the door of a house to begin your visit with a family, you cannot be sure of what they will be like. You will have to gather information about the family in order to provide the best nursing care possible.

Families share universal characteristics with every other family. These characteristics provide an important key to understanding each family's uniqueness. Five of the most important family characteristics for community health nurses to recognize are as follows:

1. Every family is a small social system.
2. Every family moves through stages in its life cycle.
3. Every family has its own cultural values and rules.
4. Every family has structure.
5. Every family has certain basic functions.

No matter how many families a nurse may visit over the course of a year, each one will have universal features; it is important for community health nurses to know each family's unique set of characteristics and their effects on family health. These five universal characteristics of family life, which provide the framework of this chapter, are based on systems theory, sociology, and family development.

Families as Social Systems

Many Americans fall into the habit of viewing families merely as individuals. This may be caused partly by the strong cultural emphasis on individualism. This error also occurs because families are often encountered through the individual members. When a community health nurse sits in a living room talking with a young mother about her new infant, it is difficult to keep in mind that all the other family members are present by way of their influence. Systems theory offers some insights about how families operate as social systems. Knowing the attributes of living systems or open systems can help strengthen understanding of family structure and function. There are five attributes of open systems that help explain how families function: (1) families are interdependent, (2) families maintain boundaries, (3) families exchange energy with their environments, (4) families are adaptive, and (5) families are goal oriented.

Interdependence among Members

All the members of a family are interdependent; each member's actions affect the other members, and what affects the family system affects each family member. For example, consider the changes a father might make to reduce his risk of coronary heart disease. If he cuts back on working overtime, the family's income will be reduced. If he begins to eat different foods, food preparation and eating patterns in the family will be altered. If he starts a new exercise program three evenings a week, this may upset other family routines. Even his ability to carry out his usual roles as husband and father may be affected if, for instance, he has less time to help his children with their homework or share household chores with his wife.

Family Boundaries

Families as systems set and maintain boundaries that can include outside influences (permeable) or not (limiting) (Wright & Leahey, 2009). These boundaries result from shared experiences and expectations and link family members together in a bond that excludes the rest of the world. Also a greater concentration of energy exists within the family than between the family and its external environment, thereby creating a **family system boundary.**

Energy Exchange

Family boundaries are semipermeable; although they protect and preserve the family unit, they also allow selective linkage with the outside world. To function adequately as open systems, families exchange materials or information with their environment (Friedman et al., 2003). This process is called **energy exchange.** This exchange promotes a healthy ecologic balance between the family system and the environment that is its immediate community. See Display 18.2.

Adaptive Behavior

Families are adaptive, equilibrium-seeking systems. Families never stay the same. They shift and change in response to internal and external forces. The family composition changes as new members are added.

> **DISPLAY 18.2 THINK OF YOUR OWN FAMILY**
>
> How do you help your family? What kind of tasks do you do to maintain your family's equilibrium? Do you care for younger siblings? Clean? Cook? Give money to the family?

Roles and relationships change as members advance in age and experience. With each new set of pressures, the family shifts and accommodates to regain balance and maintain a normal lifestyle.

Goal-Oriented Behavior

Families as social systems are goal directed. Families exist for a purpose—to establish and maintain a milieu that promotes the development of their members. To fulfill this purpose, a family must perform basic functions, such as providing love, security, identity, a sense of belonging; assisting with preparation for adult roles in society; and maintaining order and control. In addition to these functions, each family member engages in tasks to maintain the family as a viable unit.

Family Life Cycle

Many of the characteristics and defined developmental stages of individual growth also apply to families. For example, families change continuously. Families grow and develop as the individuals within them mature and adapt to changes. A family's composition, set of roles, and interpersonal relationships change with time (Friedman et al., 2003). Families, too, vary with each stage of the family life cycle.

Consider the following example. The Jordan family, a young married couple, concentrated on learning their new roles of husband and wife and building a mutually satisfying marriage. With the birth of their first child, Scott, the family composition and relationships changed and role transitions occurred. The Jordan family consists of not only a husband and wife but also a father, mother, and son; the family added three new roles. Within the next 4 years, two daughters, Lisa and Tiffany, were born. The introduction of each new member not only increased family size but significantly reorganized family living. As Duvall and Miller (1985) pointed out, no two children are born into precisely the same family. The children entered school; Mrs. Jordan went back to work, and soon, Scott was leaving for college. The Jordan family, like every family, is moving through a predictable and sequential pattern of stages known as the **family life cycle**.

Community health nurses who are knowledgeable about this cycle can provide anticipatory guidance to families. For instance, while teaching prenatal care to a pregnant teen, the nurse can help the soon-to-be mother to anticipate the responsibility and costs of raising her child by helping her calculate child care needs that must be met while she finishes school. The nurse can assist the teen in figuring out the monthly costs of breast-feeding versus buying formula; disposable diapers versus cloth or a diaper service; and the clothing, equipment, and medical costs of infant care. When working with middle-aged parents of an adult son who has had a brain injury, the nurse can discuss what arrangements the parents have made for their son's care after they are older and unable to provide care themselves, or after one or both of them die.

Stages of the Family Life Cycle

There are two broad stages in the family life cycle: one of expansion as new members are added and roles and relationships are increased, and one of contraction as family members leave to start lives of their own or age or die. Within this framework of the expanding-contracting family are more specific phases, such as launching of children and retirement of parents. In some families, expansion and contraction are repeated as various members are added, return home with their children and perhaps a partner, or leave home permanently.

Family Developmental Tasks

To progress through the stages of the life cycle, a family must carry out its basic functions and the developmental tasks associated with those functions. Unlike developmental tasks, which are specific to each age level, family developmental tasks are ongoing throughout the life cycle. All families, for instance, must provide for the physical needs of their members at every stage. The manner and degree to which each function is carried out varies depending on how well members accomplish individual developmental tasks and meet the demand of a particular stage. Physical maintenance, for example, affects the parents' ability to accept responsibility and procure the necessary resources to provide food, clothing, and shelter for their children. At early stages, children are dependent on their parents for meeting these needs; at the school, teenage, and launching stages, children may increasingly contribute to home management and family income. The responsibility for these tasks shifts from just the parents to other family members as well.

Some functions require greater emphasis at certain stages. Socialization, for example, consumes much of a family's time during the early years of child development. These same functions and their associated developmental tasks can be further broken down into actions specific to certain stages. While carrying out its function of maintaining controls, a family sets clearly defined limits for children at the preschool stage: "Do not cross the street;" "You may have dessert only after you finish your meal;" or "Bedtime is at 8 o'clock." During the school stage, control activities may center on allocating responsibilities and division of labor within the family: "Feed the dog;" "Clean your room;" or "Take out the trash." When a family reaches the teenage stage, its control function increasingly focuses on the relationships between family members and outsiders. The family may regulate some activities by setting limits: "Be home by midnight." In areas such as moral conduct, controls may involve family values and therefore may be more subtle. A family at this stage must recognize the need for young people to assume increasing responsibility for their own behavior and acknowledge its own diminishing control over members who are exploring independence. Duvall and Miller (1985) described these activities as "stage critical" family developmental tasks that must be completed before moving onto the next stage. Sample community health nursing actions with the family at different stages are presented in Table 18-1.

Table 18.1 Stage-Critical Family Developmental Tasks

Stage of Family Life Cycle	Family Position	Stage-Critical Family Developmental Tasks	Role of the Community Health Nurse
Forming a partnership	Female partner Male partner	Establishing a mutually satisfying relationship	Interact with family where they are at
Childbearing	Partner–mother Partner–father Infant child(ren)	Adjusting to pregnancy and the promise of parenthood Fitting into the kin network Having and adjusting to infants, and encouraging their development Establishing a satisfying home for both parents and infant(s)	Assist them in developing strong relationships
Preschool-age	Partner–mother Partner–father Child, siblings	Adapting to the critical needs and interests of preschool children in stimulating, growth-promoting ways Coping with energy depletion and lack of privacy as parents	Assist in preparing for family expansion through education and anticipatory guidance
School-age	Partner–mother Partner–father Child, siblings	Fitting into the community of school-age families in constructive ways Encouraging children's educational achievement	Encourage time for each other as adults in a relationship separate from parenting role
Teenage	Partner–mother Partner–father Child, siblings	Balancing freedom with responsibility as teenagers mature and emancipate themselves Establishing outside interests and careers as growing parents	Provide anticipatory guidance for the school-aged children as they grow into adulthood
Launching center	Partner–mother–grandmother Partner–father–grandfather Child, sibling, aunt or uncle	Releasing young adults into work, military service, college, marriage, etc., with appropriate rituals and assistance Maintaining a supportive home base	Provide anticipatory guidance for the contracting family as children leave home
Middle-aged parents	Partner–mother–grandmother Partner–father–grandfather	Rebuilding the relationship Maintaining kin ties with older and younger generations	Prepare adults for grandparenting role
Aging family members	Widow or widower Partner–mother–grandmother Partner–father–grandfather	Adjusting to retirement Coping with bereavement and living alone Closing the family home or adapting it to aging	Assist aging adults with emotional and financial security, as they approach retirement Prepare the aging adults with ways to cope with the losses of old age, including changes in space, work, health, status, and loss of friends and family members

Family Culture

Family culture is an acquired knowledge that family members use to interpret their experiences and generate their behaviors that in turn influence their actions. The concept of family culture arises from a significant body of literature in the social and behavioral sciences. Culture explains why families behave as they do (Leininger & McFarland, 2006; Pender, Murdaugh, & Parsons, 2010). Family culture also gives the community health nurse a basis for assessing family health and designing appropriate interventions. Three aspects of family culture deserve special consideration: (1) family members share certain values that affect family behavior, (2) certain roles are prescribed and defined for family members, and (3) a family's culture determines its distribution and use of power.

Shared Values and Their Effect on Behavior

Although families share many broad cultural values drawn from the larger society in which they live, they also develop unique characteristics. Every family has its own set of values and rules for operation that can be considered as family culture (Stewart & Goldfarb, 2007). Some values are explicitly stated: "Family matters must always stay within the family." Such values may give rise to specific operating rules: "Don't tell anyone about our problems."

Like all cultural values, many family values remain outside the conscious awareness of family members. These values, often not verbalized, become powerful determinants of what the family believes, feels, thinks, and does. Family values include those beliefs transmitted by previous generations, religious influences, immediate social pressures, and the larger society. Values become an integral part of a family's life and are difficult to change. A family that values free expression for every member engages comfortably in loud, noisy debates. Another family that values quietness, order, and control does not tolerate its members raising their voices. One family uses birth control based on beliefs about human life and parental responsibility; another family chooses not to use birth control because the members may feel it is against their religion. How a family views education, health care, lifestyle, courtship, marriage, childrearing, sex roles, or any of the myriad of other issues requiring choices depends on the cultural values of the family.

Roles

Roles, the assigned or assumed parts that members play during day-to-day family living, are bestowed and defined by the family (Kaakinen et al., 2010). For instance, the father role may be assigned as an authoritative one that includes establishing rules, judging behavior, and administering punishment for violation of rules. In another family, the father role maybe defined primarily as that of a breadwinner and supporting the mother's decisions in day-to-day childrearing. If there is an absence of a male parent, a grandfather, uncle, friend, or even the mother may take over the father role. Selection of specific roles to be played in any given family varies depending on the family's structure, needs, and patterns of functioning. In a single-parent family, the parent may need to assume the roles of mother, father, and breadwinner, as well as others.

Families distribute among their members all the responsibilities and tasks necessary to conduct family living. The responsibilities of breadwinner and homemaker, with their accompanying tasks, may belong to husband and wife, respectively, or may be shared if both husband and wife have jobs outside the home. Older children may help younger ones with homework or entertain them. This releases parents for other tasks and increases the responsibility of older children.

Family members may play several roles at the same time. This can be taxing. A woman may play the role of wife to her husband, daughter to her mother, and mother to each of her children. The mother role may involve taking on several additional roles and responsibilities, and varies with each child's needs. Parents may care for their children and also have some responsibility for aging parents. This has been recently termed the "sandwich generation.". A single parent often takes on the role of both father and mother but may distribute responsibilities and tasks more widely. A grandmother or a child may assume responsibility for some chores and thereby relieve some of the demands on the single parent. Among families, there is great variation in expectations for each role and in the degree of flexibility in divisions of roles. An example may be specific tasks given to girls versus boys within the family. Girls may be given childcare or kitchen responsibilities and boys given yard tasks. Confusion and conflict can develop unless roles are clarified.

Other roles of family may extend beyond the immediate family. There may be extended family members nearby who interact with the family on a regular basis or only on special occasions like birthdays. If both parents are employed, they may have an expansive network of folks within the neighborhood. Friendships are often made with the parents of children's friends, particularly if the children participate in the same activities. Many families enjoy the fellowship of organized religious or cultural groups. This fellowship can be a source of support or comfort, as well as an additional role function for the family members. Family members can also participate in roles outside the family. These may involve local or regional politics, community improvement, volunteerism for nonprofit groups, or other groups outside the home that the community may offer. These diverse role relationships should enrich and energize the participants. However, many people become overcommitted, creating an imbalance of role responsibilities that is draining and causes friction and stress. The community health nurse must work with families to achieve a balance of activities that promote family health.

Distribution and Use of Power

Power is the possession of control, authority, or influence over others—assuming patterns in each family. In some families, power is concentrated primarily in one member; in other families, it is distributed on a more egalitarian basis. The traditional patriarchal family, in which the father holds absolute authority over the other members, is rare in American society. However, the pattern of husband as head of the household and dominant member of the family is still frequently seen. The dominant power, whether male or female, holds the majority of the decision-making power, particularly over more important family matters such as employment, finances, and health care. Other areas of decision-making, including choices about vacations, housing, leisure activities, household purchases, and child rearing, may be shared or delegated. With changing societal influences, however, the present trend among American families is toward egalitarian power distribution.

Family Structures

Globally, families—in all varied forms—are the basic social unit. The meaning of family among the Hmong of northern Laos may include hundreds of people who make up a clan. In Mexico, families remain close, are large, and extend into multiple generations. In Germany and Japan, families are small and tend to the needs of their elders at home. In the United States, where families come from many cultural groups, many variations coexist within communities.

For many people in the United States, the term family used to evoke a picture of a husband, wife, and children living under one roof, with the man as breadwinner and the woman as homemaker. In the past, this nuclear family was often seen as the norm for everyone. Changes in social values and cultural lifestyles (i.e., women working outside the home) combined with acceptance of alternative lifestyles have changed the definition of family. Today, definitions of a family include unmarried adults living together with or without children, single-parent households, divorced couples combining households with children from previous marriages (the blended family), and gay couples with or without children.

It is a privilege to gain entry into a family's home. This is a uniquely private space belonging to the family. The people who are members of this household interact, care for one another, and bond in ways that may never be fully understood by anyone outside the family. Therefore, being granted entrance into this system gives the community health nurse an opportunity to work with the family that few other professionals experience. Each type of household requires recognition and acceptance by community health nurses, who must help families achieve optimal health.

Families come in many shapes and sizes. The varying family structures or compositions comprise the collective characteristics of individuals who make up a family unit (age, gender, and number). McGoldrick, Carter and Garcia-Preto (2011) find changes in family structure related to societal changes such as increased divorce rates, rise in single parent families, high rates of unwed childbearing, two-income households, and an increase in work time, especially for women. **Family structures** fall into two general categories: traditional and contemporary and are discussed later.

Family Functions

Families in every culture throughout history have engaged in similar functions: families have produced children, physically maintained their members, protected their health, encouraged their education or training, given emotional support and acceptance, and provided supportive and nurturing care during illness. Some societies have experimented with separation of these functions, allocating activities such as childcare, socialization, or social control to a larger group. In U.S. society, certain social institutions help perform some aspects of traditional **family functions**. Schools, for example, help socialize children, professionals supervise health care, and religious organizations influence values.

Six functions are typical of American families today and are essential for the maintenance and promotion of family health: (1) providing affection, (2) providing security, (3) instilling identity, (4) promoting affiliation, (5) providing socialization, and (6) establishing controls (Duval & Miller, 1985). See Table 18-2 for a list of tasks associated with these functions.

SOCIAL CLASS

As a community health nurse, it is important to include social class of families you are visiting in your assessment. Social class often shapes a family's access and choices to work, educational, and health care opportunities (McGoldrick et al., 2011). Their overall health is often determined by their class position. "The biggest predictor of one's health is one's wealth" (Unnatural Causes, 2011). How healthy we are and how long we live is often related to our social standing. The neighborhoods families choose to live in and the schools their children attend are often determined by social class. These decisions/choices have lifelong implications and shape the history of families.

TRADITIONAL FAMILIES

Traditional families are those that are likely most familiar to us. They include the nuclear family—husband, wife, and children living together in the same household. In nuclear families, the workload distribution between the two adults can vary. Both adults may work outside the home; one adult may work outside the home, while the other stays at home and assumes primary responsibilities for the household; or partners may alternate, constantly renegotiating work and domestic responsibilities.

According to the U.S. Census Bureau (2011) for the first time, only 48% of American households consist of a married couple. In 2010, 66% of the families with children under 18 years of age lived with two parents (ChildStats.gov, 2011). Children living in two-parent families continues to decrease.

A nuclear dyad family consists of two adults living together who have no children or who have grown

Table 18.2 Family Functions

Functions	Tasks
Providing affection	1. Meeting physical needs (food, shelter, clothing, health care) 2. Provides dependability
Providing security and acceptance	1. Provide need fulfillment 2. Offers a safe retreat
Instilling identity and satisfaction	1. Teaching roles 2. Instilling values and goals
Promoting affiliation	1. To give a sense of belonging 2. Provide a connection to a family
Providing socialization	1. Transmit their culture 2. Learn roles within the family
Establishing controls	1. Maintain order 2. Learn right and wrong 3. Teach division of labor.

From Duval, E. R., & Miller, B. C. (1985). *Marriage and family development.* New York: Harper & Row.

children living outside the home. A single adult family is one in which one adult is living alone by choice or because of separation from a spouse or children or both. Separation may be the result of divorce, death, or distance from children.

Sometimes, in close-knit ethnic communities, families form a **kin-network**, in which several nuclear families live in the same household or near one another and share goods and services. They may own and operate a family business, sharing work and child care responsibilities, income and expenses, and even meals. Variations of this trend are increasing among all groups as children postpone leaving home because of economic conditions or educational plans, or an elderly parent moves into an adult child's home to recover from a recent illness. The number of young adults who continue to live with their parents is on the rise. Nineteen percent of men and 10% of women between the ages of 25 and 34 years continue to live with their parents (U.S. Census Bureau, 2011).

Another variation of the traditional nuclear family is the blended family. In this structure, single parents marry and raise the children from each of the previous relationships together. They may be custodial parents who have the children except during planned visits with the noncustodial parent, or they may share custody, so that the children live in the blended arrangement only part time or possibly live in two separate blended homes. The family may include children from the couple, in addition to the children brought into the relationship.

CONTEMPORARY FAMILIES

The traditional nuclear family has been a fundamental part of our cultural heritage shared by many Americans, and reinforced by religion, education, and other influential social institutions. Variations from this pattern often were treated as deviant and abnormal. Walsh (2012) describes the continued diversity in types of families and foresees the possibilities of normality and healthy functioning in each of these diverse family types. McGoldrick et al. (2011) fosters the importance of putting a positive spin on the families that make up our world. The nurse is in a unique position to assess families in a strength-based model rather than viewing certain families as deviant.

Society has begun to accept contemporary definitions of family.

Divorce

Divorce changes family structures. Half of all marriages now end in divorce (the rate is higher for teen mothers), and the median duration of marriages is approximately 7 years. In the United States, the marriage rate is 6.8 per 1,000 and the divorce rate is 3.4 per 1,000 (Centers for Disease Control and Prevention [CDC], 2011). Seventy percent of divorced individuals remarry (McGoldrick et al., 2011). See Table 18-3.

Adjusting to divorce involves a series of transitions and reorganizations for all family members. For children, it may require coping with a new geographic location and a new school, as well as adjusting to changes in the mental and physical health of family members. In addition to the normal growth and developmental changes, children of divorce may face an absent father or mother, interparental conflict, economic distress, parental adjustment, multiple life stressors, and short-term crises.

Blending

Not all divorced adults stay single. Most remarry or cohabitate with another adult, who may or may not have children. This new couple may have children from their

Table 18.3 When Families Divorce

Phase	Emotional Responses	Transitional Issues
1. Stressor leading to marital differences	Reveal the fact that the marriage has major problems	Accepting the fact that the marriage has major problems
2. Decision to divorce	Accepting the inability to resolve marital differences	Accepting one's own contribution to the failed marriage
3. Planning the dissolution of the family system	Negotiating viable arrangements for all members within the system	Cooperating on custody visitation, and financial issues Informing and dealing with extended family members and friends
4. Separation	Mourning loss of intact family Working on resolving attachment to spouse	Develop coparental arrangements/relationships Restructure living arrangements Adapt to living apart Realign relationship with extended family and friends Begin to rebuild own social network
5. Divorce	Continue working on emotional recovery by overcoming hurt, anger, or guilt	Giving up fantasies of reunion Staying connected with extended families Rebuild and strengthen own social network
6. Postdivorce	Separate feelings about ex-spouse from parenting role Prepare self for possibility of changes in custody as child(ren) get older; be open to their needs Risk developing a new intimate relationship	Make flexible and generous visitation arrangements for child(ren) and noncustodial parent and extended family members Deal with possibilities of changing custody arrangements as child(ren) get older Deal with child(ren)'s reaction to parents establishing relationships with new partners

union, creating an even more complex family. Merged or blended families require considerable adjustment and relearning of roles, tasks, communication patterns, and relationships.

Identifiable phases occur in divorce, remarriage, and the blending of families; each phase has its own emotional transitions and developmental issues. We all come to new relationships with our own history from the past. McGoldrick et al. (2011) describe new relationships postdivorce as having three sets of emotional baggage: "from the family of origin, the first marriage, and the process and aftermath of separation, divorce, or death and the period between marriages" (p. 324).

Because this emerging family pattern has become so prominent in such a short period, it is very possible that the community health nurse is familiar with this pattern or lives in such a family. Nursing skills that are needed when working with divorced or blended families include the ability to listen and be empathetic, as well as a nonjudgmental attitude. The nurse can be a rich resource for the family. Support groups for adults and children are excellent resources and provide invaluable services at a time of emotional instability in the family. Peer support groups for children and adolescents and support from within the schools should be used, if available, or started if they do not exist. The community health nurse can have a significant role in community-wide planning if services are needed but unavailable. See Table 18-4.

Single-Parent Family

One of the most common contemporary family structures is the single-parent family mostly headed by a woman. Sometimes single women choose to adopt or have children without being married. Sometimes pregnancy without marriage creates this family unity. Twenty-three percent of all children live only with their mother and 3% of children live with their father (ChildStats.gov, 2011).

Over time this form of family has become more accepted by society. It is important for community health nurses to view the strengths of single-parent families. Building on their current strengths can be most helpful in terms of meeting the challenges that they may face.

Adolescent Parents

Statistics indicate that single-parent families are being headed increasingly by teenagers, some of whom become pregnant in junior high school. Although the birth rate among teens 15 to 19 years old declined between 2008 and 2009, teen birth rates remain almost nine times higher than those in other developed countries (CDC, 2011). Specific factors related to teen birth rates are poor performance in school, growing up in a single-parent family, having parents with low levels of education, living in poverty, lack of access to contraception, and being sexually active (CDC, 2011).

Table 18.4 Remarriage and Blending Families

Phase	Emotional Responses	Developmental Issues
1. Meeting new people	Allowing for the possibility of developing a new intimate relationship	Dealing with child(ren)'s and ex-family members' reactions to a parent "dating"
2. Entering a new relationship	Completing an "emotional recovery" from past divorce Accepting one's fears about developing a new relationship Working on feeling good about what the future may bring	Recovery from loss of marriage is adequate Discovering what you want from a new relationship Working on openness in a new relationship
3. Planning a new marriage	Accepting one's fears about the ambiguity and complexity of entering a new relationship such as: New roles and responsibilities Boundaries: space, time, and authority Affective issues: guilt, loyalty, conflicts, unresolvable past hurts	Recommitment to marriage and forming a new family unit Dealing with stepchild(ren) as custodial or noncustodial parent Planning for maintenance of coparental relationships with ex-spouses Planning to help child(ren) deal with fears, loyalty conflicts, and memberships in two systems Realignment of relationships with ex-family to include new spouse and child(ren)
4. Remarriage and blending of families	Final resolution of attachment to previous spouse Acceptance of new family unit with different boundaries	Restructuring family boundaries to allow for new spouse of stepparent Realignment of relationships to allow intermingling of systems Expanding relationships to include all new family members Sharing family memories and histories to enrich members' lives

Infants born to teen mothers are at risk for low birth weight, developmental delay, and death before 1 year of age. The infant mortality rate among mothers younger than 15 is twice as high as for women between the ages of 20 and 24 years, and 20% higher among teens between ages 15 and 19 years than from women in their twenties (CDC, 2011). Of all births in 2009 to 15 to 17 year olds, 94% were to unmarried mothers (ChildStats.gov, 2011).

Teen fathers are often left out of the loop for services that communities provide for the teen mother and infant. However, paternal involvement contributes positively to the physical, social, and cognitive development of children. Children with absent fathers are at increased risk for behavioral difficulties and poor academic performance. A father who is emotionally supportive of the mother and provides child care and financial support directly and indirectly affects the well-being of his child.

The implications for the role of the community health nurse are greatest with the adolescent parent population. For example, nurses work with young teens through schools, clinics, or home-visiting programs to ensure healthy pregnancies and teach parenting skills to the parents and grandparents. Nurses can also ensure that the infant receives immunizations and primary care health services and can provide family planning information to the new parents. SmithBattle (2007) suggests that teen mothers respond positively to community health nursing interventions. On a broader scale, community health nurses should collaborate with other professionals to make sure that the community has resources for all levels of prevention, with a focus on primary prevention. Nurses can play a key role in advocating for educational, health, and social policy that would most benefit teen families (SmithBattle, 2007).

Cohabitating Couples

Another form of nontraditional families are couples that form a family alliance outside of a legal marriage. Cohabitating couples may range from young adults living together to an elderly couple sharing their lives outside of marriage to avoid tax penalties or inheritance issues. Cohabitating couples may be heterosexual or gay/lesbian; they may or may not share a sexual relationship. In some instances, these couples have their own biologic or adopted children.

Gay and Lesbian Families

Although the exact number of **gay and lesbian families** is not known, this emerging family type is increasing. It is estimated that there are 600,000 to 4 million children with gay or lesbian parents in the United States (U.S. Census Bureau, 2011).

One of the new topic areas established by *Healthy People 2020* is Lesbian, Gay, Bisexual, and Transgender (LGBT) Health and speaks to the importance of understanding the discrimination and oppression that LGBT families have faced (Display 18.3). Although much progress has been made in accepting people with values and beliefs different from those of the mainstream, pervasive homophobia and heterosexism persist (U.S. Department of Health and Human Services, 2010).

Gay and lesbian families have many of the same fears and concerns regarding parenting that any family may have. In addition, they experience the stress that accompanies being stigmatized by much of a society. Lack of acceptance from their families and communities may have negative implications on their own family. The nurse can become a valued resource for the family. Through education and anticipatory guidance, the nurse can assist the family to successfully navigate the developmental stages of their children as well as the varied issues faced by families. Research has shown that the psychosocial development of the children of gay or lesbian parents is the same as children with heterosexual parents (American Academy of Pediatrics, 2011). Weber (2010) states "a challenge for nurses lies in creating an environment in which the family feels confident, relaxed, and comfortable enough to disclose and discuss their sexual orientation and family constellation" (p. 12).

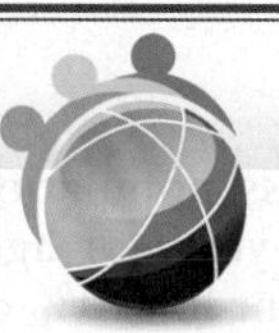

DISPLAY 18.3 *HEALTHY PEOPLE 2020 OBJECTIVES*

Selected Healthy People Goals and Objectives Related to Family Health

Goal: Improve pregnancy planning and spacing, and prevent unintended pregnancy.

Overview: Family planning is one of the 10 great public health achievements of the 20th century. The availability of family planning services allows individuals to achieve desired birth spacing and family size and contributes to improved health outcomes for infants, children, women, and families.

FP-1	Increase the proportion of pregnancies that are intended
FP-5	Reduce the proportion of pregnancies conceived within 18 months of a previous birth
FP-6	Increase the proportion of females or their partners at risk of unintended pregnancy who used contraception at most recent sexual intercourse
FP-8	Reduce pregnancy rates among adolescent females
FP-9	Increase the proportion of adolescents aged 17 years and under who have never had sexual intercourse
FP-12	Increase the proportion of adolescents who received formal instruction on reproductive health topics before they were 18 years old
FP-13	Increase the proportion of adolescents who talked to a parent or guardian about reproductive health topics before they were 18 years old

Goal: Improve the health and wellbeing of women, infants, children, and families.

Overview: Improving the wellbeing of mothers, infants, and children is an important public health goal for the United States. Their wellbeing determines the health of the next generation and can help predict future public health challenges for families, communities, and the health care system. The objectives of the Maternal, Infant, and Child Health topic area address a wide range of conditions, health behaviors, and health system indicators that affect the health, wellness, and quality of life of women, children, and families.

Morbidity and mortality

MICH-1	Reduce the rate of fetal and infant deaths
MICH-8	Reduce low birth weight (LBW) and very low birth weight (VLBW)

Infant care

MICH-21	Increase the proportion of infants who are breast-fed
MICH-22	Increase the proportion of employers that have worksite lactation support programs

Disability and other impairments

MICH-30	Increase the proportion of children, including those with special health care needs, who have access to a medical home
MICH-31	Increase the proportion of children with special health care needs who receive their care in family-centered, comprehensive, coordinated systems

Older Adults

Elderly individuals are the fastest growing segment of the population. In 2008, 38.9 million people in the United States were over the age of 65 years (CDC, 2011). Those over 85 years continue to grow and projections are estimated to increase from 5.7 million in 2008 to 19 million in 2050 (AgingStats.gov, 2011). Most elders live independently, well into their 80s, and maintain healthy contacts with family and friends. Others feel isolated because of chronic health problems that limit mobility, thereby reducing or eliminating the ability to interact or contribute meaningfully in society.

The community health nurse needs to understand the complex dynamics of such situations and offer support and encouragement as family members work through chronic health problems. Often, a nurse serves an entire community of elders in a senior apartment complex, an assisted living center, or a mobile home community, for whom maintaining wellness is the focus. Keeping physically active, eating healthy meals, receiving appropriate medical care and immunizations, and establishing and maintaining social contacts are some of the tasks elders should focus on to stay healthy well into old age; these are some of the areas in which the community health nurse can intervene (Touhy & Jett, 2012).

Foster Families

Many children are removed from their homes of origin because of abuse, violence, or neglect. In most communities, these children are housed with families known as **foster families** (Christenson & McMurty, 2009; Marcellus, 2010). These families take a variety of forms, but all foster families have formal training to accept unrelated children into their homes on a temporary basis, while the children's parents receive the help necessary to reunify the original family. Although this arrangement is not ideal, most foster families provide safe and loving homes for these children in transition. Often foster children have emotional and physical health problems, and they may never have experienced the positive structure that foster families provide. These problems, which can cause stress for everyone involved, are typically ones that the community health nurse can help to solve. See Evidence-Based Practice regarding the impact on children when a parent is unable to care for them due to incarceration.

Homeless Families

Children make up 39% of the homeless population and 42% of the children are under 5 years of age. Families with young children now account for 40% of

EVIDENCE-BASED PRACTICE

Parenting Programs for Incarcerated Parents and Their Children

Recognizing the significant public health implications of parents who are in prison and their children was the impetus for a literature review of programs targeting these vulnerable families. Newman, Fowler, and Cashin (2011) cited the intergenerational nature of criminal activity and delinquency as leading to poor choices made by these children during childhood and into their adult years. The risk that these children will themselves develop poor parenting skills and engage in criminal activity is well documented. Families with one or more parents incarcerated are a growing problem in Australia, the United States, and England, with nearly 2 million children in the United States alone with a parent in prison. The authors reviewed the literature on 11 prison programs designed to deliver some level of parenting support using a variety of methods, both short and longer term. These programs were seen to vary in both delivery methods and evaluation; most significantly few looked at the long-term impact of the programs. Using educationally based approaches covering areas of child development, communication, play skills, child safety, and discipline, they ranged from as few as 5 hours to a program lasting 24 weeks. The potential for improving child–parent relationships through increased contact and facilitation of that contact, were seen as essential to both the child's wellbeing and the recidivism of the parents. The authors stress that addressing this growing public health problem requires assurance that evidence-based approaches are used and evaluation of effectiveness is ongoing.

1. As you will see in Chapter 30, many public health nurses are employed in state and federal prisons; what challenges might they face in providing parenting support to these populations?
2. How could long-term evaluation of these programs be achieved?
3. What challenges from the prison system, the public health care system, and politicians would the public health nurse face in the implementation of a program such as these? What sources of support could be identified?
4. Aside from the literature, what other sources might provide information on parenting support (or lack of) in the prison system?

Newman, C., Fowler, C., & Cashin, A. (2011). The development of a parenting program for incarcerated mothers in Australia: A review of prison-based parenting programs. *Contemporary Nurse, 39*(1), 2–11.

the nations' homeless population and in the course of the year, more than 1.3 million children are homeless (National Law Center on Homelessness and Poverty, 2011). Of the adults in homeless families, 29% are working (National Center on Family Homelessness, 2011).

Typically **homeless families** are young single mothers with two children. Ninety-two percent of these women have experienced physical and/or sexual abuse. They typically have poorer health than other women; one half with a recent history of major depression and one third have a chronic physical condition (National Center on Family Homelessness, 2011).

Homeless families present the community health nurse with unique challenges. Primarily, the family is in crisis often not being able to provide for its most basic needs. Knowing the resources available in the community is an important first step in providing the family with the help to deal with the crisis and assist in the provision of ongoing shelter, food, health, employment, and schooling needs.

IMPLICATIONS FOR COMMUNITY HEALTH NURSES

The variety of family structures raises three important issues for consideration. First, community health nurses can no longer hold to a myth that idealizes the traditional nuclear family. They must be prepared to work with all types of families and accept them as valid. Unless the community health nurse can accept the full array of family lifestyles and address the special needs of each, they may not be able to help the family and may even create additional difficulties.

Second, the structure of an individual's family may change several times over a lifetime. A girl may be born into a nuclear family and then becomes part of a single-parent family when her parents are divorced. As she matures, she may become a single adult living alone, and then become a part of a cohabitating couple. Still later, she may marry and have children in a nuclear family. For the individual, each family form involves changes in roles, interaction patterns, socialization processes, and links with external resources. The community health nurse must learn to address clients' needs throughout these life changes equipping people with the skills needed to deal the inevitability of changing structures.

Finally, each type of family structure creates different issues and problems that, in turn, influence a family's ability to perform basic functions. Black and Lobo (2008) make the distinction with a strength-based orientation such that the nurse is able to focus on capabilities and strengths while assessing deficits. Wright and Leahey (2009) discuss the need for nurses to identify and develop strengths with families in planning nursing care. Variations in structure create variations in family strengths and needs, an important consideration for community health nurses. See Display 18.4.

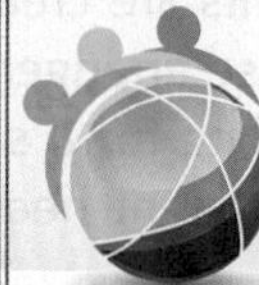

DISPLAY 18.4 QUESTIONS THE NURSE MAY ASK THE FAMILY

1. What are your strengths as a family?
2. If you had to tell me your three most favorite things about your family what would they be?
3. Name one quality about your mother that you really respect. About your partner? Your child?

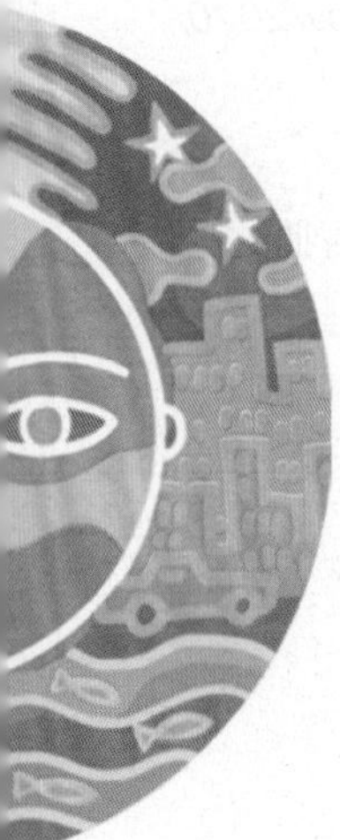

SUMMARY

The family as the unit of service has received increasing emphasis in nursing over the years. Today, family nursing has an important place in nursing practice, particularly in community health nursing. Its significance results from recognizing that the family itself must be a focus of service, that family health and individual health strongly influence each other, and that family health affects community health. A community health nurse's effectiveness in working with families depends on an understanding of family theory and characteristics, in addition to changing family structures.

Every family on the globe is unique; its needs and strengths are different from those of every other family. At the same time, each family is alike because of certain shared universal characteristics. Five of these universal characteristics have particular significance for community health nursing: every family is a small social system, has its own cultural values and rules, has structure, has certain basic functions, and moves through stages in its life cycle.

Family patterns influence the role of the community health nurse. The single adolescent parent needs the community health nurse's knowledge of family developmental theory. More complex

interaction patterns and living arrangements are created by divorce, remarriage, the blending of families, and the unique relationships these arrangements create. Gay and lesbian families with children may also have special needs calling for a sensitive understanding of society's reaction to their family. Understanding families different needs will help the nurse provide appropriate services.

The chapter ends as it begins with several important points to consider when working with families. The nurse begins where the family is and accepts the family's own definition of who their family is and listens to the family's ideas about the direction of visits and time together. The nurse should begin the work assessing the family's strengths, which will begin to build a positive relationship between the nurse and the family. This is the essential starting point in the community health nurse's work.

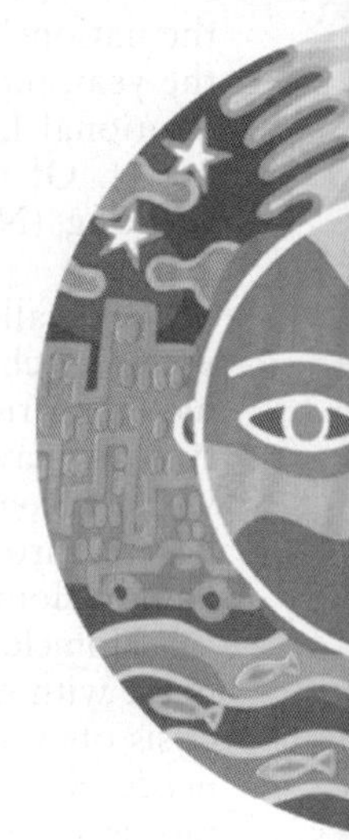

ACTIVITIES TO PROMOTE **CRITICAL THINKING**

1. Get together with a small group of your peers. Ask each of your peers to define family and then compare each of your definitions. How similar or different are each of the definitions? What in each person's own experience may account for the way they look at families?
2. Analyze two families (other than your own) that you know well, one traditional and one contemporary, and answer the following questions:

   If the major breadwinner in this family was unable to work or lost his or her job, how would the family most likely respond immediately and in the long term?

   What developmental stage is this family in and how does that affect their functioning?

   What are the strongest and weakest functions performed by this family?

   How could a nurse intervene in this situation?
3. More gay and lesbian couples are becoming parents. What are some of the needs they have in common with other parents? What would be some of the differences?
4. Talk with members of a blended family and discuss with each member his or her relationships with stepchildren, stepparents, or siblings. What strengths can they identify in their family? How has this helped them adapt to their blended family?
5. Read through the new topic areas of *Healthy People 2020* related to family at *http://healthypeople.gov/2020/about/new2020.aspx*
   - What do the new areas reflect about changes in our society?
   - How do social determinants relate to family?
   - *Healthy People 2020* calls for more research in the areas of LGBT parenting issues throughout the life course. What would you hypothesize potential areas of concern?

REFERENCES

AgingStats.gov: Federal Interagency Forum on Aging-Related Statistics. (2011). *http://www.agingstats.gov/agingstatsdotnet/Main_Site/Data/2010_Documents/Population.aspx*

American Academy of Pediatrics. (2011). Retrieved from http://www.aap.org/

Black, K., & Lobo, M. (2008). A conceptual review of family resilience factors. *Journal of Family Nursing, 14*(1), 33–55. doi: 10.1177/1074840707312237.

Campbell, T. L. (2006). Improving health through family interventions. In D. R. Crane, & E. S. Marshall (Eds.). *Handbook of families & health: Interdisciplinary perspectives* (pp. 379–395). Thousand Oaks, CA: Sage Publications.

Centers for Disease Control and Prevention. (2011). Retrieved from *http://www.cdc.gov*

ChildStats.gov: A forum on child and family statistics. (2011). Retrieved from *http://www.childstats.gov*

Christenson, B. L., & McMurty, J. (2009). A longitudinal evaluation of the preservice training and retention of kinship and nonkinship foster/adoptive families one and a half years after training. *Child Welfare, 88*(4), 5–22.

Duvall, E. M., & Miller, B. (1985). *Marriage and family development* (6th ed.). Philadelphia, PA: Lippincott Williams & Wilkins.

Friedman, M. M., Bowden, V. R., & Jones. E. G. (2003). *Family nursing: Research, theory, and practice* (5th ed.). Upper Saddle River, NJ: Prentice Hall.

Kaakinen, J. R., Gedaly-Duff, V., Coehlo, D. P., & Hanson, S. M. (2010). *Family health care nursing: Theory, practice and research* (4th ed.). Philadelphia, PA: F.A. Davis Company.

Leininger, M. M., & McFarland, M. (2006). *Culture care diversity and universality: A worldwide nursing theory* (2nd ed.). Sudbury, MA: Jones and Bartlett.

Marcellus, L. (2010). Supporting resilience in foster families: A model for program design that supports recruitment, retention, and satisfaction of foster families who care for infants with prenatal substance exposure. *Child Welfare, 89*(1), 7–29.

McGoldrick, M., Carter, B., & Garcia-Preto, N. (2011). *The expanded family life cycle: Individual, family, and social perspectives* (4th ed.). Upper Saddle River, NJ: Prentice Hall.

National Center on Family Homelessness. Retrieved from *http://www.familyhomelessness.org/families.php?p=ts*

National Law Center on Homelessness and Poverty. (2011). Retrieved from *http://www.nlchp.org/*

Pender, N. J., Murdaugh, C. L., & Parsons, M. A. (2010). *Health promotion in nursing practice* (6th ed.). Upper Saddle River, NJ: Prentice Hall.

SmithBattle, L. (2007). Legacies of advantage and disadvantage: The case of teen mothers. *Public Health Nursing, 24*(5), 409–420. doi: 10.1111/j.1525-1446.2007.00651.x

Stewart, P., & Goldfarb, K. P. (2007). Historical trends in the study of diverse families. In B. S. Trask & R. R. Harmon (Eds.). *Cultural diversity and families: Expanding perspectives* (pp. 3–19). Thousand Oaks, CA: Sage Publications.

Touhy, T. A., & Jett, K. (2012). *Ebersole & Hess' toward healthy aging: Human needs and nursing response* (8th ed.). Saint Louis, MO: Elsevier Mosby.

United Nations. (2011). Retrieved from *http://www.un.org/en/*

Unnatural Causes. (2011). Retrieved from *http://www.unnaturalcauses.org*

U.S. Census Bureau. (2011). Retrieved from *http://www.census.gov/*

U.S. Department of Health and Human Services, Office of Disease Prevention and Health Promotion. *Healthy People 2020*. Washington, DC. Retrieved from *http://www.healthypeople.gov/2020/*

Walsh, F. (2012). *Normal family processes: Growing diversity and complexity* (4th ed.). New York, NY: The Guilford Press.

Weber, S. (2010). Nursing care of families with parents who are lesbian, gay, bisexual, or transgender. *Journal of Child & Adolescent Psychiatric Nursing, 23*(1), 11–16. doi: 10.1111/j.1744-6171.2009.00211.x

World Health Organization. (1976). *Statistical indices of family health* (Rep. No. 589). Geneva, Switzerland: WHO Press. Retrieved from *http://whqlibdoc.who.int/trs/WHO_TRS_587.pdf*

Wright, L. M., & Bell, J. M. (2009). *Beliefs and illness: A model for healing*. Calgary, Alberta, Canada: Fourth Floor Press, Inc.

Wright, L. M., & Leahey, M. (2009). *Nurses and families: A guide to family assessment and intervention* (5th ed.). Philadelphia, PA: F. A. Davis.

CHAPTER

19

Working with Families: Applying the Nursing Process

"If the family were a fruit, it would be an orange, a circle of sections, held together but separable—each segment distinct."

—Letty Cottin Pogrebin

KEY TERMS

Conceptual framework
Developmental framework
Eco-map
Family health
Family nursing
Genogram
Interactional framework
Outcome evaluation
Referral
Resource directory
Strengthening
Structural–functional framework

LEARNING OBJECTIVES

Upon mastery of this chapter, you should be able to:

- Describe the components of the nursing process as they apply to enhancing family health.
- Identify the steps in a successful family health intervention.
- Describe useful activities and actions when intervening on family health visits.
- List at least six specific safety measures the community/public health nurse should take when traveling to a home or making a home visit.
- Describe the effect of family health on individual health.
- Describe individual and group characteristics of a healthy family.
- Identify five family health practice guidelines.
- Describe three conceptual frameworks that can be used to assess a family.
- Describe the 12 major assessment categories for families.
- List the five basic principles the community/public health nurse should follow when assessing family health.
- Discuss the two foci of family health visits: education and health promotion.
- Describe the three types of evaluations that are necessary after family health interventions.

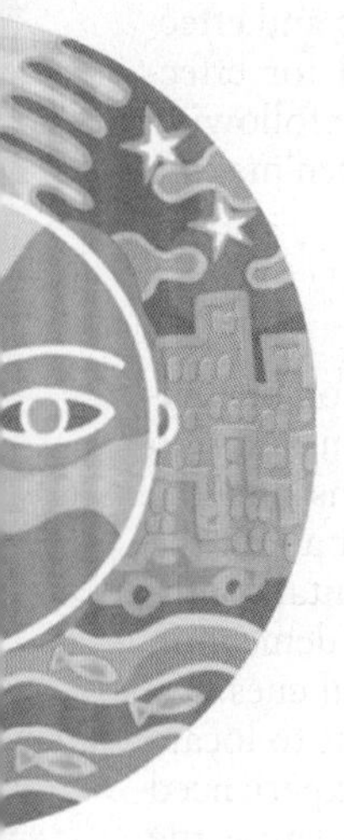

Chapter 18 explored the theoretical basis of family formation and the variety of family structures. Other chapters have stressed that families come in all sizes, consist of members of many ages and biologic relationships, and experience the world filtered through their unique cultures. There are many theoretical approaches and roles to consider when caring for families. This chapter explores the nursing process as it applies to working with families as a unit of service.

Community/public health nurses deliver care to families in their homes, their work settings, classrooms, clinics and outpatient departments, neighborhood centers, and homeless shelters. Although community health nursing emphasizes the family as a unit of service, a gap often exists between family nursing theory, development, and practice. The problem, in part, is derived from a health care system that fosters individual services, often to the exclusion of family. This is evident in many third-party payer and reimbursement policies that impose limits to the kinds of services funded, in public health agencies' tendencies to organize services around individuals, and in government requirements that agencies keep statistics for specific diseases or service categories that reflect individual rather than family or aggregate data.

The family has been the main unit of service in communities for more than a century (Schorr & Kennedy, 1999). It is with the family in mind that the bulk of health care and related services are provided in the community. Immunization programs exist for infants and children. Parks, recreational services, organized team sports, and social centers exist for the physical and emotional wellbeing of families. Pregnant women can attend childbirth education classes and receive medical care from their health care providers. Growing families can access parenting classes and support groups for help with developmental crises and in the management of chronic illness. Senior centers exist for the older adults in families, and myriad social and recreational activities offer senior discounts. What all these clients have in common is they are members of families.

Think about how your family has influenced you. Did family members sway your career choice or where you are attending school? What about your value system, or how you view your health? What about the friendships you've formed? What about the foods you eat; would those choices be different if you had grown up with vegetarian parents versus a parent who took you out every fall to hunt deer?

Just as each family is unique, so too are their homes and communities. Some families live in homes that look very much like yours, where you will feel comfortable almost immediately, whereas others live in places that may not feel so comfortable to you. To a novice community/public health nurse, it can be daunting to enter a small cluttered apartment or a sparsely furnished single room, or a home in disrepair. Families live in mobile homes, in high-rise inner-city apartments, in rural cabins, and on farm labor camps. Each home and neighborhood can bring its own set of unique challenges, as well as strengths, to the families you are visiting.

Family-level problem-solving techniques are needed to deal with important health issues including health promotion, pregnancy and childbirth, acute life-threatening illness, chronic illness, substance abuse, domestic violence, and terminal illness (Friedman, Bowden, & Jones, 2003; Shepherd, 2011; Vanderburg, Wright, Boston, & Zimmerman, 2010). The first step is to develop family assessment skills (Wright & Leahey, 2009). This is foundational to the development of a database on which to formulate nursing diagnosis, an essential step before planning, implementation, and evaluation of services can occur. This chapter focuses on the nursing process: assessing, planning, implementing, and evaluating to enhance family health.

NURSING PROCESS COMPONENTS APPLIED TO FAMILIES AS CLIENTS

Assessing, planning, implementing, and evaluating nursing care are steps used to deliver care to clients in acute care settings and in the extensive clinic system. These same steps are used with families and aggregates in community health settings. The steps do not change, but the context and client focus are different, and external variables that have not been encountered in other contexts must now be considered.

Working With Families in Community Health Settings

Family visits need not be limited to homes. Family members may be visited in school or at work during a lunch break, in a day care or senior center, in a group home, or myriad after-work or after-school and recreational settings. The nurse must be creative in accommodating various family schedules and routines. In general, if a visit is all right with the family, school, or employer, it should be all right with the nurse (see Perspectives: Voices from the Community). Families appreciate the individualized effort and respond more positively when nurses are willing to work with family member schedules.

When making visits in public places, such as worksites or schools, be mindful of confidentiality and respect the family's wishes. A client may agree to your visit during lunch break in a department store on a Tuesday, which is the boss's day off, or after the lunch crowd in a fast-food restaurant disperses and the client can take a break. Seek out a place for the visit where other employees or customers cannot overhear your conversation with the client.

Sometimes, visiting clients where they spend their time during the day helps to enhance family assessment.

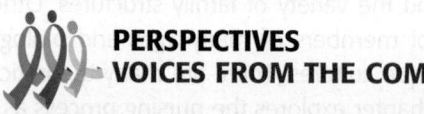

PERSPECTIVES
VOICES FROM THE COMMUNITY

"I couldn't believe it when she [the community health nurse] said she could visit me during my lunch break. I have been so worried about Ben's hearing and with my new work hours I kept missing her—I got her notes she left in the screen door. She actually drove all the way out to my work to tell me about his hearing test at school and the teacher's classroom changes. I can't afford to lose this job—and she came here!"

Beth, 34, Ben's mother

In families with a child in day care or an elderly family member in an adult day care program, your assessment of that individual's ability to manage, participate, and interact in the situation can give insight into problems the family is referring to when you make a home visit. Visiting children during the school day often gives insight into health problems the parents may be concerned about. Such visits can offer the community health nurse an excellent opportunity to consult with the principal, teachers, school nurse, counselor, and school psychologist. The community health nurse may suggest a team meeting of school professionals and the parents, coordinate the meeting, and act as liaison and client advocate during the meeting.

Working With Families Where They Live

Depending on the setting for community health nursing practice, the nurse encounters most clients in their homes and neighborhoods. Some see families in transition, who are living on the streets, in homeless shelters, or with relatives or friends. Regardless of the family's location, the client is the family; the family is the unit of service in family nursing (Kaakinen, Gadaly-Duff, Hanson, & Coehlo, 2009).

The Home Visit

Working in the community and being able to visit families in their homes is a privilege. In this unique setting you are permitted into the most intimate of spaces we, as human beings, have. Our homes are our creations, our private spaces; they hold our personal treasures and our memories. To let a stranger into our home takes a certain amount of trust. To enter a client's family home also takes trust on the part of the nurse. Once the door is shut behind you, the rules change; you are in the client's world where they are the experts, and you are the guest and may feel like a stranger.

Nursing Skills Used During Home Visits

Many skills, in addition to expert nursing skills, are needed when assessing, planning, implementing, and evaluating services in the home to families at a variety of functional levels. Expert interviewing skills and effective communication techniques are essential for effective family intervention (see Chapter 10). The following paragraphs describe special skills required when making home visits.

Acute Observation Skills

The environment is new to you, and observation of environment and client are equally important. In addition to focusing on the family members' concerns and the purpose of the visit, you need to be observant about the neighborhood, travel safety, home environmental conditions, number of household members, client demeanor, and body language, as well as other nonverbal cues.

Travel in new neighborhoods and attempts to locate a family can cause distress to even the most experienced nurse. Often clients are difficult to locate because the house or apartment number is missing. The residence may be situated behind another house, or it may be a basement apartment without a number. Many anomalies in the layout of a building or a neighborhood may make it difficult for the nurse to locate a client. Addresses on referrals may have numbers transposed such as 123 Hickory instead of 132 Hickory. Perhaps there is a North Hickory that is miles away from South Hickory, or there is a Hickory Boulevard, Drive, Road, Street, Court, Lane, or Way. There is always the chance that the address is fictitious, given by a client who, for whatever reason, prefers to remain as anonymous as possible.

Assessment of Home Environmental Conditions

Conditions in the neighborhood and home environments reveal important assessment information that can guide planning and intervention with families. While traveling to and arriving at the family home, you have been gathering information about resources and barriers encountered by the family. This information is used during planning with the family. It is important to remember that neighborhood conditions and even the physical appearance of the apartment or house may contradict the family's values, resources, and goals. They may have little control over the neighborhood or the building they live in, especially if they are renting. For instance, the family may be a young couple with a baby who can afford $475 in rent; the only apartment available to them for that amount is in a deteriorating low-income neighborhood with dilapidated buildings occupied by renters and owned by absentee landlords, who may own several buildings, mainly for profit. The manager, who may not know the landlord and is employed through the owner's management company, handles the property. Yet, when you enter the apartment, you may see a well-furnished, neat, and clean home that is opened to you with pride by the family.

In another situation, you may plan to visit an older couple who lives in their own home in an upscale suburban neighborhood. On approaching the house, however, you barely manage to squeeze through a pathway made in the living room, which is piled ceiling-high with boxes, newspapers, and furniture. This continues throughout the house and even into a back bedroom, where half the bed is covered with papers, books, and a few cats. An older woman is in the bed. The husband moves very slowly, and after showing you in, he leaves the bedroom and heads toward the backyard.

Many environmental clues in each of these situations help the nurse begin an assessment that will lead to a plan to assist each family. Most neighborhoods and homes do not present such extremes. However, if you are unprepared for the extremes, they may overwhelm you, and you may become so distracted that you cannot focus wholly on the family and incorporate these important observations into the plan.

Assessment of Body Language and Other Nonverbal Cues

After you have knocked on the door or rung the doorbell and are in the home (see *Perspectives –: Public Health Nursing Instructor*), or even while greeting the people in the doorway, you are gathering data. Being human, you may form opinions or make judgments about the family from the initial meeting. Know that they are doing the same. Be aware of all household members; acknowledge and greet them. If some are absent, inquire about them. Make this a habit on all visits. Each family member is important and has opinions and health care needs, even if you only see certain members of the family on each visit.

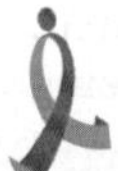

PERSPECTIVES
PUBLIC HEALTH NURSING INSTRUCTOR

How You Knock Helps Families Open The Door

At first this may seem trite, but how do you knock on the door when you visit a family? Do you use the "I don't want to be here and if they don't hear the knock I can quietly leave" type of knock that even Superman can't hear? Or do you knock like, "I'm a bill collector and YOU BETTER open this door!" During this knock, the entire family is leaving through the back door! We suggest a knock that is loud enough to be heard, yet friendly and nonthreatening. If necessary, practice "your knock" until you can create this beneficial combination.

With some families, it is helpful to call toward the door as you knock or ring the bell with, "Mrs. Smith, this is Jenny from the Health Department—remember I was coming by today" or, "Ms. Jiminez, it's the student community health nurse, Terry Guara, and I brought those pamphlets for you" or, "Hello, it's James from the neighborhood clinic, we planned to meet today." Using such a greeting allows the family to know who is at the door and choose to open the door if they want. It will get you into more homes than the "quiet-as-a-mouse" or "bill-collector" knocks.

—*Alice K. PHN*

Be observant of family body language and demeanor. These nonverbal cues provide information that must not be overlooked. Observations such as, "You seem anxious today," or "Did I come at a bad time? You seem distracted," are openings that allow family members to express what is on their minds. If you are not open to body language while making a visit, you may overlook important cues and continue with your agenda, without realizing that the family is distracted by another, more pressing issue.

On a related note, it is important to be aware of your own body language. If you fidget with car keys during the entire visit, noisily chew gum, give minimal eye contact while continuously looking at your paperwork, appear rushed, or refuse to sit on any of the furniture, your behavior with tell the family a great deal about you, including how you feel about being in their home.

PLANNING TO MEET THE HEALTH NEEDS OF FAMILIES DURING HOME VISITS

The greatest barrier to a successful family health visit is lack of planning and preparation. A visit is not successful just because the nurse enters a home or other setting where clients are present. A successful family health visit takes much planning and preparation and requires accurate documentation and follow-up. In addition, safety measures must be followed not only while traveling in the neighborhood, but also in the home.

Components of the Family Health Visit

The structure of family health visits can be divided into four components that follow the nursing process (Display 19.1). Previsit preparation steps (assessment and planning) are necessary to ensure that the actual family health visit (implementation) is complete. The documentation and planning for the next visit (evaluation) concludes the responsibilities for one visit and prepares the nurse for the next action needed.

Previsit Preparation

Community health nurses design a plan for the initial family health visit based on a referral coming into the agency. A **referral** is a request for service from another agency or person. This request is formalized by use of a form or information that the originating agency has transferred to the receiving agency. Referrals may be formal, coming from complementary agencies, or they may be informal, resulting from verbal or telephone referrals from friends or relatives who believe that someone needs help. Referrals are the source of new cases for the agencies, and they need timely responses. Referrals could be from labor and delivery units, requesting service for low-birth-weight babies and teen mothers. They could be from social service agencies, requesting a home assessment for a child being returned to parents after previous removal from the home. A referral could come

DISPLAY 19.1 GUIDELINES FOR MAKING HOME VISITS: 30 STEPS TO SUCCESS

The following guidelines can be followed to evaluate yourself after making a home visit; or it can be a tool used when you are evaluated by another nurse (peer or instructor). Rate yourself using the following scale: 0 = does not apply, 1 = unsatisfactory, 2 = satisfactory.

Rating	
	Assessment
____	1. Studies referral, record, or other available data about the family.
____	2. Gathers community resource information potentially appropriate to the family.
____	3. Obtains appropriate supplies or educational material in anticipation of family needs.
	Planning
____	4. Contacts family to set up an appropriate time for the home visit.
____	5. Ascertains correct address and directions to the family for the home visit.
____	6. Formulates a written plan for nursing intervention with each family member.
____	7. Organizes a chart with forms and charting tools based on the focus of the visit.
____	8. Plans a route to the family's home that is the most direct, being resource efficient.
	Implementation
____	9. Travels the community with safety, locating the family home with ease.
____	10. Knocks on the door loudly enough to be heard and in a friendly manner.
____	11. Introduces self to family members in an appropriate manner.
____	12. Clearly states the reason for the visit.
____	13. Allows a few moments of socialization before beginning the visit.
____	14. Smiles, speaks in a pleasant, friendly tone of voice, and maintains eye contact.
____	15. Uses aseptic technique when providing nursing care.
____	16. Respects the dignity, privacy, safety, and comfort of family members.
____	17. Listens attentively to ascertain what family members are saying or implying.
____	18. Converses with family members during the home visit.
____	19. Communicates accurate and meaningful information to family members.
____	20. Responds to family members in a way that encourages them to continue talking.
____	21. Uses appropriate words of explanation for family member understanding.
____	22. Utilizes opportunities for incidental teaching.
____	23. Commends progress made by individual family members.
____	24. Explains nursing measures before, during, and after each procedure.
____	25. Shares the results of nursing measures with family members when indicated.
____	26. Closes the home visit by summarizing the main points of the visit.
____	27. Makes plans for the next visit, considering family member wishes.
	Evaluation
____	28. Utilizes information gathered on the home visit to plan care for next visit.
____	29. Documents home visit in an appropriate and timely manner.
____	30. Completes a self-evaluation of the home visit.

via a telephone call from a woman in a city 500 miles away, requesting that a nurse check on an elderly relative who lives alone in the community and has recently exhibited slurred speech. Follow-up visits are made to these families based on need and agency protocol.

Nurses must have a physical place to work, with access to a telephone, the internet, and any other supportive resources deemed necessary, such as educational material (pamphlets, brochures, computer, and related Web site addresses to access educational information), charting tools, and other supplies required for home visits. Nurses also need a **resource directory**, which is a published list of resources for the broader community, or a nurse-made directory of resources created over years of working with people in the community. Some agencies issue a nursing bag to their nurses, but if not, many public health nurses become creative and devise their own carryall for supplies. The supplies needed depend on the type of visit; some nurses have several totes for different types of visits. Think about what basic supplies you would need to visit a new mother and her infant, or an elderly man with hypertension.

Once the nurse is prepared, contact with the family is needed. For a home visit, ideally, the referral contains a correct telephone number for the family, a relative, or a neighbor. If the referral or chart does not contain this information, the nurse makes an unannounced visit. During this visit, it is important to get a contact number for the family. When calling for the first time, introduce yourself, explain the reason for the call, and why the family was referred, what the visit consists of, and determine when a visit would be convenient for the family and the nurse. Some people become defensive or suspicious of the nurse's intentions. For example, a new young mother may think, "What did they see me doing wrong with my baby in the hospital?" In this kind of situation, it is very important that the nurse explain that:

- The visit is a service provided by the agency to all mothers.
- The visit is paid for by taxes (or donations) or by the client's health maintenance organization (if applicable), so there is no direct charge to the family.
- Young mothers often have lots of questions about their new babies. Having a nurse come to the home provides an opportunity for the mother to ask questions and for the nurse to show the mother things she may not know about her baby.

The nurse needs to ask explicit directions to where the family is staying. The referral may have a different address, and the family may forget to mention that they are staying elsewhere.

Making the Visit

On locating and meeting the family, the following guidelines for initial contact should be used (Allender, 1998):

- Introduce yourself and explain the value to the family of the nursing services provided by the agency.
- Spend the first few minutes of the visit establishing cordiality and getting acquainted (a mutual discovery or "feeling out" time).
- Use acute observational skills.
- Be sensitive to verbal and nonverbal cues.
- Be adaptable and flexible (you may be planning a prenatal visit, but the woman delivered her baby the day after you made the appointment, and now there is a newborn).
- Use your "sixth sense" as a guide regarding family responses, questions they ask, and your personal safety (trust your feelings).
- Be aware of your own personality—balance talking and listening—and be aware of your nonverbal behaviors.
- Be aware that most clients are not acutely ill and have higher levels of wellness than are generally seen in acute care settings.
- Become acquainted with all family and household members if you are making a home visit.
- Encourage each person to speak for himself.
- Be accepting and listen carefully.
- Help the family focus on issues and move toward the desired goals.
- After the body of the visit is over, review the important points, emphasizing family strengths.
- Plan with the family for the next visit.

The length and primary focus of the visit will vary depending on its purpose. As a general guide, if the visit is shorter than 20 minutes, it probably should be folded into another visit (unless you are offering a piece of very important information, are providing supplies, or have come at the family's request). On the other hand, if the visit exceeds 1 hour, it should be conducted over two visits. Families have routines that are important to them, and taking a large portion of time out of their day may lead to resentment, putting future visits in jeopardy. Similarly, if nothing of value (according to the family) occurs on a visit, family members may not continue to make themselves available for future visits. This becomes a balancing act for the family and the nurse, and it is an area in which using your sixth sense and picking up on nonverbal cues is helpful (Zerwekh, 1997). In addition, home visits are an expensive way to provide nursing services, which are community based. The outcome of better health for family members must be demonstrated in order to support the value of such costly services (see Evidence-Based Practice).

Concluding and Documenting the Visit

After planning for the next visit, saying goodbye to the family members terminates the home visit. This is a good time to put away the paperwork, materials, and supplies from this visit and retrieve items needed for the next visit on your schedule. It is always safer to open your trunk in front of this home and get out what is needed for the next family's visit than to open your trunk in front of the next family's home. You do not want to give community members information about what is stored in your car's trunk while it is unattended and you are in the family's home.

Most typically, the documentation of each home visit is completed as soon as the nurse returns to the agency. Some agencies provide their nurses with laptop computers and electronic charting forms, and charting is encouraged at the end of the visit before leaving for the next one. Sometimes, time is allowed for the nurse to chart at their own home after the last visit of the day. For the most part, you will be expected to complete the charting, using agency forms, as soon as is practically possible. Most agencies expect all charting to be completed by the end of each workday or not later than the end of the work week.

Agencies use a variety of forms that assist the nurse to document fully and succinctly. On some forms, the nurse uses code numbers, letters, or checkmarks on developmental or disease-specific care plans that are devised in a checklist format. For example, a packet of four pages may be used to document a postpartum visit and newborn assessment: two narrative forms to chart the expectations for the mother and baby and postpartum newborn assessment forms on which head-to-toe assessment information is documented. These forms contain a place to document parent or client teaching according to expected parameters and a place for listing other professional's involvement with the family. Similar developmentally focused forms may be used in the agency for

EVIDENCE-BASED PRACTICE

The Nurse–Family Partnership (NFP) has a long history of providing prenatal and infancy home visits by nurses to first-time at-risk mothers. The overall goal of this program is to prevent child abuse and neglect, children's mental health problems, and infant mortality through home visiting during the first 2 years of the child's life. The program has demonstrated positive results in various ethnic and racial groups and in a variety of living contexts through randomized trials. In order to assess other long-term benefits of the program, 19-year-olds (n = 310) were recruited from among the 400 families enrolled in the NFP between 1978 and 1980 in a semirural area of New York. Of the sample, 29% of the mothers had received nurse home visits during pregnancy and the child's first 2 years, 25% received home visits during pregnancy, and 45% did not receive either form of home visiting. These young adults completed a telephone interview that assessed high-school graduation, employment, sexual behavior, childbearing, substance use, and criminal behavior. The girls, whose mothers received both pregnancy and infancy visits by the nurse, were less likely to have been arrested or convicted, had fewer children, and less Medicaid use. With respect to the factors assessed, there were few programmatic effects demonstrated for the boys. The researchers noted that adult patterns of criminal behavior and educational attainment cannot be effectively assessed for 19-year-olds and propose further study of these individuals at 27 years of age. They further suggest examination of the coherence of intervention effects between the mothers and daughters that was not demonstrated with the sons.

Nursing Implications: Home visiting can be a costly effort for a community. The NFP has demonstrated that comprehensive home visiting by nurses can have a positive impact on both the mothers and the children. The cost savings in terms of reduced use of public assistance programs, decreased criminal behavior, reduced pregnancy rates, and delayed pregnancy can offset the operating costs of the program. In addition, the academic achievement of these children may ultimately prove beneficial to the long-term economic prospects of these at-risk children and the communities in which they live. Communities considering reducing or eliminating home visiting programs may want to consider retaining them, or possibly implementing the NFP program.

Reference: Eckenrode, J., Campa, M., Luckey, D. W., Henderson, C. R., Cole, R., Kitzman, H., et al. (2010). Long-term effects of prenatal and infancy nurse home visitation on the life course of youths, 19-year follow-up of a randomized trial. *Archives of Pediatrics & Adolescent Medicine, 164*(1), 9–15.

high-risk infants, high-risk children, adolescents, and older adults. Other packets of forms may focus on chronic illness, such as chronic obstructive pulmonary disease, hypertension, diabetes, alcoholism, acquired immunodeficiency syndrome (AIDS), or cancer that are common in the agency client base.

Focus of Family Health Visits

The focus of family health visits depends on the mission and resources of the agency providing the service and the needs of the families being served. Some agencies provide education, recreational activities such as summer camps, and support groups for families of people with specific health problems such as Alzheimer's disease, asthma, diabetes, or neurologic disorders. Other agencies provide services directed toward those with special social or economic needs, such as immigrant families, people living in poverty, or the homeless (Kneipp et al., 2011; Monsen, Sanders, Radosevich, & Geppert, 2011; Vanderburg et al., 2010). Home visits may be a part of the service being provided and are best conducted and received in the comfort and privacy of a family's home. In general, family health visits are designed to be educational, to provide anticipatory guidance, and to focus on health promotion or prevention.

Family Education and Anticipatory Guidance

Official agencies, such as county or city health departments, distribute their services based on the broader community's needs. For example, if there is a large population of teen pregnancies and high-risk infants, the health department may contract with hospitals and private doctors' offices to provide home or clinic visits to all teens and women with high-risk pregnancies and their newborns after delivery. On these visits, the community/public health nurse teaches prenatal, postpartum, and newborn care and provides anticipatory guidance (information needed in the future regarding the child and the need for regular infant health care provider visits, immunizations, and safety awareness). Another community may have a significant number of older adults who need to learn how to manage a chronic illness, enhance their nutrition, and practice safety measures to prevent injuries and falls.

Family Promotion and Illness Prevention

All populations, regardless of age, income, culture, or nation of origin, need the fundamental protection immunization gives to protect themselves and the health of the larger community. In addition, providing the means for families to receive required immunizations is a responsibility of health departments. Usually, immunization services are not brought into the home, but the nurse can provide information about immunizations, teach the importance of following an immunization schedule, and follow up with the client during home visits.

Teaching people how to prevent illness and how to remain healthy is basic to community/public health nursing (see Chapter 11). Even within the limitations of chronic illnesses, family members can be taught health promotion activities to live as healthfully as possible (Edelman & Mandle, 2010; Pender, Murdaugh, & Parson, 2011). Health promotion activities may include screening for hypertension and elevated cholesterol, performing a physical assessment, and teaching about nutrition and safety. The American Nurses Association's 2007 *Public Health Nursing: Scope and Standards of Practice* highlights this role in the following statement: "When public health nurses partner with individuals, the focus becomes the promotion of knowledge, attitudes, beliefs, practices, and behaviors that support and enhance health, with the ultimate goal of improving the overall health of the population" (p. 7). This holistic emphasis can also be found in the newest additions to the *Healthy People 2020* topics and objectives (U.S. Department of Health and Human Services [USDHHS], 2010). In particular, social determinants of health have been added with the ultimate goal of creating "social and physical environments that promote good health for all" (see Display 19.2).

Such activities can occur during a family health visit; while family members are at their place of work, school, or recreation; or at self-help group meetings. Community health nurses provide health promotion services to couples during prenatal classes by teaching about the expected changes during pregnancy and providing anticipatory guidance for safe infant care. They may also screen older adults at senior centers for hypertension or elevated cholesterol or teach family members who attend support groups, such as Alcoholics Anonymous.

Personal Safety on the Home Visit

As mentioned earlier in this chapter, personal safety while traveling throughout the community is essential. In addition, continuation of personal safety while on the home visit must be considered.

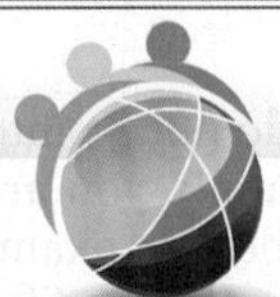

DISPLAY 19.2 *HEALTHY PEOPLE 2020*—SELECT TOPICS AND OBJECTIVES

Topic: Health-Related Quality of Life and Wellbeing

Health-related quality of life (HRQoL) is a multidimensional concept that includes domains related to physical, mental, emotional, and social functioning. It goes beyond direct measures of population health, life expectancy, and causes of death and focuses on the impact health status has on quality of life. A related concept of HRQoL is wellbeing, which assesses the positive aspects of a person's life, such as positive emotions and life satisfaction.

Objective: Social Determinants of Health

Goal: Create social and physical environments that promote good health for all. Emerging Strategies to Address Social Determinants of Health

Overview: Health starts in our homes, schools, workplaces, neighborhoods, and communities. We know that taking care of ourselves by eating well and staying active, not smoking, getting the recommended immunizations and screening tests, and seeing a doctor when we are sick all influence our health. Our health is also determined in part by access to social and economic opportunities; the resources and supports available in our homes, neighborhoods, and communities; the quality of our schooling; the safety of our workplaces; the cleanliness of our water, food, and air; and the nature of our social interactions and relationships. The conditions in which we live explain in part why some Americans are healthier than others and why Americans more generally are not as healthy as they could be.

Objective: Lesbian, Gay, Bisexual, and Transgender Health

Goal: Improve the health, safety, and wellbeing of lesbian, gay, bisexual, and transgender (LGBT) individuals.

Overview: LGBT individuals encompass all races and ethnicities, religions, and social classes. Sexual orientation and gender identity questions are not asked on most national or state surveys, making it difficult to estimate the number of LGBT individuals and their health needs. Research suggests that LGBT individuals face health disparities linked to societal stigma, discrimination, and denial of their civil and human rights.

Objective: Genomics

Goal: Improve health and prevent harm through valid and useful genomic tools in clinical and public health practices.

Overview: The new Genomics topic area and objectives for 2020 reflect the increasing scientific evidence supporting the health benefits of using genetic tests and family health history to guide clinical and public health interventions.

Source: U.S. Department of Health and Human Services. (2010). *Healthy People 2020. Topics and objectives.* Retrieved from http://www.healthypeople.gov/2020/topicsobjectives2020/default.aspx

Personal Safety While Traveling and in the Neighborhood

On leaving your "base of operation," such as the health department office, neighborhood clinic, homeless shelter, or campus classroom, have with you all the necessary tools to travel in the community with safety. Most importantly, leave an itinerary of your planned travels, the telephone numbers of families you will attempt to visit, and your cellular phone number. Traveling in the community takes a variety of forms and means different things to different people.

If you are traveling in an agency or private car, you need:

- A full gas tank
- A city/county map
- A cellular phone
- The family addresses
- Money for lunch or telephone calls (in case you are in an area where your cellular phone does not work)

If you are using public transportation, plan to

- Have exact change for each bus trip
- Carry a bus schedule
- Exit the bus as near as possible to your client's home
- Know where to get the bus for the return trip or to the next home visit
- Carry a cellular phone

If you are walking or riding a bicycle to a home visit, you still need to travel safely. In some neighborhoods, it is best to call ahead to the family you plan to visit, give them an approximate time of your arrival, and if necessary, ask them to watch out for your arrival. When walking in neighborhoods, walk with direction and purpose; do not look lost even if you are. Use neighborhood shopkeepers as resources for direction and information and as refuge if you feel uncomfortable or threatened. If you need to ask for directions, and you are not near any stores, look for another professional, such as a social worker, a public service employee (postal or utility worker), or an apartment manager. If you need to approach a stranger for information, select a woman. If you see a group of people that makes you feel uncomfortable, cross the street, limit eye contact, and continue to the home you are intending to visit. Always avoid walking through alleys or along buildings that open onto alleys, and stay in the middle of the sidewalk or closer to the street. It might be helpful to carry a whistle on your key ring.

It is always safest to avoid compromising situations by staying alert and using safe traveling methods whenever you are in public, no matter how "safe" the area appears. However, if an individual or group accosts you, immediately try to break free and run to a public place while making loud noises. Yell "Fire!" This response gets more attention than "Help!" If a criminal wants your nursing bag, purse, or wallet, freely give it up; the contents are not worth your safety. Some nurses feel safer after they have attended self-defense classes, which are offered by police departments, as employee in-service programs in some agencies, and on some university campuses.

In some rough inner-city neighborhoods, professionals visiting families travel only in pairs (usually with at least one male in the pair) or with a security guard or police escort. Know whether these resources are necessary or available to you before venturing into a crime-ridden community. In some inner-city neighborhoods, community health nurses refuse to visit people living on one block or in one apartment building. Similar issues are found in rural areas known for drug manufacturing and distribution. Know and do not challenge important safety measures that are used by expert nurses and are followed for personal safety. Safety issues are unique to each community.

Another focus of concern is the perceived risk to self when making a home visit. An individual's cognition and perception of a situation; his views on risk taking; and the time, setting, and coping process all factor into feelings of safety when traveling in a community, entering a family's home, or conducting a home visit (Kendra & George, 2001). What one person sees as a risk, another sees as a challenge or an opportunity. Yet another may see nothing. We each perceive risks differently based on knowledge, experience, and personality.

Arriving at the Home

Make sure you are at the right house, and do not go into the home until you are assured that the family you are intending to visit does live there and is home. For example, you may be planning to visit 16-year-old Jennifer and her 5-day-old infant, Marcus. However, when you knock, a 50-year-old man answers the door. Do not enter the house without asking whether Jennifer can come to the door or you can see her, even if he invites you in. Remain outside the home and go inside only after you talk to Jennifer at the door. This precaution ensures that the family members you want to visit are really home and that this is the right address.

Friction Between Family Members

During a home visit, two or more family members may begin to argue or physically fight with one another. Immediately remove yourself from the home visit and let the family know that with such distraction it is not a good time to visit and that you will return at another time. Never step in and offer to assist an adult family member when two people are physically fighting; you may be the next victim. If necessary, call 911 from your cellular phone once you are out of the house. Depending on the type of altercation, it may be appropriate to discuss the friction in the family at a later visit.

Family Members Under the Influence

If the focus of the visit is on two family members and a third member is demonstrating behaviors that indicate drug or alcohol use, you must use your judgment as to the best action to take. The agency you work for or the school you attend has guidelines you should follow. If the intoxicated person goes to another room, it might be appropriate to continue the visit and perhaps discuss your observations with the remaining family members. If the person becomes abusive, remains in the room, or interrupts the visit it is best to terminate the visit and reschedule when the family member is not under the influence or is not present. You do not want to put yourself in the middle of a situation that could deteriorate rapidly and compromise your safety.

The Presence of Strangers

In some families, the coming and going of many extended family members, neighbors, and friends is common; it is the norm and is not distracting to them, but it may be to the nurse. For example, what would you do if you arrived at a home and five teenage boys were sitting on the front porch steps, so that you had to edge your way past them to the door? What if you found three men sleeping on the living room floor in the small apartment of a teenage mother and her infant, or four neighbor children riding their tricycles inside the house during a teaching visit to two young parents who do not seem fazed by the commotion? These situations may not be indicative of danger, but they can make you feel vulnerable, uncomfortable, or distracted from the purpose of the visit. Inquire about the people you observe in the periphery of the home visit; ask about their relationship to the family and whether they should be included in the visit. The family may suggest that you ignore the other people or say they are transient family members. It may be important to learn who they are and if they have unmet health care needs or their presence influences the health of the family you are visiting.

EFFECTS OF FAMILY HEALTH ON THE INDIVIDUALS

The health of each family member affects the other members and contributes to the level of **family health**. For example, a woman whose husband has had a stroke may cope successfully with the resulting physical and emotional demands of his care but may have inadequate reserves for effectively meeting the needs of her children. The level at which a family functions—how well it is able to solve problems and help its members reach their potential—significantly affects the individual's level of health. A healthy family fosters individual growth and resistance to ill health and sustains members during times of crisis such as serious illness, emotional dilemmas, divorce, or death of a family member (Haggman-Laitila, Tanninen, & Pietila, 2010; Shin, Choi, Kim, & Kim, 2010). On the other hand, a family with limited coping skills or an underdeveloped capacity for problem solving, self-management, or self-care is often unable to promote the potential of its members or assist them in times of need.

Family health standards and practices also influence each member's health. For instance, many individuals, even as adults, adhere to cultural and family patterns of eating, exercise, and communication. Cultural (see Chapter 5) and family values influence decisions about utilizing preventative health care as well as access to services such as immunizations, regular health assessments, or family planning (Spector, 2008). Family patterns also dictate whether members participate in their own health care and how they follow through and comply with professional advice. Individuals influence family health, and the family can either obstruct or facilitate individual health. The family becomes an important focus for community health nursing assessment and intervention.

CHARACTERISTICS OF HEALTHY FAMILIES

How does the community/public health nurse determine family health status? Analysis of how basic functions are met does not give a satisfactory picture of a family's health status. More definitive criteria are needed. Although it is difficult to define a "normal" family, studies have provided some standards that characterize a healthy family (Barker, 2007; Shin et al., 2010; Thompson, 1998). Over the years, research on families and on family health behavior has produced a growing body of data with which to assess family health.

In looking at families over the years, researchers have found many similar characteristics. Otto (1973) identified characteristics of family unity, loyalty and interfamily cooperation, support and security, role flexibility, and constructive relationships with community. Olson et al. (1983) identified seven major family strengths that are important for family functioning and coping with crisis: family pride, family support, cohesion, adaptability, communication, religious orientation, and social support. Becvar and Becvar (2008) listed the following characteristics: (a) a legitimate source of authority that is supported and consistent over time, (b) a stable and consistent system of rules, (c) consistent and regular nurturing behaviors, (d) effective child-rearing practices, (e) stable and well-maintained marriages, (f) a set of agreed-upon goals toward which the family and individuals work, and (g) sufficient flexibility to change in the face of both expected and unexpected stressors. Parachin (1997) identified six signs of a healthy family: maintaining a spiritual foundation, making the family a top priority, asking for and giving respect, communicating and listening, valuing service to others, and expecting and offering acceptance. Six important characteristics of healthy families that consistently emerge in the literature (Becvar & Becvar, 2008; Freidman et al., 2003; Kaakinen et al., 2009) are the following:

1. A facilitative process of interaction exists among family members.
2. Individual member development is enhanced.
3. Role relationships are structured effectively.

4. Active attempts are made to cope with problems.
5. There is a healthy home environment and lifestyle.
6. Regular links with the broader community are established.

Healthy Interaction Among Members

Healthy families communicate. Their patterns of interaction are regular, varied, and supportive. Adults communicate with adults, children with children, and adults with children (Anderson & Sabatelli, 2010). These interactions are frequent and assume many forms. Healthy families use frequent verbal communication. They discuss problems, confront each other when angry, share ideas and concerns, and write or call each other when separated. They also communicate frequently through nonverbal means, particularly those families from cultural or subcultural groups that are less verbal. There are innumerable ways to convey feelings and thoughts without words, including smiling encouragingly, embracing warmly, frowning disapprovingly, being available, withdrawing for privacy, doing an unsolicited favor, serving refreshments, and giving a gift. The family that has learned to communicate effectively has members who are sensitive to one another. They watch for cues and verify messages to ensure understanding. This kind of family recognizes and deals with conflicts as they arise. Its members have learned to share and to work collaboratively with each other.

Effective communication is necessary for a family to carry out basic functions. Family members must communicate to demonstrate affection and acceptance, to promote identity and affiliation, and to guide behavior through socialization and social controls. Just as there is a correlation between a high degree of communication and a high degree of effectiveness in organizational functioning, facilitative communication patterns within a family promote the health and development of its members. Healthy families are more likely than unhealthy families to negotiate topics for discussion, use humor, show respect for differences of opinion, and clarify the meaning of one another's communications.

Enhancement of Individual Development

Healthy families are responsive to the needs of individual members and provide the freedom and support necessary to promote each member's growth. If a father in a healthy family loses his job, the family will work to support his ego and help him use his energy constructively to adjust and find new work. The healthy family recognizes and fosters the growing child's need for independence by increasing opportunities for the child to try new things alone. This kind of family can tolerate differences of opinion or lifestyle. Each member is accepted unconditionally, and the right to be an individual is respected. Within an appropriate framework of stability and structure, the healthy family encourages freedom and autonomy for its members (Friedman et al., 2003).

Patterns of promoting individual member development vary from one family to another depending on cultural orientation. The way in which autonomy is expressed in an Italian American family differs from its expression in a Native American family, yet each family can promote freedom and autonomy. The result is an increase in competence, self-reliance, social skills, intellectual growth, and overall capacity for self-management among family members (Wright & Leahey, 2009) (see *From the Case Files*).

Effective Structuring of Relationships

Healthy families structure role relationships to meet changing family needs over time (Kaakinen et al., 2009). In a stable social context, some families establish member roles and tasks (e.g., breadwinner, primary decision maker, or homemaker) that are maintained as workable patterns throughout the life of the family. Families in rural areas, isolated communities, or religious and subcultural groups are more likely than others to retain role consistency, because they face little or no external pressure or need to change. For example, the Amish community in Pennsylvania has maintained marked differentiation in family roles for more than 100 years.

In a technologically advanced society such as the United States, most families must adapt their roles to changing family needs created by external forces. As women enter the workforce, family roles, relationships, and tasks change to meet the demands of the new situation. Many husbands assume more homemaking responsibilities; fathers engage in child rearing, children along with adults in their families share decision making and a more equal distribution of power. The latter may be essential for the survival of a single-parent family, in which the children must assume adult responsibilities while the parent works to support the family.

Changing life-cycle stages require alterations in the structure of relationships. The healthy family recognizes members' changing developmental needs and adapts parenting roles, family tasks, and controls to fit each stage (Anderson & Sabatelli, 2010). For example, household chores of increasing complexity and responsibility are assigned as children become capable of handling them. Rules of conduct relax as members learn to govern their own behavior.

Active Coping Effort

Healthy families actively attempt to overcome life's problems and issues. When faced with change, they assume responsibility for coping and seek energetically and creatively to meet the demands of the situation (Becvar & Becvar, 2008; Olson et al., 1983). Coping skills are needed to deal with emotional tragedies such as substance abuse problems, serious illness, or death. If a family member has a substance abuse problem, the

From the **Case Files**

A Family Assessment: Meeting Hector's Needs

You are a home health nurse working in Smithville. You have been given a referral for a new client, Hector. Hector is being released from the rehabilitation unit of Metropolis Hospital. Although he lives in Smithville, Metropolis Hospital was the only facility willing to accept a Medicaid client with a severe spinal cord injury.

Hector is a 19-year-old Hispanic man who sustained major injury to his spinal cord (T-4 injury) in a motorcycle accident. The injury occurred approximately 6 weeks ago. Hector has been diagnosed as paraplegic with some residual limitation of upper body strength and mobility.

Your job is to facilitate Hector's transition from the hospital to the home environment. You will be teaching Hector and his caregivers about the following:

1. Nutrition and fluid intake
2. Signs and symptoms warranting follow-up
3. Medication administration
4. Bowel and bladder care
5. Skin care
6. Activities of daily living (ADLs), self-care with sensory–motor deficits
7. Safety/injury prevention
8. Community resources
9. Rehabilitative services
10. Anticipatory guidance about grief, anger, and suicidal ideations; sexual function; fear of abandonment, role change, and social isolation; and altered family processes

Following is a synopsis of information obtained during your initial visit with Hector and his family in their home.

Visit One. Hector lives in a migrant labor camp located on the outskirts of Smithville. His family has resided in the camp for 18 years. Living in the two-bedroom cabin like home are:

- Hector
- Hector's uncle Manuel (32 years old). Manuel's job is seasonal; he has been offered a temporary job for a much higher salary, working out of state.
- Hector's brother Efran (16 years old). Efran is considering dropping out of high school in order to assist with the care of his family. His goal is to become an auto mechanic. He is fluent in both Spanish and English.
- Manuel's wife Micaela (29 years old). Micaela was a teacher in Mexico. She is extremely supportive of her family. She is concerned about the possibility of another pregnancy but does not believe in the use of birth control.
- Manuel and Micaela's children, Arturo (5 years old) and Jasmin (6 months old). Arturo begins a Head Start Program soon and will be gone for 5 hours each day. Jasmin is a healthy baby; she continues to be breast-fed and is thriving at home.
- Hector's 74-year-old paternal grandmother (Abuela), who has recently arrived from Mexico and plans on assisting in Hector's care. Abuela has congestive heart failure and arthritis. She is not a legal resident of the United States and is not eligible for medical assistance.

The whereabouts of Hector's mother are unknown; she moved from their village in Mexico shortly after Efran was born. She has remarried and started another family. She has had no contact with Hector or Efran. Hector's father lives in their home village in Mexico. Although he lived in the migrant camp in Smithville for many years, he recently remarried and has two young daughters in Mexico. Hector's father is aware of Hector's injury and has no plans to return to the United States.

Your ability to speak fluent Spanish has enabled you to solicit the above information. Manuel has provided you with most of the information. He has been very involved in Hector's recovery through daily visits to the rehabilitation unit and frequent discussions with Hector's health care providers. Manuel tells you that "Hector is like a son to me … I have a responsibility to my older brother to watch over his son. My brother watched out for me when I was young … he even left school to work to help support our family." Manuel adds, "We don't have much but we will take care of Hector … we'll all work together."

You begin your discussion by explaining your role as home health nurse. You inform the family about the type of education and interventions you are able to provide. You ask Hector and the family to tell you what they have learned from the health care team at the rehabilitation unit and what plans have been developed by the family to address Hector's medical and psychosocial needs. As you begin the visit you notice that Hector's grandmother is sitting quietly in the corner of the room rocking Jasmin. You learn that Efran is working in the fields. Arturo is in school. Manuel, Micaela, and Abuela are participating in the home visit this morning. The conversation is as follows.

Nurse: Hector, can you tell me how you feel about being home?

Hector (looks at Micaela): Okay, I guess.

Micaela: He's a little scared, I think. He feels like it's going to be too much for us to deal with.

Nurse (looking at Hector): There's so much happening right now, so much to think about …

Hector: Uh-huh.

(Hector is maintaining eye contact with Manuel and Micaela only; since this is your initial visit to the home you feel that Hector may be more comfortable in the role of observer.)

From the Case Files I *(Continued)*

Nurse (looking at Manuel and Micaela): Do you have any questions before we begin?

Micaela: They gave us a lot of information at the hospital... I'm most afraid about if the phone doesn't work and Hector needs help. What if something happens to Hector and I can't call anyone? That's the only thing I worry about.

Abuela: If anything happens to him I'll be right here with you, "mija." We can do this, we can take care of Hector if we work together.

Manuel: There is a store with a phone only two blocks away, if you needed to you could call from there. What I want to know is how we can get Hector into school or something that will help him to be around kids his own age. His English is good enough, he even finished high school. He needs to be ready to make a future for himself.

Hector (grins and looks at Manuel): Right, uncle that is what I want, too.

You continue the conversation by revisiting Micaela's concerns about access to a telephone in case of an emergency. You ask specific questions about her concerns and use this as an opportunity to educate the family about circumstances warranting immediate follow-up. Together you decide that Micaela will develop a list of specific concerns that you will review together at a subsequent visit planned for 2 days from today. Today's visit consists of the following:

I. Assessment
   A. Home environment
      1. Safety
      2. ADLs
   B. Knowledge of disease processes
   C. Fluid volume balance
   D. Nutritional resources of family
      1. Food availability
      2. Food preparation
   E. Insurance and financial status

II. Education
   A. Medications
   B. Warning signs and symptoms and appropriate follow-up procedures
   C. Bowel and bladder care
   D. Hygiene prior to and following patient care

The plan for your visit in 2 days includes:

I. Referrals
   A. Community resources
   B. Educational opportunities
   C. Support groups (Spanish speaking)
   D. Peer group opportunities for Hector

II. Assessment
   A. Continuation of above

III. Education
   A. Continuation of above

Questions

1. What is the social structure of this family (traditional vs. nontraditional)? Be specific about the type of traditional or nontraditional family system that exists in this scenario.
2. Discuss an example of triangulation in this scenario.
3. What essential functions are present within this family system?
4. What developmental stages appear to have been achieved?
5. What steps will you take in order to empower the family to make their own decisions?
6. List the strengths of the family.
7. Prioritize Hector's issues—medical and psychosocial.
8. Prioritize issues facing the other family members.
9. Identify mutual goals for this family:
   Immediate
   Midrange
   Long-term
10. What community health nursing interventions will you utilize to achieve these mutual goals?

family may seek counseling and treatment opportunities involving all family members. If a family member is seriously ill, the family may ask for and accept assistance from extended family members or community health care workers. In the event of death in the family, receiving consolation and support from one another and from relatives and friends is an important step in the healing process. The healthy family recognizes the need for assistance, accepts help, and pursues opportunities to eliminate or decrease the stressors that affect it (Haggman-Laitila et al., 2010).

More frequently, healthy families cope with less dramatic, day-to-day changes. For instance, one family may cope with the increased cost of food by cutting down on meat consumption, substituting other protein foods, and eating in restaurants less frequently. Healthy families are open to innovation, support new ideas, and find ways to solve problems. One family may try to solve the problem of spending too much on transportation by cutting down on daily travel; this may cause additional problems if three members have jobs in different areas of town or need to go to school functions and meetings. Another family, responding to environmental concerns and a personal need for a healthier lifestyle, may explore and arrive at new ways to reach destinations by walking, bicycling, skating, or carpooling to school or work. Healthy coping may go beyond finding a simple, obvious solution. Members may try to rearrange schedules to avoid frequent trips to regular destinations and plan ahead to avoid last-minute trips to stores. Healthy families actively seek and use a variety of resources to solve problems. They may discover these resources within the family or externally; they engage in self-care. For example, a professional couple, faced with the unaffordable expense of daytime babysitting, arranged their work schedules so that they could share childcare during the first 2 years. Later, they joined a cooperative preschool that allowed their child to attend daily, but required parental participation only 1 day a week. In another example, a single parent of five children, who was also a full-time nursing student, was able to finance two or three family outings each year by recycling aluminum cans that everyone in the family collected.

Healthy Environment and Lifestyle

Another sign of a healthy family is a healthy home environment and lifestyle. Healthy families create safe and hygienic living conditions for their members. For instance, a healthy family with young children "childproofs" the home by removing potential hazards such as exposed electric outlets and cleaning solvents from the child's reach. A healthy family with an older adult who is prone to falls installs lighting and handrails. A healthy home environment is one that is clean and reduces the spread of disease-causing organisms.

A healthy family lifestyle encourages appropriate balance in the lives of its members. In an ideal family, there is activity and rest sufficient for the energy needs of daily living; the diet offered is varied and nutritionally sound, physical activity maintains ideal weight while promoting cardiac health; preventative hygiene habits are taught and followed by family members; emotional and mental health are encouraged through a support network of caring others; and family members seek out and use health care services and demonstrate adherence to recommended regimens.

The emotional climate of a healthy family is positive and supportive of growth. Contributing to this healthful emotional climate is a strong sense of shared values, often combined with a strong religious orientation (Olson et al., 1983). A healthy family demonstrates caring, encourages and accepts expression of feelings, and respects divergent ideas. Members can express their individuality in the way they dress or decorate their rooms. The home environment makes family members feel welcome and accepted.

Regular Links with the Broader Community

Healthy families maintain dynamic ties with the broader community. They participate regularly in external groups and activities, often in a leadership capacity. They may join in local politics, participate in a church bazaar, or promote the school's paper drive to raise money for science equipment. They use external resources suited to family needs. For example, a farm family with teenagers, recognizing the importance of peer group influences on adolescents, becomes very active in the local 4-H Club. Another family, in which the father is out of work, joins a job transition support group. Healthy families also know what is going on in the world around them. They show an interest in current events and attempt to understand significant social, economic, and political issues. This ever-broadening outreach gives families knowledge of external forces that might influence their lives. It exposes them to a wider range of alternatives and a variety of contacts, which can increase options for finding resources and strengthen coping skills.

An unhealthy family has not recognized the value of establishing links with the broader community. This may be because of knowledge deficits regarding community resources, previous negative experiences with community services, or a lack of connection with the community due to family expectations or cultural practices.

It is important for the community health nurse to assess the family's relationship with the broader community, in addition to structural and developmental variations, interaction, coping strategies, and lifestyle. With a comprehensive family assessment, the nurse has a base from which to begin a plan of care.

FAMILY HEALTH PRACTICE GUIDELINES

Family nursing is a kind of nursing practice in which the family is the unit of service (Friedman et al., 2003, Kaakinen et al., 2009). It is not merely a family-oriented approach, in which family concerns that affect the health of an individual are taken into account. Family nursing asks how one provides health care to a collection of people. It does not mean that nursing must relinquish the service to individuals. One of the distinct contributions of the nursing profession is its holistic approach to individual needs. Community health nurses rise to the challenge of adding a service to populations that include families.

Five principles guide and enhance family nursing practice: (1) work with the family collectively, (2) start where the family is, (3) adapt nursing interventions to the family's stage of development, (4) recognize the validity of family structural variations, and (5) emphasize family strengths.

Work with the Family Collectively

To practice family nursing, nurses must set aside their usual focus on the individual and remind themselves that several people together have a collective personality, collective interests, and a collective set of needs. Viewing a group of people as one unit may seem less strange if one considers the way in which business organizations are perceived. For example, you may think of a particular corporation as conservative or liberal. You may hear that a women's group has taken a stand on abortion or that a government agency needs to become better organized. In each case, the group is viewed collectively as a single entity with attributes and activities in common. So it is with families. A family has its own personality, interests, and needs.

As much as possible, community health nurses want to involve all the family's members during nurse–client interactions (Wright & Leahey, 2009). This approach reinforces the importance of each individual member's contributions to total family functioning. Nurses want to encourage everyone's participation in the work that the nurse and the family jointly agree to do. Like a coach, the nurse wants to help family members work together as a team for their collective benefit. Consider how a nurse might work collectively with the Beck family (Display 19.3).

Start Where the Family Is

When working with families, community health nurses begin at the present, not the ideal level of functioning. To discover where a family is, the community health nurse first conducts a family assessment to ascertain the members' needs and level of health and then determines collective interests, concerns, and priorities. The accompanying description of the Kovac family illustrates this principle (Display 19.4).

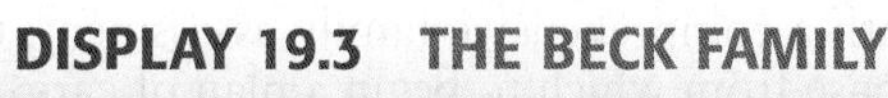

DISPLAY 19.3 THE BECK FAMILY

A community health nurse had an initial contact with Mr. and Mrs. Beck and their youngest child at the well-baby clinic. The 9-month-old child was over the 95th percentile for weight and at the 40th percentile for height. The nurse also noted that both parents were obese. The nurse asked about the eating patterns in the family and of the baby in particular and suggested a home visit to determine whether the Becks were interested in family nursing. The nurse explained the purpose of home visits (to assess all family members, coping patterns, eating patterns, and food purchasing choices) and the importance of including all family members and asked for a time that would be good for the family as a whole. The nurse explained that each person should be involved and committed to the agreed-upon goals; that, like a team of oarsmen, the family would have to pull together to accomplish the purpose of the visits. To help the Beck family improve its nutritional status, the nurse might suggest a session of brainstorming to uncover many causes of poor nutrition. More brainstorming might result in solutions and plans for action. On each visit, the nurse would view the Becks as a group. Group responses and actions would be expected. Evaluation of outcomes would be based on what the family did collectively. The Becks were interested, and a home visit date was made.

Adapt Nursing Intervention to the Family's Stage of Development

Although every family engages in the same basic functions, the tasks necessary to accomplish these functions vary with each stage of the family's development. A young family, for instance, can appropriately meet its members' affiliation needs by establishing mutually satisfying relationships and meaningful communication patterns. As the family enters later stages, bonds change with the release of some members into new families and the loss of others through death. Awareness of the family's developmental stage enables the nurse to assess the appropriateness of the family's level of functioning and to tailor interventions accordingly. Nurses are often adept at family assessment, but interventions need to be the focus (Kaakinen et al., 2009; Wright & Leahy, 2009). A nurse's work with the Ravina family illustrates this need (Display 19.5).

Recognize the Validity of Family Structure Variations

Many families seen by community health nurses are nontraditional, such as single-parent families and unmarried couples. Other families are organized around nontraditional patterns, for example both parents may have careers, a husband may care for children at home, while his wife financially supports the family, or both parents may telecommute and work at home. Such variations in structure and organizational patterns have resulted from social and technologic changes in employment practices, welfare programs, economic conditions, gender roles, status of women and minorities, birth control, incidence of divorce, and even war. Such variations in family structure and organization lead to revised patterns of family functioning. Member roles and tasks often differ dramatically from our expectations. Examples are a family with a single parent who works full-time while raising children or a dual-career marriage in which both partners have undifferentiated roles. Community health nurses, many of whom are accustomed to traditional family patterns, must learn to understand and accept these variations in family structure and organization in order to address the needs of the families.

There are two important principles to remember. First, what is normal for one family is not necessarily normal for another. Each family is unique in its combination of structures, composition, roles, and behaviors. As long as a family carries out its functions effectively and demonstrates the characteristics of a healthy family, one must agree that its form, no matter how variant, is valid.

Second, families are constantly changing. Marriage transforms two people into a married couple without

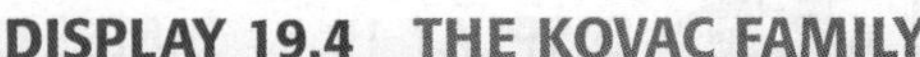

DISPLAY 19.4 THE KOVAC FAMILY

Marcia Kovac brought her baby, Tiffany, to the well-child clinic once but failed to keep further appointments. Concerned that the family might be having other difficulties, Sara Villa, a community health nurse, made a home visit. The mobile home was cluttered and dirty; the baby was crying in her playpen. Marcia seemed uninterested in the nurse's visit. She listened politely but had little to say. She repeated that everything was okay and that the baby was doing fine, explaining that she was just fussy because she was teething. As they talked, Marcia's husband Henry, a delivery van driver, stopped by to pick up a sports magazine to read on his lunch hour. The three of them discussed the problems of inflation and how expensive it was to raise a child. Sara reminded them that the clinic was free and that they could at least get good health care without extra cost. They agreed without enthusiasm. After Henry left, the nurse spent the remainder of the visit discussing infant care with Marcia, particularly emphasizing regular checkups and immunizations.

The next visit also focused on the baby, but Sara had an uncomfortable feeling that this family was not really interested in her help. After consulting her supervisor, the nurse did what she wished she had done in the first place. She asked to talk with Marcia and Henry together and explained frankly why she had come to their home and what she could offer in the way of counseling, teaching, support, and referral to other community resources. She then asked them what problems or concerns they had. The Kovacs were more than responsive and described their financial difficulties and feelings of isolation from family and friends. They were new in the city, and both their families lived some distance away on farms. The neighbors were friendly but not close enough to confide in. They believed they would eventually overcome their problems if they just had "someone to lean on," as they put it.

Now Sara could address the Kovacs' primary needs and concerns for friends and emotional support. The nurse began to address the Kovacs' social needs first and introduced them to a young couples' group that met at the community center. Sara continued to make periodic home visits and shared additional information about community services that the Kovacs might find helpful. She praised Marcia and Henry for following up on immunizations for Tiffany. Over time, Sara saw differences in the family's interest in their relationship with the community and their connection to its services. Sara realized that before she could address the issue of Tiffany's health, she needed to address the emotional health of the parents.

DISPLAY 19.5 THE RAVINA FAMILY

The Ravinas, a couple in their early 70s, recently moved to a retirement complex. They received nursing visits after Mrs. Ravina's stroke 3 years earlier but requested service now because Mr. Ravina was feeling "poorly" all the time. He though that perhaps his diet and lack of activity might be the cause and hoped the nurse would have some helpful suggestions. The couple had eagerly awaited Mr. Ravina's retirement from teaching, planning to be lazy, travel, visit all their children, and do all those things they never had time to do when they were young. Now neither of them seemed to have enough energy or the capacity to enjoy their new life. The move from their home of 28 years had been difficult: They were still trying to find space in the tiny apartment for their cherished books and mementos, although they had given many of them away.

Ronald Bell, a community health nurse, recognized that the Ravinas were experiencing a situational crisis (leaving their home of 28 years), a developmental crisis (aging and entering retirement), and perhaps some underlying health problems. Many of the Ravinas' expectations for this new life stage were unrealistic; they had not adequately prepared themselves for the adjustments that the loss of their home and retirement would demand. Through discussion Ronald was able to help the Ravinas understand their situation and express their feelings. He completed physical assessments on the Ravinas and encouraged regular follow-up with their health care provider. He also helped them join a support group of retired persons who were experiencing some of the same difficulties. Because this nurse was able to help the Ravinas through their crisis in a supportive and nonjudgmental manner, he found them receptive later to discussing preparation for the inevitable loss and bereavement that would occur when one of them died. He was adapting his nursing intervention to this family's stage of development.

children. Adding children changes the family structure. Divorce alters the structure and roles. Remarriage with the addition of children from another family changes the family again. Children grow up and leave the home while the parents, together or singly, are left to adjust to yet another family structure. Throughout the life cycle, a family seldom stays the same for very long. Each of these changes forces a family to adapt to its circumstances. Consider the young women with a baby whose husband deserts her: she has no choice but to assume a single-parent role. Each change also creates varying degrees of stress and demands considerable adaptive energy on the family's part. Many family changes are predictable and part of the normal life-cycle growth. Some changes are not predictable or may have a less traditional structure. The nurse's responsibility is to help families cope with the changes while remaining nonjudgmental and accepting of variations in family structure. For example, homosexual unions may be difficult for some nurses to deal with, particularly if they conflict with the nurse's own set of values. Yet the nurse's responsibility remains the same—to help promote the collective health of that family. The nurse should view all families as unique groups, each with its own set of needs and whose interests can best be served through unbiased care. Consider the nurse's work with James Cutler and Brian Hoag (Display 19.6).

Empowering Families

Throughout the family visit, you must remember that the ultimate goal is to assist the family in becoming independent of your services (Haggman-Laitila et al., 2010). This is accomplished through the approach used in conducting the visit. How you structure the nurse–client relationship also influences the outcomes. Four thoughts will help to clarify your working relationship with families:

- The family functioned in a manner that worked for them before you ever met them.
- If you ever feel obliged to do something for a family, consider who did this before you were available.
- Find family strengths even in the most deprived family situation.
- If you were in a similar situation, would you manage, cope, or function as well as the members of this family?

Many families have strengths that some middle-class nurses may overlook or interpret as weaknesses. It is the nurse's job to recognize the strengths in families and to help families recognize them as well. For example, some families borrow needed items (diapers, food, and clothes) from each other, whereas others do not even recognize their next-door neighbors by sight. Children from large families often learn to physically care for one another and entertain themselves, whereas in some families with only one or two children the youngsters must constantly be entertained. The members of one family may take public transportation or walk to accomplish errands.

DISPLAY 19.6 JAMES CUTLER AND BRIAN HOAG

James Cutler and Brian Hoag have a 6-year monogamous relationship. A homosexual couple, they worked with an attorney to privately adopt a child. The arrangements were completed and their 2-week-old son, Adrian, arrived in their home last week. Helen Jeffers, a community health nurse, receives a referral from the county hospital where Adrian was born. The request is for an assessment of the home situation and parenting skills. The baby tested positive for cocaine with Apgar scores of 6 and 8 and had some initial difficulty sucking. Birth weight was 2,900 g. Discharge weight, at 3 days, was 2,850 g. At her first home visit, Helen finds a neat and orderly two-bedroom condominium, well-equipped with baby supplies. The infant has gained 200 g and is being well cared for by two fatigued parents who had had limited contact with infants previously. James and Brian have many questions and are anxious learners. Helen plans with the couple to make weekly home visits to assess infant growth and development, provide support, and answer questions. She also suggests a neighborhood parenting class and finding a reliable babysitter, and she helps James and Brian develop an infant care work schedule. After 6 weeks of intervention, Adrian is thriving; Helen closes the case to home visits, feeling confident that the parents' goal of becoming knowledgeable and confident has been achieved.

Too often, community health nurses tend to focus their attention on family weaknesses, looking for and referring to them as *needs* or *problems*. This negative emphasis can be devastating to a family and can undermine any hope of a therapeutic relationship between nurse and client. Families need their strengths reinforced. Emphasizing a family's strengths fosters a positive self-image, promotes self-confidence, and often helps a family feel better able to address other problems.

At times, community health nurses want to help families by taking one of the members to a doctor or to the store or by bringing a supply of formula or diapers. It might be a simple task, because you will be driving by the clinic anyway or there are extra cans of formula in the agency office, but will it promote the family's independence and self-sufficiency? It is a much better gift to promote the skill of planning ahead, so that the family may meet its own transportation needs (neighbors, family members, loose change saved for the bus, or even walking) or find ways to use formula supplies wisely. For example, bottles can be filled with only the amount the baby consumes, so that ounces are not wasted at each feeding. Unused formula should be kept refrigerated, so that it does not spoil, and care should be taken to make sure that infants are not overfed. The amount of formula consumed in 24 hours by the baby can be determined to ensure that the correct quantity is being provided. After a child reaches the appropriate age, foods and fluids other than formula may be provided. A can of powdered formula may be kept on hand for emergencies, and families may wish to switch to powdered formula if they are using the more expensive premixed or concentrated formulas. Once families learn these skills, crises will occur less frequently or will be managed more effectively.

Finally, you should always look for ways to genuinely praise families for managing in difficult situations. On a home visit, you can empower families by pointing out the positive aspects of their self-care and care giving, rather than pointing out what they do not do or have (Renpenning, Taylor, & Eisenhandler, 2003).

One helpful communication technique is **strengthening**. Verbally list the positive aspects of an otherwise negative situation in a natural and conversational manner. For example, a young woman, who is holding her baby, greets you at the door. You note that she has a dresser drawer on the floor next to her mattress for the baby to sleep in. They live in a sparsely furnished one-room apartment. She has two baby bottles and a limited assortment of baby clothes. Later during the first visit, you say, "Carlo looks so happy when you cuddle him in your arms, and you are considering his safety by letting him sleep in the dresser drawer next to your mattress. I notice you wash each bottle before making the formula, and you keep him warm in the sleeper and blanket. I think you are managing Carlo very well." In this brief scenario, you have mentioned, in a positive way, bonding, infant health and safety, and proper infant clothing. You have not mentioned the absence of furniture, a full set of bottles, or a layette of clothing. During the remainder of the visit, you discuss the services your agency can provide and assess whether any of them would be of interest to the young mother. This strengthening technique helps the nurse approach the family positively rather than with a condescending or punitive approach. And, in the above example, you have empowered this young mother to make decisions for her family and to use you as a resource and guide (Wright & Leahey, 2009).

If there is nothing positive the nurse can honestly say, he should be able at the very least to say that the family seems to be managing as best it can. This is not to say that the nurse should ignore problems. On the contrary, assessment should explore all aspects of family functioning to determine both strengths and weaknesses. The nurse needs a total picture to achieve an adequate perspective in nursing care planning and to know when the family is ready to begin work on problems. Even as the nurse becomes more aware of a family's unhealthy behaviors, the emphasis should remain on the positive ones. Emphasizing strengths indicates to the clients they are important to the nurse.

Family strengths are traits that facilitate the ability of the family to meet the members' needs and the demands made by systems outside the family unit. Not all traits that appear positive are necessarily strengths. Before the nurse selects a trait to emphasize, the behavior should be examined closely to determine whether it is actually facilitating family functioning. A strong work orientation may be a strength when balanced with play and relaxation, but in a family obsessed by work experiences, this trait is a weakness. Whether a trait is considered a strength or weakness is determined by the amount of free choice, as opposed to compulsive drive, being exercised.

Some traits a nurse may consider as possible strengths are basic family functions, family developmental tasks, and characteristics of family health. For instance, a nurse might wish to note when a family meets its members' physical, emotional, and spiritual needs; shows respect for members' various points of view; or fosters self-discipline in its children. An illustration of this principle is found in the family nursing care of the Stevensons (Display 19.7).

FAMILY HEALTH ASSESSMENT

The focus of each family visit is different. On a first visit, initial assessment data must be obtained in addition to helping the family set goals they want to accomplish. On subsequent visits, action and activities are taken to reach the goals. To assess a family's health in a systematic way, three tools are needed: (1) a conceptual framework on which to base the assessment, (2) a clearly defined set of assessment categories for data collection, and (3) a method for measuring a family's functional level.

Conceptual Frameworks

A **conceptual framework** is a set of concepts integrated into a meaningful explanation that helps one interpret human behavior or situations. Several conceptual frameworks have been used historically to study families (Hill & Hansen, 1960; Reiss, 1981). Anderson and Sabatelli (2010) have also published models describing family functioning. Three frameworks that are particularly useful in community health nursing are presented here: the interactional, structural–functional, and developmental frameworks.

The **interactional framework** describes the family as a unit of interacting personalities and emphasizes communication, roles, conflict, coping patterns, and decision-making processes. This framework focuses on internal relationships but neglects the family's interactions with the external environment.

The **structural–functional framework** describes the family as a social system relating to other social systems in the external environment, such as church, school, work, and the health care system. This framework examines the interacting functions of society and the family, considers family structure, and analyzes how a family's structure affects its function.

The **developmental framework** studies the family from a life-cycle perspective by examining members' changing roles and the tasks in each progression of life-cycle

DISPLAY 19.7 THE STEVENSON FAMILY

The community health nurse, Keith Dow, made an initial home visit after referral by an outpatient physician who was concerned about possible child abuse. Alice Stevenson had brought her baby to the emergency room for treatment of a laceration on the baby's forehead. He had fallen off the table while she was changing him, she claimed. A bruise on his arm made the physician suspicious, but Alice explained it was caused by his older brother's rough play. The nurse opened the visit by stating that he was simply following up on the emergency room treatment and wanted to see how the baby was progressing. Keith made no mention of child abuse. He observed the mother and children closely, looking for small things to compliment Alice on (strengthening) while learning all he could about the family's background. Because the nurse appeared approving rather than suspicious or judgmental, Alice agreed to further visits. During a later visit, Alice admitted to the nurse that she had slapped the baby and her ring cut his forehead. She could not get him to stop crying, no matter what she did; she just could not endure it any longer, she said. There had been other times when she grabbed him roughly to pull him away from things he wasn't allowed to touch, causing bruises on his arms. Alice told the nurse that she had not planned this baby; when her husband found out she was pregnant, he had left her shortly before the baby was born. Like many abusive parents, Alice had unrealistic expectations of her children's behavior as well as very inadequate self-esteem. Realizing that Alice would be particularly vulnerable to any criticism, the nurse concentrated on her strengths. Keith complimented her on how well she managed her home and dressed the children, on maintaining her job, and on reading to her 3-year-old son. It took many visits before Alice trusted the nurse, but in time, they were able to discuss her feelings frankly and work toward improving this family's health. Keith got her to attend a support group for single parents and she began counseling. Emphasizing strengths had provided a bridge for Alice and assisted in bringing her into a helping relationship.

stage. This framework incorporates elements from interactional and structural–functional approaches, so that family structure, function, and interaction are viewed in the context of the environment at each stage of family development.

Others have combined these concepts in various ways to design family assessment and intervention models that focus on human–environmental interactions, interactional and structural–functional frameworks, self-care, responses to stressors, and a developmental framework.

The six characteristics of healthy families already discussed serve as an initial framework for assessing family health by a combination of interactional, structural–functional, and developmental concepts.

Data Collection Categories

When using a conceptual framework for family health assessment, the community health nurse selects specific categories for data collection. The amount of data that one can collect about any given family may be voluminous, perhaps more than necessary for the purposes of the assessment. The assessment process is lengthy, time consuming, and ongoing. The nurse must gather the most essential on the first visit. By selecting one or two priority concerns of the family and the nurse, it is possible to focus assessment on these identified areas. The nurse then uses this information as a guide to obtaining additional information needed on subsequent visits.

Certain basic information is needed, however, to determine a family's health status and to design appropriate nursing interventions. From many sources in the family health literature, particularly Edelman and Mandle (2009) and Friedman et al. (2003), a list of 12 data collection categories has been generated. Table 19-1 lists the 12 categories, each grouped into one of three data sets: family strengths and self-care capabilities, family stresses and problems, and family resources.

1. *Family demographics* refer to such descriptive variables as a family's composition, its socioeconomic status, and the ages, education, occupation, ethnicity, and religious affiliations of members.
2. *Physical environment* data describe the geography, climate, housing, space, social and political structures, food availability and dietary patterns, and any other elements in the internal or external physical environment that influence a family's health status.
3. *Psychological and spiritual environment* refers to affective relationships, mutual respect, support, promotion of members' self-esteem and spiritual development, and life satisfaction and goals.
4. *Family structure and roles* include family organization, socialization processes, division of labor, and allocation and use of authority and power.
5. *Family functions* refer to a family's ability to carry out appropriate developmental tasks and provide for members' needs.

Table 19.1 Categories of Data Collection for Family Health Assessment

Assessment Categories	Family Strengths and Self-Care Abilities	Family Stresses and Problems	Family Resources
1. Family demographics			
2. Physical environment			
3. Psychological and spiritual environment			
4. Family structure/roles			
5. Family functions			
6. Family values and beliefs			
7. Family communication patterns			
8. Family decision-making patterns			
9. Family problem-solving patterns			
10. Family coping patterns			
11. Family health behavior			
12. Family social and cultural patterns			

6. *Family values and beliefs* influence all aspects of family life. Values and beliefs might deal with raising children, making and spending money, education, religion, work, health, and community involvement.
7. *Family communication patterns* include the frequency and quality of communication within a family and between the family and its environment.
8. *Family decision-making patterns* refer to how decisions are made in a family, by whom they are made, and how they are implemented.
9. *Family problem-solving patterns* describe how a family handles problems, who deals with them, the flexibility of a family's approach to problem solving, and the nature of solutions.
10. *Family coping patterns* encompass how a family handles conflict and life changes, the nature and quality of family support systems, and family perceptions and responses to stressors.
11. *Family health behavior* refers to familial health history, current physical health status of family members, family use of health resources, and family health beliefs.
12. *Family social and cultural patterns* comprise family discipline and limit-setting practices; promotion of initiative, creativity, and leadership; family goal setting; family culture; cultural adaptations to present circumstances; and development of meaningful relationships within and outside the family.

Assessment Methods

Many different methods are used to assess families. These methods serve to generate information about selected aspects of family structure and function; the methods must match the purpose for assessment and are done in conjunction with the family. Assessing family health may be done informally through observation and occasional questioning, or it can take a more formal approach. Specific questions may be asked of each family member, and information such as health data and family history may be included. Physical data such as height, weight, pulses, temperature, and blood pressure are recorded on an assessment tool. The developmental level of the family will guide specific assessment questionnaires, tools, or tests that the community health nurse can use for gathering information on individuals within the family, for example, the use of developmental screening tests for young children or a high-risk infant flow sheet (Fig. 19-1) for a newborn with an identified or potential health problem (e.g., high-risk newborn, drug-exposed newborn, failure-to-thrive, birth-defect).

Two assessment tools are the eco-map and the genogram. The **eco-map** is a diagram of the connections between a family and the other systems in its ecologic environment. It was originally devised to depict the complexity of the client's story. Developed by Ann Hartman in 1975 to help child welfare workers study family needs, the tool visually depicts dynamic family–environment interactions (Hartman, 1978). The nurse involves family members in the map's development. A central circle is drawn to represent the family, and smaller satellite circles on the periphery represent people and systems, such as school or work, whose relationships with the family are significant. The lines to and from the central circle to the satellite circle depicts the strength of the relationship (Fig. 19-2). The map is used to discuss and analyze these relationships.

FLOW SHEET—HIGH-RISK INFANT

Pt's Name ______________________ Address ______________________________ Phone ____________

At Birth: Weight ____________ Length __________ Head Circ. ____________ APGARS __________

	Date										
Irritability											
Lethargic											
Vomiting											
Diarrhea											
Feedings											
• Amount											
• Frequency											
• Suck											
Seizures/Convulsions											
Stools											
• Color											
• Consistency											
• Frequency											
Urine Output											
Edema											
Eyes Roll											
Temperature											
Pulse											
Respiration											
Weight											
Length											
Femoral Pulses											
Reflexes											
Muscle Tone											
Skin											
• Color											
• Condition											
Auscultate Chest											
Edema											
Output-Concentration											
Respiratory Function											
• Nasal Flaring											
• Grunting											
• Sternal Retracting											
• Tachycardia											
Head Circumference											
Chest Circumference											
Initials											

O - Normal X - Problem (See Narrative) C - Counseled for prevention

FIGURE 19-1. High-risk infant flow sheet.

Immunization (Circle & Date)

DTaP 1 2 3 4 ________ PPD ________ MMR ________ Hib ________

Polio 1 2 3 ________ Hep B ________ Varicella ________ PCV ________ RV ________ Flu ________

Instruction	Instruction Date	Pt. Understanding Date	Pamphlets Given Date	Comments	Initials
Review Disease Process					
Temperature Technique					
Feeding & Technique					
Bonding					
General Care					
• Bath					
• Hygiene					
• Formula Preparation					
• Cord Care					
Prevention of Infection					
Environment—Temperature Control					
Position					
Growth & Development					
Safety					
Stimulation					
Immunizations					
Referred to:					
Medical App./Date/M.D.					
S/S of Sick Child					

Initials	Signature

FIGURE 19-1. *(Continued)*

The **genogram** displays family information graphically in a way that provides a quick view of complex family patterns. It is a rich source of hypotheses about a family over a significant period of time, usually three or more generations (McGoldrick, Gerson, & Petry, 2008). Family relationships are delineated by genealogic methods, and significant life events are included (e.g., birth, death, marriage, divorce, illness). Identifying characteristics (e.g., race, religion, social class), occupations, and places of family residence is also noted. Again, this tool is used jointly with the family. It encourages family expression and sheds light on family behavior and problems (Fig. 19-3). Recognizing the value of this type of assessment, the *U.S. Surgeon General's Family History Initiative* was launched in 2005. This ongoing initiative seeks to bring awareness of the familial links between health outcomes and the need to develop prevention strategies based on potential health risks (USDHHS, 2012). Using the downloadable materials provided on the Web site, families can create their own family heath portrait; this is also a valuable tool for the nurse to use with the family. *Healthy People 2020* builds on this theme, stressing that genetic testing and family health history should guide clinical and public health interventions (USDHHS, 2010).

Community health nurses use several different family assessment instruments to gather data on family structure, function, and development. Public health nursing agencies usually develop their own tools, often in the form of questionnaires, checklists, flow sheets, or interview guides. The format varies to fit organizational needs. For example, most agencies have changed to computerized information management systems and have adjusted data collection to be technologically compatible. Two sample assessment tools are shown in Figures 19-4 and 19-5. Figure 19-4 shows a checklist format with scores and dates of

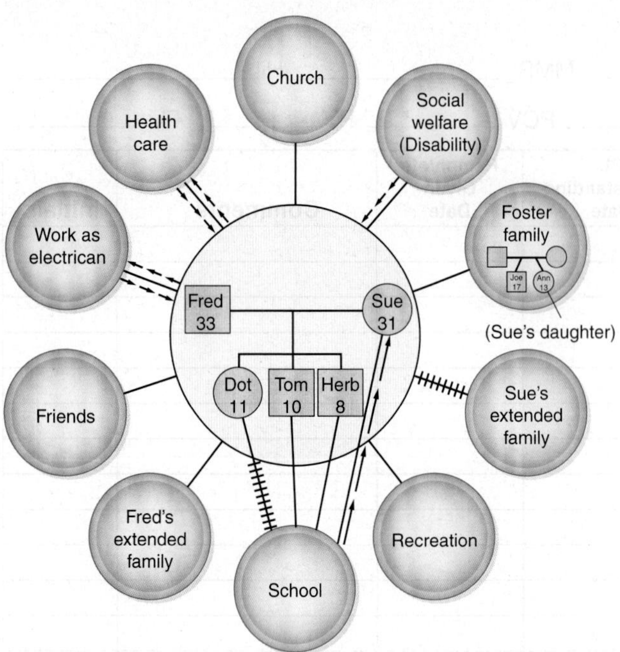

FIGURE 19-2. Eco-map of family's relationship to its environment. Lines indicate types of connections: *solid lines*, strong: *dotted lines*, tenuous; *lines with crossbars*, stressful. *Arrows* signify energy or resource flow, and absence of lines indicates no connection.

assessment gathering. It is useful over a span of time for observing family growth or decline, especially for the novice community health nurse, who can document assessment data as rapport with the family is established or as the comfort level with home visits increases.

Figure 19-5 offers an open-ended assessment tool. Such a tool may be useful in a teen perinatal program or a senior support program, in which a primary nurse makes the home visits and an additional nurse visits occasionally. The open-ended format is brief and lends itself to subjectivity. The goal is to create a document that is informative for all who use it while limiting subjective observations—a difficult task with open-ended tools. However, there may be an agency or program for which this tool fits best.

Other methods may use assessment tools or technology (e.g., videotaping family interactions, structured observation, and analysis of life-changing events). The Self-Care Assessment Guide (Cleveland & Allender, 1999) measures a family member's ability to provide self-care (Fig. 19-6). In a public health nursing agency or other community-based agency, documentation is completed for individuals after family assessment information data are gathered. Useful information can be gathered about stressors and self-care practices, including prescription medicines, over-the-counter (OTC)

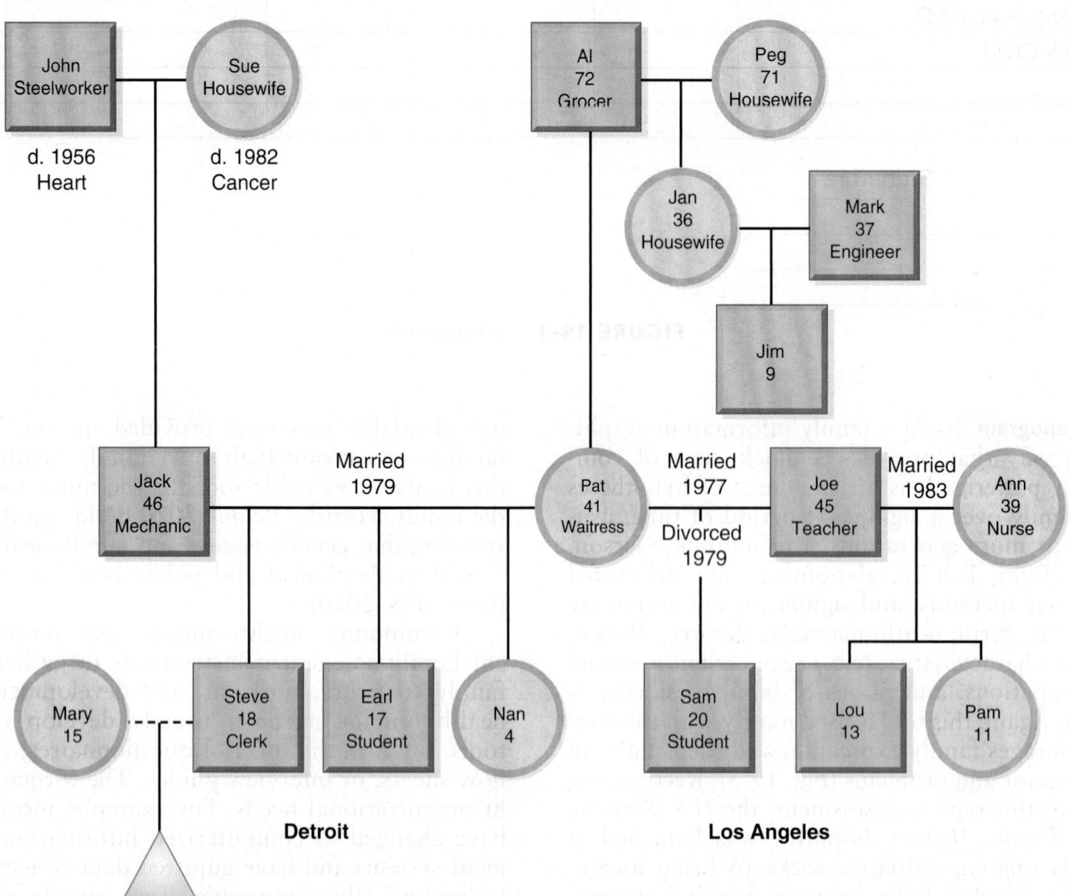

FIGURE 19-3. A genogram depicting three generations of family history. *Square*, male; *circle*, female; *triangle*, infant; *solid line*, married; *broken line*, not married.

medicines, herbal remedies, nutritional supplements, and other complementary therapies. Such tools are useful adjuncts, especially for families coming from cultural groups different from that of the health care provider. They are often used in combination with other tools to enhance the breadth of data collection and understanding of the family.

GUIDELINES FOR FAMILY HEALTH ASSESSMENT

An assessment of family health will be most accurate if it incorporates the following five guidelines:

1. Focus on the family as a total unit.
2. Ask goal-directed questions.

Family Assessment

Family Name ____________________

Family Constellation

Member	Birth Date	Sex	Marital Status	Education	Occupation	Community Involvement

Financial Status ____________________

Using the following scale, score the family based on your professional observations and judgement:

0 = Never 3 = Frequently
1 = Seldom 4 = Most of the time
2 = Occasionally N = Not observed

	score	date	score	date	score	date	score	date
Facilitative Interaction among Members								
a. Is there frequent communication among all members?								
b. Do conflicts get resolved?								
c. Are relationships supportive?								
d. Are love and caring shown among members?								
e. Do members work collaboratively?								
Comments ____________________								
Totals								
Enhancement of Individual Development								
a. Does family respond appropriately to members' developmental needs?								
b. Does it tolerate disagreement?								
c. Does it accept members as they are?								
d. Does it promote member autonomy?								
Comments ____________________								
Totals								

FIGURE 19-4. Family assessment using questions based on characteristics of healthy families.

	score	date	score	date	score	date	score	date
Effective Structuring of Relationships								
a. Is decision making allocated to appropriate members?								
b. Do member roles meet family needs?								
c. Is there flexible distribution of tasks?								
d. Are controls appropriate for family stage of development?								
Comments ______________________________								
Totals								
Active Coping Effort								
a. Is family aware when there is a need for change?								
b. Is it receptive to new ideas?								
c. Does it actively seek resources?								
d. Does it make good use of resources?								
e. Does it creatively solve problems?								
Comments ______________________________								
Totals								
Healthy Environment and Life-style								
a. Is family life-style health promoting?								
b. Are living conditions safe and hygienic?								
c. Is emotional climate conducive to good health?								
d. Do members practice good health measures?								
Comments ______________________________								
Totals								
Regular Links with Broader Community								
a. Is family involved regularly in the community?								
b. Does it select and use external resources?								
c. Is it aware of external affairs?								
d. Does it attempt to understand external issues?								
Comments ______________________________								
Totals								

FIGURE 19-4. *(Continued)*

3. Collect data over time.
4. Combine quantitative and qualitative data.
5. Exercise professional judgment.

Focus on the Family, Not the Member

Family health is more than the sum of its individual members' health. If the health of each person in a family was rated and the scores combined, the total would not show how healthy that family is. To assess a family's health, the nurse must consider the family as a single entity and appraise its aggregate behavior (Centers for Disease Control and Prevention, 2012; Wright & Leahey, 2009). As each criterion in the assessment process is considered, the community health nurse asks, "Is this typical of the family as a whole?" Assume that the nurse is assessing the communication patterns of a family. The nurse observes supportive interaction between two members in the family. What about the others? Further observation shows good communication among all but one member. It may be decided that, despite that one person, the family as a whole has good communication. If individual behavior deviates from that of the aggregate, the nurse notes the differences. They can influence total family functioning and need to be considered in nursing care planning.

FAMILY ASSESSMENT

Family Name ____________________

Family Constellation

Member names	Occupation	Educational background

Significant change in family life —

Coping ability of family —

Energy level —

Decision-making process within the family—

Parenting skills —

Support systems of the family—

Use of health care (include plans for emergencies) —

Financial status —

Other impressions —

Signature of Nurse ____________________ Date ____________

FIGURE 19-5. Open-ended family assessment.

Ask Goal-Directed Questions

The activities of any investigator, if fruitful, are guided by goal directed questions. When solving a crime, a detective has many specific questions in mind. So, too, does the physician attempting a diagnosis, the teacher trying to discern a student's knowledge level, or the mechanic repairing a car. Similarly, the nurse determining a family's level of health has specific questions in mind. It is not enough to make family visits and merely ask members how they are. If relevant data are to be gathered, relevant questions must be asked. The family assessment tool shown in Figure 19-4 provides a sample set of questions that community health nurses use to assess a family's health. Built on the framework of the characteristics of a healthy family, these questions guide thinking and observations. They direct attention to specific aspects of family behavior to facilitate the goal of discovering a family's level of health.

Consider the characteristic, "Active Coping Effort." When visiting a family, the community health nurse watches for signs of the family's response to change and its problem-solving ability. The nurse asks, "Does this family recognize when it needs to make a change?" or "How does it respond when a change is imposed?" Perhaps a health problem has arisen; for instance, the baby has diarrhea. Does the family assume responsibility for dealing with the problem? Do family members consider a variety of ways to solve it? How do they respond to the nurse's suggestions? Do they seek out resources on their own, such as reading about causes of infant diarrhea, using home remedies, or consulting with the community health nurse, the doctor, or a nurse practitioner? How well do they use resources, once identified? Do they try creative methods for solving the problem and see it through to resolution? As the nurse focuses on these behaviors, he is asking goal-directed questions aimed at finding out the family's coping skills. This investigation is one part of the nurse's assessment of the family's total health picture.

The set of questions presented in Figure 19-4 is one useful way to appraise family health. Another, more open-ended format is used by some community health nursing agencies. This approach, displayed in Figure 19-5, proposes assessment categories as stimuli for nursing questions. When exploring family support systems, for example, the nurse asks, "What internal resources or strengths does this family have?" "Who outside the family can and do they turn to for help?" "What agencies such as churches, clubs, or community services do they use?" The open-ended style of this assessment tool allows questions aimed at determining family health to be raised.

SELF-CARE ASSESSMENT GUIDE

Name ______________________ Birth date __________

Address ______________________ Phone number __________

Names of health care providers visited in past year:

Name	Discipline	Address	Phone number	Times visited past year
1.				
2.				

Surgeries (Include date)

1. ______________________
2. ______________________

Major acute illnesses (Include date; indicate whether hospitalization was necessary)

1. ______________________
2. ______________________

Chronic illnesses (Include date)

1. ______________________
2. ______________________

Age of parents (If deceased, indicate date of death, age at death, and cause of death)

Mother ______________ Father ______________

Age of grandparents (If deceased, indicate age at death and cause of death)

MGM ________ MGF ________ PGM ________ PGF ________

Natural teeth Y N

Dentures or partials Y N

Dental care: ____ Brush teeth/Frequency __________
____ Floss teeth/Frequency __________

Women/men over 50 Sigmoidoscopy/colonoscopy Date ______

Women

Breast self-exam Y N Frequency __________
Mammograms Y N Frequency __________
Pap smears Y N Frequency __________

Men

Testicular self-exam Y N Frequency __________

PSA Y N Date ______ Results ______

TB skin test (Date) __________ Results ______

Immunizations

Td/Tdap ______________________
Flu vaccine ______________________
Hepatitis vaccine ______________________
Zoster ______________________
Other ______________________

Weight (At age 25) ____Current weight ____Normal weight ____

Height (At age 25) ____Current height ____

Dietary practices (24-hour dietary recall)

First meal (Time) ____ Contents (Include amount) __________

Second meal (Time) ____ Contents (Include amount) __________

Third meal (Time) ____ Contents (Include amount) __________

Snacks (Include time, contents, and amount) __________

Usual food eaten (not mentioned above) __________

Foods not eaten at all (by preference) __________

Food allergies __________

Medicine allergies __________

Food taboos __________

Religious practices that affect health (prayer, special practices or services) __________

Exercise patterns (Include sample activities, duration, frequency, problems or side effects):

1. ______________________
2. ______________________

Medications and therapies

OTC drugs (Include name, length of treatment, frequency of use, side effects):

1. ______________________
2. ______________________
3. ______________________
4. ______________________

Prescription drugs (Include name, length of treatment, frequency of use, side effects):

1. ______________________
2. ______________________
3. ______________________
4. ______________________

Folk medicine/home remedies (e.g., postpartum isolation, mustard poultice for chest congestion):

1. ______________________
2. ______________________
3. ______________________
4. ______________________

Complementary therapies (e.g., biofeedback, imagery, herbalism)

1. ______________________
2. ______________________
3. ______________________
4. ______________________

Plan for self-care improvement

Overall goal ______________________

Areas needing modification (e.g., enhancement, moderation, deletion; include short- and long-term goal for each area):

1. ______________________
STG: ______________________
LTG: ______________________
2. ______________________
STG: ______________________
LTG: ______________________

Client role to reach long-term goals

Nurse's role(s) to reach long-term goals (e.g., collaboration, teaching, evaluation)

Others' roles in reaching goals (Include discipline, name, address and phone number)

1. ______________________
2. ______________________

Comments

FIGURE 19-6. Self-care assessment guide. Adapted from Cleveland, L., & Allender, J. A. (1999). Environment: Self-care issues. In L. Cleveland, D. S. Aschenbrenner, S. J. Veneable, & J. A. P. Yensen (Eds). *Nursing management in drug therapy*. Philadelphia, PA: Lippincott Williams & Wilkins, with permission.

Allow Adequate Time for Data Collection

Accurate family assessment takes time. The assessment initiated on the first or second visit will most likely give only a partial picture of how a family is functioning. Time is needed to accumulate observations, make notes, and see all the family members interacting together in order to make a thorough assessment. To appraise family communication patterns, for instance, the nurse needs to observe the family as a group, perhaps at mealtime or during some family activity. The family needs to feel comfortable in the nurse's presence, so that they will respond freely; time and patience are needed for such rapport to develop.

Consider one nurse's experience. Jolene Burns had talked with the Olson family twice, first in the clinic, and then at home. Because Mr. Olson had not been present either time, Jolene asked to see the family together and arranged an early evening visit. The Olsons were receiving nursing services for health promotion. They were particularly interested in discussing discipline of their young children. They contracted with Jolene for 6 weekly visits to be held in the late afternoon, when Mr. Olson was home from work. Jolene's assessment began with her first contact with the Olsons. She made notes on their chart and, guided by questions similar to those in Figure 19-5, kept a brief log. After the fourth visit, she filled out an assessment form to keep as a part of the family record. It was not until then that Jolene felt she had collected enough data to make valid judgments about this family's level of health.

Combine Quantitative With Qualitative Data

Any appraisal of family health must be qualitative. That is, the nurse must determine the presence or absence of essential characteristics in order to have a database for planning nursing actions. To guide planning more specifically, the nurse can also determine the degree to which various signs of health are present. This is a quantitative measure. The nurse asks whether a family does or does not engage in some behaviors and how often. Is this behavior fairly typical of the family, or does it occur infrequently? Figures 19-4 and 19-5 demonstrate ways to measure family health quantitatively.

For example, if the nurse were to use the tool in Figure 19-4 to assess the Beck family's ability to enhance individuality, he could score behavior on a scale from 0 (never) to 4 (most of the time). After several observations, the nurse would probably conclude that responses to the members' developmental needs were appropriate most of the time (*a* under "Enhancement of Individual Development"). Opposite *a* on the assessment form, the nurse would write the numeral 4 and the date of assessment.

The value of developing a quantitative measure is to have some basis for comparison. The nurse can assess a family's progression or regression by comparing its present score with its previous scores. For instance, had the nurse conducted a family health assessment of the Kovacs 6 months ago and compared it with their present level of health, he would probably have discovered a drop in their scores in several areas. Many of their communication patterns, role relationships, and coping skills, in particular, would show signs of deterioration. A scored assessment gives a vivid picture of exactly which areas need intervention. For this reason, it is useful to conduct periodic assessments when a case is reopened, or every 3 to 6 months if it is kept open for an extended period. The nurse can monitor the progress of high-risk families through early introduction of preventive measures when a trend or regressive behavior is observed. Periodic quantitative assessments also provide a means of evaluating the effectiveness of nursing action and can point to documented signs of growth.

Quantitative data serve another useful purpose. The nurse can compare one family's health status with that of another family as a basis for priority setting and nursing care planning. The difference in the level of health between the Becks and the Kovacs, for example, shows that the Kovacs need considerably more attention right now.

Exercise Professional Judgment

Although nurses seek to validate data, their assessment of families is still based primarily on their own professional judgment. Assessment tools can guide observations and even quantify those judgments, but, ultimately, any assessment is subjective. Even though it may be observed that a family makes good use of a community agency, the decision that use of this external resource contributes to the health of the family is a subjective one. This determination is not bad. Indeed, effective health care practice depends on sound professional judgment. However, nurses must be cautious about overemphasizing the value or infallibility of an assessment tool. It is only a tool and should be used as a guide for planning, not as an absolute and irrevocable statement about a family's health status. Caution is particularly important when dealing with quantitative scores, which may seem to be objective.

Ordinarily, assessment of a family is best conducted unobtrusively. An assessment tool used by the nurse is not a questionnaire to be filled out in the family's presence but rather a way to guide the nurse's observations and judgments. Before going into a family's home, the community health nurse may wish to review the questions. He may find it helpful to keep the assessment tool in a folder for easy reference during the visit. Depending on the nurse's relationship with the family, notes may be made during or immediately after the encounter. Like Jolene, the nurse may choose to keep a short log—an accumulation of notes—until enough data have been collected to complete the assessment form. Occasionally, a family with high self-care capability may be involved in the assessment. The nurse should introduce the idea carefully and use professional judgment to determine when the family is ready to engage in this kind of self-examination.

EDUCATION AND HEALTH PROMOTION

Teaching health promotion activities should begin only after family members express an interest and recognize a need. If the family is not at a level of functioning that enables members to use anticipatory guidance and teaching, the nurse can provide more basic services, such as gathering resources and acting as a counselor. If family members are ready to learn ways to improve their health status, the nurse needs to assess the best teaching approach to use and tailor interventions to the specific family needs and functional capability (Monsen, Radsosevich, Kerr, & Fulkerson, 2011; Monsen, Sanders, et al., 2011). Consideration of language barriers, previous knowledge and experience, family and community resources, and time available will influence the choice of approach (see Chapter 11).

EVALUATING IMPLEMENTED FAMILY HEALTH PLANS

The final step in the nursing process is evaluation. The evaluation process leads to a reassessment of your work with the family and a determination of what is needed in preparation for the next visit. This reassessment helps you in further individualizing services to the family. Evaluation of the structure-process of the visit and your self-evaluation can be done informally in a reflective manner. Outcomes are documented in the client record, and the evaluation becomes formalized. A thorough evaluation also assists you in making the most appropriate referrals and contacting key resources to meet family needs.

Types of Evaluations

Each family visit should be evaluated in three ways: structure-process, outcome, and self-evaluation. Each provides a different piece of information about the success of the visit. If the visit was not successful, what part made it less than successful? Most importantly, were the outcomes achieved? If not, is there something about the structure-process or your own preparedness or behavior that needs to be changed? When conducting an evaluation of the home visit, you are looking for answers to these questions.

Structure-Process

The structure-process of a visit should be analyzed first. Were there aspects of the organization, timing, environment, or sequencing of the components that needed to be changed or modified to make it a more effective visit? What could you have done about these factors? Were you organized? Would better preparation help with your organization? Were there distractions in the home that influenced organization? Ask yourself questions such as these, and then make plans to avoid or reduce disorganizing distractions. For example, if you made the visit based on limited information from a referral, you now have additional family data and can be better prepared for the next visit. If transportation schedules made the family late to the clinic, perhaps other transportation could be arranged. If the distraction on a home visit occurred because children were arriving home from school, visits could be made earlier in the day. If the television was playing loudly, you could make it a point to ask the family whether they would mind turning down the volume, or visit at a time when they do not watch television. Make the modifications that you can to assist with the visit process.

Outcome Evaluation

Second and most important is evaluation of the outcomes of the visit. Were the anticipated outcomes achieved? If not, why? If so, what made it possible? The **outcome evaluation**, or the assessment of change in the family's (client's) health status based on mutually agreed activities, is a formal process demonstrated in the documentation of the home visit. The agency may use the Nursing Outcomes Classification (NOC) System along with the Nursing Intervention Classification (NIC) System, or it may use the Omaha System discussed in Chapters 12 and 14. Alternatively, there may be agency-driven criteria for success and expectations for each client category or visit type. On a visit-by-visit basis, the changes observed in the family may be small; progress toward an expected outcome is noted. At the conclusion of agency services to the family, the cumulative changes in the client's health and the success or failure to achieve various outcomes are evaluated. Depending on the conclusions that can be drawn, the decision to terminate services may need to be reevaluated. It is possible that continuance of service is required, and the terms must be renegotiated. Whatever the decision, the family must be included in the decision-making process.

Self-Evaluation

The third component of evaluation is self-evaluation. What aspect of your performance as a community/public health nurse during the home visit facilitated the achievement of a desired outcome? Were you prepared? Did you gather all the data needed to assist the family on the next visit? What would you do differently if you could do the visit over? What went right? What went wrong? What are you going to do on the next visit to make it better? This closer look at yourself is important for your own growth and effectiveness as a community health nurse. Beam, O'Brien, and Neal (2010) describe how self-evaluation or reflection can be used during maternal-child home visiting to improve practice.

Sometimes, we cannot see our own strengths or flaws, and evaluations by others are helpful. In some agencies, regular peer evaluations are conducted. An agency staff nurse makes a family visit with the community health nurse and provides feedback based on her observations. This is a useful technique to use even at times other than planned evaluations of all staff members in the agency. You might ask a colleague to accompany you on a home visit to a family that has not made progress toward outcome achievement or to a family you have not been able to "reach" or find difficult to work with (Drummond, Weir, & Kysela, 2002). For a variety of reasons, consultation with peers regarding certain visits and how best to conduct them can assist you in being better prepared or more focused. It can improve your interaction with families from different cultures or in difficult situations (Spector, 2008).

Planning for the Next Visit

Part of the evaluation of one family visit is planning for the next. Use what occurred on the previous visit to guide you toward activities on subsequent visits. Goals may need to be modified, or family situations may change and specific outcomes become irrelevant. For example, you may plan to visit a prenatal family one last time before the baby is born to reinforce prior teaching about when to leave for the hospital with a second pregnancy. You intend to remind the parents to arrange babysitting for the older child and to assess the pregnant woman's rising blood pressure and complaints of backache. When you arrive for the visit, the husband is home alone with the younger child and is about to leave to bring his wife and new baby home from the hospital. He asks you about the diaper rash that just appeared on the 2-year-old. He also asks how to secure the new car seat into the car, because the instructions do not seem to make sense for his make of car. Outcomes for a problem-free pregnancy and healthy birth are no longer relevant; there are new outcomes to be formulated and worked on with this young family.

More frequently, planning for subsequent visits is relatively predictable and is done to ensure that steps toward outcome accomplishment are achieved on the visit. Being totally prepared each time is the best predictor of a successful family visit. Once you have met and gotten to know a family during a visit, the planning can be individualized and tailored to meet the family's unique needs. This information is not available from a paper referral, which makes planning for a first home visit important. The tone set during the first visit can affect your continued success with the family.

Referrals

A referral in written or verbal form (by agency-created form, telephone, fax, or e-mail) initiates contact with a family. In addition to responding to a referral, which begins the relationship with a family, the nurse makes referrals on behalf of the family. Families often need access to services beyond the agency's scope, and the nurse's knowledge of other resources can mean the difference between their having and not having access to additional services. Therefore, nurses must have information available to them about the eligibility requirements and availability of services provided by a bevy of official, voluntary, religious, and neighborhood organizations. If this information is not readily at hand, community health nurses need to know how to locate needed services. This is a daunting challenge, because the services are many, and organizations frequently change telephone numbers, Web sites, services, and the populations they serve. Networking with colleagues on a regular basis helps keep nurses up to date with community services from which they can generate referrals for clients.

Contacting Resources

At times, community health nurses implement their roles as client advocates by facilitating easier access to services for the family. Community health nurses know how to access key personnel in agencies and can eliminate some of the red tape involved in obtaining services. Nurses can provide pointers that may help families procure needed services; for example, clients may have an advantage if they go to an agency early in the morning in the middle of the week. The fact that they should have all forms completely filled out and should bring their last 3 month's rent and utility receipts, or that they should ask to speak with a certain worker, may also be helpful information.

When nurses seek informal services for families, a relationship with the director of the agency can help them gain services for the clients. For example, a client family has a personal crisis and needs a donation of food and a volunteer to stay with a handicapped child for 3 days while a spouse undergoes surgery. The nurse telephones the religious leader of a neighborhood church and shares the family's requests, clarifies the situation, and gets a donation of food from the church's food pantry. The name of a member of the church who can stay with the child is also provided. The family may not have been aware that such services were available to them, and the links provided by the nurse are as important as other community health nursing functions.

SUMMARY

The family unit remains the focus of service in community health nursing. Family health and individual health strongly influence each other, and family health also affects community health. Assessing, planning, implementing, and evaluating nursing care are steps used to deliver care to clients in acute care settings, in the extensive clinic system, and in the home.

It is important for the nurse to understand healthy family characteristics and to use a variety of tools so that family assessments are thorough.

Healthy families demonstrate six important characteristics:

1. A facilitative process of interaction exists among family members.
2. Individual member development is enhanced.
3. Role relationships are structured effectively.
4. Active attempts are made to cope with problems.
5. There is a healthy home environment and lifestyle.
6. Regular links with the broader community are established.

To assess a family's health systematically, the nurse needs a conceptual framework on which to base the assessment, a clearly defined set of categories for data collection, and a method for measuring the family's level of functioning. The six characteristics of a healthy family provide one assessment framework that community health nurses can use. Assessment tools to aid the nurse in appraising the health of families include the eco-map and the genogram.

There are 12 main categories of family dynamics for which the nurse must collect data: family demographics, physical environment, psychological/spiritual environment, family structure and roles, family functions, family values and beliefs, family communication patterns, family decision-making patterns, family problem-solving patterns, family coping patterns, family health behaviors, and family social and cultural patterns.

Community health nurses enhance their practices with families by observing five principles: work with the family collectively, start where the family is now, fit nursing interventions to the family's stage of development, recognize the validity of family structural variation, and emphasize family strengths.

During assessment, the nurse should focus on the family as a total unit, use goal-directed assessment questions, allow adequate time for data collection, combine quantitative with qualitative data, and exercise professional judgment.

Making family health visits is a unique role for nurses and is one of the activities common to most community/public health nurses. In some agencies, family health visits are conducted for only the most high-risk families. In other agencies, a visit is the method of choice for most care.

When nurses visit families, they must use acute observational skills, good verbal and nonverbal communication, assessment skills, and a "sixth sense" to guide them safely in the community and with the families they visit. Some visits are conducted with families in settings other than their homes. Neighborhood clinics, schools, work places, or recreational settings may be the preferred or the only locations in which you can gather most of the family members for the visit. Other families may be in transition and living in homeless shelters or with relatives or neighbors. These settings are familiar to the family and provide a unique environment for the nurse in which to visit the family.

Previsit preparation, conduct of the visit, and postvisit documentation are the main components of a family health visit. Each step is important and has value for the success of the next step. Being well prepared for a visit is the first concern (e.g., know the location, have family health status information and needed materials). The visit should be conducted in an orderly and organized fashion. Time should be allowed for getting acquainted, for the body of the visit, including teaching and anticipatory guidance, and for any other nursing care that may be a part of the visit. Concluding with a summary of the important parts of the visit and planning for the next visit ensures an appropriate ending.

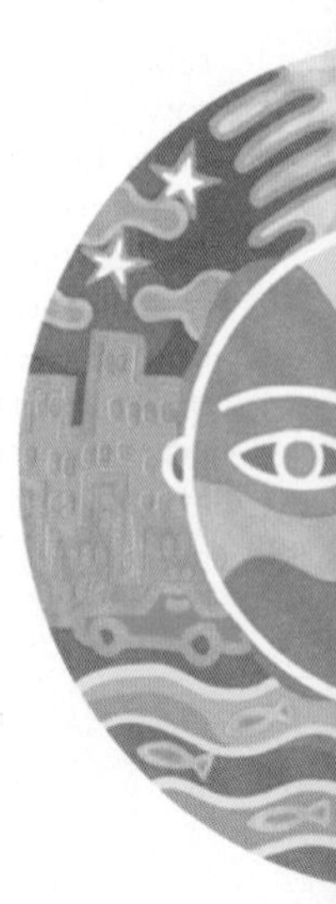

Being safe in a neighborhood is important for all people. Community health nurses spend a great part of the day in the community, and safe travel is of constant importance. Use of a personal or agency car, public transportation, or walking to visit families each has its own set of precautions for personal safety. Even in a family's home, personal safety must be a consideration. If family members are arguing or under the influence of drugs or alcohol, the situation may deteriorate rapidly and become unsafe; at this point, it is best to terminate the visit.

During the implementation phase of the family health visit, the nurse establishes a verbal or written contract with the family. This permits understanding by both the family and the nurse of the personal roles and responsibilities in the relationship. Empowerment of family members is significant for clients. People who are empowered can help themselves for a lifetime and can make independent decisions about their own health.

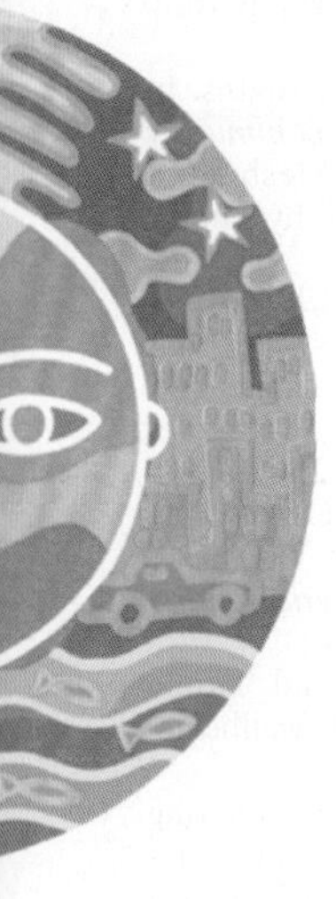

Evaluation and preparation for the next visit completes the family health visit cycle. Three types of evaluation can be conducted at the end of a visit. Recall of the structure-process assists the nurse in reflecting on the physical aspects of the visit that were positive or negative. Discovering these factors can help enhance the positive and eliminate the negative. Evaluating whether the outcomes of the visit were achieved is done in a more formal way with agency documentation. Because the purpose of conducting family health visits is to bring about positive changes in family behaviors, it is necessary to evaluate the achievement of mutual goals made by the nurse and the family. The hardest part of evaluation is looking at yourself and how you conduct home visits. Often, peer evaluation is a helpful way to obtain feedback, because people tend to minimize their own strengths and overlook their weaknesses.

Conducting family health visits involves making referrals to other agencies and services on behalf of the family. One agency cannot provide all the services that a family needs. Written or verbal forms of communicating a need involve contacting resources available in the community. Community health nurses have unique skills in knowing and locating both official and voluntary services within their community. Such skills come with experience.

ACTIVITIES TO PROMOTE **CRITICAL THINKING**

1. Construct an eco-map of your family. Ask a peer to do the same thing. Assess the balance between your family and the resources in its environment. How does your eco-map compare with that of your peer? What changes are needed in each family system? Are you able to influence the changes that are needed?
2. Draw a genogram of your family and ask a peer to discuss it with you. Make your drawing of the genogram as complete as possible. Then analyze your thoughts and feelings. How did you feel while tracing your family history? Did you learn anything new about your family? Did any family trends or traits appear? Did any uncomfortable or suppressed information come to the surface? Do you have any new insights about your family?
3. Assess a family (other than your own) that you know well by completing a family assessment guide. You may use one of the forms in this chapter or an available form from another source. Based on your assessment, determine as many nursing interventions as you can think of that could be used to promote this family's health as practically as possible.
4. Invite a peer to go on a family health visit with you, and be open to feedback regarding your strengths and weaknesses. How does it make you feel to have someone else on a family health visit with you, knowing they are observing your skills? Offer to do the same for a peer and provide him with feedback. Discuss your experience.
5. Go on several family health visits with an experienced community health nurse and observe the nurse's visiting techniques. Observe how he contacts the family; knocks on the door; greets the family; conducts, summarizes, and concludes the visit; and makes plans for the next visit. Discuss the various techniques used and ask questions about your observations to get a better idea of why things are done as they are. Use some of this information on your next home visit.
6. Initiate a small group discussion among your peers about safety on your school campus and in your community. Encourage each person to share the safety habits used. How are these techniques different from safety techniques used when making home visits in the community? If they are different, why? Should they be different?

REFERENCES

Allender, J. A. (1998). *Community and home health nursing.* Philadelphia, PA: Lippincott-Raven.

American Nurses Association. (2007). *Public health nursing: Scope and standards of practice.* Silver Spring, MD: Nursesbooks.org.

Anderson, S. A., & Sabatelli, R. M. (2010). *Family interaction: A multigenerational developmental perspective* (5th ed.). Upper Saddle River, NJ: Pearson.

Barker, P. (2007). *Basic family therapy* (5th ed.). Hoboken, NJ: Whiley-Blackwell.

Beam, R. J., O'Brien, R. A., & Neal, M. (2010). Reflective practice enhances public health nurse implementation of Nurse-Family Partnership. *Public Health Nursing, 27*, 131–139. doi: 10.1111/j.1525-1446.2010.00836.x

Becvar, D. S., & Becvar, R. J. (2008). *Family therapy: A systematic integration* (7th ed.). Columbus, OH: Allyn & Bacon.

Centers for Disease Control and Prevention—National Center for Health Statistics. (2012). *National Survey of Family Growth.* Retrieved from http://www.cdc.gov/nchs/nsfg.htm

Cleveland, L., & Allender, J. A. (1999). Environment: Self-care issues. In L. Cleveland, D. S. Aschenbrenner, S. J. Veneable, & J. A. P. Yensen (Eds.), *Nursing management in drug therapy.* Philadelphia, PA: Lippincott Williams & Wilkins.

Drummond, J. E., Weir, A. E., & Kysela, G. M. (2002). Home visitation practice: Models, documentation, and evaluation. *Public Health Nursing, 19*, 24–29.

Eckenrode, J., Campa, M., Luckey, D. W., Henderson, C. R., Cole, R., Kitzman, H., et al. (2010). Long-term effects of prenatal and infancy nurse home visitation on the life course of youths, 19-year follow-up of a randomized trial. *Archives of Pediatrics & Adolescent Medicine, 164*(1), 9–15.

Edelman, C. L., & Mandle, C. L. (Eds.). (2009). *Health promotion throughout the life span* (7th ed.). St. Louis, MO: Mosby.

Friedman, M. M., Bowden, V. R., & Jones, W. (2003). *Family nursing: Research, theory and practice* (5th ed.). Upper Saddle River, NJ: Prentice-Hall.

Haggman-Laitila, A., Tanninen, H., & Pietila, A. (2010). Effectiveness of resource-enhancing family-oriented intervention. *Journal of Clinical Nursing, 19*, 2500–2510. doi: 10.1111/j.1365-2702.2010.03288.x

Hartman, A. (1978). Diagrammatic assessment of family relationships. *Social Casework, 59*(10), 59–64.

Hill, R., & Hanson, D. (1960). The identification of conceptual frameworks utilized in family study. *Marriage and Family Living, 22*, 299–311.

Kaakinen, J., Gedaly-Duff, V., Hanson, S., & Coehlo, D. (2009). *Family health care nursing: Theory, practice, and research* (4th ed.). Philadelphia, PA: F.A. Davis.

Kendra, M. A., & George, V. D. (2001). Defining risk in home visiting. *Public Health Nursing, 18*, 128–137.

Kneipp, S. M., Kairalla, J. A., Lutz, B. J., Pereira, D., Hall, A. G., Flocks, J., et al. (2011). Public health nursing case management for women receiving temporary assistance for needy families: A randomized controlled trial using community-based participatory research. *American Journal of Public Health, 101*, 1759–1768. doi:10.2105/AJPH.2011.300210

McGoldrick, M., Gersen, R., & Petry, S. (2008). *Genograms: Assessment and intervention* (3rd ed.). New York, NY: W.W. Norton & Company.

Monsen, K. A., Radosevich, D. M., Kerr, M. J., & Fulkerson, J. A. (2011). Public health nurses tailor interventions for families at risk. *Public Health Nursing, 28*, 119–128. doi: 10.1111/j.1525-1446.2010.00911.x

Monsen, K., Sanders, A., Yu, F., Radosevich, D., & Geppert, J. (2011). Family home visiting outcomes for mothers with and without intellectual disabilities. *Journal of Intellectual Disability Research, 55*, 484–499. doi: 10.1111/j.1365-2788.2011.01402.x

Olson, D., McCubbin, H., Barnes, H., Larson, A., Muxem, A., & Wilson, M. (1983). *Families: What makes them work?* Beverly Hills, CA: Sage.

Otto, H. A. (1973). A framework for assessing family strengths. In A. Reinhardt, & M. Quinn (Eds.), *Family-centered community nursing: A sociocultural framework.* St. Louis, MO: Mosby.

Parachin, V. M. (1997, March/April). Six signs of a healthy family. *Vibrant Life*, 5–6.

Pender, N. L., Murdaugh, C. L., & Parson, M. A. (2011). *Health promotion in nursing practice* (6th ed.). Upper Saddle River, NJ: Pearson.

Reiss, D. (1981). *The family's construction of reality.* Cambridge, MA: Harvard University Press.

Renpenning, K. M., Taylor, S. G., & Eisenhandler, S. A. (2003). *Self-care theory in nursing: Selected papers of Dorothea Orem.* New York, NY: Springer.

Schorr, T. M., & Kennedy, M. S. (1999). *100 years of American nursing.* Philadelphia, PA: Lippincott Williams & Wilkins.

Shepherd, M. L. (2011). Behind the scales: Child and family health nurses taking care of women's emotional wellbeing. *Contemporary Nurse, 37*(2), 137–148

Shin, S. H., Choi, H., Kim, M. J., & Kim, Y. H. (2010). Comparing adolescents' adjustment and family resilience in divorced families depending on the types of primary caregiver. *Journal of Clinical Nursing, 19*, 1695–1706. doi: 10.1111/j.1365-2702.2009.03081.x

Spector, R. E. (2008). *Cultural diversity in health and illness* (7th ed.). Upper Saddle River, NJ: Prentice-Hall.

Thompson, P. (1998). Adolescents from families of divorce: Vulnerability to physiological and psychological disturbances. *Journal of Psychosocial Nursing and Mental Health Services, 36*(3), 34–39.

U.S. Department of Health and Human Services. (2010). *Healthy People 2020. Topics and objectives.* Retrieved from http://www.healthypeople.gov/2020/topicsobjectives2020/default.aspx

U.S. Department of Health and Human Services. (2012). *U.S. Surgeon General's Family Health History Initiative.* Retrieved from http://www.hhs.gov/familyhistory/.

Vanderburg, S., Wright, L., Boston, S., & Zimmerman, G. (2010). Maternal child home visiting program improves nursing practice for screening of woman abuse. *Public Health Nursing, 27*, 347–352. doi: 10.1111/j.1525-1446.2010.00865.x

Wright, L., & Leahey, M. (2009). *Nurses and families: A guide to family assessment and intervention* (5th ed.). Philadelphia, PA: F.A. Davis.

Zerwekh, J. V. (1997). Making the connection during home visits: Narratives of expert nurses. *International Journal for Human Caring, 1*(1), 25–29.

thePoint: Everything You Need to Make the Grade!

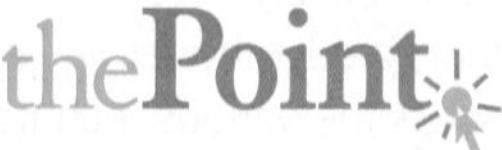

Visit http://thePoint.lww.com/Allender8e for selected readings, study aids for all learning styles, and more!

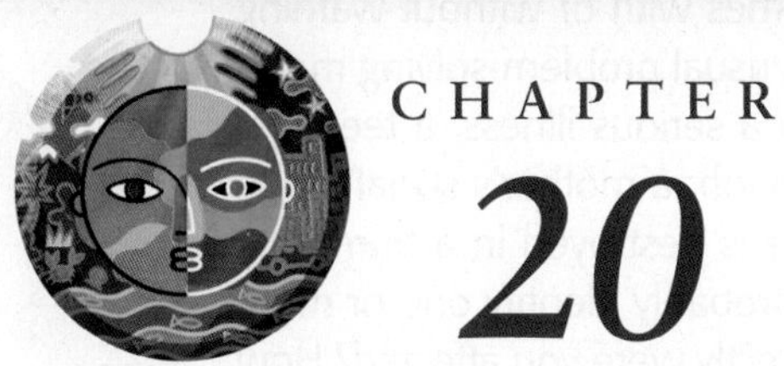

CHAPTER 20

Violence Affecting Families

"The right things to do are those that keep our violence in abeyance; the wrong things are those that bring it to the fore."

—*Robert J. Sawyer* (1960), Calculating God

KEY TERMS

Adolescent dating violence (ADV)
Battered child syndrome
Child abuse
Crisis theory
Cycle of violence
Developmental crisis
Elder abuse
Emotional abuse
Intimate partner violence (IPV)
Mandated reporters
Neglect
Physical abuse
Sexual abuse
Shaken baby syndrome
Situational crisis

LEARNING OBJECTIVES

Upon mastery of this chapter, you should be able to:

- Explain the difference between developmental crises and situational crises, and give examples of each within families.
- Discuss strategies to prevent the impact of a situational crisis and a developmental crisis at a primary, secondary, and tertiary level of prevention.
- Discuss the global incidence and prevalence of family violence.
- Describe how the United States has responded to family violence.
- Identify characteristics of abuse against infants, children, and adolescents.
- Describe the "cycle of violence" seen in intimate partner/spousal abuse.
- Explain common types of elder abuse.
- Describe the community health nurse role with families in crises at each level of prevention.
- Use the nursing process to outline nursing actions in developmental and situational crises.

A *family crisis* is a stressful and disruptive event (or series of events) that comes with or without warning and disturbs the equilibrium of the family. A family crisis can also result when usual problem-solving methods fail. All families experience periods of crisis: a toddler is diagnosed with a serious illness; a teenager discovers she is pregnant; a father and sole breadwinner in a family loses his job; a mother's social drinking becomes habitual after her children go off to college; or a family's home is destroyed in a hurricane, earthquake, flood, or fire. If you think back on your family's history, you can probably identify one or more periods of crisis that you and your family members experienced. If so, how directly were you affected? How did the crisis resolve? As a result of the crisis, did any permanent changes occur in your family's dynamics or individual behaviors?

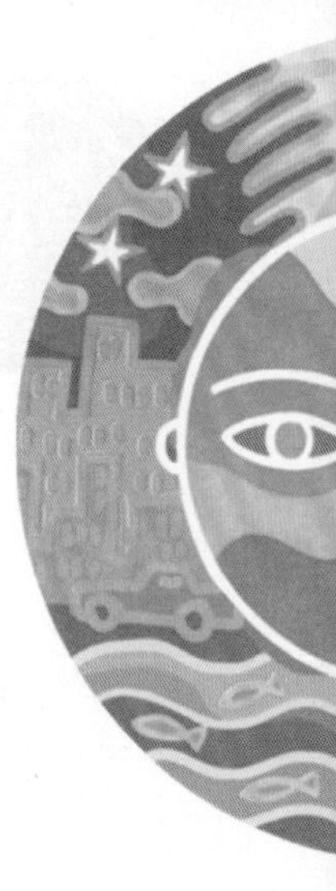

People respond to crises differently. Some people approach crisis as a challenge, an event to be reckoned with, while others may feel overwhelmed and defeated or give up. Some individuals seek help if needed and come through the experience unscathed or as survivors, perhaps even stronger than before. Other individuals who are unable to cope with the crisis, or who do not cope well, may suffer severe psychological damage or may inflict their feelings of rage, frustration, or powerlessness onto their children, partners, or elders. This chapter focuses on families that have responded to stressors with violence, neglect, or abuse and those that have experienced stress and loss as a result of violence initiated by others.

Regardless of their responses, families in crisis need help, and community health nurses have a unique opportunity and responsibility to provide that help in a broad variety of situations. For example, in one family, an 8-year-old boy begins doing poorly in school; he wets his pants during class twice in 1 week and starts a small fire in the schoolyard. The school nurse is astute enough to begin an investigation into the family dynamics that may be contributing to these symptoms. In another family, a pregnant woman reschedules her appointment at a community clinic twice and then arrives at the appointment with multiple faded bruises on her face and arms. The clinic nurse uses sensitivity and caring while screening her for domestic violence.

Primary and secondary prevention measures used by community health nurses that help prevent crises include teaching families parenting skills and coping strategies and informing them about community resources. In addition to assessment and education, community health nurses provide tertiary responses with direct assistance during times of crisis. This chapter discusses the knowledge and skills that community health nurses use in their practice of crisis prevention and intervention aimed at promoting improved health for families in the community.

DYNAMICS AND CHARACTERISTICS OF A CRISIS

Researchers have studied the nature of crises and have developed a body of knowledge called **crisis theory**. Initially limited to the field of mental health, crisis theory now influences every field of health care. The theory helps to explain why people respond in certain ways during a crisis and predicts phases people go through during and after a crisis. These responses and phases are important ideas for the community health nurse to understand before working in prevention or management of crises.

How does a crisis occur? Each of us is a dynamic system living within a given environment under circumstances unique to us alone. Our behavior—both consciously and subconsciously—is gauged to maintain a balance within ourselves and in our relations with others. When some internal or external force disrupts our system's balance and alters its functioning, a loss of equilibrium occurs. The individual then attempts to restore equilibrium by using whatever resources are available to him or her, in an effort to cope with the situation. Coping refers to those actions and ways of thinking that assist people in dealing with and surviving difficult situations. If individuals cannot readily cope with a stressful event—for example, if one's home is destroyed by fire, or one fails a final examination—the person experiences a crisis.

Crises are precipitated by a specific identifiable event that becomes too much for the usual problem-solving skills of those involved. Often, a single distressing event follows a host of previous difficulties and becomes the "straw that breaks the camel's back." For example, a wife who suffers years of spousal abuse finally becomes unable to cope and shoots her husband during a violent attack. Occasionally, tragic events occur suddenly without previous stressors, as when a father is killed in a plane crash or a child drowns in the family swimming pool.

Crises are normal in that all people feel occasionally overwhelmed. A person intervening in a crisis today may well be tomorrow's crisis victim. No individual is immune from sudden overwhelming difficulties. For example, Barbara, a hospice nurse, assists families through crises as part of her job, and suddenly, her own spouse is diagnosed with cancer. Her coping skills are strained as she feels overwhelmed with personal and increased demands that require her support and attention.

Often a crisis is not an event per se, but rather a person's perception of the event. Each person reacts in his own way. A situation that throws one person off course may merely create an interesting detour for another (see Display 20.1). It is usually the individual's interpretation of the event, rather than the event itself, that is crucial. At other times, a community crisis occurs on a large scale or is so unexpected that the crisis directly involves people who are known by others hundreds of miles away, causing distant friends and relatives shock and sorrow. Examples of such crises are Hurricane Katrina, or a night-club fire that kills dozens of people, or the terrorist attacks on September 11, 2001. Even strangers, knowing no one involved directly, are affected and experience signs and symptoms of stress (Levy & Sidel, 2002).

Crises are resolved, either positively or negatively, within a brief period, usually 4 to 8 weeks (Aguilera, 1998; Hoff, 2001). People's strong need to regain homeostasis and the intense nature of crises contribute toward making the crisis a temporary condition that will not continue indefinitely. In the family in which the wife shot her abusive husband, as shocking as the event might seem, life returns to a recognizable pattern within a few weeks. Even though family members will feel the change for years, the crisis soon subsides. The husband is hospitalized and recovers from his wound; the wife's case goes to trial, and she is sentenced to 2 years in prison; the children stay with relatives and attend school.

Crisis resolution can be an adaptive process in which growth and improved health occur, or it can be maladaptive, resulting in illness or even death. The battered wife reevaluates her life, gets divorced, learns employment skills in jail, and becomes more assertive, with stronger self-esteem; after she is paroled, she returns to her children, now able to support them financially and emotionally. She finds personal growth and health while successfully resolving the crisis. The children settle into their aunt's home with minimal difficulty, start a new school, and visit their mother and father regularly. After release, the mother finds an apartment near her sister's home, so that the children can continue in the same school district. The husband recovers from his wounds, gets counseling, relocates to another town, and sees his children frequently. The crisis situation is resolved at a higher level of wellness for all members than existed before the crisis. In this example, the members are determined to improve their situation by working with skilled health care professionals. By using the resources within the community, this family is healthier after the crisis.

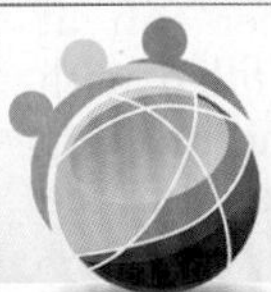

DISPLAY 20.1 TWO FAMILIES' RESPONSE TO CRISIS

The Redondos and the Fosters will be moving to a town in another state, 900 miles away, because of a job change. The Redondos are in crisis over the move. They have never lived in any other town. They will have to leave relatives and lifelong friends who live nearby and a community in which they have been very involved. Mrs. Redondo is the secretary at her family's house of worship. Their teenage daughter, a cheerleader, just started high school. Their son is in kindergarten; Grandma happily watches him in the mornings before school. Everyone is upset because of how the move will affect them. The family is stressed and argues each evening. They don't want to put their house up for sale or even to visit the new community to which they will be moving. Mr. Redondo is second-guessing his decision to move, but his choices were limited as his company is relocating. The Redondos, in crisis, are not exploring alternatives that may allow them to stay in their present community. One possible alternative might be for Mrs. Redondo to work while Mr. Redondo looks for another job. When people perceive that they are in crisis, decision making and problem solving become more difficult.

The Fosters, however, are excitedly looking forward to their move. They have two young children who are not yet in school. The move will bring them only 50 miles from old college friends. They hope to realize a significant profit on their house, which they recently remodeled. They can't wait to go "house hunting" in the new town. Everyone is enjoying planning the anticipated move; their two children, aged 3 and 4, have been playing "moving day" with their favorite toys.

Both families are experiencing the same event. The difference is each person's situation and perception of the event. The Redondos' equilibrium is being disrupted. They have not developed previous coping skills and do not see the move as a positive experience. They are at a different time in their family life cycle than are the Fosters. Although the move upsets their equilibrium, too, the Fosters experience it as an exciting event that conjures positive feelings; they are passing these feelings on to their children. They see this move as an opportunity.

Developmental Crises

Developmental crises are periods of disruption that occur at transition points during normal growth and development (see Display 20.2). When developmental crises occur, people feel threatened by the demands placed on them and have difficulty making the changes necessary to fit the new stage of development.

During the process of normal biopsychosocial growth, people go through a succession of life cycle stages, from birth through old age. Each stage differs from the previous one, and transitions from one stage to the next require changes in roles and behavior. Popular and classic authors such as Levinson (1978), Bridges (1980, 2001), Sheehy (1976, 1992, 1999), and Sheehy and Delbourgo (1996) have called these periods "passages" and "transitions." These transitions are times when developmental or maturational crises occur.

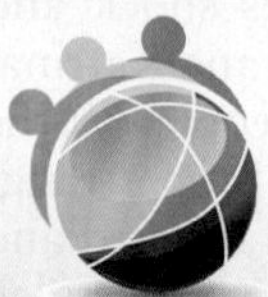

DISPLAY 20.2 MAJOR DIFFERENCES BETWEEN TYPES OF CRISES

Developmental Crisis

Part of normal growth and development that can upset normalcy
Precipitated by a life transition point
Gradual onset
Response to developmental demands and society's expectations

Situational Crisis

Unexpected period of upset in normalcy
Precipitated by a hazardous event
Sudden onset
Externally imposed "accident"

Most family developmental crises have a gradual onset. The change is evolutionary rather than revolutionary. People usually anticipate and even prepare to start school, enter adolescence, leave home, marry, have a baby, retire, or die. Individuals move into and through each transitional period knowing in advance that some kind of change will be required. In many instances, people have already seen others experience these transitions. As a result, developmental crises have a degree of predictability. These developmental crises offer a time for anticipation and adjustment.

Developmental crises arise from both physical and social changes. Each new life stage confronts people with changed relationships, responsibilities, and roles. The transition to parenthood, for example, demands a change in role from caring for oneself and one's mate to include nurturing, caring for, and protecting a completely helpless infant. Relationships with adults, children, and even one's parents also change. Parenthood is an entrance into a previously inexperienced part of the adult world. New parents may fear the unknown. Will this infant develop normally? Can I give adequate care? Parents often feel anxiety about the responsibility of shaping this new person's life, satisfying society's expectations for their child's proper education and training, or bringing children into a world that is in crisis and already overpopulated. Parents may worry about the increased financial burden while struggling with mixed feelings about giving up a large measure of freedom. These transitions put people under considerable stress, which contributes to tension, feelings of helplessness, and resultant crisis. Some people adapt quickly; others cannot cope, probably because earlier developmental crises went unresolved. If people lack a repertoire of adaptive skills, even positive and planned changes can develop into crises (Display 20.3).

DISPLAY 20.3 A DEVELOPMENTAL CRISIS

Marcia Sand is 39 years old. Married for 22 years, she has been a capable homemaker and mother of four children. Her husband, Lou, a construction worker for the past 20 years, thinks Marcia does a "super job at home." In the past, Marcia's time was filled with cooking, laundry, cleaning, shopping, and meeting the endless demands of the family. Their limited income prompted her to adopt many money-saving strategies. She made most of her own and the children's clothes, did all her own baking, and raised vegetables in her backyard garden. Now the youngest of the children, Tommy, has just left home to join the Navy. Her husband spends much of his spare time at the local bar with his friends, leaving Marcia alone. With a nearly empty house and little need for cooking, baking, and sewing, Marcia has lost her sense of usefulness. She thinks of taking a job but knows her choices are limited because she has only a high school education. Marcia has not slept well in weeks; she wakes up tired and drags through the day barely able to manage the simplest task. She cries frequently but does not know why. Her hair, always neat and attractive in the past, looks bedraggled, and her shoulders slump. "I just can't seem to get on top of things any more," she complains.

Marcia has entered a developmental crisis that is sometimes called the "empty nest syndrome." She faces a turning point in her life, a time when parenting has seemingly ended. Leaving her satisfying homemaker role, she faces a new life stage filled with unknowns, changes, and a seeming lack of purpose. The transition came about gradually, almost imperceptibly, but now she must deal with it. Yet she feels unable to cope and wishes to turn to someone who would understand and lend her strength. She can be helped, but her crisis could also have been prevented at the precrisis phase. Anticipatory planning could have prevented the dilemma Marcia finds herself in now.

Situational Crises

A **situational crisis** is a stressful, disruptive event arising from external circumstances that occur suddenly, often without warning, to a person, group, aggregate, or community. Typically, the external event requires behavioral changes and coping mechanisms beyond the abilities of the people involved.

Such events are not predicted, expected, or planned. The crisis occurs to people because of where they are in time and space. For instance, a baby grabs her mother's hot cup of tea and burns her chest; a college student is raped in the library parking lot; an older adult falls and fractures a hip; a mother with a van full of Little League baseball players has a crash at a busy intersection; or a hurricane devastates a state. These events, which involve loss or the threat of loss, represent life hazards to those affected. Some crisis-precipitating events can be positive, such as a significant job promotion or sudden acquisition of great wealth; however, the change still makes increased demands on individuals who must make major life adjustments. Even positive events involve a modified grieving process, because the individuals involved may be losing or giving up old, familiar, and comfortable situations and facing stressful changes.

Community health nurses see an almost infinite variety of situational crises, including debilitating disease, economic misfortune, unemployment, physical abuse, divorce, unwanted pregnancy, drug and alcohol abuse, sudden death of a loved one, tragic accidents such as a drowning or plane crash, and many others. In each situation, people feel overwhelmed and need help to cope. Skilled intervention can make the difference between a healthy and an unhealthy outcome.

Multiple Crises

Different kinds of crises can overlap in actual experience, compounding the stress felt by the persons involved. For example, a couple may experience a developmental crisis (birth) and a situational crisis (birth defect) simultaneously, thus compounding the resulting stress. The developmental crisis of midlife may be complicated by situational crises such as a divorce or job change. With older adults, the developmental crisis of retirement may be compounded by the situational crisis of a fire that destroys the family home. The transition a child faces entering school may occur at the same time the family moves to a new neighborhood and a new infant joins the family. The child must share the parent's attention and affection with a new sibling at a time when all the child's resources are needed to cope with starting school and adjusting to the new neighborhood. Classic research shows that accumulated stresses can lead to ill health (Holmes & Rahe, 1967). Those who normally work through one crisis in a healthy way may find that compounding events overwhelm them, causing more stress than they can handle.

HISTORY OF FAMILY VIOLENCE

Family crisis is not limited to the developmental crises people experience or the situational crises that come upon us suddenly, usually from forces—such as nature—that are external to the family. Many women and children in the world also experience the crisis of domestic violence. The terms domestic violence, family violence, and interpersonal violence refer to morbidity and mortality attributable to violence within the home setting, involving action by a family member or intimate partner. Domestic violence involves "a systematic pattern of assaultive and coercive behaviors, including physical, sexual, and psychological attacks and economic coercion, that adults or adolescents use against their intimate partner" (Kramer, 2002, p. 190). This type of violence occurs worldwide and is becoming a global public health burden.

Global History

Family violence is not new. For centuries, children were thought of as the property of their parents, and any treatment doled out by the parents was their prerogative. In fact, most countries had animal welfare laws long before child welfare laws were adopted. In addition, the ideology of childhood that emerged in the Western world in the late 1800s assumed that only "abnormal" children needed protection. These children were casualties of an urban–industrial society and were abandoned, dependent, or delinquent—the products of social dislocation such as orphans or refugee children.

In the early 1900s, sensitive leaders concerned with child welfare issues emerged. Several international agencies were created designed to positively affect the health of children. The British Children's Act was passed in 1908, and the first White House Conference on Children was held in 1909. These were early attempts to define a role for the state in the welfare of children. The U.S. conference was the forerunner of the United States Children's Bureau (USCB), and a national voluntary organization, later known as the Child Welfare League of America, was established to complement federal agency efforts (Bolen, 2001). The USCB became a model for other countries, with well-developed programs targeting infant mortality. In one innovative program of the early 1900s, a heated, mobile, child welfare center was used in rural communities and was staffed by a female physician and a public health nurse to improve health care to children.

Other international organizations emerged in the early 1900s including the International Association for the Promotion of Child Welfare (IAPCW), the League of Red Cross Societies (LRCS), the Save the Children Fund (SCF), and the Save the Children International Union (SCIU). The latter two agencies were immensely successful in raising funds for children in Germany, Austria, France, Hungary, and Serbia. As these organizations began serving the needs of children internationally, they moved from a sentimental depiction of victims to a medico-social-scientific view of children at risk, expanding and uncovering the concepts of child victimization, exploitation, and abuse (Bolen, 2001).

By the mid-1920s, the work of these agencies began to focus on children from non-European countries. The first conference on children from non-European countries focused on African children in 1931 and included such issues as infant mortality, child labor, education, and child slavery. In 1924, the League of Nations adopted the Declaration of the Rights of the Child, which would influence the League of Nation's successor, the United Nations (UN), in the years to come in the form of the Declaration of the Rights of the Child (1959) and the Convention on the Rights of the Child (1989).

The UN continues to hold annual hearings on the Rights of the Child and has addressed global concerns, such as children without parental care, indigenous children, violence against children, HIV/AIDS, children with disabilities, and the economic exploitation of children (Office of the United Nations High Commissioner for Human Rights, Committee on the Rights of the Child, 2007).

Children are not the only victims of family morbidity and mortality from violence. Historically, women were also treated as property and often suffered physical and psychological damage. Gender-based violence, or violence against women (VAW), has global public health and human rights ramifications (World Health Organization [WHO], 2007a). Worldwide, between 15% and 71% of women have experienced physical or sexual violence (WHO, 2007a). Abuse toward women is often perpetrated by an intimate partner and is not reported. Areas of war and conflict have been known to use sexual violence toward women as a war tactic (WHO, 2007a). As with children, the rights of women are socially, culturally, and religiously influenced, with change coming slowly.

United States History

The history of treatment of children, women, and elders in the United States began with emigration in the 1500s and has been influenced by the cultural and religious practices of early settlers. In addition, necessity, attitudes of the time, and the stress and hardship of life in the colonies and on the frontier influenced how people were treated.

Children were born into families to help with the chores of an agricultural society. Families had many children, infant mortality rates were high, and it was not uncommon for half of the children in a family to die before their second birthday. Older people did not retire; they contributed to family survival until they died. There were no special considerations for children, women, or elders. The best a woman could hope for was that the man she married would not abuse her emotionally, physically, sexually, or fiducially (taking advantage of a person's financial resources). Women had limited or no education, resources, or rights, and children had none. If a woman married "poorly," she would have to live with the consequences. Separation and divorce were either unheard of or were a "death sentence" for the woman and her children, because there was nowhere they could go and no way for the woman to support her family.

Public Laws and Protection

It took many years for the United States to establish laws that benefited women and children. Nonetheless, the United States began earlier than many other countries to protect children, women, and elders. The Children's Bureau began to focus on child abuse in the 1960s, supporting development of a child abuse mandatory reporting law in 1962 to be used as a model by the states. The law required health professionals and child care workers to report suspected child abuse to appropriate officials.

In 1974, the Child Abuse Prevention and Treatment Act (CAPTA) was passed, becoming Public Law 93-247 (PL 93-247). This law served to reinforce the earlier mandatory reporting law model and was aimed at solving the growing problem of child abuse in the country. PL 93-247 has been amended several times since 1974. The Child Abuse Prevention and Treatment and Adoption Reform Act of 1978 preceded the Family Violence Prevention and Services Act of 1984. Later, all three acts were consolidated into the Child Abuse Prevention, Adoption, and Family Services Act of 1988 (PL 100-294), and most recently, the Act was amended and reauthorized as the Keeping Children and Families Safe Act of 2003 (PL 108-36) (Child Welfare Information Gateway, 2004).

PL 108-36 supports funding to states in their efforts to prevent violence in families and to identify and treat victims. The funding comes in the form of the CAPTA and state grants that meet eligibility requirements (Administration for Children and Families [ACF], 2006). One aspect of the funding supports the National Child Abuse and Neglect Data System (NCANDS) that tracks reports of child abuse and neglect and all fatalities from child abuse or neglect in the United States. In 2010, NCANDS reported an estimate of 1,262 child deaths caused by injury or neglect (ACF, 2010). Information on adoption, out-of-home care for children, preventing and responding to child abuse and neglect, supporting and preserving families, and resources are available via the Child Welfare Information Gateway, a program under the U.S. Department of Health and Human Services (USDHHS), Administration of Children and Families. The Administration on Aging, also under the USDHHS, supports similar programs including the National Center on Elder Abuse (2006) that works to educate and assist families, seniors, and health care and legal providers regarding elder abuse.

Healthy People 2020 Goals

The goal for *Healthy People 2020* regarding injury and violence prevention is to prevent unintentional injuries and violence and reduce their consequences (USDHHS, 2010, 2011). Determinants that affect violence include (a) individual behavior, (b) physical environment, (c) access to services, (d) social environment, and (e) societal-level factors. Through previous tracking and program strategies, new focus areas in violence prevention have been identified. The *Healthy People 2010* final review (Centers for Disease Control and Prevention [CDC], 2010b) demonstrated declines in several areas and identification of new or modified objectives for 2020. Declines were seen in physical assaults by intimate partners from 3.6 to 2.3 per 1,000 population; rape or attempted rape declined by 66.7% from 1998 to 2009; physical assaults dropped by 47.6% between 1998 to 2009 in the 12 years and older population, while physical fighting for 9th to 12th grade students dropped by 13.9%. Homicides remained essentially unchanged at 6.0 per 100,000 population in 1999 and 6.1 per 100,000 population in 2007.

Current *Healthy People 2020* trends identified for youth involve bullying, dating violence, and sexual violence, while the rates and causes of elder abuse were also cited as areas needing more research and strategies for prevention (USDHHS, 2010).

The problem of violence is pervasive, affecting the victim directly and family members and society indirectly. Selected violence and abuse objectives for *Healthy People 2020* include the following:

- Reduce homicides from a baseline of 6.1 deaths per 100,000 population that occurred in 2007 to a target of 5.5 homicides per 100,000 population
- Reduce child maltreatment deaths from 2.4 per 100,000 children under age 18 years that occurred in 2008 to a target of 2.2 deaths per 100,000 children in 2020
- Reduce the number of adolescents carrying weapons on school property during the past 30 days from a 2009 baseline of 5.6% of students in grade 9 through 12, to a target of 4.6% (data from Youth Risk Behavior Surveillance System [YRBS], CDC, 2010d)

Social environment and societal-level determinants are expanding in the *Healthy People 2020* tracking to investigate what works in violence prevention. This tracking is multifocused through research, program development, and policy making. Education programs on conflict resolution coping and bullying provide data and strategies to reduce violence among students. Policies and legislation that affect social attitudes and regulations to deter violence, promote community involvement, and create safer communities are also being studied. Investigating individual behaviors, such as risk-taking, drug and alcohol use, or factors influencing individual development, guide further learning of risk, as well as prevention measures.

Myths and Truths About Family Violence

Many myths about family violence need to be dispelled. Strongly held myths by members of society, including community health nurses and other health care providers, may interfere with their ability to help families in crisis get the help they need. Table 20-1 displays some common myths and truths about family violence.

Table 20-1 Common Myths and Truths About Abuse in Families

Myth	Truth
Violence in families is rare.	Family violence is common and increasing.
Violence occurs most frequently among low-income families.	Family violence occurs across all incomes.
Violence occurs more frequently in some racial and cultural groups.	Family violence occurs across all racial and cultural groups.
Violence in families does not coexist with love.	Love may exist but is unable to be displayed appropriately due to conflicting emotions.
Men who batter women are mentally ill.	The percentage of batterers who are mentally ill is the same as in the general population.
Women who accept battering are mentally ill.	The percentage of battered women who are mentally ill is the same as in the general population; however, they have low-esteem and a damaged spirit.
Violence occurs only in heterosexual relationships.	Domestic violence has no gender or sexual boundaries; it can occur among all people.
Abused women instigate the battering.	Quite the contrary, they go out of their way not to agitate or confront the abuser.
Abuse occurs when the abuser is under the influence of drugs or alcohol.	It can, but many abusers do not drink or use drugs.
Children should not be taken from their parents.	In some violent families, the safest place for the child is with another family member or a foster home (temporarily or permanently).
Even abusive parents are better for a child than a child living elsewhere.	Children must be protected, and living away from abusive parents may save their lives.
Abused children become abusive adults.	Some may but most can learn how to channel their emotions positively if the cycle of violence is broken.

FAMILY VIOLENCE AGAINST CHILDREN

Communicable diseases, as a cause of morbidity among children, "are coming under control through a combination of health promotion, prevention, and simplified standard treatment regimens. At the same time, the healthy growth and development of many children is threatened because there is a combination of rapid, often disruptive social, cultural, and economic changes" (WHO, 1998, p. 71). This continuing morbidity is psychosocial in nature and is associated with behavioral problems that are more difficult to prevent than the diseases known for centuries. In 2001, the WHO's Committee on the Rights of the Child stated, "Globally, around 40 million children are subjected to child abuse each year ... violence [that] results from individual, family, community, and structural factors" (para. 5–6), yet violence directed at children is preventable. The insult of violence against a child poses a potential risk for lifelong health problems including "depression, anxiety disorders, smoking, alcohol and drug use, aggression and violence towards others, risky sexual behaviors, and post-traumatic stress disorders" (WHO, n.d. b). Therefore, ending violence against children would "contribute to preventing a much broader range of noncommunicable diseases" (WHO, n.d. b.).

Child abuse defined by the federal CAPTA (42.U.S.C.A., 5106g) from the *Keeping Children and Families Safe Act* of 2003 is "at minimum: any recent act or failure to act on the part of a parent or caretaker which results in death, serious physical or emotional harm, sexual abuse or exploitation; or an act or failure to act which presents an imminent risk of serious harm" (Child Welfare Information Gateway, 2008, para. 1). More commonly, child abuse is identified as maltreatment toward a child that may include physical, emotional, general neglect, medical or educational neglect, physical punishment or battering, emotional or sexual maltreatment and exploitation, or a combination of these mistreatments.

Child abuse and the associated psychosocial developmental problems are taking a toll globally in human costs and economically in health care services. Countries vary in risk toward children; the World Health Organization found that approximately 20% of women and 5% to 10% of men had experienced sexual abuse as a child. Youth violence, as well as homicide rates, had increased in many countries (WHO, 2002a, 2000b). Worldwide, fatal abuse of infants and very young children was nearly double that of children between 5 and 14 years old and varied with lower rates of child homicide in countries with higher levels of income (WHO, 2007b, chap. 3, p. 60). Identifying and gathering worldwide data about child abuse are difficult because many cases are not investigated and death reports may not be classified as the result of abuse or homicide.

Another concern for children is their role in families that may require very young children to aid the family financially. A child's "chores" may include spending the whole day scrounging around city dumps gathering bits of food, clothing, or other useful or saleable items. Some children are sold for sexual favors while others spend all day working in fields, home businesses, or "sweat shops" for the equivalent of pennies a day. In some societies, female children are not valued and are killed at birth, given away, or sold into slavery for a pittance.

Child abuse in the United States is most often recognized in the categories of neglect, physical abuse, sexual abuse, and emotional abuse. Often, there is an overlay of maltreatment when a report is made to Child Protective Services (CPS) or the police. The NCANDS reported 3.3 million referrals to CPS departments in 2010; three fifths of the CPS reports were made by professionals, such as teachers, law enforcement officers, and social services. Infants (birth to 1 year) had the highest victimization rate at 20.6 per 1,000 children in the same age group (ACF, 2010). Girls were victimized at a higher rate (51.2%) than boys (48.5%), while 44.8% of the victims were White, 21.9% were African American, and 21.4% were Hispanic (ACF, 2010). Neglect continued as the category of highest occurrence at 78.3%, while 17.6% of children were found to have suffered physical abuse, and sexual abuse was determined as the primary cause in 9.2% of the investigations. Of all child fatalities in the United States, 79.4% were in children 4 years of age or younger (ACF, 2010). NCANDS estimated 1,530 child fatalities in the United States in 2006 and 1,560 in 2010. The dependence of small children makes them vulnerable to abuse and neglect as shown in both the United States and worldwide child abuse data.

Nationally, measures have been taken to improve data gathering and information about violence toward children, as well as outcomes for these children. The *National Survey of Child and Adolescent Well-Being* (NSCAW) is a longitudinal study on the wellbeing of children who have encountered the child welfare system (ACF, 2007a, 2007b). Other important sources of tracking child maltreatment occur in conjunction with *Healthy People 2020*, the Youth Risk Behavior Survey, and the Child Welfare Outcomes 2006–2009: Report to Congress (ACF, 2010). The Outcomes reports describe state-level data and trends, as well as the demographic data of race, age, and ethnicity. Foster care children are also covered in the outcomes report and data.

Child Neglect

Neglect occurs when the physical, emotional, medical, or educational resources necessary for healthy growth and development are withheld or unavailable. Neglect is obvious to an observer if a very young child is playing unattended outside, is not dressed appropriately for the weather, or has an unkempt appearance. However, neglect is not always so obvious. Parents may refuse to buy eyeglasses for a child who needs them or to access dental care for severely decayed teeth (medical neglect). An 8-year-old may get to school only 3 days a week, possibly without breakfast and no lunch money or packed lunch (educational neglect). A family with three children may live in a sparsely furnished apartment with very little food available and only intermittent heat and multiple people coming and going in the residence, while the children may appear at school unwashed and without coats in winter weather (general neglect). Emotional neglect may be seen when demands placed on a child are excessive or inappropriate for her development, or the caretaker berates or verbally humiliates a child frequently and without reason.

Thousands of children in the United States experience neglect each day. They are frequently "invisible" victims. At times, sensational stories of severe child neglect are reported in the media and cause public outrage. Examples include 12 children found among piles of garbage in an abandoned apartment building during a drug raid; parents vacationing in Florida while their 2 daughters, aged 6 and 4, were left unattended at home; or 3 young children found barely alive, kept in a basement closet. However, most children suffering from neglect do not make newspaper headlines or television reports. They go to school like others. If they are fortunate, their plight is uncovered by a community health nurse, a teacher, neighbor, or counselor. Because of the invisibility of neglect, its prevalence is hard to estimate. Often cases of neglect are brought to the attention of the proper authority only during the investigation of other forms of abuse or family issues (Display 20.4).

Physical Abuse

Physical abuse is intentional harm to a child by another person that results in pain, physical injury, or death. The abuse may include striking, biting, poking, burning, shaking, or throwing the child. Corporal punishment, which involves violence against a child as a form of discipline, was an acceptable form of discipline earlier in our country's history and is still condoned in some subgroups. Many parents today were raised in families in which physical punishment was used as a form of discipline. Even today, it is not unusual to see a parent slap the hand of a toddler to get his attention after he has been told not to do something several times or to prevent him from touching something that would hurt him more than a slap on the hand. Most families know where to draw the line. Others—especially if they were raised with "the belt" or "the switch"—see no harm in using the same physical disciplinary practices with their children.

Some parents cannot control the degree of physical punishment they give their child. In one case in 2002, a mother repeatedly physically assaulted her young daughter while getting her into the car. The mother's behavior was recorded by the store's parking lot surveillance camera. Intervention and follow-up occurred, including incarceration and counseling for the mother and foster home placement for the child. If physical punishment is administered in anger, while the parent is under the influence of mind-altering substances or out of a sense of frustration, the punishment may cross over to become battering of the child.

C. Henry Kempe identified the **battered child syndrome** in the 1960s, now defined as "the collection of injuries sustained by a child as a result of repeated mistreatment or beating" (U.S. Department of Justice [USDOJ], 2002, p. 1). Battered child investigations require thorough follow-up and interviews with caretakers, medical personnel, family members, and school personnel. Investigators should be aware that "a major trait of abusive caretakers is either the complete lack of an explanation for critical injuries or explanations that do not account for the severity of injuries" (p. 4). Display 20.5 lists behavioral indicators of physical abuse (USDOJ, 2002).

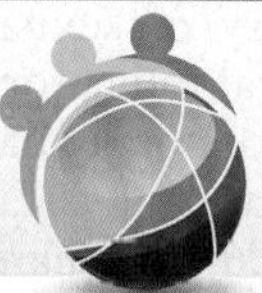

DISPLAY 20.4 SIGNS AND SYMPTOMS OF NEGLECT

Neglect may be suspected if one or more of the following conditions exist:

- The child lacks adequate medical or dental care.
- The child is often sleepy or hungry.
- The child is often dirty, demonstrates poor personal hygiene, or is inadequately dressed for weather conditions.
- There is evidence of poor or inadequate supervision for the child's age.
- The conditions in the home are unsafe or unsanitary.
- The child appears to be malnourished.
- The child is depressed, withdrawn, or apathetic; exhibits antisocial or destructive behavior; shows fearfulness; or suffers from substance abuse or speech, eating, or habit disorders (e.g., biting, rocking, whining).

Sexual Abuse

Sexual abuse of children includes acts of sexual assault or sexual exploitation of a minor and may consist of a single incident or many acts over a long period. Sexual assault includes rape, gang rape, incest, sodomy, lewd or lascivious acts with a child younger than 14 years of age (in most states), oral copulation, fondling of the child's genitals, penetration of the genital or anal opening by a foreign object, and child molestation. Sexual exploitation of children includes conduct or activities related to pornography that depict minors in sexually explicit situations and promotion of prostitution by minors (USDOJ, 2007). Incest is sexual abuse among family members who are related by blood (e.g., parents, grandparents, older siblings, aunts, and uncles); it constitutes the most hidden form of child abuse. Intrafamilial sexual abuse refers to sexual activity involving family members who are not related by blood (e.g., stepparents, boyfriends). In most reported cases, the father or male caretaker is the initiator, and the victim is a female child; however, boys are victims more often than previously believed, and adolescents were reported as "perpetrators in at

DISPLAY 20.5 SIGNS AND SYMPTOMS OF PHYSICAL ABUSE

Types of Injuries

Types of physical abuse injuries include bruises, burns, bite marks, abrasions, lacerations, head injuries, internal injuries, and fractures.

Behavioral Indicators of Physical Abuse

The following behaviors are often exhibited by physically abused children:

- The child is frightened of parents/caretakers or, at the other extreme, is overprotective of parent or caretakers.
- The child is excessively passive, overly compliant, apathetic, withdrawn or fearful or, at the other extreme, excessively aggressive, destructive, or physically violent.
- The child and/or parent or caretaker attempts to hide injuries; child wears excessive layers of clothing, especially in hot weather; child is frequently absent from school or misses physical education classes if changing into gym clothes is required; child has difficulty sitting or walking.
- The child is frightened of going home.
- The child is clingy and forms indiscriminate attachments.
- The child is apprehensive when other children cry.
- The child is wary of physical contact with adults.
- The child exhibits drastic behavioral changes in and out of parental/caretaker presence.
- The child is hypervigilant.
- The child suffers from seizures or vomiting.
- The adolescent exhibits depression, self-mutilation, suicide attempts, substance abuse, or sleeping and eating disorders.

Other indicators of physical abuse may include the following:

- A statement by the child that the injury was caused by abuse (chronically abused children may deny abuse).
- Knowledge that the child's injury is unusual for the child's specific age group (e.g., any fracture in an infant).
- Knowledge of the child's history of previous or recurrent injuries.
- Unexplained injuries (e.g., parent is unable to explain reason for injury; there are discrepancies in explanations; blame is placed on a third party; explanations are inconsistent with medical diagnosis).
- A parent or caretaker who delays seeking or fails to seek medical care for the child's injury.

least 20% of reported cases" (Kellogg, 2005). The initial sexual abuse may occur at any age, from infancy through adolescence. However, the largest number of cases involves girls younger than 11 years of age. Regardless of how gentle, trivial, or coincidental the first approach may have seemed, sexual coercion tends to be repeated and to escalate over a period of years. The child may blame himself or herself for tempting or provoking the abuser.

The mother, who is expected to protect the child, may purposely isolate herself from a problem of sexual abuse. Sometimes, the mother is distant, uncommunicative, or so disapproving of sexual matters that the child is afraid to speak up. Sometimes, she is extremely insecure and feels confrontation may cause anger or the loss of her husband or boyfriend, or the mother's economic security may depend on her partner/spouse. The mother may feel threatened or feel that she cannot allow herself to believe or even to suspect that her child is at risk. She may have been a victim herself of child abuse and may not trust her judgment or her right to challenge the man's authority in the home. Some mothers consciously acknowledge that their children are being sexually abused but, for whatever reason, choose to "look the other way." Until the victim is old enough to realize that incest or intrafamilial sexual abuse is not a common occurrence or is strong enough to obtain help outside the family, there is little chance of escape unless the abuse is reported (Crime and Violence Prevention Center, 2003b).

Indicators of sexual abuse are seen in various ways, and attention should be given to a history of sexual abuse, sexual behavior indicators, behavioral indicators in younger children and behavioral indicators of sexual abuse in older children and adolescents, and physical symptoms of sexual abuse (see Display 20.6). As mandated reporters, community health nurses should be aware that sexual abuse of a child may surface through a broad range of physical, behavioral, and social symptoms. Some of these indicators, taken separately, may not be symptomatic of sexual abuse and should be examined in the context of other behaviors or situational factors.

Community health nurses may be part of the Sexual Assault Response Team (SART). This group's responsibilities include obtaining the evidence and providing support to the victim and family after an episode of sexual abuse has been reported. SART members include nurses, physicians, social workers, police, laboratory personnel, lawyers, and district attorney staff. Care for children who have been sexually abused varies, as the duration of the molestation, the age, and symptoms of the child will influence their care measures. "Poor prognostic signs include more intrusive forms of abuse, more violent assaults, longer periods of sexual molestation, and closer relationship of the perpetrator to the victim"

DISPLAY 20.6 INDICATORS OF SEXUAL ABUSE

I. History of Sexual Abuse

- A child confides to a friend, classmate, teacher, a friend's mother, or other trusted adult that she/he has experienced sexual abuse.
- A child may disclose information indirectly by such statements as:
  "I know someone ..."
  "What would you do if ... ?"
  "I heard something about somebody..."
- The child has torn, stained, or bloody underclothing (among her/his clothing or is wearing it).
- Knowledge that a child's injury/disease (vaginal trauma, sexually transmitted disease) is unusual for the specific age group.
- Unexplained injuries/diseases (parent/caretaker unable to explain reason for injury/disease); there are discrepancies in explanation; blame is placed on a third party; explanations are inconsistent with medical diagnosis.
- A very young girl is pregnant or has a sexually transmitted disease. Pregnancy alone does not constitute sexual abuse, but if there are indications of coercion or significant age disparity between the minor and her partner, this may lead to reasonable suspicion of sexual abuse that must be reported.

II. Sexual Behavioral Indicators of Sexually Abused Children

- Detailed and age-inappropriate understanding of sexual behavior (especially among very young children)
- Sexually explicit language
- Inappropriate, unusual, or aggressive sexual behavior with peers or toys
- Compulsive indiscreet masturbation
- Excessive curiosity about sexual matters or genitalia (self or others)
- Unusually seductive or flirtatious behavior with classmates, teachers, and other adults
- Excessive concern about homosexuality, especially by boys

III. Behavioral Indicators of Sexual Abuse in Younger Children

- Enuresis (wetting pants or bedwetting)
- Fecal soiling
- Eating disturbances such as overeating or undereating
- Fears or phobias
- Overly compulsive behavior
- School problems or significant change in school performance (attitude and grades)
- Age-inappropriate behavior that includes pseudomaturity or regressive behavior such as bedwetting or thumb sucking
- Inability to concentrate
- Sleeping disturbances (nightmares, fear of falling asleep, fretful sleep pattern, sleeping long hours)
- Drastic behavior changes
- Speech disorders
- Frightened of parents/caretaker or of going home or being at home

IV. Behavioral Indicators of Sexual Abuse in Older Children and Adolescents

- Withdrawal
- Chronic fatigue
- Clinical depression, apathy
- Overly compliant behavior
- Over- or underreaction (hysteria or cavalier attitude) to a genital exam
- Poor hygiene or excessive bathing
- Poor peer relations and social skills; inability to make friends
- Acting out; running away; aggressive, antisocial, or delinquent behavior
- Alcohol or drug abuse
- Prostitution or excessive promiscuity
- School problems, frequent absences, sudden drop in school performance
- Refusal to change clothes for physical education class
- Nonparticipation in sports and social activities
- Fearful of showers or restrooms
- Fearful of home life as demonstrated by arriving at school early and leaving late
- Suddenly fearful of other things (going outside or participating in familiar activities)
- Extraordinary fear of males (in cases of male perpetrator and female victim)
- Self-consciousness of body beyond that expected for age
- Sudden acquisition of money, new clothes, or gifts with no reasonable explanation
- Suicide attempt or other self-destructive behavior
- Crying without provocation
- Setting fires

V. Physical Symptoms of Sexual Abuse

- Sexually transmitted diseases, especially in prepubescent girls
- Genital discharge or infection
- Physical trauma or irritation to the anal/genital area (pain, itching, swelling, bruising, bleeding, lacerations, abrasions), especially if injuries are unexplained or there is an inconsistent explanation
- Pain during urination or defecation
- Difficulty in walking or sitting due to genital or anal pain
- Psychosomatic symptoms (stomach aches, headaches, chronic pain)

Adapted from the Crime and Violence Prevention Center. (1996). *Child abuse: Educator's responsibilities.* Sacramento, CA: California Attorney General's Office.

(American Academy of Pediatrics, Committee on Child Abuse and Neglect, 1999, para. 24). Parents may also need counseling and support following the investigation and proceedings involving their child's victimization.

The sexual assault nurse examiner (SANE) role is more explicit in assisting the victim and appropriate family members immediately after the victim presents to the police or to an emergency department setting. The nurse has very specific actions to take to promote trust, obtain needed specimen evidence, and treat the sexual abuse victim. The victim has already been significantly traumatized, and the nurse can be effective in this role only if trust can be established during this critical time after the sexual assault. The SANE is trained to work with victims of all ages, both genders, and under all sexual abuse situations.

Although there are several classifications of child molesters, pedophiles present the greatest danger. A pedophile is an adult whose main sexual interest is a child. A pedophile tends to be well-liked by children. Pedophiles, who most often are men, frequently choose to work in professions or volunteer organizations that allow them easy access to children, where they can develop the trust and respect of children and their parents. The pedophile believes that sex with children is appropriate and often lures children into sexual relationships with love, rewards, promises, and gifts. He may be among a child's family members (e.g., grandfather, father, uncle, cousin) or a trusted community leader the child knows (e.g., next-door neighbor, teacher, coach, or religious leader). Recent reports of pedophiles among clergy in the Roman Catholic Church have clearly rocked the church's status and stability. As of July 2006, the National Sex Offender Public Registry (NSOPR), sponsored through the Department of Justice, is used in all 50 states, thereby improving efforts to safeguard all children (Rape, Abuse, & Incest National Network [RAINN], 2006). This resource provides information regarding the more than 500,000 registered sex offenders throughout the United States.

Human trafficking of children on a national and international scale is recognized by the United States in the Trafficking Victims Protection Act of 2000 (TVPA). This federal law defined "severe forms of human trafficking' as: the recruitment, harboring, transportation, provision or obtaining of a person for sex trafficking ... or for labor or services through the use of force, fraud, or coercion..." (ACF, 2009). The law specifically identified any child less than 18 years who engaged in commercial sex as a victim of trafficking (ACF, 2009). The USDHHS established a National Human Trafficking Resource Center (NHTRC), which operates a 24-hour crisis line at 1.888.3737.888 in over 170 languages.

Emotional Abuse

Emotional abuse of children involves psychological mistreatment or neglect, such as when parents do not provide the normal experiences that produce feelings of being loved, wanted, secure, and worthy (Crime and Violence Prevention Center, 2003c). This type of abuse is commonly associated with other types of abuse and may involve verbal abuse, such as name calling, belittling, or threatening. A mother may shout at the child, "You're just like your father, a good-for-nothing, lazy bum." A father may say, "You're ugly. You look just like your mother." If the child spills some juice, a parent may scream, "Everything you do, you do wrong. Can't you do anything right?"

Emotional abuse may also take the form of emotional abandonment. Some parents "shun" their children as a form of punishment. They will not speak to them and do not look at them; they behave as if their child does not exist. This behavior may continue for a day or longer, whenever a child displeases the parent. In some cases, the shunning lasts for days.

Verbal threats, although a common discipline practice, are also a form of emotional abuse. Examples of verbal threats include "Take your feet off the furniture of I'll chop your feet off" and "Do that again, and you'll really know what my belt feels like." In the first instance, the child might realize that the parent wouldn't really chop her feet off, but hearing the parent say such a violent thing can be emotionally scarring. In the second instance, the parent may have beaten the child with a belt in the past, so merely threatening to use the belt again causes emotional trauma.

Emotional abuse alone is rarely reported because it is another "hidden" form of abuse. However, **mandated reporters**, people who have a responsibility for the welfare of children and include public and private school employees; administrators and employees of youth centers and recreation programs; child welfare employees; foster parents; group home and residential facility personnel; social workers; probation workers; health care workers including nurses, doctors, and chiropractors; animal control workers; and personnel working in film development laboratories, are required by law to report *suspected* cases of severe emotional neglect or abuse or deprivation in addition to *suspected* neglect and physical or sexual abuse (Crime and Violence Prevention Center, 2003a, 2003c) (see Display 20.7).

Specific Abusive Situations

The previous information addressed the major types of child abuse in families, yet other patterns of abuse against children need to be discussed. Shaken baby syndrome, Munchausen syndrome by proxy, and maternal filicide defined as a child murdered by the mother are fairly rare, but by the time the symptoms are recognized, it is often too late, with the diagnosis made during subsequent visits to the emergency department or at autopsy.

In addition, Internet crimes against children, child abduction, and crimes against children by babysitters are an increasingly common fear of parents. These types of abuse are occurring more often as children and adolescents have increased time and access to computers and because both parents (or a single parent) must work, while children are spending more time alone or with babysitters. Community concern regarding child abductions by family members or strangers has resulted

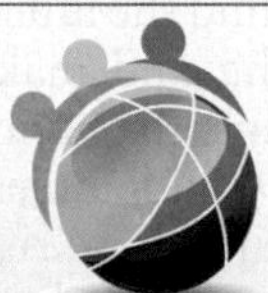

DISPLAY 20.7 SIGNS AND SYMPTOMS OF EMOTIONAL ABUSE OR DEPRIVATION

Emotional abuse should be suspected if the child displays the following behavioral indicators:

- Is withdrawn, depressed, or apathetic
- Is clingy and forms indiscriminate attachments
- "Acts out" and is considered a behavior problem
- Exhibits exaggerated fearfulness
- Is overly rigid in conforming to instructions of teachers, doctors, and other adults
- Suffers from sleep, speech, or eating disorders
- Displays signs of emotional turmoil that include repetitive, rhythmic movements (rocking, whining, picking at scabs)
- Pays inordinate attention to details or exhibits little or no verbal or physical communication with others
- Suffers from enuresis and fecal soiling
- Unwittingly makes comments such as "Mommy always tells me I'm bad"
- Experiences substance abuse problems

Emotional deprivation should be suspected if the child

- Refuses to eat adequate amounts of food and therefore is very frail
- Is unable to perform normal learned functions for a given age (e.g., walking, talking)
- Displays antisocial behavior (aggression, disruption) or obvious delinquent behavior (drug abuse, vandalism); conversely, the child may be abnormally unresponsive, sad, or withdrawn.
- Constantly "seeks out" and "pesters" other adults such as teachers or neighbors for attention and affection
- Displays exaggerated fears

in the institution of *Amber Alert* systems in many states. School violence is also an area of increasing concern for families and will be addressed.

Shaken Baby Syndrome

Shaken baby syndrome is the intentional abusive action of violently shaking an infant or toddler, usually a child of 2 years or younger (National Institute of Neurological Disorders and Stroke [NINDS], 2007). The type of damage that occurs to these infants very seldom occurs through play, as in minor falls or as a result of tossing a baby in the air. The classic medical symptoms associated with infant shaking are bilateral retinal hemorrhage, subdural or subarachnoid hematomas, absence of other external signs of abuse, and symptoms that may include breathing difficulties, seizures, dilated pupils, lethargy, and unconsciousness (USDOJ, 2002). These injuries occur from a violent, sustained action in which the infant's head, which lacks muscular control, is violently whipped forward and backward, hitting the chest and shoulders. According to experts, an observer would describe the shaking as being "as hard as the shaker was humanly capable of shaking the baby" or "hard enough that it appeared the baby's head would come off" (USDOJ, 2002). Within minutes to hours after the injury, the baby begins to show symptoms such as irritability, lethargy, vomiting, breathing problems, seizures, or unconsciousness. A typical explanation given by the parents or caretakers is that the baby was "fine" and then suddenly went into respiratory arrest or began having seizures—both common symptoms of shaken baby syndrome. Children who survive shaken baby syndrome may require lifelong care (NINDS, 2007).

Munchausen Syndrome by Proxy

Munchausen syndrome is a psychological disorder in which a client fabricates the symptoms of a disease in order to undergo medical tests, hospitalization, or even medical or surgical treatment. Clients with this disorder may intentionally injure him/herself or induce illness in him/herself. In cases of *Munchausen syndrome by proxy*, a parent or caretaker attempts to bring medical attention to herself by injuring or inducing illness in her child. The following scenarios are typical of these cases:

- The child's parent or caretaker brings the child to the emergency department or calls paramedics repeatedly for alleged problems that have no medical basis.
- The child experiences "seizures" or "respiratory arrest" only when the parent or caretaker is present—never in the presence of a neutral third party or when hospitalized, unless the parent or caretaker reports that the incident occurred in her presence alone.
- While the child is hospitalized, the parent or caretaker shuts off intravenous tubes or life-support equipment, causing the child distress, and then turns everything back on and summons help.
- The parent or caretaker induces illness by introducing a mild irritant or poison into the child's body; chronic ingestion of such substances may cause the child's death.

Health providers, mental health professionals, and attorneys may be involved in working with such cases, requiring careful attention to the history of the illness/injury, the treatment, documentation, and communication with the parent/caretaker. Attention to the child's safety is paramount, although the parent may remove the child from care or take the child to another facility if the caregiver's suspicions are aroused (Stirling & Committee on Child Abuse and Neglect, 2007).

Child Murder by Mother

A rare, yet concerning type of child death is known as *maternal filicide*, defined as child murder by the mother (Friedman & Resnick, 2007). The parent or stepparent is frequently the perpetrator when a young child is murdered; maternal filicide is known to occur in all areas of the world. In the United States, the child homicide rate is 8.0 deaths per 100,000 infants, while for preschool-aged children, the rate drops to 2.5 deaths per 100,000, and in school-aged children, the rate declines to 1.5 homicides per 100,000 (Friedman & Resnick, 2007). Research indicates five common motives when a mother murders her child. An *altruistic filicide* is defined as a situation when the mother kills her child out of love, in the belief that her child's life or fate is worse than death. A second motive that may occur is a *psychotic filicide* wherein the mother may suffer from delirium or psychosis and murder her child as a result of her unstable mental disorder. A third, and the most common, motive is *fatal maltreatment* a situation in which the child's death is an unintentional result from repeated abuse or Munchausen syndrome by proxy. *Unwanted child filicide* occurs when the child is unwanted and the mother feels the child is a hindrance. The fifth and most rare motive is a *spouse revenge filicide* when the mother murders her child as revenge toward the father (Friedman & Resnick, 2007).

Infanticide is defined as the murder of a child during the first year of life, while *neonaticide* is the murder of an infant within the first 24 hours of life (Friedman & Resnick, 2007). Neonaticides are almost always committed by mothers who have risk factors as a young, unmarried woman, with an unwanted pregnancy who received no prenatal care (Friedman & Resnick, 2007). Infanticide in the United States was found to be associated with economic stress. Other risk characteristics for maternal filicide include a mother who was (a) socially isolated, (b) poor, (c) acted as a full-time caregiver, and (d) often had a history of domestic violence or relationship problems. "Neglectful or abusive mothers were often substance abusers," while the majority of perpetrators exhibited psychosis, depression, or suicidality (Friedman & Resnick, 2007). An anecdotal note on maternal filicide is that 16% to 29% of mothers who murder their child will commit suicide (Nock & Marzuk, 1999). Measures for prevention and support to mothers include parenting classes, emotional support, providing emergency numbers for support, as well as treating maternal substance abuse.

Internet Crimes Against Children

Internet crimes are insidious because they come right into the home. Children either unintentionally or intentionally may access an Internet chat room or Web site developed or used by pedophiles. The perpetrator establishes contact, usually passing himself off as a teen or young man who has similar interests, and states affection for and understanding of the youth's "problems." Eventually, the pedophile either sets up a meeting time and place or engages in sexually explicit dialogue with the minor (USDOJ, 2001b). Many minors find the attention from this stranger inviting or exciting and make plans to meet the person. When this happens, the minor falls victim to this individual, putting the child/adolescent at great risk. This computer-based child abuse risk has led the U.S. Attorney General to authorize a federal awareness and justice program focusing solely on technology-facilitated sexual exploitation and abuse against children, named *Project Safe Childhood* (USDOJ, 2006).

Community health nurses can assist families to prevent such Internet crimes in various ways by

- Encouraging placement of "blocks" on computers via the Internet server
- Urging parents to discuss with their children the dangers of online "friendships" that seek face-to-face meetings
- Establishing parent–child contracts for Internet use
- Monitoring the time and Internet sites a child uses
- Keeping the computer in a high-traffic area in the home, affording easy observation
- Setting the Internet browser security feature to "high"
- Installing a firewall, antivirus, and anti-adware/spyware programs that increase privacy
- Discouraging downloading of games and other media that might contain Trojan or worm programs that enable remote access by unauthorized users (Dombrowski & Gischlar, 2004)

Furthermore, parents can contact the Cyber Tip Line at (800) 843-5678 or www.cybertipline.com if they suspect that an online predator has contacted their child (National Center for Missing and Exploited Children, 2011).

Child Abduction

Child abduction is a crime that every parent fears, and although stranger abduction happens infrequently, it remains the greatest fear for parents. However, intense media coverage gives the impression that such crimes occur frequently, and this causes great stress among parents and community members. Nationally, the Amber Alert program and the Child Abduction Response Teams (CART) were established to provide a prompt and professional response to child abduction (USDOJ, 2005).

Child abduction by family members or intimate partners, such as a divorced mother, father, stepparent, boyfriend, or grandparents, is more common. Nonetheless, the parent from whom the child was taken may be unaware that the abduction was by a relative or known person and may experience the same type of stress and loss as parents who lose a child by stranger abduction. In some cases, knowing the relative or person who abducted the child causes just as much fear because the abductor may have a history of violence or sexual abuse crimes.

Prevention of child abduction is difficult, and at times, parents who think they have taught their children well may have a false sense of security. Some studies assessed the effects on children of taking a "stranger awareness" class. The class included lessons on avoiding strangers, not talking to strangers, identifying who is a stranger, saying "no" to strangers, and running away and screaming if addressed by a stranger. Yet, researchers found that when the children left the classroom, if an unknown person (a stranger sent in by the researcher) asked the child to help him find a lost puppy or go help them get candy, many of the children responded readily without using any of the actions learned in the stranger awareness class. Parents who watched their children on tapes of these studies could not believe what they saw. Children are trusting and curious, and they may not consider people who look like their parents as *strangers*.

Community health nurses can help parents improve their child's safety by promoting close supervision of young children and practicing behaviors that promote anonymity. Ideas that help improve the child's safety include

- Holding the child's hand while in malls or stores
- Keeping the child in the seat of a shopping cart
- Keeping a young child in sight at all times when playing outside
- Sharing parental supervision with another mother when children play, so that an adult is always supervising the children
- Not putting the child's name or initials on clothing or backpacks
- Teaching the child a "password" that only the parents and child know to use when a different person is picking them up from a neighborhood activity

Older children and teens who go outside the home unattended by parents should be encouraged to use the following behaviors that promote safety: staying with groups of other children or teens, having a cell phone, leaving an itinerary with the parents, and not changing their plans without contacting parents. Other measures that can benefit older children and adolescents are attending a self-defense class and carrying a whistle and/or pepper spray.

Crimes Against Children by Babysitters

Crimes against infants and young children by babysitters have been reported in the media in past years (USDOJ, 2001a). Some parents who have suspected mistreatment of their children by caretakers have used hidden cameras to reveal the problem. Abuse by caretakers is a fear of parents who work and leave their children with others.

The community health nurse can help parents assess day care settings by providing them descriptors for finding good day care providers. Parents who use neighbors as babysitters should get references and should drop by the home or day care setting at various times during the day. They should assess their infants and follow up on any bruises, rashes, burns, conditions, or behaviors they observe that are not normal for their child. With older children, parents need to listen to them and ask about their day and activities. Parents must not ignore signs, such as a child's fear of going to the babysitter or reports of spankings, being shouted at, or other inappropriate treatment. Day care centers and many home day care programs are licensed by the state. Programs for which parent complaints have been filed with licensing agencies are monitored more closely, and the state is mandated to make changes or close the facility if necessary. Parents need to know that their child is safe and cared for when they leave them to pursue their employment or educational activities.

School Violence

An area of growing concern regarding violence against children has been in school settings. Violence in schools may range from bullying, slapping, or punching to weapon use (CDC, 2010c). Random shootings and hostage situations in schools over the past decade have fueled fears about the safety of students and promoted research into how to prevent this type of community violence affecting children. The U.S. Department of Education, DHHS, and DOJ have collaborated to provide funding, programs, and trainings that improve school safety through the *Safe Schools Healthy Students* initiative. Six areas identified for attention in building safe school climates are:

- Creating a safe school environment
- Providing alcohol, drug, and violence prevention and early intervention programs
- Supporting school and community mental health prevention and treatment intervention services
- Providing early childhood psychosocial and emotional development programs
- Addressing education reform
- Designing safe school policies (Safe Schools Healthy Students Initiative, 2006)

The Youth Risk Behavior Survey collects information about health and prevention issues of adolescents. Included in the survey are questions about violence risks such as fighting, use of illegal drugs, carrying a weapon, and being threatened or injured with a weapon on school property. In 2009, 22.3% of students checked that they were offered, sold, or given an illegal drug by someone on school property during the preceding 12 months; 12.4% of students reported being in a physical fight on school property during the previous 12 months, while 7.8% of students reported being threatened or injured with a weapon on school property during the preceding 12 months, and 5.9% of students reported they had carried a weapon, such as a gun, knife, or club, on school property during the 30 days before the survey (CDC, 2010d). School violence has immediate and long-term effects on students demonstrated by an increase in depression, anxiety, psychological problems, and fear (CDC, 2010c).

Risk factors surrounding youth violence can be categorized as individual risks, relationship risks, and/or community/societal risks. Individual risks for perpetrating youth violence may include a history of violent victimization; a history of early aggressive behaviors, attention deficit, hyperactivity, or learning disorders; an association with delinquent peers; gang involvement; high emotional distress; social rejection; family violence and conflict; or poor behavioral control (CDC, 2010c). Low parental involvement, parental substance abuse or criminality, poor supervision, low emotional attachment to the parent, and a harsh, lax, or inconsistent form of discipline increase a child/adolescent's risk for violence (CDC, 2010e). Community and societal risk factors for youth violence are associated with diminished economic opportunities, a high concentration of poverty, transiency, and family disruption, with low levels of community participation (CDC, 2010e). Youth development programs address these risk factors in schools and communities, as well as promoting activities that help students in meeting their individual needs. Mentoring has been identified as a beneficial program for at risk teens when effectively trained and supported mentors are utilized. Social skills, conflict resolution, and programs that support student sports, arts, and extracurricular interests decrease an individual's risk in being involved in violence. School and societal strategies include surveillance, maintenance of facilities, and consistent classroom management techniques, along with adequate student supervision (CDC, 2010e). Parent involvement and education is expanding through programs such as with *Healthy Start* and parent-participation preschools, *Loving Solutions* for elementary age students, and the *Parent Project* for parents of difficult adolescents.

PERSPECTIVES
VOICES FROM THE COMMUNITY

Family Violence

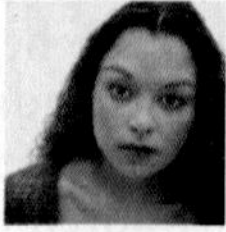

My family was always shouting at each other—it was just the way it was. The hitting—well, that happened, but it wasn't nearly as bad as all that yelling. Now here I am in the same boat all over again—the yelling, the hitting, and I've got this new baby to take care of. I'm just so tired. When the nurse showed up today to check on the baby and me, I swore to myself I wouldn't tell her about the fight we had last night (anyway it wasn't nearly as bad as the other times). Then she looked at me and asked if I felt safe and that was it . . . I said NO before I realized my mouth was even open. I told her that he punched me in the side while I was changing the baby's diaper. She was so kind—she didn't tell me how stupid I was for staying with him, but she did help me look at my options. Since I was holding the baby when he hit me, she said she was required to make a report of child abuse. That was awful news, and I started to cry; but like she said, I could have dropped her or he could have missed me and hit her. I knew he'd be furious when he found out—then I was really in a panic. Well, she told me about a place in town I can stay for a time with the baby, and she helped me make arrangements. I'm so tired and scared, but I know now that I need to keep my baby safe. I still don't know what made me tell the nurse—I guess it was because she asked. I know I'm doing the right thing for me and the baby.

PARTNER/SPOUSAL ABUSE

Adult violence is rooted in childhood violence. A father hits a mother. The mother hits her son. The son hits his sister. The sister hits her little brother. The little brother sets fire to the cat, pulls wings off butterflies, and grows up to be a spouse batterer. Although abused girls may grow up to be abusing mothers, more often they grow up to be abused wives. Researchers operationalize domestic violence as punching, grabbing, shoving, slapping, choking, kicking, biting, hitting with a fist or some other object, being beaten, or being threatened with a knife or gun by a spouse or cohabiting partner. See Perspectives: Voices from the Community.

Partner violence often begins during adolescent dating or dating at any age, with a push or shove that at first is overlooked by the girlfriend (Hanson, 2002). As these minor episodes of violence continue, the victim typically feels that she is doing something wrong and attempts to modify her behavior. She also assumes wrongly that once she and her boyfriend are married, these physical assaults will stop automatically or that in time she will be able to "change" him, yet the cycle of violence has already begun.

Cycle of Violence

The **cycle of violence** is a repetitive, cyclic pattern of abuse seen in domestic violence situations. This theory of family violence was first described as a three-phase cycle by Walker in 1979, after she studied more than 1,000 battered women and a smaller group of battering men. The cycle includes the tension-building phase, the acute battering incident, and the loving reconciliation (Jenkins & Davidson, 2001). The psychological dynamics of these three phases help explain why women feel so guilty and ashamed of their partner's violence toward them, and why they find it so difficult to leave, even when their lives are in danger (see Display 20.8). Often, as the cycle of violence continues, the frequency of the cycle increases, with the tension-building phase and the acute battering incident occurring more often and elimination of the loving reconciliation phase. Without intervention, this shorter, more violent cycle becomes increasingly risk-filled for outcomes that may lead to injury or maiming of a partner, incarceration, or death of a partner.

The Domestic Abuse Intervention Project in Duluth, Minnesota, developed a wheel of violence, identifying power and control at the center and citing eight categories of perpetrator behaviors. This model is a useful tool for visualizing the multidimensional nature of abuse in which threats, coercion, isolation, blaming, intimidation, and use of children, male privilege, and economics convene to control the victim (Fig. 20-1).

Dating Violence

Dating violence in adolescent relationships is a serious and prevalent problem. Because of its prevalence, community health nurses should include screening for dating

DISPLAY 20.8 THE CYCLE OF VIOLENCE

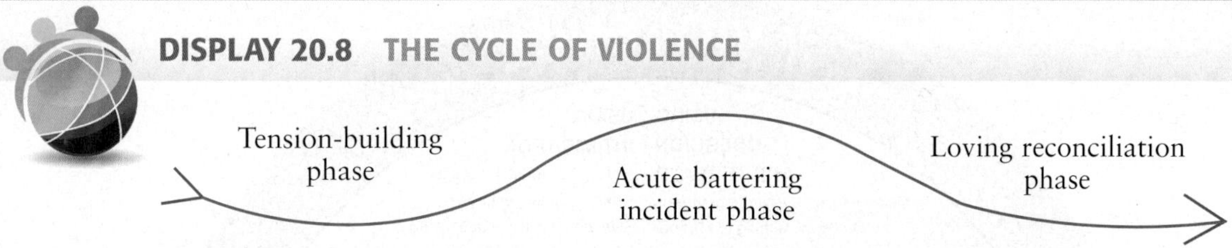

Tension-Building Phase

The woman senses her partner's increasing tension. She may or may not know what is wrong. The partner is "edgy" and lashes out in anger. He challenges her, calls her names, and tells her she is stupid, incompetent, and unconcerned about him. She "tries hard" not to make any "mistakes" that may upset him. She takes the responsibility for making him feel better and begins to set herself up to feel guilt when he eventually explodes in spite of her best efforts to calm and please him. During the increasing tension, the woman is rarely angry even at the most outrageous demands or blame. Rather, she internalizes her appropriate anger at the partner's unfairness and, instead, experiences depression, anxiety, and a sense of helplessness. As the tension in the relationship increases, minor episodes of violence increase, such as pinching, tripping, or slapping. The batterer knows his behavior is inappropriate, and he fears the woman will leave him. This fear of rejection and loss increases his rage at the woman and his need to control her.

Acute Battering Incident

The tension-building phase ends in an explosion of violence. The incident that sets off the man's violence is often trivial or unknown, leaving the woman confused and feeling helpless. The woman may or may not fight back. She may try to escape the violence or call for help. If she cannot escape the beating, she may have a sense of unreality—as if it is a dream. Following the battering, the woman is in a state of physical and psychological shock. She may be passive and withdrawn or hysterical and incoherent. She may not be aware of the seriousness of her injuries and may resist help. The man discounts the episode and also underestimates the woman's injuries. He may not summon medical help even when her injuries are life threatening.

Loving Reconciliation

The loving reconciliation phase may begin a few hours to several days following the acute battering incident. Both partners have a profound sense of relief that "it's over." Although the woman is initially angry at the man, he begins an intense campaign to "win her back." Just as his tension and violence were overdone, his apologies, gifts, and gestures of love may also be excessive. Showering her with love and praise helps her repair her shattered self-esteem. It is nearly impossible for her to leave him during this phase as he is meeting her desperate need to see herself as a competent and lovable woman. The woman's feelings of power and romantic ideals are nurtured. She believes this gentle, loving person is her "real" lover. She believes that if only she can find the key, she can stop him from further violent episodes. She believes that no matter how often it has happened before, somehow this episode seems different this time and it will never happen again.

The Increasing Spiral of Violence

One aspect of the cycle of violence of particular concern is its progressive and spiraling nature. Once violence has begun, every study indicates that it not only continues but over time increases in both frequency and severity. As the violence continues, the three-phase cycle begins to change. The tension-building phase becomes shorter and more intense, the acute battering incidents become more frequent and severe, and the loving reconciliation phase becomes shorter and less intense. After many years of battering, the man may not apologize at all.

violence in all encounters with teens. **Adolescent dating violence (ADV)** includes physical, sexual, emotional, and verbal abuse between teenagers who are or have been in a casual or serious dating relationship (Hanson, 2002). In the United States, ADV was reported by nearly 10% of students in the past 12 months; furthermore, victims of dating violence are at higher risk for dating violence in college (CDC, 2010d). Teens, male or female, who experience dating violence in adolescence, are more at risk for binge drinking, suicide attempts, doing poorly in school, physical fighting, and sexual activity (CDC, 2011b). Programs through schools and communities, such as *Choose Respect*, are part of a national effort to address harmful beliefs about dating violence and promote healthy and respectful dating relationships (CDC, 2010a).

Partner/Spousal Abuse

Spousal abuse is violence against an intimate partner and is pervasive globally. The WHO reported in a multi-study review that 10% to 52% of women reported being

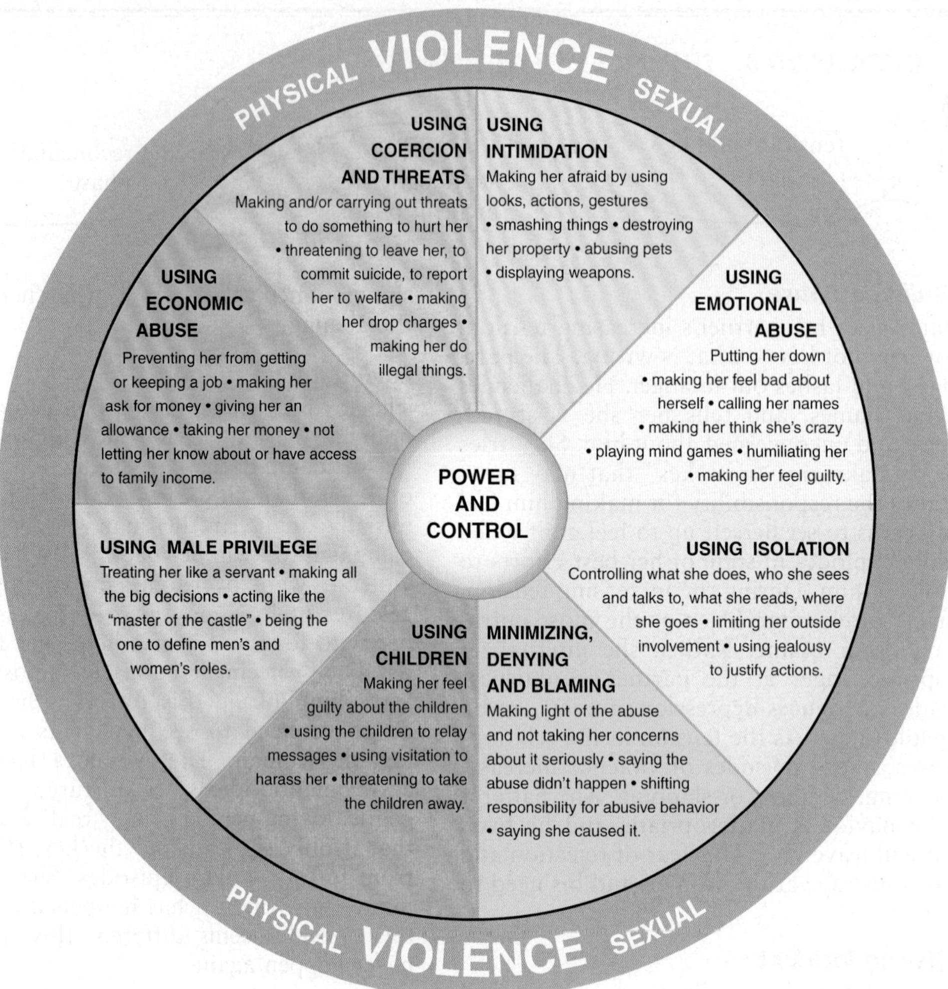

FIGURE 20-1. Wheel of violence.

physically abused by an intimate partner at some point in their lives, and 10% to 30% of women had experienced sexual violence by an intimate partner (WHO, 2005, p. 1). Because of the nature of **intimate partner violence (IPV)**, the problems are difficult to study and believed to be underreported. Much remains unknown about factors that increase or decrease the likelihood that men will behave violently toward women, factors that endanger or protect women from violence, and the physical and emotional consequences of partner violence on women and their children.

The USDOJ defines domestic violence as "a pattern of abusive behavior in any relationship that is used by one partner to gain or maintain power and control over another intimate partner" (USDOJ, Office on Violence Against Women [VAW], n.d., para. 1). Although domestic violence is categorized as physical abuse, sexual abuse, emotional abuse, economic abuse, or psychological abuse, the victim commonly experiences a combination of these abuses or threats of abuse in these areas. Intimidation and threats create an atmosphere of fear for the victim and may include humiliation, isolation, terrorizing, coercing, blaming, manipulating, stalking, and/or destruction of property or pets valued by the partner. *Stalking* may occur by either partner in a relationship, demonstrated as a "pattern of repeated and unwanted attention, harassment, contact, or any other course of conduct directed at a specific person that would cause a reasonable person to feel fear" (USDOJ, 2011). Stalking behavior may occur weekly but has been known to occur for 5 years or longer (Baum, Catalano, Rand, & Rose, 2009). Women are at greater risk as victims of stalking, while harassment occurs equally between men and women, with cyberstalking occurring in 25% of victims (Baum et al., 2009).

IPV is a leading cause of morbidity and mortality in women worldwide, as well as a public health and human rights issue (WHO, 2011). In the United States, IPV affects more than 12 million people each year; moreover, 79% of victims experienced the first rape or IPV before age 24 (CDC, 2011a). Fox and Zawitz (2004), cited by the CDC, found females accounted for 76% of IPV homicides and males were 24% of IPV homicides (CDC, 2006a). It is important to note that of those who died from IPV homicide, 44% had been to an emergency department within the last 2 years, and of those, 93% had at least one injury at that time (CDC, 2006a; Crandall, Nathens, Kernic, Holt, & Rivara, 2004). Health care providers have a responsibility and opportunity to assess and initiate a safety plan when these patients are seen in the emergency room. A compendium of assessment tools for IPV can be found on the CDC Web site.

Violence During Pregnancy

IPV during pregnancy increases a woman's vulnerability to her and her fetus; 44% to 48% of all pregnant women are abused at least once during the pregnancy (CDC, 2006a; Gazmararian et al., 2000). Abuse during pregnancy has been linked with maternal health problems such as smoking, alcohol and substance abuse, delay in prenatal care, stress, physical injuries, headaches, and lack of attachment to the infant (Campbell, 2002; Thananowan & Heidrich, 2008). The fetus is also endangered with higher rates of intrauterine growth retardation; preterm labor, resulting in low birth weight; and other neonatal risks (Altarac & Strobino, 2002), or increased risk of miscarriage and perinatal death (Janssen et al., 2003). Abuse is more likely to be reported by pregnant adolescents than pregnant adults and by women with unplanned pregnancies compared with other pregnant women. Curry, Doyle, and Gilhooley (1998) found that pregnant teens who were abused were more likely to be high school dropouts, smoked more, and experienced more second-trimester bleeding. Once born, the infant of an abused teen or adult is at risk for child abuse.

The most serious aspect of IPV as a threat to a woman's safety is the link between abuse during pregnancy and homicide, called femicide. *Femicide*, the killing of women, happens worldwide, although the link between IPV and homicide needs further study (WHO, 2011). One finding in a United States 11-city review found pregnancy significantly increased a woman's risk of IPV homicide, as men who abused their partner during pregnancy were particularly more dangerous and, therefore, more likely to commit homicide (Campbell et al., 2003).

Studies indicate that the prenatal care visit is one of the few times when women are seen by the helping professions. This visit is an important opportunity to identify women who are abused and therefore at risk for homicide. It is imperative that nurses conduct an assessment for danger and lethality, so that the women can be aware of their own level of risk and take safety precautions as needed. A series of questions requiring a "yes" or "no" response and inquiries about occurrences of abuse, escalation of abuse, frequency, severity, weapons, drugs or alcohol use by the perpetrator, and safety of other children should be incorporated into prenatal home visit assessments. This is especially important with women who have not followed through with prenatal care, thereby allowing health care professionals to monitor the progress of their pregnancies (Display 20.9).

DISPLAY 20.9 DOMESTIC VIOLENCE RISK ASSESSMENT TOOL

Frame the Questions

"Because abuse and violence are common in the lives of women, I have begun to ask about it with all women (or all pregnant women). I don't know if this is a problem for you, but I would like to ask you some questions, talk about ways to reduce your risk of being hurt, and give you some information and phone numbers that might be helpful to you."

Universal Questions

	Yes	No
1. Do you feel safe in your current relationships? Comments: ______	____	____
2. Have you ever been physically abused (pushed, shoved, hit, punched, bitten, burned, etc.)? Comments: ______	____	____
3. Have you ever been emotionally abused (neglected, called names, controlled, threatened, had your activities or decisions hindered, been denied resources to meet your physical or financial needs)? Comments: ______	____	____
4. Have you ever been sexually abused (forced to have an unwanted sexual act)? Comments: ______	____	____
5. Do you want to talk to someone about receiving help? Comments: ______	____	____

Resources

National Domestic Violence Hotline:
1-800-799-SAFE (7233)
Local Battered Women's Shelter ______
Local Department of Women's Health Services ______
Other resources ______

Adapted from Sheehy, G. (2000). *Violence against women.* Fairfax, VA: The National Women's Health Information Center; Kramer, A. (2002). Domestic violence: How to ask and how to listen. *Nursing Clinics of North America, 37*(1), 189–210; and Davis, R. E., & Harsh, K. E. (2001). Confronting barriers to universal screening for domestic violence. *Journal of Professional Nursing, 17*(6), 313–320.

Batterer Characteristics

Although men who batter come from all walks of life educationally, culturally, and socioeconomically, perpetrators have some common characteristics. The following attributes represent personal characteristics often seen in batterers:

- Low self-esteem
- Low income
- Low academic achievement
- Involvement in aggressive or delinquent behavior as youth
- Heavy alcohol and drug use
- Depression
- Anger and hostility
- Personality disorders
- Prior history of being physically abusive
- Having few friends and being isolated from other people
- Unemployment
- Emotional dependence and insecurity
- Belief in strict gender roles (e.g., male dominance and aggression in relationships)
- Desire for power and control in relationships
- Being a victim of physical or psychological abuse (consistently one of the strongest predictors of perpetration) (CDC, 2006a, para. 24).

Relationship, community, and societal factors have also been identified that affect a perpetrator's risk for battering. Identified relationship factors include marital fights and tension, divorce and separations, money problems, and problematic and difficult family relationships, as well as the male's need for dominance and control in the relationship. Societal factors associated with increased risk are strict role stereotyping about the roles the husband and wife should follow in a relationship. Aspects identified within a community that lead to increased risks for IPV may be a lack of resources in the community, a failure or unwillingness of others to intervene or contact authorities when they are aware of the abuse, and factors associated with poverty, such as overcrowding and unemployment (CDC, 2006a).

Victim Characteristics

Studies have also revealed risk factors associated with victims. Increasing the victim's abilities to manage and improve their behaviors and understanding of relationship patterns and abuse allows victims to change their risk of being a victim. Individual risk factors for IPV victims include

- A prior history of IPV
- Being female
- Young age
- Heavy alcohol and drug use
- High-risk sexual behaviors
- Witnessing or experiencing violence as a child
- Being less educated
- Unemployment
- For men, having a different ethnicity from their partner
- For women, having a greater education level than their partner
- For women, being American Indian/Alaska Native or African American
- For women, having a verbally abusive, jealous, or possessive partner (CDC, 2006a, para. 19).

Marked differences between partner's incomes, levels of education, or job status place a victim more at risk for IPV. Community characteristics are similar to those of the perpetrator, revealing that those communities with fewer available resources, in areas of poverty, and having a lack of sanctions against violent behaviors increase one's risk. Traditional gender roles, such as a belief that men work and women are submissive and should stay home, are societal risk factors associated with higher IPV risk (CDC, 2006a, para. 19).

Effects of Violence on Children

"Sixty percent of American children were exposed to violence, crime, or abuse in their homes, schools, or community" (Finkelhor, Turner, Ormrod, Hamby, & Kracke, 2009). Children who are exposed to family violence are more at risk for abuse and for violence later in their life as either a perpetrator or victim. Although domestic violence may not be directed at a child, that child may become a victim as a bystander or when trying to protect a parent. Effects of family violence are often seen in emotional, cognitive, physical, and/or behavioral manifestations of the child. Children who have been exposed to violence are more likely to (a) use drugs and alcohol, (b) experience depression anxiety and/or posttraumatic stress syndrome, (c) do poorly in school, or (d) participate in criminal activity (Finkelhor et al., 2009).

Most often, wife abuse and child abuse occur together. Literature reviews consistently suggest that a positive correlation exists between children's witnessing IPV and some aspects of impaired child development (Lemmey et al., 2001). Young children are particularly vulnerable to the effects of violence, as they lack the ability to understand the trauma and are likely to exhibit somatic complaints (headaches, eating or sleep problems) and/or behavior regression (clinging, whining, or becoming nonverbal) (Volpe, 1996). Meanwhile, school-age children and adolescents are more likely to either act out with delinquent behaviors or withdraw. It is more common for girls to become withdrawn and an important reason for health care providers to include an assessment for family violence concerns. Children in families with domestic violence are at risk for depression, negative mental health effects, and consequences that last far into their adult lives. These maladjustments may be behavioral (aggression and conduct problems), emotional (withdrawal, anxiousness, fearfulness), social, cognitive (learning disabilities), and/or physical. Providers who work with children need to listen in a sincere, nonjudgmental manner and provide

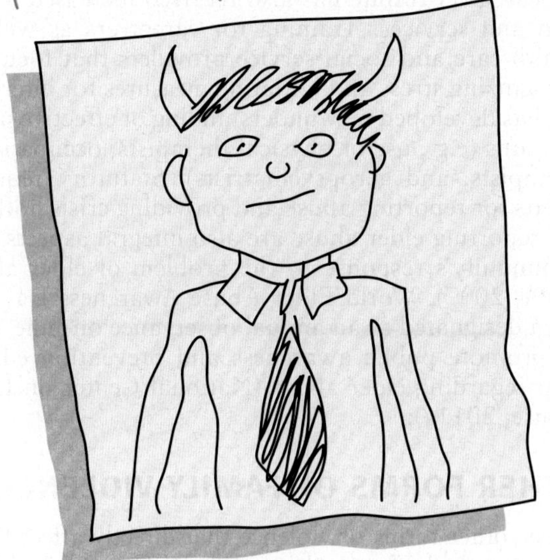
My Daddy is a Monster
He hurts my mommy
He hurts me too
Sometimes he hits
Sometimes he says things
That scare me and
make my mommy cry
after he leaves
Sometimes I wish he
won't come back ...ever.
I love my daddy.
National Coalition Against Domestic Violence • P.O. Box 34103 • Washington, DC 20043-4103 • 1-800-799-SAFE

FIGURE 20-2. Poster of "My Daddy Is a Monster."

ongoing support when assisting the child and family with resources, such as counseling, education, or community violence prevention programs (Fig. 20-2).

MISTREATMENT OF ELDERS

Elder abuse, the mistreatment or exploitation of older adults, may involve physical, sexual, or emotional or psychological abuse; neglect; abandonment; financial or material exploitation; or self-neglect (National Center on Elder Abuse, 2011b), or any combination of these mistreatments. Older women experienced abuse at a higher rate than elderly men—67% of elderly women—while only 32% of elderly men experienced abuse (Teaster et al., 2006). Caregiver neglect was found in 20% of elder abuse cases, while 15% of cases involved emotional, psychological, or verbal abuse. Another 15% of cases identified financial exploitation of the senior, with 11% identified as physical abuse, and sexual abuse was found in only 1% (Teaster et al., 2006). Thirty-three percent of elder abuse was perpetrated by adult children, while another 22% of elder abuse was committed by other family members, 16% occurred by strangers, and 11% involved the senior's spouse or intimate partner (Teaster et al., 2006).

Abuse against elders is not new, but research on elder abuse is new. Until recently, the reasons for elder abuse were extrapolated from the literature on abuse in younger populations. But by the mid-1980s, more research was being conducted about elder abuse, and the findings indicated that elder abuse results from multiple, interrelated variables associated with the perpetrator or the victim (Capezuti, Siegler, & Menzey, 2008).

Forms of physical abuse were found to include rough handling during caregiving, pinching, hitting, and slapping. Emotional abuse, which can take many forms, included being shouted at or threatened and having needed care withheld. More rarely, elders are sexually abused, which may include rape. Some elders are neglected by those they depend on to meet their caregiving needs. Elders with dementia and those requiring assistance for all activities of daily living (ADLs) are more at risk because of caregiver stress or burnout, which increases an elder's risk for abuse and neglect. With neglect, the elder may appear unwashed and unkempt or may suffer from malnutrition and dehydration, or even pressure sores. Elders who are dependent on others for their care often do not report abuse for fear of being abandoned. They feel powerless and at a loss about how to change a bad situation. They often fear reprisal from the perpetrator if they tell others about the abuse.

Older adults are frequently exploited in a variety of ways. Family members may take their Social Security retirement money, savings, or investments and use these funds on themselves. Criminals often approach elders with get-rich-quick schemes, sham investment opportunities, overpriced home repairs, or as collectors for illegitimate charities, thereby preying on the trusting nature of older adults.

Perpetrator and Victim Characteristics

The dominant underlying factors that contribute to abuse of an elder by a family member are social isolation and pathology on the part of the perpetrator. Research has identified emotional or financial dependence on the victim, alcohol use, and isolation or few external contacts as major contributing factors. Fifty-three percent of alleged perpetrators against elders were female (Teaster et al., 2006). Men are more likely to exploit or physically abuse elders, whereas women are more likely to neglect elders physically or abuse them psychologically. Because women are more frequently the caretakers of elders, they are in a position to provide either appropriate or neglectful care to frail older adults (Capezuti et al., 2008).

Some characteristics of older people appear to increase their risk of abuse. These risks include dementia and poor health (Capezuti et al., 2008). Newly diagnosed cognitive impairment correlates with occurrences of abuse. If violence or threats of violence by the elder toward the caregiver accompany dementia, this contributes to the elder's risk for abuse. The failing health of an elder may also contribute to self-neglect or diminished ability for self-defense or escape from maltreatment. Finally, if the abuser and victim live together, the close proximity can bring up unresolved family conflicts or create new conflicts and tension (Capezuti et al., 2008). Abuse in an elder often leads to a downward spiral in their life with a loss of independence, increased health complications, and potentially death (Burgess & Hanrahan, 2006).

Risk Factors

Regardless of the type of abuse an elder suffers or the motivation of the abuser, two factors are common to all elder abuse situations. The first factor is the *invisibility* of elders in general and of abused elders specifically. It is estimated that fewer than 10% of elder abuse cases are reported. In 1988, Pillemer and Finkelhor found that only one of every 14 cases of elder abuse came to public attention in Massachusetts, a state with model reporting laws. Reasons for invisibility among the elderly are multifaceted. Older people usually have less contact with the community. They are no longer in the workforce or in public on a regular basis, which keeps their problems hidden longer. In addition, older adults are reticent to admit to being abused or neglected. Because the abuser is most often a family member, the elder desires to protect the abuser; without this abusing family member, the elder may be entirely alone. On the other hand, the elder may fear reprisal from the abuser for coming forward with a self-report of abuse or telling someone about the home situation. Cultural and societal values also contribute to keeping "family matters" private, while shame and embarrassment make it difficult for many elders to tell others of the abuse (American Psychological Association [APA], 2007).

The second risk factor is the *vulnerability* of older adults. Many elders who are frail are dependent on others for some aspect of their day-to-day survival. At first, they may need to rely on others for transportation, shopping, and housekeeping. Later, they may need help with financial affairs, cooking, and laundry. In time, the elder may need help managing medications, bathing, and eating. The degree to which an elder needs assistance is often kept hidden from others because the elder fears being removed from his present living situation and being placed in a more restrictive environment. Additionally, vulnerability in elders is increased when any of the following characteristics are present: (a) impairment and isolation, (b) poverty and pathologic caregivers, (c) learned helplessness and living in a violent subculture, and (d) living in deteriorating housing and crime-ridden neighborhoods.

Prevention of Elder Abuse

Awareness of elder abuse and education about the types of abuse via media campaigns has improved community recognition of the problem. Increasing attention is now directed at the unique care needs of elders, including resources for the elderly and the need for caregiver respite has also received increased attention and services. Training for caregivers as well as health care and social service providers that focus on recognizing stress and initiating measures for intervening has developed new understanding of effective interventions (e.g., use of physical therapists, occupational therapists, and geropsychiatrists). Statutory requirements for reporting abuse and providing crisis hotlines for reporting elder abuse are also integral aspects of a community's response to the problem of elder abuse (APA, 2007). World Elder Abuse Awareness Day has been designated as an annual observance on June 15th to promote public awareness and prevention education regarding elder abuse (National Center on Elder Abuse, 2011a).

OTHER FORMS OF FAMILY VIOLENCE

Three other forms of violence that directly affect families are suicide, homicide, and rape. These three forms of violence demonstrate the ultimate extreme of violence to the victim and are the most traumatic to the surviving family members.

Suicide

Suicide is taking action that causes one's own death. In the United States, suicide is the 11th leading cause of death, as more than 31,000 people kill themselves each year (CDC, 2006b). Not all suicide attempts are successful, and each year, over 425,000 people are treated in emergency rooms from self-inflicted injuries (CDC, 2006b). These attempts to cause or actually cause self-harm are known as *parasuicidal acts*. Gender has an influence on suicide rates and fatalities—men are four times more likely than women to die, yet women are three times more likely than men to report a suicide attempt (CDC, 2006b). The *Healthy People 2010* goal was to reduce suicides to not more than 6 per 100,000 people, yet in 2004, there were 32,439 suicides, a rate of 89 suicides per day, or one suicide every 16 minutes (American Association of Suicidology [AAS], 2006).

Worldwide, the suicide rate has been increasing for the past 45 years. In 2000, "a global mortality rate of 16 per 100,000 people, or one death every 40 seconds," occurred, which translates to nearly 1 million people (WHO, n.d. a,, para. 1). The estimate for suicide attempts is up to 20 times more frequent than the fatality rate. Older men have traditionally had the highest suicide rate, although a noted increase in younger people is occurring in both developed and developing countries (WHO, n.d. b, para. 3). Ninety percent of suicides are associated with mental disorders, the most common are depression and substance abuse, which commonly occur during times of individual or family crisis (e.g., loss of a loved one, loss of employment) (WHO, n.d. b, para. 4).

It is important to be aware of warning signs of potential suicide when working with people in crisis.

Threats or comments that indicate a plan or giving personal items away are potential indicators of a person contemplating suicide. Access to guns increases one's risk regardless of age, gender, or ethnicity because firearms are the most utilized method of suicide. Health providers and others may find *IS PATH WARM*, a mnemonic from the AAS (n.d.), helpful when looking at possible warning signs for suicide. These signs are

I—ideation
S—substance abuse
P—purposelessness
A—anxiety
T—trapped
H—hopelessness
W—withdrawal
A—anger
R—recklessness
M—mood change

Completed suicides are carried out in a variety of ways, some more violent than others. Women usually choose less violent methods, such as overdosing on medications. Men choose more violent forms of suicide, such as hanging, use of firearms, or vehicle crashes. Deaths from suicide are underreported because of a tendency to group them as accidental deaths or deaths from undetermined causes.

Community awareness campaigns and education programs are needed to help a person recognize the risks and the importance of initiating prevention for someone who is suicidal. Crisis hotlines with 24-hour access are a vital resource for a distraught individual, friend, or loved one to contact and find help during a crisis and to learn about local resources to contact. Appropriate and consistent treatment, most often a combination of antidepressants and psychotherapy approach, is needed for those suffering from depression because individuals with a major depressive disorder have approximately a 20 times higher risk for suicide than the general population (AAS, 2007). The surviving loved ones require attention to their grief and bereavement. Support groups often provide benefits, allowing the bereaved to share their intense feelings of guilt and learn how to deal with any sense of a stigma, embarrassment, or shame felt by the survivors.

Homicide

Homicide is any non–war-related action taken to cause the death of another person. Violence has historically been associated with crime and is generally categorized by the method or age group affected. The WHO cites, "On an average day, 1,424 people are killed in acts of homicide, almost one person every minute" (2002b, para. 2). More shocking is the report that violence is the leading cause of death for those from ages 15 to 44 years, and precipitating factors are often fighting, bullying, and drunkenness (para. 5).

The homicide rate in the US has been fairly consistent at 6.1 per 100,000 for the past decade. The *Healthy People 2020* objective is to reduce the homicide rate by 10% to 5.5 per 100,000 (USDHHS, 2011). Within this goal is the stark realization that a 10% decline in just the homicide rate for those aged 15–44 years would mean nearly 1200 lives would be saved each year (CDC, 2012). Many homicide casualties are victims of domestic abuse as the cycle of violence escalates; a partner may be killed during a violent episode or by a recruited third party. Homicide in young infants and children is most often perpetrated by the parent, stepparent, or caregiver. Conflict between adolescent males may escalate if weapons or guns are available, resulting in homicide.

Evidence suggests that violence can be prevented by measures aimed at individuals, families, and communities. Although biologic and personal factors may influence one's predisposition to violence, an interaction between one's family, community, cultural, and other factors combine to create violence (WHO, 2002a). The WHO cites four key steps in developing a public health approach to violence; these steps are

- Uncovering as much knowledge as possible about all aspects of violence
- Investigating why it occurs
- Exploring ways to prevent violence
- Taking action, which includes disseminating information, and evaluating programs' effectiveness (WHO, 2002a, p. 1)

Prevention methods include education programs for preschool, school-aged children, and adolescents to decrease bullying and improve social skills; parent education courses and parent resources such as advice lines, support groups, or a crisis nursery; and community measures that improve firearm safety and reduce firearm injuries (WHO, 2002a).

Rape

Rape is an act of aggression in which the perpetrator is motivated by a desire to dominate, control, and degrade the victim. Once considered an act of sexuality, rape is now believed to be a combination of domination and sexuality, or defined as a "sexual expression of aggression." The National Violence Against Women Survey (NVAWS) working with the CDC and National Institute of Justice reports that 302,091 women and 92,748 men are raped each year in the United States. Furthermore, the survey estimates that one in six women and one in 33 men have been a rape victim at some time during their life, with over half of all rapes occurring before the age of 18 and one third of the rapes occurring before age 12 (CDC, 2004). Rape, in more than eight of ten cases (83%), is perpetrated by someone the victim knows (CDC, 2004).

The violence of rape creates physical and psychological harm for the victim and those close to them. Health problems for the victim may include head, pelvic, back, or facial pain; depression; suicidal ideation; eating disorders; gastrointestinal disorders; or substance abuse (CDC, 2004). Fear, anxiety, or shame may become debilitating for the victim. Counseling and professional care are necessary for the rape victim from the time the rape is reported through any legal process that may result.

Community measures useful in preventing rape include rape prevention education (RPE) programs for adolescents and college students, date rape education, hotlines staffed to provide help for victims of rape or VAW, and having trained professionals, such as a SARTs on hand (CDC, 2004). SART members are trained to understand the psychological and physical assessment needs of the victim, as well as the legal requirements for an investigation and court proceeding. Rape crisis centers and state sexual assault coalitions work together with law enforcement, health care providers, and community-based organizations (CBOs) to provide community education and care and support to victims.

LEVELS OF PREVENTION: CRISIS INTERVENTION AND FAMILY VIOLENCE

Family violence is a family crisis and needs intervention. Community health nurses are in a unique position to prevent, identify, and intervene during crisis situations. Because community health nurses encounter people in their own settings, a more accurate assessment with direct observation, discussion, and intervention can occur. The community health nurse's assessment skills, familiarity with the community, and access to resources enhance his ability to help families in crisis. By using the three levels of prevention, the nurse can begin to assist families in a variety of ways to counter problems arising from domestic violence.

Primary Prevention

The cycle of violence within the family can be interrupted. Even when partners, spouses, or parents have been brought up in violent homes by abusive parents, they can learn to rechannel and control their emotions and behaviors and use more appropriate coping strategies. Primary prevention is the most effective level of intervention in terms of promoting clients' health and containing costs. Primary prevention reflects a fundamental human concern for wellbeing and includes planned activities undertaken by the nurse to prevent an unwanted event from occurring, to protect current health and healthy functioning, and to promote improved states of health for all members of a community. For the community health nurse, any activity that fosters healthful practices will counteract unhealthful influences, thereby empowering an individual or family help prevent a crisis. Health promotion must take into account the physical, psychological, sociocultural, and spiritual needs of the individual and family.

Opportunities for families to improve relationships with their partner or spouse and children may begin with learning social problem-solving skills. Both partners benefit by participating in these learning sessions/opportunities. Assertiveness skills for women provide a foundation on which additional empowerment can build. Many people have not learned positive problem-solving skills that are socially acceptable, while women may have learned passivity and submissiveness in response to their own childhood parenting or from an abusive upbringing.

Healthy self-esteem improves education and occupational success. If poverty is a factor related to the violence, adequate educational preparation and having a successful employee role may eliminate this stressor. Violence occurs across all socioeconomic levels; however, if a family is so impoverished that its basic needs cannot be met, stress can lead vulnerable family members to seek illegal ways to solve their financial problems. Living in neighborhoods where criminal activity is common often leads to increased violence and risk of abuse.

Parenting, one of life's most difficult roles, influences children in their coping strategies, decision making, and sense of self-confidence. Parenting classes are an important resource to assist parents, particularly parents who are at high risk, such as teens, people with no exposure to children in their upbringing, and people raised in violent and abusive families. Parenting classes offer an opportunity for parents to share information and the stresses of parenting, while learning new strategies for managing their children's behaviors and appropriate physical, emotional, and developmental expectations for their children's ages.

Community health nurses often make home visits to families based on referrals from hospital perinatal departments. During the mother's postpartum stay, a nurse may have noted some inappropriate parenting behaviors or that the parents may meet high-risk parameters set by the hospital, such as being age 17 or younger, being a single parent, or having a history of substance abuse. On the first few visits to the family, the nurse can assess parenting skills and need for further teaching. If a parenting class is recommended, the course should cover age-appropriate content, such as safety, breast-feeding, formula preparation, food progression, anticipatory guidance for growth and development, discipline techniques including behavior modification and time-out, well-baby care, and immunizations. Additional benefits for the parents are the social support they receive from participating with other parents and having the opportunity to share their needs and concerns about child-rearing.

Home visiting has been formalized into public health nursing model programs around the country, based on two decades of work by David Olds and others. This evidenced-based program has shown that nurse follow-up and interventions during the pregnancy and for the first 2 years of the child's life was effective in preventing child abuse, decreasing the mother's reliance on government assistance, having mothers with longer spacing between their children and fewer subsequent pregnancies, and improving health habits, such as less smoking by mothers (Eckenrode et al., 2010; Olds, Henderson, Tatelbaum, & Chamberlin, 1988; Olds et al., 1999, 2010). In these programs, a nurse visits the mother and child on a regular basis over 1 to 3 years, teaching and role-modeling parenting techniques, providing needed support, and initiating necessary referrals.

The interrelatedness between families and communities cannot be overlooked or underestimated. Neighborhoods need to be enfranchised, developed, and attentive to the needs for health and safety for all community members. Empowered families can take back their neighborhoods from criminals, and their empowerment acts as a source of growth for other families.

Secondary Prevention

Early diagnosis and prompt treatment of the effects of family crisis or violence is the focus at a secondary level of prevention. Secondary prevention seeks to reduce the intensity and duration of a crisis and to promote adaptive behavior. By creating a positive relationship with family members and seeing them in their homes, the community health nurse can often uncover and intervene in a crisis or stop abusive situations.

People in crisis need help. Often, they desperately want help. The crisis, or violence, and its associated disequilibrium has a twofold effect on the individuals involved: it renders them temporarily helpless and unable to cope on their own, and it makes them especially receptive to outside influence. Community health nurses can implement crisis resolution models to assist clients at the secondary level. The following process has been used successfully in the mental health field by those working on crisis hot lines, in mental health centers, or in emergency departments. These steps are

1. Establish rapport.
2. Assess the individual and the problem for lethality.
3. Identify major problems and intervene.
4. Deal with feelings.
5. Explore alternatives and coping mechanisms.
6. Develop an action plan.
7. Follow up, including anticipatory planning for coping with future crises (Aguilera, 1998).

People in crisis will seek and generally receive some kind of help, but the nature of that help may act in favor of or against a healthy outcome from which the participants can grow and evolve. A client's desire for assistance gives the helping professional a prime opportunity to intervene; this opportunity also presents a challenge to make the intervention as effective as possible. Behaviors found to be helpful in these interventions include the following:

- *Respect confidentiality*. Discussions must occur in private, without other family members present or in within the proximity for hearing. Confidentiality is essential to build trust and ensure the client's safety.
- *Believe and validate the client's experiences*. Listen to and believe him. Acknowledge the client's feelings and validate that many others have had similar experiences.
- *Acknowledge any injustice*. In the case of violence, acknowledge that no one deserves to be abused.
- *Respect clients' autonomy*. Respect their right to make life decisions, particularly regarding whether to involve the police. Validate and respect clients' choices. They are the experts in their lives.
- *Help the client plan for future safety*. What past strategies have been successful for self-protection? Does the client have a safe place to escape to if necessary? If children are involved, what plans are available to protect them? Help clients to recognize danger in their lives.
- *Promote access to community services*. Know the resources in your community. Is there a shelter for battered or homeless clients? A domestic violence hotline? A rape crisis center? Give clients the appropriate phone numbers (Davis & Harsh, 2001; Kramer, 2002).

One goal of crisis intervention should be to help clients reestablish a sense of safety and security while allowing them to ventilate their feelings and have those feelings validated. This process helps reestablish equilibrium at as healthy a level as possible and can result in client change and growth. Minimally, the goal is to resolve the immediate crisis and restore clients to their precrisis level of functioning. Ultimately, however, intervention seeks to raise their functioning to a healthier, more mature level that will enable them to cope with and prevent future crises. As discussed earlier, crises tend to be self-limited; intervention time generally lasts from 4 to 8 weeks, with resolution, one way or another, within 2 or 3 months (Aguilera, 1998). The urgency of the situation represents a window of opportunity that invites prompt, focused attention by the client and nurse in working together to achieve intervention goals.

Special programs for children who live in homes where crises and violence are chronic include Head Start programs for prekindergarten children who meet certain socioeconomic characteristics. These programs are designed to give children social and academic stimulation, thereby increasing their skills for when they enter kindergarten. Other programs for social skills development may include a Special Friends program explicitly for children who have survived abusive situations, or primary intervention programs (PIP), in which the child works with a trained, supportive, and caring adult.

Abuse survivors and those living in homes with domestic violence experience multiple developmental and psychological problems. Children who are experiencing academic and social failure should receive ongoing services as needed through their elementary, middle, and high school grades. Early identification and intervention with conduct-disordered youth ensure that appropriate resources are obtained and, hopefully, that behavior outbursts and violence will be eliminated. School nurses are important interprofessional team members in providing assessments and programs for these youth.

Intervention at the secondary level for adults who experience abuse focuses on women and their children. Shelters for women and children are available in most communities and offer a variety of services, including counseling, classes in self-esteem building and assertiveness training, referrals to or programs for job training, and even money/budgeting and time management classes. Some shelters offer programs that last up to 2 years with progressive independence and employment skill development while the women and their children live in a protected home environment with their addresses kept confidential from abusers.

Depending on the situation that brings the woman to a shelter, the perpetrator may or may not be incarcerated or on probation. If arrested during the most recent violent episode, the abuser may be released, on parole, or incarcerated. Even while incarcerated, the abuser may be able to take part in an anger management class, psychological counseling, substance abuse treatment, Alcoholics Anonymous (AA) meetings, or Narcotics Anonymous (NA) meetings. Visits between the abuser and the children are supervised, if that is part of a court order.

At times, the nurse may be responding to a referral regarding suspected abuse; at other times, an abusive or neglectful situation may be uncovered on a home visit made for another reason. In any case, the community health nurse has an important role in reporting suspected abuse and encouraging the child, partner/spouse, or elder to go to the appropriate facility to seek care and to file required documentation about the abuse (see From the Case Files).

From the Case Files

Community Health Nursing and a Potential Family in Crisis

You are a community health nurse working for Smithville Health Department. You are following up on a referral from a community clinic's family planning clinic. The referral was made for a 19-year-old woman, Sandy, who presented in clinic and exhibited inappropriate behaviors with her 6-month-old daughter. In their referral, staff stated that they observed the mother shouting at the child, accusing her of "being spoiled rotten." They added that the mother appeared quite anxious and seemed to have difficulty waiting the 15 minutes for her examination. Although the behaviors described in this referral were insufficient to warrant a report to social services, the staff felt that this young mother would benefit from intervention on the part of the nurse.

You prepare for this home visit by reviewing the medical records of both Sandy and her child to determine whether the family has had previous involvement with social service agencies such as CPS. You find that the maternal grandparents made a referral to Child Welfare on behalf of Sandy when she was 15. They were concerned about the relationship between Sandy and her stepfather. The report cited suspected sexual involvement between the two. An investigation occurred but was inconclusive, and the charges were never pursued.

You also discuss the case with family planning and immunization clinic staff, since the family receives services at both clinics. The staff advises you that they are familiar with Sandy and her husband Nick. They state that their only interaction with Nick was during a family planning clinic 2 months ago. They report that Sandy appeared anxious and in a hurry on that day, stating, "I really need to hurry, Nick is waiting in the car and he gets impatient." Shortly after that, the staff tells you, Nick came running into the clinic shouting, "What the hell is taking you people so long?" He reportedly glared at Sandy, and the two quickly exited the clinic.

You phone the client and advise her that you are a nurse with the local health department. You inform her that nurses often visit new mothers to assist them in finding resources. You add that as a community health nurse, you will be available to talk with her about her child's growth and development.

The client expresses interest in the visit and states, "I want you to show me some things about feeding her and stuff. I need help figuring out what to do at night, she still isn't sleeping much and it's driving me crazy." You advise the client that you will be happy to discuss those issues with her, that you will bring information that you will review with her. You add that you noted in her medical record that the father of the baby is living in the home and assure her that she may involve other family members, including the father of the baby, in the home visit. You jointly decide that the visit will occur the following day at 10:30 AM and that the father of the baby will be present if his work schedule allows.

On the day of the visit, as you walk up the stairs toward the apartment, you notice someone looking at you through the curtains. As you near the apartment door, the curtains close. Your repeated knocking on the door is met with no response. You call the client's name but there is no answer.

Questions

1. Would this scenario provoke anxiety for you? How would you deal with your reaction?
2. How is this different from a scenario in the acute care setting in which a supervisor would be readily available?
3. Given this scenario, what actions will you take?
4. If you had been working in the family planning clinic on the day that Nick came in, what, if anything, would you have done differently?
5. As young parents, Nick and Sandy are part of an aggregate that has unique risk factors for parenting. List as many of these risk factors as you can think of and brainstorm about possible community health nursing interventions for each.
6. What methods would you suggest the clinic staff utilize to detect signs and symptoms of physical, sexual, or emotional abuse among this aggregate?

Reporting Abuse

All states have reporting laws for suspected abuse, although states differ on aspects of the timeline for reporting, who to notify, and the sequence of events. The following steps represent one state's guidelines for reporting suspected child abuse (Crime and Violence Prevention Center, 2003b):

1. All mandated reporters must report known or suspected abuse.
2. Immediately, or as soon as reasonably possible, a local child protective agency (police department after normal working hours) must be contacted and given a verbal report. During this verbal report, mandated reporters must give their name—which is kept confidential and may be revealed only in court or if the reporter waives confidentiality (others can give information anonymously)—the name and age of the child, the present location of the child, the nature and characteristics of the injury, and any other facts that led the reporter to suspect abuse or that would be helpful to the investigator.
3. Within 2 working days, a written report must be completed by the mandated reporter and filed. If a mandated reporter fails to report known or suspected instances of child abuse, they may be subject to criminal liability, punishable by up to 6 months in jail or a fine of $1,000.

Similar steps are required for nurses when reporting elder abuse. Cases of maltreatment and neglect among elders are reported to a local area agency on aging, Adult Protective Services, or to the police, and a screening/documentation form is used to gather and record pertinent information. Guidelines for filing the report and agency notification are specific within each state.

In cases of partner/spousal abuse, adults who are mentally competent cannot be removed involuntarily from the abusive situation. The community health nurse can encourage the victim to leave the perpetrator for the victim's safety until the perpetrator gets professional help and can give information regarding community resources, such as a shelter for women and children. If the adult has a life-threatening injury or illness, medical follow-up must be encouraged; however, the victim may still be reluctant to seek help. At times, another family member or neighbor who witnesses the abusive event calls 911; when the police and paramedics arrive, the victim may have support to seek care and needed protection. A domestic violence screening/documentation form is completed by the nurse as a part of the official health records for the client.

Tools

Assessment of suspected abuse cannot be overemphasized. The community health nurse may be the only person entering the home of a family in crisis where abuse is occurring. Asking the right questions, being a careful observer, and following the correct reporting process and recording procedures may mean the difference between life and death for a victim of violence.

Displays 20.10, 20.11, and 20.12 consist of three sample tools that the community health nurse and other advocates use in their role as a mandated reporter. These forms include a Suspected Child Abuse Report, a two-page Medical Report of Suspected Child Abuse, and a Domestic Violence Screening/Documentation Form.

Tertiary Prevention

Tertiary prevention focuses on the rehabilitation of the family from the violence and crisis they have sustained. The family may never again have the same connections because partners may separate—by choice, motivated by fear or hatred; by court order, if the perpetrator is incarcerated; or by death. If the family chooses to stay together, long-term intervention for all family members is needed to establish a climate more conducive to family normalcy. Many of the services discussed as part of the secondary level of prevention are continued into the tertiary prevention phase to promote healing and to restore and promote family growth.

If incarceration is a part of tertiary prevention, the effects of having one family member living in this environment must be factored into the services and support provided by the community health nurse to the family as a whole (see Chapter 30 for information on correctional facilities). Even if the partner/spouse has separated from the perpetrator emotionally and/or legally, the perpetrator usually has legal rights to see the children. This may mean that other family members, usually from the abuser's side of the family, can bring the children to the prison to visit their parent. Just making arrangements for these visits can cause stress to the visitors. The community health nurse needs to be aware of the complicated dynamics and emotional stress such difficult situations can produce for all family members. The victim–perpetrator relationship is as complex as the forces that created the violence and abuse.

FAMILIES FACING VIOLENCE FROM OUTSIDE THE FAMILY

The concern of violence coming into the family from outside the home, often beyond the family's control, is a relatively new phenomenon in the United States. There has always been some degree of violence that affects families in their homes, such as burglaries, or at times murder, or abduction. Increasingly, however, home invasion, a form of forced entry to terrorize family members, is a violent crime perpetrated most frequently by strangers. Other forms of violence of which families are more aware include the potential for terrorist activities through planned community violence (such as the plane crashes on September 11, 2001) and biologic, chemical, or radioactive actions (see Chapter 17). Communities have developed resources such as the National Organization for Victim Assistance (NOVA) and crisis response teams (CRT), to assist individuals and groups experiencing a disaster or violent event (e.g., child murder or school shootings).

Home invasion is an increasing new form of terror. It occurs mainly in large cities, although rural areas

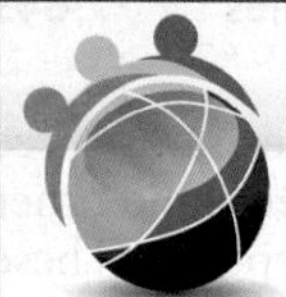

DISPLAY 20.10 SUSPECTED CHILD ABUSE REPORT

SUSPECTED CHILD ABUSE REPORT

To Be Completed by Reporting Party
Pursuant to Penal Code Section 11166

A. CASE IDENTI-FICATION — *TO BE COMPLETED BY INVESTIGATING CPA*
VICTIM NAME:
REPORT NO./CASE NAME:
DATE OF REPORT:

B. REPORTING PARTY

NAME/TITLE		
ADDRESS		
PHONE ( )	DATE OF REPORT	SIGNATURE

C. REPORT SENT TO

☐ POLICE DEPARTMENT ☐ SHERIFF'S OFFICE ☐ COUNTY WELFARE ☐ COUNTY PROBATION

AGENCY	ADDRESS	
OFFICIAL CONTACTED	PHONE ( )	DATE/TIME

D. INVOLVED PARTIES

VICTIM

NAME (LAST, FIRST, MIDDLE)	ADDRESS	BIRTHDATE	SEX	RACE
PRESENT LOCATION OF CHILD		PHONE ( )		

SIBLINGS

	NAME	BIRTHDATE	SEX	RACE		NAME	BIRTHDATE	SEX	RACE
1.					4.				
2.					5.				
3.					6.				

PARENTS

NAME (LAST, FIRST, MIDDLE)	BIRTHDATE	SEX	RACE	NAME (LAST, FIRST, MIDDLE)	BIRTHDATE	SEX	RACE
ADDRESS				ADDRESS			
HOME PHONE ( )	BUSINESS PHONE ( )			HOME PHONE ( )	BUSINESS PHONE ( )		

E. INCIDENT INFORMATION

IF NECESSARY, ATTACH EXTRA SHEET OR OTHER FORM AND CHECK THIS BOX. ☐

1. DATE/TIME OF INCIDENT — PLACE OF INCIDENT — *(CHECK ONE)* ☐ OCCURRED ☐ OBSERVED

IF CHILD WAS IN OUT-OF-HOME CARE AT TIME OF INCIDENT, CHECK TYPE OF CARE:
☐ FAMILY DAY CARE ☐ CHILD CARE CENTER ☐ FOSTER FAMILY HOME ☐ SMALL FAMILY HOME ☐ GROUP HOME OR INSTITUTION

2. TYPE OF ABUSE: *(CHECK ONE OR MORE)* ☐ PHYSICAL ☐ MENTAL ☐ SEXUAL ASSAULT ☐ NEGLECT ☐ OTHER

3. NARRATIVE DESCRIPTION:

4. SUMMARIZE WHAT THE ABUSED CHILD OR PERSON ACCOMPANYING THE CHILD SAID HAPPENED:

5. EXPLAIN KNOWN HISTORY OF SIMILAR INCIDENT(S) FOR THIS CHILD:

SS 8572 (Rev. 1/93)

INSTRUCTIONS AND DISTRIBUTION ON REVERSE

DO NOT submit a copy of this form to the Department of Justice (DOJ). A CPA is required under Penal Code Section 11169 to submit to DOJ a Child Abuse Investigation Report Form SS-8583 if (1) an active investigation has been conducted and (2) the incident is **not** unfounded.

Police or Sheriff-WHITE Copy; County Welfare or Probation-BLUE Copy; District Attorney-GREEN Copy; Reporting Party-YELLOW Copy

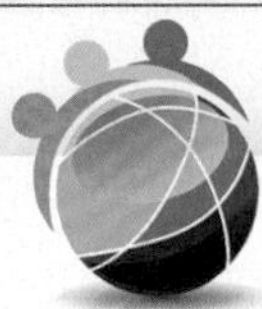

DISPLAY 20.11 MEDICAL REPORT: SUSPECTED CHILD ABUSE

DOJ 900 84 89220

MEDICAL REPORT—SUSPECTED CHILD ABUSE

HOSPITAL

INSTRUCTIONS: ALL PROFESSIONAL MEDICAL PERSONNEL ARE REQUIRED BY SECTION 11166 OF THE PENAL CODE TO COMPLETE THIS FORM IN CONJUNCTION WITH THE SS 8572 SUSPECTED CHILD ABUSE REPORT WHERE CHILD ABUSE, AS DEFINED BY SECTION 11165 OF THE PENAL CODE, IS SUSPECTED. THE REPORTS, DOJ 900 AND SS 8572, MUST BE SUBMITTED TO A POLICE OR SHERIFF'S DEPARTMENT, OR A COUNTY PROBATION OR WELFARE DEPARTMENT WITHIN 36 HOURS. PROFESSIONAL MEDICAL PERSONNEL MEANS ANY PHYSICIAN AND SURGEON, PSYCHIATRIST, PSYCHOLOGIST, DENTIST, RESIDENT, INTERN, PODIATRIST, CHIROPRACTOR, LICENSED NURSE, DENTAL HYGIENIST OR ANY OTHER PERSON WHO IS CURRENTLY LICENSED UNDER DIVISION 2 (COMMENCING WITH SECTION 500) OF THE BUSINESS AND PROFESSIONS CODE. EACH PART OF THE FORM MUST BE COMPLETED UNLESS INAPPLICABLE. IN FILLING OUT THIS FORM, NO CIVIL LIABILITY ATTACHES AND NO CONFIDENTIALITY IS BREACHED.

I. GENERAL INFORMATION Print or type

PATIENT'S NAME | HOSPITAL ID NO.

ADDRESS | CITY | COUNTY | STATE | PHONE

AGE | BIRTHDATE | RACE | SEX | DATE AND TIME OF ARRIVAL | MODE OF TRANSPORTATION | DATE AND TIME OF DISCHARGE

ACCOMPANIED TO HOSPITAL BY: NAME | ADDRESS | CITY | STATE | RELATIONSHIP

PHONE REPORT MADE TO | ID NO. | DEPARTMENT | PHONE | RESPONDING OFFICER/AGENCY

NAME OF: ☐ FATHER ☐ STEPFATHER | ADDRESS | CITY | COUNTY | HOME PHONE | BUS. PHONE | AGE/DOB

NAME OF: ☐ MOTHER ☐ STEPMOTHER | ADDRESS | CITY | COUNTY | HOME PHONE | BUS. PHONE | AGE/DOB

SIBLINGS: LAST NAME, FIRST | DOB | LAST NAME, FIRST | DOB | LAST NAME, FIRST | DOB

II. MEDICAL EXAMINATION

A. History

1. EXPLANATION OF INJURIES BY PARENT OR PERSON ACCOMPANYING CHILD (LOCATION, DATE, TIME AND CIRCUMSTANCES)
2. PATIENT'S STATEMENT EXPLAINING INJURY (PARAPHRASE)
3. PATIENT'S EMOTIONAL REACTION TO EXAMINATION (SUBMISSIVE, COMPLIANT, ETC.)
4. PREVIOUS HISTORY OF CHILD ABUSE (IF KNOWN)

B. Sexual Assault Perform exam only if necessary.

1. ACTS COMMITTED: NOTE—COITUS, FELLATIO, CUNNILINGUS, SODOMY
2. DURING ASSAULT: ☐ VAGINAL PENETRATION (HOW) | EJACULATION: ☐ VAGINAL ☐ ORAL ☐ ANAL ☐ OTHER:
   ☐ ANAL PENETRATION (HOW) | ☐ CONDOM USED ☐ VOMITED ☐ LOSS OF CONSCIOUSNESS ☐ OTHER:
3. AFTER ASSAULT: ☐ WIPED/WASHED ☐ BATHED ☐ DOUCHED ☐ VOMITED ☐ CHANGED CLOTHES ☐ BRUSHED TEETH ☐ DEFECATED ☐ OTHER:

C. Physical Examination | DATE AND TIME OF EXAM | DATE AND TIME OF ASSAULT | BP | PULSE | RESP | TEMP

HEIGHT | WEIGHT | HEAD CIRCUM | LAST TETANUS | KNOWN ALLERGIES | CURRENT MEDICATION

DIAGNOSTIC DATA

Check if indicated and incorporate results in written examination at left

- ☐ X-rays (skull, chest, longbone, full skeletal)
- ☐ Bleeding, coagulation, tourniquet, tests
- ☐ Funduscopic
- ☐ Other

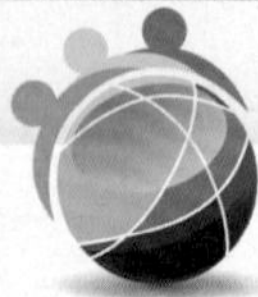

DISPLAY 20.11 MEDICAL REPORT: SUSPECTED CHILD ABUSE *(Continued)*

DOJ 900

DATE	HOSPITAL ID NO.	HOSPITAL

PHYSICAL EXAMINATION (CONTINUED) LOCATE AND DESCRIBE IN DETAIL ANY INJURIES OR FINDINGS. TRAUMA, BRUISES; ERYTHEMA, EXCORIATIONS, LACERATIONS, WOUNDS. TRACE OUTLINE USED AND INDICATE LOCATION OF WOUNDS/LACERATIONS USING 'X' FOR SUPERFICIAL, 'O' FOR DEEP; SHADE FOR BRUISES OR BURNS. BESIDE EACH INJURY INDICATED NOTE COLOR, SIZE, PATTERN, TEXTURE, AND SENSATION. WRITE OVER UNUSED OUTLINES. DESCRIBE IN DETAIL SHAPE OF ARM OR OTHER BRUISES WHICH MAY INDICATE FORCE

D. PELVIC A PELVIC EXAMINATION SHOULD NOT BE PERFORMED UNLESS THE PARENT, GUARDIAN OR MINOR CONSENT OR UNLESS NECESSARY AS PART OF TREATMENT. SEE DEPARTMENT OF HEALTH REGULATIONS TITLE 22, DIVISION 2, VICTIMS OF SEXUAL ASSAULT. SAME INSTRUCTIONS AS GENERAL PHYSICAL, IN ADDITION, NOTE PUBIC HAIR COMBINGS WHERE INDICATED, DRIED SECRETIONS AND RECENT INJURIES TO HYMEN, TRACE AND OUTLINE AS ABOVE.

III. DIAGNOSTIC IMPRESSION OF TRAUMA AND INJURIES

IV. TREATMENT/DISPOSITION OF PATIENT

A. ☐ GC CULTURE ☐ VDRL ☐ PREGNANCY TEST ☐ POST COITAL ESTROGEN ☐ VD PROPHYLAXIS ☐ OTHER:

☐ MOTILE SPERM: ☐ PRESENCE ☐ ABSENCE ☐ NOT TAKEN ☐ FAMILY ASSESSMENT BY: NOT ORDERED ☐

B. ORDERS:

C. DISPOSITION: ☐ ADMIT TRANSFERRED TO:

☐ RELEASED ACCOMPANIED BY: NAME ADDRESS RELATIONSHIP

I HAVE RECEIVED THE INDICATED ITEMS AS EVIDENCE AND A COPY OF THIS REPORT.

OFFICER: ID NO.: DATE:

NURSE SIGNATURE OF EXAMINATION PHYSICIAN

V. SPECIMENS

STAINS/FOREIGN MATERIALS (WHEN INDICATED)

LOOSE HAIR ___ FINGERNAIL SCRAPINGS ___

BLOOD ___ DIRT OR GRAVEL ___

THREADS ___ VEGETATION ___

GRASS ___ CLOTHING ___

DRIED SECRETIONS ___

	SLIDES	SWABS
VAGINAL	___	___
RECTAL	___	___
ORAL	___	___
ASPIRATES/WASHINGS	___	___
BITE MARKS	___	___
OTHER:	___	___

PATIENT'S SAMPLES. TIME OF COLLECTION AT MD DISCRETION

BLOOD ___

HAIR FROM HEAD ___

SALIVA ___

HAIR FROM PUBIC AREA ___

D. FOLLOW-UP WITHIN:

☐ MEDICAL ___ HRS ___ DAYS

☐ SOCIAL SERVICES ___ HRS ___ DAYS

☐ PRIVATE MD ___ HRS ___ DAYS

☐ OTHER ___ HRS ___ DAYS

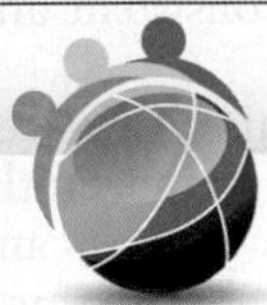

DISPLAY 20.12 DOMESTIC VIOLENCE SCREENING/DOCUMENTATION FORM

DV SCREEN

❒ Screened
- ❒ Yes
- ❒ No
- ❒ Probable/Suspected DV

❒ Not Screened

Routinely Screen at Each Visit

"Because violence is so common in women's lives, I've begun to ask about it routinely."

Ask Direct Questions

"I'm concerned that your injuries/symptoms may have been caused by someone hurting you. Is this what happened to you?"

-OR-

"Has your intimate partner or ex-partner ever physically hurt you? Have they ever *threatened* to hurt you or someone close to you?"

Assess Patient Safety

❒ Yes ❒ No Is patient afraid to go home?

❒ Yes ❒ No Has physical violence increased in severity over past years?

❒ Yes ❒ No Have threats of homicide been made?

❒ Yes ❒ No Have threats of suicide been made?

❒ Yes ❒ No Is alcohol or substance abuse also a problem?

❒ Yes ❒ No Is there a gun in the house?

❒ Yes ❒ No Is patient afraid of their partner?

❒ Yes ❒ No Was safety plan discussed?

Referrals

❒ hotline number given

❒ legal referral made

❒ shelter number given

❒ in-house referral made

❒ discharge instructions given

Date ________ Patient ID#________

Patient Name

Provider Name

Patient Pregnant? Yes ___ No ___

Describe frequency and severity of present and past abuse (use direct quotes as much as possible)

Describe location and extent of injury

Indicate where injury was observed

❒ Yes ❒ No Photographs taken?

❒ Yes ❒ No Consent to be photographed?

(Attach Photographs) + Appropriate Form

are not immune. *Home invasion* is the purposeful and sudden entry into a home by force while the family is home and awake. The effectiveness of this form of terror relies on surprise. Motivation may be material or thrill; household belongings are frequently stolen while family members are incapacitated by being bound, blindfolded, and/or gagged. In some cases, family members are killed. Often, the perpetrators are under the influence of drugs or alcohol, and at times, the violence may be gang related.

The community health nurse most likely will not encounter families who have experienced such violence. However, nurses may work with extended family members of the victims or families who have reported such a happening in their neighborhood and are now fearful of a reoccurrence. Fear of violence can create psychological and physiologic stress reactions similar to the sensations that occur when one actually experiences the violence. These fears should not be ignored. The role of the nurse includes four steps discussed in the generic approach to crisis intervention (see discussion in "Generic Approach").

METHODS OF CRISIS INTERVENTION

Crisis intervention in community health nursing uses either a generic or individual approach, or both. For the majority of crisis encounters, the generic approach is more appropriate. Family violence is a major situational crisis in which community health nurses intervene. However, many other situational and developmental crises affect families, and these families are benefited by the skills of the community health nurse. Newly recognized crises include community violence coming into the home and the potential of terrorism at home.

Generic Approach

The generic approach creates interventions to fit a particular type of crisis, focusing on the nature and course of the crisis rather than on the psychodynamic of each client (Aguilera, 1998). Crisis intervention using the generic approach is tailored to a specific kind of crisis, situational or developmental, and comprises four important elements: (1) use of adaptive behavior and coping strategies, (2) support of the individual/family, (3) preparation for the practical and emotional future, and (4) anticipatory guidance.

As an example, the generic approach is used with families experiencing child abuse. The child may be in foster care while the family receives needed services and rebuilds itself. The nurse encourages the parents to discuss and analyze their feelings, teaches stress-reduction techniques and positive coping skills, and creates a supportive, caring atmosphere, especially through self-help groups such as Parents Anonymous. The nurse can help individual family members strengthen their self-esteem by encouraging positive interpersonal relationships. The community health nurse also teaches needed parenting skills, providing anticipatory guidance, so that parents are prepared to raise their children with consistent and age-appropriate discipline techniques.

The generic approach does not require advanced professional psychotherapy skills. More importantly, this approach works well with families, groups, and even communities in crisis. The community health nurse may work with a group of cancer clients, abused elders, adolescents struggling with developmental crisis, or an entire community recovering from a natural or man-made disaster. The generic approach allows the nurse to intervene with any group of people who have a crisis in common. This approach also offers a broad base of support because the crisis group members can provide resources for one another beyond those brought by the nurse.

Individual Approach

The individual approach is used for clients who do not respond to the generic approach or who need special therapy. Individual crisis intervention should not be confused with individual psychotherapy, which tends to focus on a client's developmental past. In contrast, crisis intervention directs treatment toward the immediate state of disequilibrium, identifying its causes and developing coping mechanisms. Family members or significant others are included during the process of crisis resolution. An entire group may need this type of intervention. If this approach is needed, clients should be referred to a professional with specialized training.

ROLE OF THE COMMUNITY HEALTH NURSE IN CARING FOR FAMILIES IN CRISIS

Crisis intervention in community health assumes that clients have resources. If their potential for managing stressful events can be tapped, people in crisis will need minimal direct assistance. In accordance with the self-care concept, crisis intervention seeks to identify and build on client strengths. Aguilera (1998) outlined a series of four steps for intervention during crisis: assessment, planning, intervention, and resolution. Interventions to promote crisis resolution are presented using the three levels of prevention in Table 20-2.

Assessment and Nursing Diagnosis

Initially, the nurse must assess the nature of the crisis and the client's response to it. How severe is the problem, and what risks are the clients facing? Are other people also at risk? Assessment must be rapid but thorough and focused on specific areas.

First, the nurse concentrates on the immediate problem during the assessment. Why have clients asked for help right now? How do they define the problem? What precipitated the crisis? When did it occur? Was it a sudden accidental or situational event, or a slower developmental one?

Next, the nurse focuses on the clients' perceptions of the event. What does the crisis mean to them, and

Table 20-2 Levels of Prevention to Promote Crisis Resolution

Phase	Goals	Interventions
Primary prevention		
Precrisis	Health promotion	Anticipatory guidance
	Disease prevention	Reduce factors that increase vulnerability
	Education	Reduce hazards in some events (safety and multiplicity of stressors)
		Reinforce positive coping strategies
		Mobilize social support and other resources
Secondary prevention		
Crisis	Reduction of stress load	Assist with reaction to the event and functioning
	Cure or restoration of function	Allow behavior: dependence, grief
		Set goals with client
		Refer to resources
Tertiary prevention		
Postcrisis	Rehabilitation and maintenance	Promote adaptation to a changed level of wellness
		Promote interdependence
		Reinforce newly learned behaviors, lifestyle changes, coping strategies
		Explore application of learned behaviors to new situations
		Identification and use of additional resources

how do they think it will affect their future? Are they viewing the situation realistically? When a crisis occurs to a family or group, some members see the situation differently from others. During intervention, all family members should be encouraged to express themselves, to talk about the crisis, and to share their feelings about its meaning. Acceptance of the wide range of feelings is important.

Determine who is available to offer support to the individual or family. Consider family, friends, clergy, other professionals, community members, and agencies. Who are the clients close to, and who do they trust? One advantage of group intervention is that the members provide some of this support for one another. In subsequent sessions, the quality of support should be evaluated. Sometimes, a well-meaning individual can worsen the situation or deter clients from facing and coping with reality.

Finally, the nurse assesses the clients' coping abilities. Have they had similar kinds of experiences in the past? What techniques have they tried in this situation, and if they did not work, why not? Clients should be encouraged to think of other stress-relieving techniques, perhaps ones they have used in the past, and to try them.

The nurse gathers all of these data and mentally begins to form nursing diagnoses. As a plan of care is developed for the client, these nursing diagnoses are formalized in writing. Standardized nursing diagnoses are available for reference, or the agency where the nurse works may have a preferred format for nursing diagnoses. These nursing diagnoses are effective tools for the nurse to begin planning interventions.

Planning Therapeutic Interventions

Several factors influence clients' reaction to crises. Nurses should try to determine what factors are affecting clients before making intervention plans. The major balancing factors—clients' perceptions of the event, situational supports, human resources, and clients' coping skills—have been assessed in the first step (Aguilera, 1998). While continuing to explore these, the nurse now also considers the clients' general health status, age, past experiences with similar types of situations, sociocultural and religious influences, and the actual assets and liabilities of the situation. This assessment helps clarify the situation and gives the nurse an opportunity to further encourage the clients' participation in the resolution process. If clients are defensive, resistant, and rigid, they are not processing clearly and can complete only simple tasks. It will take time before these clients can begin to solve problems related to the effects of the crisis on themselves and the loss they are experiencing, but the nurse will want to encourage them to reach this level.

A therapeutic plan is based on multiple factors:

- The kind of crisis (situational or developmental, acute or chronically recurring)
- The effect the crisis is having on clients' lives (can they still work, go to school, and keep house, or are they secured within their home for an indefinite period, not knowing whether other family members have survived a major natural or man-made crisis?)
- Where they are in coming to resolution of the crisis

- The ways in which significant others are affected and respond
- Their level of preparation for such a crisis
- The clients' strengths and available resources

Using this problem-solving process, the nurse and clients develop a plan. They review the event that precipitated the crisis, obvious symptoms, and the disruption in the clients' lives. The plan may focus on several areas. For instance, clients may need to grasp intellectually the meaning of the crisis, to engage in greater expression of feelings, or work both on the intellectual and emotional aspects. Part of the plan may be directed toward finding appropriate and safe shelter, counseling, or physical care. Another part may focus on helping clients identify and use more effective coping techniques or locate supportive agencies and resources. The plan may also include development of realistic goals for the future.

Implementation

During implementation, communication between the nurse and clients is important. Discussions about what is happening, reviewing the family's plan and rationale for this approach, and making appropriate changes are necessary parts of this communication. Assigning definite activities at the end of each session will help clients try out different solutions and evaluate various coping behaviors. Implementation is enhanced by using the following guidelines (Levy & Sidel, 2002; Vastag, 2001):

1. *Demonstrate acceptance of clients.* A crisis often shatters the ego. Clients need to feel the support of a positive, caring person who does not judge their feelings or behavior. Some negative expressions, such as anger, withdrawal, and denial, are normal aspects of the crisis phase. Accept them as normal.
2. *Help clients confront crisis.* Clients need to face and discuss the situation. Expressing their feelings reduces tension and improves reality perception. Recounting what has actually occurred may be painful, but it helps clients confront the crisis. Do not assume that once clients have told about the event, no further recounting is necessary. Each time the story is told, the client comes closer to dealing realistically with the crisis.
3. *Help clients find facts.* Distorted ideas and unknown factors of the situation create additional tension and may lead to maladaptive responses. For instance, it would help inexperienced parents to know that children younger than 2 years of age cannot deliberately misbehave. Facts about childhood development and parenting training may be important for preventing crisis.
4. *Help clients express feelings openly.* Suppressed feelings can be harmful. For instance, a widow may feel guilty that she is glad her husband is gone. Expression of such feelings helps reduce tension and gives clients an opportunity to deal with them.
5. *Do not offer false reassurance.* Clients need to face reality, not avoid it. A statement such as "Don't worry, it will all work out" is demeaning and meaningless. Instead, make positive statements about faith in the clients' ability to cope: "It is a very difficult situation, but I believe you will be able to deal with it."
6. *Discourage clients from blaming others.* Clients often blame others as a way to avoid reality and the responsibility for problem solving. Withhold judgment when clients blame others but point out other causal factors and avenues for dealing with the situation.
7. *Help clients seek out coping mechanisms.* Explore and test old and new techniques to reduce stress and anxiety. Ask questions. What are the things that need to be done? What do clients think they can do? This assistance gives clients more adaptive energy to work toward resolution.
8. *Encourage clients to accept help.* Denial in the early phases of crisis cuts off help. Encouraging clients to acknowledge the problem is a first step toward acceptance of help. Often, clients fear the loss of their independence and the invasion of their privacy. A client may say, "We ought to be able to handle this problem." At this point, the community health nurse can reassure clients that people in a crisis of this sort almost always need help. Preparing people to accept help enables them to make the best use of what others have to offer.
9. *Promote development of new positive relationships.* Clients who have lost significant others through unintentional or intentional death, divorce, incarceration, or an act of perpetrated violence should be encouraged to find new connections, purpose, and people to fill the void and provide needed supports and satisfactions.

Evaluation of Crisis Resolution and Anticipatory Planning

In the final step, clients and the nurse evaluate, stabilize, and plan for the future. Evaluating the outcome of the intervention might address the following:

- Are the clients using effective coping skills and exhibiting appropriate behavior?
- Are adequate resources and support persons available?
- Is the diagnosed problem solved?
- Have the desired results been accomplished?

Analysis of these outcomes will provide a greater understanding for coping with future crises.

To stabilize the change that has occurred, identify and reinforce all of the positive coping mechanisms and behaviors. Discuss why they are effective, and explore ways to use them in future stressful situations. Summarize the crisis experience, emphasizing the clients' successes with coping, reconfirm their progress, and reinforce their self-confidence. It is especially important to point to the evidence that the client has reached their precrisis level, or an even higher level of functioning.

Clients' plans for the future should include setting realistic goals and means to implement them. Review with clients how their handling of the present crisis can help them cope with, minimize, or preferably prevent future crises.

SUMMARY

Crisis is a temporary state of severe disequilibrium for persons who face a threatening situation. A crisis is a state that individuals can neither avoid nor solve with their usual coping abilities and occurs when some force disrupts normal functioning, thereby causing a loss of balance or normalcy in life. Crises create tension; subsequently, efforts are made to solve the problem and reduce the tension. If such efforts meet with failure, people feel upset, redefine the situation, try other solutions, and, if failure continues, the person eventually reaches the breaking point.

Two main types of crisis are developmental and situational. Developmental crises are disruptions that occur during transitional periods in normal growth and development. These transitions usually have a gradual onset and are often predictable. Situational crises are precipitated by an unexpected external event and occur suddenly, sometimes without warning.

Family violence constitutes a unique crisis for the victim and the entire family and is becoming disturbingly prevalent in the world. Historically, family violence is not new. Only in the last half century of our nation's history have laws and societal concerns been raised about the treatment of spouse/partners, children, and seniors. Although advances in human rights have been made, abuses against women and children remain socially and culturally accepted in some countries, and attitudes have been slow to change.

Child abuse occurs among children of all ages, from infancy through the teen years, and may be physical, emotional, and/or sexual. Neglect and sexual exploitation are additional forms of child abuse. Neglect may be described as general neglect or specific, such as medical or educational neglect. Child abuse, such as shaken baby syndrome or Munchausen syndrome by proxy, is sometimes identified only on autopsy. Teen dating violence, violence during pregnancy, and VAW in general constitutes partner/spousal abuse. Finally, a most unsettling form of violence—elder abuse, neglect, and exploitation—is occurring more frequently than previously suspected.

New and unexpected forms of violence are becoming a reality in our unsettled world. Within communities, violence comes into the home in the form of Internet crimes against children, child abductions, and home invasions. Globally, terrorist groups threaten attacks on civilians in the United States and abroad. For people in the Unites States, this form of terror is a new reality. Preparation against and survival of such attacks is a new concern for most Americans, and the community health nurse has an important role to play (see Chapter 17).

Community health nurses use three levels of prevention when working with families. Primary prevention focuses on providing people with the skills and resources to prevent violent situations. Secondary prevention involves immediate intervention at the time of the violent episode. This secondary level includes providing different services for each family member, such as medical attention, emotional support, and police involvement. Tertiary prevention offers family rebuilding services and helps the family establish equilibrium with a structure that may be different, but healthier.

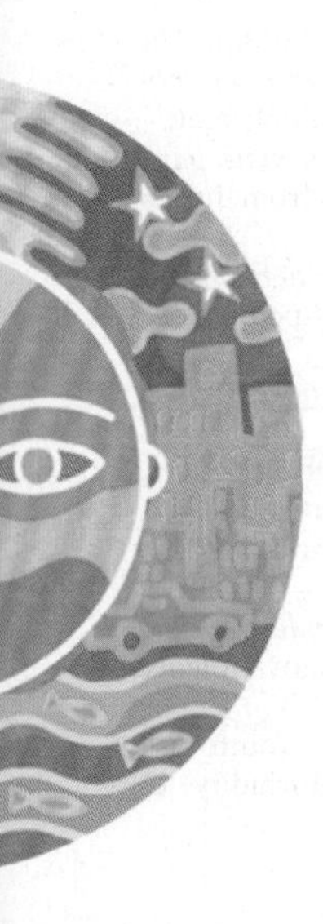

People in crisis need and often seek help. Crisis intervention builds on these two phenomena to achieve its primary goal—reestablishment of equilibrium. The two major methods of crisis intervention are the generic and the individual approaches. The generic approach is used with groups of people involved in the same type of crisis, such as rape victims, mothers who have lost children because of drunken driving, or a family experiencing child abuse. The individual approach is used if clients do not respond to the generic approach or need additional therapy. Crisis intervention begins with assessment of the situation, followed by planning a therapeutic intervention. The nurse then implements and carries out the intervention, building on the strengths and self-care ability of clients. Crisis intervention concludes with resolution and anticipatory planning to avert possible future crises.

Regardless of the method of intervention the community health nurse uses, the steps of the nursing process provide a framework within which to intervene. Assessing the family's assets and liabilities, their willingness to change, and the nature of the violence helps the nurse form a nursing diagnosis. With this diagnosis, the nurse can begin to plan appropriate interventions and implement plans in concert with the family. Evaluation of the intervention techniques provides the nurse with new data to assist with ongoing assessment of the family's progress and additional anticipatory guidance needs.

ACTIVITIES TO PROMOTE **CRITICAL THINKING**

1. What are the major differences between a developmental and a situational crisis? Give examples of each from personal experiences.
2. Describe a developmental crisis experienced by a family. What was this family's response? Describe some actions a community health nurse might have taken (alone or within an interdisciplinary team) to help the family cope with the crisis.
3. Watch a news station on television or the internet. Listen for examples of developmental or situational crises occurring to families in the world. Analyze the situations and anticipate what the role of a community health nurse would be during the crises selected.
4. Family violence is a significant public health problem. Assume that a battered wife becomes a community health nurse's client, and the nurse suspects there may be more women with this problem in the community. Describe how the nurse might provide assistance using the crisis intervention steps. Then discuss how a three-level preventive program might be instituted in the community.
5. Using the Internet, select a situational crisis, such as spousal abuse, adolescent sexual exploitation, or neglect of the elderly, and read the most current information on this topic. Depending on your personal interests or current community health nursing experiences, develop a file of articles you have uncovered using the Internet. This file can be useful to you, to agency staff in your clinical setting, and to families you visit.

REFERENCES

Administration for Children and Families. (2006). *Modifications to the CAPTA State Grant Program by the Keeping Children and Families Safe Act of 2003 (Public Law 108-36)*. Washington D.C.: U.S. Department of Health and Human Services. Retrieved http://www/acf/hhs/gov/programs/cb/laws_policies/policy/im/im0304.htm

Administration for Children and Families. (2007a). *How many children are abused and neglected each year?* Retrieved from http://faq.acf.hhs.gov/cgi-bin/acfrightnow.cfg/php/enduser/std_adp.php?p_faqid

Administration for Children and Families. (2007b). National Survey of Child and Adolescent Well-Being (NSCAW), 1997–2010. Retrieved from http://www.acf. hhs.gov/programs/opre/abuse_neglect/nscaw/nscaw_overview. html#overview

Administration for Children and Families. (2009). *Child victims of human trafficking*. Retrieved from http://www.acf.hhs.gov/trafficking

Administration for Children and Families. (2010). *Child Maltreatment 2010*. Retrieved from http://www.acf.hhs.gov/programs

Aguilera, D. C. (1998). *Crisis intervention: Theory and methodology* (8th ed.). St. Louis, MO: Mosby.

Altarac, M., & Strobino, D. (2002). Abuse during pregnancy and stress because of abuse during pregnancy and birthweight. *Journal of American Medical Women's Association, 57*(4), 208–214.

American Academy of Pediatrics, Committee on Child Abuse and Neglect. (1999). Guidelines for the evaluation of sexual abuse of children: Subject review. *Pediatrics, 103*(1), 186–191. Retrieved from http://pediatrics.aappubications.org/cgi/content/full/pediatrics;103/1/186

American Association of Suicidology. (2006). *Suicide in the U.S.A. based on current (2004) statistics*. Retrieved from http://www.suicidology.org/associations/1045/files/Suicide InThe US.pdf

American Association of Suicidology. (2007). *Facts about suicide and depression*. Retrieved from http://www.suicidology.org/associations/104/files/Depression.pdf

American Association of Suicidology. (n.d.). *Warning signs: IS PATH WARM?* Retrieved from http://www.suicidology.org/associations/1045/files/Mnemonic.pdf

American Psychological Association. (2007). *Elder abuse and neglect: In search of solutions*. Washington, DC: Office on Aging. Retrieved from http://www.apa.org/pi/aging/eldabuse.html

Baum, K., Catalano, S. M., Rand, M. R., & Rose, K. (2009). *Stalking victimization in the United States*. Retrieved from http://bjs.usdoj.gov/index.cfm

Bolen, R.M. (2001). *Child sexual abuse: Its scope and our failure*. Norwell, MA: Kluwer Plenum.

Bridges, W. (1980). *Transitions: Making sense of life's changes* (2nd ed.). Cambridge, MA: Perseus Publishing.

Bridges, W. (2001). *The way of transition: Embracing life's most difficult moments*. Cambridge, MA: Perseus Publishing.

Burgess, A., & Hanrahan, N. (2006). *Identifying forensic markers in elderly sexual abuse*. Washington, DC: National Institute of Justice.

Campbell, J. C. (2002). Health consequences of intimate partner violence. *Lancet, 359*(9314), 1331–1336.

Campbell, J. C., Webster, D., Koziol-McLain, J., Block, Campbell, D., & Curry, M. A. (2003). Risk factors for femicide in abusive relationships: Results from a multisite case control study. *American Journal of Public Health, 98*(7), 1089–1097.

Capezuti, E. A., Siegler, E. L., & Mezey, M. D. (Eds.). (2008). *The encyclopedia of elder care: The comprehensive resource on geriatric and social care* (2nd ed.). New York: Springer Publishing.

Centers for Disease Control and Prevention. (2006a). *Intimate partner violence: Overview*. Retrieved July 25, 2008 from http://www.cdc.gov/ncipc/factsheets/ipvfactshtm

Centers for Disease Control and Prevention. (2006b). *Understanding suicide*. Retrieved from http://www.cdc.gov/ncipc/pub-res/Suicide%20Fact%

Centers for Disease Control and Prevention. (2010a). *Choose respect*. Retrieved from http://www.cdc.gov/chooserespect

Centers for Disease Control and Prevention. (2010b). *Healthy People 2010 final review: injury and violence prevention*, 91–97. Retrieved from http://www.cdc.gov/nchs/data/hpdata2010/hp2010_final_review

Centers for Disease Control and Prevention. (2010c). *Understanding school violence*. Retrieved from http://www.cdc.gov/violence prevention/pdf/school violence

Centers for Disease Control and Prevention. (2010d). Youth risk behavioral surveillance—United States, 2009. Morbidity & Mortality Weekly Report 2010, 59(No.SS-5).

Centers for Disease Control and Prevention. (2010e). *Youth violence*. Retrieved from http://www.cdc.gov/violenceprevention/youth violence

Centers for Disease Control and Prevention. (2011a, November). *National Intimate Partner and Sexual Violence Survey 2010*. Retrieved from http://www.cdc.gov/violenceprevention/pdf/NISVS

Centers for Disease Control and Prevention. (2011b). *Preventing teen dating violence*. Retrieved from http://www.cdc.gov/Features/datingviolence

Centers for Disease Control and Prevention, National Center for Injury Prevention and Control. (2004). *CDC's rape prevention and education grant program: Preventing sexual violence in the United States 2004*. Retrieved from *http://www.cdc.gov/ncipc/pub-res/pdf/RPE%20AAG.pdf*

Centers for Disease Control & Prevention. (2012). Ten leading causes of death by age group, United States-2009. Retrieved from http://www.cdc.gov/injury/wisqars/LeadingCauses.html

Child Welfare Information Gateway. (2004). *About CAPTA: A legislative history*. Retrieved from http://www.childwelfare.gov/pubs/factsheets/about.cfm

Child Welfare Information Gateway. (2008). *What is child abuse and neglect?* Retrieved from http://www.childwelfare.gov/pubs/factsheets/whatiscan.pdf

Crandall, M., Nathens, A. B., Kernic, M. A., Holt. V. L., & Rivara, F. P. (2004). Predicting future injury among women in abusive relationships. *Journal of Trauma-Injury Infection and Critical Care, 56*(4), 906–912.

Crime and Violence Prevention Center. (2003a). *Child abuse: Educator's responsibilities*. Sacramento, CA: California Attorney General's Office. Retrieved from http://www.safestate.org/shop/files/CAEd.Resp.pdf

Crime and Violence Prevention Center. (2003b). *Child abuse and neglect reporting law, condensed version*. Sacramento, CA: California Attorney General's Office. Retrieved from http://www.safestate.org/shop/files/CA_Child_Abuse_ Rep.pdf

Crime and Violence Prevention Center. (2003c). *Child abuse prevention handbook*. Sacramento, CA: California Attorney General's Office. Retrieved from http://www.safestate.org/shop/files/child abuse handbook chap_1-3.pdf./child abuse handbook chap_4-6.pdf, and .../child abuse handbook appen3-7.pdf

Curry, M. A., Doyle, B. A., & Gilhooley, J. (1998). Abuse among pregnant adolescents: Differences by developmental age. *Maternal and Child Nursing, 23*(3), 144–150.

Davis, R. E., & Harsh, K. E. (2001). Confronting barriers to universal screening for domestic violence. *Journal of Professional Nursing, 17*(6), 313–320.

Dombrowski, S. C., & Gischlar, K. (2004). *Keeping children safe on the Internet: Guidelines for parents*. Retrieved from http//www.nasponline.org/publications/cq/cq342internetsafety_ho.aspx

Eckenrode, J., Campa, M., Luckey, D. W., Henderson, C. R. Cole, R., Kitzman, H., et al. (2010). Long-term effects of prenatal and infancy nurse home visitation on the life course of youths: 19-year follow-up of a randomized trial. *Archives of Pediatrics and Adolescent Medicine, 164*(1), 9–15.

Finkelhor, D., Turner, H., Ormrod, R., Hamby, S., & Kracke, K. (2009). *Children's exposure to violence: A comprehensive national survey*. Bulletin. Washington, DC: U.S. Department of Justice, Office of Justice Programs, Office of Juvenile Justice and Delinquency Prevention. Retrieved from http://www.justice.gov

Fox, J. A., & Zawitz, M. W. (2004). *Homicide trends in the United States*. Washington, DC: Department of Justice.

Friedman, S. H., & Resnick, P. J. (2007). Child murder by mothers: Patterns and prevention. *World Psychiatry, 6*(1), 137–141.

Gazmararian, J. A., Petersen, R., Spitz, A. M., Goodwin, M. M., Saltzman, L. E., & Marks, J. S. (2000). Violence and reproductive health: Current knowledge and future research directions. *Maternal and Child Health Journal, 4*(2), 79–84.

Hanson, R. F. (2002). Adolescent dating violence: Prevalence and psychological outcomes. *Child Abuse and Neglect, 26*, 449–453.

Hoff, L. A. (2001). *People in crisis: Clinical and public health perspectives* (5th ed.). Indianapolis, IN: Jossey-Bass.

Holmes, T., & Rahe, R. (1967). The social readjustment rating scale. *Journal of Psychosomatic Research, 11*, 213–217.

Janssen, P. A., Holt, V. L., Sugg, N. K., Emanuel, I, Critchlow, C.M., & Henderson, A. D. (2003). Intimate partner violence and adverse pregnancy outcomes: A population-based study. *American Journal of Obstetrics and Gynecology, 188*(5), 1341–1347.

Jenkins, P. J., & Davidson, B. P. (2001). *Stopping domestic violence: How a community can prevent spousal abuse*. Norwell, MA: Kluwer Academic/Plenum.

Kellogg, N. (2005). The evaluation of sexual abuse in children. *Pediatrics, 116*(2), 506–512.

Kramer, A. (2002). Domestic violence: How to ask and how to listen. *Nursing Clinics of North America, 37*(1), 189–210.

Lemmey, D., Malecha, A., McFarlane, J., Willson, P., Watson, K., et al. (2001). Severity of violence against women correlates with behavioral problems in their children. *Pediatric Nursing, 27*(3), 265–270.

Levinson, D. J. (1978). *The seasons of a man's life*. New York: Knopf.

Levy, B. S., & Sidel, V. W. (2002). *Terrorism and public health: A balanced approach to strengthening systems and protecting people*. New York: Oxford University Press.

National Center on Elder Abuse. (2011a). *How you can help in the fight against elder abuse*. Retrieved from http://www.ncea.aoa.gov

National Center on Elder Abuse. (2011b). *Major types of elder abuse*. Retrieved from http://www. ncea.aoa.gov

National Center on Elder Abuse. (2006). *Help for elders and families*. Washington, DC: National Center on Elder Abuse. Retrieved from http://www.elder abusecenter.org/default.cfm?p=worried.cfm

National Center for Missing and Exploited Children. (2011). *Cyber tipline*. Retrieved at http://www.missingkids.com/missingkids/servlet/PublicHomeServlet?LanguageCountry=en_US&

National Institute of Neurological Disorders and Stroke. (2007). *NINDS shaken baby syndrome information page*. Retrieved from http://www.ninds.nih.gov/disorders/shakenbaby/shakenbaby.htm

Nock, M. K., & Marzuk, P. M. (1999). Murder-suicide: Phenomenology and clinical implications. In D. G. Jacobs (Ed.), *Guide to suicide assessment and intervention* (pp. 188–209). San Francisco: Jossey-Bass.

Office of the United Nations High Commissioner for Human Rights. (2007). *Committee on the Rights of the Child*. Retrieved from http://www.ohchr.org/english/bodies/crc/discussion.htm

Olds, D. L., Henderson, C. R., Kitzman, H. J., Eckenrode, J. J., Cole, R. E., & Tatelbaum, R. C. (1999). Prenatal and infancy home visitation by nurses: Recent findings. *The Future of Children, Home Visiting: Recent Program Evaluations, 9*(1), 44–65.

Olds, D. L., Henderson, C. R., Tatelbaum, R., & Chamberlin, R. (1988). Improving the life-course development of socially disadvantaged mothers: A randomized trial of nurse home visitation. *American Journal of Public Health, 78*(11), 1436–1445.

Olds, D. L., Kitzman, H. J., Cole, R. E., Hanks, C. A., Arcoleo, K. J., Anson, E. A., et al. (2010). Enduring effects of prenatal and infancy home visiting by nurses on maternal life course and government spending: Follow-up of a randomized trial among children at age 12 years. *Archives of Pediatrics and Adolescent Medicine, 164*(5), 419–424.

Pillemer, K., & Finkelhor, A. (1988). The prevalence of elder abuse: A random sample survey. *The Gerontologist, 28*, 51–57.

Rape, Abuse, & Incest National Network. (2006). *All 50 states now included in national sex offender public registry*. Retrieved from http://www.rainn/org.news/national-sex-offender-registry.index.html

Safe Schools Healthy Students Initiative. (2006). About the Safe Schools/Healthy Students (SS/HS) initiative: A comprehensive approach to youth violence prevention. Retrieved from http://www.sshs.samhsa.gov/initiative/about.aspx

Sheehy, G. (1976). *Passages: Predictable crises of adult life*. New York: Dutton.

Sheehy, G. (1992). *The silent passage*. New York: Ballantine.

Sheehy, G. (1999). *Understanding men's passages: Discovering the new map of men's lives*. New York: Ballantine Books.

Sheehy, G., & Delbourgo, J. (1996). *New passages: Mapping your life across time*. New York: Ballantine Books.

Stirling, J., & Committee on Child Abuse and Neglect. (2007). Beyond Munchausen syndrome by proxy: Identification and treatment of child abuse in a medical setting. *Pediatrics, 119*, 1026–1030.

Teaster, P. B., Otto, J. M., Dugar, T. D., Mendiondo, M. S., Abner, E. L., & Cecil, K. A. (2006). *The 2004 survey of state Adult Protective Services: Abuse of adults 60 years of age and older.* Report to the National Center on Elder Abuse, Administration on Aging. Washington, DC. Retrieved from http://www.ncvc.org/ncvc

Thananowan, N., & Heidrich, S. M. (2008). Intimate partner violence among pregnant Thai women. *Violence Against Women, 14*(5), 509–527.

U.S. Department of Health and Human Services. (2010). *Healthy People 2020.* Retrieved from http:people.gov/2020

U.S. Department of Health and Human Services. (2011). *Injury and violence prevention—Healthy People.* Retrieved from http:people.gov/2020/topicobjectives 2020

U.S. Department of Justice (2001a). *Crimes against children by babysitters* (NCJ 189102). Washington, DC: U.S. Department of Justice, Office of Justice Programs.

U.S. Department of Justice (2001b). *Internet crimes against children* (NCJ 184931). Washington, DC: U.S. Department of Justice, Office of Justice Programs.

U.S. Department of Justice. (2002). *Battered child syndrome: Investigating physical abuse and homicide.* Retrieved from http://www.ncjrs.gov/pdffiles1/ojjdp/161406.pdf

U.S. Department of Justice. (2005). Department of Justice launches initiative to train child abduction response teams. Retrieved from http://www.ojp.gov/newsroom/2005/OJP06010.htm

U.S. Department of Justice. (2006). *Project safe childhood: Protecting children from online exploitation and abuse.* Retrieved from http://www.projectsafechildhood.gov/introductionwcover.pdf

U.S. Department of Justice. (2007). *Commercial sexual exploitation of children: What do we know and what do we do about it?* Retrieved from http://www.ojp.usdoj.gov/nij/pubs-sum/215733.htm

U.S. Department of Justice, Office on Violence Against Women. (2011). *Areas of focus.* Retrieved from http://www.ovw.usdoj.gov

U.S. Department of Justice, Office on Violence Against Women. (n.d.). *About domestic violence.* Retrieved from http://www.usdoj.gov/ovw/domviolence.htm.

Vastag, B. (2001). Experts urge bioterrorism readiness. *Journal of the American Medical Association, 285,* 30–31.

Volpe, J. S. (1996). *Effects of domestic violence on children and adolescents: An overview.* American Academy of Experts in Traumatic Stress, Inc. Retrieved from http://www.aaets.org/article8.htm

World Health Organization. (1998). *Report of the Director-General: The world health report 1998. Life in the 21st century: A vision for all.* Geneva, CH: World Health Organization.

World Health Organization. (2002a). *First ever global report on violence and health released.* Retrieved from http://www.who.int/mediacentre/news/releases/pr73/en

World Health Organization. (2002b). *Public health and violence: European facts and trends.* Retrieved from http://www.euro.who.int/document/mediacentre/fs1

World Health Organization. (2005). *WHO multi-country study on women's health and domestic violence against women: Initial results on prevalence, health outcomes and women's responses.* Retrieved from http://www.who.int/gender/violence/who_multi-country_study/summary_report/en/index. html

World Health Organization. (2007a). *Gender-based violence.* Geneva, CH: World Health Organization. Retrieved from http://www.who.int/gender/violence/en/

World Health Organization. (2007b). *World report on violence and health: Child abuse and neglect by parents and other caregivers.* Retrieved from http://www.who.int/violence_ injury_prevention/violence/global_campaign/en/chap3.pdf

World Health Organization. (2011). *Intimate partner violence during pregnancy.* Retrieved from http://whqlibdoc.who.int/hq/2011/WHO_RHR-11.35

World Health Organization. (n.d. a). *Suicide prevention (SUPRE).* Retrieved from http://www.who.int/mental_ health/prevention/suicide/suicide prevent/en/

World Health Organization. (n.d. b) *Violence and Injury Prevention and Disability (VIP): Prevention of child maltreatment.* Retrieved from http://www.who.int/violence-injury-prevention/violence/activities/child-maltreatment/en

World Health Organization, Committee on the Rights of the Child. (2001). *Prevention of child abuse and neglect: Making the links between human rights and public health.* Retrieved from http://www.who.int/child-adolescent-health/New_Publications/Rights/CRC-statement_rev_III.htm

UNIT 6

PROMOTING AND PROTECTING THE HEALTH OF POPULATIONS WITH DEVELOPMENTAL NEEDS

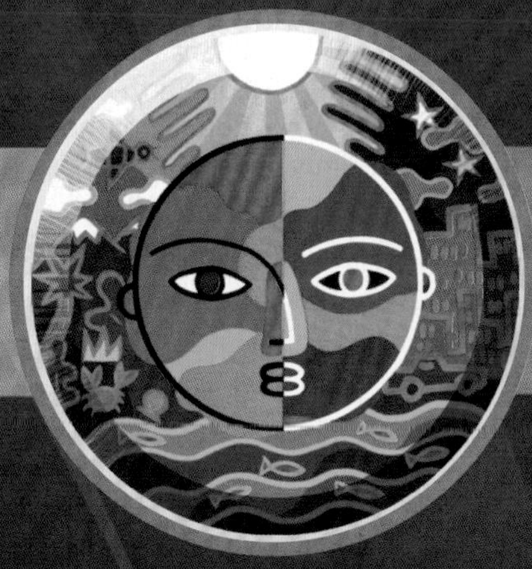

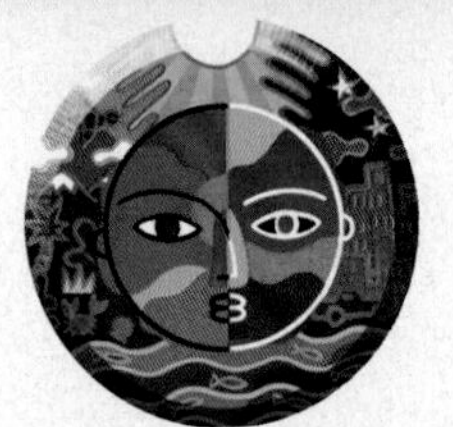

CHAPTER

21

Maternal–Child Health: Working with Perinatal, Infant, Toddler, and Preschool Clients

"Be gentle with the young."

—***Juvenal*** *(55–127 AD)*

KEY TERMS

Alcohol-related birth defects
Alcohol-related neurodevelopmental disorder
Child abuse
Environmental tobacco smoke (ETS)
Fetal alcohol effects
Fetal alcohol spectrum disorders
Fetal alcohol syndrome
Gestational diabetes mellitus (GDM)
Head Start
High-risk families
Infant
Low-birth-weight
Population health
Preconception care
Preschooler
Shaken baby syndrome
Smokeless tobacco products
Sudden infant death syndrome (SIDS)
Toddler
Very-low-birth-weight

LEARNING OBJECTIVES

Upon mastery of this chapter, you should be able to:

- Identify major health problems and concerns for childbearing women, infant, toddler, and preschool populations globally and in the United States.
- Identify the *Healthy People 2020* goals established for the maternal–child population.
- Discuss major risk factors and special complications for childbearing families.
- Describe the important considerations in developing effective health promotion programs to fit the needs of diverse maternal–child populations.
- Describe various roles of a public and community health nurse in serving the maternal–child population.
- Describe a variety of programs that promote and protect health and prevent illness and injury of infant, toddler, and preschool populations.
- State the recommended immunization schedule for infants and children, and give the rationale for the timing of each immunization.
- Give examples of methods and interventions the public and community health nurse might use in working with infants, toddlers, and preschool populations to help promote their health.

Maternal and child populations have always been priorities for public health and public and community health nursing (P/CHN). These populations consist of childbearing women, including adolescents, and infants and children through adolescence. In this chapter, the focus is on childbearing women, including adolescents and infants through age 4. Often, more than half of P/CHN practice in official public health agencies involves primary prevention work with mothers, such as **preconception care,** provision of prenatal care, and monitoring infant health. Why should maternal–infant populations require this amount of attention from P/CHN? Despite advanced technology and availability of excellent perinatal services in the United States, we often have less than optimal birth outcomes—for instance, 307,066 low-birth-weight (LBW) and 467,201 preterm infants yearly (American Pregnancy Association, 2011). Also, certain segments of the maternal and infant populations, such as adolescent mothers and those who are economically disadvantaged or women and children of color, remain at high risk for disparities in regard to maternal deaths and complications and child risk and illness. Although some women receive excellent prenatal care and benefit from diagnostic and technological resources, many others are without access to prenatal care and adequate nutrition. The Save the Children (2008, p. 31) report on maternal–child health notes that:

The United States spends more money on health care per capita than nearly any other country in the world, yet has the highest rates of child poverty and the lowest levels of child health and safety of the rich countries. As a result, infant and child mortality rates in the United States are higher than in any other industrialized country, the only exceptions being Latvia, Lithuania, and Slovakia.

For an example of a country that has implemented successful policies to eliminate maternal–child inequities, see Evidence-Based Practice: How Sweden Achieved Maternal–Child Health Equity.

Historically, the health of U.S. women and children has largely fallen under the umbrella of Title V of the Social Security Act, enacted in 1935. (For more on the Social Security Act, see Chapter 6.) Funding for state Maternal and Child Health and Crippled Children programs was part of this original legislation, as was some provision for child welfare services. Title V is "the longest-standing public health legislation in American history" and came to fruition after other legislation established a National Birth Registry; provided *Infant Care*, the first educational pamphlet; established the Children's Bureau; and enacted the first Child Labor Law of 1916 (Maternal Child Health Bureau [MCHB], n.d., para. 4). For an illustration of MCHB functions and programs, see Display 21.1.

In 1909, formal prenatal care was first provided in Boston by the Instructive District Nursing Association and spread across the country to outpatient clinics (MCHB, 2008). Since the inception of Title V, other legislation has included Emergency Maternity and Infant Care Program (1943) that funded maternity and infant care for the wives of lower-income servicemen in the early days of the baby boom and the 1970 Family Planning Act that provided the first federal funds for contraception to prevent unintended pregnancies. In 1976, the Improved Pregnancy Outcome Projects sought to decrease the levels of infant mortality by strengthening the efforts of states to better plan and implement maternal–child health programs, and Healthy Start programs were begun in 1991—starting with 15 demonstration project sites exhibiting high infant mortality rates (IMRs) and growing to 104 sites in 38 states to provide preconception, postpartum, and infant care to at-risk women (MCHB, 2011). Evaluation of Healthy Start programs reveals that almost all programs provide home visitation to prenatal clients, and most continued these visits to infants and toddlers. Health education, smoking cessation counseling, services for perinatal depression, and involvement of male partners are hallmarks of most programs.

This chapter addresses major areas of concern regarding population health for maternal–infant clients. It also explores the global needs of and related services available to the youngest and thus most vulnerable of society's members. Health services that are commonly available in the United States for pregnant and postpartum women, infants, toddlers, and the preschool population are examined, and the role of the public and community health nurse in providing those services is explored.

HEALTH STATUS AND NEEDS OF PREGNANT WOMEN AND INFANTS

Public and community health nurses constitute a key group of health care workers involved in both program planning and the actual delivery of services to mothers and babies in the community. A solid understanding of vital statistics and other data regarding mothers and infants serves nurses as they determine the appropriateness and the effectiveness of programs and services. A review of some global and national vital statistics of the past decade provides insight into the key problems facing this population.

Global Overview

One of the major indicators of **population health** is maternal health, which is often measured by the maternal mortality rate (MMR). The MMR is a measure of obstetric risk and is determined by dividing the number

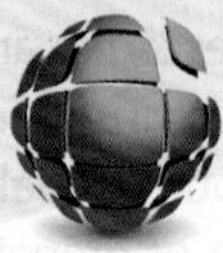

EVIDENCE-BASED PRACTICE

How Sweden Achieved Maternal Child Health Equity

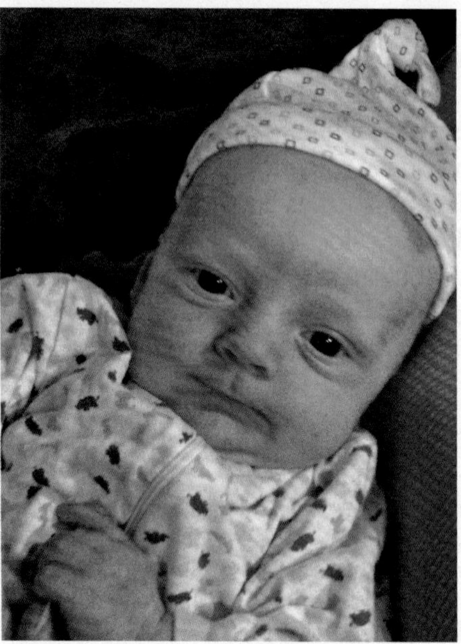

Author's private photo with permission from Deanna Rector.

For mothers and children of any income level, Sweden is a wonderful place to live. However, this was not always the case; the poorest infants were 3.5 times more likely to die before age 1 in the 1920s. In the 1930s, due to public concern about the "child survival gap" (p. 32), the government instituted a set of comprehensive new policies that included free prenatal and other maternal–child health services, along with housing reforms and welfare support—including financial support for low-income families. Around 60% of pregnant women and 80% of infants were covered by 1950. Currently, the inequity related to infant mortality rates has virtually been eliminated, and the decreases in social inequality have led to "one of the lowest rates of child mortality in the world" (p. 32). This case study highlighting how government policies can affect population health outcomes is an example for other countries, such as the United States, that struggle with less than adequate maternal–child health indicators and significant disparities in health outcomes.

Source: Save the Children. (2008). State of the world's mothers 2008. Westport, CN: Author.

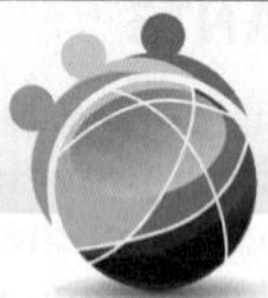

DISPLAY 21.1 TYPES OF SERVICES OFFERED THROUGH FEDERAL MATERNAL–CHILD HEALTH FUNDING

Direct Health Care Services (Gap Filling)

Examples: Basic Health Services and Health Services for CSHCN

Enabling Services

Examples: Transportation, Translation, Outreach, Respite Care, Health Education, Family Support Services, Purchase of Health Insurance, Case Management, Coordination with Medicaid, WIC, and Education

Population-Based Services

Examples: Newborn Screening, Lead Screening, Immunization, Sudden Infant Death Syndrome Counseling, Oral Health, and Injury Prevention

Infrastructure Building Services

Examples: Needs Assessment, Evaluation, Planning, Policy Development, Coordination, Quality Assurance, Standards Development, Monitoring, Training, Applied Research, Systems of Care, and Information Systems

U.S. Department of Health and Human Services. (2008). *State MCH-Medicaid Coordination: A Review of Title V and Title XIX Interagency Agreements* (2nd ed.). Retrieved from ftp://ftp.hrsa.gov/mchb/IAA/A_State_MCH_Medicaid_Intro.pdf

of maternal deaths by the number of live births per 100,000. Most maternal deaths are the result of direct causes (complications of pregnancy, labor, and delivery), hypertensive disorders, intervention omissions or incorrect treatment, the chain of events resulting from any one of these, and unsafe abortions. In 2010, more than 50% of maternal deaths occurred in sub-Saharan Africa and about 33% in South Asia. In these developing countries, the MMR is 290 per 100,000 live births. This compares to developed countries, such as Canada, Australia, New Zealand, Japan, and most European countries where the MMR is around 14 per 100,000 live births—a very wide disparity (World Health Organization [WHO], 2010). The U.S. MMR was 24 in 2008. Ireland and Greece's MMR is <4, making them very good places for expectant mothers. Although the MMR has decreased since 1990 by 34%, the worldwide goal is 5.5% decrease per year (WHO, 2008a, 2010). These goals are important because most maternal mortality can be prevented.

Infant Mortality

Another critical population health indicator is the IMR. Globally, 3.3 to 4 million neonatal deaths and 6 million deaths of children under age 1 year occurred in 2009; these deaths are primarily caused by poor maternal health, poor postnatal care of mothers and babies, poor hygiene, LBW, malnutrition, infections, such as pneumonia and sepsis, HIV/AIDS, malaria, and diarrheal infectious diseases (2008a). The lowest percent of neonatal deaths occurred in the African region; in contrast, the highest malarial and HIV/AIDS deaths for children under age 5 occurred there. In the United States, IMR for Blacks is 67% higher than for non-Hispanic White women. This compares with the total Latino (Puerto Rican, Mexican, Cuban, & Central/South American) IMR of 2.02 that is lower than non-Hispanic White women (Centers for Disease Control and Prevention [CDC], 2011a). WHO estimated in 2011 that 1.5 million infants worldwide would be saved if there were more infants exclusively breast-fed for the first 6 months of life. Currently, breast-feeding practice worldwide is at 35% (WHO, 2011a). In the United States, the highest IMRs are found among non-Hispanic Blacks (see Fig. 21-1).

HIV/AIDS

There are 34 million adults and children living with human immunodeficiency virus (HIV). Sixty percent of cases are found in sub-Saharan Africa (WHO, 2011b). Rates are rising faster in Eastern Europe and Central Asia (WHO, 2011a). In 2009, 16.6 million children were orphaned from HIV/AIDS (ChildInfo, 2011). Most

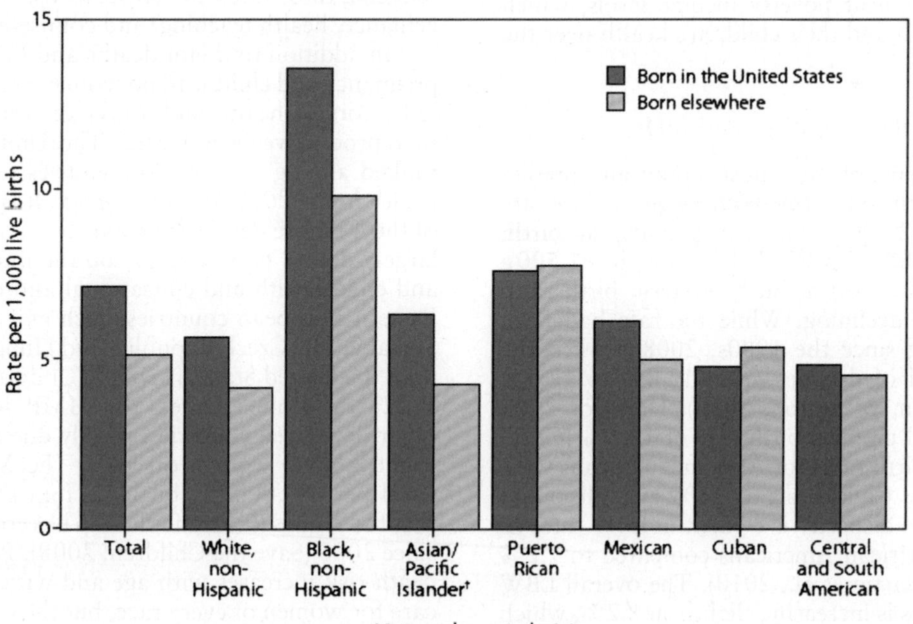

FIGURE 21-1. U.S. IMRs, by Mother's Place of Birth and Race/Ethnicity. (Source: Mathews, T. J., & MacDorman, M. F. (2011). Infant mortality statistics from the 2007 period linked to birth/infant death data set. *National Vital Statistics Report, 59*(6). Retrieved from http://www.cdc.gov/mmwr/preview/mmwrhtml/mm6026a6.htm)

children with acquired immunodeficiency syndrome (AIDS) are children of HIV-positive mothers (WHO, 2009). Mother-to-child transmission (MTCT) of HIV can be reduced by a stunning 67% with a single antiretroviral drug taken for a short time, and combination therapies are even more effective in reducing MTCT (Harris, Fowler, Sansom, Ruffo, & Lampe, 2007). To reduce MTCT, women must seek prenatal care early enough in their pregnancies for the antiretroviral drug to be effective. Antiretroviral therapy was provided to 6.6 million persons in 2010, with approximately 450,000 of them children (WHO, 2011a). Most of the population favors routine HIV testing, and women are more likely to be tested and understand that treatment can help their unborn children (Cockcroft, Andersson, Milne, Mokoena, & Masisi, 2007).

National Overview

In the United States, 4.25 million women gave birth in 2008, 2% less than in 2007 (Martin et al., 2010). The general fertility rate was 68.6 births per 1,000 women ages 15 to 44 years; the crude birth rate was 14 per 1,000 population. Birth rates declined in the three major ethnic–racial groups: African American, Caucasian, and Hispanic; American Indian/Alaska Native group birth rates were unchanged. Almost 41% of births were to unmarried women (U.S. Department of Health and Human Services [USDHHS], 2007). When unmarried women rely on a single income, financial resources are more limited, and many of these women raise their children at poverty or near poverty income levels, which impacts their health and their children's health over the life course of both.

Birth Weight and Preterm Birth

Birth weight is one of the most important predictors of infant mortality. **Low-birth-weight** babies are those weighing <2,500g (or <5.5 pounds) at birth; **very-low-birth-weight** (VLBW) babies weigh <1,500g (or <3 pounds 4 ounces) at birth. Preterm birth rates have been slowly declining. While the rate had been steadily increasing since the 1980s, 2008 marked the first 2-year period of decline—from 12.8% to 12.3% (Martin, Osterman, & Sutton, 2010). Data for 2009 indicate an overall preterm birth rate of 12.2% (CDC, 2009a). Preterm birth rates for African Americans were 17% compared to Caucasians at 11% and Hispanics at 12%. This same disparity is evident in LBW rates as well: 13.7% for African Americans compared to 7.2% for Caucasians (Martin et al., 2010). The overall LBW in the United States is increasing slightly at 8.2%, which can be somewhat explained by increased multiple births. Statistics for VLBW are 1.5% overall but 3.0% for African Americans (Martin et al., 2011). These numbers represent a significant disparity for African Americans. National trends in morbidity and mortality for VLBW infants indicate continued "neonatal and long-term morbidity" without significant increases in survival (Fanaroff et al., 2007, p. 147).

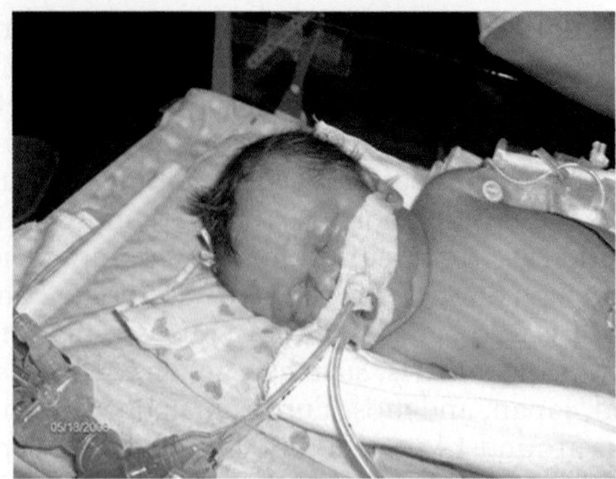

Infant in NICU. Author's private photo with permission from Danielle Rector.

Infant complications of preterm birth include hearing and vision problems; acute respiratory, gastrointestinal, and immunologic problems; and central nervous system (CNS), motor, cognitive, behavioral, and socioemotional disorders. A variety of growth concerns, as well as acute and chronic health and developmental problems, often occur, and the families of these infants are burdened with additional economic and emotional costs. As preschoolers, children born preterm were more likely than peers to have poor social, emotional, and physical functioning, indicating some continuing effects (Zwicker & Harris, 2008). Maternal mortality, LBW, and VLBW births are three areas requiring attention by health care providers and the public health system. Public and community health nurses can contribute to reducing these rates and societal costs by outreach, surveillance, health teaching, and counseling.

In addition to infant deaths and LBW, the effects of pregnancy and childbirth on women are other important indicators of health and reflect discrepancies in access to reproductive health care. The United States is not ranked among the top 10 countries in maternal–child health in the *2011 Mother's Index*. It is ranked 31st out of the 43 more developed countries. The U.S. ranking is largely due to poorer scores on the indices of maternal and child health and educational and economic status. Eastern European countries, such as Latvia, Lithuania, Slovakia, the Czech Republic, and Hungary, rank higher than the United States (Save the Children, 2011).

In the United States, the MMR is higher than in other developed countries, mostly due to the disparities found among women of color. The MMR for Blacks (36.1 per 100,000 live births) is four times greater than that for Whites (9.8), and the gap has continued to widen since 2000 (Save the Children, 2008). Pregnancy-related death risk increases with age and with lack of prenatal care for women of every race, but the risk of pregnancy-related death for U.S. Black women is three to four times greater than for White women. Even though maternal deaths are low, most maternal deaths are preventable. Gaskin (2008) believes that maternal deaths are underreported especially as they relate to medical error.

One of the maternal–child objectives for *Healthy People 2020* is to improve the proportion of infants who are breast-fed (CDC, 2011a). Breast-feeding is beneficial to both mother and infant, and currently, almost 61% of U.S. infants were breast-fed for the recommended 6-month period. Almost 82% were breast-fed in the postpartum period (CDC, 2011a). Asian–Pacific Island mothers are more likely to breast-feed (86.4%), and Black mothers are least likely to breast-feed (58.11%). Older mothers with higher household incomes are more likely to breast-feed their infants than younger mothers and are also more likely to breast-feed for a longer period of time. Even though the American Academy of Pediatrics (AAP) recommends that infants be exclusively breast-fed for the first 6 months of life, only 14.8% were in 2009 (Hamilton, Martin, & Ventura, 2010). It is estimated that if 90% of U.S. families would comply with the recommended AAP guideline regarding exclusive breast-feeding, $113 billion and 911 infant deaths would be saved (Bartick & Reinhold, 2010). See Table 21-1 for *Healthy People 2020* maternal, infant, and child health objectives.

Table 21.1 ***Healthy People 2020:*** **Summary of Objectives for Maternal, Infant, and Child Health**

Goal: Improve the health and wellbeing of women, infants, children, and families

Number	Objective
Morbidity and Mortality	
MICH-1	Reduce the rate of fetal and infant deaths
MICH-2	Reduce the 1-yr. mortality rate for infants with Down's syndrome
MICH-3	Reduce the rate of child deaths
MICH-4	Reduce the rate of adolescent and young adult deaths
MICH-5	Reduce the rate of maternal mortality
MICH-6	Reduce maternal illness and complications due to pregnancy (during hospitalized labor and delivery)
MICH-7	Reduce cesarean births among low-risk (full-term, singleton, vertex presentation) women
MICH-8	Reduce low birth weight (LBW) and very low birth weight (VLBW)
MICH-9	Reduce preterm births
Pregnancy Health and Behaviors	
MICH-10	Increase the proportion of prégnant women who receive early and adequate prenatal care
MICH-11	Increase abstinence from alcohol, cigarettes, and illicit drugs among pregnant women
MICH-12	Increase the proportion of pregnant women who attend a series of prepared childbirth classes
MICH-13	Increase the proportion of mothers who achieve a recommended weight gain during their pregnancies
Preconception Health and Behaviors	
MICH-14	Increase the proportion of women of childbearing potential with intake of at least 400 mcg of folic acid from fortified foods or dietary supplements
MICH-15	Reduce the proportion of women of childbearing potential who have low red blood cell folate concentrations
MICH-16	Increase the proportion of women delivering a live birth who received preconception care services and practiced key recommended preconception health behaviors
MICH-17	Reduce the proportion of persons aged 18 to 44 yrs. who have impaired fecundity (physical barrier preventing pregnancy or carrying to term)
Postpartum Health and Behavior	
MICH-18	Reduce postpartum relapse of smoking among women who quit smoking during pregnancy
MICH-19	Increase the proportion of women giving birth who attend a postpartum care visit with a health worker
Infant Care	
MICH-20	Increase the proportion of infants who are put to sleep on their backs
MICH-21	Increase the proportion of infants who are breast-fed
MICH-22	Increase the proportion of employers that have worksite lactation support programs
MICH-23	Reduce the proportion of breast-fed newborns who receive formula supplementation within the first 2 days of life
MICH-24	Increase the proportion of live births that occur in facilities that provide recommended care for lactating mothers and their babies
MICH-25	Reduce the occurrence of FAS
MICH-26	Reduce the proportion of children diagnosed with a disorder through newborn blood spot screening who expérience developmental delay requiring special education services

(Continued)

Table 21.1 ***Healthy People 2020:*** **Summary of Objectives for Maternal, Infant, and Child Health** ***(Continued)***

Number	Objective
***Infant Care* (Continued)**	
MICH-27	Reduce the proportion of children with cerebral palsy born as LBW infants (<2,500 g)
MICH-28	Reduce occurrence of neural tube defects
MICH-29	Increase the proportion of young children with an ASD and other developmental delays who are screened, evaluated, and enrolled in early intervention services in a timely manner
Health Services	
MICH-30	Increase the proportion of children, including those with special health care needs, who have access to a medical base
MICH-31	Increase the proportion of children with special health care needs who receive their care in family centered, comprehensive, coordinated systems
MICH-32	Increase appropriate newborn blood spot screening and follow-up testing
MICH-33	Increase the proportion of VLBW infants born at level III hospitals or subspecialty perinatal centers

Source: USDHHS. (2010). *Healthy People 2010: Maternal, infant, and child health objectives.* Retrieved from http://healthypeople.gov/2020/topicsobjectives2020/objectiveslist.aspx?topicId=26

Adolescent Mothers

In 1991, after a steady 5-year upward trend, the United States reached a 20-year high in the number of children born to teen mothers (aged 15 to 19 years). That trend then declined until 2005, when it rose ever so slightly. In 2008, there were 41.5 births per 1,000 women age 15 to 19 years. Recent findings from the National Survey of Family Growth (2006–2008) show no significant changes in adolescent sexual activity and contraception use (Martin et al., 2010). Additionally, there continues to be an increasing trend for unwed teenage mothers to keep their babies. These "children having children" with limited educational and economic advantages will affect the health of society well into the future. See Chapter 22 for more on adolescent pregnancy.

The *Healthy People 2020* (USDHHS, 2012a) document encompasses specific goals and objectives for the maternal–child population, based on the previous achievements in the same or similar areas. After years of working toward improving maternal–child health, the United States has made limited progress. One objective, however, has been met; 70% of infants are now being put to sleep on their backs, up from a 35% baseline. The rate for sudden infant death syndrome (SIDS) had dropped by over 50% since 1994. This can be attributed to the national public health education campaign known as "Back to Sleep" (Eunice Kennedy Shriver National Institute of Child Development and Health, 2012).

Risk Factors for Pregnant Women and Infants

Most pregnant women in the United States are healthy; they have normal pregnancies and produce healthy babies. Many factors contribute to the health problems of those mothers and babies who figure in the statistics on infant mortality and LBW. The factors associated with LBW and infant mortality can be grouped into three categories (CDC, 2009a; Partington, Steber, Blair, & Cisler, 2009):

1. Lifestyle: Smoking, inadequate nutrition, high alcohol consumption, substance abuse, poor prenatal care, environmental toxins, stress, violence and lack of social support, and bed sharing
2. Sociodemographic: Low maternal age, low educational level, poverty, and unmarried status
3. Medical and gestational history: Primiparity, multiple gestation, short interpregnancy intervals, premature rupture of the membranes, uterine abnormality, febrile illness during pregnancy, abortion, genetic factors, gestation-induced hypertension, less than ideal weight gain during pregnancy, and diabetes

It is in the realm of lifestyle choices that P/CHNs can have the most significant impact on pregnancy outcomes such as LBW, preterm birth, and infant mortality. However, programs that provide access to P/CHNs have decreased, and provider awareness to refer pregnant women to P/CHN programs has diminished.

Substance Use and Abuse

Another area of concern is **substance use** and abuse among the childbearing population. The range of adverse consequences associated with the use of tobacco, alcohol, and illicit drugs during pregnancy is wide and includes preterm birth, LBW, and fetal alcohol syndrome (FAS) (described later in this chapter). This puts these women and their unborn children in double jeopardy; not only are they at risk from the consequences of alcohol or drug use but they also do not receive the preventive prenatal care that can eliminate or reduce other obstetric complications. Mothers who smoke also are at risk of having premature or lower birth weight babies, along with other sequelae (Mercer, Merlino, Milluzzi, & Moore, 2008).

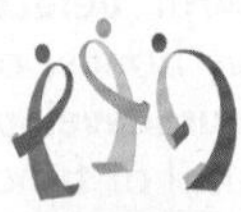

PERSPECTIVES STUDENT VOICE

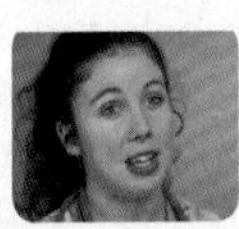

I began working as a nurse's aide at our local hospital when I started nursing school. I learned first-hand the dangers of childbirth and the long-term consequences that can result. One night, a single young female reported to the emergency room in labor and was admitted to the labor and delivery department and seen by the nurse midwife who had provided prenatal care for the mother in the clinic. The young mother-to-be was very excited. Her contractions continued, and she did not progress with the labor process, so she was to be started on oxytocin (Pitocin) to increase the effectiveness of her labor. The nurse midwife checked on her patient frequently, but problems began after the first 8 hours of labor. As the dosage was increased, the fetus reacted with bradycardia, and the nurse midwife did not notify the physician. The Pitocin dosage was decreased and then the heart rate stabilized; this process continued for three cycles. The nurse midwife signed off her 12-hour shift and handed care of the patient over to the nurse midwife coming on shift. Again, whenever the Pitocin dosage was increased to the point of becoming effective, the fetus would respond with bradycardia. Report was given, and the physician in charge was still not notified. The first two times, the fetus recovered. The third time, the fetus did not recover; instead, the bradycardia increased. By this time, the mother had been in labor for over 24 hours, and the fetus was in irreversible distress. The physician was notified of an emergency and reported to the bedside within 5 minutes. An emergency cesarian section was performed, and the Apgar scores at delivery were 0 at 1 minute, 0 at 5 minutes, 0 at 10 minutes, and 3 at 15 minutes. The infant was severely neurologically damaged. I found out later that the infant was diagnosed with severe cerebral palsy and will never walk, talk, or feed normally. She cannot swallow and will require suctioning, gastrostomy tube feeding, and total care throughout her lifetime. She is also cortically blind. The hospital and physician were sued. The nurses and the nurse midwives in the labor and delivery room were found negligent in not reporting to the physician when the patient's labor failed to progress. The nurse midwives from both shifts were found negligent for failure to recognize fetal distress and summon the physician. A multimillion dollar award was given, and the nurses and nurse midwives employed by the hospital were fired. It is sad to think that this tragedy could have been avoided with prudent nurse–patient advocacy, reporting, and appropriate documentation—the things our nursing instructors are always drumming into our heads. I know that as a new graduate, I am now in a position of responsibility to make decisions to notify the physician or not. I have decided that the choice should always be to notify the physician. Even though it may seem inconvenient, it really should be done. I will never forget this case and its long-reaching consequences for the child and family, as well as for the nursing staff and nurse midwives.

Lyndsay, Student Nurse

Substance abuse during pregnancy is a problem with staggering social and medical implications, such as preterm births, LBW, miscarriage, placental abruption, developmental delays, and child behavior and learning problems later in life (American Pregnancy Association, 2012). The precise rate of substance abuse among pregnant women is difficult to determine. In a large study (n = 27,874) of substance abuse and pregnancy, 26.3% of the women reported previous use and 2.6% current use. Adverse outcomes of these pregnancies included LBW, preterm birth, small for gestational age (SGA), and admission to the neonatal intensive care unit (NICU). The investigators also noted that many substance-using women also use tobacco and alcohol while pregnant (Hayatbakhsh et al., 2012).

In the United States, almost 90% of substance-abusing women are of reproductive age and are most commonly reported to abuse cocaine, amphetamines, opioids, alcohol, marijuana, and tobacco. Also, the use of several substances—or polysubstance abuse—is fairly common in this population (Hayatbakhsh et al., 2012). Opiate-exposed infants are at increased risk of perinatal morbidity and mortality and are more likely than healthy infants to have neurodevelopmental impairment at age 18 months and 3 years (Hunt, Tzioumi, Collins, & Jeffery, 2008). Cocaine use during pregnancy is associated with impaired fetal growth, neonatal seizures, and congenital anomalies. Cocaine-exposed infants demonstrate dysregulation of autonomic nervous system functions (e.g., heart rate, respiratory sinus arrhythmias) within the first year of life, and this alteration of response to stressors continues into later childhood (Kable, Coles, Lynch, & Platzman, 2008). A study using volumetric magnetic resonance imaging (MRI) to examine brain volumes in 10- to 14-year-old children exposed in utero to cocaine, alcohol, cigarettes, and marijuana found that each substance was individually related to decreased head circumference and cortical gray matter and that "these substances may act cumulatively during gestation to exert lasting effects on brain size and volume" (Rivkin, et al., 2008, p. 741).

Neonatal withdrawal is characterized by abnormal functions of the gastrointestinal tract, the CNS, and the respiratory system. Poor feeding, abnormal sleep patterns, long-term learning disabilities, and delayed language development may be observable results of maternal drug use. In addition, the child faces a high risk of infectious diseases, including hepatitis B and HIV (March of Dimes, 2008). Infants prenatally exposed to opiates are also more likely to succumb to SIDS (Kahlert, Rutin, Kind, 2007).

A lifestyle choice that includes the use of drugs during pregnancy has placed millions of children at risk. These children are seen in NICUs, foster care, special education programs in the public schools, and later in the juvenile court system. Family structure patterns are altered because grandparents may find themselves primary caregivers for their grandchildren. A woman who is an illicit intravenous drug user loses her inhibitions and engages in high-risk sexual behaviors introducing other public health problems; these include acquisition of sexually transmitted infections (STIs), including HIV, and possible spread of the infection to the fetus or others (De Genna, Cornelius, & Cook, 2007). The primary, secondary, and tertiary prevention roles of the P/CHN cannot be underestimated when drug use takes such a high toll on every aspect of society.

Alcohol Use

Another societal problem is the use and especially addiction to alcohol. It is difficult to establish accurate statistics on the number of women who drink during pregnancy (American Pregnancy Association, 2012). Binge drinking among women ages18 to 44 during the last 30 days ranged from 5% to 23% with the majority between 11% and 23% (National Center on Birth Defects & Developmental Disabilities [NCBDDD], 2009). More binge-drinking women with high levels of usual alcohol consumption were found in the 18- to 24-year-old age group or among women who were current smokers (Tsai, Floyd, Green, & Boyle, 2007).

Alcohol use can cause devastating effects in the fetus, even when limited to early pregnancy and in the absence of addiction, and can lead to an array of neurocognitive and behavioral disorders, sometimes with structural anomalies, now described as **fetal alcohol spectrum disorders** (FASD). For example, regular intake of alcohol during pregnancy, especially in the first trimester, can cause the most recognizable form of the disorder, **fetal alcohol syndrome**, which is characterized by structural abnormalities of the head and face (e.g., microcephaly and flattening of the maxillary area), intrauterine growth retardation, decreased birth weight and length, developmental delays related to CNS abnormalities that can cause intellectual impairment, hyperactivity, altered sleep patterns, feeding problems, perceptual difficulties, impaired concentration, mood problems, and language dysfunction (NCBDDD, 2011a). FAS is estimated to occur at a rate of 0.2 to 1.5 per 1,000 live births in selected areas of the United States (NCBDDD, 2011b). Among the Native American population, alcohol abuse is a major public health problem, and FAS rates are as high as 8.97 per 1,000. P/CHNs working collaboratively with FAS specialists among this population have been effective in preventing FAS and in helping children born with FAS (Beckett, 2011). This completely preventable leading cause of birth defects imposes major costs for educational and health care systems.

What was once termed **fetal alcohol effects** (FAEs) syndrome, characterized as causing some but not all of the symptoms of FAS, is now separated into the more descriptive categories of **alcohol-related birth defects** (ARBDs), indicating problems with hearing, bones, or heart, and kidneys, and **alcohol-related neurodevelopmental disorder** (ARND), represented by mental or functional problems, including cognitive and/or behavioral abnormalities (NCBDDD, 2011b). Recent research has helped to better classify the fetal effects of alcohol and may continue to lead to more specific classifications (Manning & Eugene-Hoyme, 2007). These conditions occur in children whose mothers have used varying amounts of alcohol while pregnant, and physical signs are often much more subtle than in cases of FAS. However, those with FASD may have one or more of the following behaviors or characteristics (NCBDDD, 2011b):

- Small size for gestational age, or small stature in relation to peers
- Facial abnormalities (e.g., smooth philtrum)
- Poor coordination
- Hyperactivity, attention problems, learning disabilities
- Difficulties in school, especially with math
- Developmental disabilities (e.g., speech and language delays)
- Intellectual disability or low IQ
- Vision and hearing problems; problems with heart, kidneys, bones
- Poor reasoning and judgment skills
- Sleep and sucking disturbances in infancy (para. 5).

It is important to provide evidence-based primary prevention before pregnancy and to reach women before a lifestyle of drinking becomes such a part of their lives that they are unable or unwilling to abstain during pregnancy. For example, the Pregnancy Risk Assessment Monitoring System (PRAMS) is a surveillance system developed by the CDC and state health departments to collect population-based information on maternal preconception, prenatal, pregnancy, and postpartum behaviors and experiences. Recent data collection revealed that prior to conception, 23% of women used tobacco and 12.8% continued to smoke while pregnant (CDC, 2012b). Only 35.1% of pregnant women took a multivitamin tablet at least 4 days a week, 10.2% were anemic, and 3.6% reported physical abuse (D'Angelo et al., 2008). Children are also at risk based on maternal alcohol use during child rearing, especially for adolescent mothers age 15 to 19 years. Combined data from 2005 to 2009 indicate that 30% of young mothers used alcohol and 12% used marijuana in the past month (Substance Abuse & Mental Health Services Administration [SAMHSA], 2011).

Working with women of childbearing age to improve their general health behaviors and promote better preparation for pregnancy is essential. For those pregnant women and mothers already using substances, maternal drug and alcohol treatment programs that focus on supportive parent–child attachment, enhancement of parenting and child-rearing capabilities, and encouragement of the use of support systems that can improve child health and cognitive development are needed. In-home family skills training and parenting education programs that are evidence-based and promote P/CHN and client rapport can be effective methods of working with substance-abusing mothers and their at-risk children; however, more studies are recommended. In a systematic review of home visitation with alcohol- and drug-using mothers, there was no significance of home visitation with mothers reducing substance use of entering drug and alcohol rehabilitation programs. However, individual studies showed significance in home visitation reducing these mothers' involvement with Child Protective Services indicating a positive effect on parenting and child care practices even if not effective on the addictive behavior (Turnbull & Osborn, 2012).

Tobacco Use

Tobacco use has increased dramatically among women, especially since the women's movement of the 1970s, inevitably affecting maternal and newborn health. The nicotine in tobacco is a major addictive substance, and smoking is an addiction that many people find difficult to stop. Although the risk factors of smoking are well documented, many pregnant women continue to smoke. Smoking during pregnancy is one of the most studied risk factors in obstetric history. It has been associated with ectopic pregnancy, spontaneous abortions, intrauterine growth retardation, preterm birth, stillbirths, higher perinatal mortality, SGA birth, LBW birth, neonatal anomalies, and lower Apgar scores (Weck, Paulose, & Flaws, 2008). For pregnant women, an education level below high school graduation and those with a current nicotine-dependence were at higher risk of smoking (90.5%) than college-educated women without nicotine dependence (3.9%), according to a study from Harvard university researchers (Gillman, Breslau, Subramanian, Hitsman, & Koenen, 2008). Smoking is "one of the strongest predictors of both LBW and preterm birth" and is "often linked to stress and depression" (Hobbell, Goldstein, & Barrett, 2008, p. 345). For instance, women who may have started smoking as adolescents often continue to smoke in response to life stressors. Health problems do not end once the infant is born. Infants of women who smoked during pregnancy continue to be at higher risk for LBW, preterm birth, poor fetal growth, SIDS, respiratory infections, asthma, ear infections, and decreased lung function (Mercer, Merlino, Milluzzi, & Moore, 2008; Wang & Pinkerton, 2008; Wigle et al., 2008).

Passive smoking or **environmental tobacco smoke (ETS)**—exposure to tobacco smoke from other people smoking in one's environment—also puts a person at risk for smoking-related disease. The Surgeon General has outlined major conclusions related to ETS based on years of research findings. One conclusion is that there is no risk-free level of secondhand smoke. Related to children and ETS, there is an increased risk of SIDS, more acute respiratory infection, ear disease, worse asthma, and risk for poor lung growth (CDC, 2012b). If a pregnant woman lives with a smoker, she and her fetus can be negatively affected by the other person's addiction. The use of **smokeless tobacco products**, such as snuff and chewing tobacco, has led to an increase in oral cancers related to tobacco exposure. Maternal smokeless tobacco use among some women has been associated with lower birth weight by an average of 78 g controlling for other factors and a mean of 331 g for pregnant women who smoke (England et al., 2012).

Public and community health nurses and other health care professionals must be involved in the control of tobacco products on many levels, especially in health policy development, community outreach, and education. It is also important to have skills in client assessment, planning, and intervention, to serve as positive role models, and to be active in research implementation. In the case of tobacco control, health policy development has made important strides at the grassroots level (see Chapter 13). A top priority of health care policy development is to reduce access of youth to tobacco products by restricting tobacco product advertising and promotion. Some significant policy steps that have been taken to discourage young people from smoking include imposing substantial cigarette excise taxes; requiring that public places, such as malls, restaurants, and even bars, be smoke-free; monitoring tobacco retailers for illegal sales to minors; and keeping cigarettes in locked cases. Most smokers become addicted to tobacco use in their early teens. If fewer adolescents begin smoking, there will be fewer women of childbearing age who smoke in the future.

An initial health history of a pregnant woman should always include the assessment of tobacco use, smoking status, and exposure to smoke in the personal environment. Stress should also be assessed (e.g., unintended pregnancy; nutrition; chronic stress and daily hassles; levels of social support; mental health issues, such as depression or anxiety, work stressors, racism, or discrimination; and any significant life events, such as death or other significant losses) (Hobbell, Goldstein, & Barrett, 2008).

The P/CHN must not only advise clients to quit smoking but also offer supportive and empathetic approaches to stress reduction and smoking cessation, including methods or interventions that can help. For example, the P/CHN may counsel clients individually, refer for behavioral therapy, provide self-help manuals, or recommend nicotine replacement therapy or medication. Other approaches, such as support groups, can be helpful. Any permanent reduction in the number of cigarettes smoked, amount of secondhand smoke inhaled, or amount of smokeless tobacco products used is helpful in improving the health of the mother and her fetus. Particular attention should be paid to adolescent mothers (15–19 years) as their rates of smoking are much higher than adolescents of those ages who are not mothers (SAMHSA, 2011).

Nurses can be positive role models for health and demonstrate health promotion strategies to clients by their own behavior—if a nurse has struggled with smoking cessation, her admission of failures or explanation of successful strategies offers an opportunity to enhance credibility with clients as they recognize that the nurse struggles with some of the same health issues.

Intimate Partner Violence

Intimate partner violence (IPV) is any coercive action taken by someone against an intimate partner (New York City Department of Health and Mental Hygiene [NYCDOHMH], 2012). Pregnancy is a vulnerable period for women and can increase their risk for IPV. IPV can range from physical abuse to woman and fetus via blows to the belly and psychological coerciveness. It is estimated that between 4% and 8% of pregnant women from all walks of life experience IPV per year (NYCDOHMH, 2012). Reasons for increased IPV during pregnancy can be an unintended pregnancy, increased stress related to supporting a child, and jealousy. One large-scale retrospective study of pregnant and postpartum women in Massachusetts from 2001 to 2005 found that in 1,675 hospital visits for assault, 1,528 physical injuries were diagnosed—largely to the head and neck (42.2%) for the total sample and torso (21.5%) in pregnant women; the percentage dropped to 8.7% in the postpartum sample (Nannini et al., 2008). Victims of IPV have high levels of stress and higher rates of smoking during pregnancy, as well as inadequate utilization of prenatal care services (Chambliss, 2008). Pregnant women who experience psychological IPV also have 25.8% higher incidence of postpartum depression (Ludermir, Lewis, Valonqueiro, Araujo, & Araya, 2010).

Sexually Transmitted Infections

In the United States, an estimated 1,080,000 pregnant women annually are infected with bacterial vaginosis, 880,000 with herpes simplex virus 2, and 100,000 have *chlamydia*. Fewer than 1,000 annually contract syphilis and 13,200 are estimated to have gonorrhea. Hepatitis B is estimated in 16,000 pregnant women, and around 6,400 women are diagnosed with HIV annually (CDC, 2012e).

STIs can pass from mother to baby. Syphilis can cross the placenta and infect the fetus, as can HIV—which can also be passed to the infant through breast-feeding (CDC, 2012e). Other STIs (e.g., gonorrhea, hepatitis B, *chlamydia*, genital herpes) can infect the baby as it passes through the birth canal during delivery. LBW, stillbirth, conjunctivitis, blindness, deafness, neurologic damage, chronic liver disease, and cirrhosis, along with neonatal sepsis and pneumonia, are possible infant complications of maternal STIs. Mothers may have premature rupture of membranes and resultant infection, or may have a premature onset of labor. Some STIs can lead to cervical and other cancers, pelvic inflammatory disease, infertility, chronic hepatitis, and many other health problems (CDC, 2009a). Research indicates that bacterial vaginosis can lead to preterm labor (American Pregnancy Association, 2012), so screening for this health problem during pregnancy is highly recommended by public health experts.

A pregnant woman who discovers she has an STI often feels ashamed, betrayed, embarrassed, and angry. Those who are asymptomatic may not realize they are infected or deny the existence of the disease and fail to carry out the treatment plan after diagnosis. Although educating the pregnant client about the effects of STIs is critical, providing information alone is not enough. The P/CHN has a pivotal role in enhancing the empowerment of women so they can act on the information they receive. The P/CHN engages with the pregnant clients and helps them understand that they have control over their bodies. Usually, STIs are first discovered in pregnancy during routine prenatal screening, which places the clinic nurse and the nurse who may make home visits in the position to take an affirmative approach to treatment and follow-up.

HIV and AIDS

The HIV epidemic is the great tragedy of the final two decades of the 20th century, but great strides are being made in the 21st century. As a result of early detection and antiviral therapy, there has been a substantial decline in the number of infants born with HIV since the height of the epidemic. Mothers who transmitted the virus to their newborn infants reported contracting it through sex with an infected partner, injection drug use, or other unspecified methods. In a large-scale New York study, 45% of mothers with infected infants had not participated in perinatal HIV prevention interventions. Prenatal, intrapartum, or neonatal antiretroviral drugs were lacking, largely due to maternal illicit drug use, and were associated with LBW babies (Peters et al., 2008). An HIV-positive woman who is pregnant or who has delivered a baby requires special nursing management of the pregnancy and of the family after the birth of the newborn. There are many teaching opportunities for the P/CHN during a high-risk pregnancy, such as helping the client identify, change, or curtail high-risk behaviors and promoting adherence to prenatal and HIV care. Success in changing behaviors often requires an interdisciplinary approach of health care, social, emotional, and financial resources.

In the United States and other developed nations, HIV-infected women are advised not to breast-feed their infants because there is a 15% chance that the infants will become infected with HIV from breast milk (Shearer, 2008); others report rates as high as 50% (Lockman, 2010). The P/CHN focuses teaching on providing a safe, available form of infant formula. In developing countries, the lack of clean water still makes formula feeding dangerous, and breast-feeding is usually recommended. The infection rate for HIV from breast-feeding and the mortality rate from formula made with impure water are about the same, resulting in a dilemma for women and health care providers in developing countries.

Poor Nutrition, Weight Gain, and Oral Health

Nutrition is very important to the unborn child, and mothers' choices, even before conception, can affect the baby's health and development. It is at about 3 weeks' gestation—often before the woman recognizes that she is pregnant—the infant's neural tube is forming. Hormones and nutrients set gene switches that affect later life.

Research has demonstrated a positive correlation between weight gain during pregnancy and normal birth weight in the babies. In 2009, the Institute of Medicine (IOM) released new guidelines for weight gain during pregnancy based on body mass indices (BMIs). Weight gain between 25 and 35 pounds during pregnancy is recommended for women with BMIs ranging from 18.5 to 24.9, and the recommendation is 28 to 40 pounds for underweight women with a BMI under 18.5; while overweight women with a BMI between 25 to 29 should gain 15 to 25 pounds, and obese women with a BMI over 30.0 should hold their weight gain to between 11 and 20 pounds (IOM, 2009).

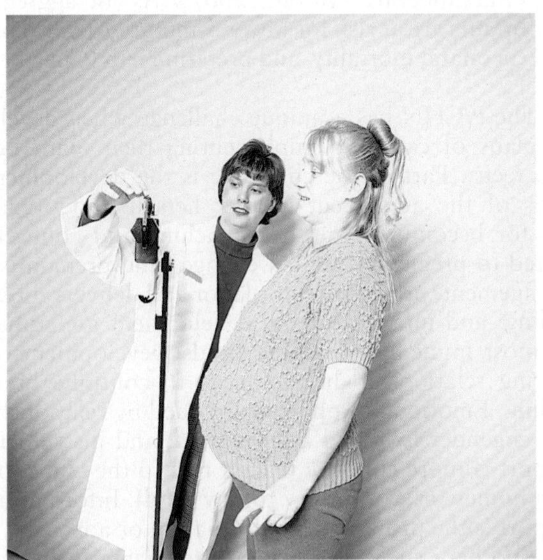

Weight gain during pregnancy should be monitored regularly.

Obesity currently affects about 20% of all pregnancies in the United States. Gestational diabetes poses the greatest risk to obese pregnant women and increases the risk or preterm birth (CDC, 2012d). P/CHNs who work with morbidly obese pregnant women can help them most by emphasizing good nutrition and by encouraging them to maintain their prepregnant weight without drastically reducing caloric intake. This can be accomplished primarily by a marked decrease in consumption of "empty calories" from junk food and replacing with increased intake of fruits, vegetables, and low-fat sources of calcium. Pregnancy is never a time for dieting. Following nutritional guidelines ensures the proper number of servings and portion sizes. Nutritional counseling can have an additional benefit in that it may ultimately decrease the risk of obesity or eating disorders in the client's children. For women who are prone to gaining too much weight, nutrition-rich, low-calorie foods are recommended. Exercise during pregnancy is essential and can reduce maternal weight gain and improve cardiovascular fitness (Gavard & Artal, 2008). After assessment, the P/CHN can determine whether the unwanted weight gain is related to the consumption of additional calories, to limited activity, or to fluid retention. Each cause must be managed differently. Underweight women have twice as many LBW babies as women whose weight is within normal range. Low maternal weight gain is associated with LBW infants who have higher incidences of growth problems, developmental delays, CNS disorders, and mental retardation (CDC, 2009a). Nutritional teaching is part of the P/CHN's role when working with a pregnant woman who has difficulty gaining the recommended weight during pregnancy. Finding ways to add calories to foods and increasing the woman's desire to eat are effective methods to improve maternal weight gain. Insufficient caloric intake in pregnant adolescents (who themselves are still growing) is an additional concern for their future health and health of the infant over the life course. Oral health during pregnancy is also very important to assess. Periodontal infection may affect around 40% of women of childbearing age and is especially common among disadvantaged and ethnic or racial minorities who may not have adequate access to dental health care (Boggess & Society for Maternal-Fetal Medicine Publications Committee, 2008). Maternal periodontal disease has also been linked to preterm birth, LBW, preeclampsia, and early fetal loss (Ferguson, Hansen, Novak, & Novak, 2007). High maternal levels of the bacteria that cause cavities have been associated with a greater chance of subsequent dental caries in the infant (Silk, Douglass, Douglass, & Silk, 2008).

Public and community health nurses should teach women of childbearing age the importance of regular dental health checkups and proper dental hygiene, along with making referrals for dental treatment when needed. Dental health procedures have generally been found to be effective and safe for pregnant women, especially during the second trimester (Dasanayake, Gennaro, Hendricks-Munoz, & Chghun, 2008; Silk et al., 2008). Sugar-free gums that contain xylitol and chlorhexidine may be helpful in reducing the maternal child transmission of caries-causing bacteria (Silk et al., 2008). Dental health is not only important during pregnancy, but poor dental hygiene and disease have been linked to health conditions, such as cardiovascular disease and diabetes. Dental health should be a part of general primary preventive education for all childbearing-age women.

Socioeconomic Status and Social Inequality

As noted earlier, poverty plays a role in pregnancy and birth outcomes. Social and economic disparities are factors in preterm birth in both developed and developing nations and reflect some of the social determinants of health. These relationships may be more indirect, as poorer women often lack health insurance, have less access to quality prenatal care services, have poorer nutrition, and are exposed to more situational and psychological stressors. Even Canada, noted for universal health care coverage, has been noted to have inadequate levels of prenatal care related to socioeconomic status

(SES) disparities (Weck et al., 2008). Prenatal stress is difficult to research, but some recent studies using animal models indicate that exposure to stress prenatally leads to learning problems, anxiety and depression, and coping problems (The Hebrew University of Jerusalem, 2008).

Prenatal care is crucial to ensure good outcomes of pregnancy. The crisis surrounding professional liability insurance has been especially critical in the case of physicians specializing in obstetrics and gynecology (OB-GYN). Over the past decade, insurance costs have risen dramatically. In some instances, premiums have equaled the obstetrician's income. OB-GYNs have either moved to states where lawsuits have limits set by legislation and insurance rates are reasonable, or they reduce the number of high-risk obstetrical cases or total deliveries in an effort to reduce their premium costs. Some of them chose to stop practicing altogether leaving many pregnant women without convenient access to appropriate prenatal care (see Perspectives: Student Voices). Other factors, outlined in more detail in Chapter 25, may also affect the health of both mothers and babies.

Adolescent Pregnancy

Pregnancy during the adolescent years (13–19) is considered a health risk because of the ongoing physical growth and the demands of psychosocial development during these years. The United States leads most developed nations in the rates of teenage pregnancy, abortion, and childbearing. There is a strong association between young maternal age and high IMR, and infants born to adolescents are at increased risk for preterm delivery and for neonatal and postneonatal mortality (Usta, Zoorob, Abu-Musa, Naassan, & Nassar, 2008). These adverse birth outcomes are independent of education level, use of cigarettes and alcohol during pregnancy, or prenatal care. Simply being an adolescent puts pregnant teens and their offspring at risk (Chen et al., 2007). Infants born to Black adolescents are more likely to be LBW babies than are infants of White teens. Infants born to very young adolescents (aged 10–14 years) are at very high risk for neonatal mortality. Adolescent mothers have increased psychological risks, such as isolation, powerlessness, depressive disorders, and increased somatic complaints. Developmental and maturational processes are disrupted or compromised, and young mothers face diminished prospects for completing their education. It is important for P/CHNs to assess each pregnant adolescent's situation in order to promote the best outcomes based on evidence including family support and living situation, relationship with the father of the baby and other supportive friends, school plans, and the ability to care for her own health and that of her infant, as well as her hopes, goals, strengths, and weaknesses, in order to effectively plan interventions (Nurse-Family Partnership, 2011).

The markers for successful pregnancy outcomes and future life events are complex and dependent on the expectant mother's health behavior, social determinants, and living environment. The mother's educational attainment, marital experiences, subsequent fertility behavior, labor force experience, occupational attainment, and experiences with poverty and public assistance are all directly related to the adolescent pregnancy and are often negatively affected (Boden, Fergusson, & Horwood, 2008). The issues of adolescent parenting are complex. They encompass many areas, including emotional, physical, and social issues, and the life experiences of adolescent mothers often are characterized as unequal to those of their peers who delayed childbirth (Smithbattle, 2007).

Pregnant adolescents are less likely to receive early and continuous prenatal care, and they are more likely to use alcohol and to smoke during their pregnancies. Moreover, their diets are often lacking in essential vitamins and minerals (Moran, 2007). As an aggregate, their infants are at risk for lower 5-minute Apgar scores, LBW, neonatal mortality, and preterm birth (Chen et al., 2007).

The P/CHN has a unique challenge when developing plans of care and implementing them with pregnant teens. Part of the challenge is the developmental needs of the adolescent mother herself and preparation for becoming a mother. Teaching and counseling related to pregnancy-related changes and prenatal self-management, preparation for labor and delivery, breastfeeding, and infant care and development are some of the most immediate learning needs Development of a trusting relationship helped teens to continue breastfeeding. Emotional support is provided by relationships that engender love and appreciation, and instrumental support is more concrete (e.g., a ride to the clinic, help with homework, or money to buy food). Informational support is the provision of information or advice.

Another issue with pregnant adolescents is the problem of repeated pregnancies. One Texas study found that 42% of teen mothers had another pregnancy within 2 years' time, 73% of them went on to deliver an infant (Raneri & Wiemann, 2007). Predictors identified in the study included "not being in a relationship with father of the first child three months later," being more than 3 years younger than the father of the first baby, "experiencing intimate partner violence" within 3 months of the first birth, not being in school 3 months after the first child's birth, and "having many friends who were adolescent parents" (p. 39). Second pregnancies during adolescence have been associated with "worse outcomes" when compared to first-time teen mothers (Reime, Schucking, & Wenzlaff, 2008, p. 4). Public and community health nurses can provide interventions that may help postpone subsequent pregnancies such as counseling, referral, and intensive case management (Nurse-Family Partnership, 2011).

Emotional Needs

Teenagers who become pregnant deal with this change in their life in a variety of ways. Some have such a strong denial system that they deny the pregnancy, even to themselves. They may be 3 or 4 months into the pregnancy before they can admit it and seek a pregnancy confirmation. Often, their parents are the last to know. What is difficult about this scenario is that prenatal care is delayed into the second or third trimester of pregnancy. If the teen chooses to continue with the pregnancy, the delayed prenatal care could compromise the wellbeing of both the young mother and the fetus. Holub et al. (2007) studied the effects of prenatal and parenting stress on a large group of 14- to 19-year-olds and found that those who had high levels of both stressors exhibited lower maternal adjustment (i.e., positive attitude toward being a mother, care of the infant, competent parenting) and higher emotional distress after giving birth. They concluded that early interventions for both prenatal and parenting support are needed. It takes time for adolescent mothers to begin to understand the role of parent and to get to "know their baby" (Smithbattle, 2007, p. 261).

Caring and supportive parents, P/CHNs, and school nurses can be instrumental in guiding an adolescent through this difficult time. Adolescent parents have difficult choices to make, including decisions about continuing with the pregnancy, keeping the baby, or finding adoptive parents. Some may choose abortion. These choices are difficult, may be strongly influenced by peer opinions and social pressure, and are fraught with emotion. Adolescents and supportive parents, in consultation with professionals, can explore all options. This may be the time that the P/CHN first begins to work with the teen, perhaps at school or in a school-based clinic. First contact may also occur in a clinic or physician's office, or on a home visit resulting from a referral from a health care provider. Home visiting programs for adolescent mothers have been effective in improving prenatal care, parenting scores, and school continuation rates. They have also contributed to reducing preterm births (Barnet, Liu, DeVoe, Alperovitz-Bichell, & Duggan, 2007; Flynn, Budd, & Modelski, 2008). The nurse can offer educational services, emotional support, and referrals for services as needed. Because postpartum depression is not uncommon, and adolescents are at increased risk, it may be important for P/CHN contact to continue periodically for 1 to 2 years postpartum (Mayberry, Horowitz, & Declercq, 2007; Reid & Meadows-Oliver, 2007).

The goal of any pregnancy is positive maternal–infant outcomes, including a positive relationship. For some adolescent mothers, positive relationships are more difficult to achieve than for older mothers. Positive relationships and self-esteem have an impact on the quality of mothering and positive responses to infant distress. In classic studies home visitation studies conducted by Olds et al. (2007), Nurse-Family Partnership (2011), and by Koniack-Griffin, Anderson, Verzemnieks & Brecht (2000) and Koniack-Griffin et al. (2002 & 2003), intensive intervention programs improved parenting outcomes, including self-esteem and self-confidence. Public and community health nurses who have special training in the evidenced-based home visitation models for high-risk maternal–child populations can provide each participant with services that promote the overall health of the mother and maternal–infant bonding. Results of these studies can further guide nurses in their work with pregnant adolescents.

Physical Needs

Pregnant teens have a gamut of physical needs that can be addressed by routine prenatal care and education, but there is need for continuity if such endeavors are to be successful. Routine prenatal care is one of the most important needs, and adolescents may require assistance in recognizing the value of health professionals monitoring the pregnancy. Some may feel embarrassed and uncomfortable with male health care providers and refuse to keep appointments or may want to be accompanied by the baby's father or a girlfriend. Whatever it takes to get the teen to prenatal appointments should be encouraged, including making arrangements for transportation (e.g., procuring bus tokens, calling a taxi, or arranging for a friend or social worker to drive the teen to her appointments). Where feasible, specialty-focused clinics for pregnant and parenting teens may be most effective. School-based clinics have shown promise in providing easily accessible prenatal care, lowering the risk of giving birth to LBW infants, and reducing school dropout rates (Strunk, 2008).

The pregnant adolescent needs education regarding changes in her emotional state and her body, the growth and development of the fetus, dietary requirements, and rest and relaxation needs. She also needs anticipatory guidance for caregiving and parenting. Teaching can take place as part of each prenatal appointment, in specific classes at school for pregnant teens, in the health department clinic, or during home visits. In each setting, the P/CHN can modify the teaching methods to the setting and the individual needs of the adolescent. Studies show that P/CHN home visits and preparation-for-motherhood classes are effective in promoting better outcomes for adolescents and their infants, including better use of resources (e.g., prenatal visits), fewer hospital days, lower school dropout rates, fewer repeat pregnancies 2 years postpartum, and decreased infant mortality (Flynn et al., 2008).

Changing adolescent behavior during pregnancy can be challenging, and P/CHNs must keep in mind the developmental differences between early, middle, and late adolescents with regard to intentions and health habits (Phipps, Rosengard, Weitzen, Meers, & Billinkoff, 2008). The P/CHN may focus on one important and seemingly less complex issue of nutrition during pregnancy. However, it is a more difficult task to change the eating habits of teens than it is to change those of adults. In their stage of development, adolescents usually are more concerned with body image than with fetal growth and development. Fad diets, peer pressure, and personal control are all issues with which the pregnant adolescent is struggling. If a teen has been raised in poverty, a multiplicity of other issues can affect her motivation to make dietary changes during pregnancy. Adolescents are more often concerned with present needs and respond better to relaxed, informal group approaches to education that involve topics of their choosing and do not resemble the school setting. Pregnancy diaries, creative activities (crafts, drawing, making snacks), small group activities and games, videos with discussions, social media and computer-assisted interventions, and visits to local community resources (hospital delivery rooms, social services, lactation counselors) are more appealing than classroom lectures. Programs that offer empowerment and group prenatal care are helpful. Also, teaching and support groups may be helpful in promoting healthy prenatal behaviors and preparing for motherhood (National Clearinghouse on Families & Youth, n.d.).

Social Needs

Peer support and acceptance is an expected part of adolescent development but can also influence the stress level of the teen. There may be changes in acceptance by social groups or in types of activities (e.g., surfboarding, mountain climbing) based on the pregnancy. The group may participate in behaviors that the pregnant adolescent should not participate in, such as smoking, drinking, or taking illicit drugs. This causes conflict for a pregnant teen who has a strong need to be accepted by her peer group and who also knows that she has a responsibility to her unborn child. The P/CHN can facilitate help for the adolescent client to problem solve her dilemma by providing a social support system among the attendees at prenatal classes. The nurse can also convince the teen's parents or other adults in her life to offer her more support. Often, a developmental crisis such as an adolescent pregnancy can help cement the mother–daughter relationship. It takes time and work on the part of the parents and the teen. The adolescent will need the support of her parents after the baby is born, and strengthening the relationship during pregnancy is an important start.

Another social outlet and an important resource is school. The teen should be encouraged to continue her studies, with the goal of graduation. The health and welfare of children are related to the educational levels of their parents. Internet support groups organized and monitored by nurses are beginning to provide another means of social support for pregnant and parenting adolescents (Hudson, Campbell-Grossman, Keating-Lefler, & Cline, 2008). Computer and Internet-based interventions have demonstrated success in providing knowledge and promoting delayed sexual activity in Appalachian high schools (Roberto, Zimmerman, Carlyle, & Abner, 2007). Greater self-efficacy in negotiating condom use was also noted in participants, and the majority of high school students (88.5%) participated in at least one activity aimed at preventing adolescent pregnancy and transmission of STIs and HIV. Teen pregnancy and education are discussed more thoroughly in Chapter 22.

Maternal Developmental Disability

For couples who are developmentally disabled, having a child puts increased stress on a system that is already burdened. Parenting requires attending to not just the child's physical care but socialization and developmental stimulation, well child and illness health care, emotional nurturing, and age-appropriate supervision. Depending on the social support, and coping skills of the developmentally delayed parent, the stress and need for emotional control and positive decision making can be monumental. Evidence from a large cohort study in Britain found that, for 4- to 6-year-olds, there was "no association of parental IQ with conduct or emotional problems" in the children; however, for children age 7 into adolescence, "strong evidence was observed" between lower parental IQ and child "conduct, emotional, and attention problems" (Whitley, Gale, Deary, Kivimaki, & Batty, 2011, p. 1032). Confounding variables included the environment of the home, parental affect, and child IQ. Even though there may not be strong evidence for these problems, children are still at risk for understimulation and environmental insecurity. Parent training/child care skills programs, peer to peer support groups, community agencies, and careful home monitoring can reduce the risk of **child abuse** and neglect and promote more effective parenting (Promising Practices Network, 2012).

Much of the pediatric literature discusses the needs of developmentally disabled infants and children and the roles of nurses and health care professionals in assisting the families of these children. Developmentally disabled adults, however, are rarely represented in studies of disability, so there is limited information about their experiences and success as parents. Sometimes bizarre behaviors can occur because the parent does not understand basic concepts regarding normal child development. As with nondevelopmentally delayed parents, more responsive and involved developmentally disabled parents have better parenting outcomes. Periodic developmental screening, infant stimulation and home visitation programs, and special health care instruction have demonstrated some evidence-based results (Promising Practices Network, 2012), but there is a great need for more research. How does the P/CHN work with developmentally disabled parents effectively? Most importantly, nursing support must enhance the natural resilience of the family. Extended family support systems, along with community agencies and religious organizations that provide services for mentally disabled adults and children, can improve the outcomes for these families. The success of family support depends on immediate and continuing health promotion visits by multidisciplinary providers. The goal is to establish safe parenting routines that will serve as a foundation for parenting skills needed when the infant begins to walk and explore—a time when the infant's safety is more in jeopardy.

The establishment of a trusting relationship between the nurse and the family is of foremost importance. Teaching by demonstration with many visual aids and prompts, along with games and creative approaches to engage and sustain attention, can challenge the nurse's creativity. Modeling of appropriate parenting behavior needs to occur on each visit. Supervision and monitoring of family functioning must continue until the child reaches adulthood. Many agencies employing P/CHNs cannot provide the intensive follow-up that such a family requires. It is then necessary to make referrals to organizations that can provide support, such as the American Association of Retarded Citizens (AARC) or Exceptional Parents Unlimited. The nurse may stay involved as a consultant to the paraprofessionals or make periodic home visits at times of developmental or situational crisis.

Complications of Childbearing

Some maternal deaths are not preventable (e.g., amniotic fluid embolism). Morbidity is also a factor, and although some major risk factors among pregnant women and infants have been discussed, several common complications of childbearing bear mentioning. The effects of hypertensive disease in pregnancy, gestational diabetes, postpartum depression, and grief in families who have lost a child are important areas in which the P/CHN can intervene effectively.

Hypertensive Disease in Pregnancy

Blood pressure measurements in all people show daily variation, regardless of physical and mental activities. Hypertension in pregnancy may be chronic or related specifically to pregnancy. In a 13-year study (1995–2008) reviewing primary and secondary chronic hypertension in pregnancy, the prevalence almost doubled (0.90%–1.52%), and this was shown to contribute to adverse maternal outcomes of renal failure, pulmonary edema, preeclampsia, and in-hospital mortality (Bateman, Bansil, Hernandez-Diaz, Myhre, et al., 2012).

Preeclampsia results in new-onset high blood pressure and protein in the urine, along with nondependent edema, and can result in eclampsia (characterized by convulsions and/or coma), pulmonary edema, liver rupture, renal failure, disseminated intravascular coagulopathy (DIC), and cortical blindness. The effects from pregnancy-induced hypertension on infants are often serious because placental health is associated with fetal growth (Mistry & Williams, 2011), but long-term maternal consequences, especially cardiovascular, can also be significant. Low-dose aspirin therapy also can prevent preeclampsia and subsequent infant complications (Meads et al., 2008). Various methods are employed to attempt to prevent and control hypertension during pregnancy, namely, a diet rich in fresh fruits and vegetables, adequate fluid intake, weight gain limitations, rest, and regular exercise. These remain the most common preventive suggestions that P/CHNs, in collaboration with the clients' primary health care providers, can give to their pregnant clients. A calm environment, periods of rest, and the pregnant woman either elevating her feet or reclining in a left side-lying position are also recommended. Additional assessment data may guide the nurse to focus teaching on stress reduction techniques and modification or elimination of smoking. Public and community health nurses can provide frequent monitoring of blood pressure and other symptoms and encourage the client to be vigilant in keeping prenatal appointments. However, medication or even hospitalization may be necessary. The P/CHN can offer support and understanding while continuing to be a resource for the client as the pregnancy progresses and the infant is born.

Gestational Diabetes

Gestational diabetes mellitus (GDM) occurs in pregnant women who have never had a problem with high blood glucose but do during pregnancy. The average onset for GDM is around the 24th week of pregnancy (American Diabetes Association [ADA], 2011). GDM is estimated to occur in about 18% of pregnancies and is estimated to cost $623 million (ADA, 2011). For the mother with GDM, there is a higher risk of hypertension, preeclampsia, urinary tract infections, cesarean section, and future risk of type 2 diabetes. Pathophysiologically, GDM is similar to type 2 diabetes, and more than one third of women with GDM eventually develop type 2 diabetes during their lifetimes. Although type 2 diabetes prevalence is higher in some racial and ethnic groups, for GDM the effects of poorer pregnancy outcomes are spread out across ethnic and racial groups with similar rates of complications of pregnancy-induced hypertension and preterm birth (Mocaski & Savitz, 2012). Because growth and maturation of the fetus are closely associated with the delivery of maternal nutrients, particularly glucose, maintenance of appropriate glucose levels is essential to the health of the fetus. Daily self-monitoring of blood glucose levels is recommended. Women should be encouraged to monitor blood glucose levels regularly 6 weeks postpartum and periodically throughout their life.

The infant is at increased risk for fetal death because GDM has been associated with macrosomia large-for-gestational-age (LGA) babies, birth injuries such as broken shoulders, breathing problems, and abnormally high blood sugars at birth (ADA, 2011). An Iranian study using a 75-g glucose tolerance testing (GTT) protocol found a 6.1% incidence of GDM and a correlation between 1-hour blood glucose levels and neonatal birth weights (Shirazian et al., 2008).

The public and community health nurse can help in the control of GDM by encouraging early prenatal care, adequate nutrition, rest and exercise, and adherence to the particular dietary, activity, and blood glucose monitoring regimen suggested by the woman's health care provider. A structured walking program was shown to regulate glucose levels in women with GDM effectively, while reducing daily insulin levels (Davenport, Mottola, McManus, & Gratton, 2008). Although earlier recommendations were restricted to human insulin, a comprehensive review of current research on GDM management and outcomes found both maternal and infant benefits and a low likelihood of fetal harm with either the use of insulin or oral diabetes medications (Nicholson et al., 2008). Waist circumference measurements and a family history of diabetes along with GDM are associated with development of later type 2 diabetes (Nicholson et al., 2008; Lee, Jang, Park, Metzger, & Cho, 2008).

Those P/CHNs working with pregnant women should provide education on early warning signs for GDM and the importance of regular prenatal care, reminder about getting the glucose tolerance test around the 24th week of pregnancy, and follow-up.

Postpartum Depression

Although most people recognize the common fleeting mood swings immediately after childbirth known as "baby blues," high-profile cases like Andrea Yates, who suffered from postpartum psychosis and drowned her five small children, are rare (1 or 2 per 1,000 births) but nonetheless tragic. The actress Brooke Shields discussed her postpartum depression and treatment with antidepressant medications, making this condition more visible and less stigmatizing.

Depressive disorders during a woman's lifetime are fairly common phenomena; 20.6% of women and 11% of men were diagnosed in 2006 (Heo, Murphy, Fontaine, Bruce, & Alexopoulos, 2008). Also, depression and posttraumatic stress disorder (PTSD) have been found in both mothers and fathers subsequent to a healthy birth following a prior perinatal loss (Armstrong, Hutti, & Myers, 2009). It is estimated that about 11% of postpartum woman experience postpartum depression (American Pregnancy Association, 2012). Meta-analyses have indicated that risks for postpartum depression include a family history of psychiatric illness, poor social support, stressful life events, anxiety during pregnancy, the personality traits of neuroticism, and more recently perfectionism (Gelabert et al., 2012). Depression can affect anyone, even women without a history of prior depression. Perinatal depressive symptoms may not indicate major clinical depression. Nevertheless, symptoms may cause considerable psychological distress, such as irritability and restlessness; feeling hopeless, sad, and overwhelmed; having little energy or motivation and crying unexpectedly; sleeping and eating too little or too much; problems with cognition (memory, decision making, focus); loss of pleasure or interest in usually pleasant activities; and withdrawal from family and friends.

The value of confidants to new mothers is evident, and mothers should be encouraged to ask for help from family and friends or to talk with other new mothers or join support groups. Group and individual therapy are helpful, as is medication. P/CHNs can encourage new mothers with depressive symptoms to get adequate rest (nap while baby is sleeping), be realistic and not try to be the perfect homemaker, ask for help from her partner with feedings during the night and with household chores, get out of the house periodically, and spend quality time with her partner. They can also refer them for a mental health evaluation.

There are several nonpharmacologic interventions the P/CHN can initiate in addition to the ones mentioned above. First, caffeine can lead to sleep disturbance, and alcohol is a depressant that has been implicated in depression. A simple yet helpful suggestion is the elimination of both. Getting adequate sleep is important because sleep deprivation exacerbates psychiatric symptoms. Napping when the baby naps, resting when possible throughout the day, and going to bed early (albeit with the knowledge that sleep may be interrupted two or more times to feed the infant) will provide more hours of rest and sleep. Anxiety symptoms often coexist with depression. Relaxation techniques that reduce anxiety can be helpful, including listening to relaxing music, doing yoga, or performing a simple exercise routine. Participation in a support group allows women to identify with others who may be experiencing similar difficulties. Through discussion, women provide each other with both emotional and practical support.

A final area of assistance is client education. A woman with postpartum depression is more likely to manage her depression successfully if she is aware of the symptoms of depression; the need for a support system; the importance of adequate rest, sleep, and nutrition; and the possibility of supportive psychological or pharmacologic therapy. The critical nature of postpartum depressive symptoms and the potential negative ramifications for mothers and their children are evident. Depression during pregnancy can result in lower birth weight or premature infants. Moreover, postpartum depression can affect parenting and infant stimulation that can lead to delays in infant language development and emotional bonding, lower activity levels, and behavior and sleep problems. Untreated depression can lead to substance abuse, inadequate prenatal care and nutrition, poor pregnancy outcomes, family disruption, and inadequate mother–infant bonding. However, the safety of antidepressants in pregnant and breast-feeding women is not clear (Boucher, Bairam, & Beaulac-Baillargeon, 2008; Maschi et al., 2008; Oberlander et al., 2008; Pearson et al., 2007).

Even though psychotropic medications have been shown to cross the placental barrier and have been found both in amniotic fluid and breast milk, the American College of Obstetricians and Gynecologists (ACOG) cautions against leaving mental illnesses untreated and recommends that the use of antidepressants be individualized and that further research be conducted (ACOG Committee on Practice Bulletins, 2008).

Public and community health nurses can intervene by initiating primary preventive mental health and coping measures that promote mental health throughout pregnancy and the postpartum period. If women with compromised mental health resources can be identified, then positive mental health outcomes may be fostered by supporting their self-esteem, optimizing the quality of their primary intimate relationships, anticipatory guidance on issues that may arise during pregnancy and the postpartum period, and reducing day-to-day stressors. At times, the nurse's efforts alone are not sufficient, and a referral to community mental health services for early detection and treatment is essential for the women and their children.

Fetal or Infant Death

An infrequent role for P/CHNs in maternal–child health is that of grief counselor. A couple may experience a miscarriage or ectopic pregnancy, stillbirth, or the death of an infant from **sudden infant death syndrome (SIDS)**, which is "the unexpected, sudden death of a child under age 1 in which an autopsy does not show an explainable cause of death" (Pub Med Health, 2011, para. 1). The exact cause of SIDS is not certain, but it is believed to be associated with carbon dioxide regulation and sleep arousal problems. It is more common in boys and during winter months and most often occurs in infants between 2 and 4 months of age (Pub Med Health, 2011a). Increased rates of SIDS are associated with stomach sleeping position, exposure to cigarette smoke, premature birth, cosleeping, having a sibling that died of SIDS, and soft bedding in the crib. SIDS is the leading cause of death for infants from 1 to 12 months of age; more than 2,250 infants die annually from SIDS. Since 1990, the SIDS rate has dropped more than 50%, but the rates for Black and American Indian/Alaska Native infants are disproportionately higher (CDC, 2011c).

In each situation of loss, the P/CHN has an important supportive role. People respond to grief in a variety of ways: Some express deep sadness, shock, or disbelief; some weep and are unable to talk; and others talk incessantly about regrets or guilt. Even if a miscarriage occurs early in a pregnancy, the bonding between the mother and fetus has begun, and expressions of grief may be as intense as with the loss of an infant or child. Women often have feelings of abandonment, bereavement, and guilt, thinking that they did something wrong. When parents are unable to identify the exact cause of their fetal loss, they have a more difficult time letting go of grief and anxiety (Nikcevi, Kuczmierczyk, & Nicolaides, 2007). Although grief reactions vary, women experiencing grief after miscarriage have been described as "similar in intensity to grief after other types of major losses" (p. 283). The sense of grief usually begins to diminish by around 6 months (Brier, 2008). Increased anxiety levels are also found, sometimes more frequently than depression, and can last for about the same amount of time, leaving some women more at risk for PTSD and obsessive-compulsive disorder (OCD) (Cumming et al., 2007). Psychological counseling has been associated with greater decreases over time in levels of worry, grief, and self-blame (Nikcevi et al., 2007; Swanson, Chen, Graham, Wojnar, Petras, 2009). For couples who have delivered a stillborn baby, the shock is compounded by the experience of carrying the pregnancy to full term, along with the anticipation of an imminent delivery and the expectation of an addition to the family. This is especially true if all signs before the birthing event itself were positive. They may say such things as, "We felt him move just yesterday and now he's dead—what did I do wrong?" or "I did everything right during this pregnancy. Why did this happen?" These are questions for which there may be no answers, even from the family's health care provider. Frequently, a stillbirth is related to birth defects (15%–20%), fetal entanglement in the umbilical cord (15%), placental problems (10%–20%), reduced fetal growth (20%), or to an infection (10%–20%). Trauma and *Rh* disease can also lead to stillbirths (March of Dimes, 2012).

Mothers who experience stillbirths recognize the need for spiritual and psychosocial support from professional caregivers and relate that they struggle to find meaning through their grief, which is often "emotionally complex" and long-lasting (Cacciatore & Bushfield, 2007). Families must acknowledge the death of the child and integrate the loss into their family lives. Home visitation and simply being there for the family and listening well are invaluable nursing interventions. Referral to mental health counseling or support groups specific to parents of stillborn children where they can share their feelings may be very helpful (March of Dimes, 2012). Providing continuity and support to the family for months after the death of an infant gives the P/CHN an opportunity to assess the family for signs of unresolved grief. Grieving families may find comfort, support, and helpful information from support groups and resources such as Compassionate Friends or First Candle. When a family experiences loss of an infant after the baby has been brought home from the hospital, grief and guilt are compounded by the loss of an anticipated future and the disrupted continuity in family life. An infant may die of SIDS, a congenital anomaly, an infection, or an accident. There are constant reminders of the infant's presence in the home from memories, photos, videos, and accumulated possessions. This death disrupts family homeostasis and the psychological and physiologic equilibrium of the family. In many cases, the police are involved and an autopsy is required, contributing to the anguish of the grieving family. This promotes both guilt and loss of self-esteem and can even threaten the marriage. The lack of a clear causative factor, especially in the case of SIDS, can be frightening to parents (Yiallourou, Walker, & Horne, 2008).

INFANTS, TODDLERS, AND PRESCHOOLERS

Healthy children are a vital resource to ensure the future wellbeing of nations. They are the parents, workers, citizens, leaders, and decision makers of tomorrow, and their health and safety depend on today's decisions and actions. Their futures lie in the hands of those people responsible for their wellbeing, including the P/CHN, whose dominant responsibility is to the community as an entity.

The wellbeing of children has been a subject of great public health concern globally and in the United States. Its importance has been emphasized through development of numerous laws and services, yet the needs of many children continue to go unmet. Young children (up to age 4) are totally dependent on their caregivers. This contributes to their vulnerability during these years. Many young children often go to bed hungry; some infants and toddlers do not receive even the most basic immunizations before they reach school age. Accidents and injuries are a leading cause of death; preventable communicable diseases increase mortality among the very young.

Whereas the United States provides leadership in many arenas, its failure to protect and promote the health of its youngest citizens represents a significant breakdown. However, in many other nations—mostly less-developed countries—child health and wellbeing are in even greater jeopardy.

Global History of Children's Health Care

Only recently in the history of the world have children been considered valuable assets, even in countries where there are now well-developed programs of infant health promotion and protection, infant and child day care services, and strict educational expectations for all children. In some countries today, however, female infants and children or those born with congenital anomalies are not valued. Countries, such as India and China, provide inequitable care for male and female children. Gender-selective abortions or infanticide also occur. Some birth, growth, and developmental rituals are harsh and would be considered illegal if judged by Western standards. Cultural practices that are fostered by political forces prevent many countries from improving the health of infants and young children (Save the Children, 2011). For these reasons, there are great differences globally in child health care systems.

The health of children in one country can affect that of children in other countries, including the United States. Major natural disasters place whole populations at risk, especially the very young and the very old. Examples include the severe acute respiratory syndrome (SARS) epidemic in 2003; the 2004 earthquake and tsunami that affected families from Sri Lanka, India, Indonesia, and Somalia to Thailand; and the Chinese earthquake of 2008 (International Save the Children Alliance, 2008).

NATIONAL PERSPECTIVE ON INFANTS, TODDLERS, AND PRESCHOOLERS

The **infant** (birth to 1 year), **toddler** (ages 1 and 2 years), and **preschooler** populations (ages 3 and 4 years) are generally healthy years. Most U.S. children have a usual source of health care (95%), and their parents report them to be in excellent or very good health (Bloom, Cohen, & Freeman, 2011). Growth and development of infants and young children should be monitored regularly. Pediatricians and P/CHNs often provide anticipatory guidance for parents so that they better understand what to expect as their child grows and can plan for safety issues that may arise. See "Internet Resources" posted on thePoint (http://thepoint.lww.com/Allender8e) for growth charts and educational resources.

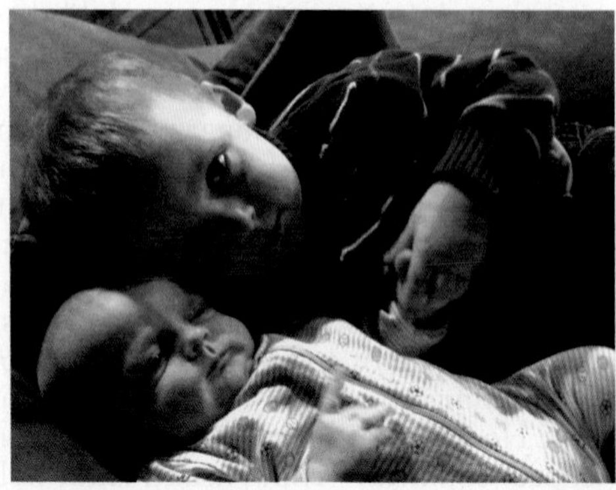

Author's private photo with permission from Deanna Rector.

The mortality rate for children ages 1 to 4 years is 29.2 per 100,000. Major causes of death for children ages 1 to 19 years are unintentional injuries (motor vehicle crashes, falls, drowning, fires, and burns) and homicide (Mathews, Minino, Osterman, Strobino & Guyer, 2011). Among infants aged 1 year or younger, American Indian/Alaska Natives and Blacks have had higher total injury death rates over the past few years than other racial and ethnic populations—two times the rate of injury death compared with White infants. Black infants were affected by the highest rate of homicide (Bernard, Paulozzi, Wallace, & CDC, 2007). The percentage of children under age 1 year who have died violent deaths is 1.6%, almost twice the percentage for children below age 15 years (Karch, Lubell, Friday, Patel, & Williams, 2008). Almost 20% of child maltreatment deaths occur to infants under age 1 year (CDC, 2008).

Accidents and Injuries

Toddlers and preschoolers are at risk for many types of accidents and unintentional injuries, such as those caused by unsafe toys, falls, burns or scalding, drowning, motor vehicle crashes, and poisonings. These unintentional injuries are the leading cause of death for children from age 1 to 14 years (Bloom et al., 2011). The loss of children's lives resulting from all injuries combined represents a staggering number of productive life years lost to society. Childhood injuries lead to almost 23,000 deaths annually (Mathews et al., 2011), and 40% of these are the result of unintentional injuries.

To prevent infant suffocation and SIDS, infants should go to sleep on their backs, in a crib or child-friendly bed without soft bedding or pillows, and parents should be cautioned about risk factors for SIDS and the potential dangers of sleeping with their babies. Information about the SIDS prevention campaign *Back to Sleep*, sponsored by the Association of Maternal and Child Health Programs and many other organizations, should be provided to all parents of infants, and education should begin with hospital nurses and continue with P/CHNs in the community.

Burn injuries can affect children of all ages. Bath water that is too hot can also cause serious scalding injuries. Cigarette lighters and matches are fascinating to young children. Toddlers or preschoolers may be able to start a flame, injuring or killing themselves or others. The sound of a smoke alarm may frighten young children, and it is important for P/CHNs to instruct parents not only to teach their young children about fire prevention but also to be aware of the sound of the alarm and know what actions to take when they hear it, such as the *Stop Drop and Roll* program taught in Head Start and other preschool programs. The P/CHN should also take every opportunity on home visits and in other health education settings to ask or observe if parents have a functional smoke detector in their home. Most community fire departments will install and test smoke detectors for free. Preventing the sources of injury or death from burns may be accomplished by eliminating opportunity and source. Through child supervision, safe storage of matches and lighters, and keeping children away from stoves and electrical outlets, burns and fires can be prevented.

Drowning is another category of unintentional injury in children. Brief lapses in supervision can have disastrous consequences. Young children are at risk for drowning wherever water occurs in depths exceeding a few inches—such as in toilet bowls, bathtubs, mop buckets or cans filled with rainwater, puddles, ponds, spas, and swimming pools. Lakes, rivers, streams, and irrigation ditches or canals are other water hazards. Infants, toddlers, and preschool-aged children are especially vulnerable because they are not aware of water dangers and they explore without fear. Poor children, especially children of color, are at higher risk for drowning because of lack of access to swimming lessons. The P/CHN can work with community groups and recreation centers to promote swimming for children. Parents need to provide a drown-free environment. Guidelines include the following:

- Bathe young children in shallow water.
- Never leave young children unattended during a bath.
- Keep toilet lids down and bathroom doors closed—preferably secured with childproof safety handles.
- Never leave full mop buckets unattended.
- Eliminate water-collection sites around the home by turning over or removing empty buckets, containers, flower pots, and other items that can collect rainwater.
- Fence swimming pool areas and install childproof locks or alarm devices that sound when the water is disturbed.
- Promote water safety measures, including teaching young children to swim.
- Vigilant supervision of young children at play to prevent involvements with neighborhood water sources

Supervising children in or around bathtubs, spas, pools, or other water receptacles is critical and requires close (arm's length) distances. The real dangers of accidental drowning are related in From the Case Files I.

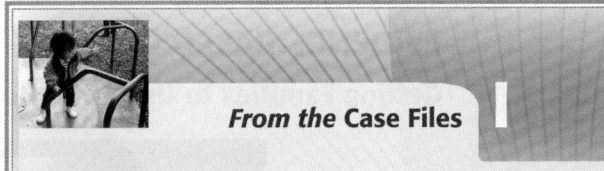

Mop Bucket Drowning

I am a Head Start nurse, and one of my assigned centers is located within a farm-labor camp. There are many large, hardworking families in the camp. Older siblings often watch over young children and help with household chores. Most families keep their cinder block homes tidy and clean, and floors are constantly being mopped (no one has carpeting—it is a bare-minimum type of accommodation). One day, several children were absent from school, and when I made home visits to determine the cause of the absences, I discovered that one of the Garcia family's children, a toddler named Miguel, had unexpectedly died. Because many of the absent children were cousins, parents had kept them home while attending to the family. I knew the Garcia family well, and when I stopped by to check on them, they told me that Miguel had fallen into a large mop bucket the older sister had been using to clean the kitchen floor. She had gone outside for just a minute to separate the 5-year-old twins who were fighting, and when she returned, she found Miguel head first in the bucket. She tried to revive him but could not. The parents were working, trying to earn extra money for an elderly grandmother who needed surgery, and only learned of the tragedy when they returned home at the end of a long day. It was a very sad situation, and it reminded me of how even an everyday item can become deadly. Safety and prevention of unintentional injuries, especially with curious toddlers and preschoolers, is extremely important to teach all families.

Myra, Head Start Nurse

Injuries and deaths from motor vehicle crashes continue to be a major safety problem in the United States. Although 84% of United States families use safety belts (Pickrell & Ye, 2011), some families do not use infant safety seats or child booster seats consistently, even though for decades the law has required their use. Other families have them and use them regularly, but do not install them properly, placing the child at as much risk as if there were no restraint. The most current recommendations for safety seat use are categorized by age. For children birth to 1 year, a rear-facing seat should be used; 1 to 3 years, child should continue in rear-facing seat until reaching the height or weight limit of the seat placed in the back seat; 4 to 7 years, keep child in back seat with a harness-type car seat until they reach weight or height limits; and 8 to 12 years, child should be in a booster seat until back seat safety lap belt fits properly (National Highway Traffic Safety Administration, 2011). There is much opportunity in this area for the P/CHN to educate the public and ensure that parents have the information and skills to secure their children properly when traveling by car. Safety seat clinics, where installations are checked and corrected, can help to promote the proper use of age-appropriate child restraints. See Evidence-Based Practice: Getting Families to Use Child Booster Seats for an example of effective interventions.

Poisoning is a constant safety concern for young children, and toddlers are most often at risk. Sources of poisoning include household plants, prescription medications, over-the-counter drugs, unintentional medication overdoses, household cleaning products, other chemicals stored within a child's reach, and lead. P/CHNs can provide parents with the number for the Poison Help Hotline (1-800-222-1222) and encourage them to post it next to each telephone and call immediately in the event of a suspected poisoning or overdose (American

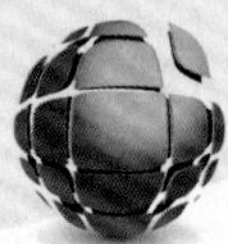

EVIDENCE-BASED PRACTICE

Getting Families to Use Child Booster Seats (Carrot or Stick?)

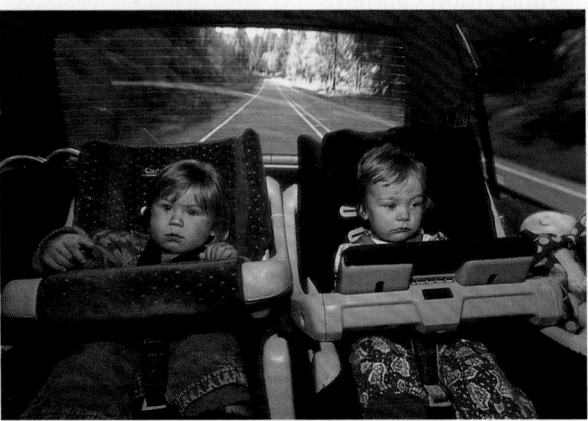

Many health departments, law enforcement, and social service agencies educate parents about the laws and benefits related to the use of child safety seats. Still, not every family consistently uses them. What is the best method to use to ensure compliance with laws? Should we offer incentives (carrots), or should we rely on citations and fines (sticks)?

Researchers conducted a systematic review involving the "acquisition and use of booster seats," those child safety seats that should be used for children up to 80 pounds and 58 inches tall. They found five quality studies with a total of 3,070 participants and concluded that interventions, which included incentives—like gift certificates or discount coupons for booster seats—or gifts of booster seats, along with education about their proper use, were the most effective. They found only one study that looked at enforcement of laws related to use of booster seats, and it was without significant findings. Therefore, researchers concluded that public health professionals could be more effective using carrots rather than sticks when promoting the use of booster seats or, possibly, other child safety seats or restraints.

Source: Ehiri, J., Ejere, H., Magnussen, L., Emusu, D., King, W., & Osberg, W. (2009, January 21). Interventions for promoting booster seat use in four to eight year olds traveling in motor vehicles: How effective are they? *Cochrane Summaries*. Retrieved from http://summaries.cochrane.org/CD004334/interventions-for-promoting-the-use-of-booster-seats-in-four-to-eight-year-olds-travelling-in-motor-vehicles-how-effective-are-they

Association of Poison Control Centers [AAPCC], n.d. a). They can also educate and demonstrate for parents how to childproof the home by eliminating major sources of poisoning. This includes keeping plants out of a child's reach or eliminating them from the home until the child is older, locking up household chemicals (e.g., toilet bowl cleaner, bleach, mouthwash, oven and drain cleaners, pesticides, gasoline, paint thinner, hair products) and storing them out of a child's sight and reach, using childproof medication containers, and storing all medicines in a locked box with a key that is kept out of reach (AAPCC, n.d. b). Alcoholic beverages should also be kept out of reach, as should tobacco products. Outside hazards, such as wild mushrooms and poisonous plants, flowers, and berries, must also be considered (AAPCC, n.d. b). It is also important to eliminate sources of lead in and around the home.

Lead Poisoning

Lead poisoning historically resulted in encephalopathy and death. Today, morbidity from lead poisoning is subtle and most often affects the CNS with long-term changes in behavior and IQ. The CDC estimates that 250,000 children between the ages of 1 and 5 years have elevated blood lead levels, or 10 μg of lead per deciliter of blood (CDC, 2012a). Lead in paint, dust, and soil can be inadvertently consumed, and lead also crosses the placental barrier. It can be transferred in breast milk and is also found in some infant formulas (AAP, 2009). Lead is one cause of childhood poisoning. There is no safe level of lead, and the elimination of elevated blood lead levels in children is a U.S. health goal. The primary sources of lead exposure in preschool-aged children continue to be lead-based paint and lead-contaminated soil and house dust. The critical age of exposure (or peak level) is thought to be between ages 18 and 36 months. Levels generally begin to decline after age 3 years. Children who live in poverty and play in substandard housing areas remain at risk for direct exposure to significant sources of lead. Lead safety and housing code enforcement, along with periodic monitoring to detect new lead hazards, can help prevent future lead exposures. Public and community health nurses, working together with environmental health sanitarians, should promote opportunities for blood lead screening, especially if it is suspected that children in certain homes, apartments, or neighborhoods are at risk for lead poisoning. Children have also been exposed to lead in some toys, candies, cosmetics, traditional medicines, and eating or drinking utensils imported from other countries. Many of these have been tested and revealed to have high levels of lead. Education and public awareness campaigns can help prevent this type of lead poisoning. In 2007, the large American toy manufacturer Fisher-Price recalled almost 100,000 toys, and millions of other toys made in China were also recalled due to unacceptable lead levels (New York State Department of Health, 2007).

Cost-benefit analysis has estimated a return of between $17 and $221 for every dollar spent in lead paint hazard control (Gould, 2009). The incidence of elevated blood lead levels in children has dropped significantly from 20% in 1990 to 1.6% in 2000 (Levin et al., 2008), but some communities, especially those with older housing units, continue to have concerns. One example is Rochester, NY; the city passed a comprehensive rental housing-based lead law in 2005. Researchers subsequently evaluated its effects by reviewing city inspections of housing and health department data on child blood lead levels and discussed the new law with landlords. They noted reduced lead hazards in housing and decreased blood lead levels in children (Korfmacher, Ayoob, & Morley, 2012). PHNs can alert clients to the dangers of lead and work as an advocate for policies to reduce this childhood danger.

Child Maltreatment

Child maltreatment is a major public health concern for the United States. It is any type of abuse directed at a child under 18 years old. Child maltreatment can be physical, emotional, and sexual abuse and child neglect (e.g., withholding feeding or medical care). Neglect is more an act or acts of omission in which a child's basic needs are not met. Children under age 4 years are at the greatest risk for severe abuse and neglect (CDC, 2010b). Abuse and neglect comprise the third leading cause of death for young children under age 3 years and the fifth leading cause of death for those between the ages of 1 and 9 years. Almost 20% of child maltreatment deaths occur to infants under age 1 (CDC, 2008). In 2008, approximately 772,000 children were found by child protective workers to be abused or neglected, and 1,740 died of neglect or abuse (CDC, 2010a). Exposure of infants to drugs in utero is a form of neglect (Reinberg, 2008). In recent years, there has been an increase in reported cases of physical and sexual abuse in day care centers, nursery schools, children's organizations, and churches. However, only about 10% of abuse cases involve nonparental perpetrators, such as foster care staff or day care personnel—80% of child abuse perpetrators are parents (USDHHS, 2008).

A large, national prospective cohort study following at-risk children from birth to age 8 years recently determined that children who are victims of neglect in the first 2 years of life are more likely to have symptoms of childhood aggression than those who were physically abused or neglected later in life (Kotch et al., 2008). It is believed that many more children also suffer from forms of abuse and neglect, but thousands of cases are not reported and not reflected in the statistics. The problem is often difficult to detect and is underreported (ScoutNews, 2008). One example of an often overlooked form of abuse is shaken baby syndrome. **Shaken baby syndrome**, suspected in infants or toddlers who exhibit traumatic brain injuries caused by violent shaking or impact, is characterized by a triad of symptoms: retinal hemorrhage, subdural hemorrhage, and/or subdural hemorrhage with few signs of external trauma (Altimer, 2008). The soft brain tissues are injured as they move violently against the rough cranial bones as the infant is shaken or thrown against a hard object.

Failure to thrive (FTT) can be related to many behavioral or physiological etiologies for infants but can also be related to child neglect. Child neglect differs from child abuse in that the action of the parent, or guardian, is more one of omission as in neglect, rather than commission as in an injury. Risk factors that point to child neglect as the basis for FTT include those most often cited for abuse and neglect, along with specific concerns about parents intentionally withholding food, being resistant to recommended interventions, and having rigid beliefs about nutrition and health regimens that may jeopardize the infant. Growth problems in the first 2 months of life may result in IQ deficits in later childhood, and early intervention programs that involve home visitation have been effective in attenuating the long-term effects of FTT (Black, Dubowitz, Krishnakumar, & Starr, 2007; Emond, Blair, Emmett, & Drewett, 2007).

Child maltreatment is seldom the result of any single factor but rather a combination of chaotic environments, stressful situations, and parents who have difficulty coping with problems and stress. Risk factors for child maltreatment are found in four areas:

- Parent or caregiver behaviors
- Family characteristics
- Child factors
- Environment

Parental factors may include personality characteristics that include an external locus of control and poor self-esteem, along with problems with impulse control and antisocial behavior. Depression and anxiety may also play a role, and parents who had a childhood history of abuse or neglect may maltreat their children. Substance abuse is often a factor in child abuse and neglect cases. Alcohol and drug abuse often lead to neglect, as parents use money meant for household expenses on substances. Little knowledge of normal age-appropriate child development can result in unrealistic expectations. Holding negative attitudes toward their children, viewing them as property, exhibiting harsh parenting styles and verbal aggression, not knowing how to handle children's behaviors, and being easily frustrated are parental characteristics that have also been associated with risk of child maltreatment. Young parental age is also a factor, although this may be because it is also associated with poverty, lower levels of social support, and higher levels of stress. Cohabitation or sharing child supervision with a nonbiological parent can also increase the risk of child maltreatment under certain conditions.

Family characteristics that include IPV and marital conflict, financial stress and unemployment, and social isolation may lead to increased risk of child maltreatment. Children living with single parents (most often mothers) are at higher risk of physical and sexual abuse, as well as neglect; they are also more likely to live in poverty. Single parents have the sole caretaker burden and experience more stress than parents who have joint responsibilities. Children from single parent homes are 77% more likely than those living with both parents to experience physical abuse and are 80% more at risk of a resultant injury. Families in which child neglect occurs often are characterized by greater numbers of children or report a larger number of people living in the household. The household is frequently more chaotic, with constantly changing players—for example, mothers and children living on and off with grandmothers, aunts, boyfriends, or others. Families at high risk for child abuse may be those that are either chronically troubled or temporarily stressed (USDHHS, 2008).

Slightly more girls than boys were reported to be victims of maltreatment in 2006 (51.5% vs. 48.2%), and rates were highest for the youngest children (24.4 per 1,000 for birth to age 1; 14.2 for ages 1–3; 13.5 for ages 4–7). Almost 75% of children from birth to age 3 were neglected, and American Indian/Alaska Native and Black children had the highest rates of maltreatment (15.9/15.4 and 19.8, respectively) when compared to White and Hispanic children (10.7 and 10.8 per 1,000) (USDHHS, 2008). Children who are premature or LBW may be at greater risk of maltreatment because of the greater parental stress engendered by more demands on the caregiver. Children with difficult temperaments or behavior problems, or whose parents perceive them to have problems, including disabled children, could be at greater risk for abuse or neglect.

The environment can play a part, along with parental, family, and child factors, in determining risk for child abuse and neglect. Parents who maltreat their children have reported more loneliness, greater isolation, and lower levels of social support. Social isolation may indicate a lack of positive role models to help them better understand parenting and the consequences of child maltreatment. Unemployment, poverty, and neighborhood factors such as crime, violence, and substance use play a part in the stress placed on families. Strong, significant relationships have been found between unemployment, poverty, and child maltreatment, especially child neglect. The availability of affordable, quality, licensed day care facilities is recognized as one long-term solution for the prevention of child abuse. When their young children are safely cared for, two parents or a single parent can work and provide more resources for the family, thereby decreasing the stress that may precipitate abuse. Although poverty and lack of education are often linked with child abuse and neglect, no socioeconomic level is immune. Parent training programs can help teach parents to cope with fussy infants and difficult toddlers, and child sexual abuse prevention programs may also be helpful. However, P/CHN home visitation programs, like the Nurse-Family Partnership, have been researched and found to be "the most effective and longest enduring intervention for high-risk families" (Krugman, Lane, & Walsh, 2007, p. 711). See Display 21.2. See also Chapters 20 and 22 for more on child abuse and neglect.

Communicable Diseases

Infants, toddlers, and preschool-aged children experience a high frequency of acute illnesses, more than any other age group. Common types of acute conditions seen from birth to age 5 include fever, respiratory infections (including ear infections, colds, influenza), conjunctivitis (pink eye), and gastrointestinal problems. Communicable diseases are prevalent in these age groups, as very young children are building an immune system and are just beginning to come in contact with a greater number of people outside their families. In 2008, Yorita, Holman, Sejvar, Steiner, and Schonberger found that almost 43% of infant hospitalizations were due to infectious diseases; about 1 in every 14 infants was hospitalized. Males and non-White infants were most at risk, and the annual cost of hospitalization of U.S. infants was almost $700 million. The most common diagnoses were infections of the lower respiratory tract (59%) and upper respiratory tract (6.5%), septicemia (6.5%), and urinary tract, kidney, and bladder infections (76%). The incidence of pneumonia in North America is about 35 to 40 cases per 1,000 children under age 5, but most are handled with outpatient care and medication (Durbin & Stille, 2008).

Acute respiratory illnesses (ARIs) are common in children under age 5. In a community-based prospective cohort study tracking children from birth through age 5, researchers found that before age 2, an average of four ARIs occurred each year. Between ages 2 and 5, the number of ARIs dropped to two or three episodes yearly. Most of the infections were upper respiratory, but about half of the children had at least one lower respiratory infection during their first year of life. They also noted that symptoms generally lasted for 4 weeks and resolved with or without the use of cough and cold medications and antibiotics (Kusel, de Klerk, Holt, Landau, & Sly, 2007). This information is especially helpful for P/CHNs who need to emphasize that over-the-counter cough and cold medications should not be used for children under age 2. The U.S. Food and Drug Administration (FDA) questioned their safety and effectiveness at a hearing in October 2007, and manufacturers removed medication targeted to infants and toddlers; they also changed labels all cold and cough medications to read that they should not be used in children under age 4 (CDC, 2009c). This

DISPLAY 21.2 REPORTS OF AN EMERGENCY FOSTER HOME

The following are examples of the various situations from which abused and neglected children come, as reported by a couple who had an emergency foster home for the county department of social services. The examples represent children placed with them over a 2-year period in which they cared for 256 children.

- Two-week-old Jose was taken to their home because the parents (under the influence of drugs) were found swinging Jose upside down in circles in an infant carrier as they walked along a downtown street at 3 AM. After being returned to his parents, he returned to foster care 1 month later after being found abandoned in an infant carrier at the county fair.
- Andre, Otis, and Selma, ages 8, 5, and 4, went to the foster home when the social services agency discovered they had been living with their father in an abandoned car for 2 years. They stayed for 3 weeks while the social worker found suitable housing for this family and counseling for the father.
- Victoria, 5 years old, a loving and passive child, arrived wearing a diaper and appeared developmentally delayed. She had a history of being physically and sexually abused. Her family was very dysfunctional, and it took the social worker several weeks to sort out relatives and their intentions before placing Victoria in a long-term foster home.
- Ronald and Randall, 6-year-old twin boys who were forced to "sexually please their mother" for several years, came to the emergency foster home before being placed with relatives while their mother underwent psychiatric treatment. The boys began counseling during their stay in the emergency foster home.
- Antoinette, age 7, had severe asthma and was very withdrawn. She came to the emergency foster home because her mother (and the mother's boyfriend) refused to care for her. The child came with every photograph of herself and personal mementos because the mother wanted no reminders of the child. The social worker located a grandmother who would be the child's guardian.
- Thirteen-year-old Robert came home from school one day and found his mother and all their furniture gone. After a few weeks of Robert living in the basement of the apartment building, someone alerted the social services agency, and he was placed in the emergency foster home for 2 months. His mother finally called social services after 6 weeks, saying Robert was too difficult for her to handle, but she may want to see him again someday. Robert was eventually placed in a group home for boys.
- Quyn, a 17-year-old Laotian girl, came into foster care after being referred by the school nurse because of wounds observed on her wrists and ankles. Quyn reported being strapped to a chair for 12 or more hours at a time by her father because she was not following the old ways and was shaming the family by being seen in public, unchaperoned, with a boy. Several meetings were held between the parents, a Southeast Asian community leader, and the social worker to resolve this situation so that Quyn could go home safely.

was in response to emergency room visits and deaths linked to their toxic effects. In 2011, the U.S. FDA formally recommended that the drugs not be used in children under age 2 as they had "serious and potentially life-threatening side effects" (2011, para. 1). They are continuing to study the effectiveness and safety in children between the ages of 2 and 11. However, parents may be uninformed about this and may use old bottles or try to give smaller doses of adult medications to their infants and toddlers. Public and community health nurses should inform parents of the dangers and suggest safer interventions that may help alleviate symptoms, such as use of a bulb syringe and saline nose drops, a cool-mist humidifier, or petroleum jelly under the nose, as well as acetaminophen/ibuprofen for fever (Cincinnati Children's Hospital Medical Center, 2010).

Bronchiolitis is the most common type of lower respiratory infection among infants. It is the leading cause of hospitalization in this age group. The majority of hospitalizations for bronchiolitis are for infants 6 months and younger. Respiratory syncytial virus (RSV) is the cause in 70% of cases and can rise to 100% during winter epidemics. Although wheezing, tachypnea, and chest retractions can be frightening to parents, most healthy infants survive (95%). However, P/CHNs working with at-risk infants need to work with parents and pediatricians to ensure that palivizumab (monoclonal antibody) or RSV immunoglobulin is given to preterm infants, or those born closer to term but exposed to environmental pollution or to other children (Worrall, 2008). An effective RSV vaccine has not yet been found, but palivizumab (Synagis) can be used to help prevent the most severe cases of RSV in high-risk infants (e.g., premature, congenital heart problems) and is given monthly by injection during RSV season (Mersch & Nettleman, 2011).

As with older children and adults, air pollution may make infants and children under age 5 more susceptible to bronchitis and other respiratory illness. Preschool-age children are thought to be especially "vulnerable to air pollution-induced illnesses" (Hertz-Picciotto, et al., 2007, p. 1510). Public and community health nurses can inform families who live in areas where air pollution is significant to take the necessary precautions.

Vaccines are one of the greatest achievements of public health. The number of childhood vaccines increased from 5 in 1961 to 16 in 2011 (Hinman, Orenstein, & Schuchat, 2011). Since 1980, there has been a 99% or greater decrease in deaths due to the vaccine-preventable diseases of mumps, pertussis, tetanus, and diphtheria and 80% or greater decline in deaths associated with vaccines instituted since 1980: hepatitis A and B, *Haemophilus influenzae* type B (HiB), and varicella (Roush, Murphy, & The Vaccine-Preventable Disease Table Working Group, 2007). Smallpox has been eradicated worldwide, and the viruses for polio, rubella, and measles are no longer endemic in the United States. The decline in the number of cases of measles, mumps, rubella, pertussis, and tetanus has been dramatic (99.9%, 95.9%, 99.9%, 92.2%, and 92.9%, respectively), and cases of varicella have declined 88%. Intensive campaigns have promoted immunizations that stimulate "protective immune responses against acute and chronic infectious diseases, as well as some infectious diseases that result in cancer" (Roush et al., 2007, p. 2155). It is estimated that the childhood series of vaccines (DTP, polio, MMR, Hib, hepatitis B, and varicella) saves almost $10 billion in direct costs, $33 billion in indirect costs, 14 million infections, and 33,000 premature deaths for each fully vaccinated U.S. birth cohort (Schuchat, 2011).

Their immature immune systems and lack of exposure to antigens, along with somewhat porous physical barriers to microbes, put infants at high risk of infection. By 4 to 6 months, however, a brisker antibody response to vaccines becomes possible (Nadel, 2009). Successful infant and childhood immunization programs have been responsible for high vaccine coverage and the subsequent decline in morbidity and mortality from these preventable diseases (Roush et al., 2007).

The CDC's Advisory Committee on Immunization Practices develops policies and guidelines, based on review of current scientific research, recommending "specific licensed vaccines for infants, children, adolescents, and adults" (Roush et al., 2007, p. 2156). The committee provides suggestions for available immunizations for the 17 vaccine-preventable diseases through the Vaccines for Children Program, a federal program providing uninsured and low-income families with vaccines at no charge through their primary care providers and local health department clinics. The National Immunization Survey provides surveillance for this program, and the *Healthy People 2010* goal regarding immunization administration was met and exceeded in 2004 when more than 80% of children received all recommended vaccines (CDC, 2008). State-level immunization registries help track vaccine coverage at all age levels. Because day care centers and schools require proof of immunization, vaccination rates have improved over the last two decades (Roush et al., 2007).

The financing of immunizations for infants and children has significantly improved as a result of two major initiatives. The Vaccines for Children Program and the Child Health Insurance Program (CHIP) cover children on Medicaid, uninsured children, and American Indian/Alaska Native children. In addition, underinsured children who receive immunizations at federally qualified health centers and rural health clinics are covered. Additional state programs and funds help provide free or low-cost vaccines for children who are not covered by the other programs. There are several ways for P/CHNs to help all families obtain free or low-cost immunizations and contribute to maintaining adequate levels of community immunity to communicable disease.

Even if financial barriers are removed, there are other barriers. Transportation is a significant problem for some parents, especially in rural areas and for families in urban areas who have several children and need to take public transportation. All 50 states provide for medical exceptions to mandatory vaccination, and 49 allow religious exemptions; 20 permit philosophical or personal exemptions (National Conference of State Legislatures, 2010). Despite public health announcements in the media, some mothers remain unaware of the disabling consequences of diseases such as polio and do not realize the importance of fully vaccinating their children. Also, as more vaccines become available and the deadly diseases they prevent become a distant memory in the public's mind, more concerns about the safety of vaccines emerge. The link between thimerosal, a vaccine preservative, and autism has not been verified; a large case–control study found no increased risk for autism spectrum disorder (ASD) and thimerosal (Price et al., 2010). The use of thimerosal has been reduced, or completely curtailed; single-dose packaging does not require the ethyl mercury preservative (Hinman et al., 2011). Numerous websites have emerged that advise against childhood immunization and provide graphic horror stories about the handful of severe reactions to vaccination. Media coverage about vaccine adverse events also contributes to decreased compliance on the part of parents in getting their children immunized. In the recent past, antivaccine individuals and groups have been very vocal and appeared on the now-defunct television programs *Oprah* and *Larry King Live* to "make strong emotional appeals" against vaccinating children (Parikh, 2008, p. 622). They have linked childhood immunizations to their children's autism, even though extensive scientific research has failed to find any significant association. Parikh (2008) notes that, logical or not, people "do not forget this kind of emotional prowess" and notes that scientific and medical experts only counter these emotion-laden arguments with dry evidence and statistics that "do not resonate with many parents" (p. 622). Public and community health nurses and other health professionals are encouraged to provide parents of very young children with meaningful stories of preventable deaths due to these diseases and to "defend our beliefs... more strongly" rather than relying solely on dispassionate facts and figures (Parikh, 2008, p. 622).

At the start of the 21st century, some resurgence of pertussis, varicella, and mumps was noted, and changes were made to vaccination recommendations. Pertussis immunity was found to wane with age, and a reformulated vaccine was recommended for adolescents and adults (Tdap) so that pertussis was not inadvertently spread among infants who had not yet received their full vaccine series (Hinman et al., 2011). A two-dose varicella series is now recommended over the single-dose vaccine, and measles outbreaks were found in populations where parents had refused MMR vaccination and received personal belief exemptions (Hinman et al., 2011). Greater education and improved education is needed to overcome this concern.

Worldwide, vaccine coverage has increased due to effects of manufacturers and philanthropists (e.g., Bill & Melinda Gates Foundation). The WHO has specific disease eradication and vaccine promotion programs around the world (see Chapter 16).

Chronic Diseases

Infants and young children can be afflicted with chronic diseases that affect their quality of life. For instance, the most common chronic disease among the 6 to 11 age group is *dental caries* (CDC, 2010a). Some children begin to show signs and symptoms of cavities by the age of 10 months, and decay can begin to develop as soon as teeth erupt. Enamel defects, and subsequent caries, are more prevalent in children living in poverty and in preterm or LBW infants. One study of kindergarteners in San Francisco found that almost half of the 5-year-olds had dental caries, and lower SES was associated with higher numbers of cavities (Boyce et al., 2010). Dental sealants are helpful in preventing further cavities; children receiving sealants in school-based programs report 60% fewer new cavities in back molars, where most decay begins (CDC, 2010a).

Asthma symptoms may begin in infants and toddlers. Asthma is considered by some to be the most common chronic disease of childhood, with 14% (10 million) of children younger than age 18 years diagnosed with asthma in 2010 (Bloom et al., 2011). Inner-city, low-income, and minority children are disproportionately affected, and asthma hospitalizations are common (Jacobson et al., 2008). Public and community health nurses can assist families in finding appropriate health care providers and encourage proper administration of asthma medications and treatments. They can also teach families to reduce the presence of asthma triggers in their homes (see Chapter 22 for more information on asthma and other chronic diseases of childhood and adolescence).

Autism is a developmental spectrum disorder that is often first noticed in toddlers. Parents become aware that the child's communication and interaction with others is different and that the child may also display obsessive and narrow interests. The CDC estimates the prevalence of autism at 1 in 110 children, and boys are four times more likely than girls to develop autism. An average of 41% of children with ASD also have intellectual disabilities (NCBDDD, 2012). What causes autism is unclear, but some theories suggest faulty early neural patterning and overgrowth as a possible explanation (Courchesne et al., 2007). The CDC is conducting multistate research, the Study to Explore Early Development (SEED), to get a clearer picture of the number of children with ASD, "discover the risk factors and causes, and raise awareness of the signs and symptoms" (NCBDDD, n.d., para. 6). Families may need to be referred to early educational intervention programs and social service agencies for assistance.

Sickle cell anemia, an inherited blood disorder, affects thousands of children in the United States, most often those of African or Hispanic Caribbean ancestry. The characteristic chronic and severe anemia is common in young children with this condition, and it can affect memory, learning, and behavior (Schatz & Roberts, 2007). When both parents have the genetic mutation, the newborn will be afflicted with the disease. Those with the sickle cell trait have no symptoms of the disease but can pass it on to their offspring. In many states, routine newborn screening for sickle cell anemia is offered. Because sickle cell anemia can lead to splenic sequestration (or pooling of blood in the spleen), many children have either nonfunctioning spleens or have had them surgically removed. Risk of infection is always a concern when this occurs before age 5 (University of Chicago Medical Center, 2012). Public and community health nurses working with populations at risk for this disease can educate and refer families for diagnosis and treatment.

The incidence of *food allergies* is increasing in the population. Infants with close family members who have atopic diseases are at risk for development of allergies. Prolonged breast-feeding for 1 year is recommended for these infants, or the use of hypoallergenic infant formula. The National Institute of Allergy and Infectious Diseases (2010) does not recommend a delay in the introduction of the most allergic foods (milk, eggs, and peanuts) for infants past the usual 4 to 6 month of age as this will not prevent a child from developing an allergy. Fortunately, once allergies are diagnosed, they can be managed through dietary changes and by avoidance of allergy-producing foods. Parents need to be educated, so that they can consistently read food labels and alert family members to the young child's allergy so that inappropriate foods are avoided.

Other chronic illnesses can have a profound effect on child and family. *Muscular dystrophy* (MD) and *cystic fibrosis* (CF) are two diseases that not only affect quality of life but also severely shorten the child's life. MD is a constellation of genetic disorders characterized by progressive atrophy and weakening of skeletal muscles. The onset of some forms of MD begins in infancy or early childhood, and MD is more common in boys than in girls (1 of more than 3,600 infants are males). *Duchenne MD* usually begins before age 6 and progresses rapidly until most boys are wheelchair bound and require a ventilator (Pub Med Health, 2010). Genetic testing can determine who is a carrier of the gene and can aid in confirming the clinical diagnosis.

CF usually begins in infancy and is characterized by a persistent cough or wheeze, shortness of breath, poor weight gain despite a good appetite, and a salty taste to the skin. Sticky, thick mucus builds up in the lungs and digestive tract. Respiratory infections become increasingly more frequent as the child ages. It is the major cause of severe chronic lung disease in children. Chest physiotherapy to help mobilize secretions is performed daily, usually by the parents. Aerosolized antibiotic treatments and mucus-thinning medications help to improve lung function and reduce respiratory infections (Pub Med Health, 2011). Public and community health nurses reinforce these techniques and teach the family to avoid exposure to respiratory infections and to initiate prescribed antibiotic prophylaxis promptly. As much as feasible, the young child should be involved in his own care, offered valid choices, and encouraged to participate in decision making. The family needs emotional support as members work through feelings of anticipatory grief.

Antecedents for a number of chronic diseases that develop in adolescence and adulthood may be found in infancy and early childhood. Recent research has noted that genetics may account for 30% to 40% of risk, but environment (e.g., diet) may be responsible for 60% to 70% of risk of *diabetes*. Further, there are some early indications that breast-feeding and refraining from giving infants cow's milk until after age 1 year may result in less risk of type 1 diabetes. Vitamin D deficiency has also been implicated (Dada, 2010). More epidemiologists are beginning to recognize the importance of a life course approach to chronic disease and the societal costs of disadvantaged fetal and child health and development (Guyer et al., 2008). Among other variables, diet and nutrition play an important role in later health, and more and more research about these health connections are being released every year.

Poor Nutrition and Dental Hygiene

Other health problems found in the birth to preschool-age group include nutritional problems (underfeeding or overfeeding, overeating, and inappropriate food choices) and poor dental health. Nutritional and dental health needs are great during this period of rapid growth. Many factors contribute to early nutritional and dental problems.

A healthy start is foundational to wellbeing later in life. Nutrition is basic in strengthening this foundation. Bonding between mother and infant and overall maternal health are predictors of infant weight gain. Both nutrition and bonding can be accomplished by breast-feeding. Some of the benefits of breast-feeding include (Goldman, Hopkinson, & Rassin, 2007):

Convenience: Milk is always at the perfect temperature, and no preparation is needed; the infant can instantly begin feeding when hungry.

Cost: No formula or bottles to buy; costs are limited to healthful diet for the mother, breast pads, nursing bras, and (possibly) a breast pump.

Nutrition: Breast milk is species specific; the proteins are easily digested, and fats are well absorbed; it is the most complete form of nutrition for human infants.

Anti-infective and antiallergic properties: Breast milk contains immunoglobulins, enzymes, and leukocytes that protect against pathogens, and it decreases the incidence of allergy by eliminating exposure to potential antigens. Babies exclusively breast-fed for 6 or more months have fewer respiratory illnesses, ear infections, and cases of diarrhea.

Infant growth: Breast-fed babies usually gain weight at a more moderate rate and are leaner than bottle-fed babies; rapid weight gain in infancy has been associated with later chronic diseases.

Long-term health effects: Breast-feeding exclusively for at least 6 months is associated with reduced risk of overweight in later life, and breast-fed infants have slightly higher IQ scores.

Benefits for mothers: Breast-feeding burns extra calories, helps to reduce postpartum bleeding, and delays ovulation and menstruation; it also lowers the risk of later ovarian and breast cancers.

The benefits of breast-feeding for the infant are well established and include protection against respiratory infections and diarrhea, long-term increased cognitive development through adolescence, and some improvement in blood pressure and total cholesterol (Klein et al., 2008; Turck, 2007). Higher levels of docosahexaenoic acid, important to brain development, are found in breast milk, and its benefits are correlated with the duration of breast-feeding (Turck, 2007). Several systematic reviews have found that the longer a mother breast-feeds her infant, the greater the protection against later obesity. This is thought to be due to the "growth acceleration hypothesis" that associates faster growth in infancy with later obesity levels and the fact that breast milk permits slower growth when compared to infant formulas (Singhal, 2007, p. 15).

Public and community health nurses can encourage pregnant women to consider the benefits of breast-feeding their infants carefully and provide education and interventions to assist them with the most common barriers: concern about insufficient supply of breast milk, problems with the baby latching onto the breast, painful nipples, and scheduling problems (McCann, Baydar, & Williams, 2007). Women often choose to breast-feed their babies when they fully understand the health effects for their infants and themselves and when they receive positive influence from family and friends (Brodribb, Fallon, Hegney, & O'Brien, 2007). The public and community health nurse can join with labor and delivery nurses and lactation consultants in promoting breast-feeding among mothers in the community. Nurses can lobby local hospitals to educate new mothers about the benefits of breast-feeding and stop the routine distribution of free samples of infant formula (Kaplan & Graff,

2008). It is important to establish breast-feeding early, as 70% of women in a nationwide study made the same feeding choice (bottle or breast) for subsequent infants (Taylor, Geller, Risica, Kirtania, & Cabral, 2008).

Overfeeding of an infant can lead to childhood obesity and becomes a risk factor for heart disease, hypertension, and diabetes. The propensity for obesity begins as early as infancy and by childhood for most people. Breast-feeding until 6 to 12 months of age is thought to provide some protection against obesity. However, most of the factors influencing obesity are thought to be behavioral and environmental, such as less physical activity and nutrition high in fats, salt, and sugar (Taveras, Gillman, Klein, Rich-Edwards, & Rifas-Shiman, et al., 2010; USDHHS, 2012b).

Child and adolescent obesity prevalence in 2009 to 2010 was 16.9%, with 9.7% of infants and toddlers characterized as overweight. A significant trend in obesity prevalence was found for males between the ages of 2 and 19 over the previous 12-year period; this was not the case for females (Ogden, Carroll, Kit, & Flegal, 2012). A study of 4-year-old children found an obesity prevalence of 18.4%, with racial/ethnic differences noted. The highest prevalence was for American Indian/Alaska Native children at 31.2%, but Hispanic children (22%) and non-Hispanic black children (20.8%) also had higher rates of obesity than the overall average (Anderson & Whitaker, 2009). Another large study of 4-year-olds found prenatal and early childhood risk factors to be more prevalent among Black and Hispanic populations (e.g., maternal depression, rapid infant weight gain, higher sugar-sweetened beverage intake, and higher intake of fast foods). There were also lower rates of breast-feeding among those populations (Taveras et al., 2010).

Childhood obesity is thought to contribute to the rise in type 2 diabetes (Morrison, Glueck, Horn, & Wang, et al., 2010). Although overfeeding can lead to problems, poor infant growth is also problematic. The pattern of growth may also be important, such as growth problems in infancy along with overweight in later childhood. The most common sources of energy and nutrients for infants and toddlers are breast milk, formula, and milk. Fortified foods (e.g., grain-based foods with added vitamin A, folate, and iron) become increasingly more significant in toddler diets. In general, most nutrition recommendations include providing for a wide variety of foods for children. Public and community health nurses can encourage parents to continue to introduce new healthy foods to their toddlers and not give up or give in too soon. Home visiting programs that promote fruit and vegetable consumption in preschoolers have been shown to be effective in increasing the number of servings for both children and parents (Haire-Joshu et al., 2008).

Young children's diets, often unreasonably high in sugar, increase the incidence of dental caries in this population group. The practice of allowing infants to feed from the bottle beyond 15 to 16 months, or to fall asleep with a bottle, can lead to *baby bottle tooth decay* or *nursing caries*. Mothers may persist in giving toddlers and preschoolers bottles filled with milk, juice, or sugared drinks in an effort to buy time by assuaging crying children, who often cease crying when they see the bottle (Freeman & Stevens, 2008). Frequent snacking and sippy cups filled with juice or sugary drinks can also lead to cavities. It is recommended that sugary foods be eaten at mealtimes and not as snacks and that regular snack times be established. Also, between ages 6 and 12 months, sippy cups are often used to wean infants from the breast or bottle, but between-meal drinks should consist of water or milk. Parents of infants older than 6 months who have several erupted teeth should be instructed to rub the infant's gums with a damp, clean cloth and to begin toothbrushing, using a soft pediatric toothbrush with a very small amount of fluoride toothpaste—about the size of a grain of rice. It is also important to address parents' misconceptions about dental health and question them about their cultural beliefs and practices related to dental health and hygiene (Horton & Barker, 2008; Schroth, Brothwell, & Moffatt, 2007).

Fluoride supplementation may be needed by 6 months of age if local water supplies are not fluoridated. Generally, breast-feeding infants do not require supplemental fluoride, and liquid or chewable fluoride supplements should not be given with formula or milk because absorption will be decreased. As children reach the toddler years, they are able to brush their own teeth with enthusiasm. Toothpaste should be used sparingly, and adults should continue to supervise toothbrushing. Children of this age can get overzealous with the amount of toothpaste they use and it should not be ingested. The American Academy of Pediatric Dentistry (2011) recommends an initial dental visit no later than 12 months of age. Medicaid benefits among states have varied dental benefits.

Dental caries is a preventable condition that can be addressed with proper nutrition and hygiene. The younger the age when dental caries first appear, the more the child is at risk for future tooth decay that sets up inflammatory responses leading to chronic health conditions, such as heart disease and stroke, in adulthood (Yost & Li, 2008). Untreated dental caries can also lead to serious infections. Pain can interfere with learning at school. Many health departments are using fluoride varnishes as a means of preventing dental caries in young children. Dental hygienists and P/CHNs may be trained to apply the varnishes while making home visits, or children and families may visit clinics for treatment.

HEALTH SERVICES FOR INFANTS, TODDLERS, AND PRESCHOOLERS

A variety of programs that directly or indirectly serve the health needs of very young children may be found in most communities. Public and community health nurses play a major and vital role in delivering these services. In public and community health, programs fall into three categories, which approximate the three priorities of P/CHN practice: prevention, protection, and promotion.

Preventive Health Programs

Neighborhood community centers found in urban and rural settings provide families with parenting education, health and safety education, immunizations, various screening programs, and family planning services. In some areas, nurse-run clinics are established at local schools or community centers to assist in outreach services to the community. Public and community health nurses, in collaboration with an interdisciplinary team, are often the primary care providers in these programs. The major goals are to keep communities healthy by focusing on primary and secondary prevention services. Three examples of preventive health programs for infants and young children are immunization programs, parent training programs, and quality day care services.

Immunization Programs

Health departments, community clinics, and private health care providers continue to offer immunizations against the major childhood infectious diseases—measles, mumps, rubella, varicella, polio, diphtheria, tetanus, pertussis, hepatitis A and B, and HiB—some of which can cause permanent disability and even death. Pneumococcal, meningococcal, and influenza vaccines are also recommended, as is the vaccine for rotavirus (CDC, 2012c; Committee on Infectious Diseases, 2008). Many of these diseases no longer plague infants and children, and newer vaccines offer even greater promise of health. Pneumococcal conjugate vaccine has been associated with reductions in the incidence of otitis media and insertion of pressure-equalizing tubes in children under age 5, resulting in reduced expense for antibiotic prescriptions and ambulatory medical visits (Poehling et al., 2007; Zhou, Shefer, Kong, & Nuorti, 2008). See Chapter 22 for the recommended schedule for 0 to 6 years.

Although the threat of these diseases has been substantially reduced, vigilance is still essential. Low immunization levels in many areas, particularly among the poor and medically underserved, and increased disease rates signal the need for constant surveillance, outreach programs, and innovative educational efforts (Roush et al., 2007). A study comparing vaccination coverage among 19- to 35-month-old children found that those children with special health care needs had roughly the same rate of coverage as children in the general population. However, White, affluent children were more likely to be underimmunized, and poor, Hispanic children receiving Medicaid were more likely to be immunized (O'Connor & Bramlett, 2008). This was one case of disadvantaged populations having an advantage over those with access to private health care and insurance. One large study, examining the rates of underimmunization of 3 month olds in underserved areas of Manhattan, Detroit, San Diego, and rural Colorado, found that vaccination coverage varied between 70.5% and 82.4%. Whenever infants and young children come in contact with public health and other community clinics, it is always important to check immunizations and provide the necessary vaccines. Public and community health nurses are deeply involved in preventive activities that promote immunizations. One important intervention is to provide each parent with immunization record that they can keep so that they have a record of their children's immunizations. This is very important until a national immunization registry is implemented. Health departments and day care centers often work collaboratively to provide vaccinations. However, a study of inner-city, subsidized child care centers found that only 73.3% of 3-month-olds were up to date on vaccines, and 12-month-olds had even worse compliance at 44.2% (McCaskill et al., 2008). A compulsory immunization law, varying in its application from state to state, has enabled public health personnel to carry out these preventive services.

Parent Training Programs

Parent education and training programs have been useful in providing parents with the tools needed to deal with the stresses and challenges of parenting effectively. A meta-analysis of 77 program evaluations revealed that effective programs consist of teaching parents to use time-out rather than corporal punishment as a means of discipline, promoting consistency in discipline, encouraging emotional communication skills and positive parent–child interaction, and requiring that parents practice these skills during classroom sessions (Kaminski, Valle, Filene, & Boyle, 2008). An effective training program for parents of preschool children is the Incredible Years Parent Training Program. Parent participants report decreased levels of stress and positive changes in their children after participating in this program (Levac, McCay, Merka, & Reddon-D'Arcy, 2008). Some health and social service agencies offer this program for high-risk families of young children, and some evaluation studies have found this program to improve behavior and reduce symptoms of attention deficit hyperactivity disorder (ADHD) in preschool-age children (Jones, Daley, Hutchings, Bywater, & Eames, 2007, 2008).

Quality Day Care and Preschool Programs

In 2010, nonrelative child providers cared for approximately 52% of children (birth to 4 years) of working mothers (Federal Interagency Forum on Child and Family Statistics, 2010). About 24% spent time in center-based child care. The National Institutes of Health funded a longitudinal national study to research quality child care and early education. They studied cognitive and language development, health and physical growth, social behavior, and emotional development. The findings indicated that children in quality child care environments had better cognitive and language development and school readiness at 4.5 years than those in less than quality centers This was attributed to better stimulation techniques, such as asking questions and repeating vocalizations to the children (Federal Interagency Forum on Child and Family Statistics, 2011).

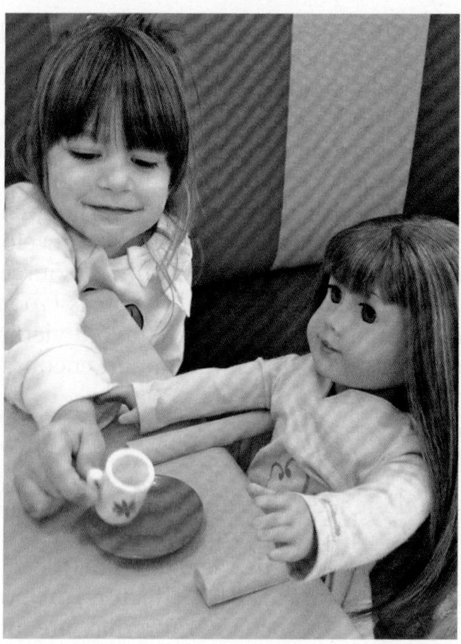

Author's private photo with permission from Danielle Rector.

Although safe, affordable child care is important, the long-term benefits of early childhood education are numerous. They include higher rates of high school completion, college attendance, and full-time employment; lower rates of felony arrests, convictions, and incarcerations; and fewer reports of depressive symptoms (Reynolds et al., 2007). **Head Start**, a federally funded program that offers early childhood education to low-income children between ages 3 and 5, has consistently demonstrated significant improvements in preschoolers' social, emotional, and cognitive development, and those attending Head Start do better on several developmental and educational measures. Head Start children are also more likely to receive dental and health screenings, to have up-to-date immunization coverage, to have better school attendance, and to be less likely to be held back in school. The benefits of Head Start extend to families because more Head Start parents read more frequently to their children than do parents of children not enrolled in the program. Because parents of preschoolers in Head Start must demonstrate parent involvement in the program, they are more likely to demonstrate upward mobility and positive growth. Many states provide preschool programs, but Head Start programs generally offer numerous benefits to society in the areas of education, health, economics, and crime prevention (National Head Start Association [NHSA], n.d.). The quality of day care and preschool programs varies considerably; licensing laws can regulate only minimum safety and health standards. In addition, numerous child care operations are too small to require licensing, leaving quality and compliance unevaluated. Public and community health nurses can influence the quality of day care and preschool programs through active child care consultation efforts that focus on health educational efforts for staff, monitoring of health and safety standards, and working to improve the state's or community's role in passing stronger licensing laws. They can also work with parents and communities providing referral to regulatory agencies and teaching about what characteristics to look for in a quality child care center.

Health Protection Programs

Health protection programs for infants and young children are designed to protect them from illness and injury. Ultimately, these programs may even protect their lives.

Safety and Injury Protection

Accident and injury control programs serve a critical role in protecting the lives of children. Efforts to prevent motor vehicle crashes, a major cause of death, may include driver education programs, better highway construction, improved motor vehicle design and safety features, and continuing research into the causes of various types of crashes. Injury prevention and reduction have been addressed through strategies such as state laws requiring the use of safety restraints (e.g., seatbelts, child safety seats), availability of front and side driver and passenger airbags, substitution of other modes of travel (air, rail, or bus), lower speed limits, stricter enforcement of drunk driving laws, safer automobile design, and helmets for motorcyclists, bicycle riders, and skaters.

For infants, toddlers, and preschool-aged children to be safe when traveling in vehicles, they must be restrained in an approved infant carrier, child restraint seat, or booster seat. These must be positioned and secured as described by the manufacturer; used at all times, even for the shortest distances; placed in the back seat, never in the front seat; and installed in the appropriate position (facing rear or front) based on the weight or age of the infant or young child. Programs that provide training, education, and child safety seats have been shown to improve child safety seat use (Letourneau, Crump, Bowling, Kullinski, & Allen, 2008).

Lead poisoning prevention programs can be found in most state and local health departments. The Lead Contamination Control Act of 1988 provided for CDC funding and programs to eliminate childhood lead poisoning (CDC, 2009b). The CDC provides technical assistance, training, and surveillance at a national level. P/CHNs can help with targeted screening and case management and provide education to clients and communities about lead poisoning.

Protection From Child Abuse and Neglect

Services to protect children from abuse are not as well developed or effective as safety and injury prevention programs, an observation accounted for by a variety of factors. Most child abuse occurs in the home, so only the most blatant situations become evident to outsiders. Public and community health nurses and physicians who see injured children may find parents' explanations plausible and may not suspect or want to believe that abuse might be responsible. Avoidance of legal involvement keeps others from reporting suspected cases. Fortunately, this attitude is changing among professionals who work with children and other community members.

For many years, states have had mandatory reporting laws. The Child Abuse Prevention and Treatment Act, enacted in 1974, provides funding to states to aid in preventing and investigating child abuse and neglect. Over the years, numerous amendments have expanded the definition of child abuse and the persons who are required to report. People mandated to report suspected child abuse include all those who work with children: day care providers, teachers, social workers, nurses, doctors, clergy, coaches, and so forth. In addition, animal humane workers and commercial photograph developers are mandated reporters. Procedures for reporting categories of child abuse have also been clarified, and 1990 updates included services for homeless children and families. Today, professionals and the public are more aware of the problem, and there has been an increase in reporting. In 1974, the National Center for Child Abuse and Neglect was established as a result of the Child Abuse Prevention and Treatment Act. The center collects and analyzes information on child abuse and neglect, serves as an information clearinghouse, publishes educational materials on the subject, offers technical assistance, and conducts research into the problem. The Adoption and Safe Families Act, enacted in 1997, gives further direction in working with families and promotes the safety of children, while recognizing the child's need for a permanent home.

In addition, these acts spurred all of the states to pass mandatory reporting laws and design procedures for investigation of suspected cases of child abuse and neglect. All states have some form of child protective services or family services, whose charge is to protect children and strengthen families. They often work with law enforcement and the judicial system, but health professionals and educators are also important team members. The basic dilemma facing those who work in this area is maintaining the family unit, if possible while at the same time keeping children safe. Most professionals adopt the *levels of prevention* model to describe child abuse and neglect prevention efforts.

Primary Prevention

Primary prevention measures include the use of public service announcements that promote positive parenting, family support groups, and public awareness campaigns about child maltreatment and how to report it, along with establishing community education to enhance the general wellbeing of children and their families. Educational-type services are designed to enrich the lives of families, to improve the skills of family functioning, and to prevent the stress and problems that might lead to dysfunction and abuse or neglect (Feinberg & Kan, 2008; Melnyk et al., 2007). The Safe Environment for Every Kid (SEEK) program has been effective in helping to prevent child maltreatment (Dubowitz, Feigelman, Lane, & Kim, 2009).

Primary prevention also focuses on parent preparation during the prenatal period; practices that encourage parent–child bonding during labor, delivery, the postpartum period, and early infancy; and provision of information regarding support services for families with newborns. It is also helpful to provide parents of children of all ages with information regarding child-rearing strategies, anticipatory guidance for developmental milestones and tasks, and community resources. Child sexual abuse prevention curricula, such as *Good Touch/Bad Touch*, teach children skills to avoid victimization, promote discussion with children, and encourage them to tell an adult.

Secondary Prevention

Services are designed to identify and assist families who may have risk factors for impaired parenting to prevent abuse or neglect. **High-risk families** are those families that exhibit the symptoms (risk factors) of potentially abusive or neglectful behavior or that are under the types of stress associated with abuse or neglect. These can include families living in poverty, substance abuse or mental health problems, parents who were abused when they were children, and parents or children with developmental disabilities. Early intervention with high-risk families can improve emotional and functional coping and help prevent further problems. High school parent education programs for pregnant adolescents, home visitation programs targeted to at-risk families, and respite care for families with special needs children are all examples of secondary prevention actions. Family resource centers in schools or community centers located in low-income neighborhoods can offer resource and referral services to families who may be dealing with multiple sources of stress. Home visitation programs, such as the Nurse-Family Partnership, Early Head Start, and Healthy Families America, provide parent support and education and promote healthier family functioning. Some home visitation programs to high-risk mothers and families have demonstrated decreased rates of child abuse and neglect (Black et al., 2007).

Tertiary Prevention

Intervention and treatment services are designed to assist a family in which abuse or neglect has already occurred, so that further abuse or neglect may be prevented and the consequences of abuse or neglect may be minimized. Often, families are referred to mental health counselors to improve family communication and functioning. Some families may require crisis respite when they feel they cannot manage the stresses of child care. Role models, through the use of parent mentor programs, provide support and nonjudgmental coaching to parents who have sometimes been the victims of abuse themselves. Some programs have shown promise in preventing recurrence of physical abuse, although not with neglect (MacMillan et al., 2009).

The public and community health nurse has a major role in all levels of prevention of child maltreatment. In addition, the nurse is in a unique position to detect early signs of neglect and abuse. The P/CHN must establish rapport with families and assist with appropriate interventions and referrals at the secondary and tertiary levels of prevention. The advanced practice P/CHN may also work with abused and neglected families as part of an interdisciplinary approach with teachers, the department of social services, the judicial system, foster families, and other health care providers is needed. The effectiveness of local programs depends, in large measure, on the willingness of health professionals to increase their awareness and work as a team to detect, report, develop, and evaluate interventions for the perpetrators and victims of abuse and neglect. Ongoing education of health care providers is recommended to increase awareness of changing child abuse patterns, new reporting laws, and resources available to families.

Health Promotion Programs

Early childhood development and intervention programs are designed to have positive effects on the outcomes of children's cognitive and social development. Some health promotion programs have considered children's physical health, and fewer have focused on parent–child interaction and child social development. All are considered important health promotion programs from birth through preschool years.

Infant Brain Development Research and Parent–Child Interactions

New research into the normal brain development of infants and toddlers has revealed that brain maturation in the first few years of life is very rapid: The brain grows to 80% of adult size by age 3, and the myelination pattern of an 18- to 24-month-old child is similar to that of an adult (Almli, Rivkin, McKinstry, & Brain Development Cooperative Group, 2007; Zero to Three, 2012). The prefrontal cortex of 4-year-olds is already functional and becomes more organized throughout later adolescence (Tsujimoto, 2008). Early environment exerts a lasting influence on brain development, even in the womb (Nava-Ocampo & Koren, 2007). Appropriate early environment and stimulation promotes healthy development.

Because brain development is thought to be "activity-dependent," and *pruning* or selection of only the most active neural circuits occurs in early childhood, parents are encouraged to provide appropriate nutrition, avoid potentially harmful substances, and provide appropriate stimulation for their infants, toddlers, and preschoolers (Zero to Three, 2012). During the first 2 years, when rapid myelination is taking place, 50% of total calories should come from fat, but after age 2, 1% or 2% milk should be the norm. Harmful substances, such as tobacco (cigarettes), chemicals, and radiation, should be avoided during pregnancy, as should contact with people who have infectious diseases. Meaningful parent–child interactions should be established early; they include holding, rocking, comforting, touching, talking, and singing. When parents talk to infants and read to young children, children later demonstrate more advanced language and literacy skills. Providing a caring and supportive environment, with opportunities to learn and explore, is supportive of healthy brain development and promotes secure infant attachment (Duursma, Augustyn, & Zuckerman, 2008; Roisman & Fraley, 2008; Zero to Three, 2012).

Young children who do not have early exposure to this type of environment—for example, those who are in institutional care—exhibit delays in cognitive and social development, as well as attachment disorders (van IJzendoorn et al., 2011). However, when placed with foster families who provide a warm, stimulating environment, children's cognitive development improves—especially for those who made the change at younger ages (Nelson et al., 2007).

Gazing into an infant's eyes, paying attention to and interacting with toddlers, and listening to and answering preschoolers' questions are important parental behaviors that promote social development (Chouinard, 2007; Grossman & Johnson, 2007). Providing infants and young children with secure, learning-rich environments where they can use their senses to discover new things helps them to maximize their potential. Emotional comfort and a secure environment ensure that young children will better deal with their feelings. Public and community health nurses can provide information to parents on the most current research results about brain development as well as tangible suggestions such as low-cost brain stimulating toys and community resources to encourage quality parent–child interactions that promote appropriate physical growth and cognitive and social development.

Developmental Screening

With the emphasis on infant and early childhood development, P/CHNs often routinely carry out developmental screenings. Tools such as the Ages and Stages Questionnaire (ASQ), Parents' Evaluation of Developmental Status (PEDS), and the Denver II are often used by P/CHNs as they make routine home and child care center visits to follow at-risk infants, children, and families or as outreach interventions during special events such as community health fairs. Those working with high-risk or medically vulnerable infant programs periodically screen their clients to determine gaps in development and provide suggestions to parents that promote advancement.

Developmental screening tools are also helpful in educating parents about normal child development and can provide a means of anticipatory guidance on developmental milestones and future safety issues. *Bright Futures*, an important resource for nurses and parents, provides tools to help families determine appropriate developmental milestones and expected behaviors, along with suggestions about when to seek help from professionals. A variety of screening tools available to nurses and other health professionals, ranging from parent report instruments to those that involve direct assessment of behaviors and skills, can examine overall physical and cognitive development, or screen for such things as temperament, behavior, autism, and speech and language problems. It is important for the P/CHN to use tools that have reported validity and reliability. Early identification of problems can lead to interventions such as enrollment in early intervention programs and help children with school readiness (Wold & Nicholas, 2007). A study of preschool children born to low-risk mothers concluded that 10% of the children screened were at high risk for developmental problems, indicating that routine developmental screening can not only promote health for those at risk but for those with few risk factors. By educating parents and care providers on expected developmental milestones, the P/CHN can provide secondary prevention through early detection of potential problems (Tough et al., 2008). In the last decade, more than 70% of children with disabilities were not first detected by their health care providers, and the AAP first recommended developmental screening and surveillance during preventive health care visits in 2001 (AAP, 2006).

Programs for Children with Special Needs

Many children have special needs. They may have a congenital or acquired developmental disability, birth defect, or a chronic emotional, mental, or physical disease. The CDC conducts a periodic randomized national survey on children with special health care needs, with the most recent data available for analysis being 2009 to 2010 (CDC, 2011b). About 120,000 U.S. infants are born with a birth defect each year (March of Dimes, 2011). Some children suffer injuries after birth (see From the Case Files II). Autism and other mental or behavioral disorders develop after infancy and may require special services. Educational, health, and social or recreational services should be available for all children.

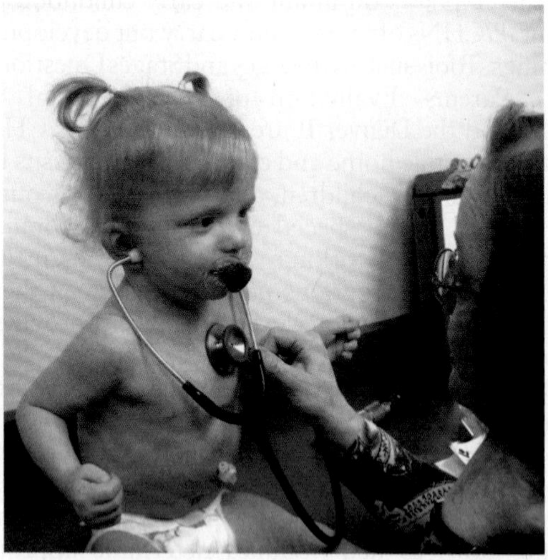

Private author's photo used with permission of Tamara Harris and Lisa Sharp, APRN, BC.

Federal law mandates early identification and intervention services for those with a variety of developmental disabilities. Developmental delays are characterized by slower development in one or more areas. The Individuals with Disabilities Education Act (IDEA) provides early intervention services, usually at home, for those from birth to age 2 who have developmental delays in physical, cognitive, communication, emotional, social, and adaptive development. Intervention services are also available to children with a mental or physical problem that is likely to result in a developmental delay. Newborns can receive infant stimulation services at home or in some schools specially designed to meet the needs of the very young. These programs are offered on a part-time basis for 1 to 2 hours, two to three times a week. Special education preschools are available for young children from ages 3 to 5. By preschool age, children may advance to half-day programs. Additional services can be provided to assist the families in getting children to the programs. Door-to-door bus service in specially equipped small buses or vans safely transports young children who arrive at school in wheelchairs or with other assistive devices. Early stimulation programs, such as the Infant Health and Development Program targeted to preterm and LBW infants, have demonstrated improved parent–child interactions, along with greater motor skill and cognitive development (Bonnier, 2008).

Availability of health services for children with special needs varies with the size of the community. In small rural communities, children and their parents may have to travel long distances to receive specialized services, and in inner-city neighborhoods, lack of money for transportation can make even nearby services equally inaccessible. Accessibility is also influenced by lack of knowledge, attitudes, and prejudices. Another area of concern for special needs children is quality day care for their child. In a statewide study in Nebraska, in both rural and urban areas, 30% of licensed child care providers felt they had inadequate training to care for children with special needs (Kaiser, Kaiser & Likness, 2010). This training may be an area where the P/CHN can provide intervention. Public and community health nurses must recognize the power of these immobilizing factors and be able to deal with them effectively to make positive changes. See Chapter 25 for more on barriers to health care.

Most communities offer additional social and recreational programs for children with special needs. For example, American Lung Association affiliate offices sponsor camping programs for children with asthma or other lung diseases. Often, these are camps for school-aged children that may last up to 1 week and be located in mountain or beach areas, but they may also be day camps, with parents in attendance for preschoolers. Nationwide programs, such as the Special Olympics, offer recreational competition for children with special needs in a variety of sports, such as bowling, track and field, skiing, and swimming. The P/CHN best serves families as a resource for such programs. Some parents are not aware of the rights or services available for their special needs children. Nurses can advocate for parents and help establish services in communities where needed services are lacking.

Nutritional Programs

Adequate nutrition must begin before birth. One of the most productive health promotion programs is the Special Supplemental Food Program for Women, Infants, and Children (WIC). In addition to supporting

From the Case Files 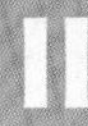

A Case of Kernicterus

A young mother was hospitalized for the birth of her second daughter, a beautiful little girl born without incident. The infant was taken to the mother for feeding and care by the nursing staff, and the mother noticed that her daughter was not very active. The infant had difficulty latching on for breast-feeding. The mother told her obstetrical nurse that the infant seemed very different from her first child. The infant was irritable, but the nurse reassured the mother that the baby was fine and "not all babies are alike." Still, the new mother was concerned.

By the second day, the mother noticed that the baby was not very alert and did not want to feed. She also noticed that the baby's color was "yellowish," and the mother notified the nurse. Again, the nurse reassured the mother that this was "normal" for infants of Asian descent. The baby still was not feeding well, and there was yellowish-orange color stool in the baby's diaper. The mother notified the nurse and asked the nurse to call the doctor. The nurse refused and told the mother that she was "overreacting." The nurse again reassured the mother that the baby was "fine" and no action was taken. The mother felt that the nurse was not listening to her concerns. The baby continued to be irritable, and the nurse said that the baby just needed to breast-feed and was insistent that the new mother was "not breast-feeding properly." The new mother was instructed not to give the baby water or additional fluids, so that the baby would breast-feed. No additional fluids were offered. The young mother was not satisfied with the nursing care and was offended that the nurse would not listen to her. A referral was made to the breast-feeding specialist at the hospital to help the new mother feed her infant. There were no phone calls documented to the physician nor was there documentation of the "yellowish-orange" stool. (The young mother kept the diaper for further proof of her concerns, though.) There was no documentation of irritability, inability to breast-feed, lethargy, or jaundiced appearance of the skin. The physician discharging the infant did not receive any information regarding irritability or yellowish stool. The nursing emphasis postpartum was on breast-feeding, and the nurses documented that the young mother had an "uncooperative attitude."

The young mother and infant were discharged home on the second postpartum day. No blood work was done for the "yellowish" color of the baby's skin, even though the yellowish tone to lower extremities and abdomen was documented in the nurse's notes and on the discharge summary. No referrals were made to Home Health or Public Health for follow-up.

Within 48 hours of discharge, the young mother brought her lethargic baby to the hospital's emergency room. On day 4 of life, the infant's bilirubin was 46. The infant was severely neurologically damaged, and the brain damage that resulted was irreversible. She was diagnosed with severe cerebral palsy, secondary to kernicterus (excessive bilirubin). The child will never be able to walk or talk. She will be fed through a gastrostomy tube for the rest of her life. She has normal intelligence, but it is locked into a dysfunctional body. The patient and family were devastated.

The physician and hospital (nurses) were sued. The nurses on duty could not defend their actions with their charting, or lack thereof. The attorneys for the hospital, representing the physician and nurses, could not defend the actions of their clients. A multimillion dollar settlement was granted, and the nurses were fired. Unfortunately, this is not an isolated case. The irreversible brain damage that occurs as a result of untreated hyperbilirubinemia should not occur in the 21st century. This was a no-win situation that could have been avoided with proper nursing intervention. Hyperbilirubinemia should always be in the forefront of newborn assessment during the first few days of life.

The nurses involved in this case were not acting as the patient's advocate. The young mother tried to tell the nurses, and the nurses should have listened to their patient. The physician should have been notified immediately when signs and symptoms were first noted. Incorrect assumptions were made due to the nationality of the patient, an indication of lack of cultural competence. Home health nursing or public health nursing care should have been arranged for infant follow-up after discharge, but these interventions did not happen.

Linda O., Certified Life Care Planner, Nurse Consultant

women and young children with nutritious foods and achieving the initial goals of decreasing the rates of preterm and LBW babies, increasing the length of pregnancy, and reducing the incidence of infant and child iron deficiency anemia, WIC also improves pregnant women's nutritional status. WIC is not an entitlement program, but rather, Congress sets funding and eligibility requirements yearly (U.S. Department of Agriculture [USDA], 2012).

WIC provides information to parents about eating healthfully and promoting healthy rates of growth. Parents become more aware of the need to reduce consumption of saturated fat, salt, sugar, and overprocessed foods. The P/CHN, through nutrition education, reinforcement of positive practices, and referral, plays a significant role in promoting the health of infants and young children (see Levels of Prevention Pyramid). For more information about WIC, see Chapter 22.

LEVELS OF PREVENTION PYRAMID

SITUATION: Desire for a healthy, full-term infant

GOAL: Using the 3 levels of prevention, negative health conditions are avoided, promptly diagnosed, and treated, and/or the fullest possible potential is restored.

TERTIARY PREVENTION

<table>
<tr><th rowspan="2">Rehabilitation</th><th colspan="2">Primary Prevention</th></tr>
<tr><th>Health Promotion & Education</th><th>Health Protection</th></tr>
<tr>
<td>• The parents and significant others begin to bond with the newborn.
• Parents get to know the newborn and establish a successful breast- or bottle-feeding routine.
• The infant returns home in an age-appropriate infant car seat, which is used properly when traveling.
• The infant's birth is celebrated according to cultural and religious preferences.
• Parents resume sexual intercourse using a family planning method of their choice.
• The parents enjoy the new life they have created.</td>
<td>• Educate about benefits of early postpartum care.
• Set goals with client to make and keep appointments for postpartum and newborn visits to health care providers.</td>
<td>• Educate to avoid exposure to people with infectious diseases.
• Educate and follow up to assure that infant immunization schedule begins on time and continues through childhood.</td>
</tr>
</table>

SECONDARY PREVENTION

Early Diagnosis	Prompt Treatment
• The mother starts prenatal care early in the first trimester and continues care at regular intervals throughout the pregnancy.	• The mother does not use alcohol, tobacco, or other mood-altering substances during the pregnancy. • The mother takes a daily prenatal vitamin with folic acid. • Parents avoid exposure to people with infectious disease. • The mother has adequate nutrition, rest, sleep, and exercise. • The mother begins supportive services if eligible (WIC, Temporary Assistance for Needy Families). • Family and significant others continue to be supportive. • The parents attend labor preparation, infant care, and parenting classes. • Name(s) is selected for the infant. • Delivery method and location are selected. • The home is prepared for the infant: e.g., adequate infant furnishings and supplies are acquired within the parents' budget. • Preparations and plans are made regarding breast- or bottle-feeding. • A pediatrician or pediatric nurse practitioner is selected. • An infant car seat is acquired and properly installed. • Plans are made to get to the chosen health care facility when in labor.

PRIMARY PREVENTION

Health Promotion and Education	Health Protection
• The pregnancy is planned. • Pregnancies are spaced 2 years (or more) apart. • Mother has a positive attitude going into the pregnancy. • A health care provider is chosen. • There are financial resources to meet the expanding family's needs. • Family and significant others are supportive. • Mother's weight is as close to ideal as possible before conception.	• Parents do not use alcohol, tobacco, or other mood-altering substances when planning to conceive. • The mother begins a vitamin regimen containing folic acid before the pregnancy.

ROLE OF THE PUBLIC AND COMMUNITY HEALTH NURSE

Public and community health nurses face the challenge of continually assessing each population's current health problems as well as determining available and needed services. P/CHN interventions with maternal, infant, toddler, and preschool populations are focused on health promotion, health protection, and early intervention. They may include work in family planning or high-risk clinics, telephone information services and hotlines, outreach interventions, child care consultation, or home visitation programs. The nurse uses educational and health coaching interventions when teaching family planning, nutrition, safety precautions, and appropriate health-seeking or child care skills. Such interventions involve providing information and encouraging client groups (parents and young children) to participate in their own health care. Other interventions include strategies in which the nurse uses a greater degree of persuasion or positive manipulation, such as conducting voluntary immunization programs, working in a lead screening program, encouraging smoking cessation during pregnancy, preventing communicable diseases, and encouraging appropriate use of child safety devices such as car seats. Finally, the nurse may use interventions that motivate people into adherence with laws that require certain immunizations or mandate reporting of suspected child abuse and environmental health standards violations, such as sanitation issues.

The P/CHN acts as an advocate and a resource for childbearing women and couples and families of young children. The P/CHN may be called upon to provide information to young mothers about infant temperament, sleep schedules, colic, parenting, discipline, toilet training, television or video choices, and nutrition and feeding (Dopkins-Stright, Canley-Gallagher, & Kelley, 2008). The P/CHN should be aware of federal, state, and local laws that preserve and protect the rights of children and families. Availability of educational, medical, social, and recreational services needed by young families is a necessity. The nurse helps to secure these services in the community she or he serves. Ensuring that families have the resources to provide a safe and healthy environment for their children can take many forms. The nurse may lobby to change existing laws, initiate the effort needed to establish programs and services in the community, and teach families about infant safety or the importance of immunizations.

SUMMARY

Maternal–child health clients are an important population group to P/CHNs because their physical and emotional health is vital to the future of society. The United States does not fare well in comparison to other developed nations on maternal–child health indicators.

Problems of substance abuse, sexually transmitted diseases, and teen pregnancy can lead to less than optimal outcomes for newborns. Complications of pregnancy and childbirth, such as hypertension, gestational diabetes, postpartum depression, and fetal or infant death, offer opportunities for P/CHNs to provide education, outreach, and support.

IMRs are no longer declining. Toddler and young child mortality and morbidity are often related to unintentional injuries. Worldwide, toddlers and preschoolers are at risk for accidents (falls, drowning, burns, and poisoning); acute illnesses, particularly respiratory illnesses; and nutritional, dental, and emotional ailments. Violence against children and deaths from homicide elicit valid concerns. These problems create major challenges for the P/CHN who seeks to prevent illness and injury among children and to promote and protect their health.

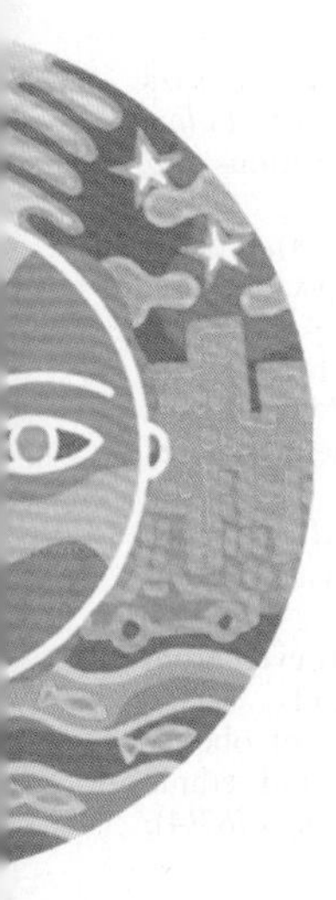

Health services for children span three categories: preventive, health protecting, and health promoting. The P/CHN plays a vital role in each. Preventive services include immunization programs, along with quality day care and preschool. Health protection services include accident and injury prevention and control, as well as services to protect children from child abuse. Health promotion services include infant development through effective parent–child interaction, developmental screening, and services to children with special needs.

The role of P/CHNs include providing interventions to serve young children's health needs, such as educational interventions for the young child that include nutrition teaching to provide information and encourage parents to act responsibly on behalf of their children to assist in healthy habit formation for a lifetime. Other interventions involve encouraging age-appropriate immunizations or cessation of smoking during pregnancy, and P/CHNs may employ persuasive tactics to move clients toward more positive health behaviors. With reporting and intervening in child abuse, nurses practice a form of professional coercion to protect children from threats to their health.

ACTIVITIES TO PROMOTE **CRITICAL THINKING**

1. What specific objectives has your local health department developed for mothers and infants to help achieve the goals listed in the ***Healthy People 2020*** document? How do your county's statistics compare with those of others in your state on (1) IMRs (collectively and by specific ethnic groups), (2) incidence of LBW and VLBW infants, and (3) incidence of birth defects?
2. Using the Internet, locate national websites that give you current information about progress toward meeting some of the ***Healthy People 2020*** goals with infants, toddlers, and preschool-aged children. Are we making progress? What can a P/CHN do locally to promote meeting these goals? What needs to be done on the regional, state, or national level?
3. Describe three different maternal–child populations in your county. What are their most pressing health needs? Do any existing services target these populations? How well, in your judgment, are clients' needs being met? Interview a city or county P/CHN and other public health professionals to help you find answers.
4. Sonia, an 18-year-old woman, is single and 14 weeks pregnant. Her first prenatal visit was made at the urging of her aunt, who uses the clinic. Sonia reluctantly admitted to the clinic nurse that the pregnancy was unplanned. She consumes alcohol two to three times a week, frequently as much as six 12-ounce cans of beer and 16 ounces of wine, and she smokes one pack of cigarettes a day. She has tried a variety of street drugs in the last 3 months but does not use any on a regular basis. The clinic nurse believed that Sonia might not return for regular prenatal care and made a referral to the P/CHN for follow-up home visits to assess Sonia's home environment and teach prenatal care and preparation for the infant. You have been assigned the case. Design a plan of care to address Sonia's needs. What specific services and programs might you recommend? What barriers might exist? How would the prenatal and postpartum teaching delivered to Sonia differ from care needed by other single teens?
5. What is the major cause of death among infants, toddlers, and preschool-aged children? What community-wide interventions could be initiated to prevent these deaths? Select one intervention for each age group, and describe how you and a group of community health professionals might develop this preventive measure.
6. Describe one health promotion program that you as a P/CHN could initiate and carry out to improve the health of children in a day care center or preschool program.
7. Look at the MMR and child health vital statistics in your county or community. What do these statistics tell you about your community's health? What other related statistics are important to gather to determine if your community is a positive and healthy place for childbearing women and young children?
8. Go to the ***Centers for Disease Control*** website (www.cdc.gov) and look up the current childhood immunization schedule for children ages 0 to 4 years. How would you determine how to modify the schedule for a 30-month-old who is missing his last set of immunizations?

REFERENCES

ACOG Committee on Practice Bulletins. (2008). ACOG practice bulletin: Clinical management guidelines for obstetrics & gynecology No. 92. Use of psychiatric medication during pregnancy and lactation. *Obstetrics and Gynecology, 111*, 1001–1020.

Almli, C., Rivkin, M., McKinstry, R., & Brain Development Cooperative Group. (2007). The NIH MRI study of normal brain development (objective-2): Newborns, infants, toddlers, and preschoolers. *NeuroImage, 35*, 308–325.

Altimer, L. (2008). Shaken baby syndrome. *Journal of Perinatal and Neonatal Nursing, 22*(1), 68–76.

American Academy of Pediatric Dentistry. (2012). *Frequently asked questions.* Retrieved from http://www.aapd.org/pediatricinformation/faq.asp

American Academy of Pediatrics (AAP). (2006). *Developmental surveillance and screening of infants and young children: Policy statement with 2006 revision.* Retrieved from http://aappolicy.aappublications.org/cgi/content/full/pediatrics;108/1/192

American Academy of Pediatrics (AAP). (2009). *Lead exposure in children: Prevention, detection, and management. Policy Statement.* Retrieved from http://aappolicy.aappublications.org/cgi/content/full/pediatrics;116/4/1036

American Association of Poison Control Centers. (n.d. a). *Poison centers can help.* Retrieved from http://www.aapcc.org/dnn/PoisoningPrevention/FAQ/tabid/117/Default.aspx

American Association of Poison Control Centers. (n.d. b). *You can prevent poisonings at home.* Retrieved from http://www.aapcc.org/dnn/PoisoningPrevention/PoisonProofYourHome/tabid/118/Default.aspx

American Diabetes Association. (2011). *Gestational diabetes.* Retrieved from http://www.diabetes.org/diabetes-basics/prevention/checkup-america/gdm.html

American Pregnancy Association. (2012). *Statistics.* Retrieved from http://www.americanpregnancy.org/main/statistics.html

Anderson, S. E., & Whitaker, R. C. (2009). Prevalence of obesity among US preschool children in different racial and ethnic groups. *Archives of Pediatrics and Adolescent Medicine, 163*(4), 344–348.

Armstrong, D. S., Hutti, M. H., & Myers, J. (2009). The influence of prior perinatal loss on parents' psychological distress after the birth of a subsequent healthy infant. *Journal of Obstetric, Gynecologic, &and Neonatal Nursing*, *38*(6), 654–666.

Barnet, B., Liu, J., Devoe, M., Alperovitz-Bichell, K., & Duggan, A. (2007). Home visiting for adolescent mothers: Effects on parenting, maternal life course, and primary care linkage. *Annals of Family Medicine*, *5*(3), 224–232.

Bartick, M., & Reinhold, A. (2010). The burden of suboptimal breastfeeding in the United States. *Pediatrics*, 125(5), E1048–E1056.

Bateman, B. T., Bansil, P., Hernandez-Diaz, S., Myhre, J. M., et al. (2012). Prevalence trends, and outcomes of chronic hypertension: A nation-wide sample of delivery admissions. *American Journal of Obstetrics and Gynecology*, *206*(2), 134.e1–134.e8.

Beckett, C. D. (2011). Fetal alcohol spectrum disorders: A Native American journey to prevention. *Family and Community Health*, *34*(30), 242–245.

Bernard, S., Paulozzi, L., Wallace, D., & Centers for Disease Control and Prevention (CDC). (2007). Fatal injuries among children by race and ethnicity—United States, 1999–2002. *MMWR Surveillance Summary 18*, *56*(5), 1–16.

Black, M., Dubowitz, H., Krishnakumar, A., & Starr, R. (2007). Early intervention and recovery among children with failure to thrive: Follow-up at age 8. *Pediatrics*, *120*(1), 59–69.

Bloom, B., Cohen, R. A., Freeman, G. (2011). Summary health statistics for U.S. children: National Health Interview Survey, 2010. National Center for Health Statistics. *Vital Health Statistics*, *10*(250). Retrieved from http://www.cdc.gov/nchs/data/series/sr_10/sr10_250.pdf

Boden, J. M., Fergusson, D. M., & Horwood, L. J. (2008). Cigarette smoking and suicidal behaviour: results from a 25-year longitudinal study. *Psychological Medicine*, *38*(3), 433–439.

Boggess, K., & Society for Maternal-Fetal Medicine Publications Committee. (2008). Maternal oral health in pregnancy. *Obstetrics and Gynecology, 111*(4), 976–986.

Bonnier, C. (2008). Evaluation of early stimulation programs for enhancing brain development. *Acta Paediatrica*, *97*(7), 853–858.

Boucher, N., Bairam, A., & Beaulac-Baillargeon, L. (2008). A new look at the neonate's clinical presentation after in utero exposure to antidepressants in late pregnancy. *Journal of Clinical Psychopharmacology*, *28*(3), 334–339.

Boyce, W. T., Den Besten, P. K., Stamperdahl, J., Zhan, L., Jiang, Y., Adler, N. E., et al. (2010). Social inequalities in childhood dental caries: The convergent roles of stress, bacteria, and disadvantage. *Social Science and Medicine*, *71*(9), 1644–1652.

Brier, N. (2008). Grief following miscarriage: A comprehensive review of the literature. *Journal of Women's Health*, *17*(3), 451–464.

Brodribb, W., Fallon, A., Hegney, D., & O'Brien, M. (2007). Identifying predictors of the reasons women give for choosing to breastfeed. *Journal of Human Lactation*, *23*(4), 338–344.

Cacciatore, J., & Bushfield, S. (2007). Stillbirth: The mother's experience and implications for improving care. *Journal of Social Work in End-of-Life and Palliative Care*, *3*(3), 59–79.

Centers for Disease Control and Prevention (CDC). (2008). Nonfatal maltreatment of infants: United States, October 2005–September 2006. *Morbidity and Mortality Weekly Report*, *57*(13), 336–339.

Centers for Disease Control and Prevention (CDC). (2009a). *Birth outcome and risk factor analysis*. Retrieved from http://www.cdc.gov/pednss/how_to/read_a_data_table/prevalence_tables/birth_outcome.htm

Centers for Disease Control and Prevention (CDC). (2009b). *CDC's lead poisoning prevention program*. Retrieved from http://www.cdc.gov/nceh/lead/about/program.htm

Centers for Disease Control and Prevention (CDC). (2009c). *Cold and cough medicines: Information for parents*. Retrieved from http://www.cdc.gov/Features/pediatriccoldmeds/

Centers for Disease Control and Prevention (CDC). (2009d). *Trends in sexually transmitted diseases in the United States: 2009 National Data for gonorrhea, chlamydia and syphilis*. Retrieved from http://www.cdc.gov/std/stats09/tables/trends-table.htm

Centers for Disease Control and Prevention (CDC). (2010a). *Preventing dental caries with community programs*. Retrieved from http://www.cdc.gov/oralhealth/publications/factsheets/dental_caries.htm

Centers for Disease Control and Prevention (CDC). (2010b). *Understanding child maltreatment*. Retrieved from http://www.cdc.gov/violenceprevention/pdf/CM-FactSheet-a.pdf

Centers for Disease Control and Prevention (CDC) (2011a) *Breastfeeding Report Card: United States, 2011*. Retrieved from http://www.cdc.gov/breastfeeding/data/reportcard.htm

Centers for Disease Control and Prevention (CDC). (2011b). *State and local area integrated telephone survey (SLAITS): National survey of children with special health care needs*. Retrieved from http://www.cdc.gov/nchs/slaits/cshcn.htm#09-10

Centers for Disease Control and Prevention (CDC). (2011c). *Sudden unexpected infant death and sudden infant death syndrome*. Retrieved from http://www.cdc.gov/sids/

Centers for Disease Control and Prevention (CDC). (2012a). *Lead*. Retrieved from http://www.cdc.gov/nceh/lead/

Centers for Disease Control and Prevention (CDC). (2012b). *PRAMS and smoking*. Retrieved from http://www.cdc.gov/prams/TobaccoandPRAMS.htm

Centers for Disease Control and Prevention (CDC). (2012c). *Recommended immunization schedule for persons aged 0 through 6 years—United States, 2012*. Retrieved from http://www.cdc.gov/vaccines/recs/schedules/downloads/child/0-6yrs-schedule-pr.pdf

Centers for Disease Control and Prevention (CDC). (2012d). *Diabetes and Pregnancy*. Retrieved from http://www.cdc.gov/Features/DiabetesPregnancy/

Centers for Disease Control and Prevention (CDC). (2012e). *STDs & pregnancy: CDC fact sheet*. Retrieved from http://www.cdc.gov/std/pregnancy/STDFact-Pregnancy.htm

Chambliss, L. R. (2008). Intimate partner violence and its implication for pregnancy. *Clinical Obstetrics and Gynecology*, *51*(2), 385–397.

Chen, X., Wen, S., Fleming, N., Demissie, K., Rhoads, G., Walker, M., et al. (2007). Teenage pregnancy and adverse birth outcomes: A large population-based retrospective cohort study. *International Journal of Epidemiology*, *36*(2), 368–373.

ChildInfo. (2011). *Orphan estimates*. Retrieved from http://www.childinfo.org/search.php?q=orphan+estimates&Go.x=9&Go.y=8

Chouinard, M. M. (2007). Children's questions: A mechanism for cognitive development. *Monographs of the Society for Research in Child Development*, *72*(1), vii–ix, 1–112; discussion 113–126.

Cincinnati Children's Hospital Medical Center. (2010). *Cough and cold remedies for children under two*. Retrieved from http://www.cincinnatichildrens.org/health/c/cough-cold/

Cockcroft, A., Andersson, N., Milne, D., Mokoena, T., & Masisi M., (2007). Community views about routine HIV testing and antiretroviral treatment in Botswana: Signs of progress from a cross sectional study. *BMC: International Health and Human Rights*, *7*, *5*.

Committee on Infectious Diseases. (2008). Prevention of influenza: Recommendations for influenza immunization of children, 2007–2008. *Pediatrics*, *121*(4), 1016–1031.

Courchesne, E., Pierce, K., Schumann, C., Redcay, E., Buckwalter, J. A., Kennedy, D. P., et al. (2007). Mapping early brain development in autism. *Neuron*, *56*(2), 399–413.

Cumming, G., Klein, S., Bolsover, D., Lee, A. J., Alexander, D. A., Maclean, M., et al. (2007). The emotional burden of miscarriage for women and their partners: Trajectories of anxiety and depression over 13 months. *BJOG: British Journal of Obstetrics and Gynecology, 114*(9), 1139–1145.

Dada, H. G. (2010). Nutrition and type 1 diabetes—can diet reduce risk? *Today's Dietician*, *12*(8), 36.

D'Angelo, D., Williams, L., Morrow, B., Cox, S., Harris, N., Harrison, L., et al. (2008). Preconception and interconception health status of women who recently gave birth to a live-born infant: Pregnancy Risk Assessment Monitoring System (PRAMS), United States, 26 reporting areas, 2004. *Morbidity and Mortality Weekly Report, Surveillance Summaries*, *56*(10), 1–35.

Dasanayake, A., Gennaro, S., Hendricks-Munoz, K., & Chun, N. (2008). Maternal periodontal disease, pregnancy, and neonatal outcomes. *MCN: American Journal of Maternal and Child Nursing*, *33*(1), 45–49.

Davenport, M., Mottola, M., McManus, R. & Gratton, R. (2008). A walking intervention improves capillary glucose control in women with gestational diabetes mellitus: A pilot project. *Applied Physiology, Nutrition and Metabolism*, *33*(3), 511–517.

De Genna, N., Cornelius, M., & Cook, R. (2007). Marijuana use and sexually transmitted infections in young women who were teenage mothers. *Women's Health Issues, 17*(5), 300–309.

Dopkins-Stright, A., Cranley-Gallagher, K., & Kelley, K. (2008). Infant temperament moderates relations between maternal parenting in early childhood and children's adjustment in first grade. *Child Development, 79*(1), 186–200.

Dubowitz, H., Feigelman, S., Lane, W., & Kim, J. (2009). Pediatric primary care to help prevent child maltreatment: The Safe Environment for Every Kid (SEEK) model. *Pediatrics, 123*(3), 858–864.

Durbin, W., & Stille, C. (2008). Pneumonia. *Pediatrics in Review, 29*, 147–160.

Duursma, E., Augustyn, M., & Zuckerman, B. (2008). Reading aloud to children: The evidence. *Archives of Disease in Childhood*, doi:10.1136/adc.2006.106336.

Emond, A., Blair, P., Emmett, P., & Drewett, R. (2007). Weight faltering in infancy and IQ levels at 8 years in the Avon Longitudinal Study of Parents and Children. *Pediatrics, 120*(4), E1051–E1058.

England, L. J., Kim, S. Y., Shapiro-Mendoza, C. K., Wilson, H. G., Kendrick, J. S., Satten, G. A., et al. (2012). Maternal smokeless tobacco use in Alaska Native women and singleton infant birth size. *Acta Obstetricia et Gynecologica Scandinavica, 91*(1), 93–103; PMID: 21902677.

Eunice Kennedy Shriver National Institute of Child Development and Health. (2012). *Back to Sleep public education* campaign. Retrieved from http://www.nichd.nih.gov/sids/

Fanaroff, A. A., Stoll, B. J., Wright, L. L., Carlo, W. A., Ehrenkranz, R. A., Stark, A. R., et al. (2007). Trends in neonatal morbidity and mortality for very low birthweight infants. *American Journal of Obstetrics and Gynecology, 196*(2), 147–154.

Federal Interagency Forum on Child and Family Statistics. (2011). *America's Children: Key National Indicators of Well-Being, 2011*. Washington, DC: U.S. Government Printing Office.

Feinberg, M., & Kan, M. (2008). Establishing family foundations: Intervention effects on coparenting, parent/infant well-being, and parent-child relations. *Journal of Family Psychology, 22*(2), 253–263.

Ferguson, J., Hansen, W., Novak, K., & Novak, M. (2007). Should we treat periodontal disease during gestation to improve pregnancy outcomes? *Clinical Obstetrics and Gynecology, 50*(2), 454–467.

Flynn, L., Budd, M., & Modelski, J. (2008). Enhancing resource utilization among pregnant adolescents. *Public Health Nursing, 25*(2), 140–148.

Freeman, R., & Stevens, A. (2008). Nursing caries and buying time: An emerging theory of prolonged bottle feeding. *Community Dental and Oral Epidemiology, 36*(5), 425–433.

Gaskin, I. M. (2008). Maternal death in the United States: a problem solved or a problem ignored? *The Journal of Perinatal Education, 17*(2), 9–13.

Gavard, J., & Artal, R. (2008). Effect of exercise on pregnancy outcome. *Clinical Obstetrics and Gynecology, 51*(2), 467–480.

Gelabert, E., Subira, S., Garcia-Esteve, L., Navarro, P., Plaza, A., Cuyas, E., et al. (2012). Perfectionism dimensions in major postpartum depression. *Journal of Affective Disorders, 136*(1–2), 17–25.

Gillman, S., Breslau, J., Subramanian, S., Hitsman, B., Koenen, K. (2008). Social factors, psychopathology, and maternal smoking during pregnancy. *American Journal of Public Health, 98*(3), 448–453.

Goldman, A., Hopkinson, J., & Rassin, D. (2007). Benefits and risks of breastfeeding. *Advances in Pediatrics, 54*, 275–304.

Gould, E. (2009). Childhood lead poisoning: Conservative estimates of the social and economic benefits of lead hazard control. *Environmental Health Perspectives, 117*(7), 1162–1167.

Grossman, T., & Johnson, M. (2007). The development of the social brain in human infancy. *European Journal of Neuroscience, 25*(4), 909–919.

Guyer, B., Ma, S., Grason, H., Frick, K., Perry, D., Wigton, A., et al. (2008). Investments to promote children's health*: A systematic literature review and economic analysis of interventions in the preschool period*. Baltimore, MD: Johns Hopkins Bloomberg School of Public Health.

Haire-Joshu, D., Elliott, M., Caito, N., Hessler, K., Nanney, M. S., Hale, N., et al. (2008). High 5 for kids: The impact of a home visiting program on fruit and vegetable intake of parents and their preschool children. *American Journal of Preventive Medicine, 47*(1), 77–82.

Hamilton B. E., Martin J. A., & Ventura S. J. (2010). *Births: Preliminary data for 2009. National vital statistics reports*. Retrieved from http://www.cdc.gov/nchs/data/nvsr/nvsr59/nvsr59_03.pdf

Harris, N., Fowler, M., Sansom, L., Ruffo, N., Lampe, M. A. (2007). Use of enhanced perinatal human immunodeficiency virus surveillance methods to assess antiretroviral use and perinatal human immunodeficiency virus transmission in the United States, 1999–2001. *American Journal of Obstetrics and Gynecology, 197*(3 Suppl), S33–S41.

Hayatbakhsh, M. R., Fenady, V. J., Gibbons, K. S., Kingsbury, A. M., Hurrion, E., Mamun, A. A., et al. (2012). Birth outcomes associated with cannabis use before and during pregnancy. *Pediatric Research, 71*(2), 215–219.

Heo, M., Murphy, C., Fontaine, K., Bruce, M., Alexpoulos, G. (2008). Population projection of U.S. adults with lifetime experience of depressive disorder by age and sex from year 2005 to 2050. *International Journal of Geriatric Psychiatry, 23*(12), 1266–1270.

Hertz-Picciotto, I., Baker, R., Yap, P., Dostal, M., Joad, J. P., Lipsett, M., et al. (2007). Early childhood lower respiratory illness and air pollution. *Environmental Health Perspectives, 115*(19), 1510–1518.

Hinman, A. R., Orenstein, W. A., & Schuchat, A. (2011). Vaccine-preventable diseases, immunizations, and *MMWR*—1961–2011. *Morbidity and Mortality Weekly Report (MMWR), 60*(4), 49–57.

Hobbell, C., Goldstein, A., & Barrett, E. (2008). Psychosocial stress and pregnancy outcome. *Clinical Obstetrics and Gynecology, 51*(2), 333–348.

Holub, C., Kershaw, T., Ethier, K., Lewis, J., Milan, S., & Ickovics, J. (2007). Prenatal and parenting stress on adolescent maternal adjustment: Identifying a high-risk subgroup. *Maternal Child Health Journal, 11*(2), 153–159.

Horton, S., & Barker, J. (2008). Rural Latino immigrant caregivers' conceptions of their children's oral disease. *Journal of Public Health Dentistry, 68*(1), 22–29.

Hudson, D., Campbell-Grossman, C., Keating-Lefler, R., & Cline, P. (2008). *Issues in Comprehensive Pediatric Nursing, 31*(1), 23–35.

Hunt, R., Tzioumi, D., Collins, E., & Jeffery, H. (2008). Adverse neurodevelopmental outcome of infants exposed to opiate in-utero. *Early Human Development, 84*(1), 29–35.

International Save the Children Alliance. (2008). *Three years on from the tsunami: Rebuilding lives: Children's road to recovery*. London, UK: Author.

Institute of Medicine (IOM). (2009). *Weight gain during pregnancy: Reexamining the guidelines*. Retrieved from http://www.iom.edu/Reports/2009/Weight-Gain-During-Pregnancy-Reexamining-the-Guidelines.aspx

Jacobson, J., Goldstein, I., Canfield, S., Ashby-Thompson, M., Husain, S. A., Chew, G. L., et al. (2008). Early respiratory infections and asthma among New York City Head Start children. *Journal of Asthma, 45*(4), 301–308.

Jones, K., Daley, D., Hutchings, J., Bywater, T., & Eames, C., (2007). Efficacy of the Incredible Years Basic Parent Training Programme as an early intervention for children with conduct problems and ADHD. *Child Care, Health and Development, 33*(6), 749–756.

Jones, K., Daley, D., Hutchings, J., Bywater, T., & Eames, C. (2008). Efficacy of the Incredible Years Programme as an early intervention for children with conduct problems and ADHD: Long-term follow-up. *Child Care, Health and Development, 34*(3), 380–390.

Kable, J., Coles, C., Lynch, M., & Platzman, K. (2008). Physiological responses to social and cognitive challenges in 8-year olds with a history of prenatal cocaine exposure. *Developmental Psychobiology, 50*(3), 251–265.

Kahlert, C., Rudin, C., Kind, C. (2007). Sudden infant death syndrome in infants born to HIV-infected and opiate-using mothers. *Archives of Diseases in Children, 92*(11), 1005–1008.

Kaiser, M., Kaiser, K. L., & Likness, S. (2010). Child care provider needs assessment: Caring for Nebraska children with special needs. *Nebraska Department of Health and Human Services*. Lincoln, NE: Author

Kaminski, J., Vale, L., Filene, J., & Boyle, C. (2008). A meta-analytic review of components associated with parent training program effectiveness. *Journal of Abnormal Child Psychology, 36*(4), 567–589.

Kaplan, D., & Graff, K. (2008). Marketing breastfeeding: Reversing corporate influence on infant feeding practices. *Journal of Urban Health*, doi: 10.1007/s11524-008-9279-6.

Karch, D., Lubell, K., Friday, J., Patel, N., & Williams, D. D. (2008). Surveillance for violent deaths: National Violent Death Reporting System, 16 states, 2005. *Morbidity and Mortality Weekly Report, Surveillance Summaries, 57*(SS03), 1–43, 45.

Klein, M., Bergel, E., Gibbons, L., Coviello, S., Bauer, G., Benitez, A., et al. (2008). Differential gender response to respiratory infections and to the protective effect of breast milk in preterm infants. *Pediatrics, 121*(6), E1510–E1516.

Koniack-Griffin, D., Anderson, N. L. R., Verzemnieks, I., & Brecht, M. L. (2000). A public health nursing early intervention program for adolescent mothers: Outcomes from pregnancy through 6 weeks postpartum. *Nursing Research, 49*, 130–138.

Koniack-Griffin, D., Anderson, N. L. R., Brecht, M. L., Verzemnieks, I., Lesser, J., Kim, S. (2002). Public health nursing care for adolescent mothers: Impact on infant health and selected maternal outcomes at 1 year post-birth. *Journal of Adolescent Health, 30*, 44–54.

Koniack-Griffin, D., Verzemnieks, I. L., Anderson, N. L. R., Brecht, M. L., Lesser, J., Kim, S., et al. (2003). Nurse visitation for adolescent mothers: Two-year infant health and maternal outcomes. *Nursing Research, 52*(2), 127–136.

Korfmacher, K. S., Ayoob, M., & Morley, R. (2012). Rochester's lead law: Evaluation of a local environmental health policy innovation. *Environmental Health Perspectives, 120*(2), 309–315.

Kotch, J., Lewis, T., Hussey, J., English, D., Thompson, R., Litrownik, A. J., et al. (2008). Importance of early neglect for childhood aggression. *Pediatrics, 121*(4), 725–731.

Krugman, S., Lane, W., & Walsh, C. (2007). Update on child abuse prevention. *Current Opinions in Pediatrics, 19*(6), 711–718.

Kusel, M., de Klerk, N., Holt, P., Landau, L. I., & Sly, P. (2007). Occurrence and management of acute respiratory illnesses in early childhood. *Journal of Paediatrics and Child Health, 43*(3), 139–146.

Lee, H., Jang, H., Park, H., Metzger, B. E., & Cho, N. H. (2008). Prevalence of type 2 diabetes among women with a previous history of gestational diabetes mellitus. *Diabetes: Research and Clinical Practice, 81*(1), 124–129.

Letourneau, R., Crump, C., Bowling, J., Kullinski, D., & Allen, C. (2008). Ride Safe: A child passenger safety program for American Indian/Alaska Native children. *Maternal Child Health Journal, 12*(Suppl 1), 55–63.

Levac, A., McCay, E., Merka, P., & Reddon-D'Arcy, M. (2008). Exploring parent participation in a parent training program for children's aggression: Understanding and illuminating mechanisms of change. *Journal of Child and Adolescent Psychiatric Nursing, 21*(2), 78–88.

Levin, R., Brown, M. J., Kashtock, M., Jacobs, D., Whelan, E. A., Rodman, J., et al. (2008). Lead exposures in U.S. children, 2008: Implications for prevention. *Environmental Health Perspectives, 116*(10), 1285–1293.

Lockman, S. (2010). Acute maternal HIV infection during pregnancy and breastfeeding: Preventing mother-to-child transmission in resource-limited settings. *Medscape Nurses News*. Retrieved from http://www.medscape.com/viewarticle/718849

Ludermir, A. B., Lewis, G., Valangueiro, S. A., de Araujo, T. V. B., & Araya, R. (2010). Violence against women by their intimate partner during pregnancy and postnatal depression: A prospective cohort study. *Lancet, 376*(9744), 903–910.

MacMillan, H. L., Wathen, C. N., Barlow, J., Fergusson, D. M., Leventhal, J. M., Taussiq, H. N. (2009). Interventions to prevent child maltreatment and associated impairment. *The Lancet, 9659*(17), 250–266.

Manning, M., & Eugene-Hoyme, H. (2007). Fetal alcohol spectrum disorders: A practical clinical approach to diagnosis. *Neuroscience and Biobehavioral Reviews, 31*(2), 230–238.

March of Dimes. (2008). *Databook for policymakers: Maternal, infant and child health in the United States 2008*. Washington, DC: Author.

March of Dimes. (2011). *Birth defects*. Retrieved from http://www.marchofdimes.com/baby/birthdefects.html

March of Dimes. (2012). *Loss and grief: Stillbirth*. Retrieved from http://www.marchofdimes.com/baby/loss_stillbirth.html

Martin, J. A., Hamilton, B. E., Ventura, S. J., Osterman, M. J., Kirmeyer, S., Mathews, T. J., et al. (2011). Births: Final data for 2009. *National Vital Statistics Reports*, 60(1). Retrieved from http://www.cdc.gov/nchs/data/nvsr/nvsr60/nvsr60_01.pdf

Martin, J. A., Hamilton, B. E., Sutton, P. D., Ventura. S. J., Mathews, T. J., & Oesterman, M. (2010). Births: Final Data for 2007. *National Vital Statistics Report*. Retrieved from http://www.cdc.gov/nchs/data/nvsr/nvsr58/nvsr58_24.pdf

Martin, J. A., Osterman, M., & Sutton, P. D. (2010). Are preterm births on the decline in the United States? Recent data from the National Vital Statistics System. *NCHS Data Brief No. 39*. Retrieved from http://www.cdc.gov/nchs/data/databriefs/db39.pdf

Maschi, S., Clavenna, A., Campi, R., Schiavetti, B., Bernat, M., Bonati, M. (2008). Neonatal outcome following pregnancy exposure to antidepressants: A prospective controlled cohort study. *BJOG: British Journal of Obstetrics and Gynecology, 115*(2), 283–289.

Maternal Child Health Bureau (MCHB). (n.d.). *Historical timeline*. Health Resources and Services Administration. Retrieved from http://www.mchb.hrsa.gov/timeline/.

Maternal Child Health Bureau (MCHB). (2011). Programs A–Z. Retrieved from http://mchb.hrsa.gov/AZ/azdescriptions.html

Mathews, T. J., & Macdorman, M. F. (2011). Infant mortality statistics from the 2007 period linked birth/infant death data set. *National Vital Statistics Report*. Retrieved from http://www.cdc.gov/nchs/data/nvsr/nvsr59/nvsr59_06.pdf

Mathews, T. J., Minino, A. M., Osterman, M., Strobino, D. M., & Guyer, B. (2011). Annual summary of vital statistics: 2008. *Pediatrics, 127*(1), 146–157.

Mayberry, L., Horowitz, J., & Declercq, E. (2007). Depression symptoms prevalence and demographic risk factors among U.S. women during the first 2 years postpartum. *Journal of Obstetrical, Gynecological and Neonatal Nursing, 36*(6), 542–549.

McCann, M., Baydar, N., & Williams, R. (2007). Breastfeeding attitudes and reported problems in a national sample of WIC participants. *Journal of Human Lactation, 23*(4), 314–324.

McCaskill, Q., Livingood, W., Crawford, P., Dekle, A. M., Hou, T., Wood, D. L. (2008). Immunization levels among inner city children enrolled in subsidized childcare. *Journal of Healthcare for the Poor and Underserved, 19*(2), 596–610.

Meads, C., Cnossen, J., Meher, S., Juarez-Garcia, A., ter Riet, G., Duley, L., et al. (2008). Methods of prediction and prevention of preeclampsia: Systematic reviews of accuracy and effectiveness literature with economic modeling. *Health and Technology Assessment, 12*(6), 1–270.

Melnyk, B., Feinstein, N., Alpert-Gillis, L., Fairbanks, E., Crean, H. F., Sinkin, R. A., et al. (2007). Reducing premature infants' length of stay and improving parents' mental health outcomes with the Creating Opportunities for Parent Empowerment (COPE) neonatal intensive care unit program: A randomized, controlled trial. *Pediatrics, 118*(5), E1414–E1427.

Mercer, B., Merlino, A., Milluzzi, C., & Moore, J. (2008). Small fetal size before 20 weeks' gestation: Associations with maternal tobacco use, early preterm birth, and low birthweight. *American Journal of Obstetrics and Gynecology, 198*(6), 673–678.

Mersch, J., & Nettleman, M. D. (2011). *Respiratory syncytial virus (RSV)*. Retrieved from http://www.medicinenet.com/respiratory_syncytial_virus/page4.htm

Mistry, H. D., & Williams, P. J. (2011). The importance of antioxidant micronutrients in pregnancy. *Oxidative Medicine and Cellular Longevity*, doi: 10.1155/2011/841749.

Moran, V. H. (2007). A systematic review of dietary assessments of pregnant adolescents in industrialized countries. *British Journal of Nutrition, 97*(3), 411–425.

Morrison, J. A., Glueck, C., Horn, P., & Wang, P. (2010). Childhood predictors of adult type 2 diabetes at 9- and 26-year follow-ups. *Archives of Pediatrics and Adolescent Medicine, 164*(1), 53–60.

Moscaski, M., & Savvitz, D. A. (2012). Ethnic differences in association between gestational diabetes and pregnancy outcomes. *Maternal Child Health Journal, 16*(2), 64–373.

Nadel, S. (Ed.). (2009). *Infectious diseases in the pediatric intensive care unit* (2nd ed.). London, UK: Springer Publishing.

Nannini, A., Lazar, J., Berg, C., Barger, M., Tomashek, K., Cabral, H., et al. (2008). Physical injuries reported on hospital visits for assault during the pregnancy-associated period. *Nursing Research, 57*(3), 144–149.

National Center on Birth Defects & Developmental Disabilities (NCBDDD). (n.d.). *CDC's study to explore early development*. Retrieved from http://www.cdc.gov/ncbddd/autism/documents/SEED_10yrs.pdf

National Center on Birth Defects & Developmental Disabilities (NCBDDD). (2009). *Reducing alcohol-exposed pregnancies*. Retrieved from http://www.cdc.gov/ncbddd/fasd/documents/redalcohpreg.pdf

National Center on Birth Defects & Developmental Disabilities (NCBDDD). (2011a). *Fetal alcohol spectrum disorders (FASD): Data & statistics*. Retrieved from http://www.cdc.gov/ncbddd/fasd/data.html

National Center on Birth Defects & Developmental Disabilities (NCBDDD). (2011b). *Fetal alcohol spectrum disorders (FASD): Facts about FASDs*. Retrieved from http://www.cdc.gov/ncbddd/fasd/facts.html

National Center on Birth Defects & Developmental Disabilities (NCBDDD). (2012). *How many children have autism?* Retrieved from http://www.cdc.gov/ncbddd/features/counting-autism.html

National Clearinghouse on Families & Youth. (n.d.). *YES! Youth empowerment strategies for all working with pregnant and parenting youth*. Retrieved from http://ncfy.acf.hhs.gov/publications/youth-empowerment-strategies/pregnant-parenting

National Conference of State Legislatures. (2010). *States with religious and philosophical exemptions from school immunization requirements*. Retrieved from http://www.ncsl.org/issues-research/health/school-immunization-exemption-state-laws.aspx

National Head Start Association (NHSA). (n.d.). *Benefits of Head Start and Early Head Start programs*. Retrieved from http://www.nhsa.org/files/static_page_files/399E0881-1D09-3519-AD-56452FC44941C3/BenefitsofHSandEHS.pd

National Highway Traffic Safety Administration (NHTSA). (2011). *Traffic safety facts: Child safety seat recommendations*. Washington, DC: Author.

National Institute of Allergy and Infectious Diseases. (2010). *Food allergy: Pregnancy, breastfeeding and introducing solid foods to your baby*. Retrieved from http://www.niaid.nih.gov/topics/foodAllergy/understanding/Pages/Pregnancy.aspx

Nava-Ocampo, A., & Koren, G. (2007). Human teratogens and evidence-based teratogen risk counseling: The Motherisk approach. *Clinical Obstetrics and Gynecology, 50*(1), 123–131.

Nelson, C., Zeanah, C., Fox, N., Marshall, P. J., Smyke, A. T., Guthrie, D. (2007). Cognitive recovery in socially deprived young children: The Bucharest Early Intervention Project. *Science, 318*(5858), 1937–1940.

New York City Department of Health and Mental Hygiene (YCDHMH). (2012). *Intimate partner violence*. Retrieved from http://www.nyc.gov/html/doh/html/epi/domviol.shtml

New York State Department of Health. (2007). *Lead in children's toys: Questions and answers for parents*. Retrieved from http://www.health.ny.gov/environmental/lead/recalls/questions_and_answers.htm

Nicholson, W., Wilson, L., Witkop, C., Baptiste-Roberts, K., Bennett, W. L., Bolen, S., et al. (2008). Therapeutic management, delivery, and postpartum risk assessment and screening in gestational diabetes. *Evidence Report/Technology Assessment AHRQ, 162*, 1–96.

Nikcevi, A., Kuczmierczyk, A., & Nicolaides, K. (2007). The influence of medical and psychological interventions on women's distress after miscarriage. *Journal of Psychosomatic Research, 63*(3), 283–290.

Nurse-Family Partnership. (2011). *Proven effective through extensive research*. Retrieved from http://www.nursefamilypartnership.org/proven-results

Oberlander, T., Warburton, W., Misri, S., Riggs, W., Aghajanian, J., Hertzman, C. (2008). Major congenital malformations following prenatal exposure to serotonin reuptake inhibitors and benzodiazepines using population-based health data. *Birth Defects Research B: Developmental and Reproductive Toxicology, 83*(1), 68–76.

O'Connor, K., & Bramlett, M. (2008). Vaccination coverage by special health care needs status in young children. *Pediatrics, 121*, E768–E774.

Ogden, C. L., Carroll, M. D., Kit, B., & Flegal, K. (2012). Prevalence of obesity & trends in body mass index among US children & adolescents, 1999–2010. *JAMA, 307*(5), 483–490.

Olds, D., Kitzman, H., Hanks, C., Cole, R., Anson, E., Sidora-Arcoleo, K., et al. (2007). Effects of nurse home-visiting on maternal and child functioning: Age 9 follow-up of a randomized trial. *Pediatrics, 120*(4), E832–E845.

Parikh, R. K. (2008). Fighting for the reputation of vaccines: Lessons from American politics. *Pediatrics, 121*, 621–622.

Partington, S., Steber, D., Blair, K., & Cisler, R. (2009). Second births to teenage mothers: Risk factors for low birth weight and preterm birth. *Perspectives on Sexual and Reproductive Health, 41*(2), 101–109.

Pearson, K., Nonacs, R., Viguera, A., Heller, V. L., Petrillo, L. F., Brandes, M., et al. (2007). Birth outcomes following prenatal exposure to antidepressants. *Journal of Clinical Psychiatry, 68*(8), 1284–1289.

Peters, V., Liu, K., Robinson, L., Dominguez, K. L., Abrams, E. J., Gill, B. S., et al. (2008). Trends in perinatal HIV prevention in New York City 1994–2003. *American Journal of Public Health*, doi: 10.2105/AJPH.2007.110023.

Phipps, M., Rosengard, C., Weitzen, S., Meers, A., Billinkoff, Z., et al. (2008). Age group differences among pregnant adolescents: Sexual behavior, health habits and contraceptive use. *Journal of Pediatric and Adolescent Gynecology, 21*(1), 9–15.

Pickrell, T. M., & Ye, J. Y. (2011, November). *Seat belt use in 2011 – Overall results*. (Traffic Safety Facts Research Note. Report No. DOT HS 811 544). Washington, DC: National Highway Traffic Safety Administration.

Poehling, K., Szilagyi, P., Grijalva, C., Martin, S. W., LaFleur, B., Mitchel, E., et al. (2007). Reduction of frequent otitis media and pressure-equalizing tube insertions in children after introduction of pneumococcal conjugate vaccine. *Pediatrics, 119*(4), 707–715.

Price, C. S., Thompson, W. W., Goodson, B., Weintraub, E. S., Croen, L. A., Hinrichsen, V. L., et al. (2010). Prenatal and infant exposure to thimerosal from vaccines and immunoglobulins and risk of autism. *Pediatrics*, doi: 10.1542/peds.2010-0309.

Promising Practices Network. (2012). *Infant health and development programs*. Retrieved from http://www.promisingpractices.net/program.asp?programid=136

Pub Med Health. (2010). *Muscular dystrophy (MD): Inherited myopathy*. Retrieved from http://www.ncbi.nlm.nih.gov/pubmedhealth/PMH0002172/

Pub Med Health. (2011). *Cystic fibrosis*. Retrieved from http://www.ncbi.nlm.nih.gov/pubmedhealth/PMH0001167/

Pub Med Health. (2011a). *Sudden infant death syndrome: SIDS*. U.S. National Library of Medicine. Retrieved from http://www.ncbi.nlm.nih.gov/pubmedhealth/PMH0002533/

Raneri, L., & Wiemann, C. (2007). Social ecological predictors of repeat adolescent pregnancy. *Perspectives in Sexual and Reproductive Health, 39*(1), 39–47.

Reid, V., & Meadows-Oliver, M. (2007). Postpartum depression in adolescent mothers: An integrative review of the literature. *Journal of Pediatric Health Care, 21*(5), 289–298.

Reime, B., Schucking, B., & Wenzlaff, P. (2008). Reproductive outcomes in adolescents who had a previous birth or an induced abortion compared to adolescents' first pregnancies. *BMC Pregnancy and Childbirth, 8*(4). Retrieved from http://www.biomedcentral.com/1471-2393/8/4

Reinberg, S. (2008, April 3). More than 90,000 U.S. infants are victims of abuse of neglect. *U.S. News and World Report*. Retrieved from http://health.usnews.com/usnews/health/healthday/080403/more-than-90000-us-infants-are-victims-of-abuse-or-neglect.htm

Reynolds, A., Temple, J., Suh-Ruu, O., Robertson, D. L., Mersky, J. P., Topitzes, J. W., et al. (2007). Effects of a school-based, early childhood intervention on adult health and wellbeing. *Archives of Pediatrics and Adolescent Medicine, 161*(8), 730–739.

Rivkin, M., Davis, P., Lemaster, J., Cabral, H., Warfield, S., Mulkern, R., et al. (2008). Volumetric MRI study of brain in children with intrauterine exposure to cocaine, alcohol, tobacco, and marijuana. *Pediatrics*, *121*(4), 741–750.

Roberto, A., Zimmerman, R., Carlyle, K., & Abner, E. (2007). A computer-based approach to preventing pregnancy, STD, and HIV in rural adolescents. *Journal of Health in the Community*, *12*(1), 53–76.

Roisman, G., & Fraley, R. (2008). A behavior-genetic study of parenting quality, infant attachment security, and their covariation in a nationally representative sample. *Developmental Psychology*, *44*(3), 831–839.

Roush, S., Murphy, T., & The Vaccine-Preventable Disease Table Working Group. (2007). Historical comparisons of morbidity and mortality for vaccine-preventable diseases in the United States. *The Journal of the American Medical Association*, *298*(18), 2155–2163.

Save the Children. (2008). *State of the world's mothers 2008*. Westport, CN: Author.

Save the Children. (2011). *State of the world's mothers: 2011*. Retrieved from http://www.savethechildren.org/site/c.8rKLIXMGIpI4E/b.6743707/k.219/State_of_the_Worlds_Mothers_2011.htm

Schatz, J., & Roberts, C. (2007). Neurobehavioral impact of sickle cell disease in early childhood. *Journal of the International Neuropsychological Society*, *13*, 933–943.

Schroth, R., Brothwell, D., & Moffatt, M. (2007). Caregiver knowledge and attitudes of preschool oral health and early childhood caries (ECC). *International Journal of Circumpolar Health*, *66*(2), 153–167.

Schuchat, A. (2011). Human vaccines and their importance to public health. *Procedia in Vaccinology*, *5*, 120–126.

ScoutNews. (2008). *Study links spanking to physical abuse*. Retrieved from http://www.consultaspecialist.com/backup/show_news.php?news_id=2358

Shearer, W. T. (2008). Breastfeeding and HIV infection. *Pediatrics*, *121*(5), 1046–1047.

Shirazian, N., Mahboubi, M., Emdadi, R., Yousefi-Nooraie, R., Fazel-Sarjuei, Z., Sedighpour, N., et al. (2008). Comparison of different diagnostic criteria for gestational diabetes mellitus based on the 75-g glucose tolerance test: A cohort study. *Endocrinology Practice*, *14*(3), 312–317.

Silk, H., Douglass, A., Douglass, J., & Silk, L. (2008). Oral health during pregnancy. *American Family Physician*, *77*(8), 1139–1144.

Singhal, A. (2007). Does breastfeeding protect from growth acceleration and later obesity? *Nestle Nutrition Workshop Series: Pediatric Program*, *60*, 15–25 (discussion 25–29).

Smithbattle, L. (2007). Learning the baby: An interpretive study of teen mothers. *Journal of Pediatric Nursing*, *22*(4), 261–271.

Strunk, J. A. (2008). The effect of school-based health clinics on teenage pregnancy and parenting outcomes: An integrated literature review. *Journal of School Nursing*, *24*(1), 13–20.

Substance Abuse & Mental Health Services Administration (SAMHSA). (2011). Substance abuse among young mothers. *The National Survey on Drug Use and Health*. Retrieved from http://www.oas.samhsa.gov/2k11/196/YoungMothers.htm

Swanson, K., Chen, H., Graham, J., Wojnar, D., Petras, A. (2009). Resolution of depression and grief during the first year after miscarriage: A randomized controlled clinical trial of couples-focused interventions. *Journal of Women's Health*, *18*(8), 1245–1257.

Taveras, E. M., Gillman, M., Klein, K., Rich-Edwards, J., & Rifas-Shiman, S. (2010). Racial/ethnic differences in early-life risk factors for childhood obesity. *Pediatrics*, *125*(4), 686–695.

Taylor, J., Geller, L., Risica, P., Kirtania, U., & Cabral, H. J. (2008). Birth order and breastfeeding initiation: Results of a national survey. *Breastfeeding and Medicine*, *3*(1), 20–27.

The Hebrew University of Jerusalem. (2008, October 27). Stress during pregnancy has detrimental effect on offspring. *Science Daily*. Retrieved from http://www.sciencedaily.com/releases/2008/10/081027140724.htm

Tough, S., Siever, J., Leew, S., Johnston, D. W., Benzies, K., Clark, D. (2008). Maternal mental health predicts risk of developmental problems at 3 years of age: Follow up of a community based trial. *BMC: Pregnancy and Childbirth*, *8*(1), 16–20.

Tsai, J., Floyd, R., Green, P., & Boyle, C. (2007). Patterns and average volume of alcohol use among women of childbearing age. *Maternal and Child Health Journal*, *11*, 437–445.

Tsujimoto, S. (2008). The prefrontal cortex: Functional neural development during early childhood. *Neuroscientist*, doi: 10.1177/1073858408316002.

Turck, D. (2007). Later effects of breastfeeding practice: The evidence. *Nestle Nutrition Workshop Series: Pediatric Program*, *60*, 31–39 (discussion 39–42).

Turnbull, C., & Osborn, D. A. (2012). Home visits during pregnancy and after birth for women with an alcohol or drug problem. *Cochrane Summaries*, *1*(1). PMID 22258956.

United States Department of Agriculture (USDA). (2012). About WIC. *USDA Food & Nutrition Service*. Retrieved from http://www.fns.usda.gov/wic/aboutwic/

United States Department of Health and Human Services (USDHHS). (2007). Women's Health USA 2007. *Health Resources and Services Administration*. Rockville, MD: Author.

United States Department of Health and Human Services (USDHHS). (2008). Child maltreatment 2006. *Administration on Children, Youth and Families*. Washington, DC: Author.

United States Department of Health and Human Services (USDHHS). (2012a). *Healthy People 2020*. Retrieved from http://www.healthypeople.gov/2020/default.aspx

United States Department of Health and Human Services (USDHHS) (2012b). *Child Obesity*. Retrieved from http://aspe.hhs.gov/health/reports/child_obesity/

United States Food & Drug Administration (FDA). (2011). *Public health advisory: FDA recommends that over-the-counter (OTC) cough and cold products not be used for infants and children under 2 years of age*. Retrieved from http://www.fda.gov/drugs/drugsafety/postmarketdrugsafetyinformationforpatientsandproviders/drugsafetyinformationforheathcareprofessionals/publichealthadvisories/ucm051137.htm

University of Chicago Medical Center. (2008). *Sickle cell disease*. Retrieved from http://www.uchospitals.edu/online-library/content=P00101

Usta, I., Zoorob, D., Abu-Musa, A., Naassan, G., & Nassar, A. (2008). Obstetric outcome of teenage pregnancies compared with adult pregnancies. *Acta Obstetrics and Gynecology Scandinavia*, *87*(2), 178–183.

Van IJzendoorn, M. H., Palacios, J., Sonuga-Barke, E., Gunnar, M., Vorria, P., et al. (2011). Children in institutional care: Delayed development and resilience. *Monographs of the Society for Research in Child Development*, *76*(4), 8–30.

Wang, L., & Pinkerton, K. (2008). Detrimental effects of tobacco smoke exposure during development on postnatal lung function and asthma. *Birth Defects Research. Part C, Embryo Today: Reviews*, *84*(1), 54–60.

Weck, R., Paulose, T., & Flaws, J. (2008). Impact of environmental factors and poverty on pregnancy outcomes. *Clinical Obstetrics and Gynecology*, *51*(2), 349–359.

Whitley, E., Gale, C., Deary, I., Kivimaki, M., & Batty, D. (2011). Association of maternal and paternal IQ with offspring conduct, emotional, and attention problem scores: Transgenerational evidence from the 1958 British Birth Cohort Study. *Archives of General Psychiatry*, *68*(10), 1032–1038.

Wigle, D., Arbuckle, T., Turner, M., Bérubé, A., Yang, Q., Liu, S., et al. (2008). Epidemiologic evidence of relationships between reproductive and child health outcomes and environmental chemical contaminants. *Journal of Toxicology and Environmental Health. Part B, Critical Reviews*, *11*(5–6), 373–517.

Wold, C., & Nicholas, W. (2007). Starting school healthy and ready to learn: Using social indicators to improve school readiness in Los Angeles. *Preventing Chronic Disease*, *4*(4). Retrieved from http://www.cdc.gov/pcd/issues/2007/oct/pdf/07_0073.pdf

World Health Organization. (2008a). *Maternal mortality in 2005*. Retrieved from http://www.who.int/reproductivehealth/publications/monitoring/9789241596213/en/index.html

World Health Organization. (2009). *HIV/AIDS Health Topic*. Retrieved from http://www.who.int/hiv/en/index.html

World Health Organization. (2010). *Media centre: Maternal mortality*. Retrieved from http://www.who.int/mediacentre/factsheets/fs348/en/index.html

World Health Organization. (2011a). *Exclusive breastfeeding for six months best for babies everywhere*. Retrieved from http://www.who.int/mediacentre/news/statements/2011/breastfeeding_20110115/en/

World Health Organization. (2011b). *HIV/AIDS*. Retrieved from http://www.who.int/mediacentre/factsheets/fs360/en/index.html

Worrall, G. (2008). Bronchiolitis. *Canadian Family Physician, 54*(5), 742–743.

Yiallourou, S., Walker, A., & Horne, R. (2008). Effects of sleeping position on development of infant cardiovascular control. *Archives of Disease in Childhood*, doi: 10.1136/adc.2007.132860.

Yorita, K., Holman, R., Sejvar, J., Steiner, C. A., Schonberger, L. B. (2008). Infectious disease hospitalizations among infants in the United States. *Pediatrics, 121*(2), 244–252.

Yost, J., & Li, Y. (2008). Promoting oral health from birth through childhood; Prevention of early childhood caries. *MCN: American Journal of Maternal Child Nursing, 33*(1), 17–23.

Zero to Three. (2012). *Early experiences matter*. Retrieved from http://www.zerotothree.org/site/PageServer?pagename=ter_key_brainFAQ

Zhou, F., Shefer, A., Kong, Y., & Nuorti, J. (2008). Trends in acute otitis media-related health care utilization by privately insured young children in the United States, 1997–2004. *Pediatrics, 121*(2), 253–260.

Zwicker, J., & Harris, S. (2008). Quality of life of formerly preterm and very low birth weight infants from preschool age to adulthood: A systematic review. *Pediatrics, 121*(2), E366–E376.

CHAPTER

22

School-Age Children and Adolescents

"Youth isn't always all it's touted to be."

—*Lawana Blackwell, The Dowry of Miss Lydia Clark, 1999*

KEY TERMS

Anorexia nervosa
At risk of overweight
Attention deficit hyperactivity disorder (ADHD)
Autism spectrum disorder (ASD)
Binge eating
Bulimia
Food insufficiency
Learning disability
Overweight
Pediculosis

LEARNING OBJECTIVES

Upon mastery of this chapter, you should be able to:

- Identify major health problems and concerns for U.S. school-age children and adolescent populations.
- Explain how health status can influence academic achievement.
- State the recommended immunization schedule for school-age children and adolescents.
- Examine the trends in mortality and injury among school-age children and adolescents and identify the most important areas needing intervention.
- Discuss *Healthy People 2020* objectives affecting adolescents and the barriers that may be involved in attaining these objectives.
- Describe types of programs and services that promote health and prevent illness and injury of school-age children and adolescent populations.

According to Erick Erickson's developmental framework, the school age and adolescent years are a time of task mastery and development of competence and self-identity. During these years, children grow physically, as well as emotionally and socially. They move from the total control of parents and families during infant and toddler years to deriving more and more influence from outside the home–from school, teachers, peers, and other groups.

The challenges of childhood and adolescence include developmental issues, school concerns, behavioral and learning problems, emotional and mental health issues, and the risk behaviors characteristic of teenage years. This chapter explores the health needs of school-age children and adolescents and describes various services that address those needs, along with the community health nurse's role in assisting families with children.

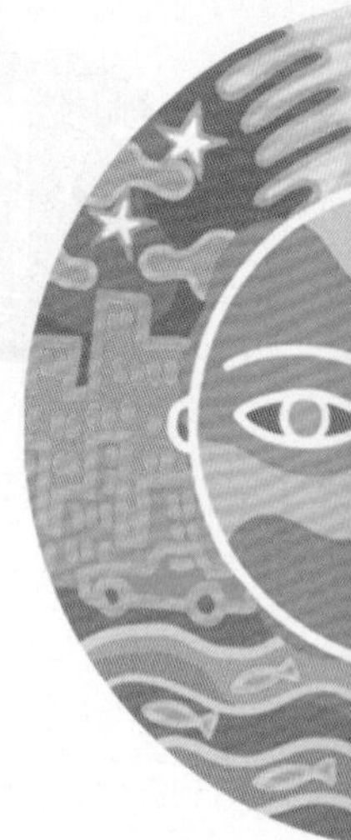

SCHOOL—CHILD'S WORK

In the United States in 2010, about 55 million school-age children and adolescents (5–18 years old) attended more than 132,000 public, private, and charter schools (National Center for Education Statistics [NCES], 2011; National Clearinghouse for Educational Facilities, 2012). In 2010, the U.S. population aged 0 to 17 was composed of 53.5% White/non-Hispanic, 14% Black, 4.3% Asian, 23.1% Hispanic, and 5.2% all other groups (Forum on Child and Family Statistics [FCFS], 2011b).

Children and adolescents spend most of their waking hours in school. Their academic success can predict future education, employment, and income. The quality of their educational experiences (e.g., teacher–child interactions) can influence learning (Pianta, Belsky, Vandergrift, Houts, & Morrison, 2008; Quan-McGimpsey, 2011). These children are the parents, workers, leaders, and decision makers of tomorrow, and their future success depends in good measure on achievement of their educational goals today. Child health has been linked to school success—healthy children are found to be more motivated and prepared to learn (Centers for Disease Control and Prevention [CDC], 2008a; Pati, Hasheem, Brown, Fiks, & Forrest, 2009), and coordinated school health programs are linked to academic achievement (Murray, Low, Hollis, Cross, & Davis, 2007). This is well-known to school nurses and public health nurses (PHNs) working in schools.

HEALTH PROBLEMS OF SCHOOL-AGE CHILDREN

The wellbeing of children has been a subject of great concern in the United States since the days of Lillian Wald. For many years, international organizations, including the World Health Organization (WHO), the United Nations International Children's Education Fund (UNICEF), and U.S. governmental agencies, nonprofit groups, and charitable foundations have focused their resources on improving the health and wellbeing of children. Nonetheless, the needs of millions of children in the United States and worldwide remain unmet. The *Healthy People 2020* document has four objectives for early (birth to age 8) and middle childhood (aged 6–12):

- Increase the proportion of children who are ready for school in all five domains of healthy development (physical and social–emotional development, approaches to learning, language, and cognitive development).
- Increase the proportion of parents who use positive parenting and communicate with their health care professionals about positive parenting.
- Decrease the proportion of children who have poor quality of sleep.
- Increase the proportion of elementary, middle, and senior high schools that require health education (U.S. Department of Health and Human Services [U.S. DHHS], 2012).

Even in the wealthiest nations, many children face complex and often chronic health problems that cause them to miss school days or participate only marginally in the classroom. Because childhood is a critical period during which certain behaviors or health conditions are known to lead to more serious adult illnesses, it is vital for community health nurses and school nurses to screen children and identify problems early (Haines et al., 2011; Nauta, Byrne, & Wesley, 2009). The chronic health problems of children younger than age 18 are often characterized by severity (e.g., persistence of symptoms and impact on social functioning) and duration (usually longer than 3 to 12 months) and often include:

- Diabetes
- Asthma
- Autism spectrum disorders (ASDs)
- Cystic fibrosis
- Spina bifida
- Neuromuscular disorders
- Juvenile rheumatoid arthritis
- Seizure disorders
- Hemophilia
- Congenital heart disease
- Attention deficit hyperactivity disorder (ADHD)

- Nutritional problems—anemia or obesity/overweight
- Cerebral palsy
- Mental illnesses (Torpy, Campbell, & Glass, 2010).

Other conditions may also be defined as chronic, such as allergies, ear infections, and sinusitis; and hearing or speech disorders. Some chronic conditions may affect a child socially and emotionally, as well as physically. School attendance and relationships with family and peers may be affected.

Chronic Diseases

Stomachaches, headaches, colds, and flu are frequent complaints of school-age children, but it is not uncommon for this same age group to be afflicted with some type of chronic disease. Common chronic problems include hay fever, sinusitis, dermatitis, tonsillitis, asthma, and hearing difficulties. Chronic health problems such as these can affect a child's ability to learn and/or his or her physical and social development. Other more serious conditions, such as diabetes, sickle cell anemia, or seizure disorders, have definite effects on academic achievement (Currie, 2009).

A national, prospective, longitudinal study of U.S. children and youth examined the prevalence of chronic illness in three cohorts of children (aged 2 through 8) followed for 6-year intervals. For the first cohort period ending in 1994, 12.8% of children had a chronic illness; for the second cohort period, 25.1% reported a chronic illness; and for the third cohort, the number with at least one chronic illness rose to 26.6%. Chronic illness was defined in the study as lasting for at least 12 months and requiring medication, specialized health services, special equipment, or limiting activities/schooling; they were grouped under four categories (obesity, behavior/learning problems, asthma, other physical conditions). The researchers also noted higher rates of chronic illness for males and Hispanic and Black children (Van Cleave, Gortmaker, & Perrin, 2010). The numbers of children with chronic conditions are increasing, and more children with significant health problems are present in schools (Castillo, 2008). In the school setting, some children require specialized physical health care procedures, such as catheterization, suctioning, or ventilator care. The U.S. Supreme Court ruled that even complex nursing services (i.e., ventilator care) must be provided by schools, even though school nurses are not always present in each school building every day (American Academy of Pediatrics [AAP], 2008). (See Chapter 30 for more on school nursing.) The Individuals with Disabilities Education Act (IDEA) and Section 504 of the Rehabilitation Act of 1973 mandate that services must be provided for children identified as *disabled*. Many conditions may be characterized as disabling under these two laws, including autism, deafness or hearing impairment, blindness or vision impairment, emotional disturbances, mental retardation, specific learning disabilities (LDs), speech or language impairments, or other health impairments (e.g., ADHD, asthma). Once they have been characterized as disabled, children may qualify for special educational services. Children with chronic health conditions that can affect learning (e.g., diabetes, seizure disorders) may receive medications or other related services while in school, to maintain their health and promote their ability to learn.

Chronic diseases of childhood and adolescence affect the entire family and can lead to developmental and social issues for children, as well as missed school days and eventual school failure (CDC, 2008a).

Asthma

Asthma is the most common chronic disease of childhood. In 2009, it was estimated that 14% of children younger than age 18 have at some time been diagnosed with asthma, and the asthma rates have been steadily increasing over the last two decades; Black, non-Hispanic children exhibited the highest asthma attack rates at 17%, compared with 9% for White, non-Hispanic children and 8% for children of Mexican heritage. Overall, about 5% of children reported an episode within the past year (FCFS, 2011e).

Although reasons for the increasing cases of asthma are somewhat unclear, experts speculate that better recognition and diagnosis of the disease; overcrowded conditions; and exposure to air pollution (indoor or outdoor), allergens, and irritants in the environment are probable culprits and may trigger asthma attacks. Many schools have high levels of allergens and irritants. Children and adolescents with asthma may have attacks triggered by infections, exposure to cigarette smoke, stress, strenuous exercise, or weather changes (e.g., cold, wind, rain) (Sleath et al., 2011).

Pediatric asthma is among the respiratory system ailments (including pneumonia and acute bronchitis) that were the top cause of hospital stays for children in 2009 at over 510,000 (Clark, 2011). Treatment for chronic asthma usually includes cromolyn sodium, leukotriene modifiers, inhaled and oral corticosteroids or long-acting beta agonists and anti-IgE therapy, but acute symptoms may involve inhaled $beta_2$ agonists and sometimes anticholinergics (Asthma & Allergy Foundation of America [AAFA], 2011; Drotar & Bonner, 2009). Parent and child education, along with adherence to oral corticosteroid regimens, can help decrease the number of emergency room visits and hospitalizations due to asthma attacks (Self, Chrisman, Jacobs, Vo, & Winton, 2010).

Teaching families to reduce allergens in their homes by controlling dust mites, vacuuming frequently, preventing animal dander and the entry of pollen into the home, and avoiding mold and mold spores may help minimize asthma symptoms for many children. In addition, families should be educated on the danger of indoor environments with mold and mold spores, and the use of household items or products (e.g., furniture, flooring, and paints) made from volatile organic compounds (VOCs) (AAFA, 2011). School nurses and PHNs often work with students, families, and physicians to develop an asthma action plan to control, prevent, or minimize the untoward effects of acute asthma episodes. The goal is to control asthma symptoms and minimize school absences resulting from asthma (Basch, 2011a). Asthma triggers are noted, and school staff members are taught to assist the child in avoiding these triggers. Peak flow meters can be used to determine early signs of asthma problems and to facilitate early interventions; asthma action plans and holding chambers/spacers are used. While only one third of schools have a full-time school nurse (viewed as vital to the success of an asthma control program), 80% allowed students to self-administer their inhalable asthma medications (Wheeler, Buckley, Gerald, Merkle, & Morrison, 2009).

Monitoring asthma medications and teaching proper methods of inhaler use are also vital school nursing or PHN functions. Although the link between asthma and academic achievement is not definitive, some evidence exists that school nurse case management of asthmatic children can lead to fewer absences and contribute to better overall asthma control (Millard, Johnson, Hilton, & Hart, 2009).

Autism

Autism spectrum disorders (ASDs) are complex developmental disorders often originally noticed within the first few years of life. There are three types of ASDs: (1) autistic disorder, (2) Asperger's syndrome, and (3) pervasive developmental disorder/not otherwise specified, or "atypical autism" (CDC, 2010a). A child's communication skills and interaction with others is most often affected, along with obsessive behavior and narrowed interests. Behaviors associated with autism include:

- Language problems (no language, delay in language, repetitive use of language)
- Motor mannerisms (often repetitive rocking, hand flapping, object twirling)
- Fixation on objects (restricted interests)
- No spontaneous play or make-believe play; no interest in peers (problems making friends)
- Little or no eye contact (may also resist hugging)

Autism prevalence has been calculated at approximately 1 out of every 110 births (CDC, 2010a). The estimated lifetime expense for an autistic child averages $3.5 to $5 million (Autism Society of America [ASA], n.d.). Autism is not a new disorder—descriptions of autistic behavior have been identified in 18th century writings. Currently, early detection and intervention therapies focusing on speech, coordination, and interaction skills can help to improve development. Boys are four times more likely than girls to have the disorder (CDC, 2010a). Because autism is a "spectrum disorder" that presents differently among individuals, behaviors and severity can vary widely (ASA, n.d.).

The cause of autism is not clear—some genetic links have been found, but environment may also be a factor. There is a higher risk of subsequent children having autism in a family with one autistic child or a parent with ASD (CDC, 2010a; National Institute of Neurological Disorders and Stroke [NINDS], 2012). It is often associated with other disorders (e.g., congenital rubella syndrome, Down syndrome, fragile X syndrome, tuberous sclerosis), but the exact causes are not fully understood (CDC, 2010a; NINDS, 2012).

PHNs may come in contact with families dealing with autism through work in well-child or immunization clinics. It is important to educate parents that parenting practices are now known *not* to be a cause of autism and that multiple, large-scale research studies on childhood immunizations have shown no relationship between immunization and autism (National Vaccine Information Center, 2012; CDC, 2010a; NINDS, 2012). The CDC is conducting a multiyear study to identify risk factors for autism, the Study to Explore Early Development (SEED), in an effort to better understand the causes of autism. It is also important to assist families in accessing services for their children, as early intervention is most helpful.

Diabetes

Diabetes is another common chronic illness in children, with type 1 being the leading cause of diabetes in all children (National Diabetes Education Program [NDEP], n.d.). Both type 1 (T1DM) and type 2 diabetes (T2DM) are found in school-age children, with T2DM rising almost exponentially in this age group, leading some scientists to call this a major public health crisis. T2DM in children and adolescents, virtually nonexistent before 1999, now comprises about half of new cases in many communities (Dietz, 2009). This epidemic is thought to stem from increasing rates of childhood obesity, sedentary lifestyle, and the predisposition of certain ethnic groups (e.g., American Indian, Mexican American) to the disease. A family history of T2DM may also play a role; in over 75% of cases the child or adolescent has a first- or second-degree relative with T2DM (Rosenbloom, Silverstein, Amemiya, Zeitler, & Klingensmith, 2009). A longitudinal study of 699 10- to 17-year-olds with recent-onset T2DM, the Treatment Options for Type 2 Diabetes in Adolescents and Youth (TODAY) study, concluded that the disease progression for children and youth is different than for adults and that it progresses more rapidly than originally expected. Early results revealed that 50% of participants required insulin within only a few years of diagnosis and, by the end of the 4-year study, almost one third had hypertension, 17% had early signs of kidney disease, and 13% demonstrated signs of visual problems. Early and aggressive treatment is recommended, as 50% of participants responded to metformin therapy and were able to maintain glycemic control over the time period of the study (TODAY Study Group, Zeitler, Hirst, Pyle et al., 2012).

Another recent national study with shocking results found an increase in the prevalence of prediabetes/diabetes from a rate of 9% in 1999 to 23% in 2008 (May, Kuklina, & Yoon, 2012). This study included youth aged 12 to 19 years, and researchers found that those who were more overweight or obese had greater increased prevalence of cardiovascular disease (CVD) risk factors (e.g., hypertension, higher LDL cholesterol).

Approximately 37% of those of normal weight, 49% of those considered overweight, and 61% of obese adolescents had at least one CVD risk factor.

A more recent category of diabetes, double diabetes, is found when a child or adolescent presents features of both T1DM and T2DM. For instance, when a child with T2DM develops antibodies to β-cells or when an adolescent with T1DM becomes overweight or obese, they may be characterized as having double diabetes (Pozzilli, Guglielmi, Caprio, & Buzzetti, 2011).

Younger children with T1DM, especially those who use insulin pumps, may need careful monitoring, something that is not always possible for the school nurse, who is often assigned to several school sites and may not be present when problems arise. A multidisciplinary team approach to care is needed, coordinating family, school staff, and physician collaboration. See Chapter 30 for more on the school nurse's role with school-age children with diabetes.

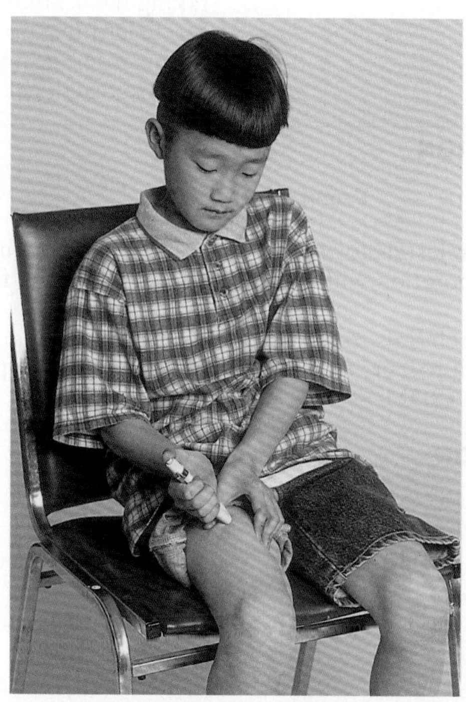

PHNs and school nurses work with diabetic school-age children to assure proper glucose monitoring and insulin administration.

Children and adolescents with diabetes may be reluctant to comply with medical regimens, although strict adherence has proved to reduce later microvascular complications. Intensive treatment control has reduced clinical neuropathy by 60%, retinopathy by 53%, and microalbuminuria by 54%, as well as HbA1c levels, and at a 17-year follow-up, cardiovascular events were 50% lower in those adhering to stricter control (Donaghue, Chiarelli, Trotta, Aligrove, & Dahl-Jorgensen, 2009). Testing blood glucose levels and taking insulin at school can be frustrating and cause children to feel singled out or different from their peers. Adolescents with T1DM or T2DM have higher rates of depression than those without diabetes (Monaghan, Singh, Streisand, & Cogen, 2010), and one study found that blood glucose monitoring had a mediating effect on depression related to high HgA_1C levels (McGrady, Laffel, Drotar, Repaske, & Hood, 2009). It is important for school nurses and PHNs to understand each child's unique concerns and to alert teachers and school personnel to the signs and symptoms (as well as treatment) of hypoglycemia.

In addition to the obvious emergency health-related concerns for diabetic children, a meta-analytic study of children with T1DM found "mild cognitive impairments and subtly reduced overall intellectual functioning" that could affect their school achievement (Naguib, Kulinskaya, Lomax, & Garralda, 2009, p. 271). Fluctuations between hyperglycemia and hypoglycemia affected math performance and mental efficiency in another study of children with T1DM (Gonder-Frederick et al., 2009). Moreover, the youth's own perception of obesity and overweight have been found to correlate with lower academic performance (Florin, Shults, & Stettler, 2011). Alerting teachers to these concerns may help them better understand the academic complications of this disease.

It is imperative to teach children and families that proper diet, oral antidiabetic medications or insulin administration, physical activity, and blood glucose testing are vital strategies to keep blood glucose levels as close to normal as possible. The prevention of T2DM through education and improvement in exercise, nutrition, and lifestyle can be one of the most important areas of focus for health professionals who work with the school-age population—including PHNs who may come into contact with them during immunization or child health clinics. Health education and health promotion to decrease childhood obesity and sedentary lifestyles may help stem the tide of T2DM in children and adolescents (see Levels of Prevention Pyramid).

Juvenile Rheumatoid Arthritis

Juvenile rheumatoid arthritis is a painful autoimmune disorder characterized by persistent joint swelling and stiffness with periods of remission and flare-up. It is often diagnosed between the ages of 6 months and 16 years. It is treated with nonsteroidal anti-inflammatory drugs (NSAIDs), disease-modifying antirheumatic drugs (DMARDs), such as methotrexate, and sometimes corticosteroids or newer biologic response modifiers (Pub Med Health, 2011). Exercise is often an important component of therapy, and an adapted physical education program may be developed for these children. Long-term sequelae may result, such as slow rate of growth or uneven growth of arm or leg, as well as pericarditis and joint destruction. Many adolescents with this disorder require additional support and counseling (Pub Med Health, 2011). Once again, the school nurse or PHN can serve as a liaison between the health care and education communities and advocate for any necessary accommodations.

Seizure Disorders

Seizure disorders are not uncommon in the school-age population. Epilepsy is a disorder of the brain in which neurons sometimes transmit abnormal signals. Epilepsy

LEVELS OF PREVENTION PYRAMID

SITUATION: The public health nurse and children with type 2 diabetes (T2DM)

GOAL: By using the three levels of prevention, negative health conditions are avoided, promptly diagnosed and treated, and/or the fullest possible potential is restored.

TERTIARY PREVENTION		
Rehabilitation	**Primary Prevention**	
	Health Promotion & Education	*Health Protection*
• Monitor the child's health • Work closely with the child, family, physician, and teacher to ensure proper follow-up • Be alert to monitor for any possible complications (e.g., medication side effects)	• Continue to promote a healthy lifestyle that includes appropriate food choices and daily physical activity within the limitations of T2DM	• Educate the teachers on safety precautions for children in their classroom diagnosed with T2DM • Monitor children taking medications for T2DM (e.g., over- or underdosage and adverse reactions)

SECONDARY PREVENTION	
Early Diagnosis	**Prompt Treatment**
• Teach older children to calculate their body mass index (BMI) • Monitor BMI scores • Yearly screenings for height and weight (calipers are useful) • Complete health histories on at-risk children	• Initiate referrals for health care provider follow-up in collaboration with parents of students at risk for T2DM • Initiate referrals to health care providers in collaboration with parents of students with signs and symptoms of T2DM

PRIMARY PREVENTION	
Health Promotion & Education	**Health Protection**
• Educate to promote good nutrition and a physically active lifestyle • Provide classroom contact in the early primary grades to encourage children to make good food choices • Limit passive activities and increase sports and physical activity • Teach older children how to make better food choices at fast food restaurants	

is considered to be one of the most common disabling neurologic conditions, and it is most common in the very young and in elderly populations. Over 300,000 children under age 15 and more than 570,000 older adults have epilepsy; more than 90,000 children may have treatment-resistant seizures (Epilepsy Foundation, n.d.). About 50% of children will have a second seizure, so treatment with medications is often postponed to determine if it is really needed; intractable epilepsy is thought to occur in only 5% to 15% of children (Arts & Geerts, 2009). Many children diagnosed with epilepsy can have their seizures controlled with medications, such as Tegretol, Dilantin, Depakote, Neurontin, Topamax, and Lamictal (WebMD, 2012). Vagus nerve stimulators are used in some cases after other treatments have failed (Elliott et al., 2011). Rectal diazepam is commonly prescribed for younger children and those with developmental disabilities, yet nurses are not always available to make an appropriate nursing assessment of the child before the drug is given to stop a seizure

(Klimach, 2009). Often, school secretaries or health aides are trained to give the emergency medication—highlighting the conflict between education laws and nurse practice acts (see more on this in Chapter 30). Treatment of epilepsy has been greatly enhanced by the use of newer antiepilepsy drugs (AEDs) specific to the pediatric population and, in some cases, by a diet rich in proteins and fats and low in carbohydrates—a *ketogenic diet* (Neal et al., 2009).

It is important to monitor medication compliance and teach school staff about first-aid measures for seizure victims. When teachers are anxious about having a child with epilepsy in the classroom, educational programs for them and other school staff members can be provided. Community health nurses or school nurses can help allay fears and promote appropriate and timely care.

Family dynamics are also a consideration, as behavior problems can arise (Rodenburg, Wagner, Austin, Kerr, & Dunn, 2011). Children and adolescents with seizure disorders may feel embarrassed or be the victims of teasing or bullying (Hamiwka et al., 2009). They may exhibit signs of school avoidance, or they may have problems learning. Seizure activity, along with the side effects of antiepileptic medications, may lead to problems with memory and learning, as well as changes in behavior (Loring, 2010). Moreover, seizures can affect short-term memory or language functions (WebMD, 2009). It is important for school nurses to work with children with epilepsy and to teach all students about the disease process and the need for empathy and understanding.

Childhood Cancers

In 2011, cancer was the leading cause of death from disease among U.S. children between infancy and age 15. Leukemias, brain, and central nervous system cancers are the most common types of childhood cancers (National Cancer Institute [NCI], 2011a). Childhood cancers, especially leukemias, now have better outcomes than ever before. Five-year survival rates for childhood cancers increased from <50% in the 1970s to 80% in the 2010s, generally as a result of treatment advances and participation in clinical trials (NCI, 2011b). More children are surviving childhood cancers, and concern has shifted to later complications of treatment rather than about cancer recurrence. Survivors are at greater risk of gastrointestinal, auditory, and cardiovascular complications (Goldsby et al., 2011; Mulrooney et al., 2009; Whelan et al., 2011). Also, children who have been treated with chemotherapy and/or radiation may develop a second primary cancer, and the risk of leukemia may be increased (NCI, n.d). White children, more than children from any other racial/ethnic group, are more likely to develop a childhood cancer (NCI, 2011a).

Acquired immune deficiency syndrome (AIDS), high levels of ionizing radiation, Down syndrome, and other genetic syndromes (e.g., Gorlin syndrome) have been linked to a higher risk for some childhood cancers. Pesticide exposure may be a factor, but research findings have not been decisive. Parental smoking may be linked to an increased cancer risk, but evidence for this is also inconclusive (NCI, n.d.).

Because many children return to school after initial hospitalization and treatment for cancer, school nurses or PHNs can help make this transition easier by educating classmates about cancer (e.g., it is not contagious), helping the children make necessary adjustments, and vigilantly protecting any immunocompromised students from communicable diseases (Moore et al., 2009).

Behavioral and Learning Problems

Other childhood health problems, less easy to detect and measure but often just as debilitating, are those of emotional, behavioral, and intellectual development. Although these problems are not new, awareness and concern have increased as the rates of occurrence for other life-threatening childhood diseases have diminished. Emotional or behavior problems and LDs are prevalent in childhood. One classic study of national data found a lifetime prevalence of LD at 9.7% (Altarac & Saroha, 2007). In a national survey, 5.4 million (9.5%) of 4- to 17-year-olds reported ever being diagnosed with ADHD. Parent report of ADHD was 22%, with rates increasing 3% annually from 1997 to 2006. Approximately 5.6% of girls and 13.2% of boys reported having been diagnosed with ADHD. LDs, along with ADHD, were reported in 4% of children; and this was more commonly found in the older age group of 12 to 17 years (CDC, 2011a).

Learning Disabilities

Children and adults who have average or above-average intelligence and who demonstrate significant difficulties in one or more areas of learning (e.g., reading, writing, mathematics, attention, coordination) may have a **learning disability**. Thinking and organization skills can also be affected. LDs may occur in one area or be overlapping—they are often lifelong conditions (NINDS, 2011). LDs, or learning disorders, are often recognized as the child progresses in school, and special education services may be needed. Causes of LDs and emotional behavioral problems appear to have genetic, environmental, and cultural influences. Approximately 8% to 10% of students have an LD, formally defined as a "neurologically based processing disorder" (Silver, 2011, para 5). About two thirds of learning disabled students receiving special education services are male (National Center for Learning Disabilities [NCLD], 2011). The number of children with LDs in the lowest economic group is twice that in the highest economic group (CDC, 2011a). Children characterized as being in fair or poor health were more than four times as likely to have a LD and three times as likely to have ADHD as children with excellent, very good, or good health status (CDC, 2011a).

Children with LDs can be helped through special education services. In fact, about 41% of children receiving special education services have an LD

(NCLD, 2011). Students must first be carefully diagnosed through psycho-educational testing (IQ testing, achievement tests, and measures of processing abilities); then, special education or resource teachers can build on the child or adolescent's strengths while working to compensate for weaknesses (NINDS, 2011). Some LDs are apparent in early school years, whereas others do not present problems until early adolescence. Battles over homework, poor grades, acting out in school, or frequent child complaints about school, teachers, or schoolwork are often harbingers of LDs. Common signs of LDs are (Silver, 2011):

- Reading problems
- Writing problems (fine-motor control and handwriting; problems with spelling, grammar, punctuation, capitalization; difficulty controlling flow of thoughts)
- Math problems (problems learning and understanding concepts, missing steps or sequencing of problems, and placement of numbers in columns)
- Language problems (cannot quickly process what is heard, problems with multiple instructions, difficulty organizing thoughts and speaking in classroom situations)
- Motor problems (problems with fine-motor planning activities, such as tying, cutting, coloring, and gross-motor planning, such as jumping and running; trouble with visual–motor activities, such as hitting or catching a ball)
- Sequencing (getting letters or numbers out of order; organization (messy binders)
- Memory (difficulty retaining what was learned); abstraction (confused, or not understanding what was said)

If LDs are not dealt with in childhood and adolescence, they can lead to later, more serious, problems related to employment, relationships, and quality of life in adulthood. Approximately 55% of adults (18–64 years) with LD, compared with 76% of those without LD, reported that they were employed. Children can receive services in schools, based on IDEA and Section 504; provisions of the Americans with Disabilities Act (ADA) provide protections for adults with LD (NCLD, 2011). The PHN and school nurse can assist individuals and families in recognizing LDs and locating necessary resources. Some students with significant LDs may qualify for special education services, and school nurses can be helpful in facilitating this process along with teachers and learning specialists.

Attention Deficit Hyperactivity Disorder

Attention deficit hyperactivity disorder (ADHD), a common childhood disorder, is a cluster of problems related to hyperactivity, impulsivity, and inattention. Its estimated prevalence has ranged from 3% to 5%, representing about 2 million children (National Institute of Mental Health [NIMH], n.d.). As mentioned earlier, there is an overall 9.5% lifetime prevalence of ADHD, with one study indicating 9% lifetime prevalence for 13- to 18-year-olds; 1.8% for severe ADHD (Merikangas et al., 2010). One study found the rate of ADHD diagnosis increased from 7% to 9% from 1998 to 2009, with the largest increase among low-income and poor children, and higher prevalence among non-Hispanic White children (Akinbami, Kuym Oastirm, & Reuben, 2011). Along with the increase in ADHD diagnosis, there has been a rise in prescriptions to treat this disorder; there has also been a rise in ADHD stimulant medication abuse by adolescents. Calls to poison control centers rose over a 7-year period by 76%—a rate much higher than for overall substance abuse calls. ADHD prescription estimates over the same time period showed increases of 133% for amphetamines, 52% for methylphenidates, and 80% for combined medications (Setlik, Bond, & Ho, 2009). In fact, a recent survey of college students found 5.4% of respondents admitted use of ADHD medications to enhance studying and improve attention problems, although they had no medical justification for use (Rainer et al., 2009). While research has shown medications to be effective in controlling behavioral issues, and with less success improve academic achievement, medication titration is a trial-and-error proposition (Hale et al., 2011). Boys are often recognized as having ADHD in early elementary grades, because they most often exhibit hyperactivity symptoms. Girls, on the other hand, are at increased risk for not receiving appropriate services because they often do not exhibit the hyperactivity component and may not be appropriately diagnosed and treated for ADHD.

Although a number of parents believe that sugar, food coloring agents, or other food additives may worsen ADHD symptoms in their children, research shows no behavioral or learning differences in double-blind studies using sugar and sugar substitutes. And, additive-free or non-Western diets are difficult to achieve (Millichap & Yee, 2012). Some research shows that prenatal exposure to nicotine and psychosocial adversity are associated with ADHD (CDC, 2011a). Symptoms of ADHD may be related to such diverse causes as lead poisoning and traumatic brain injuries, but new research focuses on the inherited tendencies for problems with dopamine receptors and transporter genes, along with evidence of decreased blood flow in the prefrontal regions of the brain (Byrnie, 2008). These findings support a neurobiological basis for the condition. Some evidence indicates that children with ADHD who are medicated properly later show peak cortical thickness in the frontal areas of the brain consistent with control subjects without ADHD, indicating that medication can restore brain development to a more normal rate, rather than the 3-year delay seen in previous studies (NIMH, n.d.; Pantoine, 2009). Some classic family and twin studies reveal a higher heritability factor (0.8) for ADHD and its symptoms of inattention (71% of variance) and hyperactivity (73% of variance) than for other psychiatric disorders, and researchers consider ADHD a "familial and highly heritable disorder" (Bezdjian, Baker, & Tuvblad, 2011; Thapar, Langley, O'Donovan, & Owen, 2006, p. 714; Wood & Neale, 2010). In families that have children with ADHD, about 25% of close relatives also had ADHD (NIMH, n.d.).

Not all behaviors related to ADHD, such as hyperactivity, may truly be ADHD. Health and psychological professionals must take a careful history and note if sudden family changes may have recently occurred (e.g., divorce, death, family crises) that may cause children to behave erratically. Untreated chronic middle ear infections, undetected temporal lobe seizures, and anxiety or depression can also be the source of some behavior problems that mimic ADHD, as can other brain disorders (NIMH, n.d.). Although some health professionals believe that many of the symptoms found in people with ADHD are part of the normal spectrum of human behavior, others note that people with ADHD have functional impairment in academic, social, or occupational areas resulting from their problem behaviors. Noted differences have even been reported in the results of electroencephalograms between children with and without ADHD, possibly due to cortical hypoarousal in children with ADHD (Nazari, Wallois, Aarabi, & Berquin, 2011). Nursing researchers have documented qualitative data from children and adolescents who described their difficulties, as well as mother's parenting experiences (Kendall, Hatton, Beckett, & Leo, 2003; Peters & Jackson, 2009). This disorder can be very disruptive for children and families, and additional support and counseling is often needed.

At each stage of development, those with ADHD are presented with distinct challenges. For example, children in elementary school are often involved in conflicts with peers and have problems organizing tasks. They may be more prone to accidents, and may have more school-related problems, such as grade retention and suspension or expulsion. They often have problems with grooming and handwriting, and they exhibit difficulty sleeping and making friends. As adolescents, 80% still exhibit symptoms of inattentiveness, hyperactivity, and impulsiveness. Compared with non-ADHD teens, they may have more conflict with their parents, poorer social skills, and ongoing problems at school. They may face more difficulty driving and are more prone to injury while driving, biking, or walking than their peers. They are also more likely to use tobacco and alcohol, spend less time with their families, and more often experience negative moods. As young adults, they are less likely to be enrolled in college, more likely to have begun sexual activity at an earlier age and to have been treated for a sexually transmitted infection (STI), and more likely to experience lower job performance ratings than their peers. In adulthood, they tend to have more marital and occupational problems. They often have less formal education and lower levels of savings. Poor social skills may also continue to be an issue (NIMH, n.d.). About half of adults with ADHD were first diagnosed as children. Adult ADHD is thought to affect 4.4% of U.S. adults, and it often goes undiagnosed and untreated; only 10% to 25% of those having adult ADHD have been diagnosed and are receiving treatment. Almost 95% of them continue to have attention deficit problems, but about one third report symptoms of hyperactivity (Kessler et al., 2010).

ADHD is sometimes found with associated disorders, such as communication or language disorders and LDs. About half of ADHD children and adolescents have learning or other mental disorders. Common comorbid conditions are bipolar, depressive, and anxiety disorders, Tourette's syndrome, as well as conduct disorders and oppositional-defiant disorder (Brown, 2009). At an earlier age of onset, ADHD is associated with more parental reports of child aggressive behavior, and some researchers have noted that about one third of males who exhibited severe ADHD in preschool also developed early-onset conduct disorder later in childhood and adolescence (Beauchaine, Hinshaw, & Pang, 2010). Differentiating between ADHD and bipolar condition can be difficult in early childhood, as bipolar disorder in children can present as a chronic mood problem, with some symptoms related to depression, irritability, and elation (Brown, 2009).

Collaboration among the child's family, school, and physician is needed to diagnose ADHD and to plan appropriate interventions and educational accommodations. Although parents have a wealth of knowledge about the child, teacher confirmation of ADHD-related behaviors is very important. School nurses and PHNs can assist parents in recognizing the symptoms of ADHD and in obtaining appropriate treatment and follow-up. A multimodal treatment approach is recognized as most effective. This includes medication, usually methylphenidate (Ritalin, Metadate, or Concerta), dextroamphetamine (Dexedrine or Dextrostat), or combined dextroamphetamine and amphetamine (Adderall); school accommodations for learning problems; and social skills training for the child with ADHD (NIMH, n.d.). Family and individual counseling, parent support groups, and training in behavior management techniques, as well as family education about the condition, are also essential features of this treatment method. Not all children and adolescents respond to medication and a good number do not fully comply with their medication regimen; medication dosage must be carefully monitored and adjusted (Molina et al., 2009).

The main goal of medical treatment for school-age children is academic improvement. If this does not occur, medication may need to be changed or discontinued. Parental response, severity of ADHD symptoms in children, and types of treatment plans are all important factors in the success of interventions for ADHD children and families. School nurses and community health nurses can work closely with school staff, parents, and physicians in determining the efficacy of treatment regimens.

Parents often voice concern about giving their children a stimulant medication to treat ADHD, and some families pursue alternative treatments (Patoine, 2009). Families may use some type of complementary and alternative medicine (e.g., acupuncture, nutritional supplements, diet), and they may not discuss this fact with health care providers. Some promising results with neurofeedback were found in one meta-analysis (Arns, Ridder, Strehl, Breteler, & Coenen, 2009). Newer nonstimulant medications, such as atomoxetine (Strattera) and guanfacine hydrochloride (Intuniv), have been used in children and adolescents.

Parental resistance to treatment may result from side effects (e.g., problems with sleep, appetite, greater anxiety) or stem from fears about later abuse of substances. As adolescents, those with ADHD may experiment with alcohol and other substances earlier than non-ADHD teens do, while concurrent hyperactivity has been shown to predict low self-esteem, leading to social withdrawal and abuse of substances (Tarter, Kirisci, Feske, & Vanyukov, 2007). One large-scale Finnish study found that symptoms of inattentiveness and hyperactivity in childhood were more predictive of alcohol use disorders and illicit drug use in later adolescence than an ADHD diagnosis (Sihvola et al., 2011). Some pediatricians are recommending supplementation with omega-3 fish oils when parents refuse medication, as there has been some evidence that this may be beneficial in reducing symptoms (Millichap & Yee, 2012).

Behavioral and Emotional Problems

The lifetime prevalence of any mental disorder among 13- to 18-year-olds is 46.3% (Merikangas et al., 2010). It is estimated that 5.4% of children between the ages of 6 and 17 have ever been diagnosed with a behavioral or conduct problem (Ghandour, Kogan, Blumberg, Jones, & Perrin, 2012). About 10% of children and adolescents have been diagnosed at some point with anxiety or depression. Around 20% of school-age children display behaviors consistent with oppositional-defiant disorder (e.g., hostile, stubborn, disobedient, belligerent, defiant), and 2.1% of children have been diagnosed with conduct disorder characterized by a persistent violation of norms/rules and others' rights (American Academy of Child & Adolescent Psychiatry [AACAP], 2011a). Symptoms of conduct disorder, sometimes thought to be a more severe form of antisocial behavior than oppositional-defiant disorder, is often characterized by behaviors that may include destruction of property, fire setting, cruelty to animals or people, and/or bullying and threatening behavior. Schizophrenia in childhood affects 1 in 40,000 children under age 12, and adult schizophrenia, which affects 1 in 100 people, usually begins in young adulthood (age 18 for males, age 25 for females). Bipolar disorder, most often found in adults, is also found in children and adolescents. Early identification of children and adolescents at risk for developing bipolar disorder may be accomplished through the use of behavior checklists and other psychometric tools that reveal higher scores related to aggression, delinquent behavior, and attention problems, or withdrawal and anxiety/depression (Giles, DelBello, Stanford, & Strakowski, 2007). It is important to find referral sources for these children and their families, and this may be difficult in more rural or outlying areas.

School-age problem behaviors stem from many causes, some of them genetic and others environmental. Corporal punishment may be a risk factor for antisocial behavior (Taylor, Manganella, Lee, & Rice, 2010), and several studies have noted a link between corporal punishment and restricted development of cognitive ability and increased externalizing behaviors (Gershoff et al., 2012; Straus & Paschall, 2009). Physical punishment (e.g., slapping, spanking, pinching, pulling ears) is thought both to trigger and maintain child behavior problems, and decreasing this parental behavior could be associated with better child mental health and lower levels of behavior problems (Mulvaney & Mebert, 2007).

Children are barometers of their environment. The current rate of divorce in the United States is double what it was in the 1950s. Over the last 30 years, the percentage of children living with two married parents decreased from close to 80% to 66% in 2010; about 4% of children lived with two unmarried parents. Four percent of children did not live with either parent, and 54% of those children lived with grandparents. The majority of children living with one parent live with their mother. Children of divorce are more likely to exhibit behavior problems, with children who are products of highly contentious divorces most at risk (FCFS, 2011d). School nurses can be alert to early symptoms and refer parents to marital counseling or suggest family therapists. Some schools also offer support groups for children of divorce.

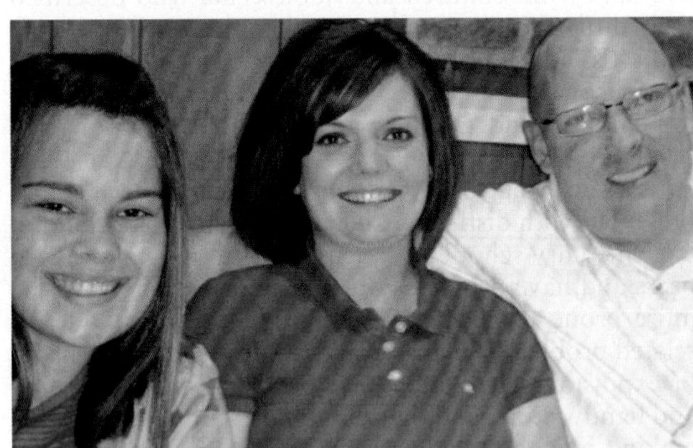

Fewer children now live in two-parent homes. Author's private photo with Permissions of Merysa Schultz, Deanna Rector, Jon Rector

School refusal, where a child develops a pattern of refusing to go to school or remain in school for the entire school day, is found in 2% to 5% of school-age children and differs from truancy. Unlike truancy, school refusal is commonly associated with symptoms of emotional distress—usually anxiety or depression—but may also be associated with oppositional-defiant disorder, ADHD, or other disruptive behavior disorders. Often, the children complain of headaches, stomachaches, or other physical ailments, but some are motivated to miss school to gain parental attention (Anxiety Disorders Association of America [ADAA], 2012; Dube & Orpinas, 2009). School refusal (formerly called school phobia) is most commonly found in children between ages 5 and 6 or ages 10 and 11. Transitional periods, such as school entry or moving to middle school or high school, are often the most difficult. Rates are generally reported by parents to be higher for girls and younger children (ADAA, 2012; Allen, Lavallee, Herren, Ruthe, & Schneider, 2010). Children usually present to the school nurse or PHN with headaches and/or abdominal pains. They may throw tantrums, cry, or exhibit panic and fear to their parents in an attempt to stay home from school. Sometimes, children are afraid of something in the school environment (e.g., bullies, teachers, test taking), or they may have a type of separation anxiety. Family enmeshment or detachment, or high levels of family conflict, may contribute to school refusal problems. The best interventions include early return to school, with parental involvement in school, systematic desensitization (graded exposure to the classroom), relaxation training, and counseling being the most effective (ADAA, 2012). Occasionally, antidepressant medications are used as well. PHNs and school nurses can serve as a liaison with the child, family, school, and health care/mental health care providers to promote a positive outcome.

Disabled Children

Children with disabilities accounted for almost 6% of the total school-age population in 2010. Cognitive and self-care difficulties were the two most common disabilities reported, followed by vision, ambulatory, and hearing problems (Brault, 2011). Between 2008 and 2009, almost 6.5 million students were classified as disabled, or 13.2% of school-age students; this was down slightly from 2003 to 2004 (13.7%). The most commonly cited disabilities are specific LD, speech or language disability, intellectual disability, emotional disturbance, and other health impairments (NCES, 2011). The prevalence of developmental disabilities in children aged 3 to 17 increased from 12.84% to 15.04% between 1997 and 2008. Hispanic children had the lowest prevalence, and boys had higher overall prevalence than girls. Rates for autism and ADHD, along with other developmental delays, increased; hearing loss declined (Boyle, Boulet, Schieve, Cohen, 2011).

Many children with perceived disabilities or problems are referred for assessment and possible placement in special education programs each year. School nurses often serve as a liaison between parents, physicians, and educators and are part of the team developing an individualized education plan (IEP) for children who qualify for special education services. Most children receive special services in a regular classroom because *full inclusion* or *mainstreaming* legislation mandates that fewer children be segregated into special classes or separate schools. See Chapter 26 for more on clients with disabilities, and Chapter 30 for more on school nursing.

Problems Associated with Economic Status

After reaching a low point (16.2%) in 2000, childhood poverty in the United States rose to 20.7% in 2009 (FCFS, n.d.d.). This increase in poverty did not vary by parents' place of birth, employment status, or educational level, leading many to speculate that this jump in the poverty rate reflects overall economic conditions. According to the Children's Defense Fund (CDF, 2011), 1 in 6 Black and 1 in 7 Hispanic children live in extreme poverty, as does 1 in 20 White children. About 1 in 3 Black and Hispanic children lives in poverty, along with 1 in 10 White children. Overall, children make up 24% of the U.S. population, but they represent 34% of all those in poverty (Addy & Wight, 2012). While the United States ranked number one among industrialized nations in gross domestic product (GDP), health expenditures, defense expenditures, and military technology, it ranked 17th in reading scores and 30th in infant mortality. It ranked last because of high rates of relative child poverty and adolescent birth mothers (aged 15–19), and was also last in protecting children against gun violence (CDF, 2011). It is in society's best economic interest to care for its children, because they will become the taxpayers of tomorrow. Historically, experts posited that single-parent families (usually without an adult man present), welfare reform, and economic trends that kept less well-educated populations from entering all but the most menial jobs combined to produce a powerful synergistic effect on children and adolescents.

Poverty has profound and lasting effects on children. A classic study found that more than 20% of low-income children between the ages of 6 and 17 have some type of mental health problem (Chau & Douglas-Hall, 2007). A large birth cohort study found that family poverty predicted increased rates of depression and anxiety in adolescents and young adults, and that an increased frequency of child poverty exposure, or repeated exposures, was associated with poorer mental health and reduced levels of cognitive development (Najman et al., 2009, 2010). Childhood poverty, leading to high levels of chronic stress and allostatic load, is inversely associated with adult working memory levels (Evans & Schamberg, 2009). Children living in poverty have poorer health and are more likely to suffer from a chronic health condition (e.g., asthma, anemia), as well as injuries and accidents (Moore, Redd, Burkhauser, Mbwana, & Collins, 2009). As adolescents, they more often experience depression and mental health problems and engage in more health-risk behaviors (e.g., smoking, early sexual activity), and more externalizing/adolescent delinquent behaviors (Child Trends Databank, 2012a).

As adults, these children will be more likely to have lower occupational status and lower wages. Poor children and adolescents are at higher risk for negative cognitive outcomes and learning problems, resulting in fewer school days, lower math and reading scores, more grade failures, and earlier high school dropout (Child Trends Databank, 2012a). One study found family wealth as a significant partial predictor of test scores in school-age children. The disparity in this study was stunning—White families owned more than 10 times the assets of Black families and White children's test scores were significantly higher than those of Black children (Yeung & Conley, 2008). Parental education level and employment status play large roles in childhood poverty. For children with parents having less than a high school diploma, 85% live in low-income families; and 73% of children with one parent who works less than full time annually live in poverty (Addy & Wight, 2012).

The social, emotional, and behavioral problems of some poor children may be the end result of disproportionate exposure to environmental toxins, parental substance abuse, maternal depression, trauma and abuse, divorce, violent crime, low-quality child care, inadequate nutrition, and decreased cognitive stimulation and exposure to vocabulary in early childhood and infancy (Child Trends Databank, 2012a).

The relationship between lower socioeconomic status (SES) and poor health persists throughout childhood and adolescence into adulthood (Conroy, Sandel, & Zuckerman, 2010), and, conversely, childhood health is strongly associated with lower SES during adulthood (Smith, 2009). A population-based cohort study found that lower childhood SES was significantly related to obesity and higher systolic blood pressure in women, and some association was found for men and smoking. These outcomes are cardiovascular risk factors, and even when social inequalities level off with age, early poverty may affect cardiovascular health by these risk factors (Schumann et al., 2011).

Welfare reforms enacted in 1996 (i.e., The Personal Responsibility and Work Opportunity Reconciliation Act [PRWORA]) have been successful in moving many families from welfare to work. With a combination of welfare time limits, increasing work requirements/sanctions, and reducing financial disincentives for work, welfare reform and work success programs were projected to lead to greater employment. By 2000, the number of families receiving cash assistance (now with a 5-year lifetime limit) fell to half the number served in 1996; however, many of those continuing to work still earn wages below the poverty level (Martin & Caminada, 2009; Shields & Behrman, 2002). The Earned Income Tax Credit (EITC) was provided as an incentive for low-income wage earners, and employment rates for single mothers of children did increase from 1987 to 2006 by 11%. During the economic expansion of the 1990s, single mothers with less than a high school education had an employment rate that rose 20% between 1992 and 1999; and many believe that this tax change was largely responsible (Hoynes, 2008). However, employment rates that increased during the mid-1990s have once again fallen in the face of a declining job market in the mid-2000s (Parrott & Sherman, 2006). A study of Wisconsin welfare leavers found that those who left before the recession had less difficulty finding jobs and child care, while those exiting the welfare system during the recession had lower employment rates and more difficulty with child care due to sporadic employment (Kwon & Meyer, 2011). More than 1 million single mothers are now thought to be in the "no work, no welfare" group—with no jobs and no government support. While welfare reform was found to reduce the probability of high school dropout by 15% for adolescents from disadvantaged families, it also decreased the probability of college enrollment for adult women eligible for welfare by 20% (Dhaval, Corman, & Reichman, 2012). Long-term welfare dependency has been reduced, with little or slightly positive effects on child behavioral and academic outcomes and small or negative outcomes for adolescents, depending upon the state (Ziliak, 2009). As part of welfare reform, the mission of case workers changed from eligibility verification/payments to service delivery/promoting client self-sufficiency; the decline in social worker caseloads by over half has been linked to a drop in service to qualifying families, rather than a reduction in the numbers of poor families (Godfrey & Yoshikawa, 2011; Hoynes, 2008; Parrott & Sherman, 2006). Also, employment and earnings success is often tied to client–caseworker interaction and personalized client attention, with great variation among states and counties (Godfrey & Yoshikawa, 2011).

Funding cuts to the Food Stamp Program, decreased benefits to legal immigrants, and reductions in Medicaid eligibility have impacted many poor families. Reduced allotments of food stamps to households with mixed citizens/noncitizens have led to persistent and higher levels of food insecurity among very young child citizens of noncitizen parents compared to those of U.S.-born mothers (Chilton et al., 2009). Some affected by welfare reform decreased their food stamp participation while turning more to the special supplemental food program for Women, Infants, and Children (WIC), or the National School Lunch/Breakfast Program, as a source of essential food items for their children. Safety-net programs—specifically, WIC and the food stamp program—have been shown to reduce the risk of nutrition-related problems (e.g., anemia, nutritional deficiency, failure-to-thrive). They have also been associated with a reduction in the risk of child abuse and neglect (Slack et al., 2011). Children in families in which welfare benefits were reduced or terminated due to sanctions (usually related to inability to find work or comply with program rules) had greater odds of hospitalizations and food insecurity. One longitudinal study found that, after 3 years, children in the child welfare or child protective system had stable insurance coverage, a finding partially attributable to the persistence of social workers finding available coverage for children in this vulnerable group or the movement of the children into the foster care system (Raghavan, Aarons, Rosch, & Leslie, 2008).

The PRWORA did provide needed changes in child support enforcement—in 2005, over 50% of families in programs received child support, up from 20% in 1996 (Parrott & Sherman, 2006). Another study noted increased income from child support postwelfare reform and suggested that the mandatory policy of establishing paternity prior to receipt of welfare benefits aided greatly in this endeavor (Lee, 2009). And, despite problems with welfare reform, some studies noted earlier show that school-age children in families that participate in these programs do better in school and exhibit fewer behavior problems than those from families that do not participate. More negative outcomes, however, were found for adolescents, even though employment and income levels increased (Ziliak, 2009). Some studies indicate that about half the families who leave welfare for work actually have fewer economic resources than they had while on welfare.

Although almost 21% of children live below the federal poverty level ($23,050 for family of four in 2012), economists note that families need about twice the income of the federal poverty level to survive (Coverage for All, 2012; Fass & Cauthen, 2008). These families are characterized as low-income, and more than 28 million children live in these circumstances. Millions more children live in moderate-income families that have inadequate child care, limited health insurance, limited access to higher education, and poor housing. Almost 20% of children live in distressing situations and are at risk of being homeless. About 19% of poor children have no health insurance; overall, 11.7% of children are uninsured (Fass & Cauthen, 2008). In some states, this figure is 30%, even though more than 90% of uninsured children have one or more parents who work, and more than 66% have family incomes greater than the poverty level (see Chapters 6 and 25). Since the recession, student homeless rates have increased across rural, suburban, and urban school districts (Miller, 2011).

Some specific physical health problems are related to poverty (e.g., lead poisoning, iron deficiency anemia, increased susceptibility to illness). Children living in poorer neighborhoods are exposed to higher levels of community violence and may be more prone to seeing the world as a hostile and dangerous place; they are often also exposed to higher levels of family violence and are more at risk of subsequent mental health issues (Linares, 2008). A longitudinal study of childhood poverty and its relationship to health status found that "the greater the number of years spent living in poverty, the more elevated was overnight cortisol and the more dysregulated was the cardiovascular response" (Evans & Kim, 2007, p. 953). This study demonstrated the physiologic effects of poverty, mediated by increased social and physical risk factors (e.g., substandard housing, environmental toxins, crowding, noise, greater family conflict, harsher parenting styles). Earlier research showed an association between crowding and noisy conditions and hypertension. The results reported by Evans and Kim (2007) align with previous research demonstrating that exposure to early childhood poverty leads to later morbidity in adulthood—"an early history of poverty appears to set children on a life-course trajectory of ill health" (p. 956). It is important to put in place programs and safeguards to reduce child poverty and its long-term negative effects (Anthony, King, & Austin, 2011).

Many school-age children suffer from the effects of poverty-related hunger. It is difficult to concentrate and learn properly if meals are often skipped or if food consistently does not provide enough nourishment (Kursmark & Weitzman, 2009). **Food insufficiency** is defined as not having enough food to eat, while food insecurity is characterized by "reduced quality, variety, or desirability" of one's diet, but there may be no real indication of a reduction of food intake (U.S. Department of Agriculture [USDA], 2011b, para. 5). In the USDA survey (2010), rates of food insecurity have been rising since 2007, but leveled off in 2010. About 14.5% of U.S. households reported some degree of food insecurity in 2010, representing 48.8 million people. Variation among states occurs, with North Dakota reporting 2.7% and Mississippi 19.4%. In December 2011, more than 46.5 million Americans participated in the Supplemental Assistance Nutrition Program (SNAP, or food stamps); this represents an increase of 2.4 million over the previous year (Food Research & Action Council [FRAC], 2011). About 30% of those who are eligible use any of the largest federal food assistance programs, such as food stamps, free or reduced school lunches, and WIC. Thus, children go hungry because many eligible families do not use these services. In 2011, about 20% of Americans surveyed reported a hardship providing food for their families (FRAC, 2011). Those children who participate in school lunch and breakfast programs suffer fewer of the side effects of hunger that affect learning; however, not all schools participate in these programs. For more on poverty, see Chapter 25.

Injuries

The loss of children's lives that results from all injuries combined suggests a staggering loss to society in the number of years of productive life lost. Injuries that require medical attention or result in restricted activity occur at a rate of 250 out of 1,000 U.S. children and adolescents. The annual cost of medical treatment is $17 billion. According to the CDC, an injury is "unintentional or intentional damage to the body" (2010c, para. 2), but use of the word accident is considered incorrect, as injuries may be prevented through environmental, individual behavioral, legislative, and institutional policy changes. For children and adolescents (aged 5–19 years), 67% of all deaths are the result of injury-related causes, 48% from motor vehicles (as pedestrians or occupants), 21% from all other unintentional injuries, 16% from homicides, and 14% from suicides (CDC, 2010a, 2010c). For adolescents, injuries are responsible for 80% of deaths (FCFS, 2011a, 2011c).

The death rate for adolescents (15–19 years) dropped to 53.4 per 100,000 in 2009 from 61.9 in 2007. Almost 260 injury-related emergency department (ED) visits and 12 hospitalizations occur for every fatal adolescent injury (FCFS, 2011a, 2011c). For children aged 5 to 14, the death rate in 2009 was 14 per 100,000, with the death rate dropping by half since 1980 (FCFS, 2011c). Black children had the highest death rates at 20. Unintentional injury and injury death rates were 4 and 6 per 100,000 overall, and this was the leading cause of death in children aged 1 to 14. For the 5- to 14-year-olds, this was followed by cancer (2), homicide (1), and birth defects (1). Injury death rates have dropped over the past two decades (FCFS, 2011c).

For all racial and ethnic groups, death rates were higher for infants and late adolescents, and dropped during the middle years. Homicide rates were highest for Black children in all age groups (Bernard, Paulozzi, & Wallace, 2007). Injuries not resulting in death often cause permanent disabilities, or emotional and physical consequences for children and their families.

Each year, about 4 million children and adolescents are injured at school, and over 1 million sports-related injuries occur in 10- to 17-year-olds (CDC, 2010c). Nonfatal injuries among adolescents most often involve being struck by or against an object or person, but for younger children the cause is most often a fall (FCFS, 2011c).

A large-scale study examining the risk factors for passenger deaths in fatal motor vehicle crashes found that in more than 21% of cases of child passenger fatalities, alcohol was a factor. When drivers were younger than age 18, the greatest risk factors for death were most often associated with drivers younger than age 16, failure to use seat belts or other restraints, and driving on high-speed roads (Winston, Kallan, Senserrick, & Elliott, 2008). Suicides in the 10- to 19-year-old group more commonly involved firearms for Whites and Blacks, but suffocation/hanging was more prevalent for Alaska Natives/American Indians, Asian/Pacific Islanders, and Hispanics.

Another, more recent, danger for adolescents is use of cell phones while driving. While not only a concern among adolescents, among the general population cell phone usage while driving leads to distractions and has been estimated to lead to a four times greater risk of crashing (Farmer, Braitman, & Lund, 2010). One study found that drivers under age 30 used cell phones 16% of the time while driving; the average use for the population was 7% (Farmer et al., 2010). The use of cell phones can lead to injury in younger populations, as many school-age children now have them. One study of 10- to 11-year-olds found that cell phone use while crossing the street led to greater distraction and potential for injury (Stavrinos, Byington, & Schwebel, 2009). Legislation in many states has banned the use of cell phones (talking and/or texting) while driving, but one North Carolina study found that a newly enacted law had "little or no effect on teenage drivers' use of cell phones shortly after the law took effect" (Foss, Goodwin, McCartt, & Hellinga, 2009, p. 419). A larger, seven-state study on the long-term effects of cell phone laws found reductions in cell phone use, maintained over time, but noted that further research was needed to determine if a reduction in crashes could be attributed to these laws (McCartt, Hellinga, Strouse, & Farmer, 2010).

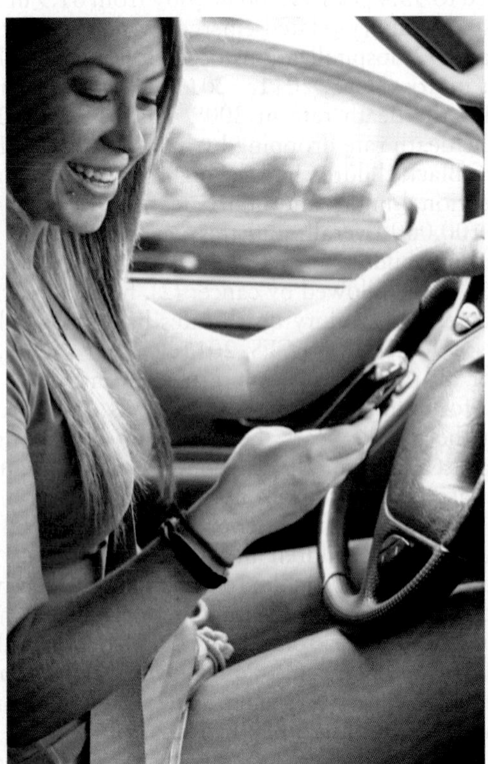

Cell phone use while driving is dangerous, especially for inexperienced adolescent drivers.

For children and adolescents, aged 6 to 19, unintentional strangulation deaths from the "choking game" are often misreported (CDC, 2008b). This behavior involves self-strangulation, or strangulation by a friend through the use of hands or a noose, causing a brief euphoric high due to cerebral hypoxia. Most of the victims are male (estimated at almost 87%), and the average age is estimated at 13.3 years. Survivors may have serious neurological impairments, concussions/broken bones, or eye hemorrhages (CDC, 2009b). Most parents were unaware of this potentially fatal activity until a child's death occurred, but warning signs, such as bloodshot eyes; disorientation after being alone; belts, scarves, and ropes tied to doorknobs or bedroom furniture; and marks on the neck should lead parents to suspect this dangerous activity (CDC, 2008b).

Community health nurses can promote injury prevention and control through education, promotion of engineering and environmental protection strategies, and legislative advocacy (Philbrook, Richardson, & Kriel, 2009). (See From the Case Files.) PHNs can advance the prevention of unintentional injuries and deaths by working with families to initiate consistent use of seat belts and child safety seats in vehicles, and the use of helmets and other protective gear for children riding bikes and skateboarding. Where water is a natural hazard, wearing life jackets while boating and swimming can help decrease accidental drowning. Promotion of smoke and carbon monoxide detectors, poison prevention, and sudden infant death syndrome (SIDS) education can help to further decrease injury death rates. Teaching parents about presetting hot-water heaters to lower than 130°F, recognizing the hazards of infant walkers, storing matches and lighters safely, and using pool fencing can help to prevent common unintentional injuries (Safe Kids USA, 2009). Advocacy for stricter seat belt and child safety seat enforcement, as well as programs to provide child safety seats and bicycle helmets, has been shown to positively affect mortality and injury rates (Du et al., 2010).

Community health nurses can work with their local health departments and community action groups to provide seats and helmets to families who cannot afford them, organize clinics to educate about proper installation and use, and encourage local police to enforce seat belt and safety seat laws.

Communicable Diseases

The mortality rates of school-age children 5 to 14 years old are comparatively low and have decreased substantially over the last century, a reduction that can be attributed to the effective prevention and control of the acute infectious diseases of childhood, "one of the greatest achievements of the 20th century" (Brunham, 2009, p. 5). Although mortality rates are low in this country, worldwide mortality due to communicable diseases is 6 million deaths annually; morbidity due to communicable diseases among school children worldwide is also high. Tuberculosis (TB) HIV, and malaria are common,

From the Case Files I

The use of restraints (seatbelts, infant car seats, child booster seats) has been shown to be an effective population-level intervention that reduces fatalities and serious injuries (Du et al., 2010). I was part of a group of pediatric nurses, epidemiologists, health educators, and physicians from a large mid-Western medical center who worked with 20 elementary schools to evaluate the most effective way to provide information on booster seat use in kindergarten children. Because we understood that most children use a seatbelt and not a car or booster seat, increasing their chances of injury, we wanted to address this issue even though our state did not have any specific regulation about booster seats at that time. Our group designed three interventions: (1) a group receiving information only, (2) a group receiving a 1-hour class for parents offered at the school, or (3) a classroom presentation for children about proper booster seat use with a follow-up letter to parents about the presentation. Three to six months later, telephone follow-up was made. Parents in all three groups did not report the 70% goal of knowledge that booster seat use could protect their children in an automobile crash. The group with the greatest improvement in booster seat use was the one receiving a parent presentation and a booster seat. It was difficult to determine the best educational approach, because the demographics of the three groups were too different (language spoken, immigrant status, reading level), but we believed that the gift of a booster seat, along with personal contact and interaction, was most effective. Involving both parents and children was thought to be a better way to go in future research. The use of written educational material alone did not increase use of booster seats. Written information alone is often not effective—a good thing to keep in mind when you drop off pamphlets to clients and don't spend time going over them and answering questions.

—Julie, RN

Adapted from Philbrook, J., Kiragu, A., Geppert, J., Graham, P., Richardson, L., & Kriel, R. (2009). Pediatric injury prevention: Methods of booster seat education. *Pediatric Nursing, 35*(4), 215–220.

as is pneumonia due to upper respiratory infections and parasitic infections (World Bank, 2011). Among school children, the incidence rates of measles, rubella (German measles), pertussis (whooping cough), infectious parotitis (mumps), and varicella (chickenpox) have dropped considerably because of widespread immunization efforts (see Fig. 22-1 for childhood immunization schedule).

Over the past several decades, the incidence of vaccine-preventable diseases has generally decreased, although in 2006 and 2009, measles outbreaks were reported. In 2005, hepatitis A immunization was recommended to begin at age 1 year. The reported cases of mumps, hepatitis A, and meningococcal disease decreased in the under age 5 population between 2007 and 2009 (Maternal and Child Health Bureau, 2011). Some of these communicable illnesses carry potentially serious complications, such as birth defects from rubella and nerve deafness from mumps. Cases of pertussis in the birth to age 4 group increased by more than 1,000 from 2007 to 2008, and the highest increase was in infants under age 6 months who had not yet received the scheduled doses of the vaccine (Maternal and Child Health Bureau, 2011).

One Wisconsin study found 261 cases of rubella and mumps in one county, and 47% of the children with confirmed cases reported using the weight room in a particular high school. An important finding was that 84% of children with reported vaccine histories had received five or more doses of pertussis vaccine, further indicating that booster vaccinations may be required for adolescents and adults (Sotir et al., 2008).

Vigorous campaigns have been undertaken by health departments to get children immunized. Along with the standard diptheria, tetanus, and pertussis vaccine, an immunization for mumps, measles, and rubella (MMR) has been available for more than 25 years, and newer vaccines for *Haemophilus influenzae* type b (Hib), hepatitis A and B, and varicella have been developed and are now included in the childhood immunization schedule. Meningococcal, pneumococcal, and rotavirus vaccines have also been added, along with yearly influenza vaccines for all children younger than age 5 (Barclay, 2012). Human papillomavirus (HPV) for girls aged 11 and above was recommended in 2009, and in 2011 the Advisory Committee on Immunization Practices recommended routine use for 11- and 12-year-old males. It recommended that previously unvaccinated 13- to 21-year-olds also receive the vaccine, noting that males up to age 26 may be safely vaccinated (Dunne et al., 2011).

As increasing numbers of school-age children must show proof of required vaccinations before they are allowed to enroll in school, the percentages of children in this age group who are immunized against specific diseases may continue to rise. But, more parents of young children are choosing not to immunize their children, invoking religious or personal belief exceptions. This practice has led to outbreaks of vaccine-preventable diseases: More than 214 children (mostly unvaccinated) were infected with measles in a large outbreak related to high numbers of unvaccinated children and overseas travelers (Reinberg, 2011). However, immunization compliance for adolescents has often been problematic due to lack of sufficient insurance coverage and poor systems for tracking and recall, as well as fewer well-child visits to health care providers among this age group. This has improved in recent years, though. Results from a 2009 national

FIGURE 1: Recommended immunization schedule for persons aged 0 through 6 years—United States, 2012 (for those who fall behind or start late, see the catch-up schedule [Figure 3])

Vaccine ▼ Age ►	Birth	1 month	2 months	4 months	6 months	9 months	12 months	15 months	18 months	19–23 months	2–3 years	4–6 years
Hepatitis B[1]	Hep B	HepB			HepB							
Rotavirus[2]			RV	RV	RV[2]							
Diphtheria, tetanus, pertussis[3]			DTaP	DTaP	DTaP		see footnote[3]	DTaP				DTaP
Haemophilus influenzae type b[4]			Hib	Hib	Hib[4]		Hib					
Pneumococcal[5]			PCV	PCV	PCV		PCV				PPSV	
Inactivated poliovirus[6]			IPV	IPV	IPV							IPV
Influenza[7]					Influenza (Yearly)							
Measles, mumps, rubella[8]							MMR		see footnote[8]			MMR
Varicella[9]							Varicella		see footnote[9]			Varicella
Hepatitis A[10]							Dose 1[10]				HepA Series	
Meningococcal[11]						MCV4 — see footnote [11]						

Range of recommended ages for all children

Range of recommended ages for certain high-risk groups

Range of recommended ages for all children and certain high-risk groups

This schedule includes recommendations in effect as of December 23, 2011. Any dose not administered at the recommended age should be administered at a subsequent visit, when indicated and feasible. The use of a combination vaccine generally is preferred over separate injections of its equivalent component vaccines. Vaccination providers should consult the relevant Advisory Committee on Immunization Practices (ACIP) statement for detailed recommendations, available online at http://www.cdc.gov/vaccines/pubs/acip-list.htm. Clinically significant adverse events that follow vaccination should be reported to the Vaccine Adverse Event Reporting System (VAERS) online (http://www.vaers.hhs.gov) or by telephone (800-822-7967).

1. **Hepatitis B (HepB) vaccine.** (Minimum age: birth)
   At birth:
   - Administer monovalent HepB vaccine to all newborns before hospital discharge.
   - For infants born to hepatitis B surface antigen (HBsAg)–positive mothers, administer HepB vaccine and 0.5 mL of hepatitis B immune globulin (HBIG) within 12 hours of birth. These infants should be tested for HBsAg and antibody to HBsAg (anti-HBs) 1 to 2 months after completion of at least 3 doses of the HepB series, at age 9 through 18 months (generally at the next well-child visit).
   - If mother's HBsAg status is unknown, within 12 hours of birth administer HepB vaccine for infants weighing ≥2,000 grams, and HepB vaccine plus HBIG for infants weighing <2,000 grams. Determine mother's HBsAg status as soon as possible and, if she is HBsAg-positive, administer HBIG for infants weighing ≥2,000 grams (no later than age 1 week).

   Doses after the birth dose:
   - The second dose should be administered at age 1 to 2 months. Monovalent HepB vaccine should be used for doses administered before age 6 weeks.
   - Administration of a total of 4 doses of HepB vaccine is permissible when a combination vaccine containing HepB is administered after the birth dose.
   - Infants who did not receive a birth dose should receive 3 doses of a HepB-containing vaccine starting as soon as feasible (Figure 3).
   - The minimum interval between dose 1 and dose 2 is 4 weeks, and between dose 2 and 3 is 8 weeks. The final (third or fourth) dose in the HepB vaccine series should be administered no earlier than age 24 weeks and at least 16 weeks after the first dose.
2. **Rotavirus (RV) vaccines.** (Minimum age: 6 weeks for both RV-1 [Rotarix] and RV-5 [Rota Teq])
   - The maximum age for the first dose in the series is 14 weeks, 6 days; and 8 months, 0 days for the final dose in the series. Vaccination should not be initiated for infants aged 15 weeks, 0 days or older.
   - If RV-1 (Rotarix) is administered at ages 2 and 4 months, a dose at 6 months is not indicated.
3. **Diphtheria and tetanus toxoids and acellular pertussis (DTaP) vaccine.** (Minimum age: 6 weeks)
   - The fourth dose may be administered as early as age 12 months, provided at least 6 months have elapsed since the third dose.
4. ***Haemophilus influenzae* type b (Hib) conjugate vaccine.** (Minimum age: 6 weeks)
   - If PRP-OMP (PedvaxHIB or Comvax [HepB-Hib]) is administered at ages 2 and 4 months, a dose at age 6 months is not indicated.
   - Hiberix should only be used for the booster (final) dose in children aged 12 months through 4 years.
5. **Pneumococcal vaccines.** (Minimum age: 6 weeks for pneumococcal conjugate vaccine [PCV]; 2 years for pneumococcal polysaccharide vaccine [PPSV])
   - Administer 1 dose of PCV to all healthy children aged 24 through 59 months who are not completely vaccinated for their age.
   - For children who have received an age-appropriate series of 7-valent PCV (PCV7), a single supplemental dose of 13-valent PCV (PCV13) is recommended for:
     — All children aged 14 through 59 months
     — Children aged 60 through 71 months with underlying medical conditions.
   - Administer PPSV at least 8 weeks after last dose of PCV to children aged 2 years or older with certain underlying medical conditions, including a cochlear implant. See *MMWR* 2010:59(No. RR-11), available at http://www.cdc.gov/mmwr/pdf/rr/rr5911.pdf.
6. **Inactivated poliovirus vaccine (IPV).** (Minimum age: 6 weeks)
   - If 4 or more doses are administered before age 4 years, an additional dose should be administered at age 4 through 6 years.
   - The final dose in the series should be administered on or after the fourth birthday and at least 6 months after the previous dose.
7. **Influenza vaccines.** (Minimum age: 6 months for trivalent inactivated influenza vaccine [TIV]; 2 years for live, attenuated influenza vaccine [LAIV])
   - For most healthy children aged 2 years and older, either LAIV or TIV may be used. However, LAIV should not be administered to some children, including 1) children with asthma, 2) children 2 through 4 years who had wheezing in the past 12 months, or 3) children who have any other underlying medical conditions that predispose them to influenza complications. For all other contraindications to use of LAIV, see *MMWR* 2010;59(No. RR-8), available at http://www.cdc.gov/mmwr/pdf/rr/rr5908.pdf.
   - For children aged 6 months through 8 years:
     — For the 2011–12 season, administer 2 doses (separated by at least 4 weeks) to those who did not receive at least 1 dose of the 2010–11 vaccine. Those who received at least 1 dose of the 2010–11 vaccine require 1 dose for the 2011–12 season.
     — For the 2012–13 season, follow dosing guidelines in the 2012 ACIP influenza vaccine recommendations.
8. **Measles, mumps, and rubella (MMR) vaccine.** (Minimum age: 12 months)
   - The second dose may be administered before age 4 years, provided at least 4 weeks have elapsed since the first dose.
   - Administer MMR vaccine to infants aged 6 through 11 months who are traveling internationally. These children should be revaccinated with 2 doses of MMR vaccine, the first at ages 12 through 15 months and at least 4 weeks after the previous dose, and the second at ages 4 through 6 years.
9. **Varicella (VAR) vaccine.** (Minimum age: 12 months)
   - The second dose may be administered before age 4 years, provided at least 3 months have elapsed since the first dose.
   - For children aged 12 months through 12 years, the recommended minimum interval between doses is 3 months. However, if the second dose was administered at least 4 weeks after the first dose, it can be accepted as valid.
10. **Hepatitis A (HepA) vaccine.** (Minimum age: 12 months)
    - Administer the second (final) dose 6 to18 months after the first.
    - Unvaccinated children 24 months and older at high risk should be vaccinated. See *MMWR* 2006;55(No. RR-7), available at http://www.cdc.gov/mmwr/pdf/rr/rr5507.pdf.
    - A 2-dose HepA vaccine series is recommended for anyone aged 24 months and older, previously unvaccinated, for whom immunity against hepatitis A virus infection is desired.
11. **Meningococcal conjugate vaccines, quadrivalent (MCV4).** (Minimum age: 9 months for Menactra [MCV4-D], 2 years for Menveo [MCV4-CRM])
    - For children aged 9 through 23 months 1) with persistent complement component deficiency; 2) who are residents of or travelers to countries with hyperendemic or epidemic disease; or 3) who are present during outbreaks caused by a vaccine serogroup, administer 2 primary doses of MCV4-D, ideally at ages 9 months and 12 months or at least 8 weeks apart.
    - For children aged 24 months and older with 1) persistent complement component deficiency who have not been previously vaccinated; or 2) anatomic/functional asplenia, administer 2 primary doses of either MCV4 at least 8 weeks apart.
    - For children with anatomic/functional asplenia, if MCV4-D (Menactra) is used, administer at a minimum age of 2 years and at least 4 weeks after completion of all PCV doses.
    - See *MMWR* 2011;60:72–6, available at http://www.cdc.gov/mmwr/pdf/wk/mm6003. pdf, and Vaccines for Children Program resolution No. 6/11-1, available at http://www. cdc.gov/vaccines/programs/vfc/downloads/resolutions/06-11mening-mcv.pdf, and *MMWR* 2011;60:1391–2, available at http://www.cdc.gov/mmwr/pdf/wk/mm6040. pdf, for further guidance, including revaccination guidelines.

This schedule is approved by the Advisory Committee on Immunization Practices (http://www.cdc.gov/vaccines/recs/acip), the American Academy of Pediatrics (http://www.aap.org), and the American Academy of Family Physicians (http://www.aafp.org).
Department of Health and Human Services • Centers for Disease Control and Prevention

FIGURE 22-1. Childhood immunization schedule.

immunization survey revealed that by age 11, most adolescents had received their childhood vaccines, and the rate of HPV vaccination among 11- to 12-year-old girls rose significantly from 11.1% to 30.5% within the previous 2 years. Results, however, also showed continuing problems with providers not offering all recommended vaccines when adolescents presented for vaccination visits (Stokley, Cohn, Jain, & McCauley, 2011). One study comparing vaccination rates of 12- to 18-year-olds at school-based health centers (SBHCs) and community health centers found significantly higher completion rates for most vaccines, even in populations with inadequate insurance coverage (Federico, Abrams, Everhart, Melinkovich, & Hambidge, 2010). Other considerations regarding communicable diseases involve their seasonality (e.g., mumps and varicella peak in April, pertussis and typhoid fever peak in August) and how climate change may affect the incidence and distribution of communicable diseases, especially vector- and water- and food-borne diseases (Greer, Ng, & Fisman, 2008). See Figure 22-2, adolescent immunization schedule.

With the marked rise in community-acquired methicillin-resistant *Staphylococcus aureus* (CA-MRSA), PHNs and school nurses must be alert when skin infections or other conditions do not resolve quickly in children and adolescents (Pallin et al., 2008). Sports teams, for instance, may spread this infection, along with others like molluscum contagiosum, as participants come into close contact. Referral to an infectious disease specialist may need to be considered.

Head Lice

Pediculosis (head lice) is a frustrating and common problem for many preschool and school-age children, and the incidence has been increasing with approximately 6 to 12 million 3- to-11-year-olds infected annually (CDC, 2010b). A classic study conducted by a school nurse in California found the highest incidence of head lice in her school district occurred among early elementary children, and that girls were three times more likely to have head lice than boys. Hispanic and White children had the highest rates, and Black children had the lowest rate (Estrada & Morris, 2000). Girls are thought to be at higher risk due to social behavior (closer contact, sharing of items), and close crowded conditions can also be a risk factor (CDC, 2010b). An infestation of *Pediculus humanus* var. *capitis*, the parasite that lives and feeds on the human scalp, can be an embarrassing nuisance to families of any socioeconomic level. These very tiny, wingless insects need blood to survive and can cause itching and skin irritation. They do not transmit disease, but secondary bacterial infections can occur from children scratching their scalps (CDC, 2010b). They are most often found toward the nape of the neck, where hair is usually thickest, but their pearly white eggs (nits) are distributed all over the head. They are attached to the hair shaft with a glue-like substance and can be detected by careful examination of the scalp. Because nits hatch within 10 days, and the immature louse can reach reproductive maturity within 8 to 9 days, recurring cycles of infestation are common. Without treatment, the cycle repeats every 3 weeks (Frankowski, Bocchini, & Council on School Health & Committee on Infectious Diseases, 2010). Complete eradication generally requires that all nits be removed along with lice.

Head lice are most often transmitted by direct contact (head-to-head) or may be passed from infected to uninfected children through shared items such as combs and brushes, hats, scarves, sheets, and towels (items called *fomites*). Contrary to some popular myths, lice do not fly or jump, and they cannot be contracted from animals—they live only on humans. They do not survive long off the human head, <3 days (CDC, 2010b; Frankowski et al., 2010). Schools may have recurring outbreaks of head lice that can be traced back to particular families who have failed to completely eradicate an infestation. Because of perceived social stigma, some families are defensive and unresponsive to attempts at education and intervention. Some schools resort to "no nit" policies and establish routine head lice examinations, with a goal of early detection and treatment. However, the American Academy of Pediatrics calls for abandonment of such policies because they have not been effective in curbing head lice infestations, they often result in significant lost school days and negative social impact, and they may lead to misdiagnosis and unnecessary treatment (Frankowski et al., 2010).

Treatment of head lice has been estimated to cost over $1 billion annually in direct and indirect costs (Frankowski et al., 2010). Treatment commonly includes over-the-counter insecticide shampoos, such as pyrethrin-based *RID*, *R&C*, *Pronto*, or *A200*. Malathion (*Ovide*) and benzyl alcohol lotion (Ulesfia lotion) are also recommended treatments. Lindane (*Kwell*) is no longer a recommended treatment for head lice (CDC, 2010b). Oral antibiotic and anthelmintic agents, such as Septra and Ivermectin, and natural products (*Hair-Clean 1-2-3; Clear Lice Egg Remover Gel*), as well as occlusive agents, such as petroleum jelly or essential oils, may also be used (Frankowski et al., 2010). Solvents that aid in dissolving the "cement" that holds the nit in place have been shown to be helpful when using fine-tooth combs (e.g., Lice Meister)—these include white vinegar and formic acid (Guenther, 2012). In some cases, resistance to topical pediculicides may necessitate the use of other measures. A custom machine, blasting hot air for 30 minutes (*Louse Buster*), has shown some promising results, but is expensive and requires training for operators. Frustrated families, having repeated problems with head lice infestations, have tried such unusual remedies as kerosene, acetone, bleach, vodka, and other extreme measures to try to kill lice and nits without success (Frankowski et al., 2010).

School nurses and PHNs also need to educate families about reducing reinfestation by careful cleaning and treatment of any fomites (e.g., combs, hats, towels, sheets, clothing, upholstered furniture) and scrupulous nit removal. Placing pillows and stuffed animals in

FIGURE 2: Recommended immunization schedule for persons aged 7 through 18 years—United States, 2012 (for those who fall behind or start late, see the schedule below and the catch-up schedule [Figure 3])

Vaccine ▼ Age ►	7–10 years	11–12 years	13–18 years
Tetanus, diphtheria, pertussis[1]	1 dose (if indicated)	1 dose	1 dose (if indicated)
Human papillomavirus[2]	see footnote[2]	3 doses	Complete 3-dose series
Meningococcal[3]	See footnote[3]	Dose 1	Booster at 16 years old
Influenza[4]	Influenza (yearly)		
Pneumococcal[5]	See footnote [5]		
Hepatitis A[6]	Complete 2-dose series		
Hepatitis B[7]	Complete 3-dose series		
Inactivated poliovirus[8]	Complete 3-dose series		
Measles, mumps, rubella[9]	Complete 2-dose series		
Varicella[10]	Complete 2-dose series		

Range of recommended ages for all children

Range of recommended ages for catch-up immunization

Range of recommended ages for certain high-risk groups

This schedule includes recommendations in effect as of December 23, 2011. Any dose not administered at the recommended age should be administered at a subsequent visit, when indicated and feasible. The use of a combination vaccine generally is preferred over separate injections of its equivalent component vaccines. Vaccination providers should consult the relevant Advisory Committee on Immunization Practices (ACIP) statement for detailed recommendations, available online at http://www.cdc.gov/vaccines/pubs/acip-list.htm. Clinically significant adverse events that follow vaccination should be reported to the Vaccine Adverse Event Reporting System (VAERS) online (http://www.vaers.hhs.gov) or by telephone (800-822-7967).

1. **Tetanus and diphtheria toxoids and acellular pertussis (Tdap) vaccine.** (Minimum age: 10 years for Boostrix and 11 years for Adacel)
   - Persons aged 11 through 18 years who have not received Tdap vaccine should receive a dose followed by tetanus and diphtheria toxoids (Td) booster doses every 10 years thereafter.
   - Tdap vaccine should be substituted for a single dose of Td in the catch-up series for children aged 7 through 10 years. Refer to the catch-up schedule if additional doses of tetanus and diphtheria toxoid–containing vaccine are needed.
   - Tdap vaccine can be administered regardless of the interval since the last tetanus and diphtheria toxoid–containing vaccine.
2. **Human papillomavirus (HPV) vaccines (HPV4 [Gardasil] and HPV2 [Cervarix]).** (Minimum age: 9 years)
   - Either HPV4 or HPV2 is recommended in a 3-dose series for females aged 11 or 12 years. HPV4 is recommended in a 3-dose series for males aged 11 or 12 years.
   - The vaccine series can be started beginning at age 9 years.
   - Administer the second dose 1 to 2 months after the first dose and the third dose 6 months after the first dose (at least 24 weeks after the first dose).
   - See *MMWR* 2010;59:626–32, available at http://www.cdc.gov/mmwr/pdf/wk/mm5920.pdf.
3. **Meningococcal conjugate vaccines, quadrivalent (MCV4).**
   - Administer MCV4 at age 11 through 12 years with a booster dose at age 16 years.
   - Administer MCV4 at age 13 through 18 years if patient is not previously vaccinated.
   - If the first dose is administered at age 13 through 15 years, a booster dose should be administered at age 16 through 18 years with a minimum interval of at least 8 weeks after the preceding dose.
   - If the first dose is administered at age 16 years or older, a booster dose is not needed.
   - Administer 2 primary doses at least 8 weeks apart to previously unvaccinated persons with persistent complement component deficiency or anatomic/functional asplenia, and 1 dose every 5 years thereafter.
   - Adolescents aged 11 through 18 years with human immunodeficiency virus (HIV) infection should receive a 2-dose primary series of MCV4, at least 8 weeks apart.
   - See *MMWR* 2011;60:72–76, available at http://www.cdc.gov/mmwr/pdf/wk/mm6003.pdf, and Vaccines for Children Program resolution No. 6/11-1, available at http://www.cdc.gov/vaccines/programs/vfc/downloads/resolutions/06-11mening-mcv.pdf, for further guidelines.
4. **Influenza vaccines (trivalent inactivated influenza vaccine [TIV] and live, attenuated influenza vaccine [LAIV]).**
   - For most healthy, nonpregnant persons, either LAIV or TIV may be used, except LAIV should not be used for some persons, including those with asthma or any other underlying medical conditions that predispose them to influenza complications. For all other contraindications to use of LAIV, see *MMWR* 2010;59(No.RR-8), available at http://www.cdc.gov/mmwr/pdf/rr/rr5908.pdf.
   - Administer 1 dose to persons aged 9 years and older.
   - For children aged 6 months through 8 years:
     — For the 2011–12 season, administer 2 doses (separated by at least 4 weeks) to those who did not receive at least 1 dose of the 2010–11 vaccine. Those who received at least 1 dose of the 2010–11 vaccine require 1 dose for the 2011–12 season.
     — For the 2012–13 season, follow dosing guidelines in the 2012 ACIP influenza vaccine recommendations.
5. **Pneumococcal vaccines (pneumococcal conjugate vaccine [PCV] and pneumococcal polysaccharide vaccine [PPSV]).**
   - A single dose of PCV may be administered to children aged 6 through 18 years who have anatomic/functional asplenia, HIV infection or other immunocompromising condition, cochlear implant, or cerebral spinal fluid leak. See *MMWR* 2010:59(No. RR-11), available at http://www.cdc.gov/mmwr/pdf/rr/rr5911.pdf.
   - Administer PPSV at least 8 weeks after the last dose of PCV to children aged 2 years or older with certain underlying medical conditions, including a cochlear implant. A single revaccination should be administered after 5 years to children with anatomic/functional asplenia or an immunocompromising condition.
6. **Hepatitis A (HepA) vaccine.**
   - HepA vaccine is recommended for children older than 23 months who live in areas where vaccination programs target older children, who are at increased risk for infection, or for whom immunity against hepatitis A virus infection is desired. See *MMWR* 2006;55(No. RR-7), available at http://www.cdc.gov/mmwr/pdf/rr/rr5507.pdf.
   - Administer 2 doses at least 6 months apart to unvaccinated persons.
7. **Hepatitis B (HepB) vaccine.**
   - Administer the 3-dose series to those not previously vaccinated.
   - For those with incomplete vaccination, follow the catch-up recommendations (Figure 3).
   - A 2-dose series (doses separated by at least 4 months) of adult formulation Recombivax HB is licensed for use in children aged 11 through 15 years.
8. **Inactivated poliovirus vaccine (IPV).**
   - The final dose in the series should be administered at least 6 months after the previous dose.
   - If both OPV and IPV were administered as part of a series, a total of 4 doses should be administered, regardless of the child's current age.
   - IPV is not routinely recommended for U.S. residents aged18 years or older.
9. **Measles, mumps, and rubella (MMR) vaccine.**
   - The minimum interval between the 2 doses of MMR vaccine is 4 weeks.
10. **Varicella (VAR) vaccine.**
    - For persons without evidence of immunity (see *MMWR* 2007;56[No. RR-4], available at http://www.cdc.gov/mmwr/pdf/rr/rr5604.pdf), administer 2 doses if not previously vaccinated or the second dose if only 1 dose has been administered.
    - For persons aged 7 through 12 years, the recommended minimum interval between doses is 3 months. However, if the second dose was administered at least 4 weeks after the first dose, it can be accepted as valid.
    - For persons aged 13 years and older, the minimum interval between doses is 4 weeks.

This schedule is approved by the Advisory Committee on Immunization Practices (http://www.cdc.gov/vaccines/recs/acip), the American Academy of Pediatrics (http://www.aap.org), and the American Academy of Family Physicians (http://www.aafp.org).
Department of Health and Human Services • Centers for Disease Control and Prevention

FIGURE 22-2. Adolescent immunization schedule.

airtight bags, drying sheets, blankets and towels on high heat, and washing all hats and clothing are effective measures. It is not necessary to use fumigant sprays, as they can be toxic (CDC, 2010b). It is difficult, however, to prevent children—who are social creatures—from coming into close contact with one another and becoming reinfected. In some larger cities, entrepreneurs have started nit removal businesses (e.g., Nit Pickers, Hair Fairies) to assist parents with this tedious task.

Other Health Problems

Other health problems found in this age group are nutritional problems (primarily overeating and inappropriate food choices) and poor dental health. Obesity often begins in childhood and becomes a risk factor for CVD and diabetes later in life (Dietz, 2009; Dixon, Pena, & Taveras, 2012; Nadeau, Maahs, Daniels, & Eckel, 2011). The percentage of children who are obese has risen over 13% between 1980 and 2008, with 19.2% of children aged 6 to 17 considered obese in 2007–2008 (Fig. 22-3), despite the fact that 24% of American children lived in households characterized by food insecurity at some time during the year with rates steadily rising since the recent recession (Child Trends Databank, 2012b).

Food allergies can also play a role in poor nutritional status, especially with school-age children and adolescents. Although 20% of children and adolescents may report a food allergy (Noimark & Cox, 2008), one classic study in England noted that only 2.3% of 11- and 15-year-old children actually demonstrated sensitivity upon skin testing and double-blind food challenges (Pereira et al., 2005). Food allergies can be especially problematic in the school setting (see Chapter 30), and new food labeling initiated in 2006 makes identification of the eight most common food allergens (i.e., milk, eggs, fish, shellfish, tree nuts, peanuts, wheat, soybeans) a much easier process (U.S. Department of Agriculture (USDA)., 2011a).

Dental caries is another common problem among school-age children. Over 16% of U.S. schoolchildren have untreated cavities, but the rate for children living below the poverty level is much higher at 26% (FCFS, n.d.c).

Childhood Obesity

About one third of U.S. children are classified as overweight or at risk of becoming overweight (FCFS, n.a.a). The CDC uses the term **overweight**, rather than obese, in defining children who have a body mass index (BMI) at or above the 95th percentile. Children with a BMI between the 85th and 94th percentile are defined as **at risk of overweight** (Ogden & Carroll, 2010). (See Display 22.1 for an explanation and examples.) The obesity rate has tripled for children and adolescents, and about 17% of children aged 2 to 19 are obese. Obese children are more likely to become obese adults. A classic Surgeon General's report states that there is a 70% chance of adult overweight or obesity if an adolescent is overweight; if at least one parent is overweight, the risk jumps to 80% (2007). Results of a recent Youth Risk Behavior Survey (YRBS) indicated that almost 78% of high school students surveyed ate fewer than five servings of fruits and vegetables the day before, and almost 30% drank soda at least once a day (CDC, 2011g).

The poor eating habits that develop during childhood are generally thought to persist into adulthood, contributing to the leading causes of death and disability—CVD, cancer, and diabetes. Treating hypertension and high cholesterol, stopping tobacco use, controlling diabetes, reducing obesity, and improving physical activity are all helpful in reducing CVD. Evidence of early atherosclerosis and fatty streaks has been found in autopsy studies of children as young as 6 years, and many now acknowledge the need to prevent cumulative cardiac risk factors (Masia et al., 2009). Preventive measures and early management of cardiovascular risk factors is now considered a more effective form of treatment than just clinical treatment of the disease complications after the fact. Aside from its relationship with inactivity, television viewing and other sedentary behaviors have been associated with higher intake of fats, sweet and salty snacks, and carbonated drinks, as well as lower intakes of fruits and vegetables in a systematic review of studies with children, adolescents, and adults (Pearson & Biddle, 2011). Watching television while eating meals has been shown to lead to increased frequency of poor food choices, and food is the most heavily advertised product on children's television. Highly sweetened products (e.g., sweetened beverages and sugar-rich cereals), as well as fast food, are the most frequently advertised foods. American children and adolescents watch more than 3 to 4 hours of television daily, and increased television watching has been associated with less exercise, increased overweight, lower grades, and less time spent reading (AACAP, 2011b). Perhaps due to recent public scrutiny and concern, one study found that overall food ads dropped among the 2- to 11-age group. However, these ads increased among adolescents (12–17 years). While ads for sugar-sweetened beverages (fruit drinks, sodas) dropped in younger children, fast food ads increased for all age groups (Powell, Szczypka, & Chaloupka, 2010).

As children move from elementary to middle school, their food choices change dramatically. Fad diets and peer pressure become more of an issue. Media fast food promotion, targeted to middle and high school students, is common. Diets most often include fast food French fries and hamburgers, pizza, and sweetened carbonated beverages. The average adolescent diet consists of excess fat and added sugars, and often is lacking in micronutrients, such as calcium, iron, and zinc, as well as many vitamins and folic acid. Deficits in micronutrients can compromise development; some people advocate multiple food fortification to improve nutritional status and reduce anemia, but unequivocal evidence is lacking (Best et al., 2011). This is a time when school-based nutrition education programs can have an influence, and a national study found some decrease in low-nutrition/high sugar/high-fat foods in middle and high schools. Some high school à la carte menus now offer reduced-fat

FIGURE 3. Catch-up immunization schedule for persons aged 4 months through 18 years who start late or who are more than 1 month behind —United States • 2012
The figure below provides catch-up schedules and minimum intervals between doses for children whose vaccinations have been delayed. A vaccine series does not need to be restarted, regardless of the time that has elapsed between doses. Use the section appropriate for the child's age. **Always use this table in conjunction with the accompanying childhood and adolescent immunization schedules (Figures 1 and 2) and their respective footnotes.**

Persons aged 4 months through 6 years					
Vaccine	Minimum Age for Dose 1	Minimum Interval Between Doses			
		Dose 1 to dose 2	Dose 2 to dose 3	Dose 3 to dose 4	Dose 4 to dose 5
Hepatitis B	Birth	4 weeks	8 weeks and at least 16 weeks after first dose; minimum age for the final dose is 24 weeks		
Rotavirus[1]	6 weeks	4 weeks	4 weeks[1]		
Diphtheria, tetanus, pertussis[2]	6 weeks	4 weeks	4 weeks	6 months	6 months[2]
Haemophilus influenzae type b[3]	6 weeks	4 weeks if first dose administered at younger than age 12 months 8 weeks (as final dose) if first dose administered at age 12–14 months No further doses needed if first dose administered at age 15 months or older	4 weeks[3] if current age is younger than 12 months 8 weeks (as final dose)[3] if current age is 12 months or older and first dose administered at younger than age 12 months and second dose administered at younger than 15 months No further doses needed if previous dose administered at age 15 months or older	8 weeks (as final dose) This dose only necessary for children aged 12 months through 59 months who received 3 doses before age 12 months	
Pneumococcal[4]	6 weeks	4 weeks if first dose administered at younger than age 12 months 8 weeks (as final dose for healthy children) if first dose administered at age 12 months or older or current age 24 through 59 months No further doses needed for healthy children if first dose administered at age 24 months or older	4 weeks if current age is younger than 12 months 8 weeks (as final dose for healthy children) if current age is 12 months or older No further doses needed for healthy children if previous dose administered at age 24 months or older	8 weeks (as final dose) This dose only necessary for children aged 12 months through 59 months who received 3 doses before age 12 months or for children at high risk who received 3 doses at any age	
Inactivated poliovirus[5]	6 weeks	4 weeks	4 weeks	6 months[5] minimum age 4 years for final dose	
Meningococcal[6]	9 months	8 weeks[6]			
Measles, mumps, rubella[7]	12 months	4 weeks			
Varicella[8]	12 months	3 months			
Hepatitis A	12 months	6 months			
Persons aged 7 through 18 years					
Tetanus, diphtheria/ tetanus, diphtheria, pertussis[9]	7 years[9]	4 weeks	4 weeks if first dose administered at younger than age 12 months 6 months if first dose administered at 12 months or older	6 months if first dose administered at younger than age 12 months	
Human papillomavirus[10]	9 years	Routine dosing intervals are recommended[10]			
Hepatitis A	12 months	6 months			
Hepatitis B	Birth	4 weeks	8 weeks (and at least 16 weeks after first dose)		
Inactivated poliovirus[5]	6 weeks	4 weeks	4 weeks[5]	6 months[5]	
Meningococcal[6]	9 months	8 weeks[6]			
Measles, mumps, rubella[7]	12 months	4 weeks			
Varicella[8]	12 months	3 months if person is younger than age 13 years 4 weeks if person is aged 13 years or older			

1. **Rotavirus (RV) vaccines (RV-1 [Rotarix] and RV-5 [Rota Teq]).**
   - The maximum age for the first dose in the series is 14 weeks, 6 days; and 8 months, 0 days for the final dose in the series. Vaccination should not be initiated for infants aged 15 weeks, 0 days or older.
   - If RV-1 was administered for the first and second doses, a third dose is not indicated.
2. **Diphtheria and tetanus toxoids and acellular pertussis (DTaP) vaccine.**
   - The fifth dose is not necessary if the fourth dose was administered at age 4 years or older.
3. ***Haemophilus influenzae* type b (Hib) conjugate vaccine.**
   - Hib vaccine should be considered for unvaccinated persons aged 5 years or older who have sickle cell disease, leukemia, human immunodeficiency virus (HIV) infection, or anatomic/functional asplenia.
   - If the first 2 doses were PRP-OMP (PedvaxHIB or Comvax) and were administered at age 11 months or younger, the third (and final) dose should be administered at age 12 through 15 months and at least 8 weeks after the second dose.
   - If the first dose was administered at age 7 through 11 months, administer the second dose at least 4 weeks later and a final dose at age 12 through 15 months.
4. **Pneumococcal vaccines.** (Minimum age: 6 weeks for pneumococcal conjugate vaccine [PCV]; 2 years for pneumococcal polysaccharide vaccine [PPSV])
   - For children aged 24 through 71 months with underlying medical conditions, administer 1 dose of PCV if 3 doses of PCV were received previously, or administer 2 doses of PCV at least 8 weeks apart if fewer than 3 doses of PCV were received previously.
   - A single dose of PCV may be administered to certain children aged 6 through 18 years with underlying medical conditions. See age-specific schedules for details.
   - Administer PPSV to children aged 2 years or older with certain underlying medical conditions. See *MMWR* 2010:59(No. RR-11), available at http://www.cdc.gov/mmwr/pdf/rr/rr5911.pdf.
5. **Inactivated poliovirus vaccine (IPV).**
   - A fourth dose is not necessary if the third dose was administered at age 4 years or older and at least 6 months after the previous dose.
   - In the first 6 months of life, minimum age and minimum intervals are only recommended if the person is at risk for imminent exposure to circulating poliovirus (i.e., travel to a polio-endemic region or during an outbreak).
   - IPV is not routinely recommended for U.S. residents aged 18 years or older.
6. **Meningococcal conjugate vaccines, quadrivalent (MCV4).** (Minimum age: 9 months for Menactra [MCV4-D]; 2 years for Menveo [MCV4-CRM])
   - See Figure 1 ("Recommended immunization schedule for persons aged 0 through 6 years") and Figure 2 ("Recommended immunization schedule for persons aged 7 through 18 years") for further guidance.
7. **Measles, mumps, and rubella (MMR) vaccine.**
   - Administer the second dose routinely at age 4 through 6 years.
8. **Varicella (VAR) vaccine.**
   - Administer the second dose routinely at age 4 through 6 years. If the second dose was administered at least 4 weeks after the first dose, it can be accepted as valid.
9. **Tetanus and diphtheria toxoids (Td) and tetanus and diphtheria toxoids and acellular pertussis (Tdap) vaccines.**
   - For children aged 7 through 10 years who are not fully immunized with the childhood DTaP vaccine series, Tdap vaccine should be substituted for a single dose of Td vaccine in the catch-up series; if additional doses are needed, use Td vaccine. For these children, an adolescent Tdap vaccine dose should not be given.
   - An inadvertent dose of DTaP vaccine administered to children aged 7 through 10 years can count as part of the catch-up series. This dose can count as the adolescent Tdap dose, or the child can later receive a Tdap booster dose at age 11–12 years.
10. **Human papillomavirus (HPV) vaccines (HPV4 [Gardasil] and HPV2 [Cervarix]).**
    - Administer the vaccine series to females (either HPV2 or HPV4) and males (HPV4) at age 13 through 18 years if patient is not previously vaccinated.
    - Use recommended routine dosing intervals for vaccine series catch-up; see Figure 2 ("Recommended immunization schedule for persons aged 7 through 18 years").

Clinically significant adverse events that follow vaccination should be reported to the Vaccine Adverse Event Reporting System (VAERS) online (http://www.vaers.hhs.gov) or by telephone (800-822-7967). Suspected cases of vaccine-preventable diseases should be reported to the state or local health department. Additional information, including precautions and contraindications for vaccination, is available from CDC online (http://www.cdc.gov/vaccines) or by telephone (800-CDC-INFO [800-232-4636]).

FIGURE 22-3. Catch-up schedule for immunizations.

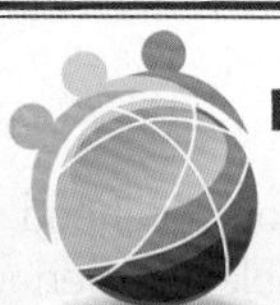

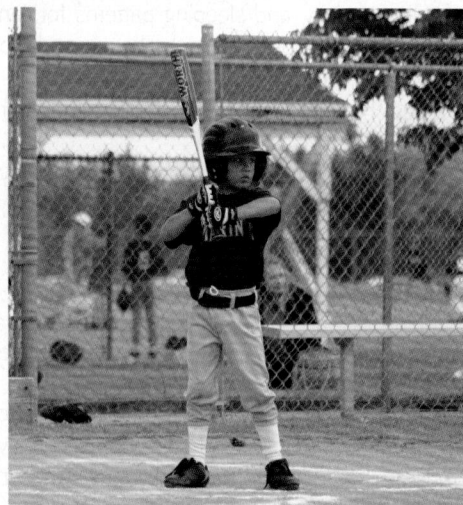

DISPLAY 22.1 EXPLANATION AND EXAMPLES OF OVERWEIGHT CLASSIFICATION FOR CHILDREN AND TEENS

Body mass index (BMI) is used as a screening tool to identify weight problems in children and teens. The criteria are different from those used for adults, as body fat differs between boys and girls, and the amount of body fat changes with age. BMI-for-age growth charts for boys and girls are available at http://www.cdc.gov/growthcharts.

Weight Status Category	***Percentile Range***
Underweight	Less than the 5th percentile
Healthy weight	5th percentile to less than the 85th percentile
At risk of overweight	85th to less than the 95th percentile
Overweight	Equal to or greater than the 95th percentile

Source: Centers for Disease Control and Prevention. (2011). *About BMI for Children & Teens.* From http://www.cdc.gov/healthyweight/assessing/bmi/childrens_bmi/about_childrens_bmi.html

items, and a small association was found between school food environment and types of food consumed/student BMIs (Terry-McElrath, O'Malley, Delva, & Johnston, 2009). See Using the Nursing Process.

For many years, research studies have examined childhood obesity and its causes, even examining infant temperament and eating style with later weight gains (Faith & Hittner, 2010). In longitudinal research, preschool children whose BMI was greater than the 85th percentile were five times more likely to continue to be overweight at age 12. Children younger than age 9 with a BMI between the 75th and 85th percentiles have been shown to have a 40% to 50% greater chance of being overweight by age 12 (Nader et al., 2006). A longitudinal cohort study found that failure to self-regulate, or control impulsive behaviors, in 3- to 5-year-old children predicted higher BMI and most rapid BMI gains over the 9 years of the study (Francis & Susman, 2009). In another long-term study following children from age 5 to age 15, intake of sweetened beverages (not fruit juice or milk) was associated with greater adiposity and higher body fat percentages, and waist circumference at age 15 (Fiorito, Marini, Francis, Smiciklas-Wright, & Birch, 2009). Parents can help their younger children develop better habits by implementing suggestions recommended by the American Heart Association (2011), for example:

- Serve a variety of fruits and vegetables. Limit juice to 4 to 6 oz. per day.
- Keep fat intake between 25% and 35% of total daily calories (aged 4 to 18).
- Provide foods low in saturated fat, trans fat, cholesterol, added sugar, and salt.
- Encourage kids to eat only enough calories to maintain healthy weight.
- Help kids be physically active at least 60 minutes each day.
- Serve whole-grain/high-fiber cereals and breads.
- Serve low-fat and fat-free dairy products (two to three cups of milk daily).
- Serve fish more often, but avoid fried fish.
- Keep introducing a variety of healthy foods, but don't overfeed your child.

Physical activity is important in preventing childhood obesity. Author's private photo with Permission of Holly Raphael.

Inadequate Nutrition

Poor nutritional status of schoolchildren is a global issue, but also a problem in this country (Best et al., 2010). Undernutrition can also have serious consequences, including effects on the cognitive development and academic performance of children and chronic health (Kirkpatrick, McIntyre, & Potestio, 2010; Weitzman & Zhou, 2012). Classic research indicates that food insecurity in kindergarten is associated with poorer mathematics performance in children and in delayed reading performance and social skills for girls (Jyoti, Frongillo, & Jones, 2005). Irritability, lack of energy, and difficulty concentrating are only some of the problems that arise from skipped meals or consistently inadequate nutrition. Infection and illness that lead to loss of school days can affect academic progress and interfere with the acquisition of basic skills, such as reading and mathematics. Food insecurity has been associated with child development problems, psychological and social issues, and poor general health (Weitzman & Zhou, 2012).

About 14.5% of U.S. households reported some degree of food insecurity in 2010, representing 48.8 million people. Over 20% of households with children were

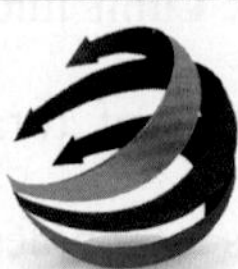

USING THE NURSING PROCESS

James Lopez is entering third grade. His teacher comes to you, the school nurse, because she is concerned about his poor performance in school. He frequently comes to school late and often puts his head on his desk and appears to be falling asleep. You notice that James has gained a significant amount of weight over the summer. His face is much fuller now than in his second-grade picture.

Assessment (Initial Visits)

You call James' mother and make an appointment for a home visit.

You do a health history, noting family history of diabetes, current eating, activity, and sleeping patterns for James and the family, and determine whether he has a regular physician and insurance or Medicaid.

You assess his vital signs, height and weight, hearing, and vision.

You talk more with his teacher about his activity on the playground and any signs of excessive thirst, hunger, or general fatigue.

Nursing Diagnoses

After a home visit, a meeting with James' teacher, and two observations and interviews with James, you decide on the following nursing diagnoses:

1. Nutrition: More than Body Requirements related to James' eating as a way of coping and his sedentary lifestyle.
2. Altered Family Process related to mother's recent change from being a stay-at-home single mom to attending truck driving school (necessitating absences of several days at a time, with James cared for by a married teenage sister and her husband).

Findings, Plan, and Implementation

James has been eating large quantities of snack food and fast food meals for the last 3 months, since his mother started her training. He has also quit participating in soccer and baseball, because his mother can no longer provide transportation. His bicycle was recently stolen, and he spends a lot of time playing video and computer games. James misses his mother when she is away and says that he "stays up late watching television" and has "trouble getting up for school" when he is at his sister's house.

You plan to work with the family to refer James to his physician to rule out diabetes. A family meeting is scheduled so that you can provide some health education on childhood obesity and inactivity. You discuss some possible interventions that the family can put into place:

- Decrease reliance on fast food meals.
- Have a regular evening mealtime and encourage less snacking.
- Provide fresh fruit and vegetable snacks and decrease purchases of high-calorie, high-fat snack foods.
- Decrease sedentary activity (e.g., video and computer games, television viewing) and increase physical activity (e.g., team sports, walking, bicycling, active outdoor games).
- Establish a reasonable bedtime and consistently enforce it.
- Offer referral for family counseling so that James can discuss his feelings in a safe environment.
- With the family's input, seek ways for James and his mother to keep in better contact and for his sister to gain a greater understanding of good parenting practices.
- Meet with the teacher, the family, and James to discuss ways to help with his school performance.
- Continue to monitor James' progress with monthly height and weight checks, personal interviews, home visits, and teacher conferences.

Evaluation

The physician reported that James does not have diabetes; however, if he continues to gain weight and remains inactive he is at a higher risk for type 2 diabetes. Evaluation of nursing diagnoses 1 and 2 includes the following goals:

- The family will report less reliance on fast food and more meals cooked at home.
- The family will report more purchases of fresh fruits and vegetables and fewer purchases of high-calorie, high-fat snacks.
- James will report more physical exercise (by the use of a calendar) and fewer hours spent in sedentary activity (corroborated by family).
- James will exhibit less tardiness and fewer signs of sleep deprivation at school, and his school performance will improve.
- James and his family will complete sessions with a family counselor.
- James' weight will remain stable or will decrease as his height increases over time.

food insecure, and of those headed by single women with children, 35.1% reported food insecurity (FRAC, 2011). A national study of food insecurity found that it was associated with overweight status in children between the ages of 12 and 17, especially girls and children living in poverty (Casey Jones, & Hare, 2006). However, reviews of research studies done over the past 15 years have shown mixed results with the association of food insecurity and childhood obesity (Eisenmann, Gundersen, Lohman, Garasky, & Stewart, 2011; Larson, & Story, 2011). There is some indication that there is a significant relationship between food insecurity and increased BMI in young adult females, and a growing consensus that both problems warrant further research (Gooding, Walls, & Richmond, 2011; Gunderson, Garasky, & Lohman, 2009).

An analysis of data from the Panel Study of Income Dynamics found that poverty during the earliest stages of life was "significantly associated with increased adult body mass index" for both males and females (Ziol-Guest, Duncan, & Kalil, 2009, p 527). An earlier study by Olson, Bove, and Miller (2007) conducted a qualitative and quantitative study to examine how childhood poverty-associated food deprivation may lead to adult obesity. They found that, in some cases, early deprivation influenced later food choices and that there was an active drive to avoid food insecurity. Women in their study also developed patterns of emotional eating, and they concluded that attitudes and behaviors toward food were formed in childhood as a response to deprivation. Food insecurity in childhood has been linked to both undernutrition and overnutrition, and is most harmful during critical periods of development; it is also linked to postponed medical care and medications, lack of routine well-child medical visits, and absence of a usual source of health care for children (Ma, Gee, & Kushel, 2008). Because poor households around the world often spend 50% to 80% of their income on food, and with concerns about cuts to nutrition programs and higher food prices, concerns are growing about the development of an entire generation (De Pee et al., 2010).

Undernutrition is frequently associated with poverty and hunger, but social pressure to be thin can also spark purposeful undernutrition. Because prepubertal children often exhibit a period of adiposity before a growth spurt, they are at risk for developing eating disorders (Culbert et al., 2009). Along with childhood obesity, prevention of eating disorders is also a high priority in this age group (Neumark-Sztainer, 2009). A 5-year study of the frequency of reading magazine articles about dieting and weight loss found that girls who frequently read these magazines were two times more likely to engage in unhealthful weight-control measures (e.g., skipping meals, smoking more cigarettes, fasting) than those who did not read magazine articles about dieting and weight loss. Extreme weight-control measures (e.g., laxative use, vomiting) were found three times more often in high-frequency readers versus nonreaders (van den Berg, Neumark-Sztainer, Hannan, & Haines, 2007). The recent YRBS found that almost 11% of high school students reported not eating for 24 hours or more in order to keep from gaining or lose weight; vomiting and laxatives were used by 4% (CDC, 2011g). DeLeel, Hughes, Miller, Hipwell, and Theodore (2009) found that 11% of 9-year-old girls scored in the anorexic range on body image and eating disturbance measures among a racially and SES study population. Body image and dieting behaviors are prevalent among younger children. While there has been some concern about the possibility that obesity prevention measures may lead to eating disorders, no real evidence of that has surfaced, and experts feel that both problems can be effectively addressed through evidence-based interventions. Suggestions include stressing family meals and physical activities, promoting a positive body image, and decreasing media focus. More specific suggestions include:

- Foods to *encourage* (fruits, vegetables) versus foods to *limit* (high-fat/high-sugar/low nutritional value), rather than *good* or *bad* foods.
- A focus on dietary restraint/portion size rather than dieting or deprivation.
- More research on the continuum of mindless eating to obsessive preoccupation with food intake and on helping individuals better use internal cues for hunger or satiety.
- Simultaneous promotion of healthy eating behaviors while protecting positive body images in children (Schwartz & Henderson, 2009).

It is important to talk with overweight children and adolescents about their experiences of being mistreated due to their problems with weight, and to encourage families to not just talk about weight, but to do more together to promote healthy eating and increased physical activity (Neumark-Sztainer, 2009). A randomized controlled trial found that efforts to retrain eating behaviors (e.g., slowing down eating speed, reducing total food intake, lifestyle modification) were helpful in reducing BMI in obese adolescents (Ford et al., 2010). A systematic review of school-based physical activity programs for children and adolescents found some evidence of positive effects, and physical activity promotion in schools is recommended (Dobbins, DeCorby, Robeson, Husson, & Tirilis, 2009). School nurses and PHNs can provide families with necessary information to promote healthful eating and exercise.

Inactivity

An association between poor eating habits and physical inactivity has been found in numerous research studies (Sallis & Glanz, 2009). More television watching, fewer family meals eaten together at home, and living in an unsafe neighborhood were shown to be associated with overweight (Gable, Chang, & Krull, 2007). The YRBS revealed that 66.7% of children surveyed who were enrolled in physical education classes did not attend class on a daily basis. In addition, fewer than 19% of respondents stated that they were physically active for 60 minutes daily. Almost 33% watched three or more hours of television daily and just below 25% used a computer (other than for schoolwork) or played a video game on a daily basis (CDC, 2011g). Children who watched television and were less physically active during after-school hours were more likely to become overweight by age 12 in one 12-year longitudinal study of almost 1,000 children (O'Brien et al., 2007). One study noted that television advertising, not just television viewing, was associated with obesity in children (Zimmerman & Bell, 2010).

In a study of adolescent girls and their families, researchers found that parents' modeling of physical activity, television viewing, fruit and vegetable consumption, and use of soft drinks were significantly associated with the teens' behaviors, indicating that improvements in parent behaviors can affect adolescents (Bauer, Neumark-Sztainer, Fulkerson, Hannan, & Story, 2011). School nurses and PHNs can work with families to increase their levels of physical activity and to encourage limited television viewing for school-age children. They can also advocate for increased physical education in the school setting, and for increased safe recreational opportunities in all neighborhoods.

Dental Health

Dental caries affects 42% of children between the ages of 2 and 11, with 23% having untreated cavities in primary (baby) teeth. About 21% of children (6–11 years of age) have dental caries in their permanent teeth and 8% have untreated caries. Mexican American children have the highest rates of decay in both primary and permanent teeth (National Institute of Dental & Craniofacial Research [NIDCR], 2011). In a classic study, comparing African refugee children with U.S. children, the rate of dental caries for refugee children was half that of U.S. children (Cote et al., 2004). Poor children report twice the rate of untreated dental caries than do children from higher-income families (Division of Oral Health, 2008). One twin study found that traits for dental caries and sucrose sweetness preference exhibit an independent "genetic contribution" (Bretz et al., 2006, p. 1,156), and later research identified genetic variation in three taste pathway genes and found two of these significantly associated with risk of dental caries (Wendell et al., 2010).

The prevalence of dental caries in school-age children has decreased significantly since the early 1970s because of community fluoridation projects and the use of fluoride toothpaste (FCFS, n.d.c). Fluoridated drinking water, the availability of school-provided fluoride rinse or gel, and dental sealant programs are cost-effective, proven methods of reducing dental caries in school-age children (Lam, 2008). Between 11% and 72% of poor children have been found to have early childhood caries, an infectious disease thought to be caused by *Streptococcus mutans* and exacerbated by poor dietary practices. Topical antimicrobial therapies show some promise in these cases (Kroll & Nedley, 2007).

The peak incidence of dental caries is found among school-age children and adolescents, although the effects of decay are observed in adulthood as caries activity recurs or various restorations fracture or wear out and must be replaced. In 2009, 84% of school-age children visited a dentist in the past year, but for children living in poverty, only about 75% did, and a little of 50% of uninsured children saw a dentist (FCFS, n.d.d). These rates have improved slightly with coverage through the State Children's Health Insurance Program (SCHIP), and the rate of caries in permanent teeth of school children also decreased from 75% in 2000 to 85% in 2007 over the decade of *Healthy People 2010* with the expansion of sealant programs (Edelstein & Chinn, 2009; Tomar & Reeves, 2009). Yet, access to dental care is still problematic. Barriers to dental care are more prevalent among the poor and those who are institutionalized.

Financial barriers and lack of education lead to poor dental health values and adversely affect the appropriate use of early dental services and conscientious personal oral health care. School-based dental sealant program research was reviewed and found to be effective in managing cavities in this age group (Gooch et al., 2009). A systematic review of evidence for the use of prescription fluoride supplements noted that these should be prescribed when drinking water is deficient in fluoride and children are at high risk of developing cavities (Rozier et al., 2010). PHNs and other community health nurses working with school-age children and families can promote good dental health through education and advocacy, as well as through collaboration to provide adequate dental services to uninsured children and promotion of fluoridation and sealant programs.

ADOLESCENT HEALTH

Adolescence is a time of self-discovery, movement toward self-reliance, increasing opportunities, and pivotal choices that can affect the remainder of an individual's life. Adolescence generally begins with puberty and encompasses the ages between 10 and 24; it consists of early adolescence (aged 10–14), middle adolescence (15–17), and late adolescence (18 to mid-20s). Adult society largely segregates adolescents and often has ambiguous expectations for them (Damon & Lerner, 2008). Adolescents are part of a subculture, one with its own language, dress, social mores, and values. The tasks of adolescence remain fairly constant: Adolescents must become autonomous, come to grips with their emerging sexuality and the skills necessary to attract a mate, and acquire skills and education that can prepare them for adult roles, all while resolving identity issues and developing values and beliefs (Damon & Lerner, 2008; Dayan, Bernard, Olliac, Mailhes, & Kermarrec, 2010). The search for and expression of developing identity, along with the strong drive for social acceptance, are evident in the personal home pages and blogs of adolescents on social networking Internet sites such as Twitter and Facebook (Schmitt, Dayanim, & Matthias, 2008).

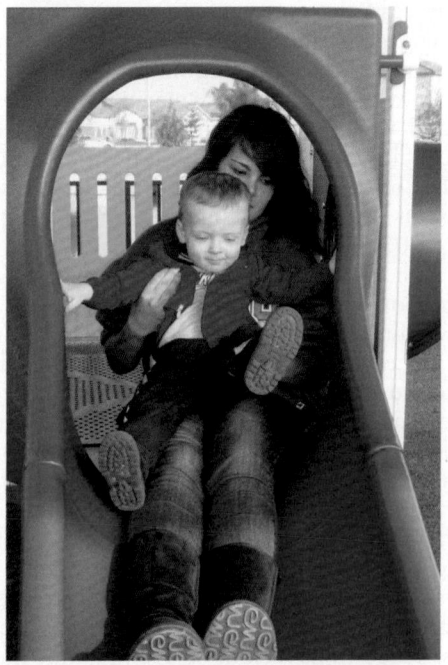

Common first jobs for adolescents include babysitting and yard work. Author's private photo with Permissions of Merysa Schultz, Deanna Rector, Jon Rector.

Adolescents are generally healthy, but parents and teens may differ in their perceptions of the adolescent's health. Adolescents from lower-income brackets frequently report poorer health than those from higher-income groups (Johnson & Wang, 2008). As with other population groups, socioeconomic level and health are inversely related for adolescents. Adolescents also exhibit inverse relationships between income level and school achievement, most likely due to a lack of successful strategies for academic success (Oyserman, Johnson, & James, 2011). Parental long-term unemployment is also negatively associated with adolescent self-reported health status and depressive symptoms and psychosomatic complaints. These, along with poor health behaviors related to lack of physical activity and drug use or smoking, contribute to self-perceived poor or fair health (Piko, 2007). Social stressors and strained relations with peers and parents are also related to health complaints, including psychosomatic complaints (Damon & Lerner, 2008; Hjern, Alfven, & Ostberg, 2008). Common complaints of adolescents include sleep deprivation, fatigue, chronic insomnia, acne, and concerns about weight and body image (Chung & Cheung, 2008; Koch, Ryder, Dziura, Njike, & Antaya, 2008). As children become adolescents, their sleep patterns change—they move from early risers/sleepers to staying up later and sleeping in later, or catching up on sleep over weekends. This transition becomes more apparent through high school. Scientists believe that these changes in circadian and homeostatic sleep regulation support this delayed sleep phase, and there are concerns about consistent lack of sleep (Hagenauer, Perryman, Lee, & Carskadon, 2009). A national survey of adolescents revealed that 68.9% reported getting insufficient sleep and this was associated with higher odds of several risk behaviors such as use of cigarettes, alcohol, and tobacco, as well as current sexual activity, physical fighting, and physical inactivity (McKnight-Eily et al., 2011). Another U.S. survey of over 14,000 adolescents corroborated the association of short sleep duration and high cholesterol, with "each additional hour of sleep ... associated with ... significantly decreased odds of being diagnosed with high cholesterol in young adulthood" for females (Gangwisch, Malaspina, Babiss, Opler, 2010, p. 956). Lytle, Pasch, and Farbakhsh (2011) found a relationship between sleep duration and BMI in middle school students, but did not find the same results among high school students. They noted that waking up later on weekends was related to lower body fat and healthier weight for girls, but not for boys, and warned "inadequate sleep is a risk factor for early adolescent obesity" (p. 324). Sleep deprivation, along with television viewing time, has been related to increased BMI and blood pressure, and a poor body weight perception (being overweight or underweight) has predicted problem behaviors in both male and female adolescents (Wells et al., 2008). A small (n = 201) study examining the effects of moving the start of school from 8 AM to 8:30 AM found that more adolescents reported getting 8 hours of sleep (16.4%–54.7%) and there were significant improvements in health, mood, and alertness with the delayed start time (Owens, Belon, & Moss, 2010).

In the past, routine health care visits by adolescents were not commonplace. However, newer recommended vaccines and better awareness of the health needs of adolescents have led to improvement, but concerns remain. In 2006, over 84% of 10- to 17-year-olds had a physician visit within the past year, but only 66.2% had a well-child checkup (Mulye et al., 2009). Irwin, Adams, Park, and Newacheck (2009) evaluated data from a national survey and found that 38% of adolescents had a visit for preventive care within the last year, but only 40% spent time alone with their health care provider. Sadly, only 10% had all areas of recommended anticipatory guidance addressed (e.g., healthy diet, seat belt/helmet use, smoking/secondhand smoke), and teens from low-income or uninsured families were at greater risk of not having any preventive health care visits. Most health care visits for adolescents were for female reproductive health care, and birth control was a common prescription written at outpatient visits.

While hospitalization rates for adolescents are low, the leading cause of hospitalization in 15- to 24-year-olds is pregnancy related. Trauma and mental disorders were the next two causes of hospitalization, and trauma-related disorders are the leading reason for emergency room visits. Almost 17% of adolescents have some special health care need (Mulye et al., 2009). About 20% of 12- to 17-year-olds with special health care needs do not get the health care services they need. About 87% of adolescents (aged 12–17) had insurance coverage in 2006; but the number drops to <77% for those in poverty. Hispanic adolescents have the least proportion of health insurance—public or private—and were the least likely (along with Asians) to have had a health care visit in the past year (Mulye et al., 2009).

Health literacy during adolescence is an important consideration. Teens are frequent users of mass media (Internet, television, radio, text messaging), and specific health-related educational interventions can be targeted to them by using these media. One study found that 56% of high school students in an online sample had heard of MedlinePlus, and 52% had "adequate levels of health literacy" as measured by an online test (Ghaddar, Valerio, Garcia, & Hansen, 2012). Community health nurses can help young people find reliable sources of information, as well as work with families to ensure proper monitoring of Internet use. Sexual predators, pornography, and cyber bullying are among the Internet dangers encountered by adolescents (Pujazon-Zazik & Park, 2010).

During the period that roughly encompasses the teen years, adolescents encounter many complex changes, physically, emotionally, cognitively, and socially (Damon & Lerner, 2008). Rapid and major developmental adjustments create a variety of stresses with concomitant problems that have an impact on health. More recent advanced neuroimaging techniques have demonstrated marked changes in the adolescent brain, especially related to white and gray matter and the prefrontal cortex (Blakemore, 2008; Blakemore, den Ouden, Choudhury, & Frith, 2007; Casey, Jones, & Hare, 2008; Johnson, Blum, & Giedd, 2009), along with other regions of the brain related to "attention, reward evaluation, affective discrimination, response inhibition, and goal-directed behavior," that help explain the cognitive and affective peculiarities of this developmental period (Yurgelun-Todd, 2007, p. 251).

The uneven changes in brain development may also help explain the risk-taking behaviors and higher incidence of unintentional injuries found in this population (Johnson et al., 2009). Unintentional injuries were the leading cause of death in the 10- to 19-year-old age group. Most deaths in this adolescent/young adult age group are due to preventable causes. The overall injury death rate in 2009 for adolescents 10 to 14 years of age was 17.9 per 100,000 and for 15- to-19-year-olds it was 69.7, indicating a dramatic rise as teens gain more freedom and begin to drive (Kochanek, Kirmeyer, Martin, Strobino, & Guyer, 2012). The overall unintentional death rate for only motor vehicle–related injuries was 14.9 (Bernard et al., 2007). The death rate from motor vehicle–related injuries for this age group peaked during the 1970s and 1980s, then declined throughout the next two decades, although motor vehicle–related injuries remain the number one cause of injury mortality for this age group (Bernard et al., 2007). Gender differences are also apparent: girls are much less likely than boys to engage in behaviors that put them at risk for injuries, resulting in twice the rate of unintentional injury death rate for male than female adolescents. This gender difference has persisted over three decades and is greater than age or ethnic differences in both unintentional and violence-related injury deaths (Sorenson, 2011). See Figure 22-4.

Unintentional injuries also cause the greatest level of morbidity, and the largest cause is transportation (drivers and passengers; bicyclists; pedestrians). Other causes include drowning, poisoning, fires, sports, and recreation, and work-related injuries (Sleet, Ballesteros, & Borse, 2010). Almost 175,000 sports- and recreation-related injuries (aged 1–19) are treated annually in EDs. The causes of most injuries requiring treatment include bicycling, playground activities, football, basketball, and soccer. Football and girl's soccer have the highest injury rates among youth sports (0.47 and 0.36 per 1,000 exposures), and the incidence of traumatic brain injury (TBI)/concussion ED visits has risen 60% over the last decade (CDC, 2011b).

Health Objectives For Adolescents

Healthy People 2020 objectives are focused on improving the health of all Americans. Goals and objectives for adolescent health have been developed. Because much of the mortality and morbidity in this age group stems from risk-taking behaviors, many objectives addressing alcohol-related unintentional injuries, violent behaviors, and suicide and mental health issues, as well as more responsible reproductive health behaviors, are included throughout the document under Substance Abuse, Mental Health, etc. (Jain, Kolbe, Seo, Kay, & Brindis, 2011) (see Table 22-1). The 2007 midcourse review of these critical objectives found overall mortality trends at two times the 2010 target rate, although the 10- to 14-year-old rate is "on pace to reach the 2010 target" (p. 331). Unintentional injury results are mixed; motor vehicle–related crashes (with and without alcohol) increased slightly, but seat belt use also increased, and the number of adolescents reporting that they rode with a driver who had been drinking alcohol decreased. The objectives

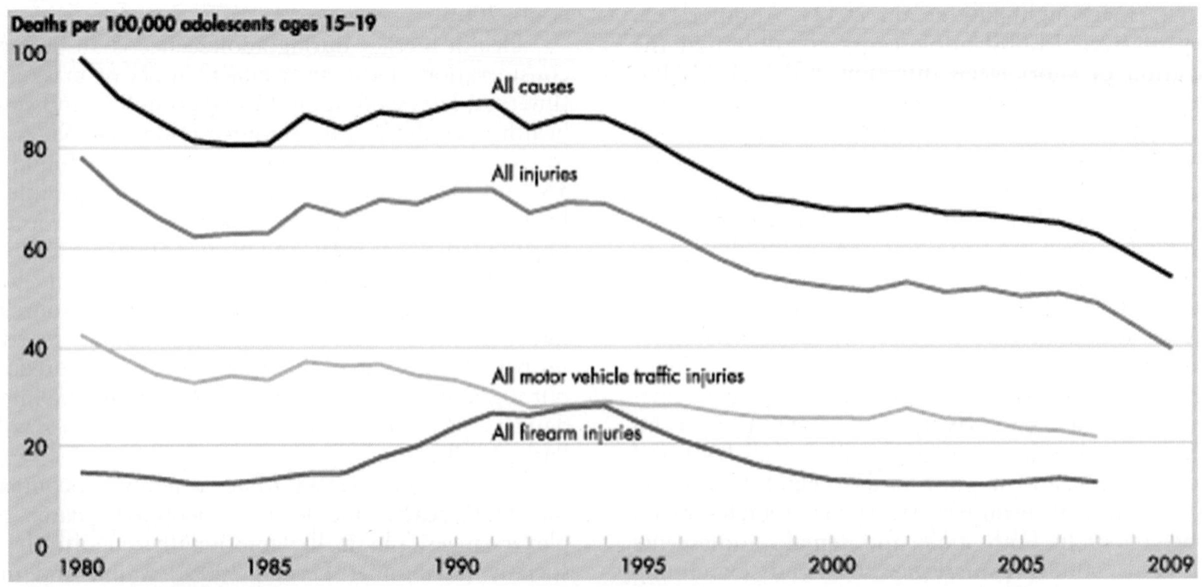

FIGURE 22-4. Death rates among adolescents aged 15 to 19 by all causes and all injury causes and selected mechanisms of injury, 1980–2009. (From http://www.childstats.gov/americaschildren/phenviro8.asp)

Table 22.1 ***Healthy People 2020:*** **21 Critical Health Objectives for Adolescents and Young Adults**

Goal: Improve the healthy development, health, safety, and wellbeing of adolescents and young adults.

Number	Objective
AH-1	Increase the proportion of adolescents who have had a wellness checkup in the past 12 mo.
AH-2	Increase the proportion of adolescents who participate in extracurricular and out-of-school activities.
AH-3	Increase the proportion of adolescents who are connected to a parent or other positive adult caregiver.
AH-4	Increase the proportion of adolescents who and young adults who transition to self-sufficiency from foster care.
AH-5	Increase the proportion of schools with a school breakfast program.
AH-7	Reduce the proportion of adolescents who have been offered, sold, or given an illegal drug on school property.
AH-8	Increase the proportion of adolescents whose parents consider them to be safe at school.
AH-9	Increase the proportion of middle and high schools that prohibit harassment based on student's sexual orientation or gender identity.
AH-10	Decrease the proportion of public schools with a serious violent incident.
AH-11	Reduce adolescent and young adult perpetration of, as well as victimization by, crimes.

From U.S. DHHS (2012). Adolescent health. Retrieved from http://healthypeople.gov/2020/topicsobjectives2020/objectiveslist.aspx?topicId=2

related to "homicide, physical fighting, and carrying a weapon have shown little or no improvement" (p. 331), and mental health objectives have shown mixed results. Suicide rates and reported attempted suicides are not significantly improved, and only modest increases are found in other objectives related to mood and treatment. Binge drinking and marijuana use demonstrate small decreases, and vigorous physical activity reports are basically unchanged. Tobacco use has gone down considerably, but obesity and overweight figures increased by more than 50%. The adolescent pregnancy rate decreased 34%—the best results of all 21 objectives—almost achieving the 2010 target rate, and related objectives are on pace to reach targets (e.g., never having sex, used a condom with last sexual contact). Chlamydia infection rates have increased, but may be an artifact of more sensitive testing and improved reporting (Park, Brindis, Chang, & Irwin, 2008). Analysis of the *21 Critical National Health Objectives for 2010* relating to adolescents and young adults revealed that only 2 targets had been met (i.e., rode with a driver who had drunk alcohol, physical fighting) and progress had been made toward 12 of the objectives. Jiang, Kolbe, Seo, Kay, & Brindis (2011) reported that no progress was made on four objectives and two objectives actually showed worse results (i.e., rates of Chlamydia infection and overweight).

Because adolescents have less contact with the health care system than children, many conditions may go undetected. Also, a shift occurs from a childhood preponderance of physical conditions to more social behavioral problems in adolescence. Risk behaviors become much more evident, along with their attendant outcomes: unsafe sexual activity, substance use, violence, and motor vehicle–related issues (Michaud, 2008). Also, the transition from high school into early adulthood is often difficult and those individuals with mental health issues often have worse outcomes than those with physical conditions (Park, Adams, & Irwin, 2011).

Emotional Problems and Suicide

The adolescent years are a time of rapid growth and change. Hormonal influences may cause a teen to be emotional and unpredictable at times (Damon & Lerner, 2008). The influence of peers increases, and peer pressure may influence behavior. Teens test family rules and generally search for their own identity and individuality apart from the family. Most parents and teens ride out this period with love and understanding and no long-term negative effects. For some children, however, a real or perceived lack of emotional support can lead to temporary or permanent emotional problems. A large national study linked adolescent maltreatment with delinquent behaviors and substance abuse (Hollist, Hughes, & Schaible, 2009). Also, gender differences in types and trajectories of emotional and behavioral problems have been noted, with more females developing adolescent-onset depression and males demonstrating more conduct problems at an earlier age of onset (Zahn-Waxler, Shirtcliff, & Marceau, 2008).

Depression, schizophrenia, and eating disorders may first appear during adolescence. About 50% of mental health conditions begin before age 14, and 75% by age 21 (Knopf, Park, & Mulye, 2008). It is estimated through parent ratings that approximately 12% of 12- to 17-year-olds have a serious behavioral or mental health problem (12% of females and 12.3% of males), and low-income youth were rated at almost

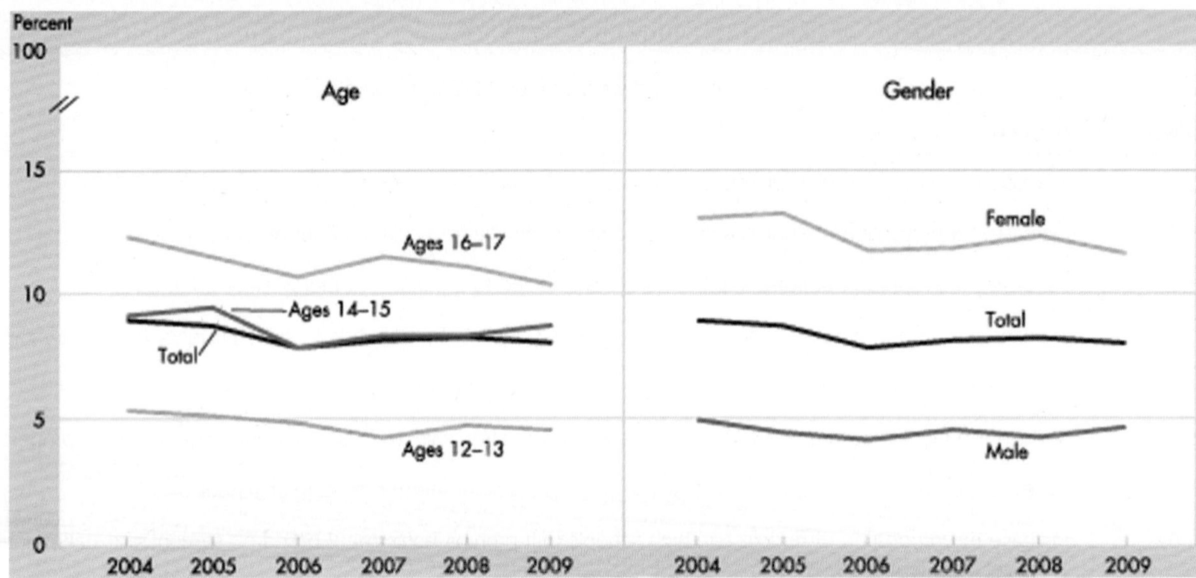

FIGURE 22-5. Percentage of youth aged 12 to 17 who experienced a major depressive episode (MDE) in the past year by age and gender, 2004–2009. (From http://www.childstats.gov/americaschildren/health4.asp)

18% (Knopf et al., 2008). Common adolescent mental health problems include depression, anxiety disorders, ADHD, and substance abuse problems. Mild depression affects over 25% of adolescents, but prevalence rates vary (Fig. 22-5). Depression is two times more likely among females (aged 15–20), and comorbidities (e.g., anxiety disorder, and addictive and conduct disorders) are not uncommon (Knopf et al., 2008). Researchers have concluded that between 20% and 25% of adolescents display symptoms of emotional distress, and about 10% have moderate to severe symptoms (Knopf et al., 2008). Adolescent brain maturation may explain susceptibility to depression during this period of development (Andersen & Teicher, 2008).

Many adolescents are reluctant to seek help for emotional problems, or help may not be readily available to them. Most research shows that many adolescents with "significant emotional distress" fail to receive mental health treatment—estimates have ranged from 10% to <40% (Knopf et al., 2008, p. 9). Survey results have found that 21.3% of youth aged 12 to 17 have been given some type of mental health services, but the usual disparities apply (e.g., ethnicity, income level, rural vs. urban locale). Treatment for serious mental health problems may include hospitalization or placement in a group home. However, primary care providers commonly evaluate children and adolescents for psychosocial problems in their everyday practice. Pediatricians report that almost 19% of patient visits concerned conduct or emotional problems or ADHD (Knopf et al., 2008). Secondary data analysis of a national longitudinal survey found "low rates of mental health counseling persist from adolescence to young adulthood" (Yu, Adams, Burns, Brindis, & Irwin, 2008, p. 268). School-based programs to educate adolescents about depression and suicide prevention have been useful (Swartz et al., 2010). For some, more universal approaches are viewed as more effective in preventing a wider range of social and emotional problems (Durlak, Weissberg, Dymnicki, Taylor, & Schellinger, 2011). PHNs and school nurses often participate in the development or administration of these types of programs.

Suicide is the third leading cause of death in adolescents and young adults, with a death rate of 6.9 per 100,000 for 15- to-19-year-olds that is down from the peak rate in the early 1990s. In this age group, five times more males than females died by suicide (NIMH, 2010). A classic study found that a psychiatric diagnosis is noted in 90% of suicide victims, with depression reported in over 50% of all cases (National Alliance for Mental Illness [NAMI], 2011; Shaffer, Gould, & Hicks, 2007). Untreated depression is often a factor in adolescent suicide and should be screened for and evaluated (Dudley, Goldney, & Hadzi-Pavlovic, 2010; Pelkonen, Karlsson, & Marttunen, 2011). Although questions have been raised and the FDA issued a black box warning that adolescents beginning treatment may be at increased for suicidal ideation, selective serotonin reuptake inhibitors (SSRIs) among the more commonly prescribed antidepressant medications are almost never found during autopsy of teen suicide victims (Liberzon & George, 2010; Shaffer et al., 2007). In 2009, almost 14% of high school students reported that they seriously considered suicide in the previous 12 months (down from 29% in 1991), and 6.3% made at least one suicide attempt. Almost 2% made an attempt that required medical attention (CDC, 2011g). Geographically, higher suicide rates occur in the West (e.g., Alaska, New Mexico, Montana), and the lowest rates are found in the northeastern United States (Shaffer et al., 2007). As adolescents grow older, they are more at risk for suicide: the rate increases from 1.5 per 100,000 for ages 10 to

14 to 8.2 for ages 15 to 19. It is 12.8 for older adolescents (20–24), and about 2 million adolescents attempt suicide each year (NAMI, 2011). While adolescent suicide rates have declined between 1992 and 2006 and deaths by poisoning and firearms have also decreased, an alarming finding is that suicide deaths by hanging or suffocation have dramatically increased. This is especially true for girls (Bridge et al., 2010).

It is important to question a teen about her history of depression or feelings of hopelessness, as well as the quality and quantity of her social support systems and the availability of means to follow through on suicide threats; it is also helpful to have intensive therapy visits early on and discussions about safety planning (Bethell & Rhodes, 2008; Pelkonen et al., 2011). School and discipline problems, family discord, and depression, as well as drug and alcohol abuse can increase the risk of suicide (NIMH, 2010). Recent stressful events and preoccupation with suicide, as well as substance use, are also important to note. Being bullied, a history of sexual or physical abuse, aggressive conduct disorders, and personality disorders are risk factors for adolescent suicide attempts (Greydanus, Patel, & Pratt, 2010). In a classic treatise, Shaffer et al. (2007) note that gay, lesbian, and bisexual youth have high rates of suicidal ideation and suicide attempts, and for all youth, having a close family member who committed suicide doubles the risk. Greydanus et al. (2010) noted a relationship between chronic illness (e.g., diabetes, epilepsy) in adolescents and suicide risk, often due to high rates of depression. *Suicide contagion* refers to copycat suicides, especially among high school students, after a highly publicized suicide. This can lead to suicide clusters—deaths of three to seven adolescents over a 3- to 9-month period (Shaffer et al., 2007).

Suicide hotlines are often ineffective for adolescents, as they are infrequently used (Shaffer et al., 2007). Suicide prevention programs and direct intervention by counselors or school nurses to determine an adolescent's suicide intentions may be effective school-based interventions. It is important for counselors to identify markers for attempted suicide, such as a precipitating event, intense affective state, suicide ideation or actions, deterioration in social or academic functioning, or increased substance abuse. Community health nurses and community mental health counselors may serve as consultants to schools in the development of sound prevention programs. Hallmarks of good prevention programs include student education on suicide awareness and intervention; coping and problem-solving skills training; skill building by reinforcement of strengths/protective factors while dealing with risk-taking behaviors; teaching about the association between suicide and mental health (especially depression). Suicide screening is often thought to be effective in reducing suicidal ideation, but there is limited research to substantiate this (Miller, Eckert, & Mazza, 2009). One longitudinal study of the effectiveness of a school district's suicide prevention and intervention program found that, over 18 years, the rate of suicide dropped from 5.5 per 100,000 to 1.4, and attempts during the same period also dropped (Zenere & Lazarus, 2009). A comprehensive review of school-based suicide prevention programs found few studies with statistically significant results (7.6%) and none that supported program effect replication. Some examples of programs used in high schools include *Lifelines* and *SOS: Signs of Suicide* (Miller et al., 2009). Depression prevention programs have had better outcomes with one meta-analysis finding that 41% of depression prevention programs demonstrated significantly reduced symptoms of depression (Stice et al., 2009). Skills-training programs that target a broader range of problems (e.g., depression, anxiety, negative self-perceptions) have been effective in teaching adolescents how to monitor feelings, identify triggers, avoid and reframe negative thoughts. Relaxation skills training, learning how to seek out help from others, and promoting healthier responses to stress have also been successful in impacting internalizing behaviors (Terzian, Hamilton, & Ericson, 2011).

A behavior that can sometimes accidentally result in suicide is *self-injury* or *cutting*. Adolescents with this abnormal behavior who overdose, head bang, cut, burn, brand, mark, or otherwise dangerously harm themselves are attempting to find relief from profound psychological pain. The physical injury distracts them from these painful emotions, possibly giving them a feeling of control or providing a means of feeling emotions when they are cut off from them. Scars often remain long after the behavior has stopped (AACAP, 2009). Peer influence is often a factor for girls, and longitudinal research has demonstrated a "socialization effect" with self-injurious behavior that also includes suicide (Prinstein et al., 2010). A large study of almost 2,000 adolescents found an 8% rate of self-harm, and a reduction in frequency of self-injury with age (7% no longer self-harmed as young adults). Adolescent self-harming behaviors were associated with use of marijuana, alcohol, and cigarettes, as well as higher rates of depression and anxiety symptoms and antisocial behavior (Moran et al., 2012). One smaller longitudinal study found that over the 2.5 years data were collected, 18% of 11- to 14-year-olds engaged in nonsuicidal self-injury, with 14% reported as new cases (Hankin & Abela, 2011). This behavior most often begins in early adolescence or late childhood. It can continue into adulthood. It is more common in girls and in those with a family history of suicide, self-injury, or maternal depression. Isolation, neglect, or abuse may predispose an adolescent to this behavior. Depression, poor quality of relationships, excessive seeking of reassurance, and eating disorders are commonly associated with self-injury. PHNs and school nurses can provide education to adolescents and families about this condition, and can work with schools to promote prevention strategies, such as early detection and referral to mental health providers.

Violence

The total costs of youth violence (e.g., quality of life, medical costs, lost productivity) are more than $158 billion each year (Hammond & Arias, 2011). Violence is costly in many other ways, not just for those involved, but also for those who witness it. A national survey of almost 5,000 children and adolescents found that 60.6% had personally experienced or witnessed violence in the past year. Physical assault was reported by 46.3% of respondents, and 6.1% experienced sexual victimization. Over 10% suffered an injury or had 5 or more instances of victimization (Finkelhor, Turner, Ormrod, & Hamby, 2009).

Homicide is the second leading cause of death for adolescents (aged 10–24), it is more common in males than females, and in 84% of cases it involved the use of a firearm. In 2007, an average of 16 adolescents were murdered each day (CDC, 2010d). Firearm-related homicide rates are higher in urban areas, but suicides and unintentional firearm deaths are more prevalent in rural counties (Nance, Carr, Kallan, Branas, & Wiebe, 2010). The homicide rate among African American adolescents is 60.7 per 100,000, and for Hispanic males it is 20.6; it is only 3.5 among White males, indicating a wide disparity. In 2008, over 656,000 adolescents were treated for violence-related injuries in EDs (CDC, 2010d). Almost 1,580 homicides of school-age youth occurred in the 2008–2009 school year, but only 17 of these occurred on school grounds (Robers, Zhang, & Truman, 2012).

Delinquency is thought to peak during middle adolescence—around age 16. Analysis of longitudinal data revealed that 60% of adolescents were generally not engaged in delinquent acts, and 27.7% had low levels in early adolescence increasing to more moderate levels. About 5% of those with early moderate levels of delinquency reported increases and then decreases during later adolescence. Only 1.3% of males who were chronic offenders had high levels initially and increased levels of delinquency over time (Pepler, Jiang, Craig, & Connolly, 2010). Children assault and kill other children at school and on the streets. Eight percent of high school students reported being injured or threatened with a weapon, such as a gun, knife, or club, on school grounds. Four percent of students (aged 12–18) reported victimization during the 6 months prior to the survey, and public school students had twice the rate of those in private schools (Robers et al., 2012).

Gangs are often associated with teen violence. U.S. gangs are now found in communities across the country, with a rise in gang membership to more than 1 million members. Authorities believe that gangs are responsible for up to 80% of crimes and are the primary distributor of most illegal drugs; there has been a rise in gang presence in rural and suburban schools (Johnson, 2009). Mexican drug gangs were found to be in every region of the United States (BBC News, 2010). The 2009 National Youth Gang Survey reported an increase in gang activity from 2008, 34.5% versus 32.4%, respectively. While youth gangs may not effectively manage drug distribution as well as more established, older gangs, they are involved in various forms of violence that often includes intergang conflict (Egley & Howell, 2011). Public schools reported gang activity at 16% in 2009–2010, down from 20% 2 years earlier; but 20% of students reported gang presence at their schools with more high school students than sixth graders noting gangs being present (Robers et al., 2012). While gang members may engage in violence and intimidation, other instances of school violence have captured greater media attention. Incidents of high school shootings, such as the one at Columbine High School, have raised concerns among parents and teachers. These high-profile events are rare, but they bring attention to the need for change. School violence has been linked to bullying and the overall school environment, and should be addressed quickly. However, the incidence of homicides on school property has actually decreased over the past 15 years (Virginia Youth Violence Project, n.d.). Comprehensive school safety and crisis response plans are needed, and threat assessment may be helpful in preventing this type of violence (Borum, Cornell, Modzeleski, & Jimerson, 2010).

Bullying can result in depression, social anxiety, internalizing and psychosomatic symptoms, loneliness, and poor school performance (Arseneault et al., 2008). Daily or weekly bullying incidents were reported by 23% of public schools during the 2009–2010 school year, and 28% of students reported bullying at school; cyber bullying was reported by 6% of students (Robers et al., 2012). The percentage of young adolescents who do not feel safe at school decreased slightly over the past 5 years. In 2009, 17.5% of adolescents reported carrying a weapon to school during the past month (5.9% carried a gun), and more than 31.5% were involved in physical fights in the last year (11.1% on school property). Males were more likely to be involved in carrying weapons and fighting (CDC, 2010d). Another form of violence found among adolescents and young adults is dating violence (or date rape), and females can also be the perpetrators of this although it is more common among males (Foshee, Reyes, & Ennett, 2010).

Cultural and environmental influences on youth include the violence to which children and adolescents are exposed. Increased aggressive behavior among children and teens has been attributed to violence in the environment, the home (spousal and child abuse), and the community, as well as to what children see on television and in movies. The effects of family violence (domestic violence, child maltreatment) can lead to internalizing and externalizing behaviors among youth (Moylan et al., 2010). Personally experiencing violence or witnessing it as a child are risk factors for adolescent behaviors such as school dropout, running away from home, attempting suicide, and delinquency (Haynie, Petts, Maimon, & Piquero, 2009). Violence is an increasing threat as students move from elementary school into middle and high school. Ninth-grade students reported the highest rate of physical fights in a study of high school students (Robers et al., 2012). However, adolescents who are better connected to school are less likely to engage in violent behaviors. A longitudinal study of early adolescents found links between poor school engagement and delinquency, as well as depression and substance use (Li & Lerner,

2011). School climate is important in reducing the levels of violence in this age group, as is adequate parental support (Krohn, Lizotte, Bushway, Schmidt, & Phillips, 2010). Family cohesion can also be a mediating factor for delinquency as a consequence of childhood effects of violence (Barr et al., 2011).

Following the lead of the federal government with the implementation of the Gun-Free School Act and the Safe and Drug-Free Schools and Communities Act, most schools developed *zero-tolerance policies* to counteract and prevent violence and substance use (Peterson & Schoonover, 2008). These policies "mandate typically harsh consequences or punishments, such as suspensions and expulsions, for a wide range of rule violations" (Evenson, Justinger, Pelischek, & Schultz, 2009, p. 6). In 2009–2010, 39% of public schools took serious disciplinary action against youth accused of specific offenses (Robers et al., 2012). Many schools now have metal detectors and security guards, and some schools conduct random searches of students' lockers in an effort to prevent violence. However, the American Psychological Association Zero Tolerance Task Force (2008) examined 20 years of research studies, and found little evidence of effectiveness and some indication that these policies actually may be worse than ineffective. They noted that these policies actually lead to increased violent and disruptive behavior and higher dropout rates. The task force found that a disproportionate number of Black and Hispanic students were expelled or suspended from school, and that zero-tolerance policies do not consider children's lapses in judgment as a normal aspect of development. They recommended adaptations to zero-tolerance policies to make them more flexible and individualized to students, school sites, and situations. Students with disabilities are also disproportionately affected and this type of school discipline is seen as reactive, rather than proactive, and punitive, rather than corrective (Evenson et al., 2009). Others call for a "firm but fair and supportive approach" that provides assistance for struggling students and positive adult role models (Gregory & Cornell, 2009).

Community efforts, youth development and violence prevention programs, and parenting education have been used to address youth violence, and a multimodal approach is often most effective (Allison, Edmonds, Wilson, Pope, & Farrell, 2011). Because family cohesion has been found to be a moderating influence for adolescents who witness community violence, programs that improve parenting practices and promote family cohesion are needed (Barr et al., 2011). Focusing on high-risk youth to improve parenting, peer relationships, academic achievement, and social cognition may be an effective means of preventing adolescent conduct disorder and delinquency (Dodge & McCourt, 2010).

Substance Abuse

Substance abuse among young people was almost unknown before 1950, and rare before 1960, but exploded in the mid-1960s; by 1981, 66% of high school students had ever tried an illicit drug and this dropped to 47% by 2008 (Johnston, O'Malley, Bachman, & Schulenberg, 2009). Adolescent drug experimentation and use pose serious physical and psychological threats. The YRBS, a national survey of high school students, found that 36.7% of teens report having tried marijuana, and 72.5% consumed alcohol at least once. Almost 21% used marijuana within the past 30 days, and 11.7% reported ever using inhalants like glue or aerosols (CDC, 2011g). A more recent survey reported that 47% of high school seniors have tried an illicit drug, which reflects a slight improvement over earlier surveys. The use of narcotics other than heroin (e.g., Vicodin, Oxycontin) has generally risen with 2008 prevalence for high school seniors at close to 10% for Vicodin (Johnston et al., 2009). The most recent YRBS results indicated that almost one fourth of high school students engaged in binge drinking (five or more drinks within a couple of hours), and 4.5% drank alcohol on school property at least once (CDC, 2011g).

Why do adolescents turn to alcohol or illicit drugs? Acosta, Manubay, and Levin (2008) have described parallels between addictive behavior and obesity—especially related to personality, environmental risk factors, genetic predisposition, and common neurobiologic brain pathways. A large-scale, 25-year prospective longitudinal study in New Zealand found that gender, novelty-seeking behaviors, childhood conduct disorder, and parental illicit drug use predicted use of illicit drugs in 16- to 25-year-olds. Marijuana use, substance-using peers, and alcohol use were also factors (Fergusson, Boden, & Horwood, 2008; Fergusson, Horwood, & Ridder, 2007). Depression has also been linked to alcohol and substance use (Fig. 22-6). Can peers lure adolescents into alcohol and drug use? Most evidence reveals both genetic and environmental influences—in other words, those who were more prone by genetics to use substances "were more vulnerable to adverse influences of their best friends" (Harden, Hill, Turkheimer, & Emery, 2008).

Alcohol is the most frequently used substance for U.S. adolescents—it is often their first drug of choice. In one large study the reasons cited by adolescents for trying alcohol included such things as "to find out what effect it would have," "to have more fun at a party," and "because it was exciting." Teens drinking for the last two reasons were more likely to engage in risky drinking, and those with symptoms of depression were three times more likely to binge drink (Kuntsche & Muler, 2012, p. 34). Early drinkers more often report academic problems, use of other substances, and delinquent behavior in middle and high school. Analysis of national survey data found that adolescents who begin first alcohol use before the age of 13 had significantly more involvement in violent behaviors and suicide attempts than those who delayed the initiation of alcohol (Swahn, Bossarte, & Sullivent, 2008). Early use of alcohol was found to be a marker for later alcohol and drug dependence in one classic longitudinal study (King & Chassin, 2007), and age of alcohol initiation for Whites was earlier than for Blacks and

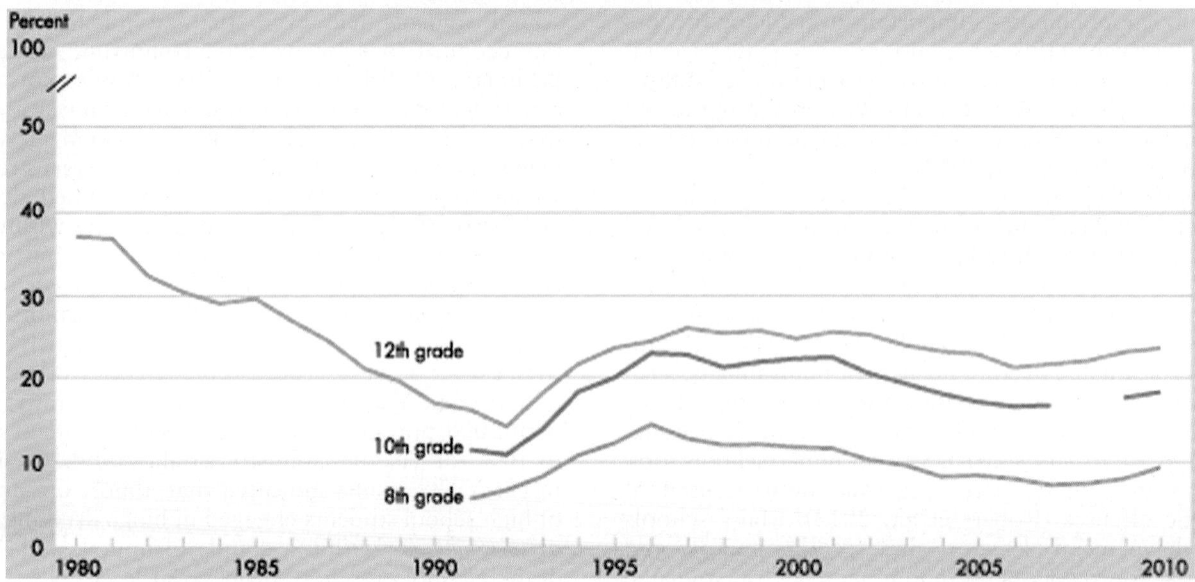

FIGURE 22-6. Percentage of 8th-, 10th-, and 12th-grade students who reported using illicit drugs in the past 30 days by grade, 1980–2010. (From http://www.childstats.gov/americaschildren/beh3.asp)

Hispanics and more quickly progressed to alcohol dependence in a recent national survey (Alvanzo et al., 2011). It is important to stress education and prevention in late childhood to delay the initiation of alcohol use.

More than $1.7 billion was spent on alcohol advertising in 2009, and some feel that this influences adolescent drinking (Moreno, 2011). A classic study on the effects of alcohol advertising on youth drinking rates (Snyder, Milici, Slater, Sun, & Strizhakova, 2006) found that youth (aged 15–26) who saw more advertising for alcohol drank more on average (each dollar spent per capita on alcohol advertising raised the number of drinks consumed by 3%). Alcohol promotional items (e.g., clothing, posters) have been associated with binge drinking (Fisher, Miles, Austin, Camargo, & Colditz, 2007). Binge drinking is generally defined as having five or more drinks at one time—usually within a couple of hours—and it often increases as adolescents get older (CDC, 2011g). Binge drinking has been associated with poor academic achievement and other risk behaviors (e.g., sexual activity, smoking, using illicit drugs, riding with a driver who had been drinking, attempting suicide), and the more adolescents binge drink, the more they engage in risk behaviors (Miller, Naimi, Brewer, & Jones, 2007). Adolescent binge drinking was associated and parental alcoholism was influential in later adult substance use disorders (Haller, Handley, Chassin, & Bountress, 2010).

Family drinking and perceived family norms related to drinking have been found to affect adolescents' perceptions of the benefits of drinking. This perception, in turn, predicts their drinking behavior (Epstein, Griffin, & Botvin, 2008). Parenting practices (e.g., monitoring, discipline, enforcing rules related to alcohol use) have also been found to have an influence on adolescent drinking behavior (Latendresse et al., 2008). Factors prevalent during adolescence, such as divorce, parental trust, social class and relationships, along with depressive symptoms and poor impulse control and self-esteem, were associated with excessive alcohol use in adults (Huurre et al., 2010).

Adolescents who are engaged emotionally and connected to school generally have better outcomes; lower levels of engagement were linked to substance use and delinquency in one longitudinal study (Li & Lerner, 2011). Family meal times have been shown to promote family cohesion and problem- and emotion-focused coping by encouraging parents to help their children feel part of the family and allowing them valuable time to coach them in effective methods for dealing with daily stresses and problems (Franko, Thompson, Affenito, Barton, & Striegel-Moore, 2008). To promote the health and welfare of adolescent children, it is vital to stress to families with young children the continued importance of family meals throughout adolescence.

Marijuana is the most commonly used illicit drug among 14- to 17-year-olds—42.6% of high school seniors reported ever using marijuana. Bureau of Justice Statistics. (n.d.). Use of marijuana by early adolescents fell, but middle to late adolescent use remained the same (Johnston et al., 2009). This is an important finding, because early marijuana use (before age 15) has been associated with a much greater likelihood of adult cocaine and heroin use and drug dependency (Office of National Drug Control Policy [ONDCP], 2012). Marijuana use has negative health effects, including anxiety, panic attacks, increased heart rate, frequent respiratory infections, impaired memory and learning, and tolerance. Regular marijuana smokers often have respiratory complications similar to those of tobacco smokers—cough, phlegm, respiratory infections, and airway obstruction (ONDCP, 2012).

Inhalant abuse is very common, and shows signs of resurgence (Johnston et al., 2009). Inhalant use begins in early adolescence—more 12- and 13-year-olds reported using inhalants than any other illicit drug. The most commonly reported inhalants used were shoe polish, glue or toluene, spray paints, and lighter fluid or gasoline (NSDUH, 2008). Other inhalants commonly used include amyl nitrite "poppers"; locker room deodorizers or "rush"; cleaning fluid, degreasers, or correction fluid; halothane, ether, or other anesthetics; lacquer thinner or other paint solvents; butane or propane gases; nitrous oxide or "whippets"; and other aerosol sprays (NSDUH, 2008). Inhalant abuse can result in severe nervous system damage or death. Control of legal products, such as spray paint, lighter fluid, household solvents, gasoline, and glue, is difficult, making this problem almost impossible to monitor adequately.

Other drugs that are used by adolescents and young adults include "club drugs" such as MDMA (Ecstasy), a synthetic drug with amphetamine and hallucinogenic properties; Rohypnol (the date rape drug that is often mixed with alcohol to produce sedative hypnotic effects); ketamine (a rapid-acting anesthetic); lysergic acid diethylamide (LSD), a hallucinogen originally popularized in the 1960s; and gamma hydroxybutyrate (GHB, a drug that is touted as a synthetic steroid in fitness clubs and that has been associated with sexual assaults). Rates of use for ketamine, Rohypnol, and GHB have declined over the past few years, but psilocybin or "magic mushrooms" are still widely used. Ecstasy use has generally declined but may become popular again among younger adolescents. Over-the-counter cold and cough medications containing the cough suppressant dextromethorphan are sometimes used to produce a "high," and between 4% and 7% of adolescents are reported to have used them (Johnston et al., 2009). Visits to the ED and deaths have occurred from the use of many of these drugs.

Cocaine use has remained steady in recent years, after peaking in the late 1990s. Heroin use fell below peak levels reached in 2001 but continues to remain steady. Smoking or snorting of heroin, which is popular among adolescents and young adults because they mistakenly believe it precludes the strong physical addictiveness of this drug, has been found to lead to injection drug abuse (Johnston et al., 2009). A systematic review of studies on the health outcomes among adolescents (10–24 years) found consistent associations between meth and "depression, suicidal ideation, and psychosis," as well as an increased risk of HIV and other STIs (Marshall & Werb, 2010, p. 991). Methamphetamine may be smoked, along with marijuana, or injected. Methamphetamine labs are a public health hazard and can often be found in rural areas. PHNs should be aware of this when making home visits in outlying areas.

Another drug used by adolescents is anabolic steroids. The illicit use of anabolic steroids is difficult to monitor; however, 0.8% of 8th graders, 1.1% of 10th graders, and 1.4% of 12th graders reported using steroids in a national survey (Johnston et al., 2009). A survey of high school students noted use was higher in males, especially those participating in sports, and 49% of students believed that athletic performance could be improved with steroid use; 38% thought that use improved appearance (Lorang, Callahan, Cummins, Achar, & Brown, 2011). Some coaches have, at times, turned a blind eye to steroid abuse, but educational campaigns to fight the rising level of abuse in adolescents have led to decreases in use since peak levels were reached in 2000. Sato, Schulz, Sisk, and Wood (2008, p. 647) report that animal models show "adolescent anabolic–androgenic steroid exposure increases aggression, and causes lasting changes in neurotransmitter systems." Other symptoms include irritability, increased risk-taking behavior, extreme mood swings, and euphoria, as well as psychiatric conditions that may be intensified or induced. Because steroids are often readily available through Internet pharmacies, policymakers and health educators must make adolescents aware of the dangers, such as altered serotonin levels and increased aggression (Lumia & McGinnis, 2010).

Adolescents are becoming more involved with prescription drugs, often found in their parents' medicine cabinets, purchased on the Internet, or bought from friends at school (McCabe, West, Morales, Cranford, & Boyd, 2007; McCabe et al., 2012). Teens may have "pharming parties," in which medication bottles are emptied onto tables and selected like candy. Medications are often mixed with alcohol, and adolescents often mistakenly believe prescription medications are safer than street drugs when used to produce a high. Ritalin, prescribed to students with ADHD, may be given or sold to others, but the most commonly used medications are Oxycontin, Vicodin, tranquilizers, and sedatives. One in 20 high school seniors has tried Oxycontin, and almost 10% of high school seniors have used Vicodin (Johnston et al., 2009). This trend is very disturbing because of society's nonchalant, casual attitude toward prescription medications and their easy access. Early onset (before age 13) of nonmedical use of prescription medications is a predictor of later prescription drug abuse and drug dependence (McCabe et al., 2007). A large survey of over 3,600 12- to 17-year-olds found a significant association with nonmedical use of prescription drugs and delinquent behavior, history of witnessed violence and PTSD, as well as other types of substance use and abuse. Among those interviewed, 6.7% admitted using drugs that were not prescribed to them for medical conditions (McCauley et al., 2010).

Tobacco products are also easily acquired, often from parents. About $10 billion is spent annually on marketing tobacco products (Koch, 2012). In the YRBS, high school students were asked if they had ever tried cigarettes, and the rates were similar for males and females at 46.3% and 46.1%. When asked about smoking a whole cigarette for the first time before age 13, 11.8% of boys and 9.4% of girls responded positively (CDC, 2011g). But, nearly 20% of high school seniors regularly smoke cigarettes, indicating that the efforts to reduce smoking rates in this age group are slowing. The use of smokeless tobacco, or "chew," is on the rise, with 15% now reporting regular use from a low of around 11% in 2003 (Koch, 2012). Social disapproval and heightened perception of health risks were thought to help contribute to the previous downward trend of smoking and smokeless tobacco use, along with price increases and advertising bans (Johnston et al., 2009). But, tobacco marketing continues to be problematic, as the tobacco industry has joined with convenience stores to more prominently display tobacco products, and even though state and federal taxes comprise about half the cost of a pack of cigarettes states have not always sufficiently invested these funds in adolescent tobacco prevention (Koch, 2012). In a study of adolescents who use tobacco, addictive symptoms have been shown to begin to appear within the first few weeks of initiating smoking, highlighting the need to continue to attack this problem (DiFranza, 2008). One longitudinal study found that adolescents who had low academic aspirations, perceived themselves to be unconventional, and had internalizing behaviors (e.g., depressive symptoms) were less likely to participate in smoking-cessation programs. Parental smoking also was a negative influence, and other research demonstrated less effective quit attempts for adolescents with at least one smoking parent (Brook et al., 2010; Kong, Carmenga, & Krishnan-Sarin, 2012). An Internet-based virtual reality world, along with real-time motivational interviewing by experienced smoking-cessation counselors, is an innovative program showing promise with adolescent smokers (Woodruff, Conway, Edwards, Elliott, & Crittenden, 2007). In addition, parental disapproval was related to a greater number of attempts at abstinence for boys, but not for girls (Kong et al., 2012).

Primary health care providers do not always question adolescents about smoking, drinking, and use of other substances. Some evidence highlights the effectiveness of brief interventions by health care providers in encouraging smoking cessation, and improvement in other risk behaviors (Heikkinen, Broms, Pitkaniemi, Koskenvuo, & Meurman, 2009). But, the long-term effectiveness of this type of intervention was not demonstrated in a Finnish cohort study (Saari, Kentala, & Mattila, 2012). PHNs and community health nurses can provide information to teens about smoking cessation programs and promote primary prevention by educating children and adolescents to choose not to smoke or engage in other health-risk behaviors. They can also encourage physicians and parents to question and monitor adolescents about smoking and the use of tobacco products.

Teen Sexuality and Pregnancy

Teenage pregnancies, sexually transmitted diseases (STDs), and HIV/AIDS are public health concerns associated with the sexual activity of adolescents. In the 2009 YRBS, 46% of high school students reported ever having sexual intercourse, and 61.1% used a condom during their last sexual intercourse. Almost 14% reported having had sexual intercourse with four or more persons, and 22.9% used birth control pills to prevent pregnancy (CDC, 2011d). In 2008, teens (aged 15–19) experienced 733,000 pregnancies and those under age 14 had 13,500 pregnancies. Adolescents aged 15 to 19 have the highest unintended pregnancy rates—about 7% became pregnant in 2008 (Finer, 2010; Kost & Henshaw, 2012). Early sexual debut has been associated with delinquency, as well as with other negative outcomes, so this public health problem can lead to other more serious consequences than pregnancy (Armour, 2007). Early puberty was related to greater sexual activity and higher rates of delinquency in a large study of 9- to-13-year-olds (Negriff, Susman, & Trickett, 2011).

The United States leads most developed nations in rates of teenage pregnancy, abortion, and childbearing. The teen birth rate in this country declined to its lowest level in 70 years from 1991 to 2009; yet the U.S. rate is six to nine times higher than that of "developed countries with the lowest birth rates" (Pazol et al., 2011, p. 419). Despite a slight increase in 2006–2007, since 1991, pregnancy and birth rates for 15- to 19-year-old girls have declined by 37%. In 2009, the rate was 39.1 births per 1,000 females. The rate for Hispanic adolescent girls was 70.1 per 1,000; for Blacks the rate was 59 per 1,000. For non-Hispanic Whites, the rate was 25.6 per 1,000. There is a wide discrepancy between states, with rates varying from 16.4 to 64.2, and southern states having higher numbers of teen pregnancies and births (Pazol et al., 2011). Some research has indicated that shared social norms about adolescent pregnancy may vary among racial/ethnic groups, and this may account for a larger amount of influence than religious or socioeconomic factors (Mollborn, Domingue, & Boardman, 2011). An examination of state-level characteristics found that those states with higher rates in 1991 and sharper increases through 2007 were more likely to have higher rates of unemployment, unmarried births, violent crime, and a higher proportion of Hispanic and Black residents than lower birth rate states. They were also less likely to have public funding for abortion (Terzian & Moore, 2012). The downward trend for teen birth rates is thought to be associated with a drop in the percentage of students who had sexual intercourse and those having sex without contraception. The use of two forms of birth control (i.e., condoms together with birth control pills or Depo-Provera) increased from 5% to 9% in the decade preceding 2009 (Pazol et al., 2011). The rate of teenage abortion was 17.8 per 1,000 in 2008, the lowest since abortions became legal. The highest rate was in 1988 at 43.5 (Kost & Henshaw, 2012). The rate of adolescent fatherhood also declined; between 1990 and 2006, it dropped from 24 to 18 per 1,000 males. Almost half of male teens state they would be very upset if they were responsible for a pregnancy (Guttmacher Institute, 2012a, 2012b).

The babies of adolescent mothers are more likely to die during infancy and school-age years, and are at higher risk for academic failure, poor social outcomes, and hospitalization, according to a population-based retrospective cohort study (Jutte et al., 2010). Young mothers are more likely to smoke tobacco and are at high risk of bearing infants with low birth weights. They are also less likely to receive adequate prenatal care or to gain the recommended weight during pregnancy. Adolescent mothers are at a greater risk than mothers over age 20 to experience a complication of pregnancy (e.g., anemia, hypertension, premature labor), and the risk increases for those under age 15 (Briggs, Hopman, & Jamieson, 2007; Usta, Zoorob, Abu-Musa, Naassan, & Nassar, 2008). Adolescent mothers are also at risk for a greater number of physical, psychological, and social problems, including dropping out of high school, reliance on public assistance, limited earning potential, social isolation, and mental disorders (Boden, Fergusson, & Horwood, 2008; East, Reyes, & Horn, 2007; Reid & Meadows-Oliver, 2007). Compared with women giving birth at age 30, teen mothers can expect 2 years less education and they are 10% to 12% less likely to finish high school and are less likely to attend college (Basch, 2011b). The consequences can continue long after adolescence. A longitudinal study found that "teen mothers' life trajectories reflected legacies of unequal life chances that began in childhood and persisted into their 30s," but that those who were from higher socioeconomic groups "fared better over time" (Smithbattle, 2007, p. 409). Adolescent girls living with a single parent or not living with either parent have higher teen birth rates than those who live with both parents (Wildsmith, Manlove, Jekielek, Moore, & Mincieli, 2012). Adolescents report positive outcomes, but also that teen parenting is "hard," and they recognize that their current and future lives are profoundly affected (Herrman, 2008, p. 42). A retrospective cohort study of women in their 70s and 80s found that those who had been teenage mothers had a higher risk of death than women who bore children after age 20, and they also had a higher prevalence of heart and lung disease, and cancer (Henretta, 2007). Also, those who choose to end their pregnancies by abortion may encounter other physical and psychosocial complications.

By 19 years of age, 7 out of 10 males and females have had sexual intercourse. Only 13% of teens have had sex by age 15 (Guttmacher Institute, 2012a). As such, it would behoove U.S. society to provide effective sexuality education. There is often debate about the virtues of comprehensive versus abstinence-only educational programs. Despite the contentiousness about the subject, in 2006, 87% of private and public schools in the United States required health education, most of it at the high school level. Most adolescents (age 15–19) received education about STIs (93%) and abstinence (84%), but about 33% were not instructed about contraception. Many sexually active teens have no instruction on contraception before their first sexual experience (33% girls, 46% boys) (Fields, 2012; Guttmacher Institute, 2012b). Teaching about contraception did not increase the risk of adolescent sexual activity or STIs, but it did decrease the risk of pregnancy in a study of abstinence-only versus comprehensive sexual education programs among a national sample of adolescents (Kohler, Manhart, & Lafferty, 2008). Analysis of data from a national survey found that sex education, of any type, when compared to no education was associated with delayed sexual intercourse for both adolescent males and females. When education included instruction in birth control, along with abstinence, adolescents were more likely to use contraception (birth control pills or condom) at first sexual intercourse and less likely to have a much older partner (Lindberg & Maddow-Zimet, 2012). Besides formal education through schools, adolescents note that peers, the media, and parents are also sources of information on sexual health. Between 70% and 79% of teens report talking with a parent about sex, although girls more often talk with parents about how to say no to sex or use birth control (Guttmacher Institute, 2012a, 2012b).

Pregnancy prevention programs can be effective in reducing teen pregnancy and birth rates, as well as in reducing the number of second births to teenage mothers. A prospective cohort study found that increased levels of sexuality education within schools was associated with decreased teen birth rates, although the reverse was found in some states with higher religiosity and political conservatism (Cavazos-Rehg et al., 2012). A small study of mostly African American 14- to 19-year-old, abstinent girls found four themes: self-respect (I am worth it), potential negative consequences of sex (Hold on, there's a catch), impact of mothers (Mama says ... think before you let it go), and influence of boys/other peers (Boys will be boys). Building on self-esteem and family influences, researchers cited the need to develop interventions to help adolescents maintain abstinence and delay sexual activity (Morrison-Beedy et al., 2008). Positive youth development (PYD) programs have been found to promote adolescent sexual and reproductive health by focusing on social and cognitive competence, prosocial bonding, future orientation, and self-determination. A systematic review found that PYD programs that were skill building, and enhanced bonding/strengthened families, while empowering youth and engaging them in real-world activities and roles, were the most effective (Gavin et al., 2010). These programs focus on overall youth development, not just sexuality.

Primary care providers often miss opportunities to provide counseling on prevention of pregnancy, HIV, and STDs, as well as other risk factors for unintentional injury (Ozer et al., 2011). Nurses can provide information and counseling on emergency contraception and collaborate with schools to promote effective pregnancy prevention programs (Haynes, 2007). It is important for community health nurses to provide education and health counseling on these subjects.

Sexually Transmitted Infections

STI and HIV infections are epidemic among adolescents worldwide (Sales & DiClemente, 2010). More than 20 diseases can be transmitted sexually; only the most common are reportable. Each year, about half of the STI cases occur among the 15- to 24-year-old age group, even though they represent only 25% of the population of sexually active individuals. These diseases include syphilis, gonorrhea, chlamydia, HPV, and herpes simplex virus. Approximately 30 of the 100 known types of HPV strains are sexually transmitted; some of these are related to cervical cancer, and others lead to genital warts. Described earlier in this chapter, Gardasil, a vaccine effective against some forms of HPV-related disease, can be administered in three doses to 11- to 12-year-old females and now to males as well (Dunne et al., 2011).

Chlamydia, gonorrhea, and syphilis are other STDs found in the adolescent population. Of the 19 million new cases of STIs annually, about half are among adolescents (15–24 years old), and more than 8,300 of 13- to 24-year-olds in reporting states had HIV infection in 2009 (CDC, 2011d). In the adolescent population, STIs are more common among those engaging in sexual risk behaviors. In 2009, 46% of high school students reported ever having sexual intercourse and 34% were active within the previous 3 months. Almost 15% had sex with four or more partners, and 39% did not use a condom with their last sexual contact (CDC, 2011d). Chlamydia is the most common STI; adolescent girls 15 to 19 years of age had the highest reported cases of chlamydia and gonorrhea (409,531 out of 1.5 million cases). Adolescent males are reported to have a similar prevalence, but do not experience symptoms in the same way as females; so infection may go undetected for longer periods of time (CDC, 2009a).

About one in four adolescent females (aged 14–19) have an STI; and that number increased to about half for African American girls (Sales & DiClemente, 2010). Compared with adults, adolescents (10–19 years) and young adults (20–24 years) are at increased risk for acquiring STIs. Reasons for this may include a greater likelihood of multiple sex partners, unprotected intercourse, and selection of higher-risk partners, as well as immature biology making them more vulnerable to infection and earlier sexual initiation. Barriers to improvement include lack of health insurance and transportation, concerns about confidentiality, and lack of quality STI prevention services or clinics targeted to younger age groups (CDC, 2009a; Sales & DiClemente, 2010). Adolescent girls also have a physiologically amplified susceptibility to chlamydia infection because of increased cervical ectopy (Monroy et al., 2010). Serious complications from STIs include pelvic inflammatory disease (PID), sterility, increased risk of cancers of the reproductive system, and, with syphilis, blindness, mental illness, and death. There are also complications for the unborn children of those infected with STIs. In one study on follow-up for adolescents with STIs diagnosed in EDs, a large number did not receive appropriate treatment. Of those who did, 25% did not realize they had an STI, which put them at risk of avoiding reinfection and nontreatment of sexual partners (Reed & Huppert, 2011).

Even though death rates from HIV/AIDS have dramatically fallen, new HIV infections reported annually do not reflect the same steep decline. Also, some research indicates that 21% of U.S. adolescents and adults with HIV may be undiagnosed (Campsmith, Rhodes, Hall, & Green, 2010). Adolescents and young adults (aged 13–29) comprised 39% of all new cases of HIV infection in 2009. There was a 48% increase in new HIV infections among young Black men having sex with men between 2006 and 2009 (CDC, 2011c). New medications are thought to be the cause of the declining death rate, whereas new cases are increasing within adolescent and young adult populations. Females, males having sex with other males, injection drug users, and racial minorities have higher rates of STI/HIV during adolescence (Sales & DiClemente, 2010). Also, those experiencing childhood sexual abuse are more at risk for HIV/AIDS risk behaviors as adolescents (Jones et al., 2010).

As noted earlier, sex education is effective at both delaying the onset of sexual activity and increasing the use of contraception in adolescents who are already sexually active. It is also effective in increasing safer-sex practices, knowledge of birth control method efficacy, and overall sexual knowledge when that content is taught (Lindau, Tetteh, Kasza, & Gilliam, 2008). Prevention strategies, identified by systematic review of research, found the best strategies to reduce sexual risk behaviors included targeting behaviors that are most easily amenable to change (e.g., condom use, decreased number of sexual partners, abstinence), tailoring programs to the target population (e.g., subgroups such as African American females, gay/bisexual males), using theory as a guide in development of programs (e.g., modeling discussions with partners about condom use, skill building by role playing situations, increasing self-efficacy), and addressing a broader content than just STI/HIV prevention education (e.g., problem solving, social skills, gender pride, capacity building). Evidence-based interventions are the most effective (Sales & DiClemente, 2010). See Chapter 30 for the school nurse's role with STI/HIV.

Acne

About 80% of individuals between the ages of 11 and 30 have acne. Most of these are adolescents, although pediatric acne (ages 7–11) cases are growing (Mancini, Baldwin, Eichenfield, Friedlander, & Yan, 2011). The precise cause of acne is not fully understood. It is generally related to several factors. Genetics plays a part (there is often a family history of acne), and hormonal influences are also at play (especially an increase in male hormones), and greasy cosmetics may plug cells of follicles, producing a plug (National Institute of Arthritis and Musculoskeletal and Skin Diseases [NIAMSD], 2010). Acne generally begins during puberty (10–12 years of age) with the increase in circulating male hormones that stimulate sebaceous glands in the skin. The excess sebum (oil) causes irritation in the pores and results in a buildup of cells, leading to whiteheads. Open pores are known as blackheads. A red and inflamed pustule can develop or, in serious cases of acne, cysts or nodules can form. Untreated, this can lead to pitting and scarring.

It is now known that greasy foods and chocolate do not cause acne but may be aggravating factors (along with stress, environmental irritants, and certain cosmetics) in susceptible adolescents. Abrasive scrubbing of the skin, pressure from backpacks, tight collars, or sports helmets, and picking or squeezing blemishes may make acne worse (NIAMSD, 2010). Common treatment regimens include skin cleansers, peelers, and medications to decrease sebaceous gland activity. Topical retinoids are the first-line drugs of choice due to their anti-inflammatory properties. Benzoyl peroxide is used to kill bacteria on the skin and in the pores. It may be sold over the counter (OTC) or by prescription. Other OTC medications include salicylic acid and resorcinol. Retin A (a topical vitamin A ointment), glycolic acid, and alpha-hydroxy acids help to peel the impacted cells from the pores. Antibiotics (oral or topical), such as tetracycline (Ala-Tet) or doxycycline (Adoxa), may be prescribed to help control bacteria on the skin. Isotretinoin (Accutane) reduces the size and activity of sebaceous glands but can cause liver or kidney dysfunction. Because of an extremely high risk of birth defects, female adolescents taking Accutane are prescribed oral contraceptives; these may also be prescribed for girls not taking this drug who have hormonally influenced acne (NIAMSD, 2010; Ramanathan & Hebert, 2011). Sun sensitivity is another side effect of this medication. Corticosteroids may be injected directly into the comedones. Dapsone gel (Aczone) can be applied twice daily to the face, and some adolescents choose to try coplemenary therapies such as tea tree oil, aloe vera, or witch hazel, as well as biofeedback and hypnosis (Ramanathan & Hebert, 2011).

The best preventive measures are keeping the skin clean, eating a balanced diet that includes fresh fruits and vegetables, drinking lots of water, and getting adequate sleep. It is important for male adolescents to shave carefully and for all teens with acne to avoid touching their faces or picking at their blemishes. They may want to use skin and hair products that are noncomedogenic. Adolescents with severe acne may need to be referred to dermatologists who specialize in this skin disorder.

Poor Nutrition and Eating Disorders

Poor nutrition and obesity are not uncommon among adolescents, whose diets often consist of snacks with limited nutritional value interspersed among unhealthful meals. Increased fast food consumption has been tied to poor diets and the increase in obesity in the United States (Li Harmer, Cardinal, Bosworth, & Johnson-Shelton, 2009; Moore, Roux, Nettleton, Jacobs, & Franco, 2009). The eating behavior of adolescents is influenced by many things, among them psychosocial factors, family and peers, availability of fast food, and mass media marketing (Davis & Carpenter, 2009; Kremer, Leslie, Berk, & Toumbourou, 2010). Girls are more at risk for problems with nutrition for several reasons: they tend to diet inappropriately, to have more finicky eating habits, and to be less physically active than teenage boys. Boys typically eat large quantities of food, which increases the likelihood of obtaining adequate nutrients, and they also tend to be more physically active than girls. The quality of an adolescent's diet has implications for later health, as evidenced by a study of fruit and vegetable consumption among 13- to 17-year-olds. The beneficial effects of vegetable and fruit intake on inflammatory and oxidative stress markers were already evident in these adolescents, indicating a good basis for future health (Holt et al., 2009).

Issues with body image and control are at the heart of anorexia nervosa and bulimia nervosa, common problems for adolescent girls. Eating disorders are considered psychiatric conditions, but there is a continuum of altered eating that does not fall within the diagnostic guidelines of an eating disorder (American Dietetic Association, 2011). **Anorexia nervosa** is an eating disorder with an emotional etiology that is characterized by body image disturbance (i.e., girls see themselves as fat although they may be extremely thin), an intense fear of becoming fat or gaining weight, and refusal to maintain adequate body weight (i.e., BMI of 18 or greater). **Bulimia** is an eating disorder characterized by recurrent episodes of binge eating with repeated compensatory mechanisms to prevent weight gain, such as vomiting (purging type) and fasting or exercise (nonpurging type). Lifetime prevalence of anorexia nervosa is 0.3%, and bulimia is 0.9% (Swanson, Crow, LeGrange, Swendsen, & Merikangas, 2011).

Binge eating, also a recognized eating disorder, involves recurrent episodes of binge eating without fasting, self-induced vomiting, or other compensatory measures, and lifetime prevalence of this disorder is 1.6% (Swanson et al., 2011). Self-esteem, depressive symptoms, and emotional eating are very sensitive predictors of binge eating, 34% of adolescents have reported secretive eating (Knatz, Maginot, Story, Neumark-Sztainer, & Boutelle, 2011). Low levels of support from peers can also be linked to binge eating, and binge eating is associated with an increased risk of becoming overweight or obese (Knatz et al., 2011).

These diseases have emotional causes that are often associated with role impairment, other psychiatric conditions, along with suicidality, and pose complex challenges to treatment (Swanson et al., 2011). A review of current research on eating disorders notes how environmental factors (e.g., nutrition, stress) may lead to epigenetic changes that affect the risk of developing an eating disorder (Campbell, Mill, Uher, & Schmidt, 2011). There is some evidence of mother and peer attitudes and behaviors increasing the risk of later escalations of symptoms among adolescents. The transition from adolescence into young adulthood is an important one as "eating disorder risk factors and symptoms increase over time" (Linville, Stice, Gau, & O'Neill, 2011, p. 749). Nutrition education, psychological counseling, and cognitive-behavioral techniques that teach clients how to control stimuli, substitute alternative behaviors, and use positive visualization are all part of treatment; development of a support network is also important. Family and individually based treatments are most often used for severe cases of adolescent eating disorders and have been studied most often. Self-concept is often distorted and self-esteem is low; therefore, activities are initiated to improve the adolescents' feelings about themselves and to bolster their coping mechanisms. Medications (e.g., antidepressants) have been used to treat some adolescents with eating disorders, but there is little evidence of their effectiveness (Lock, 2011). In a sample of adolescents enrolled in a treatment program for bulimia nervosa, 62% had a comorbid diagnosis—generally a major mood disorder. Over 65% had consumed alcohol and 30% had used an illicit drug (Fisher & le Grange, 2007).

The key to prevention may be tied to girls' perceptions of their appearance and education about the risks of dieting. One classic study indicated that adolescent girls who were severe dieters were 18 times more likely to develop an eating disorder than those who did not diet. Even moderate dieters were at risk; they were five times more likely to develop an eating disorder. Psychiatric morbidity was also a factor; it increased risk sevenfold. Exercise is seen as a more viable alternative than extreme dieting for adolescents who want to control their weight. Adolescents who use unhealthy and extreme weight-control behaviors (e.g., binge eating, fasting, skipped meals) continue these behaviors into adulthood. This is more common for females, but one third of males reported these behaviors in a recent study (Pedersen, 2011).

HEALTH SERVICES FOR SCHOOL-AGE CHILDREN AND ADOLESCENTS

A number of programs serve the health needs of school-age children and adolescents. Community health nurses play a major and vital role in delivering these services. Such programs fall into three categories that approximate the three practice priorities of community health nursing practice: illness prevention, health protection, and health promotion.

Preventive Health Programs

Among programs to prevent physical illness and other health problems among adolescents are immunizations and TB testing, as well as school- and community-based education and support programs. Private and public counseling programs and other social services are also geared to promote health and prevent illness.

Immunizations and Tuberculosis Testing

Low immunization levels for adolescents, particularly among the poor, and increased disease rates signal the need for constant surveillance, outreach programs, and better documentation and educational efforts (Vandermeulen et al., 2008). Community health nurses are deeply involved in each of these preventive activities. Health departments and schools often work collaboratively to provide immunization services. Compulsory immunization laws are helpful in carrying out these preventive services, but recent survey results reveal that not all adolescents are fully covered. A national immunization survey revealed mixed results for achievement of *Healthy People 2010* goals for adolescent vaccination (90% coverage). While there were significant increases in vaccination rates for hepatitis B, varicella, tetanus/diphtheria/acellular pertussis (Tdap), meningococcal conjugate vaccine, and HPV, only hepatitis B and varicella rates met or slightly exceeded the 90% goal. MMR vaccination was at 89%, but Tdap was further behind at 74.7%; problematic pertussis outbreaks have been reported in several states. For instance, California had a fivefold increase in only the first 6 months of 2010 compared to the total for 2009 (Dorrell, Stokley, Yankey, & Cohn, 2010; Hitt, 2010). It is important for adolescents, as well as adults, to get a single dose of Tdap to protect themselves and infants who may be around them from whooping cough. While pertussis in adolescents or adults often manifests as an upper respiratory infection with a chronic cough, for infants who have not yet been fully immunized it can lead to serious complications. A systematic review examining diagnosis of pertussis in older children/adolescents and adults based on inspiratory whoop, postpertussive emesis, and paroxysmal cough found reliance on these classic symptoms is of limited use indicating that physicians may not recognize milder symptoms experienced beyond infancy (Cornia, Hersch, Lipsky, Newman, & Gonzales, 2010).

In the recent past, adolescents were only given "catch-up" vaccinations (those missed in childhood), except for a tetanus/diphtheria booster. Now, recommended immunizations include Tdap, meningococcal vaccine (MCV4), pneumococcal polysaccharide vaccine (PPV), both hepatitis A and B, influenza vaccine, and HPV vaccine for both boys and girls—along with any missed vaccines, for example, polio and varicella (see Figs. 22-2 and 22-3). Often, school nurses and community health nurses work with nurse volunteers to provide immunization clinics at elementary and middle schools; these are convenient for adolescents and their parents. School-based clinics are also great places to catch adolescents who need updated immunizations. One study of vaccine completion rates for teens (16–18 years) compared results from community health clinics (CHCs) and SBHCs and found significantly higher rates for most vaccines at SBHCs (Federico et al., 2010). There is some evidence that adolescent vaccinations may become more available at retail pharmacies—much like flu shots for older adults (Skiles, Cai, English, & Ford, 2011). Researchers note, however, that higher levels of medical and dental health needs are met when children and adolescents have a *medical home* (or regular source of primary care). But, only 56.9% of 1- to 17-year-olds did in 2007, and adolescents were less likely than younger children to have a medical home (Strickland, Jones, Ghandour, Kogan, & Newacheck, 2011).

Although immunization clinics may improve rates of compliance, it is recommended that 11- and 12-year-olds be scheduled for routine health care visits to their physicians, so that immunizations can be administered, checked, and updated. Adolescents who have not had chickenpox, and have not received prior vaccination, should be given the varicella virus vaccine. Routine visits give the health care provider an opportunity to discuss risk behaviors and health concerns with adolescents, and to intervene early as problems arise.

In addition to immunizations required for school entry, many states or local school districts now require

TB skin tests for school-age children and adolescents. Children have a much higher risk of disease progression than do adults. Annual testing is often recommended for children and adolescents from high-risk populations. A large retrospective study of TB cases and rates between 1994 and 2007 found that 31% of reported TB cases were among foreign-born children and adolescents. For adolescents, TB rates were almost 20 times higher than for U.S.-born teens. When the month of entry to this country was known, it was determined that over 20% of foreign-born children and adolescents with TB were first diagnosed within 3 months of entry (Menzies, Winston, Holtz, Cain, & McKenzie, 2010). Targeted TB skin testing identifies adolescents and children at risk for latent TB who could benefit from treatment to prevent progression of the disease. The following questions should be asked to determine risk:

- Was the child born outside the United States? If so, where? (Children born in Asia, Africa, Latin America, and Eastern Europe require TB skin testing.)
- Has the child traveled outside the United States? If so, where and with whom? (If child stayed with friends/family in Latin America, Asia, Africa, or Eastern Europe for 1 week or more, TB skin testing should be done.)
- Has the child been exposed to anyone with TB? Who? Did contact person have active or latent TB? When was child exposed and what was the nature of contact? (Notify the local health department if the child had contact with a person having TB.)
- Does the child have close contact with a person who had a positive TB skin test? (Other questions may relate to contact with persons who have HIV, have been in jail or shelters, or are injection drug users; or if the child ingested raw milk/products? Does the child live in a household with member(s) who were born or traveled outside the United States?)
- Positive skin tests for children and adolescents have three cutoff points (CDC, 2011e):
    - Induration ≥5 mm (if child has close contact with known or suspected TB, if child or adolescent is suspected of having TB disease, if child or adolescent's immune system is suppressed).
    - Induration ≥10 mm (if child or adolescent is at an increased risk of disseminated disease or if child or adolescent has been exposed to cases of TB disease).
    - Induration ≥15 mm (if child is 4 years old or older and has no known risk factors).

Education and Social Services

The health education of school-age children and adolescents includes a wide variety of approaches and can range from the basics of handwashing for elementary school students (Lecky et al., 2011) to hearing conservation for students who like to listen to loud music (Blood & Blood, 2011).

Parental support services are commonly available through many public and private agencies, including churches. These services can have long-range effects on the health of school-age children, because emotionally healthy parents and stable families offer a healthful environment and support system for children and can facilitate their progress in school. In most states, community health nurses provide teaching and counseling services to parents in their homes and in groups. School nurses, school mental health counselors, and school psychologists also organize parent support groups in local schools. This is particularly important during periods of transition (e.g., from elementary to middle school, from middle to high school). Discussing parenting concerns and increasing parents' understanding of normal child growth and development helps to allay fears and prevent problems. Through such efforts, family violence and abuse can be averted. Reduction in rates of divorce and the attendant consequences may also be a benefit of strengthening family resilience.

Family planning programs, often stationed strategically in inner cities, near schools, or in school-based clinics, provide birth control information and counseling to young people. In some communities, the school-based clinic dispenses condoms. In most states, adolescents have the right to consent for sexual and reproductive health care without parental permission (Burstein & English, 2010; English, 2007). Community health nurses, in collaboration with an interdisciplinary team, are usually the primary care providers in these programs. Their major goals are to prevent teenage pregnancy, educate teens about reproduction and contraception, and encourage responsible sexual behavior. Teaching parents about adolescent sexuality is important, as parents can influence their child's sexual behavior (Morrison-Beedy et al., 2008). A review of studies examining caregiver-targeted interventions that address adolescent risk/protective behaviors noted that personal contact targeting parents and other caregivers leads to effective improvements in adolescent health (Burrus et al., 2012). Other forms of contact were not as effective (e.g., Internet), but person-to-person interventions were the most effective.

Providing STI services and HIV/AIDS education can be a daunting task. Many young people with STIs are often afraid or embarrassed to seek help, and others who have been exposed to the HIV virus may not know that they are infected. Gay and bisexual young men are particularly at risk, as are youth who have been sexually abused (Jones et al., 2010). Furthermore, community health professionals receive very little training in these areas and may be uncomfortable and judgmental in their approaches. Quality services that are easily accessible, provide anonymity for clients, are age-appropriate or targeted to adolescents, and are staffed with health care providers who exhibit nonjudgmental attitudes are better able to attract young people who need help (Sales & DiClemente, 2010). Some argue that drastic changes in the provision of services to young people are needed to effect change, as adolescents often feel more comfortable when services are targeted to them rather than the general population.

One review of studies found that integrated STI/HIV prevention, treatment, and family planning services were effective for the majority of the population, but found inconclusive results among males and adolescents (Church & Mayhew, 2009).

Vulnerable groups, particularly minority youth, inner-city residents, incarcerated youth, and homosexuals, may be best reached at targeted sites (e.g., STD clinics, HIV testing sites in clinics and health departments, family planning clinics, private health care providers, schools, juvenile rehabilitation facilities, employers). PHNs are available in most of these settings; they are usually the professionals who deal most directly with these clients. An open, matter-of-fact, yet respectful, demeanor is helpful in reaching adolescents and establishing rapport and trust with them. This is especially helpful when dealing with sexual issues. Improved public awareness and education, screening of high-risk groups, appropriate treatment of infected people, and identification and treatment of sexual partners can reduce the threat of STIs.

Community health nurses should educate parents about the effects of smoking in the home and its relationship to adolescent smoking. A national survey on tobacco use among youth found that smoking at home was associated with current smoking across all of adolescence, while smoking decreased as adolescents moved from early to middle stages in relationship to peer smoking influences (Villanti, Boulay, & Juon, 2011). Media campaigns for tobacco use prevention have been successful, as have some school-based education programs (Wakefield, Loken, & Hornik, 2010). Targeted smoking cessation messages from peers that emphasized benefits of quitting were the most effective for adolescents in one evaluative study (Latimer et al., 2012). Social marketing campaigns to decrease drug use have also shown some effectiveness among adolescents (Scheier & Grenard, 2010). Community health nurses often work with law enforcement officials, school district administrators, and other community agencies to ensure compliance with local regulations and prevent or delay the use of tobacco products (Villanti, McKay, Abrams, Holtgrave, & Bowie, 2010). Information on smoking cessation and resources to help prevent tobacco use by children and adolescents is available through the Foundation for a Smokefree America (for more information, see the Internet Resources found on thePoint).

Health Protection Programs

Safety and Injury Prevention

Accident- and injury-control programs serve a critical role in protecting the lives of school-age children and adolescents. They are cost-effective: Seat belt laws, child safety seats, and helmet laws have saved millions of dollars in medical care. Efforts to prevent motor vehicle accidents, a major cause of death, include driver education programs, better highway construction, improved motor vehicle design and safety features, and continuing research into what causes various types of crashes. Injury prevention and reduction have been addressed through strategies such as state laws requiring the use of safety restraints, installation of driver and front passenger airbags, substitution of other modes of travel (air, rail, or bus), lower speed limits, stricter enforcement of drunk driving laws, graduated drivers licenses (GDLs) for teenagers, safer automobile design, and helmets for motorcyclists, bicycle riders, and skaters. While adolescents may have negative attitudes toward GDLs and learner supervision requirements, these have been effective in reducing deaths and injuries (Brookland & Begg, 2011).

In developing interventions, community health nurses need to recognize that adolescents are prone to risk-taking/novelty-seeking behaviors as a result of their cognitive, physical, and psychosocial developmental stage (Johnson & Jones, 2011). Students Against Drunk Driving (SADD) and Friday Night Live activities can promote more responsible driving habits among teens. Communities can also work with law enforcement officials to ensure compliance with mandatory seat belt laws and to promote safe speeds and appropriate driving behaviors near schools.

Safety programs also seek to protect school-age children and adolescents from the hazards of poisonings, ingestion of prescription or OTC drugs, product-related accidents (unsafe toys, bicycles, skateboards, skates, play ground equipment, and furniture), and recreational accidents, including drowning and sports-related injuries. Safety services assume various forms. Poison control centers in many localities offer information and emergency assistance. Whereas the federal Consumer Product Safety Commission monitors the safety of products, education programs in schools or through local fire or police departments teach school-age children about bicycle and water safety, fire dangers, and hazards related to poisoning. Generally, the community health nurse can educate families to recognize potentially hazardous situations and encourage efforts to eliminate them. Working with school nurses and school district officials to reduce playground hazards can contribute to the reduction of school-related injuries.

Environmental hazards and other dangers await school-age children and adolescents in the workforce. There were over 17 million workers under age 24 in 2010, and 359 workers under age 24 died from a work-related injury in 2009. Hospitals treated almost 800,000 work-related injuries that occurred to adolescent workers between 1998 and 2007, almost twice the rate for workers over age 25. One *Healthy People 2020* objective seeks to reduce the number of ED-treated occupational injuries among 15- to 19-year-olds (CDC, 2011f). Because often work in restaurants where floors can be slippery and kitchen equipment can be hazardous, they have a higher frequency of workplace injuries. The federal government notes that fatal occupational injuries among adolescents are most often in the service sector (32%), construction (28%), wholesale/retail trade (10%), and agriculture (10%). The highest death rates in mining, agriculture, and construction were among younger workers (Estes, Jackson, & Castillo, 2010). Community health nurses can join with occupational health nurses and school nurses to teach parents and children about the dangers and risks inherent in the workplace, and they can work with local employers to ensure safe working conditions and reasonable hours of employment that do not interfere with school. Adolescent workers, depending upon social class and income backgrounds, may accrue either benefits or harm to their future education and employment because of high school jobs (Staff & Mortimer, 2008). One study noted that 17- and 18-year-old students working an average of 14.7 hours weekly who experienced lack of adequate sleep, psychological distress, and higher physical work had greater levels of fatigue (Laberge et al., 2011).

Infectious Diseases

Programs that protect school-age children and adolescents against infectious diseases encompass such efforts as closing swimming pools that have unsafe bacteria counts, conducting immunization campaigns in conjunction with influenza or measles outbreaks, and working with hospital pediatric units to reduce the incidence and threat of iatrogenic disease. Prevention of community-acquired MRSA is a new challenge for public schools, and PHNs may work with school nurses or others to provide educational programs covering a variety of infectious diseases (Alex & Letizia, 2007). Epidemiologic investigations, especially with school sports teams, may be necessary to determine the cause of outbreaks (Pallin et al., 2008).

Child Protective Services

In 1974, the National Center for Child Abuse and Neglect was established as a result of the Child Abuse Prevention and Treatment Act. The center collects and analyzes information on child abuse and neglect, serves as an information clearinghouse, publishes educational materials on the subject, offers technical assistance, and conducts research into the problem (Administration on Children & Families, 2011b).

In 2010, an estimated 3.3 million referrals were made alleging child abuse and/or neglect of approximately 5.9 million children. Over 60% of these referrals were screened and almost 2 million cases had Child Protective Services (CPS) responses. Over 436,000 cases of child abuse or neglect were substantiated (ACF, 2011a). Most victims suffered from neglect (78.3%), but approximately 17.6% were physically abused, and 9.2% were sexually abused. There were 2.07 deaths per 100,000 children, and 79.4% of children were under age 4. More than 32% of deaths were attributed to neglect, and more than 40% due to multiple types of maltreatment. Most perpetrators of child abuse and maltreatment—more than 80%—were parents (Administration for Children & Families [ACF], 2011a). Fathers or male caretakers are most often perceived to be perpetrators for physical abuse fatalities; mothers are more often thought to be associated with deaths stemming from neglect. Consequences for affected children include lower self-esteem, depression, suicide, self-abuse, substance abuse, eating disorders, less empathy for others, antisocial behavior, delinquency, aggression, violence, low academic achievement, and sexual maladjustment (Eaves, Prom, & Silberg, 2010; Haynie et al., 2009; Hollist et al., 2009; Moylan et al., 2010). Long-term emotional, social, cognitive, and physical consequences often follow abused children into adolescence and adulthood—post-traumatic stress disorder, poor attachment and problems with trust, difficulties with language development and abstract reasoning, high-risk health behaviors, and abusive or violent behavior (Heim, Shugart, Craighead, & Nemeroff, 2010; Wang & Holton, 2007).

Neglectful families are generally profiled as having high levels of problems among adults, reports of stressful life events, and a higher incidence of maternal depression, and these families often live at or below the poverty level. Children and adolescents who are raised in blended homes (where one parent is not their biologic parent) are at greater risk of physical or sexual abuse (McRee, 2008). Adolescents who run away, act out at school, commit illegal acts, or engage in high-risk behaviors (e.g., drug abuse, sexual promiscuity) may be exhibiting externalizing behaviors in response to years of abuse and neglect (Lansford, Dodge, Pettit, & Bates, 2010). Young adults who have been arrested for general or violent offenses and those who use illicit drugs are more likely to have been abused or neglected in adolescence (Lansford et al., 2010; Moylan et al., 2010; Williams, Van Dorn, Bright, Jonson-Reid, & Nebbitt, 2010).

The average lifetime cost per child nonfatal victim of maltreatment is estimated in 2010 at $210,012, and for each child death, it is $1,272,900 including the loss of productivity (Fang, Brown, Florence, & Mercy, 2012). Services to protect children from abuse are not as well-developed or as effective as safety and injury-protection programs, for a variety of reasons. Most child abuse occurs in the home, so only the most blatant situations become evident to outsiders (Spivey et al., 2008). Child social workers are also often unable to assess recurrent risk of child maltreatment, even when families continue in their caseloads (Dorsey, Mustillo, Farmer, & Elbogen, 2008). A wish to avoid legal involvement keeps others from reporting suspected cases, although this attitude is changing among professionals who work with children and other community members. Teachers (16.4%), legal and law enforcement personnel (16.7%), and social services staff (11.5%) were the three highest reporters of child abuse in 2010; others reporting maltreatment include anonymous sources (9%), other relatives (7%), parents (68%), and neighbors (4.4%) (ACF, 2011a).

In some areas, community health nurses are working together with social workers, mental health workers, and substance abuse counselors as part of a team that provides services to families. Improved training of mandated reporters, such as teachers and physicians, has led to better reporting of abuse; as professionals and the public become more aware of the problem, an increase in reporting has occurred. Child abuse prevention education programs can be found in many public health departments and through some school districts as a primary preventive intervention. Primary prevention of child maltreatment can also occur through home visiting programs utilizing PHNs. These visits can also help to connect high-risk families to the community and promote better child outcomes, as noted in class research by Russell, Britner, and Woolard (2007).

Families often have many time constraints that can lead to difficulties in providing adequate social support and sufficient opportunities for teaching children socialization skills and appropriate methods of coping with stress. Family stressors can cause parental conflict and lead to disruptions in parent–child relationships. Outcomes for children are worse when these situations occur early in childhood and continue for longer periods of time. Programs that target at-risk families, especially adolescent mothers and young couples prone to partner violence or harsh parenting practices, may help to prevent later child abuse (Moore & Florsheim, 2008). PHNs, school nurses, and other nurses working in the community setting must be vigilant for signs of family stress, harsh parenting practices, family violence, and other risk factors for child abuse and neglect and provide resources and respite as needed (Taylor, Baldwin, & Spencer, 2008).

Child death review teams are found at state and local levels and, through their work, improvements in interagency collaboration, procurement of more comprehensive data sets, and identification of gaps in CPS have led to better services for families and prosecution of abusers, along with improvements in child protective and other community supportive services (Christian & Sege, 2010; Keleher & Arledge, 2011).

Oral Hygiene and Dental Care

School-based programs that provide fluoride rinses and dental sealants and promote tooth brushing and nutrition education for dental health can be found in most areas of the country. Fluoridation of community water supplies is considered the most effective, safe, and low-cost means of protecting the dental health of children and adolescents. Fluoridation of drinking water, school-provided fluoride rinse or gel, and dental sealant programs are cost-effective and can reduce dental caries (Edelstein & Chinn, 2009; FCFS, n.d.b; Lam, 2008).

Fluoride makes teeth less susceptible to decay by increasing the resistance of tooth enamel to the bacterially produced acid in the mouth. Since 1945, public water supplies have been fluoridated at relatively low cost to communities. Water fluoridation has been ranked as one of the 10 greatest public health achievements of the 20th century (Division of Oral Health, 2012).

Some individuals and groups oppose fluoridation because of possible adverse effects (including fluorosis, which can cause mottling of tooth enamel). Research results have been mixed, although most studies have supported the low risk of water fluoridation and the benefits of decreased caries. In the United States, because of children's potential for multiple exposures to fluoride through drinking water, processed foods and beverages, toothpaste, gels, and rinses, physicians may prescribe lower doses of fluoride supplements or deem that they are not needed (Rozier et al., 2010). While most dental care is focused on children, adolescents remain in need of dental health services. A large study of high school students found that lower SES was significantly associated with a higher prevalence of severe dental caries and also with lower rates of sealants, dental services, and brushing, although these behaviors were less significant than SES (Polk, Welyant, & Manz, 2010). In addition to regular dental care, good nutrition, and proper oral hygiene, community health nurses can promote public water fluoridation as an important program for protecting children's dental health.

Health Promotion Programs: Nutrition and Exercise

Nutrition and weight-control programs form another important set of health promotion services. Children need to learn sound dietary habits early in life to establish healthy lifelong patterns. Being overweight during childhood or adolescence may persist into adulthood and may increase the risk for some chronic diseases later in life (Dixon et al., 2012; Nadeau et al., 2011). Some school programs teach and provide good nutrition and encourage eating patterns that prevent obesity (Food & Nutrition Service, 2008). A number of weight-control programs for overweight children and adolescents are available through schools, health departments, community health centers, health maintenance organizations, and private groups.

Children and adolescents are particularly vulnerable to media and peer pressures with regard to their food choices. Because of increased rates of childhood obesity and a greater awareness of the need for better nutrition in adolescence, legislative support to limit soft drink sales at public schools is growing. Parents and children are becoming more aware of the need to cut consumption of saturated fat, salt, sugar, and overprocessed foods, and increase fruit and vegetable consumption in order to feel and look better. The community health nurse, through nutrition education and reinforcement of positive practices, plays a significant role in promoting the health of children.

SUMMARY

Physical health and illness, developmental issues, schooling, behaviors, and emotional and mental problems are major concerns for all Americans and especially for U.S. school-age and adolescent populations. Children and adolescents are important population groups to community health nurses, because their physical and emotional health can affect not only their academic achievement but also the future of society. This population particularly needs the guidance and direction that can be provided by community health nurses. Among the health problems that affect learning and achievement in school-age children are chronic diseases, such as asthma, autism, and diabetes; behavioral and learning problems, such as ADHD and learning and other disabilities; poverty; injuries; communicable diseases, such as measles and mumps; and dietary problems involving inadequate nutrition, obesity, inactivity, and poor dental health.

One nationwide measure to prevent communicable diseases is the federally and state-mandated immunization program for school-age children and adolescents. Among vaccines given on schedule throughout childhood are those that prevent polio, smallpox, diphtheria, tetanus, typhoid, and many other diseases, so that these diseases will not be passed from one person to another in epidemic proportion.

Mortality rates for children and adolescents have decreased dramatically since the early 1900s, but morbidity rates remain high. Children and adolescents are vulnerable to many illnesses, injuries, and emotional problems, often as a result of a complex and stressful environment. Violence against children and deaths due to homicide occur in the United States at alarming rates. Unintentional injuries, suicide, and homicide are the leading threats to life and health for adolescents. Other health problems include alcohol and drug abuse, unplanned pregnancies, STIs and HIV/AIDS, and poor nutrition. All of these problems create major challenges for the community health nurse who seeks to prevent illness and injury among children and adolescents and to promote their health.

Among the objectives for children and adolescents proposed by *Healthy People 2020*, some key goals are reduction of alcohol-related unintentional injuries; declines in violent behaviors, suicide, and mental health issues; and more responsible reproductive health behaviors. Barriers to achieving these goals vary. Some include economic inequities; lack of sufficient immunization, educational, and community-supported health programs; and the presence of risk behaviors typical among developing youth. Community health nurses play a large role in promoting the health of young people, their families, and communities through education programs and by developing strategies to support healthy growth and development and prevent risky behaviors that lead to injury, teen pregnancy, and sometimes death.

Health services for children and adolescents span three categories: prevention, health protection, and health promotion. The community health nurse plays a vital role in each. Preventive services may include immunization programs, parental support services, family planning programs, services for those with STIs, and alcohol and drug abuse prevention programs. Health protection services often include accident and injury control, programs to reduce environmental hazards and control infectious diseases, and services to protect children and adolescents from child abuse and neglect. Health promotion services may include programs in nutrition and weight control, along with HIV/AIDS prevention, and smoking, alcohol, and drug abuse education. PHNs are integral to the health and wellbeing of children and adolescents, through their work with families, schools, and other community agencies.

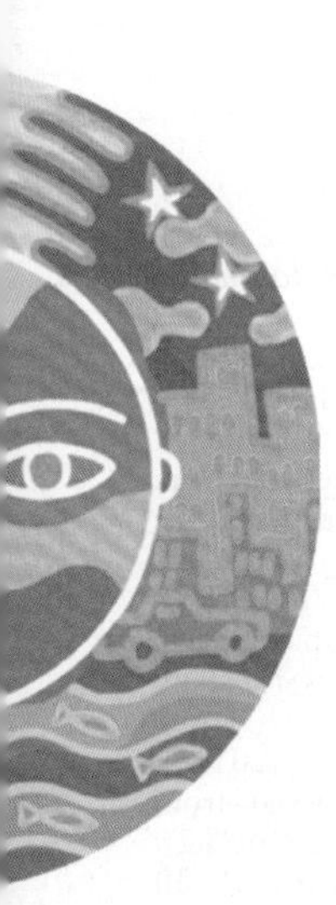

ACTIVITIES TO PROMOTE CRITICAL THINKING

1. You are a community health nurse assigned to work at a school. You learn that more than 20% of the students in this school district are receiving Ritalin, Adderall, or some other medication for treating ADHD. What issues should you consider in determining whether these medications are being appropriately prescribed?
2. What is the major cause of death among younger school-age children? Adolescents? What community-wide interventions could be initiated to prevent these deaths? Select one intervention for children and one for adolescents and describe how you and a group of community health professionals might develop effective preventive measures.
3. A 14-year-old girl from a middle-class family and a 14-year-old girl from a poor family both come to the health department clinic where you work. The girls have similar symptoms that suggest gonorrhea. Would your assessment and intervention be the same for the two girls? What are your values and attitudes toward people with infections that are sexually transmitted? Does social class, race, age, or sex make any difference in how you feel about them? What is one action the community health nurse can take to prevent such infections in this population group?
4. Discuss possible methods of doing nutritional assessments in school-age children and adolescents. What programs could be instituted to encourage healthier diets and increased exercise? What other factors might need to be considered? How could you, as a community health nurse, work with schools and parents to increase physical activity and improve nutrition for school-age children and adolescents?
5. A new elementary school to which you have been assigned has repeated outbreaks of head lice and very limited access to health care. Using the Internet, research causes for recurrent head lice infestations and effective over-the-counter treatment products. Are "no-nit" policies effective? Why or why not? Discuss possible education programs you might implement or other innovative methods of treatment and control you might be able to institute.

REFERENCES

Acosta, M., Manubay, J., & Levin, F. (2008). Pediatric obesity: Parallels with addiction and treatment recommendations. *Harvard Review of Psychiatry*, *16*(2), 80–96.

Addy, S., & Wight, V. R. (2012). *Basic facts about low-income children, 2010: Children under age 18*. National Center for Children in Poverty [NCCP]. Retrieved from http://www.nccp.org/publications/pub_1049.html

Administration for Children & Families. (2011). *Child maltreatment 2010*. Retrieved from http://www.acf.hhs.gov/programs/cb/stats_research/index.htm#can

Administration for Children & Families. (2011). *Organization structure*. Retrieved from http://www.acf.hhs.gov/programs/cb/aboutcb/org.htm#ocan

Akinbami, L. J., Liu, X., Pastor, P. N., & Reuben, C. A. (2011). Attention deficit hyperactivity disorder among children aged 5–17 years in the United States, 1998–2009. *NCHS Data Brief*, 70. Retrieved from http://www.toxicpsychiatry.com/storage/ADHD%20NCHS%20stats%20age%205-17%20years%20US%2098-2009%20Akinbami%20et%20al.pdf

Alex, A., & Letizia, M. (2007). Community-acquired methicillin-resistant *Staphylococcus aureus*: Considerations for school nurses. *Journal of School Nursing*, *23*(4), 210–214.

Allen, J. L., Lavallee, K., Herren, C., Ruthe, K., & Schneider, S. (2010). DSM-IV criteria for childhood separation anxiety disorder: Informant, age, and sex differences. *Journal of Anxiety Disorders*, *24*(8), 946–952.

Allison, K. W., Edmonds, T., Wilson, K., Pope, M., & Farrell, A. D. (2011). Connecting youth violence prevention, positive youth development, and community mobilization. *American Journal of Community Psychology*, *48*(1–2), 8–20.

Altarac, M., & Saroha, E. (2007). Lifetime prevalence of learning disability among US children. *Pediatrics*, *119*(Suppl. 1), s77–s83.

Alvanzo, A., Storr, C., La Flair, L., Green, K., Wagner, F., & Crum. R. (2011). Race/ethnicity and sex differences in progression from drinking initiation to the development of alcohol dependence. *Drug and Alcohol Dependence*, *118*(2–3), 375–382.

American Academy of Child & Adolescent Psychiatry. (2009). *Self-injury in adolescents*. Retrieved from http://aacap.org/page.ww?name=Self-Injury+in+Adolescents§ion=Facts+for+Families

American Academy of Child & Adolescent Psychiatry. (2011a). *Children with oppositional defiant disorder*. Retrieved from http://www.aacap.org/page.ww?section=Facts%20for%20Families&name=Children%20With%20Oppositional%20Defiant%20Disorder

American Academy of Child & Adolescent Psychiatry. (2011b). *Children and watching TV*. Retrieved from http://www.aacap.org/cs/root/facts_for_families/children_and_watching_tv

American Academy of Pediatrics. (2008). *Policy statement: The role of the school nurse in providing school health services*. Retrieved from http://aappolicy.aappublications.org/cgi/content/full/pediatrics;108/5/1231

American Dietetic Association. (2011). Position of the American Dietetic Association: Nutrition intervention in the treatment of eating disorders. *Journal of the American Dietetic Association, 111*, 1236–1241.

American Heart Association. (2011). *Understanding childhood obesity*. Retrieved from http://www.heart.org/idc/groups/heart-public/@wcm/@fc/documents/downloadable/ucm_428180.pdf

American Psychological Association Zero Tolerance Task Force. (2008). Are zero tolerance policies effective in the schools? An evidentiary review and recommendations. *American Psychologist, 63*(9), 852–862.

Andersen, S., & Teicher, M. (2008). Stress, sensitive periods and maturational events in adolescent depression. *Trends in Neuroscience, 31*(4), 183–191.

Anthony, E., King, B., & Austin, M. J. (2011). Reducing child poverty by promoting child well-being: Identifying best practices in a time of great need. *Children and Youth Services Review, 33*, 1999–2009.

Anxiety Disorders Association of America (ADAA). (2012). *School refusal*. Retrieved from http://www.adaa.org/living-with-anxiety/children/school-refusal

Armour, S. (2007). *Delaying sex can have positive effects for adolescents*. Medical News. Retrieved from http://www.news-medical.net/news/2007/02/27/22218.aspx?page=2

Arns, M., Ridder, S., Strehl, U., Breteler,M., & Coenen, A. (2009). Efficacy of neurofeedback treatment in ADHD: The effects on inattention, impulsivity and hyperactivity. A meta-analysis. *Clinical EEG and Neuroscience, 40*(3), 180–189.

Arseneault, L., Milne, B., Taylor, A., Adams, F., Delgado, K., Caspi, A., et al. (2008). Being bullied as an environmentally mediated contributing factor to children's internalizing problems: A study of twins discordant for victimization. *Archives of Pediatric and Adolescent Medicine, 162*(2), 145–150.

Arts, W., & Geerts, A. T. (2009). When to start drug treatment for childhood epilepsy: The clinical-epidemiological evidence. *European Journal of Paediatric Neurology, 13*(2), 93–101.

Asthma & Allergy Foundation of America (AAFA). (2011). *Asthma overview*. Retrieved from http://www.aafa.org/display.cfm?id=8

Autism Society of America. (n.d.). *About autism*. Retrieved from http://www.autism-society.org/about-autism/

Barclay, L. (2012). AAP updates childhood and adolescent immunization schedules. *Medscape Medical News*. Retrieved from http://www.medscape.com/viewarticle/757879

Barr, S., Hanson, R., Begle, A., Kilpatrick, D., Saunders, B., et al. (2011). Examining the moderating role of family cohesion on the relationship between witnessed community violence and delinquency in a national sample of adolescents. *Journal of Interpersonal Violence*, doi: 10.1177/0886260511416477.

Basch, C. E. (2011a). Asthma and the achievement gap among urban minority youth. *Journal of School Health, 81*(10), 606–613.

Basch, C. E. (2011b). Teen pregnancy and the achievement gap among urban minority youth. *Journal of School Health, 81*(10), 614–418.

Bauer, K., Neumark-Sztainer, D., Fulkerson, J., Hannan, P., & Story, M. (2011). Familial correlates of adolescent girls' physical activity, television use, dietary intake, weight, and body composition. *International Journal of Behavioral Nutrition and Activity, 8*, 25. Retrieved from http://www.ijbnpa.org/content/8/1/25

BBC News. (2010). *Mexican drug gangs spread to every region of US*. Retrieved from http://news.bbc.co.uk/2/hi/8588509.stm

Beauchaine, T. P., Hinshaw, S., & Pang, K. (2010). Comorbidity of attention-deficit/hyperactivity disorder and early-onset conduct disorder: Biological, environmental, and developmental mechanisms. *Clinical Psychology: Science and Practice, 17*(4), 327–336.

Bernard, S., Paulozzi, L., & Wallace, L. J. D. (2007). Fatal injuries among children by race and ethnicity: United States, 1999–2002. *Morbidity and Mortality Weekly Report (MMWR)*. Retrieved from http://www.cdc.gov/mmwr/PDF/ss/ss5605.pdf

Best, C., Neufingerl, N., Del Rosso, J., Transler, C., van den Briel, T., & Osendarp, S. (2011). Can multi-micronutrient food fortification improve the micronutrient status, growth, health, and cognition of schoolchildren? A systematic review. *Nutrition Reviews, 69*(4), 186–204.

Best, C., Neufingerl, N., van Geel, L., van den Briel, T. & Osendarp, S. (2010). The nutritional status of school-aged children: Why should we care? *Food and Nutrition Bulletin, 31*(3), 400–417.

Bethell, J., & Rhodes, A. (2008). Adolescent depression and emergency department uses: The roles of suicidality and deliberate self-harm. *Current Psychiatry Reports, 10*(1), 53–59.

Bezdjian, S., Baker, L. A., & Tuvblad, C. (2011). Genetic and environmental influences on impulsivity: a meta-analysis of twin, family and adoption studies. *Clinical Psychology Review, 31*(7), 1209–1223.

Blakemore, S. J. (2008). The social brain in adolescence. *Nature Reviews: Neuroscience, 9*(4), 267–277.

Blakemore, S. J., den Ouden, H., Choudhury, S., & Frith, C. (2007). Adolescent development of the neural circuitry for thinking about intentions. *Social, Cognitive and Affective Neuroscience, 2*(2), 130–139.

Blood, I. M., & Blood, G. W. (2011). Podcasts, Google, and YouTube—oh my! An innovative online course for university students on preventing hearing loss. *Perspectives on Public Health Issues Related to Hearing and Balance, 1*(1), 4–12.

Boden, J., Fergusson, D., & Horwood, J. (2008). Early motherhood and subsequent life outcomes. *Journal of Child Psychology and Psychiatry, 49*(2), 151–160.

Borum, R., Cornell, D., Modzeleski, W., & Jimerson, S. (2010). What can be done about school shootings? A review of the evidence. *Educational Researcher, 39*(1), 27–37.

Boyle, C. A., Boulet, S., Schieve, L., Cohen, R. (2011). Trends in the prevalence of developmental disabilities in US children 1997–2008. *Pediatrics, 127*(6), 1034–1042.

Brault, M. W. (2011). School-aged children with disabilities in U.S. metropolitan statistical areas: 2010. *American Community Survey Briefs*. Retrieved from http://www.census.gov/prod/2011pubs/acsbr10-12.pdf

Bretz, W. A., Corby, P. M., Melo, M. R., Coelho, M., Costa, S., Robinson, M. et al. (2006). Heritability estimates for dental caries and sucrose sweetness preference. *Journal of Evidence Based Dental Practice, 51*(12), 1156–1160.

Bridge, J. A., Greenhouse, J., Sheftall, A., Fabio, A., Campo, J., & Kelleher, K. (2010). Changes in suicide rates by hanging and/or suffocation and firearms among young persons aged 10–24 years in the United States: 1992–2006. *Journal of Adolescent Health, 46*(5), 503–505.

Briggs, M., Hopman, W., & Jamieson, M. (2007). Comparing pregnancy in adolescents and adults: Obstetric outcomes and prevalence of anemia. *Journal of Obstetrics and Gynecology, Canada, 29*(7), 546–555.

Brook, J. S., Marcus, S., Zhang, C., Stimmel, M., Balka, E., & Brook, D. (2010). Adolescent attributes and young adult smoking cessation behavior. *Substance Use and Misuse, 45*(13), 2172–2184.

Brookland, R., & Begg, D. (2011). Adolescent, and their parents, attitudes towards graduated driver licensing and subsequent risky driving and crashes in young adulthood. *Journal of Safety Research, 42*(2), 109–115.

Brown, T. (Ed.). (2009). *ADHD comorbidities: Handbook for ADHD complications in children and adults*. Washington, DC: American Psychiatric Publishing, Inc.

Brunham, R. C. (2009). Infectious disease prevention and control: Remembering 1908 and imagining 2108. *Canadian Journal of Public Health, 100*(1), 5–6.

Bureau of Justice Statistics. (n.d.). *Drugs and crime facts*. Retrieved from http://bjs.ojp.usdoj.gov/content/dcf/du.cfm

Burrus, B., Leeks, K., Sipe, T., Dolina, S., Soler, R., Elder, R. et al. (2012). Person-to-person interventions targeted to parents and other caregivers to improve adolescent health: A community guide systematic review. *American Journal of Preventive Medicine, 42*(3), 316–326.

Burstein, G., & English, A. (2010). Pediatricians should become familiar with state consent laws for minors. *AAP News, 31*(6), 17.

Byrnie, F. H. (2008, May 27). *"Go/no go" task reveals brain anomalies in children with ADHD*. The Dana Foundation. Retrieved from http://www.dana.org/news/features/detail.aspx?id=12468

Campbell, I. C., Mill, J., Uher, R., & Schmidt, U. (2011). Eating disorders, gene-environment interactions and epigenetics. *Neuroscience and Biobehavioral Reviews, 35*(3), 784–793.

Campsmith, M. L., Rhodes, P., Hall, H. I., & Green, T. (2010). Undiagnosed HIV prevalence among adults and adolescents in the United States at the end of 2006. *Journal of Acquired Immune Deficiency Syndromes, 53*(5), 619–624.

Casey, B. J., Jones, R., & Hare, T. (2008). The adolescent brain. *Annals of the New York Academy of Science*, *1124*, 111–126.

Casey, P. H., Pippa, M. S., Gossett, J. M., et al. (2006). The association of child and household food insecurity with childhood overweight status. *Pediatrics*, *118*(5), E1406–E1413.

Castillo, C. L. (Ed.). (2008). *Children with complex medical issues in schools: Neuropsychological descriptions and interventions*. New York: Springer Publishing.

Cavazos-Rehg, P., Krauss, M., Spitznagel, E., Iguchi, M., Schootman, M., Cottler, L. et al. (2012). Associations between sexuality education in schools and adolescent birthrates. *Archives of Pediatrics and Adolescent Medicine*, *166*(2), 134–140.

Centers for Disease Control and Prevention (CDC). (2008a). *Student health and academic achievement*. Retrieved from http://www.cdc.gov/HealthyYouth/health_and_academics/index.htm

Centers for Disease Control and Prevention (CDC). (2008b). Unintentional strangulation deaths from the "choking game" among youths aged 6–19 years: United States, 1995–2007. *Morbidity and Mortality Weekly Report*, *57*(6), 141–144.

Centers for Disease Control and Prevention (CDC). (2009a). *CDC report finds adolescent girls continue to bear a major burden of common sexually transmitted diseases: Press release*. Retrieved from http://www.cdc.gov/nchhstp/newsroom/STDsurveillancepressrelease.html

Centers for Disease Control and Prevention (CDC). (2009b). *Research update. The choking game: CDC's findings on a risky youth behavior*. Retrieved from http://www.cdc.gov/homeandrecreationalsafety/Choking/choking_game.html

Centers for Disease Control and Prevention (CDC). (2010a). *Autism spectrum disorders*. Retrieved from http://www.cdc.gov/ncbddd/autism/index.html

Centers for Disease Control and Prevention (CDC). (2010b). *Head lice*. Retrieved from http://www.cdc.gov/parasites/lice/head/index.html

Centers for Disease Control and Prevention (CDC). (2010c). *Healthy youth! Unintentional injuries, violence and the health of young people*. Retrieved from http://www.cdc.gov/healthyyouth/injury/facts.htm

Centers for Disease Control and Prevention (CDC). (2010d). *Youth violence: Facts at a glance*. Retrieved from http://www.cdc.gov/ViolencePrevention/pdf/YV-DataSheet-a.pdf

Centers for Disease Control and Prevention (CDC). (2011a). *Attention-deficit/hyperactivity disorder (ADHD)*. Retrieved from http://www.cdc.gov/ncbddd/adhd/data.html

Centers for Disease Control and Prevention (CDC). (2011b). *Concussion in sports and play: Get the facts*. Retrieved from http://www.cdc.gov/concussion/sports/facts.html

Centers for Disease Control and Prevention (CDC). (2011c). *HIV among youth*. Retrieved from http://www.cdc.gov/hiv/youth/

Centers for Disease Control and Prevention (CDC). (2011d). *Sexual risk behavior: HIV, STD, and teen pregnancy prevention*. Retrieved from http://www.cdc.gov/HealthyYouth/sexualbehaviors/

Centers for Disease Control and Prevention (CDC). (2011e). *Tuberculin skin testing*. Retrieved from http://www.cdc.gov/tb/publications/factsheets/testing/skintesting.htm

Centers for Disease Control and Prevention (CDC). (2011f). *Young worker safety and health*. Retrieved from http://www.cdc.gov/niosh/topics/youth/

Centers for Disease Control and Prevention (CDC). (2011g). *Youth Risk Behavior Surveillance system*. Retrieved from http://www.cdc.gov/HealthyYouth/yrbs/

Chau, M., & Douglas-Hall, A. (2007). *Low-income children in the United States: National and state trend data, 1996–2006*. National Center for Children in Poverty. Colombia University Mailman School of Public Health.

Child Trends Databank. (2012a). *Children in poverty*. Retrieved from http://www.childtrendsdatabank.org/?q=node/221

Child Trends Databank. (2012b). *Food insecurity*. Retrieved from http://www.childtrendsdatabank.org/alphalist?q=node/36

Children's Defense Fund. (2011). *The state of America's children, 2011*. Retrieved from http://www.childrensdefense.org/child-research-data-publications/data/state-of-americas-2011.pdf

Chilton, M., Black, M., Berkowitz, C., Casey, P., Cook, J., Cutts, D. et al. (2009). Food insecurity and risk of poor health among US-born children of immigrants. *American Journal of Public Health*, *99*(3), 556–562.

Christian, E. W., Sege, R. D.; The Committee on Child Abuse and Neglect, The Committee on Injury, Violence, and Poison Prevention, & The Council on Community Pediatrics. (2010). Child fatality review: Policy statement. *Pediatrics*, *126*(3), 592–596.

Chung, K., & Cheung, M. (2008). Sleep-wake patterns and sleep disturbance among Hong Kong Chinese adolescents. *Sleep*, *31*(2), 185–194.

Church, K., & Mayhew, S. H. (2009). Integration of STI and HIV prevention, care, and treatment into family planning services: A review of the literature. *Studies in Family Planning*, *40*, 171–186.

Clark, C. (2011). *Top 10 reasons for pediatric hospitalizations*. Health Leaders Media. Retrieved from http://www.healthleadersmedia.com/page-1/LED-269728/Top-10-Reasons-For-Pediatric-Hospitalizations

Conroy, K., Sandel, M., & Zuckerman, B. (2010). Poverty grown up: How childhood socioeconomic status impacts adult health. *Journal of Developmental and Behavioral Pediatrics, 31*(2), 154–160.

Cornia, P., Hersch, A., Lipsky, B., Newman, T., & Gonzales, R. (2010). Does this coughing adolescent or adult patient have pertussis? *JAMA*, *304*(8), 890–896.

Cote, S., Geltman, P., Nunn, M., Lituri, K., Henshaw, M., & Garcia, R. (2004). Dental caries of refugee children compared with U.S. children. *Pediatrics, 114*(6), E733–E740.

Coverage for All. (2012). *2012 federal poverty level*. Retrieved from http://coverageforall.org/pdf/FHCE_FedPovertyLevel.pdf

Culbert, K., Burt, S., McGue, M., Iacono, W., & Klump, K. (2009). Puberty and the genetic diathesis of disordered eating attitudes and behaviors. *Journal of Abnormal Psychology*, *118*(4), 788–796.

Currie, J. (2009). Healthy, wealthy, and wise: Socioeconomic status, poor health in childhood, and human capital development. *Journal of Economic Literature*, *47*(1), 87–122.

Damon, W., & Lerner, R. (Eds.). (2008). *Child and adolescent development: An advanced course*. Hoboken, NJ: John Wiley & Sons, Inc.

Davis, B., & Carpenter, C. (2009). Proximity of fast-food restaurants to schools and adolescent obesity. *American Journal of Public Health*, *99*(3), 505 510.

Dayan, J., Bernard, A., Olliac, B., Mailhes, A. S., & Kermarrec, S. (2010). Adolescent brain development, risk-taking, and vulnerability to addiction. *Journal of Physiology—Paris*, *104*(5), 279–286.

DeLeel, M., Hughes, T., Miller, J., Hipwell, A., & Theodore, L. (2009). Prevalence of eating disturbance and body image dissatisfaction in young girls: An examination of the variance across racial and socioeconomic groups. *Psychology in the Schools*, *46*(8), 767–775.

De Pee, S., Brinkman, H. J., Webb, P., Godfrey, S., Darnton-Hill, I., Aldeman, H. et al. (2010). How to ensure nutrition security in the global economic crisis to protect and enhance development of young children and our common future. *The Journal of Nutrition*, *140*(1), 1385–1425.

Dhaval, M. D., Corman, H., & Reichman, N. E. (2012). Effects of welfare reform on education acquisition of adult women. *Journal of Labor Research*, doi: 10.1007/s12122-012-9130-4.

Dietz, W. H. (2009, March 26). *CDC Congressional testimony: Current status and activities to decrease the prevalence of obesity among U.S. children and adolescents*. Retrieved from http://www.cdc.gov/washington/testimony/2009/t20090326.htm

DiFranza, J. (2008). Hooked from the first cigarette. *Scientific American*, *298*(5), 82–87.

Division of Oral Health. (2012). *Community water fluoridation*. Centers for Disease Control. Retrieved from http://www.cdc.gov/fluoridation/

Dixon, B., Pena, M., & Taveras, E. (2012). Lifecourse approach to racial/ethnic disparities in childhood obesity. *Advances in Nutrition: An International Review Journal, 3*, 73–82.

Dobbins, M., DeCorby, K., Robeson, P., Husson, H, & Tirilis, D. (2009). School-based physical activity programs for promoting physical activity and fitness in children and adolescents aged 6–18. *The Cochrane Collaboration*, doi: 10.1002/14651858.CD007651.

Dodge, K. A., & McCourt, S. N. (2010). Translating models of antisocial behavioral development into efficacious intervention policy to prevent adolescent violence. *Developmental Psychobiology*, *52*(3), 277–285.

Donaghue, K. C., Chiarelli, F., Trotta, D., Aligrove, J., & Dahl-Jorgensen, K. (2009). Microvascular and macrovascular complications associated with diabetes in children and adolescents. *Pediatric Diabetes, 10*(s12), 195–203.

Dorrell, C., Stokley, S., Yankey, D., & Cohn, A. (2010). National, state, and local area vaccination coverage among adolescents aged 13–17 years—United States, 20009. *Morbidity and Mortality Weekly (MMWR), 59*(2), 1018–1023.

Dorsey, S., Mustillo, S., Farmer, E., & Elbogen, E. (2008). Caseworker assessments of risk for recurrent maltreatment: Association with case-specific risk factors and reports. *Child Abuse and Neglect, 32*(3), 377–391.

Drotar, D., & Bonner, M. (2009). Influences on adherence to pediatric asthma treatment: A review of correlates and predictors. *Journal of Developmental and Behavioral Pediatrics, 40*(6), 574–582.

Du, W., Finch, C., Hayen, A., Bilston, L., Brown, J., & Haatfield, J. (2010). Relative benefits of population-level interventions targeting restraint-use in child car passengers. *Pediatrics, 125*(2), 304–312.

Dube, S. R., & Orpinas, P. (2009). Understanding excessive school absenteeism as school refusal behavior. *Children and Schools, 31*(2), 87–95.

Dudley, M., Goldney, R., & Hadzi-Pavlovic, D. (2010). Are adolescents dying by suicide taking SSRI antidepressants? A review of observational studies. *Australasian Psychology, 18*(3), 242–245.

Dunne, E., Markowitz, L., Chesson, H., Curtis, C. R., Saraiya, M., Gee, J., et al. (2011). Recommendations on the use of quadrivalent human papillomavirus (HPV) vaccine in males: Advisory Committee on Immunization Practices (ACIP), 2011. *Morbidity and Mortality Weekly Report (MMWR), 60*(50), 1705–1708.

Durlak, J. A., Weissberg, R. P., Dymnicki, A. B., Taylor, R., & Schellinger, K. (2011). The impact of enhancing students' social and emotional learning: A meta-analysis of school-based universal interventions. *Child Development, 82*(1), 405–432.

East, P., Reyes, B., & Horn, E. (2007). Association between adolescent pregnancy and a family history of teenage births. *Perspectives on Sexual and Reproductive Health, 39*(2), 108–115.

Eaves, L. J., Prom, E. C., & Silberg, J. L. (2010). The mediating effect of parental neglect on adolescent and young adult anti-sociality: A longitudinal study of twins and their parents. *Behavior Genetics, 40*(4), 425–437.

Edelsteink, B., & Chinn, C. (2009). Update on disparities in oral health and access to dental care for America's children. *Academic Pediatrics, 9*(6), 415–419.

Egley, A., & Howell, J. (2011, June). *Highlights of the 2009 National Youth Gang Survey*. Washington, DC: U.S. Department of Justice.

Eisenmann, J. C., Gundersen, C., Lohman, B., Garasky, S., & Stewart, S. (2011). Is food insecurity related to overweight and obesity in children and adolescents? A summary of studies, 1995–2009. *Obesity Reviews, 12(5)*, e73–e83.

Elliottt, R., Rodgers, S., Bassani, L., Morsi, A., Gelle, E., Carlson, C. et al. (2011). Vagus nerve stimulation for children with treatment-resistant epilepsy: A consecutive series of 141 cases. *Journal of Neurosurgery: Pediatrics, 7*(5), 491–500.

English, A. (2007). Sexual and reproductive health care for adolescents: Legal rights and policy challenges. *Adolescent Medicine: State of the Art Reviews, 18*(3), 571–581, viii–ix.

Epilepsy Foundation. (n.d.). *About epilepsy*. Retrieved from http://www.epilepsyfoundation.org/aboutepilepsy/

Epstein, J., Grifin, K., & Botvin, G. (2008). A social influence model of alcohol use for inner-city adolescents: Family drinking, perceived drinking norms, and perceived social benefits of drinking. *Journal of Studies on Alcohol and Drugs, 69*(3), 397–405.

Estes, C., Jackson, L., & Castillo, D. (2010). Occupational injuries and deaths among young workers—United States, 1998–2007. *Morbidity & Mortality Weekly (MMWR), 59*(15), 449–455.

Estrada, J. S., & Morris, R. I. (2000). Pediculosis in a school population. *Journal of School Nursing, 16*(3), 32–38.

Evans, G., & Kim, P. (2007). Childhood poverty and health: Cumulative risk exposure and stress dysregulation. *Childhood Poverty and Health, 18*(11), 953–957.

Evans, G. W., & Schamberg, M. A. (2009). Childhood poverty, chronic stress, and adult working memory. *Proceedings of the National Academy of Sciences, 106*(16), 6545–6549.

Evenson, A., Justinger, B., Pelischek, E., & Schultz, S. (2009). Zero tolerance policies and the public schools: When suspension is no longer effective. *National Association of School Psychologists Communique, 37*(5), 6–7.

Faith, M. S., & Hittner, J. B. (2010). Infant temperament and eating style predict change in standardized weight status and obesity risk at 6 years of age. *International Journal of Obesity, 34*, 1515–1523.

Fang, X., Brown, D., Florence, C., & Mercy, J. (2012). The economic burden of child maltreatment in the United States and implications for prevention. *Child Abuse and Neglect, 36(2)*, 156–165.

Farmer, C. M., Braitman, K., & Lund, A. K. (2010). Cell phone use while driving and attributable crash risk. *Traffic Injury Prevention, 11*(5), 466–470.

Fass, S., & Cauthen, N. K. (2008, October). *Who are America's poor children?* National Center for Children in Poverty. Retrieved from http://www.nccp.org/publications/pdf/text_843.pdf

Federico, S., Abrams, L., Everhart, R., Melinkovich, P., & Hambidge, S. (2010). Addressing adolescent immunization disparities: A retrospective analysis of school-based health center immunization delivery. *American Journal of Public Health, 100*(9), 1630–1634.

Fergusson, D., Boden, J., & Horwood, L. (2008). The development of antecedents of illicit drug use: Evidence from a 25-year longitudinal study. *Drug and Alcohol Dependence, 96*(1–2), 165–177.

Fergusson, D., Horwood, L., & Ridder, E. (2007). Conduct and attentional problems in childhood and adolescence and later substance use, abuse and dependence: Results of a 25-year longitudinal study. *Drug and Alcohol Dependence, 88*(Suppl. 1), S14–S26.

Fields, J. (2012). Sexuality education in the United States: Shared cultural ideas across a political divide. *Sociology Compass*, 6(1), 1–14.

Finer, L. B. (2010). Unintended pregnancy among U.S. adolescents: Accounting for sexual activity. *Journal of Adolescent Health, 47*(3), 312–314.

Finkelhor, D., Turner, H., Ormrod, R., & Hamby, S. (2009). Violence, abuse, and crime exposure in a national sample of children and youth. *Pediatrics, 124(5)*, 1411–1423.

Fiorito, L., Marini, M., Francis, L., Smiciklas-Wright, H., & Birch, L. (2009). Beverage intake of girls at age 5 y predicts adiposity and weight status in childhood and adolescence. *The American Journal of Clinical Nutrition, 90*(4), 935–942.

Fisher, S., & le Grange, D. (2007). Comorbidity and high-risk behaviors in treatment-seeing adolescents with bulimia nervosa. *International Journal of Eating Disorders, 40*(8), 751–753.

Fisher, L., Miles, I., Austin, S., Camargo, C., & Colditz, G. (2007). Predictors of initiation of alcohol use among US adolescents: Findings from a prospective cohort study. *Archives of Pediatric and Adolescent Medicine, 161*(10), 959–966.

Florin, T. A., Shulte, J., & Stettler, N. (2011). Perception of overweight is associated with poor academic performance in US adolescents. *Journal of School Health, 81*(11), 663–670.

Food & Nutrition Service. (2008, April). *School lunch & breakfast; Cost study II final report.* U.S. Department of Agriculture. Retrieved from http://www.fns.usda.gov/Ora/menu/Published/CNP/FILES/MealCostStudy.pdf

Food Research & Action Council (FRAC). (2011). *SNAP food stamp participation 2011.* Retrieved from http://frac.org/reports-and-resources/snapfood-stamp-monthly-participation-data/#1dec

Ford, A., Bergh, C., Sodersten, P., Sabin, M., Hollinghurst, S., Hunt, L., (2010). Treatment of childhood obesity by retraining eating behaviour: Randomised controlled trial. *Medscape Nurses News*. Retrieved from http://www.medscape.com/viewarticle/715470

Forum on Child and Family Statistics (FCFS). (2011a). *Adolescent injury and mortality*. Retrieved from http://www.childstats.gov/americaschildren/phenviro8.asp

Forum on Child and Family Statistics (FCFS). (2011b). *America's children: Racial and ethnic composition (0–17)*. Retrieved from http://www.childstats.gov/americaschildren/tables.asp

Forum on Child and Family Statistics (FCFS). (2011c). *Child injury and mortality*. Retrieved from http://www.childstats.gov/americaschildren/phenviro7.asp

Forum on Child and Family Statistics (FCFS). (2011d). *Family structure and children's living arrangements*. Retrieved from http://www.childstats.gov/americaschildren/famsoc1.asp

Forum on Child and Family Statistics (FCFS). (2011e). *Indicator health 8: Percentage of children 0–17 with asthma, 1997–2009*. Retrieved from http://www.childstats.gov/americaschildren/health_fig.asp

Forum on Child and Family Statistics (FCFS). (n.d.a). *Obesity: Percentage of children 6–17 who are obese. Health 7*. Retrieved from http://www.childstats.gov/americaschildren/tables.asp

Forum on Child and Family Statistics (FCFS). (n.d.b). *Oral health, 2011*. Retrieved from http://www.childstats.gov/americaschildren/care4.asp

Forum on Child and Family Statistics (FCFS). (n.d.c). *Oral health: Percentage of children ages 5–17 with untreated dental caries. Table HC4.C*. Retrieved from http://www.childstats.gov/americaschildren/tables.asp

Forum on Child and Family Statistics (FCFS). (n.d.d). *Percentage of all children and related children living below selected poverty levels by selected characteristics, 1980–2009*. ECON1-A. Retrieved from http://www.childstats.gov/americaschildren/tables/econ1a.asp

Foshee, V., Reyes, H., & Ennett, S. (2010). Examination of sex and race differences in longitudinal predictors of the initiation of adolescent dating violence perpetration. *Journal of Aggression, Maltreatment and Trauma, 19*(5), 492–516.

Foss, R. D., Goodwin, A., McCartt, A. T., & Hellinga, L. A. (2009). Short-term effects of a teenage driver cell phone restriction. *Accident Analysis and Prevention, 41*(3), 419–424.

Francis, L. A., & Susman, E. J. (2009). Self-regulation and rapid weight gain in children from age 3 to 12 years. *Archives of Pediatrics and Adolescent Medicine, 163*(4), 297–302.

Franko, D., Thompson, D., Affenito, S., Barton, B., & Striegel-Moore, R. (2008). What mediates the relationship between family meals and adolescent health issues. *Health Psychology, 27*(2 Suppl.), S109–S117.

Frankowski, B., Bocchini, J., & Council on School Health & Committee on Infectious Diseases. (2010). Head lice. *Pediatrics*, doi: 10.1542/peds.2010-1308.

Gable, S., Chang, Y., & Krull, J. (2007). Television watching and frequency of family meals are predictive of overweight onset and persistence in a national sample of school-aged children. *Journal of the American Dietetic Association, 107*(1), 53–61.

Gangwisch, J., Malaspina, D., Babiss, L., Opler, M. (2010). Short sleep duration as a risk factor for hypercholesterolemia: Analyses of the National Longitudinal Study of Adolescent Health. *Sleep, 33*(7), 956–961.

Gavin, L. E., Catalano, R., David, G., Ferdon, C., Gloppen, K., & Markham, C. (2010). A review of positive youth development programs that promote adolescent sexual and reproductive health. *Journal of Adolescent Health*, 46(3 Suppl.), s75–s91.

Gershoff, E., Lansford, J., Sexton, H., Davis-Kean, P., & Sameroff, A. (2012). Longitudinal links between spanking and children's externalizing behaviors in a national sample of white, black, Hispanic, and Asian American families. *Child Development*, doi: 10.1111/j.1467-8624,2911.01732.x.

Ghaddar, S., Valerio, M., Garcia, C., & Hansen, L. (2012). Adolescent health literacy: The importance of credible sources for online health information. *Journal of School Health, 82*(1), 28–36.

Ghandour, R., Kogan, M., Blumberg, S., Jones, J., & Perrin, J. (2012). Mental health conditions among school-aged children: Geographic and sociodemographic patterns in prevalence and treatment. *Journal of Developmental and Behavioral Pediatric, 33*(1), 42–54.

Giles, L., DelBello, M., Stanford, K., & Strakowski, S. (2007). Child Behavior Checklist profiles of children and adolescents with and at high risk for developing bipolar disorder. *Child Psychiatry and Human Development, 38*(1), 47–55.

Godfrey, E. B., & Yoshikawa, H. (2011). Caseworker-recipient interaction: Welfare office differences, economic trajectories, and child outcomes. *Child Development, 83*(1), 382–398.

Goldsby, R., Chen, Y., Raber, S., Li, L., Diefenbach, K., Shnorhavorian, M. et al. (2011). Survivors of childhood cancer have increased risk of gastrointestinal complications later in life. *Gastroenterology, 140*(5), 1464–1471.

Gonder-Frederick, L., Zrebiec, J., Bauchowitz, A., Ritterbrand, L., Magee, J., Cox, D., et al. (2009). Cognitive function is disrupted by both hypo- and hyperglycemia in school-aged children with Type 1 diabetes: a field study. *Diabetes Care, 32*(6), 1001–1006.

Gooch, B., Griffin, S., Gray, S. K., Kohn W., Rozier, R. G., Siegal, M. et al. (2009). Preventing dental caries through school-based sealant programs: Updated recommendations and reviews of evidence. *The Journal of the American Dental Association, 140*(11), 1356–1365.

Gooding, H. C., Walls, C., & Richmond, T. (2011). Food insecurity and increased BMI in young adult women. *Epidemiology*, doi: 10.1038/oby.2011.233.

Greer, A., Ng, V., & Fisman, D. (2008). Climate change and infectious diseases in North America: The road ahead. *Canadian Medical Association Journal, 178*(6), 715–722.

Gregory, A., & Cornell, D. (2009). "Tolerating" adolescent needs: Moving beyond zero tolerance policies in high school. *Theory Into Practice, 48*(2), 106–113.

Greydanus, D., Patel, D., & Pratt, H. (2010). Suicide risk in adolescents with chronic illness: Implications for primary care and specialty pediatric practice. A review. *Developmental Medicine and Child Neurology, 52*(12), 1083–1087.

Guenther, L. (2012). *Pediculosis*. Retrieved from http://www.emedicine.com/med/topic1769.htm

Gunderson, C., Garasky, S., & Lohman, B. (2009). Food insecurity is not associated with childhood obesity as assessed using multiple measures of obesity. *The Journal of Nutrition, 139*(6), 1173–1178.

Guttmacher Institute. (2012a, February). *Facts on American teens' sexual and reproductive health*. Retrieved from http://www.guttmacher.org/pubs/FB-ATSRH.html

Guttmacher Institute. (2012b, February). *Facts on American teens' sources of information about sex*. Retrieved from http://www.guttmacher.org/pubs/FB-Teen-Sex-Ed.html

Hagenauer, M. H., Perryman, J., Lee, T., & Carskadon, M. (2009). Adolescent changes in the homeostatic and circadian regulation of sleep. *Developmental Neuroscience, 31*(4), 276–284.

Haines, J., Ziyadeh, N., Franko, D., McDonald, J., Mond, J., & Austin, S. B. (2011). Screening high school students for eating disorders: Validity of brief behavioral and attitudinal measures. *Journal of School Health, 81*(9), 530–535.

Hale, J., Reddy, L., Semrud-Clikeman, M., Hain, L., Whitaker, J., Morley, J. et al. (2011). Executive impairment determines ADHD medication responses: Implications for academic achievement. *Journal of Learning Disabilities, 44*(2), 196–212.

Haller, M., Handley, E., Chassin, L., & Bountress, K. (2010). Developmental cascades: Linking adolescent substance use, affiliation with substance use promoting peers, and academic achievement to adult substance use disorders. *Development and Psychopathology, 22*, 899–916.

Hamiwka, L., Yu, C., Hamiwka, L., Sherman, M., Anderson, B., & Wirrell, E. (2009). Are children with epilepsy at greater risk for bullying than their peers? *Epilepsy and Behavior, 15*(4), 500–505.

Hammond, W. R., & Arias, I. (2011). Broadening the approach to youth violence prevention through public health. *Journal of Prevention and Intervention in the Community, 39*(2), 167–175.

Hankin, B. L., & Abela, J. R. (2011). Nonsuicidal self-injury in adolescence: Prospective rates and risk factors in a 2 1/2 year longitudinal study. *Psychiatry Research, 186*(1), 65–70.

Harden, K., Hill, J., Turkheimer, E., & Emery, R. (2008). Gene-environment correlation and interaction in peer effects on adolescent alcohol and tobacco use. *Behavior Genetics*. doi: 10.1007/s10519-008-9202-7.

Haynes, K. (2007). An update on emergency contraception use in adolescents. *Journal of Pediatric Nursing, 22*(3), 186–195.

Haynie, D. L., Petts, R. J., Maimon, D., & Piquero, A. R. (2009). Exposure to violence in adolescence and precocious role exits. *Journal of Youth and Adolescence, 38*(3), 269–286.

Heikkinen, A., Broms, U., Pitkaniemi, J., Koskenvuo, M., & Meurman, J. (2009). Key factors in smoking cessation intervention among 15–16-year-olds. *Behavioral Medicine, 35*(3), 93–99.

Heim, C., Shugart, M., Craighead, W. E., & Nemeroff, C. (2010). Neurobiological and psychiatric consequences of child abuse and neglect. *Developmental Psychobiology, 52*(7), 671–690.

Henretta, J. (2007). Early childbearing, marital status, and women's health and mortality after age 50. *Journal of Health and Social Behavior, 48*(3), 254–266.

Herrman, J. (2008). Adolescent perceptions of teen births. *Journal of Obstetrical, Gynecological and Neonatal Nursing, 37*(1), 42–50.

Hitt, E. (2010, August 20). CDC: Adolescent vaccinations increased substantially from 2008 to 2009, reaching several Healthy People 2010 immunization goals. *Medscape Medical News*. Retrieved from http://www.medscape.com/viewarticle/727269

Hjern, A., Alfven, G., & Ostberg, V. (2007). School stressors, psychological complaints and psychosomatic pain. *Acta Paediatrica, 97*, 112–117.

Hollist, D. R., Hughes, L. A., & Schaible, L. M. (2009). Adolescent maltreatment, negative emotion, and delinquency: An assessment of general strain theory and family-based strain. *Journal of Criminal Justice, 37*(4), 379–387.

Holt, E. M., Steffen, L., Moran, A., Basu, S., Steinberger, J., Ross, J. et al. (2009). Fruit and vegetable consumption and its relation to markers of inflammation and oxidative stress in adolescents. *Journal of the American Dietetic Association, 109*(3), 414–421.

Hoynes, H. (2008). *The Earned Income Tax Credit, welfare reform, and the employment of low-skilled single mothers*. Federal Reserve Bank of Chicago Conference. Retrieved from http://www.econ.ucdavis.edu/faculty/hoynes/working_papers/Chicago-Fed-Final.pdf

Huurre, T., Lintonen, T., Kaprio, J., Pelkonen, M., Martthunen, M., & Aro, H. (2010). Adolescent risk factors for excessive alcohol use at age 32 years. A 16-year prospective follow-up study. *Social Psychiatry and Psychiatric Epidemiology, 45*(1), 125–134.

Irwin, C., Adams, S., Park, M. J., & Newacheck, P. (2009). Preventive care for adolescents: Few get visits and fewer get services. *Pediatrics, 123*(4), e565–e572.

Jaing, N., Kolbe, L., Seo, D. C., Kay, N. S., & Brindis, C. (2011). Health of adolescents and young adults: Trends in achieving the 21 Critical National Health Objectives by 2010. *Journal of Adolescent Health, 49*(2), 124–132.

Johnson, K. (2009, January 29). FBI: Burgeoning gangs behind up to 80% of U.S. crime. *USA Today*. Retrieved from http://www.usatoday.com/news/nation/2009-01-29-ms13_N.htm

Johnson, S. B., & Jones, V. C. (2011). Adolescent development and risk of injury: Using developmental science to improve interventions. *Injury Prevention, 17*, 50–54.

Johnson, S., & Wang, C. (2008). Why do adolescents say they are less healthy than their parents think they are? The importance of mental health varies by social class in a nationally representative sample. *Pediatrics, 121*(2), 307–313.

Johnson, S., Blum, R., & Giedd, J. (2009). Adolescent maturity and the brain: The promise and pitfalls of neuroscience research in adolescent health policy. *Journal of Adolescent Health, 45*(3), 216–221.

Johnston, L. D., O'Malley, P. M., & Bachman, J. G., Schulenberg, J. E. (2009). Monitoring the future: National results on adolescent drug use. *Overview of key findings, 2008*. (NIH Publication No. 09-7401). Bethesda, MD: National Institute on Drug Abuse.

Jones, D. J., Runyan, D., Lewis, T., Litrownik, A., Black, M., Wiley, T., et al. (2010). Trajectories of childhood sexual abuse and early adolescent HIV/AIDS risk behaviors: The role of other maltreatment, witnessed violence, and child gender. *Journal of Clinical Child and Adolescent Psychology, 39*(5), 667–680.

Jutte, D. P., Roos, N., Brownell, M., Briggs, G., MacWilliams, L., & Roos, L. (2010). The ripples of adolescent motherhood: Social, educational, and medical outcomes for children of teen and prior teen mothers. *Academic Pediatrics, 10*(5), 293–301.

Jyoti, D. F., Frongillo, E. A., & Jones, S. J. (2005). Food insecurity affects school children's academic performance, weight gain, and social skills. *Journal of Nutrition, 135*(12), 2831–2839.

Keleher, N., & Arledge, D. N. (2011). Role of child death review team in a small rural county in California. *Injury Prevention, 17*, i19–i22.

Kendall, J., Hatton, D., Beckett, A., & Leo, M. (2003). Children's accounts of attention-deficit/hyperactivity disorder. *Advances in Nursing Science, 26*(2), 114–130.

Kessler, R. C., Green, J., Adler, L., Barkley, R., Chatterji, S., Faraone, S. et al. (2010). Structure and diagnosis of adult attention-deficit/hyperactivity disorder: Analysis of expanded symptom criteria from the Adult ADHD Clinical Diagnostic Scale. *Archives of General Psychiatry, 67*(11), 1168–1178.

King, K., & Chassin, L. (2007). A prospective study of the effects of age of initiation of alcohol and drug use on young adult substance dependence. *Journal of Studies on Alcohol and Drugs, 68*(2), 256–265.

Kirkpatrick, S., McIntyre, L., & Potestio, M. (2010). Child hunger and long-term adverse consequences for health. *Archives of Pediatrics and Adolescent Medicine, 164*(8), 754–762.

Klimach, V. J. (2009). The community use of rescue medication for prolonged epileptic seizures in children. *Seizure, 18*(5), 343–346.

Knatz, S., Maginot, T., Story, M., Neumark-Sztainer, D., & Boutelle, K. (2011). Prevalence rates and psychological predictors of secretive eating in overweight and obese adolescents. *Childhood Obesity, 7*(1), 30–35.

Knopf, D., Park, M. J., & Mulye, T. P. (2008). *The mental health of adolescents: a national profile, 2008*. Retrieved from http://nahic.ucsf.edu/wp-content/uploads/2008/02/2008-Mental-Health-Brief.pdf

Koch, W. (2012, March 13). Teen tobacco 'epidemic' shocks Surgeon General. *USA Today*. Retrieved from http://yourlife.usatoday.com/health/story/2012-03-08/Teen-tobacco-epidemic-shocks-surgeon-general/53404520/1

Koch, P., Ryder, H. F., Dziura, I., Njike, V., & Antaya R. J. (2008). Educating adolescents about acne vulgaris: A comparison of written handouts with audiovisual computerized presentations. *Archives of Dermatology, 144*(2), 208–214.

Kochanek, K., Kirmeyer, S., Martin, J., Strobino, D., & Guyer, B. (2012). Annual summary of vital statistics: 2009. *Pediatrics, 129*(2), 338–351.

Kohler, P., Manhart, L., & Lafferty, W. (2008). Abstinence-only and comprehensive sex education and the initiation of sexual activity and teen pregnancy. *Journal of Adolescent Health, 42*(4), 344–351.

Kong, G., Carmenga, D., & Krishnan-Sarin, S. (2012). Parental influence on adolescent smoking cessation: Is there a gender difference? *Addictive Behaviors, 37*(2), 211–216.

Kost, K., & Henshaw, S. (2012, February). *U.S. teenage pregnancies, births and abortions, 2008: National trends by age, race and ethnicity*. Washington, DC: Guttmacher Institute.

Kremer, P. J., Leslie, E., Berk, M., & Toumbourou, J. (2010). Associations between diet quality and depressed mood in adolescents: Results from the Australian Healthy Neighbourhoods Study. *Australian and New Zealand Journal of Psychiatry, 44*(5), 435–442.

Krohn, M., Lizotte, A., Bushway, S., Schmidt, N., & Phillips, M. (2010). Shelter during the storm: A search for factors that protect at-risk adolescents from violence. *Crime and Delinquency*. doi: 10.177/0011128710389585.

Kroll, D., & Nedley, M. (2007). Dental caries: State of the science for the most common chronic disease of childhood. *Advances in Pediatrics, 54*(1), 215–239.

Kuntsche, E., & Muller, S. (2012). Why do young people start drinking? Motives for first-time alcohol consumption and links to risky drinking in early adolescence. *European Addiction Research, 18*(1), 34–39.

Kursmark, M., & Weitzman, M. (2009). Recent findings concerning childhood food insecurity. *Current Opinion in clinical Nutrition and Metabolic Care, 12*(3), 310–316.

Kwon, H. C., & Meyer, D. R. (2011). How do economic downturns affect welfare leavers? A comparison of two cohorts. *Children and Youth Services Review, 33*, 588–597.

Laberge, L., Ledoux, E., Auclair, J., Thuilier, C., Gaudreault, M. Gaudreault, M., et al. (2011). Risk factors for work-related fatigue in students with school-year employment. *Journal of Adolescent Health, 48*(3), 289–294.

Lam, A. (2008). Increase in utilization of dental sealants. *Journal of Contemporary Dental Practice, 9*(3), 81–87.

Lansford, J. E., Dodge, K., Pettit, G., & Bates, J. (2010). Does physical abuse in early childhood predict substance use in adolescence and early adulthood? *Child Maltreatment, 15*(2), 190–194.

Larson, N., & Story, M. (2011). Food insecurity and weight status among U.S. children and families. *American Journal of Preventive Medicine, 40*(2), 166–173.

Latendresse, S., Rose, R., Viken, R., Pulkkinen, L., Kaprio, J., & Dick, D. (2008). Parenting mechanisms in links between parents' and adolescents' alcohol use behaviors. *Alcoholism, Clinical and Experimental Research, 32*(2), 322–330.

Latimer, A., Kerishnan-Sarin, S., Cavallo, D., Duhig, A., Salovey, P., & O'Malley, S. (2012). Targeted smoking cessation messages for adolescents. *Journal of Adolescent Health, 50*(1), 47–53.

Lecky, D., McNulty, C., Adriaenssens, N., Herotova, T., Holt, J., Touboul, P. et al. (2011). What are school children in Europe being taught about hygiene and antibiotic use? *Journal of Antimicrobial Chemotherapy, 66*(Suppl. 5), v13–v21.

Lee, K. (2009). Impact of the 1996 welfare reform on child and family well-being. *Journal of Community Psychology, 37*(5), 602–617.

Li, F., Harmer, P., Cardinal, B., Bosworth, M., & Johnson-Shelton, D. (2009). Obesity and the built environment: Does the density of neighborhood fast-food outlets matter? *American Journal of Health Promotion, 23*(3), 203–209.

Li, Y., & Lerner, R. M. (2011). Trajectories of school engagement during adolescence: Implications for grades, depression, delinquency, and substance use. *Developmental Psychology, 47*(1), 233–247.

Liberzon, I., & George, S. (2010). SSRI-enhanced locus coeruleus activity and adolescent suicide: Lessons from animal models. *Neuropsychopharmacology, 35*, 1619–1620.

Linares, L. O., Stovall-McClough, K. C., Li, M., Morin, R., Silva, A., & Albert, M. (2008). Salivary cortisol in foster children: A pilot study. *Child Abuse and Neglect, 32*, 665–670.

Lindau, S., Tetteh, A., Kasza, K., & Gilliam, M. (2008). What schools teach our patients about sex: Content, quality and influences on sex education. *Obstetrics and Gynecology, 111*(2 Pt 1), 256–266.

Lindberg, L. D., & Maddow-Zimet, I. (2012). Consequences of sex education on teen and young adult sexual behaviors and outcomes. *Journal of Adolescent Health*. doi: 10.1016/j.jadohealth.2011.12.028.

Linville, D., Stice, E., Gau, J., & O'Neill, M. (2011). Predictive effects of mother and peer influences on increases in adolescent eating disorder risk factors and symptoms: A 3-year longitudinal study. *International Journal of Eating Disorders, 44*(8), 745–751.

Lock, J. (2010). Treatment of adolescent eating disorders: Progress and challenges. *Minerva Psichiatrica, 51*(3), 207–216.

Lorang, M., Callahan, B., Cummins, K., Achar, S., & Brown, S. (2011). Anabolic androgenic steroid use in teens: Prevalence, demographics, and perception of effects. *Journal of Child and Adolescent Substance Abuse, 20*(4), 358–369.

Loring, D. W. (2010). Teaching the teachers: Data to benefit school systems and doctors about children with newly diagnosed epilepsy. *Epilepsy Currents, 10*(2), 38–39.

Lumia, A. R., & McGinnis, M. Y. (2010). Impact of anabolic androgenic steroids on adolescent males. *Physiology and Behavior, 100*(3), 199–204.

Lytle, L., Pasch, K., & Farbakhsh, K. (2011). The relationship between sleep and weight in a sample of adolescents. *Behavior and Psychology, 19*(2), 324–331.

Ma, C., Gee, L., & Kushel, M. (2008). Associations between housing instability and food insecurity with health care access in low-income children. *Ambulatory Pediatrics, 8*(1), 50–57.

Mancini, A. J., Baldwin, H. E., Eichenfield, L., Friedlander, S., & Yan, A. (2011). Acne life cycle: The spectrum of pediatric disease. *Seminars in Cutaneous Medicine and Surgery, 30*(3 Suppl.), s2–s5.

Marshall, B., & Werb, D. (2010). Health outcomes associated with methamphetamine use among young people: A systematic review. *Addiction, 105*(6), 991–1002.

Martin, M., & Caminada, K. (2009). *Welfare reform in the United States: A descriptive policy analysis*. Department of Economics Research Memorandum 2009.03. Retrieved from http://papers.ssrn.com/sol3/papers.cfm?abstract_id=1553811

Masia, S., Charakida, M., Wang, G., O'Neill, F., Taddei, S., & Deanfield, J. (2009). Hope for the future: Early recognition of increased cardiovascular risk in children and how to deal with it. *European Journal of Cardiovascular Prevention and Rehabilitation, 16*(2, Suppl.), s61–s64.

Maternal and Child Health Bureau. (2011). Vaccine-preventable diseases. *Child Health USA, 2011*. Retrieved from http://mchb.hrsa.gov/chusa11/hstat/hsc/pages/209vpd.html

McCabe, S. E., West, B. T., Morales, M., Cranford, J. A., & Boyd, C. J. (2007). Does early onset of non-medical use predict prescription drug abuse and dependence? Results from a national study. *Addiction, 102*, 1920–1930.

McCabe, S. E., West, B., Teter, C., Cranford, J., Ross-Durow, P., & Boyd, C. (2012). Adolescent nonmedical users of prescription opioids: Brief screening and substance use disorders. *Addictive Behaviors*, in press (available online February 7, 2012).

McCartt, A. T., Hellinga, L., Strouse, L., & Farmer, C. M. (2010). Long-term effects of handheld cell phone laws on driver handheld cell phone use. *Traffic Injury Prevention, 11*(2), 133–141.

McCauley, J., Danielson, C., Amstadter, A., Ruggiero, K., Resnick, H., Hanson, R. et al. (2010). The role of traumatic history in nonmedical use of prescription drugs among a nationally representative sample of US adolescents. *Journal of Child Psychology and Psychiatry, 51*(1), 84–93.

McGrady, M., Laffel, L., Drotar, D., Repaske, D., & Hood, K. (2009). Depressive symptoms and glycemia control in adolescents with Type 1 diabetes: Mediational role of blood glucose monitoring. *Diabetes Care, 32*(5), 804–806.

McKnight-Eily, L., Eaton, D., Lowry, R. Croft, J., Presley-Cantrell, L., & Perry, G. (2011). Relationships between hours of sleep and health-risk behaviors of US adolescent students. *Preventive Medicine, 53*(4–5), 271–273.

McRee, N. (2008). Child abuse in blended households: Reports from runaway and homeless youth. *Child Abuse and Neglect, 32*(4), 449–453.

Menzies, H. J., Winston, C., Holtz, T., Cain, K., & McKenzie, W. (2010). Epidemiology of tuberculosis among US- and foreign-born children and adolescents in the United States, 1994–2007. *American Journal of Public Health, 100*(9), 1724–1729.

Merikangas, K. R., He, J., Burstein, M., Swanson, S. A., Avenevoli, S., Cui, L. et al. (2010). Lifetime prevalence of mental disorders in U.S. adolescents: Results from the National Comorbidity Study—Adolescent Supplement (NCS-A). *Journal of the American Academy of Child and Adolescent Psychiatry 49*(10), 980–989.

Michaud, P. A. (2008). Adolescent medicine: From clinical practice to public health. *Georgian Medical News, 156*, 61–65.

Millard, M. W., Johnson, P., Hilton, A., & Hart, M. (2009). Children with asthma miss more school: fact or fiction? *Chest, 135*, 303–306.

Miller, D., Eckert, T., & Mazza, J. (2009). Suicide prevention programs in the schools: A review and public health perspective. *School Psychology Review, 38*(2), 168–188.

Miller, J., Naimi, T., Brewer, R., & Jones, S. (2007). Binge drinking and associated health risk behaviors among high school students. *Pediatrics, 119*(1), 76–85.

Miller, P. M. (2011). A critical analysis of the research on student homelessness. *Review of Educational Research, 81*(3), 308–337.

Millichap, J. G., & Yee, M. W. (2012). The diet factor in attention-deficit/hyperactivity disorder. *Pediatrics, 129*(2), 330–337.

Molina, B., Hinshaw, S., Swanson, J., Arnold, E., Vitiello, B., Jensen, P. et al. (2009). The MTA at 8 years: Prospective follow-up of children treated for combined-type ADHD in a multisite study. *Journal of the American Academy of Child and Adolescent Psychiatry, 48*(5), 484–500.

Mollborn, S., Domingue, B. W., & Boardman, J. D. (2011, November). *Racial, socioeconomic, and religious influences on school-level teen pregnancy norms and behaviors: Working paper*. Boulder, CO: Institute of Behavioral Science, University of Colorado.

Monaghan, M., Singh, C., Streisand, R., & Cogen, F. (2010). Screening and identification of children and adolescents at risk for depression during a diabetes clinic visit. *Diabetes Spectrum, 23*(1), 25–31.

Monroy, O. L., Aguilar, C., Lizano, M., Cruz-Tatonia, F., Cruz, R., & Rocha-Zavaleta, L. (2010). Prevalence of human papillomavirus genotypes, and mucosal IgA anti-viral responses in women with cervical ectopy. *Journal of Clinical Virology, 47*(1), 43–48.

Moore, D., & Florsheim, P. (2008). Interpartner conflict and child abuse risk among African American and Latino adolescent parenting couples. *Child Abuse and Neglect, 32*(4), 463–475.

Moore, K. A., Redd, Z., Burkhauser, M., Mbwana, K., & Collins, A. (2009, April). *Children in poverty: Trends, consequences, and policy options*. Washington, DC: Child Trends Research Brief.

Moore, L., Roux, A., Nettleton, J., Jacobs, D., & Franco, M. (2009). Fast-food consumption, diet quality, and neighborhood exposure to fast food: The multi-ethnic study of atherosclerosis. *American Journal of Epidemiology, 170*(1), 29–36.

Moran, P., Coffey, C., Romaniuk H., Olsson, C., Borschmann, R., Carlin, J., & Patton, G. (2012). The natural history of self-harm from adolescence to young adulthood: A population-based cohort study. *The Lancet, 379*(9812), 21–27.

Moreno, M. A. (2011). Advice for parents: Media influence on adolescent alcohol use. *Archives of Pediatric & Adolescent Medicine, 165*(7), 680.

Morrison-Beedy, D., Carey, M., Cote-Arsenault, D., Seibold-Simpson, S., & Robinson, K. (2008). Understanding sexual abstinence in urban adolescent girls. *Journal of Obstetrical, Gynecological and Neonatal Nursing, 37*(2), 185–195.

Moylan, C. A., Herrenkohl, T., Sousa, C., Tajima, E., Herrenkohl, R., & Russo, M. J. (2010). The effects of child abuse and exposure to domestic violence on adolescent internalizing and externalizing behavior problems. *Journal of Family Violence, 25*(1), 53–63.

Mulrooney, D. A., Yeazel, M., Kawashima, T., Mertens, A., Mitby, P., Stovall, M. et al. (2009). Cardiac outcomes in a cohort of adult survivors of childhood and adolescent cancer: Retrospective analysis of the Childhood Cancer Survivor Study cohort. *BMJ, 339*, b4606. Retrieved from http://www.bmj.com/content/339/bmj.b4606.full

Mulvaney, M., & Mebert, C. (2007). Parental corporal punishment predicts behavior problems in early childhood. *Journal of Family Psychology, 21*(3), 389–397.

Mulye, T. P., Park, M. J., Nelson, C., Adams, S., Irwin C., & Brindis, C. (2009). Trends in adolescent and young adult health in the United States. *Journal of Adolescent Health, 45*, 8–24.

Murray, N., Low, B., Hollis, C., Cross, A., & Davis, S. (2007). Coordinated school health programs and academic achievement: A systematic review of the literature. *Journal of School Health, 77*(9), 589–600.

Nadeau, K., Maahs, D., Daniels, S., & Eckel, R. (2011). Childhood obesity and cardiovascular disease: Links and prevention strategies. *Nature Reviews Cardiology, 8*, 513–525.

Nader, P., O'Brien, M., Houts, R., Bradley, R., Belsky, J., Crosnoe, R. et al. (2006). Identifying risk for obesity in early childhood. *Pediatrics, 118*(3), E594–E601.

Naguib, J. M., Kulinskaya, E., Lomax, C., & Garralda, E. M. (2009). Neuro-cognitive performance in children with Type 1 diabetes—a meta-analysis. *Journal of Pediatric Psychology, 34*(3), 271–282.

Najman, J. M., Hayatbakhsh, M., Clavarino, A., Bor, W., O'Callaghan, M., & Williams, G. (2010). Family poverty over the early life course and recurrent adolescent and young adult anxiety and depression: A longitudinal study. *American Journal of Public Health, 100*(9), 1719–1723.

Najman, J. M., Hayatbakhsh, M., Herson, M., Bor, W., O'Callaghan, M., & Williams, G. (2009). The impact of episodic and chronic poverty on child cognitive development. *The Journal of Pediatrics, 154*(2), 284–289.

Nance, M. L., Carr, B., Kallan, M., Branas, C., & Wiebe, D. (2010). Variation in pediatric and adolescent firearm mortality rates in rural and urban US counties. *Pediatrics, 125*(6), 1112–1118.

National Alliance for Mental Illness (NAMI). (2011). *Suicide in youth*. Retrieved from http://www.nami.org/Template.cfm?Section=By_Illness&template=/ContentManagement/ContentDisplay.cfm&ContentID=10210

National Cancer Institute (NCI). (n.d., 2011a). *Fact sheet: Childhood cancers*. Retrieved from http://www.cancer.gov/cancertopics/factsheet/Sites-Types/childhood

National Cancer Institute (NCI). (2011b). *A snapshot of pediatric cancers*. Retrieved from http://www.cancer.gov/aboutnci/servingpeople/snapshots/pediatric.pdf

National Center for Education Statistics (NCES). (2011). *Digest of education statistics, 2010* (NCES 2011-015), Chapter 2. Retrieved from http://nces.ed.gov/fastfacts/display.asp?id=64

National Center for Learning Disabilities (NCLD). (2011). The state of learning disabilities. Retrieved from http://www.fmptic.org/download/2011_state_of_ld_final.pdf

National Clearinghouse for Educational Facilities. (2012). *How many schools are there in the U.S.?* Retrieved from http://www.ncef.org/ds/statistics.cfm#

National Diabetes Education Program (NDEP). (n.d.). *The facts about diabetes: A leading cause of death in the U.S.* Retrieved from http://ndep.nih.gov/diabetes-facts/index.aspx

National Institute of Arthritis and Musculoskeletal & Skin Diseases. (2010). *Questions and answers about acne*. Retrieved from http://www.niams.nih.gov/Health_Info/Acne/default.asp

National Institute of Dental & Craniofacial Research (NIDCR). (2011). *Dental caries (tooth decay) in children (age 2 to 11)*. Retrieved from http://www.nidcr.nih.gov/DataStatistics/FindDataByTopic/DentalCaries/DentalCariesChildren2to11

National Institute of Mental Health (NIMH). (n.d.). *NIMH pages about attention deficit hyperactivity disorder (ADHD)*. Retrieved from http://www.nimh.nih.gov/topics/topic-page-adhd.shtml

National Institute of Mental Health (NIMH). (2010). *Suicide in the U.S.: Statistics and prevention*. Retrieved from http://www.nimh.nih.gov/health/publications/suicide-in-the-us-statistics-and-prevention/index.shtml

National Institute of Neurological Disorders and Stroke (NINDS). (2011). *NINDS learning disabilities information page*. Retrieved from http://www.ninds.nih.gov/disorders/learningdisabilities/learningdisabilities.htm

National Institute of Neurological Disorders and Stroke (NINDS). (2012). *Autism fact sheet*. Retrieved from http://www.ninds.nih.gov/disorders/autism/detail_autism.htm? css=print

National Vaccine Information Center. (2012). *Introduction to autism information*. Retrieved from http://www.nvic.org/vaccines-and-diseases/Autism.aspx

Nauta, C., Byrne, C., & Wesley, Y. (2009). School nurses and childhood obesity: An investigation of knowledge and practice among school nurses as they relate to childhood obesity. *Issues in Comprehensive Pediatric Nursing, 32*(1), 16–30.

Nazari, M. A., Wallois, F., Aarabi, A., & Berquin, P. (2011). Dynamic changes in quantitative electroencephalogram during continuous performance test in children with attention-deficit/hyperactivity disorder. *International Journal of Psychophysiology, 81*(3), 230–236.

Neal, E., Chaffe, H., Schwartz, R., Lawson, M., Edwards, N., Fitzsimmons, G. et al. (2009). A randomized trial of classical and medium-chain triglyceride ketogenic diets in the treatment of childhood epilepsy. *Epilepsia, 50*(5), 1109–1117.

Negriff, S., Susman, E., & Trickett, P. (2011). The developmental pathway from pubertal timing to delinquency and sexual activity from early to late adolescence. *Journal of Youth and Adolescence, 40*(10), 1343–1356.

Neumark-Sztainer, D. (2009). Preventing obesity and eating disorders in adolescents: What can health care providers do? *Journal of Adolescent Health, 44*, 206–213.

Noimark, L., & Cox, H. (2008). Nutritional problems related to food allergy in childhood. *Pediatric Allergy and Immunology, 19*(2), 188–195.

O'Brien, M., Nader, P. R., Houts, R. M., Bradley, R., Friedman, S., Belsky, J. et al. (2007). The ecology of childhood overweight: A 12-year longitudinal analysis. *International Journal of Obesity, 31*(9), 1469–1478.

Office of National Drug Control Policy. (2012). *Marijuana: Know the facts*. Retrieved from http://www.whitehouse.gov/sites/default/files/page/files/marijuana_fact_sheet_3-28-12.pdf

Ogden, C. & Carroll, M. (2010). *Prevalence of obesity among children and adolescents: United States trends 1963–1965 through 2007–2008*. Retrieved from http://www.cdc.gov/nchs/data/hestat/obesity_child_07_08/obesity_child_07_08.htm

Olson, C., Bove, C., & Miller, E. (2007). Growing up poor: Long-term implications for eating patterns and body weight. *Appetite, 49*(1), 198–207.

Owens, J., Belon, K., & Moss, P. (2010). Impact of delaying school start time on adolescent sleep, mood, and behavior. *Archives of Pediatrics and Adolescent Medicine, 164*(7), 608–614.

Oyserman, D., Johnson, E., & James, L. (2011). Seeing the destination but not the path: Effects of socioeconomic disadvantage on school-focused possible self content and linked behavioral strategies. *Self and Identity, 10*(4), 474–492.

Ozer, E. M., Adams, S., Orrell-Valente, J. K., Wiobbelsman, C., Lustig, J. L., Millstein, S., Garber, A., & Irwin, C. (2011). Does delivering preventive services in primary care reduce adolescent risky behavior? *Journal of Adolescent Health, 49*(5), 476–482.

Pallin, D. J., Egan, D., Pelletier, A., Espinola, J., Hooper, D., & Camargo, C. (2008). Increased U.S. emergency department visits for skin and soft tissue infections, and changes in antibiotic choices, during the emergence of community-associated methicillin-resistant *Staphylococcus aureus*. *Annals of Emergency Medicine, 51*(3), 291–298.

Pantoine, B. (2009, March 17). *ADHD studies target circuitry, stimulants' effects*. The Dana Foundation. Retrieved from http://www.dana.org/news/brainwork/detail.aspx?id=19826

Park, M., Adams, S., & Irwin, C. (2011). Health care services and the transition to young adulthood: Challenges and opportunities. *Academic Pediatrics, 11*(2), 115–122.

Park, M., Brindis, C., Chang, F., & Irwin, C. (2008). A midcourse review of the *Healthy People 2010* critical health objectives for adolescents and young adults. *Journal of Adolescent Health, 42*, 329–334.

Parrott, S., & Sherman, A. (2006, August 17). *TANF at 10: Program results are more mixed than often understood*. Washington, DC: Center on Budget & Policy Priorities.

Pati, S., Hasheem, K., Brown, B., Fiks, A., & Forrest, C. (2009). Project report: Early childhood predictors of early school success. *Child Trends*. Retrieved from http://www.childtrends.org/Files/Child_Trends-2009_05_26_FR_EarlySchoolSuccess.pdf

Pazol, K., Warner, L., Gavin, L., Callaghan, W. M., Spitz, M., Anderson, J. et al. (2011). Vital signs: Teen pregnancy—United States, 1991–2009. *Morbidity and Mortality Weekly Report (MMWR), 60*(13), 414–420.

Pearson, N., & Biddle, S. (2011). Sedentary behavior and dietary intake in children, adolescents, and adults. *American Journal of Preventive Medicine, 41*(2), 178–188.

Pedersen, T. (2011, June 26). *Teens' unhealthy eating behaviors continue into adulthood*. Retrieved from http://psychcentral.com/news/2011/06/26/teen-unhealthy-eating-behaviors-continue-into-adulthood/27252.html

Pelkonen, M., Karlsson, L., & Marttunen, M. (2011). Adolescent suicide: Epidemiology, psychological theories, risk factors, and prevention. *Current Pediatric Reviews, 7*(1), 52–67.

Pepler, D. J., Jiang, E. Craig, W., & Connolly, J. (2010). Developmental trajectories of girls' and boys' delinquency and associated problems. *Journal of Abnormal Child Psychology, 38*(7), 1033–1044.

Pereira, B., Venter, C. Grundy, J., Clayton, C. B., Arshad, S. H., & Dean, T. (2005). Prevalence of sensitization to food allergens, reported adverse reaction to foods, food avoidance, and food hypersensitivity among teenagers. *Journal of Allergy and Clinical Immunology, 116*(4), 884–892.

Peters, K., & Jackson, D. (2009). Mothers' experiences of parenting a child with attention deficit hyperactivity disorder. *Journal of Advanced Nursing, 65*(1), 62–71.

Peterson, R. L., & Schoonover, B. (2008). *Fact sheet #3: Zero tolerance policies in schools*. Muncie, IN: Consortium to Prevent School Violence. Retrieved from http://www.ncsvprp.org/resources_assets/CPSV-Fact-Sheet-3-Zero-Tolerance.pdf

Philbrook, J. K., Kiragu, A. Geppert, J., Graham, P., Richardson, L., & Kriel, R. (2009). Pediatric injury prevention: Methods of booster seat education. *Pediatric Nursing, 35*(4), 215–220.

Pianta, R., Belsky, J., Vandergrift, N., Houts, R. & Morrison, F. J. (2008). Classroom effects on children's achievement trajectories in elementary school. *American Educational Research Journal*. doi: 10.3102/ 0002831207308230.

Piko, B. (2007). Self-perceived health among adolescents: The role of gender and psychosocial factors. *European Journal of Pediatrics, 166*(7), 701–708.

Polk, D. E., Weyant, R., & Manz, M. (2010). Socioeconomic factors in adolescents' oral health: Are they mediated by oral hygiene behaviors of preventive interventions? *Community Dentistry and Oral Epidemiology, 38*(1), 1–9.

Pozzilli, P., Guglielmi, C., Caprio, S., & Buzzetti, R. (2011). Obesity, autoimmunity, an double diabetes in youth. *Diabetes Care, 34*(Suppl 2), x166–s170.

Powell, L. M., Szczypka, G., & Chaloupka, F. (2010). Trends in exposure to television food advertisements among children and adolescents in the United States. *Archives of Pediatrics and Adolescent Medicine, 164*(9), 794–802.

Prinstein, M., Heilbron, N., Guerry, J., Franklin, J., Rancourt, D., Simon, V., et al. (2010). Peer influence and nonsuicidal self injury: Longitudinal results in community and clinically-referred adolescent samples. *Journal of Abnormal Child Psychology, 38*(5), 669–682.

Pub Med Health. (2011). *Juvenile rheumatoid arthritis*. Retrieved from http://www.ncbi.nlm.nih.gov/pubmedhealth/PMH0001487/

Pujazon-Zazik, M., & Park, M. J. (2010). To Tweet or not to Tweet: Gender differences and potential positive and negative health outcomes of adolescents' social Internet use. *American Journal of Men's Health, 4*(1), 77–85.

Quan-McGimpsey, S. (2011). Early education teachers' conceptualizations and strategies for managing closeness in childcare: The personal domain. *Journal of Early Childhood Research, 9*(3), 232–246.

Rabiner, D., Anastopoulos, A., Costello, E., Hoyle, R., McCabe, S., & Swartzwelder, H. (2009). Motives and perceived consequences of nonmedical ADHD medication use by college students: Are students treating themselves for attention problems? *Journal of Attention Disorders. 13*(3), 259–270.

Raghavan, R., Aarons, G., Rosch, S., & Leslie, L. (2008). Longitudinal patterns of health insurance coverage among a national sample of children in the child welfare system. *American Journal of Public Health, 98*(3), 478–484.

Ramanathan, S., & Hebert, A. A. (2011). Management of acne vulgaris. *Journal of Pediatric Health Care, 25*(5), 332–337.

Reed, J. L., & Huppert, J. S. (2011). Adolescent sexually transmitted infections: A community epidemic. *Journal of Prevention and Intervention in the Community, 39*(3), 243–255.

Reid, V., & Meadows-Oliver, M. (2007). Postpartum depression in adolescent mothers: An integrative review of the literature. *Journal of Pediatric Health Care, 21*(5), 289–298.

Reinberg, S. (2011). *Unvaccinated kids behind largest U.S. measles outbreak in years: Study*. U.S. News & World Report. Retrieved from http://health.usnews.com/health-news/family-health/childrens-health/articles/2011/10/20/unvaccinated-kids-behind-largest-us-measles-outbreak-in-years-study

Robers, S., Zhang, J., & Truman, J. (2012). *Indicators of school crime and safety: 2011*. Washington, DC: National Center for Education Statistics.

Rodenburg, R., Wagner, J., Austin, J., Kerr, M., & Dunn, D. (2011). Psychosocial issues for children with epilepsy. *Epilepsy and Behavior, 22*(1), 47–54.

Rosenbloom, A. L., Silverstein, J. H., Amemiya, S., Zeitler, P., & Klingensmith, G. J. (2009). Type 2 diabetes in children and adolescents. *Pediatric Diabetes, 10*(s12), 17–32.

Rozier, R. G., Adair, S., Gralham, F., Iafolla, T., Kingman, A., Kohn, W. et al. (2010). Evidence-based clinical recommendations on the prescription of dietary fluoride supplements for caries prevention. *The Journal of the American Dental Association, 141*(12), 1480–1489.

Russell, B., Britner, P., & Woolard, J. (2007). The promise of primary prevention home visiting programs: A review of potential outcomes. *Journal of Prevention and Intervention in the Community, 34*(1–2), 129–147.

Saari, A. J., Kentala, J., & Mattila, K. (2012). Long-term effectiveness of adolescent brief tobacco intervention: A follow-up study. *BMC Research Notes, 5*, 101. Retrieved from http://www.biomedcentral.com/content/pdf/1756-0500-5-101.pdf

Safe Kids USA. (2009, March). *Raising safe kids: One stage at a time*. Retrieved from http://www.safekids.org/assets/docs/ourwork/research/research-report-safe-kids-week-2009.pdf

Sales, J. M., & DiClemente, R. J. (2010). *Adolescent STI/HIV prevention programs: What works for teens?* Retrieved from http://www.actforyouth.net/resources/rf/rf_sti_0510.pdf

Sallis, J. F., & Glanz, K. (2009). Physical activity and food environment: Solutions to the obesity epidemic. *Milbank Quarterly, 87*(1), 123–154.

Sato, S., Schulz, K., Sisk, C., & Wood, R. (2008). Adolescents and androgens, receptors and rewards. *Hormones and Behavior, 53*(5), 647–658.

Scheier, L. M., & Grenard, J. L. (2010). Influence of a nationwide social marketing campaign on adolescent drug use. *Journal of Health Communication: International Perspectives, 15*(3), 240–271.

Schmitt, K., Dayanim, S., & Matthias, S. (2008). Personal homepage construction as an expression of social development. *Developmental Psychology, 44*(2), 496–506.

Schumann, B., Kluttig, A., Tiller, D., Werdan, K., Haerting, J., & Greiser, K. (2011). Association of childhood and adult socioeconomic indicators with cardiovascular risk factors and its modification by age: the CARLA Study, 2002–2006. *BMC Public Health, 11*, 289.

Schwartz, M., & Henderson, K. (2009). Does obesity prevention cause eating disorders? *Journal of the American Academy of Child and Adolescent Psychiatry, 48*(8), 784–786.

Self, T., Chrisman, C., Jacobs, A., Vo, N., & Winton, J. (2010). Preventing emergency department visits and hospitalizations for asthma by use of oral corticosteroids at home: Are we adhering to national guidelines? *Journal of Asthma, 47*(10), 1123–1127.

Setlik, J., Bond, G. R., & Ho, M. (2009). Adolescent prescription ADHD medication abuse is rising along with prescriptions for these medications. *Pediatrics, 124*(3), 875–880.

Shaffer, D., Gould, M., & Hicks, R. (March 14, 2007). *Teen suicide fact sheet*. New York: Columbia University.

Shields, M. K., & Behrman, R. E. (2002). Children and welfare reform: Analysis and recommendations. *The Future of Children, 12*(1), 5–26.

Sihvola, E., Rose, R., Dick, D., Korhonen, T., Pulkkinen, L., Raevuori, A., et al. (2011). Prospective relationships of ADHD symptoms with developing substance use in a population-derived sample. *Psychological Medicine, 41*, 2615–2623.

Silver, L. (2011). Doctor to doctor: Information learning disabilities for pediatricians and other physicians. *Learning Disabilities Association of America*. Retrieved from http://www.ldaamerica.org/aboutld/professionals/doctor_to_doctor.asp

Skiles, M. P., Cai, J., English, A., & Ford, C. A. (2011). Retail pharmacies and adolescent vaccination: An exploration of current issues. *Journal of Adolescent Health, 48*(6), 630–632.

Slack, K. S., Berger, L., DuMont, K., Yang, M. Y., Kim, B., Erhard-Eietzel, S., et al. (2011). Risk and protective factors for child neglect during early childhood: A cross-study comparison. *Children and Youth Services Review, 33*(8), 1354–1363.

Sleath, B., Carpenter, D., Saynor, R., Ayala, G., Williams, D., Davis, S. et al. (2011). Child and caregiver involvement and shared decision-making during asthma pediatric visits. *Journal of Asthma, 48*(10), 1022–1031.

Sleet, D. A., Ballesteros, M. F., & Borse, N. N. (2010). A review of unintentional injuries in adolescents. *Annual Review of Public Health, 31*, 195–212.

Smith, J. P. (2009). The impact of childhood health on adult labor market outcomes. *The Review of Economics and Statistics, 91*(3), 478–489.

Smithbattle, L. (2007). Legacies of advantage and disadvantage: The case of teen mothers. *Public Health Nursing, 34*(5), 409–420.

Snyder, L., Milici, F., Slater, M., Sun, H., & Strizhakova, Y. (2006). Effects of alcohol advertising exposure on drinking among youth. *Archives of Pediatrics and Adolescent Medicine, 160*(1), 18–24.

Sorenson, S. B. (2011). Gender disparities in injury mortality: Consistent, persistent, and larger than you'd think. *American Journal of Public Health, 101*(Suppl. 1), s353–s358.

Sotir, M. J., Cappozzo D. L., Warshauer D. M., Schmidt, C., Monson, T., Berg, J. et al. (2008). A countywide outbreak of pertussis: Initial transmission in a high school weight room with subsequent substantial impact on adolescents and adults. *Archives of Pediatric and Adolescent Medicine, 162*(1), 79–85.

Spivey, M., Schnitzer, P., Kruse, R., Slusher, P., & Jaffe, D. (2008). Association of injury visits in children and child maltreatment reports. *Journal of Emergency Medicine*. doi: 10.1016/j.jemermed. 2007.07.025.

Staff, J., & Mortimer, J. (2008). Social class background and the 'school to work' transition. *New Directions for Child and Adolescent Development, 119*, 55–69.

Stavrinos, D., Byington, K., & Schwebel, D. (2009). Effect of cell phone distraction on pediatric pedestrian injury risk. *Pediatrics, 123*(2), e179–e185.

Stice, E., Shaw, H., Bohon, C., Marti, C., & Rohde, P. (2009). A meta-analytic review of depression prevention programs for children and adolescents: Factors that predict magnitude of intervention effects. *Journal of Consulting and Clinical Psychology, 77*(3), 486–503.

Stokley, S., Cohn, A. Jain, N., & McCauley, M. (2011). Compliance with recommendations and opportunities for vaccination at ages 11 to 12 years. *Archives of Pediatrics and Adolescent Medicine, 165*(9), 813–818.

Straus, M. A., & Paschall, M. J. (2009). Corporal punishment by mothers and development of children's cognitive ability: A longitudinal study of two nationally representative age cohorts. *Journal of Aggression, Maltreatment and Trauma, 18*(5), 459–483.

Strickland, B. B., Jones, J., Ghandour, R., Kogan, M., & Newacheck, P. (2011). The medical home: Health care access and impact for children and youth in the United States. *Pediatrics, 127*(4), 604–611.

Swahn, M., Bossarte, R., & Sullivent, E. (2008). Age of alcohol use initiation, suicidal behavior, and peer and dating violence victimization and perpetration among high-risk, seventh-grade adolescents. *Pediatrics, 121*(2), 297–305.

Swanson, S. A., Crow, S., LeGrange, D., Swendsen, J., & Merikangas, K. (2011). Prevalence and correlates of eating disorders in adolescents. *Archives of General Psychiatry, 68*(7), 714–723.

Swartz, K. L., Kastelic, E., Hess, S., Cox, T., Gonzales, L., Mink, S., & DePaulo, J. (2010). The effectiveness of a school-based adolescent depression education program. *Health Education and Behavior, 37*(1), 11–22.

Tarter, R., Kirisci, L., Feske, U., & Vanyukov, M. (2007). Modeling the pathways linking childhood hyperactivity and substance use disorder in young adulthood. *Psychology of Addictive Behaviors, 21*(2), 266–271.

Taylor, C., Manganello, J., Lee, S., & Rice, J. (2010). Mothers' spanking of 3-year-old children and subsequent risk of children's aggressive behavior. *Pediatrics, 125*(5), e1057–e1065.

Taylor, J., Baldwin, N., & Spencer, N. (2008). Predicting child abuse and neglect: Ethical, theoretical and methodological challenges. *Journal of Clinical Nursing, 17*(9), 1193–1200.

Terry-McElrath, Y., O'Malley, P., Delva, J., & Johnston, L. (2009). The school food environment and student body mass index and food consumption: 2004 to 2007 national data. *Journal of Adolescent Health, 45*(3, Suppl.), s45–s56.

Terzian, M., Hamilton, K., & Ericson, S. (2011). *What works to prevent or reduce internalizing problems or socio-emotional difficulties in adolescence*. Washington, DC: Child Trends.

Terzian, M., & Moore, K. A. (2012). *Examining state-level patterns in teen childbearing: 1991 to 2009*. Washington, DC: Child Trends.

Thapar, A., Langley, K., O'Donovan, M., & Owen, M. (2006). Refining the attention deficit hyperactivity disorder phenotype for molecular genetic studies. *Molecular Psychiatry, 11*(8), 714–720.

TODAY Study Group, Zeitler, P., Hirst, K., Pyle, L., et al. (2012). A clinical trial to maintain glycemic control in youth with type 2 diabetes. *New England Journal of Medicine, 366*, 2247–2256.

Tomar, S. L., & Reeves, A. F. (2009). Changes in the oral health of US children and adolescents and dental public health infrastructure since the release of the Healthy People 2010 objectives. *Academic Pediatrics, 9*(6), 388–395.

Torpy, J. M., Campbell A., & Glass, R. M. (2010). Patient page: Chronic diseases of children. *JAMA, 303*(7), 682.

U.S. Department of Agriculture (USDA). (2010). *Food security status of U.S. households, 2010*. Retrieved from http://www.ers.usda.gov/Briefing/FoodSecurity/stats_graphs.htm#food_secure

U.S. Department of Agriculture (USDA). (2011a). *Food labeling*. Retrieved from http://fnic.nal.usda.gov/nal_display/index.php?info_center=4&tax_level=2&tax_subject=273&topic_id=1317

U.S. Department of Agriculture (USDA). (2011b). *Food security in the United States: Definitions of hunger and food security*. Retrieved from http://www.ers.usda.gov/briefing/foodsecurity/labels.htm

U.S. Department of Health and Human Services (U.S. DHHS). (2012). *Early and middle childhood: Healthy People 2020*. Retrieved from http://healthypeople.gov/2020/topicsobjectives2020/objectiveslist.aspx?topicId=1

Usta, I., Zoorob, D., Abu-Musa, A., Naassan, G., & Nassar, A. H. (2008). Obstetric outcome of teenage pregnancies compared with adult pregnancies. *Acta Obstetricia et Gynecologica Scandinavica, 878*(2), 178–183.

Van Cleave, J., Gortmaker, S., & Perrin, J. (2010). Dynamics of obesity and chronic health conditions among children and youth. *JAMA, 303*(7), 623–630.

van den Berg, P., Neumark-Sztainer, D., Hannan, P., & Haines, J. (2007). Is dieting advice from magazines helpful or harmful? Five-year associations with weight-control behaviors and psychological outcomes in adolescents. *Pediatrics, 119*(1), E30–E37.

Vandermeulen, C., Roelants M., Theeten, H., Depoorter, A. M., Van Damme, P., & Hoppenbrouwers, K. (2008). Vaccination coverage in 14-year-old adolescents: Documentation, timeliness, and sociodemographic determinants. *Pediatrics, 121*(3), 428–434.

Villanti, A., Boulay, M., & Juon, H. S. (2011). Peer, parent and media influences on adolescent smoking by developmental stage. *Addictive Behaviors, 36*(1–2), 133–136.

Villanti, A. C., McKay, H., Abrams, D., Holtgrave, D., & Bowie, J. (2010). Smoking-cessation interventions for U.S. young adults: A systematic review. *American Journal of Preventive Medicine, 39*(6), 564–574.

Virginia Youth Violence Project. (n.d.). *School violence myths.* Retrieved from http://youthviolence.edschool.virginia.edu/violence-in-schools/survey-hoax.html

Wakefield, M., Loken, B., & Hornik, R. (2010). Use of mass media campaigns to change health behaviour. *The Lancet, 376*(9748), 1261–1271.

Wang, C. T., & Holton, J. (2007). *Total estimated cost of abuse and neglect in the United States. Economic impact study.* Retrieved from http://member.preventchildabuse.org/site/DocServer/cost_analysis.pdf?docID=144

WebMD. (2012). *Drugs for children with epilepsy.* Retrieved from http://www.webmd.com/epilepsy/medicines-for-children-with-epilepsy

Weitzman, M., & Zhou, S. (2012). Commentary on household hardships, public programs, and their associations with the health and development of very young children: Insights from Children's HealthWatch. *Journal for Applied Research on Children, 3*(1), article 13.

Wells, J., Hallal, P. C., Reichert, F. F., Menezes, A., Araujo, C., & Victora, C. (2008). Sleep patterns and television viewing in relation to obesity and blood pressure: Evidence from an adolescent Brazilian birth cohort. *International Journal of Obesity.* doi: 10.1038/ijo.2008.37.

Wendell, S., Wang, X., Brown, M., Cooper, M. E., DeSensi, R, Weyant, R., et al. (2010). Taste genes associated with dental caries. *Journal of Dental Research, 89*(11), 1198–1202.

Wheeler, L., Buckley, R., Gerald, L. B., Merkle, S., & Morrison, T. A. (2009). Working with schools to improve pediatric asthma management. *Pediatric Asthma, Allergy and Immunology, 22*(4), 197–206.

Whelan, K., Stratton, K., Kawashima, T., Leisenring, W., Hayashi, S., Waterbor, J., et al. (2011). Auditory complications in childhood cancer survivors: A report from the childhood cancer survivor study. *Pediatric Blood and Cancer, 57*(1), 126–134.

Wildsmith, E., Manlove, J., Jekielek, S., Moore, K. A., & Mincieli, L. (2012). Teenage childbearing among youth born to teenage mothers. *Youth & Society, 44*(2), 258–283.

Williams, J. H., Van Dorn, R., Bright, C., Jonson-Reid, M., & Nebbitt, V. (2010). Child maltreatment and delinquency onset among African American adolescent males. *Research on Social Work Practice, 20*(3), 253–259.

Winston, F., Kallan, M., Senserrick, T., & Elliott, M. (2008). Risk factors for death among older child and teenaged motor vehicle passengers. *Archives of Pediatric and Adolescent Medicine, 162*(3), 253–260.

Wood, A. C., & Neale, M. C. (2010). Twin studies and their implications for molecular genetic studies: Endophenotypes integrate quantitative and molecular genetics in ADHD research. *Journal of the American Academy of Child and Adolescent Psychiatry, 49*(9), 874–883.

Woodruff, S., Conway, T., Edwards, C., Elliott, S. P., & Crittenden, J. (2007). Evaluation of an internet virtual world chat room for adolescent smoking cessation. *Addictive Behavior, 32*(9), 1769–1786.

World Bank. (2011). *Health, nutrition, and population.* Retrieved from http://web.worldbank.org/WBSITE/EXTERNAL/TOPICS/EXTSOCIALPROTECTION/EXTDISABILITY/0,,contentMDK:20208203~menuPK:418901~pagePK:148956~piPK:216618~theSitePK:282699,00.html

Yeung, W., & Conley, D. (2008). Black-White achievement gap and family wealth. *Child Development, 79*(2), 303–324.

Yu, J., Adams, S., Burns, J., Brindis, C., & Irwin, C. (2008). Use of mental health counseling as adolescents become young adults. *Journal of Adolescent Health, 43*(3), 268–276.

Yurgelun-Todd, D. (2007). Emotional and cognitive changes during adolescence. *Current Opinions in Neurobiology, 17*(2), 251–257.

Zahn-Waxler, C., Shirtcliff, E., & Marceau, K. (2008). Disorders of childhood and adolescence: Gender and psychopathology. *Annual Review of Clinical Psychology, 27*(4), 275–303.

Zenere, F. J., & Lazarus, P. J. (2009). The sustained reduction of youth suicidal behavior in an urban, multicultural school district. *School Psychology Review, 18*(2), 189–199.

Ziliak, J. P. (Ed.). (2009). *Welfare reform and its long-term consequences for America's poor.* Cambridge, UK: Cambridge University Press.

Zimmerman, F., & Bell, J. (2010). Associations of television content type and obesity in children. *American Journal of Public Health, 100*(2), 334–340.

Ziol-Guest, K., Duncan, G., & Kalil, A. (2009). Early childhood poverty and adult body mass index. *American Journal of Public Health, 99*(3), 527–532.

CHAPTER

23

Adult Women and Men

"Male and female represent the two sides of the great radical dualism. But in fact they are perpetually passing into one another. Fluid hardens to solid, solid rushes to fluid. There is no wholly masculine man, no purely feminine woman."

—***Margaret Fuller*** **(1810–1850), Woman in the Nineteenth Century, 1845**

KEY TERMS

Adult
Anorexia nervosa
Binge eating
Bisexual
Bulimia nervosa
Cancer
Cardiovascular disease
Chronic fatigue and immune dysfunction syndrome (CFIDS)
Chronic lower respiratory disease
Diabetes mellitus
Erectile dysfunction
Gay
Health disparities
Health literacy
Life expectancy
Menopause
Obesity
Osteoporosis
Prostate
Substance use
Transgender
Unintentional injuries

LEARNING OBJECTIVES

Upon mastery of this chapter, you should be able to:

- Identify key demographic characteristics of women and men throughout the adult lifespan.
- Provide a health profile of adult women and men living in the United States.
- Discuss the major chronic illnesses found in adult women and men in the United States.
- Compare and contrast the manifestations of chronic illnesses in adult women and men.
- Identify primary, secondary, and tertiary health promotion activities designed to improve the health of women and men.
- Describe the role of the community health nurse in promoting the health of adult women and men across the lifespan.

The term *adult* has many different meanings in society. To children, an adult is anyone in authority, including a 14-year-old babysitter. As people age, they tend to redefine the term upward. It is not unusual, for example, to hear an elderly person describe a couple in their mid-30s as "kids." The United States Criminal Justice System distinguishes between adults and juveniles for purposes of delimiting types of crimes and possibilities for punishment, and labor legislation provides different protections for children than for adult workers. Even hospitals and health care systems vary somewhat as to the ages at which they distinguish pediatric and geriatric clients from middle-aged adults.

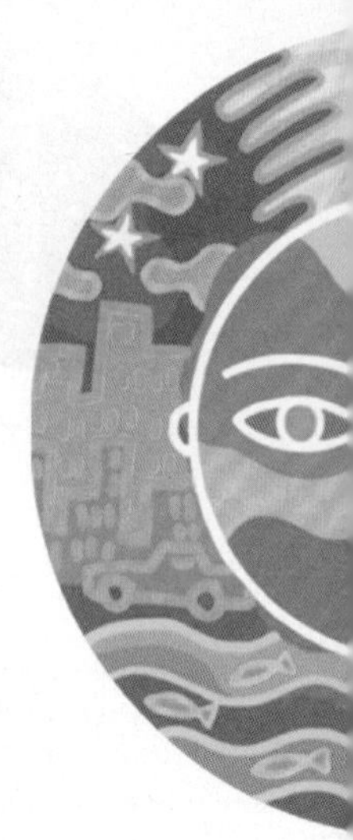

How would you characterize an adult? Does your definition rest solely on age, or is it influenced by other factors, such as marital status, employment status, financial independence, amount of responsibility for self and others, and so on? For the purposes of this chapter, an **adult** is defined as anyone 18 years of age or older. Obviously, there are tremendous differences in health profiles and health care needs as people age. As adults enter their middle years (35–65), they experience many normal physiologic changes. However, some changes are the result of disease, environment, or lifestyle and can be modified through behavior change. A physical profile of middle-aged adults is organized by body systems and can be found in Display 23.1.

DISPLAY 23.1 PHYSICAL PROFILE OF MIDDLE-AGED ADULTS BY BODY SYSTEM

Body System	***Physical Characteristic***
Skeletal system	Intervertebral disks flatten over time.
Integumentary system	Decreased secretions by sebaceous glands lead to drier skin.
	Sweat glands diminish in size and number.
	Skin loses elasticity and is more prone to wrinkles.
	Hair bulbs lose melanin usually resulting in gray hair by age 50.
Muscular system	Muscle fibers decrease by approximately 10%.
	Lean body mass is replaced by adipose tissue.
	Decreased grip strength occurs at this age.
Endocrine and reproductive system	Menses stops.
	Synthesis of estrogen decreases.
	Tissues of the reproductive system (e.g., cervix and uterus) gradually atrophy.
	Uterine changes make pregnancy less likely.
	Intercourse may be more painful due to diminishing natural lubrications.
	Less frequent erections
	Testosterone levels decline gradually.
Neurologic system	Nerve impulses are conducted 5% slower.
	Cognition is unaffected, although there is a gradual loss of neurons.
	Eyesight is poorer due to loss of elasticity in the lens.
	Auditory discrimination of certain tones and consonants gradually decreases.
Cardiovascular system	By age 50, the heart's efficiency may be only 80%.
	Elasticity of heart and blood vessels decreases.
	Cardiac output decreases.
Respiratory system	Elasticity of lungs decreases.
	Breathing capacity decreases to 75% due to diminished strength of chest wall muscles.
Urinary system	Decreased glomerular filtration rate appears in women.
	Loss of bladder tone and tissue atrophy may lead to incontinence or possibly prolapse.
	In men, an enlarged prostate may result in nocturia or dribbling.

Throughout history, the health care needs of women and men have differed more often than they have been alike. Many health promotion and health protection programs are designed specifically for women or for men. Mammography screening programs and prenatal clinics are designed with women's health in mind. Teaching testicular self-examination (TSE) and prostate cancer screening are health promotion programs for men. Programs in many areas, such as cardiac rehabilitation, stress management, and dating violence prevention, may have had one gender in mind at one time but are now established as programs for both genders. Nevertheless, morbidity and mortality statistics, historical development of research foci, and workforce changes required that the health care needs of women and men be examined separately. This chapter focuses on the health of women and men across the adult lifespan.

DEMOGRAPHICS OF ADULT WOMEN AND MEN

Mortality statistics are considered the most reliable indicator of the health status of a population. In 2007, a total of 2,423,712 people died in the United States (Xu, Kochanek, Murphy, & Tejada-Vera, 2010). The crude death rate was 760.2 per 100,000 for all ages. Causes of death varied by age, gender, and ethnicity, but the 10 leading causes of death for all people in rank order included the following:

1. Diseases of the heart 616,067
2. Malignant neoplasms 562,875
3. Cerebrovascular diseases 135,952
4. Chronic lower respiratory diseases (CLRDs) 127,924
5. Accidents (unintentional injuries) 123,706
6. Alzheimer's disease 74,632
7. Diabetes mellitus 71,382
8. Influenza and pneumonia 52,717
9. Nephritis, nephritic syndrome, and nephrosis 46,448
10. Septicemia 34,828

Diseases of the heart and malignant neoplasms accounted for 48.6% of deaths in 2007, and these diseases are the top two causes of death for both women and men. However, cerebrovascular diseases were the third leading cause of death for women, and unintentional injuries were the third leading cause of death in men. Mortality from heart disease has exhibited a downward trend since 1950, but cancer mortality did not begin to decline until the 1990s (Kochanek, Xu, Murphy, Miniño, & Kung, 2011).

Since the beginning of the 21st century, the major causes of death have remained fairly consistent. This was a major shift from the turn of the 20th century, when communicable diseases such as tuberculosis and pneumonia were leading causes of death. The shift from communicable to chronic illness can be attributed to the significant advances in public health, prevention, technology, pharmacotherapy, and biomedical research.

LIFE EXPECTANCY

Life expectancy is the average number of years that an individual member of a specific cohort (usually a single birth year) is projected to live. It is another standard measurement that is used to compare the health status of various populations, typically calculated from age-specific death rates. Health statistics often report life expectancy figures from birth to 65 years of age (see Table 23-1).

In the United States, life expectancy has increased consistently over time. Between 1990 and 2007, life expectancy at birth increased 3.6 years for men and 1.8 years for women. The gap between men and women narrowed from 6.8 years in 1990 to 5.0 years in 2007.

Table 23.1 Life Expectancy at Birth and 65 Years of Age According to Sex: United States, Selected Years, 1900–2007

	At Birth			At 65 Years		
Year	Both Sexes	Male	Female	Both Sexes	Male	Female
1900	47.3	46.3	48.3	–	–	–
1950	68.2	65.6	71.1	–	12.8	15.1
1960	69.7	66.6	73.1	14.4	12.9	15.9
1970	70.8	67.1	74.7	15.2	13.1	17.1
1980	73.7	70.0	77.4	16.5	14.2	18.4
1990	75.4	71.8	78.8	17.3	15.2	19.1
2000	76.8	74.1	79.3	17.7	16.1	19.1
2007	77.9	75.4	80.4	18.7	17.3	19.9

–, data not available.

Extracted from National Center for Health Statistics. (2011). *Health, United States, 2010: With special feature on death and dying* (DHHS Pub. No. 1232). Hyattsville, MD: Public Health Service.

Table 23.2 Life Expectancy at Birth for Selected Countries by Sex

	Female	Male	Disparity
Japan	86.0	79.2	6.8
France	84.4	77.5	6.9
Switzerland	84.4	79.5	4.9
Spain	84.3	77.8	6.5
Australia	83.7	79.0	4.7
Iceland	82.9	79.4	3.5
Germany	82.7	77.4	5.3
Greece	82.0	77.0	5.0
United States	80.4	75.4	5.0
Hungary	77.3	69.2	8.1

Extracted from National Center for Health Statistics. (2011). *Health, United States, 2010: With special feature on death and dying* (DHHS Pub. No. 1232). Hyattsville, MD: Public Health Service.

There are, however, differences in the life expectancy between Whites and Blacks for both genders. In 2007, life expectancy at birth for White males was 6 years greater than Black males, and White females' life expectancy was 4 years greater than Black females (National Center for Health Statistics [NCHS], 2011).

Globally, the life expectancy in the United States trails that of more than 25 other countries (Table 23-2). Japan reports the highest life expectancy. In all countries, disparities exist between female and male life expectancy, some as much as 8 years. The smallest disparity can be found between women and men living in Iceland (NCHS, 2011).

HEALTH DISPARITIES

One of the goals of *Healthy People 2020* is to eliminate **health disparities.** A health disparity is defined as a difference in health status that occurs by gender, race/ethnicity, education or income, disability, geographic location, or sexual orientation (U.S. Department of Health and Human Services [USDHHS], 2010a). Disparities in health occur when one segment of the population has a higher incidence of disease or mortality rate than another, or when survival rates are less for one group than another (Truman et al., 2011). Often, persons with the greatest health burden have the least access to information, communication technologies, health care, and supporting social services. Interdisciplinary, collaborative, public, and private approaches, as well as public–private partnerships are needed to develop strategies to address the health disparity goal of *Healthy People 2020.*

HEALTH LITERACY

Health literacy is defined as the degree to which individuals have the capacity to obtain, process, and understand basic health information and services needed to make appropriate health decisions. The ability to read and understand health information is key to managing health problems. Low health literacy contributes to health disparities and has been documented as an increasing problem among certain racial and ethnic groups, non-English speaking populations, and persons over 65 years of age in the United States (Bennett, Chen, Soroui, & White, 2009; White, Chen, & Atchison, 2008). See Chapter 11 for additional information on health literacy.

MAJOR HEALTH PROBLEMS OF ADULTS

Morbidity and mortality among adults vary substantially by age, gender, and race/ethnicity. The six leading causes of death are presented in this section. Diseases of the heart and cerebrovascular diseases are the first and third causes of death in adults and are discussed together. Malignant neoplasms, CLRDs, unintentional injuries, and diabetes mellitus are discussed separately. Other selected additional major causes of death are covered in detail in other chapters: suicide (Chapter 27), Alzheimer's disease (Chapter 24), and homicide (Chapters 17 and 20).

Coronary Heart Disease and Stroke

Cardiovascular disease (CVD), the leading cause of death in the United States, is responsible for 17% of national health expenditures (Heidenreich et al., 2011). More than 34% of all deaths in the United States are due to CVD, primarily coronary heart disease (CHD) and stroke. An estimated 1 in 3 adults (81 million) is living with one or more types of CVD. It is estimated that every 25 seconds, an American will have a coronary event, and every day, nearly 2,200 will die of CVD. In 2010, CVD was projected to cost more than $503 billion, which

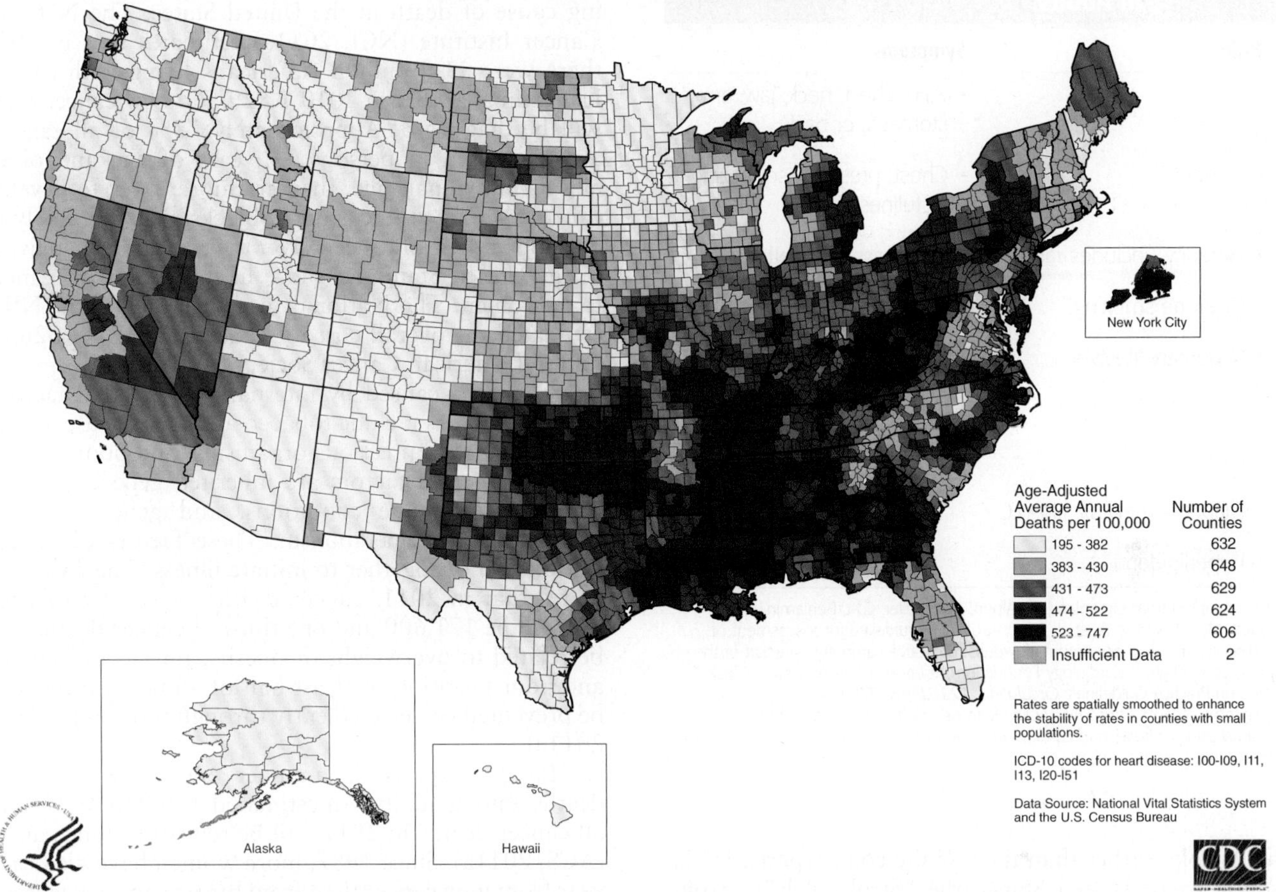

FIGURE 23-1. Heart disease death rates, 2000–2006 adults ages 35+ by county. (Retrieved from http://www.cdc.gov/dhdsp/maps/national_maps/hd_all.htm)

includes health services, medications, and lost productivity (Centers for Disease Control and Prevention [CDC], 2010c; Roger et al., 2011) (Fig. 23-1).

Risk factors contributing to CHD can be separated into two categories: personal and hereditary. Personal risk factors include gender, age, race/ethnicity, cholesterol level (specifically the ratio of low-density to high-density lipoproteins), diabetes, obesity, physical inactivity, high blood pressure, and cigarette smoking. The most modifiable of these factors are cholesterol, high blood pressure, cigarette smoking, obesity, and physical inactivity. Heredity obviously cannot be changed. The likelihood of heart disease or stroke multiplies with the increasing number of risk factors present (Table 23-3).

We now know that CVD affects more women than men, but the race/ethnicity disparities in heart disease have remained consistent over time. The incidence of CVD is higher in the Black population than the White. Death rates (per 100,000) in 2007 were 294.0 for White males and 405.9 for Black males. White females had a death rate of 205.7 compared to the rate for Black females, 86.1. Except for a relatively small increase in 1993, mortality from heart disease has steadily declined since 1980. From 1997 to 2007, death rates from CVD declined by 27.8% (Roger et al., 2011; Xu et al., 2010).

Disparities exist in cardiovascular treatment outcomes based on gender. Since 1984, more women than men have died each year from heart disease. When compared to men, women have poorer health outcomes after a cardiac event; 23% of women who have a heart attack die within 1 year, compared with 18% of men. Women are also two to three times more likely to die following heart bypass surgery (Lloyd-Jones et al., 2010; Roger et al., 2011; Women's Heart Foundation, n.d.).

Approximately 795,000 Americans suffer strokes each year, and strokes account for almost 1 in 18 deaths in the United States (American Heart Association [AHA], 2011a) (see Fig. 23-2). Disparities also exist among people who have had a stroke. In 2007, women accounted for 60.6% of all stroke deaths in the United States. Each year, approximately 55,000 more women than men have a stroke. Men are at a greater risk of having a stroke at a younger age than women; however, this difference dissipates with age. Blacks are twice as likely to have their

Table 23.3 Primary Risk Factors for Coronary Heart Disease and Symptoms of Heart Attack in Adults

Risks	Symptoms
• Age	• Pain: chest, neck, jaw, arm, stomach, or back
• Gender	• Chest: pressure, squeezing, or fullness
• Heredity (includes race)	• Shortness of breath
• Cigarette smoking	• Cold sweat
• Sedentary lifestyle	• Nausea
• Excess body weight	• Lightheadedness
• Hypertension	
• Diabetes mellitus, HbA1C	
• Hyperlipidemia	

Risks: Adapted from Greenland, P., Alpert, J. S., Beller, G.A., Benjamin, E. J., Budoff, M. J., Fayad, Z. A, et al. 2010 ACCF/AHA guideline for assessment of cardiovascular risk in asymptomatic adults: Executive summary: A report of the American College of Cardiology Foundation/American Heart Association Task Force on Practice Guidelines. *Circulation, 122*, 2748–2764.
Symptoms: Adapted from American Heart Association. (2011c). *Warning signs of heart attack, stroke, and cardiac arrest.* Retrieved from http://www.heart.org/HEARTORG/Conditions/Conditions_UCM_305346_SubHomePage.jsp

first stroke earlier than their White counterparts. In the southeastern United States (the "Stroke Belt"), stroke death rates for both Blacks and Whites are higher than in any other part of the country (Glasser et al., 2011; Liao, Greenlund, Croft, Kennan, & Giles, 2009).

The hallmark Framingham Heart Study identified major risk factors associated with the development of CVD and the effects of related factors such as blood triglycerides, gender, and psychosocial issues. The study began in 1948 under the direction of National Heart Institute, now known as the National Heart, Lung, and Blood Institute (NHLBI). At that time, the death rates from CVD were rising, but little was known about the general causes of heart disease and stroke. The Framingham Heart Study researchers recruited 2,336 men and 2,873 women between the ages of 30 and 62 in an effort to identify common factors or characteristics that contribute to CVD. Every 2 years, these individuals were scheduled for an extensive medical history, physical examination, and laboratory tests. In 1971, the study enrolled 5,124 of the original participants' adult children and their spouses, and in 2002, a third generation (the children of the Offspring Cohort) were recruited and examined. Findings from the Framingham Heart Study continue to make important scientific contributions regarding the development and treatment of CVD and related health issues. Recently, the investigators expanded their research into the role of genetics and CVD (NHLBI, 2011).

Cancer

Cancer is a major chronic illness and the second leading cause of death in the United States. The National Cancer Institute (NCI, 2011a) estimates that in 2008 there were 11.9 million Americans living with cancer. It is estimated that in 2010 1,529,560 new cancer cases will be diagnosed. Approximately 78% of all cancers are diagnosed in persons 55 years of age and older, and as individuals age, they are more likely to develop cancer. Among ethnic groups, Blacks are more likely to develop and die of cancer. Over their lifetime, men living in the United States are more likely to develop cancer than women. The National Institutes of Health (NIH) estimated the overall cost for cancer in 2010 at $263.8 billion (American Cancer Society [ACS], 2011a).

Cancer is caused by internal and external factors. External factors include tobacco and alcohol use, chemicals, radiation, infectious organisms, and poor lifestyle choices. Internal factors are inherited gene mutations, hormones, immune conditions, and gene mutations that occur from metabolism. These factors can occur in isolation or together to initiate illness. The ACS estimates that in 2011, cancer deaths caused by tobacco use will be 171,600 and one third of cancer deaths will be related to overweight or obesity, physical inactivity, and poor nutrition. At least half of all new cancers can be prevented or detected early through screenings (ACS, 2011a).

Lung cancer is the number one cause of cancer deaths among adults. An estimated 156,940 or 27% of all cancer deaths in 2011 will be related to lung cancer (ACS, 2011a). Since 1987, more women have died each year from lung cancer than from breast cancer. Cigarette smoking is the predominant risk factor for lung cancer. Quantity of cigarettes smoked and the number of years smoking increase an individual's risk of developing lung cancer. Other risk factors include occupational or environmental exposure to secondhand smoke, radon, asbestos, genetic susceptibility, and a history of tuberculosis. Current efforts to reduce mortality by early detection have been unsuccessful. Early detection of lung cancer by chest x-ray, analysis of cells in sputum, and fiber-optic examination of the bronchial passages has shown limited effectiveness in reducing lung cancer deaths. However, low-dose spiral computerized tomography (CT) scans and molecular markers in sputum have produced more promising results in detecting lung cancers at an earlier stage of the disease (ACS, 2011a).

Colon and rectal cancers are the third most common cancers in adults. Among adults, an estimated 102,340 cases of colon and 39,879 cases of rectal cancers are expected to occur in 2011 and 49,380 deaths. The risk of developing colorectal cancer increases with age, and 90% of all cases are diagnosed in individuals 50 years of age or older. There are several modifiable factors associated with the increased risk of colorectal cancer. These factors include obesity, physical inactivity, a diet high in red or processed meat, alcohol consumption, long-term smoking, and inadequate intake of fruits and vegetables. Other risk factors include certain

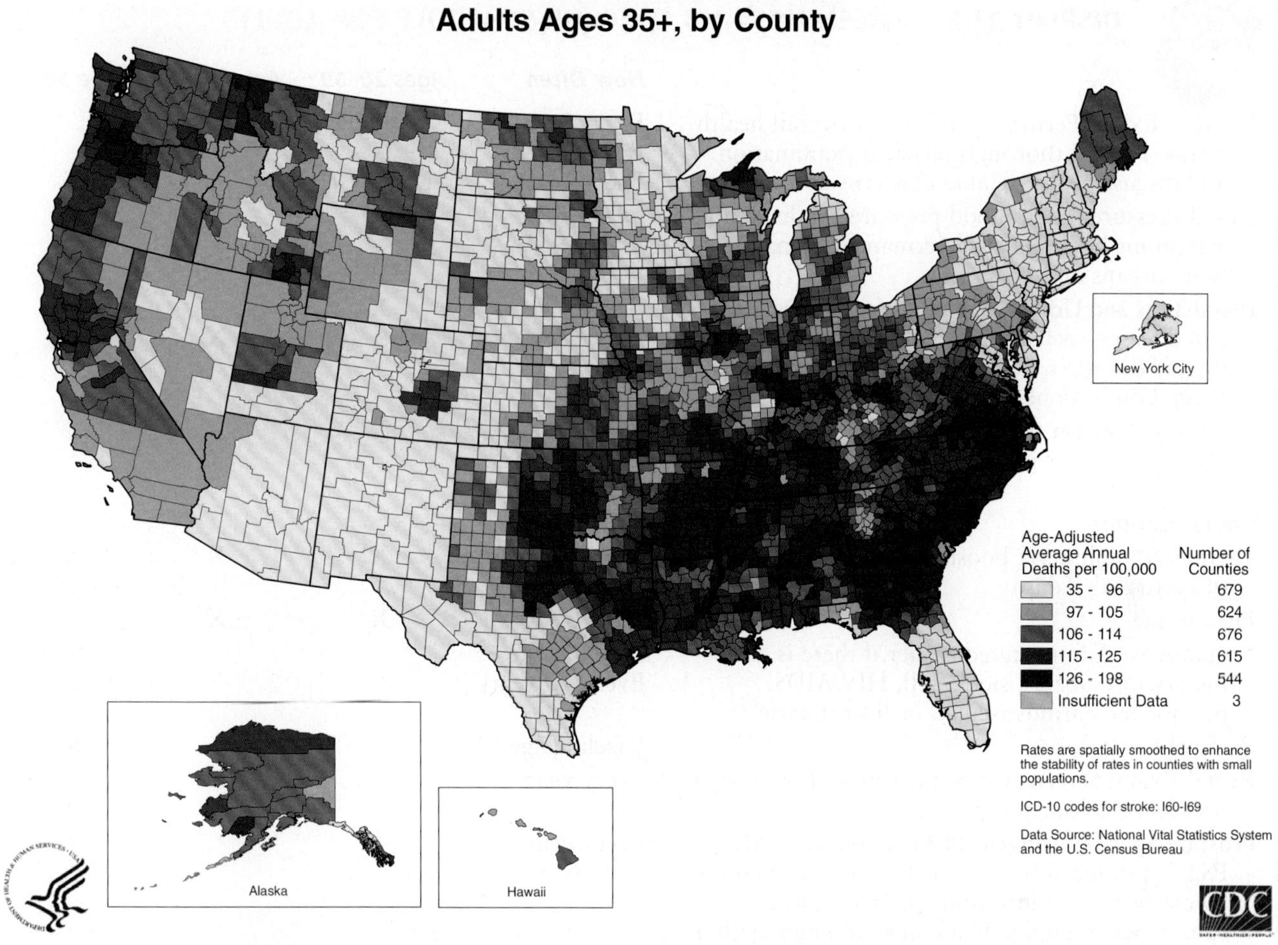

FIGURE 23-2. Stroke death rates, 2000–2006 adults ages 35+ by county. (Retrieved from http://www.cdc.gov/dhdsp/maps/GISX/mapgallery/maps/pdf/stroke_mortality.pdf)

inherited genetic mutations, personal or family history of polyps or colorectal cancer, and personal history of chronic inflammatory bowel disease. Screening for colon and rectal cancer should begin at age 50 for men and women who are at average risk (ACS, 2011a) (see Display 23.2).

Chronic Lower Respiratory Diseases

Chronic lower respiratory disease comprises three major conditions: chronic bronchitis, emphysema, and asthma. CLRD is the fourth leading cause of death in the United States. The term chronic obstructive pulmonary disease (COPD) includes emphysema and chronic bronchitis. COPD is a major cause of disability, and over 12.1 million adults in the United States (aged 18 and over) are estimated to have the disease. However, approximately 24 million adults in the United States demonstrate evidence of impaired lung function, which could indicate an underdiagnosis of COPD (American Lung Association [ALA], 2008). In 2010, approximately $49.9 billion was spent on direct and indirect health care costs related to COPD (ALA, 2011).

Tobacco smoking is the major risk factor for developing COPD, accounting for more than 85% of cases. Smokers are 12 to 13 times more likely to die from COPD compared to nonsmokers. The remaining COPD cases are attributable to environmental exposures and genetic factors (ALA, 2011). Since 2000, the number of women dying from COPD surpassed the number of men. This rise is probably related to the increase in smoking among women after World War II and the difference in how cigarette smoke is metabolized by women as compared to men. Research suggests that women are at higher risk for DNA damage from cigarette smoke and are less able to repair this damage.

Chronic bronchitis sufferers are more likely to be between 18 and 44 years of age and female, whereas emphysema sufferers are usually 45 years of age and older and male. Both conditions are more commonly found among Whites than Blacks (ALA, 2008, 2011; CDC, 2008).

The exact cause of asthma is unknown, but research indicates that both genetic and environmental factors contribute to its cause. In adults, the prevalence rate among women is 60% greater than the rate among

DISPLAY 23.2 SCREENINGS AND CHECKUP SCHEDULE FOR ADULTS

	How Often	*Ages 20–39*	*Ages 40–49*	*Age 50+*
Physical Exam: Performed to review overall health status. Have a thorough physical examination and discuss health-related concerns and topics.	Every 3 years Every 2 years Every year	X 	 X 	 X
Blood Pressure: High blood pressure can have no symptoms but can cause permanent damage to body organs and systems.	Every year	X	X	X
Blood Tests and Urinalysis: Screens for various illnesses and diseases, such as high cholesterol, kidney, or thyroid disorders, before problems or symptoms occur. Can be done at time of physical exam	Every 3 years Every 2 years Every year	X 	 X 	 X
Electrocardiogram (EKG): EKG screens for heart abnormalities or problems.	Baseline–age 30 Every 4 years Every 3 years	X 	 X 	 X
Immunizations				
Tetanus & diphtheria booster (plus 1-time booster of pertussis - Tdap)	Every 10 years	X	X	X
Flu vaccine	Every year	X	X	X
Pneumovax: Administered earlier if there is a history of diabetes, sickle cell, HIV/AIDS, pulmonary, cardiovascular, or liver disease	Baseline age 65 Every 10 years			X X
Zostavax	Baseline age 65			X
Rectal Exam: Screens for hemorrhoids, lower rectal problems, colon, and prostate cancer	Every year	X	X	X
Prostate-Specific Antigen (PSA) Blood Test (Men): PSA is produced by the prostate. Levels increase when there is an infection, enlargement, or cancer. Screening for Black men and men with a family history should start at age 45.*	Every year		*	X
Clinical Breast Exam (Women): Breast exam by health care provider	Every year	X	X	X
Mammography (Women): Screening should begin at age 40 unless high risk.*	Every year		*	X
Pelvic Exam and Pap Smear (Women):	Every year	X		
A pelvic exam is performed to evaluate the size and position of the vagina, cervix, uterus, fallopian tubes, and ovaries. A Pap test is performed to look for changes in the cells of the cervix, such as dysplasia or cancer.	Every 3 years after 3 consecutive negative Pap smears		X	X
Self-Exams: *Testicles* are examined to find lumps. *Skin* is checked to look for signs of changing moles, freckles, or early skin cancer. *Breasts* are examined to find abnormal lumps in their early stages.	Monthly	X	X	X
Hemoccult: Screens the stool for microscopic amounts of blood that can be the first indication of polyps or colon cancer	Every year		X	X
Colon Rectal Health: A flexible endoscope is used to examine the rectum, sigmoid, and descending colon for cancer at its earliest stages. The exam also detects polyps that can progress to cancer if not found early.	Every 3–4 years			X
Chest X-Ray: Should be considered in smokers over the age of 45	Discuss with physician		X	X
Bone Health: Bone mineral density is measured.	Baseline As needed		X 	 X

Adapted from Brott, A., & The Blueprint for Men's Health Advisory Board. (2008). *Blueprint for men's health: A guide to healthy lifestyle* (2nd ed.). Retrieved from http://www.blueprintformenshealth.com/blueprint/

men. Asthma prevalence rates in the Black population are 24% higher than in the White population. Among employed adults, over 10 million days of work are lost each year due to asthma (ALA, 2008; CDC, 2011k).

Unintentional Injuries

Unintentional injuries refer to any injury that results from unintended exposure to physical agents, including heat, mechanical energy, chemicals, or electricity. They are the fifth leading cause of death overall and the leading cause of death for persons 44 years of age and younger (CDC, 2007). In 2007, a total of 182,479 Americans died of injuries from a variety of causes. The top three causes of unintentional injuries include motor vehicle crashes, poisoning, and falls (CDC, 2010b, 2011b, 2011f, 2011h).

In the United States, unintentional mortality increased by 11% between 1999 and 2005, from 35.3 per 100,000 persons to 39.0 in 2005. Among racial/ethnic groups, only White persons had a significant increase, 15% for males and 20% for females. Overall, the greatest increases in mortality were seen in poisoning and falls, an 86% and 36% increase, respectively (Hu & Baker, 2009).

Mortality from unintentional injuries in the United States based on age:

- Motor vehicle accidents are the leading cause of death among persons 34 years of age and younger.
- Homicide is the second leading cause of death, and suicide is the third leading cause among persons 15 to 24 years of age.
- Suicide is the second leading cause of death, and homicide is the third leading cause among persons 25 to 34 years of age.
- Falls are the leading cause of death from unintentional injury among persons 65 years of age and older.

In 2009, there were 30,797 motor vehicle related fatalities (U.S. Department of Transportation, National Highway Traffic Safety Administration [NHTSA], n.d.). The average cost per fatal incident was $1,290,000. The costs related to these deaths take into account wages and productivity losses, medical expenses, administrative expenses, motor vehicle damage, and employer's uninsured costs (National Safety Council, n.d.).

A *disabling injury* is one that results in restriction of normal activities of daily living (ADLs) beyond the day on which the injury occurred. Disabling injuries occur disproportionately among the young and the elderly. Seat belts, helmets, smoke detectors, and poison control centers save billions of dollars in direct and indirect medical costs. These primary and secondary prevention strategies save lives and money.

An *unsafe condition* is any environmental factor, either social or physical, that increases the likelihood of an unintentional injury. An icy walkway is an example of an unsafe condition; although it poses a hazard, it does not cause an injury but makes it more likely that an injury will occur. *Injury prevention* and *injury control* refer to any effort to prevent injuries or lessen their severity. These efforts often focus on assessment of the environment for unsafe conditions, such as loaded guns in the home or asbestos in school buildings and workplaces.

Diabetes Mellitus

Diabetes mellitus is the seventh leading cause of death in the United States. According to the CDC, nearly 25 million Americans have diabetes, and it is estimated that 79 million have prediabetes. Prediabetes is a condition in which blood sugar levels are higher than normal but not enough to be diagnosed as diabetes (CDC, 2011g). Diabetes affects 11.3% of Americans 20 years of age and older and 26.9% of Americans 65 years of age and older. Among individuals 20 years of age and older with diabetes (diagnosed and undiagnosed), 12.6 million (10.8%) are women and 13.0 million (11.8%) are men (see Table 23-4). After adjusting for population age differences, minorities continue to have higher rates of diabetes. Among individuals 20 years of age or older, 7.1% of Whites, 8.4% of Asian Americans, and 12.6% of Blacks had been diagnosed with diabetes. Compared to non-Hispanic White adults, the risk of diagnosed diabetes was 18% higher among Asian Americans, 66% higher among Hispanics/Latinos, and 77% higher among non-Hispanic Blacks. In 2010, there were 1.9 million new cases of diabetes diagnosed in people 20 years of age and older (CDC, 2011g) (see Fig. 23-3).

Diabetes is a major chronic health condition that puts individuals at risk for other serious health conditions including heart disease, stroke, hypertension, blindness, kidney disease, and nervous system disease

Table 23.4 Diagnosed and Undiagnosed Diabetes Among People Ages 20 Years or Older, United States, 2010

Group	Number or Percentage Who Have Diabetes
Ages 20 y or older	25.6 million, or 11.3%, of all people in this age group
Ages 65 y or older	10.9 million, or 26.9%, of all people in this age group
Men	13.0 million, or 11.8%, of all men ages 20 y or older
Women	12.6 million, or 10.8%, of all women ages 20 y or older
Non-Hispanic Whites	15.7 million, or 10.2%, of all non-Hispanic Whites ages 20 y or older
Non-Hispanic Blacks	4.9 million, or 18.7%, of all non-Hispanic Blacks ages 20 y or older

From National Diabetes Information Clearinghouse. (2011). *Diagnosed and undiagnosed diabetes among people ages 20 years or older, United States, 2010*. Retrieved from http://diabetes.niddk.nih.gov/dm/pubs/statistics/#Diagnosed20

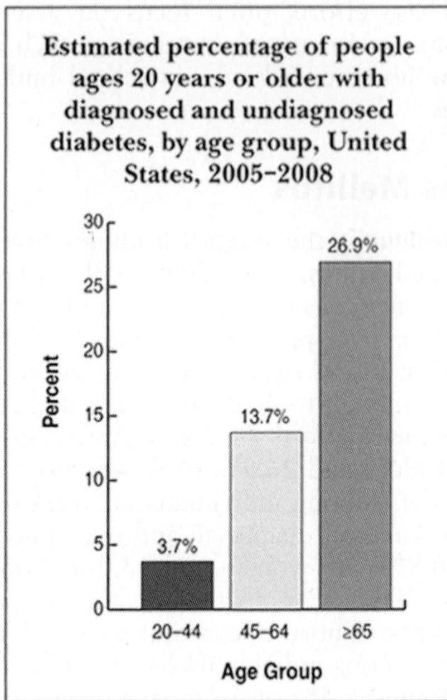

FIGURE 23-3. Diagnosed and undiagnosed diabetes. (From National Health and Nutrition Examination Survey. (2011). *Diagnosed and undiagnosed diabetes*. Retrieved from http://diabetes.niddk.nih.gov/dm/pubs/statistics/#Diagnosed20)

(i.e., neuropathy, which is a loss of sensation or pain in the feet or hands). Because diabetes can affect any part of the body, damage to other body systems can be minimized by good blood glucose control (assessed by hemoglobin A1C). In 2007, the estimated direct and indirect costs for individuals diagnosed with diabetes were $174 billion. Direct costs represented medical care, and indirect costs were for disability, work loss, and premature mortality. After adjusting for population age and gender differences, people diagnosed with diabetes had expenditures that were 2.3 times greater than individuals who did not have diabetes (CDC, 2011g).

Substance Use

According to the Substance Abuse and Mental Health Services Administration (SAMHSA), **substance use** refers to the selected use of potentially dangerous substances including alcohol, tobacco products, drugs, inhalants, and other substances that can be consumed, inhaled, injected, or otherwise absorbed into the body with possible damaging effects. It is a serious and continuing problem among adult women and men living in the United States. In 2009, an estimated 22.5 million persons (ages 12 and older) were classified with substance dependency or abuse in the past 12 months (SAMHSA, 2010a, 2010b).

In the United States, a third of lifestyle-related deaths annually are attributed to excessive alcohol use, heavy drinking (more than two drinks per day on average for men or more than one drink per day on average for women) or binge drinking (five or more drinks during a single occasion for men or four or more drinks during a single occasion for women). In addition, approximately 79,000 deaths are attributed to alcohol use each year (CDC, 2011a). In 2009, 52% of adults, 18 years of age and older, reported being a current regular drinker (at least 12 drinks in the past year). Among males, 61% reported being a current regular drinker as compared to females at 43%. Whites (58%) are also more likely to be current drinkers than other ethnic groups, Hispanics/Latinos 42% and Blacks 39%, respectively. More than 32% of automobile fatalities were alcohol related in 2009. The social and economic costs of alcohol abuse exceeds $184 billion annually in the United States (NHTSA, 2010; Pleis, Ward, & Lucas 2010; World Health Organization, 2004).

Tobacco use is a significant public health and financial cost to persons living in the United States. It increases the number of deaths due to CVD and cancer annually. In 2009, approximately 20.6% of adults in the United States were current cigarette smokers, 5.4% cigar smokers, and 3.5% used smokeless tobacco (primarily chewing tobacco and snuff). Among cigarette smokers, more men smoke (23%) than women, (18%). American Indians and Alaska Natives (23.2%) smoke more cigarettes than Whites (22.1%), Blacks (21%), and Hispanics/Latinos (14.5%). Eighteen of the *Healthy People 2020* objectives are related to tobacco use; unfortunately, the tobacco objectives for *Healthy People 2010* were not met. Annually, smoking across the United States costs $193 billion in health care costs and lost productivity, and smoking-related diseases claim an estimated 443,000 lives—1 in every 5 deaths. Currently, at least 8.6 million people in the United States have 1 serious illness caused by smoking, and 88 million are exposed to secondhand smoke (CDC, 2010f, 2010g, 2011i; NCHS, 2010; Pleis, et al., 2010; USDHHS, 2010a, 2010b).

Illicit drug use refers to use and misuse of illegal and controlled drugs. The primary illicit drugs used in the United States are cocaine, ecstasy, heroin, marijuana, and methamphetamine. In 2009, 8.7% of persons 12 years and older reported use of illicit drugs, with the highest percentage among individuals aged 18 to 20 years (22.2%). The second highest percentage was 18.4% among young adults between the ages of 21 and 25. In general, drug use declined with age. American Indians and Alaska Natives (18.3%) used more illicit drugs than other racial/ethnic groups, Blacks (9.6%), Whites (8.8%), and Hispanics/Latinos (7.9%) (SAMHSA, 2010a).

Abuse of prescription drugs is the misuse of these drugs for nonmedical reasons. The illegal use of prescription drugs is one of the fastest-growing forms of drug abuse and is becoming a major public health concern. A recent study showed that the estimated number of emergency department visits for nonmedical use of opioid analgesics increased 111%, 144,600 to 305,900 visits between 2004 and 2008. Oxycodone, hydrocodone, and methadone represented the most frequently misused medications. In 2009, about 7 million persons aged 12 or older (2.7%) had misused prescription drugs (pain relievers, tranquilizers, stimulants, and sedatives).

Young adults aged 18 to 25 had a higher prevalence of dependence on or abuse of prescription drugs (6.3%) compared to persons in other age groups. Men generally have higher rates than women for misuse (CDC, 2010a; SAMHSA, 2010a). This issue is covered in greater detail in Chapter 27.

Obesity

Obesity is defined as having a body mass index (BMI) of 30 or greater and is recognized as a national health threat and a major public health challenge. Individuals who have a BMI of 40 or greater or are more than 100 pounds overweight are considered to have *morbid obesity* (NIH, 2010). Obesity is a major risk factor for CVD, certain types of cancer, type 2 diabetes, obstructive sleep apnea, and premature death (Finkelstein, Brown, Wrage, Allaire, & Hoerger, 2010). One of the *Healthy People 2020* objectives is to decrease the proportion of adults who are obese by 10% (USDHHS, 2010a). In 2007 to 2008, the age-adjusted prevalence of obesity in the United States was 33.8%, 32.2% among men and 35.5% among women. Obesity was greatest among Blacks (44.1%) and Hispanics/Latinos (38.7%) (Flegal, Carroll, Ogden, & Curtin, 2010).

Over the past 20 years, there has been a dramatic increase in obesity in the United States. In 2009, only Colorado and the District of Columbia had a prevalence of obesity <20%, and 33 states had a prevalence ≥25%. Nine of these 33 states had a prevalence of obesity ≥30% (CDC, 2011j). In 2008, medical care costs related to obesity in the United States were estimated to be $147 billion (Finkelstein, Trogdon, Cohen, & Dietz, 2009). This high prevalence and cost of disease underscore the need for additional measures to educate persons regarding healthier lifestyle choices, increasing physical activity, and decreasing caloric intake.

Bariatric surgery is a clinically and cost-effective intervention for moderately to severely obese individuals (Picot et al., 2009). However, socioeconomic factors have been found to play a major role in determining who undergoes surgery. In the United States, the bariatric patient is most likely to be White, female, privately insured, and have a high median income (DeMaria, Pate, Warthen, & Winegar, 2010; Martin, Beekley, Kjorstad, & Sebesta, 2010). The average cost of a bariatric procedure is $20,000 to $25,000, and about $1.5 billion are spent annually. Since 2003, the number of bariatric surgeries has plateaued at approximately 113,000 surgeries per year (Livingston, 2010; NIH, 2009).

WOMEN'S HEALTH

Women have not been the focus of medical attention throughout the centuries. Health benefits achieved by women were incidental compared to men. Advances in women's health are very recent and primarily an advantage for women living in Western countries, where the women's or feminist movement has made major inroads.

Overview of Factors Influencing Women's Health

Women's rights in the United States started in the second half of the 19th century and over time addressed issues directly or indirectly impacting the health of women: voting rights, labor laws, reproductive rights, and violence against women (Imbornoni, 2007; Stone, 2011). This section of the chapter examines women's health concerns over the adult lifespan and the major causes of acute and chronic illness and death and the issues, trends, and policies that have and currently affect women.

Women's health is still overlooked in much of the world. Only in the past few decades has the health of women been a formidable issue in the United States, coming not so coincidently with the modern women's feminist movement that began in the 1960s. The landmark publication *The Feminine Mystic* (Friedan, 1997) helped launch the modern women's movement by critically examining the role of women in American society (Fox, 2006). The Boston Women's Health Book Collective (2011), *Our Bodies, Ourselves* (initial release 1973), represented the first book to explore women's health issues, exclusively written by and for women. This publication "created new possibilities and expectations for the relationship between women and their bodies" (Kline, 2010, p. 3) and resulted in more female researchers and women as participants in research.

Feminists paved the way for women to have their voices heard on many health, social, and political issues. Women sought out higher education opportunities in greater numbers and entered workplaces once solely occupied by men, especially during and after World War II. These positive changes escalated women toward greater equality and, with equality, came the freedom—and pressure—for women to compete with men in their social and work settings. Issues in women's health were discovered as a result of research that now more regularly includes women. The importance of women's research was reaffirmed in the NIH Revitalization Act of 1993, Subtitle B—Clinical research equity regarding women and minorities to "identify projects for research on women's health that should be conducted or supported by the national research institutes; identify multidisciplinary research relating to research on women that should be so conducted or supported ..." (Section 486).

Women's Health Research

In response to changing priorities, researchers have designed and implemented major studies that focus exclusively on women. Five significant studies have and continue to provide important health information about women: *The Women's Health Initiative* (WHI; a major 15-year research program addressing the most common causes of death, disability, and poor quality of life in postmenopausal women—CVD, cancer, and osteoporosis), *The Women's Health Study (WHS)* (evaluating

What do *you* think?

A woman's dressing style that included a tightly laced corset was popular from the late 1700s throughout the late 1800s in Germany, England, and the United States. It was brought into question by an anatomist, S. T. von Soemmerring in 1793. He identified compression of rib cages and internal organs as contributing to digestive problems, fainting, and shortness of breath. For the next century, dress reformers advocated looser lacing and clothes that allowed for a more natural movement. However, these reformers belonged to the "radical fringe" of the feminist movement, and the tiniest waists, regardless of their impact on health, continued to be in vogue as the "hourglass" figure was sought by middle class and upper class women. More recently, hiatal hernias caused by overly tight girdles and corsets have been termed "Soemmerring's syndrome" in tribute to the first physician to warn of the dangers, more than 200 years ago.

Adapted from Fee, E., Brown, T. M., Lazarus, J., & Theerman, P. (2002). The effects of the corset. *American Journal of Public Health, 92,* 1085.

the effects of vitamin E and low-dose aspirin therapy in primary prevention of CVD and cancer in apparently healthy women), *The Nurses' Health Study I* (investigating the potential long-term consequences of the use of oral contraceptives), *The Nurses' Health Study II* (studying oral contraceptives, diet, and lifestyle risk factors in a population younger than the original Nurses' Health Study cohort), and *The Nurses' Health Study III* (learning more about how women's lifestyles during their 20s, 30s, and 40s can influence disease risk later in life).

The WHI addressed CVD, cancer, and osteoporosis and was one of the largest prevention studies of its kind in the United States, starting in 1991 and spanning 15 years. The three major components of the WHI were a randomized controlled clinical trial of promising but unproven approaches to prevention, an observational study to identify predictors of disease, and a study of community approaches to developing healthful behaviors. This study was sponsored by the NIH and the NHLBI involving 161,808 women ages 50 to 79 and was considered to be one of the most far-reaching clinical trials for women's health ever undertaken. Enrolled women participated in a follow-up phase of this study until 2010. To date, more than 616 publications have been associated with findings from this study, which address coronary artery calcium, breast cancer risk, colorectal cancer, venous thrombosis, peripheral arterial disease risk, risk of CHD, dementia and cognitive function, and the effects of estrogen alone in reducing the risk of CHD (NHLBI, 2010).

The *WHS* was a randomized, double-blind, placebo-controlled clinical trial sponsored by the NHBLI and the NCI. It was the first large clinical trial to study the use of low-dose aspirin to prevent heart attack and stroke in women 45 years of age and older. This study began in 1991 and continued through March 2009 for additional observation and follow-up of the original 28,345 participants. Current findings indicate that low-dose aspirin does not prevent first heart attacks or death from cardiovascular causes in women; however, stroke was found to be 17% lower in the aspirin group. More than 104 professional articles are associated with this investigation. Recent publications have addressed the relationship of dietary omega-3 fatty acids and fish consumption with the risk of type 2 diabetes and caffeine consumption with the incidence of atrial fibrillation (WHS, 2011).

The *Nurses' Health Studies* (three separate phases) represent the longest running study related to women's health in the world, investigating factors that influence the health of women. *The Nurses' Health Study I*, a prospective study that began in 1976, enrolled 122,000 registered nurses ages 30 to 55 from 11 states, who responded to 170,000 mailed questionnaires. Every 2 years, participants received a follow-up questionnaire with questions about diseases and health-related topics including smoking, hormone use, and menopausal status. Later in the study, questions regarding diet and nutrition and quality of life were added. *The Nurses' Health Study II* represented women who started using oral contraceptives in adolescence, a population with long-term exposure during early reproductive years. Participants were between 25 and 42 years of age, and 116,686 women were enrolled and followed forward in time. Every 2 years, participants received a follow-up questionnaire and were surveyed about diseases and health-related topics including smoking, hormone use, pregnancy history, and menopausal status. These women also received nutrition and quality-of-life assessments later in the study. *The Nurses' Health Study III* began recruitment in 2010 and will continue until 100,000 nurses (registered and licensed practical, 22 to 45 years of age) are enrolled. This investigation is supported by major nursing organizations. Overall, as of 2010, outcomes from phases I and II have spawned 1,245 professional publications (Harvard Medical School, 2010a; Nurses' Health Study, n.d; Nurses' Health Study: Phase 3, n.d.).

Women's Health Promotion Across the Lifespan

What health care needs do women have that are different from those of men? Is there a need to look at health promotion throughout the life cycle of adult women? How is the health of an 18-year-old different from that of a 50-year-old woman? Most of us would have no trouble agreeing that women have different health care needs that must be considered and that these needs vary with age. Knowing what the needs are is essential to knowing how to help women promote their health.

Healthy People 2020 Goals for Women

As a nation, we have been focusing on improving the health of all citizens through the Healthy People initiatives, commencing with the 1979 Surgeon General's report, *Healthy People: The Surgeon General's Report on Health Promotion and Disease Prevention*, providing measurable population objectives. *Healthy People 2000* set a standard for change and improvement in objectives that were met or exceeded in some areas and were far from being reached in others. In that initiative, objectives in 14 areas focused specifically on women's health. *Healthy People 2010* focused on two overarching goals: increasing the quality of life and eliminating health disparities, containing 25 objectives relating to women. *Healthy People 2020* reaffirmed the goals of *2010* and added two additional goals: quality of life, healthy development, and healthy behaviors across the life span and creating social and physical environments that promote good health (Koh, 2010; USDHHS, 2010a). In the nation's fourth generation of health planning, 27 objectives pertain to the health of women (Display 23.3). As the community health nurse works with women at various stages in the life cycle, the objectives in *Healthy People 2020* can give structure to program planning and services offered to women in the community at the primary, secondary, and tertiary levels of prevention.

Young Adult Women (18 to 35 Years)

Women in the earlier years of adulthood have different tasks to accomplish and issues to address than do women in later adulthood, and the transition from adolescence to adulthood can be stressful. According to Erik H. Erikson (Stevens, 1983), the major developmental tasks that young women need to accomplish are forming an identity and the development of intimacy. Behaviors associated with young adulthood include attracting and choosing a significant other for the long-term and establishing a home. This task is phrased as such to include lesbians—women who have sex with other women. However, not all lesbians in this age group have "come out" or revealed to others that they are lesbian or **bisexual**—having sex with people of both genders. Young women during this stage also prepare and choose a life's work that is personally satisfying, plan for children by using a variety of parenting models (childbirth, adoption, foster parenting), and develop a personal philosophy that encompasses meaningful and comforting spiritual beliefs that are consistent with day-to-day living.

Women in this age group tend to be healthy. Unfortunately, during this period, many women engage in health-risk behaviors such as physical inactivity, eating poorly, participating in unprotected sexual intercourse, and smoking. Some, if not all, of these behaviors may have been established in adolescence and represent modifiable behaviors. If not addressed, these behaviors can contribute significantly to the leading causes of morbidity and mortality: diseases of the heart and vascular systems, cancers, chronic respiratory diseases, and diabetes (Health Resources and Services Administration, 2010; O'Dougherty, Arikawa, Kaufman, & Kurzer, 2009). The majority of health concerns for many of these women are related to eating disorders, reproductive health and sexually transmitted infections (STIs), physical activity, mental health and mood disorders, and substance use.

Eating Disorders

Eating disorders are complex, chronic illnesses primarily affecting young women. The cause of these disorders is not clear; however, the incidence is on the rise in the United States and other parts of the world. The three most common are anorexia nervosa, bulimia nervosa, and binge eating. **Anorexia nervosa** is an eating disorder that is marked by weight loss, emaciation, a disturbance in body image, and a fear of weight gain. Persons affected lose weight either by excessive dieting or by purging themselves of ingested calories. This illness is typically found in industrialized nations and usually begins in the teen years. Young women are 10 to 20 times more likely than young men to suffer from the disorder. The young woman claims to feel fat even when she is emaciated. Refusal to maintain body weight can be life-threatening due to electrolyte disturbances, anemia, and secondary cardiac arrhythmias. Affected women need to understand that low body weight can cause the body to stop producing estrogen, which leads to amenorrhea (absent menstrual periods). Low estrogen levels contribute to losses in bone density. If anorexia nervosa is suspected, the client must be referred to a health care provider for follow-up as soon as possible (Office on Women's Health, 2009a; NIH, 2011).

A related disorder, **bulimia nervosa**, is marked by recurrent episodes of binge eating, self-induced vomiting and diarrhea, excessive exercise, strict dieting or fasting, and an exaggerated concern about body shape and weight. In many ways, anorexia and bulimia are similar; except, women with anorexia nervosa rarely binge eat. Females in careers in which low weight is required (e.g., modeling, entertainment), individuals who have been sexually abused or come from families with a history of eating disorders, and individuals with low self-esteem and a history of not being "in control" or with communication and emotional difficulties are at greater risk for either disorder. The community health nurse should refer a woman suspected of practicing bulimic behaviors to an appropriate health care provider (Office on Women's Health, 2009b).

Binge eating is an eating disorder characterized by repeated episodes of uncontrolled eating. It is the newest clinically recognized eating disorder. The onset is usually in late adolescence and the early 20s, and starts following significant weight loss from dieting. However, many binge eaters are obese because they usually do not induce vomiting and diarrhea or engage in excessive exercise. Typically, individuals with this disorder eat quickly, eat until they are uncomfortably full, eat when they are not hungry, eat large amounts of food alone, have difficulty expressing their feelings, have difficulty controlling impulses and stress, and feel depressed

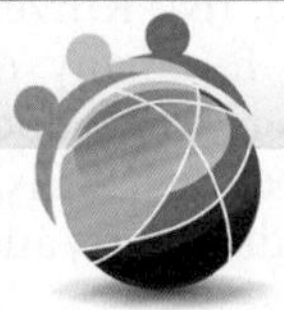

DISPLAY 23.3 *HEALTHY PEOPLE 2020* OBJECTIVES FOR WOMEN

1. Reduce the breast cancer death rate, from 22.9 deaths per 100,000 women to 20.6 deaths per 100,000
2. Reduce the death rate from cancer of the uterine cervix, from 2.4 deaths per 100,000 to 2.2 deaths per 100,000 women
3. Reduce invasive uterine cervical cancer from 7.9 new cases per 100,000 females to 7.1 new cases per 100,000 females
4. Reduce late-stage female breast cancer from 43.2 new cases per 100, 000 females to 41.0 new cases per 100,000 females
5. Increase the proportion of women who receive a cervical cancer screening based on the most recent guidelines from 84.5% of women aged 21 to 65 years to 93% of women aged 21 to 65 years
6. Increase the proportion of women who receive a breast cancer screening based on the most recent guidelines from 73.7% of females aged 50 to 74 years to 81.1% of females aged 50 to 74 years
7. Increase the proportion of pregnancies that are intended, from 51% to 56%
8. Reduce the proportion of females experiencing pregnancy despite use of a reversible contraceptive method from 12.4% to 9.9%
9. Reduce the proportion of pregnancies conceived within 18 months of a previous birth from 35.3% to 31.7%
10. Increase the proportion of females or their partners at risk of unintended pregnancy who used contraception at most recent sexual intercourse from 83% to 91.3%
11. Reduce pregnancy rates among adolescent females aged 15 to 17 years from 40.2 pregnancies per 1,000 to 36.2 pregnancies per 1,000
12. Increase the proportion of females in need of publically supported contraceptives services and supplies who receive those services and supplies from 53.8% to 64.5%
13. Increase the proportion of women with a family history of breast and/or ovarian cancer who receive genetic counseling from 23.3% to 25.6%
14. Reduce the rate of maternal mortality from 12.7% to 11.4%
15. Reduce maternal illness and complications due to pregnancy (complications during hospitalized labor and delivery) from 31.1% to 28%
16. Reduce cesarean births among low-risk (full-term, singleton, vertex presentation) women from 26.5% to 23.9%
17. Increase the proportion of pregnant women who receive early and adequate prenatal care form 70.8% to 77.9%
18. Increase abstinence from alcohol, cigarettes, and illicit drugs among pregnant women from 89.4% to 98.3%
19. (Developmental) Increase the proportion of pregnant women who attend a series of prepared childbirth classes
20. (Developmental) Increase the proportion of mothers who achieve a recommended weight gain during their pregnancies
21. Increase the proportion of women of childbearing potential with intake of at least 400 μg of folic acid from fortified foods or dietary supplements from 23.8% to 26.2%
22. Reduce the proportion of women of childbearing potential who have low red blood cell folate concentrations from 24.5% to 22.1%
23. Increase the proportion of women delivering a live birth who received preconception care services and practiced key recommended preconception health behaviors (took multivitamins/folic acid every day in the month prior to pregnancy) from 30.1% to 33.1%
24. (Developmental) Reduce postpartum relapse of smoking among women who quit smoking during pregnancy
25. (Developmental) Increase the proportion of women giving birth who attended a postpartum care visit with a health worker
26. Reduce iron deficiency among young children and females of childbearing age (12 to 49 years) from 10.4% to 9.4%
27. Reduce iron deficiency among pregnant females form 16.1% to 14.5%

Adapted from U.S. Department of Health and Human Services. (2010a). *Healthy people 2020: Understanding and improving health*. Retrieved from http://www.healthypeople.gov/2020/default.aspx

about overeating. This disorder also puts these women at increased risk for type 2 diabetes, high cholesterol, gallbladder disease, depression, heart disease, and some cancers (Mond, Peterson, & Hay, 2010; Office on Women's Health, 2009c).

Overall, eating disorders are not gender specific, as some men are affected—more than a million males affected daily. Currently, the perception is that White females are affected more than other ethnic groups; however, trends indicate that individuals from other ethnic groups also suffer from eating disorders (National Eating Disorders Association, 2011; Office on Women's Health, 2009b). The community health nurse can play a vital role in identifying persons affected and refer them to appropriate health care providers or self-help groups. A screening tool that may be helpful in this effort is the Malnutrition Universal Screening Tool, a 5-step tool to identify adults who are malnourished, at risk of malnutrition (undernutrition), or obese (Malnutrition Advisory Group, 2008).

Reproductive Health

By age 25, at least 50% of childbearing women have given birth once. Women need to be as healthy as possible to have positive pregnancy outcomes. Based on published research and the input of experts, the CDC has put forth recommendations for preconception care. The main goal of preconception care is to "provide health promotion, screening, and interventions for women of reproductive age to reduce risk factors that might affect future pregnancies" (Johnson et al., 2006, p. 3). Recommendations for preconception care address consumer awareness, individual responsibility, minimizing health problems, access to care, disparities, and research. Although *Healthy People 2020* addresses preconception care, many of the preconception objectives are related to family planning and maternal health (see Display 23.3). Community health nurses have been at the forefront of maternal and child health care for decades, and they must continue to strive to incorporate components of preconception care into their practices. Nurses must advocate for clients to influence public policy, which has the potential to improve access to care for many women and improve pregnancy outcomes (Jack, Atrash, Bickmore, & Johnson, 2008).

Sexual health and STIs are important health concerns for young women. Sexual activity typically commences in adolescence and continues throughout the lifespan. STIs are epidemic in the United States, especially among young adults (see Chapter 8). Many of the common infections are asymptomatic, but not always. The two most common STIs affecting women are chlamydia and gonorrhea. It is estimated that approximately 2.8 million cases of chlamydia occur in the United States each year and is the most reported notifiable disease. Females 20 to 24 years of age have the second highest rate, preceded by 15- to 19-year-old adolescents. gonorrhea rates have reached a plateau in recent years, but the prevalence is still 111.6 cases per 100,000 persons. Historically, gonorrhea rates for men were higher than women, but they are now very similar. Both chlamydia and gonorrhea are underdiagnosed, which can have deleterious consequences for women. If treatment is delayed, women can develop pelvic inflammatory disease, chronic pelvic pain, ectopic pregnancy, and infertility (CDC, 2009b, 2011c).

Community health nurses working with females need to provide factual information to increase women's knowledge of STI risk. This information should be a part of frank discussions regarding condom use, sexual partners (male and female), type of sexual activity (oral, anal, vaginal), life-threatening consequences of an undiagnosed STI, and undesirable pregnancy outcomes. Outside of abstinence, condom use is the first line of prevention against STIs.

Adult Women (35 to 65 Years)

Women in the adult age group of 35 to 65 years have established themselves into patterns of living that have served them well or ill. During this period, the results of years of choices may present themselves in the form of chronic illnesses. Nevertheless, many women in this age group have time to change their health habits to possibly reverse encroaching chronic illnesses. For other women, lifestyle choices and undetected diseases have shortened their lifespans, and large numbers of women in this age group are dying prematurely.

EVIDENCE-BASED PRACTICE

Bridging Financial Gaps

A two-group pretest/posttest experiment was designed and implemented to examine the effect of an education program on knowledge and perceived risk of sexually transmitted infections (STIs). The sexually transmitted infection knowledge survey and the perceived risk of sexually transmitted infection survey were used to measure knowledge and perceived risk among 104 women of childbearing age at two universities. The education program included a presentation on condoms, dental dams, and instructions on proper use. In addition, an informational brochure was provided. No education intervention or brochure was provided for the comparison group. Outcomes indicated that participants in the intervention group improved their STI knowledge and perceived risk from participating in a 30-minute educational intervention ($p = 0.0001$).

STIs are a major burden on the already overtaxed public health system. More than 12 million new cases are diagnosed annually, and more than $8 billion is spent to diagnose and treat STIs and their complications in the United States. When interacting with clients who are sexually active, nurses need to consider incorporating brief educational interventions about STIs into client care; nurses cannot assume that persons are knowledgeable. The more informed individuals are about STI transmission and prevention, the more likely they are to protect themselves.

Johnson-Mallard, C. A., Kromrey, J. D., Kromrey, J. D., Campbell, D. W., Jevitt, C. M., et al. (2007). Increasing knowledge of sexually transmitted infection risk. *The Nurse Practitioner*, *32*(2), 26–32.

Menopause and Hormone Replacement Therapy

Women in this age group experience **menopause**, a time that marks the permanent cessation of menstrual activity, usually occurring between the ages of 45 and 55 years. However, it can occur as early as age 30. Natural menopause is defined as cessation of menstrual periods for 12 consecutive months, with no other apparent cause. Surgical removal of the ovaries produces menopause, and 600,000 total hysterectomies are performed each year in the United States. At least one in three women has had a hysterectomy by the age of 60 and is the second most common surgery among women preceded only by cesarean delivery. Symptoms of menopause differ among women and last from months to years. They range from hardly noticeable in some women to very severe in others. Symptoms include nervousness, hot flashes (flushes), chills, excitability, fatigue, mood disorders (apathy, mental depression, crying episodes), insomnia, palpitations, vertigo, headache, numbness, tingling, myalgia, urinary disturbances, and vaginal dryness (Office on Women's Health, 2009d).

In 2002, researchers found an increased rate of breast cancer, ovarian cancer, heart disease, and stroke among healthy women in the *WHI* study who were taking combined estrogen and progestin hormone replacement therapy (HRT). The initial reaction to this information was a dramatic decline in prescribing by physicians, which included both combined HRT and estrogen alone. The debate over the risk versus benefit of long-term HRT is ongoing, and there is strong agreement HRT should not be used for the primary or secondary prevention of CVD. However, it is clear that postmenopausal women should discuss the risks of HRT with their primary care provider (LaCroix et al., 2011; Mosca et al., 2011; National Institutes of Health News, 2010).

Osteoporosis

A gradual loss in bone density is **osteoporosis**. Typically, bone density peaks about age 25, and over time, bones become fragile and easily facture. It is estimated that 1 out 5 women in the United States has *osteoporosis*. Therefore, it is important for women to build strong bone early. Bone density is influenced by many factors such as heredity, race/ethnicity, physical activity, and nutrition. It is important for women of all ages to maintain a healthy diet and engage in physical activity. Medications such as bisphosphonates (Fosamax, Boniva, Reclast, and Actonel) can improve bone density. Every woman 65 years of age or older should be screened for osteoporosis (Office on Women's Health, 2009e).

Heart Disease

Diseases of the heart are the number one killer of women. Based on preliminary data for 2009, a total of 598,607 persons in the United States died of heart disease and 50% of these were women. A racial disparity exists, with death rates related to CVD for Black women at 204.5 per 100,000 compared to 150.5 per 100,000 for White women. The most common heart problem, CHD, is underdiagnosed, undertreated, and under-researched in women. In addition, women have higher mortality after heart attack and poorer outcomes than do men, which may be related to delayed diagnosis and treatment. Risk factors for heart disease in women are age, family history, race/ethnicity, physical inactivity, obesity, diabetes mellitus, high blood pressure, high cholesterol, and cigarette smoking (Kochanek et al., 2011; Mosca et al., 2011; NCHS, 2011).

Family history, race/ethnicity, and advancing age cannot be changed, but women can make lifestyle changes to alter other risk factors. The remaining risk factors are issues that the community health nurse can discuss with female clients in this age group. Community health nurses can help raise awareness regarding heart disease when working with women at the individual, family, or aggregate levels. Some important facts that can be shared are:

- According to a recent survey, 36% of women did not perceive themselves to be at risk for heart disease.
- Two thirds of women who die suddenly from CHD have had no previous symptoms.
- 9 out of 10 heart disease patients have at least 1 risk.
- Heart disease is sometimes thought of as a "man's disease," but about the same number of women and men die each year of heart disease.
- Women have atypical heart symptoms or less acute chest pain, which may delay them from seeking care.
- Women are less likely to complete secondary prevention programs,
- Hormone therapy does not reduce coronary events.
- 1 in 2.6 female deaths are from CVD, compared with 1 in 30 from breast cancer.

An excellent lay resource is "*Go Red for Women*," a public awareness program of the AHA to help improve knowledge (AHA, 2011b). Also, the *Well-Integrated Screening and Evaluation for Women across the Nation* (WISEWOMAN), a CDC program that helps women with little or no health insurance reduce their risk for heart disease, stroke, and other chronic diseases (located in 21 sites across 19 states), can be helpful. The program assists women ages 40 to 64 in improving their diet, physical activity, and other behaviors. This program also provides cholesterol tests and other screening (CDC, 2010h; Mosca et al., 2011).

Cancer

Cancer is the second leading cause of death for women, estimated to kill 271,520 females in the United States in 2011. Genetic abnormality plays a role in cancer (possibly linked to environmental exposures), but only 5% of cancers are hereditary. Thus, the vast majority of cancers are random, and the majority occurs in persons 55 years of age and older. The lifetime risk of a woman getting cancer is 1 in 3. To help address this disparity, community health nurses can provide more opportunities for education and screening for this population. Screening has reduced the deaths for cancers of the breast, colon, rectum, and cervix (ACS, 2010a, 2011a).

Breast cancer is the most common cancer among women; however, more women die of lung cancer. In 2010, it is estimated that 39,840 breast cancer–related deaths will occur (NCI, 2011b). Overall, the death rates from breast cancer have declined since 1990, and the biggest decline was among women under 50 years of age. This can be attributed to early detection and improvements in treatment. The sooner breast cancer is discovered, the more successfully it is treated. By engaging in routine breast self-examinations (BSE), having regular mammograms, eating a diet low in fat and high in fruits and vegetables, breast-feeding (if possible), and avoiding prolonged use of estrogen replacement therapy, a woman is doing what she can to promote breast health. The community health nurse has many resources available to provide information and to teach BSE individually to women in their homes, small groups in clinics, or in various other community settings (see Chapter 12) (ACS, 2011a). See Table 23-5.

Women should begin BSE at age 20 and continue monthly for the remainder of their lives. Clinical breast examination, conducted by a health care provider, should be done as a part of routine gynecologic or health examinations every 3 years for women 20 to 40 years of age and then annually. Mammography is not usually recommended for women younger than 40 years of age but is recommended annually thereafter. Women who have a first-degree relative with breast cancer (mother, sister), a breast cancer gene (BRCA 1 or BRCA 2), or have had previous breast cancer are at a higher risk for developing the disease than other women in the general population. Therefore, these individuals need to consult their physicians regarding timelines for screenings (ACS, 2011a).

Table 23.5 Breast Cancer Death Rates Among All Women: 2003–2007

(Age-Adjusted Rates per 100,000)

Women	Rate
All women	24.0
Black	32.4
White	23.4
American Indian/Alaska Native	17.6
Hispanic	15.3
Asian/Pacific Islander	12.2

Extracted from National Cancer Institute. (2011b). *SEER stat fact sheets: Breast.* Retrieved from http://seer.cancer.gov/statfacts/html/breast.html

Papanicolaou (Pap) smears have improved early detection and prevention of cervical cancer dramatically. Both the incidence and the death rates for cervical cancer have declined in recent decades due to treatment of preinvasive cervical lesions. The major risk factors for this disease are infection with certain types of the human papillomavirus (HPV), unprotected intercourse at an early age, and multiple sex partners. In 2011, it was estimated that 12,710 new cases of invasive cervical cancer will be diagnosed in the United States, contributing to 4,290 deaths among women from this disease. The 5-year survival rate for this cancer if prompt treatment is initiated is 70% for all stages and 91% for local infiltration, making it one of the most successfully treated cancers. Community health nurses can continue to improve screening and early diagnosis through education and advocating for low-cost screening, which will allow many at-risk elderly, low-income, and rural women access to regular Pap screenings. In addition, making women aware of the HPV vaccines Gardasil (given between the ages of 9 to 26 years) and Cervarix (given between the ages of 10 to 25 years) may reduce the incidence of cervical cancer in upcoming decades. Of note in 2010, Gardasil was approved for use in males 9 to 26 years of age to prevent anal cancer (ACS, 2011a).

Ovarian cancer contributes to more deaths than any other cancer of the female reproductive system. Death rates have steadily declined by 1.7% each year since 2002. In 2010, 13,850 deaths were anticipated and in 2011, 15,460 deaths are expected. The primary risk factor for this disease is heredity, a strong family history of breast or ovarian cancer. For this reason, it is imperative that women have annual pelvic exams. The 5-year survival rate is 46% compared to cervical (70%) and breast (89%). Women at high risk should receive a pelvic exam, transvaginal ultrasound, and a blood test for the tumor marker CA 125. An ongoing clinical trial in the United Kingdom is examining the efficacy of screening, using the serial values of CA 125 to estimate risk and referring women with high risk for ultrasound examination to improve survival. Therefore, community health nurses need to continue to stress the importance of early detection. (ACS, 2011a; Hartge, 2011; NCI, 2011c).

Chronic Fatigue and Immune Dysfunction Syndrome

Chronic fatigue and immune dysfunction syndrome (CFIDS) is characterized by persistent and debilitating fatigue and additional nonspecific symptoms such as sore throat, headache, painful muscles, joint pain, difficulty thinking, and loss of short-term memory. CFIDS affects as many as 500,000 persons in the United States, and 80% of those diagnosed with the syndrome are women between 25 and 45 years of age. Rest does not relieve the fatigue. Symptoms may wax and wane and are difficult to validate objectively, but they are subjectively debilitating. Symptoms can last for months or years. Because the cause is unknown, there is no specific treatment and no prevention suggestions. Treatment is focused on supportive care for the associated pain, depression, and insomnia. The CFIDS Association of America provides support and information for women and is one of seven organizations that contributed to the newly released paper *Chronic Pain in Women: Neglect, Dismissal and Discrimination* (Chronic Pain Research Alliance, 2011), a report that raises awareness of chronic pain conditions that disproportionately impact women. The community health nurse can assess activity level and degree of fatigue, emotional response to the illness, and coping ability. Emotionally supportive family members and health care providers are helpful. Referring women to mental health counseling or a local support group is useful for many women and within the role of the community health nurse (CDC, 2011d).

MEN'S HEALTH

Gender is among the numerous factors that influence health. More male neonates die at birth, and men are more likely to die earlier from a chronic illness than women. This is evidenced by the difference in life expectancy between men and women: in the United States, women survive an average of 5 years longer than men (Pinkhasov et al., 2010).

Overview of Factors Influencing Men's Health

The concept of masculinity is an influencing factor in men's health. Men are socialized to be independent and conceal their vulnerability. Therefore, even when they are aware of personal physical or mental health problems, they are less likely to access the health care system. How the male identity is maintained can include activities that are hazardous to their health, and the result is a high death rate from unintentional injuries among young men. Examples of these activities include working in dangerous jobs, engaging in behaviors that lead to increased risk of homicide or car crashes, excessive alcohol consumption, smoking, substance use, and unsafe sex practices (Courtenay, 2011; Creighton & Oliffe, 2010; Sloan, Gough, & Conner, 2010).

In 2009, legislation to create an Office on Men's Health in the USDHHS was introduced. The office was designed to mirror the work of the existing Office on Women's Health and be responsible for coordinating men's health awareness, prevention, and research efforts conducted by federal and state governments. However, the bill did not progress out of the congressional subcommittee on health and has not been reintroduced (Murphy, 2009). See chapter 13 regarding the role of the community health nurse in public health policy efforts.

Factors that contribute to the deteriorating state of men's health include a lack of quality health education programs for men, health care services that are only accessed half as much by men when compared to women, and a lack of male gender-specific research (Harvard Medical School, 2010b). Considering all of these factors, the community nurse must determine the health care needs of men at various stages and how nurses can best meet these needs throughout the adult lifespan.

Men's Health Promotion Across the Adult Lifespan

In the early years of young adulthood (between 18 and 35 years), men continue to grow and mature. Adult men aged 35 to 65 years have reached maturity, the peak of their physical and intellectual development, and their greatest earning power. What specific needs do men in these age groups have? Are their needs being met through services provided?

Healthy People 2020 Goals for Men

Although *Healthy People 2020* has 27 health objectives specifically for women and seven specifically for men, many apply to both women and men of all ages. The seven men's objectives focus on prostate health, reproductive health, and disease prevention among men, especially men who have sex with men (MSM) (see Display 23.4).

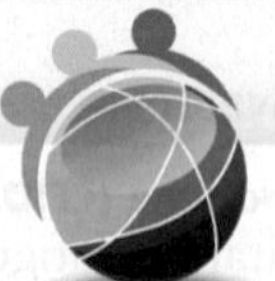

DISPLAY 23.4 *HEALTHY PEOPLE 2020* OBJECTIVES FOR MEN

1. Reduce the number of prostate cancer death rates from 23.5 deaths per 100,000 to 21.2 deaths per 100,000
2. (Developmental) Increase the proportion of men who have discussed with their health care provider whether or not to have a prostate-specific antigen (PSA) test to screen for prostate cancer
3. Increase the proportion of sexually active males aged 15 to 44 years who received reproductive health services by 10%, from 14.9% to 16.4%
4. Reduce the number of new AIDS cases among adolescents and adult men who have sex with men (MSM) by 10%, from 16,749 new cases to 15,074 new cases
5. Increase the proportion of adolescents and adults who have been tested for HIV in the last 12 months among (developmental) MSM
6. (Developmental) Decrease the proportion of MSM who reported unprotected anal sex in the past 12 months
7. Increase the proportion of sexually active unmarried males 15 to 44 years of age who used a condom at last intercourse by 10%, from 60.7% to 55.2%

Adapted from U.S. Department of Health and Human Services. (2010a). *Healthy people 2020*. Retrieved from http://www.healthypeople.gov/2020/default.aspx

Young Adult Men (18 to 35 Years)

The young adult male has many tasks to accomplish. These tasks include the acquisition of training or education that will lead to a personally and financially rewarding career, selecting a compatible lifetime companion and establishing a life together, finding comfort with and meaning to existence through practicing and internalizing a belief and value system that works for him, actively planning for having (or not having) children, and participating in the betterment of the greater community, both actively (volunteering, committee work, leadership positions) and passively (voting, being a good citizen, obeying laws).

Depending on his attitudes and practices before a man enters young adulthood, he may or may not be enticed to experiment or continue with the use of tobacco, alcohol, or illicit drugs. Experimentation or usage of these substances can occur in college, the military, or working at a full-time job. Young men also engage in behaviors or take risks without thinking about the consequences. They respond to challenges such as drag racing, exceeding speed limits, and binge drinking. This is an important age group for the community health nurse to reach with health information because the decisions made in these formative years affect how these young men live the rest of their lives. The nurse can meet with young adult men in work settings, college campuses, military bases, health clubs and bars, and at single-adult groups sponsored by religious communities and other organizations.

Another issue to address during the early years is the young man's attitudes and beliefs toward sex and sexual experimentation. Young men may question their sexuality as they mature, and during this stage, some men come to the realization that they are homosexual. **Gay** is the commonly accepted term for a homosexual—a person who has sexual interest in or has sexual intercourse exclusively with members of his or her own gender. Some men who have sex with men, women, or both often do not consider themselves to be gay or bisexual. They are categorized as MSM. When taking a sexual history, community health nurses must ask men if they have sex with women, men, or both.

Transgender, another term associated with sexuality, is used to describe individuals who experience and/or express their gender differently from what people might expect. These individuals express characteristics that do not correspond with the person's apparent or presumed gender. An example is when a presumed male chooses to put on makeup and clothes that a female would traditionally wear. Some transgender individuals define themselves as *female-to-male* or *male-to-female* and may take hormones and/or undergo medical procedures to enhance or make permanent their gender selection, including gender reassignment surgery. Others prefer to simply be called *male* or *female*—the gender they present to others, whether or not they have undergone medical or surgical reassignment.

Sexual experimentation, whether heterosexual or homosexual, can place young men at risk for diseases that affect long-term health or are life-threatening. Men who are sexually active can reduce the possibility of being infected with a STI by limiting the number of sexual partners and using condoms consistently and correctly. Condoms also serve as a form of birth control for men. *Monogamy*, having sex with only one partner, and abstinence can further reduce or eliminate the chance of contracting an STI. Community health nurses can serve as a resource for young men and can help them obtain free or low-cost condoms and treatment for STIs.

Human Immunodeficiency Virus and Men

Despite advances in the prevention and treatment of human immunodeficiency virus (HIV), the disease continues to disproportionately impact men in the United States. At the end of 2008, the CDC estimated 679,590 adults and adolescents were living with HIV in the 40 states and 5 United States–dependent areas with confidential name-based reporting. Men accounted for 76% of all diagnoses of HIV infection among adults and adolescents, and 65.7% of those males were men who had sex with men (MSM). In 2009, the rate of HIV infection among men was 32.9 per 100,000 persons compared to 9.8 in women. The rate of HIV infection was highest among persons 20 to 24 years of age, 36.9 cases per 100,000 persons. When examining trends in the disease based on race/ethnicity, the burden of the disease is highest among men of color. The rate of new HIV infections among Black men is 6 times higher than White men and nearly 3 times higher than Hispanic/Latino men (CDC, 2010d, 2011e).

Alcohol and illicit drug use are known to decrease social inhibitions and increase the risk for HIV transmission through risky sexual behaviors (i.e., lack of condom use) and the sharing of needles or other injection equipment. Community health nurses must be able to talk openly and nonjudgmentally with men about their use of substances and sexual relationships. These conversations can be challenging, but they have to occur if the number of HIV infections is to be reduced (CDC, 2009a, 2010e; Woolf & Maisto, 2009).

Testicular Cancer

The risk for testicular cancer is a health problem that young men should be aware of even before early adulthood. The disease occurs most often in men between 20 and 39 years of age. Men with a personal history of undescended testicles or a family history of testicular cancer have the highest risk of developing this cancer (ACS, 2011b; Townsend, Richardson, & German, 2010). It is a rare form of cancer and is not on the list of objectives for men in *Healthy People 2020*. However, if detected early, this cancer is highly curable. It is beneficial to the overall health of a young man to know how to perform a TSE, and teaching men how to do this exam appropriately is an important role for the community health nurse (see Display 23.5).

EVIDENCE-BASED PRACTICE

The Global Community

The human immunodeficiency virus (HIV)/AIDS epidemic in South Africa has resulted in the need for older adults, particularly women, to provide care for sick adult children and orphaned grandchildren. Based on a community needs assessment, a health education intervention program was designed to improve skills and knowledge that could be used by older people in their caregiving tasks. The intervention consisted of four workshops and was piloted using a longitudinal, one-group study design. Some of the topics included in the intervention were HIV/AIDS knowledge, effective intergenerational communication, providing home-based basic nursing care, accessing social services and grants, and relaxation techniques. A pretest was done prior to implementing the interventional program, a posttest was conducted immediately after the program, and a follow-up test was done 3 months after the program ended. One-on-one interviews were used for data collection at each of the three time intervals. The study included 202 adult caregivers who were 60 years of age or older, the majority (81.7%) being female. Of the 202 participants, 141 completed all four of the program's workshops.

Results from this study found that participants who completed all four workshops had a more positive attitude toward people living with HIV, perceived more control over nursing activities provided, and were more likely to improve their knowledge about HIV/AIDS. In addition, participants who completed all four workshops perceived themselves more capable of providing nursing care than those who did not attend all of the workshops. The results found no changes in the perceived ability to communicate with older children and grandchildren or attitudes toward communication. These results indicate that the interventions had a positive effect on assisting older adults in providing care to their sick children and orphaned grandchildren. However, additional research is needed to gain a better understanding of the social and cultural relationship between generations and how to assist older caregivers in addressing structural needs, such as financial assistance and generation of income that can be used in caring for themselves and their dependents.

Boon, H., Ruiter, R. A., James, S., Van Den, B., Willims, E., & Reddy, P. (2009). The impact of a community-based pilot health education intervention for older caregivers of orphaned and sick children as a result of HIV and AIDS in South Africa. *Journal of Cross-Cultural Gerontology, 24*, 373–389.

The choices a young adult man makes during these years establish healthy eating, work, rest, and exercise habits that will benefit him for a lifetime. A man should follow the dietary food guidelines that are recommended by U.S. Department of Agriculture (2010) when considering personal likes and dislikes. He and his family will benefit if he is able to balance work and home, doing his best in both settings. Establishing a pattern of rest that allows his body to recover and refresh from a day full of meaningful activities will help him look forward to each day. He should establish an exercise routine that meets his personal needs, fits his skills and talents, and includes some physical activities that involve his family. These choices provide him with the knowledge that he is doing everything he can to keep himself healthy and to prevent the two major killers of men—heart disease and cancer. However, there are additional considerations. Typically, young adult clients have few interactions with health care providers in any given year. It is often assumed that young adult males in this age range are not at risk for physical or psychological disease. This is a myth. It is important for people in this age group to have regular health checkups, be assessed for early signs of disease, and engage in health promotion activities.

Adult Men (35 to 65 Years)

Men in the developmental stage between 35 and 65 years of age are often faced with caring for both their own children and aging parents and in-laws. The physical, economic, and emotional demands can be great: Older adults may have extended care needs while, simultaneously, the family must bear the economic burdens of putting children through college. Meanwhile, men are adjusting to the reality that their career path is probably set and many of their life choices have been made.

The term "midlife" is applied to the first half of this age period, 35 to 49 years. It is a time when many men focus on a reappraisal of values, priorities, and personal relationships. As the term "midlife crisis" implies, this can be one of the more difficult stages of life. It can be an emotional time of doubt and anxiety when a man becomes uncomfortable with the idea that his life is half over. He may believe that he has not accomplished enough, or he may struggle to find new meaning or purpose in his life. Men may experience boredom with their personal life, job, or partners, and a desire to make changes in these areas may occur (Freund & Ritter, 2009).

The later years in this stage, ages 50 to 64, involve preparation for retirement. In anticipation of retirement, these years are marked by expanded social relationships and pursuit of new hobbies to fill increased leisure time, along with anticipating finishing a career and accumulation of the best retirement benefits. The decisions made during these years will play out over the rest of a man's life and could alter how a spouse or long-term partner lives out their years. Health problems that were left undiagnosed when the man was younger begin to emerge.

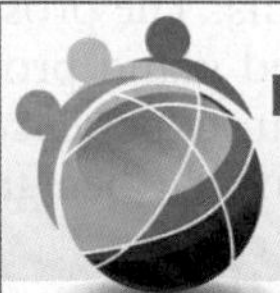

DISPLAY 23.5 PERFORMING TESTICULAR SELF-EXAMINATION (TSE)

- TSE should be performed monthly.
- TSE should be done right after a hot shower or bath. The scrotum is most relaxed then, which makes it easier to examine the testicles.
- Examine one testicle at a time. Use both hands to gently roll each testicle (with slight pressure) between your fingers. Place your thumbs over the top of your testicle, with the index and middle fingers of each hand behind the testicle, and then roll it between your fingers.
- The epididymis, which feels soft, rope-like, and slightly tender to pressure, is located at the top of the back part of each testicle. This is a normal lump.
- One testicle (usually the right one) is slightly larger than the other; this is normal.
- When examining each testicle, feel for any lumps or bumps along the front or sides. Lumps may be as small as a piece of rice or a pea.
- If there are any swellings, lumps, or changes in the size or color of a testicle, or if there is any pain or achy area in your groin, let your doctor know right away.
- Lumps or swelling may not be cancer, but a physician should be consulted.

Adapted from Testicular Cancer Resource Center. (2009). *How to do a testicular self-examination*. Retrieved from http://tcrc.acor.org/tcexam.html

Peers may be suffering and succumbing to diseases, and a man begins to adjust to the potential loss of loved ones, particularly a spouse or long-term companion (Beutel, Glaesmer, Wiltink, Marian, & Brahler, 2010).

Successful navigation of this stage can be fulfilling but may require a man to enhance his self-care skills. This includes having a positive attitude toward aging, one that examines the benefits of maturity, finds a balance between work and home, and maintains a healthy lifestyle by eating balanced meals and obtaining regular exercise. The community health nurse can provide anticipatory guidance to men approaching this stage and help them with ways to manage life more effectively.

Reproductive Health

During this stage, especially when a man has decided that his family is complete, he may choose a permanent form of birth control. For men, permanent birth control can be obtained through a surgical procedure called a *vasectomy*. A vasectomy includes removal of all or a segment of the vas deferens, so that sperm cannot be released. The procedure is routinely conducted on an outpatient basis, minimally invasive, and takes about 30 minutes. Vasectomies are considered permanent; however, with the advent of microsurgical techniques, vasectomy reversals are now possible.

In the United States, approximately 20% of couples that use some form of contraception rely on a vasectomy. The number of vasectomies performed grew steadily during the 1990s, but recent data suggest that the number of vasectomies has flattened or declined while the number of female sterilizations has increased (Pile & Barone, 2009). The National Survey of Family Growth data estimate that between 1998 and 2002, 175,000 to 354,000 vasectomies were performed annually in the United States (Eisenberg & Lipshultz, 2010; Grober, Jarvi, Lo, & Shin, 20011).

Erection problems are common among men of all ages but especially in men as they age. **Erectile dysfunction** (ED), sometimes called "impotence," is the repeated inability to get or keep an erection firm enough for sexual intercourse. The word "impotence" may also be used to describe other problems that interfere with sexual intercourse, such as lack of sexual desire and problems with ejaculation or orgasm. Using the term *erectile dysfunction* makes it clear that these other problems are not involved (American Urological Association [AUA], 2009b).

Since an erection requires a specific sequence of events, ED can occur when any of the associate events are disrupted. The sequence includes nerve impulses in the brain, spinal column, areas around the penis, and response in muscles, fibrous tissues, veins, and arteries in and near the corpora cavernosa. Damage to nerves, arteries, smooth muscles, and fibrous tissues, often as a result of disease, are the most common causes of ED. Comorbidities such as diabetes, kidney disease, chronic alcoholism, multiple sclerosis, atherosclerosis, vascular disease, and neurologic disorders are primary risk factors for ED (Albersen, Mwamukonda, Shindel, & Lue, 2011; Thorve et al., 2011).

Lifestyle choices that contribute to heart disease and vascular problems also increase the risk of ED. Smoking, being overweight, and lack of exercise are possible causes of ED. Surgery (especially radical prostate and bladder surgery for cancer) can injure nerves and arteries near the penis, causing ED. Injury to the penis, spinal cord, prostate, bladder, and pelvis can lead to ED by harming nerves, smooth muscles, arteries, and fibrous tissues of the corpora cavernosa. In addition, many common medicines—antihypertensives, antihistamines, antidepressants, tranquilizers, appetite suppressants, and cimetidine—can produce ED as a side effect (Albersen et al., 2011; AUA, 2009b; Kupelian, Araujo, Chiu, Rosen, & McKinlay, 2010).

In diagnosing ED, the medical history should include whether or not erections occur at other times. If an erection can be achieved with masturbation or upon awakening, the problem is probably not physical and is related to stress or an emotional problem. Treatment for ED usually proceeds from least to most invasive. For some men, making a few healthy lifestyle changes may solve the problem. Smoking cessation, weight loss, and increased physical activity may help some men regain sexual function. Cutting back on any drugs with harmful side effects is considered next. For example, drugs for high blood pressure work in different ways. If a particular drug is causing problems with erection, a different class of blood pressure medicine might work just as well. Psychotherapy and behavior modifications in some men should also be considered (AUA, 2009b; Kupelian et al., 2010).

Drugs for treating ED can be taken orally, injected directly into the penis, or inserted into the urethra at the tip of the penis. In March 1998, the US Food and Drug Administration (FDA) approved sildenafil citrate (Viagra), the first pill to treat ED. Since that time, vardenafil hydrochloride (Levitra [oral], Staxyn [sublingual]) and tadalafil (Cialis) have also been approved. Viagra, Levitra, Staxyn, and Cialis all belong to a class of drugs called phosphodiesterase (PDE) type 5 inhibitors. These drugs work by relaxing smooth muscles in the penis during sexual stimulation and allow increased blood flow. They can be taken as needed before sexual activity, up to once a day. Low-dose daily dosing rather than "on-demand" dosing has been found to be beneficial for some couples (Sadovsky, Brock, Gutkin, & Sorsaburu, 2009).

Heart Disease and Men

Cardiovascular disease is a term that refers to the broadest category of diseases that affect the heart and blood vessels. Despite a decline in the death rate from CVD, the burden of disease among men remains high. About one in three adult men has some form of CVD. In 2007, CVD caused 391,886 deaths in men, a death rate of 251.2 per 100,000 (AHA, 2011a). It was estimated in 2007 that 6.8 million inpatient cardiovascular operations and procedures were performed in the United States; 3.9 million of those were performed on men (Roger et al., 2011).

Approximately 70% to 89% of sudden cardiac events occur in men, and 50% of these men have no previous symptoms of disease. The average age of a first heart attack for men is 64.5 years. For men 55 to 64 years of age, the median survival time after a first heart attack is 17 years. If all forms of major CVD were eliminated, life expectancy would increase by almost 7 years (Roger et al., 2011).

Major risk factors for heart disease in men include hypertension, hyperlipidemia, tobacco use, diabetes, lack of physical activity, excessive alcohol consumption, and low daily fruit and vegetable consumption. When working with adult men, the community health nurse should educate men about the importance of modifying factors that increase their risk of developing CVD. Knowing the signs and symptoms of a heart attack and how to access emergency medical treatment are also important topics that the community health nurse should discuss with adult males.

Prostate Health

Prostate health is another concern that may occur later in this life stage. The **prostate** is a doughnut-shaped gland located at the bottom of the bladder, about halfway between the rectum and the base of the penis. The prostate encircles the urethra. The walnut-sized gland produces most of the fluid in semen. Men can experience infection (prostatitis), prostate enlargement (benign prostatic hyperplasia [BPH]), and prostate cancer.

BPH is very common among men. The primary risk factor for developing BPH is age. Nearly 50% of men >50 years of age report symptoms that are related to prostate gland enlargement. Symptoms of BPH are caused by an obstruction of the urethra and gradual loss of bladder function, which results in incomplete emptying of the bladder. The most commonly reported symptoms of BPH involve lower urinary tract symptoms (LUTS), such as hesitant, interrupted, or weak urinary stream; urgency or leaking of urine; and more frequent urination, especially at night. Men often report the symptoms of BPH before the physician diagnoses it through a digital rectal examination (DRE). Treatment for BPH can include medication or surgery to reduce the size of the prostate (AUA, 2010; Black, Grove, & Morrill, 2009).

Prostate cancer is the most frequently diagnosed cancer in men and the second leading cause of cancer death. According to the ACS (2010b), 1 man in 6 will get prostate cancer during his lifetime and 1 man in 36 will die from the disease. More than 2 million men in the United States who have had prostate cancer at some point are still alive today. Prostate cancer is very rare before the age of 40, but the chance of having prostate cancer rises rapidly after age 50. Almost 2 out of 3 prostate cancers are found in men over the age of 65. Age is the strongest risk factor for prostate cancer, but family history and ethnicity also need to be considered. Prostate cancer occurs more often in Black men than in men of other races and occurs less often in Asian and Hispanic/Latino men. The reasons for these racial and ethnic differences are not clear. The ACS recommends that screening of men who are at average risk should begin at age 50 and should include a blood test to assess levels of prostate-specific antigen (PSA) and a DRE. Individuals at higher risk for developing the disease (Black men or men with a first-degree relative diagnosed with prostate cancer before age 65) should begin screening at age 45. For men who have several first-degree relatives diagnosed with prostate cancer, a discussion about screening should occur at age 40 (ACS, 2010b; AUA, 2009a).

Treatment for prostate cancer depends on the man's age, overall health status, and stage of disease. Treatment options include surgery to remove all or part of the prostate (prostatectomy), radiation, and hormone therapy. Surgery, radiation, and hormone therapy all have the potential to disrupt sexual desire and performance, temporarily or permanently. Urinary dysfunction and urinary incontinence are common side effects that can occur after surgery or radiation. Rather than immediate treatment, watchful waiting or active surveillance is an option that may be appropriate for older men with limited life expectancy and/or less aggressive tumors (AUA, 2009a). A community health nurse can reinforce or clarify information shared with the man by his health care provider, discuss his treatment options with him and his family, and provide the support they may need if prostate cancer is diagnosed.

ROLE OF THE COMMUNITY HEALTH NURSE

The community health nurse works with adults in all age groups using the three levels of prevention—primary, secondary, and tertiary—as a guide. Interventions are conducted at the individual, family, group, and aggregate levels to make progress toward the *Healthy People 2020* objectives (see Levels of Prevention Pyramid).

Client teaching by the community health nurse is a major factor in preventing and managing chronic diseases. The challenge to the nurse is to be prepared to discuss issues, backed up with knowledge of and access to the appropriate community resources, to meet client needs. What the nurse can accomplish can be quite dramatic in terms of reducing days in the hospital because of chronic disease, improving quality of life for the chronically ill person, and preventing a combination of unhealthful habits from becoming causative factors in new cases of chronic disease. A nursing care plan matrix can guide the community health nurse in discussing

LEVELS OF PREVENTION PYRAMID

SITUATION: Breast cancer

GOAL: Using the three levels of prevention, negative health conditions are avoided or promptly diagnosed and treated, and the fullest potential is restored.

TERTIARY PREVENTION

Rehabilitation	Primary Prevention: *Health Promotion & Education*	Primary Prevention: *Health Protection*
• Recovery at home with return to activities of daily living within 2 weeks	• Maintains periodic follow-up with health care provider, follow-up mammogram at 6 and 12 months, and as recommended by health care provider • Education regarding risk for other cancers (cervical, ovarian, uterine, etc.)	• Continues to practice breast self-examination (BSE) and receive mammograms as required; receives screening for ovarian cancer—transvaginal ultrasonography and blood test for tumor marker CA 125

SECONDARY PREVENTION

Early Diagnosis	Prompt Treatment
• Identification of lump in left breast, appointment made with health care provider for evaluation • Receives mammogram and sonogram	• Needle aspiration of lump followed by cytologic studies • Lumpectomy with removal of two suspicious lymph nodes • Low-dose radiation

PRIMARY PREVENTION

Health Promotion and Education	Health Protection
• Education regarding how to perform the BSE • Education regarding timelines for BSE and mammograms • Education regarding environmental exposure and breast cancer (smoking, alcohol, chemicals) • Education regarding low-fat diet and maintaining a body mass index <29	• Avoidance of environmental exposures that may contribute to cancer • Performs monthly BSE and obtains mammogram as appropriate

DISPLAY 23.6 NURSING CARE PLAN MATRIX FOR HEALTH PROMOTION, YOUNG ADULTS: 18–35

Community health nurses can use this matrix to individualize teaching, services, and/or care to young adult clients. Use the questions to stimulate the development of an individualized approach that is client-focused and client-driven with the community health nurse acting as the catalyst. In any or all of these areas, the community health nurse may (1) discuss issues and commend the client for positive attitudes and behaviors (e.g., when the client is making healthful decisions, such as condom use for his/her health and the health of significant others), (2) discuss the issues and guide the client to resources that will enhance more positive behaviors and decisions (e.g., flu shot clinic or healthy lifestyle program for adults), or (3) discuss the issues and inform the client that immediate changes must be made to protect the health of self or others and inform/utilize the appropriate resources as soon as possible (e.g., follow-up for symptoms related to suspected STI).

1. *Life partner.* Ascertain whether the client is looking for a life partner or is choosing to live a single life. Discuss how the single life is satisfying for the client and ways to make it richer.
   Discuss settings in which client can meet others (male or female, based on sexual preference) with similar interests, philosophy, and outlook, such as work settings, school settings, faith communities, recreational communities, and the like.
   Discuss what the client is looking for in a potential life partner, expectations for the relationship, what the client contributes, how the client compromises and resolves conflict, and other issues. If in a relationship, what is good, what needs improving, and how to initiate change.
2. *Life's work.* How is the client preparing for his/her life's work (education, formal training, on the job training)? Will the life's work provide resources for client's life plans? Will the work choice provide long-term satisfaction? Is the work choice a "stepping stone" to another work role? How will/does he handle work and rearing children? What needs changing or can be improved in the work/children arrangement?
3. *Planning for children.* What knowledge does he/she have about family planning? What methods fit best with his/her philosophy, religious beliefs, and lifestyle? What are the long-term effects of the choices? How many children is the client planning to rear? Has he/she thought through the ramifications of this number? If choosing not to have (or unable to have) children, how will he/she deal with this? Does he/she want alternative suggestions for raising a child (adoption, foster parenting) or information about interacting with children (volunteering)?
4. *Maintaining physical and mental health.* In this area, the community health nurse needs to explore all areas of health promotion and protection. This will include discussions regarding primary and secondary prevention. Primary prevention discussions could include:
   - Diet and nutrition
   - Physical and leisure activities
   - Safe sex practices
   - Periodic health examinations
   - Personal safety—seat belts, protective helmets, dating violence, etc.
   - Immunizations
   - Regular use of sunscreen
   - Stress reduction activities

   Secondary prevention discussions could include:
   - Breast self-examination
   - Testicular self-examination
   - Smoking cessation
   - Pelvic exams and Pap smears
   - Counseling and support at times of stress
5. *Developing a life's philosophy.* Discuss client's personal life satisfaction, which may include religiosity and spirituality, living in congruence with cultural/ethnic/family beliefs and expectations, and coming to a comfortable level of satisfaction with life choices, having few regrets.

areas of health promotion and protection with the client. An example of a nursing care plan matrix for young adults can be found in Display 23.6.

Primary Prevention

Primary prevention activities focus on education to promote a healthy lifestyle. Much of the community health nurse's time is spent in the educator role. When working with individuals, the community health nurse should encourage routine health examinations, healthy eating habits, adequate sleep, moderate drinking, and no smoking. Among aggregates, the community health nurse focuses on community needs for services and programs that will keep that population healthy, such as providing flu clinics, teaching sexual responsibility, and preventing STIs.

The community health nurse may collaborate with community leaders and other stakeholders in designing programs, work with committees to secure funding, or approach the state legislature to lobby for needed changes to state laws and policies governing the health of adults. At other times, the nurse works with small groups of adults who could benefit from making healthy choices in diet, relaxation, and physical activity. Likewise, it is not unusual for the community health nurse to work with an individual to promote healthy living.

Secondary Prevention

Secondary prevention focuses on screening for early detection and prompt treatment of diseases. Throughout the lifespan, screening tests can help adults identify disease early (see Display 23.2). A significant amount of the community health nurse's time is spent in assessing the need for planning, implementing, or evaluating programs that focus on the early detection of diseases. This is followed with teaching to prevent further damage from the disease in progress or to prevent the spread of the disease, if it is communicable. Examples of secondary prevention programs include establishing mammography clinics, teaching breast and TSE, and screenings—blood pressure, blood glucose, BMI, and cholesterol. Wherever adults gather in groups, this is a good place to provide both primary and secondary health care and prevention services.

Tertiary Prevention

The tertiary level of prevention focuses on rehabilitation and preventing further damage to an already compromised system. Many adults that a community health nurse works with have chronic diseases, conditions resulting from another disease, or long-standing injuries with resulting disability. Ideally, negative health conditions can be prevented. If not, the next best thing is for them to be diagnosed early, without damage to an individual's health. But if negative health conditions have not been treated or brought under control, then the individual is at a tertiary level of prevention. At this level of prevention, the nurse focuses on maintaining quality of life.

Depending on the client's age, tertiary prevention can be simple or very complicated. A 19-year-old man who breaks his leg while skiing needs information about using crutches safely, a reminder to eat protein foods for bone healing, and an appointment to return to his health care provider to get the cast removed or if he experiences various symptoms. He needs no additional help from others. Tertiary prevention in this case is easy. On the other hand, a 62-year-old woman who is 70 pounds overweight with out-of-control blood glucose levels, symptoms of congestive heart failure, and difficulty walking more than 20 feet has much to accomplish in order to feel healthy. Can the nurse help the woman lose weight? Will weight loss bring her diabetes under control and alleviate congestive heart failure symptoms? With some weight reduction, will she be able to walk more easily? Or, will the woman feel better with physical therapy and a different medication regimen? Is there a quicker, safer, and better approach? On assessment, the nurse discovers that the woman has been as much as 80 pounds overweight for 40 years. Will this information alter the nurse's approach to helping this woman? What additional information does the nurse need?

Caring for people at the tertiary level of prevention can become quite complicated because many body systems may be involved. In addition, all people function within many social systems, which may include family expectations, roles people have within the family, expected behaviors, community system knowledge and involvement, personal expectations, motivation, and support. Working at the tertiary level involves all of the nurse's skills in addition to community resources and a client who can be or wants to be motivated.

SUMMARY

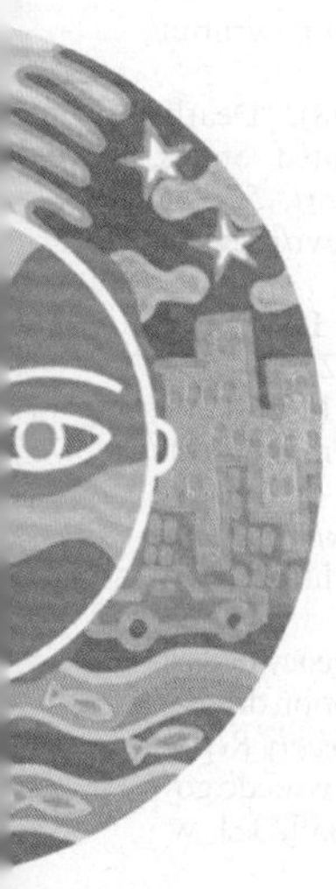

The 20th century saw a shift in the leading causes of death, from communicable to noncommunicable diseases. Currently, the five leading causes of death in adults are diseases of the heart, malignant neoplasms, cerebrovascular diseases, CLRDs, and unintentional injuries—none of which are communicable. The health care needs of adults are of great concern. Many needs are the same for both women and men, but the important differences were addressed in this chapter.

Adults have health care needs that change as they age. Diet and exercise, obesity, substance use, safety, and healthy lifestyle choices are issues that adults must consider throughout their lives. Heart disease and cancers remain important concerns for both men and women, and health decisions made as a young adult can have a major impact on persons as they age.

Chronic illness is an issue of increasing concern for both men and women as life expectancies increase. Community health nurses should use the three levels of prevention to promote health across the lifespan. Primary prevention activities focus on education to promote a healthy lifestyle. Secondary prevention focuses on screening for early detection and prompt treatment of diseases. The community health nurse's role at this stage is to assess needs, plan, implement, or evaluate programs that focus on the early detection of diseases and to educate clients to prevent further damage from or spread of disease. The tertiary level of prevention focuses on rehabilitation and prevention of further damage to an already compromised system. At this level of prevention, the nurse focuses on maintaining quality of life.

ACTIVITIES TO PROMOTE **CRITICAL THINKING**

1. Using the local newspaper, select three articles that relate to a preventable chronic disease. For each article, summarize the content, identify the likely cause, and describe how the disease may have been prevented.
2. You are asked to offer a weight control program for 12 young adults who are residents in an apartment complex that has monthly programs related to health and wellness. The ages of the intended participants range from 20 to 35. What steps would you take to develop a successful program?
3. Using the Internet and school library, research a chronic disease associated with men or women aged 35 to 65. Write a two-page paper in which you identify selected concerns and discuss both personal responsibility and societal responsibility regarding management of this health problem.
4. Access the website for the Nurses' Health Study 3 at: *http://www.nhs3.org/*. If you were to join the study what would be the benefits to you personally and to your nursing practice? How would you encourage other nurses to participate? What strategies might you use to encourage participation?

REFERENCES

Albersen, M., Mwamukonda, K. B., Shindel, A. W., & Lue, T. F. (2011). Evaluation and treatment of erectile dysfunction. *Medical Clinics of North America, 95*, 201–212. doi:10.1016/j.mcna.2010.08.016

American Cancer Society (2010a). *Lifetime risk of developing or dying from cancer*. Retrieved from http://www.cancer.org/Cancer/CancerBasics/lifetime-probability-of-developing-or-dying-from-cancer

American Cancer Society. (2010b). *Prostate cancer*. Retrieved from http://www.cancer.org/acs/groups/cid/documents/webcontent/003134-pdf.pdf

American Cancer Society. (2011a). *Cancer facts and figures: 2011*. Atlanta, GA: American Cancer Society. Retrieved from http://www.cancer.org/acs/groups/content/@epidemiologysurveilance/documents/document/acspc-029771.pdf

American Cancer Society. (2011b). *Testicular cancer*. Retrieved from http://www.cancer.org/acs/groups/cid/documents/webcontent/003142-pdf.pdf

American Heart Association. (2011a). *Men & cardiovascular diseases—2011 update*. Retrieved from http://www.heart.org/idc/groups/heart-public/@wcm/@sop/@smd/documents/downloadable/ucm_319573.pdf

American Heart Association. (2011b). *Go Red for Women*. Retrieved from http://www.goredforwomen.org/about_the_movement.aspx

American Heart Association. (2011c). *Warning signs of heart attack, stroke, and cardiac arrest*. Retrieved from http://www.heart.org/HEARTORG/Conditions/Conditions_UCM_305346_SubHomePage.jsp

American Lung Association. (2008). *Lung disease data: 2008*. Retrieved from http://www.lungusa.org/assets/documents/publications/lung-disease-data/LDD_2008.pdf

American Lung Association. (2011). *Chronic obstructive pulmonary disease (COPD) fact sheet*. Retrieved from http://www.lungusa.org/lung-disease/copd/resources/facts-figures/COPD-Fact-Sheet.html

American Urological Association. (2009a). *Management of clinically localized prostate cancer*. Retrieved from http://www.auanet.org/content/guidelines-and-quality-care/clinical-guidelines/main-reports/proscan07/content.pdf

American Urological Association. (2009b). *Management of erectile dysfunction, an update*. Retrieved from http://www.auanet.org/content/guidelines-and-quality-care/clinical-guidelines.cfm?sub=ed

American Urological Association. (2010). *Management of benign prostatic hypertrophy (BPH), update 2010*. Retrieved from http://www.auanet.org/content/guidelines-and-quality-care/clinical-guidelines.cfm?sub=bph

Bennett, I. M., Chen, J., Soroui, J. S., & White, S. (2009). The contribution of health literacy disparities in self-rated health status and preventive health behaviors in older adults. *Annals of Family Medicine, 7*(3), 204–211. doi:10.1370/afm.940

Beutel, M. E., Glaesmer, H., Wiltink, J., Marian, H., & Brahler, E. (2010). Life satisfaction, anxiety, depression, and resilience across the life span of men. *The Aging Male, 13*(1), 32–39. doi:10.3109/13685530903296698

Black, L., Grove, A., & Morrill, B. (2009). The psychometric validation of a US English satisfaction measure for patients with benign prostatic hyperplasia and lower tract symptoms. *Health and Quality of Life Outcomes, 7*(55). doi: 10.1186/1477-7525-7-55

Boon, H., Ruiter, R. A., James, S., Van Den, B., Willims, E., & Reddy, P. (2009). The impact of a community-based pilot health education intervention for older caregivers of orphaned and sick children as a result of HIV and AIDS in South Africa. *Journal of Cross-Cultural Gerontology, 24*, 373–389. doi 10.1007/s10823-009-9101-2

Boston Women's Health Book Collective. (2011). *Our bodies, ourselves* (9th ed.). New York, NY: Simon and Schuster.

Brott, A., & The Blueprint for Men's Health Advisory Board. (2008). *Blueprint for men's health: A guide to healthy lifestyle* (2nd ed.). Retrieved from http://www.blueprintformenshealth.com/blueprint/

Centers for Disease Control and Prevention. (2007). State-specific unintentional injury deaths – United States, 1999–2004. *Morbidity and Mortality Weekly Report, 56*(43), 1137–1140. Retrieved from http://www.cdc.gov/mmwr/preview/mmwrhtml/mm5643a4.htm

Centers for Disease Control and Prevention. (2008). Deaths from chronic obstructive pulmonary disease—United States, 2000–2005. *Morbidity and Mortality Weekly Report, 57*(45), 1229–1232. Retrieved from http://www.cdc.gov/mmwr/preview/mmwrhtml/mm5745a4.htm

Centers for Disease Control and Prevention. (2009a). HIV infection among injection drug users – 34 States, 2004–2007. *Morbidity and Mortality Weekly Report, 58*(46), 1291–1295. Retrieved from http://www.cdc.gov/mmwr/preview/mmwrhtml/mm5846a2.htm

Centers for Disease Control and Prevention. (2009b). *Sexually transmitted diseases surveillance, 2008*. Retrieved from http://www.cdc.gov/std/stats08/chlamydia.htm

Centers for Disease Control and Prevention. (2010a). Emergency department visits involving nonmedical use of selected prescription drugs—United States, 2004–2008. *Morbidity and Mortality Weekly Report (MMWR), 59*(23), 705–709. Retrieved from http://www.cdc.gov/mmwr/preview/mmwrhtml/mm5923a1.htm?s_cid=mm5923a1_w

Centers for Disease Control and Prevention. (2010b). *Falls among older adults*. Retrieved from http://www.cdc.gov/HomeandRecreationalSafety/Falls/adultfalls.html

Centers for Disease Control and Prevention. (2010c). *Heart disease and stroke prevention: Addressing the nation's leading killers. At a glance, 2010*. Retrieved from http://www.cdc.gov/chronicdisease/resources/publications/AAG/dhdsp.htm

Centers for Disease Control and Prevention. (2010d) *HIV among African Americans*. Retrieved from http://www.cdc.gov/hiv/topics/aa/pdf/aa.pdf

Centers for Disease Control and Prevention. (2010e). Prevalence and awareness of HIV infection among men who have sex with men—21 cities, United States 2008. *Morbidity and Mortality Weekly Report, 59*(37), 1201–1207. Retrieved from http://www.cdc.gov/mmwr/preview/mmwrhtml/mm5937a2.htm?s_cid=mm5937a2_w

Centers for Disease Control and Prevention. (2010f). Vital signs: Current cigarette smoking among adults aged ≥18 years – United States, 2009. *Morbidity and Mortality Weekly Report (MMWR), 59*(35), 1135–1140. Retrieved from http://www.cdc.gov/mmwr/preview/mmwrhtml/mm5935a3.htm?s_cid=mm5935a3_w

Centers for Disease Control and Prevention. (2010g). *Vital signs: Tobacco use & secondhand smoke*. Retrieved from http://www.cdc.gov/vitalsigns/TobaccoUse/Smoking/index.html

Centers for Disease Control and Prevention. (2010h). *Women and Heart Disease Fact Sheet*. Retrieved from http://www.cdc.gov/dhdsp/data_statistics/fact_sheets/docs/fs_women_heart.pdf

Centers for Disease Control and Prevention. (2011a). *Alcohol & public health*. Retrieved from http://www.cdc.gov/alcohol/

Centers for Disease Control and Prevention. (2011b). *The burden of injury and violence: A pressing public health concern*. Retrieved from http://www.cdc.gov/injury/overview/index.html

Centers for Disease Control and Prevention. (2011c). *Chlamydia fact sheet*. Retrieved from http://www.cdc.gov/std/chlamydia/chlamydia-fact-sheet-August-2011.pdf

Centers for Disease Control and Prevention. (2011d). *Chronic fatigue syndrome*. Retrieved from http://www.cdc.gov/cfs/

Centers for Disease Control and Prevention. (2011e). *HIV Surveillance Report*, 2009, Vol. 21. Retrieved from http://www.cdc.gov/hiv/surveillance/resources/reports/2009report/index.htm#cover

Centers for Disease Control and Prevention. (2011f). *Injuries and violence are leading causes of death: Key data and statistics*. Retrieved from http://www.cdc.gov/injury/overview/data.html

Centers for Disease Control and Prevention. (2011g). *National diabetes fact sheet: National estimates and general information on diabetes and prediabetes in the United States, 2011*. Atlanta, GA: U.S. Department of Health and Human Services. Retrieved from http://www.cdc.gov/diabetes/pubs/pdf/ndfs_2011.pdf

Centers for Disease Control and Prevention. (2011h). *Poisoning in the United States: Fact sheet*. Retrieved from http://www.cdc.gov/HomeandRecreationalSafety/Poisoning/poisoning-factsheet.htm

Centers for Disease Control and Prevention. (2011i). *Smoking and tobacco use*. Retrieved from http://www.cdc.gov/tobacco/data_statistics/index.htm

Centers for Disease Control and Prevention. (2011j). *U.S. obesity trends*. Retrieved from http://www.cdc.gov/obesity/data/trends.html#State

Centers for Disease Control and Prevention. (2011k). Vital signs: Asthma prevalence, disease characteristics, and self management education—United States, 2001–2009, *Morbidity and Mortality Weekly Report, 60*(17), 547–552. Retrieved from http://www.cdc.gov/mmwr/preview/mmwrhtml/mm6017a4.htm

Chronic Pain Research Alliance. (2011). *Chronic pain in women: Neglect, dismissal and discrimination*. Retrieved from http://endwomenspain.org/sites/default/files/WIP%202011%20Report%20FINAL%20high%20res_1.pdf

Courtenay, W. (2011). *Dying to be men: Psychosocial, environmental, and biobehavioral directions in promoting the health of men and boys*. New York, NY: Routledge

Creighton, G., & Oliffe J. (2010). Theorising masculinities and men's health: A brief history with a view to practice. *Health Sociology Review, 19*(4), 409–418. doi:10.5172/hesr.2010.19.4.409

DeMaria, E. J., Pate, V., Warthen, M., & Winegar, D. A. (2010). Baseline data from American Society for Metabolic and Bariatric Surgery – designated Bariatric Surgery Centers of Excellence using the Bariatric Outcomes Longitudinal Database. *Surgery for Obesity and Related Diseases, 6*(4), 347–355. doi:10.1016/j.soard.2009.11.015

Eisenberg, M. L., & Lipshultz, L. I. (2010). Estimating the number of vasectomies performed annually in the United States: Data from the National Survey of Family Growth. *The Journal of Urology, 184*, 2068–2072. doi:10.1016/j.juro.2010.06.117

Fee, E., Brown, T. M., Lazarus, J., & Theerman, P. (2002). The effects of the corset. *American Journal of Public Health, 92*, 1085. Retrieved from http://ajph.aphapublications.org/cgi/reprint/92/7/1085.pdf

Finkelstein, E. A., Brown, D. S., Wrage, L. A., Allaire, B. T., & Hoerger, T. J. (2010). Individual and aggregate years-of-life-lost associated with overweight and obesity. *Obesity, 18*(2), 333–339. doi:10.1038/oby.2009.253

Finkelstein, E. A., Trogdon, J. G., Cohen, J. W., & Dietz, W. (2009). Annual medical spending attributable to obesity: Payer- and service-specific estimates. *Health Affair, 28*(5), 822–831. doi:10.1377/hlthaff.28.5.w822

Flegal K. M., Carroll, M. D., Ogden, C. L., & Curtin, L. R. (2010). Prevalence and trends in obesity among US adults 1999–2008. *Journal of the American Medical Association, 303*(3), 235–241. doi:10.1001/jama.2009.2014

Fox, M. (2006, February 5). Betty Friedan, who ignited cause in 'feminine mystique,' dies at 85. *New York Times*. Retrieved from http://www.nytimes.com/2006/02/05/national/05friedan.html

Freund, A. M., & Ritter, J. (2009). Midlife crisis: A debate. *Gerontology, 55*, 582–591. doi: 10.1159/000227322

Friedan, B. (1997). *The feminine mystique*. New York: W.W. Norton.

Glasser, S. P., Judd, S., Basile, J., Lackland, D., Halanysch, J., Cushman, M., et al. (2011). Prehypertension, racial prevalence and its association with risk factors: Analysis of the REasons for Geographic and Racial Differences in Stroke (REGARDS) study. *American Journal of Hypertension, 24*(2), 194–199. doi:10.1038/ajh.2010.204

Greenland, P., Alpert, J. S., Beller, G. A., Benjamin, E. J., Budoff, M. J., Fayad, Z. A, et al. (2010). 2010 ACCF/AHA guideline for assessment of cardiovascular risk in asymptomatic adults: Executive summary: A report of the American College of Cardiology Foundation/American Heart Association Task Force on Practice Guidelines. *Circulation, 122*, 2748–2764. doi:10.1161/CIR.0b013e3182051bab

Grober, E. D., Jarvi, K., Lo, K. C., & Shin, E. J. (2011). Mini-incision vasectomy reversal using no-scalpel vasectomy principles: Efficacy and postoperative pain compares with traditional approaches to vasectomy reversal. *Urology, 77*(3), 602–606. doi:10.1016/j.urology.2010.09.051

Hartge, P. (2011). Reducing cancer death rates through screening. *Cancer, 17*, 449–450. doi10.1002/cncr.25622

Harvard Medical School. (2010a). *Join the Nurses' Health Study III*. Retrieved from http://www.nhs3.org/files/NHS3pressrelease.pdf

Harvard Medical School. (2010b). Mars vs. Venus: The gender gap in health. *Harvard Men's Health, 14*(6), 1–4. Retrieved from http://www.health.harvard.edu/newsletters/Harvard_Mens_Health_Watch/2010/January/mars-vs-venus-the-gender-gap-in-health

Health Resources and Services Administration. (2010). *Women's health USA 2010*. Retrieved from http://mchb.hrsa.gov/whusa10/index.html

Heidenreich, P. A., Trogdon, J. G., Khavjou, O. A., Butler J., Dracup, K., Ezekowitz, M. D., et al. (2011). Forecasting the future of cardiovascular disease in the United States: A policy statement from the American Heart Association, *Circulation, 123*(8), 933–944. doi: 10.11661/CIR.0b013e31820a55f5

Hu, G. & Baker, S. (2009). Trends in unintentional injury deaths, U.S., 1999–2005: Age, gender, and racial/ethnic differences. *American Journal of Preventive Medicine, 37*(3), 188–194. doi: 10.1015/j.amepre.2009.04.023

Imbornoni, M. (2007). *Women's rights movement in the United States: Timeline of key events in the American Women's Rights Movement*. Retrieved from http://www.infoplease.com/spot/womenstimeline1.html

Jack, B. W., Atrash, H., Bickmore, T., & Johnson, K. (2008). The future of preconception care: A clinical perspective. *Women's Health Issues, 18S*, S19–S25. doi:10.1016/j.whi.2008.09.004

Johnson, K., Posner, S. F., Biermann, J., Cordero, J. F., Atrash, H. K., Parker, C. S., et al. (2006). Recommendations to improve preconception health and health care: United States. *Morbidity and Mortality Weekly Report, 55*(RR06), 1–23. Retrieved from http://www.cdc.gov/mmwr/pdf/rr/rr5506.pdf

Johnson-Mallard, V., Lengacher, C. A., Kromrey, J. D., Kromrey, J. D., Campbell, D. W., Jevitt, C. M., et al. (2007). Increasing knowledge of sexually transmitted infection risk. *The Nurse Practitioner, 32*(2), 26–32 .

Kline, W. (2010). *Bodies of knowledge: Sexuality, reproduction, women's health in the second wave.* Chicago, IL: University of Chicago Press.

Kochanek, K. D., Xu, J., Murphy, S. L., Miniño, A. M., & Kung, H. (2011). Deaths: Preliminary date for 2009. *National Vital Statistics Report, 59*(4), 1–51. Retrieved from http://www.cdc.gov/nchs/data/nvsr/nvsr59/nvsr59_04.pdf

Koh, H. K. (2010). A 2020 vision for Healthy People. *New England Journal of Medicine, 362*, 1653–1656. doi: 10.1056/NEJMp1001601

Kupelian, V., Araujo, A. B., Chiu, G. R., Rosen, R. C., & McKinlay, J. B. (2010). Relative contributions of modifiable risk factors to erectile dysfunction: Results from the Boston Are Community Health (BACH) Study. *Preventive Medicine, 50*(1–2), 19–25. doi: 10/1016/j.pmed.2009.11.006

LaCroix, A. Z., Chlebowski, R. T., Manson, J. E., Aragaki A. K., Johnson, K. C., Martin, L., et al. (2011). Heath outcomes after stopping conjugated equine estrogens among postmenopausal women with prior hysterectomy: A randomized clinical trial. *Journal of the American Medical Association*, 305, 1305–1314. doi: 10.1001/jama.2011.382

Liao, Y., Greenlund, K. J., Croft, J. B., Keenan, N. L., & Giles, W. H. (2009). Factors explaining excess stroke prevalence in the US stroke belt. *Stroke, 40*, 3336–3341. doi: 10.1161/STROKEAHA.109.561688

Livingston, E. H. (2010).The incidence of bariatric surgery has plateaued in the U. S. *The American Journal of Surgery, 200*(3), 378–385. doi:10.1016/j.amjsurg.2009.11.007

Lloyd-Jones, D., Adams, R. J., Brown, T. M., Carnethon, M., Dai, S. De Simone, G., et al. (2010.) Heart disease and stroke statistics—2010 update: A report from the American Heart Association. *Circulation, 121*, e46–e215. doi: 10.1161/CIRCULATIONAHA.109.192667

Malnutrition Advisory Group. (2008). *Malnutrition Universal Screening Tool.* Retrieved from http://www.health.vic.gov.au/older/toolkit/05Nutrition/docs/Malnutrition%20Universal%20Screening%20Tool%20%28MUST%29%20.pdf

Martin, M., Beekley, A., Kjorstad, R., & Sebesta, J. (2010). Socioeconomic disparities in eligibility and access to bariatric surgery: A national population-based analysis. *Surgery for Obesity and Related Diseases*, 6(1), 8–15. doi:10.1016/j.soard.2009.07.003

Mond, J. M., Peterson, C. B., & Hay P. J. (2010). Prior use of extreme weight-control behaviors in a community sample of women with binge eating disorder or subthreshold binge eating disorder: A descriptive study. *International Journal of Eating Disorders*, *43*, 440–446. doi: 10.1002/eat.20707

Mosca, L., Bejamin, E. J., Berra, K., Bezanson, J. L., Dolor, R. J., Lloyd-Jones, D. M, et al. (2011). Effectiveness-based guidelines for the prevention of cardiovascular disease in women – 2011 update: A guideline from the American Heart Association. *Circulation*, 123, 1243–1262. doi: 10.1161/CIR.0b013e31820faaf8

Murphy, T. (2009). *Murphy brings men's health issues to the federal stage.* Retrieved from http://murphy.house.gov/s2009/murphy-brings-mens-health-issues-to-the-federal-stage/

National Cancer Institute. (2011a). *SEER stat fact sheets: All sites.* Retrieved from http://seer.cancer.gov/statfacts/html/all.html

National Cancer Institute. (2011b). *SEER stat fact sheets: Breast.* Retrieved from http://seer.cancer.gov/statfacts/html/breast.html

National Cancer Institute. (2011b). *SEER stat fact sheets: Ovary.* Retrieved from http://seer.cancer.gov/statfacts/html/ovary.html

National Center for Health Statistics. (2011). *Health, United States, 2010: With special feature on death and dying* (DHHS Pub. No. 1232). Hyattsville, MD: Public Health Service. Retrieved from http://www.cdc.gov/nchs/data/hus/hus10.pdf

National Diabetes Information Clearinghouse. (2011). *Diagnosed and undiagnosed diabetes among people ages 20 years or older, United States, 2010.* Retrieved from http://diabetes.niddk.nih.gov/dm/pubs/statistics/#Diagnosed20

National Eating Disorders Association. (2011). *Find specific information regarding eating disorders in men and boys.* Retrieved from http://www.nationaleatingdisorders.org/information-resources/men-and-boys.php

National Health and Nutrition Examination Survey. (2011). *Diagnosed and undiagnosed diabetes.* Retrieved from http://diabetes.niddk.nih.gov/dm/pubs/statistics/#Diagnosed20

National Heart, Lung, and Blood Institute. (2010). *Women's Health Initiative.* Retrieved from http://www.nhlbi.nih.gov/whi/

National Heart, Lung, and Blood Institute. (2011). *Framingham Heart Study.* Retrieved from http://www.framinghamheartstudy.org/index.html

National Institutes of Health. (2009). *Bariatric surgery and obesity* (NIH Publication No. 08-4006). Retrieved from http://win.niddk.nih.gov/publications/gastric.htm

National Institutes of Health. (2010). Obesity. *Medline Plus Encyclopedia.* Retrieved from http://www.nlm.nih.gov/medlineplus/ency/article/007297.htm

National Institutes of Health. (2011). *What people with anorexia nervosa need to know about osteoporosis.* Retrieved from http://www.niams.nih.gov/Health_Info/Bone/Osteoporosis/Conditions_Behaviors/anorexia_nervosa.asp

National Institutes of Health News. (2010). *WHI study data confirm short-term heart disease risks of combination hormone therapy for postmenopausal women.* Retrieved from http://www.nih.gov/news/health/feb2010/nhlbi-15.htm

National Institutes of Health Revitalization Act of 1993, PL 103-43, *Subtitle B—Clinical research equity regarding women and minorities.* Retrieved from http://grants.nih.gov/grants/funding/women_min/guidelines_amended_10_2001.htm

National Safety Council. (n.d.). *The cost of injuries: How much do you really pay?* Retrieved from http://www.nsc.org/news_resources/injury_and_death_statistics/Pages/EstimatingtheCostsofUnintentionalInjuries.aspx

Nurses' Health Study. (n.d.). Retrieved from http://www.channing.harvard.edu/nhs/

Nurses' Health Study: Phase 3. (n.d.). Retrieved from http://nhs2survey.org/NHS3/

O'Dougherty, M., Arikawa, A., Kaufman, B. C., & Kurzer, M. S. (2009). Purposeful exercise and lifestyle physical activity the lives of young adult women: Findings from a diary study. *Women & Health, 49*, 642–661. doi: 10.1080/03630240903496150

Office on Women's Health. (2009a). *Anorexia.* Retrieved from http://www.womenshealth.gov/publications/our-publications/fact-sheet/anorexia-nervosa.pdf

Office on Women's Health. (2009b). *Bulimia.* Retrieved from http://www.womenshealth.gov/publications/our-publications/fact-sheet/bulimia-nervosa.pdf

Office on Women's Health. (2009c). *Binge eating.* Retrieved form http://www.womenshealth.gov/publications/our-publications/fact-sheet/binge-eating-disorder.pdf

Office on Women's Health. (2009d). *Hysterectomy.* Retrieved from http://www.womenshealth.gov/publications/our-publications/fact-sheet/hysterectomy.cfm

Office on Women's Health. (2009e). *Osteoporosis.* Retrieved from http://www.womenshealth.gov/publications/our-publications/fact-sheet/osteoporosis.pdf

Picot, J., Jones, J., Colquitt, J. L., Gospodarevskaya, E., Loveman, E., Baxter, L., et al. (2009). The clinical effectiveness and cost-effectiveness of bariatric (weight loss) surgery for obesity: A systematic review and economic evaluation. *Health Technology Assessment, 13*(41), 1–190, 215–357. doi: 10.33310/hta13410

Pile, J. M., & Barone, M. A. (2009). Demographics of vasectomy – USA and international. *Urology Clinics of North America, 36*, 295–305. doi: 10.1016/j.ucl.2009.05.006

Pinkhasov, R. M., Shteynshlyuger, A., Hakimian, P., Lindsay, G. K., Samadi, D. B., & Shabsigh, R. (2010). Are men shortchanged on health? Perspective on life expectancy, morbidity, and mortality in men and women in the United States. *The International Journal of Clinical Practice, 64*(4), 465–474. doi: 10.1111/l.1742-1241.2009.02289x

Pleis, J. R., Ward, B. W., & Lucas, J. W. (2010) *Summary health statistics for U.S. adults: National Health Interview Survey, 2009. National Center for Health Statistics. Vital Health Statistics, 10*(249). Retrieved from http://www.cdc.gov/nchs/data/series/sr_10/sr10_249.pdf

Roger, V. L., Go, A. S., Loyd-Jones, D. M., Adams, R. J., Berry, J. D., Brown, T. M., et al. (2011). Heart disease and stroke statistics—2011 update: A report from the American Health Association. *Circulation, 123*, e18–e209. doi: 10.1161/CIR.0b013e3182009701

Sadovsky, R., Brock, G. B., Gutkin, S. W., & Sorsaburu, S. (2009). Toward a new 'EPOCH': Optimising treatment outcomes with phosphodiesterase type 5 inhibitors for erectile dysfunction. *The International Journal of Clinical Practice, 63*(8), 1214–1230. doi: 10.1111/j.1742-12411.2009.02119.x

Sloan, C., Gough, B., & Conner, M. (2010). Healthy masculinities? How ostensibly healthy men talk about lifestyle, health, and gender. *Psychology & Health, 25*(7), 783–803. doi: 10.1080/08870440902883204

Stevens, R. (1983). *Erik Erikson: An introduction*. New York, NY: St. Martin's Press

Stone, G. (2011). *About International Women's Day (8 March)*. Retrieved from http://www.internationalwomensday.com/

Substance Abuse and Mental Health Services Administration. (2010a). *Results from the 2009 National Survey on Drug Use and Health: Volume I. Summary of National Findings* (Office of Applied Studies, NSDUH Series H-38A, HHS Publication No. SMA 10-4856 Findings). Retrieved from http://oas.samhsa.gov/NSDUH/2k9NSDUH/2k9Results.htm#Ch1

Substance Abuse and Mental Health Services Administration. (2010b). *Results from the 2009 National Survey on Drug Use and Health: Volume II. Technical Appendices and Selected Prevalence Tables* (Office of Applied Studies, NSDUH Series H-38B, HHS Publication No. SMA 10-4856 Appendices). Retrieved from http://oas.samhsa.gov/NSDUH/2k9NSDUH/2k9ResultsApps.htm#AppC

Testicular Cancer Resource Center. (2009). *How to do a testicular self-examination*. Retrieved from http://tcrc.acor.org/tcexam.html

Thorve, V. S., Kshirsagar, A. D., Vyawahare, N. S., Joshi, V. S., Ingale, K. G., & Mohite, R. J. (2011). Diabetes-induced erectile dysfunction: Epidemiology, pathophysiology, and management. *Journal of Diabetes and Complications, 15*, 129–136. doi: 10.1016/j.diacomp.2010.03.003

Truman, B. I., Smith, C. K., Roy, K., Chen, Z., Moonesingh, R., Ahu, J., et al. (2011). CDC health disparities and inequalities report – United States, 2011. *Morbidity and Mortality Weekly Report, 60*(Suppl.). Retrieved from http://www.cdc.gov/mmwr/pdf/other/su6001.pdf

Townsend, J. S., Richardson, L. C., & German, R. R. (2010). Incidence of testicular cancer in the United States, 1999–2004. *American Journal of Men's Health, 4*(4), 353–360. doi: 10.1177/1557988309356101

U.S. Department of Agriculture and U.S. Department of Health and Human Services. (2010). *Dietary guidelines for Americans, 2010* (7th ed.). Washington, DC: U. S. Printing office. Retrieved from http://www.cnpp.usda.gov/Publications/DietaryGuidelines/2010/PolicyDoc/PolicyDoc.pdf

U.S. Department of Health and Human Services, Office of Disease Prevention and Health Promotion. (2010a). *Healthy People 2020*. Washington, DC: Author. Retrieved from http://www.healthypeople.gov/2020/default.aspx

U.S. Department of Health and Human Services. (2010b). *How tobacco smoke causes disease: The biology and behavioral basis for smoking-attributable disease: A Report of the Surgeon General*. Atlanta, GA, Retrieved from http://www.surgeongeneral.gov/library/tobaccosmoke/report/full_report.pdf

U.S. Department of Transportation, National Highway Traffic Safety Administration. (2010). *Alcohol impaired driving*. Retrieved from http://www.nhtsa.gov/

U.S. Department of Transportation, National Highway Traffic Safety Administration. (n.d.). *Traffic safety facts 2009*. Retrieved from http://www-nrd.nhtsa.dot.gov/Pubs/811402EE.pdf

White, S., Chen, J., & Atchison, R. (2008). Relationship of preventive health practices and health literacy: A national study. *American Journal of Health Behavior, 32*(3), 227–242. doi:10.3163/1536-5050.97.3.013

Women's Health Study (WHS): A randomized trial of low-dose aspirin and vitamin E in the primary prevention of cardiovascular disease and cancer. (2011). Retrieved from http://clinicaltrials.gov/show/NCT00000479

Women's Heart Foundation. (n.d.). *Women and heart disease facts*. Retrieved from http://www.womensheart.org/content/HeartDisease/heart_disease_facts.asp

World Health Organization. (2004) *Global statistics: Report on alcohol*. Retrieved from http://www.who.int/substance_abuse/publications/global_status_report_2004_overview.pdf

Woolf, S. E, & Maisto, S. A. (2009). Alcohol use and risk of HIV infection among men who have sex with men. *AIDS Behavior, 13*, 757–782. doi: 10.1007/s10461-007-9354-0

Xu, J., Kochanek, M. A., Murphy, S. L., & Tejada-Vera, B. (2010). Deaths: Final data for 2007. *National Vital Statistics Report, 58*(2). Retrieved from http://www.cdc.gov/nchs/data/nvsr/nvsr58/nvsr58_19.pdf

CHAPTER

24

Older Adults: Aging in Place

"We are always the same age inside."

—Gertrude Stein

KEY TERMS

Ageism
Aging in place
Alzheimer's disease (AD)
Assisted living
Case management
Centenarians
Continuing care retirement communities (CCRCs)
Custodial care
Elder abuse
Geriatrics
Gerontology
Hospice
Long-term care
Nursing home
Oldest old
Osteoporosis
Palliative care
Polypharmacy
Respite care
Senility
Skilled nursing facilities

LEARNING OBJECTIVES

Upon mastery of this chapter, you should be able to:

- Describe the global and national health status of older adults.
- Identify and refute at least three common misconceptions about older adults.
- Describe characteristics of healthy older adults.
- Provide an example of primary, secondary, and tertiary prevention practices in the older adult population.
- Identify four chronic conditions most commonly found in the older adult population.
- Identify four types of elder abuse.
- Discuss four primary criteria for effective programs for older adults.
- Describe various types of living arrangements and care options as older adults age in place.
- Describe the difference between hospice and palliative care.
- Describe the future of an aging America and the role of the community health nurse.

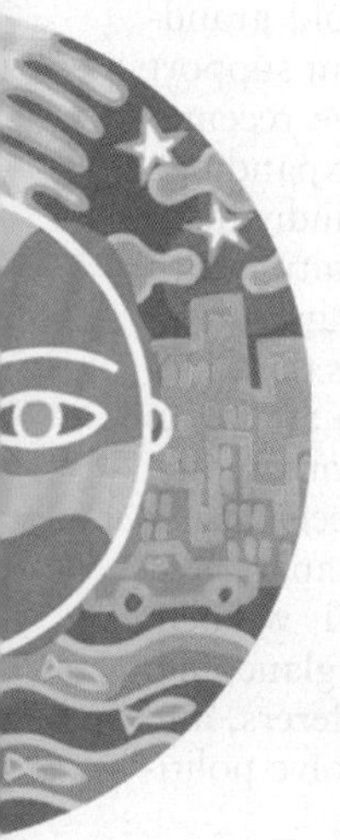

Older Americans constitute a large and rapidly growing population group. If you aren't already part of it, you will be in the future. Perhaps your parents and grandparents are in that group now. Improved medical care, advances in public health standards, and focus on prevention have contributed to dramatic increases in life expectancy in the United States. An American born in 1900 could expect to live 47.3 years. By 2050, life expectancy will rise to 82.6 (Centers for Disease Control and Prevention [CDC], 2010n). A second reason for a huge growth in the number of older adults began in 2011 as the baby boomers (people born after World War II between the years of 1946 and 1964) reached age 65.

- **Baby boomers comprise 28% of the US population, nearly 3 in 10 Americans (The Corporation for National and Community Service, 2011a).**
- **Every 7 seconds, one of these baby boomers becomes age 60.**
- **The result is that in the time period between 2011 and 2029, when the last of the baby boomers turns 65, there will be an era of unprecedented growth in the older population.**
- **By 2050, there will be 80 million American older adults.**
- **While in 1994 older adults accounted for 1 in 8 Americans, by 2030 they will account for 1 in 5 of the population (CDC, 2010n).**

Looking forward to the changing health needs of the nation, *Healthy People 2020*, the roadmap for health in the United States, lists four overarching goals. They are:

1. Attain high-quality, longer lives free of preventable disease, disability, injury, and premature death
2. Achieve health equity, eliminate disparities, and improve the health of all groups
3. Create social and physical environments that promote good health for all
4. Promote quality of life, healthy development, and healthy behaviors across all life stages (*Healthy People 2020, 2011a*)

Recognizing the need to focus more on the growing population of older adults, *Healthy People 2020* added older adults as a new topic area (*Healthy People 2020, 2011c*).

The future older population is expected to be better educated than the current one. The increased levels of education will most likely accompany better health, higher incomes, more wealth, and consequently a higher standard of living in retirement. As people retire at younger ages and in better health, they will require programs and services that support preventive health measures. The programs provide opportunities for continued wellbeing and enhanced quality of life and contribute to overall longevity. This group's potential for longevity could result in impending poor retirement planning and dwindling finances, increased living costs, increasing chronic disease and disability, diminishing functional capacity, and ongoing losses.

- Health care costs in the United States will continue to rise, surpassing $2.3 trillion in 2008. Half of this spending (51%) was for hospitals and physician visits, 10% on medications, 6% for nursing homes, and 3% for home health (KaiserEDU, 2010).
- The cost of providing health care for an American 65 years and older is three to five times greater than the cost for someone younger (CDC, 2011c).
- The number of people over the age of 65 who will require health care services will create challenges, as well as opportunities, for our already overburdened, understaffed, and ever changing health care system. Although tremendous efforts have been made to develop and promote preventive health programs and services, the outcomes and benefits of these efforts may not be evident for many years.

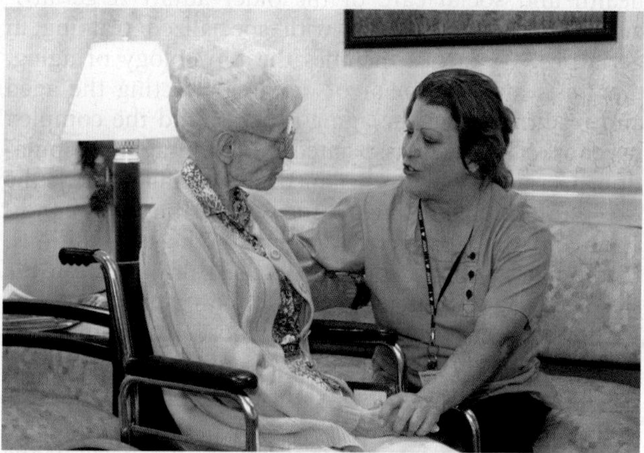

The cost of providing health care for those over age 65 is three to five times higher than for younger populations.

For community health nursing, growth in the aging population will present opportunities for nurses to work with communities to strengthen and build programs and services that focus on supporting the aging population's highest functional level. Like other nursing specialty areas, the community health nurse (CHN) will be in the position to advocate for the needs of an aging population and work with other agencies and organizations involved with health care delivery to ensure that seniors have access to high-quality health care and comprehensive services that address their unique and complex problems.

This chapter focuses on population-based nursing for the older adult. There are four fundamental requirements for effective nursing with any population:

1. Know the characteristics of the population.
2. Set aside stereotypes based on misconceptions about the population.
3. Know the health needs of the population as a basis for nursing intervention.
4. View the population from an aggregate, public health perspective that emphasizes health protection, health promotion, and disease prevention.

This chapter first examines the characteristics of the aging population in the United States and the global challenge of an aging society. Some myths and misconceptions about older adults are described, and ageism is discussed. Next, the primary, secondary, and tertiary health needs of older adults are explored. Diseases common among older adults are reviewed. Several types of elder abuse are described along with factors that contribute to the abuse of seniors. Finally, population-based health services and nursing interventions applied to the health of the aging population are discussed in light of cost containment and comprehensive care at the beginning of the new millennium.

GERIATRICS AND GERONTOLOGY

Geriatrics is the medical specialty that deals with the health and social care of the older adult. A geriatrician is a medical doctor with specialized training in geriatrics. Geriatrics includes the physiology of aging, diagnosis and treatment of diseases affecting the aged and resulting from the aging process, and the complex psychosocial issues associated with the aging population. Geriatrics, like other medical specialties with the exception of palliative care, focuses on abnormal conditions and the treatment and cure of those conditions. In the past, geriatric nursing focused primarily on the sick aged. As the nursing profession has grown, its scope has broadened. Many nurses choose to be involved with community-based nursing, focusing on prevention and improved health behaviors for the growing aging population.

Gerontology refers to the study of all aspects of the aging process, including economic, social, clinical, and psychological factors, and their effects on the older adult and on society. Gerontology is a broad, multidisciplinary practice, and gerontologic nursing concentrates on promoting the health and maximum functioning of older adults.

CHNs work with many types of older people. In one instance, the nurse may work to promote and maintain the health of a vigorous 80-year-old man who lives alone in his home. As another example, the nurse may give postsurgical care at home to a 69-year-old woman, teaching her husband how to care for her and helping them contact community resources for assistance with shopping, meals, housekeeping, and transportation services. Perhaps, nursing intervention focuses on teaching nutrition and maintaining a healthful lifestyle for an extended family that includes a 73-year-old grandmother. The nurse may also lead a bereavement support group for senior citizens whose spouses have recently died. The possibilities are limitless and ever expanding.

A CHN works with older adults at the individual, family, and group levels. However, a community health perspective must also concern itself with the aggregate of older adults. There are many groups of seniors the CHN may choose to work with, such as those who attend an adult day care center, belong to a retirement community, live in a nursing home, or use Meals on Wheels. Other groups include residents of a senior citizens' apartment building, retired business and professional women, older postcataract surgery patients at risk for glaucoma, the older poor, Alzheimer's disease (AD) sufferers, and the homeless. Work with clients can also involve political advocacy.

HEALTH STATUS OF OLDER ADULTS

As noted earlier, the growth in the number and proportion of older adults living in the United States is unprecedented in our nation's history. The proportion of individuals aged 65 and older is projected to increase from 12.4% in 2000 to 20.23% by the year 2050 (Administration on Aging, 2010b). People are living longer as a result of improved health care, eradication and control of many communicable diseases, use of antibiotics and other medicines, healthier dietary practices, safer global water supplies, regular exercise, and accessibility to a better quality of life including education and social services. Increased life expectancy reflects, in part, the success of public health interventions, but public health programs must now respond to new challenges including the growing burden of chronic illness, injuries, disabilities; increasing concerns about future caregiving; and rapidly rising health care costs (CDC, 2010d).

The rising number of older adults increases demands on the public health system and on medical and social services and health care delivery. Currently, 50 million older adults have some type of disability (*Healthy People 2020, 2010a*). Chronic diseases, which affect older adults disproportionately, contribute to disability, diminish quality of life, and increase health care costs.

- Of those, over 65, 59% report arthritis as the leading cause of disability (CDC, 2011a).
- Diabetes and AD affect one in four and one in eight of those age 65 and older, respectively, and are expected to have even greater effects on the US health care system in the next few decades (Alzheimer's Association, 2011a; American Diabetes Association, 2011).

Two key challenges that are new to the public health arena, although they have long been the target of health care and aging services professions, are preventing and treating cognitive decline and addressing end-of-life issues. Meeting these challenges, along with the increasing number of individuals with chronic conditions, is critical to ensuring that the aging population can look forward to their later years. As more and more Americans reach age 65, society is increasingly challenged to help them grow old with dignity and comfort.

Global Demographics

The unprecedented growth in older adults is not limited to the United States but is happening worldwide. Almost 500 million people were 65 and older in 2008. By 2030, the world's older adults are projected to reach 1 billion. This means that one person out of every eight will be an older adult (Administration on Aging, 2010a). In most of the world, the population of those over 85 years of age is the fastest growing part of the population and is projected to increase 2.3% between 2008 and 2030 (U.S. Census Bureau, 2008).

Because of this demographic shift along with altered societal expectations, changes in attitudes and social policies worldwide are needed; many countries have few or no social programs, pensions, or health care services available for their older adults populations.

Life expectancy at birth around the world now is 67 (Central Intelligence Agency [CIA], 2011). Life expectancy has increased in developing countries since 1950, although the amount of increase varies. A higher life expectancy at birth for females compared with males is almost universal, with the average gender differential estimated at approximately 4 years worldwide (69 years for females, 65 for males) in 2011 (CIA, 2011). The high percentages are in part the result of a longer lifespan, but they also reflect low birth rates in many countries.

- Presently, the world population is at roughly 6.6 billion people, but population projections continue to predict increases (from 9.3 billion in 2050 to 10.1 billion by the end of this century) (United Nations, 2011).
- The median age of the world's population is 28 years, and this has been increasing due in part to declining fertility and a 20-year increase in the average lifespan during the second half of the 20th century (CIA, 2011).

National Demographics

As a result of demographic transitions including declining infant and childhood mortality, lower fertility rates, and improvements in adult health, the shape of the global age distribution is changing. The age distribution in developed countries, such as the United States, represents a larger proportion of older to younger populations. By 2025, the United States is expected to have 80% more older adults than in 2000, but working-age adults will grow by only 15% (Atlas.gov, 2011).

There are disparities in life expectancy among various subgroups in the population. Life expectancy is highest for White Americans and lowest for Black Americans, who have the highest death rates of any of America's racial and ethnic groups (CDC, 2011c). Although life expectancies have been increasing for all Americans in general, a variety of factors have caused those figures to level off in recent years. These factors include unhealthy lifestyles; societal problems, such as deaths caused by firearms, substance abuse, and human immunodeficiency virus/acquired immunodeficiency syndrome (HIV/AIDS); and the rise of AD among older adults.

The Hispanic, Black, and Asian populations have been expanding and are projected to grow substantially through 2025 (U.S. Census Bureau, 2011). The health status of racial and ethnic minorities of all ages lags far behind that of nonminority populations. For a variety of reasons, older adults may experience the effects of health disparities more dramatically than any other population group. In an effort to help address these health disparities, the Racial and Ethnic Approaches to Community Health (REACH, 2010) Program supports community-based coalitions in the design, implementation, and evaluation of innovative strategies to reduce or eliminate health disparities among racial and ethnic minorities (Administration on Aging, 2010a). Methods utilized include "capacity building, targeted actions, community/system change, widespread risk/protective behavior change, and health disparity reduction" (p. 2). An example of one of these programs is highlighted in Display 24.1. The goal is to achieve health equity, eliminate disparities, and improve the health of all groups (U.S. Department of Health and Human Services, 2011).

Current research has shown that although many efforts—such as aspirin use for high-risk adults, tobacco-use screening and brief intervention, colorectal cancer screening for adults over age 50, and immunization for pneumococcal disease for those age 65 and older—can be very effective, they are not always implemented or consistently utilized. Nevertheless, older people are healthier than ever before. Increasing numbers of capable older adult people are living independently. Hearty older adults—people older than 65 years of age who maintain a level of wellness and activity, well above present expectations for that age—are increasing in number. Many continue to work and stay involved in community programs and activities. Some have become valuable volunteers, helping others in such community activities as hospice and literacy programs for adults, serving as foster grandparents, working in libraries and homeless shelters, or providing services such as Meals on Wheels. Research has shown a connection between positive health effect and community involvement/participation, volunteering, and other forms of social capital (Barron et al., 2009).

Not only are more people living into old age but also, once they get there, they are living longer. Because of this expansion, subcategories of the over-65 age group are being used (CDC, 2010n). **Oldest old** refers to people who are 85 and above (Segen's Medical Dictionary, 2011). However, some organizations use 80 as the cutoff for oldest old. This is the fastest growing age group in the United States and worldwide. Those 100 years old or older are called **centenarians**.

DISPLAY 24.1 RACIAL AND ETHNIC APPROACHES TO COMMUNITY HEALTH (REACH)—DETROIT, MICHIGAN

High rates of diabetes-related hospital discharges and diabetes-related mortality were noted in both southwest and eastern areas of Detroit, Michigan. Public health nurses and other officials also checked statistical data and found that 43% of African Americans in Detroit were overweight, whereas 33% of Whites were overweight. Almost half of all residents reported that they had a sedentary lifestyle, and one third stated that they engaged in no physical activities during their leisure time. Many of these people were older adults and elderly.

It was decided that this problem had to be addressed at multiple levels: with individuals and families (changing behaviors), social support systems, community agencies and services, and by making changes in policies and programs offered by Detroit Community Health and Social Services. They formed a partnership, based upon the principles of community-based participatory research (see Chapter 4). They began by collecting additional data on the prevalence of diabetes, the accessibility of quality health care services, and what community resources were available that promoted healthy lifestyles. They also looked for acceptable models of community-based interventions and gathered perspectives from members of the community by holding family focus groups.

They began educating their target population and conducted diabetes education and self-management classes over a period of 5 to 6 weeks. They had good results with retention of REACH participants (80%) and significant improvements in both physical activity and dietary knowledge and behavior. Self-care behaviors and diabetes problem areas were also significantly improved ($p < .05$), as were levels of hemoglobin A_1C. Hypertension was also decreased, from a baseline of 54.1% of REACH participants to 42.4% at the 6-month mark.

This multilevel, community-based intervention made marked improvements on several outcome measures for the targeted population. What type of disease or problem is most prevalent in your area? With whom could you collaborate to design interventions? Which levels would you want to address? How would you measure success (which outcomes would you select)?

Two Feathers, J., Kieffer, E. C., Palmisano, G., Anderson, M., Sinco, B., Janz, N., et al. (2005). Racial and ethnic approaches to community health (REACH). Detroit partnership: Improving diabetes-related outcomes among African American and Latino adults. *American Journal of Public Health, 95*(9), 1552–1560.

Growth in the number of older adults will significantly affect health care resources, housing options for older adults, and national longevity statistics. As the number of older people increases, so, too, will their need for assistance with activities of daily living (ADLs) and other services. Many people will be involved with the care of a family member who needs assistance in attending to ADLs such as dressing, eating, toileting, and bathing, and researchers are seeking effective methods of providing respite to caregivers and reducing costs (CDC, 2010d).

In the United States, approximately 80% of older adults have one chronic condition and half of older adults have two chronic conditions. It is estimated that health care costs for chronic disease treatment account for more than 75% of national health expenditures (NHEs) (KaiserEDU, 2010). Approximately 7 of 10 deaths are from chronic conditions. Heart disease, cancer, and stroke cause half the total deaths (CDC, 2010f). Death is only part of the picture of the burden of chronic disease among older Americans. These conditions can cause years of pain, disability, and loss of function and independence before resulting in death. In addition to chronic conditions that require ongoing monitoring and management, the CHN should anticipate the needs of many older adults who will face the loss of a spouse, helpmate, or companion and who may experience loneliness, social isolation, and depression.

Many older adults live in poverty. In 2009, the Administration on Aging reported that 8.9% of older adults (3.4 million) lived below the poverty line and another 5.4% (2 million) were "near poor" living under 125% of the poverty level. More old women are poor (10.7%) than men (6.6%). Those living alone are more likely to live in poverty (15.6%) than those who live with family (5.4%) (Administration on Aging, 2010a). Older African Americans have the highest rate of poverty (20%) followed by Hispanics (18%), Asians (16%), and White older adults (7%) (Administration on Aging, 2010a).

The education level of the older population is increasing. The percentage of older adults who have completed high school increased between 1970 and 2001 (from 28% to 78%). There is considerable variability among those of different races or ethnic origins. In 2009, 83.1% of White older adults had finished high school compared to 71.9% of Asian, 63.8% of Blacks, and 45% of Hispanics (Administration on Aging, 2010a). These figures are predicted to change as the United States witnesses a trend toward a more educated senior population because of the significant number of baby boomers who completed high school and entered college during and since the 1960s. The number of seniors with bachelor's degrees increased from 28% in 1970 to 78.3% in 2009 (CDC, 2010n). With higher levels of education should come broader health consumerism and improved quality of life.

DISPELLING AGEISM

Ageism is a term that describes negative stereotyping of older adults and discrimination because of older age. In America, ageism is a major problem (McGuire, Klein, & Chen, 2008). These stereotypes often arise from negative personal experiences, myths shared throughout the ages, and a general lack of current information. Unfortunately, health concerns and symptoms in older adults are often overlooked or dismissed as part of the normal aging process. By becoming more aware of myths and realities of CHNs can improve the health and quality of life of the growing population of older adults. Ageism can interfere with effective practice and prevent the kind of comprehensive and interdisciplinary services and care that aging persons need and deserve (Allen, Cherry, Palmore, 2009). Ageism has an impact on both society and culture, even though most individuals are not aware of it. Ageism creates needless fear, waste, illness, and misery (Palmore, 2005).

Myths Regarding Older Adults

Most people know little about aging and may have negative stereotypes about older adults. CHNs must guard against ageism in their practice by dispelling common myths and misconceptions.

The Myth of Senility

Myth: It is normal for older adults to become more confused and childlike, forgetful, and lose contact with reality as they age. They become "senile."

Reality: **Senility** is an obsolete term used to describe deterioration in the mental functions of some older people. The word implies that with growing old come symptoms of forgetfulness, confusion, and changes in behavior and personality. This term is stereotypical, implying that older people are mentally deficient. Memory loss is *not* an inevitable part of the aging process. The brain is capable of producing new brain cells at any age, so significant memory loss is *not* an inevitable result of aging. But, just as it is with muscle strength, you have to use it or lose it. Lifestyle, health habits, and daily activities have a huge impact on the health of the brain. At any age, there are many ways you can improve your cognitive skills, prevent memory loss, and protect your gray matter (HelpGuide, 2011f).

Certainly, AD and arteriosclerosis cause memory loss and altered behavior in the older adult, but many older adults have similar symptoms as a result of anxiety, loss, depression, or grief, or simply from side effects of medications or changes in their routines. These reactions need to be diagnosed by health care providers and differentiated from disease processes. A recent review of the available literature on the relationship between exercise and cognition indicates that social engagement and physical activity may help maintain cognitive functioning in older adults (Angevaren, Aufdemkampe, Verhaar, Aleman, & Vanhees, 2008; McAuley et al., 2009).

Age-related memory loss can be the result of several physiological factors.

First, the hippocampus, a region of the brain involved in the formation and retrieval of memories, often deteriorates with age. Second, growth factors—hormones and proteins that protect and repair brain cells and stimulate neural growth—decline with age. Third, older people often experience decreased blood flow to the brain. This can impair memory and lead to changes in cognitive skills (HelpGuide, 2011f).

Intelligence, learning ability, and other intellectual and cognitive skills do not decline with age. Cognitive deficits are often caused by reversible factors. Sometimes, even what looks like significant memory loss can be caused by treatable conditions and reversible external factors such as medication side effects, depression, vitamin B_{12} deficiency, thyroid problems, alcohol abuse, or dehydration (HelpGuide, 2011f). Generally, older people are capable of making their own decisions; they want and need the freedom to make choices and to be as independent as their limitations will allow.

The Myth of the Rocking Chair

Myth*: As age increases older adults withdraw, become inactive, and cease being productive.*

Reality: While some older adults do become disengaged, many remain active for as long as possible. Diminished capabilities and personal preferences affect the level of activity. As age advances, older adults do not necessarily become inactive and sit in rocking chairs on the porch. The average American retires at age 63. Prior to the 1990s, the average age of retirement had been declining. Now, it is moving upward. A recent trend has been for retirees to return to work; 11% in one survey reported they are not retired (Pew Research Center, 2009).

Labor force participation rates of those over 60 (not retired) have been increasing over the past decade for men and women age 62 to 64 (4% increase for men and 12% increase for women). Millions of Americans older than age 65 work full- or part-time, and many others, who are not included in labor statistics, work but do not report their earnings. An example is the grandmother who chooses to give up full-time employment in an unsatisfying job to babysit for three preschool grandchildren and is paid in cash by her two children. The grandmother gets to spend time with growing grandchildren and supplement her retirement income, the parents feel comfortable that their mother is caring for their children, and the grandchildren are experiencing the joy of being with their grandparent. In another situation, active retired older adults assist with their two children's businesses. The mother types legal documents for the son's law practice during busy times, and the father helps out on Saturdays at the daughter's pool supply store. Everyone wins in these situations.

Meaningful activity remains important to seniors. Healthy older people usually do not disengage or withdraw and isolate themselves from society; rather, they are active and involved. Remaining active—through a daily routine, purposeful behavior, and a positive view of life—produces the best psychological climate.

The Myth of Homogeneity

Myth: As older adults age, they lose their individual differences and become progressively more alike.

Reality: As a person ages, his/her personality remains fairly constant. Not only are individual differences retained, these differences become even more pronounced with age. Generally, an older adult becomes more like the person he or she was in youth (i.e., a talkative teenager, e.g., becoming a talkative older person or a stubborn youngster carrying the trait of stubbornness into old age). Except for changes in physical appearance and experiencing more physical problems, being "old" feels no different from how we feel now or when we were young. In reality, an old person is a young person who has just lived longer.

The aging process is quite distinct among older people, and they age at widely disparate rates. Some people still play golf, drive a car, and participate in social and community activities at age 85; others are frail and cannot move about well, needing assistance with their ADLs. Some prefer to equate "real age" with biological age, not chronological age; this depends on how well an individual takes care of himself or herself physically and mentally. Exercise, nutrition, vitamins, seat belt use, and other factors are thought to play a role in healthy aging. Physical, social, and mental health parameters; life experiences; and genetic traits all combine to make aging an individualized process (see Levels of Prevention Pyramid).

LEVELS OF PREVENTION PYRAMID

SITUATION: Making a healthy transition into a satisfying old age

GOAL: Using the three levels of prevention: health promotion improves overall health and wellbeing, and prevents or delays chronic diseases, while secondary prevention ensures prompt early diagnosis and treatment of conditions, and tertiary prevention aids in rehabilitation and continuing health promotion. preventing or delaying chronic diseases, promptly diagnose, and treat conditions, until the fullest possible potential is restored.

TERTIARY PREVENTION

Rehabilitation	Primary Prevention	
	Health Promotion & Education	*Health Protection*
• Adapt to changed roles with spouse and significant others. • Maintain health while assessing increasing dependency needs, including alternative housing, modifications in transportation, and changing health care needs.	• Periodically review and update will, insurances, and other important documents as needed. • Keep beneficiaries or executors aware of changes in and location of documents and personal wishes regarding end-of-life care and funeral/burial arrangements.	

SECONDARY PREVENTION

Early Diagnosis	Prompt Treatment
• Follow the U.S. Task Force Recommendations for regular screening of potential health problems. • Reflect on past successes and contributions to the workforce.	• Allow time for adaptation to this life transition. • Organize new free time into satisfying and enriching activities.

PRIMARY PREVENTION

Health Promotion and Education	Health Protection
• Early preparation—emotionally and financially • Plan ahead for changes in health status and potential need for long-term care. • Complete documents, such as a will and a living will.	• Regularly assess health status. • Follow the U.S. Task Force Recommendations for immunizations. • Implement a health-promoting regimen that includes diet and exercise. • Assess living environment for safety hazards.

The Myth of Inability

Myth: Older adults are forgetful, unable to learn new thing, and are set in their old ways of doing things.

Reality: Learning is a lifetime ability that continues into old age. While older adults may experience some difficulty with short-term (or working) memory as they get older, their long-term memory generally remains sound. People at any age can learn new information and skills. Research indicates that older people can learn new skills and improve old ones, including how to use a computer and the Internet. Learning occurs best in a self-paced, supportive environment. Studies have demonstrated that exercising the brain improves memory (Li et al., 2008). Older adults have spent a lifetime adapting to change, with varying measures of success. People older than 65 years grew up in an age when having an automobile was a luxury, and many did not have a microwave oven, video recorder, or DVDs until they were in middle adulthood. Elders learned to adapt to these changes, and they are becoming increasingly computer literate today. The ability to change does not depend on age but rather on personality traits acquired throughout life or, sometimes, because of socioeconomic difficulties. For example, elders living on fixed incomes may be faced with inflationary costs. This may cause them to vote against a school levy that would increase taxes, although they otherwise would be very supportive of schools because they value education.

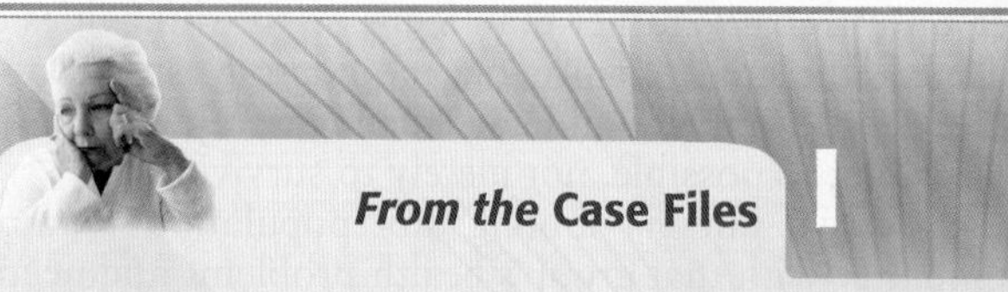

From the Case Files I

I am a PHN and live next door to Minerva Blackstone, affectionately called Minnie by her friends. Minnie is a lively 87-year-old woman who enjoys life. Every day, except in bad weather, she walks a half mile to visit her granddaughter Karen. There, she works on the quilt she is making for Karen. In addition, twice a week, Minnie takes the city bus to the senior citizens' center to join her friends in an exercise class. Although her eyesight has somewhat diminished, Minnie enjoys reading in the evening or crocheting while she watches television. Mysteries and comedies are her favorite kinds of stories.

Minnie is a happy person but is not content unless she is up on the latest political developments. She always has opinions on current events and expresses them with vigorous shakes of her curly white hair at her monthly group meeting on women and politics. She has a good appetite and generally sleeps well. Minor arthritis does not hamper her activities, nor does the hypertension that she controls by taking her medication with conscientious regularity. Minnie is enjoying a healthy, successful old age.

Carole Stokes, District PHN

MEETING THE HEALTH NEEDS OF OLDER ADULTS

No one knows conclusively all of the variables that influence healthy aging, but it is known that a lifetime of healthy habits and circumstances, a strong social support system, and a positive emotional outlook all significantly influence the resources people bring to their later years. Most people recognize a healthy older person when they meet one. See From the Case Files I for an example of healthy aging.

What is healthy old age? As was mentioned earlier, the vast majority (94%) of our older adult, even those with chronic diseases or other disabilities, are living outside institutions and are relatively independent. Their ability to function is a key indicator of health and wellness and is an important factor in understanding healthy aging. Good health in the older adult means maintaining the maximum possible degree of physical, mental, and social vigor. It means being able to adapt, to continue to handle stress, and to be active and involved in life and living. In short, healthy aging means being able to function, even when disabled, with a minimum of help from others.

Wellness among the older population varies considerably. It is influenced by many factors, including personality traits, life experiences, current physical health, and current societal supports and personal health behaviors including smoking, obesity, and excessive alcohol use. One way to measure healthy aging on a large scale is the degree to which states have met or exceeded targets on 11 of the *Healthy People 2010* older adult health indicators (CDC, 2010i). For instance, we have already exceeded the goal of 70% of the population receiving mammograms within the past 2 years by achieving 79.1% (CDC, 2008c). Colorectal screenings also achieved higher than expected results (actual 66.6% with a goal of 50%) (CDC, 2008a). Checks for cholesterol in the past 5 years were 94.7% (with a goal of 80%), exceeding its goal (CDC, 2009a). The number of people who currently smoke has also dropped to 8%, less than the 12% goal set by *Healthy People 2010* (CDC, 2009b). Other actions that can increase healthy aging include addressing health disparities among older adults, encouraging people to plan for end-of-life care and communicate their wishes through advance directives, improving oral health and increasing physical activity among seniors by promoting environmental changes, increasing adult immunization levels, and preventing falls. Some older adults demonstrate maximum adaptability, resourcefulness, optimism, and activity. Others, often those from whom we tend to draw our stereotypes, have disengaged and present a picture of dependence and resignation. Most older adults fall somewhere in between these two extremes. Although the level of wellness varies among older adults, that level can be raised. The goals in community health nursing are to maximize the wellness potential of older adult clients and to support their highest level of functional ability enabling them to remain independent. Nurses must analyze and build on an older person's strengths rather than focus on the difficulties or deficits. The goal for an aging population is to enable older people to thrive and have the highest quality of life for as long as possible, not merely to survive.

Effective nursing among any population requires familiarity with that group's health problems and needs. Aging, in and of itself, is not a health problem. Rather, aging is a normal, irreversible physiologic process. Its pace, however, can sometimes be slowed, as researchers are discovering, and many of the problems associated with aging can be prevented. The aging process is subtle, gradual, and lifelong. One can see remarkable differences among individuals in the rate of aging. Even in a single individual, various systems of the body age at different rates. Therefore, chronologic age cannot readily be a reliable indicator of health needs. Methods for calculating your "real age" can give you a better picture of your body's true state of health (see www.realage.com for a calculator you can use for yourself and your clients).

However, the proportion of people with health problems increases with age, and as a group, older adults are more likely than younger ones to suffer from multiple, chronic, and often disabling conditions requiring ongoing care and management.

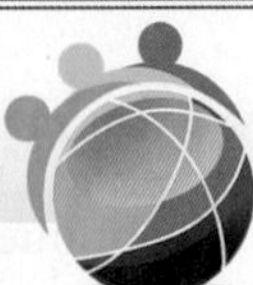

DISPLAY 24.2 STRATEGIES FOR SUCCESSFUL AGING

- Do at least 30 minutes of sustained, rhythmic, vigorous exercise four times a week.
- Eat "like a bushman" (a healthy diet of fruits, whole grains, vegetables, and lean meat).
- Get as much sleep and rest as needed.
- Maintain a sense of humor and deflect anger.
- Set goals and accept challenges that force you to be as alive and creative as possible.
- Don't depend on anyone else for your well-being.
- Be necessary and responsible; live outside yourself (give to others, become involved).
- Don't slow down. Stick with the mainstream. Avoid the shadows. Stay together. Maintain energy flow in a purposeful direction; aging need not be characterized by losses. Maintain contacts with family and friends, and stay active through work, recreation, and community.
- Get regular checkups.
- Don't smoke—it's never too late to quit.
- Practice safety habits at home to prevent falls and fractures. Always wear seat belts when traveling by car.
- Avoid overexposure to the sun and the cold.
- If you drink, moderation is the key—when you drink, let someone else drive.
- Keep personal and financial records in order to simplify budgeting and investing—plan long-term housing and financial needs.
- Keep a positive attitude toward life—do things that make you happy.

LEVELS OF PREVENTION

Older adults, like any age group, have certain basic needs: physiologic and safety needs, as well as the needs for love and belonging, self-esteem, and self-actualization. Their physical, emotional, and social needs are complex and interrelated. The following sections discuss these needs according to primary, secondary, and tertiary prevention activities.

Primary Prevention

As discussed previously in this text, primary prevention activities involve those actions that keep one healthy. Such primary prevention activities as health education, follow-through of sound personal health practices (e.g., flossing, seat belt use, exercise), recommended routine screenings, and maintenance of an appropriate immunization schedule ensure that older adults are doing all that they can to maintain their health. The list in Display 24.2 includes strategies for successful aging. Taken from a variety of sources, it provides primary prevention activities the CHN can use when working with older adults, either individually or in groups.

Nutrition and Oral Health Needs

People who have maintained sound dietary habits throughout their life have little need to change in old age. The USDA recently replaced the food pyramid with My Plate as a visual to guide the food intake of Americans (U.S. Department of Agriculture, 2011). Tufts University has modified My Plate for older adults (see Fig. 24-1). The modifications include an emphasis on drinking plenty of fluids such as water and/or fat-free milk, high fiber intake, as well as adding multivitamins to the diet. Also emphasized is the importance of regular exercise with icons depicting common activities that include daily errands and household chores (Tufts University, 2011).

Many older adults have not established such habits but may be required to do so because of disease processes such as diabetes or cardiovascular disease. It is generally believed that older people need to maintain their optimal weight by eating a diet that is low in fats, moderate in carbohydrates, and high in proteins with a daily calorie count of 1,200 to 1,600. Foods with "empty calories," such as salty snacks, candy, fatty foods, and alcohol, should be limited; they meet hunger needs by satisfying appetite only, while providing little nutrition. Cereals and whole grains, dried beans, and nuts can provide fiber needed by seniors, and eating colorful fruits and vegetables (rather than fruit juice) also contributes to fiber and may help to prevent macular degeneration. Another important thing to remind older adults to do is to drink adequate amounts of liquids, especially water. Eight glasses a day are recommended, and many older adults have a diminished

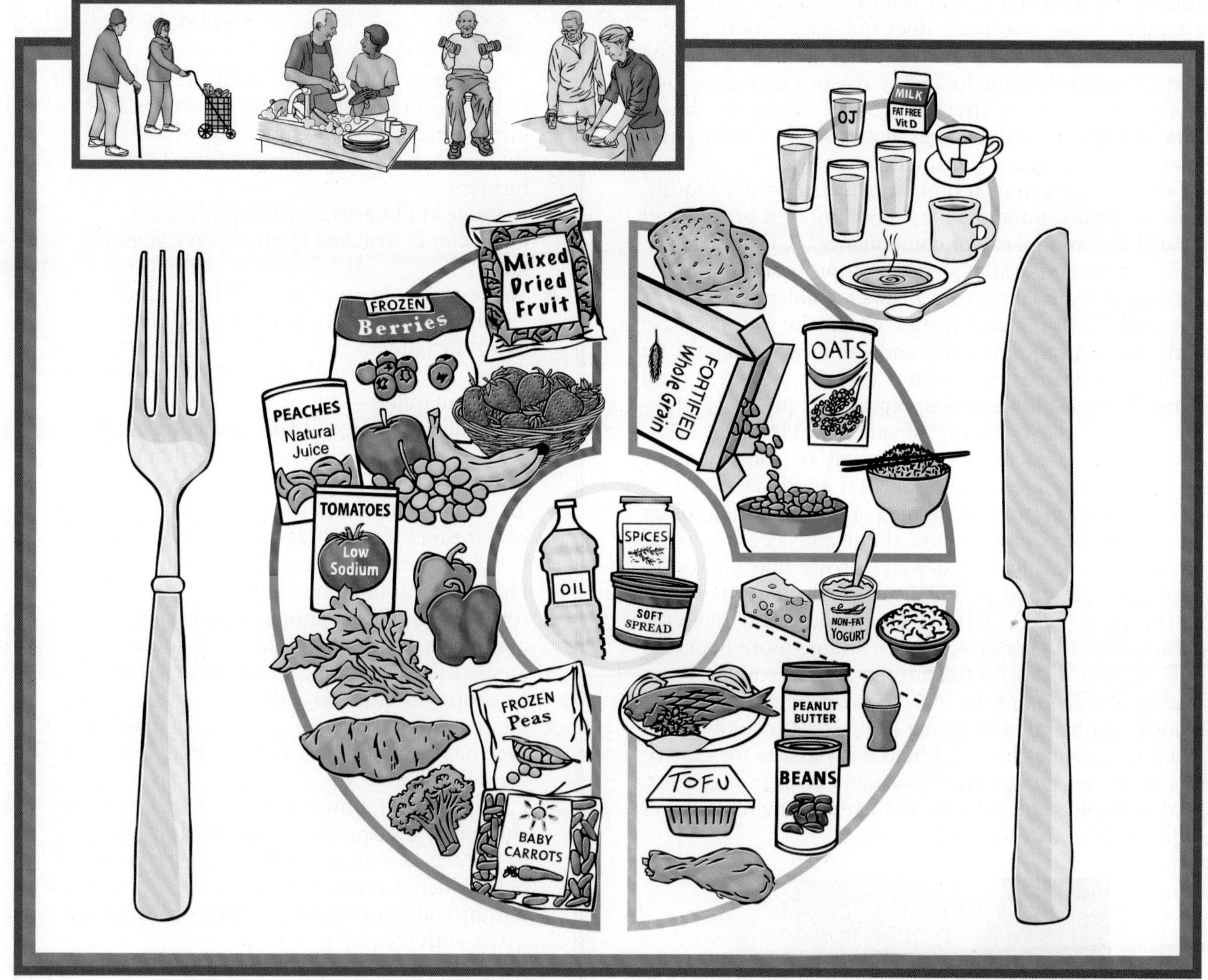

FIGURE 24-1. Myplate for older adults. Copyright Tufts University, 2011. Used with permission.

feeling of thirst and can easily become dehydrated if they do not purposefully plan their fluid intake. Older adults need less vitamin A but more calcium and vitamin D (for healthy bones), more folic acid, and more vitamins B_6 and B_{12} (for cognitive health) than younger adults (Slavin, 2008). Many communities offer meals to seniors, either at senior centers or by way of Meals on Wheels, through grants provided by the Older Adult Nutrition Program (Administration on Aging, 2011a).

Major advances in the field of oral health including community water fluoridation, advanced dental technology, better oral hygiene, and more frequent use of dental services have had a substantial impact on the number of older adults who retain their natural teeth. Before the time of widespread fluoride use, it was common for people to lose most or all of their teeth by midlife. The percentage of older adults who have lost all their natural teeth has declined to 18%, surpassing the *Healthy People 2010* target of no more than 20% (CDC, 2008b, 2010i). Severe tooth loss in older adults compromises their food quality (Savoca et al., 2010). Most people can keep their natural teeth for a lifetime with preventive practices. Oral health is integral to general health and wellbeing throughout one's life. A good deal of research has demonstrated the connection between oral health and general health due to chronic inflammation that releases cytokines and C-reactive protein causing endothelial damage and cholesterol plaque attachment in cardiovascular disease and stroke. Poor oral health has also been associated with peripheral vascular disease, diabetes, and risk for death caused by pneumonia in nursing homes (American Geriatric Society Foundation for Healthy Aging, n.d.). Even those with dentures must be vigilant in maintaining oral health, as they are still at risk from inflammatory processes leading to diseases like pneumonia (American Dental Association, 2011).

The oral health of older adults, however, is often neglected. Many older adults, especially those with limited or fixed incomes or cognitive limitations, are not able to maintain their oral health or visit a dentist on a regular basis. Medicare does not cover routine dental services. Maintaining oral health during the senior years is more difficult for many reasons including lack of dental insurance after retirement, economic disadvantages and limited incomes, decreased nutritional and fluid intake, changes in gums and increased periodontal disease, as well as a higher incidence of dry mouth. Saliva contains minerals for rebuilding of tooth enamel as well as "antimicrobial components" (CDC, 2010m). Fluid intake and oral hygiene are appropriate topics for anticipatory guidance from PHNs for older adults.

Oral health and hygiene needs do not decrease with age. Eating, chewing, and swallowing should be an uncomplicated and natural process. Eating should remain a pleasurable social experience, preferably taking place in the company of others. CHNs can assist older adults with meal management by following the suggestions outlined in Display 24.3 and Figure 24-1.

In addition to maintaining a healthy diet, older adults are cautioned to limit the use of alcohol, avoid tobacco, drink fluoridated water or use fluoride toothpaste, practice good oral hygiene and have regular dental checkups (CDC, 2010m). They should also avoid the habitual use of laxatives, instead adding more fiber and bulk to their diet with fresh fruits and vegetables. Also, inadequate fluid intake can contribute to bowel and bladder problems. Following a diet that includes eight or more 8-ounce glasses of fluid daily assists the gastrointestinal and genitourinary systems in their functions. Increased physical activity and exercise helps keep an older adult's bowel patterns regular.

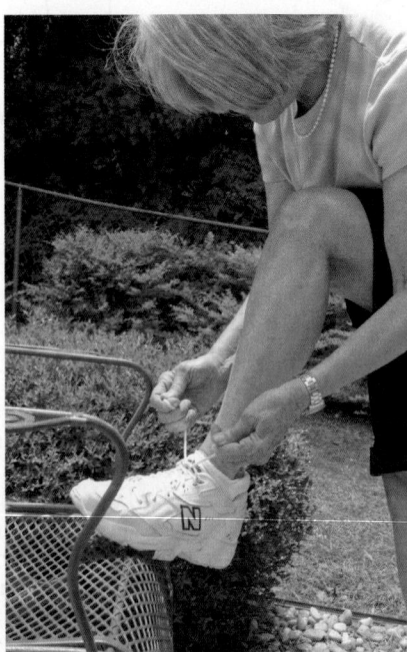

Physical activity, drinking plenty of water, and adding fiber and bulk to their diet with fresh fruits and vegetables are healthy ways seniors can assure good bowel patterns.

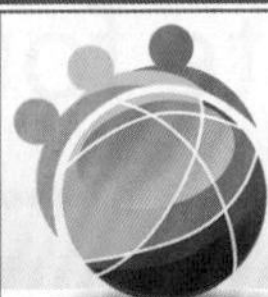

DISPLAY 24.3 MEAL MANAGEMENT CONSIDERATIONS

- Complete a safety check with the older adult to assess the ability to operate stoves and microwave ovens. Include the elder's ability to reach and put things on and off stove burners.
- Arrange cupboards so commonly used items can be reached from an easy standing level.
- Suggest use of turntables and long-handled "grabbers" while discouraging use of step stools or ladders.
- Assess the elder's typical meal for quality and availability—can be accomplished for all meals by doing a 24-hour dietary recall —begin with the most recent meal and work backward.
- To ensure that elders eat an appropriate number of times a day, suggest that they "eat by the clock" or with a certain TV show.
- Help older adults build support system for sharing grocery shopping, cooking, and meals.
- Suggest they bake once a week for an activity or shop with another elder.
- Suggest buying convenience foods, making sure they have nutritional value, such as frozen vegetables or dinners.
- Consider community resources to assist with shopping, transportation, or meal preparation as needed. Keeping a continuous shopping list helps elders to remember needed grocery items and provides a reference if someone offers to assist with shopping.
- Help elders consider increasing socialization by eating together with friends—rotating among three to four friends each week or eating out with friends and selecting restaurants that are physically and financially accessible.

Exercise Needs

Older adults need to exercise; in fact, they thrive when exercise is incorporated into their daily routine (National Institute on Aging, 2010a). Research demonstrates that exercise and increased physical activity have multiple benefits for the older adult including arthritis relief, restoration of balance and reduction of falls, strengthening of bone, proper weight maintenance, and improved glucose control. It also contributes to a healthy state of mind, improved sleep, and reduces the risk of heart disease. (CDC, 2011i).

Aging does not and should not involve passivity; instead, physical activity and movement contribute to the quality of intellectual and physical performance in old age. Exercise, such as a daily walk, can keep muscles in good tone, enhance circulation, and promote mental health and adequate sleep (CDC, 2011e; Healthfinder.gov, 2011). Exercise may occur in connection with such activities as homemaking chores, gardening, hobbies, or recreation and sports. Often, such physical outlets are enjoyed in the company of other people, meeting social and emotional needs as well as physical ones. Even among the very old, an exercise routine that includes activities that improve strength, flexibility, and coordination may indirectly, but effectively, decrease the incidence of osteoporotic fractures by lessening the likelihood of falling. Resistance training (with small dumbbells or resistance bands), along with either tai chi or regular walking, has been shown to increase muscle strength, stability, and functional ability among seniors (Healthfinder.gov, n.d.).

Public health nurses can encourage exercise among clients and examine factors that prevent them from regularly exercising. Physical disabilities need not be a barrier to exercise CDC, 2011f).

Sleep

Sleep is another new area of focus in *Healthy People 2020*. Sleep is essential for health, productivity, energy, and emotional balance. In older adults, adequate sleep is necessary to fight off infection and support the metabolism of sugar to prevent diabetes or to work effectively and safely. Sleep timing and duration affect a number of endocrine, metabolic, and neurological functions that are critical to the maintenance of individual health. Untreated, sleep disorders and chronic short sleep are associated with an increased risk of heart disease, high blood pressure, obesity, diabetes, and all-cause mortality.

Some changes in sleep are natural with aging. The body produces lower levels of growth hormone, resulting in a decrease in slow wave or deep sleep. Illness often means more fragmented sleep (more rapid sleep cycles) and more awakenings between sleep cycles. As circadian rhythms (the internal clock that tells you when to sleep and when to wake up) change, the older adult may want to go to sleep earlier in the evening and wake up earlier in the morning. If bedtimes are not adjusted to these changes, the older adult may find it difficult to fall and stay asleep.

Older adults also tend to wake up more often during the night. Consequently, they may have to spend longer in bed at night to get the hours of sleep needed, or may have to make up the shortfall by taking a nap during the day. In most cases, such sleep changes are normal and don't indicate a sleep problem (HelpGuide, 2011j). While sleep requirements vary from person to person, most healthy adults tend to require between 7.5 to 9 hours of sleep per night to function at their best (HelpGuide, 2011j).

The cognitive and medical consequences of untreated sleep disorders decrease health-related quality of life, contribute to functional limitations and loss of independence, and are associated with an increased risk of death from any cause (*Healthy People 2020, 2010b*).

Economic Security Needs, Poverty

Economic security is another major need for older adults. Worrying about finances is often one of the most debilitating factors of old age. Fearing the potential cost of major illness and not wanting to be a burden on family or friends, many older people conserve their limited finances by establishing frugal eating patterns, using health resources sparingly, not taking their medications or only taking medications in partial doses, reducing costs for home heating and cooling, and, in general, spending little on themselves. People sometimes have to choose between food, housing, and medications. Another factor that is driving up the cost of health care for the aging population is that many clients wait until they are truly ill before seeking health care. In waiting for conditions to improve or go away, they often miss out on important preventive health measures and community-based programs that can maximize function and help the client maintain health at a higher level. Too often, the fear—let alone the reality—of financial difficulties prevents older adults from leading full and active lives.

For older adults today who have lived many years past retirement and perhaps have not planned for sufficient financial security to maintain them throughout these additional, unexpected years, the fears are not unfounded. Putting older people in touch with appropriate community resources can do much to relieve the source of that stress and anxiety. The CHN can also provide information about potential consumer fraud (e.g., telemarketing schemes) targeted to elderly. This is a form of financial abuse perpetrated by criminals who have no personal relationship with the victims, and seniors with retirement income, savings accounts, or property are disproportionately targeted. Losses from this type of fraud can wipe out a lifetime of savings and leave the older adult feeling foolish and helpless.

Psychosocial Needs

All human beings have psychosocial needs that must be met for their lives to be rich and fulfilling. Without healthy relationships with other people, life can be very lonely and lacking in quality. With advancing age, the psychosocial issues are many. A major issue that confronts the majority of our aging population is coping with multiple losses. In addition, maintaining independence, social interaction, companionship, and purpose is necessary for a healthy old age. Older adults who have maintained good health and have developed a supportive system of family and friends have more fulfilled lives. Programs such as Friendly Visitors, where volunteers regularly meet with isolated seniors either in their homes or long-term care facilities, can be an effective method of increasing social support for those who have no family members nearby.

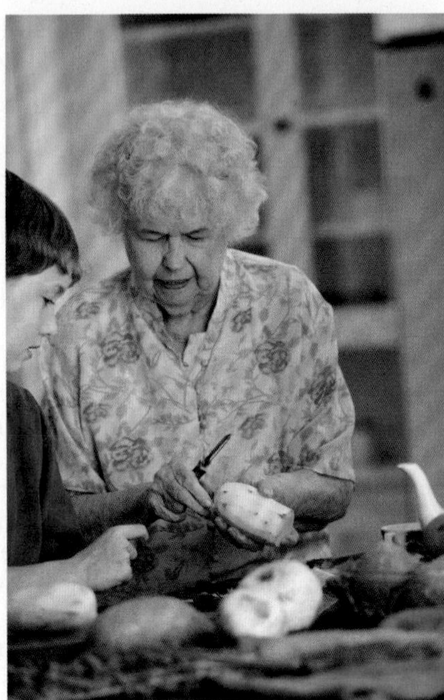

A supportive system of family and friends helps older adults meet their psychosocial needs.

Spiritual Needs

Holistic nursing is a hallmark of community and public health nursing. This means a focus on body, mind, and spirit. The word spirit comes from the Latin meaning "breath" and refers to the core of an individual, the part that gives meaning to life (New World Encyclopedia, 2011). Spirituality is far more encompassing than religion, though we often see the two used interchangeably. Many people think that spirituality and religion are the same. Religion and spirituality may exist together, but as Twycross (1988) wrote "everyone has a spiritual component, but not everyone is religious" (as cited in Center on Aging Studies Without Walls, n.d., para. 4.). Religion is generally recognized to be the practical expression of spirituality, or the organization, rituals, and practice of one's beliefs. Religion includes specific beliefs and practices, while spirituality is far broader.

Religion and associated activities are common among older adults. Older adults may turn to spirituality and religion when they meet difficult life-changing events and experience personal losses. Their reaction to these events and losses may cause distress and temporary or chronic psychological conditions. Many older persons report that religion helps them cope or adapt with losses or difficulties. While other sources of well-being decline, religion may become more important over time. At the time when religious support is most needed, older persons are less able to access it (because of failing health, immobility, or lack of transportation).

Different individuals within cultures have differing philosophies and practices of spirituality but derive similar positive outcomes. For many, old age may be a time of life review. These years become a time of redefining self without the association of lifelong friends, spouses, or work that helped define the self during decades of adult life. This may be a time of reevaluation of what give meaning and satisfaction.

Faith-based nursing is one of the community nursing roles that epitomizes this holistic approach of caring for their clients, many of whom are older adults (see Chapter 31). As Ebersole (1998) elucidates in a classic text, nurses can support the spiritual dimension of clients in times of difficulty by developing the following skills:

- Listening
- Being aware of signs of mental health problems and urge professional help
- Sharing concern and observations
- Providing privacy
- Reassuring the value of the person
- Allowing decisions to be made
- Accepting without judgment
- Helping express religious, spiritual, or social needs
- Recognizing cultural differences
- Keeping separate values and spiritual beliefs that are different
- Referring to professionals when needs are beyond listener's ability to help
- Using humor as appropriate

Coping with Multiple Losses

Older adults may experience multiple losses, including loss of income and prestige from a career once practiced or the economic stability of an enjoyable job, loss of space due to replacement of a larger residence by a much smaller home or apartment, and reductions in health and vitality that may result in limited movement or pain as a daily concern or may necessitate another move to a more dependent living environment. Repetitive losses occur as significant others, relatives, friends, and acquaintances die. There are no right or wrong ways to grieve, but there are healthy ways to cope with the pain. Assisting older adults to cope with these losses is an important role of the public health nurse. To do this, PHNs need to be aware of some of the facts about grief.

First, it is not true that ignoring pain will help it go away faster. In the long run, ignoring pain will only make it worse. It is necessary to face grief and deal with it in order to experience real healing. Feeling sad, frightened, or lonely is a normal reaction to loss. Second, crying does not mean you are weak or do not feel a loss. Crying is a normal response to loss, but this does not mean that someone who does not cry does not feel the loss. It may just be shown in a different way. Third, there is no set time for grieving. It will differ from person to person (HelpGuide, 2011c).

The most important tip for assisting older adults in coping with grief and loss is making sure they have the support of other people. Wherever it comes from, connecting with others helps the healing process.

There are five stages of grief: denial, anger, bargaining, depression, and finally acceptance. Inadequate coping with the compounding losses can make an older person believe that life holds no meaning. Depression may be a difficult problem for older adults. Social and emotional withdrawal can often occur, as can suicide. Although older populations have a much lower rate of suicide attempts than younger age groups do, the rate of completed suicide is high. As mentioned earlier, White men have the highest rate of suicide death. Although they comprise only 12% of the US population, people age 65 and older accounted for 16% of suicide deaths in 2004. More than 14.3 of every 100,000 people age 65 and older died by suicide in 2004, higher than the rate of about 11 per 100,000 in the general population (National Institute of Mental Health, 2007). Because most persons who commit suicide have visited their primary care provider in the last month of their lives, recognition and treatment of depression in health care settings is a promising way to prevent suicide in this age group.

Mortality after bereavement is high and can sometimes be prevented through nursing intervention. Loss and the mourning process among elders have been examined in many studies. It has been found that the ability to mourn prior states of one's self and the past is crucial to successful aging. Life review can be liberating and can provide energy for current living, including planning for the future. In one study, higher levels of self-affirmation, confidence, self-esteem, and life satisfaction were noted (Chiang, Lu, Chu, Chang, & Chou, 2008). Although men and women experience similar levels of depression during early bereavement, it is often more difficult for men to seek and receive social support. Depression has been found to increase the risk of death for those who have lost a spouse, independent of age or bereavement. The death of a spouse has effects upon the health of the surviving spouse, and depression can exacerbate these effects. In addition to preventing early deaths after the loss of a spouse, the greater goal for the nurse in promoting successful aging can be accomplished when the nurse recognizes the significance of accepting all the losses of aging. The loss of a spouse is much more frequent for women than for men. With this knowledge, a woman can age more successfully by planning for the future through anticipatory guidance, with the help of a CHN. Many women can expect to live alone for up to 20 years at the end of their life for several reasons. Women have a longer life expectancy than men, and in most cultures, they marry men older than themselves. The nurse can help widowed seniors make these years meaningful and as healthy as possible.

Maintaining Independence

Relatively few (4.1%) older adults are institutionalized in nursing homes. The vast majority live in the community setting, with more than half (58.4%) living with their spouse and another 30.1% living alone. With increasing age, women are more likely to live alone. By age 75, 49% of women live alone. The proportion of those requiring nursing home care also increases with age; 0.9% of persons 65 to 74 live in nursing homes, compared to 3.5% of those 75 to 84, and the percentage rising to 14.3% for those 85 and older (Administration on Aging, 2010a). Alternative housing arrangements are also available (e.g., group-living situations for older adults in which many types of housing and care possibilities are offered). This concept is not new, but these centers are being built now in greater numbers to meet the needs of a growing segment of the older adult population. These situations are well suited to those who desire such comprehensive living choices and have the financial means for the housing and care arrangements provided.

The average age of older adults in residential care is getting higher and is currently about 85 years. Such facilities typically are not chosen by the hardy older adult or by totally independent young elders, who prefer to receive services that allow them to remain in their own homes—commonly referred to as *aging in place* (Pynoos, Nishita, Cicero, & Caraviello, 2008; Sabia, 2008). Despite popular notions, only a small minority of older Americans move to warmer climates after retirement (National Association of Area Agencies on Aging, 2010). Many older adults who are vigorous and functioning independently live in their own homes. Only about 4.1% live in places such as skilled nursing facilities, extended care facilities, supervised living facilities, and AD centers, and not all of these are permanent residents (Administration on Aging, 2010a). Many are recovering from illnesses or undergoing rehabilitation after an injury or surgery and will return to their living situation in the community within a matter of weeks.

Older people need independence. As much as possible, they need to make their own decisions and manage their own lives. Those who stay independent are happier. Even those with activity limitations because of disability can still exercise decision-making options about many, if not most, aspects of their daily living. Unfortunately, because many older adults have chronic diseases, it can be more difficult for them to maintain their independence. It is estimated that 75% of those over age 65 have one chronic illness, and 50% have at least two chronic illnesses (CDC, 2011d). The need for autonomy—to be able to assert oneself as a separate individual—is important for all people. Independence helps to meet the need for self-respect and dignity. A self-management program, developed by a federal agency, is being utilized to prevent or delay disability among older adults. The Chronic Disease Self-Management Program teaches patients to better manage their medications and symptoms and to maintain greater functional ability. Those who have participated in this program have shown better communication with their physicians and fewer physician visits and hospitalizations, as well as better coping and symptom management and more energy and increased exercise 6 months later (CDC, 2010e). This program has shown beneficial results for nearly a decade (Jerant, Kravitz, Moore-Hill, & Franks, 2008). The good news is that the percentage of older adults becoming severely disabled has been gradually declining for over a decade, thought to be due to better awareness of the dangers of smoking, the need for better diet and exercise, new medications for cardiovascular and other diseases, and advances in eye surgery.

Maintaining Independence

Older people need independence, and those who stay independent are happier. As much as possible, they need to make their own decisions and manage their own lives. Even those with activity limitations because of disability can still exercise decision-making options about many, if not most, aspects of their daily living. Unfortunately, because many older adults have chronic diseases, it can be more difficult for them to maintain their independence.

The number of US adults reporting a disability is increasing; 47.5 million US adults report a disability. More than one third of these are aging baby boomers. Arthritis is the most common cause of disability. The number of people reporting a disability increases with age, with women having a higher prevalence of disability than men at all ages. Given the size of the baby boomer generation, the number of adults with disability is likely to increase dramatically as the baby boomers enter into higher-risk age groups over the next 20 years (CDC, 2009c).

The need for autonomy—to be able to assert oneself as a separate individual—is important for all people. Independence helps to meet the need for self-respect and dignity. They need to have their ideas and suggestions heard and acted upon, and they ought to be addressed by their preferred names in a respectful tone of voice. Respect for the older adult is not a strong value in American society, but it is highly valued in Asian, Italian, Hispanic, and Native American cultures. Older people represent a rich resource of wisdom, experience, and patience that is often unacknowledged in the United States.

Interaction, Companionship, and Purpose

Older people need companionship and social interaction, particularly if they live alone. The company of other people and the companionship of a household pet offer avenues for expression and response and add meaning to life (Owen, 2007). As people age, their social networks weaken, and CHNs and others can help to improve their psychosocial health by working at individual, family, and community levels (Chong, 2007). The problem is of greatest significance for women, who outnumber men considerably in the later years and who more frequently live alone.

It is also important for older adults without companions to discover and develop a friendship with someone who can be considered a *confidante*, someone in whom the older adult can confide, share reflections on the past, and trust. It could be a close friend, a sibling, a son or daughter, or an acquaintance. This person is usually seen daily or talked with on the telephone each week. In particular, mothers and daughters form confidant bonds. Many women consider a sibling a confidant, especially if that person lives close by; this is especially true for childless and single women.

Meaningful activity is another need of the older adult that adds purpose to life. Some kind of active role in community life is essential for mental health, satisfaction, and self-esteem. These activities can range from involvement in hobbies, such as gardening or crafts, to volunteer work or even full-time employment. Examples include the federally supported Foster Grandparents and Senior Companions programs, which engage more than 5 million Americans in service (The Corporation for National and Community Service, 2011b). These older adults work part-time offering companionship and guidance to handicapped children, the terminally ill, and other people in need.

Additional volunteering opportunities abound. Internationally, many older professionals join the Peace Corps, which was initiated in the early 1960s. In this program, people of all ages work for 2-year periods in global communities that are in need of services to improve personal health, education, environment, and the larger community (Peace Corps, 2009). On the national level, the AmeriCorps program is similar but with a 10-month commitment volunteering with local and national nonprofit and government agencies. Retired people can volunteer to help others, donating their skills at a time in their lives when they are in transition from employment to retirement or to fill active retirement years (AmeriCorps, 2011). Through the Corporation for National and Community Service, older adults can volunteer in the Retired and Senior Volunteer Program (RSVP), or the Foster Grandparent Program. The Senior Companion Program engages seniors in a bevy of activities designed to improve people's lives and the environment (Senior Corps, 2011; The Corporation for National and Community Service, 2011b). Environmental Alliance for Senior Involvement (EASI) is a nonprofit coalition of aging, volunteer, and environmental organizations that began in 1991. It sponsors various environmentally focused programs, such as assisting the Hawk Mountain Sanctuary to protect birds of prey, or monitoring streams and other waterways for cleanliness.

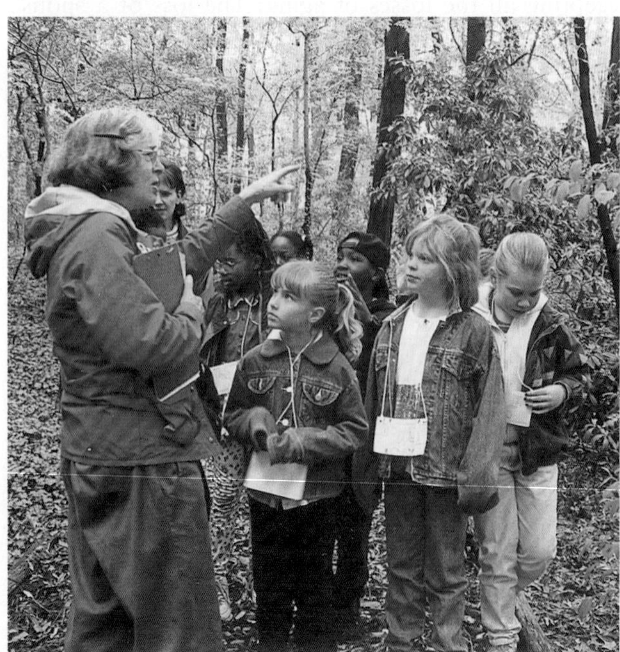

Volunteering can be a rewarding experience for older adults.

Many older adults choose not to engage in long-term volunteering, and other programs are more appropriate for them. Elderhostel, Inc., the not-for-profit world leader in lifelong learning since 1975, is the creator of Road Scholar educational adventures providing high-quality, affordable, educational adventures for adults who are 55 years of age and older. It is the nation's first and the world's largest education and travel organization for older adults, offering "more than 7,000 learning adventures in all 50 states and more than 150 countries" (Road Scholar, 2011, para. 1). Their theme-based, short-term (3 days to 3 weeks) educational programs are infused with a spirit of camaraderie and adventure. The success of this program is based on recognizing that learning is a lifelong process that is rewarding at any age—and it is learning without any test or term papers! Elderhostel is inspired by the youth hostels and folk schools of Europe but guided by the needs and interests of older citizens.

Safety Needs

People of all ages have safety needs, and safety issues are a major concern for older adults and the CHNs who work with them. Several areas of focus are discussed here: personal health and safety, home safety, and community safety.

Personal health and safety includes three major areas: immunizations, prevention of falls, and drug safety. Immunizations are not just for children. Older adults are at risk not only of contracting influenza or pneumonia but also of dying from them. According to the CDC, in 2007, influenza accounted for close to 46,000 annual deaths among those aged 65 and above (CDC, 2011c). Although the overall influenza immunization rate among older adults has steadily increased from between 15% and 20% before 1980 to 68.9% in 2007, some seniors still refuse to have yearly vaccinations for a disease that causes more than 200,000 Americans to be hospitalized and about 36,000 deaths (National Foundation for Infectious Diseases, 2008).

Immunizations

The CDC recommends that all adults over 50 receive three immunizations, for influenza, pneumonia, and shingles (CDC, 2010k, n.d.). While influenza does kill an estimated 36,000 per year, in older adults it is the exacerbating effect on other conditions (e.g., pneumonia, congestive heart failure, or chronic obstructive pulmonary disease [COPD]) that makes flu of great concern in older adults (CDC, 2011b). In 2008, 67% of older adults reported having a flu shot. There remain, however, racial and ethnic disparities in senior vaccination rates. While 70% of non-Hispanic Whites received flu shots, 55% of Hispanics and only 50% of non-Hispanic Blacks received flu shots (The Federal Interagency Forum on Aging Related Statistics, 2010). These racial and ethnic disparities were found even in groups who are usually most likely to avail themselves of health care services (e.g., those with higher education levels, those who have more frequent visits to health care providers). The reasons for the continuing disparity are not well understood but are thought to be related to differences in care settings (e.g., lower vaccination rates with particular providers), lack of trust in providers, and communication problems, especially with those who do not speak English well. When PHNs work with seniors, it is important to include outreach efforts, such as culturally targeting communication, reaching out to those providers serving this population, and offering vaccination clinics in underserved sections of the community.

Pneumococcal vaccine coverage rates have also increased steadily from 38.4% in 1995 to 66.8% in 2009, but improvement is still needed (CDC, n.d.). While this is a great improvement, it does not reach the *Healthy People 2010* goal of 90% vaccine coverage for a disease that causes more than 200,000 Americans to be hospitalized and about 36,000 deaths (CDC, 2010i, 2010j; National Foundation of Infectious Diseases, 2008). In 2008, 60% of older adults had never received a pneumonia vaccine. Similar to flu vaccination, certain racial and ethnic groups remain substantially below those of the general population. For instance, only 45% of African Americans and 36% of Hispanics had a pneumonia vaccination (The Federal Interagency Forum on Aging Related Statistics, 2010). Attempts to improve immunization coverage involve changing provider knowledge, attitudes, and behavior through reminders and standing orders, so that "missed opportunities" when seeing clients are prevented. One simple method is to ask clients about their beliefs and fears related to immunizations and then to address them directly and honestly. Additional opportunities for vaccinating people exist beyond the primary care setting, as CHNs are well aware. People can be reached during emergency department visits, at neighborhood and senior centers, at religious facilities, and in other settings where elders may gather. Regardless of the site, a method for tracking and communicating vaccinations is needed so that vaccination information may be documented and shared with the elder's primary care provider. Clinicians often fail to document immunizations for adult patients. Immunizations protect more than the at-risk population; they protect society as a whole. People of any age with a chronic illness, such as heart disease, diabetes, or chronic respiratory disease, and people older than 65 years of age should be encouraged to receive an annual flu vaccine and the pneumonia vaccine every 5 years.

Shingles is caused by the varicella zoster virus (VZV), the same virus that causes chickenpox. Anyone who has had chickenpox can develop shingles because VZV remains in the nerve cells of the body after the chickenpox infection clears, and VZV can reappear years later causing shingles. Shingles is a painful localized skin rash often with blisters. The disease most commonly occurs in people 50 years old or older, people who have medical conditions that keep the immune system from working properly, or people who receive immunosuppressive drugs (CDC, 2011h). CDC recommends Zostavax for use in people 60 years old and older to prevent shingles. This is a one-time vaccination. There is no maximum age for getting the shingles vaccine (CDC, 2011h).

Fall Prevention

Each year, approximately one third of people over age 65 experience a fall (CDC, 2010h). Falls and the resulting injuries can have a dramatic impact on self-confidence and independence, often leading to decreased mobility, increased debility, and diminished quality of life, as well as additional strain on health services. The injuries received from a fall can result in death, disability, nursing home admission, and direct medical costs. In 2007, a total of 18,000 older adults died from injuries related to falls (CDC, 2010h). This rate of death from falls has risen sharply in the last decade. In 2009, 2.2 million falls in older adults required visits to the emergency room. The cost of these falls was over $19 billion in 2000, $179 million for fatal falls and $19 billion for the nonfatal ones (CDC, 2010h). Falls cause the majority of hip fractures, which can often result in long-term functional impairments that may require admission to a nursing home for up to a year or more. Causative factors involve both environmental hazards (e.g., lack of handrails and nonslip surfaces) and host issues (e.g., cognition, vision). Fall prevention that involves education, strengthening and balance exercises, medication evaluation, and environmental improvements is an important function of the CHN. Use of a home safety checklist can give the nurse a baseline of information from which to begin teaching and providing interventions to ensure continued safety for many independent seniors who choose to remain in their homes (see Display 24.4).

Medications

Medications are often prescribed to control the effects of chronic conditions, and older adults' bodies can react differently than those of younger people (on whom most new drugs are tested). A significant safety issue for the older adult arises from the use of prescription and over-the-counter (OTC) drugs. Problems can arise from a single problem or a combination of issues such as (1) number of medications taken daily, (2) absorption rate of medications, (3) drug interactions, and (4) side effects.

Older adults often have multiple chronic diseases for which they take prescription medications. It is not unusual for older people to be taking 4 to 6 medications daily and fill 13 prescriptions or more each year. While older adults comprise only 13% of the population, they account for approximately one third of all medications prescribed in the United States (National Institute on Drug Abuse [NIDA], 2011). In addition, many older adults take OTC medications and/or dietary supplements.

Older adults often receive multiple prescriptions from multiple providers and sometimes from multiple pharmacies. This puts them in danger of receiving double doses of the same or similar medications. This can happen, for instance, when one health care provider prescribes a name-brand medication and a second one writes a prescription for the same medication but in generic form. Often, the person has no idea that they are taking two doses of the same medication Also, common medications like acetaminophen can be found in a variety of OTC and prescription medications (e.g., cold remedies, arthritis topical ointments), and inadvertent overdosing can be a real problem.

Absorption time is usually slower in older adults, and distribution changes as drugs may stay in the body longer due to a higher percentage of fat stores, along with reduced liver and kidney function that affect clearance time.

Most adverse drug events (ADEs) are due to drug interactions. The greater number of medications taken, the more likely there will be side effects. Multiple medications or complicated drug regimens for many older people can lead to unexpected and dangerous drug interactions or drug–disease interactions; sometimes, medications are prescribed for symptoms that may actually be a side effect of an original medication.

Medication side effects or drug interactions can lead to falls and further disability. Older adults need education about the drugs they take and their possible effects. They also need proper supervision of their overall medication intake, including complementary and alternative therapies (e.g., herbal treatments) and OTC drugs. It is also important for all seniors to keep a list of their current medications and doses and to have this available in the event of an emergency. However, many hospitals and providers prefer the "brown bag method" of determining accurate medication information; patients are asked to bring everything they take with them. This is an area in which the CHN can intervene very effectively and with much success (see Display 24.5).

The consequences of polypharmacy are enormous. Approximately 30% of hospital admissions of older adults are drug related (Marek & Antle, 2011). Each year, in hospitals alone, there are 28,000 cases of life-threatening heart toxicity from adverse reactions to digoxin, the most commonly used form of digitalis (i.e., drug that regulates the speed and strength of heart beats) in older adults. Since as many as 40% or more of these people are using this drug unnecessarily, many of these injuries are preventable (Public Citizen's Health Research Group, 2011). Each year 41,000 older adults are hospitalized—and 3,300 of these people die—from ulcers caused by NSAIDs (i.e., nonsteroidal anti-inflammatory drugs, usually for treatment of arthritis). Each year 32,000 older adults suffer from hip fractures attributable to drug-induced falls, resulting in more than 1,500 deaths. A study in long-term care showed that polypharmacy was a risk factor for falls (Baranzini et al., 2009). In another study, the main categories of drugs responsible for the falls leading to hip fractures were sleeping pills and minor tranquilizers (30%), anti-psychotic drugs (52%), and antidepressants (17%). All of these categories of drugs are often prescribed

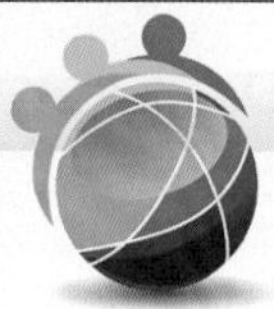

DISPLAY 24.4 GUIDELINES FOR ASSESSING THE SAFETY OF THE ENVIRONMENT

Illumination and Color Contrast

- Is the lighting adequate but not glare producing?
- Are the light switches easy to reach and manipulate?
- Can lights be turned on before entering rooms?
- Are night-lights used in appropriate places?
- Are there working flashlights close by (bedroom, kitchen, bath, living room)?
- Is color contrast adequate between objects such as a chair and floor?

Hazards

- Are there throw rugs, highly polished floors, or other hazardous floor coverings?
- If area rugs are used, do they have a nonslip backing and are the edges tacked to the floor?
- Are there cords, clutter, or other obstacles in pathways?
- Is there a pet that is likely to be running underfoot?

Furniture

- Are chairs the right height and depth for the person?
- Do the chairs have armrests?
- Are tables stable and of the appropriate height?
- Is small furniture placed well away from pathways?

Stairways

- Is lighting adequate?
- Are there light switches at the top and bottom of the stairs?
- Are there securely fastened handrails on both sides of the stairway?
- Are all the steps even?
- Are the treads nonskid?
- Should colored tape be used to mark the edges of the steps, particularly the top and bottom steps?

Bathroom

- Are grab bars placed appropriately for the tub and toilet?
- Does the tub have skid-proof strips or a rubber mat in the bottom?
- Has the person considered using a tub seat?
- Is the height of the toilet seat appropriate?
- Has the person considered using an elevated toilet seat?
- Does the color of the toilet seat contrast with surrounding colors?
- Is toilet paper within easy reach?

Temperature

- Is the temperature of the room(s) comfortable?
- Can the person read the markings on the thermostat and adjust it appropriately?
- During cold months, is the room temperature high enough to prevent hypothermia?
- During hot weather, is the room temperature cool enough to prevent hyperthermia?

Overall Safety

- How does the person obtain objects from hard-to-reach places?
- How does the person change overhead light bulbs?
- Are doorways wide enough to accommodate assistive devices?
- Do door thresholds create hazardous conditions?
- Are telephones easily accessible, especially for emergency calls?
- Would it be helpful to use a cordless portable phone or a cellular phone?
- Would it be helpful to have some emergency call system available?
- Does the person wear sturdy shoes with nonskid soles?
- Are smoke alarms present and operational?
- Is there a carbon monoxide detector (if the house has gas appliances)?
- Does the person keep a list of emergency numbers by the phone?
- Does the person have an emergency exit plan in the event of fire?

Bedroom

- Is the height of the bed appropriate?
- Is the mattress firm at the edges to provide enough support for sitting?
- If the bed has wheels, are they locked securely?
- Would side rails be a help or a hazard?
- When side rails are in the down position, are they completely out of the way?
- Is the pathway between the bedroom and bathroom clear of objects and adequately illuminated, particularly at night?
- Would a bedside commode be useful, especially at night?
- Does the person have sufficient physical and cognitive ability to turn on a light before getting out of bed?
- Is furniture positioned to allow safe use of assistive devices for ambulation?
- Is a telephone situated near the bed?

Kitchen

- Are storage areas used to the best advantage (e.g., are objects that are most frequently used in the most accessible places)?
- Are appliance cords kept out of the way?
- Are nonslip mats used in front of the sink?
- Are the markings on stoves and other appliances clearly visible?
- Does the person know how to use the microwave oven and other appliances safely?

Assistive Devices

- What assistive devices are used?
- Is a call light available, and does the person know how to use it?
- Would the person benefit from any assistive devices that are not being used?
- Are assistive devices being used safely and properly, or do they present additional hazards?

Adapted from Miller, C. A. (2008). *Nursing for wellness in older adults* (5th ed.). Philadelphia, PA: Lippincott, Williams & Wilkins.

DISPLAY 24.5 PROMOTING POLYPHARMACY SAFETY IN THE OLDER ADULT THROUGH MEDICATION REVIEW

- Ask the client to bring all of his or her medications for you to examine.
- List all medications, along with dosage and time taken.
- Note the pharmacy or pharmacies where each prescription originates. Has more than one physician prescribed medications for the client?
- Ask about medical conditions and diseases for which he or she takes medications. Does the client have a clear understanding of each medication and its benefits and potential side effects?
- Ask the client for which condition or disease each medication is prescribed. Does the client understand the basic disease process and how the prescribed medication works?
- Are there duplicate medications (e.g., contain the same active ingredient, both a generic and a proprietary form)?
- What are the most common side effects of each medication?
- Is the dosage prescribed within the recommended range?
- Is the client experiencing any symptoms of potential drug interactions (e.g., nausea, headaches, dizziness)?
- Is one medication being used to treat possible side effects of another medication?
- Ask if the client takes all medications as prescribed. Are any doses or medications skipped?
- Does the client use a daily or weekly pill box? Does the client have some system of checking off when medications have been taken each day?
- Is the client taking any medications that were prescribed for someone else?
- Is the client taking any over-the-counter or herbal remedies?

Adapted from: Hanlon, J., & Schmader, K. (2010). What types of inappropriate prescribing predict adverse drug reactions in older adults? *The Annals of Pharmacotherapy, 44*(6), 1110–1111; Wooten, J., & Galavis, J. (2005). *Polypharmacy: Keeping the older adult safe.* RNWeb. http://www.rnweb.com/rnweb/content/printContentPopup.jsp?id=172920; Bushardt, R., & Jones, K. (2005). Nine key questions to address polypharmacy in the older adult. *Journal of the American Academy of Physician Assistants.* Retrieved from http://jaapa.com/issues/j20050501/articles/polypharm0505.htm

unnecessarily, especially in older adults (Public Citizen's Health Research Group, 2011).

Two million older Americans are addicted or at risk of addiction to minor tranquilizers or sleeping pills because they have used them daily for at least one year, even though there is no acceptable evidence that the tranquilizers are effective for more than 4 months (Public Citizen's Health Research Group, 2011).

Safety in the Community

Safety can involve many things, such as pedestrian and driving issues, crime and fear of crime against elders, and environmental factors such as sun exposure, pollution, heat, and cold.

Because of age-related changes in vision, hearing, mobility, and the effects of polypharmacy, elders are at risk in the community as pedestrians and as drivers. Automobile crashes and pedestrian injuries can be life-threatening events when elders are involved. As pedestrians, elders must be increasingly vigilant to traffic patterns, sidewalk irregularities, and the possibility of being a victim of street crime. Often out of necessity and pride, elders drive longer than their abilities permit. As people age, they are more prone to lapses in memory and attention, problems with depth perception and gauging distance of cars in traffic, reduced manual dexterity and reaction time, and impairment of other skills critical to driving safety (HelpGuide, 2011h). Older adults are more likely to receive traffic citations and be involved in an automobile accident than younger people. Fatal car crashes rise sharply after a person turns 70 (HelpGuide, 2011h). In 2008, more than 5,500 older adults were killed and more than 183,000 were injured in motor vehicle crashes. This amounts to 15 older adults killed and 500 injured in crashes on average every day. There were 33 million licensed older drivers in 2009, which is a 23% increase from 1999 (CDC, 2011g). Per mile traveled, fatal crash rates increase starting at age 75 and rise more notably after age 80. This is largely due to increased susceptibility to injury and medical complications among older drivers rather than an increased tendency to get into crashes (CDC, 2011g).

Because they generally have chronic diseases and are often frail, elder drivers are more susceptible to injury than younger drivers (American Occupational Therapy Association, 2011). Stopping driving is usually a difficult and painful decision for the elder to make. Some communities offer specialized driving classes for elders who want to continue to drive for as long as possible. At times, the car keys may have to be taken from the elder for his or her own safety and that of others. This may be necessary especially with elders who have dementia, AD, uncorrectable vision problems, or stroke-related physical or cognitive after effects. Only 10 states require mandatory eye testing for drivers over age 65, just 5 states require seniors to renew their drivers' licenses in person, and 2 states require a mandatory road test. Public health nurses may need to consult with older adults and their families about determining when it is time for elders to stop driving.

DISPLAY 24.6 REDUCING THE FEAR OF CRIME

- Allow elder adults time to discuss their fears of crime.
- Facilitate a realistic self-assessment of their ability to avoid crime and to defend themselves.
- Teach basic safety and security techniques.
- Correct the elder's sensory losses if possible, such as by getting a hearing aid or glasses.
- Correct a physical disability if possible, such as by treating the pain of arthritis or obtaining physical therapy.
- Facilitate access to safe, reliable, and affordable transportation.
- Identify family members, friends, neighbors, or caregivers who can support efforts to leave the home on a more regular basis.
- Encourage an elder to make a daily telephone or e-mail contact with at least one supportive person.
- Encourage the elder to get to know his or her neighbors.
- Encourage elders to travel and conduct community activities and errands together.
- Encourage participation in local senior centers and other community-based programs.
- Refer to alternative housing options available for older adults.
- Provide information on local services that assist and support crime victims.

Actual crime against older adults in the community is lower than any other age group of the population: 2.8 per 1,000 cases for those 65 and over versus 12 to 48.4 per 1,000 for those 50 to 64 years old and 20 to 24 years old, respectively (U.S. Department of Justice, 2008). However, the general public often perceives elders' fear of crime as a major issue. Display 24.6 lists client-centered nursing interventions designed to reduce fear among older adults and empower them to feel safer in their communities.

Environmental factors can have an effect on the health and safety of elders when they are outside. Sun exposure, pollution, and exposure to heat and cold can have negative effects on older adults. They are vulnerable, as are infants and children, to climatic changes and should take a variety of preventive measures. These may include use of a sunblock when gardening, reading, or walking outside for longer than 10 minutes, even on days with an overcast sky. Other measures include staying indoors on days when the air quality is poor or there is an air safety alert. Drinking additional fluids, wearing protective covering, and limiting outdoor activities and exposure on days with elevated temperatures are also warranted. Conversely, limiting outdoor exposure time and wearing appropriate winter clothing, especially layers of clothes, on cold, snowy, or icy days are important. Although sun exposure is beneficial for vitamin D production, older adults need to be careful about limiting their exposure. Teaching geographically and seasonally appropriate safety precautions is the responsibility of the CHN providing services to groups of older adults in the community.

Secondary Prevention

Secondary prevention focuses on early detection of disease and prompt intervention (see Chapter 1). Much of the CHN's time is spent in educating the community on preventive measures and positive health behaviors. This includes encouraging individuals to obtain routine screening for diseases such as hypertension, diabetes, or cancer, which, if identified early, can be treated successfully. Many nurses, working in collaboration with community agencies, are in positions to establish screening programs based on the desires and demographics of the community and agency focus, making them accessible to the population being served.

Older adults need to be encouraged to follow the routine health screening schedule prescribed by their clinic or health care provider. The health screening schedule described in Table 24-1 was developed by the largest health maintenance organization (HMO) in the world, serving millions of clients, and is presented here as a guide. The United States Preventive Services Task Force (USPSTF) (U.S. Preventive Services Task Force, 2010b) proposed a more comprehensive view of interventions and recommendations for the periodic health examination of people older than 65 years of age. They have identified age-specific evidence-based preventive services guidelines that are outlined in Display 24.7.

Diseases Common in Old Age

Alzheimer's Disease

Alzheimer's disease (AD) is the most common form of dementia in older adults: It was first described by Dr. Alois Alzheimer in 1907. He described the symptoms that are now known as AD. Although much is still unknown about this devastating disease, we do know that today, one in eight Americans live with AD. The number of people developing this disease doubles every 5 years as people live beyond age 65, until at age 85 an individual has a 50% risk of developing this disease (Alzheimer's Association, 2011c). Every 59 seconds, another person develops AD, and this will change to every 33 seconds by the year 2050. Age is the greatest risk factor for AD. Most individuals with AD are over age 65 (Alzheimer's Association, 2011c). AD increased 66% in the years between 2000 and 2008. It is the only major disease that increased during that timeframe. Because of this growth, *Healthy People 2020* designated dementias, including AD, as one of the new focus areas (*Healthy People 2020, 2011b, 2011c*).

Table 24.1 Recommended Health Screening/Immunizations for Older Adults

Adult Health Screenings and Immunizations Schedule

Test	Who Needs It	How Often	Comments
General Health			
Height	All adults	Every year	
Weight	All adults	Every year	
Physical examination	All adults	Every year	
Advance directives	All adults	Every year	
Heart Health			
Blood pressure	All	Every year	
Cholesterol	All	At least every 2 yrs.	
Diet review	All adults with high cholesterol levels and those at risk for diabetes and heart disease	Ask your doctor	
Diabetes HgA_1C	All adults over age 45	Every 3 yrs.	
Cancer			
BREAST			
Clinical breast examination	All adult women starting at 40	Clinical breast examination yearly	Start sooner if at risk
Mammogram	After age 50 every year	Every year after age 50	
CERVICAL			
Pap test	All women	Every 1–3 yrs.	Normally be able to stop after age 65 if all PAP tests have been negative
Pelvic exam	All women	Ask your doctor	
PROSTATE			
Digital rectal examination	All men over 50	Every year	
COLORECTAL			
Fecal occult blood	Adults starting at 50	Every year	
BONE HEALTH			
Bone mass density	Starting at 65	Ask your doctor	
SENSORY			
Hearing	All adults	Every 1–2 yrs.	
Vision	All adults	Every 1–2 yrs.	
Glaucoma	Adults over age 65	Every 1–2 yrs.	
BEHAVIORAL			
Depression	All adults	Discuss with your doctor	
Obesity	All adults		
Tobacco use	All adults		
Alcohol use	All adults		
STIs AND HIV			
HIV	Both partners	Talk to your doctor	

Table 24.1 Recommended Health Screening/Immunizations for Older Adults *(Continued)*

Adult Health Screenings and Immunizations Schedule

Test	Who Needs It	How Often	Comments
IMMUNIZATIONS			
Diphtheria–tetanus	All adults	Every 10 yrs.	
Influenza	Adults over 50	Every year	
Pneumococcus	All adults 65 and over	Once	
Hepatitis B	Ask your doctor		
Herpes zoster to prevent shingles	All adults starting at 60	Once	

Adapted from: Scan Health Plan (2009).

The occurrence of AD is not a normal development in the aging process. It is characterized by a gradual loss of memory, decline in ability to perform routine tasks, disorientation, difficulty in learning, loss of language skills, impaired judgment and ability to plan, and personality changes. As the disease progresses, these changes become so severe that they interfere with the individual's daily functioning, resulting in total dependence on others for care and eventually in death. Although most people live from 4 to 10 years, some people live 20 years after the onset of symptoms (Alzheimer's Association, 2011c). AD is the seventh leading cause of death among all Americans and the fifth leading cause of death for those over 65 (CDC, 2010a). Most people diagnosed with AD are older than 65 (called late-onset AD); however, it is possible for the disease to occur in people between the ages of 30 and 60, but early onset AD is usually considered an inherited form of the disease, another risk factor for Alzheimer's (Alzheimer's Association, 2011c).

There is a simple way to describe the difference between the normal forgetfulness of aging and AD. From time to time, we all forget where we have put our keys, but people with early stage AD may notice that they tend to forget things more often—especially recent activities or events, or names of familiar things or people (Alzheimer's Association, 2011d; 2012). Although these symptoms are bothersome, they are usually not serious enough to cause alarm. As the disease advances, the symptoms become serious enough to cause people with AD or their family members to recognize that things are not right and that help is needed. In the middle stages of AD, people eventually forget how to do simple tasks like brushing their teeth or combing their hair, and they begin to no longer be able to think clearly. They eventually have problems speaking, understanding, reading or writing, or recognizing people they have known for years. People who suffer from AD may become anxious or aggressive and may wander away from home, thus requiring the need for total care (Alzheimer's Association, 2011d).

There is no single test to identify AD (Alzheimer's Association, 2011b). It is recommended that health care providers offer a comprehensive exam including a complete health history; physical exam; lab tests; neurologic, functional, and mental status assessments; and possible brain scans (Alzheimer's Association, 2011a). A comprehensive assessment is needed because many conditions, including some that are treatable or reversible (e.g., thyroid disease, depression brain tumors, drug reactions), may cause dementia-like symptoms. Physicians are now able to accurately diagnose 80% to 90% of people who show symptoms, but the only definitive diagnosis of AD is done at autopsy by the examination of brain tissue (Administration on Aging, 2011b; National Institute on Aging, 2011). Probable causes of AD are many. Promising leads involve the role of neurotransmitters, proteins, metabolism, environmental toxins, and genes. Research has shown links between some genes and AD, with three gene variants identified for early onset AD and one that boosts risk for late-onset type. A recent study showed that disrupted sleep can lead to the buildup of brain plaques—a hallmark of AD—in mice. However, mouse studies are preliminary, and additional research will be needed to clarify if lack of sleep actually plays a role in the development of amyloid plaques in humans (Contie, 2009).

Discovering the cause and a means of preventing AD, as well as better methods of earlier diagnosis, will be a significant achievement that may be realized in this century (National Institute on Aging, 2011). The current costs of AD to Americans total $183 billion annually. Medicare expenses make up $93 billion of this total (Alzheimer's Association, 2011b). Currently, 16 different agents are under study relative to AD, compared with 90 for cardiovascular disease; the medical community is not putting the same amount of effort into research for AD as it does for other diseases.

Several medications have been approved for use with Alzheimer's patients. Medications called cholinesterase inhibitors are prescribed for mild to moderate AD. However, these drugs only delay the progression of symptoms for a limited time (National Institute on Aging, 2010b). At best, available medications "turn back the clock somewhat" with the disease worsening at a slower rate, or the drugs control some of the client's behaviors that jeopardize safety, thereby promoting caregiver management.

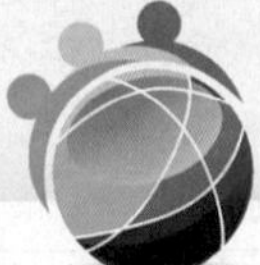

DISPLAY 24.7 HEALTH MAINTENANCE PROGRAMS AND SERVICES FOR OLDER ADULTS

Resources for Community Health Nurses to Utilize With Clients

- Communication services (phones, emergency access to health care)
- Dental care services
- Dietary guidance and food services (such as Meals on Wheels, commodity programs, or group meal services)
- Escort and protective services
- Exercise and fitness programs
- Financial aid and counseling
- Friendly visiting and companions
- Health education
- Hearing tests and hearing aid assistance
- Home health services (including skilled nursing and home health aide services)
- Home maintenance assistance (housekeeping, chores, and repairs)
- Legal aid and counseling
- Library services (including tapes and large-print books)
- Medical supplies or equipment
- Medication supervision
- Podiatry services
- Recreational and education programs (community centers, Elderhostel)
- Routine care from selected health care practitioners
- Safe, affordable, and ability-appropriate housing
- Senior citizens' discounts (food, drugs, transportation, banks, retail stores, and recreation)
- Social assistance services offered in conjunction with health maintenance
- Speech or physical therapy
- Spiritual ministries
- Transportation services
- Vision care (prescribing and providing eye glasses, diagnosis and treatment of glaucoma and cataracts)
- Volunteer and employment opportunities (Vista, RSVP)

Adapted from *Guide to clinical preventive services* (U.S. Preventive Services Task Force, 2010a).

How does this disease affect the role of the community health nurse? Often, the person with AD is cared for at home until very late in the disease course. Perhaps more than any other disease, AD is responsible for enormous caregiver burden. In 2010, over 17 billion hours were provided by family members caring for a person with AD. The economic value placed on this unpaid care totaled $202.6 billion for that year (Alzheimer's Association, 2011b). The intense care given to these clients can be a constant drain on the emotional and physical reserves of their families, which highlights the need for respite care. The client exhibits depression, agitation, sleeplessness, and anxiety, which can greatly upset the family's normal routine. In many situations, the main caregiver is an aged spouse. The stress of providing care puts the caregiver's health at risk, as well. In 1992, Congress created the Alzheimer's Disease Supportive Program to encourage states to provide support for persons and families with Alzheimer's. The intensity of caregiving is aptly described in a book written for AD family members, *The 36-Hour Day* (Mace & Rabins, 2006). Another good book is *Staying Connected While Letting Go: The Paradox of Alzheimer's Caregiving* (Braff & Olenik, 2003) (see What Do You Think?).

Because so many elders afflicted with AD reside at home with their family members providing care, it is important for the CHN to monitor and assess the levels

What do *you* think?

Have you heard of the *Best Friends* approach to Alzheimer's care? The approach has changed the caregiving approach to AD and is changing the lives of caregivers, families, and clients. It improves the quality of life not only for clients with AD but also for those providing care. *Best Friends* is a groundbreaking and uplifting method for the care of people with AD. It builds on the essential elements of friendship: respect, empathy, support, trust, and humor. These are the building blocks of a care model that is both effective and flexible enough to adapt to each person's remaining strengths and abilities. The *Best Friends* approach does not just prevent catastrophic episodes; it makes every day consistently reassuring, enjoyable, and secure.

From: Bell, V., & Troxel, D. (2011). *An overview of the Best Friends™ approach to Alzheimer's care*. Baltimore, MD: Health Professions Press. Retrieved from http://www.healthpropress.com/sos/BestFriends_Overview.pdf (*Best Friends™* is a trademark of Health Professions Press, Inc.)

of stress on family members. The nurse can intervene as necessary and provide caregivers with methods to cope and adapt as needed, making applicable referrals. The nurse can assist with planning and preparing the caregiver for what lies ahead (HelpGuide, 2011d). Most communities have resources for clients and their families. They may provide family and caregiver support groups, respite care, counseling, and legal or financial consultation. These services are available through local agencies, such as the Area Agency on Aging, but there are also government-sponsored national resources that offer information, referral services, and educational materials (e.g., Alzheimer's Association) all of which can be accessed by the CHN or the families in need. Some may find online support groups helpful. The nurse needs to know what resources are available in order to guide families to them (see Using the Nursing Process).

Arthritis

Arthritis encompasses more than 100 diseases and conditions that affect joints, surrounding tissues, and other connective tissues and is the leading cause of disability for adults in the United States (CDC, 2011c). Common forms include osteoarthritis (OA), rheumatoid arthritis (RA), gout, and fibromyalgia. OA is the most common

USING THE NURSING PROCESS WHEN WORKING WITH OLDER ADULTS

Assessment

Mr. and Mrs. Boxwell are in their late 70s and have lived modestly on a fixed income since Mr. Boxwell's retirement. However, their budget has been strained this year as they have had $300 to $400 a month in out-of-pocket expenses for prescription medications. Mrs. Boxwell confessed to you (the community health nurse visiting them after receiving a referral from the coordinator of the senior center they attend) that at times they will skip medication doses to "make ends meet" in some months. They both take drugs for high blood pressure; also, Mrs. Boxwell is diabetic and Mr. Boxwell has heart failure. They live in a small, older home, and their older model car is seldom driven as they report "the traffic is getting worse" and they have "come close to having a car crash two times" while they were driving in the past 3 months. They are receptive to your suggestions and are trying to stay healthy and independent.

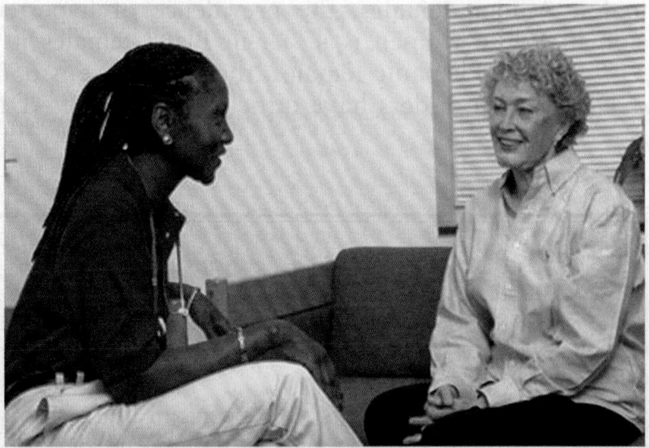

Nursing Diagnoses

1. The clients are at risk for an alteration in their health status due to insufficient finances to purchase needed medications for chronic diseases.
2. The clients are at risk for altered safety when driving related to chronic health problems, diminished driving skills, and a history of near automobile crashes.

Plan and Implementation

DIAGNOSIS 1

The community health nurse will explore the clients' eligibility for Medicare Part D and Medicaid. It is possible these clients are eligible, yet unaware of these programs.

The community health nurse will consult with the clients' primary health care provider and ask for a change in prescriptions from brand names to generic. Also, ordering some medications in larger doses that come in scored tablets may be less expensive, and the client can safely break the larger pills in half. Mrs. Boxwell will check with her present distributor of diabetic supplies about getting larger quantities, generic brands of syringes, alcohol pads, etc.

DIAGNOSIS 2

Mr. Boxwell will look into selling the car and exploring the bus schedule and other senior shuttle services that can be used to travel to the doctor and grocery store. Mr. and Mrs. Boxwell's daughter spends a day with them monthly and takes them wherever they want to go, as long as it is "a fun outing," and they will look into coordinating errands with her.

Evaluation

The couple is eligible for Medicare Part D, and this will help defray the out-of-pocket costs for medications. They have reduced medication costs as much as possible and report not missing any prescribed medications.

They sold their car and are negotiating the bus in good weather and using a taxi in the winter or when it is raining (they figured they save $1,000 a year in auto insurance, auto maintenance, and gasoline, while the bus and taxi costs them about $22 a month).

Since the couple is receptive to the help you have provided, you initiate a discussion regarding their long-term plans for housing needs as they get older. They are not opposed to a senior housing option and have been talking about it with their daughter. They are going to talk with a realtor about selling their house, explore some senior apartments with their daughter on her monthly visits, and review their budget.

form of arthritis affecting both young and old, with two thirds of sufferers younger than age 65. However, the incidence increases with age. For those aged 18 to 44, 7.6% report physician-diagnosed arthritis. For those 45 to 64, the incidence rises to 29.8% and for those 65 and older, 50% report physician-diagnosed arthritis (CDC, 2011c). By 2030, it is estimated that 25% of the total adult population will have physician-diagnosed OA (CDC, 2011c).

With OA, the number of cartilage cells diminishes, cartilage becomes ulcerated and thinned, subchondral bone is exposed, and boney surfaces rub together resulting in joint destruction. This disease is no longer considered to be only a normal consequence of aging. Risk factors include obesity, repetitive mechanical overuse of a joint, and heredity. For those underweight or of normal weight, 16.4% have arthritis. Among those who are overweight, 21.4% have arthritis, and this increases to 66% for those who are obese (CDC, 2010b). Classic symptoms include aching, stiffness, and limited motion of the involved joint. Discomfort increases with overuse and during damp weather. Acetaminophen is the first drug of choice; however, clients often find a combination of medications and daily routines that helps them the most. The nurse can best assist these clients by assessing the safety of a particular regimen and suggesting treatment changes as new research becomes available, including new medications, surgical options for joint replacement, and dietary changes (e.g., vitamins, foods high in essential fatty acids) (National Institute of Arthritis and Musculoskeletal and Skin Diseases [NIAMS], 2010). Arthritis limits ADLs and quality of life and is a costly disability. Forty two percent of those with arthritis report activity limitations (CDC, 2010b). In 2003, arthritis-related costs totaled $218 billion. This included $81 billion for medical costs and $47 billion in lost earnings (CDC, 2010b).

RA is a progressive chronic condition that begins during young adulthood and becomes disabling as the disease continues, attacking tissues of the joints and causing systemic damage in the later years. It affects diarthrodial (synovial-line) joints. This form of arthritis is an autoimmune disease that causes inflammation, deformity, and crippling. RA is treated with anti-inflammatory agents, corticosteroids, antimalarial agents, gold salts, and immunosuppressive drugs. Joint discomfort is often relieved by gentle massage, heat, and range-of-motion exercises (NIAMS, 2009).

The CHN needs to be aware of the major differences between these two prevalent forms of arthritis. Recommended treatments, including physical therapy, diet, and medication, change as more evidence-based research is conducted on arthritis. It is important to keep up-to-date on treatments, as these conditions are treated in the community and affect a large portion of the midlife and older populations that a PHN may carry in his or her caseload. Cancers, which are characterized by the uncontrolled growth and spread of abnormal cells, steadily increase in incidence in aging adults. Cancer causes 13% (7.6 million) of deaths worldwide. Age is a fundamental risk factor of cancer with the incidence of cancer rising dramatically with age. The leading types of cancers are lung, stomach, liver, colorectal, and breast (WHO, 2011). One popular theory is that as the body ages, the immune system declines, losing its ability to serve as a buffer against abnormal cancer cells that have been forming in the body throughout life. Tobacco use is a major risk factor for cancer. Harmful alcohol use, poor diet, and physical inactivity are other main risk factors (WHO, 2011).

It is particularly important for the CHN to be aware of the increased incidence of cancer in older clients because older people often under report symptoms that may be early signs of cancer. It is vital for PHNs, through assessments at clinics, on home visits, or during participation in screening programs, to encourage clients to report untoward symptoms in order to promote early detection, which gives clients their best chance of survival. Adherence to the health care practitioner's recommended schedule for health screening should be encouraged. In addition, being aware of and educating clients about the American Cancer Society's *Seven Warning Signals of Cancer* can possibly save their lives (Display 24.8).

Cardiovascular Disease

Following arthritis and hearing impairment, hypertension is the third most frequent chronic condition for people older than age 65. About 66% of those between 65 and 75 have been diagnosed with hypertension, as have about 75% of those 75 years and older (CDC, 2011c). Hypertension increases with age and affects men more frequently than women. Hypertension is more prevalent in minorities. For example, hypertension in White adult males is 61%, while the prevalence in Black males is 71% and 69% in Hispanic males. Among females, the prevalence of hypertension in White women is 47%, in Black females it is 51%, and in Hispanic females, the prevalence is 65% (CDC, 2011c). Elders have difficulty managing ADLs

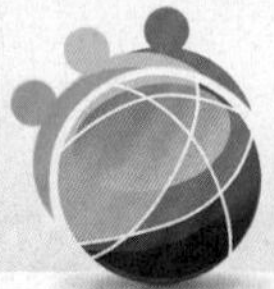

DISPLAY 24.8 CAUTION: SEVEN WARNING SIGNS OF CANCER

The seven warning signs of cancer can be remembered through the use of the mnemonic device, *CAUTION*, as follows:

1. Change in bowel or bladder habits
2. A sore or sore throat that does not heal
3. Unusual bleeding or discharge
4. Thickening or lump in breast or elsewhere
5. Indigestion or difficulty in swallowing
6. Obvious change in wart or mole
7. Nagging cough or hoarseness

Source: The American Cancer Society

if antihypertensive medications lower their blood pressure too dramatically. Hypotension leads to problems of safety, including a higher risk of falls, and blood pressure should be monitored by the PHN. Both hypertension and hypotension can have significant detrimental effects on the health of older adults.

Heart disease is the leading cause of death for both men and women in the United States (CDC, 2011c). Risk factors in the aging population associated with cardiovascular disease include tobacco use or exposure to tobacco smoke, inappropriate nutritional patterns, diabetes, high cholesterol, and lack of exercise. There are also regional differences in the pattern of deaths from heart disease: The southeastern coastal plains (Appalachia) and lower Mississippi River Valley (southern parts of Georgia and Alabama) have the highest death rates, and Blacks and Whites generally have higher rates of heart disease death than Hispanics or Asians and other races/ethnicities (CDC, 2011c).

Disease prevention is an important role for the CHN. Based on the knowledge of the prevalence of hypertension in older adults, the CHN can provide primary prevention by teaching community groups and individuals about this condition and ways to prevent its occurrence and can provide secondary prevention by screening seniors on a regular basis.

Depression

Depression is not a normal part of growing older, yet it is one of the most common, and most treatable, of all the mental disorders in older adults (CDC, 2010g). It is a major health concern in this population and can be life-threatening if unrecognized and untreated. Research has shown that medical costs are much higher for older adults who have medical conditions plus depression (National Institute of Mental Health, 2009). Biological, psychological, and social changes place older adults at high risk for the development and recurrence of depression. It is frequently related to multiple losses, such as retirement, a health change, or the death of a significant other. Depression is reported to be more common in women than in men (Barry, Allore, Guo, Bruce, & Gill, 2008). However, as mentioned earlier in this chapter, depression in men is more severe, resulting in suicide at a higher rate than among women. Higher levels of perceived social support are related to lower instances of depression among all people, and women especially seem to make these supportive connections throughout life more effectively than men do. The nurturance, reassurance, and support women get from intimate relationships with other women are not often as highly developed in men, and for this reason, men display more symptoms of depression after a loss.

The nurse needs to keep in mind the many potential causes of depression. Medical conditions, such as stroke, cancer, vitamin B_{12} deficiency, diabetes, chronic pain with dependence on prescription painkillers, or insomnia, may lead to depressive symptoms. Many prescription drugs can trigger or exacerbate depression. These include blood pressure medications, sleeping pills, calcium channel blockers, ulcer medications, and painkillers. Dementia and depression can be confused. Never assume that loss of mental sharpness is just a sign of old age. It may be difficult to differentiate whether an older adult is suffering from grief or depression or dementia (National Institute of Mental Health, 2009). CHNs can help elders prevent the overwhelming signs and symptoms of depression related to losses by working with aggregates of elders in the community. Through senior centers, adult housing units, senior day care centers, or men's and women's groups at religious centers, the CHN can meet with seniors to offer support, teach strategies to improve the quality and quantity of support systems, invite mental health speakers to discuss the topic of depression prevention, and generally assess the holistic health status of the elders in that setting. The increased years added to life through the advances of the past few decades in medications and treatment should lead to healthy and happy later life for seniors, filled with activities that bring joy and contentment. Years lost to depression are a wasted resource that could be prevented through early intervention and medical management.

Diabetes

According to the American Diabetes Association, 13% of all Americans had diabetes in 2010. For those age 65 or older, the percentage jumps to 26.9%, or 10.9 million (American Diabetes Association, 2011). Diabetes mellitus (DM) affects the health of older people and limits their ability to perform activities. Among people 65 years and older in 1999 to 2000, 15.1% of men and 13.0% of women reported having diabetes. The prevalence of diabetes tends to be higher among Hispanics and non-Hispanic Blacks. The number of people with DM has increased sixfold since 1958, and 95% of these have type 2 diabetes. Type 2 diabetes can often be prevented with adherence to proper diet and regular exercise with the addition of oral medications, when needed.

More Americans than ever suffer from various forms of DM, and the resulting rates of death and serious complications, such as adult blindness, kidney disease, and foot or leg amputations, are especially high for elders and racial/ethnic minority populations (Nwasuruba, Khan, & Egede, 2007). In the past, DM was not always managed effectively; fear and misinformation about the disease may hinder today's elders from getting an early diagnosis or from participating in effective teaching and instruction on how to manage DM.

Being diagnosed with DM can cause depression or anger, and the CHN must tailor educational programs to meet individual client needs. The plan should be comprehensive, with special emphasis placed on the areas in which each client needs information. For example, a spouse may be concerned about preparing meals that meet her husband's needs, whereas the husband may be more concerned with how the disease will affect his long days on the golf course or sexual functioning; in contrast, a single older woman may worry whether she can see well enough to draw up her insulin or can afford to pay for diabetic supplies and special foods. All newly diagnosed diabetics need a comprehensive overview of the disease process followed by an individualized approach for ongoing control and management of the disease.

Self-care behaviors (e.g., appropriate diet, glucose monitoring, medication management, foot care) are not often consistently practiced, yet they are necessary to promote good health and fewer complications (Hornick, & Aron, 2008; Nwasuruba et al., 2007). CHNs are ideally situated to meet group and individual needs. They have the resources and skills to plan and implement diabetic education classes for groups of elders, in addition to making home visits to address specific learning deficits that impact an individual's ability to manage their diabetes properly. The group setting allows elders to share their experiences, learn from each other, and benefit from the support of the group. Home visits permit the nurse to focus on an assessment of the client, home, family support, diabetic supplies and technique, and overall health management.

Osteoporosis

Osteoporosis is a disease of bone in which the amount of bone is decreased and the strength is reduced. Osteoporosis is a generalized, persistent, and disabling disease that can overshadow every facet of an elder's overall functional level and independence. It causes acute and chronic pain, subsequent fractures, decreased physical activity, limited mobility, changes in body image, role changes, a reduction in ability to perform ADLs, and depression.

Researchers estimate that one in five women in the United States have osteoporosis and that half the women over 50 will have a fracture of the hip, wrist, or vertebrae (National Center for Biotechnology Information, 2010). In osteoporosis, calcium leaches from the bone mass and results in small holes forming in the bones. These empty spaces within the bone increase susceptibility to fractures of hip, wrist, or vertebra (National Center for Biotechnology Information, 2010). The risk of osteoporosis increases with age. As the disease progresses, other characteristics appear (e.g., compression of the vertebrae results in loss of height and the hunched back deformity known as dowager's hump).

Proper diet and exercise throughout life are now recognized as the most effective measure to maintain bone health. There is growing evidence that vitamin D supplementation can prevent fractures and that calcium supplementation is also crucial (National Center for Biotechnology Information 2010). There are many FDA-approved drugs to treat osteoporosis that can be prescribed by a primary care provider. Therefore, identification of risk factors and regular screenings are essential to prevent the progression of this debilitating disease.

CHNs can focus their teaching on primary prevention and ensure that people eat diets rich in vitamin D and calcium and include calcium supplements as needed. Not smoking, maintaining a healthy weight, participating in weight-bearing activities, and receiving ongoing bone density screenings are positive health behaviors that can contribute to strong bones throughout life. The value of hormone replacement therapy (HRT) in women—its benefits and possible long-term side effects—must be considered on the advice of the primary care provider, whose judgment should be based on the latest research findings along with the individual woman's needs.

Tertiary Prevention

Tertiary prevention involves follow-up and rehabilitation after a disease or condition has occurred or been diagnosed and initial treatment has begun. Chronic diseases that are common among older adults, such as heart failure, stroke, diabetes, cognitive impairment, or arthritis, cannot always be prevented but can frequently be postponed into the later years of life through a lifetime of positive health behaviors. However, when they occur, the debilitating symptoms and damaging effects can be controlled through healthy choices encouraged by the CHN and recommended by the primary care practitioner.

Although many older adults are considered generally healthy, 80% have at least one chronic condition and 50% have at least two (CDC, 2011d). A small proportion suffer more disabling forms of disease, such as COPD, cerebral vascular accidents (CVAs), cancer, or DM, the latter two requiring extensive care and ongoing medical management. The most common health problems of older people in the community are arthritis, reduced vision, hearing loss, heart disease, peripheral vascular disease, and hypertension. In 2002, the top three causes of death for US adults aged 65 or older were heart disease (32% of all deaths), cancer (22%), and stroke (8%). These accounted for 61% of all deaths in this age group. The tragedy of these leading killers is that they are often preventable. Although the risk for disease and disability clearly increases with advancing age, poor health is not always an inevitable consequence of aging. Although many older adults experience relatively good health, almost all may expect to be chronically ill for an extended amount of time at the end of their lives. Chapter 26 expands on clients with disabilities and chronic illnesses and the role of the CHN working with these populations in the community.

HEALTH COSTS FOR OLDER ADULTS: MEDICARE AND MEDICAID

As the number of older adults grows, so do costs for health care. In 2009, the NHEs grew to $2.9 trillion, or $8,088 per person. This accounted for 17.6% of the gross domestic product (GDP), as discussed in Chapter 6. Medicare spending was $502.3 billion (20% of NHE) and Medicaid grew to $373.9 billion (15% of NHE). In 2010, Medicare benefits totaled $509 billion or 23% of the nation's health care spending (Kaiser

Family Foundation, 2008). However, it is a myth that Medicare or Medicaid covers all health care costs for older adults. In actuality, an older adult spends a great deal out-of-pocket for health care. Individuals and their families cover 52% of long-term care costs out of pocket. The cost of paid long-term care is only the tip of the iceberg. Approximately 75% of long-term care services and support are provided on an unpaid basis by family members. This is often done at a heavy physical and financial cost, including lost opportunities for employment, health insurance, and retirement savings.

Services for older adults are very expensive. Some examples of average costs in the United States (Our Parents, 2009) for health care services are:

- $64 per day for an adult day care services
- $19 per hour for a home health aide
- $21 per day for a certified nursing assistant (CNA)
- $3,131 per month for care in an assisted living facility
- $198 per day for a semiprivate room in a nursing home

Most nursing home stays do not qualify for Medicare coverage. The average cost of a stay in a nursing home is $70,000 annually. In many areas it costs much more. Over the past few years, nursing home rates have risen 30% while assisted living rates increased 41% (Our Parents, 2009). Medicaid is the primary payer for long-term services, covering 40% of all spending for long-term care services (Kaiser Commission on Medicaid Facts, 2011).

Medicare

While Medicare does cover many services for older adults, there can be significant out-of-pocket costs. Some examples follow (Medicare.gov, n.d.):

Part A (hospital insurance) covers:

- Inpatient care in hospitals (such as critical access hospitals, inpatient rehabilitation facilities, long-term care hospitals)
- Inpatient care in a skilled nursing facility (limitations apply)
- Hospice care services
- Home health services
- Religious nonmedical health care institution

Services not covered by Part A:

- Custodial care (or long-term care): If beneficiaries are hospitalized, they pay a $1,132 deductible. If their stay lasts longer than 60 days, they are billed $283 per day for days 61 through 90.

Hospitalizations and rehospitalizations are a significant expense for the Medicare program. A major theme of health care reform was the prevention of hospitalizations by providing more supportive care at home, care that is generally covered by the Medicaid programs.

Part B (supplementary medical insurance for physician visits) covers:

- Essential coverage for physicians

Services not covered by Part B:

- Beneficiaries pay 20% of the Medicare-approved amount for any visits to their doctor.
- Medicare premiums for medical insurance (part B) are $1,380 per person per year for most beneficiaries and are higher for those with incomes above $80,000.

Part C (Medigap—private health plans)
Part D (prescription drug benefits):

The Part D national base beneficiary premium for prescription drug coverage is $388 per person per year. A beneficiary's actual costs depend on the plan to which he or she belongs. For more on Medicare, see Chapter 6.

Medicaid

While the majority of people enrolled in Medicaid are children and families, most Medicaid spending goes for services provided to people aged 65 and over and people with disabilities (Kaiser Commission on Medicaid Facts, 2011).

For seniors, one of the most significant gaps in Medicare coverage is the cost of "custodial care," or help with ADLs like bathing, dressing, eating, getting into or out of a chair, or using the bathroom. Contrary to what many people believe, Medicare does not cover this kind of care, either in a nursing home or in the beneficiary's own home. Funding for this type of care is generally covered by Medicaid waiver programs and Older Americans Act funds.

It is another myth that Medicaid is a program for the poor while Medicare is for those who are financially secure. Nearly half of all Medicare beneficiaries had incomes below twice the federal poverty level (FPL) in 2008 ($20,800 for an individual and $28,000 for a couple). Poverty rates vary greatly among different segments of the Medicare population, with higher rates for females, non-older adult beneficiaries with disabilities, those age 85 or older, and Black and Hispanic beneficiaries. More than two thirds of Black and Hispanic beneficiaries live on incomes below twice the poverty level, compared to 41% of Whites. More than half of all beneficiaries ages 85 and older, and more than two thirds of the under 65 disabled, live on incomes below two times the poverty level (Kaiser Family Foundation, 2010).

Medicare and Medicaid are integral programs that provide quality health care for older adults across the country. Further cuts to these programs will affect the livelihood of many individuals. Given our current economic state, increased spending in these programs is not feasible, nor sustainable. Our only chance to continue to help older adults live healthier and happier lives is to create innovations in Medicare and Medicaid that result in savings to both programs and increased efficiency and quality in the care that these programs provide.

If seniors' health and long-term services and support needs are not met, their condition ultimately can deteriorate to the point where they need to be hospitalized or admitted to a skilled nursing facility where cost of care is markedly higher.

ELDER ABUSE

Elder abuse is a problem that is under recognized and underreported. And it has devastating consequences. Current data on the prevalence of elder abuse are scarce and dated because it is largely underreported. Therefore, the complexity of defining elder abuse, and the debate over classification of types of mistreatment, compounds the task of evaluating the magnitude of the problem. Some of the risk factors for elder mistreatment, such as isolation, add to its "invisibility." The National Research Council reports that no survey of the US population has ever been undertaken that can provide a true national estimate for the incidence of elder mistreatment. The victims are often isolated older women who are difficult to access. Inadequate funding for research and state-to-state incompatibilities in tracking protective service statistics also contribute to the paucity of national studies (National Center on Elder Abuse, 2005; n.d.c). The National Institute of Justice (2010) conducted a large survey of older adults. In this study 1.6% of the respondents reported physical abuse, but only 31% had reported the incident. When other forms of abuse were included, 11% of those surveyed had some kind of mistreatment in the previous year, with over 5.2% reporting financial abuse, 5.1% emotional mistreatment, and 5.1% experienced potential neglect.

Older adults are at increased risk for abuse due to social isolation, mental impairment, and dependence on others. **Elder abuse** is defined by the National Center on Elder Abuse as "intentional or neglectful acts by a caregiver or any other person that causes harm or a serious risk of harm to a vulnerable adult" (2011, para. 1). Physical abuse, neglect, emotional or psychological abuse, verbal abuse and threats, financial abuse and exploitation, sexual abuse, and abandonment are considered forms of elder abuse (National Center on Elder Abuse, n.d.a). In some states, self-neglect is also considered a form of mistreatment (National Center on Elder Abuse, 2010). This occurs when an older adult neglects to take care of his or herself in a way that leads to illness or injury. Self-neglect includes such behaviors as failing to take medications, refusal to seek medical attention for a serious illness, leaving a burner on the stove on and unattended, poor hygiene, dressing inappropriately for the weather, or confusion. Self-neglect is the form of abuse most commonly reported to Adult Protective Services (National Center on Elder Abuse, n.d.b). It is notable that financial abuse often accompanies one of the other forms of abuse. The financial abuse of seniors is a growing problem, often called the "crime of the 21st century." It is one of the most sinister forms of abuse. A senior can be financially stable and living independently one day and become destitute and forced to live in a facility the next as a result of abuse. Sadly, most elder abuse occurs in the elder's own home, and the abuser is usually a family member. In states reporting on the *2004 Survey of State Adult Protective Services*, almost half of all cases investigated were substantiated. Most victims of elder abuse are White (77.1%), and the majority of victims are reported to be over age 80 and female (National Center on Elder Abuse, 2006). The most common perpetrators of elder abuse are spouses or partners of elders, often in a relationship with long-term domestic violence. Family members account for 76% of reported mistreatment, while strangers account for only 3% (National Institute of Justice, 2010). Abusers, particularly adult children, are often dependent on the victim for financial assistance, housing, or because of personal problems such as mental illness, alcohol, or drug abuse (National Center for Elder Abuse, 2010). An elder person in immediate danger should be removed from his or her environment; however, elder abuse does not often come to the attention of PHNs or other providers of services to older adults. It is estimated that five occurrences of neglect, abuse, exploitation, or self-neglect go unreported for every case that is reported. Therefore, nurses working in the community with older adults must be vigilant for signs of elder abuse and knowledgeable about reporting laws.

Various state, local, and county agencies investigate and enforce elder abuse laws. The first agency to respond to a report of elder abuse in most states is APS. In some states, certain professionals are required or encouraged to report elder abuse. The people required to report elder abuse are generally doctors and nurses, psychologists, police officers, social workers, and employees of banks and other financial institutions. The National Institute of Justice (2008) has identified four areas that are potential markers for identifying elder abuse:

- Physical condition and quality of care (e.g., unreported injuries, malnourishment)
- Facility/housing characteristics (e.g., unchanged linens, strong odors)
- Inconsistencies in statements/records (e.g., statements given vs. what you see)
- Staff/family member behaviors (e.g., evasiveness, lack of knowledge or concern)

APPROACHES TO OLDER ADULT CARE

In general, nursing service to seniors can be divided into two approaches: geriatrics and gerontology. In addition, healthy older adults can be effectively cared for in the community through case management approaches, which focus on all three types of services: primary, secondary, and tertiary. The ultimate goal of community-based case management for the aging population is to enhance the quality of care by decreasing fragmentation, maximizing resources, and providing the highest quality of care possible.

Case Management and Needs Assessment

Case management involves assessing needs, planning and organizing services, and monitoring responses to care throughout the length of the caregiving process, condition, or illness. This concept, which has been practiced by CHNs for many years, focuses primarily on the health needs of clients. Social workers use case management to address their clients' social needs, including their financial problems. Some HMOs provide a coordinated system of services for their enrolled clients. However, many communities provide no such advocate for their older residents, and a more comprehensive, community-wide system approach needs to be developed in order to serve the entire older population. Such a system might be based in an agency specifically designed to serve as case manager or agent to assess clients' needs and assemble existing agencies and services to meet those needs.

Various techniques or tools are available to assess the needs of older adults:

- The Older Americans Resources and Services Information System (OARS), developed by Duke University Center for the Study of Aging and Human Development, utilizes two sections of one tool—OARS Multidimensional Functional Assessment Questionnaire (OMFAQ)—to determine levels of functioning in five areas (mental health, physical health, economic resources, social resources, and ability to perform ADLs), along with the extent and intensity of utilization, as well as perceived need, of services. Administration time is about 45 minutes, and this tool is commonly used in research and to determine effectiveness of services, as well as assessment of functional status.
- The Barthel Index assesses functional independence and is often used to determine levels of disability or dependence of stroke victims with respect to ADLs. The Modified Rankin Scale (MRS) is another common tool used for this purpose (Sulter, Steen, & De Keyser, 1999).
- The Katz Index of ADLs is based on an evaluation of the functional independence or dependence of clients with respect to bathing, dressing, toileting, and related tasks (Hartford Institute for Geriatric Nursing, 2007). The Instrumental Activities of Daily Living Scale looks at an older adult's ability to perform such activities as using the telephone, shopping, doing laundry, and handling finances.
- Other tools sometimes used with clients include the Stanford 7-day Physical Activity Recall questionnaire (PAR) (Sallis, Buono, Roby, Micale, & Nelson, 1993) and the Physical Activity Scale for the Elderly (PASE) (Washburn, Smith, Jette, & Janney, 1993). All of these tools measure physical activity and functioning.

A frequently overlooked area of assessment is the client's spiritual needs (Hoffert, Henshaw, & Mvududu, 2007). Religious dedication and spiritual concern often increase in later years. Limited ability or lack of transportation may prevent older people from attending religious services or engaging in spiritually enhancing activities. Self-health ratings, including clients' reports on their spiritual needs, provide another useful assessment technique.

HEALTH SERVICES FOR OLDER ADULT POPULATIONS

How well are the needs of older adults being met? To answer this question, other questions must be raised. Do health programs for older adults encompass the full range of needed services? Are programs both physically and financially accessible? Do they encourage clients to function independently? Do they treat senior citizens with respect and preserve their dignity? Do they recognize older adults' needs for companionship, economic security, and social status? If appropriate, do they promote meaningful activities instead of overworked games or activities such as bingo, shuffleboard, and ceramics? Are health care services and other social services provided based on evidence and research?

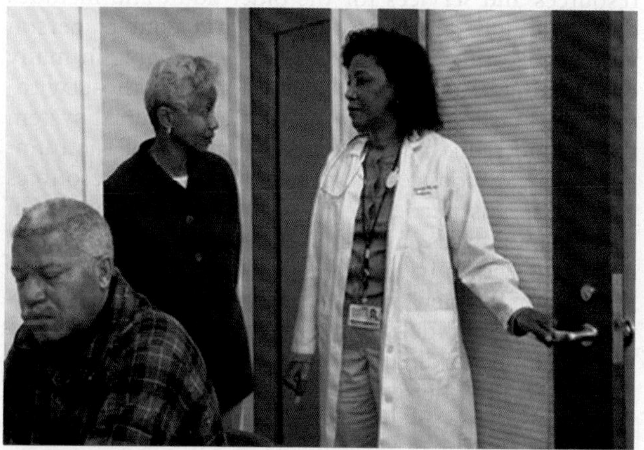

Effective services for older adults should be comprehensive, coordinated, accessible, and demonstrate evidence-based quality.

Criteria for Effective Service

Several criteria help to define the characteristics of an effective community health service delivery system. Four, in particular, deserve attention. For the delivery system of a community health service to be effective, it should be *comprehensive*. Many communities provide some programs, such as limited health screening or selected activities, but do not offer a full range of services to more adequately meet the needs of their senior citizens. Gaps and duplication in programs most often result from poor or nonexistent community-wide planning. Furthermore, such planning should be based on thorough assessment of the needs of the population in that community. A comprehensive set of services should provide the following:

- Adequate financial support
- Adult day care programs
- Access to high-quality health care services (prevention, early diagnosis and treatment, rehabilitation)
- Health education (including preparation for retirement)

- In-home services
- Recreation and activity programs that promote socialization
- Specialized transportation services

A second criterion for a community service delivery system is *coordination*. Often, older people go from one agency to the next. After visiting one place for food stamps, they go to another for answers to Medicare questions, another for congregate dining, and still another for health screenings. Such a patchwork of services reflects a system organized for the convenience of providers rather than consumers. It encourages misuse and discourages effective use. Instead, there should be coordinated, community-wide assessment and planning. Communities must consider alternatives that can meet many needs in one location, such as multiservice agencies and interdisciplinary collaborative programs.

A coordinated information and referral system provides another link. Most communities need this type of information network, which contains a directory of all resources and services for the older adult and includes the name and telephone number of a contact person with each listing. Such a network is available in many communities and should be developed in those without one. A simplified information and referral system that includes one number, such as an 800 phone number, that can connect seniors with available resources and services is particularly helpful to older people. In most communities, coordination is not present, or it is not done with any regularity or thoroughness. Many agencies in a given community do not coordinate services but instead deliver their own services in a patchwork and uncoordinated fashion. Collaboration among those who provide services to seniors can provide vital information for planning and implementing needed programs.

A third criterion is *accessibility*. Too often, services for seniors are inconveniently located or are prohibitively expensive. Some communities are considering multiservice community centers to bring programs and services for elderly closer to home. The Program of All-Inclusive Care of the older adult (PACE) is one example of this. Comprehensive services are offered to eligible nursing home patients, including personal, health care, and housing services (e.g., adult day care, meals, social workers, nurses, primary care physicians, dentists, podiatrists, optometrists, prescriptions, medical specialists, and acute and nursing home care). More convenient, and perhaps, specialized transportation services and more in-home services, such as home health aides, homemakers, and Meals on Wheels, may further solve accessibility problems for many older adults. Federal, state, and private funding sources can be tapped to ease the burden on the economically pressured population.

Finally, an effective community service system for older people should promote *quality* programs. This means that services should truly address the needs and concerns of a community's senior citizens and be based on scientific evidence. Evaluation of the quality of a community's services for the older adult is closely tied to their assessed needs. What are the needs of this specific population group in terms of nutrition, exercise, economic security, independence, social interaction, meaningful activities, and preparation for death? Planning for quality community services depends on having adequate, accurate, and current data. Periodic needs assessment is a necessity to ensure updated information and initiate and promote quality services.

Services for Older Adults by Level of Care Required

Most older adults want to remain in their own homes for the remainder of their lives and be as independent and in control of their lives as possible (HelpGuide, 2011i). The National Association of Area Agencies on Aging has created a blueprint for developing livable communities where people can live in their own communities and grow old with all the services necessary (National Association of Area Agencies on Aging, 2010). **Aging in place** is a term used for seniors who choose to remain in their own homes. To successfully remain at home, the older adults need transportation, a home that can be modified if moving up and down steps becomes a problem, a yard that can be maintained, personal care if needed, a way to safely take medications, live in a safe neighborhoods, and have family or friends who can help when needed (HelpGuide, 2010a).

Maintaining functional independence should be the primary goal of services for the older population. Assessment of needs and the ability to function and use of techniques such as OARS, the Instrumental Activities of Daily Living Scale, or other previously mentioned tools form the basis for determining appropriate services. Although many of the well seniors can assess their own health status, some are reluctant to seek needed help. Therefore, outreach programs serve an important function in many communities. They locate people in need of health or social assistance and refer them to appropriate resources.

Health screening is another important program for early detection and treatment of health problems among older adults. Conditions to screen for include hypertension, glaucoma, hearing disorders, cancers, diabetes, anemia, depression, mild cognitive impairment, and nutritional deficiencies. At the same time, assessment of clients' socialization, housing, and economic needs, along with proper referrals, can prevent further problems from developing that would compromise their health status. Health maintenance programs may be offered through a single agency, such as an HMO, or they may be coordinated by a case management agency with referrals to other providers. These programs should cover a wide range of services needed by the senior population, such as those listed in Display 24.7.

At times, seniors who remain in their own homes or apartments need home care services brought to them. Other seniors live with family members and go to an adult day care center during the day. The third category of living arrangements includes those that are short-term. It may be a rehabilitation hospital for recovery and physical therapy related to a hip fracture, or respite care, which gives the usual caregiver a much-needed rest from 24-hour-a-day caregiving and helps prevent "burnout." Families of terminally ill clients and those with severe dementia cared for at home often use respite services.

To meet the multiple housing and caregiving needs of today's elders and in anticipation of the larger numbers to come, many options are becoming available. A range of housing types, from luxurious retirement communities with all amenities for the active and healthier senior to secure and more modestly priced or low-income apartments for independent senior living, are being built in most communities.

The concept of **continuing care retirement communities (CCRCs)**, sometimes referred to as total life centers, allows seniors to "age in place," with flexible accommodations designed to meet their health and housing needs as these needs change over time (American Association of Retired Persons [AARP], 2011a). CCRCs are the most expensive long-term care solution available to seniors; however, they provide all levels of living, from total independence to the most dependent, and are designed to meet the continuous living needs of older aging adults. Residents entering CCRCs sign a long-term contract that provides for housing, services, and nursing care, usually all in one location. Many seniors enter into CCRC contracts while they are healthy and active, knowing they will be able to stay in the same community and receive nursing care should this become necessary. Seniors who invest in a CCRC have adequately planned for housing and care for the remainder of their life and have the financial means to support it. Entrance fees can range from $100,000 to $1,000,000 and monthly fees from $3,000 to $5,000 (AARP, 2011b). Others may choose to remain in their own home because they do not desire consolidated living arrangements that include only older adults, or because they have not planned adequately for the expense. Nevertheless, demand is increasing for this type of housing option. Adults nearing retirement today are investigating this concept as a viable option as they actively plan for their retirement.

Although only 6% of the population lives in **skilled nursing facilities**, such organizations remain the most visible type of health service for older adults. These facilities provide skilled nursing care along with personal care that is considered nonskilled or **custodial care**, such as bathing, dressing, feeding, and assisting with mobility and recreation. Currently, approximately 2 million people are receiving nursing home care.

Some struggle to maintain the appearance of doing well in order to maintain their independence. Often, they fear that their children or others will make decisions for them that include leaving their homes. Home, whatever form it takes, is where these people believe they are the happiest.

There is increased emphasis on providing needed services for elders at home. This trend started several years ago when it became evident that people improved more quickly and at lower cost when they were cared for as outpatients in their own homes. Today's heightened emphasis on health care cost control gives added support for providing services at home. Given the increase in longevity, the potential for cost savings appears significant if dependent older people can be maintained at home. Doing so encourages functional independence as well as emotional wellbeing.

Adult Day Care

Day care services offer a place where older adults can go during the day for social activities, nutrition, nursing care, and physical and speech therapies. They can be publically or privately funded, nonprofit or for-profit. The average price for adult day care is $64.00 per day (HelpGuide, 2011a). Medicare does not cover adult day care. The most recent nationwide survey of adult day centers confirmed more than 4,600 centers operating in the United States (National Adult Day Care Services Association, n.d.).

Home Care Services

Home care provides services, such as skilled nursing care, psychiatric nursing, physical and speech therapies, homemaker services, social work services, and dietetic counseling (see Chapter 32). These services are useful for families who are caring for an older person, especially if the caregivers work and no one is at home or available during the day. One disadvantage to those remaining in their homes is that services for the dependent older adults in the community are often fragmented, inadequate, and inaccessible, and at times, they operate with little or no maintenance of standards or quality control.

Independent Living

This is a general term for any housing arrangement designed exclusively for seniors. Types of independent living facilities include subsidized senior housing, retirement communities, and senior apartments restricted to those who are older (usually 55+) (HelpGuide, 2010b). These facilities provide minor assistance with ADLs and maintenance for the housing facility.

The *Village Concept* is a relatively new solution for independent living in which older adults live in their own homes in a village, giving them access to services such as transportation and grocery shopping or helping with household chores provided by the village. This means that the older adult is not dependent on family or friends. This option requires a membership fee, often more than $500 a year, based on services needed (HelpGuide, 2011i)

The dependent older adult needs someone in the community to assess their particular needs; assemble, coordinate, and monitor the appropriate resources and services; and serve as their advocate. Some communities have ombudsmen to serve in this role. But CHNs can easily fill the role of case manager for clients. This case management approach tailors services to the long-term needs of clients and enables them to function longer outside of institutions.

Assisted Living

Assisted living or assisted living facilities (residences) provide supervision or assistance with ADLs, coordination of services by outside health care providers, and monitoring of resident activities to help to ensure their health, safety, and wellbeing (Administration on Aging, 2011c). Assistance may include the administration or supervision of medication, or personal care services provided by trained staff.

Assisted living as it exists today emerged in the 1990s as an alternative on the continuum of care for older adults. Usually, it includes seniors for whom independent living is no longer appropriate but who do not need the 24-hour medical care provided by a nursing home. Assisted living is a philosophy of care and services promoting independence and dignity.

Other names for assisted living are residential care, board and care, congregate care, sheltered housing, adult congregate living care, adult living facilities, supported care, enhanced care, adult homes, retirement residences, adult foster care, and community-based retirement facilities. There is no nationally recognized definition of assisted living. Regulation and licensing of these facilities occurs at the state level. More than two thirds of the states use the licensure term "assisted living." Other licensure terms used for this type of care include residential care home, assisted care living facilities, and personal care homes. Each state's licensing agency has its own definition of the term it uses to describe assisted living. Because the term assisted living has not been defined in some states, it is often a marketing term used by a variety of senior living communities, licensed or unlicensed. The difference in licensing is usually based on the size of the facility or the services it can offer. Services that are provided include help with ADLs, health care management and monitoring, housekeeping and laundry, transportation, security, recreation, and either reminders or help with medications (Administration on Aging, 2011c). Although skilled nursing care is not provided, assisted living is an expensive option ranging in cost from less than $10,000 to over $50,000 a year with an average rate of $1,800.00 per month (Administration on Aging, 2011c). Medicare does not cover the costs of assisted living; therefore, almost all of the expenses must be paid for out-of-pocket (HelpGuide, 2011b).

Medicare only pays for medical care, not housing costs. Medicaid may help pay some assisted living costs and limited custodial home care, but not generally for housing costs related to personal care homes. Those facilities focusing on the care of people with AD are physically designed with clients' safety and individual needs considered and are staffed with paraprofessionals trained to meet each person's needs.

Nursing homes/long-term care/skilled nursing facilities include those services that provide care for people at different stages of dependence for extended periods of time. New choices are now available and provide housing for larger number of elders than do nursing homes. The average nursing home cost is around $75,000 (HelpGuide, 2011e). Medicare only covers limited stays in long-term care. For 100 days following a hospital stay, Medicare covers a nursing or rehabilitation center. Medicare does not, however, pay for custodial care (care that includes help with ADLs but not skilled nursing care). Medicaid will pay for nursing home care for those with limited assets (HelpGuide, 2011e).

Medicare and Medicaid generally pay only for care in skilled nursing facilities. Medicaid may pay for care in intermediate care facilities but only after the client meets income and asset tests that leave them essentially indigent. Medicaid coverage of assisted living services is available in a few states that can grant Medicaid waivers. The average length of time a senior remains in an assisted living residence is about 28.3 months (National Center for Assisted Living, 2011). Due to licensing restrictions, when someone becomes bedridden or needs additional assistance or skilled nursing care, they generally must move from assisted care into another facility.

Nursing home reform was promoted in 1987 with passage of the Omnibus Budget Reconciliation Act (OBRA), putting increased demands on facilities to provide competent resident assessment, timely care plans, quality improvement, and protection of resident rights (OBRA, 1987). This increased complexity of services has resulted in increased costs in these facilities. Staffing needs increase as care becomes more complex and the resident population grows. Licensed personnel must be knowledgeable decision-makers, managers of unskilled staff, staff educators, and role models, as well as efficient and effective administrators in an essentially autonomous practice setting. And, as the population grows, the need for greater number of both licensed and attendant staff becomes more evident. Because many of these jobs offer low pay and are without substantial benefits or a career ladder, it is projected that it will be difficult to find enough staff to meet the growing demands.

In the past, nursing homes had stigmas attached to them. Many people saw them as places that enforced dehumanizing and impersonal regulations, such as segregation of sexes, strict social policies, and sometimes overuse of chemical and physical restraints. Media attention to such conditions, together with current licensing regulations, should make these types of practices the rare exception. Gradually, the fear and despair associated with such facilities will begin to dissipate. In addition, as competition comes from facilities offering lower levels of care (e.g., assisted living centers), residents in nursing homes who are receiving more minimal care may be attracted to move to other types of housing.

Even in institutions in which the quality of care is outstanding, costs are so high that family resources are soon depleted if not planned for long in advance of the need. Although Medicaid pays for skilled nursing costs if the client meets low-income and asset requirements, and Medicare pays for a limited period of care, clients and families pay more than half of the total costs. Life savings that older parents had hoped to leave to their children may be quickly consumed, forcing them into indigence.

END OF LIFE: ADVANCE DIRECTIVES, HOSPICE, PALLIATIVE CARE

A final need of older adults is preparing for a dignified death. In her classic work, Elisabeth Kübler-Ross (1975) described death as the final stage of growth and one that deserves the same measure of quality as other stages of life. Although death is a natural part of life, many older people fear death as an experience of pain, humiliation, discomfort, or financial concern for loved ones. Sometimes, very aggressive and heroic medical treatments are offered to those near the end of their lives, often at the urging of family members. Planning for a dignified death is an important issue for many older people, and PHNs can facilitate conversations among family members and provide necessary information and resources.

Advance Directives

Living wills and advance health care directives (AHCD), sometimes referred to as *advance directives*, are legal documents that instruct others about end-of-life choices should an individual be unable to make decisions independently. The forms for advance directives are available for every state online at http://www.nhpco.org/i4a/forms/form.cfm?id=88 (National Hospice and Palliative Care Organization, 2011). An AHCD only becomes effective under the circumstances specified in the document. This document allows for appointment of a health care agent who will have the legal authority to make health care decisions on behalf of the patient and for specific written instructions for future health care in the event of any situation in which the patient can no longer speak for himself or herself. Examples include:

- The use of dialysis and breathing machines
- Use of resuscitation if breathing or heartbeat stops
- Tube feeding
- Organ or tissue donation

Having such documents prepared and making them known to significant others can ensure that wishes will be honored. These documents can provide clear directions for families and health care professionals and are gaining more recognition and importance as a result of increasing ethical dilemmas and challenges brought on by advances in technology (Medline Plus, 2011). Advance directives can be revoked or replaced at any time as long as the individual in question is capable of making his or her own decisions. It is recommended that these documents be reviewed every 2 years or so, or in the event of a change in health status, and revised to ensure that they continue to accurately reflect an individual's wishes.

Hospice

Hospice is an option that takes a multidisciplinary approach to end-of-life care and needs. Hospice is more a concept of care than a specific place, although some hospice organizations provide individuals with a place to die with dignity if they have no home or choose not to die at home. Hospice is an option for people with a "projected" life expectancy of 6 months or less and often involves palliative care (pain and symptom relief) as opposed to ongoing curative measures.

In 2009, about one and a half million people received services from hospice. The Medicare hospice benefit, enacted by congress in 1982, is the predominant source of payment for hospice. In 2009, 83% of hospice patients were age 65 or older—and more than one third of all hospice patients were age 85 or older. The number of hospice programs nationwide continues to increase—from the first program that opened in 1974 to approximately 5,000 programs today. The majority of hospices are independent, freestanding agencies, while the remaining agencies are either part of a hospital system, home health agency, or nursing home. Hospices may range in size from small all-volunteer agencies that care for fewer than 50 patients per year to large, national corporate chains that care for thousands of patients each day (National Hospice and Palliative Care. Organization, 2010).

Hospice enables many clients to live their end days to the fullest, with purpose, dignity, grace, and support; in fact, one recent large-scale study found that hospice patients survived 29 days longer than nonhospice patients (National Hospice and Palliative Care Organization, 2010). Hospice care focuses on all aspects of an individual's life and wellbeing: physical, social, emotional, and spiritual (Administration on Aging, 2011d). Individuals are permitted to go on and off hospice care as needed, or if they change their mind and decide to return to curative treatment. Some community health nursing agencies offer hospice programs staffed by their nurses. It is a service that has been well received by older adults, meets important needs, and is growing in use. (See Chapter 32 for more on hospice.)

Palliative Care

Palliative care consists of comfort and symptom management and does not provide a cure. For most chronic ongoing health conditions—such as diabetes, high blood pressure, congestive heart failure, arthritis, and COPD—there are no cures, only symptom relief. Relative to the senior population, which suffers from more chronic conditions than the rest of the population, palliative care should not be viewed as synonymous with hospice or end-of-life care. Rather, palliative care should be viewed as any care primarily intended to relieve the burden of physical and emotional suffering that often accompanies the illnesses associated with aging. Palliative care should be a major focus of care throughout the aging process, regardless of whether death is imminent within 6 months (Administration on Aging, 2011d). Many seniors are now "preplanning" their funerals. This option is gaining momentum in the senior population and allows individuals to make arrangements with a funeral home of their choice, selecting interment or cremation, a memorial service or a celebration of life gathering, music to be played, and other personal details. All options are chosen by the senior rather than leaving these choices and decisions solely to their family members. Other older adults may place less emphasis on the rituals, as was demonstrated by one older adult who left these choices to her children by telling them, "Surprise me!"

CARE FOR THE CAREGIVER

The burden of caregiving is receiving more attention in recent years because it is such a demanding and costly role. An increasing number of older people are cared for in their home by a spouse or other family member on an unpaid basis. Almost 75% of persons receiving care at home rely exclusively on informal caregivers, usually women between the ages of 45 and 64. The demands of caregiving exact a toll on the caregiver, who not only may miss important screening and health care visits for themselves but often gives up a social life. These demands exact a toll on the health of the caregiver. Caregiving has been associated with increased levels of depression and anxiety, as well as increased use of psychoactive medications, poorer levels of self-reported health, compromised immune function, and increased mortality (CDC, 2010c). For example, there are nearly 15 million Alzheimer's and dementia caregivers providing 17 billion hours of unpaid care valued at $202 billion (Alzheimer's Association, 2011a). These caregivers not only suffer emotionally but also physically. Because of the toll of caregiving on their own health, caregivers for those with AD and dementia had $7.9 billion in additional health care costs in 2010. More than 60% of family caregivers report high levels of stress because of the prolonged duration of caregiving and 33% report symptoms of depression (Alzheimer's Association, 2011a). Their own decline in health compromises their ability to be a caregiver unless they get some relief (see Chapter 32).

Respite care is a service that is receiving increasing attention. It provides time off for caregivers, including family members, who care for someone who is ill, injured, or frail. Respite care can take place in an adult day center, in the home of the person being cared for, or even in a residential setting such as an assisted living facility or nursing home. Although there are different approaches to respite care, all have the same basic objective: to provide caregivers with planned temporary, intermittent, substitute care, allowing for relief from the daily responsibilities of caring for the care recipient (ElderCare, 2010; HelpGuide, 2011g). Respite care is sometimes available through agencies that provide volunteers to relieve caregivers; neighbors, churches, or volunteer organizations may be potential sources of assistance. Some skilled nursing facilities provide an extra room to give temporary institutional housing for the older adults while caregivers take a break over a weekend, for instance. Clients may also need a change from the constant interaction with their caregivers. Long-term care insurance may cover some costs of respite care. The 2000 Older Americans Act Amendments provided funding for states to work through the National Family Caregiver Support Program (NFCSP) to address respite care specifically on the local level (ElderCare, 2010).

THE COMMUNITY HEALTH NURSE IN AN AGING AMERICA

CHNs can make a significant contribution to the health of older adults. Because these nurses are in the community and already have contact with many seniors, they are in a prime position to begin needs assessments and mutual planning for the health of this group. Case management is often a critical aspect of the nurse's role because the CHN must know what resources are available and when and how to make referrals for these older clients (see From The Case Files II).

Older adults are changing dramatically. The numbers and types of home care services, for example, are mushrooming. Many entrepreneurs, including nurses, who recognize the potential of this growing market, have begun offering goods and services targeted to older adults. CHNs must keep abreast of new developments, programs, regulations, and social and economic forces, along with their potential impacts on the provision of health services.

More importantly, CHNs need to be proactive, designing interventions that maximize nursing's resources and provide the greatest benefit to clients. For example, CHNs might develop a case management program for older adults that comprises a community-wide assessment, information, and referral service. Such a program might contract with existing agencies to serve as a clearinghouse for the older adult and to channel clients to appropriate services. Financing of such a program might be based on tax dollars (if it is a public agency), grants, or some innovative fee-for-service reimbursement system.

Many of the older population's health problems can be prevented and their health promoted. Changing to a healthier lifestyle is one of the most important preventive measures the nurse can emphasize. Education and support are key to the success of these changes.

The role of the CHN as a teacher is an important one. Educating the about their health conditions, safety, and use of medications is another important way to prevent problems. Influenza and pneumonia can be prevented through regular health maintenance, which includes immunizations. Other problems associated with environmental conditions and the aging process, such as arthritis, diabetes, and some cancers, can be diagnosed and treated early, thereby minimizing their deleterious effect on functional independence.

Many types of accidents that frequently happen to older adults are preventable. CHNs can make a difference through their work with individuals, families,

PERSPECTIVES VOICES FROM THE COMMUNITY

Continuing Care Centers—A Solution for Aging Adults

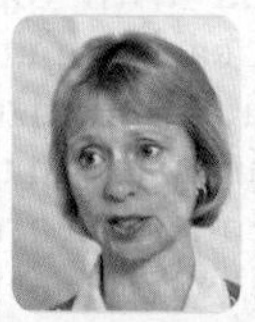

I am really sold on continuing care retirement communities! We have one in our area that is a big hit with our middle- and upper-income folks. The Otterbein Lebanon Retirement Community is a model continuing care center and is one of five Otterbein homes located in Ohio. With housing options for 1,200 residents on a 1,500-acre campus in rural southeastern Ohio, older adults can choose housing options that include freestanding two- and three-bedroom homes, one-bedroom cottages, or apartment-style one- or two-bedroom or one-room studio units, where they live independently.

They are licensed for 296 beds, including assisted living options from one-room studio apartments (with limited facilities for meal preparation) to semiprivate rooms in which nurses oversee medication and staff is available to assist with personal care. If caregiving needs become greater, additional services are available. Both skilled nursing services and a freestanding 30-bed Alzheimer's living unit exist for the frailest older adults. This is a real advantage for my clients who want to remain in the same place, even as their physical condition may worsen.

Regardless of the living arrangement, the residents are free to come and go as they wish and all have access to congregate dining in their large and attractive restaurant-style dining room.

The retirement community is expanding. One hundred and ten patio homes were built in 1999–2000 with additional expansion planned.

The Otterbein Lebanon Retirement Community also provides a health clinic, adult day care, and the other usual services found in a community: a bank, post office, ice cream parlor, a small convenience store, hairdresser, library, a church (with a 70-member choir, a bell choir, and men's and women's clubs), a thrift shop, and an arts and crafts shop open to the public. Because of the popularity of this Otterbein Lebanon community, there is a waiting list for some independent living areas.

Many of the assisted living and skilled nursing beds are occupied by residents who moved into the independent living areas 10 to 15 years ago while they were in their 70s or 80s. Their ages now range from the late 80s to older than 100, and care needs have increased. This is wonderful because, in this type of setting, frail people do not have to leave their community to get the care they need, and longtime friends are nearby to care for them or offer companionship. It is not unusual to see many of the independent seniors volunteering to help feed the frail patients in the skilled nursing care units. In fact, residents volunteer more than 85,000 hours a year to the Otterbein Lebanon Retirement Community. They know that when they need the care, a senior friend will be there for them.

Judy, PHN

and aggregates in promoting and teaching safety measures to prevent such accidents. As discussed earlier, falls are a leading cause of injury and death for the older adult and result from a combination of internal factors (e.g., diseases, effects of medicines) and external factors (e.g., lighting, area rugs, lack of handrails) that are preventable or controllable. Nurses can make a difference in the lives of older clients by using available materials and their own resources when teaching safety.

CHNs face a serious challenge in addressing the needs of the growing and aging population. At the same time, nursing can be at the forefront of developing innovative health services for seniors, rising to meet the opportunity and the challenge.

The number of older adults (age 65 and older) is increasing and becoming a larger percentage of the overall population. Women commonly outlive men by a number of years, making women a larger part of this older population. With improved medicines and medical technology, many people are now living into their 80s and 90s in relatively good health. They are able to enjoy these later years and still make contributions to their families and society. This extended life expectancy is, of course, good news; however, it has also created a myriad of new health needs and concerns, not only for the older population but also for health care facilities and professionals who deliver services to older adults.

Healthy longevity is the goal for the aging population and is a focus of *Healthy People 2020*. This means being able to function as independently as possible; maintaining as much physical, mental, and social vigor as possible; and adapting to life's changes while coping with the stresses and losses and still being able to engage in meaningful activity.

To promote and maintain health and prevent illness, older people need to be educated about their own health care needs. In particular, they should understand the potential hazards of drug interactions if they are taking multiple medications. They also need good nutrition and adequate exercise; they need to be as independent and self-reliant as possible; they need coping skills to face the possibility of financial insecurity and the loss of a spouse or other loved ones; they need social interaction, companionship, and meaningful activities; and they need to resolve anxieties regarding their own eventual death.

The most common health problems of older adults are chronic and often progressive conditions such as arthritis, vision and hearing loss, heart disease, hypertension, and diabetes, all of which can become disabling

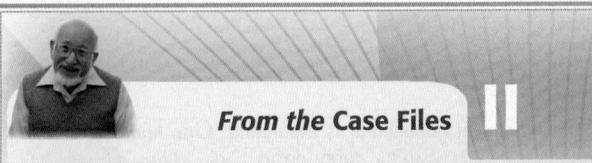

From the Case Files II

Johnny Jessup is 94 years old and lives with his wife, age 86, in a small mobile home on some acreage in a rural area of our county. He had mastoiditis as a child and lost a good deal of hearing. His vision is good, though, and he only wears glasses for reading. He was diagnosed with prostate cancer 20 years ago and still suffers from the radiation treatments he had at that time. He wears a protective "diaper" because he is often bowel incontinent. He is generally in good health, with no hypertension or evidence of heart disease. He spends most of his days outside, watering his berries, flowers, and fruit trees. He worked as a farmer and laborer—always outside—and he enjoys being in the sun and away from the television that his wife, Maude, likes to watch. He has difficulty hearing it, and when he turns up the volume, it "hurts her ears" and they argue over that. They have one son who lives in the same town, but he works long hours at his job. They speak by phone every other day, and he comes by to visit when he can. Their three grandsons are all away at college and they rarely see them.

As a young man, Johnny liked to dance, and he occasionally will go to the local senior center dances. Maude does not like to dance and will not accompany him there. Sometimes, this is a source of stress. Johnny likes to drink an "occasional cold beer," but he never drinks "hard liquor." He quit smoking 25 years ago, but he had been a heavy smoker from the age of 20. His appetite has usually been good, but he sometimes has difficulty eating fresh fruit or nuts because of his bowel problems. Maude has recently been having memory lapses and some difficulty remembering to turn off the stove and close the refrigerator door. She has trouble with a number of daily tasks. She likes to have someone bring them fast food as a treat every week, and they now require assistance with errands and most housekeeping tasks.

Recently, Johnny noticed that he was having more difficulty doing his outside chores. He seems more "weak" and "tired" and he has recently had quite a bit of "nausea and vomiting." Maude and Johnny's son took them for an appointment with his urologist, and it was determined that his prostate-specific antigen (PSA) was elevated.

You are a district PHN and have recently been assigned to the Jessup family to assess their functional limitations and provide them with information on resources they might need over the next few months. How would you begin your visit? How can you best determine their functional and physical limitations? What other assessments could be helpful (social, spiritual, mental/cognitive, etc.)? What resources and services might be helpful to them?

conditions. Other major causes of death or disability are cancer, CVSs, AD, and accidents and injuries resulting from falls, fires, or automobile crashes. Older adults also often suffer adverse side effects from **polypharmacy** (multiple medications prescribed for various chronic conditions), making polypharmacy a danger. Many of these health problems associated with old age are preventable to some extent, and early diagnosis and treatment of some conditions can minimize their adverse effects. Many accidents and injuries that render older adults unable to live independently are preventable.

Too frequently, older adults suffer from the emotional side effects of aging, such as feelings of distress and anxiety regarding their future, loneliness and social isolation when loved ones or friends die, and even depression, feeling that life is over and they have no purpose or meaningful function in life. However, older people can also enter this phase of life determined to keep physically and mentally healthy, interacting with others and making viable contributions to others and society.

Many programs are available to older adults, both for those who are healthy, hearty, and active, and for those needing some level of dependent or semidependent care. Programs for hearty older people include health maintenance programs that cover a wide range of health services, wellness programs, health screening, outreach programs, social assistance programs, and information about volunteering and educational opportunities in the community. A variety of living arrangements and care options are available from which to choose and can be tailored to the older person's desires and needs. These include the newest concepts of continuing care centers, which offer a full range of living arrangements—from totally independent living to skilled nursing services—all within one community. There are also facilities that provide skilled nursing and custodial care, assisted living, home care, day care, respite care, and hospice.

The community health perspective includes a case management approach that offers a centralized system for assessing the needs of older people and then matching those needs with the appropriate services. The CHN should also seek to serve the entire older population by assessing the needs of the population, examining the available services, and analyzing their effectiveness. The effectiveness of programs can be measured according to four important criteria (targeted to the specific needs of the population): comprehensiveness, effective coordination, accessibility, and quality.

The CHN can make significant contributions to the health of the older population as a whole by being aware of new developments and programs that become available, new regulations, and innovative social and economic forces and their impacts on the provision of health services. More importantly, the CHN can design interventions that maximize nursing resources and provide the greatest benefit to the older adult population.

ACTIVITIES TO PROMOTE **CRITICAL THINKING**

1. On the Internet, go to http://www.caringinfo.org/i4a/pages/index.cfm?pageid=3287 and download instructions for filling out your own advance directive. Complete the form for your state and discuss your wishes with someone who is likely to be involved in your health care.
2. Picture a person who you know well or know a great deal about. Make a list of characteristics that describe this person. How many of these characteristics fit your picture of most senior citizens? What are your biases (ageisms) about them?
3. If you were Minnie Blackstone's community health nurse (see From the Case Files I), what interventions would you consider using to maintain and promote her health? Why?
4. As part of your regular community health nursing workload, you visit a senior day care center one afternoon each week. You take the blood pressures of several people who are taking antihypertensive medications and do some nutrition counseling. The center accommodates 60 senior clients, and you would like to serve the health needs of the aggregate population. List potential health needs of this group. What actions might you consider taking at an aggregate level? With whom would you consult as you plan programs at the center?
5. Assume that you have been asked by your local health department to determine the needs of the population in your community. How would you begin conducting a needs assessment? What data might you want to collect? How would you find out what services are already being offered and whether they are adequate?
6. Visit a continuing care center in your community. Assess the housing options, services, and health care provisions. Would you live here when you are older? How would you feel about a family member living here? What would you change if you could?
7. Using the Internet, locate innovative programs for elders in the community at the primary, secondary, and tertiary levels of care. Determine whether such programs could work in your community.
8. How can you assist older adults with their spiritual health? What are important considerations to keep in mind? With another student, practice how you would open a conversation about this with an elderly client.
9. In From the Case Files II, how would you address the subject of advance directives? Where could you locate information specific to your state? Who else should you include in this conversation? Why is it important to have current advance directives in place?

REFERENCES

Administration on Aging. (2010a). *A profile of older Americans: 2010*. Retrieved from http://www.aoa.gov/AoAroot/Aging_Statistics/Profile/2010/index.aspx

Administration on Aging. (2010b). *Projected future growth of the older population*. Retrieved from http://www.aoa.gov/AoARoot/Aging_Statistics/future_growth/future_growth.aspx#age

Administration on Aging. (2011a). *Elderly nutrition program*. Retrieved from http://www.aoa.gov/aoaroot/Press_Room/Products_Materials/index.aspx

Administration on Aging. (2011b). *Facts: Alzheimer's disease*. Retrieved from http://www.aoa.gov/aoaroot/Press_Room/Products_Materials/fact/pdf/Alzheimers_Disease.pdf

Administration on Aging. (2011c). *Facts: Assisted living*. Retrieved from http://www.aoa.gov/aoaroot/Press_Room/Products_Materials/fact/pdf/Assisted_Living.pdf

Administration on Aging. (2011d). *Facts: Hospice care*. Retrieved from http://www.aoa.gov/aoaroot/Press_Room/Products_Materials/pdf/Hospice_Care.pdf

Allen, P. D., Cherry, K. E., & Palmore, E. (2009). Self-reported ageism in social work practitioners and students. *Journal of Gerontological Social Work, 52*(2), 124–134.

Alzheimer's Association. (2012). *Alzheimer's myths*. Retrieved from http://www.alz.org/alzheimers_disease_myths_about_alzheimers.asp

Alzheimer's Association. (2011a). *2011 Alzheimer's disease facts and figures*. Retrieved from http://www.alz.org/alzheimers_disease_facts_and_figures.asp

Alzheimer's Association. (2011b). *Fact sheet*. Retrieved from http://www.alz.org/documents_custom/2011_Facts_Figures_Fact_Sheet.pdf

Alzheimer's Association. (2011c). *Risk factors*. Retrieved from http://www.alz.org/alzheimers_disease_causes_risk_factors.asp?WT.mc_id=risk_factors_02&gclid=CPyM2-aoxKkCFQsj7AodlA1Vkw

Alzheimer's Association. (2011d). *Stages of Alzheimer's*. Retrieved from http://www.alz.org/alzheimers_disease_stages_of_alzheimers.asp

American Association of Retired Persons (AARP) (2011a). *Assessing housing options*. Retrieved from http://assets.aarp.org/aarp.org_/web/marketing/membership/membership1.htm?p=membership1.0.7.1.html

American Association of Retired Persons (AARP). (2011b) *Continuing care retirement communities: What they are and how they work*. Retrieved from http://www.aarp.org/relationships/caregiving-resource-center/info-09-2010/ho_continuing_care_retirement_communities.html

American Dental Association. (2011). *Oral health topics*. Retrieved from http://www.ada.org/2996.aspx

American Diabetes Association. (2011). *Diabetes statistics*. Retrieved from http://www.diabetes.org/diabetes-basics/diabetes-statistics/

American Geriatrics Society Foundation for Health in Aging. (n.d.). *Disorders of the mouth*. Retrieved from http://www.healthinaging.org/agingintheknow/chapters_print_ch_trial.asp?ch=46

American Occupational Therapy Association. (2011). *Myths and realities about older drivers*. Retrieved from http://www.aota.org/Older-Driver/Consumer/Myths.aspx

AmeriCorps. (2011). *About AmeriCorps*. Retrieved from http://www.americorps.gov/about/media_kit/factsheets.asp

Angevaren, M., Aufdemkampe, G., Verhaar, H. J., Aleman, A., & Vanhees, L. (2008). Physical activity and enhanced fitness to improve cognitive function in older people without known cognitive impairment. *Cochrane Database Systematic Reviews, 16*(2).

Atlas.gov. (2011). *The United States population in international context: 2000*. Retrieved from http://www.nationalatlas.gov/articles/people/a_international.html

Baranzini, F., Poloni, N., Diurni, M., Ceccon, F., Colombo, D., Colli, C., et al. (2009). Polypharmacy and psychotropic drugs as risk factors for falls in long-term care settings for elderly patients in Lombardy. *Recent Progress in Medicine, 100*(1), 9–16.

Barron, J., Tan, E. J., Yu, Q., Song, M., McGill, S., Fried, L. P. (2009). Potential for intensive volunteering to promote the health of older adults in fair health. *Journal of Urban Health, 86*(4), 641–653.

Barry, L. C., Allore, H. G., Guo, Z., Bruce, M. L., & Gill, T. M. (2008). Higher burden of depression among older women: the effect of onset, persistence, and mortality over time. *Archives of General Psychiatry, 65*(2), 172–178.

Braff, S., & Olenik, M. R. (2003). *Staying connected while letting go: The paradox of Alzheimer's caregiving*. New York: M. Evans & Co.

Center on Aging Studies Without Walls. (n.d.). *Spirituality and aging*. Retrieved from http://cas.umkc.edu/casww/sa/spirituality.htm

Centers for Disease Control and Prevention (CDC). (n.d.). *Ever had Pneumonia vaccine*? Retrieved from http://apps.nccd.cdc.gov/SAHA/Default/IndicatorDetails.aspx?IndId=EPV~N

Centers for Disease Control and Prevention (CDC). (2008a). *Colorectal cancer screening*. Retrieved from http://apps.nccd.cdc.gov/SAHA/Default/IndicatorDetails.aspx?IndId=ESC~N

Centers for Disease Control and Prevention (CDC). (2008b). *Indicator summary: Oral health: Complete tooth loss*. Retrieved from http://apps.nccd.cdc.gov/SAHA/Default/IndicatorDetails.aspx?IndId=CTL~N

Centers for Disease Control and Prevention (CDC). (2008c). *Mammogram within past 2 years*. Retrieved from http://apps.nccd.cdc.gov/SAHA/Default/IndicatorDetails.aspx?IndId=MPY~N

Centers for Disease Control and Prevention (CDC). (2009a). *2009 state-by-state report card: Cholesterol checked in past 5 years (%)*. Retrieved from http://apps.nccd.cdc.gov/SAHA/Default/IndicatorDetails.aspx?IndId=CCY~N

Centers for Disease Control and Prevention (CDC). (2009b). *Current smoking*. Retrieved from http://apps.nccd.cdc.gov/SAHA/Default/IndicatorDetails.aspx?IndId=CS ~N

Centers for Disease Control and Prevention (CDC). (2009c). *Number of U. S. adults reporting a disability is increasing*. Retrieved from http://www.cdc.gov/media/pressrel/2009/r090430.htm

Centers for Disease Control and Prevention (CDC). (2010a). *Alzheimer's disease*. Retrieved from http://www.cdc.gov/aging/aginginfo/alzheimers.htm

Centers for Disease Control and Prevention (CDC). (2010b). *Arthritis related statistics*. Retrieved from http://www.cdc.gov/arthritis/data_statistics/arthritis_related_stats.htm

Centers for Disease Control and Prevention (CDC). (2010c). *Caregiving*. Retrieved from http://www.cdc.gov/aging/caregiving/index.htm

Centers for Disease Control and Prevention (CDC). (2010d). *Caregiving: A public health priority*. Retrieved from http://www.cdc.gov/aging/caregiving/

Centers for Disease Control and Prevention (CDC). (2010e). *Chronic disease self-management program (CDSMP)*. Retrieved from http://www.cdc.gov/arthritis/interventions/self_manage.htm

Centers for Disease Control and Prevention (CDC). (2010f). *Chronic diseases are the leading causes of death and disability in the U.S.* Retrieved from http://www.cdc.gov/chronicdisease/overview/index.htm

Centers for Disease Control and Prevention (CDC). (2010g). *Depression is not a normal part of growing older*. Retrieved from http://www.cdc.gov/aging/mentalhealth/depression.htm

Centers for Disease Control and Prevention (CDC). (2010h). *Falls among older adults: An overview*. Retrieved from http://www.cdc.gov/homeandrecreationalsafety/falls/adultfalls.html

Centers for Disease Control and Prevention (CDC). (2010i). *Healthy People 2010 targets*. Retrieved from http://apps.nccd.cdc.gov/SAHA/Default/HealthyTargets.aspx

Centers for Disease Control and Prevention (CDC). (2010j). *Healthy People 2010 targets*. Retrieved from http://apps.nccd.cdc.gov/SAHA/Default/HealthyTargets.aspx

Centers for Disease Control and Prevention (CDC). (2010k). *Key facts about flu vaccine*. Retrieved from http://www.cdc.gov/flu/protect/keyfacts.htm

Centers for Disease Control and Prevention (CDC). (2010l). *NHIS arthritis surveillance*. Retrieved from http://www.cdc.gov/arthritis/data_statistics/national_nhis.htm

Centers for Disease Control and Prevention (CDC). (2010m). *Oral health. Preventing cavities, gum disease, tooth loss, and oral cancers: At a glance 2010*. Retrieved from http://www.cdc.gov/chronicdisease/resources/publications/AAG/doh.htm

Centers for Disease Control and Prevention (CDC). (2010n). *Population profile of the United States*. Retrieved from http://www.census.gov/population/www/pop-profile/natproj.html

Centers for Disease Control and Prevention (CDC). (2011a). *Arthritis: Meeting the challenge at a glance 2011*. Retrieved from http://www.cdc.gov/chronicdisease/resources/publications/aag/arthritis.htm

Centers for Disease Control and Prevention (CDC). (2011b). *Estimating seasonal influenza-associated deaths in the United States: CDC study confirms variability of flu. Questions and answers*. Retrieved from http://www.cdc.gov/flu/about/disease/us_flu-related_deaths.htm

Centers for Disease Control and Prevention (CDC). (2011c). *Health, United States, 2010 with special features on death and dying*. Retrieved from www.cdc.gov/nchs/data/hus/hus10.pdf

Centers for Disease Control and Prevention (CDC). (2011d). *Healthy aging: Helping people to live long and productive lives and enjoy a good quality of life*. Retrieved from http://www.cdc.gov/chronicdisease/resources/publications/aag/aging.htm

Centers for Disease Control and Prevention (CDC). (2011e). *How much physical activity do older adults need?* Retrieved from http://www.cdc.gov/physicalactivity/everyone/guidelines/olderadults.html

Centers for Disease Control and Prevention (CDC). (2011f). *Making physical activity a part of an older adult's life*. Retrieved from http://www.cdc.gov/physicalactivity/everyone/getactive/olderadults.html

Centers for Disease Control and Prevention (CDC). (2011g). *Older adult drivers data & statistics*. Retrieved from http://www.cdc.gov/Motorvehiclesafety/Older_Adult_Drivers/data.html

Centers for Disease Control and Prevention (CDC). (2011h). *Shingles vaccination: What you need to know*. Retrieved from http://www.cdc.gov/vaccines/vpd-vac/shingles/vacc-need-know.htm

Centers for Disease Control and Prevention (CDC). (2011i). *Why strength training*? Retrieved from http://www.cdc.gov/physicalactivity/growingstronger/why/

Central Intelligence Agency (CIA). (2011). *CIA world factbook*. Retrieved from https://www.cia.gov/library/publications/the-world-factbook/geos/xx.html

Chiang, K., Lu, R., Chu, H., Chang, Y., & Chou, K. (2008). Evaluation of the effect of a life review group program on self-esteem and life satisfaction in the elderly. *International Journal of Geriatric Psychiatry, 23*(1), 7–10.

Chong, A. M. (2007). Promoting the psychosocial health of the elderly- the role of social workers. *Social Work in Health Care, 44*(1–2), 91–109.

Contie, V. (2009). Lack of sleep linked to *Alzheimer's plaques in mice. National Institutes of Health*. Retrieved from http://www.nih.gov/researchmatters/october2009/10052009sleep.htm

Ebersole, P. (1998). *Toward healthy aging: Human needs and nursing response* (5th ed.). St. Louis, MO: Mosby.

ElderCare. (2010). *Respite care*. Retrieved from http://www.eldercare.gov/ELDERCARE.NET/Public/Resources/Factsheets/Respite_Care.aspx

Hartford Institute for Geriatric Nursing. (2007). *Try this series: Katz index of independence in activities of daily living*. Retrieved from http://consultgerirn.org/uploads/File/trythis/try_this_2.pdf

healthfinder.gov. (n.d.). *Lower your risk of falling*. Retrieved from http://healthfinder.gov/prevention/ViewTopic.aspx?topicID=17&cnt=1&areaID=5

healthfinder.gov. (2011). *Stay active as you get older: Quick tips*. Retrieved from http://healthfinder.gov/prevention/ViewTool.aspx?toolId=4

Healthy People 2020. (2010a). *Disability and health*. Retrieved from http://healthypeople.gov/2020/topicsobjectives2020/overview.aspx?topicid=9

Healthy People 2020. (2010b). *Sleep*. Retrieved from http://www.healthypeople.gov/2020/topicsobjectives2020/overview.aspx?topicid=38

Healthy People 2020. (2011a). *About Healthy People*. Retrieved from http://www.healthypeople.gov/2020/about/default.aspx

Healthy People 2020. (2011b). *Dementias, including Alzheimer's disease*. Retrieved from http://www.healthypeople.gov/2020/topicsobjectives2020/overview.aspx?topicid=7

Healthy People 2020. (2011c). *New topic areas*. Retrieved from http://www.healthypeople.gov/2020/about/new2020.aspx

HelpGuide. (2010a). *Home care services for seniors: Services to help you stay at home*. Retrieved from http://helpguide.org/elder/senior_services_living_home.htm

HelpGuide. (2010b). *Independent living for seniors*. Retrieved from http://helpguide.org/elder/independent_living_seniors_retirement.htm

HelpGuide. (2011a). *Adult day care centers*. Retrieved from http://www.helpguide.org/elder/adult_day_care_centers.htm

HelpGuide. (2011b). *Assisted living facilities: Tips for choosing a facility and making the transition*. Retrieved from http://www.helpguide.org/elder/assisted_living_facilities.htm

HelpGuide. (2011c). *Coping with grief and loss*. Retrieved from http://helpguide.org/mental/grief_loss.htm

HelpGuide. (2011d). *Dementia and Alzheimer's care: Planning and preparing for the road ahead*. Retrieved from http://www.helpguide.org/elder/alzheimers_disease_dementias_caring_caregivers.htm

HelpGuide. (2011e). *A guide to nursing homes, skilled nursing facilities and convalescent homes*. Retrieved from http://helpguide.org/elder/nursing_homes_skilled_nursing_facilities.htm

HelpGuide. (2011f). *Memory loss and aging: Causes, treatment, and help for memory problems*. Retrieved from http://www.helpguide.org/life/prevent_memory_loss.htm

HelpGuide. (2011g). *Respite care*. Retrieved from http://helpguide.org/elder/respite_care.htm

HelpGuide. (2011h). *Senior driving: Safety tips, warning signs, and knowing when to stop*. Retrieved from http://www.helpguide.org/elder/senior_citizen_driving.htm

HelpGuide. (2011i). *Understanding senior housing options*. Retrieved from http://helpguide.org/elder/senior_housing_residential_care_types.htm

HelpGuide. (2011j). *Sleeping well as you age: Helpful sleep tips for seniors*. Retrieved from http://www.helpguide.org/life/sleep_aging.htm

Hoffert, D., Henshaw, C., & Mvududu, N. (2007). Enhancing the ability of nursing students to perform a spiritual assessment. *Nurse Educator*, *32*(2), 66–72.

Hornick, R., & Aron, D. (2008). Preventing and managing diabetic complications in elderly patients. *Cleveland Clinic Journal of Medicine*, *75*(2), 153–158.

Jerant, A., Kravitz, R., Moore-Hill, M., & Franks, P. (2008). Depressive symptoms moderated the effect of chronic illness self-management training on self-efficacy. *Medical Care*, *46*(5), 523–531.

Kaiser Commission on Medicaid Facts. (2011). *Medicaid and long-term care services and supports*. Retrieved from http://www.kff.org/medicaid/upload/2186-08.pdf

KaiserEDU. (2010). *U.S. health care costs*. Retrieved from http://www.kaiseredu.org/Issue-Modules/US-Health-Care-Costs/Background-Brief.aspx

Kaiser Family Foundation. (2008). *Medicare fact sheets*. Retrieved from http://www.kff.org/medicare/factsheets.cfm

Kaiser Family Foundation. (2010). *Poverty among the Medicare population, 2008*. Retrieved from http://facts.kff.org/chart.aspx?ch=1722

Li, S. C., Schmiedek, F., Huxhold, O., Röcke, C., Smith, J., & Lindenberger, U. (2008). Working memory plasticity in old age: practice gain, transfer, and maintenance. *Psychology & Aging*, *23*(4), 731–742.

Mace, N. L., & Rabin, P. (2006). *The 36-hour day*. Baltimore, MD: The Johns Hopkins University Press.

Marek, K., & Antle, L. (2011). Medication management of the community-dwelling older adult. In R. G. Hughes (Ed.). *Patient safety and quality: An evidence-based handbook, for nurses*. Rockville, MD: Agency for Healthcare Research & Quality. Retrieved from http://www.ncbi.nlm.nih.gov/books/NBK2670/

McAuley, E., Hall, K. S., Motl, R. W., White, S. M., Wójcicki, T. R., Hu, L., et al. (2009). Trajectory of declines in physical activity in community-dwelling older women: social cognitive influences. *Journal of Gerontology, Psychological Sciences & Social Sciences*, *64*(5), 543–550.

McGuire, S. L., Klein, D. A., & Chen, S. L. (2008). Ageism revisited: a study measuring ageism in East Tennessee, USA. *Nursing & Health Sciences*, *10*(1), 11–16.

Medicare.gov. (n.d.). *Medicare benefits*. Retrieved from http://www.medicare.gov/navigation/medicare-basics/medicare-benefits/medicare-benefits-overview.aspx

Medline Plus. (2011). *Advance directives*. Retrieved from http://www.nlm.nih.gov/medlineplus/advancedirectives.html

National Adult Day Care Services Association. (n.d.). *Overview and facts*. Retrieved from http://www.nadsa.org/?page_id=80

National Association of Area Agencies on Aging. (2010). *A blueprint for action: Developing a livable community for all ages*. Retrieved from www.n4a.org/pdf/07-116-n4a-blueprint4actionwcovers.pdf

National Center for Assisted Living. (2011). *Assisted living: Resident profile*. Retrieved from http://www.ahcancal.org/ncal/resources/Pages/ResidentProfile.aspx

National Center for Biotechnology Information. (2010). *Osteoporosis*. Retrieved from http://www.ncbi.nlm.nih.gov/pubmedhealth/PMH0001400/

National Center on Elder Abuse. (n.d.a). *The scope of elder abuse*. Retrieved from http://www.ncea.aoa.gov/ncearoot/main_site/library/cane/CANE_Series/CANE_EAScope.aspx

National Center on Elder Abuse. (n.d.b). *Self-neglect. An update of the literature 2000–2005*. Retrieved from http://www.ncea.aoa.gov/main_site/library/cane/CANE_Series/CANE_selfneglectupdate.aspx

National Center on Elder Abuse. (n.d.c). *Statistics at a glance*. Retrieved from http://www.ncea.aoa.gov/ncearoot/main_site/library/statistics_research/abuse_statistics/statistics_at_glance.aspx

National Center on Elder Abuse. (2005). *Fact sheet: Elder abuse prevalence and incidence*. Retrieved from http://www.ncea.aoa.gov/main_site/pdf/publication/FinalStatistics050331.pdf

National Center on Elder Abuse. (2006). *The 2004 survey of state adult protective services: Abuse of adults 60 years of age and older*. Retrieved from http://www.ncea.aoa.gov/Main_Site/pdf/2-14-06%20FINAL%2060+REPORT.pdf

National Center on Elder Abuse. (2010). *Why should I care about elder abuse?* Retrieved from http://www.ncea.aoa.gov/ncearoot/main_site/pdf/publication/NCEA_WhatIsAbuse-2010.pdf

National Center on Elder Abuse. (2011). *Frequently asked questions. What is elder abuse?* Retrieved from http://www.ncea.aoa.gov/Main_Site/FAQ/Questions.aspx

National Foundation for Infectious Diseases. (2008). *Influenza*. Retrieved from http://www.nfid.org/influenza/

National Hospice and Palliative Care Organization. (2010). *Hospice care in America 2010*. Retrieved from http://www.nhpco.org/files/public/Statistics_Research/Hospice_Facts_Figures_Oct-2010.pdf

National Hospice and Palliative Care Organization. (2011). *Caring connections: Download your state's advance directives*. Retrieved from http://www.caringinfo.org/i4a/pages/index.cfm?pageid=3289

National Institute of Arthritis and Musculoskeletal and Skin Diseases (NIAMS). (2009). *Rheumatoid arthritis*. Retrieved from http://www.niams.nih.gov/Health_Info/Rheumatic_Disease/default.asp

National Institute of Arthritis and Musculoskeletal and Skin Diseases (NIAMS). (2010). *Arthritis*. Retrieved from http://www.niams.nih.gov/Health_Info/Arthritis/default.asp

National Institute of Justice. (2008). *Potential markers for elder mistreatment*. Retrieved from http://www.nij.gov/nij/topics/crime/elder-abuse/potential-markers.htm

National Institute of Justice. (2010). *The prevalence of elder abuse*. Retrieved from http://www.nij.gov/journals/265/elder-abuse-prevalence.htm

National Institute of Mental Health. (2007). *Older adults: Depression and suicide facts (fact sheet)*. Retrieved from http://www.nimh.nih.gov/health/publications/older-adults-depression-and-suicide-facts-fact-sheet/index.shtml

National Institute of Mental Health. (2009). *Health care costs much higher for older adults with depression plus other medical conditions*. Retrieved from http://www.nimh.nih.gov/science-news/2009/health-care-costs-much-higher-for-older-adults-with-depression-plus-other-medical-conditions.shtml

National Institute on Aging. (2010a). *Exercise and physical activity for older adult: Benefits of exercise*. Retrieved from http://nihseniorhealth.gov/exerciseforolderadults/benefitsofexercise/02.html

National Institute on Aging. (2010b). *Alzheimer's disease medications fact sheet*. Retrieved from http://www.nia.nih.gov/Alzheimers/Publications/medicationsfs.htm

National Institute on Aging. (2011). *Diagnosis of Alzheimer's*. Retrieved from http://www.nia.nih.gov/Alzheimers/Alzheimers Information/Diagnosis/

National Institute on Drug Abuse (NIDA). (2011). *Trends in prescription drug abuse*. Retrieved from http://www.drugabuse.gov/publications/research-reports/prescription-drugs

New World Encyclopedia. (2011). *Spirit*. Retrieved from http://www.newworldencyclopedia.org/entry/Spirit

Nwasuruba, C., Khan, M., & Egede, L. E. (2007). Racial/ethnic differences in multiple self-care behaviors in adults with diabetes. *Journal of General Internal Medicine*, *22*(1), 115–120.

Omnibus Budget Reconciliation Act. (1987). *Federal nursing home reform act from the Omnibus Budget Reconciliation Act of 1987*. Retrieved from www.ncmust.com/doclib/OBRA87summary.pdf

Our Parents. (2009). *Comparing costs for in-home care, nursing homes, assisted living, and adult day care*. Retrieved from http://www.ourparents.com/articles/comparing_costs_in_home_care_nursing_homes_and_assisted_living_and_adult_day_care

Owen, T. (2007). Working with socially isolated older people. *British Journal of Community Nursing*, *12*(3), 115–116.

Palmore, E. (2005). Three decades of research on ageism. *Generations*, *29*(3), 87–90.

Peace Corps. (2009). *Online information for 50+ applicants*. Retrieved from http://www.peacecorps.gov/index.cfm?shell=meet.regrec.event&eventid=84989

Pew Research Center. (2009). *Growing old in America: Expectations vs. reality*. Retrieved from http://pewresearch.org/pubs/1269/aging-survey-expectations-versus-reality

Public Citizen's Health Research Group. (2011). *Drug-induced diseases*. Retrieved from http://www.worstpills.org/public/page.cfm?op_id=5

Pynoos, J., Nishita, C., Cicero, C., & Caraviello, R. (2008). Aging in place, housing, and the law. *Elder Law Journal*, *77*. Retrieved from http://heinonline.org/HOL/LandingPage?collection=journals&handle=hein.journals/elder16&div=6&id=&page=

Racial & Ethnic Approaches to Community Health (REACH). (2011). About REACH. Retrieved from http://www.cdc.gov/reach/about.htm

Road Scholar. (2011). *Explore the world with Road Scholar*. Retrieved from http://www.roadscholar.org/

Sabia, J. (2008). There's no place like home: A hazard model analysis of aging in place among older homeowners in the PSID. *Research on Aging*, *30*(1), 3–35.

Sallis, J. F., Buono, M. J., Roby, J. J., Micale, F. G., & Nelson, J. A. (1993). Seven-day recall and other physical activity self-reports in children and adolescents. *Medicine & Science in Sports & Exercise*, *25*(1), 99–108.

Savoca, M. R., Arcury, T. A., Leng, X., Chen, H., Bell, R. A., Anderson, A. M., et al. (2010). Severe tooth loss in older adults as a key indicator of compromised dietary quality. *Public Health Nutrition*, *13*(4), 466–474.

Scan Health Plan. (2009). *Adult health screenings and immunization schedule*. Retrieved from www.scanhealthplan.com/arizona/…/

Segen's Medical Dictionary. (2011). *Oldest old*. Retrieved from http://medical-dictionary.thefreedictionary.com/Oldest+Old

Senior Corps. (2011). *About Senior Corps*. Retrieved from http://www.seniorcorps.gov/

Slavin, J. L. (2008). Position of the American Dietetic Association: health implications of dietary fiber. *Journal of the American Dietetic Association*, *108*(10), 1716–1731.

Sulter, G., Steen, C., & De Keyser, J. (1999). Use of the Barthel index and modified Rankin scale in acute stroke trials. *Stroke*, *30*(8), 1538–1541.

The Corporation for National and Community Service. (2011a). *About baby boomers*. Retrieved from http://www.getinvolved.gov/newsroom/programs/factsheet_boomers.asp

The Corporation for National and Community Service. (2011b). *Our programs and initiatives*. Retrieved from http://www.getinvolved.gov/newsroom/programs/index.asp

The Corporation for National and Community Service. (2011c). *The corporation: About us*. Retrieved from http://www.nationalservice.gov/about/overview/index.asp

The Federal Interagency Forum on Aging Related Statistics. (2010). *Older Americans 2010: Key indicators of well-being*. Retrieved from http://www.aoa.gov/agingstatsdotnet/Main_Site/Data/2008_Documents/OA_2008.pdf

Tufts University. (2011). *MyPlate for older adults*. Retrieved from http://now.tufts.edu/news-releases/tufts-university-nutrition-scientists-unveil-

Two Feathers, J., Kieffer, E. C., Palmisano, G., Anderson, M., Sinco, B., Janz, N., et al. (2005). Racial and Ethnic Approaches to Community Health (REACH) Detroit partnership: improving diabetes-related outcomes among African American and Latino adults. *American Journal of Public Health*, *95*(9), 1552–1560.

United Nations. (2011). *U.N. forecasts 10.1 billion people by century's end*. Retrieved from http://www.nytimes.com/2011/05/04/world/04population.html

U.S. Census Bureau. (2008). *An aging world: 2008*. Retrieved from www.census.gov/prod/2009pubs/p95-09-1.pdf

U.S. Census Bureau. (2010). *The next four decades: The older population in the United States 2010 to 2050*. Retrieved from http://www.census.gov/prod/2010pubs/p25-1138.pdf

U.S. Department of Agriculture. (2011). *MyPlate*. Retrieved from http://www.choosemyplate.gov/

U.S. Department of Health and Human Services. (2011). *Healthy people 2020*. Retrieved from http://www.healthypeople.gov/2020/about/default.aspx

U.S Department of Justice. (2008). *Criminal victimization in the United States, 2008—statistical tables*. Retrieved from http://bjs.ojp.usdoj.gov/index.cfm?ty=pbdetail&iid=2218

U.S. Preventive Services Task Force. (2010a). *Guide to clinical preventive services, 2010–2011*. Retrieved from http://www.ahrq.gov/clinic/pocketgd.htm

U.S. Preventive Services Task Force. (2010b). *Recommendations*. Retrieved from http://www.uspreventiveservicestaskforce.org/recommendations.htm

Washburn, R. A., Smith, K. W., Jette, A. M., & Janney, C. A. (1993). The Physical Activity Scale for the Elderly (PASE): development and evaluation. *Journal of Clinical Epidemiology*, *46*(2), 153–162.

WHO. (2011). *Key facts about cancer*. Retrieved from http://www.who.int/cancer/about/facts/en/

thePoint: Everything You Need to Make the Grade!

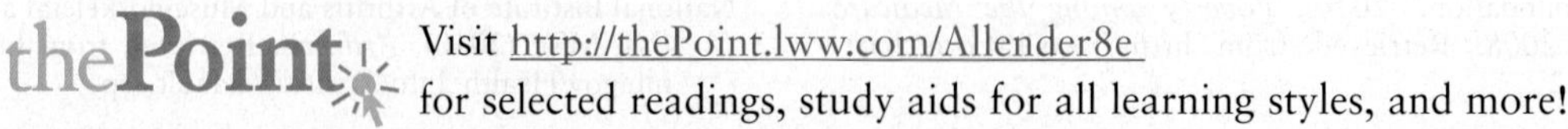

thePoint
Visit http://thePoint.lww.com/Allender8e
for selected readings, study aids for all learning styles, and more!

UNIT 7

PROMOTING AND PROTECTING THE HEALTH OF VULNERABLE POPULATIONS

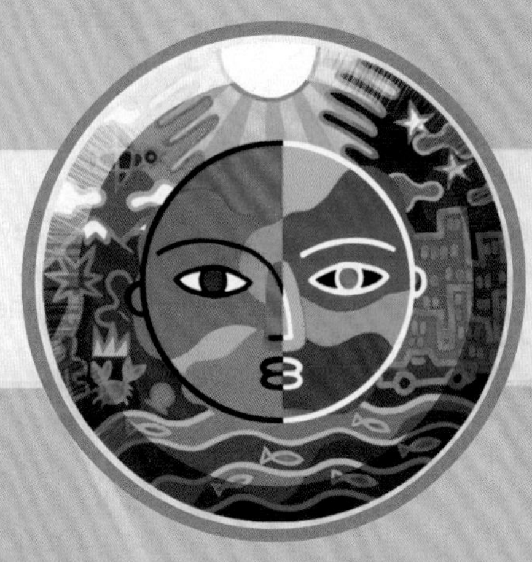

CHAPTER 25

Working With Vulnerable People

"How far you go in life depends on your being tender with the young, compassionate with the aged, sympathetic with the striving, and tolerant of the weak and the strong—because someday you will have been all of these."

—George Washington Carver

KEY TERMS

Differential vulnerability hypothesis
Environmental resources
Health disparity
Human capital
Relative risk
Social capital
Social determinants of health
Socioeconomic gradient
Socioeconomic resources
Vulnerability
Vulnerable populations

LEARNING OBJECTIVES

Upon mastery of this chapter, you should be able to:

- Describe the term "vulnerable populations."
- Describe and explain a conceptual model of vulnerability.
- Discuss the effects of vulnerability and relative risk.
- Differentiate between the concepts of social capital and human capital.
- Identify the key premise of the differential vulnerability hypothesis.
- List three of the most common factors related to vulnerability.
- Explain the socioeconomic gradient in health.
- Describe three types of health disparities.

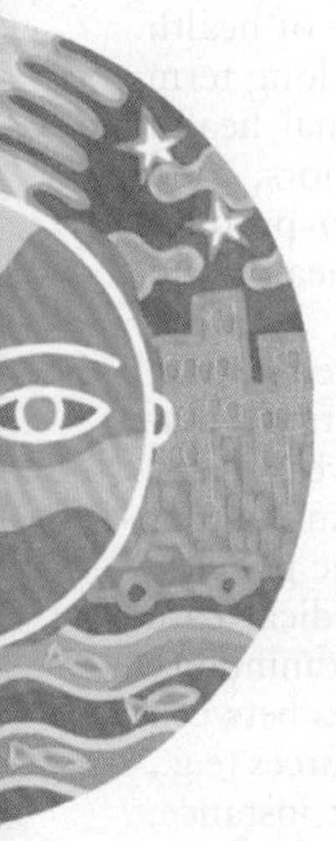

Vulnerability is susceptibility to poor health (Shi & Stevens, 2010). The public health nurse (PHN) caseload often consists largely of vulnerable populations. Often, **vulnerable populations** are subpopulations, such as ethnic or racial minorities, the uninsured, those with acquired immune deficiency syndrome (AIDS), children, the elderly, the poor, and those who are homeless (Shi & Stevens, 2010). These subpopulations often have higher morbidity and mortality rates, less access to health care (and disparities in outcomes of health care), shorter life expectancy, and an overall diminished quality of life than the population in general (Shi & Stevens, 2010; University of California Los Angeles [UCLA] Center for Vulnerable Populations Research, 2007).

In this chapter, we examine popular models and theories of vulnerability, important concepts, and contributing factors. We also briefly discuss health disparities that are more common among vulnerable members of society and the role of PHNs working with these groups. This chapter provides an overview of this subject and lays the foundation for other chapters in this section.

THE CONCEPT OF VULNERABLE POPULATIONS

Models and Theories of Vulnerability

A popular conceptual framework of vulnerability contains three related concepts: resource availability, relative risk, and health status (Flaskerud & Winslow, 1998). The authors posited that a lack of resources (e.g., socioeconomic and environmental) increases a population's exposure to risk factors and reduces their ability to avoid illness. A community's health status can be observed by noting disease prevalence along with morbidity and mortality rates. Within this framework, the more risk a population faces, the greater the impact on their health status (e.g., higher morbidity and mortality rates). A feedback loop exists from health status to resource availability as higher morbidity and mortality further deplete community resources (Fig. 25-1). The central point of the model demonstrates the importance of nursing research and practice, along with ethical and policy analysis, in affecting resources, relative risk, and health status. This can occur by direct interaction with one or more of these three factors (e.g., reducing risk factors through education) or indirectly through intervention at the junction of two factors (e.g., working to minimize morbidity related to a specific risk factor such as encouraging the consistent use of statins for hypercholesterolemia).

To further define model components, Flaskerud and Winslow (1998) explained that **socioeconomic resources** include such items as human capital (e.g., jobs, income, housing, education), social connectedness or integration (e.g., social networks or ties, social support or the lack of it, characterized by marginalization), and social status (e.g., position, power, role). **Environmental resources** deal mostly with access to health care and the quality of that care. The authors noted the differential access to health care among the poor, different ethnic and racial groups, and other underserved populations. Limited access or lack of access to care can arise from many sources, including crime-ridden neighborhoods, insufficient transportation systems, lack of adequate numbers and types of providers, and limited choices of health care plans or no health insurance. **Relative risk** refers to exposure to risk factors identified by a substantial body of research as lifestyle, behaviors and choices (e.g., diet, exercise, use of tobacco, alcohol and other drugs, sexual behaviors), use of health screening services (e.g., mammogram, colonoscopy), and stressful events (e.g., crime, violence, abuse, firearm use). The authors noted, for instance, that in populations of single-parent female-headed homes in poverty with little or no access to social programs, violence and homicide are more prevalent. Flaskerud and Winslow provided evidence of the link between poor health status and socioeconomic resource availability through the loss of income, jobs, and health insurance. In the case of environmental resources, high morbidity in an already underserved population will only exacerbate access problems. See Figure 25-1 for Flaskerud and Winslow's Vulnerable Populations Conceptual Model.

This conceptual model has generated a large body of research, including longitudinal, community-based studies of low-income Latina women receiving human

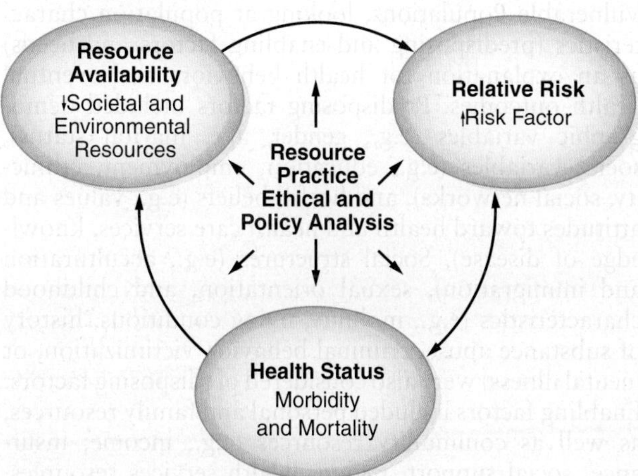

FIGURE 25-1. Vulnerable populations conceptual model. (Adapted from Flaskerud, J. & Winslow, B. (1998). Conceptualizing vulnerable populations health-related research. *Nursing Research, 47*(2), 69–78.)

immunodeficiency virus (HIV) education, counseling, and antibody testing (Flaskerud & Nyamanthi, 2000); nursing interventions with special medical needs evacuees during Hurricane Gustav (Missildine et al., 2009); public health planning for socially isolated populations in Canada (Cloutier-Fisher & Kobayashi, 2009); health promotion intervention for African American men (Scott, 2009); conceptualizing family members of the violent mentally ill as a vulnerable population (Copeland, 2007); predicting posttraumatic stress disorder symptoms in low-income pregnant and postpartum Latinas (Sumner, Wong, Schetter, Myers, & Rodriguez, 2011); community and cultural assessment of Somali Bantu refugees in Idaho (Springer, Black, Martz, Deckys, & Soelberg, 2011); administrative perspectives of vulnerable populations in an academic nursing center for the homeless (Strehlow & Fongwa, 2005); vulnerability of African American grandmother caregivers (Carr, 2006); enhancing utilization of resources among pregnant adolescents (Flynn, Budd, & Modelski, 2008); relationship among resource availability, intimate partner violence, and depression among Hispanic women (Gonzalez-Guarda et al., 2009); review of literature on HIV and Mexican migrant workers in the United States as a vulnerable population (Albarran & Nyamathi, 2001); assessment of cultural and environmental barriers to making necessary asthma-focused changes for children in homes of Latino families (Kueny, Berg, Chowdhury, & Anderson, 2011); and vulnerability of medically underserved, rural populations (Rawlett, 2011). Adaptations of the model and extensions to newer conceptual frameworks include working with traumatic brain-injured patients (Bay, Kreulen, Shaves, & Currier, 2006); framework to develop advocacy and promote empowerment in African American grandmothers caring for their grandchildren (Carr, 2011); living with spinal cord injury (Fyffe, Botticello, & Myaskovsky, 2011); and developing a Caregiver Empowerment Model for family members caring for aging parents (Jones, Winslow, Lee, Burns, & Esther-Zhang, 2011).

Gelberg, Andersen, and Leake (2000) advanced another classic model, The Behavioral Model for Vulnerable Populations, looking at population characteristics (predisposing and enabling factors and needs) as an explanation for health behaviors and eventual health outcomes. Predisposing factors included demographic variables (e.g., gender, age, marital status), social variables (e.g., education, employment, ethnicity, social networks), and health beliefs (e.g., values and attitudes toward health and health care services, knowledge of disease). Social structures (e.g., acculturation and immigration), sexual orientation, and childhood characteristics (e.g., mobility, living conditions, history of substance abuse, criminal behavior, victimization, or mental illness) were also considered predisposing factors. Enabling factors included personal and family resources, as well as community resources (e.g., income, insurance, social support, region, health services resources, public benefits, transportation, telephone, crime rates, social services resources). Perceived health needs and population health conditions also were considered, as were health behaviors including diet, exercise, tobacco use, self-care, and adherence to care. The use of health services (e.g., ambulatory and inpatient care, long-term care, and alternative health care) and personal health practices (e.g., hygiene, unsafe sexual behaviors, food sources) combined with the other factors to produce outcomes such as perceived and evaluated health and general satisfaction with health care services.

LuAnn Aday (2001) developed the well-known Framework for Studying Vulnerable Populations that includes both macro- and microperspectives. Aday described the effects of policies on both communities and individuals, including social and economic policies, community-oriented health policies, and medical care and public health policies. She noted that community resources (e.g., strong neighborhoods, close ties between citizens) have a direct effect on individual resources (e.g., social status, social ties, human capital). For instance, a community with a high proportion of children, adolescents, and elderly and a majority of single female-headed households will likely also be characterized by lower education levels, higher unemployment, and lower income levels along with a subsequently higher relative risk of poor health status. When strong social networks are present and housing is adequate, the relative risk of poor psychological, social, or physical health decreases.

Aday (2001) subscribed to a **differential vulnerability hypothesis** that "negative or stressful events (such as unemployment, divorce, or death of a loved one) hurt some people more than others" (p. 4). Even though we all are subjected to stressful events (nursing school, for instance), Aday cited research showing that low socioeconomic status (SES) groups, for example, are more adversely affected by stressful or negative events than those with higher SES. The "chronic psychosocial stresses" manifested by the lack of material resources and social marginalization experienced in childhood and early adolescence can make real physical changes by influencing "gene expression via neuroendocrine regulatory dysfunction" and are the basis of vulnerability to poor health in adulthood (Furumoto-Dawson, Gehlert, Sohmer, Olopade, & Sacks, 2007, p. 1238). The expression and interaction of these developmental genes with physical and social environments can produce long-term poor health outcomes. In other words, early chronic stressors can induce physiological changes that lead to later negative health outcomes.

Like Flaskerud and Winslow (1998), Aday noted that social status (e.g., age, gender, race, and ethnicity) affects social capital and human capital. **Social capital** consists of marital status, family structure, social ties and networks, and membership in voluntary organizations, such as a church or clubs. Aday linked **human capital** to investments in individuals' capabilities and skills (e.g., education, job training) and noted that human capital comprises jobs, income, housing, and education. Aday (2001) described research showing that better health status is associated with higher education levels and noted that the personal and political power of individuals and communities differentially affect their efforts to gain access to adequate schools, housing, and employment. "The social status and social capital resources of individuals and groups in a community influence the level of investments that are likely to be made in the schools, jobs, housing, and associated earning potential of the families and individuals living within it" (p. 8).

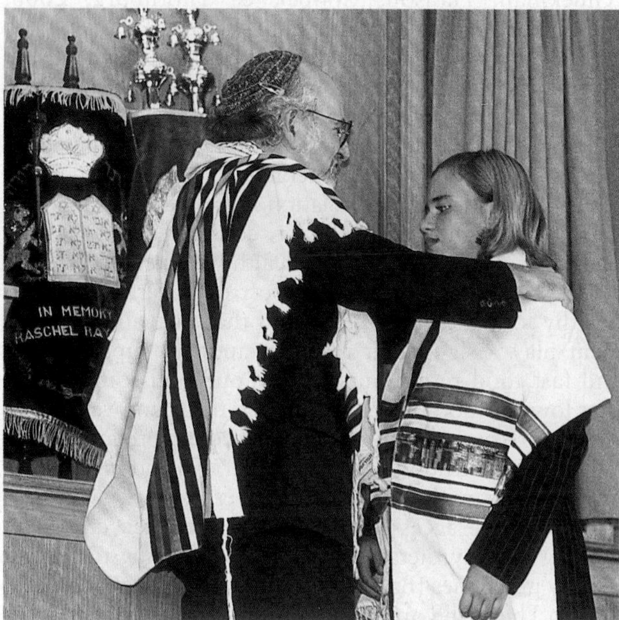

Social capital can include social ties and networks afforded by religious affiliations.

The importance of social capital is sometimes missed, as it can be subtle and less obvious than the lack of money or jobs. But the presence of friends and family or someone to rely on in case of an emergency can be invaluable in assisting individuals through many of life's difficulties. Social support, or a close confidant, can promote social and psychological health and help counteract the effects of stressful events. In our mobile society, many people live great distances from family members and have difficulty establishing new friendships. Those who live alone or who are socially isolated are at greatest risk (Aday, 2001); PHNs should be aware of this and strive to provide additional support and resources.

A General Model of Vulnerability helps to explain individual and community risk factors that lead to vulnerability, as well as problems with access to care and quality of care received that impact health outcomes on both an individual and community level (Shi, Stevens, Lebrun, Faed, & Tsai, 2008). Vulnerable populations often experience clusters of risk factors, and these are viewed as cumulative. The specific combinations of risks (e.g., low income, low education) are more detrimental to health outcomes, as is the greater number of risk factors that accumulate over time.

Most nursing students are familiar with Maslow's Hierarchy of Needs (1987) with physiological needs (e.g., water, food, air) as the base of a pyramid with the needs for safety, belonging, esteem, and self-actualization building from that most basic need. Chronic poverty, environments of crime and violence, or disenfranchisement and discrimination (vulnerability) can keep people from meeting these higher needs.

Who Is Considered Vulnerable?

In her classic book, Aday (2001) included the following factors and populations in her description of who is considered vulnerable:

- Income and education
- Age and gender
- Race and ethnicity
- Chronic illness and disability
- HIV/AIDS
- Mental illness and disability
- Alcohol and substance abuse
- Familial abuse
- Homelessness
- Suicide and homicide risk
- High-risk mothers and infants
- Immigrants and refugees

Other authors considered the uninsured and underinsured as vulnerable populations due to their difficulties with health care access and the potential for poor health outcomes (Pauly & Pagan, 2007; Shi & Stevens, 2010). Single parents and those living in violent environments may also be recognized as vulnerable populations (Johnson et al., 2009). Evans (2006) noted that those without liberty (e.g., prisoners, detainees) and rural populations, or those living in areas prone to natural disasters, are also vulnerable. The very young and the very old have particular risk factors that increase their chances of poor health, as well as unique issues with access to health care. An extensive body of research substantiates the reality of higher morbidity and mortality rates for racial and ethnic minorities than for the White population (Aday, 2001; D'Avolio, Feldman, Mitchell, & Strumpf (2008); Institute of Medicine [IOM], 2003; Meyers, 2009; Shi et al., 2008).

Prevalence of Vulnerable Populations and Causative Factors

Because many of the previously listed conditions and categories have overlapping populations, it is difficult to access accurate data and statistics for each group or category. For example, someone with little education and low income may also be a member of a racial or ethnic minority and may have inadequate housing along with a chronic illness and high-risk births. Aday (2001) noted that rates of low birth weight and infant mortality, along with teenage pregnancy and inadequate prenatal care for mothers, are indicators of substantial problems in that particular area.

Root causes of vulnerability, such as low SES, lack of insurance coverage, and race or ethnicity, have been widely researched. Which factor is considered most important? The exact weight of the interaction of these variables has been difficult to ascertain. The current approach to understanding the complex interrelationships among the factors related to vulnerability is to examine multiple determinants of health (Freudenberg & Olden, 2010); this chapter focuses on the social determinants of health.

Poverty

If only one indicator is measured—poverty—it is evident that vulnerability touches a large segment of the American population, as well as the global one. An estimated 420 million people worldwide live in chronic absolute poverty (Braunholtz-Speight, 2007). Data indicated that in 2009 about 42.9 million (14.3%) people in the United States lived below the federal poverty thresholds (Bishaw & Macartney, 2010). For 2009, the poverty thresholds were $11,161 for a single individual under 65 years of age, $14,767 for a single parent with one child, and $21,756 for a family of two adults and two children (University of Michigan, n.d.). Almost one third of those in deep poverty were under the age of 17, and about two thirds were female and White. However, Blacks are 300% more likely to live in deep poverty than Whites (Pugh, 2007).

How does poverty make one vulnerable to poor health outcomes? The answer to this question has not been adequately addressed, thus far, to provide a complete answer. However, one theory is that having less money means being less able to afford most aspects of a quality life including adequate housing in a safe neighborhood. This may lead to fewer opportunities for exercise, especially if walking outside puts one at risk of becoming a victim of violence. Fewer community resources are usually available, such as grocery stores, quality schools, recreation facilities, and health care providers. Lower income level is associated with less education and often results in a person having to work at jobs in which she or he is exposed to higher risks (e.g., mining), or the need to work at more than one job in order to make ends meet and often without health insurance coverage (Centers for Disease Control & Prevention [CDC], 2011). Because of the lack of free time, one may be less likely to shop for fresh fruits and vegetables and to cook healthy meals, with a consequent reliance on fast foods. Inadequate childcare, lower social class, and stigmatization can cause ongoing psychological stress. There may be less control over transportation and work schedules, along with a greater degree of stress on the job and at home. Chronic stress takes a toll on one's body as it "can lead to health damage through neuroendocrine, sympathetic nervous system, vascular, and immune pathways" (Braveman, 2007, p. 2). The resulting consequences of chronic stress may lead to rapid aging and "induce health-damaging behaviors such as smoking" (Aday, 2005, p. 195) (see Perspectives: Student Voices). Neighborhood characteristics (e.g., high levels of deprivation and problems, low levels of safety) have been linked to inflammatory markers for atherosclerosis in one multiethnic study, indicating neighborhood differences in cardiovascular disease risk (Nazmi, Roux, Ranjit, Seeman, & Jenny, 2010).

Research has shown that poverty and low education levels are associated with greater functional losses, certain diseases, more incidences of physical and cognitive impairment, and higher mortality rates (Adler & Rehkopf, 2008; Crimmins, Hayward, & Seeman, 2004). Lower SES can affect health outcomes throughout life as different life trajectories encompass prenatal care, childhood learning activities, family experiences, educational and career opportunities, neighborhood environment, and opportunities for health care (Blackwell, Hayward, & Crimmins, 2001; Chen, Martin, & Matthews, 2007). As one example, poor prenatal nutrition can lead to type 2 diabetes and cardiovascular disease in later life (Gluckman, Hanson, Cooper, & Thornburg, 2008; Martin-Gronert & Ozanne, 2010).

Poverty and race/ethnicity are often intertwined, but SES may be a better predictor of health outcomes in Whites than it is within other racial or ethnic groups (Adler & Rehkopf, 2008; Crimmins et al., 2004). Poor White populations suffer poor health outcomes, but in other racial or ethnic minorities, the association is much less straightforward. Although, overall, SES is considered a consistent and robust variable related to health (Chen et al., 2007).

If we examine just one aspect of poverty, access to healthy food, research has found that race and environment play a significant role. An audit of supermarkets and fast food restaurants in St. Louis, Missouri, found that low-fat food options and fresh fruits and vegetables were more often found in higher-income, predominately White neighborhoods. African American and mixed-race areas, along with White high-poverty areas, were less likely to have access to foods that are often crucial in making healthy dietary choices and adhering to federal dietary guidelines (Baker, Schootman, Barnidge, & Kelly, 2006). These SES and racial differences in fruit and vegetable availability and intake were also noted in a large-scale nationwide study (Dubowitz et al., 2008). Other researchers have noted, for instance, the lack of supermarkets or grocery stores in African American and Latino neighborhoods in Harlem (Galvez et al., 2007) and the association of greater access to supermarkets (and limited access to convenience stores) with healthier diets and lower rates of obesity (Larson, Story, & Nelson, 2009).

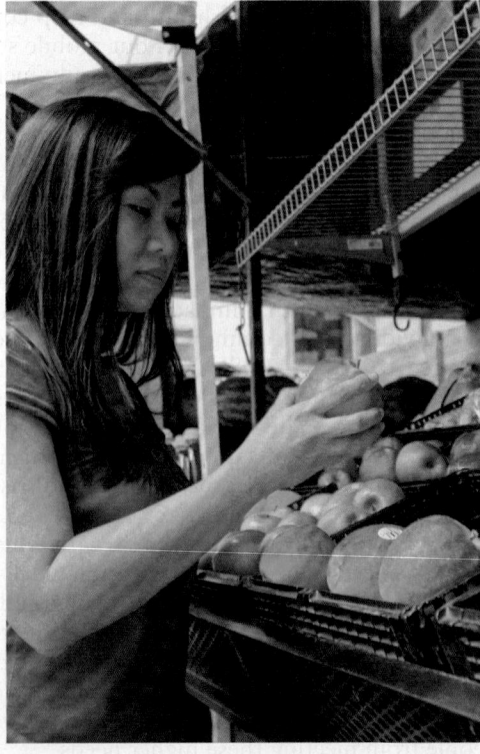

Income and race/ethnicity influences access to healthy food.

PERSPECTIVES STUDENT VOICE

A Nursing Student's View of the Aftermath of Hurricane Katrina

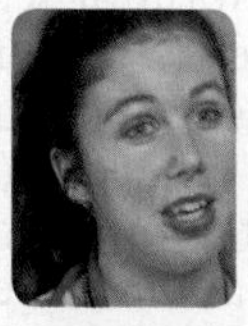

I was beginning my last year of nursing school when Hurricanes Katrina and Rita hit the Gulf Coast of Louisiana and Mississippi. Like most people, I was fixated on the television coverage of this natural disaster. A lot of the round-the-clock coverage focused on New Orleans, and much of that city seemed to be under water. People in flooded areas were stranded on housetops, while families could be seen walking on highways to get to Red Cross shelters. A horrifying image that I recall clearly was one of yellow school buses, mostly underwater, that were a key part of the city's disaster plan and were supposed to be used to assist those without personal means of transportation to move to higher ground.

It was like watching a very bad dream. We have had disasters in this country, but I did not expect to witness the lack of organization and preparation that seemed to abound with Katrina. I couldn't understand why masses of people didn't leave the area before the storms hit and why it took so long for the federal government to respond to the needs of American citizens. Those people who tried to leave found themselves delayed by the slowly moving parking lots that had once been interstate freeways. Even with personal transportation, evacuation was difficult!

What seemed very clear after Katrina was that there are large numbers of poor and vulnerable people in this country; I had not been previously aware of this. Did you know that most of those who died were poor and Black? This doesn't seem right. Didn't we abolish segregation and advance civil rights? In our community health nursing class, we discussed vulnerable populations and read some articles about this disaster. We talked about health disparities. I had never really thought about that before, but it rings true to me now. Some groups of people have higher numbers of deaths and more problems with certain diseases than other groups. We do have different levels of health care for different groups, and some people can only access the health care system by coming to the ED.

I now have a better understanding of how things happened with Katrina. When you have little money, no reliable transportation, no extended support systems, and inadequate information about an impending disaster, you are vulnerable and at the mercy of government systems that often cannot respond quickly. I often wonder how I would fare if something happened suddenly, and I couldn't access cash from my bank account, or my car was low on gas, and I hadn't bought groceries in a couple of weeks. Would I be able to survive a natural disaster like an earthquake? I have family close by and many friends, some in nursing school, who could help me. That makes me less vulnerable, but I still should do a better job of being prepared.

Brooke, Nursing Student

Another risk factor for the poor is the finding that the highest amount of pollution is most often found in neighborhoods where there is more poverty, lower education levels, and higher rates of unemployment (CDC, 2011; Evans, 2006; Havard, Degun, Zmirou-Navier, Schillinger, & Bard, 2009). Others noted an association between SES and poorer respiratory health, often due to living conditions (i.e., ambient air pollution, occupational exposure, smoking) (Schikowski et al., 2008), and of a difference in air pollution–associated mortality between those living in public versus private housing and those working a blue-collar job rather than professional, or white-collar workers (Ou et al., 2008). Also, interventions like smoking cessation have been shown to more often be accepted and successful among populations with higher levels of education, which are most often associated with higher income levels (Bulatao & Anderson, 2004), although more current research noted that lower SES groups are as likely as higher ones to attempt smoking cessation. They are, however, 50% less likely to be successful in their efforts (Kotz & West, 2009).

At the population level, increases in total income and reductions in poverty levels are "strongly associated with subsequent improvements in population health" (Aday, 2005, p. 190). Income affects health, and poor health can affect the income of an individual as well as that of a nation (see Chapter 6).

Uninsured and Underinsured

If the uninsured is also classified as a vulnerable population, even more Americans join the ranks, because the majority of those without health insurance are working adults who are not eligible for Medicaid or Medicare. In 2009, 50.7 million people in the United States were without health insurance, an increase of 4.3 million from 2008 (Sherman, Trisi, Greenstein, & Broadden, 2010). The percentage of Whites who are uninsured is estimated at 12%, Blacks at 19%, and Latinos/Hispanics at 34%, indicating racial and ethnic disparity in this area. In addition, about two thirds of those who are uninsured are living in poverty, with many of them classed as the *working poor* (Collins, 2007). However, research has indicated that disparities in access to health care and sometimes health outcomes, independent of SES or race, are often found in uninsured populations (Lillie-Blanton, 2008).

An estimated 25 million Americans with health insurance could be classified as underinsured (Schoen, Collins, Kriss, & Doty, 2008). When that number is added to the uninsured population, 75.7 million of the total US population could be characterized as vulnerable.

How does having inadequate or no health insurance lead to poor health outcomes? As explained in Chapter 6, those with few or no resources in this area do not utilize early screenings and preventive measures, and they delay getting treatment in an effort to save money. Uninsured individuals may lack a medical "home" or a consistent health care provider (Collins, 2007). They only receive care for the problem at hand and not always for underlying causes. They do not get regular physical examinations and may be inadequately immunized against common diseases. Thus, they are at risk for poorer general health as well as financial insecurity (Himmelstein, Thorne, Warren, & Woolhandler, 2009; Himmelstein, Warren, Thorne, & Woolhandler, 2005). Also, when examination and subsequent treatment are delayed, diseases, such as cancer or cardiovascular illness, may result in earlier death.

Race and Ethnicity

The United States is a multiracial, multiethnic country. About one third of the population belongs to a racial or ethnic minority group, and this proportion will continue to increase, as minorities are projected to comprise more than half of all children by 2023 (U.S. Census Bureau, 2008). Hispanics represent the largest minority group (about half of the 98 million total), and they are also the fastest-growing group, with a fertility rate of 2.80 (Population Reference Bureau, 2006; U.S. Census Bureau, 2007).

Blacks and Hispanics report higher levels of metabolic and vascular diseases, as well as cognitive impairment (Apridonidze, Shaqra, Ktaich, Liu, & Bella, 2011; Crimmins et al., 2004). In 2005, Blacks represented 12.3% of the population, but they have accounted for 40% of the total AIDS cases since the epidemic began in this country in 1981 (Andriote, 2005). Hispanics report higher incidences of diabetes but are more often found to be obese, a condition that is linked closely with type 2 diabetes. A study found an increased incidence of pulmonary embolism for Blacks, but no differences in hospital fatality rates (Schneider, Lilienfeld, & Im, 2006), whereas no racial or ethnic differences were noted in a study of interventions postmyocardial infarction (Jacobi et al., 2007). Low birth weights are more prevalent among Blacks (Nanyonjo, Montgomery, Modeste, & Fujimoto, 2007), and infant mortality rates for Blacks have been consistently almost twice the rate for Whites. However, the infant mortality rate for Cuban women was 4.42 in 2005, the only group to reach the *Healthy People 2010* goal of 4.5 deaths per 1,000 live births (MacDorman & Matthews, 2008). Life expectancy for all minority races has been consistently lower than that of Whites since 1901. Life expectancy for Blacks was only 33.7 years in 1901, whereas for Whites it was 49.4 years. The gap narrowed to 5.5 years by 2001, and to 4.7 years by 2004, but the racial/ethnic disparity still exists (CDC, 2004, 2007).

Why does simply being a member of a racial/ethnic minority group make someone vulnerable? The reasons are complex and not well understood. Poorer health outcomes for Blacks have been attributed to cultural barriers, discrimination, and lack of access to appropriate health care (Adler & Rehkopf, 2008; Evans, 2006). Others note that Black neighborhoods have lower quality health facilities and less competent practitioners, along with greater levels of pollution and "poorer built environments" (e.g., greater access to fast food, less access to supermarkets and recreational facilities)—three pathways that result in a form of segregation leading to poorer health outcomes (Landrine & Corral, 2009, p. 179). Some believe, as stated earlier, that race or ethnicity and poverty are related. But even when SES is controlled, racial disparities in health remain, especially among the Black population (Adler & Rehkopf, 2008; Crimmins et al., 2004; Chandra & Skinner, 2004; Williams & Mohammed, 2009). Some believe that the childhood experiences of the Black population may explain the disparity in mortality rates (Mechanic & Tanner, 2007; Warner & Hayward, 2002) or that disparities may be related to differing cultural norms and values (Mechanic & Tanner, 2007; Winkleby & Cubbin, 2004). Recent immigrants (e.g., foreign-born Mexican Americans) have healthier exercise and dietary patterns than those born inside the United States (Winkleby & Cubbin, 2004). For Asian Americans, one study found that native language retention was associated with lower rates of obesity in first- and second-generation participants when compared with those who become fully acculturated (Wang, Quong, Kanaya, & Fernandez, 2011). Others note the generational link between minority group membership and low educational attainment (e.g., father's education level) and the tie between education and health (Crimmins et al., 2004; Cutler & Lleras-Muney, 2010). A majority of Hispanics and Blacks have spent a lifetime at a lower level of educational attainment.

In examining racial and ethnic differences in the health of older people, Bulatao and Anderson (2004) noted differential health and risk behaviors. For instance, Whites are less likely to get mammograms and Pap smears and more likely to smoke, whereas Blacks and Hispanics have more problems with obesity and report less physical activity or exercise. SES did not explain these exercise differences. Of note, health behaviors have been found to differ within racial and ethnic groups, especially by age, income, education, country of origin, and language spoken in the home. A high prevalence of unhealthy behaviors could be predicted for Hispanics born in the United States and/or those who spoke English when compared with Hispanics born in Mexico and/or speaking Spanish. They also differed by gender; women (Hispanic and Black) are more strongly affected than men, largely resulting from greater disparity in physical inactivity and obesity (Winkleby & Cubbin, 2004; Winston, Barr, Carrasquillo, Bertoni, & Shea, 2009).

Some research has demonstrated racial differences in genetics that could offer an additional explanation for health disparities, whereas some subscribe to the mechanism of genetic risk and environmental risk exposure (Olden & White, 2005; Sanoff, Sargent, Green, McLeod, & Goldberg, 2009). Racial and ethnic genetic predisposition for disease development may be set in play by environmental triggers. Because multiple risk factors may react in a synergistic manner to cause disease, research is lacking to fully explain or predict this possible phenomenon. However, large, randomized trials have shown "race-specific drug response differences between Blacks and Whites" (Olden & White, 2005, p. 721).

VULNERABILITY AND INEQUALITY IN HEALTH CARE

Social Determinants of Health

The World Health Organization has defined the social determinants of health as "the conditions in which people are born, grow, live, work, and age," including the health system (Commission on the Social Determinants of Health, 2008, p. 5). Commonly acknowledged factors, such as social norms or attitudes (e.g., discrimination), exposure to crime, violence, and social disorder; and concentrated poverty, are associated with health outcomes, and are recognized as **social determinants of health** (CDC, 2011; U.S. Department of Health and Human Services [USDHHS], n.d.). The unequal distribution of these factors among certain groups is thought to contribute to health disparities that are persistent and pervasive. The IOM's report, *For the Public's Health: The Role of Measurement in Action and Accountability*, calls for addressing the underlying factors not only the data on morbidity/mortality (2010). When we address health disparities, we must consider these social determinants and work on all levels—individual, aggregate, community, and population—to reduce them (Marmot & Wilkinson, 2006; Williams & Sternthal, 2010). For instance, a safe and nourishing diet is needed to be healthy. Safe and accessible drinking water is also required, as are adequate housing, a supportive environment, and appropriate levels of exercise. Political resources and social structures can also influence health, and multiple inequities and disadvantages are associated with poorer health (Baker, Metzler, & Galea, 2006; Williams & Sternthal, 2010). You can check your own county's health ranking at: http://www.countyhealthrankings.org/

Social determinants of health are related to both morbidity and mortality. Quantified deaths that could be attributed to social factors in the United States were recently reported. The authors found that in 2000 about 245,000 deaths were attributable to low education, 176,000 to racial segregation, 162,000 to low social support, 133,000 to individual-level poverty, 119,000 to income inequality, and 39,000 to area-level poverty (Galea, Tracy, Hoggatt, DeMaggio, & Karpati, 2011). Moreover, it is estimated that only 10% to 15% of the increase in length of life in Western nations can be attributed to improved medical care, according to Raphael's classic treatise (2003).

In an effort to improve the health of disadvantaged groups, early public health efforts addressed determinants of health such as sanitation and poverty, along with living conditions and other environmental issues (Metzler, 2007). The present need to address underlying social conditions to improve health status is borne out by current research on race and socioeconomic class (Isaacs & Schroeder, 2004; Satcher et al., 2005; Williams & Sternthal, 2010). It is now widely acknowledged that to have an impact on the health of the population, there is a need to improve social conditions (IOM, 2003; Raphael, 2003; Williams & Sternthal, 2010). Political action and participatory action research are vital tools in reducing the effects of these conditions, as are methods of community empowerment (Metzler, 2007) (see Chapters 4 and 13).

Socioeconomic Gradient of Health

A series of large-scale, longitudinal studies in England, the now classic Whitehall studies, divided British civil servants into socioeconomic groups based upon their occupational status (e.g., executives to unskilled workers). What they discovered, over time, was an improvement in mortality and morbidity rates as the level of occupation and pay increased. Those at the lowest levels had the poorest health, but as they moved up the salary scale and occupational level, their health improved. What makes this so interesting is that all of the workers had basic health insurance coverage and free medical care—no real problems with access to health care existed. Although less pronounced, even when the researchers adjusted for diet, exercise, and smoking, the gradient persisted (Marmot, Ryff, Bumpass, Shipley, & Marks, 1997). One of the studies found higher prevalence of heart disease for all participants at the lower end of the social stratus. The researchers also found death rates for diabetic participants to be about 200% higher in the lowest social group when compared to the highest (Chaturvedi, 1998). A U.S. study, following up on children of Framingham study subjects found the association between lower socioeconomic position and coronary heart disease (Loucks et al., 2009).

This inverse relationship between social class or income and health has been termed the **socioeconomic gradient** (Kimbro, Bzotek, Goldman, & Rodriguez, 2008). It has been found in populations around the world, although not always unfailingly, and has been related to poor health outcomes regarding incidence of stroke in Swedish women (Kuper, Adami, Theorell, & Weiderpass, 2007); cardiovascular disease among the Greek population (Naska, Katsoulis, Trichopoulos, & Trichopoulou, 2011); cancer rates among the US population (Clegg et al., 2009); South Korean adolescent mortality rates, especially by suicide, circulatory disease, and "transport accident death" (Cho, Khang, Yang, Harper, & Lynch, 2007, p. 50); injury rates (i.e., blunt and penetrating injuries) (Zarzaur, Croce, Fabian, Fischer, & Magnotti, 2010); disability and functional limitation in the US population (Minkler, Fuller-Thomson, & Guralnik, 2006); increased burden of chronic illness among Argentine citizens, especially those in urban areas (Fleischer, Roux, Alazraqui, Spinelli, & De Maio, 2011); colds and flu (Stone, Krueger, Steptoe, & Harter, 2010); and neurocognitive abilities including linguistic ability and executive functions (Noble, McCandliss, & Farah, 2007).

The socioeconomic gradient has also been noted in behaviors, such as smoking, which is highest among those who are from the working class and who have low income and low educational levels (Yarnell et al., 2010). The gradient is also apparent in studies of hospital deaths. A large-scale study of hospitalized Medicare patients found higher rates of operative mortality with lower SES (Birkmeyer, Gu, Baser, Morris, & Birkmeyer, 2008). Low birth weights and breast-feeding also demonstrate a socioeconomic gradient. Lower levels of education and income are associated with higher rates of low birth weight, while those at the higher levels of occupation and income are more likely to breast-feed their infants than those at the lower levels (Heck, Braveman, Cubbin, Chavez, & Kiely, 2006; Nettle, 2010).

Health Disparities

Health disparities are differences in the quantity of disease, burden of disease, and other adverse health conditions present in different groups (Pamies & Nsiah-Kumi, 2009). Health disparities may be unavoidable, such as health-damaging behaviors that are chosen by an individual despite health education and counseling efforts, but most are thought to be due to inequities than can be corrected (Carter-Porras & Baquet, 2002; Williams & Sternthal, 2010). A long-held belief about health inequities, adopted by the World Health Organization, is that health differences that are avoidable and unnecessary are patently unfair and unjust (Whitehead, 1991). Health disparities can be objectively viewed as a disproportionate burden of morbidity, disability, and mortality found in a specific portion of the population in contrast to another.

One *Healthy People 2010* goal was the elimination of health disparities among segments of our population (USDHHS, 2000a, 2000b). The 2006 *National Health Care Disparities Report* revealed that disparities "remain prevalent" and that, while some disparities are decreasing, others are increasing (Agency for Healthcare Research and Quality [AHRQ], 2006, p. 2). Reported disparities exist in the areas of quality of health care, access to care, levels and types of care, and care settings; they exist within subpopulations (e.g., elderly, women, children, rural residents, disabled) and across clinical conditions. Thus, to continue the work on eliminating health disparities, one overarching goal for *Healthy People 2020* is to achieve health equity, eliminate disparities, and improve the health of all groups (USDHHS, 2010).

Poor access to quality care and overt discrimination are examples of disparities under investigation (Flores & Tomany-Korman, 2008; Hausmann, Jeong, Bost, & Ibrahim, 2008). Discrimination can occur during service delivery if health care providers are biased against a specific group or hold stereotypical beliefs about that group. Providers may also not be confident about providing care for a racial or ethnic group with whom they are unfamiliar. Language may be a problem, as can cultural values and norms that are unfamiliar to providers. Patients can also react to providers in a way that promotes disparities; they may not trust the information given to them and may not follow it as explained, leading to inadequate care (IOM, 2003). A survey conducted in 2006 found that in a sample of over 4,000 US adults from 14 racial and ethnic groups many of the minority respondents viewed their health care as more negative than the care received by Whites. A good number of them reported discrimination in the health care setting and did not think that they would be able to receive the best care if they became ill. These differences persisted despite controlling for socioeconomic variables, although a good deal of variation occurred across the racial and ethnic groups (Blendon et al., 2007). Another study involving "severely disadvantaged people with HIV infection" found that almost 40% reported "experiencing discrimination in the health care system" (Sohler, Li, & Cunningham, 2007, p. 347). Higher perceived discrimination was associated with HIV infection, homelessness, drug use, and race/ethnicity, emphasizing the perceived poor quality of care and difficulties with access to care.

Access to Care

The IOM (2003) report *Unequal Treatment: Confronting Racial and Ethnic Disparities in Health Care* noted a large body of research highlighting the higher morbidity and mortality rates among all racial and ethnic minority groups when compared with Whites. Differences in health care access were also explained—be it in the form of inadequate or no health insurance, problems getting health care, the quality of that care, fewer choices in where to go for care, or the lack of a regular health care provider. For instance, because there are fewer numbers of health care providers in minority neighborhoods, finding a primary care provider is more difficult for those living in these areas. Often, sufficient transportation is not available or clinic hours may be unrealistic for individuals working long hours (IOM, 2003; Landrine & Corral, 2009).

Residential segregation, although illegal, still exists and can play a role in health disparities. People of color often live in poorer areas where alcohol and tobacco are more heavily marketed (Kwate, Jernigan, & Lee, 2007). Many vulnerable populations, especially racial and ethnic minority groups and low-income populations, find health care at safety-net hospitals and community clinics, where they are at the mercy of balanced budgets and vast bureaucratic systems (IOM, 2003; Landrine & Corral, 2009). Other geographic factors can affect access to health care services (Coberley et al., 2007). For example, only 25% of pharmacies in non-White neighborhoods, compared with 72% in predominately White neighborhoods, stocked sufficient opioid drugs to meet the needs of palliative care patients in different New York neighborhoods (IOM, 2003). This lack of access to proper medication represents a disparity in health care. In a Canadian study (Lemstra, Neudorf, & Opondo, 2006), significantly different patterns of health care utilization were found in neighborhoods characterized as low income, and differences were noted for a wide variety of conditions (e.g., all-cause mortality, coronary heart disease, diabetes, poisonings, and injuries). In 2004, a survey of medical directors at all federally qualified community health clinics revealed that it was more difficult for uninsured patients to obtain access to specialty services outside the clinics (e.g., diagnostic tests, referrals to specialists) than for Medicare and Medicaid patients or those with private health insurance (Cook et al., 2007).

Health care access is also problematic for other vulnerable groups. For example, services and resources for the mentally ill and substance abusers are often fragmented and inadequate, as are those for abusing families and homeless persons. Refugees and immigrants may have difficulty finding affordable and easily accessible health care, largely due to their lack of health insurance and the need to find care at free clinics or emergency rooms (Aday, 2001; Edberg, Cleary, & Vyas, 2011). When vulnerable individuals cannot get appropriate health care or treatment for illness or disease, for whatever reason, they are more likely to have health deficits.

Quality of Care

Quality of care should result in an "increased likelihood of desired health outcomes" and should be "consistent with current professional knowledge" (IOM, 2003, p. 31). Care quality can include areas, such as patient safety issues, timeliness and effectiveness of patient care, and patient centeredness (AHRQ, 2006). Research indicates that racial and ethnic minority clients feel more comfortable and satisfied with care from a health care provider who comes from the same racial and/or ethnic group (IOM, 2003). However, a shortage exists of ethnically diverse health care providers. Despite racial and ethnic minorities comprising 34% of the US population, only 16.8% of registered nurses (RNs) are of minority racial and ethnic groups (U.S. Department of Health and Human Services, Health Resources Services Administration, 2010).

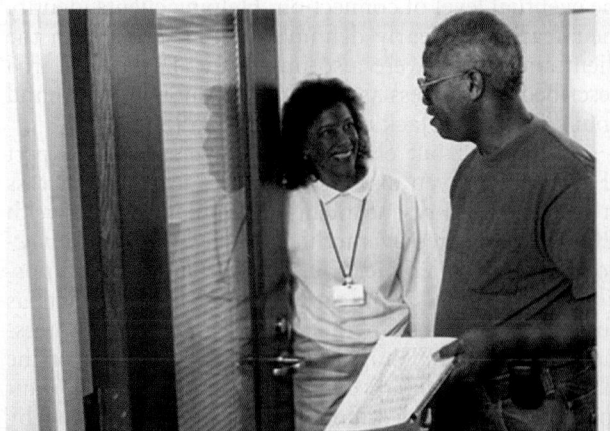

Racial and ethnic minority clients often prefer health care providers from the same racial and ethnic background.

Lack of access to quality health care services is common among racial and ethnic minority groups. A large study of over 2.3 million racial and ethnic minority patients receiving care in 4,450 hospitals for myocardial infarction, heart failure, and/or pneumonia found that significant disparities existed in quality of care most likely from receipt of care in "lower-performing hospitals" (Hasnain-Wynia et al., 2010, p. 629). Other measures, such as poor control of hypertension and cholesterol levels, were thought to be due to disparities in care within the same facilities as Whites and not an indication of the inadequacies of the health care agency. One 3-year study of more than 400 clinic patients with diabetes found improvements for hemoglobin A1c levels and no significant differences related to race or gender. Lee, Palacio, Alexandraki, Stewart, and Mooradian (2011) posited that having a medical home was the critical factor in decreasing health disparities for this population.

Communication can be a factor in poor quality of care. The authors of a study reported between 24% and 36% of low-income parents of children felt that the communication they had with their child's health care provider in a Spanish interview was "poor" (Clemans-Cope & Kenney, 2007, p. 206). Marginalized vulnerable populations, such as substance abusers, at-risk mothers and infants, abusing families, suicide- and homicide-prone individuals, and the mentally ill or disabled, may feel they are treated as "second class citizens," and cultural barriers and misunderstandings can lead to a discontinuation of recommended regimens. Poor health outcomes may result as effectiveness of health care for vulnerable populations is not often considered or even well defined (Aday, 2001; Nanyonjo et al., 2007).

WORKING WITH VULNERABLE POPULATIONS

The Role of Public Health Nurses

Community and PHNs often focus their efforts on the most vulnerable populations. In Lillian Wald's time, PHNs worked and lived among tenements (see Chapter 2). Today, most PHNs travel a good distance to reach the homes of vulnerable clients, knowing that they can leave and go back to their own circumstances. Recognizing that demeaning or dehumanizing behaviors or language directed toward clients or neighborhoods exemplifies disrespect and is often fear-based can help us all to focus our efforts (see Fig. 25.2 Dimensions of Meaning). One PHN succinctly described this fear:

> All of us, at some level, have a fear of the disenfranchised, whether it's because we could be in that place or because there may be potential harm to us. But I seek to break that fear and see someone as a human. The more I work with her, the more I see her as human. (Zerwekh, 2000, p. 47)

Working with vulnerable clients is an important component of students' clinical experiences, and necessary to better understand client circumstances and needs, as well as to be competent as nurses. It is also part of our rich nursing heritage, exemplified by Lillian Wald and others. What, then, is the PHN's role, and how can nurses be most effective when working with vulnerable groups?

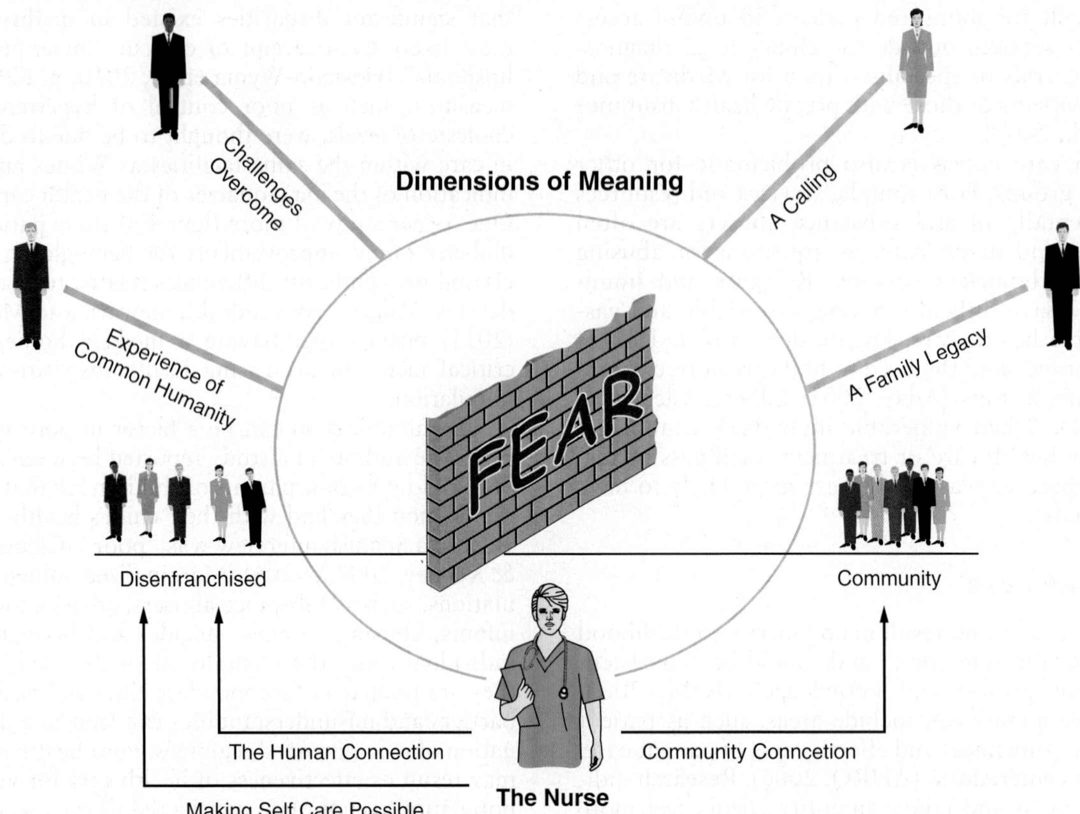

FIGURE 25-2. Breaking through the wall. Fearless caring with separated and often frightened clients has 10 themes that can be organized into three metathemes: the human connection, the community connection, and making self-care possible. The nurse goes around the separating wall of fear. (Adapted from Zerwekh, J. (2000). Caring on the ragged edge: Nursing persons who are disenfranchised. *Advances in Nursing Science, 22*(4), 47–61.)

Effective Caring

One nursing goal for clients is to help them develop their capabilities to "take charge of their own lives and make their own choices" by helping them identify all possible choices, guiding them to think through all of the issues and possible consequences, providing honest feedback, and affirming their reality (Zerwekh, 2000, p. 48). Achieving this goal can be challenging when working with the most vulnerable clients as they are often the most disenfranchised and fearful of others. PHNs often must tailor interventions to vulnerable client's specific needs and these clients often require periods of intense support (Monsen, Radosevich, Kerr, & Fulkerson, 2011). One nurse described vulnerable individuals as being behind a locked door—"the door is shut and you can't get back in" (Zerwekh, 2000, p. 50). Opening that door is the first step to working effectively with these clients. Engagement and development of rapport are essential. Because vulnerability often equates with feelings of powerlessness, the actions of PHNs can either promote engagement or destroy any chances for rapport. A Canadian study found three phases of PHN–client engagement: getting past the fear, working to build trust, and "seeking mutuality" (Jack, DiCenso, & Lohfeld, 2005, p. 182). The personal values, experiences, characteristics, and actions of both nurses and clients influenced the speed at which this process took place and the eventual level of connection. Helping clients identify their fears and clearly defining the PHN role with the client and family were also important. Earlier research described the process as "finding common ground" and "building trust" (Jack et al., 2002, p. 59).

In a small, but classic, qualitative study of expert PHNs with proven experience and a degree of success in working with disenfranchised populations, Zerwekh (2000) found three overarching themes: *human connection*, *community connection*, and *making self-care possible*. Those PHNs who can see the worth of clients as human beings and share their own humanity by expressing themselves and staying connected were part of the main theme of *human connection*. Another important component was becoming familiar with a client by learning about his past, his patterns, and the most effective means of communicating with him to draw him out. For the theme of *community connection*, subthemes of connecting clients to each other and to the community, as well as mediating bureaucratic red tape and occasionally making exceptions, were foremost, as was "haunting the case" or being a persistent advocate to get the client's needs met (p. 57). The metatheme of *making self-care possible* was characterized by "getting them through emotionally" (p. 59) or being able to listen to and counsel clients who are often on the edge with their emotions (e.g., fear, anger). Additional components of this theme included teaching clients to have self-awareness and to better understand their bodies and their feelings and coaching them to take control and foster their strengths. Confronting fear at the community level was another subtheme, as PHNs worked to break down barriers and work through long-standing prejudices and fears. Some authors believe that advocacy for vulnerable populations is an ethical responsibility for nurses who may need to help individuals and families find needed assistance (Cohen & Reutter, 2007; Erlen, 2006).

Working with disadvantaged populations can be challenging and exhausting, and the psychic distress should be "anticipated and addressed" (Beauchesne & Patsdaughter, 2005; Beidler, 2005, p. 759). Often, novice community health nurses feel overwhelmed and suffer "compassion fatigue" when confronted with the crushing realities that their vulnerable, disenfranchised clients face on a daily basis. Feelings of guilt sometimes surface when nurses contrast their own life experiences with those of their clients. To be effective in working with vulnerable populations, it is often more helpful to donate money and items on a group level rather than an individual level and to work for substantial changes in community attitudes. Also, it is vital to remain grounded to continue to have the necessary energy and compassion.

Empowerment

In Chapter 13, the author discussed the concept of empowerment and applied it to the PHN's role when working with communities. When dealing with individual clients, empowerment is defined as "an active, internal process of growth" that is reached by actualizing the full potential inherent within each client and occurring "within the context of a nurturing nurse–client relationship" in Falk-Raphael's classic article (2001, p. 4). PHNs described the process of empowerment as a two-way street, with clients gaining knowledge and skills and "acting on informed choices," but also further empowering the nurse to continue the work of empowerment (p. 6). Client empowerment is a vital role of PHNs (Mulcahy & McCarthy, 2008).

Which community health nursing activities/actions are most effective in promoting empowerment among their vulnerable clients? In Falk-Raphael's (2001) well-known qualitative study of PHNs and their clients, several themes were noted:

- *Having a client-centered approach*, denoted by flexibility in dealing with clients, for example, "meeting them where they are"; "communicating at their level"; and "backing off and following client's agenda" (p. 6).
- *Developing a trusting relationship* based on mutual respect and dignity, for example, clients as active partners with the PHN assuming more or less responsibility as needed; being empathetic, nonjudgmental, and "creating a safe environment" (p. 7).
- *Employing advocacy*, both at an individual level as well as political advocacy, for example, using their role and power as a professional to cut through bureaucratic red tape, connecting clients with available community resources, supporting clients in reaching their health goals, making their expertise available, and being a client resource as someone who is open and "available" (p. 8).
- *Being a teacher and role model*, using a variety of strategies and providing opportunities for clients to safely practice new skills, for example, teaching classes, providing individual coaching, providing positive reinforcement and support, demonstrating skills such as assertiveness and community action/participation.
- *Capacity building* through encouraging and supporting of clients' work toward attaining health goals, for example, "reflective listening and an empathetic approach" focusing on strengths, not limitations; facilitating client "self-exploration" and providing encouragement for them to "act on their choices" while being "realistic about barriers to success"; or having expectations for client accountability regarding their decisions and actions (p. 9).

Outcomes of empowerment for clients included increased self-esteem and confidence, improved self-efficacy, and the ability to "reframe situations in a positive way" (Falk-Raphael, 2001, p. 10). Clients also subsequently made better choices regarding their health and utilized resources more appropriately. They were better able to seek information and services and became more politically active. Clients' focus became more proactive than reactive, and they felt that they could communicate more effectively to define boundaries or express feelings. Consequently, clients were also better able to collaborate with their health care providers, becoming more trusting partners in care by "taking ownership for their health" (p. 10). Some clients noted a newfound ability to see their communities in a more holistic way and looked for ways to change things for the better. Both the client and the PHN undergo a "transformation" when empowerment strategies are employed (Dowling, Cooney, & Casey, 2011, p. 476).

Making a Difference

External support, along with temperament and other individual factors, has been associated with coping with stress and adverse situations. The support can be from family members, neighbors, friends, teachers, or others. PHNs can provide external support at both the individual and population levels (see Perspectives: Voices From the Community). For example, research has shown the effectiveness of social support, provided by nurses and health visitors, in promoting consistent program participation and positive social and health outcomes among low-income pregnant women (Olds et al., 2010; Shepard, Williams, & Richardson, 2004). Nurse visitation and support can also "successfully address informational needs and increase the likelihood that women will use existing community-based resources" (Tough et al., 2006, p. 183). PHNs can assist vulnerable individuals in several ways.

PERSPECTIVES
VOICES FROM THE COMMUNITY

A View of Katrina's Aftermath—Nurse Volunteer

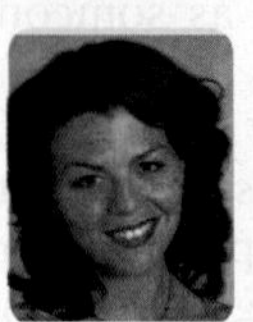

I had never been a Red Cross volunteer before, but Katrina touched my heart, and I signed up. Suddenly, I was headed to New Orleans to help in a shelter. The sheer number of people streaming into the shelter astounded me—people who had lost everything. Some of these people had waited on housetops to be rescued. Others had walked for hours to reach the shelter. A common theme among them was their vulnerability. Many were members of vulnerable populations even before Katrina struck.

At first, most were relieved to be safe and dry. However, that changed as they realized what they had lost and how uncertain their futures were. Many of the older people and those with chronic illnesses had significant health problems that worsened while they were residents of the shelter. Although they were provided with food, it was sometimes difficult for them to get the exact food they needed for their special diets. Some of them did not have all of their medications, and it took some time to complete health histories and secure necessary prescriptions. The weather was very muggy and hot, and there was little privacy. Even though the governor had called out the National Guard, people had to protect their few belongings, as theft was rampant. Toilet and bathing facilities were inadequate, space was limited, and fights often broke out between people who had been pushed to the limits of their composure.

People had to show identification to apply for emergency loans or to receive other assistance. Some of them had lost all documents in the flooding or had lost things on the way to the shelter. Standing in line was physically difficult for many people, but lines were long and standing was necessary in order to get assistance.

Many people were displaced, and a good number of them were separated from their families and friends, with no idea whether they were dead or alive. It was difficult to reconnect people, as individuals were evacuated to diverse locations. Communication was often a problem until phone lines and cell towers were back up and running.

I was there to help and to listen and provide care, but sometimes I felt frustrated and ineffective. I wanted to advocate for people and improve on systems of care, but this was almost impossible in such an erratic and crisis-driven system. Better systems need to be in place before the next disaster strikes, especially for the most vulnerable. All in all, it was a rewarding experience, and I was able to make a difference for some people on an individual basis. But there were so many who needed significant and long-term assistance!

Helena, RN, PHN, Red Cross Volunteer

Adapted from Saunders, J. M. (2007). *Vulnerable populations in an American Red Cross shelter after hurricane Katrina. Perspectives in Psychiatric Care, 43*(1), 30–37.

Through work with individual clients, PHNs can expand their own empowerment strategies to serve the community. Being aware of the community's pulse is vital and can be accomplished not only through home visits but also by attending community-level meetings and through the development of partnerships organized around specific health issues or community problems. Particularly in areas with high-risk vulnerable populations, community collaboratives can be formed to address needs identified by the members of that community (Campbell-Grossman, Brage-Hudson, Keating-Lefler, & Ofe-Fleck, 2005; Kapucu, 2008). Early detection of problems at the community level can lead to the development of programs and services to provide early intervention and avert costly tertiary care (Kapucu, 2008; Penprase, 2006; Salinsky & Gursky, 2006) or to actively meet the needs of specific groups, such as low-income elderly or diabetics (Artis, 2005; Chin et al., 2007).

Using Evidence to Reduce Vulnerability

Community health nurses can assist vulnerable populations, communities, individuals, and families to reduce their vulnerability by using evidence from research, expert opinion, and best practices (see Chapter 4 on Evidence-Based Practice). Often, evidence is embedded in policies, procedures, and clinical guidelines as demonstrated in a survey of local health departments in the state of Michigan. Almost 78% of nursing administrators reported that evidence was used for the development of practice and other agency guidelines (Ervin, Bell, & Bickes, 2009). Thus, the first place to locate evidence for practice is in the specific agency documentation for nursing practice.

Many areas for improvement of the lives of vulnerable populations lie in areas related to prevention and health promotion. Primary prevention is readily available in the form of immunizations for children, adolescents, and adults. Nursing activities to promote increasing immunization levels among vulnerable people will result in greater economic and social returns for the whole community. Similar is the involvement of nurses in smoking prevention and smoking cessation activities. In addition to immunizations and smoking cessation, the following areas are highlighted as evidence-based areas shown to improve the health status of vulnerable populations: health literacy, access to nursing services, and policy.

Improving Health Literacy

Low-income communities often have low educational levels that are related to low literacy and low health literacy levels. An estimated 80 million Americans have limited health literacy. Research demonstrates that low health literacy is associated with poorer health outcomes and poorer use of health care services (Berkman, Sheridan, Donahue, Halpern, & Crotty, 2011). In addition, low literacy or illiteracy is a contributing factor to unemployment and underemployment within vulnerable groups, thus increasing risk for low income and poverty.

Assisting vulnerable groups and communities to improve health literacy is one approach for reducing vulnerability and improving health outcomes. Many cities have literacy programs that use volunteers to provide tutoring. This is an excellent way for nurses to give back to the community. Literacy training contributes to health literacy by improving reading, writing, and comprehension skills. A crucial aspect of improving health literacy is to improve public schools so that more students graduate with adequate skills for higher education and employment (Freudenberg & Ruglis, 2007).

A first step in addressing health literacy is to assess an individual's literacy level. Tools, such as the Test of Functional Health Literacy in Adults, using hospital-written material to test reading comprehension and basic computational skills (Chew, Bradley, & Boyko, 2004) can be helpful when assessing where to start with a specific client. One question used for screening ("How confident are you filling out forms by yourself?") was found to be the best predictor of low literacy (Chew et al., 2008).

Some research shows that low-literacy clients may learn better with the use of multiple methods for teaching, such as pictures, small group classes, and audiovisual materials (Wolf et al., 2009). Written material should be carefully reviewed for reading level before it is given to clients. Many tools, such as SMOG and FOG, are available for testing reading levels of written material (Smarty, 2009).

A special challenge for nurses is preparing or locating material for clients who do not speak English. Health care agency resources need to be devoted to meeting the needs of clients who have no or few skills in English. This area of need is usually beyond the ability of the individual nurse, but the need can be made known to agency administration.

Improving Access to Nursing Services

Results from over 3 decades of research have demonstrated that home visiting by RNs is effective in improving outcomes for low-income women and children. David Olds and his research team, including Harriet Kitzman, an RN, have conducted much of the work done to demonstrate these dramatic results. Studies show that home visiting to low-income women and their children results in fewer cases of child abuse and neglect, longer spacing between pregnancies, avoidance of substance abuse and criminal behavior, and less dependence on government assistance. For the children of low-income, unmarried women, the children had fewer arrests and convictions, smoked and drank alcohol less, and had fewer sexual partners than the children who did not have nurse home visits (Olds et al., 1997, 1999). More recently, the Olds team found that families who were visited in their homes by PHNs demonstrated lasting positive effects (Olds et al., 2010).

Home visiting for other vulnerable populations demonstrated positive outcomes for Mexican mothers and their children (Cowell, McNaughton, Ailey, Gross, & Fogg, 2009) and decreasing readmissions (Ervin, Scrivener, & Simons, 2004; Paul et al., 2011). Nurse specialists and advanced practice nurses have been effective in decreasing readmissions for older patients (Naylor et al., 2004; Ornstein, Smith, Foer, Lopez-Cantor, & Soriano, 2011) and decreasing risk of infant death (Donovan et al., 2007).

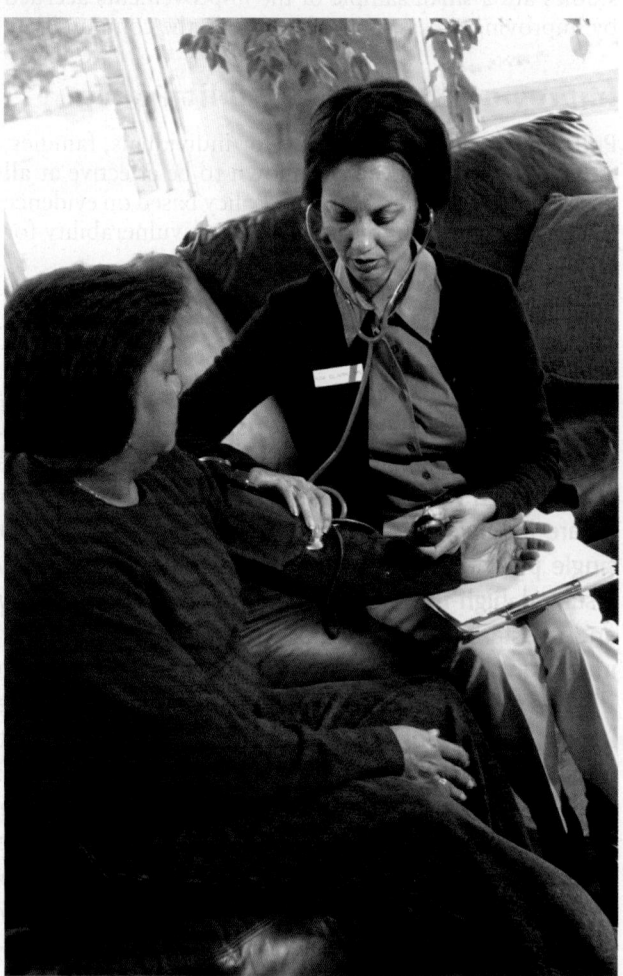

Home visiting has been shown to have positive outcomes for a variety of vulnerable populations.

Home visiting can be provided from almost any setting that provides services to communities. The usual settings are local health departments, home health care agencies, community-based hospice agencies, and visiting nurse associations. In addition, school nurses, ambulatory nurses, parish or faith-based nurses, and community health nurses have recently provided limited home visiting services to clients or families seen in a variety of settings, including outpatient clinics, Head Start programs, places of worship, and health centers. Expanding home visiting to all vulnerable groups holds promise for improving the health of many individuals and communities.

Access to nursing care through school-based clinics, community nursing centers, academic nurse-managed centers, and nurse-managed clinics has improved immunization rates in low-income children (Ervin & Young, 1996; Hull, Frauendienst, Gunderson, Monsen, & Fischbein, 2008), assisted with follow-up of children with lead poisoning (Ervin, Nelson, & Shaeff, 1999), provided good quality of care for chronic care management (Barkauskas, Pohl, Tanner, Onifade, & Pilon, 2011), and increasing access to care for communities (Pohl, Barkauskas, Bendert, Breer, & Bostrom, 2007). These studies are a small sample of the improvements accrued by improving access to nursing care in the community.

Improving Health and Public Policy

Policies to reduce vulnerability for individuals, families, and communities have been shown to be effective at all levels: local, state, and national. Policy based on evidence is an important component of reducing vulnerability for communities and individuals. This section of the chapter addresses health and public policy, including policy in schools, cities, counties, and health care settings. Policy includes social, economic, environmental, and health aspects. See Chapter 13 for an expansive discussion of policy.

Small changes in policy can make a big difference in outcomes for vulnerable communities. For example, policies to provide healthy foods in school vending machines provide healthier choices for all students, not just those considered vulnerable. Mandatory activity time for all school children contributes to preventing obesity and enhancing learning in all children as well as those who are most vulnerable because of low income and ethnicity (Beets, Tilley, Kim, & Webster, 2011; Cradock et al., 2011).

Communities that lack safe places for physical activities need to have attention directed to the appropriate governing bodies, such as the city council or the department of recreation. Community residents can be effective in bringing about change that improves a total community (Gortmaker et al., 2011).

SUMMARY

Vulnerable populations are at risk for poor health outcomes. Various models or theoretical frameworks examine personal and environmental resources and risks relative to vulnerability. Vulnerability is associated with increased risk for morbidity and mortality. Poverty, age, gender, and race or ethnicity are leading factors that make aggregates vulnerable, as can being uninsured or underinsured, a single parent, and those with little or no education. Vulnerable groups can include chronically ill or disabled, high-risk mothers and infants, those with HIV/AIDS, and the mentally ill or disabled. Alcohol and substance abusers, those prone to suicide and homicide, the homeless, abusing families, and immigrants or refugees can also be characterized as vulnerable.

It is difficult to calculate the exact numbers of Americans who are members of vulnerable groups, largely because of the overlap in populations, but it involves a significant proportion of the total population. As an example of overlap in populations, low-income status is often associated with underinsurance or race and ethnicity and may also be related to homelessness and high-risk births.

Social determinants of health are strongly associated with health outcomes. Examples of social determinants of health are social norms or attitudes, such as discrimination; exposure to crime, violence, and social disorder; and concentrated poverty. The socioeconomic gradient—an inverse relationship between social class/income and health—has been repeatedly demonstrated in research conducted around the world.

Health disparities are defined as differences in access to quality health care and in health outcomes and are usually characterized as avoidable and unfair. One of the goals of *Healthy People 2020* is to achieve health equity, eliminate disparities, and improve the health of all groups. Many disparities occur along income/class or racial/ethnic lines. A good deal of research is under way to determine more specifically the causes and consequences of health disparities.

Community health nurses often work with vulnerable populations, and nurses must learn to break through barriers of fear—their own and that of their clients. To be effective, PHNs must establish a sense of trust and rapport with their clients by finding common ground. Connecting with clients and connecting clients to the community and available resources are key factors in successful PHN–client relationships. Coaching and mentoring clients to solve their own problems and make necessary changes are also effective behaviors of PHNs.

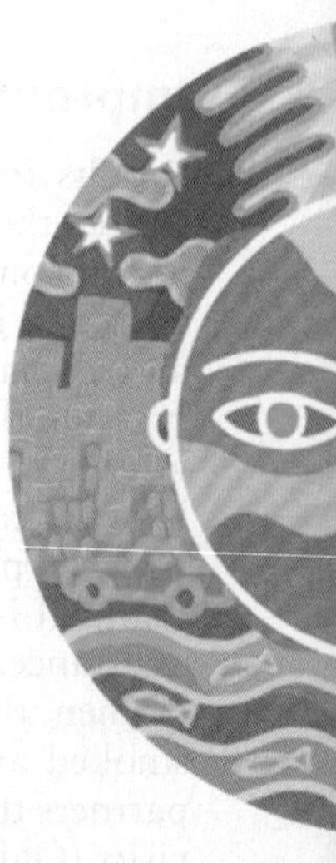

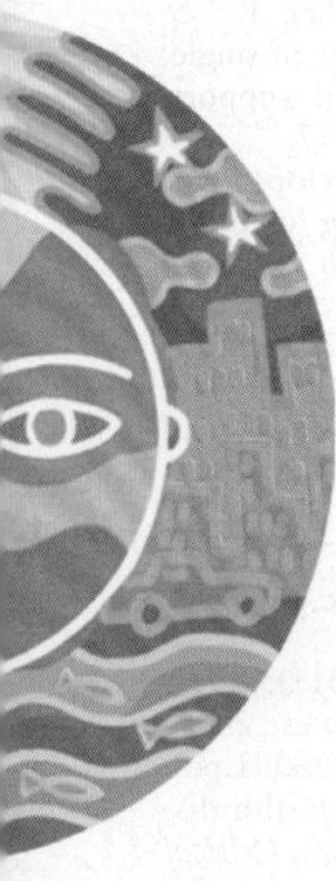

Empowerment strategies with individual clients can help them to meet their full potential, while also providing empowerment to the nurses working with them. Flexible, client-centered approaches, based on trust and mutual respect, have been found to be most effective. A nonjudgmental attitude and openness with clients lays the foundation for development of mentoring relationship. Community health nurses who work at empowering clients are advocates at the individual as well as political levels. They are a resource to clients without being paternalistic. They provide a safe place for clients to try to out skills and demonstrate new, healthier behaviors. They build capacity through active, reflective, empathetic listening, and serve as role models and teachers. Empowered clients have greater self-confidence and are better able to collaborate with health care providers. Often, empowered clients become more engaged with their communities and neighborhoods.

Community health nurses can provide individual support as well as support and leadership for vulnerable communities. Political action can involve not only health policy issues, but also political activism on the part of underserved populations to improve housing, education, and employment. Action at the community or population level is an effective and efficient way to have the "biggest bang for the buck" when improving the health of vulnerable populations.

ACTIVITIES TO PROMOTE **CRITICAL THINKING**

1. Identify at least four vulnerable groups within your community. Using the Flaskerud and Winslow's (1998) model depicted in this chapter, determine the health status for each of these groups. Describe the relative risk for each group.
2. Find available community resources for each of the identified groups. Where are they located? How easily accessible are they? What outreach services do they provide for the vulnerable population they serve? Describe some socioeconomic resources. What areas are most deficient?
3. Pick a client from your community health nursing clinical assignment. In a respectful way, discuss your fears of working in the community and ask about any fears she or he may have experienced in permitting you access to her or his home. Outline ways in which you could build upon this mutual sharing to achieve mutual trust and rapport.
4. Talk to two expert PHNs and discuss the concept of empowerment with them. What strategies have they used with clients? Ask each to share an example in which they feel that they made a real difference in the lives of their clients.
5. Locate a community collaborative that is addressing the needs of vulnerable groups in your community. Who are the members? Note the agencies represented. Are there any community members present? If possible, attend a meeting and determine the types of issues being discussed. Is there a sense of community involvement and participation?

REFERENCES

Aday, L. A. (2001). *At risk in America: The health and health care needs of vulnerable populations in the United States.* (2nd ed.). San Francisco, CA: Jossey-Bass.

Aday, L. A. (Ed.). (2005). *Reinventing public health: Policies and practices for a healthy nation.* San Francisco, CA: Jossey-Bass.

Adler, N., & Rehkopf, D. (2008). U.S. disparities in health: Descriptions, causes, and mechanisms. *Annual Review of Public Health, 29*, 235–252.

Agency for Healthcare Research and Quality (AHRQ). (2006). *National healthcare disparities report.* Retrieved from http://www.ahrq.gov/qual/nhdr06/nhdr06high.pdf

Albarran, C. R., & Nyamathi, A. (2001). HIV and Mexican migrant workers in the United States: a review applying vulnerable populations conceptual model. *Journal of the Association of Nurses in AIDS Care, 22*(3), 173–185.

Andriote, J. M. (2005, May). *HIV/AIDS and African Americans: A state of emergency.* Population Reference Bureau. Retrieved from http://www.prb.org/Articles/2005/%20HIVAIDSandAfricanAmericansAStateofEmergency.aspx

Apridonidze, T., Shaqra, H., Ktaich, N., Liu, J., & Bella, J. (2011). Relation of components of the metabolic syndrome to left ventricular geometry in Hispanic and non-Hispanic Black adults. *American Journal of Cardiovascular Disease, 1*(1), 84–91.

Artis, B. (2005). Promoting health, building community. *Health Progress, 86*(2), 27–31.

Baker, E. A., Schootman, M., Barnidge, E., & Kelly, C. (2006). The role of race and poverty in access to foods that enable individuals to adhere to dietary guidelines. *Prevention of Chronic Disease.* Retrieved from http://www.cdc.gov/pcd/issues/2006/jul/05_0217.htm

Barkauskas, V. H., Pohl, J. M., Tanner, C., Onifade, T. J., & Pilon, B. (2011). Quality of care in nurse-managed health centers. *Nursing Administration Quarterly, 35*(1), 34–43.

Bay, E., Kreulen, G. J., Shavers, C. A., & Currier, C. (2006). A new perspective: a vulnerable population framework to guide research and practice for persons with traumatic brain injury. *Research and Theory for Nursing Practice, 20*(2), 141–157.

Beauchesne, M., & Patsdaughter, C. (2005). Primary care for the underserved conference: The evolution of an emerging professional culture. *Journal of Cultural Diversity, 12*(3), 77–88.

Beets, M. W., Tilley, F., Kim, Y., & Webster, C. (2011). Nutritional policies and standards for snacks served in after-school programmes: A review. *Public Health Nutrition, 1*, 1–9.

Beidler, S. M. (2005). Ethical considerations for nurse-managed health centers. *Nursing Clinics of North America, 40*(4), 759–770.

Berkman, N. D., Sheridan, S. L., Donahue, K. E., Halpern, D. J., & Crotty, K. (2011). Low health literacy and health outcomes: An updated systematic review. *Annuals of Internal Medicine, 155*(2), 97–107.

Birkmeyer, N., Gu, N., Baser, O., Morris, A., & Birkmeyer, J. (2008). Socioeconomic status and surgical mortality in the elderly. *Medical Care, 46*(9), 893–899.

Bishaw, A., & Macartney, S. (2010). Poverty: 2008 and 2009. *American Community Service Briefs.* Retrieved from http://www.census.gov/prod/2010pubs/acsbr09-1.pdf

Blackwell, D., Hayward, O., & Crimmins, E. (2001). Does childhood health affect chronic morbidity in later life? *Social Science and Medicine, 52*, 1269–1284.

Blendon, R., Buhr, T., Cassidy, E., Perez, D. J., Hunt, K. A., Fleischfresser, C., et al. (2007). Disparities in health: Perspectives of a multi-ethnic, multi-racial America. *Health Affairs, 26*(5), 1437–1447.

Braunholtz-Speight, T. (2007). *Chronic poverty: An introduction.* London: Chronic Poverty Research Centre.

Braveman, P. (2007). Do we have real poverty in the United States? *Preventing Chronic Disease, 4*(4). Retrieved from http://www.cdc.gov/pcd/issues/2007/.oct/07_0124.htm

Bulatao, R., & Anderson, N. (Eds.). (2004). *Understanding racial and ethnic differences in health in late life: A research agenda.* Washington, DC: The National Academies Press.

Campbell-Grossman, C., Brage-Hudson, D., Keating-Lefler, R., & Ofe-Fleck, M. (2005). Community leaders' perceptions of single, low-income mothers' needs and concerns for social support. *Journal of Community Health Nursing, 22*(4), 241–257.

Carr, G. F. (2011). Empowerment: A framework to develop advocacy in African American grandmothers providing care for their grandchildren. *International Scholarly Research Network (ISRN) Nursing.* [Epub ahead of print.]

Carter-Porras, O., & Baquet, C. (2002). What is a "health disparity"? *Public Health Reports, 117*, 426–434.

Centers for Disease Control & Prevention (CDC). (2004). *National Vital Statistics Reports,* Vol. 52, No. 14, February 18, 2004. Retrieved from www.cdc.gov/nchs/data/dvs/nvsr52_14t12.pdf

Centers for Disease Control & Prevention (CDC). (2007). *Health, United States, 2006.* Retrieved from http//www.cdc.gov/nchs/data/hus/hus06/pdf#027

Centers for Disease Control & Prevention (CDC). (2011). *CDC health disparities and inequalities report, United States, 2011.* Retrieved from http://www.cdc.gov/mmwr/pdf/other/su6001.pdf

Chandra, A., & Skinner, J. (2004). Geography and racial health disparities. In N. Anderson, R. Bulatao, & B. Cohen (Eds.), *Critical perspectives on racial and ethnic differences in health in late life* (pp. 604–640). Washington, DC: The National Academies Press.

Chaturvedi, N. (1998). Socioeconomic gradient in morbidity and mortality in people with diabetes: Cohort study findings from the Whitehall study and the WHO multinational study of vascular disease in diabetes. *British Medical Journal, 316*(7125), 100–105.

Chen, E., Martin, A., & Matthews, K. (2007). Trajectories of socioeconomic status across children's lifetime predict health. *Pediatrics, 120*, e297. Retrieved from http://pediatrics.aappublications.org/content/120/2/e297.full.pdf+html

Chew, L. D., Bradley, K. A., & Boyko, E. J. (2004). Brief questions to identify patients with inadequate health literacy. *Family Medicine, 36*(8), 588–594.

Chew, L. D., Griffin, J. M., Partin, M., Noorbaloochi, S., Grill, J. Snyder, A., et al. (2008). Validation of screening questions for limited health literacy in a large VA outpatient population. *Journal of General Internal Medicine, 23*(5), 561–566.

Chin, M., Drum, M., Guillen, M., Remington, A., Levie, J., Kirchoff, A., et al. (2007). Improving and sustaining diabetes care in community health centers with health disparities collaboratives. *Medical Care 45*(12), 1135–1143.

Cho, H., Khang, Y., Yang, S., Harper, J., & Lynch, J. W. (2007). Socioeconomic differentials in cause-specific mortality among South Korean adolescents. *International Journal of Epidemiology, 36*(1), 50–57.

Clegg, L., Reichman, M., Miller, B, Hankey, B., Singh, G., Lin, Y., et al. (2009). Impact of socioeconomic status on cancer incidence and stage at diagnosis: Selected findings from the surveillance, epidemiology, and end results: National Longitudinal Morality Study. *Cancer Causes Control. 20*, 417–435.

Clemans-Cope, L., & Kenney, G. (2007). Low-income parents' reports of communication problems with health care providers: Effects of language and insurance. *Public Health Reports, 122*(2), 206–216.

Cloutier-Fisher, D., & Kobayashi, K. (2009). Examining social isolation by gender and geography: Conceptual and operational challenges using population health data in Canada. Gender, *Place, and Culture, 16*(2), 181–199.

Coberley, C., Puckrein, G., Dobbs, A., McGinnis, M. A., Coberley, S. S., Shurney, D. W. (2007). Effectiveness of disease management programs on improving diabetes care for individuals in health-disparate areas. *Disease Management, 19*(3), 147–155.

Cohen, B., & Reutter, L. (2007). Development of the role of public health nurses in addressing child and family poverty: A framework for action. *Journal of Advanced Nursing, 60*(1), 96–107.

Collins, S. (2007). Congressional testimony. Universal health insurance: Why it is essential to a high performing health system and why design matters. The Commonwealth Fund. Retrieved from http://www.commonwealthfund.org/publications/publications_show.htm?doc_id=506778#areaCitation

Commission on the Social Determinants of Health. (2008). *Closing the gap in a generation: Health equity through action on the social determinants of health*. Final report of the Commission on the Social Determinants of Health, World Health Organization.

Cook, N., Hicks, L., O'Malley, J., Keegan, T., Guadagnoli, E., & Landon, B. (2007). Access to specialty care and medical services in community health centers. *Health Affairs, 26*(5), 1459–1468.

Copeland, D. (2007). Conceptualizing family members of violent mentally ill individuals as a vulnerable population. *Issues in Mental Health Nursing, 28*(9), 943–975.

Cowell, J. M., McNaughton, D., Ailey, S., Gross, D., & Fogg, L. (2009). Clinical trial outcomes of the Mexican American Problem Solving Program (MAPS). *Hispanic Health Care International, 7*(4), 179–189.

Cradock, A. L., McHugh, A., Mont-Ferguson, H., Grant, L., Barrett, J. L., Want, Y. C., et al. (2011). Effect of school district policy change on consumption of sugar-sweetened beverages among high school students, Boston, Massachusetts, 2004–2006. *Preventing Chronic Disease, 8*(4), A74. [Epub 2011 June 15.]

Crimmins, E., Hayward, M., & Seeman, T. (2004). Race/ethnicity, socioeconomic status, and health. In N. Anderson, R. Bulatao, & B. Cohen (Eds.), *Critical perspectives on racial and ethnic differences in health in late life* (pp. 310–352). Washington, DC: The National Academies Press.

Cutler, D., & Lleras-Muney, A. (2010). Understanding differences in health behaviors by education. *Journal of Health Economics, 29*(1), 1–28.

D'Avolio, D., Feldman, J., Mitchell, P., & Strumpf, N. (2008). Access to care and health-related quality of life among older adults with nonurgent emergency department visits. *Geriatric Nursing, 29*(4), 240–246.

Donovan, E., Ammerman, R., Besl, J., Atherton, H., Atherton, H., Khoury, J. C., Altaye M, et al. (2007). Intensive home visiting is associated with decreased risk of infant death. *Pediatrics, 119*(6), 1145–1151.

Dowling, M., Cooney, A., & Casey, D. (2011). A concept analysis of empowerment in chronic illness from the perspective of the nurse and the client living with chronic obstructive pulmonary disease. *Nursing and Healthcare of Chronic Illness, 3*(4), 476–487.

Dubowitz, T., Heron, M., Bird, M., Lurie, N., Finch, C., Basturo-Davila, R., et al. (2008). Neighborhood SES and fruit and vegetable intake among whites, blacks, and Mexican-Americans in the United States. *American Journal of Clinical Nutrition, 87*(6), 1883–1891.

Edberg, M., Cleary, S., & Vyas, A. (2011). A trajectory model for understanding and assessing health disparities in immigrant/refugee communities. *Journal of Immigrant and Minority Health, 13*(3), 576–584.

Erlen, J. A. (2006). Who speaks for the vulnerable? *Orthopedic Nursing, 25*(2), 133–136.

Ervin, N. E., Bell, S. E., & Bickes, J. T. (2009). Evidence-based nursing practice in local public health. *Michigan Journal of Public Health, 3*(1), 33–46.

Ervin, N. E., Nelson, L. L., & Sheaff, L. (1999). Preventing adverse outcomes: A population focus. *Journal of Nursing Care Quality, 13*(6), 25–31.

Ervin, N. E., Scrivener, K., & Simons, T. (2004). Using the linkage model for integrating evidence into nursing practice. *Home Healthcare Nurse, 22*(9), 606–611.

Ervin, N. E., & Young, W. B. (1996). Model for a nursing center: Spanning boundaries. *Journal of Nursing Care Quality, 11*(2), 16–24.

Evans, D. P. (2006). *The calm before the storm: Addressing race as a vulnerability before and after hurricane Katrina.* Retrieved from http://www.medscape.com/viewarticle523436

Falk-Raphael, A. R. (2001). Empowerment as a process of evolving consciousness: A model of empowered caring. *Advances in Nursing Science, 24*(1), 1–16.

Flaskerud, J. H., & Nyamanthi, A. M. (2000). Collaborative inquiry with low-income women. *Journal of Health Care for the Poor and Underserved, 11*(3), 326–342.

Flaskerud, J. H., & Winslow, B. J. (1998). Conceptualizing vulnerable populations health-related research. *Nursing Research, 47*(2), 69–78.

Fleischer, N., Roux, A., Aazraqui, M. Spinelli, H., & De Maio, F. (2011). Socioeconomic gradients in chronic disease risk factors in middle-income countries: Evidence of effect modification by urbanicity in Argentina. *American Journal of Public Health, 101*(2) 294–301.

Flores, G., & Tomany-Korman, S. C. (2008). Racial and ethnic disparities in medical and dental health, access to care, and use of services in U.S. children. *Pediatrics, 121(2),* e286–e298.

Flynn, L., Budd, M., & Modelski, J. (2008). Enhancing resource utilization among pregnant adolescents. *Public Health Nursing, 25*(2), 140–148.

Freudenberg, N., & Olden, K. (2010). Finding synergy: Reducing disparities in health by modifying multiple determinants. *American Journal of Public Health, 100*(S1), S25–S31.

Freudenberg, N., & Ruglis, J. (2007). Reframing school dropout as a public health issue. *Preventing Chronic Disease, 4*(4). Retrieved from http://www.cdc.gobv/pcd/issues/2007/oct/07_0063.htm

Furumoto-Dawson, A., Gehlert, S., Sohmer, D., Olopade, O., & Sacks, T. (2007). Early-life conditions and mechanisms of population health vulnerabilities. *Health Affairs, 26*(5), 1238–1248.

Fyffe, D., Botticello, A., & Myaskovsky, L. (2011). Vulnerable groups living with spinal cord injury. *Topics in Spinal Cord Injury Rehabilitation, 17*(2), 1–9.

Galea, S., Tracy, M., Hoggatt, K. J., DiMaggio, C., & Karpati, A. (2011). Estimated deaths attributable to social factors in the United States. *American Journal of Public Health, 101*(8), 1456–1465.

Galvez, M., Morland, K., Raines, C., Kobil, J., Siskind, J., Godbold, J., et al. (2007). Race and food store availability in an inner-city neighbourhood. *Public Health Nutrition, 11*(6), 624–631.

Gelberg, L., Andersen, R., & Leake, B. (2000). The Behavioral Model for Vulnerable Populations: Application to medical care use and outcomes for homeless people. *Health Services Research, 34*(6), 1273–1302.

Gluckman, P., Hanson, M., Cooper, C., & Thornburg, K. (2008). Effect of in utero and early life conditions on adult health and disease. *The New England Journal of Medicine, 359*, 61–73.

Gonzalez-Guarda, R. M., Peragallo, N., Vasquez, E. P., Urrutia, M. T., & Mitrani, V. B. (2009). Intimate partner violence, depression, and resource availabiity among a community sample of Hispanic women. (2009). *Issues in Mental Health Nursing,* 30(4), 227–236.

Gortmaker, S. L., Swinburn, B. A., Levy, D., Carter, R., Mabry, P. L., Finegood, D. T., et al. (2011). Changing the future of obesity: Science, policy, and action. *Lancet, 378*(9793), 838–847.

Hasnain-Wynia, R., Kang, R., Landrum, M. B., Vogeli, C., Baker, D., & Weissman, J. (2010). Racial and ethnic disparities within and between hospitals for inpatient quality of care: An estimation of patient-level hospital quality alliance measures. *Journal of Health Care for the Poor and Underserved, 21*(2), 629–648.

Hausmann, L., Jeong, K., Bost, J., & Ibrahim, S. (2008). Perceived discrimination in health care and health status in a racially diverse sample. *Medical Care, 46*(9), 905–914.

Havard, S., Deguen, S., Zmirou-Navier, D., Schillinger, C., & Bard, D. (2009). Traffic-related air pollution and SES: A spatial autocorrelation study to assess environmental equity on a small area scale. *Epidemiology, 20*(2), 223–230.

Heck, K., Braveman, P., Cubbin, C., Chavez, G., & Kiely, J. (2006). Socioeconomic status and breastfeeding initiation among California mothers. *Public Health Reports, 121*(1), 51–59.

Himmelstein, D. A., Thorne, D., Warren, E., & Woolhandler, S. (2009). Bankruptcy in the US, 2007: Results of a national study. *American Journal of Medicine, 122*(8), 741–746.

Himmelstein, D., Warren, E., Thorne, D., & Woolhandler, S. (2005, February 2). Market watch: Illness and injury as contributors to bankruptcy. *Health Affairs*. doi: 10.1377/hlthaff w5.63

Hull, H., Frauendienst, R., Gunderson, M., Monsen, S., & Fischbein, D. (2008). School-based influenza immunization. *Vaccine, 26*(34), 4312–4313.

Institute of Medicine. (2003). *Unequal treatment: Confronting racial and ethnic disparities in healthcare*. Washington. DC: The National Academies Press.

Institute of Medicine. (2010). *For the Public's Health: The Role of Measurement in Action and Accountability*. Washington, DC: The National Academies Press.

Isaacs, S., & Schroeder, S. (2004). Class: The ignored determinant of the nation's health. *New England Journal of Medicine, 351*(11), 1137–1142.

Jack, S., DiCenso, A., & Lohfeld, L. (2002). Opening doors: Factors influencing the establishment of a working relationship between paraprofessional home visitors and at-risk families. *Canadian Journal of Nursing Research, 34*(4), 59–69.

Jack, S. M., DiCenso, A., & Lohfeld, L. (2005). A theory of maternal engagement with public health nurses and family visitors. *Journal of Advanced Nursing, 49*(2), 182–190.

Jacobi, J., Parikh, S., McGuire, D., Delemos, J. A., Murphy, S. A., Keeley, E. C. (2007). Racial disparity in clinical outcomes following primary percutaneous coronary intervention for ST elevation myocardial infarction: Influence of process of care. *Journal of Interventional Cardiology, 20*(3), 182–187.

Johnson, S. L., Solomon, B. S., Shields, W. C., McDonald, E. M., McKenzie, L. B., & Gielen, A. C. (2009). Neighborhood violence and its association with mothers' health: Assessing the relative importance of perceived safety and exposure to violence. *Journal of Urban Health, 86*(4), 538–550.

Jones, P., Winslow, B., Lee, J., Burns, M., & Esther-Zhang, X. (2011). Development of a caregiver empowerment model to promote positive outcomes. *Journal of Family Nursing, 17*(1), 11–23.

Kapucu, N. (2008). Collaborative community management: Better community organizing, better public preparedness and response. *Disasters, 32*(2), 239–262.

Kimbro, R., Bzostek, S., Goldman, N., & Rodriguez, G. (2008). Race, ethnicity, and the education gradient in health. *Health Affairs, 27*(2), 361–372.

Kotz, D., & West, R. (2008). Explaining the social gradient in smoking cessation: It's not in the trying, but in the succeeding. *Tobacco Control, 18*, 43–46.

Kueny, A., Berg, J., Chowdhury, Y., & Anderson, N. (2011). Poquito a poquito: How Latino families with children who have asthma make changes in their home. *Journal of Pediatric Health Care. Published online May 13.* doi: 10.1016/j.pedhc.2011.01.007

Kuper, H., Adami, H., Theorell, T., & Weiderpass, E. (2007). The socioeconomic gradient in the incidence of stroke: A prospective study in middle-aged women in Sweden. *Stroke, 38*(1), 4–5.

Kwate, N., Jernigan, M., & Lee, T. (2007). Prevalence, proximity and predictors of alcohol ads in central Harlem. *Alcohol and Alcoholism, 42*(6), 635–640.

Landrine, H., & Corral, I. (2009). Separate and unequal: Residential segregation and Black health disparities. *Ethnicity and Disease, 19*, 179–184.

Larson, N., Story, M., & Nelson, M. (2009). Neighborhood environments: Disparities in access to healthy foods in the U.S. *American Journal of Preventive Medicine, 36*(1), 74–81.

Lee, K., Palacio, C., Alexandraki, I., Stewart, E., & Mooradian, A. (2011). Increasing access to health care providers through medical home model may abolish racial disparity in diabetes care: Evidence from a cross-sectional study. *Journal of the National Medication Association, 103*(3), 250–256.

Lemstra, M., Neudorf, C., & Opondo, J. (2006). Health disparity by neighbourhood income. *Canadian Journal of Public Health, 97*(6), 435–439.

Lillie-Blanton, M. (2008, June 10). *Addressing disparities in health and health care: Issues for reform.* Testimony before the Congress of the United States. Henry J. Kaiser Family Foundation. Retrieved from http://www.kff.org/minorityhealth/upload/7780.pdf

Loucks, E., Lynch, J., Pilote, L., Fuhrer, R., Almeida, N., Richard, H., et al. (2009). Life-course socioeconomic position and incidence of coronary heart disease: The Framingham Offspring Study. *American Journal of Epidemiology, 169*(7), 829–836.

MacDorman, M. F., & Matthews, T. J. (2008). Recent trends in infant mortality in the United States. *NCHS Data Brief, no. 9.* Hyattsville, MD: National Center for Health Statistics.

Marmot, M., Ryff, C. D., Bumpass, L. L., Shipley, M., & Marks, N. F. (1997). Social inequalities in health: Next questions and converging evidence. *Social Science and Medicine, 44*(6), 901–910.

Marmot, M., & Wilkinson, R. (Eds.). (2006). *Social determinants of health.* Oxford, UK: Oxford University Press.

Martin-Gronert, M., & Ozanne, S. (2010). Mechanism linking early suboptimal nutrition and increased risk of type 2 diabetes and obesity. *The Journal of Nutrition, 140*(3), 662–666.

Maslow, A. (1987). *Motivation and personality* (3rd ed.). New York: Addison-Wesley.

Mechanic, D. & Tanner, J. (2007). Vulnerable people, groups, and populations: Societal view. *Health Affairs, 26*(5), 1220–1230.

Metzler, M. (2007). Social determinants of health: What, how, why, and now. *Preventing Chronic Disease, 4*(4). Retrieved from http://www.cdc.gov/pcd/issues/2007/oct/07_0136.htm

Minkler, M., Fuller-Thomson, E., & Guralnik, J. (2006). Gradient of disability across the socioeconomic spectrum in the United States. *New England Journal of Medicine 355*(7), 695–703.

Missildine, K., Varnell, G., Williams, J., Grover, K., Ballard, N., & Stanley-Hermanns, M. (2009). Comfort in the eye of the storm: A survey of evacuees with special medical needs. *Journal of Emergency Nursing, 35*(6), 515–520.

Monsen, K., Radosevich, D., Kerr, M., & Fulkerson, J. (2011). Public health nurses tailor interventions for families at risk. *Public Health Nursing, 28*(2), 119–128.

Mulcahy, H., & McCarthy, G. (2008). Participatory nurse/client relationships: Perceptions of public health nurses and mothers of vulnerable families. *Applied Nursing Research, 21*(3), 169–172.

Nanyonjo, R., Montgomery, S., Modeste, N., & Fujimoto, E. (2007). A secondary analysis of race/ethnicity and other maternal factors affecting adverse birth outcomes in San Bernardino County. *Maternal and Child Health Journal.* doi: 10.1007/s10995-007-0260-x

Naska, A., Katsoulis, M., Trichopoulos, D., & Trichopoulou, A. (2011). The root causes of socioeconomic differentials in cancer and cardiovascular mortality in Greece. *European Journal of Cancer Prevention.* doi: 10.1097/CEJ.0b013e32834ef1be

Naylor, M. D., Brooten, D. A., Campbell, R. L., Jacobsen, B. S., Mezey, M. D., Pauly, M. V., et al. (1999). Comprehensive discharge planning and home follow-up of hospitalized elders: A randomized clinical trial. *Journal of the American Medical Association, 281*(7), 613–620.

Naylor, M. D., Brooten, D. A., Campbell, R. L., Maislin, G., McCauley, K. M., & Schwartz, J. S. (2004). Transitional care of older adults hospitalized with heart failure: A randomized, controlled trial. *Journal of the American Geriatrics Society, 52*(5), 675–684.

Nazmi, A., Roux, A., Ranjit, N., Seeman, T., & Jenny, N. (2010). Cross-sectional and longitudinal associations of neighborhood characteristics with inflammatory markers: Findings from the multi-ethnic study of atherosclerosis. *Health and Place, 16*(6), 1104–1112.

Nettle, D. (2010). Dying young and living fast: Variation in life history across English neighborhoods. *Behavioral Ecology, 21*(2), 387–395.

Noble, K., McCandliss, B., & Farah, M. (2007). Socioeconomic gradients predict individual differences in neurocognitive abilities. *Brain and Behavior, 10*(4), 464–480.

Olden, K., & White, S. L. (2005). Health-related disparities: Influence of environmental factors. *Medical Clinics of North America, 89*(4), 721–738.

Olds, D. L., Eckenrode, J., Henderson, C. R., Jr., Kitzman, H., Powers, L, Cole, R., et al. (1997). Long-term effects of home visitation on maternal life course and child abuse and neglect. Fifteen-year follow-up on a randomized trial. *Journal of the American Medical Association, 278*(8), 637–643.

Olds, D. L., Henderson, C. R., Jr., Kitzman, H. J., Eckenrode, J. J., Cole R. E., & Tatelbaum, R. C. (1999). Prenatal and infancy home visitation by nurses: Recent findings. *Future Child, 9*(1), 44–65.

Olds, D. L., Kitzman, H. J., Cole, R. E., Hanks, C. A., Arcoleo, K. J., Anson, E. A., et al. (2010). Enduring effects of prenatal and infancy home visiting by nurses on maternal life course and government spending: Follow-up of a randomized trial among children at age 12 years. *Archives of Pediatric and Adolescent Medicine, 164*(5), 419–424.

Ornstein, K., Smith, K., Foer, D., Lopez-Cantor, M., & Soriano, T. (2011). To the hospital and back home again: A nurse practitioner-based transitional care program for hospitalized homebound people. *Journal of the American Geriatrics Society, 59*(3), 544–551.

Ou, C., Hedley, A., Chung, R., Thach, T., Chau, Y. K., Chan, K. P., et al. (2008). Socioeconomic disparities in air pollution-associated mortality. *Environmental Research, 107*(2), 237–244.

Pamies, R. J., & Nsiah-Kumi, P. A. (2009). Addressing health disparities in the 21st century. In S. Kosoko-Laski, C. T. Cook, & R. L. O'Brien (Eds.), *Cultural proficiency in addressing health disparities* (pp. 1–35). Sudbury, MA: Jones and Bartlett.

Paul, I., Beiler, J., Schaefer, E., Hollenbeak, C., Alleman, N., Sturgis, S., et al. (2011). A randomized trial of single home nursing visits vs. office-based care after nursery/maternity discharge. *Archives of Pediatric and Adolescent Medicine.* doi:10.1001/archpediatrics.2011.198

Pauly, M. V., & Pagan, J. A. (2007). Spillovers and vulnerability: The case of community uninsurance. *Health Affairs, 26*(5), 1281–1292.

Penprase, B. (2006). Developing comprehensive health care for an underserved population. *Geriatric Nursing, 27*(1), 45–50.

Pohl, J. M., Barkauskas, V. H., Bendert, R., Breer, L., & Bostrom, A. (2007). Impact of academic nurse-managed centers on communities served. *Journal of the Academy of Nurse Practitioners, 19*(5), 268–275.

Population Reference Bureau. (2006, May). *In the news: U.S. population is now one-third minority.* Retrieved from http://www.prb.org/Articles/2006/IntheNewsUSPopulationIsNowOneThirdMinority.aspx?p=1

Pugh, T. (2007, May 25). U.S. *economy leaving record numbers in severe poverty.* McClatchy Washington Bureau. Retrieved from http://www.commondreams.org/headlines07/0223-09.htm

Raphael, D. (2003). A society in decline. In R. Hofrichter (Ed.), *Health and social justice: Politics, ideology, and inequity in the distribution of disease* (pp. 59–88). San Francisco: Jossey-Bass.

Salinsky, E., & Gursky, E. (2006). The case for transforming governmental public health. *Health Affairs, 25*(4), 1017–1028.

Sanoff, H., Sargent, D., Green, E., McLeod, H., & Goldberg, R. (2009). Racial differences in advanced colorectal cancer outcomes and pharmacogenetics: A subgroup analysis of a large randomized clinical trial. *Journal of Clinical Oncology, 27*(25), 4109–4115.

Satcher, D., Fryer, G., McCann, J., Troutman, A., Woolf, S. H., Rust, G. (2005). What if we were equal? A comparison of the black-white mortality gap in 1960 and 2000. *Health Affairs, 24*(2), 459–464.

Saunders, J. M. (2007). Vulnerable populations in an American Red Cross shelter after hurricane Katrina. *Perspectives in Psychiatric Care, 43*(1), 30–37.

Schikowski, T., Sugiri, D., Reimann, V., Pesch, B., Ranft, U., & Kramer, U. (2008). Contribution of smoking and air pollution exposure in urban areas to social differences in respiratory health. *BMC Public Health, 8,* 179. Retrieved from http://www.biomedcentral.com/1471-2458/8/179

Schneider, D., Lilienfeld, D., & Im, W. (2006). The epidemiology of pulmonary embolism: Racial contrasts in incidence and in-hospital case fatality. *Journal of the National Medical Association, 98*(12), 1967–1972.

Schoen, C., Collins, S. R., Kriss, J. L., & Doty, M. M. (2008). How many are underinsured: Trends among U.S. adults, 2003 and 2007. *Health Affairs, 102,* w298–w309.

Scott, T. (2009). Utilization of the natural helper model in health promotion targeting African American men. *Journal of Holistic Nursing, 27*(4), 282–292.

Shepard, V., Williams, K., & Richardson, J. (2004). Women's priorities for lay health home visitors: Implications for eliminating health disparities among underserved women. *Journal of Health and Social Policy, 18*(3), 19–35.

Sherman, A., Trisi, D., Greenstein, R., Broadden, M. (2010). *Census data show large jump in poverty and the ranks of the uninsured.* Center on Budget & Policy Priorities. Retrieved from http://www.cbpp.org/cms/index.cef?fa=view&id=3294

Shi, L., & Stevens, G. D. (2010). *Vulnerable populations in the United States* (2nd ed.). San Francisco: Jossey-Bass.

Shi, L., Stevens, G., Lebrun, L., Faed, P., & Tsai, J. (2008). Enhancing the measurement of health disparities for vulnerable populations. *Journal of Public Health Management and Practice, November (Suppl.),* s45–s52.

Smarty, A. (2009, December 8). Resource for checking your SEO content readability. *Search Engine Journal.* Retrieved from http://www.searchenginejournal.com/readability-tools/15189/

Sohler, N., Li, X., & Cunningham, C. (2007). Perceived discrimination among severely disadvantaged people with HIV infection. *Public Health Reports, 122*(3), 347–355.

Springer, P., Black, M., Martz, K., Deckys, C., & Soelberg, T. (2010). *Somali Bantu refugees in southwest Idaho: A community and cultural assessment.* Presentation at the Western Institute for Nursing. Abstract retrieved from http://www.nursinglibrary.org/vhl/handle/10755/157369

Stone, A., Krueger, A., Steptoe, A., & Harter, J. (2010). The socioeconomic gradient in daily colds and influenza, headaches, and pain. *Archives of Internal Medicine, 170*(6), 570–572.

Strehlow, A., & Gongwa, M. (2005). *Innovative models of practice in vulnerable populations: Administrative perspective of the vulnerable populations model.* Presentation at the Western Institute for Nursing. Abstract retrieved from http://www.nursinglibrary.org/vhl/handle/10755/157991

Sumner, L., Wong, L., Schetter, C., Myers, H., & Rodriguez, M. (2011). Predictors of posttraumatic stress disorder symptoms among low-income Latinas during pregnancy and postpartum. *Psychological Trauma: Theory, Research, Practice, and Policy.* doi: 10.1037/a0023538.

Tough, S., Johnston, D., Siever, J., Jorgenson, G., Slocombe, L., Lane, C., et al. (2006). Does supplementary prenatal nursing and home visitation support improve resource use in a universal health care system? A randomized controlled trial in Canada. *Birth, 33*(3), 183–194.

University of California Los Angeles (UCLA) Center for Vulnerable Populations Research. (2007). *Who are vulnerable populations?* Retrieved from http://www.nursing. ucla.edu/orgs/cvpr/who-are-vunerable.html

University of Michigan National Poverty Center. (n.d.). *Poverty in the United States frequently asked questions.* Retrieved from http://npc.umich.edu/poverty/

U.S. Census Bureau. (2007). *Minority population tops one million.* (Press Release). Retrieved from http://www.certsus.gov/Press-Release/www/releases/archives/population/010048.html

U.S. Census Bureau. (2008). An older and more diverse nation by midcentury. (Press Release). Retrieved from http://www.census.gov/ewsroom/releases/archives/population/cb08-123.html

U.S. Department of Health and Human Services (USDHHS). (2000a). *Healthy people 2010: Understanding and improving health* (2nd ed.). Washington, DC: U.S. Government Printing Office.

U.S. Department of Health and Human Services (USDHHS). (2000b). *Healthy people 2010* (Conference ed., Vols. 1 & 2). Washington, DC: Author.

U.S. Department of Health and Human Services (USDHHS). (2007). *The 2005 HHS poverty guidelines.* Retrieved from http://aspe.hhs.gov/poverty/05poverty.shtml

U.S. Department of Health and Human Services (USDHHS). (2010). *Healthy people 2020.* Retrieved from http://www.healthypeople.gov/2020/TopicsObjectives.

U.S. Department of Health and Human Services (USDHHS). (n.d.). Determinants of health. *Healthy People 2020.* Retrieved from http://www.healthypeople.gov/2020/about/DOHAbout.aspx

U.S. Department of Health and Human Services (USDHHS). Health Resources Services Administration. (2010). *The registered nurse population: Findings from the 2008 National Sample Survey of Registered Nurses.* Washington, DC: Author.

Wang, S., Quong, J., Kanaya, A., & Fernandez, A. (2011). Asian Americans and obesity in California: A protective effect of biculturalism. *Journal of Immigrant and Minority Health, 13*(2), 276–283.

Warner, D. F., & Hayward, M. D. (2002). *Race disparities in men's mortality: The role of childhood social conditions in a process of cumulative disadvantage*. Paper presented at the annual meetings of the Population Association of America, Atlanta, May 9–11.

Whitehead, M. (1991). *The concepts and principles of equity and health*. Copenhagen, Denmark: WHO/EURO.

Williams, D., & Mohammed, S. (2009). Discrimination and racial disparities in health: Evidence and needed research. *Journal of Behavioral Science, 32*(1), 20–47.

Williams, D., & Sternthal, M. (2010). Understanding racial-ethnic disparities in health. *Journal of Health and Social Behavior, 51*(Suppl. 1), s15–s27.

Winkleby, M., & Cubbin, C. (2004). Racial/ethnic disparities in health behaviors: A challenge to current assumptions. In N. Anderson, R. Bulatao, & B. Cohen (Eds.), *Critical perspectives on racial and ethnic differences in health in late life* (pp. 450–483). Washington, DC: The National Academies Press.

Winston, G., Barr, R., Carrasquillo, O., Bertoni, A., & Shea, S. (2009). Sex and racial/ethnic differences in cardiovascular disease risk factor treatment and control among individuals with diabetes in the Multi-ethnic Study of Atherosclerosis (MESA). *Diabetes Care, 32*(8), 1467–1469.

Wolf, M., Wilson, E., Rapp, D., Waite, K., Boccini, M., Davis, T., et al. (2009). Literacy and learning in health care. *Pediatrics, 124*(Suppl. 3), s275–s281.

Yarnell, J., Patterson, C., Arveiler, D., Amouyel, P., Ferrieres, J., Woodside, J., et al. (2010). Contribution of lifetime smoking habit in France and Northern Ireland to country and socioeconomic differentials in mortality and cardiovascular incidence: the PRIME study. *Journal of Epidemiology and Community Health*. doi: 10.1136/jech.2010.123943

Zarzaur, B., Croce, M., Fabian, T., Fisher, P., & Magnotti, L. (2010). A population-based analysis of neighborhood socioeconomic status and injury admission rates and in-hospital mortality. *Journal of the American College of Surgeons, 211*(2), 216–223.

Zerwekh, J. (2000). Caring on the ragged edge: Nursing persons who are disenfranchised. *Advances in Nursing Science, 22*(4), 47–61.

thePoint: Everything You Need to Make the Grade!

thePoint Visit http://thePoint.lww.com/Allender8e for selected readings, study aids for all learning styles, and more!

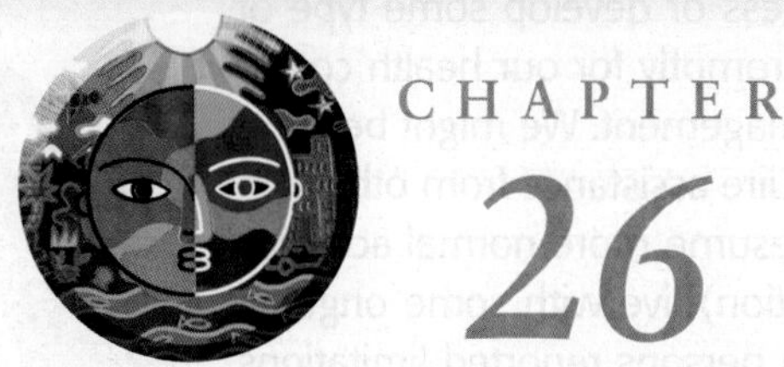

CHAPTER 26

Clients with Disabilities and Chronic Illnesses

"It was ability that mattered, not disability, which is a word I'm not crazy about using."

—***Marlee Matlin,*** Deaf Academy Award–Winning Actress

KEY TERMS

Activity
Activity limitations
American Sign Language
Americans with Disabilities Act
Assistive devices and technology
Body functions
Body structures
Braille
Chronic disease
Disability
Environmental factors
Functioning
Handicap
Health promotion
Impairments
Participation
Participation restrictions
People with disabilities
Personal factors
Secondary conditions
Universal design

LEARNING OBJECTIVES

Upon mastery of this chapter, you should be able to:

- Discuss the national and global implications of disability and chronic illness.
- Describe the economic, social, and political factors affecting the wellbeing of individuals with disabilities and chronic illness.
- Provide an example of primary, secondary, and tertiary prevention practices for disabled individuals.
- Describe the Americans with Disabilities Act.
- Discuss the benefits of universal design for all persons.

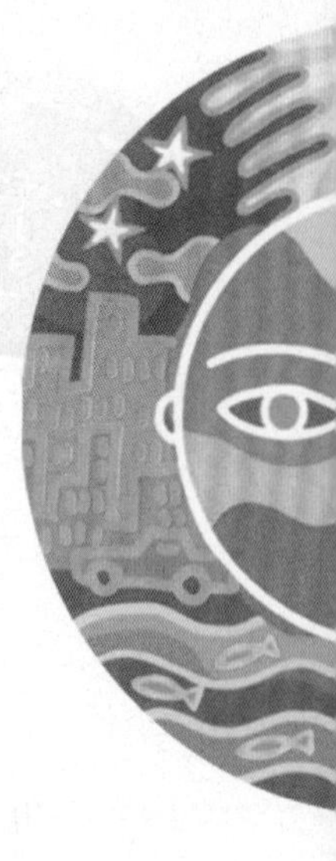

At some point in our lives, most of us will be diagnosed with a chronic illness or develop some type of disability. We may be fortunate enough to be diagnosed early and treated promptly for our health conditions and followed up with sufficient and effective disease and symptom management. We might become temporarily incapacitated, become unable to manage our daily lives, and require assistance from others. In each of these situations, we will hope that a swift recovery will assist us to resume more normal activities quickly. But an estimated 36 million Americans (almost 12% of the population) live with some ongoing level of disability (U.S. Census Bureau, 2012). In 2010 alone, over 38 million persons reported limitations in their usual activities as the result of chronic conditions (Adams, Martinez, Vickerie, & Kirzinger, 2011).

In addition to the human costs of disability and chronic illness, the related costs of direct medical care and indirect annual costs related to disability are significant burdens on those affected and on public and private payers of health and social insurance. A 2011 report found the total national disability-associated health care expenditures were $397.9 billion in 2006, or 26.7% of all U.S. national spending for health (Anderson, Wiener, Finkelstein, & Armour, 2011). Individuals with disabilities have higher health care costs as they have more chronic conditions, and their poorer health status requires more health care services. It is difficult to separate the costs of disability from the costs of chronic conditions as it is often difficult to identify which occurs first. But it is clear that reducing both types of costs will be facilitated by improved health promotion and preventive services, as well as by expanding coordinated care and targeted disease management programs (Anderson et al., 2011).

Healthy People 2020 details the continued impact of chronic and disabling diseases and conditions. For instance, arthritis remains the leading cause of disability in the United States. It affects approximately 43 million individuals and more than 20% of the adult population (U.S. Department of Health and Human Services [USDHHS], Office of Disease Prevention and Health Promotion [ODPHP], 2012b). Asthma remains a national health concern for all ages, especially for those under 18 years of age, and represents one of the four most common causes of chronic illness in children. Of particular concern are health disparities in asthma morbidity and mortality, particularly for low-income and minority populations (USDHHS, ODPHP, 2012g). The prevalence of chronic kidney disease (CKD) and end-stage kidney disease (ESKD) continues to increase; diabetes is the most common cause of kidney failure. Treatment of CKD and ESKD is expensive, with nearly 25% of the Medicare budget needed to treat Americans with these two diseases (USDHHS, ODPHP, 2012e). Back pain will fully impact the lives of 80% of all Americans, with risk factors including age, fitness level, race, ethnicity, and occupation. Three to four percent of the population is temporarily disabled due to back pain. Among those 50 years and older, 16.5% are estimated to have osteoporosis, a risk factor for additional serious injury or death following a fall (USDHHS, ODPHP, 2012b). The need to address health issues of disability and chronic illness is vital to the wellbeing of affected individuals and families and crucial to the financial health of the country.

This chapter discusses important and necessary health promotion and preventive efforts at every level. Although the treatment of chronic conditions has long been a mainstay of health care in the United States and globally, limited attention has been paid to health promotion approaches required to prevent, maintain, and improve overall wellbeing of individuals with chronic conditions and those at risk for these conditions. In addition, too little attention has been directed to health promotion approaches for those with physical or psychological disabilities. This chapter begins with an overview of disabilities and chronic illnesses, followed by a discussion of current national and global trends in addressing these issues. The various organizations that focus on improving the wellbeing of those affected by chronic and disabling conditions, the impact on their families, and the role of the community/public health nurse in addressing the related needs of individuals, families, and aggregates are discussed. The benefits of universal design and issues of easy access for all ages and abilities are also explained.

PERSPECTIVES ON DISABILITY, CHRONIC ILLNESS, AND HEALTH

What does the word *disabled* mean to you? What thoughts come to mind when you think about the word as it applies to an individual? It is defined in one dictionary as "the incapacity to do something because of a handicap—physical, mental, etc." (Morehead & Morehead, 1995). Disability is linked with *inability,* which is defined as "the lack of ability to do something, whatever the reason, but usually through incompetence, weakness, lack of training, etc.," while **handicap** is explained in the same volume as "any encumbrance or disadvantage" (Morehead & Morehead, 1995). **Chronic disease** is any illness that is prolonged, does not resolve spontaneously, and is rarely cured completely; these diseases are often preventable, and they pose a significant burden in terms of mortality, morbidity, and personal and societal cost (Centers for Disease Control and Prevention [CDC], 2007). Each of these definitions suggests connotations that are negative and evokes prevalent societal views and stereotypes faced daily by **people with disabilities.**

Chronic illness and disability-related needs differ from one individual to another, and an individual's needs may require different degrees or modes of accommodation. Long-held negative views of disabled persons and their conditions have been challenged by persons with disabilities, their families, and their allies. New and more positive approaches are emerging that view individuals and their needs from a more person-centered, holistic standpoint.

International Classification of Functioning, Disability, and Health

The *International Classification of Functioning, Disability, and Health* (ICF), published by the World Health Organization (WHO) in 2001, reflects the emerging, more positive approaches to chronic and disabling conditions. This classification system replaced the *International Classification of Impairments, Disabilities, and Handicaps* (ICIDH) (WHO, 1980). Modifying the terminology of the classification's title concretely shows the dramatic shift in thinking through which both *impairments* and *handicaps* were removed. In the newer, 2001 document, **disability** serves as a broad term for impairments, activity limitations, or participation restrictions and is linked to **functioning**, a term that encompasses all body functions, activities, and participation.

The ICF is a universal classification system with standardized language and a way to view the domains of health from a holistic vantage point. It takes into account body functions and structures, activities and participation, environmental factors, and personal factors. This allows a multidimensional evaluation of an individual's circumstances in terms of functioning, disability, and health. Through melding the "medical model" of health and health care for disabled persons with the "social model," the ICF provides a biopsychosocial approach for assessing people with disabilities that emphasizes the observation that no two people with the same disease or disability have the same level of functioning.

The specific aims of the document are (WHO, 2001, p. 5) the following:

- Provide a scientific basis for understanding and studying health and health-related states, outcomes, and determinations.
- Establish a common language for describing health and health-related states to improve communication between different users such as health care workers, researchers, policy makers, and the public, including people with disabilities.
- Permit comparison of data across countries, health care disciplines, services, and time.
- Provide a systematic coding scheme for health information systems.

Table 26-1 shows the current and potential uses of the ICF by various entities ranging from insurance companies and health care providers to policy makers and educators.

Table 26.1 Applications of the International Classification of Functioning, Disability, and Health

Statistical tool	Collection and recording of data: • Population studies and surveys • Management information systems
Research tool	Measure: • Outcomes • Quality of life • Environmental factors
Clinical tool	• Needs assessment • Matching treatments with specific conditions • Vocational assessment • Rehabilitation • Outcome evaluation
Social policy tool	• Social security planning • Compensation systems • Policy design and implementation
Educational tool	• Curriculum design • Raising awareness • Undertaking social action

From World Health Organization. (2001). *International classification of functioning, disability and health*. Geneva, Switzerland: Author.

Contributing to these emerging perspectives, the following concepts describe the ICF in relation to health (WHO, 2001, p. 10):

- **Body functions** are the physiologic functions of body systems and include psychological functions.
- **Body structures** are anatomic parts of the body such as organs, limbs, and their components.
- **Impairments** are problems in body function or structure, such as a significant deviation or loss.
- **Activity** is the execution of a task or action by an individual.
- **Participation** is involvement in a life situation, including personal and interpersonal roles and activities.
- **Activity limitations** are difficulties an individual may have in executing activities.
- **Participation restrictions** are problems an individual may experience when involved in life situations.
- **Environmental factors** make up the physical, social, and attitudinal environments in which people live and conduct their lives.
- **Personal factors** are the features of an individual's background, life, and living that are not part of a health condition or health status, such as gender, race, age, other health conditions, fitness, lifestyle habits, upbringing, coping styles, social background, education, profession, past and current experience, overall behavior pattern and character style, individual psychological assets, and other characteristics—all or any of which may play a role in disability at any level.

For the public health nurse, the ICF facilitates assessment of an individual client based on a wide range of factors. Disability or disease is just one factor to be considered in planning and implementing a care plan for clients in the community. Two individuals may have the same disability, such as a below-the-knee amputation, but their health and wellbeing can be quite different. One may have a more positive outlook, one may have more social support than the other, or one may suffer more than the other from additional health issues that impede rehabilitation. The public health nurse must always consider the totality of the situation, including the biologic, psychological, sociocultural, and environmental realms. Diseases and disabilities are conditions, yet a client may often be referred to inappropriately as "the paraplegic" or "the amputee" and not by her name. This type of designation or stereotype should be avoided: A disease or disability is something one has, not something one is. Figure 26-1 depicts the interactions among the various components addressed by the ICF in the evaluation and assessment of clients with disabilities. It can serve as a useful model for community/public health nursing practice in the overall assessment of people with disabilities.

The World Health Report

The release of the 2002 annual report for the WHO, *The World Health Report 2002: Reducing Risks, Promoting Healthy Life,* set a new standard for addressing global health. It challenged the world community to focus more attention on unhealthy behaviors that lead ultimately to chronic disease, disability, and early mortality. The report stressed that, although infectious diseases and malnutrition require ongoing vigilance because they continue to plague many parts of the world, they are not the only threat. Lifestyle choices are also one of the key contributors to morbidity and mortality levels in both affluent and poor countries. Targeting interventions at local, national, regional, and international levels is a high priority. In focusing on this new reality, the 2002 *Report* reflected a twofold purpose: to quantify the most important risks to health and to assess the cost-effectiveness of interventions designed to reduce those risks. In this context, the WHO's overall goal was "to help governments of all countries lower these risks and raise the healthy life expectancy of their populations" (WHO, 2002, p. 7).

Health care providers across the globe should broaden their practice beyond a narrow focus on acute illness to attend to lifestyle and behavioral changes that will have a key impact on increasing healthy years of life. The risks to health detailed in 2002 and the more recent 2009 WHO report include many factors that are the direct result of poverty, but other factors are more connected to excesses, especially among populations in more affluent countries. The WHO identified 10 leading health risks: (1) underweight; (2) unsafe sex; (3) high blood pressure; (4) tobacco consumption; (5) alcohol consumption; (6) unsafe water, sanitation, and hygiene; (7) iron deficiency; (8) indoor smoke from solid fuels; (9) high cholesterol; and (10) obesity (WHO, 2002, 2009). Globally, these 10 health risks are responsible for more than 33% of all deaths and a significant proportion of disability. Half of these risk factors—tobacco and alcohol consumption, high blood pressure, high cholesterol, and obesity—are directly related to lifestyle and behavioral choices (WHO, 2009).

As nutrition is vitally linked to health, nutritional imbalances can lead to severe chronic illness, disability, and premature death. Of the leading 10 health risks, five are directly related to consumption: underweight, hypertension, iron deficiency, high cholesterol, and obesity (WHO, 2009). The worldwide prevalence of adult overweight is estimated at 1.8 billion, including 500 million adults classified as obese (WHO, 2012b). Being overweight increases the risk of coronary heart disease, stroke, diabetes, and some types of cancer.

In stark contrast, in 2010 an estimated 103 million children under 5 years of age (18%) were underweight in developing countries, even though the number of affected children had decreased 11% between 1990 and 2010 (WHO, 2012c). For underweight children, malnutrition and deficits of important nutrients can lead to

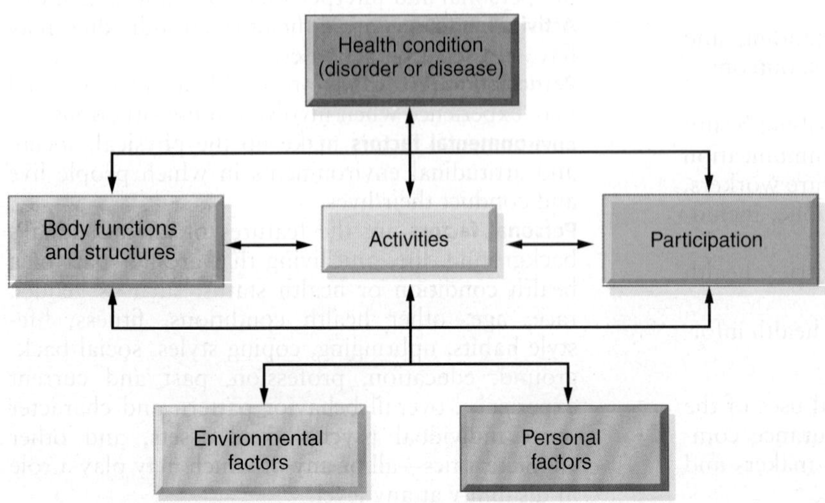

FIGURE 26-1. Model of functioning and disability. From the World Health Organization (WHO). (2001 *ICF introduction.* Geneva, Switzerland: Author.

a wide array of preventable disabilities. For example, the leading cause of acquired blindness in children is vitamin A deficiency, and the leading cause of mental retardation and brain damage is iodine deficiency (WHO, 2002).

Globally, if national and local governments can make even minimal strides toward improving the health of their citizens, a dramatic improvement in health outlook can occur for these populations and worldwide. Governments must take a proactive role in addressing the preventive health care needs of their citizens (Display 26.1). A shift in intervention focus away from a narrow focus on the most high-risk individuals to the general population is essential. For decades, public health care professionals have stressed that the main focus should be on primary and secondary prevention. As difficult as it has been in the United States to implement a shift in emphasis from treatment to health promotion efforts, it will be interesting to see if advocacy, education, and global health interventions can rebalance efforts between primary and secondary prevention against tertiary prevention. Preventing chronic disease and limiting disabilities are vital to improving global health. The cost of health care treatment is high, but the cost in terms of lost productivity and decreased quality of life is even higher. The traditional adage, "An ounce of prevention is worth a pound of cure," is a most appropriate aspiration for the years ahead.

United Nations' Convention on the Rights of Persons with Disabilities

An estimated 1 billion people across the globe (15%) live with disabilities, with between 110 and 190 million (2.2% to 3.8%) people 15 years and older having significant difficulties in functioning (WHO, 2012a). Factoring in the more than 2 billion family members affected by disability, the WHO stressed that almost one-third of the world population is directly impacted by disabilities. The sheer magnitude of this issue, and the recognition that people with disabilities are a "significantly overlooked development challenge" across the world, led to the 2006 United Nations (UN) Convention on the Rights of Persons with Disabilities. Ultimately 127 countries were signatories to the Convention or its Optional Protocol (UN, 2012).

Specific principles of the Convention include (UN, 2007b) the following:

- Respect for inherent dignity and individual autonomy, including the freedom to make one's own choices and independence of persons
- Nondiscrimination
- Full and effective participation and inclusion in society
- Respect for difference and acceptance of persons with disabilities as part of human diversity and humanity
- Equality of opportunity
- Accessibility
- Equality between men and women
- Respect for evolving capacities of children with disabilities and respect for the right of children with disabilities to preserve their identities

Despite a wide variety of legislation and program development at the national level (see Table 26-3: Disability Rights Laws), the United States has been reluctant to ratify the Convention, at least partially due to concerns about national sovereignty (U.S. Mission to the United Nations, 2006). The National Council on Disability (NCD) has advocated for US ratification of the Convention to provide "clear support for the principles of this landmark treaty and to continue our country's tradition as a world leader for people with disabilities" (NCD, 2008, Preamble). The US Congress passed a bill in support of the Convention in 2009, although this did not include the more complex step of ratifying the Convention. In his remarks at signing the bill supporting the Convention, President Barack Obama recalled his father-in-law's battle with disability

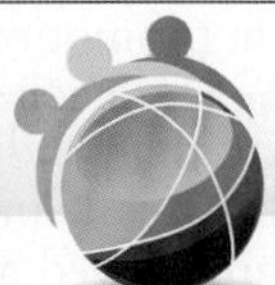

DISPLAY 26.1 2002 WORLD HEALTH ORGANIZATION RECOMMENDATIONS TO IMPROVE GLOBAL HEALTH

- Government/health ministry support for scientific research, improved surveillance systems, and better access to global information
- Development of effective, committed policies for the prevention of health risks such as tobacco consumption, unsafe sex associated with human immunodeficiency virus/acquired immune deficiency syndrome, and unhealthy diet and obesity
- Implementation of cost-effectiveness analysis to identify the most cost-effective and affordable interventions to reduce priority health risks
- Collaborative efforts (intersectoral and international) to reduce major extraneous risk to health caused by unsafe water, poor sanitation, or lack of education
- Supportive and balanced approach in addressing these major health risks that includes government, community, and individual action
- Empowerment and encouragement of individuals to make positive, life-enhancing health decisions (such as eliminating tobacco use, excessive alcohol consumption, unhealthy diet, and unsafe sex)

Adapted from World Health Organization. (2002). *The world health report 2002: Reducing risks, promoting healthy life.* Geneva, Switzerland: Author.

due to multiple sclerosis, and the beneficial outcomes of the Americans with Disability Act (Obama, 2009). In mid-2012, the US Senate was still discussing the Convention's ratification (McCain, 2012). A positive step in the progress toward equality, the Convention's broader impact in the United States will only be realized in the coming years.

The World Report on Disability

In 2011, The WHO and the World Bank reassessed global progress on addressing disability in light of the 2006 *Convention on the Rights of Persons with Disabilities* (UN, 2007a, 2007b). Not only must governments seek improvement in the lives of individuals and families living with disability, but every citizen needs to participate in their country's development. People living with disabilities must advocate to remove barriers that prevent their full participation in their communities, including access to health, education, employment, transportation, and information services. With the active participation of people with disabilities, stakeholders in each country—and globally—must establish an inclusive world characterized by enabling environments, rehabilitation and support services, adequate social protection, and relevant policies, programs, standards, and legislation (WHO & World Bank, 2011).

Recommendations of the 2011 *World Report on Disability* include the following:

- Enable access to all mainstream systems and services.
- Invest in specific programs and services for people with disabilities.
- Adopt a national disability strategy and plan of action.
- Involve people with disabilities.
- Improve human resource capacity.
- Provide adequate funding and improve affordability.
- Increase public awareness and understanding.
- Improve disability data collection.
- Strengthen and support research on disability (WHO & World Bank, 2011).

No less than other countries, Americans at every level can become engaged in translating these recommendations into action. Government at every level may play a most significant role, but there are important roles for service providers, academic institutions, the private sector, communities, and especially people with disabilities and their families.

Healthy People 2020

Healthy People is the most influential document addressing health promotion and disease prevention in the United States in order to improve the health of all Americans. It strives toward a vision of a society in which all people live long, healthy lives. Through its clearly delineated, science-based, and measurable objectives, Healthy People has had a far-reaching influence on national and state health initiatives, health care policy, research priorities, and funding since its beginning in 1979. Changing American perspectives on disability and chronic illness are reflected in the changing focus of the every-decade Healthy People plan. Following the decades of *Healthy People 1990* and *Healthy People 2000*, *Healthy People 2010* influenced the decade of the 2000s, and *Healthy People 2020* will guide public health interventions in the 2010s (USDHHS, ODPHP, 2012a).

The four overarching goals for *Healthy People 2020* are the following:

- Attain high-quality, longer lives free of preventable disease, disability, injury, and premature death.
- Achieve health equity, eliminate disparities, and improve the health of all groups.
- Create social and physical environments that promote good health for all.
- Promote quality of life, healthy development, and healthy behaviors across all ages (USDHHS, ODPHP, 2012a).

A comparison among Healthy People plans over the last decades underscores the emergence of new approaches to identifying priority areas and planning to improve the health of individuals with disabilities and chronic illness. In *Healthy People 2000*, only one priority area was devoted to disability and chronic illness: "Diabetes and Chronic Disabling Conditions," emphasized diabetes, with only limited attention to the broader range of other disabilities (asthma, CKD, arthritis, deformities or orthopedic impairments, mental retardation, peptic ulcer disease, visual and hearing impairments, and overweight) (USDHHS, 1991). *Healthy People 2010* focused directly on chronic illness and disability in the section on "Disability and Secondary Conditions," with frequent attention to these issues across almost all *Healthy People 2010* focus areas. In terms of disability and chronic illness, *Healthy People 2010* increased emphasis on conditions expected to take a toll on the nation's health in the coming years, as well as those expected to become an economic burden on the nation. In *Healthy People 2020*, the section "Disability and Health" repositions the approach to disability as now emphasizing the principles of health promotion and disease prevention for those currently experiencing disabilities and/or chronic illnesses. Rather than individuals with disabilities and/or chronic illnesses being defined by their limiting conditions, they are viewed as having the potential to meet and exceed health promotion and disease prevention goals set for the nation's population as a whole.

Interest in disability accelerated with the development of *Healthy People 2010* (prepared during the late 1990s and implemented in 2001–2010). The definition of "disability" in *Healthy People 2010* is "the general term used to represent the interactions between individuals with a health condition and barriers in their environment" (USDHHS, 2000, p. 25), and people with disabilities are those "identified as having an activity limitation or who use assistance or who perceive themselves as having a disability" (USDHHS,

2000, p. 6–25). *Healthy People 2010* also noted a lack of parity between disabled and nondisabled populations in terms of several selected objectives: leisure-time activity, use of community support programs, and receipt of clinical preventive services. For example, a lower percent of people with disabilities reported engaging in some type of leisure-time activity compared to any other group (including even those older than 65 years of age and low-income persons). Progress on this measure was noted from the 1985 level of 35% to the 1995 level of 29%, although it was still far short of the 2000 target of 20% reporting engagement in some type of leisure-time activity. People with disabilities also have an increased likelihood of being overweight, increased adverse effects from stress, and reduced rates of preventive services (e.g., tetanus boosters, Pap tests, breast examinations, and mammograms). Recognition that the health needs of disabled persons were not receiving needed attention resulted in increasing the priority of improving the health of people with disabilities.

Halfway between *Healthy People 2010* and *Healthy People 2020*, the 2005 Midcourse Review analyzed changes since implementation of *Healthy People 2010*. It recognized the "insufficient inclusion of persons with disabilities in disaster management processes, training for first responders, county-level data to locate and evacuate persons with disabilities, and resources to meet disability needs during a disaster" (USDHHS, 2005, p. 6–7). Of additional concern was the finding that two objectives moved away from their 2010 targets. A 7% increase occurred in the proportion of adults who expressed that negative feelings were impacting their lives—32% in 2003 versus the 28% level reported in 1997. With respect to employment, the proportion of adults with disabilities who were employed dropped between 1997 and 2003. As with the recession of 2001, the disproportionate impact of the economic instability beginning in 2008 on persons with disabilities reflected decreased progression toward the employment goals set for 2010.

Healthy People 2020 was released in late 2011. Based on earlier decades of Healthy People and timely perspectives, this document provides the vision, mission, goals, focus areas, and objectives for health promotion and disease prevention in the United States over the next decade. The basis for this blueprint for the nation's health into the first quarter of the 21st century was an extensive review of up-to-the-minute and evolving research and national surveys, as well as public and professional reviews and input.

Improving the health of the nation requires a multifaceted approach focused on improving parity across all groups and among all individuals. The goal of "Disability and Health" in *Healthy People 2020* is to "promote the health and wellbeing of people with disabilities" (USDHHS, ODPHP, 2012c). Twenty main objectives were identified in four broad categories, including (1) systems and policies; (2) barriers to heath care; (3) environment; and (4) activities and participation (see Table 26-2).

Table 26.2 ***Healthy People 2020:*** **Disability and Health–Objectives**

Systems and policies

- Include in the core of *Healthy People 2020* population data systems a standardized set of questions that identify "people with disabilities."
- Increase the number of Tribes, States, and the District of Columbia that have public health surveillance and health promotion programs for people with disabilities and caregivers.
- Increase the proportion of U.S. master of public health (M.P.H.) programs that offer graduate-level courses in disability and health.

Barriers to health care

- Reduce the proportion of people with disabilities who report delays in receiving primary and periodic preventive care due to specific barriers.
- Increase the proportion of youth with special health care needs whose health care provider has discussed transition planning from pediatric to adult health care.
- Increase the proportion of people with epilepsy and uncontrolled seizures who receive appropriate medical care.
- Reduce the proportion of older adults with disabilities who use inappropriate medications.

Environment

- Reduce the proportion of people with disabilities who report physical or program barriers to local health and wellness programs.
- Reduce the proportion of people with disabilities who encounter barriers to participating in home, school, work, or community activities.
- Reduce the proportion of people with disabilities who report barriers to obtaining the assistive devices, service animals, technology services, and accessible technologies that they need.
- Increase the proportion of newly constructed and retrofitted U.S. homes and residential buildings that have visitable features.
- Reduce the number of people with disabilities living in congregate care residences.

(Continued)

Table 26.2 *Healthy People 2020:* Disability and Health—Objectives *(Continued)*

Activities and participation
• Increase the proportion of people with disabilities who participate in social, spiritual, recreational, community, and civic activities to the degree that they wish. • Increase the proportion of children and youth with disabilities who spend at least 80% of their time in regular education programs. • Reduce unemployment among people with disabilities. • Increase employment among people with disabilities. • Increase the proportion of adults with disabilities who report sufficient social and emotional support. • Reduce the proportion of people with disabilities who report serious psychological distress. • Reduce the proportion of people with disabilities who experience nonfatal unintentional injuries that require medical care. • Increase the proportion of children with disabilities, birth through age 2 yrs, who receive early intervention services in home- or community-based settings.

From U.S. Department of Health and Human Services. (2012c). *Healthy people 2020, topics and objectives: Disability and health*. Retrieved from http://www.healthypeople.gov/2020/topicsobjectives2020/overview.aspx?topicid=9

These objectives indicate a growing emphasis on a holistic approach that recognizes that life satisfaction is just as important to health and wellbeing as preventive services (USDHHS, ODPHP, 2012f). It also indicates a growing realization that healthy life-years for persons with disabilities equate to decreased health costs at local, state, and national levels, just as they do for persons without disabilities.

The health of people with disabilities is influenced by many social and physical factors. Using the ICF and the WHO principles of action for addressing health determinants, Healthy People identified three areas for public health action for the year 2020:

1. Improve the conditions of daily life by:
   - Encouraging communities to be accessible so all can live in, move through, and interact with their environment.
   - Encouraging community living.
   - Removing barriers in the environment using both physical universal design concepts and operational policy shifts.
2. Address the inequitable distribution of resources among people with disabilities and those without disabilities by increasing:
   - Appropriate health care for people with disabilities.
   - Education and work opportunities.
   - Social participation.
   - Access to needed technologies and assistive supports.
3. Expand the knowledge base and raise awareness about determinants of health for people with disabilities by increasing:
   - The inclusion of people with disabilities in public health data collection efforts across the lifespan.
   - The inclusion of people with disabilities in health promotion activities.
   - The expansion of disability and health training opportunities for public health and health care professionals (USDHHS, ODPHP, 2012c).

HEALTH PROMOTION AND PREVENTION NEEDS OF THE DISABLED AND CHRONICALLY ILL

Misconceptions Impede Improvement

One of the most influential aspects of *Healthy People 2010* was that it prompted a change in thinking within the health care community about the health promotion and disease prevention needs of people with disabilities. This shift was essential to remedy the lack of health promotion and disease prevention activities for this population which have led to an increase in the number and extent of **secondary conditions**, defined as "medical, social, emotional, mental, family, or community problems that a person with a disabling condition likely experiences" (USDHHS, 2000, p. 6–25). Approaching the health needs of disabled persons from the traditional standpoint of asking what medical, rehabilitative, or long-term care is needed has failed to reduce illness or improve the overall wellbeing of the disabled or chronically ill. Moreover, a number of misconceptions have resulted that impede progress in this area: (a) that all people with disabilities have poor health, (b) that public health activities need to focus only on preventing disability, (c) that there is no need for a clear definition of "disability" or "people with disabilities" in public health practice, and (d) that environment does not play a significant role in the disability process. Increased national attention to the needs of the disabled (those needs specific to disabled persons as well as needs that are universal to all) have and should greatly improve the outlook. This change of focus in public perspectives on disability and health is clearly evident in the definition of **health promotion** used in *Healthy People 2010*: "efforts to create healthy lifestyles and a healthy environment to prevent medical and other secondary conditions, such as teaching people how to address their health care needs and increasing opportunities to participate in usual life activities" (USDHHS, 2000, p. 6–25). *Healthy People 2020* does not separate out "health promotion" as its planning committee found that the entire document related to health promotion; to define health promotion within the document might constrain its meaning, when the committee believed that health promotion should be viewed quite broadly (USDHHS, ODPHP, 2009).

The emphasis on "secondary conditions" in *Healthy People 2010* has been replaced in *Healthy People 2020* with a concern for health disparities for people with disabilities. Compared with people without disabilities, people with disabilities are more likely to: "Experience difficulties or delays in getting the health care they need; not have had an annual dental visit; not have had a mammogram in past 2 years; not have had a Pap test within the past 3 years; not engage in fitness activities; use tobacco; be overweight or obese; have high blood pressure; experience symptoms of psychological distress; receive less social-emotional support; and have lower employment rates" (USDHHS, ODPHP, 2012d). Key to addressing these barriers is for people with disabilities to: "(1) be included in public health activities; (2) receive well-timed interventions and services; (3) interact with their environment without barriers; and (4) participate in everyday life activities. Without these opportunities, people with disabilities will continue to experience health disparities, compared to the general population" (USDHHS, ODPHP, 2012d).

Missed Opportunities by Health Care Providers or Missed Opportunities to Affect Quality of Life

All of us, whether healthy, disabled, or chronically ill, require basic elements to maintain health, including clean air and water, a safe place to live, sunshine, exercise, nutritious food, socialization, and the opportunity to be successful in life's pursuits. As self-evident as these health-promoting elements may seem, for the millions of persons who deal with disability, chronic disease, or both, such basic needs may too often take second place to other issues. It is equally problematic that health promotion and disease prevention measures, most notably at the primary and secondary levels, are often nonexistent or lacking.

The issue of missed opportunities in health promotion and prevention is depicted in Figure 26-2. The focus of the health care delivery system is increasingly skewed toward secondary and tertiary prevention efforts, and limited emphasis is placed on the health promotion and primary prevention needs of the population. Although this is a concern for all persons, it is of particular importance for persons with disabilities and chronic illnesses because they are more likely to have these needs ignored altogether. As Figure 26-2 shows, an entire area of issues may be addressed with a basically healthy person but not with a disabled or chronically ill individual. Some areas of secondary and tertiary prevention unique to persons with disabilities or chronic illnesses may be completely ignored. This nonreceipt of health-promoting or preventive education, or actions vital to the health and well-being of those with disabilities or chronic illnesses, is of grave concern. For example, issues such as sexuality are often not explored with the disabled or chronically ill.

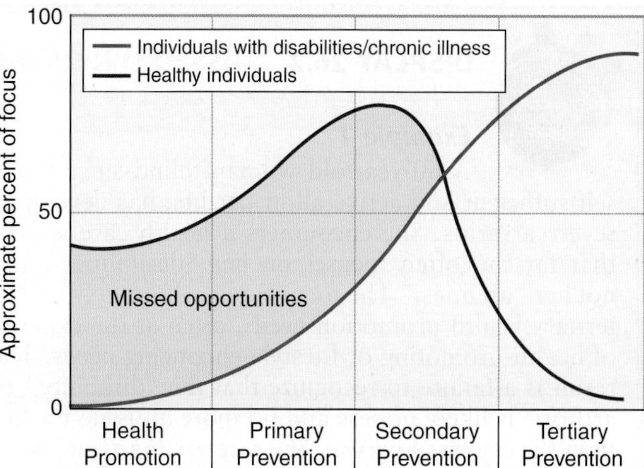

FIGURE 26-2. Difference in client focus between individuals with and without a chronic illness or disability.

This skewed view of the lifestyles, behaviors, and needs of the disabled as "different" from those of the "able-bodied" is a clear example of lack of understanding by health professionals and the public alike and leads directly to health disparities between the able-bodied and the disabled populations.

It is likely that disability or chronic illness serves as the presenting reason for an individual's encounter with the health care community, including the public health nurse. As a result, the disability or illness often drives the selection of prevention efforts, to the possible exclusion of other, equally important health issues. For example, for an individual with a primary diagnosis of Type 2 diabetes, secondary prevention efforts often center on that disease (e.g., screening for diabetic retinopathy). The need to refer the client for a Pap test or a baseline mammogram may be overlooked. Likewise, the treatment plan may include a consultation with a dietitian but fail to address the basic needs for leisure-time activities, regular physical activity, a varied and interesting diet, fresh air and sunshine, and socialization—all of which may help prevent the development of depression, a common result of chronic illness. Display 26.2 offers several examples of missed opportunities in the areas of primary and secondary prevention. It is of particular concern to the practice of community/public health nursing that the broad range of health promotion and prevention needs of all clients be addressed.

A study by Wei, Findley, and Sambamoorthi (2006) demonstrated the risk for missed opportunities for clinical preventive services among women. Of the 3,183 individuals sampled in this study, 23% were disabled. When compared to the other study participants, the disabled women were less likely to receive cancer screening (mammograms and Pap smears) within the recommended intervals. Interestingly, this group was more likely to receive influenza vaccination, cholesterol screening, and colorectal screenings as recommended. The researchers found that, overall, having a usual source of care and health insurance were predictive of preventive service receipt. In addition, they stressed the need for improving

DISPLAY 26.2 MISSED OPPORTUNITIES

Example 1

A 60-year-old woman, blind since birth, self-sufficient and active all of her life, has developed severe arthritis. She encounters a health care system that far too often focuses on her "disabilities" and not her "abilities." The focus is placed squarely on her tertiary health promotion needs, often at the expense of health-promoting or lifestyle-enhancing needs. The result is a failure to recognize that the "disability" of arthritis is likely no less and no more an issue for her than for a sighted person. She receives the same medication therapy as a sighted person but may not be offered a physical therapy program due to her disability. Her need for physical therapy is no less important, but locating an appropriate, safe, and easily accessible program requires some additional work on the part of her provider. At issue is that options potentially discussed with a sighted person are more apt to be omitted completely, which may negatively affect the client's overall health and wellbeing.

Example 2

A 20-year-old man with learning disabilities, who is employed at a local factory, receives a regularly scheduled physical examination with a new provider. He lives in a congregate care facility, which is an out-of-home facility that provides housing for people with disabilities in which rotating staff members provide care for 16 or more adults or any number of children/youth younger than 21 years of age. It excludes foster care, adoptive homes, residential schools, correctional facilities, and nursing facilities (U.S. Department of Health and Human Services [USDHHS], 2000). The major finding of the examination is that he is due for a tetanus booster and should also begin the series for hepatitis A, because he lives in a high-risk area of the western United States. He takes the referral slip and leaves the office. One year later, at his regularly scheduled visit, it becomes clear that he never received his immunizations. Apparently, he didn't know what he was supposed to do with the paper, because he has difficulty reading, and he had no idea where to go to get his "shots." The primary prevention elements were provided, but clearly not in a manner appropriate for this individual. With additional explanation and follow-up, perhaps the outcome would have been quite different.

Example 3

A 34-year-old woman who has been severely obese since the birth of her last child (4 years ago) has not had a gynecologic examination since that birth. She is aware of the need to have regular examinations, yet she cannot bring herself to make an appointment. The reason is that she knows she will have to be weighed, and this terrifies her, especially because it is done in an open area where others can see. She finally gets the courage to call for an appointment and tells the clerk that she does not want to be weighed. The clerk's response is less than helpful and she is essentially told that it is "policy." She makes the appointment but does not keep it. This situation could have been handled in a compassionate manner, recognizing the painful experience that weighing is for many individuals and suggesting alternatives, one of which could have been simply to bypass the scales until after the interview and examination. At that point, the woman may have been more amenable to the measurement and a more discrete area could have been offered. In this case, the opportunities to provide primary, secondary, and tertiary prevention were lost.

women's health care by identifying those who are most at risk and targeting efforts to reduce disparities.

Fitzmaurice, Kanarek, and Fitzgerald (2011) identified specific lifestyle risk factor behaviors in working-age adults with disabilities. Using data from the 2003 Behavioral Risk Factor Surveillance System (BRFSS), the authors explored smoking status, weight, diet, alcohol use, physical activity, and influenza and pneumococcal vaccination among approximately 200,000 community dwelling working-age adults. Their findings suggest that adults with disabilities with activity limitations and use of assistive devices may be at increased risk for poor lifestyle behaviors related to weight and physical activity, but to have lower use of alcohol consumption and increased vaccination rates than the nondisabled respondents. With the challenges faced by those with disabilities to maintain employment, the need to include screening for lifestyle behavioral risks in all routine health care visits is seen as vital. Both studies point out the need for ongoing attention to the health promotion needs of these vulnerable individuals and to take every opportunity to address those needs.

Health Care Disparities and Discrimination

It is a growing concern to those who are disabled, and to their families and advocates, that the type and quality of the health-related services, referrals, and care that they receive may not be appropriate to their circumstances. This results in increased illness and disability and potentially decreased quality or length of life. One pointed example of this disparity involved a national sample of low-income female Medicaid recipients. Women with disabilities in this sample had lower rates of receipt of medical services and were much less likely to receive cervical cancer screenings (Parish & Ellison-Martin, 2007). Although the women each had similar access to health care services, the disparities were of concern. Not surprisingly, those women with disabilities were less likely to report satisfaction with their care.

Additional disparities may exist in services received by those with chronic illness and disabilities. Racial and ethnic differences in immunization rates were found in a study analyzing data from the National Health Interview Survey of almost 2,000 individuals with diabetes (Egede & Zheng, 2003). Even after controlling for access, health care coverage, and socioeconomic status, the rates of influenza and pneumococcal immunization were lower for certain racial/ethnic groups, primarily Blacks. What is not known from these results is whether the inadequate immunization rates resulted from client acceptance issues, differential provider recommendations, or some combination of these factors.

In a more recent example, Haviland, Elliot, Hambarsoomian, and Lurie (2011) examined immunization disparities among older Hispanics and non-Hispanic Whites. Using data from the 2008 Medicare Consumer Assessment of Healthcare Providers and Systems survey, a random sample of nearly 250,000 respondents aged 65 years and older were analyzed. For Spanish- and English-speaking Hispanics, the rates for pneumococcal immunization were significantly lower than those for non-Hispanic Whites—40% and 50%, respectively compared with 74% for the non-Hispanic Whites. The lower rates persisted with the influenza vaccination with Spanish-speaking (64%) and English-speaking Hispanics (68%), compared to non-Hispanic Whites (76%). Among the findings was a higher rate of immunization for Hispanic seniors enrolled in a Medicare-managed care program rather than traditional fee-for-service Medicare. These findings point out the need to target Hispanic seniors, especially those with limited English skills to increase immunization rates.

It is discriminatory practice when an individual receives unequal, inappropriate, or limited services compared with those offered to others. Although the difference in treatment is often due to lack of understanding of the needs of disabled persons, it is nonetheless discriminatory. Such bias may not be intentional, but it can dramatically affect the health of clients and must be improved. The good news is that the incidence of unequal and inappropriate practices can be reduced with education and training of health care providers, agency staff, and insurance carriers. A crucial aspect of community/public health practice is to ensure that those individuals with disabilities or chronic illnesses are afforded the best possible care, treatment options, and opportunities to improve their health—the same options as are provided for nondisabled persons and those who do not suffer from chronic illness.

Health promotion and primary, secondary, and tertiary prevention activities are essential aspects of quality care for all persons. Those with disabilities require specialized attention to needs resulting from or related to their disabilities, yet they also require the same attention to health and wellbeing as the rest of the population. Public health nurses are in a prime position to advocate needed changes for those with disabilities and chronic illnesses. Such changes can include increased attention to health promotion and disease prevention needs, accessible and appropriate delivery of those services, and specialized treatment plans that incorporate the latest knowledge of a specific illness or disability (see Perspectives: Student Voices).

PERSPECTIVES STUDENT VOICES

For as long as I can remember, I have wanted to work with children. When I was finally accepted into the nursing program, I was so disappointed when I learned that we would only have 7 weeks in our pediatric rotation. Then, I found out about an opportunity to work with children at a school in my community health practicum—marvelous I thought. I just knew I'd be giving immunizations, physical assessments, and performing hearing checks. Then I found out that I would actually be working with school-aged children with disabilities and their parents in a special after-school health promotion program. The nurse I was assigned to asked me to come in before the program started, so that she could fill me in on the program and my role. It actually sounded great, and I was confident that I could handle this. Then she asked me something that made me worried; she asked if I had ever worked with a child who used a wheelchair, or had a continuous insulin pump, or had seizures. I told her that I had some experience in the hospital, and that I was sure that I would be prepared for any health care issues that might occur. "You misunderstand," she said, "that's not what I meant. Have you ever gotten to know a child with a disability?" I really hadn't, and it suddenly made me a bit worried. She explained to me that many people don't treat children with disabilities just like any other child. They also don't always know how to talk to the parents about their child. She suggested that one way to give me a bit of information was to go home and do some reading and look at some Web sites she recommended. One in particular, the National Organization on Disability (http://www.nod.org/), had a great feature called "Disability Etiquette Tips" that I have already found to be a big help with the kids and their parents. She also directed me to the Easter Seals Disability Services (http://www.easter-seals.com), which has a great deal of information on programs that are currently available for children and adults. I even learned that this organization used to be called the National Society for Crippled Children … I'm sure glad they changed the name.

Eileen S.

CIVIL RIGHTS LEGISLATION

Policies such as *Healthy People 2020* are important elements in addressing the health and overall needs of people with disabilities and chronic diseases in the United States. Although it has a great deal of influence on the direction and type of programs initiated, health policies alone cannot assure that individuals with disabilities will find and receive needed services and accommodations. An act of legislation is vital to ensure that every individual's rights are protected and that there is legal recourse to secure needs that have been denied. As is often true for other issues of equality, legislation is only one of many steps that must be taken. The struggle for civil rights for disabled persons in this country is gaining momentum but still lacks the influence and public attention of other civil rights efforts.

The **Americans with Disabilities Act** (ADA) was signed into law in 1990 to protect the civil liberties of the many Americans living with disabilities. This legislation was the result of a long and difficult struggle. Individuals with disabilities and their advocates made their voices heard by repeatedly demanding an end to inferior treatment and lack of equal protection under the law, which have impeded their daily lives. The ADA has set the standard for a number of subsequent laws which, together with pre-ADA legislation, have become a broad spectrum of protections for people with disabilities. These laws are listed in Table 26-3 and cover a variety of issues, including telecommunications, architectural barriers, and voter registration.

The ADA essentially "prohibits discrimination on the basis of disability in employment, state and local government, public accommodations, commercial facilities, transportation, and telecommunications [and] also applies to the United States Congress" (U.S. Department of Justice [USDOJ], 2009). For individuals to be protected under the ADA, they must have

Table 26.3 Disability Rights Laws

Law	Summary	Contact
Americans with Disabilities Act (ADA)	Prohibits discrimination in (1) employment, (2) state and local government, (3) public accommodations, commercial facilities, transportation, and telecommunications	(1) U.S. Equal Opportunity Commission; (2) Civil Rights Division, (3) U.S. Department of Justice (USDOJ); Office of Civil Rights, Federal Transit Administration, USDOJ
Telecommunications Act of 1996	Telecommunication equipment and services are accessible	Federal Communications Commission (FCC)
Fair Housing Act (amended 1988)	Prohibits housing discrimination	U.S. Department of Housing and Urban Development (HUD)
Air Carrier Access Act	Prohibits discrimination in air transportation by domestic and foreign carriers	U.S. Department of Transportation
Voting Accessibility for the Elderly and Handicapped Act of 1984	Requires polling places to be physically accessible for federal elections	USDOJ—Civil Rights Division
National Voter Registration Act of 1993	"Motor Voter Act"—makes it easier to vote by increasing low registration rates by minorities and persons with disabilities	USDOJ—Civil Rights Division
Civil Rights of Institutionalized Persons Act (CRIPA) 1997	Right to receive care in the least restrictive setting	USDOJ
Individuals with Disabilities Education Act	Make available free public education in the least restrictive environment for all children with disabilities	U.S. Department of Education—Office of Special Education Programs
Rehabilitation Act	Prohibits discrimination in all federal programs or programs receiving federal financial assistance	Agency's Equal Employment Opportunity Office U.S. Department of Labor—Office of Federal Contract Compliance Programs USDOJ
Architectural Barriers Act	Buildings constructed or altered with federal funds must meet federal accessibility standards	U.S. Architectural and Transportation Barriers Compliance Board

From U.S. Department of Justice, Civil Rights Division, Disability Rights Section. (2009). ***A guide to disability rights law***. Retrieved from http://www.ada.gov/cguide.htm

a disability or some type of relationship or association with an individual who has a disability. Under the ADA, the definition of a disability in regard to an individual is "(a) a physical or mental impairment that substantially limits one or more major life activities of such individual; (b) a record of such an impairment; (c) or being regarded as having such an impairment" (ADA, 2009). A listing of the specific diagnoses covered under the law is absent, but general major life activities related to disability are described as including "caring for oneself, performing manual tasks, seeing, hearing eating, sleeping, walking, standing, lifting, bending, speaking, breathing, learning, reading, concentrating, thinking, communicating, and working" (ADA, 2009). Major life activities that include the operation of a major bodily function related to disability include (but are not limited to) "functions of the immune system, normal cell growth, digestive, bowel, bladder, neurological, brain, respiratory, circulatory, endocrine, and reproductive functions" (ADA, 2009). Despite this specificity, there remains a broad range of interpretations and legal challenges with respect to who is actually covered by the ADA.

In addition to this uncertainty as to who is actually protected by the ADA, there can also be confusion as to who is required to comply with the provisions of the act and what specific remedial actions are necessary. The ADA currently applies to all employers with 15 or more employees (including religious organizations) and all activities of state and local governments irrespective of their size. Public transportation, businesses that provide public accommodation, and telecommunications entities are all required to provide access for individuals with disabilities. It is important to note that the ADA does not override federal and state health and safety laws. However, successful legal challenges to those statutes have been made when they were clearly outdated or when it could be argued that the public safety was not actually at risk in a specific situation. Yet considerable gray areas exist in the application of the ADA, leaving open the prospect of challenges by those who are subject to the law and those who are protected by it.

Individuals who believe that their legal rights under the ADA have been violated may seek remedy by filing a lawsuit or submitting a complaint to one of four federal offices, depending on the specific type of alleged violation: (1) the USDOJ–Civil Rights Division; (2) any U.S. Equal Employment Opportunity Commission field office; (3) the Office of Civil Rights-Federal Transit Administration; or (4) the Federal Communications Commission. The process for filing a complaint is not a simple task, and many seek the assistance of attorneys, legal aid societies, or various private organizations, some of which are discussed later in this chapter (see Display 26.3).

In 1999, the NCD found that many of the federal agencies charged with protecting the civil rights of disabled persons were limited by insufficient funding and lack of a coherent and unifying national strategy (NCD, 2000). The NCD recommended clarification of the basis for evaluating agency performance to improve the intended full expression of the law. Criteria identified to evaluate performance of the ADA include (1) proactive and reactive strategies, (2) communication with consumers and complainants, (3) policy and subregulatory guidance, (4) enforcement actions, (5) strategic litigation, (6) timely resolution of complaints, (7) competent and credible investigative processes, (8) technical assistance for protected persons and covered entities, (9) adequate agency resources, (10) interagency collaboration and coordination, and (11) outreach and consultation with the community.

In the NCD's follow-up report in 2005, the *ADA Impact Study*, progress was reported in the following areas:

- Telephone relay services were being used at high levels, and changes in technology are making usage higher.
- Public transit systems in the United States had made dramatic progress in becoming more accessible, especially to wheelchair users.
- The percentage of Americans with disabilities voting in 2004 increased dramatically.

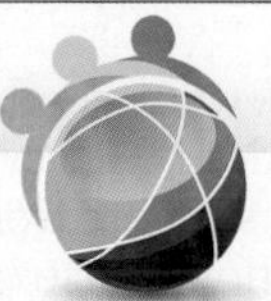

DISPLAY 26.3 OFFICE OF CIVIL RIGHTS: COMPLIANCE WITH ADA

The responsibility of the U.S. Department of Justice, Office of Civil Rights (OCR), is to investigate complaints of alleged violations of the Americans with Disabilities Act (ADA). An example of one of those complaints involved a 22-year-old Connecticut woman with cerebral palsy. She had been placed in a nursing home because of changes in her living situation and health care status, but wanted to move back into the community. The OCR intervened to ensure that the woman secured appropriate housing and that counseling and intensive case management services were in place when she moved back into the community. Without the protection afforded under the ADA, the outcome could have been much different.

Source: USDHHS, Office for Civil Rights. (2006, September). *Delivering on the promise: OCR's compliance activities promote community integration.* Retrieved from http://www.hhs.gov/ocr/civilrights/resources/specialtopics/community/deliveringonthepromisereport.html

- The education gap between people with disabilities and people without disabilities was shrinking, and people with disabilities were attending postsecondary institutions in record numbers.
- People with disabilities were experiencing less discrimination in employment (NCD, 2005, p. 3).

In a 2007 analysis, *The Impact of the Americans with Disabilities Act: Assessing the Progress Toward Achieving the Goals of the ADA*, NCD continued to find that many people with disabilities, businesses, and employers still did not understand the requirements of the ADA in relation to employment. And Americans with disabilities continued to face barriers to becoming economically self-sufficient. The NCD also found many areas of optimism: Public transportation was more accessible, especially for wheelchair users. Ramps and sidewalks had been made more accessible, although full access still lagged. Access in public accommodations continued to improve, as did public attitudes toward those with disabilities. Many people with disabilities perceived improved quality of life, which they attributed to the ADA (NCD, 2007, pp. 9–12).

It is important to those with disabilities, their families, and the professionals who serve them that a structure is in place to provide protection under the ADA, but a law does not prevent discrimination, nor does the existence of a structure such as the ADA provide immediate remedies. The most challenging aspect of providing services for persons with disabilities is to alter the perceptions and misunderstandings of others about people with disabilities. The perspective of one community member offers one such example (see Perspectives: Voices from the Community).

PERSPECTIVES
VOICES FROM THE COMMUNITY

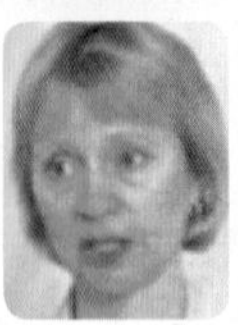

I was always such an active and healthy person, so when I was diagnosed with multiple sclerosis it hit me like a ton of bricks. Here I was with two small children and I was only 30 years old; it just wasn't fair. Some days are good and some days are just awful. I finally broke down and applied for one of those disabled parking stickers. The doctor had to approve it, and he said it was a good thing to help me save my energy for the important things, like taking care of my family. I hated to use it, but I was just getting so tired. What is so awful are the looks on people's faces when I park in the special areas near the door. I know I don't look like I'm sick. I just hate those looks—I can hear them saying under their breath, "She can't be sick . . . I'll bet that sticker is for a family member and she's just abusing it—how lazy!" If I wasn't so tired I'd park in the regular parking places.

Pat N., Tampa, Florida

FAMILIES WITH A DISABLED OR CHRONICALLY ILL MEMBER

The Family's Role in Advocacy

Families that include a member with a chronic illness or disability face many challenges. They are required to navigate a health care system that they may know little about and with which they often feel at odds. They serve as advocates for their family member in need (whether child, spouse, or parent) and may become exhausted or frustrated with their efforts, especially if they have been less than successful in achieving their goals. Many are forced to ask for or demand assistance from health care agencies, social services, or transportation sources to achieve the level of care needed by the family member. Many are required to open their home to others (e.g., community/public health nurses, social workers) to access the services. Families may have little understanding of what services they are entitled to because of language barriers, difficult agency policies, or disjointed service delivery.

The public health nurse is usually not the first health care professional that the family encounters. They may already have been through a lengthy struggle to receive assistance. In these circumstances, the nurse often is confronted by a frustrated family that distrusts yet another "professional." The nurse must gain the trust and confidence of the family by practicing consistency, following through with promised actions, and always being truthful. Not all problems that the family faces can be remedied, and even for problems that do have solutions, time and effort may be needed to obtain the desired result.

The Impact on Families

A literature review of the needs of parents with chronically ill children reported a number of common themes in the studies surveyed, among them the need for normalcy and certainty, the need for information, and the need for partnership (Fisher, 2001). Although these needs were associated with the presence of a chronically ill child in the family, the same needs are likely to occur in other families. These are certainly areas that can be addressed by the public health nurse in a practical way.

Wong and Heriot (2007) found somewhat similar results in their study of 35 parents of children with cystic fibrosis (CF). The parents who sought support from family and friends experienced less emotional distress than those who didn't, analogous to the need for partnership noted by Fisher (2001). Additional findings revealed that parents who used self-blame as a coping strategy were also more likely to report experiencing depression and were more likely to report lower levels of mental health in their children. Suggestions to assist the family included parental counseling to reduce self-blame, encouraging the children's important life goals, and providing information on available supportive social networks. With the current median life expectancy of patients with CF at well above 30 years, the issue of long-term family support is vital.

One major obstacle for families with a disabled or chronically ill member may be obtaining needed **assistive devices and technology**. These are defined in *Healthy People 2010* as "any item, piece of equipment, or product system, whether acquired commercially, modified, or customized, that is used to increase, maintain, or improve the functional capabilities of individuals with disabilities" (USDHHS, 2000, p. 6–25). An objective under Disability and Health (DH-10) in *Healthy People 2020* directly addresses obstacles to obtaining assistive devices and technologies:

> DH-10: Reduce the proportion of people with disabilities who report barriers to obtaining the assistive devices, service animals, technology services, and accessible technologies that they need (USDHHS, ODPHP, 2012c).

With constant changes in available equipment, financing, and technology, it is little wonder that families struggle to find the best alternatives. Just because a technology exists does not mean that it can be obtained. Often, the insurance carrier, whether private or governmental, sets limits on which products can be obtained or which brands are acceptable. The overriding issue of financing is no small hurdle. It is often left up to the family to learn about options and legal rights through a process of trial and error. Interventions by the community/public health nurse can greatly reduce the burden on the family. With so many product lines available on the Web, the nurse can assist families to weigh and select among options, especially with families with limited access or experience with the internet. It is equally helpful for the nurse to intervene with insurance providers if coverage of equipment is not easily obtained or to find sources of funding for the equipment from private agencies if possible. Referring families to community groups or organizations that provide specific assistance can be very helpful. Other families that share similar struggles can provide a vital link to needed services and can be contacted through self-help groups or other sources. Here, the community/public health nurse can provide expertise on available community resources and referral processes.

Respite care is another area of great importance for families of the disabled and the chronically ill. It can be emotionally draining to meet the daily needs of a member who cannot perform self-care and can lead to increased caregiver fatigue and stress. It is also important to recognize the effect of the situation on noncaregivers in the family, particularly nondisabled siblings of a disabled child. When focus is placed on the needs of one family member, other children may feel that their own needs are not as important. This can lead to behavioral and health-related problems. Respite care offers some needed relief to the family and allows for uninterrupted attention to the nondisabled children. This service can occur within the home or at an outside facility. Respite care may be provided by a private organization at little or no cost to the family, or it may be quite expensive and require financing by the insurance company or by the family itself. Whatever the source, some type of respite care is often vital to the family's health and should be a priority in the overall treatment plan of the family (see *Using the Nursing Process*).

The issue of employment is generally of great significance to families of the disabled and chronically ill, as employment options may be quite limited when a family member has special needs. The family may have to remain in a particular location to access needed health and social services, reducing the possibility of increased earning potential at a different location or in another field of employment. Family members who are working may choose less favorable employment options because the position is convenient or has more flexible hours. For instance, a person may take a part-time position at a local convenience store that does not pay particularly well in preference to a higher-paying, full-time factory position because the store is close to home and allows for frequent adjustments in schedule.

Having a chronically ill family member often means that working individuals must take time off from work. Although some legal protections are provided under the Family and Medical Leave Act of 1993, the Act does not apply in all situations. More importantly, it allows only for time off; it does not mandate payment during those periods. Family members may have to choose between taking unpaid time off and continuing to work while dealing with the needs of the family member as best they can. Some individuals choose to work part-time or not to work at all, so that they can care for family members. At a time when many families have two earners to help meet financial commitments, these families may have to rely on only one income. Limitations in income are particularly difficult when one considers the myriad needs of the disabled and chronically ill, many of which may not be covered by insurance.

Families receiving financial and other assistance from Temporary Assistance for Needy Families (TANF) also face work-related pressures. The 1996 welfare reform legislation (the Personal Responsibility and Work Opportunity Reconciliation Act) introduced regulations that potentially affect families with a chronically ill child, especially those families living in poverty. Those now receiving TANF have a 5-year lifetime limit on receipt of benefits (and states may opt to reduce years of eligibility further), institution of work requirements, and elimination of entitlement to cash benefits (USDHHS, Administration for Children and Families, 2010). The impact of these changes is of growing concern within the public health community. Following implementation of the regulatory changes, Smith, Wise, and Wampler (2002) explored the impact of TANF rules in a study of knowledge of welfare reform among families with a chronically ill child. They found that respondents often had incomplete knowledge of work requirements, even if they were entitled to exemptions because their children received Supplemental Security Income. In those cases, 37% of the respondents were

USING THE NURSING PROCESS WITH VULNERABLE POPULATIONS

Assessment

Anna Lopez is a mother of three children aged 2 to 9 years old. The eldest, Ernesto, was diagnosed with severe Down syndrome at birth. He is confined to a wheelchair, requires total care, and remains at home with his mother and younger siblings, who are not yet in school. Anna's husband works long hours as a computer repairman for a large company. They have health insurance, but it does not cover additional expenses, such as day care for Ernesto. The family has done very well in providing for Ernesto's needs, and they receive periodic visits from you, the community health nurse, to evaluate his condition and check on the feeding tube used for his nourishment. Physically, Ernesto is stable, but you notice that Anna has been increasingly withdrawn at the visits, rarely offering information, but responding to questions appropriately. She seems less engaged with her other children as well, only occasionally smiling at them.

Nursing Diagnoses

1. At risk for depression related to ongoing caregiver demands and lack of respite care
2. At risk for altered health status due to limited focus on self-care needs

Plan/Implementation

DIAGNOSIS 1

The community health nurse will discuss with the client the need for a thorough physical assessment, including an evaluation for depression. The community health nurse will contact the insurance provider to discuss day care/respite options for Ernesto. If unavailable, local community organizations will be contacted for appropriate referrals. In addition, the need for more frequent visits to the family will be discussed with the insurance carrier to address the needs of the mother as caregiver.

DIAGNOSIS 2

The community health nurse will discuss with the client her concerns about her overall physical and mental health and discuss some self-care options that may improve her wellbeing: improved nutrition, physical activity, leisure time options, and adjustment of family schedule to accommodate more free time for self-care.

Evaluation

The client was at first very reticent to make an appointment for an evaluation, but after thinking it over for a week and discussing it with her husband, she did so. Her husband was relieved that she had suggested the appointment, because he was growing increasingly concerned over her withdrawal but did not know how to bring up the subject. The family physician referred Anna to a psychologist for evaluation of the depression. The insurance carrier agreed to increase home visits on a short-term basis but did not have a respite care option available for Ernesto. Fortunately, a local faith-based community group was able to provide limited assistance to the family. They identified several members who had raised children with similar disabilities and were willing to stay with Ernesto and the other children once a week for 4 hours. This allowed Anna some free time to make appointments with her psychologist, shop, or visit friends. After several months, Anna has begun to smile more and seems much more relaxed at the home visits. The children are all doing fine, and the respite care is expected to continue for at least the next 6 months. The need for ongoing attention to her own self-care needs is emphasized with Anna by the community health nurse.

unaware that they qualified for work exemptions, and 70% had not applied for the exemptions. This indicated that eligible families with a disabled child may not have received the exemptions to which they were entitled, adding additional and unnecessary burdens to families already at risk.

The relationship between welfare status, health insurance status, and the health and medical care received by children with asthma was also studied (Wood et al., 2002). The most significant findings were (a) children of parents who had been denied TANF experienced more severe asthma symptoms and had more acute care visits than children in families that did not access the welfare system; (b) children of recent TANF applicants were more likely to be uninsured or transiently insured than those who had not applied; and (c) recent TANF applicants had the poorest mental health scores. This study underscored the high-risk status of those families with a chronically ill child and the need to provide access to health insurance and health services.

Caregiver health needs and mental health status are yet another area of concern for families who must provide for a disabled or chronically ill member. One of the largest longitudinal studies in the United States, the Nurses' Health Study, provided the data for an investigation of the impact of informal caregiving on the mental health status of caregivers (Cannuscio et al., 2002). Using data collected over a 4-year period (1992–1996), the study found that women who provided 36 or more hours per week of care for a disabled spouse were six times more likely than noncaregivers to report depressive or anxious symptoms. The frequency of symptoms was elevated but less dramatic if the women cared for a disabled or ill parent as opposed to a spouse. The findings supported the necessity of attention to the needs of caregivers, the majority of whom are women. A follow-up study by Cannuscio et al. (2004) found that higher weekly time commitment to informal care was associated with an increased risk of depression, regardless of the level of social support. For those with few social ties and high spousal time commitment, the level of depressive symptoms was much higher. Although employment status didn't appear to have an impact on depressive symptoms of caregivers, access to social ties was strongly correlated with more positive health outcomes in the caregivers (Cannuscio et al., 2004). Poor health outcomes, both physical and mental, are of growing concern as the population ages and the need for family caregiving rises. Recognizing that caregivers within a family are at increased risk for poor health outcomes, the public health nurse must select appropriate interventions to address the health needs of all family members.

Families of individuals with a disability or chronic illness are at increased risk for a number of negative consequences. Although families vary in the level of risk or disruption, the public health nurse should recognize the potential impact of the dependent member's needs on the entire family. Families may suffer from financial difficulties, poor physical or mental health, and a variety of other challenges. They are often ill prepared to deal with the complicated systems that must be accessed to obtain needed care. The public health nurse is in an optimal position to interpret those systems to the families and to advocate for the needed care, services, and equipment. The nurse must view the family holistically, recognizing additional needs that may develop as a result of the situation they currently face. The nurse should include an assessment of caregiver and family work patterns when caring for families with a disabled or chronically ill family member.

ORGANIZATIONS SERVING THE NEEDS OF THE DISABLED AND CHRONICALLY ILL

The impact of civil rights legislation would not have been achieved without the chorus of voices from advocates who deal on a daily basis with the issue of disability—the individuals themselves, their families, coworkers, employers, and advocates. Much of the credit for the legislative successes belongs to advocacy groups. This section provides an overview of some of the advocates for disabled and chronically ill individuals and their families. In addition to serving these specific populations, they also provide others opportunities to learn more about the lives and struggles of disabled persons. Each of the organizations noted offers a wide range of information, much of which can be accessed online. These organizations provide community/public health nurses with a starting point for exploring specific topics pertinent to practice. As clients and families may also be accessing online content through personal or public internet access, it is important for nurses to prescreen and make recommendations to clients and families about reliable and accurate sites.

Government

The NCD is a small, independent federal agency tasked with making recommendations to the President, Congress, and other federal agencies about issues facing Americans with disabilities. The NCD staff is led by 15 Presidential appointees, who are all confirmed by the U.S. Senate. In 1986, the NCD recommended that Congress enact a civil rights law for people with disabilities and provide the initial draft legislation, which led to the ADA in 1990. NCD currently fulfills its advisory roles regarding disability policies, programs, procedures, and practices that enhance equal opportunity by "(1) Convening stakeholders to acquire timely and relevant input for recommendations and action steps; (2) Gathering and analyzing data and other information; (3) Engaging and influencing current debates and agendas; (4) Identifying and formulating solutions to emerging and long-standing challenges; and (5) Providing tools to facilitate effective implementation" (NCD, 2012).

Private

Many private organizations—local, national, and international—address a variety of disabilities and chronic diseases. Many of the better-known organizations such as the American Heart Association and the American Cancer Association are discussed in other chapters of this book and therefore are not covered here. This discussion includes examples of groups that deal most directly with disability and chronic illness. The reader is encouraged to search internet or print resources for additional groups and organizations dedicated to specific disabilities or chronic illnesses.

The National Association of the Deaf (NAD), headquartered in Washington, DC, is a private, nonprofit organization established in 1880. As the oldest U.S. organization serving the deaf community, its mission is to "preserve, protect and promote the civil, human and linguistic rights of all deaf Americans" (NAD, 2012a). NAD's Vision 2020 Strategic Plan articulated the organization's beliefs and decade-focused goals, including ensuring that "American Sign Language is the birthright of every deaf and hard of hearing person" (NAD, 2012b). NAD's programs include advocacy, captioned media, certification of **American Sign Language** (ASL) professionals and interpreters, legal assistance, and policy development and research (NAD, 2012a). ASL uses "handshapes" to communicate ideas and concepts; it is used primarily in America and Canada by the deaf community (Grayson, 2003). Display 26.4 offers a brief summary of the purpose and use of ASL and other signed languages.

The National Organization on Disability (NOD), headquartered in Washington, DC, acts on a mission statement "to expand the participation and contribution of America's 54 million men, women, and children with disabilities in all aspects of life" (NOD, 2012). The NOD Web site connects visitors to a rich variety of sources on community involvement, economic/employment topics, and access issues (http://www.nod.org/). With its sixth national survey in 2010, an important contribution of NOD is the periodic *Kessler Foundation/NOD Survey by Harris Interactive*

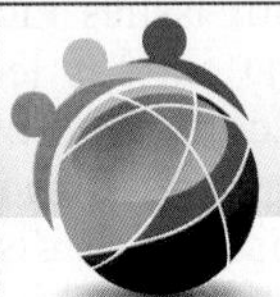

DISPLAY 26.4 SIGN LANGUAGES IN BRIEF

- Sign language is the use of "handshapes" and gestures to communicate ideas or concepts.
- American Sign Language is a unique language with its own rules of grammar and syntax.
- American Sign Language is primarily used in America and Canada and is the natural language of the deaf community.
- Sign languages are not universal.
- International Sign Language (Gestuno) is composed of vocabulary signs from various sign languages for use at international events or meetings to aid communication.
- Systems of Manually Coded English (i.e., Signed English, Signing Exact English) are not natural languages but systems designed to represent the translation of spoken language word for word.

From Grayson G. (2003). *Talking with your hands, listening with your eyes. A complete photographic guide to American Sign Language.* Garden City Park, NY: Square One Publishers; National Institute on Deafness and Other Communication Disorders. (2011). *American sign language* [NIH Pub. No. 11-4756]. Retrieved from http://www.nidcd.nih.gov/health/hearing/pages/asl.aspx

(NOD, 2010), the successor to the earlier *NOD/Harris Survey of Americans with Disabilities*, initiated in 1986 (NOD, 2004). These surveys seek to describe the gaps between people with and without disabilities in terms of employment, income, education, health care, access to transportation, entertainment or going out, socializing, attending religious services, political participation/voter registration, life satisfaction, and trends. Although improvements in all indicators have been demonstrated over the 24-year period of survey activity, progress is described as both slow and modest. The 2010 survey found that access to employment remained one of the largest gaps, with only 21% of disabled adults reporting employment compared to 59% of adults without disabilities. People with disabilities are still more likely to live in poverty. Internet access also varies greatly, with 54% of adults with disabilities having access, compared to 85% of adults without disabilities (NOD, 2010).

The American Council of the Blind (ACB) was founded in 1961 and has a current purpose "to work toward independence, security, equality of opportunity, and improved quality of life for all blind and visually impaired people" (ACB, 2011). As an organization "of the blind," rather than "for the blind," ACB is directed both literally and through its core principles by blind and visually impaired people (ACB, 2011). Services noted by the organization include information and referral, scholarship assistance, public education, and industry consultation, as well as governmental monitoring, consultation, and advocacy. Some of the major issues currently being pursued by the organization include improved education and rehabilitation for the blind and increased production and use of reading materials for the blind and visually impaired.

Guide Dogs for the Blind is a nonprofit charitable organization established to train and make available guide dogs for the visually impaired, especially in the western United States. Its mission is to provide "enhanced mobility to qualified individuals through partnership with dogs whose unique skills are developed and nurtured by dedicated volunteers and a professional staff" (Guide Dogs for the Blind, 2011). Both the dogs and services are free (with an adoption fee of $750), and the organization relies substantially on donations. It currently has two training sites, one in California and one in Oregon, with puppy raisers located throughout the Western states. The organization can be reached through its Web site (http://www.guidedogs.com/site/PageServer).

Another organization dealing with issues affecting the blind and visually impaired is the National Federation of the Blind (NFB). Founded in 1940, its purpose is "the complete integration of the blind into society on a basis of equality. This objective involves the removal of legal, economic, and social discriminations; the education of the public to new concepts concerning blindness; and the achievement by all blind people of the right to exercise to the fullest their individual talents and capacities" (NFB, 2012). Citing the need for assistance to the more than 1.1 million people in the United States who are blind, the organization provides public education, information and referral, and support for increased availability of materials in **Braille** (Display 26.5).

The oldest organization devoted to eliminating barriers for the blind and visually impaired is the American Foundation for the Blind (AFB), founded in 1921. The AFB advocates for the visually impaired through increased funding at the federal and state levels

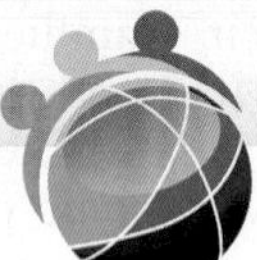

DISPLAY 26.5 WHAT IS BRAILLE?

Braille takes its name from Louis Braille, an 18-year-old blind Frenchman who created a system of raised dots on paper for reading and writing by modifying a system used on-board sailing ships for night reading. The six raised dots of each Braille "cell" vary to form palpable letters and punctuation. Persons experienced in Braille can read at speeds of 200 to 400 words per minute, comparable to print readers. Braille text can be written (1) by hand with a slate and stylus, (2) with a Braille writing machine, or (3) with specialized computer software and a Braille embossing device attached to the printer.

Source: National Federation of the Blind. (2012). *Braille–What is it? What does it mean to the blind?* Retrieved from http://www.nfb.org/images/nfb/Publications/fr/fr15/Issue1/f150113.html
More information about Braille is available at: http://nfb.org/search/node/braille

in areas such as rehabilitation research for older, visually impaired persons; improved literacy for the visually impaired, including use of Braille and assistive technology; improved employment opportunities; and increased accessibility of technology. In addition, AFB houses the Helen Keller Archives, which contain her correspondence, photographs, and various personal items and documents (AFB, 2012).

The Obesity Society seeks to promote "research, education and advocacy to better understand, prevent, and treat obesity and improve the lives of those affected" (Obesity Society, 2010). The organization addresses such issues as the need for attention to the impact of obesity on death and disability and for increased research, improved insurance coverage, and elimination of discrimination and mistreatment of people with obesity. The Society's Web site (http://www.obesity.org/) offers informational literature ranging from the global problem of obesity to treatment of obesity-related disability.

With growing awareness that human immunodeficiency virus (HIV)/acquired immune deficiency syndrome (AIDS) has become a chronic condition for most individuals affected, their long-term needs are gaining increased attention. Hundreds of Web sites and organizations are available to provide information, assistance, and support. One Web site, (http://www.thebody.com/) *The Body: The Complete HIV/AIDS Resource* (2012), offers state-by-state links to a variety of Internet and print resources. The site also includes resources in Canada and specific sites for American Indians and Alaskan Natives.

Begun in the aftermath of World War I, the Disabled American Veterans organization has provided free services to military veterans seeking to obtain benefits for service-related injuries (Disabled American Veterans, 2012). The organization is not a government agency and receives no federal funds, instead providing services through membership dues and public contributions. The mission of the organization is to help disabled veterans build better lives for themselves and their families. With the growing number of military injuries resulting from the Iraq and Afghanistan conflicts, the organization finds its service delivery even more stretched. The volunteers provide transportation to Veterans Administration (VA) medical facilities and provide ongoing service at VA hospitals, clinics, and nursing homes. The organization's homepage can be accessed at http://www.dav.org/

Universal Design

For those living with a disability or chronic disease and their family members, the issue of access is of utmost importance. As noted earlier, the cost to a family to accommodate the needs of a disabled person can be enormous. Considering that as the U.S. population ages, more and more of us will have need of accessibility in housing, business, and recreation in order to remain active and healthy as long as possible. In the concept of **universal design**, accessibility has been extended toward making tools, houses, and workplaces accessible to all. The cost of building our environments in a way that promotes access for all can be far less than the cost of remodeling those environments after the fact.

"Universal design is the design of products and environments to be usable by all people, to the greatest extent possible, without the need for adaptation or specialized design" (Mace, n.d.). The term "Universal Design" has been attributed to Ron Mace, founder of the Center for Universal Design (North Carolina State University). Mace, who had suffered from polio as a child, died suddenly in 1998, leaving behind a long legacy of advocacy on behalf of accessibility in design (Center for Universal Design, 2010).

The issue of accessibility is not new. The ADA (discussed earlier) addresses issues of access in employment, governmental building, and public accommodations. The Fair Housing Accessibility Guidelines (USDHUD, 2012), effective beginning in 1991, provide for design and construction of multifamily dwellings (four or more units) in accordance with accessibility requirements. The specific provisions include the following:

- Public use and common use portions of the dwellings are readily accessible to and usable by persons with handicaps.
- All doors within such dwellings that are designed to allow passage into and within the premises are sufficiently wide to allow passage by persons in wheelchairs.
- All premises within such dwellings contain the following features of adaptive design:
    1. An accessible route into and through the dwelling
    2. Light switches, electrical outlets, thermostats, and other environmental controls in accessible locations (see Fig. 26-3)

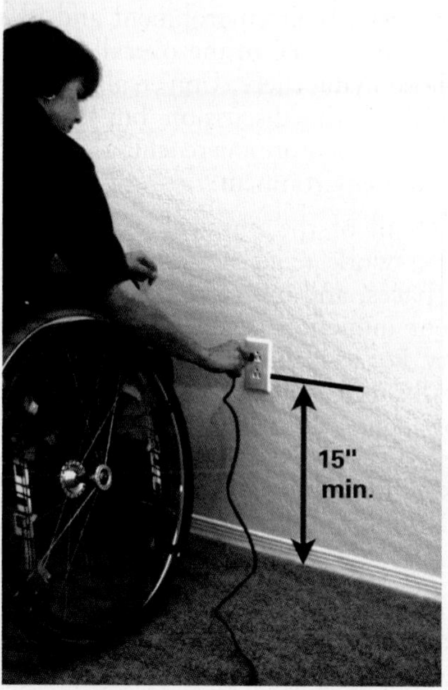

FIGURE 26-3. Recommended height of electrical outlet for ease of access for wheelchair–seated person. (Source: Center for Universal Design. (1997). Image 9267. Atlanta, GA: CDC Image Library. Retrieved from http://phil.cdc.gov/Phil/quicksearch.asp.)

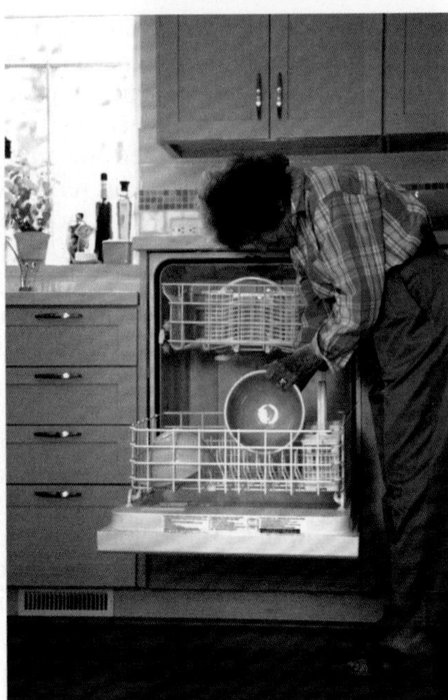

FIGURE 26-4. Universally designed raised dishwasher. (Source: Center for Universal Design. (2000). Image 9383. Atlanta, GA: CDC Image Library. Retrieved from http://phil.cdc.gov/Phil/quicksearch.asp.)

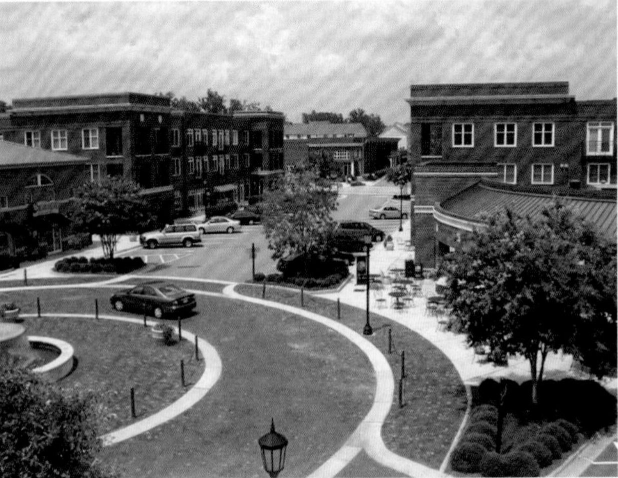

FIGURE 26-5. Planned mixed-use development with curb cuts, well-marked crossings, sidewalks, and accessible commercial and public spaces. (Source: Center for Universal Design. (2005). Image 9104. Atlanta, GA: CDC Image Library. Retrieved from http://phil.cdc.gov/Phil/quicksearch.asp.)

3. Reinforcements in bathroom walls to allow later installation of grab bars
4. Usable kitchens and bathrooms such that an individual in a wheelchair can maneuver about the space (USDHUD, 2012) (see Fig- 26-4)

Universal design incorporates access, but access does not necessarily imply universal design. The design of a community's built environment and its impact on individuals plays a role in the overall health and well-being of those living there. Universal design and access play a key role in this discussion, but the importance of accessible design is more far-reaching. According to the CDC, the built environment:

> includes all of the physical parts of where we live and work (e.g., homes, buildings, streets, open spaces, and infrastructure). The built environment influences a person's level of physical activity. For example, inaccessible or nonexistent sidewalks and bicycle or walking paths contribute to sedentary habits. These habits lead to poor health outcomes such as obesity, cardiovascular disease, diabetes, and some types of cancer. (CDC, 2006, p. 1)

For those with existing disabilities, assuring ease of access to all types of recreation and exercise options is of paramount importance. For those who may develop disabilities or chronic illnesses, having the opportunities for healthy participation in physical activity may forestall or prevent the development of illness. For the community, having an environment that promotes rather than restricts a healthy lifestyle can be economically advantageous (see Fig. 26-5). Even schools have a role to play (CDC, 2008). Building new schools away from residential areas decreases opportunities for exercise and after-school activities. As parents are increasingly forced to drive their children to school, the children remain sedentary, the pollution from cars is increased, and the risk of automobile accidents increases. Community design is a complicated and evolving issue, but the point remains: A healthier population may be achieved with attention to the environmental barriers that impede healthy lifestyles for all persons, including those with chronic or disabling conditions.

THE ROLE OF THE COMMUNITY/PUBLIC HEALTH NURSE

This chapter has discussed a number of areas in which the community/public health nurse plays a key role. It is important to review those roles in the context of the individual, the family, and the community as prime areas for nursing intervention. Chapter 3 first examined the broad spectrum of roles that the professional nurse takes on within the community. It is helpful to review those roles and think about their application to disabled and chronically ill clients, their families, and the communities in which they live.

Table 26-4 provides a grid on which to record specific examples of the roles that public health nurses assume in relation to disabilities and chronic illnesses. Take note of each role that you participate in or observe while completing your clinical experience. If you cannot find examples of the various roles at each level, perhaps

Table 26.4 Roles of the Community Health Nurse

Role	Individual	Family	Community
Clinician			
Educator			
Advocate			
Manager			
Collaborator			
Leaders			
Researcher			

you can interview a public health nurse during your clinical experience and find examples of how the nurse performs activities in each of those roles. You will probably find that, while addressing a single issue with a client, the public health nurse serves in a variety of roles and at different levels.

Consider an example of the variety of roles and multilevel practice that the public health nurse assumes with respect to a 55-year-old female client who uses a wheelchair. The client has difficulty obtaining a gynecologic examination because of the lack of accessible examination tables at the local clinic; as a result, she has not had an examination for more than 20 years. Recognizing the need for a complete examination, the public health nurse arranges with the clinic to find appropriate alternatives that will aid the client in receiving the needed examination, possibly by ensuring that additional personnel are provided (Advocate Role–Individual Level).

Because this solution is temporary and less than optimal, the nurse contacts a number of clinics in neighboring communities and finds one that has appropriate equipment for people who have difficulty transferring to a standard examination table. Unfortunately, this clinic is 1 hour away. The nurse then contacts a number of other community/public health nurses and discovers that they also have a significant number of women clients with this problem who have not received a gynecologic examination in many years (Research Role–Community Level).

Through a coordinated effort with a local transportation company and the clinic, the nurse is able to arrange a twice-yearly gynecologic screening program for women in the community who require special accommodations (Advocate and Coordinator Roles–Community Level). Information sheets that discuss the need for annual gynecologic examinations and advertise the program are distributed to area public health nurses, employers, and health clinics (Educator Role–Community Level). Data collection on examinations provided over the next few years shows a 65% increase in the number of women with special needs who have received a gynecologic examination within the past year (Research Role–Community Level).

This is not an uncommon scenario in the practice of community/public health nursing. Often, the needs of an individual open the door to areas of concern for many in a community and provide a basis for intervention that can benefit a larger population.

Like nursing practice in general, the role of the public health nurse with respect to disabilities and chronic illness requires broad and holistic practice. The complexity of issues surrounding these conditions requires creativity, tenacity, honesty, and, most of all, knowledge. Public health nurses who are informed about the issues that affect the disabled and chronically ill at local, state, and national levels are prepared to offer assistance to their clients and to their communities. Knowledge of civil rights for these individuals is crucial in serving as advocates.

The issues facing individuals and families with disabilities require strong and sustained efforts to achieve results. Although successes at the individual level are laudable, the extent to which the health and wellbeing of those affected is improved must be the ultimate goal. Community/public health nursing is in a prime position to initiate and support efforts to improve the health status of those populations. We can either leave the issues to other professionals or use our expertise and long history of caring for those less fortunate to make major and lasting changes. It is up to us.

SUMMARY

The issues of disability and chronic illness are of growing importance in public health and to community/public health nursing, both nationally and internationally. Through the efforts of the WHO, the international community has been challenged to provide increased attention to health promotion and disease prevention. Even in less developed countries, behavioral patterns linked to excesses in consumption (overweight and tobacco/alcohol use) have an impact on the quality and quantity of healthy years of life. The health promotion and disease prevention needs of the disabled and chronically ill must be given the same emphasis as the needs of those who are not disabled or ill.

The aging of the U.S. population and the rise in lifestyle-related illnesses such as diabetes and obesity are often linked with increasing rates of disability. Prevention of disability and disease is emphasized in *Healthy People 2020*, which alerts Americans over the decades about the need to give serious attention to health-promoting and disease prevention activities. Healthy People has placed increasing focus on health promotion and disease prevention needs of those with disabilities and chronic illness. It is no longer acceptable that these individuals receive care solely for tertiary health needs. Research has shown that when health-promoting (lifestyle) issues are addressed with these clients, the rates of secondary conditions are reduced, including medical, social, emotional, mental, family, and community problems. Disabilities and chronic conditions are not universally debilitating, and the overall wellbeing and health of these individuals must be a priority.

Legislation is but one step toward equality for those affected by disabilities and chronic illnesses. The ADA secured many improvements in accessibility and specific legal protections for the disabled, but it is only the beginning. Discrimination can occur at many levels; some is hurtful and intentional, but most results from misunderstanding of the needs and desires of disabled persons and their families. This may even occur in relation to the provision of health care because of lack of education. Improvement can be found only with increased community education programs for professionals and the public that target the myths and misunderstandings about those with disabilities and chronic illnesses.

Public health nurses are in a prime position to advocate for the health needs of the disabled and chronically ill. With a long history of serving those who are most vulnerable, public health nurses can help make needed changes at the individual, family, and community levels. Although it is often easier to focus on the needs of the individual, those needs are most often shared by many others. Nurses have long recognized the need to collaborate with other professionals in reaching the goal of improved health care for their clients; this continues to be an important aspect of successful efforts on behalf of the disabled and the chronically ill. It will take the concerted efforts of many to implement the changes necessary to improve the lives of those most affected, their families, and the communities in which they live.

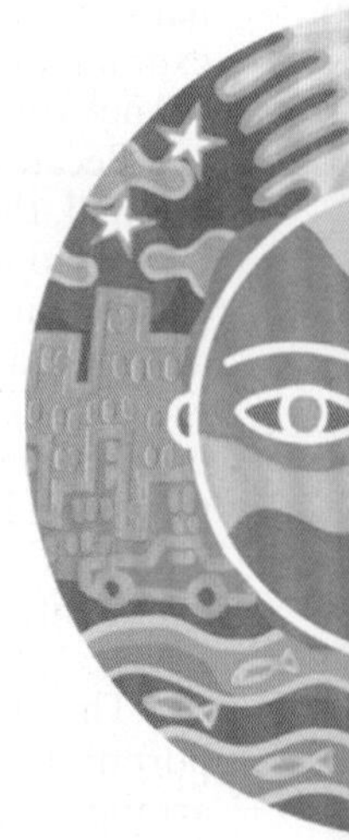

The next time you have difficulty opening a door that is unusually heavy or struggle to open the lid of a jar or feel that you were treated differently than someone else in the receipt of services, take a moment to think. Think about the challenges, struggles, and pain that face so many citizens. Consider the impact of universal design at improving your life or the life of a family member or friend. Although many argue against improving accessibility of city streets and sidewalks because of the expense, those same people may one day find that they, too, are faced with trying to master a curb that is just a bit too high.

ACTIVITIES TO PROMOTE **CRITICAL THINKING**

1. Arrange to interview an individual with a disability (e.g., hearing, vision, mobility) about the challenges that he has faced in interactions with nondisabled persons.
2. Visit some of the nongovernmental sites listed under Internet Resources and read some of the personal stories that are included.
3. Take an inventory of your house or apartment and make a list of modifications you would need to make if you were suddenly confined to a wheelchair. Would you even be able to stay in your current residence?
4. As part of your regular clinical assignment in community/public health nursing, look at those clients and families who are dealing with either a disability or chronic illness and assess how often you or other public health nurses have addressed health promotion activities (e.g., healthy eating, physical activity, leisure-time activities) with those clients.
5. Review your family history for chronic health conditions. Are you at risk? If so, what have you done to reduce your risk over the past 12 months?

REFERENCES

Adams, P. F., Martinez, M. E., Vickerie, J. L., & Kirzinger, W. K. (2011, December). Summary health statistics for the U.S. population: National Health Interview Survey, 2010. *Vital and Health Statistics*, Series 10, No. 251 [DHHS Pub. No. (PHS) 2012–1576]. Retrieved from www.cdc.gov/nchs/data/series/sr_10/sr10_251.pdf

American Council of the Blind. (2011). *Frequently asked questions*. Retrieved from http://www.acb.org/node/16

American Foundation for the Blind. (2012). *About Us: Leading the vision loss community*. Retrieved from http://www.afb.org/section.aspx?FolderID=1

Americans with Disabilities Act, U.S. Department of Justice (USDOJ). (2009). *The Americans with Disabilities Act of 1990, as amended: Section 12102: Definition of disability*. Retrieved from http://www.ada.gov/pubs/ada.htm

Anderson, W. L., Wiener, J. M., Findelstein, E. A., & Armour, B. S. (2011). Estimates of national health care expenditures associated with disability. *Journal of Disability Policy Studies, 21* (4), 230–240.

Cannuscio, C. C., Colditz, G. A., Rimm, E. B., Berkman, L. F., Jones, C. P., & Kawachi, I. (2004). Employment status, social ties, and caregivers mental health. *Social Science & Medicine, 58*, 1247–1256.

Cannuscio, C. C., Jones, C., Kawachi, I., Colditz, G. A., Berkman, L., & Rimm, E. (2002). Reverberations of family illness: A longitudinal assessment of informal caregiving and mental health status in the Nurses' Health Study. *American Journal of Public Health, 92*, 1305–1311.

Center for Universal Design. (2010). *About*. Retrieved from http://www.ncsu.edu/project/design-projects/udi/

Centers for Disease Control and Prevention. (2006). *Impact of the built environment on health*. Retrieved from http://www.cdc.gov/nceh/publications/factsheets/Impactof theBuiltEnvironmentonHealth.pdf

Centers for Disease Control and Prevention. (2007). *Chronic disease prevention*. Retrieved from http://www.cdc.gov/nccdphp/

Centers for Disease Control and Prevention. (2008). *Children's health and the built environment*. Retrieved from http://www.cdc.gov/healthyplaces/healthtopics/children.htm

Disabled American Veterans. (2012). *Building better lives for disabled American veterans and their families*. Retrieved from http://www.dav.org/

Egede, L. E., & Zheng, D. (2003). Racial/ethnic differences in adult vaccination among individuals with diabetes. *American Journal of Public Health, 93*, 324–329.

Fisher, H. R. (2001). The needs of parents with chronically sick children: A literature review. *Journal of Advanced Nursing, 36*, 600–607.

Fitzmaurice, C., Kanarek, N., & Fitzgerald, S. (2011). Primary prevention among working age USA adults with and without disabilities. *Disability and Rehabilitation, 33*(4), 343–351. doi: 10.3109/09638288.2010.490869

Grayson, G. (2003). *Talking with your hands, listening with your eyes. A complete photographic guide to American Sign Language*. Garden City Park, NY: Square One.

Guide Dogs for the Blind. (2011). *Our mission*. Retrieved from http://www.guidedogs.com/site/PageServer?pagename=about_overview_mission

Haviland, A. M., Elliot, M. N., Hambarsoomian, K., & Lurie, M. (2011). Immunization disparities by Hispanic ethnicity and language preference. *Archives of Internal Medicine, 171*(2), 158–165.

Mace, R. (n.d.). *About universal design: The Center for Universal Design*. Retrieved from http://design.ncsu.edu/cud/index.htm

McCain, J. (2012, May 25). *Press release: Bipartisan group of senators announce support for disability treaty*. Retrieved from http://www.mccain.senate.gov/public/index.cfm?FuseAction=PressOffice.PressReleases&ContentRecord_id=84b3c564-d49f-0cf5-7742-9ff158d8ef7e&Region_id=&Issue_id=

Morehead, P., & Morehead, A. (Eds.). (1995). *The new American Webster handy college dictionary*. New York, NY: Penguin Books.

National Association of the Deaf. (2012a). *About us*. Retrieved from http://www.nad.org/about-us

National Association of the Deaf. (2012b). *Vision 2020 strategic plan*. Retrieved from http://nad.org/about-us/vision-2020-strategic-plan

National Council on Disability. (2000). *Promises to keep: A decade of Federal enforcement of the Americans with Disabilities Act*. Retrieved from www.ncd.gov/publications/2000/June272000

National Council on Disability. (2005). *NCD and the Americans with Disabilities Act: 15 years of progress*. Retrieved from www.ncd.gov/publications/2005/06262005

National Council on Disability. (2007). *The impact of the Americans with Disabilities Act: Assessing the progress toward achieving the goals of the ADA*. Retrieved from www.ncd.gov/publications/2007/07262007

National Council on Disability. (2008). *Finding the gaps: A comparative analysis of disability laws in the United States to the United Nations Convention on the Rights of Persons with Disabilities (CRPD)*. Retrieved from www.ncd.gov/publications/2008/May122008

National Council on Disability. (2012). *About us*. Retrieved from http://www.ncd.gov/about

National Federation of the Blind. (2003). *What is Braille and what does it mean to the blind?* Retrieved from http://nfb.org/images/nfb/publications/fr/fr15/issue1/f150113.html

National Federation of the Blind. (2012). *What is the National Federation of the Blind?* Retrieved from http://nfb.org/who-we-are

National Organization on Disability. (2004). *Key findings: 2004 NOD/Harris Survey documents trends impacting 54 million Americans*. Retrieved from www.at508.com/040624_national_press_club.cfm

National Organization on Disability. (2010). *Kessler/NOD Surveys by Harris Interactive*. Retrieved from http://nod.org/what_we_do/research/surveys/kessler/

National Organization on Disability. (2012). *About us: Our mission and vision*. Retrieved from http://nod.org/about_us/our_mission_vision

Obama, B. (2009, July 24). *Remarks by the President on signing the U.N. Convention on the Rights of Persons with Disabilities Proclamation*. Retrieved from http://www.whitehouse.gov/the-press-office/remarks-president-rights-persons-with-disabilities-proclamation-signing

Obesity Society. (2010). *About us: Mission and vision*. Retrieved from http://www.obesity.org/about-us/mission-and-vision.htm

Parish, S. L., & Ellison-Martin, M. J. (2007). Health-care access of women Medicaid recipients: Evidence of disability-based disparities. *Journal of Disability Policy Studies, 18,* 109–116.

Smith, L. A., Wise, P. H., & Wampler, N. S. (2002). Knowledge of welfare reform program provisions among families of children with chronic conditions. *American Journal of Public Health, 92,* 228–230.

The body: The complete HIV/AIDS resource. (2012). Retrieved from http://www.thebody.com/

United Nations. (2007a). *Relationship between development and human rights*. Retrieved from http://www.un.org/esa/socdev/enable/convinfodevhr.htm.

United Nations. (2007b). *Secretariat for the Convention on the Rights of Persons with Disabilities*. Retrieved from http://www.un.org/disabilities/default.asp?id=17

United Nations. (2012). *Convention on the Rights of Persons with Disabilities*. Retrieved from http://www.un.org/disabilities/default.asp?id=150

U.S. Census Bureau. (2012). *American fact finder. Disability characteristics: 2010 American Community Survey 1-year estimates.* Retrieved from http://www.census.gov/acs/www/index.html

U.S. Department of Health and Human Services. (1991). *Healthy People 2000: National health promotion and disease prevention objectives* (S/N 017-001-00474-0). Washington, DC: U.S. Government Printing Office.

U.S. Department of Health and Human Services. (2000). *Healthy People 2010: Understanding and improving health*. Washington, DC: Government Printing Office. Retrieved from http://www.health.gov/healthypeople/ Document/

U.S. Department of Health and Human Services. (2005). *Midcourse review: Healthy People 2010*. Washington, DC: Government Printing Office. Retrieved from http://www.healthypeople.gov/data/midcourse/

U.S. Department of Health and Human Services, Administration for Children and Families. (2010). *Office of Family Assistance: Temporary Assistance for Needy Families Program*. Retrieved from http://www.acf.hhs.gov/opa/fact_sheets/tanf_factsheet.html

U.S. Department of Health and Human Services, Office for Civil Rights. (2006). *Delivering on the promise: OCR's compliance activities promote community integration*. Retrieved from http://www.hhs.gov/ocr/complianceactiv.html

U.S. Department of Health and Human Services. Office of Disease Prevention and Health Promotion. (2012a). *Healthy People 2020: About Healthy People*. Retrieved from http://www.healthypeople.gov/2020/about/default.aspx

U.S. Department of Health and Human Services, Office of Disease Prevention and Health Promotion. (2012b). *Healthy People 2020: Arthritis, osteoporosis, and chronic back conditions.* Washington, DC. Retrieved from http://www.healthypeople.gov/2020/topicsobjectives2020/overview.aspx?topicid=3

U.S. Department of Health and Human Services, Office of Disease Prevention and Health Promotion. (2012c). *Healthy people 2020: Disability and health*. Retrieved from http://www.healthypeople.gov/2020/topicsobjectives2020/overview.aspx?topicid=9

U.S. Department of Health and Human Services, Office of Disease Prevention and Health Promotion. (2012d). *Healthy people 2020: Disparities*. Retrieved from http://www.healthypeople.gov/2020/about/DisparitiesAbout.aspx

U.S. Department of Health and Human Services, Office of Disease Prevention and Health Promotion. (2012e). *Healthy People 2020: Chronic kidney disease*. Washington, DC. Retrieved from http://www.healthypeople.gov/2020/topicsobjectives2020/overview.aspx?topicid=6

U.S. Department of Health and Human Services, Office of Disease Prevention and Health Promotion. (2012f). *Healthy People 2020: Health-related quality of life and well-being.* Retrieved from http://www.healthypeople.gov/2020/about/QoLWBabout.aspx

U.S. Department of Health and Human Services, Office of Disease Prevention and Health Promotion. (2012g). *Healthy People 2020: Respiratory diseases*. Washington, DC. Retrieved from http://www.healthypeople.gov/2020/topicsobjectives2020/overview.aspx?topicid=36

U.S. Department of Health and Human Services, Office of Disease Prevention and Health Promotion, Secretary's Advisory Committee the National Health Promotion and Disease Prevention Objectives for 2020. (2009, April 20). *Eleventh meeting: Meeting minutes.* Retrieved from http://healthypeople.gov/2020/about/advisory/FACA11Minutes.aspx?page=1

U.S. Department of Housing and Urban Development. (2012). *Fair housing accessibility guidelines*. Retrieved from http://portal.hud.gov/hudportal/HUD?src=/program_offices/fair_housing_equal_opp/disabilities/fhefhag

U.S. Department of Justice. (2009). *A guide to disability rights laws.* Retrieved from http://www.ada.gov/cguide.htm

U.S. Mission to the United Nations. (2006). *Explanation of Position by Ambassador Richard T. Miller, U.S. Representative to the UN Economic and Social Council, on the Convention on the Rights of Persons with Disabilities, Agenda Item 67(b), in the General Assembly.* [USUN Press Release # 396(06)]. Retrieved from http://www.usunnewyork.usmission.gov/press_releases/20061213_396.html

Wei, W., Findley, P. A., & Sambamoorthi, U. (2006). Disability and receipt of clinical preventive services among women. *Women's Health Issues, 16,* 286–296.

Wong, M. G., & Heriot, S. A. (2007). Parents of children with cystic fibrosis: How they hope, cope and despair. *Child: Care, Health and Development*, *34,* 344–354.

Wood, P. R., Smith, L. A., Romero, D., Bradshaw, P., Wise, P. H., & Chavkin, W. (2002). Relationships between welfare status, health insurance status, and health and medical care among children with asthma. *American Journal of Public Health, 92,* 1446–1452.

World Health Organization. (1980). *International classification of impairments, disabilities, and handicaps.* Geneva, Switzerland: Author.

World Health Organization. (2001). *International classification of functioning, disability and health*. Geneva, Switzerland: Author.
World Health Organization. (2002). *The World Health Report 2002. Reducing Risks, promoting healthy life*. Geneva, Switzerland: Author.
World Health Organization. (2009). *Global health risks: Mortality and burden of disease attributable to major risks*. Retrieved from http://www.who.int/healthinfo/global_burden_disease/global_health_risks/en/index.html
World Health Organization. (2012a). *Disability and health: Fact sheet*. Retrieved from http://www.who.int/mediacentre/factsheets/fs352/en/index.html
World Health Organization. (2012b). *Obesity and overweight*. Retrieved from http://www.who.int/mediacentre/factsheets/fs311/en/
World Health Organization. (2012c). *Underweight in children*. Retrieved from http://www.who.int/gho/mdg/poverty_hunger/underweight_text/en/
World Health Organization and the World Bank. (2011). *World report on disability: Summary.* Retrieved from http://www.who.int/disabilities/world_report/2011/report/en/

CHAPTER

27

Behavioral Health in the Community

"Make your own recovery the first priority in your life."

—*Robin Norwood,* Author

"Part of being sane is being a little bit crazy."

—*Janet Long*

KEY TERMS

Addiction
Alcohol use disorders (AUD)
Community mental health
Community mental health centers
Community mental health nurse
Dependence
Mental health
Mental health care system
Mental illness
Relapse
Screening
Serious mental illness (SMI)
Serious and persistent mental illness (SPMI)
Substance use disorders (SUDs)
Tolerance

LEARNING OBJECTIVES

Upon mastery of this chapter, you should be able to:

- Discuss the incidence and prevalence of mental illness and substance use in the United States.
- Compare and contrast various theories on the etiology of substance use disorders (SUDs).
- Discuss the treatment approaches at the community level related to behavioral health.
- Describe community behavioral health resources.
- Identify the *Healthy People 2020* objectives for reducing substance use and addressing mental health needs.
- Discuss health-promoting interventions for community behavioral health.
- Describe the role of the community health nurse in the prevention of substance use and early identification and treatment of mental health disorders.

This chapter describes the role behavioral health plays in the overall health of a community and provides an overview of behavioral health prevention and treatment from the perspective of community health nursing practice with a focus on community-level interventions. A discussion is given regarding community health nursing practice in helping individuals, families, and communities to promote optimal mental health and responsible substance use and thereby decrease the prevalence and incidence of mental illness and substance use disorders (SUDs). See Display 27.1: Behavioral Health Terminology.

A NEW ERA IN MENTAL HEALTH

Entering this decade of global economic constraints, challenges in mental health nursing practice remain. Perseverance and resourcefulness are necessary to ensure quality care outcomes. The advances in research are incremental and facilitate best evidence-based practice models of mental health care. The science on brain structure functions and how learning occurs over time has impacted mental health services by expanding the possibilities of available therapies. Genetic factors continue to be an important health determinant. Populations evolve from birth through life stages, and they attend school, play, work, and age in diverse settings. Also known as social and physical determinants of health, these things impact a wide range of health, functioning, and quality of life outcomes. The physical and social determinants of health, in addition to neurophysiologic, neurochemical, and endocrine factors, are essential considerations in the care process. Community health nurse approaches require a multifaceted assessment that integrates biogenetic, physical, behavioral, and sociocultural knowledge.

The care setting is also complicated by natural uncertainties. There is the possibility of natural disasters such as earthquakes, hurricanes, or tsunamis. Environmental dangers such as nuclear plant meltdowns, terrorism, and political instability complicate health program planning. With end of the wars in Iraq and Afghanistan, returning military personnel will change the demands for resources at all fronts. The continued global economic instability and high levels of unemployment present challenges to family and community system's stability. Loss of jobs, the threat of losing one's home, rising food prices, and declining availability of publicly funded assistance bring uncertainty and stress. The full effects of these events are yet to be characterized and quantified. Going forward, community health organizational systems play crucial roles in meeting the complex population health needs with scant resources.

Several documents address the need for prevention and treatment of mental health disorders, such as *Healthy People 2020* (U.S. Department of Health and Human Services [USDHHS], 2012), *Mental Illness Surveillance Among Adults in the United States* (Centers for Disease Control and Prevention [CDC], 2011), and the classic *Report of the Surgeon General on Mental Health*, submitted by David Satcher (USDHHS, 1999). The health care goals addressed within *Healthy People 2020* (USDHHS, 2012) are relevant to community mental health nursing (see Table 27-1). Noted are improvements in mental health, including reduction of suicide rates in the general population, reduction of suicide attempts by adolescents, reduction in the number of homeless persons with severe mental illness, and increase in employment of persons with serious mental illness (SMI). Several objectives focusing on treatment expansion for the mentally ill include the following:

1. Reduction of relapse rates for persons with eating disorders
2. Increase in mental health screening and assessment in primary care settings
3. Increase in the numbers of children and adults with mental illness who receive treatment
4. Increase in treatment for persons with dual diagnosis (including substance abuse)
5. Increase in treatment for mentally ill persons in juvenile justice facilities and jails

The Report of the Surgeon General on Mental Health (USDHHS, 1999) was the first Surgeon General's report ever published on the topic of mental health and mental illness. The report concluded that effective treatments are available for most adults with an SMI who are age 18 and older and who currently, or at any time during the past year, have had a diagnosable mental, behavioral, or emotional disorder of sufficient duration to meet diagnostic criteria specified within DSM-IV, TR (Diagnostic and Statistical Manual for Mental Disorders, Text Revision) (American Psychiatric Association [APA], 2000; note that the new DSM-V is due for release 2013). The focus on the promotion of increased access to educational and employment opportunities for people with disabilities (both physical and psychiatric) was evident in President George W. Bush's New Freedom Initiative. The initiative also noted the need to increase access to assistive and universally designed technologies (The President's New Freedom Commission on Mental Health [TPNFCMH], 2003). This group identified three impediments to the provision of quality mental health care (2003):

1. Stigma that surrounds mental illnesses
2. Unfair treatment limitations and financial requirements placed on mental health benefits in private health insurance
3. Fragmented mental health service delivery system

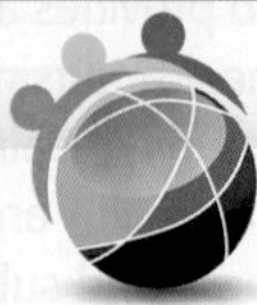

DISPLAY 27.1 BEHAVIORAL HEALTH TERMINOLOGY

- **Addiction:** A complex neurobiobehavioral disorder characterized by impaired control, compulsive use, dependency, and craving for the activity, substance, or food. Relapses are possible even after long periods of abstinence (Armstrong, Feigenbaum, Savage, & Vourakis, 2006).
- **Alcohol use disorders:** A continuum of disorders related to abuse of alcohol

  Levels of alcohol use (National Institute on Alcohol Abuse and Alcoholism [NIAAA], n.d. b):

  Moderate or Low-risk drinking: Low-level alcohol use that is not problematic (for men no more than 4 drinks/day and no more than 14 drinks/week; for women no more than 3 drinks/day and no more than 7 drinks/week)

  Heavey or At-Risk drinking: Pattern of alcohol consumption that increases the risk of harmful consequences for the user or others (more than the daily or weekly amounts listed above)

  Binge drinking: Alcohol consumption that results in consequences to physical and mental health (alcohol consumption within 2 hours that results in blood alcohol concentration of 0.08 g/dL–generally 4–5 drinks)
- **Community mental health nurse:** An individual whose practice is centered on the mental health needs of the populations served
- **Community mental health:** A field of practice that seeks to promote the mental health of the community by preventing mental illness and addressing the needs of the mentally ill
- **Community mental health centers (CMHCs):** Facilities that provide comprehensive, publicly funded services to the mentally ill population
- **Dependence:** An adaptive physiological state that includes craving, loss of control, and physical dependence characterized by withdrawal symptoms of shakiness, sweating, nausea, anxiety, and usually tolerance (NIAAA, n.d. a)
- **Mental health care system:** The collective programs designed for anyone with a mental illness. These programs may include treatments, services, or other types of supports, such as housing, employment, or disability benefits through government, private nonprofit, or private for-profit systems.
- **Mental health:** As defined in *Healthy People 2020*, mental health is "a state of successful mental functioning, resulting in productive activities, fulfilling relationships, and the ability to adapt to change and cope with adversity" (U.S. Department of Health and Human Services [USDHHS], 2012, para. 2)
- **Mental disorders:** "Health conditions that are characterized by alterations in thinking, mood, and/or behavior that are associated with distress and/or impaired functioning. Mental disorders contribute to a host of problems that may include disability, pain, or death" (USDHHS, 2012, para. 3).
- **Serious mental illness (SMI):** Mental illness that has compromised both the client's level of function and his or her quality of life is known as SMI **Serious and persistent mental illness (SPMI)** is the preferred term for SMI of a chronic nature. For example, schizophrenia is usually classified as an SPMI.
- **Substance use disorders:** The spectrum of disorders that include substance abuse and dependence and are attributed to problematic consumption or illicit use of alcohol, tobacco, illicit, and legal drugs (Armstrong et al., 2006)
  - *Alcoholism:* Also known as "alcohol dependence," a disease that includes four symptoms: craving, loss of control, physical dependence, and tolerance
- **Screening:** A mechanism used to evaluate the presence of substance use problems and to estimate the probability of a specific disorder. This may include evaluation of a client's blood alcohol level or other tools, such as questionnaires
- **Tolerance:** The need for significantly increased amounts of alcohol or drug to achieve intoxication or the desired effect or a markedly diminished effect with the continued use of the same amount of alcohol or drug (Armstrong et al., 2006)
- **Relapse:** Return to heavy alcohol, tobacco, or drug use after a period of abstinence or moderate use

Armstrong, M., Feigenbaum, J., Savage, C. L., & Vourakis, C. (Eds.). (2006). *Addictions nursing, core curriculum* (2nd ed.). Raleigh, NC: International Nurses Society on Addiction; NIAAA. (n.d. a). Alcohol use disorders. Retrieved from http://www.niaaa.nih.gov/alcohol-health/overview-alcohol-consumption/alcohol-use-disorders; NIAAA. (n.d. b). *Moderate and binge drinking*. Retrieved from http://www.niaaa.nih.gov/alcohol-health/overview-alcohol-consumption/moderate-binge-drinking; USDHHS. (2012). *Healthy People 2020: Mental health and mental disorders*, para. 2. Retrieved from http://www.healthypeople.gov/2020/topicsobjectives2020/overview.aspx?topicId=28

Table 27.1 ***Healthy People 2020*–Summary of Objectives for Mental Health and Mental Disorders (MHMD)**

Goal: Improve mental health through prevention and by ensuring access to appropriate, quality mental health services

Number	Objective
Mental Health Status Improvement	
MHMD-1	Reduce the suicide rate
MHMD-2	Reduce the suicide attempts by adolescents
MHMD-3	Reduce the proportion of adolescents who engage in disordered eating behaviors in an attempt to control their weight
MHMD-4	Reduce the proportion of persons who experience major depressive episode (MDE)
Treatment Expansion	
MHMD-5	Increase the proportion of primary care facilities that provide mental health treatment on-site or by paid referral
MHMD-6	Increase the proportion of children with mental health problems who receive treatment
MHMD-7	Increase the proportion of juvenile justice facilities that screen admissions for mental health problems
MHMD-8	Increase the proportion of persons with serious mental illness (SMI) who are employed
MHMD-9	Increase the proportion of adults with mental health disorders who receive treatment
MHMD-10	Increase the proportion of persons with co-occurring substance abuse and mental disorders who receive treatment for both disorders
MHMD-11	Increase depression screening by primary care providers
MHMD-12	Increase the proportion of homeless adults with mental health problems who receive mental health services

From Department of Health and Human Services (USDHHS). (2012b). *Healthy People 2020: Mental health & mental disorders objectives*. Retrieved from http://www.healthypeople.gov/2020/topicsobjectives2020/objectiveslist.aspx?topicId=28

Our past knowledge base relative to mental health service needs pales in the context of proposed public support cutbacks in the light of the U.S. budget deficit. We cautiously look toward the future with the realization that community health nurses in today's era of government belt-tightening will need to be creative and resourceful.

Incidence and Prevalence of Mental Disorders

Mental illness is a worldwide problem. In the *Global Burden of Disease Study*, mental illness, including suicide, accounts for more than 15% of all deaths (World Health Organization [WHO], 2007). Mental disorders are one of the strongest predictors for suicide; people with anxiety disorders and poor impulse control lead to more suicide attempts than other disorders (Nock et al., 2009). In 2004, one quarter of U.S. adults reported a mental illness in the previous year. Almost half of all Americans will develop a mental illness during their lifetime. In an examination of current national surveys, it was noted that around 16% of respondents had a diagnosis of depression sometime during their life and around 12% had some type of anxiety disorder. Those reporting bipolar disorder diagnoses or schizophrenia over their lifetime were 1.7% and 0.6%, respectively (CDC, 2011).

In a national survey, an estimated 7.5% of the adults 18 or older (16.5~16.4 million adults in 2007) reported at least 1 major depressive episode during the past year (Office of Applied Studies [OAS], 2009). More than 19 million Americans older than 18 years of age will suffer from a depressive illness at some time during their lives, and many of these individuals will be incapacitated for significant lengths of time by their illness. Over two thirds of suicides in the United States each year are caused by major depression. The age-adjusted suicide rate per 100,000 was 15.2% for men and 3.6% for women, with almost half of these having a diagnosed mental disorder (CDC, 2006). CDC notes the overall incidence of suicides as 10.95 per 100,000 (CDC, 2007). At 12%, it is the third leading cause of death among 15- to 24-year-olds; for adults 75–84 years, it accounteds for 16.3% of deaths in 2007 (CDC, 2011). For all ages, suicide is the 11th leading cause of death. Male suicides represent 79% of all suicides in the United States. However, women attempt suicide two to three times as often as men. Suicide rates are generally higher in adolescents and the elderly; however, a 16% increase in suicide rates for adults between ages 40 and 64 was found by researchers examining data from 1999 to 2005 (Hu, Wilcox, Wissow, & Baker, 2008). An interesting study by Luo, Florences, Quispe-Agnoli, Ouyang, and Crosby (2011) found an association between overall suicide rates and economic downturns; rates increased during bad economic times and dropped during more stable times.

The poor, undereducated, and the unemployed typically experience higher rates of mental illness than the general population. The poor, disproportionately representative of racial and ethnic minorities, are even more vulnerable due to the lack of access to care and the questionable quality of the care that is received (Cunningham, 2009). Also, the mentally ill are at greater risk of premature death from cardiovascular disease and other physical problems, often due to behaviors related to their mental illness. Death from cardiovascular disease has been found to be two to three times higher among those with mental illness than for the general population (Morden, Mistler, Weeks, & Bartels, 2009). A large portion of the mentally ill population, many of which are homeless, remain untreated in the community (Larimer et al., 2009). The homeless are more likely to experience behavioral health issues, such as SUDs and mental illness. One third of sheltered homeless persons have a chronic substance abuse issue, and one quarter report a severe mental illness (U.S. Department of Housing and Urban Development [USDHUD], 2010). In a survey of 2 million US adults who had a minimum of 1 homeless episode in the previous year, 46% of them reported having a mental health problem (with or without substance abuse) within that time period (TPNFCMH, 2003). **Alcohol use disorders (AUDs)** among the homeless population are reported to range between 58% and 84%, and SUDs from 27% to 57%. One survey of over 110 homeless adults found one third of them had comorbidity for both problems (Savage & Gillespie, 2008). The majority of hospital admissions among the homeless are for treatment of substance use or mental illness. They also often seek care through emergency departments (EDs) for infectious diseases, asthma, trauma, and hypertension (Savage & Gillespie, 2008).

Age influences the patterns of mental illness in the community (Copeland et al., 2009). Each year, about one of every five children and adolescents has the signs and symptoms of a mental health disorder described and defined by the APA in the fourth edition of DSM-IV, TR. The most commonly occurring conditions among American children ages 9 to 17 years are anxiety disorders, disruptive disorders, mood disorders, and SUDs. In a national study of adolescents 13 to 18 years, anxiety disorders (31.4%), behavior disorders (19.1%), mood disorders (14.3%), and SUDs (11.4%) were most common (Merikangas et al., 2010; Robert, Roberts, & Chan, 2009; Willcutt et al., 2008). Attention deficit hyperactivity disorder (ADHD) affects approximately 3% to 7% of U.S. schoolchildren, with lifetime prevalence for 13- to 18-year-olds estimated at 9%. Boys are two to three times more likely to be affected than girls (Kaufmann, Goldberg-Stern, & Shuper, 2009; Merikangas et al., 2010). ADHD continues on into adulthood for many individuals; lifetime prevalence is estimated at 8.1% of U.S. adults (NIMH, n.d. a). Autism, a developmental disorder often termed *autism spectrum disorder* or (ASD), is four times more common in boys than in girls. These pervasive developmental disorders (PDD), including autism and Asperger's disorder, as well as childhood disintegrative disorder, are projected to occur in 60 to 70 of every 10,000 children, but one large-scale study found the rate for non-Hispanic White children to be 1 in 101 eight-year-old children (Fombonne, 2009; NIMH, n.d. b).

For American adults, the most prevalent mental disorders are anxiety disorders (28.8% lifetime prevalence), followed by mood disorders (20.8%), especially major depression (16.5%) and bipolar disorder (3.9%). Anxiety, depression, and schizophrenia present special problems for this age group—anxiety and depression because they contribute to such high rates of suicide, and schizophrenia because it is so persistently disabling (NIMH, n.d.c). For the growing number of older adults, there is increased incidence of Alzheimer's disease (8% to 15% of adults age 65 and over), major depression (8% to 20%), anxiety (11.4%), and other disabling mental disorders.

Gender differences also arise in the prevalence of certain mental disorders. Anxiety disorders and mood disorders, including major depression, occur twice as frequently in women as in men (Beesdo et al., 2010). Women of color, women on welfare, poor women, and uneducated women are more likely to experience depression than women in the general population. The three main types of eating disorders (anorexia, bulimia nervosa, and binge eating) also affect more women than men (Hudson, Hiripi, Pope, & Kessler, 2007).

Mental illness, as well as substance abuse, greatly affects families; approximately 1 in 5 families are touched by mental illness. People may exhibit signs of mental illness gradually over time, or may seem to suddenly act in an erratic manner. This can be very frightening to family members, who may feel that the person is being reckless or selfish, rather than recognize the signs and symptoms of bipolar disorder or schizophrenia. To make matters worse, often the person needing treatment doesn't feel that there is "anything wrong" with them and may refuse medication or only take it sporadically. Families frequently must deal with the criminal justice system, in addition to health care and mental health treatment personnel. And, parents commonly feel that they are to blame for their child's illness, or that others believe that to be the case. When a loved one is hospitalized for a stroke, friends call and bring in food; but when it is an SMI, there are often no "casseroles" or sympathetic calls (Kornblum, 2008). The National Alliance on Mental Illness (NAMI) offers the Family-to-Family Education Program to assist caregivers of family members with an SMI (2011a). The 12-week class offers current information about common mental illnesses, common medications, current brain research, and support for problem solving, dealing with crises, and how to find local resources and support. Trained family members lead the program and provide empathy and personal knowledge about dealing with mental illness from a caregiver's perspective.

Cost of Mental Health Disorders

Adding to the heavy toll that mental illness exacts is the financial burden it creates. Costs associated with treatment of mental disorders—poor productivity, lost work time, and disability payments—are astronomical. The direct and indirect costs of mental illness and addictive disorders in the United States are >$273 billion annually. Furthermore, the cost to society when treatment is

DISPLAY 27.2 EFFORTS TO IMPROVE HEALTH BENEFITS COVERAGE AND TRANSFORM BEHAVIORAL HEALTH CARE

The existing, often intimidating maze of behavioral health services needs transformation into a more coordinated, consumer-centered, recovery-oriented system. Historically, Americans have assumed responsibility locally and regionally for working together to meet challenges and support their neighbors and communities. However, this has left many people without access to necessary services.

Mental illness is the only category of illness for which state and local governments operate distinct treatment systems, making comprehensive care unavailable in the larger health care system. With health care reform, this system will change.

Health care in America is at a pivotal point, and reform is taking place; this includes changes in coverage and access for behavioral health. Health care reform brings *essential health benefits (EHB)* in 2014 that includes at least the following:

- Ambulatory patient services
- Emergency services
- Hospitalization
- Maternity and newborn care
- Mental health and substance use disorder services, including behavioral health treatment
- Prescription drugs
- Rehabilitative and habilitative services and devices
- Laboratory services
- Preventive and wellness services and chronic disease management
- Pediatric services, including oral and vision care (Farley, 2011)

Behavioral health is included in this package of EHB, but states can choose their own benchmark plans, so coverage may vary somewhat. The 2008 Mental Health Parity and Addictions Equity Act will apply to both group and individual health plans, however, so compliance with this parity legislation will provide some assurance of minimum benefits.

From Farley, R. (2011). *Essential health benefits: What does the new HHS guidance mean for behavioral health?* National Council for Community Behavioral Healthcare. Retrieved from http://mentalhealthcarereform.org/essential-health-benefits-what-does-the-new-hhs-guidance-mean-for-behavioral-health/

not provided for these illnesses is three times the cost of direct treatment (National Alliance on Mental Illness [NAMI], 2007). As with other health issues, individuals with mental illness also are among the uninsured; 22% of adults with mental illness or SUDs have no health insurance, and 30% of those with co-occurring conditions (i.e., both mental illness and SUDs) lack coverage (National Council for Community Behavioral Health, 2012). Certainly, these facts have policy implications and suggest the need for greater preventive and mental health–promoting efforts. Display 27.2 notes governmental efforts to improve behavioral health benefits coverage as part of health care reform.

Treatment of Mental Health Disorders

Far from the history of institutionalization and inhumane treatment often noted during the first half of the 20th century (Frank & Glied, 2006), mental health treatment today is most often accomplished through the use of medications and outpatient services, such as mental health counseling (52.6%; 40.5% in 2008). Rarely, inpatient services are utilized; only 7.5% of persons getting services in 2008 received this type of care (NIMH, n.d.c). Employee assistance programs (EAPs) can be found in most large companies or agencies. Mental health services are available in many outpatient settings (e.g., community health centers, school-based clinics, college health centers) and have demonstrated effective results (Walter et al., 2011). Mental health services are often provided to the homeless, as well as residents of battered women's shelters and adolescent group homes. Group therapy is commonplace, and some feel that this type of contact is helpful not only in promoting mental health but also in breaking through the stigma of mental illness (Corrigan & Wassel, 2008). Support groups for single parents, divorced individuals, those with eating disorders, and other issues are found in most communities. These may be led by a mental health professional.

Types of therapies include psychotherapy (either individual or group) and behavioral, cognitive, or cognitive–behavioral approaches are most often used. Psychoanalysis, often with a psychiatrist, is characterized by free association and delving into the unconscious mind. Family therapy is considered helpful, especially when SUDs are also involved. Cognitive approaches involve helping clients change their negative thought patterns, and behavioral therapies use positive and negative reinforcement to change problem behaviors. Cognitive–behavioral therapy is a combination of the two. These types of therapies are of shorter duration than psychoanalysis, which can take place over several years (Doebbeling, 2007).

Geographic differences exist in prevalence and treatment of mental health disorders. One national survey found state-level estimates of parent-reported depression or anxiety among children ranged from 4.8% in Georgia to 14.4% in Vermont. Behavioral problems were lower in California (3.2%) compared to Louisiana (9.2%). However, differences in treatments had more to do with factors related to health and socioeconomic status (SES) than state of residence (Ghandour, Kogan, Blumberg, Jones, & Perrin, 2012). Like physical health care, the effectiveness of mental health care is also affected by perceived discrimination and English proficiency, highlighting the need for more bilingual services in mental health (Spencer et al., 2010). Minorities may have overall better mental health than the White population, but disparities in both physical and mental health care exist; a workforce that is more ethnically diverse is needed for more effective mental health treatment (McGuire & Miranda, 2008). However, the results of a national study found that 18% of counties had shortages of mental health professionals (e.g., nonprescribing psychologists, licensed clinical social workers) and 96% reported a shortage in prescribing mental health professionals (e.g., psychiatrists, mental health nurse practitioners). Shortages were most pronounced in rural and low-income areas (Thomas, Ellis, Konrad, Holzer, & Morrissey, 2009). Common mental health professionals include psychiatrists (M.D.), psychologists (master's or Ph.D.), psychiatric or clinical social workers (master's or Ph.D., often with specialized training in marriage and family issues), and advanced practice psychiatric nurses or mental health nurse practitioners (master's degree or higher) (Doebbeling, 2007).

States most often regulate licensing of mental health professionals and programs. Cities, counties, and states often levy taxes in order to pay for mental health care. Some seriously disabled individuals may receive assistance through federal Social Security Disability Insurance (SSDI), and the Veteran's Administration provides mental health services to the nation's veterans.

SUBSTANCE USE AND THE COMMUNITY HEALTH NURSE

Substances used in the United States that have the potential for dependence include alcohol, tobacco, and other drugs both legal and illegal. Substance use occurs across a continuum that includes abstinence, low-risk use, risky/hazardous use, harmful use, and dependence (Martin, Chung, & Langenbucher, 2008) (Fig. 27-1). From a community perspective, all substance use other than abstinence or low-risk use poses a threat to the overall health of the community as well as individuals and families. Reductions in substance use (including tobacco) are 2 of the 44 focus areas in *Healthy People 2020* (USDHHS, 2012b). (See Table 27-2 for a list of substance abuse objectives.) The community health nurse plays a vital role in developing successful prevention and treatment programs related to substance use in a community. These prevention programs are not limited to prevention of dependence but rather include the entire spectrum of use. The community health nurse focuses on the target population. For instance, *Monitoring the Future* is a yearly survey of drug and alcohol use among 8th, 9th, and 12th graders. Existing data such as these tell us the magnitude of the problem. Given a defined target geographic area, local health departments may have county-specific prevalence rates. The *Healthy People 2020* objectives set target benchmarks that can be used during the planning and program development process.

The community health nurse must begin with a basic understanding of the differences between substances of abuse. Various substances pose different threats to the health of a community. This understanding can help the community health nurse select an effective community intervention best suited to meet the particular needs of the target population. For example, the development of a tobacco smoking prevention program in adolescents is quite different from a program to reduce drug-related intentional injuries.

Table 27-3 lists some of the substances that have addictive potential. This helps public health nurses understand the issues related to a specific substance of abuse (e.g., tobacco vs. alcohol or vs. cocaine) and conceptualize the desired outcomes related to a treatment or prevention program. Examples of different overarching goals include increasing access to treatment for SUDs, reducing alcohol-related motor vehicle crashes, reducing illicit drug–related crime, or reducing secondary smoke exposure in public areas.

The key to successful community health interventions is to know initially what the overarching goal of the intervention is. The target benchmarks proposed for each category may be gleaned from Table 27-2, showing substance abuse objectives.

Trends of Substance Use

Healthy People 2020 (USDHHS, 2012a) objectives focus on tobacco, alcohol, and illicit drug use education. There are three steps in this process: (1) identifying trends, (2) differentiating legal versus illegal use, and (3) consequences of use. Community health nurses utilize the trends (as noted in Fig. 27-4) related to substance use across different populations and communities. This information is useful to the community health nurse when developing a prevention program. If the target population is young adults, prevention of heavy episodic

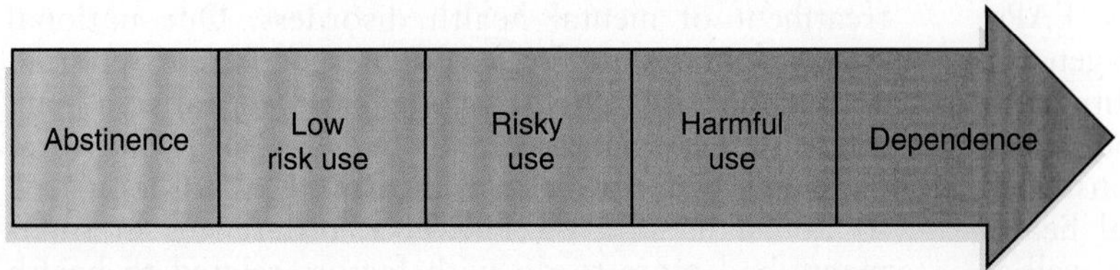

FIGURE 27-1. Continuum of substance use.

PERSPECTIVES
VOICES FROM THE COMMUNITY

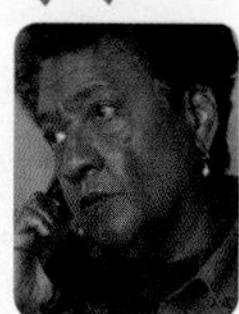

I have been a nurse for a long time. Even though I don't work in behavioral health nursing, per se, I have had many experiences throughout the years related to both mental health and substances. When I was a student in the 1970s, I remember doing a rotation in a locked mental health facility and feeling that it was just a "revolving door." Now there are so many medications available that can quickly address symptoms, and prevention and early intervention are the focus. Then, the same patients came back over and over again, and all staff could offer them was counseling, a few medications (mostly Thorazine), and electroconvulsive therapy (ECT). They had a "rubber room"—a padded room where they would place patients who were dangerous to themselves or others. It seemed so futile to me, at the time.

Years later, a close friend I had known since childhood was hospitalized for a suicide attempt. She had always been charming and outgoing, often talking excitedly about things and using her hands to punctuate her thoughts. She seemed to have boundless energy and there was nothing she couldn't do. I was shocked to learn that she had been suffering from a terrible depression and had tried to overdose on prescription medications. She was subsequently diagnosed with bipolar disorder and began a long road to recovery with many medication changes and years of hard work in therapy with a very kind, patient counselor. Her marriage didn't survive and her children suffered during her so-called crazy years, but she made it through to the other side and learned a lot from her experience. I learned a lot from that "personal" experience with mental illness.

I have also worked with many public health clients who have battled various types of mental illness (often postpartum depression, or eating disorders with new moms or teens), as well as bipolar and schizophrenia with drug users and homeless. I have seen firsthand the problem of alcohol and substance use disorders (not only alcohol and illicit drugs, but misuse of prescription medications or **huffing** *glue or aerosols). I have struggled to help them and their families find resources, or advocated on their behalf with landlords, the school system, or the sheriff as their illnesses led to problems in all areas of their lives.*

While I am not a mental health nurse practitioner, I feel that I have an understanding of the problems in the community, with families, and with individual clients. I realize the responsibility I have to reinforce with my students the human side of mental illness or substance abuse and to break through the fears they have to help them look at the client in a different way. Brain chemistry is a powerful thing—people cannot just "will" themselves to be more cheerful/less depressed, or to stop craving heroin (or chocolate, for that matter). Seeing each client as an individual and joining with them to address their issues is the best approach—that's community health nursing!

Lori, Community Health Nursing Professor

(binge) drinking may be a top concern because of the high prevalence of this type of behavior in this population (Toumbourou, Stocwell, Neighbors, Marlatt, & Rehm, 2007). If the target population is the homeless adult, then the community health nurse will need to know about chronic alcohol, cocaine, and heroin use in the local homeless community because of the high prevalence of SUDs in this population (Savage & Gillespie, 2008). Cultural and ethnic differences in alcohol and SUDs are noted, for instance, in American Indian populations, along with increased rates of fetal alcohol syndrome (FAS) (see Chapter 5). SUDs are also common in prison and jail populations, with drug offenders constituting 20% of state prison inmates (Peterselia, 2011). (See Chapter 30 for more on corrections nursing.)

Difference Between Legal and Illegal Substance Use

The second step for the community health nurse is to appreciate the difference between legal and illegal substance use. Alcohol and tobacco are legal substances in the United States, but other drugs such as marijuana, heroin, and cocaine are illegal. Use of illegal drugs affects the community not only in relation to the morbidity associated with drug use in individuals but also in relation to problems of drug trafficking and other illegal activities engaged in by the user and the seller. Thus, cultural, environmental, and pharmacological differences related to a specific substance influence the type of community health interventions needed as well as the planned outcomes.

Consequences of Substance Use

The third step is to understand the consequences of substance use that affect a community as a whole. These consequences include violence, as well as motor vehicle crashes and injuries, especially related to alcohol and illicit drug use (Cherpitel, 2007). These risks are present in all age groups. For example, alcohol use, as well as use of benzodiazepines, increases the risk for fall injury in the elderly (Bartlett, Abrahamowicz, Grad, Sylvestrre, & Tambly, 2009).

Another serious consequence to the community is the increased risk of morbidity and mortality related to substance use. This affects the community by decreasing the healthy workforce and increasing the cost of providing health care. For example, although protective at low levels of use, alcohol in excess of recommended levels increases the risk of developing serious health consequences, such as cancer or heart disease (Chen, Hankinson, Colditz, &

Table 27.2 ***Healthy People 2020*–Summary of Objectives for Substance Abuse**

Goal: Reduce substance abuse to protect the health, safety, and quality of life for all, especially children

Number	Objective
Policy and Prevention	
SA-1	Reduce the proportion of adolescents who report that they rode, during the previous 30 d, with a driver who had been drinking alcohol
SA-2	Increase the proportion of adolescents never using substances
SA-3	Increase the proportion of adolescents who disapprove of substance abuse
SA-4	Increase the proportion of adolescents who perceive great risk associated with substance abuse
SA-5	(Developmental) Increase the number of drug, driving while impaired (DWI), and other specialty courts in the United States
SA-6	Increase the number of states with mandatory ignition interlock laws for first and repeat impaired driving offenders in the United States
Screening and Treatment	
SA-7	Increase the number of admissions to substance abuse treatment for injection drug use
SA-8	Increase the proportion of persons who need alcohol and/or illicit drug treatment and received specialty treatment for abuse or dependence in the past year
SA-9	(Developmental) Increase the proportion persons who are referred for follow-up care for alcohol problems, drug problems after diagnosis, or treatment for one of these conditions in a hospital emergency department
SA-10	Increase the number of Level I and Level II trauma centers and primary care settings that implement evidence-based alcohol screening and brief intervention (SBI)
Epidemiology and Surveillance	
SA-11	Reduce cirrhosis deaths
SA-12	Reduce drug-induced deaths
SA-13	Reduce past-month use of illicit substances
SA-14	Reduce the proportion of persons engaging in binge drinking of alcoholic beverages
SA-15	Reduce the proportion of adults who drank excessively in the previous 30 d
SA-16	Reduce average annual alcohol consumption
SA-17	Decrease the rate of alcohol-impaired driving (0.08 + blood alcohol content [BAC]) fatalities
SA-18	Reduce steroid use among adolescents
SA-19	Reduce the past-year nonmedical use of prescription drugs
SA-20	Decrease the number of deaths attributable to alcohol
SA-21	Reduce the proportion of adolescents who use inhalants

From Department of Health and Human Services (USDHHS). (2012b). *Healthy People 2020: Substance abuse objectives*. Retrieved from http://www.healthypeople.gov/2020/topicsobjectives2020/objectiveslist.aspx?topicId=40

Willett, 2011; Room & Rehm, 2011). There is no safe level of alcohol consumption during pregnancy; women who drink alcohol during pregnancy are at increased risk for having a baby with fetal alcohol spectrum disorder (FASD) or FAS (NIAAA, 2006a). Members of the community with FASD and FAS require lifelong support, resulting in increased costs related to education, health care, and social services (Lupton, 2011).

Family consequences of alcohol and substance abuse can be very tragic. Alcohol and drug use has a genetic component, and family dynamics can be negatively influenced throughout many generations. All family members may be impacted, but children and adolescents are often the most affected by alcohol and drug abuse. The National Council on Alcoholism and Drug Dependence (n.d., para 7) reminds us "alcoholism and drug abuse is a family disease and affects everyone close to the person." All family members need education and support, and professionally directed interventions are sometimes necessary in order to break through the denial surrounding alcohol and substance abuse. Alcoholics Anonymous, Al-Anon (for family members), or the corresponding Narcotics Anonymous and Nar-Anon, may be helpful for both those in treatment and family members trying to break free from codependence and enabling behaviors. Recovery from abuse and addiction is a family affair, and PHNs can work with family members to provide information and support.

Substance Use and the Environment

The impact of substance use varies based on the substance. Tobacco is an environmental pollutant. Exposure to secondary tobacco smoke increases the risk for health

Table 27.3 Drugs Involved in Substance Abuse

Drug Type	Facts	Possible Signs of Use/Abuse	Possible Health Risks of Use/Abuse
Cannabis			
Hashish (hash, herb, kif) Hashish oil (hash oil, honey) Marijuana (grass, weed, dope, ganja, reefer, pot, Acapulco gold, Thai sticks)	Cannabis is made from the hemp plant, *Cannabis sativa*. When smoked or ingested, produces mild euphoria, relaxation, and intense sensory perception. Users may develop tolerance and physical dependence. Sinsemilla is a highly potent form of marijuana.	Relaxation and euphoria Altered perceptions of time and space Hallucinations or anxiety attacks with sinsemilla use	Damage to heart and lungs Damage to brain nerve cells Memory disorders Temporary loss of fertility Psychological dependence
Depressants			
Alcohol (brew, juice, liquor) Barbiturates (downers, barbs) Benzodiazepines (Valium, Librium, tranquilizers) Chloral hydrate (knockout, Mickey Finn) Glutethimide (Doriden) Methaqualone (Quaalude, Ludes) Other depressants (Equanil, Miltown, Noludar, Placidyl, Valmid)	Depressants depress or slow down the central nervous system by relaxing muscles, calming nerves, and producing sleep. Alcohol is a depressant. Depressants are composed of sedative–hypnotic and tranquilizer drugs. Depressants are addictive. Users of depressants develop a tolerance to the drugs, meaning larger doses must be taken each time to produce the same effect.	Relaxation and drowsiness; lack of concentration; disorientation; loss of inhibitions; lack of coordination; dilated pupils; slurred speech; weak and rapid pulse; distorted vision; low blood pressure; shallow breathing; staggering; clammy skin; fever, sweating; stomach cramps; hallucinations, tremors; and delirium	Liver damage; convulsions; addiction with severe withdrawal symptoms; coma; death due to overdose. For pregnant women: the newborn may be dependent and experience withdrawal or suffer from birth defects and behavioral problems
Hallucinogens			
Lysergic acid diethylamide (LSD) Phencyclidine (PCP, angel dust) Mescaline and peyote (Mesc, buttons, cactus) Psilocybin (mushrooms) Amphetamine variants (MDMA/Ecstasy, MDA/love drug, TMA, DOM, DOB, PMA, STP, 2.5-DMA) PCP analogues (PCE, PCPy, TCP) Other hallucinogens (bufotenine, ibogaine, DMT, DET)	Hallucinogens are psychedelic, mind-altering drugs that affect a person's perception, feelings, thinking, self-awareness, and emotions. A "bad trip" may result in the user's experiencing panic, confusion, paranoia, anxiety, unpleasant sensory images, feelings of helplessness, and loss of control. A "flash back" is a reoccurrence of the original drug experience without taking the drug again.	Dilated pupils, increased body temperature, heart rate, and blood pressure; sweating; loss of appetite; sleeplessness; dry mouth; tremors; hallucinations; disorientation; confusion; paranoia; violence; euphoria; anxiety; and panic	Agitation; extreme hyperactivity; psychosis; convulsions; mental or emotional problems; death
Inhalants			
Amyl nitrate (poppers, snappers) Butyl nitrate (rush, bolt, bullet) Chlorohydrocarbons (aerosol sprays, cleaning fluids) Hydrocarbons (solvents, airplane glue, gasoline, paint thinner) Nitrous oxide (laughing gas, whippets)	Inhalants are substances that are breathed or inhaled through the nose. Inhalants are depressants and depress or slow down the body's functions. Inhalants are normally not thought of as drugs because they are often common household or industrial products. However, inhalants are often the most dangerous drugs per dose.	Euphoria and lightheadedness; excitability; loss of appetite; forgetfulness; weight loss; sneezing; coughing; nausea and vomiting; lack of coordination; bad breath; red eyes; sores on nose and mouth; delayed reflexes; decreased blood pressure; flushing (skin appears to be reddish); headache; dizziness; and violence	Depression; damage to the nervous system and body tissues; damage to liver and brain; heart failure; respiratory arrest; suffocation; unconsciousness; seizures; heart failure; sudden death from sniffing

(Continued)

Table 27.3 Drugs Involved in Substance Abuse *(Continued)*

Narcotics			
Codeine (school boy) Heroin (H, harry, junk, brown sugar, smack) Meperidine (doctors) Methadone (dollies, methadose) Morphine (morpho, Miss Emma) Opium (Dover's powder) Other narcotics (Percodan, Talwin, Lomotil, Darvon, Numorphan, Percocet, Tylox, Tussionex, fentanyl)	Narcotics are composed of opiates and synthetic drugs. Opiates are derived from the seed pod of the Asian poppy. Synthetic drugs called opioids are chemically developed to produce the effects of opiates. Initially, narcotics stimulate the higher centers of the brain, but then slow down the activity of the central nervous system. Narcotics relieve pain and induce sleep. Narcotics, such as heroin, are often diluted with other substances (i.e., water, sugar) and injected. Other narcotics are taken orally or inhaled. Narcotics are extremely addictive. Users of narcotics develop a tolerance to the drugs, meaning larger doses must be taken each time to produce the same effect.	Euphoria; restlessness and lack of motivation; drowsiness; lethargy; decreased pulse rate; constricted pupils; flushing (skin appears to be reddish); constipation; nausea and vomiting; needle marks on extremities; skin abscess at injection sites; shallow breathing; watery eyes; and itching	Pulmonary edema; respiratory arrest; convulsions; addiction; coma; death due to overdose. For users who share or use unsterile needles to inject narcotics: tetanus, hepatitis, HIV/AIDS. For pregnant women: premature births; stillbirth, and acute infections among newborns
Steroids			
Anabolic–androgenic (roids, juice, D-ball)	Steroids may contribute to increases in body weight and muscular strength. The acceleration of physical development is what makes steroids appealing to athletes and young adults. Anabolic–androgenic steroids are chemically related to the male sex hormone testosterone. Anabolic means to build up the muscles and other tissues of the body. Steroids are injected directly into the muscle or taken orally.	Sudden increase in muscle and weight; increase in aggression and combativeness; violence ("roid rage"); hallucinations; jaundice; purple or red spots on body, inside mouth, or nose; swelling of feet or lower legs (edema); tremors; and bad breath. For women: breast reduction, enlarged clitoris, facial hair and baldness, deepened voice. For men: enlarged nipples and breasts, testicle reduction, enlarged prostate, baldness	Acne; high blood pressure; liver and kidney damage; heart disease; increased risk of injury to ligaments and tendons; bowel and urinary problems; gallstones and kidney stones; liver cancer. For men: impotence and sterility. For women; menstrual problems. For users who share or use unsterile needles to inject steroids: hepatitis, tetanus, AIDS
Stimulants			
Amphetamines (uppers, pep pills) Cocaine (coke, flake, snow) Crack (rock) Methamphetamines (ice, crank, crystal) Methylphenidate (Ritalin) Phenmetrazine (Preludin, Preludes) Other stimulants (Adipex, Cylert, Didrex, Lonamin, Melfiat, Plegine, Sanorex, Tenuate, Tepanil, Prelu-2)	Stimulants stimulate the central nervous system, increasing alertness and activity. Users of stimulants develop a tolerance, meaning larger doses must be taken to get the same effect. Stimulants are psychologically addictive.	Increased alertness; excessive activity; agitation; euphoria; excitability; increased pulse rate, blood pressure, and body temperature; insomnia; loss of appetite; sweating; dry mouth and lips; bad breath; disorientation; apathy; hallucinations; irritability; and nervousness	Headaches; depression; malnutrition; hypertension; psychosis; cardiac arrest; damage to the brain and lungs; convulsions; coma; death

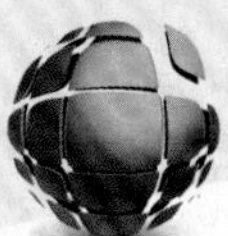

EVIDENCE-BASED PRACTICE

Substance Use Prevention with Adolescents: What Works and What Does Not Work?

As nurses, when we move from an individual-based approach to a community-based approach we need to evaluate evidence from a population perspective. A major step in preventing Substance use disorders (SUDs) is to focus on substance use in adolescents. An article by Toumbourou et al. (2007) provides us with a well conducted systematic review of the literature related to the effectiveness of interventions aimed at reducing harm associated with adolescent substance use. A systematic review should be comprehensive and unbiased; it should use a strict scientific design to select and assess research articles. This article is a good example of a rigorous review, and provides a broad overview of what works and what does not.

The authors examined evidence related to public health policies, harm reduction, prevention, screening, brief intervention, and treatment related to adolescents. They reported that public health policies related to substance use do work, such as taxation and ignition interlocks. They also reported that prevention interventions were more successful when the intervention was maintained over several years and used more than one strategy. They stated that screening and brief intervention holds promise as an effective means of reducing harmful alcohol or tobacco use and there is growing evidence that it may work with other drugs. They concluded that harm reduction strategies were also effective in reducing harmful substance use.

A meta-analytic review of 16 studies utilizing 26 outcome measures was accomplished to determine the best interventions used to reduce adolescent alcohol abuse (Tripodi, Bender, Litschge, & Vaughn, 2010). Researchers found that treatments had a medium effect on reducing use of alcohol, with larger effect sizes found for individual treatments (e.g., cognitive-behavioral therapy, motivational interviewing, brief interventions) when compared with family-based treatments (e.g., multidimensional family therapy). The behavior-oriented treatments showed greater promise in reaching long-term effects.

Sources: Toumbourou, J. W., Stocwell, T., Neighbors, C., Marlatt, G. A., & Rehm, J. (2007). Interventions to reduce harm associated with adolescent substance use. *Lancet, 369*, 1391–1401; Tripodi, S., Bender, K., Litschge, C., & Vaughn, M. (2010). Interventions for reducing adolescent alcohol abuse: A meta-analytic review. *Archives of Pediatric and Adolescent Medicine, 164*(1), 85–91.

issues related to tobacco use including cancer and respiratory complications. Alcohol interacts with the environment in relation to point of sale. Sociologic studies have demonstrated an increase in motor vehicle crashes related to the location of bars and liquor stores, especially drive-through stores (Gruenewald & Johnson, 2010).

The health care objectives addressed within *Healthy People 2020* (USDHHS, 2012b) relevant to substance use are listed under Focus Area 26 (Table 27-2). The goal is to "reduce substance abuse to protect the health, safety, and quality of life for all, especially children." Among the 25 objectives listed are reducing the consequences of use, reducing actual use, reducing risk factors associated with harmful use, increasing access to treatment, and supporting policy initiatives.

Prevalence of Substance Use and Substance Use Disorders

This section discusses the prevalence of substance use and SUDs. Different levels of use across populations are described based on the quantity, frequency, duration, and pattern of the use, as well as levels related to the prevalence of dependence. To obtain prevalence data related to substance use, surveys are conducted nationwide on a regular basis.

The community health nurse can easily get updates on the results of surveys by accessing the Web sites of both the NIDA and NIAAA. Prevalence data are reported in different ways, and it is important to distinguish between the types of reports. Some reports focus on consumption rates based on gender, ethnic/racial group, or age group. Others focus on the prevalence of SUDs.

Alcohol

Over 50% of the adult population report current alcohol use. Alcohol is an integral part of the American culture, with 80% of adults reporting use of alcohol over their lifetime. In the United States and other countries, people use alcohol in religious ceremonies, celebrations, and sporting events and as the beverage of choice at a meal. Unlike other drugs of abuse, alcohol can be consumed in moderation without resulting in alcohol dependence. To help distinguish risky and harmful use from responsible use of alcohol, NIAAA has published recommended drinking limits. For the general male adult population, the recommended drinking limits are fewer than five standard drinks daily or 14 weekly. For the general female adult population, the recommended drinking limits are fewer than four standard drinks daily or eight weekly, and for people age 65 and older, recommended drinking limits are no more than one standard drink daily or seven standard drinks weekly. The NIAAA recommends that pregnant women and women who may become pregnant abstain from alcohol (NIAAA, 2007).

12 oz. of beer or cooler	8-9 oz. of malt liquor	5 oz. of table wine	3-4 oz. of fortified wine	2-3 oz. of cordial, liqueur, or aperitif	1.5 oz. of brandy	1.5 oz. of spirits
	8.5 oz. shown in a 12-oz. glass that, if full, would have about about 1.5 standard drinks of malt liquor		(such as sherry or port) 3.5 oz. shown	2.5 oz. shown	(a single jigger)	(a single jigger at 80-proof gin, vodka, whisky, etc.) Shown straight and in a highball glass with ice to show level before adding mixer
12 oz.	8.5 oz.	5 oz.	3.5 oz.	2.5 oz.	1.5 oz.	1.5 oz.

NOTE: People buy many of these drinks in containers that hold multiple standard drinks. For example, malt liquor is often sold in 16-22, or 40 oz. containers that contain between two and five standard drinks, and table wine is typically sold in 25 oz. (750 ml) bottles that hold five standard drinks.

FIGURE 27-2. Standard drink. Adapted from NIAAA (2007).

A standard drink contains about 14 g of alcohol (0.6 fluid ounces or 1.2 tablespoons), which is equivalent to one 12-oz. bottle of beer or wine cooler; 8 to 9 oz. of malt liquor; one 5-oz. glass of table wine; 3 to 4 oz. of fortified wine; 2 to 3 oz. of cordial, liqueur, or aperitif; 1.5 oz. of brandy; or 1.5 oz. of 80-proof distilled spirits (Fig. 27-2). Heavy use is defined as drinking more than the recommended limits per drinking day, at least five different days in a month. Episodic heavy drinking (binge drinking) is defined as drinking above the recommended limits per drinking occasion at least once in the past month (NIAAA, 2007).

Trends in alcohol use in the United States differ across subsets of the population. Young adults (age 18–25) have the highest incidence of problem drinking, with binge drinking reaching a peak between ages 21 and 25 (Bernstein et al., 2010). A 2011 survey of U.S. adolescents found 5-year trends for alcohol use significantly decreased from earlier studies; binge drinking (five or more drinks in a row during the past 2 weeks) decreased for 8th, 10th, and 12th graders (NIDA, 2011). Based on recently published information, about 14% of those who use alcohol meet the criteria for alcohol dependence at some time during their lifetime (Beirut et al., 2010). In the most recent overall national survey, the highest percentage for alcohol abuse was in the 18- to 29-year age group (6.95%), and the lowest (1.21%) was in those over age 65 (Grant et al., 2004). Figure 27-3 depicts this age range of peak consumption.

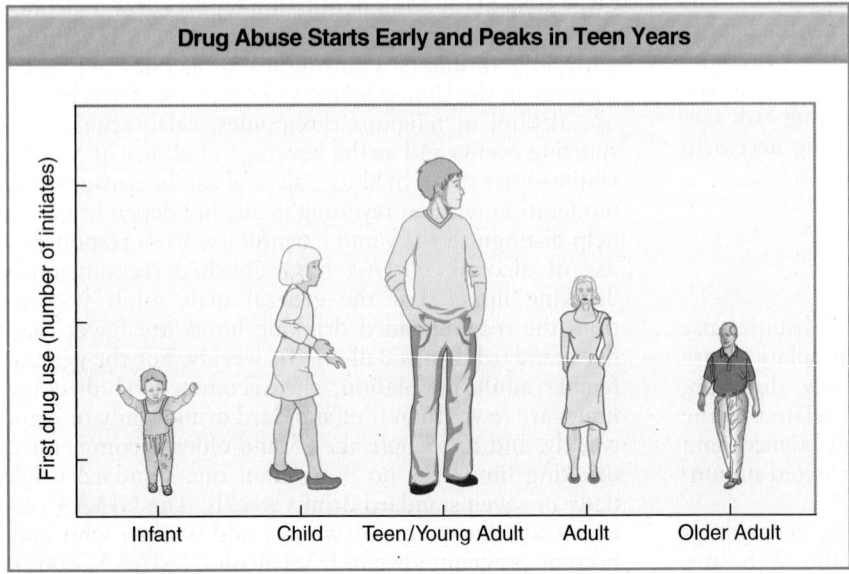

FIGURE 27-3. Prevalence of drug abuse across the lifespan. (Adapted from Grant, B. F., Dawson, D. A., Stinson, F. S., Chou, S. P., Dufour, M. C., & Pickering, R. P. (2004). The 12-month prevalence and trends in DSM-IV alcohol abuse and dependence: United States, 1991–1992 and 2001–2002. *Drug Alcohol Dependence, 74*(3), 223–234.)

Although the reported prevalence of AUDs in the elderly is low, the prevalence of AUDs and alcohol-related consequences in the elderly may increase over the next few decades due to a cohort effect. A national epidemiological survey found that, over their lifetime, 74% of adults over age 65 have used alcohol (Moore et al., 2009). Over the previous 12 months, 45% reported using alcohol. Lifetime prevalence of AUD was found to be 16.1% (Lin et al., 2011). Those over age 65 take more medications, on average, than younger populations. Alcohol consumption may increase risks of accidental death.

One population with a high prevalence of AUDs is the homeless. This high prevalence in a population most likely to experience problems with access to treatment can result in increased use of EDs and hospital admissions as well as increased alcohol-related morbidity (Ku, Scott, Kertes, & Pitts, 2010).

Tobacco

In 2008, a national survey found that 28.4% of Americans over the age of 12 (almost 71 million people) had used a tobacco product at least one time in the previous month. For 12- to 17-year-olds, the percentage was 11.4%. Almost one fourth of the population is estimated to be current cigarette smokers, with fewer people smoking cigars or using smokeless tobacco (chew) or tobacco pipes (National Institute on Drug Abuse [NIDA], 2010). Tobacco use is the primary cause of one in every five deaths in this country and is the most prevalent addictive disorder. It is related to 33% of all cancers and 90% of cases of lung cancer. Smokers have been reported to die, on average, 14 years earlier than nonsmokers. Encouragingly, there has been an overall decline in tobacco use over the past decade, but this decline is not consistent across age groups and genders. Current rates of smoking for 8th to 12th grade students hit a low point in 2009, from the record high levels of the 1990s (NIDA, 2010). The high prevalence of tobacco use among youth is a gloal concern. Also, there is no decline in tobacco use among those with mental illness. Persons with a mental illness have reported twice the rate of cigarette smoking than the general population (NIDA, 2009b).

Secondhand smoke is a significant health concern, causing serious illnesses and death. Annually, about 126 million individuals are regularly exposed to this health hazard at home or at work, and about 50,000 nonsmokers die from diseases related to this exposure. There is about a 25% to 30% increased risk of developing heart disease and 20% to 30% increased risk of lung cancer for nonsmokers exposed to secondhand smoke (NIDA, 2010). (See Table 27-4 for tobacco-related objectives.)

Table 27.4 ***Healthy People 2020*–Summary of Objectives for Tobacco (Selected)**

Goal: Reduce illness, disability, and death related to tobacco use and secondhand smoke exposure

Number	Objective
Tobacco Use	
TU-1	Reduce tobacco use by adults
TU-2	Reduce tobacco use by adolescents
TU-3	Reduce the initiation of tobacco use among children, adolescents, and young adults
TU-4	Increase the smoking cessation attempts by adult smokers
TU-5	Increase recent smoking cessation success by adult smokers
TU-6	Increase smoking cessation during pregnancy
TU-7	Increase smoking cessation attempts by adolescent smokers
Health Systems Changes	
TU-8	Increase the comprehensive Medicaid insurance coverage of evidence-based treatment for nicotine dependency in states and the District of Columbia
TU-9	Increase tobacco screening in health care settings
TU-10	Increase tobacco cessation counseling in health care settings
Social and Environmental Changes	
TU-11	Reduce the proportion of nonsmokers exposed to secondhand smoke.
TU-14	Increase the proportion of smoke-free homes.
TU-17	Increase the Federal and State tax on tobacco products.
MHMD-11	Increase depression screening by primary care providers.
MHMD-12	Increase the proportion of homeless adults with mental health problems who receive mental health services.

From USDHHS. (2012a). *Healthy People 2020: Mental health & mental disorders objectives*. Retrieved from http://www.healthypeople.gov/2020/topicsobjectives2020/objectiveslist.aspx?topicId=28; Department of Health and Human Services (USDHHS). (2012b). *Healthy People 2020: Tobacco objectives*. Retrieved from http://www.healthypeople.gov/2020/topicsobjectives2020/objectiveslist.aspx?topicId=41

Other Drugs

The overall national statistics related to illicit drug use are encouraging. In a survey of students in the 8th, 10th, and 12th grades, reported use of any illicit drug in the past month was 8.5%, 19.2%, and 25.2%, respectively. This represents little change from the previous year but is higher than the dip in use reported in 2007 (Johnston, O'Malley, Bachman, & Schulenberg, 2012). However, illicit drug use continues in the United States especially among those aged 18 to 25 (see Fig. 27-4).

Marijuana

Marijuana is the most frequently reported illicit drug. The annual prevalence rate for marijuana (cannabis) use in 2009 was 11.3%; this compares with a worldwide prevalence rate of 2.8% to 4.5%. Past month prevalence for those aged 12 and older increased to 6.6% from 6.1% the previous year (United Nations Office on Drugs & Crime [UNODC], 2010). Daily use for 8th, 10th, and 12th graders rose steadily from 2005 levels, with an attendant decline in perceived risk of use (Johnston et al., 2011). Among older groups, aged 50 to 59, the rate of current illicit drug use (including marijuana) increased to 6.2% from 2.7% in 2002 (UNODC, 2010). An explanation for the increase in use by older Americans may be a possible cohort effect among baby boomers; the public debate about marijuana legalization may be a factor in increased rates for adolescents. A recent Gallup poll found that a record 50% of Americans were in favor of legalizing marijuana; this is up markedly from 12% in favor of legalization in 1969 (Newport, 2011).

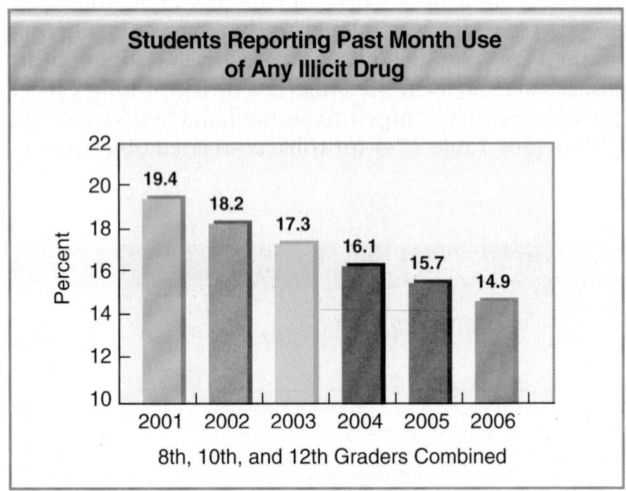

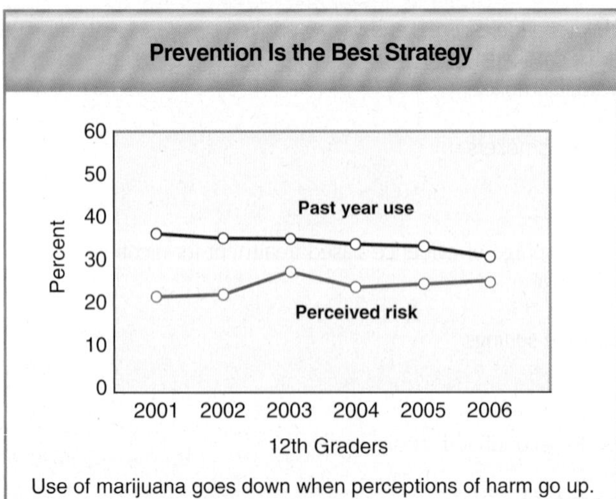

FIGURE 27-4. Trends in illicit drug use in youth. (Adapted from Johnston, L. D., O'Malley, P., Bachman, J., & Schulenberg, J. (2012). *Marijuana use continues to rise among U.S. teens, while alcohol use hits historic lows.* Retrieved from http://monitoringthefuture.org/pressreleases/11drugpr_complete.pdf)

Despite the belief that marijuana use has no serious harmful effects, increasing numbers of marijuana users are entering treatment programs, and these are generally unemployed adolescent or young adult males. More than half of them had begun using marijuana by age 14, with 90% starting by age 18. Over 90% have 12 or fewer years of formal schooling, and only 19.2% are employed full time. Most have never been married (80.5%). The majority of these clients were given a DSM diagnosis of marijuana dependence (41%) or abuse (28.8%). In addition to their problems with marijuana, 23.2% also had a psychiatric problem (UNODC, 2010). Heavy marijuana use in adolescence may lead to drug/property crime and arrests (but not violent crimes) in adulthood (Green, Doherty, Stuart, & Ensminger, 2010). Health effects associated with marijuana use include respiratory system problems (e.g., chronic cough, bronchitis, emphysema), respiratory system cancers, and cardiovascular system problems (e.g., triggering myocardial infarctions [MIs]). It has also been associated with immune system problems leading to increased vulnerability to infections (Han, Gfroerer, & Colliver, 2010).

Cocaine

Cocaine is a powerful addictive stimulant that directly affects the brain. In 2008, approximately 5.3 million Americans used cocaine in the previous year; this is about half the number of users found in 1982. The annual prevalence of cocaine use among 15- to 64-year-olds was 2.8% in 2008, but 3.4% among 12th grade students. The average 2009 price of a gram of cocaine (price adjusted for purity) was around $174 (UNODC, 2010). Use of cocaine dropped for 8th and 10th graders in 2011, but remained steady for 12th graders (Johnston et al., 2011).

The United States uses a public health surveillance system, the Drug Abuse Warning Network (DAWN), to monitor drug-related ED visits and determine the impact of drug use and associated conditions. Approximately 182 ED visits per 100,000 in 2006 were related to cocaine use; this represents about 31% of all drug-related ED visits that year. Cocaine use can have gastrointestinal, cardiovascular, and neurological effects and can lead to immune suppressive effects (Han et al., 2010). Arrhythmias, hypertension, and acute MI are possible acute cardiac complications, but cocaine toxicity can also lead to noncardiac conditions such as aggression, agitation, seizures, hyperthermia, and intracerebral infarctions (Wood & Dargan, 2010).

Opiates/Heroin

Worldwide, an estimated 15 million people use opiates (UNODC, 2010). Heroin is a very potent, addictive product of the opium poppy. Heroin use in the United States has remained fairly stable over the past decade (between 0.2% and 0.58%), but use of painkillers (often opiate derivatives or synthetic opioids) has been steadily rising to 4.8% in 2008; this is more than twice the rate for cocaine use. Admissions for drug treatment have been consistently higher for opioids than heroin over the past decade (UNODC, 2010). It was estimated that 6.2 million people age 12 and older had used a prescription medication, like oxycodone or hydrocodone, in the previous month, and deaths from opioid analgesic poisoning increased threefold from 4,000 to 13,800 deaths between 1999 and 2006 (UNODC, 2010). Use of Vicodin by 8th, 10th, and 12th grade students in 2011 was 2.1%, 5.9%, and 8.1%, respectively; this represents a drop over previous highs (Johnston et al., 2011). Lifetime use of heroin in American youth is estimated at 2%, and 20% of high school students reported having ever taken a drug such as Vicodin or Adderall without a physician's prescription (CDC, 2010).

Over 145,000 ED visits (21% of all illicit drug–related visits by males) were related to heroin use in males between 2004 and 2009 (Substance Abuse and Mental Health Services Administration [SAMHSA], 2011b). Injected drugs, like heroin, lead to the spread of HIV/AIDS, hepatitis B and C, as well as liver and kidney disease and increased risk of stroke or MI (Han et al., 2010). Because of the variability in purity of street heroin, a recreational dose can become lethal. Death rates for dependent heroin users are 6 to 20 times higher than for the general population (UNODC, 2010).

Methamphetamine, Ecstasy (MDMA), and PCP

There are numerous other drugs of abuse. Examples include methamphetamine (meth), MDMA (methylenedioxymethamphetamine or Ecstasy), phencyclidine (PCP), and inhalants. Methamphetamine use is spreading geographically especially into nontraditional drug use areas, such as the suburban and rural Midwest, with an increase in "mom and pop" labs. Methamphetamines comprised 8.8% of all ED visits for males with illicit drugs use between 2004 and 2008; other amphetamines were 2.8% (SAMHSA, 2011b). Worldwide, the prevalence for amphetamine-type substances in 2008 ranged between rates of 0.3% and 1.2%. Annual prevalence rates between 2001 and 2008 were estimated at 0.3% for methamphetamine and 1.1% for other stimulants among U.S. individuals 12 years and older. Purity levels of methamphetamine have risen to 69% in late 2009, while cost dropped to about $127 per gram (UNODC, 2010). Cessation of meth use can lead to depression (63%), headaches (39%), hallucinations (30%), chest pains (23%), paranoia (23%), and hyperthermia, fatigue, or aggression (Dobkin & Nicosia, 2009; Mooney, Glasner-Edwards, Rawson, & Ling, 2009). Along with the adverse health effects, including dental caries/excessive tooth wear of "meth mouth," meth often leads to violent behaviors and has far-reaching social costs (e.g., crime, child abuse/neglect, environmental effects) (Hamamoto, & Rhodus 2009).

MDMA/Ecstasy has spread outside the club scene with an increase in ED visits related to MDMA. About 14% of adults reported the use of MDMA in the previous year, and 24% of these respondents had a previous history of use. Co-occurrence of MDMA use with alcohol (41%), marijuana (30%), cocaine (10%), and painkillers (8%) or tranquilizers (3%) was also reported in a national drug use survey. Seven out of ten recent users experienced an SUD in the previous year (Wu et al., 2009). Adolescent MDMA users are at an increased risk for hallucinogen dependence and other SUDs (Wu, Ringwalt, Weiss, & Blazer, 2009).

The use of PCP (phencyclidine or angel dust), a white crystalline power popularly in use during the late 1980s and early 1990s, has reemerged. This dissociative drug, first introduced as an IV anesthetic, induces feelings of disengagement and distorts sounds and sights for users. Side effects can include delusions, disordered thinking, hallucinations, extreme anxiety, and other schizophrenia-like symptoms. In 2009, over 122,000 people aged 12 and older had used PCP at least one time, and in 2010, 1% of 12th graders had abused this drug at least once in the previous year (NIDA, 2009a). Other hallucinogens, like peyote (from a cactus plant), psilocybin (from certain mushrooms), and lysergic acid diethylamide (LSD), also have unpredictable effects. Long-term use of these drugs may lead to memory loss, depression, flashbacks, and addictive behavior (NIDA, 2009a).

Prescription Drugs

Abuse of prescription drugs occurs across all age groups, and there has been a rise in prescription drug abuse among Americans over the last several years; an estimated 2.4 million people in the past year used these drugs for nonmedical purposes. Over 50% were females; one third of them were between 12 and 17 years of age (NIDA, 2011). Of 18- to 25-year-olds, 5.9% of them reported abuse within the past month. Prescription drugs for managing pain, especially, can be misused. As mentioned earlier, these may include oxycodone (OxyContin), a medication designed to alleviate pain related to cancer; hydrocodone (Vicodin); and meperidine (Demerol). Stimulant drugs such as methylphenidate (Ritalin) are also misused. Although not quantified and fully characterized, sharing prescription drugs such as benzodiazepines (Xanax, Klonopin, or Valium) or hypnotics (Ambien or Restoril) with others is ill advised. This complicates the problem of drug abuse further. High school students often abuse over-the-counter (OTC) drugs (e.g., cold/cough remedies, sleep aids). They are also known to raid family medicine cabinets.

THEORETICAL FRAMEWORKS

Effective community- and population-based interventions begin with the application of specific frameworks that help the planners identify why and how the intervention will work. Two theoretical frameworks used in community/public health science are *process theory* and *effect theory*. They are both part of the Model of Program Theory and are used to plan, deliver, and evaluate the program (Issel, 2009). In relation to behavioral health, process theory helps the community health nurse identify the resources and structure needed to develop, implement, and evaluate the program. Effect theory provides the rationale for why the intervention will work.

Process Theory: Component of Program Theory

Three components comprise process theory: (1) an organizational plan that includes information on personnel and resources to be used (e.g., fiscal, information technology, supplies), (2) a service utilization plan that specifies how the program will reach its targeted client population (e.g., social marketing, screening procedures, logistics of availability/access), and (3) specifications of their outputs (e.g., expected outcomes). These things continually develop throughout the process and each affects the other (Issel, 2009).

Effect Theory: Component of Program Theory

The challenge for the community health nurse in developing interventions related to behavioral health is the fact that both mental health and substance use have a strong behavioral component. Effect theory is a useful framework for behavioral health. There are four components to the theory: determinant theory, intervention theory, impact theory, and outcome theory (Issel, 2009). Determinant theory relates to what contributes to the health problem. This is an essential component since an intervention usually focuses on one or more determinants of the health problem, either by reducing risk or providing protection against the risk. Intervention theory relates to what is actually being done (see From the Case Files).

From the Case Files

Smoking Cessation Program for Mothers in a Rural County

You have been working in the public health department well-child clinic in a rural Appalachian county and noticed that more than one-third of the mothers you are seeing are smokers and that their babies seem to be smaller than the babies of moms who do not smoke. When you mention smoking to individual mothers, they tell you they want to stop, but just are not able to. You are interested in putting together a smoking cessation program. You decide to use Issel's (2009) effect theory as a framework for building your intervention and convincing the county to fund the program. What data do you need before you begin to look at interventions (see Strategy 1 below)? What data can you get using existing databases, and what data will you need to collect yourself? Once you have reviewed the data, you decide that you want to include smoking cessation as part of well-baby visits for all mothers who are current smokers. What do you need to do before you put together the program (see Strategy 2 below)? After you have gathered all this information, what final piece is needed before you present your proposal to your public health department (see Strategy 3 below)? If you are able to implement the program what immediate impact do you expect to have and what long-term outcomes are you hoping for?

Strategies

1. Preliminary data needed:
   a. Low-birth-weight rates compared to state and national rates. (Available vital statistics public health data.)
   b. Low-birth-weight rates for smokers versus nonsmokers in your county, compared with the state and the nation. (Protected vital statistics public health data that will need approval from the state for you to access and analyze.)
   c. Comparison of asthma rates in children in your county with smoke-free homes versus homes with a parent smoking. (Available survey data using prior studies, but may not be current. Will most likely need to conduct a survey at the county level. Check with state public health department for state level data.)
   d. County tobacco use rates based on gender and age, and trends among adolescent girls in your county schools compared to state and national rates. (Available public health survey data at state and national levels. May need to conduct a survey at the county level.)
2. A review of the evidence related to smoking-cessation interventions with women of childbearing age. Were any of the studies conducted with Appalachian women? Will you need to make some adjustments to interventions that work based on culture? Are there possible economic constraints for this population in relation to pharmacologic interventions? Are the time frames reasonable in your setting?
3. You need to do an analysis of the cost to implement the program, complete a cost–benefit projection, have clear program goals and objectives, and formulate a plan to evaluate the effectiveness of the program.

The desired health impact refers to the immediate impact expected from the program. For example, if the health problem is heavy episodic (binge) alcohol consumption among college students, a logical approach may be to institute an alcohol-screening program. For such a program, the immediate *impact* for the program may be that 25% of students are screened and 75% of those who require a brief intervention (BI) and/or a referral for further assessment receive those interventions. However, the desired *outcome* of the program is an overall reduction in heavy episodic alcohol consumption on campus over a specified time period—for instance, the next 2 years. Remember that not all desired impact is related to change. The goal may be to stabilize, prevent, or maintain a health state or problem. Having a clear understanding of what a behavioral program can actually accomplish and what long-term goal it hopes to achieve prior to implementing the program will provide a clearer picture of how to proceed with the program.

When using effect theory to design a prevention program for behavioral health, a good place to start is to identify the specific health problem and then the desired health problem impact and health problem outcome. As the program is developed, the community health nurse starts by identifying the antecedent factors that led to behavioral health problems. This provides a clear rationale for why the intervention should provide the desired impact.

Public Health Prevention Theory and Behavioral Health

Three public health models of prevention provide the nurse with a guide to decide what level of prevention is the focus of the program, the type of intervention to use, and the target population. The CDC (1992) presented two complementary prevention models: the primary, secondary, and tertiary prevention model based on the natural history of disease and the behavioral, clinical, and environmental model based on how the prevention technology is delivered (CDC, 1992; Savage, 2006).

Primary prevention is conducted when no disease is present in the target population, the primary goal being prevention of disease development. Secondary prevention is conducted when the disease is subclinical with no symptoms or early symptoms present, the goal being early identification and treatment. Tertiary prevention is conducted when disease is present with symptoms, the goal being to prevent consequences of the disease, such as disability or death.

Behavioral prevention includes a broad array of strategies aimed at changing lifestyles (e.g., exercise, smoking cessation, balanced nutrition). It is a complex, sequential process targeted at individuals or groups. The goal of the intervention is to change behaviors that put the person at risk for developing the disease or to prevent consequences of the disease. Clinical prevention is based on the medical model for preventive services. It relies on one-to-one, provider-to-patient interaction and occurs within the traditional health care delivery system. Environmental prevention relies on a societal commitment for the implementation of the interventions and aims to alter the environment by reducing risk (e.g., community-wide decrease in availability of the substance, underage drinking law enforcement).

Another model used in the behavioral health field for developing prevention programs is the model used by the Institute of Medicine (IOM) based on Gordon's classic model: Classification of Disease Prevention (1987). This model helps to frame the focus of the intervention, relying on three levels of prevention: universal, selected, and indicated. Universal prevention strategies address the entire population (national, local community, school, neighborhood), with messages and programs aimed, for example, at preventing or delaying the abuse of alcohol or drugs. Selective prevention strategies target subsets of the total population that are deemed to be at risk for alcohol abuse by virtue of their membership in a particular population segment. Indicated prevention strategies are designed to prevent the onset of abuse in individuals who do not meet DSM-IV, TR criteria for addiction, but who are showing early danger signs, such as falling grades and consumption of alcohol and other gateway drugs. Other theories focus on problem behaviors and tailor interventions around that concept (Jessor, 2008).

One example of the application of this model is a description of different interventions aimed at prevention of FAS. Universal prevention strategies would address the entire population of women of childbearing age (national, local community, school, neighborhood), with messages and programs aimed at preventing the use of alcohol if pregnancy is a possibility. Selective prevention strategies would target subsets of women of childbearing age who are deemed to be at risk for alcohol use by virtue of their membership in a particular population segment. Indicated prevention strategies would be designed to prevent the use of alcohol in pregnant women who had screened positive for alcohol use during pregnancy or already had a child diagnosed with FAS or FASD.

DETERMINANTS OF BEHAVIORAL HEALTH

What determines a person as mentally healthy or mentally ill, or as a casual substance user or a serious substance abuser, is complex. There are numerous factors to consider: genetics, environment, and ethno-cultural-spiritual contexts. The individual developmental process of evolving, becoming, and maturing across the life continuum coupled with biophysiological adaptation are complex interacting variables in pinpointing determinants of mental health.

Determinants of Mental Health

Characterizing mental health versus mental illness is difficult because human beings evolve over the years with varied developmental tasks to achieve at each life stage while confronting day-to-day stressors associated with one's role functions. Complicating the issue is the frame of reference used in each society. Cultural beliefs differ regarding what one's behavior should or should not be and the level of tolerance for certain actions. There are expectations, standards, or legal parameters that put one's actions or behavior in a particular context that suggests health or illness. David Satcher, the former surgeon general, defined mental health as:

> The successful performance of mental functions, resulting in productive activities, fulfilling relationships with other people, and the ability to adapt to change and to cope with adversity; from early childhood until late life, mental health is the springboard of thinking and communication skills, learning, emotional growth, resilience, and self-esteem. (USDHHS, 1999)

The process of adaptation can be a source of stress. Several factors influence each individual's perception of stress and subsequent response. Lazarus and Folkman (1984) classically defined stress as the person's appraisal of the environment as "taxing" or endangering well-being. This implies that an event's significance is an individual personal experience. Certain elements are involved in this process: genetic factors, such as physical and psychological characteristics; learned patterns of coping or adaptation reinforced over time; and prevailing circumstances in each person's life. Correspondingly, the responses evoked may reflect adaptive or maladaptive functioning as evidenced by thoughts, feelings, and behaviors that are age-appropriate and congruent with sociocultural mores or standards. Take for instance "*resilience*."

Resilience is a dynamic process whereby individuals exhibit positive behavioral adaptation when they encounter significant life stress, adversity, trauma, tragedy, or threats. This an important human factor in coping with loss and traumatic life events. It is essential that individual coping mechanisms enable the person to function appropriately at home, work, and in various social settings. At times, the situation experienced may be perceived as overwhelming without adequate family or social support systems, thus creating a fertile ground for alcohol or drug dependency as a way of dysfunctional coping (Bottrell & Armstrong, 2012; Larimer et al., 2009).

Determinants of Substance Use Disorders

Determining the etiology of SUDs has challenged researchers for decades. The debate has centered on *nature versus nurture*, that is, how much is related to genetics (nature) and how much to the environment (nurture) (Dick, Riley, & Kendler, 2010). With the mapping of the human genome, hope has increased that the genes related to SUDs could be identified. Genetics has a major role in the development of alcohol dependence, which is thought to be a multigenomic disorder influenced by the environment (gene–environment interaction) (Hardie, 2007). Both alcohol and drug dependence share common genetic risk factors, and heritability may be in the range of 50% to 60% (Dick et al., 2010). In addition to genetic heritability, both personal and environmental factors are involved comparably in the etiology and course of SUDs (Dick et al., 2010).

Researchers have made significant progress in understanding the determinants of SUDs. Environmental influences connected to development of SUDs include influence of peers, lower SES, partner use, and substance use by family members (Kendler, Schmigtt, Aggen, & Prescott, 2008). Individual factors associated with the development of AUDs include problems with academic engagement/achievement, antisocial peer affiliations, problems in the mother–child/father–child relationship, and other stressful life events (Hicks, South, DiRago, Iacono, & McGue, 2009). The prevalence of nonmedical use of pain relievers, stimulants, tranquilizers, and sedatives among individuals 12 years and older has not changed. There is a need to continue preventive efforts and support further research in this area.

SCREENING AND BRIEF INTERVENTION IN BEHAVIORAL HEALTH

This section discusses the use of screening in behavioral health as a means for preventing development of mental health and SUDs and for providing early intervention. As mentioned earlier, screening is the presumptive identification of an unrecognized disease or defect by the application of tests, examinations, or other procedures that can be applied rapidly. From an apparently well population, screening tests sort out persons who potentially have or are at increased risk for a disease from those who probably do not have the disease. Screening is the first step in a process that may or may not lead to a diagnosis of disease; it is not intended to be diagnostic. If a screening test result is positive, a diagnostic work-up should follow. Treatment should be initiated after a disease state is diagnosed.

Screening for Mental Health Disorders: BPRS, MADRS, and CES-D

The Mental Health Parity and Addiction Equity Act (2008) and the Affordable Care Act (ACA, 2010) provide better coverage and access for those with mental disorders (see Chapter 6 for more on this). Of the large number of Americans who will be covered by the ACA, about 20% to 30% will have a mental disorder or SUD. The need for early detection has been highlighted in the New Freedom Commission on Mental Health Report (2003), mentioned earlier. The report calls for early mental health screening, assessment, and referral to mental health service programs. Prevention and early treatment are cost effective; for every dollar spent, between $2 and $10 are saved in health expenditures, court and educational costs, and lost productivity.

In 2008, an estimated 9.8 million adults reported an SMI, and 2 million youth (ages 12–17) had a major depressive episode the previous year. In 2009, 12 million adults (5.3%) reported a need for mental health care that was unmet, with about half this number not receiving any services during the previous year. This was most often due to lack of health insurance coverage, cost, or lack of knowledge about how to access services. Only half of children with common mental disorders (e.g., ADHA, anxiety, eating disorders, depression, conduct disorders) receive the professional services they require; again, most often due to lack of coverage or to costs. Many people turn first to their primary care providers. Currently, about 70% of prescriptions for antidepressants are written in private physician offices, outpatient clinics, and hospitals. Primary care physicians have often been found to fail to diagnose substance abuse, in some cases, as high as 94% (SAMHSA, 2011b).

It is critical that community health nurses focus on early detection and treatment of mental illness in this vulnerable population. Notably, suicide in the United States represents a major public health problem. In 2008, 8.3 million adults (3.7%) seriously considered suicide in the past year and 1.1 million attempted suicide (SAMHSA, 2009a). In 2010, the rate for Army suicides reached an all-time high (SAMHSA, 2011a). Reducing suicide among youth requires mental health screening, and effective programs are available (see Internet Resources found on thePoint).

The National Depression and Anxiety Screening Day is an example of community-level mental health awareness, disease-prevention program. The resources and supplies, such as a comprehensive kit of materials, promotional information, media campaign, training, and technical assistance, are available by visiting the mental health screening Web site (see Internet Resources found on thePoint).

Every community health clinic can implement a routine screening program to capture mental illness problems early. Standardized screening tools for anxiety or depression are also available, and include:

- Brief Psychiatric Rating Scale (BPRS) (Overall & Gorham, 1988)
- Beck Depression Inventory
- Montgomery-Ashberg Depression Rating Scale (MADRS).

The MADRS is known for its utility of administering the instrument from the practitioner standpoint given time constraints in the clinic. A commonly used screening instrument for depression developed in the late 1970s is the Center for Epidemiologic Studies Depression Scale (CES-D) (Radloff, 1977) (see Fig. 27-5). The CES-D and the shorter version, the CES-D 10, have established reliability and validity across populations and cultures and are widely used clinically to screen for depression (Dozeman et al., 2010; Grzywacz et al., 2010; Milette et al., 2010; Pettit et al., 2008). A newer, computer-administered version of the CES-D: SF is being validated (Blum, 2011).

Tools also exist for postpartum depression screening (Edinburgh Postnatal Depression Scale), the elderly (Geriatric Depression Scale—Short Form; Cornell Scale for Depression in Dementia), and for children (Children's Depression Inventory). Examples of these tools can be easily accessed (Sharp & Lipsky, 2002).

Screening for Substance Use and Substance Use Disorders

When screening for substance use, there are three aspects of screening: screening for actual consumption, screening for at-risk drinking, and screening for SUDs. The use of substances represents a continuum of levels of consumption and associated risks for SUDs as well as health and social consequences related to substance use.

Level of Risk

Essentially, the continuum of use is based on the level of consumption (Fig. 27-1). This model is well developed in relation to alcohol consumption and serves as a model for understanding risk and how to interpret the screening results (Martin et al., 2008).

Screening Instruments: Self-Reports

The recommendations for screening are well developed and validated in relation to alcohol use and tobacco use. There is less evidence to support the use of a specific screening approach related to other drug use, both illicit and licit. However, the evidence is growing and a growing body of literature supports screening for substance use as a standard of care for all health professionals (Lanier & Ko, 2008). The difficulty is to choose a screening instrument that will allow the clinician to screen for consumption, pattern, duration of use, and SUDs, but not all screening instruments include all elements. The other difficulty is determining whether the screening instrument has known sensitivity and specificity in the target population. For most screening instruments, the sensitivity and specificity information is based on a general population and may not be as reliable for populations such as pregnant women or the elderly (Smith, Schmidt, Allensworth-Davies, & Saitz, 2010).

Health researchers began developing and testing screening instruments aimed at identifying SUDs in the 1970s. Examples of these instruments include:

- Michigan Alcoholism Screening Test (MAST) (Selzer, 1971)
- Drug Abuse Screening Test (DAST) (Skinner, 1982)
- Cut Down, Annoyed, Guilty, Eye-Opener (CAGE) Questionnaire (Ewing, 1984).

Center for Epidemiologic Studies Depression Scale (CES-D)

Below is a list of some of the ways you may have felt or behaved. Please indicate how often you have felt this way during the **past week**: *(circle **one** number on each line)*

During the past week...	**Rarely or none of the time** (less than 1 day)	**Some or a little of the time** (1-2 days)	**Occasionally or a moderate amount of time** (3-4 days)	**All of the time** (5-7days)
1. I was bothered by things that usually don't bother me	0	1	2	3
2. I did not feel like eating; my appetite was poor	0	1	2	3
3. I felt that I could not shake off the blues even with help from my family	0	1	2	3
4. I felt that I was just as good as other people	0	1	2	3
5. I had trouble keeping my mind on what I was doing	0	1	2	3
6. I felt depressed	0	1	2	3
7. I felt that everything I did was an effort	0	1	2	3
8. I felt hopeful about the future	0	1	2	3
9. I thought my life had been a failure	0	1	2	3
10. I felt fearful	0	1	2	3
11. My sleep was restless	0	1	2	3
12. I was happy	0	1	2	3
13. I talked less than usual	0	1	2	3
14. I felt lonely	0	1	2	3
15. People were unfriendly	0	1	2	3

FIGURE 27-5. The Center for Epidemiologic Studies Depression Scale (CES-D). (From Radloff, L. (1977). The CES-D Scale: A self-report depression scale for research in the general population. *Applied Psychological Measurement, 1,* 385–401; Stanford Patient Education Research Center. (n.d.). *Center for Epidemiologic Studies Depression Scale (CES-D)*. Retrieved from http://cdn.bmedreport.netdna-cdn.com/wp-content/uploads/2009/11/CES-D-Standford-Version.pdf)

During the past week...	Rarely or none of the time (less than 1 day)	Some or a little of the time (1-2 days)	Occasionally or a moderate amount of time (3-4 days)	All of the time (5-7days)
16. I enjoyed life	0	1	2	3
17. I had crying spells	0	1	2	3
18. I felt sad	0	1	2	3
19. I felt that people disliked me	0	1	2	3
20. I could not "get going"	0	1	2	3

Scoring

Item Weights	Rarely or none of the time (less than 1 day)	Some of a little of the time (1-2 days)	Occasionally or a moderate amount of the time (3-4 days)	All of the time (5-7 days)
Items 4, 8, 12, & 16	3	2	1	0
All other items:	0	1	2	3

Score is the sum of the 20 item weights. If more than 4 items are missing, do not score the scale. A score of 16 or greater is considered depressed.

FIGURE 27-5. *(Continued)*

These self-report instruments were developed for general adult populations with a focus on dependence. They were designed to distinguish persons who probably *are* dependent from those who apparently *are not*. If the clinician only uses a tool that screens for dependence and does not screen for consumption or onset of consumption, then valuable clinical information may be missing since consumption in general puts a person at risk for negative consequences, such as injury and the potential of negative interactions with other medications. Thus, levels and patterns of consumption are as important as early identification of an SUD.

For the community health nurse, screening programs can be a valuable prevention tool. Prior to developing a screening program, it is important to establish a clear purpose for the screening (consumption and/or SUDs) and the target population as well. Then an appropriate screening tool can be chosen.

Two main methods of screening for substance use are self-report and biologic markers. Self-report relies on the person to complete a screening instrument or provide information to a health care provider. Screening instruments determined by systematic review to be effective for primary care providers in screening for illicit drug use are (Lanier & Ko, 2008):

- Alcohol, Smoking, and Substance Involvement Screening Test (ASSIST)
- Cut Down, Annoyed, Guilty, Eye-Opener—Adapted to Include Drugs (CAGE-AID)
- Car, Relax, Alone, Forget, Friends, Trouble (CRAFFT)
- DAST
- Drug Use Disorders Identification Test (DUDIT)
- Relax, Alone, Forget, Friends, Trouble (RAFFT)
- Reduce, Annoyed, Guilty, Start (RAGS)
- Rapid Drug Problems Screen (RDPS)
- Simple Screening Instrument for Substance Abuse (SSI-SA)

For alcohol use, the screening instrument recommended by the National Institute on Alcohol Abuse and

Alcoholism is the Alcohol Use Disorders Identification Test (AUDIT) (NIAAA, 2007) (see Display 27.3). The WHO developed this instrument for use across populations, and it has established high reliability and validity across ethnic groups (Reinhart & Allen, 2007). The MAST and CAGE tools are often used. Another screening tool, T-ACE (Tolerance, Annoyed, Cut Down, Eye-Opener, 2005), is based on the CAGE tool and is helpful in determining range of use; it is used with prenatal clients. The Young Adult Alcohol Problems Screening Test (YAAPST) is often used with college students, a population with known binge drinking behaviors (NIAAA, 2005).

Biologic Screenings

Biologic markers used to detect substance use include urine, blood, hair, saliva, breath, and meconium. In contrast to self-report, biologic markers provide either direct or indirect evidence of use (Pragst, 2010; Whitford,

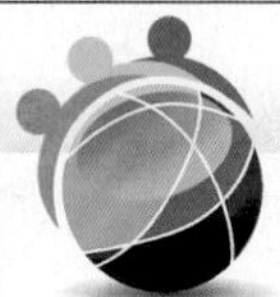

DISPLAY 27.3 ALCOHOL USE DISORDERS IDENTIFICATION TEST (AUDIT)

Please circle the answer that is correct for you.

1. How often do you have a drink containing alcohol?
   Never (0)
   Monthly or less (1)
   Two to four times a month (2)
   Two to three times per week (3)
   Four or more times per week (4)
2. How many drinks containing alcohol do you have on a typical day when you are drinking?
   1 or 2 (0)
   3 or 4 (1)
   5 or 6 (2)
   7 to 9 (3)
   10 or more (4)
3. How often do you have six or more drinks on one occasion?
   Never (0)
   Monthly or less (1)
   Two to four times a month (2)
   Two to three times per week (3)
   Four or more times per week (4)
4. How often during the last year have you found that you were not able to stop drinking once you had started?
   Never (0)
   Monthly or less (1)
   Two to four times a month (2)
   Two to three times per week (3)
   Four or more times per week (4)
5. How often during the last year have you failed to do what was normally expected from you because of drinking?
   Never (0)
   Monthly or less (1)
   Two to four times a month (2)
   Two to three times per week (3)
   Four or more times per week (4)
6. How often during the last year have you needed a first drink in the morning to get yourself going after a heavy drinking session?
   Never (0)
   Monthly or less (1)
   Two to four times a month (2)
   Two to three times per week (3)
   Four or more times per week (4)
7. How often during the last year have you had a feeling of guilt or remorse after drinking?
   Never (0)
   Monthly or less (1)
   Two to four times a month (2)
   Two to three times per week (3)
   Four or more times per week (4)
8. How often during the last year have you been unable to remember what happened the night before because you had been drinking?
   Never (0)
   Monthly or less (1)
   Two to four times a month (2)
   Two to three times per week (3)
   Four or more times per week (4)
9. Have you or someone else been injured as a result of your drinking?
   No (0)
   Yes, but not in the last year (2)
   Yes, during the last year (4)
10. Has a relative or friend, or a doctor or other health worker, been concerned about your drinking or suggested you cut down?
    No (0)
    Yes, but not in the last year (2)
    Yes, during the last year (4)

The AUDIT can detect alcohol problems experienced in the last year. A score of 8+ on the AUDIT generally indicates harmful or hazardous drinking. Questions 1–8 = 0, 1, 2, 3, or 4 points. Questions 9 and 10 are scored 0, 2, or 4 only. From National Institute on Alcohol Abuse and Alcoholism. (2005). Screening for alcohol use and alcohol related problems. *Alcohol Alert, No. 65.* National Institutes of Health. Retrieved from http://pubs.niaaa.nih.gov/publications/aa65/AA65.htm

Widner, Mellick, & Elkins, 2009). They are used with self-report and collateral report from family and friends, as a means of providing corroborating evidence of use (Whitford et al., 2009). Factors that influence sensitivity and specificity of biologic markers include other metabolic disorders or other diseases, medication use, and reliability of the method (Whitfield et al., 2008). They are rarely used in a community-based screening program due to the cost and the problems with obtaining biologic specimens. Various groups, such as legal authorities, employers, or sports programs, use biologic markers to verify alcohol or drug use.

When developing a screening program for substance use, the community health nurse must take a number of things into account. First, a screening program has to be prepared to provide or be able to refer persons who have a positive screen to the appropriate level of services. Since substance use occurs across a continuum, a screening program may identify persons with risky use who may not have an SUD. Therefore, a program should have links to clinically appropriate treatment services for nondependent substance users as well as for dependent substance users. This usually involves having linkages with community agencies that provide substance abuse treatment. Therefore, it is important to know communities' treatment capacity.

Brief Intervention for Positive Screens

When planning a screening program related to substance abuse, some of the participants in the program will screen positive for risky or hazardous use and are candidates for a BI. A BI for alcohol use can be done by any trained health care provider and can be completed in a short time. A BI generally lasts from 5 to 15 minutes, usually over one to three sessions. Strong research evidence exists for the use of BI for heavy or excess nondependent drinkers, especially those identified in primary care settings (NIAAA, 2007). As a whole, providing a BI is generally more effective in the year after delivery than if no intervention is given at all (Sommers, 2007). Less work has been done with other substances.

COMMUNITY-LEVEL INTERVENTIONS

As described in Chapter 15, the community health nurse begins with a community assessment in order to complete a community diagnosis. Once the nurse establishes a diagnosis, the next step is to decide on an intervention that can address the specific public health issue identified in the diagnosis. A good starting point in the development of community/public health intervention is to begin with the *Healthy People 2020* objectives (Tables 27-1, 27-2, and 27-4). The nurse can review the objectives and locate the specific focus area that matches the community diagnosis. For example, if the community diagnosis relates to an increase in alcohol-related motor vehicle crashes in adolescents, there are two specific *Healthy People 2020* objectives related to that issue: reduction in motor vehicle crashes and deaths and reduction in adolescents riding with a driver who has been drinking. Note that for each objective, target benchmarks and data derivation have been identified. These can be used to guide program development.

Level of Intervention from a Community Health Perspective

Once the nurse identifies the focus of the intervention, the next step is to determine the level of prevention (see Chapter 14 for more information on theoretical frameworks). First, the natural history of disease provides the framework for the traditional public health model of primary, secondary, and tertiary prevention. The next step is to decide on the type of intervention: clinical, environmental, or behavioral. The final model relates to the scope of the intervention: universal, selected, or indicated. Because a motor vehicle crash is an event rather than a disease, the desired outcome is to reduce the number of those events related to a behavior rather than a disease. Thus, the prevention of SUDs is not the focus but rather the behavior of drinking while driving. Therefore, neither a screening program (secondary prevention) nor an alcohol treatment program (tertiary prevention) is needed. Considering also that almost all adolescents either drive or ride with other adolescents, a primary behavioral intervention using a universal approach would probably work best to address this problem. For instance, social marketing focused toward adolescent drivers or those beginning to drive that focus on the behavior of drinking and driving.

Mental Health Community Interventions

"Integrative health assessment" has gained momentum in various health centers as a method for decreasing utilization of unwarranted procedures. The underlying premise here is that a person experiencing some personal trials and tribulations may manifest the stress through physical manifestations. There is greater recognition of the mind and body interaction. Accordingly, approaches to mental health promotion encompass physical, emotional, sociocultural, and intellectual considerations. Integrative health assessment is the process of identifying relevant factors, such as the following:

1. Treatment history relative to mental or emotions issues. This includes the visit to a psychologist or mental health professional for complaints of anxiety or periods of loneliness.
2. Personal life stressors. Each day, there are daily tasks relative to one's age and appropriate role function. This may be as a parent, provider, or employee. Some subtle manifestations include irritability, impulsiveness, or frustration intolerance that the individual cannot cope with in a socially appropriate manner.
3. Disturbances in sleep, appetite, or energy level that are not attributable to a rational explanation given the person's daily lifestyle

4. Complaints of chronic pain of somatic nature that is not attributable to a physical dysfunction
5. History of abuse, trauma, substance use, and family history of mental illness

One best practice of note is the Intermountain Healthcare program at Salt Lake City, Utah. Information about "mental health integration" can be accessed via the center's Web site (see Internet Resources).

Today, the community population is subjected to many uncertainties through instantaneous worldwide communication systems. Threats to personal or family safety are basic to mental health. Problems in global peace, the possibility of bioterrorism, or threats of natural disasters or calamities are unsettling. The exposure to fear and anxiety from disseminated information has untold psychological implications. For instance, the tragic news of the death in 2008 of Caylee Marie Anthony, the 3-year-old Florida girl who had been missing for months and believed by many to have been killed by her mother, is a recent example. Word of the discovery immediately reached the global population via the Internet and was repeatedly aired via television and radio, as was her mother's trial in 2011. Everyone felt shock and sorrow, although indirectly. It is clear that the psychological trauma imposed by events of this nature has implications for everyone's mental wellbeing.

Mental Health Promotion

As the field of mental health services has matured through advances in epidemiologic methods, research, and treatment, interest in illness prevention and health promotion has increased. Treatment and prevention of mental illness are important and ongoing priorities in community mental health, but promoting mental health, which is essential to healthier people for the future, needs greater emphasis.

Anticipated Outcomes of Mental Health Promotion

Mental health includes the successful performance of mental function that results in (1) productive activities, (2) fulfilling relationships, (3) the ability to adapt to change, and (4) the ability to cope with adversity. Targeting of these areas becomes a way of prioritizing in planning for health-promoting interventions. Designing programs in community mental health settings encourage productive activities (e.g., sports, hobbies), fulfilling relationships (e.g., foster grandparenting), adapting to change (e.g., volunteering), and coping with adversity (e.g., preparing for developmental crises) (SAMHSA, 2011b).

Interventions for Mental Health Promotion

Several different approaches can be used in designing interventions for mental health promotion. Two of them are discussed here: development of interventions to protect people who are potentially at risk for mental disorders and promotion of healthy activities and lifestyles to the general public.

Risk-Protective Activities

Epidemiologic data, along with the results of a growing body of other kinds of research, provide the community mental health nurse with increasing information about the factors that place people at risk for mental disorders. Targeting at-risk individuals with health promotion interventions gives them the resources needed to raise their own levels of health and protects them from mental disorders. It is known, for example, that consumption of alcohol, illegal drugs, and tobacco during pregnancy can damage the fetus. Consequently, extensive prenatal education and support programs can promote parental health and reduce this risk for the next generation. It also is known that abuse and neglect during childhood are risk factors for certain mental disorders. Promoting healthy parenting and stress-reducing activities through classes, group work, and other means can promote the health of parents and protect the health of their children.

Lifestyle and Behavior Activities

To promote the wellbeing of the public, health promotion interventions that are both life sustaining and life enhancing can be planned. Life-sustaining activities include proper nutrition and exercise, healthy sleep patterns and adequate rest, healthy coping with stress, and the ability to use family and community supports and resources. Health promotion programs in the community may address any or all of these. An example is educating schoolchildren about the food guide pyramid and encouraging healthy snacks and well-balanced meals in the home. Other examples include fitness programs for all ages, promotion of community playgrounds and walking or biking trails, and establishing networks of support in the community such as Meals on Wheels and other volunteer programs.

Life-enhancing activities include meaningful work, whether through or outside of employment; creative outlets; interpersonal relationships; recreational activities; and opportunities for spiritual and intellectual growth. Again, mental health promotion interventions can address any or all of these areas. For example, arts and crafts classes and fairs encourage creative expression, community sports events promote social outlets, participation in Elderhostel and other kinds of learning experiences can promote spiritual and intellectual stimulation, volunteer programs encourage community participation, and classes to develop new skills promote meaningful vocation.

Role of the Community Mental Health Nurse

The nurse's role in community mental health is multifaceted involving advocacy, education, case management, collaboration, and community involvement; this has been evident throughout the chapter. The *access and use of epidemiologic data* to understand and serve the mentally ill population are primary. This means identifying the incidence and prevalence of mental disorders, examining the causes and risk factors associated with mental illness, and identifying the needs of people with mental disorders. Nurses sometimes serve as part of the epidemiologic investigative team to conduct surveys and assist with data collection. However, not all data are accurate. For instance, in the older adult population, one study found that only half of those with a mental disorder used treatment services. Also, fewer than 50% with depression or anxiety perceived that they had a need for mental health care (Garrido, Kane, Kaas, & Kane, 2009).

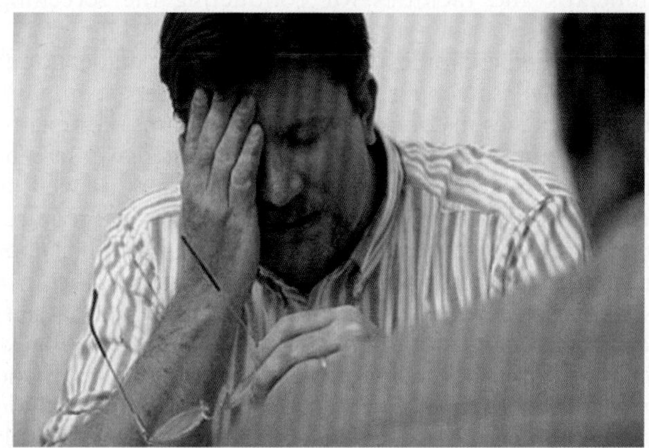

There are effective treatments for most mental illnesses, yet there often remains a stigma surrounding mental illness.

Advocacy

Next, an important part of the nurse's role with the mentally ill is *advocacy*. In this role, the nurse seeks to increase client access to mental health services, to reduce stigma and promote improved public understanding of this population, and to improve services in community mental health. The advocacy role requires being politically involved by serving on decision-making boards and committees, lobbying for legislative changes, and helping to influence mental health policy development that will better serve this population. Membership in state and national nursing organizations can be helpful in establishing collaborative partnerships to benefit the mentally ill. Membership in the National Alliance in Mental Illness (NAMI, 2011b) or other advocacy groups can also effect positive change.

In any of these venues, the vision and expertise of the community mental health nurse can be used to advocate for enhancing existing services, developing new services, and increasing access for the mentally ill to all services. PHNs can also work toward fighting stigma. For instance, when mentally ill persons commit high-visibility crimes, the media often describe them with disparaging descriptors such as psycho, lunatic, or crazy. We can help bring awareness to the plight of the mentally ill and advocate for needed services.

Education

Another aspect of the nurse's role is *education*. The community mental health nurse teaches clients individually and in groups about their mental health conditions, their treatment protocols, ways to function more independently in the community, prevention and health-promoting strategies, and much more. The nurse also teaches the public through community education programs and has an educational role with caregivers, family and community members, and health care decision makers by providing information for service planning.

Case Management

Case management for persons with SMIs is also part of the community mental health nurse's role. This includes screening, assessment, care planning, arranging for service delivery, monitoring, reassessment, evaluation, and discharge. It is often offered within the context of a community mental health center (CMHC). Case management helps the person with an SMI to access services and live as independently as possible.

The nurse's role also involves *case finding and referral*. This means early identification of persons with mental disorders who are in need of treatment and referral of those persons to the appropriate resources for treatment. The purpose of this role is secondary prevention, because early identification and treatment help to ameliorate the severity of the mental disorder and promote a speedier recovery.

Collaboration

Finally, the nurse's role includes *collaboration*. Whether serving individual clients, groups, or populations, the nurse is part of the larger community mental health team and works in collaboration with many people to accomplish the goals of community mental health. The composition of the team—made up of clients, psychiatric nurses, physicians, social workers, nutritionists, epidemiologists, psychologists, health planners, and many more—is diverse and varies depending on the community health nurse's work setting. Collaboration allows for a pooling of professional expertise that enhances the quality and effectiveness of services for the mentally ill.

When working with the mentally ill, the nurse must be aware of issues of personal safety. Although most mentally ill clients are no more prone to violence than the population at large, conditions involving paranoia, hallucinations, or mania can increase clients' tendency toward physical violence. There are situations in which psychotic clients have harmed social workers, physicians, or nurses. Clients who are under the influence of drugs or alcohol pose a potentially serious threat to the nurse's safety. The nurse should be prepared for this eventuality and plan on how to best deal with those clients suffering from addictions. Nurses working with this population must use caution in any situation that suggests danger and must take action immediately to protect themselves and their clients. This may require the nurse to take self-defense classes or assertiveness training or to carry protective gear. It may help to use an escort from a security service, collaborate with the police, or establish a "buddy system" in which two nurses work together in isolated or dangerous homes or areas. Additionally, the public health agency may consider hiring risk-management consultants to examine dangerous situations and recommend actions to preserve safety.

The nurse serving in community mental health plays many roles that are practiced in a variety of settings in collaboration with other members of the community mental health team. It is the challenge of this role and the opportunity to assist in raising the level of mental health for individuals and communities that make this field of practice so rewarding.

In this century (and beyond), community living is characterized by heightened stress and anxiety levels with daily life impacted by traffic congestion, rising fuel costs, threats of global warming and environmental pollution, increased divorce rates, deterioration of the basic family as a unit, continued reliance on the judicial system to resolve family and social conflicts, and incidence of crimes via the Internet. Indeed, individually and collectively, mental health and wellness must be a *national priority*. Healthy bodies necessitate a healthy mind.

Community organizations, religious groups, and educational institutions play critical roles in enhancing mental wellness by helping each person through the provision of family support as the basic unit of the community. The National Alliance on Mental Illness (NAMI, 2011a; b). is a nationwide organization with chapters in each state and county. NAMI's Web site contains extensive information that can be utilized by both consumer and care provider. As a national organization, NAMI is committed to enhance the care of those with mental illness and improve the quality of life of those who are affected. NAMI has the "Families to Families" program designed to provide education to families and help them learn the requisite skills in caring for a mentally ill family member. Another NAMI program is called "Peer to Peer." This is a support group designed to help the consumers cope with the illness and live productive lives.

Nonprofit organizations focus on advocacy, education, service, and funding research endeavors. Mental Health America (formerly known as the National Mental Health Association [NMHA]) is a leading nonprofit organization that promotes mental health. In its position statement, the organization urged the federal government to address the need for comprehensive, community- and strengths-based, consumer- and family-driven mental health programs. The organization was established in 1909 as a reform movement by former psychiatric patient Clifford W. Beers who experienced abuse during his stay in public and private mental institutions.

Substance Use and Community-Level Interventions

The National Alcohol Screening Day (NASD) is an example of a population-based nationwide screening program aimed at identifying persons with AUDs. The program is designed for implementation on the community level in settings such as primary care, college campuses, the work place, or faith-based agencies (O'Connor et al., 2011). For a small registration fee, NASD supplies community organizations with a screening kit that provides all the necessary information needed to conduct the screening program. This model has the national organization providing the media support and the tools for conducting a community-screening program while the agency supplies the clinicians and facilities for conducting the screening program.

Another example of obtaining ready-made population-based screening programs is to use a company that specializes in conducting such programs. For example, an employer may need a more intensive screening program that includes biologic markers as well as self-report. These programs follow current legal requirements for screening and have higher costs. Another population-based approach to screening for substance use is online screening. A participant can complete a self-report screening tool online and receive rapid feedback. Such an approach helps protect the anonymity of the participant. To be effective, the program should include a means to connect those who screen positive to health care providers.

Two government agencies provide a major resource for the community health nurse in the development, implementation, and evaluation of programs aimed at the prevention and treatment of SUDs: the Center for Substance Abuse Prevention (CSAP) and the Center for Substance Abuse Treatment (CSAT). They are both divisions of SAMHSA and have user-friendly Web sites. Their published programs are evidence-based and often include resources needed to implement the programs, such as brochures.

Community efforts are essential because often only a small percentage of persons who are in need of treatment seek it. Using a broader community approach can result in reducing harm to the community, preventing the development of SUDs, and reducing the burden of disease on the population.

Policy-Based Interventions

Not-for-profit, private for-profit, and governmental agencies play crucial roles in community health care. The provision of health care to the population requires multidisciplinary approaches that are driven by monetary reimbursements based on health care problems. Local governments may institute community mental health care policies relative to administrative processes or procedural mechanisms. Policies at the community or state levels aim to ensure the rights of individuals and public safety. Thus, cities or counties with appropriate jurisdiction over a geographic area develop policies and guidelines necessary to encourage mental health program development and implementations that address the needs of the community population.

Depending on each county, certain rules or regulations apply. It is important to learn about the community agencies and interrelationships to other county service providers to ensure the coordination of care. At the local level are freestanding programs that focus on support for individuals, families, the indigent, or the homeless. Funding may come from charitable organizations or from local governments through grant monies obtained from periodic requests for proposals (RFPs) or requests for applications (RFAs) issued by the local governing body. Other governmental agencies have roles in mental health by encouraging employee wellness in the workplace or through rules and regulations that encourage employers to provide benefits, such as mental health insurance, bereavement leave, or stress leave. The incidence of violence in the workplace has necessitated policy initiatives within the business community to respond by developing strategic plans and providing educational programs that address these issues.

Mental Health Policy and Research

The WHO, at the international level, provides assistance to each country's policy makers and planners in developing a plan for the population's mental health by utilizing available resources including promoting human rights, enhancing health, and minimizing debility from mental disorders. Many projects involve technical assistance training on comprehensive strategic planning. The WHO Mental Health in Development (MIND) project (2012) is comprised of four core themes:

1. Action in countries (support to improve the lives of those with mental disorders)
2. Mental health policy, planning, and service development (coordinate services)
3. Mental health, human rights, and legislation (reduce human rights violations)
4. Mental health, poverty, and development (mental health is vital to achieving developmental priorities)

When all of these intersect, the basic focus of the program is to act, unite, and empower people and countries to promote human rights for the mentally ill and improve the quality of their care.

Global mental health research priorities include health policy and systems research, mental health delivery systems, and cost-effective interventions especially in countries with few resources. Epidemiological research on child and adolescent mental disorders, as well as alcohol and SUDs, was also a high priority. New pharmacological treatments and other interventions, along with vaccines and other technologies, were lower priority (Tomlinson et al., 2009).

At the national level, mental health policy and research is focused on funding of services and grants to address fragmentation and gaps in care, as well as elimination of disparities and promotion of mental health screenings and early treatment (TPNFCMH, 2003). Surveillance is also done at the national level, and evidence-based best practices are outlined, along with free resources (CDC, 2011; Lanier & Ko, 2008). Recent legislation has provided greater access and coverage, with the ACA (2010) and the Mental Health Parity and Addiction Equity Act (2008). Because of this legislation increasing access along with staff reductions due to state and local budget cuts, some feel that the increased number of people seeking services will place lead to a greater gap in behavioral health services (Larrison et al., 2011). Individuals, professional nursing organizations, and other NGOs often lobby for improved policies related to mental health (Nelson & Mann, 2011).

However, most policy and funding decisions for mental health treatment and services are made at the local or state level. State psychiatric hospitals and local mental health services, as well as mental health planning and regulation, are not functions of the federal government but rather states and counties or cities. While Medicaid and Medicare funds may be used, states may also need to provide matching funds or seek federal grant funding.

Substance Use Policy

Policy related to substance use is defined broadly as any purposeful act on the part of a governmental or nongovernmental group to minimize or prevent adverse consequences related to use of potentially addictive substances. Specific strategies include implementing a law aimed at reducing use, such as taxation, or a means to allocate resources related to prevention and/or treatment priorities (Babor et al., 2010).

One consistently used policy approach involves regulating the availability of the substance (Casswell & Thamarangsi, 2009; Manubay, Muchow, & Sullivan, 2011). In relation to illicit drugs, laws are in place restricting availability through the classification of the drug (e.g., schedule II opioids). For alcohol and tobacco, there are regulations on who may buy and who may sell the products (e.g., the legal age to purchase may be 21). Other examples of governmental regulations related to alcohol and tobacco include drinking and driving laws, regulation of alcohol and tobacco promotion, regulations pertinent to bars, interlocks for individuals who drive drunk repeatedly, and limits on product outlet density (Toumbourou et al., 2007).

Policies in relation to alcohol and tobacco have a similar approach. Communities set policies that restrict both alcohol availability and consumption; this is done by controlling the number of alcohol outlets, regulating the current outlets, and setting laws that will allow the community to close problem outlets. These measures are implemented through policies related to zoning and the licensing of establishments that sell alcohol. Another measure has been to require responsible alcohol-service training for bartenders. Other examples include keg registration, stricter enforcement of underage sales of alcohol and tobacco, and controlling alcohol outlet density. Major efforts in relation to tobacco consumption in public areas have resulted in a drastic restriction of locations where tobacco users can smoke outside of their own home.

The focus of most policies related to illicit drugs has been to enact laws that criminalize the possession and sale of these substances. Other types of policies that have relevance, for example, are those enacted to prevent methamphetamine use. A number of states have restricted the sale of OTC medications that can be used to manufacture methamphetamine in home laboratories. The government enacted a major initiative when federal funding was linked to a drug-free workplace. That is, any organization that receives federal funds, such as health care facilities that receive Medicare payments, must follow the SAMHSA guidelines (SAMHSA, 2009b).

SUMMARY

Behavioral health is a key component in the health of a community. Three of the top ten leading health indicators from *Healthy People 2020* are closely linked to behavioral health issues: tobacco use, substance use, and mental health (see Display 27.4). Objectives, health indicators, and target outcomes for tobaccco, illicit substances, and alcohol use guide the PHN in program planning. In every community in the United States and the world, behavioral health directly or indirectly affects every other indicator of health. Harmful substance use overburdens the medical, social, economic, and criminal justice systems of communities and governments, thus reiterating the need for vigilance.

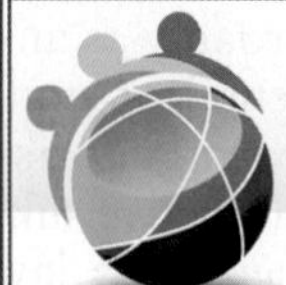

DISPLAY 27.4 *HEALTHY PEOPLE 2020* LEADING HEALTH INDICATORS

Top 10 Health Indicators

1. Physical Activity
2. Overweight and Obesity
3. Tobacco Use
4. Substance Abuse
5. Responsible Sexual Behavior
6. Mental Health
7. Injury and Violence
8. Environmental Quality
9. Immunization
10. Access to Health Care

Researchers have devoted decades to determining the etiology of SUDs specifically with regard to *nature versus nurture*—in other words, whether SUDs occur as a result of genetics or environment. Both alcohol and drug dependence share common genetic risk factors, but are also influenced by environmental factors (influence of peers, lower SES, partner use, and substance use by family members) and personal factors (high antisocial behavior, high impulsivity, major depression, social anxiety problems, a history of childhood sexual abuse, hyperactivity, attention problems, and seminal events).

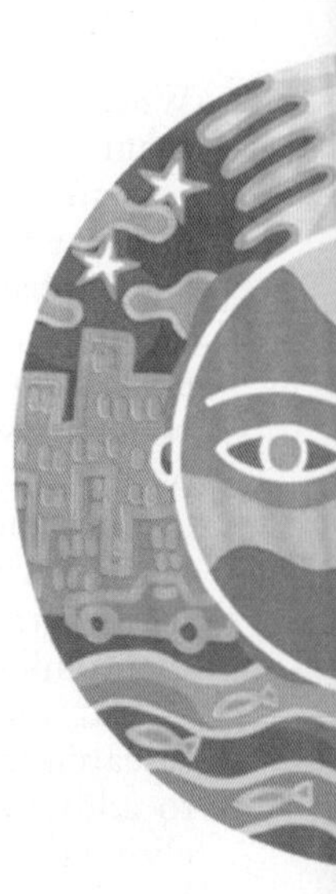

Treatment related to behavioral health at the community level begins with a community assessment in order to establish a community diagnosis, followed by intervention that can address the specific public health issue identified in the diagnosis. The community health nurse can use *Healthy People 2020* objectives as a starting point in the development of an intervention.

The community health nurse must incorporate behavioral health in the assessment, planning, and developing of community health interventions and in the evaluation of outcomes. With this comes the need for administrative, managerial, or supervisory support with commitment not only from a philosophical perspective but from a resource perspective as well. Success comes with a unified approach to mental health and substance use, requiring application of research, utilization of best practice models at the clinical level, and education of all concerned.

ACTIVITIES TO PROMOTE **CRITICAL THINKING**

1. As a community health nurse, you have been asked to design and present a 2-hour program on suicide prevention to the entire student body of the local high school. This activity is representative of which level of prevention? What are some of the considerations involved in planning this program to promote optimal success? How might you measure the effectiveness of this intervention?
2. You are part of a multidisciplinary team whose goal is to identify families in your city who are at risk for crisis (e.g., single parent, divorce, teen pregnancy, loss of job) and develop a set of interventions. How would you determine who these families are? What interventions would be appropriate to meet their needs? What level of prevention would you be targeting?
3. You have met a few elderly men in your area who live alone and are widowed, and you have heard that there are others. Assuming your advocacy role in community mental health, you decide to take some action to ensure that their needs are being met. How would you determine the risks and needs for this group? What interventions would be appropriate to meet their needs?
4. Select a problem that places people at risk for mental disorders (e.g., child abuse and neglect, drug abuse) and do a search on the Internet to learn all you can about it. What is the incidence and prevalence of this problem? What interventions are most effective in addressing it? What can be done to prevent it?
5. Search for local treatment facilities and resources for alcohol and drug abuse clients. Call a few of them to inquire about cost, access, and types of assistance available. How many people can they serve? How does this compare to the numbers of reported alcohol and drug users in your area?
6. Talk with a public health nurse working in your community. How does she see the problems of substance abuse and mental health in your area? Does she feel there are adequate resources available? How would she advocate on behalf of these clients?

REFERENCES

American Psychiatric Association. (2000). *Diagnostic and statistical manual of mental disorders*. [Text revision (DSM-IV-TR), (4th ed.)]. Washington, DC: Author.

Babor, T. F., Caetano, R., Casswell, S., Edwards, G., Giesbrecht, N., Graham, K. et al. (2010). *Alcohol: No ordinary commodity: Research and public policy* (2nd ed.). Oxford, England: Oxford University Press.

Bartlett, G., Abrahamowicz, M., Grad, R., Sylvestre, M. P., & Tamblyn, R. (2009). Association between risk factors for injurious falls and new benzodiazepine prescribing in elderly persons. *BMC Family Practice, 10*(1). Retrieved from http://www.biomedcentral.com/1471–2296/10/1/

Beesdo, K., Pine, D., Lieb, R., & Wittchen, H. (2010). Incidence and risk patterns of anxiety and depressive disorders and categorization of generalized anxiety disorder. *Archives of General Psychiatry, 67*(1), 47–57.

Beirut, L. J., Agrawal, A., Bucholz, K., Doheny, K., Laurie, C., Pugh, E. et al. (2010). A genome-wide association study of alcohol dependence. *Proceedings of the National Academy of Sciences, 107*(11), 5082–5087.

Bernstein, J., Heeren, T., Edward, E, Dorfman, D., Bliss, C., Winter, M. et al. (2010). A brief motivational interview in a pediatric emergency department, plus 10-day telephone follow-up, increases attempts to quit drinking among youth and young adults who screen positive for problematic drinking. *Academic Emergency Medicine, 17*(8), 890–902.

Blum, D. (2011). *Validation of a computer-administered version of the IRT-based Center for Epidemiologic Studies Depression Scale short form*. (Doctoral dissertation). Alliant International University. (ProQuest Publication No. 3487307).

Bottrell, D., & Armstrong, D. (2012). Local resources and distal decisions: The political ecology of resilience. *The Social Ecology of Resilience, 5*, 247–264.

Casswell, S., & Thamarangsi, T. (2009). Reducing harm from alcohol: Call to action. *The Lancet, 373*(9682), 2247–2257.

Centers for Disease Control and Prevention (CDC). (1992). A framework for assessing the effectiveness of disease and injury prevention. *Morbidity and Mortality Weekly Report, 41*(RR-3), (inclusive page numbers).

Centers for Disease Control and Prevention (CDC). (2006). Homicides and Suicides: National Violent Death Reporting System, United States, 2003–2004. *Mortality and Morbidity Weekly Report, 55*(26), 721–724.

Centers for Disease Control and Prevention (CDC). (2010). *Health topics: Alcohol and drug use*. Retrieved from http://www.cdc.gov/healthyyouth/alcoholdrug/index.htm

Centers for Disease Control and Prevention (CDC). (2011). *Health, United States 2010: with special feature on death and dying*. Retrieved from http://www.cdc.gov/nchs/data/hus/hus10.pdf

Centers for Disease Control and Prevention (CDC). (2011). Mental illness surveillance among adults in the United States. *Morbidity and Mortality Weekly Report (MMWR), 60*(Suppl.), S1–S29. Retrieved from http://www.cdc.gov/mmwr/pdf/other/su6003.pdf

Chen, W., Hankinson, S., Colditz, G., & Willett, W. (2011). Moderate alcohol consumption during adult life, drinking patterns, and breast cancer risk. *JAMA, 306*(17), 1884–1890.

Cherpitel, C. J. (2007). Alcohol and injuries: A review of international emergency room studies since 1995. *Drug and Alcohol Review, 26*, 201–214.

Copeland, W., Shanahan, L., Costello, J., & Angold, A. (2009). Childhood and adolescent psychiatric disorders as predictors of young adult disorders. *Archives of General Psychiatry, 66*(7), 764–772.

Corrigan, P., & Wassel, A. (2008). Understanding and influencing the stigma of mental illness. *Journal of Psychosocial Nursing and Mental Health Services, 46*(1), 42–48.

Cunningham, P. J. (2009). Beyond parity: Primary care physicians' perspectives on access to mental health care. *Health Affairs, 28*(3), 490–501.

Dick, D. M., Riley, B., & Kendler, K. S. (2010). Nature and nurture in neuropsychiatric genetics: Where do we stand? *Dialogues in Clinical Neuroscience, 12*(1), 7–23.

Dobkin, C., & Nicosia, N. (2009). The war on drugs: Methamphetamine, public health, and crime. *American Economic Review, 99*(1), 324–349.

Doebbeling, C. (2007). Treatment of mental illness. *The Merck manual home health handbook.* Retrieved from http://www.merckmanuals.com/home/mental_health_disorders/overview_of_mental_health_care/treatment_of_mental_illness.html

Dozeman, E., van Schaik, D., van Marwijk, H., Stek, M., van der Horst, H., & Beekman, A. (2010). The center for epidemiological studies depression scale (CES-D) is an adequate screening instrument for depressive and anxiety disorders in a very old population living in residential homes. *International Journal of Geriatric Psychiatry, 26*(3), 239–246.

Ewing, J. A. (1984). Detecting Alcoholism: The CAGE Questionnaire. *Journal of the American Medical Association, 252*, 1905–1907.

Farley, R. (2011, December 22). *Essential health benefits: What does the new HHS guidance mean for behavioral health?* Retrieved from http://mentalhealthcarereform.org/essential-health-benefits-what-does-the-new-hhs-guidance-mean-for-behavioral-health/

Fombonne, E. (2009). Epidemiology of pervasive developmental disorders. *Pediatric Research, 65*(6), 591–598.

Frank, R. G., & Glied, S. A. (2006). *Better but not well: Mental health policy in the United States since 1950.* Baltimore, MD: The Johns Hopkins University Press.

Garrido, M., Kane, R., Kaas, M., & Kane, R. (2009). Perceived need for mental health care among community-dwelling older adults. *The Journals of Gerontology Series B: Psychological Sciences and Social Sciences, 64B*(6), 704–712.

Ghandour, R., Kogan, M., Blumberg, S., Jones, J., & Perrin, J. (2012). Mental health conditions among school-aged children: Geographic and sociodemographic patterns in prevalence and treatment. *Journal of Developmental and Behavioral Pediatrics, 33*(1), 42–54.

Gordon, R. (1987). An operational classification of disease prevention. In J. Steinberg & M. Silverman (Eds.), *Preventing mental disorders: A research perspective* (pp. 20–26). Rockville, Maryland: U.S. Department of Health and Human Services: National Institute of Mental Health.

Grant, B. F., Dawson, D. A., Stinson, F. S., Chou, S. P., Dufour, M. C., & Pickering, R. P. (2004). The 12-month prevalence and trends in DSM-IV alcohol abuse and dependence: United States, 1991–1992 and 2001–2002. *Drug Alcohol Dependence, 74*(3), 223–234.

Green, K., Doherty, E., Stuart, E., & Ensminger, M. (2010). Does heavy adolescent marijuana use lead to criminal involvement in adulthood? Evidence from a multiwave longitudinal study of urban African Americans. *Drug and Alcohol Dependence, 112*(1–2), 117–125.

Gruenewald, P., & Johnson, F. (2010). Drinking, driving, and crashing: A traffic-flow model of alcohol-related motor vehicle accidents. *Journal of Studies on Alcohol and Drugs, 71*(2), 237–248.

Grzywacz, J., Alterman, T., Muntaner, C., Shen, R., Gabbard, S., Nakamoto, J. et al. (2010). Mental health research with Latino farmworkers: A systematic evaluation of the short CES-D. *Journal of Immigrant and Minority Health, 12*(9), 652–658.

Hamamoto, D., & Rhodus, N. (2009). Methamphetamine abuse and dentistry. *Oral Diseases, 15*(1), 27–37.

Han, B., Gfroerer, J., & Colliver, J. (2010). Associations between duration of illicit drug use and health conditions: Results from the 2005–2007 national surveys on drug use and health. *Annals of Epidemiology, 20*(4), 289–297.

Hardie, T. (2007). Module 1: Alcohol and genetics. In C. L. Savage (Ed.). *A nursing education model for the prevention and treatment of alcohol use disorders.* Rockville, MD: National Institute on Alcohol Abuse and Alcoholism.

Hicks, B., South, S., DiRago, A., Iacono, W., & McGue, M. (2009). Environmental adversity and increasing genetic risk for externalizing disorders. *Archives of General Psychiatry, 66*(6), 640–648.

Hu, G., Wilcox, H., Wissow, L., & Baker, S. (2008). Mid-life suicide: An increasing problem in U.S. Whites, 1999–2005. *American Journal of Preventive Medicine, 35*(6), 589–593.

Hudson, J. I., Hiripi, E., Pope, H. G., & Kessler, R. C. (2007). The prevalence and correlates of eating disorders in the National Comorbidity Survey Replication. *Biologic Psychiatry, 61*, 348–358.

Issel, L. M. (2009). *Health planning and evaluation* (2nd ed.). Boston: Jones and Bartlett Publishers.

Jessor, R. (2008). Description versus explanation in cross-national research on adolescence. *Journal of Adolescent Health, 43*(6), 527–528.

Johnston, L. D, O'Malley, P., Bachman, J., & Schulenberg, J. (2012). *Marijuana use continues to rise among U.S. teens, while alcohol use hits historic lows.* Ann Arbor, MI: University of Michigan News Service. Retrieved from http://monitoringthefuture.org/pressreleases/11drugpr_complete.pdf

Kaufmann, R., Goldberg-Stern, H., & Shuper, A. (2009). Attention-deficit disorders and epilepsy in childhood: Incidence, causative relations and treatment possibilities. *Journal of Child Neurology, 24*(6), 727–733.

Kendler, K. S., Schmitt, E., Aggen, S. H., & Prescott, C. A. (2008). Genetic and environmental influences on alcohol, caffeine, cannabis, and nicotine use from early adolescence to middle adulthood. *Archives of General Psychiatry, 65*(6), 674–682.

Kornblum, J. (2008). Families often 'lost' in trauma of mental illness. *USA Today.* Retrieved from http://www.usatoday.com/news/health/2008-02-04-mental_n.htm

Ku, B., Scott, K., Kertesz, S., & Pitts, S. (2010). Factors associated with use of urban emergency departments by the U.S. homeless population. *Public Health Reports, 125*(3), 398–405.

Lanier, D., & Ko, S. (2008). Screening in primary care settings for illicit drug use: Assessment of screening instruments—a supplemental evidence update for the U.S. Preventive Services Task Force. *Evidence Synthesis No. 58, Part 2.* Rockville, MD: Agency for Healthcare Research and Quality.

Larimer, M., Malone, D., Garner, M., Atkins, D., Burlingham, B., Lonczak, H., et al. (2009). Health care and public service use and costs before and after provision of housing for chronically homeless persons with severe alcohol problems. *JAMA, 301*(13), 1349–1357.

Larrison, C., Hack-Ritzo, S., Koerner, B., Schoppelrey, S., Ackerson, B., & Korr, W. (2011). Economic grand rounds: State budget cuts, health care reform, and a crisis in rural community mental health agencies. *Psychiatric Services, 62*(11), 1255–1257.

Lazarus, R. S., & Folkman, S. (1984). *Stress, appraisal and coping.* New York: Springer Publishing.

Lin, J., Mitchell, K., Grella, C., Warda, U., Liao, D., Hu, P., et al. (2011). Alcohol, tobacco, and nonmedical drug use disorders in U.S. adults aged 65 years and older: Data from the 2001–2002 National Epidemiologic Survey of Alcohol and Related Conditions. *American Journal of Geriatric Psychiatry, 19*(3), 292–299.

Luo, F., Florence, C., Quispe-Agnoli, M., Ouyang, L., & Crosby, A. (2011). Impact of business cycles on US suicide rates, 1928–2007. *American Journal of Public Health, 101*(6), 1139–1146.

Lupton, C. (2011). *The financial impact of fetal alcohol syndrome.* Fetal Alcohol Spectrum Disorders Center for Excellence, USDHHS. Retrieved from http://fasdcenter.samhsa.gov/publications/cost.cfm

Manubay, J., Muchow, C., & Sullivan, M. (2011). Prescription drug abuse: Epidemiology, regulatory issues, chronic pain management with narcotic analgesics. *Primary Care: Clinics in Office Practice, 38*(1), 71–90.

Martin, C., Chung, T., & Langenbucher, J. (2008). How should we revise diagnostic criteria for substance use disorders in the DSM-V? *Journal of Abnormal Psychology, 117*(3), 561–575.

McGuire, T., & Miranda, J. (2008). New evidence regarding racial and ethnic disparities in mental health: Policy implications. *Health Affairs, 27*(2), 393–403.

Merikangas, K., He, J., Burstein, M., Swanson, S., Avenevoli, S., Cui, L., et al. (2010). Lifetime prevalence of mental disorders in U.S. adolescents: results from the National Comorbidity Survey Replication—Adolescent Supplement (NCS-A). *Journal of the American Academy of Child and Adolescent Psychiatry, 49*(10), 980–989.

Milette, K., Hudson, M., Baron, M., Thombs, B., & Canadian Scleroderma Research Group. (2010). Comparisons of the PHQ-9 and CES-D depression scales in systematic sclerosis: Internal consistency reliability, convergent validity and clinical correlates. *Rheumatology, 49*(4), 789–796.

Mooney L. J., Glasner-Edwards, S., Rawson, R. A., & Ling, W. (2009). Medical effects of methamphetamine use. In J. Roll, R. Rawson, & W. Ling (Eds.). *Methamphetamine addiction: From basic science to treatment* (pp. 117–142). New York: Guilford Press.

Moore, A., Karno, M., Grella, C., Lin, J., Warda, U., Liao, D., et al. (2009). Alcohol, tobacco, and nonmedical drug use in older U.S. adults: Data from the 2001–2002 National Epidemiologic Survey of Alcohol and Related Conditions. *Journal of the American Geriatric Society, 57*(12), 2275–2281.

Morden, N., Mistler, L., Weeks, W., & Bartels, S. (2009). Health care for patients with serious mental illness: Family medicine's role. *The Journal of the American Board of Family Medicine, 22*(2), 187–195.

National Alliance on Mental Illness (NAMI). (2011a). *Family-to-family: Education program*. Retrieved from http://www.nami.org/Template.cfm?Section=Family-to-Family&lstid=605

National Alliance on Mental Illness (NAMI). (2011b). *How you can help: Become a member*. Retrieved from http://www.nami.org/Template.cfm?section=Take_Action

National Alliance on Mental Illness. (2007). *State mental health parity laws 2007*. Retrieved from http://www.nami.org/Content/ContentGroups/Policy/Issues_Spotlights/Parity1/State_Mental_Health_Parity_Laws1.htm

National Council for Community Behavioral Healthcare. (2012). *Policy issues and resources: Healthcare reform*. Retrieved from http://www.thenationalcouncil.org/cs/healthcare_reform#FactSheets

National Council on Alcoholism and Drug Dependence. (n.d.). *Alcohol and drug abuse affects everyone in the family*. Retrieved from http://www.ncadd.org/index.php/get-help/family-information-and-education/144-family-education

National Institute on Alcohol Abuse and Alcoholism (NIAAA). (2005, April). Screening for alcohol use and alcohol-related problems. *Alcohol Alert, no. 65*. Rockville, MD: Author.

National Institute on Drug Abuse. (2009a, June). *InfoFacts: Hallucinogens—LSD, peyote, psilocybin, and PCP*. Retrieved from http://www.drugabuse.gov/publications/infofacts/hallucinogens-lsd-peyote-psilocybin-pcp

National Institute on Drug Abuse. (2009b). *Report discusses co-occurrence of drug abuse with other mental disorders*. Retrieved from http://www.drugabuse.gov/news-events/nida-notes/2009/12/report-discusses-co-occurrence-drug-abuse-other-mental-disorders

National Institute on Drug Abuse. (2010). *InfoFacts: Cigarettes and other tobacco products*. Retrieved from http://www.drugabuse.gov/publications/infofacts/cigarettes-other-tobacco-products

National Institute on Drug Abuse. (2011). *Monitoring the Future survey: Overview of findings 2011*. Retrieved from http://www.drugabuse.gov/related-topics/trends-statistics/monitoring-future/overview-findings-2011

National Institute of Mental Health. (n.d.a). *Attention-deficit/hyperactivity disorder among adults*. Retrieved from http://www.nimh.nih.gov/statistics/1ADHD_ADULT.shtml

National Institute of Mental Health. (n.d.b). *Autism*. Retrieved from http://www.nimh.nih.gov/statistics/1AUT_CHILD.shtml

National Institute of Mental Health. (n.d.c). *Statistics*. Retrieved from http://www.nimh.nih.gov/statistics/index.shtml

Nelson, F., & Mann, T. (2011). Opportunities in public policy to support infant and early childhood mental health: The role of psychologists and policymakers. *American Psychologist, 66*(2), 129–139.

Newport, F. (2011). *Record-high 50% of Americans favor legalizing marijuana use*. Gallup Politics. Retrieved from http://www.gallup.com/poll/150149/record-high-americans-favor-legalizing-marijuana.aspx

Nock, M., Hwang, I., Sampson, N., Kessler, R., Angermeyer, M., Beautrais, A. et al. (2009). Cross-national analysis of the associations among mental disorders and suicidal behavior: Findings from the WHO World Mental Health Surveys. *PLoS Medicine, 6*(8), doi: 10.1371/journal.pmed.1000123.

O'Connor, P., Nyquist, J., & McLellan, A. (2011). Integrating addiction medicine into graduate medical education in primary care: The time has come. *Annals of Internal Medicine, 154*(1), 56–59.

Office of Applied Studies (OAS). (2009). *The national survey on drug use and health*. Retrieved from http://www.samhsa.gov/data/2k9/149/MDEamongAdults.pdf

Overall, J. E., & Gorham, D. R. (1988). The brief psychiatric rating scale (BPRS): Recent developments in ascertainment and scaling. *Psychopharmacology Bulletin, 24*, 97–99.

Peterselia, J. (2011). Beyond the prison bubble. *NIJ Journal, 268*, 26–31.

Pettit, J., Lewinsohn, P., Seeley, J., Roberts, R., Hibbard, J., & Hurtado, A. (2009). Association between the Center for Epidemiological Studies Depression Scale (CEDS-D) and mortality in a community sample: An artifact of the somatic complaints factor? *International Journal of Clinical and Health Psychology, 8*(2), 383–397.

Pragst, F., Rothe, M., Moench, B., Hastedt, M., Herre, S., & Simmert, D. (2010). Combined used of fatty acid ethyl esters and ethyl glucuronide in hair for diagnosis of alcohol abuse: Interpretation and advantages. *Forensic Science International, 196*(1), 101–110.

Radloff, L. (1977). The CES-D Scale: A self report depression scale for research in the general population. *Applied Psychological Measurement, 1*, 385–401.

Reinhart, D. F., & Allen, J. P. (2007). The Alcohol Use Disorders Identification Test: An update of research findings. *Alcoholism Clinical and Experimental Research, 31*(2), 185–199.

Roberts, R., Roberts, C., & Chan, W. (2009). One-year incidence of psychiatric disorders and associated risk factors among adolescents in the community. *Journal of Child Psychology and Psychiatry, 50*(4), 40–415.

Room, R., & Rehm, J. (2011). Alcohol and non-communicable diseases—cancer, heart disease and more. *Addiction, 106*(1), 1–2, doi: 10.1111/j.1160-0443.2010.03223.x.

Savage, C., & Gillespie, G. (2008). Health status and access to care for homeless adults with problem alcohol and drug use. *Journal of Addictions Nursing, 19*, 27–33.

Savage, C. L. (Ed.). (2006). Chapter IV: Health promotion and risk reduction. In M. Armstrong, J. Feigenbaum, C. Savage, & C. Vourakis (Eds.). *Addictions nursing, core curriculum* (2nd ed). Raleigh, NC: International Nurses Society on Addiction.

Selzer, M. L. (1971). The Michigan Alcoholism Screening Test: The quest for a new diagnostic instrument. *American Journal of Psychiatry, 127*, 1653–1658.

Sharp, L., & Lipsky, M. (2002). Screening for depression across the lifespan: A review of measures for use in primary care settings. *American Family Physician, 66*(6), 1001–1009.

Skinner, H. A. (1982). The drug use screening test. *Addictive Behaviors, 7*, 363–371.

Smith, P., Schmidt, S., Allensworth-Davies, & Saitz, R. (2010). A single-question screening test for drug use in primary care. *Archives of Internal Medicine, 170*(13), 1155–1160.

Sommers, M. S. (2007). Module IV: Treatment of hazardous (risky) or harmful alcohol use. In C. L. Savage (Ed.). *A nursing education model for the prevention and treatment of alcohol use disorders*. Rockville, MD: National Institute on Alcohol Abuse and Alcoholism.

Spencer, M., Chen, J., Gee, G., Fabian, C., & Takeuchi, D. (2010). Discrimination and mental health—related service use in a national study of Asian Americans. *American Journal of Public Health, 100*(12), 2410–2417.

Substance Abuse and Mental Health Services Administration (SAMHSA). (2009a, September 17). *The NSDUH report: Suicidal thoughts and behaviors among adults*. Rockville, MD: Author.

Substance Abuse and Mental Health Services Administration (SAMHSA). (2009b). Transforming mental health care in America: the federal action agenda, first steps. Retrieved from http://www.samhsa.gov/federalactionagenda/NFC_FMHAA.aspx

Substance Abuse and Mental Health Services Administration (SAMHSA). (2011a). *SAMHSA's strategic initiatives.* Retrieved from http://store.samhsa.gov/shin/content//SMA11-4666/SMA11-4666.pdf

Substance Abuse and Mental Health Services Administration (SAMHSA). (2011b, December 8). *Drug abuse warning network: The DAWN report.* Retrieved from http://www.samhsa.gov/data/2k11/WEB_DAWN_017_new/ED_Visit_IllicitDrugs_Males.pdf

The President's New Freedom Commission on Mental Health. (2003). *Achieving the promise: Transforming mental health care in America.* Retrieved from http://www.nami.org/Template.cfm?Section=Policy&Template=/ContentManagement/ContentDisplay.cfm&ContentID=16699

Thomas, K., Ellis, A., Konrad, T., Holzer, C., & Morrissey, J. (2009). County-level estimates of mental health professional shortage in the United States. *Psychiatric Services, 60*(10), 1323–1328.

Tomlinson, M., Rudan, I., Saxena, S., Swartz, L., Tsai, A., & Patel, V. (2009). Setting priorities for global mental health research. *Bulletin of the World Health Organization, 87*(6). ISSN 0042-9686.

Toumbourou, J. W., Stocwell, T., Neighbors, C., Marlatt, G. A., & Rehm, J. (2007). Interventions to reduce harm associated with adolescent substance use. *Lancet, 369*, 1391–1401.

United Nations Office on Drugs & Crime (UNODC). (2010). *World drug report 2010.* (United Nations Publication, Sales No. E.10.XI.13). Retrieved from http://www.unodc.org/documents/wdr/WDR_2010/World_Drug_Report_2010_lo-res.pdf

U.S. Department of Health and Human Services (USDHHS). (1999). *Mental health: A report of the Surgeon General.* Substance Abuse and Mental Health Services Administration, Center for Mental Health Services, National Institutes of Health, National Institute of Mental Health, Rockville, MD: Author.

U.S. Department of Health and Human Services (USDHHS). (2012a). *Healthy People 2020.* Retrieved from http://www.healthypeople.gov/2020/default.aspx

U.S. Department of Health and Human Services (USDHHS). (2012b) *Healthy People.gov: 2020 Topics And Objectives.* Retrieved http://www.healthypeople.gov/2020/topicsobjectives2020/default.aspx

U. S. Department of Housing and Urban Development (USDHUD). (2010). *The 2009 annual homeless assessment report.* Retrieved from http://www.hudhre.info/documents/5thHomelessAssessmentReport.pdf

Walter, H., Gouze, K., Cichetti, C., Arend, R., Mehta, T., Schmidt, J. et al. (2011). A pilot demonstration of comprehensive mental health services in inner-city public schools. *Journal of School Health, 81*(4), 185–193.

Whitfield, J., Dy, V., Madden, P., Health, A., Martin, N. et al. (2008). Measuring carbohydrate-deficient transferring by direct immunoassay: Factors affecting diagnostic sensitivity for excessive alcohol intake. *Clinical Chemistry, 54*(7), 1158–1165.

Whitford, J., Widner, S. Mellick, D., & Elkins, R. (2009). Self-report of drinking compared to objective markers of alcohol consumption. *The American Journal of Drug and Alcohol Abuse, 35*(2), 55–58.

Willcutt, E., Sonuga-Barke, E., Nigg, J., & Sergeant, J. (2008). Recent developments in neuropsychological models of childhood psychiatric disorders. In T. Banaschewski, & L. Rohde (Eds.). *Biological child psychiatry: trends and developments* (pp. 195–226). Basel, Switzerland: Karger.

Wood, D., & Dargan, P. (2010). Putting cocaine use and cocaine-associated cardiac arrhythmias into epidemiological and clinical perspective. *British Journal of Clinical Pharmacology, 69*(5), 443–447.

World Health Organization (WHO). (2012). *WHO MIND: Mental health in development.* Retrieved from http://www.who.int/mental_health/policy/en/

Wu, L., Parrott, A., Ringwalt, C., Patkar, A., Mannelli, P., & Blazer, D. (2009). The high prevalence of substance use disorders among recent MDMA users compared with other drug users: Implications for intervention. *Addictive Behaviors, 34*(8), 654–661.

Wu, L., Ringwalt, C., Weiss, R., & Blazer, D. (2009). Hallucinogen-related disorders in a national sample of adolescents: The influence of ecstasy/MDMA use. *Drug and Alcohol Dependence, 104*(1–2), 156–166.

thePoint: Everything You Need to Make the Grade!

thePoint Visit http://thePoint.lww.com/Allender8e
for selected readings, study aids for all learning styles, and more!

CHAPTER

28

Working with the Homeless

"Mid pleasures and palaces though we may roam, be it ever so humble, there's no place like home."

–*John Howard Payne* (1791–1852)

KEY TERMS

Chronically homeless
Continuum of care
Deinstitutionalization
Doubling up
Homeless
Housing First
Point-in-time counts
Period prevalence counts
Single room occupancy (SRO) housing
Survival sex
Unaccompanied youth
Unsheltered (hidden) homeless

LEARNING OBJECTIVES

Upon mastery of this chapter, you should be able to:

- Define the concept of homelessness.
- Describe the demographic characteristics of the homeless living in the United States.
- Discuss factors predisposing persons to homelessness.
- Examine the effects of homelessness on health.
- Compare and contrast the unique challenges confronting selected subpopulations within the homeless community.
- Analyze the extent and adequacy of public and private resources to combat the problem of homelessness.
- Assess your beliefs and values toward homelessness.
- Propose community-based nursing interventions to facilitate primary, secondary, and tertiary prevention in addressing the problem of homelessness.

What was once considered unthinkable in a prosperous nation is now an expected occurrence in towns and cities across the United States. Drive through an inner city or suburban community on any given day and you will see people on street corners holding signs "Hungry and homeless." Where is the public outcry in response to this scene? Has the American conscience been anesthetized to this form of human suffering? Or is the need simply too overwhelming and the problems too far-reaching to mount an effective campaign to prevent such a tragedy?

This chapter aims to define the concept of homelessness, examine the factors contributing to homelessness, analyze the major issues confronting the homeless, and examine the role of the community health nurse in addressing the needs of the homeless.

The McKinney–Vento Homeless Assistance Act (Title 42 of the U. S. Code) defines a person as **homeless** who lacks a fixed, regular, adequate nighttime residence including supervised public or private shelters that provide temporary accommodations, institutional settings providing temporary shelter, or public or private places that are not designed for or used as a regular sleeping accommodation for human beings (e.g., cars, parks, campgrounds). Incarcerated individuals, however, are not considered homeless under this definition (National Coalition for the Homeless [NCH], 2009p).

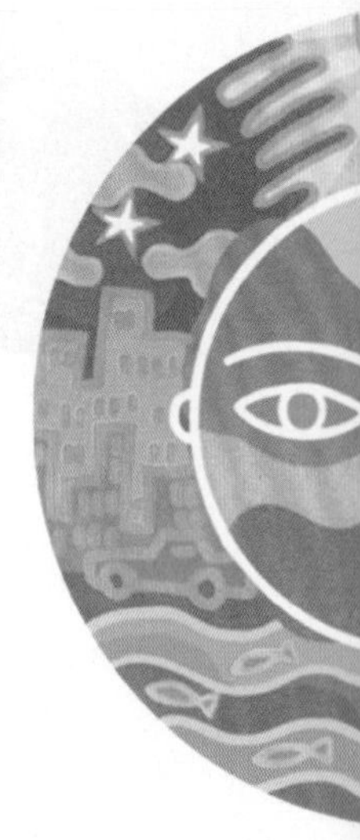

The education subtitle of the McKinney–Vento Homeless Assistance Act expands on the definition of homelessness when addressing homeless children and youth. The act includes as homeless those children who share housing with others due to economic hardship or loss of housing, are abandoned in hospitals, are awaiting placement in foster care, or are living in motels, trailer parks, or camping grounds (United Stated Department of Education, 2004).

The Department of Housing and Urban Development interprets the McKinney–Vento definition of homeless to include only people living on the streets or in shelters or those facing imminent eviction (within 1 week). While this definition may be appropriate for the urban homeless who are more likely to live on the street or in shelters, persons living in rural areas tend to cohabit with relatives or friends in overcrowded, substandard housing (NCH, 2009p). Table 28-1 outlines selected *Healthy People 2020* goals that relate to the homeless population.

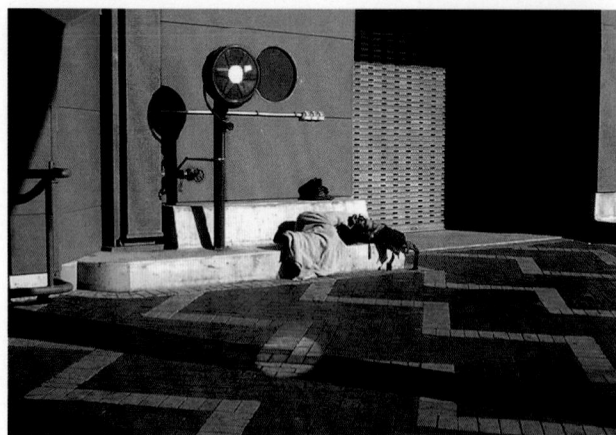

Most people think that homeless means only those living on the streets.

SCOPE OF THE PROBLEM

Poverty is directly related to homelessness. The increase in poverty and the growing shortage of affordable rental housing have led to a dramatic rise in homelessness over the past two decades (NCH, 2009p). It is difficult to estimate the number of people who are homeless, since homelessness is a temporary condition. Rather than trying to count the number of homeless people on a given day or week (**point-in-time counts**), it may be more prudent to measure the number of people who have been homeless over a longer time frame such as over the course of a year (**period prevalence counts**) (NCH, 2009j).

It is also difficult to locate and account for people who are homeless. Most estimates are based upon the number of people served in shelters or soup kitchens or the number of people who can easily be located on the streets. People who frequent places that are difficult to reach (e.g., cars, campgrounds, caves, boxcars) are considered **unsheltered (hidden) homeless**. Many people are unable to access shelters because of overcrowding and limited capacity. In rural areas, there are fewer housing options and resources for the homeless. As a result, people are forced to live temporarily with friends or family (a practice known as **doubling up**). While still experiencing homelessness, these individuals may not be counted in homeless statistics or considered eligible for homeless services (NCH, 2009j).

The United States Department of Housing and Urban Development (USDHUD), in its Annual Homeless Assessment Report to Congress, publishes the latest counts of homelessness nationwide. In 2009, on a single night in January, there were an estimated 643,067 sheltered and unsheltered homeless people across the nation. Approximately 1.56 million people used an emergency shelter or a transitional housing program during the 12-month period from October 1, 2008, to September 30, 2009. Homeless single adults represented 63% of the homeless population while 37% of the population was homeless families (USDHUD, 2010). Because of the transient nature of homelessness and the difficulty involved in locating and counting the homeless, it is unlikely that researchers will ever be able to estimate the exact magnitude of homelessness in America (NCH, 2009j).

In 2009, the United States Conference of Mayors' Task Force on Hunger and Homelessness reported its

Table 28.1 Selected *Healthy People 2020* Goals Related to Homelessness

Overarching goals	Attain high-quality, longer lives free of preventable disease, disability, injury, and premature death. Achieve health equity, eliminate disparities, and improve the health of all groups. Create social and physical environments that promote good health for all. Promote quality of life, healthy development, and healthy behaviors across all life stages.
Related access to care objectives	Increase the proportion of insured persons with coverage for clinical preventive services. Increase the proportion of persons with a usual primary care provider. Increase the number of practicing primary care providers. Increase the proportion of persons who have a specific source of ongoing care. Reduce the proportion of individuals who are unable to obtain or delay in obtaining necessary medical care, dental care, or prescription medicines. Increase the proportion of persons who receive appropriate evidence-based clinical preventive services. Increase the proportion of persons who have access to rapidly responding prehospital emergency medical services. Reduce the proportion of hospital emergency department visits in which the wait time to see an emergency department clinician exceeds the recommended time frame.

Source: *Healthy People 2020* (n.d. a). *Healthy People goals.* Retrieved from http://www.healthypeople.gov/2020/

survey findings of 27 cities across the nation. Sixteen cities, or 64% of respondents, reported a leveling off or a decrease in the number of homeless individuals over the past year. This decline is attributed to the success of public policies aimed at ending chronic homelessness among single adults and individuals with disabilities. Nineteen cities, or 76% of respondents, reported an increase in the number of families who were homeless. This finding was attributed to the economic recession and a lack of affordable housing (U.S. Conference of Mayors, 2009). Similar findings were reported in the 2009 Annual Homeless Assessment Report to Congress with the number of sheltered homeless families increasing and the number of sheltered homeless individuals declining (USDHUD, 2010).

DEMOGRAPHICS

Poverty is directly linked to homelessness. Demographic groups more likely to be poor are also at greater risk of becoming homeless.

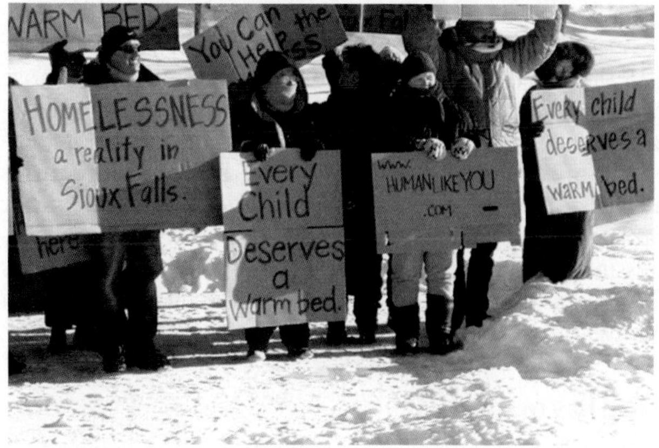
HOMELESSNESS
a reality in
Sioux Falls.
Every
Child
Deserves
a
Warm bed.
www.
HUMANLIKEYOU
.COM
Every child
deserves a
WARM bed.

Homelessness affects a wide variety of people, and support is needed from community members to address this issue. (Photo courtesy of USA. gov.)

Age

In 2009, 78% of all sheltered homeless persons were adults age 18 and older. Thirty-eight percent were between 31 and 50 years old. Only 2.8% of the sheltered homeless population was 62 years old or older. Even so, there was a slight increase in the percentage of homeless adults over age 50. This finding is consistent with the aging baby boomer population. The array of social safety net programs for the elderly may help older persons retain stable housing and avoid the need for emergency or transitional shelter. Homeless children residing in shelters tend to be young. More than half are <6 years old (USDHUD, 2010).

Gender

The majority of homeless individuals are unaccompanied adult men. Single homeless adults are more likely to be male. Approximately 64% of sheltered homeless adults are men and 36% are women. The large proportion of adult men in homeless shelters may be attributed to the inability of men to qualify for publicly funded safety net programs that are designed to target the needs of families with children and the elderly, the lack of unemployment insurance protection, the high rate of substance abuse, and the increased likelihood of incarceration. However, 80% of adults who are homeless with children are women. Women in families with incomes below poverty level are twice as likely to use a shelter as their male counterparts (USDHUD, 2010).

Ethnicity

The racial and ethnic makeup of the homeless population varies based upon geographic location. Nationally, approximately 38% of the sheltered homeless are White, non-Hispanic while approximately 38% are Black or

African American. When compared to their housed counterparts nationwide, the sheltered homeless are more likely to be adult males, African Americans, veterans, unaccompanied, and disabled (USDHUD, 2010). In rural areas, the homeless are more likely to be White, Native American, or migrant workers (NCH, 2009p).

Families

Families with children constitute the fastest-growing segment of the homeless population. Families with children represent 34% of the homeless sheltered population in the United States. Sixty-one percent of homeless people in families are children under 18. The increase in families seeking shelter is attributed to the ongoing effect of the economic recession. While most sheltered homeless families are headed by single women, in 2009, there was a slight increase in the percentage of men in homeless families. Because of the recession, more two-parent families and families headed by single fathers are becoming homeless. Since most homeless provider organizations serving families are geared to serving single women with children, it can be harder for intact families and families headed by men to access shelter (USDHUD, 2010).

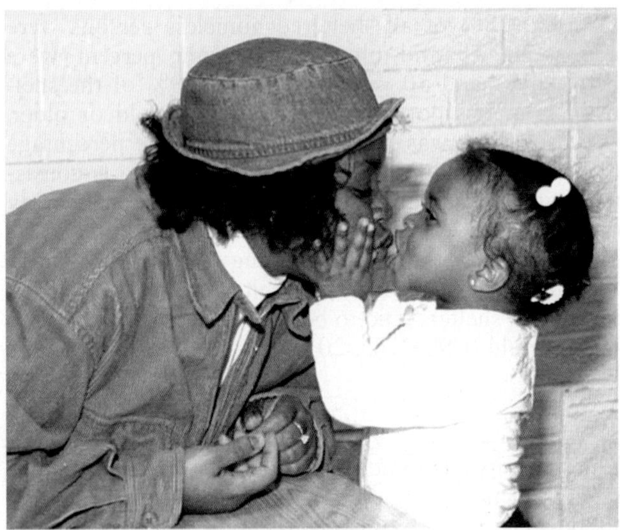

Most families seeking shelter most often comprise single mothers with children. (Photo courtesy of USA. gov.)

CONTRIBUTING FACTORS

Persons are predisposed to homelessness because of a complex array of factors that result in individuals having to choose between necessities of daily living. Scarce resources limit choices. What would you do if you had to choose between eating and buying your child's medication? Housing consumes a huge portion of one's income and is often the first asset to be lost. Many families find they are only a paycheck away from homelessness.

Poverty

In 2007, 12.5% of the US population (37.3 million people) lived in poverty. Thirty-six percent of these individuals were children. The increase in poverty rates over recent years may be attributed to declining wages, loss of jobs that offer security and carry benefits, an increase in temporary and part-time employment, erosion of the true value of the minimum wage, a decline in manufacturing jobs in favor of lower paying service jobs, globalization and outsourcing, and a decline in public assistance. As wages drop, the potential to secure adequate housing wanes (NCH, 2009c, 2009q).

The problem is compounded by a lack of affordable housing (particularly **single room occupancy (SRO) housing** or housing units intended to be occupied by one person) and limited funding for housing assistance. The USDHUD estimates that the 2010 Fair Market Rent for a two-bedroom apartment in the United States has increased 45% since the 2000 census. A household seeking to rent a two-bedroom apartment needs to earn at least $18.44 per hour to afford the unit. The federal minimum wage was $7.25 in 2010 (National Low Income Housing Coalition, 2010). As rental costs have increased and the number of available low-rent units declined and as federal support for housing assistance has dropped off, the housing gap has widened. People have been forced to pay high rents to obtain shelter. This situation leads to overcrowding and substandard housing (NCH, 2009d).

People applying for public housing must often wait years before a rental unit becomes available. In major cities, individuals may wait up to 10 years to secure housing (NCH, 2009d). As a result, people remain in shelter situations for a longer period of time. With the reduced turnover of shelter beds, shelters running at capacity are forced to turn people away.

Lack of Affordable Health Care

In the absence of affordable health care coverage a serious illness or disability can lead to job loss, savings depletion, and even eviction. Slightly over two thirds of sheltered homeless adults report having a disability. One third of sheltered homeless persons have a chronic substance abuse issue, and one quarter report a severe mental illness (USDHUD, 2010).

In 2007, approximately 45.7 million Americans (15.3% of the population) were without health care coverage. Fewer than 25% of people with salaries under $25,000 have health insurance (NCH, 2009e). Those who can qualify for medical assistance may be reluctant to seek employment, fearing termination of benefits. Many others have limited coverage, which requires higher copays or deductibles and does not cover major catastrophic illnesses. Half of all personal bankruptcies in the United States are a result of health problems (NCH, 2009e). A catastrophic adverse health event can plunge one into a homeless condition.

Employment

Many low-wage earners hold jobs with nonstandard work arrangements. Temporary employees, day laborers, independent contractors, and part-time employees are examples of work arrangements that tend to pay lower wages, offer little or no benefits, and have less job security. For persons with little or no job skills, it is virtually impossible to compete for jobs that offer a living wage. Barriers to employment among the homeless include lack of education and job skills; lack of transportation, day care, or other supportive services; lack of access to technology; and disabilities that make it difficult to pursue or retain employment. To overcome homelessness and maintain employment, one must not only obtain a job that pays a living wage but also must have access to supportive services such as child care and transportation (NCH, 2009c).

Domestic Violence

For victims of domestic violence, often the choice is between living in an abusive situation or leaving and facing life on the streets. Approximately 63% of homeless women have experienced domestic violence (NCH, 2009a). Twelve percent of the US homeless sheltered population reported being victims of domestic violence (USDHUD, n.d. a, 2010). Women who are victims of domestic violence may lack the resources needed to become independent and escape an abusive environment. The lack of affordable housing, long waiting lists for housing and social services, and limited capacity of shelters to accommodate families in crisis only serve to exacerbate the problem (NCH, 2009a).

Mental Illness

Twenty-five percent of the sheltered homeless report a severe mental illness (USDHUD, 2010). **Deinstitutionalization** (being released from institutions into the community), limited access to services, difficulty carrying out essential activities of daily living, and difficulty maintaining stable relationships contribute to the number of severely mentally ill persons represented in the homeless population (NCH, 2009m).

Poor mental health adversely affects an individual's ability to make sound judgments, solve problems effectively, and make wise decisions. Persons with mental illness may neglect to take the necessary precautions to avoid or reduce their risk of illness. Some mentally ill persons self-medicate their disturbing symptoms using street drugs, placing them at increased risk of addictions and diseases transmitted through injection drug use. Mental illness and substance abuse are often comorbid conditions, which, coupled with poor physical health, make it especially difficult to secure employment and safe, affordable housing (NCH, 2009m).

Addictions Disorders

Rates of alcohol and drug abuse are disproportionately high among the homeless; one third of the sheltered homeless in the United States report substance abuse problems (USDHUD, 2010). For persons already at risk for homelessness, the behaviors associated with an addictive disorder can create instability and jeopardize family and employment support nets. Once homeless, persons may resort to drugs or alcohol to dull the pain of being homeless and ease the feelings of hopelessness that accompany such a desperate state. They may also turn to chemical substances in an attempt to self-medicate the disturbing symptoms of an untreated mental illness.

While some homeless individuals may desire treatment to overcome their addictions, they often encounter obstacles that undermine their recovery and prevent them from obtaining the treatment they need. Limited access to care and lack of community resources make it difficult if not impossible to receive the services needed to achieve a successful recovery. There may be long waiting lists for addictions treatment, and homeless people who do not have a phone and are difficult to locate may be dropped from the waiting list. Lack of transportation and lack of documentation needed to access programs (i.e., birth certificates, social security cards) further exacerbate the problem. Denial of Supplemental Security Income (SSI) or Social Security Disability Insurance (SSDI) and Medicaid to persons with substance abuse–related disabilities creates a huge barrier to achieving recovery support, proper medical care, and housing and income assistance. Moreover, the federal programs targeting homelessness, mental health, and addictions services lack the extent of funding necessary to exert an impact that would effectively address this problem on a national level (NCH, 2009o).

Additional Variables

Additional variables impacting homelessness include personal or financial crisis, natural disasters, or personal choice. For example, Hurricanes Katrina and Rita, which devastated portions of the Gulf Coast in 2005, displaced many previously independent and self-sufficient individuals and families, rendering many homeless and in need of emergency shelter.

HOMELESS SUBPOPULATIONS

While many of the struggles facing the homeless are universal, there are subpopulations within the homeless community that are uniquely vulnerable. Often, these groups face additional burdens because of their special needs and challenges.

Homeless Men

Approximately 64% of homeless adults are men (USDHUD, 2010). The majority of homeless men are single adults. Homeless men are more likely to be employed than their homeless female counterparts. However, they usually hold temporary, low-wage jobs that offer little security. They are also more likely than homeless women to have uncontrolled substance abuse issues. This makes it more difficult for them to access shelters that require abstinence for admission (NCH, 2009o; National Health Care for the Homeless Council (NHCHC), 2001; USDHUD, 2010).

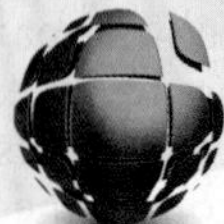

EVIDENCE-BASED PRACTICE

End-of-Life Care for the Homeless

How do we prepare homeless persons to make end-of-life decisions? Is it important for the homeless to complete advance directives?

Song and colleagues (2008), in a prospective, randomized pilot trial, compared whether a homeless population was more likely to complete an advance directive after receiving one-on-one guidance from a counselor or from using self-guided materials. They also studied whether the completion of an advance directive resulted in a change in attitudes and beliefs regarding end-of-life care among the homeless population. A convenience sample of 59 homeless individuals aged 18 or older with a high school education or higher participated in the study. The sample was obtained from a drop-in center for homeless individuals in Minnesota.

Participants completed a baseline survey regarding their knowledge, attitude, and behaviors surrounding end-of-life care and advance care planning. Subjects were randomized into two groups: one group received self-guided materials on advance directives while the second group received one-on-one guidance from a counselor. A 3-month follow-up study was conducted to determine whether study participants had completed an advanced directive.

The study found that persons who received one-on-one counseling were more likely to complete an advance directive than persons who received self-guided materials. Moreover, subjects who completed an advance directive were more likely to believe that an advance directive would ensure that their end-of-life wishes were fulfilled in the health care setting and were more likely to voice plans to document and discuss their wishes about end-of-life care with others.

What can the community health nurse do to increase awareness among health and social service providers of the need to promote end-of-life planning with homeless clients? What would you say to a colleague who believes it is a waste of time because of the "poor rates of document completion" among the homeless or because "it is difficult for a homeless person to keep track of such paperwork"? How could an intervention, such as providing end-of-life advance care planning, empower persons who are alienated from loved ones and more fearful of how they will be cared for by health professionals? What additional research is needed in this area? Do you believe that improved advance directive completion rates in the homeless will ultimately result in better end-of-life care?

Song, J., Wall, M., Ratner, E., Bartels, D. M., Ulvestad, N., & Gelberg, L. (2008). Engaging homeless persons in end-of-life preparations. *Journal of General Internal Medicine*, 23(12), 2031–2045.

Some men find themselves in a cycle of intermittent homelessness as they move back and forth between prisons, treatment centers, shelters, temporary housing, and the streets. Other men are at risk for becoming **chronically homeless**. These men may have significant health problems due to chronic substance abuse, lack of shelter, and poor access to health and social services (National Alliance to End Homelessness, 2010a; NHCHC, 2001). A chronically homeless adult is someone who has been homeless for long periods of time or has experienced repeated episodes of homelessness. In 2009, the Annual Homeless Assessment Report to Congress identified 110,917 chronically homeless individuals in its point-in-time count. Fifty-eight percent of these individuals were unsheltered (i.e., living on the street or in places not fit for human habitation). Overall, 27% of all homeless individuals experience chronic homelessness (USDHUD, 2010).

Homeless men are more likely to be treated with disdain than other homeless subgroups. Some people perceive the homeless male as largely to blame for his plight, believing that he is able bodied and should be able to work. Moreover, homeless men may not suffer from disabilities severe enough to warrant eligibility for health and social services. Often, health and social programs give priority to women and children. Single, low-income men do not qualify for medical assistance unless they are disabled (NHCHC, 2001).

Homeless Women

Thirty-six percent of all sheltered homeless persons in the United States in 2009 were women. In 2009, nearly 80% of sheltered adults in families with children were women (USDHUD, 2010). Many homeless women have experienced physical or sexual assault at some point in their lives. Domestic violence is a cause for homelessness among women. Approximately 63% of homeless women have experienced domestic violence (NCH, 2009a). Twelve percent of the homeless sheltered population in the United States reported being victims of domestic violence (USDHUD, 2010).

Lack of affordable housing forces many women to choose between living in an abusive home or facing life on the streets. Domestic violence victims often have poor credit and employment records due to the disruption caused by family violence. If violence is discovered in the home, landlords may evict tenants, forcing the family onto the streets (NCH, 2009a). Once on the street, a woman faces the risk of greater abuse. Moreover, the potential for exposure to violence and sexual assault on the streets increases the risk for sexually transmitted infections and traumatic injuries.

Homeless Children

Three of every two hundred children in America are homeless (NCH, 2009b). Homeless families are one of the fastest growing segments of the homeless population. Most of these families are headed by single female head of households. Poverty, lack of affordable housing, domestic violence, mental illness, and substance abuse contribute to the growing trend in family homelessness. Nearly 53% of homeless children in shelters are under age 6 (USDHUD, 2010). Much of the increase in family homelessness over recent years is from families who have become homeless for the first time (USDHUD, 2010).

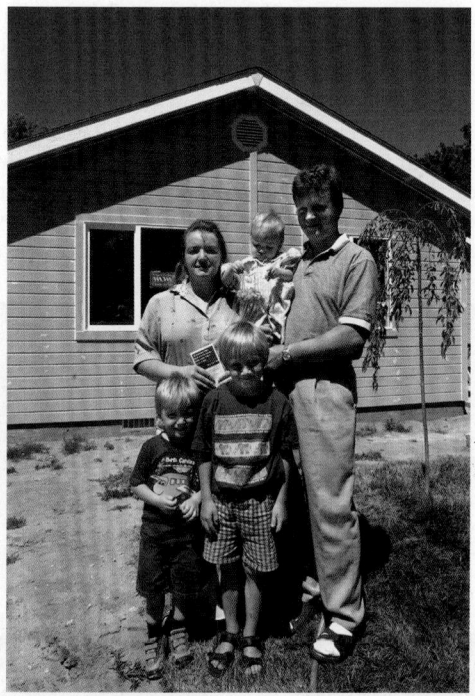

Promoting affordable housing is one area in which communities can be helpful in preventing homelessness. (Photo courtesy of USA. gov.)

The majority of homeless children and youth live in shelters, share housing with friends or relatives, or live in motels or campgrounds. When compared to their housed counterparts, homeless children are four times more likely to become ill, are twice as likely to go hungry, and have three times the rate of emotional and behavioral problems. They are four times more likely to be developmentally delayed and twice as likely to have learning disabilities. By age 12, the majority of homeless children have been exposed to violence and 25% have witnessed violent acts within their own families (National Center on Family Homelessness [NCFH], 2010; NCH, 2009g).

One in six homeless children has suffered emotional disturbances, often due to the effects of traumatic stress and violence. Depression, anxiety, fear, and aggressive and antisocial behavior are common among homeless children who are victims of violence (NCFH, 2009).

Education is compromised when one is homeless (NCH, 2009b). Although approximately 87% of homeless children are enrolled in school, only about 77% attend regularly. Barriers to education include transportation to and from the shelter, lack of academic and medical records required for registration, unstable living arrangements necessitating multiple moves, and urgent needs for food and shelter that take priority over education (NCH, 2009b).

Homeless children are more likely to get sick than other children. They have lower birth weights as infants and often require specialty care at birth. Common health complaints include ear infections, asthma, stomach problems, and speech difficulties. Homeless children experience high rates of obesity due to nutritional deficiencies and have poorer access to medical and dental care. They are twice as likely as their housed counterparts to repeat a grade in school, be expelled or suspended, or drop out of high school. Fewer than 25% of homeless children graduate from high school (NCFH, 2010).

Homeless Youth

Homeless youth are persons under 18 who lack parental, foster, or institutional care. Homeless adolescents are sometimes referred to as **unaccompanied youth** (NCH, 2008). The National Alliance to End Homelessness estimates that as many as 50,000 US youth are living on the streets (National Alliance to End Homelessness, 2010b).

Factors contributing to youth homelessness include physical and sexual abuse, family addiction, parental neglect, strained relationships, or family financial crises that lead to family separation due to inadequate shelter, housing, or child welfare resources. A history of foster care placement is positively correlated with homelessness among youth. Moreover, some youth who are discharged from residential or foster care with inadequate housing or income support may find themselves homeless (NCH, 2008).

Homeless adolescents may have difficulty accessing emergency shelter because of shelter policies that prohibit older youth from the facility or because of a lack of bed space. Due to lack of education or job training skills, many resort to prostitution or **survival sex** (exchanging sex for food, shelter, or other basic necessities). As a result, homeless youth are at higher risk for HIV, hepatitis, and sexually transmitted infections. Homeless youth also suffer disproportionately from anxiety, depression, malnutrition, conduct disorders, posttraumatic stress, and low self-esteem (NCH, 2008).

It is not uncommon for homeless youths to be arrested for running away, breaking curfews, or being without supervision. As young people age out of the foster care system or are released from juvenile detention facilities, they find themselves on the street with inadequate support systems and little opportunity for housing or employment (National Alliance to End Homelessness, 2010b).

Homeless Families

Poverty and the lack of affordable housing place families at risk of becoming homeless. Declining wages, changes in welfare programs, unstable employment, domestic violence, and a struggling economy have all contributed to the rise in family homelessness.

Nearly 80% of sheltered homeless families are headed by women. Homelessness often breaks up the family unit. Families may be separated by shelter policies that prohibit admission to older boys or men. Sometimes, parents are forced to leave their children with family or friends or to place them in foster care to shelter them from becoming homeless (NCH, 2009g).

A child is at greater risk for homelessness if his father becomes injured or ill, experiences a job loss, has a substance abuse issue, or becomes involved with the criminal justice system. Fifty percent of fathers of homeless children are unemployed, and forty-three percent have problems with drugs or alcohol. Homeless children are at a high risk of being placed in foster care, and a personal history of foster care predicts family homelessness during adulthood. To assist homeless families, attention must be focused on promoting affordable housing; supporting education, job training, and child care for parents; promoting access to school; expanding violence prevention and treatment services; and preventing unnecessary separation of families (NCFH, 2009; NCH, 2009g).

Homeless Veterans

According to the 2009 Annual Homeless Assessment Report to Congress, 13% of sheltered homeless adults are veterans (USDHUD, 2010). The National Coalition for the Homeless reports that 23% of the homeless population is veterans. On a given night, between 130,000 and 200,000 veterans are homeless (NCH, 2009h).

Female homeless veterans represent about 3% of the homeless veteran population. They are more likely to be married and have serious psychiatric illnesses but less likely to be employed or have addictions disorders than their homeless male counterparts. There is no difference in rates of mental illness or addictions between veteran and nonveteran homeless women (NCH, 2009h).

The U.S. Department of Veteran Affairs administers the Domiciliary Care for Homeless Veterans Program, which provides long-term care to homeless veterans and provides shelter, 2-year transitional housing, group homes, and work therapy for homeless veterans. These programs provide case management, residential treatment, and other services to homeless veterans and improve housing, employment, and access to care for the homeless veteran population. Unfortunately, the programs are often unable to keep pace with existing needs (NCH, 2009h).

The Rural Homeless

Homeless people in rural areas are more likely to be White, female, married, working, homeless for the first time, and homeless for a shorter length of time. Because there are fewer shelters in rural areas, they are also less likely to live in shelters or in the streets. They are more likely to be found in cars or campers or living with relatives in substandard or overcrowded housing. As a result, they may not be considered "homeless" for reporting purposes. Moreover, the communities in which they live may not be able to access as much federal funding, because the statistics do not adequately reflect the magnitude of the problem. Families with single mothers and children comprise the largest segment of the rural homeless population. Native Americans and migrant workers are more likely to be among the rural homeless. Like urban homelessness, rural homelessness is largely a result of poverty and lack of affordable housing. While housing costs are lower in rural areas, incomes are also lower (NCH, 2009n).

Homelessness in rural areas may be precipitated by structural or physical housing problems that force families to relocate to safer but more expensive housing. In addition, the lack of job opportunities, the distance between low-income housing and job sites, the lack of transportation, rising rents, geographic isolation, and lack of resources compound the problem. To address the needs of the rural homeless, the definition of homelessness needs to be expanded to include people living in temporary or substandard housing (NCH, 2009n).

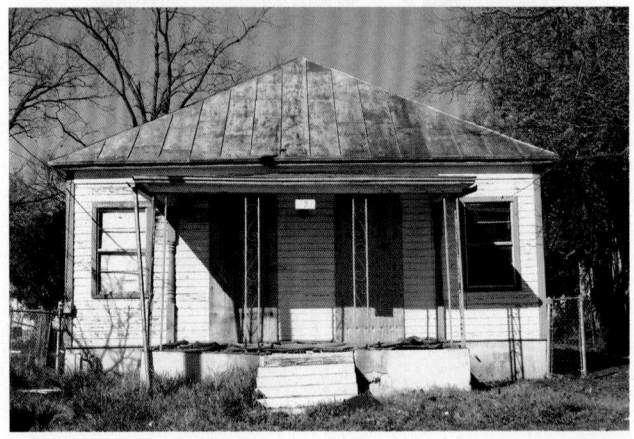

In rural areas of the country, housing may be substandard, and affordable housing may be lacking. (Photo courtesy of USA.gov.)

The Older Homeless

As with other groups, the increase in homelessness among older Americans is due in part to poverty and the lack of affordable housing. Many older people live on a fixed income. This renders them more vulnerable to unexpected financial crisis and even homelessness. Isolation also contributes to homelessness. Many older people live alone and lack a support network. Some researchers define the "older homeless" as homeless persons age 50 and older because of the declining physical health that accompanies street living. Approximately 17% of sheltered homeless persons are age 51 or older (USDHUD, 2010). Since older persons tend to distrust crowds at shelters and clinics, they are more likely to stay on the streets. They are prone to criminal victimization and suffer from a variety of health conditions including chronic diseases and functional disabilities. The Social Security benefits to which many are entitled are inadequate to cover housing costs. They may also encounter difficulties applying for benefits (NCH, 2009i).

Lesbian, Gay, Bisexual, and Transgender Homeless

Lesbian, gay, bisexual, and transgender (LGBT) persons often experience difficulty finding shelters that accept them. They are sometimes required to identify themselves as a particular gender. Transgender individuals may be turned away from shelters or subjected to physical, sexual, or verbal abuse. Twenty percent of homeless youth are LGBT. LGBT youth are twice as likely to experience sexual abuse before the age of 12 when compared with their heterosexual, homeless counterparts. They are over seven times more likely to experience sexual violence and commit suicide at much higher rates (62%) than heterosexual homeless youth (29%) (NCH, 2009l).

HEALTH CARE AND THE HOMELESS

Acute and chronic health problems are prevalent among the homeless population. Chronic health conditions such as HIV/AIDS, diabetes, hypertension, addictions, and mental disorders require ongoing monitoring and are often difficult to treat in a population that is transient and lacks stable housing (NCH, 2009e). It is difficult for the homeless to adhere to complex treatment regimens. For example, where would a homeless person find a refrigerator to store insulin? Where would someone keep supplies for dressings? How could someone with no access to transportation keep regular appointments with health care providers? How does a homeless person keep track of multiple appointment dates? How is a shelter resident who receives the typical shelter diet high in carbohydrates, fats, and sodium to adhere to a low-salt or diabetic diet?

Many homeless people expend their time and energy trying to meet basic survival needs. Health care may take a back seat to finding food, clothing, or shelter. High costs and limited access to health care and negative experiences with the health care system can also result in avoidance or delays in seeking treatment (NHCHC, n.d.).

Frostbite, leg ulcers, and upper respiratory tract infections result from chronic exposure to adverse environmental conditions. The homeless are also at higher risk of trauma and criminal victimization including muggings, beatings, and rape. When one is homeless, it is difficult to maintain adequate nutrition or personal hygiene or to have access to basic first aid (NCH, 2009e, 2009f, 2010a, 2010b, 2010c). Communicable diseases such as TB, HIV, hepatitis, and other infections threaten not only the homeless but also the public in general.

Poverty, substance abuse, poor nutrition, and coexisting medical and psychiatric illnesses also predispose the homeless to severe oral health problems. Persons with poor access to dental treatment and preventive services have higher rates of oral disease. Poor oral health is also associated with lower levels of education and income (*Healthy People 2020*, n.d. b.).

Persons with HIV/AIDS are at higher risk of homelessness, because HIV-related illness can impact job stability. Moreover, health care costs associated with treating the illness can exact an enormous financial burden on a low-income family. Insufficient funds to adequately house the poor with HIV/AIDS may also contribute to homelessness among HIV-infected individuals. The prevalence of HIV among the homeless is three times greater than that of the general population. Homeless women and adolescents are at risk of acquiring HIV infection due to the high incidence of sexual abuse and exploitation in this population (NCH, 2009f).

"Health Care for the Homeless" was a model for homeless health care developed in 1985 through a 19-city demonstration project funded by the Robert Wood Johnson Foundation and the Pew Memorial Trust. In 1987, federal legislation (the McKinney Homeless Assistance Act) was passed that authorized federal funding for these programs (NHCHC, n.d.). Grants are awarded to community-based organizations that deliver high-quality health care to homeless populations. Health Care for the Homeless projects still exist across the nation to address significant gaps in health care delivery for this vulnerable group in society.

RESOURCES TO COMBAT HOMELESSNESS

Both public and private sectors have promoted a variety of initiatives to address the problem of homelessness. These initiatives are intended to impact homelessness on the local, state, and national level and to insure a coordinated, comprehensive, and systematic approach to addressing the problem of homelessness.

Public Sector

The McKinney–Vento Homeless Assistance Act (PL100-77) was the first and only major piece of federal legislation intended to address the problem of homelessness on a national level. This landmark legislation act, passed by congress in 1987, originally consisted of 15 programs to address the major, pressing needs of the homeless. These needs included emergency shelter, transitional housing, job training, primary health care, education, and housing (NCH, 2006, 2010c). The current act has been amended four times in an effort to expand its scope and strengthen its impact. In particular, the amendments made to the act in 1990 represented significant milestones in advocating for the needs of the homeless. These amendments included the creation of the Shelter Care Plus Program, which provided for housing assistance for persons with disabilities, mental illness, AIDS, and drug and alcohol addiction. Another amendment created a demonstration program within the Health Care for the Homeless Program to provide primary care and outreach to at-risk and homeless children. In addition, the Community Mental Health Services Program was amended and retitled the Projects for Assistance in Transition from Homelessness (PATH). Finally, the amendments made in 1990 strengthened access to public education for homeless children and youth. For example, states were required to provide grant funding to local educational institutions to insure access to a free, appropriate education for homeless youth and children (NCH, 2006).

Over the years, congress has appropriated funding to enable implementation of this federal legislation. The extent of federal funding has fluctuated over the years. In recent years, some of the programs have been repealed or restructured in an effort to contain costs. While homeless advocates acknowledge that the act was an important step in addressing homelessness, the lack of adequate funding over recent years threatens its impact on a national level. Moreover, some homeless advocates feel that the legislation focuses more on emergency measures to address the crisis of homelessness rather than on promoting a proactive agenda to address the causes of homelessness (e.g., lack of good paying jobs with benefits, lack of access to affordable health care) (NCH, 2006).

The USDHUD oversees a number of programs that provide supportive housing for elderly, low-income, and disabled persons. The department also funds programs to build, buy, or rehabilitate affordable housing units for rent or ownership (NCH, 2009d; USDHUD, n.d. b). In many communities, housing is based on a **continuum of care** model where programs are developed to assist persons to transition from emergency to transitional to permanent housing. In recent years, a **Housing First** philosophy has guided much of the publicly funded housing initiatives. In a Housing First approach, housing is viewed as an immediate priority. The goal of Housing First is to prevent homelessness or to rapidly rehouse individuals who have become homeless. Housing or supportive services are not contingent upon adherence to rigid rules or policies or to the maintenance of sobriety (U.S. Interagency Council on Homelessness, 2010b).

Under the Obama administration, several important pieces of federal legislation impacting the homeless were passed. The American Recovery and Reinvestment Act of 2009 established a $1. 5 billion Homelessness Prevention and Rapid Re-housing Program (HPRP), which was enacted to assist those who are homeless, or at risk of becoming homeless, to pay rent and other housing expenses (NCH, 2010a). The Homeless Emergency Assistance and Rapid Transition to Housing (HEARTH) Act of 2009 increased funding for McKinney–Vento Programs, which provide emergency, transitional, and permanent housing and supportive services to the homeless.

On March 23, 2010, President Barack Obama signed federal health care reform legislation into law that extends health insurance coverage to 32 million uninsured Americans by 2019. This legislation will enable homeless individuals to secure health care coverage (NCH, 2010d).

Another significant milestone in federal initiatives to reduce homelessness occurred in 2001 when the federal government adopted the goal of ending chronic homelessness in 10 years. To meet this goal, annual funding was appropriated to create new permanent supportive housing. These resources helped to stimulate the production of housing. Many communities followed the lead of the federal government and developed their own 10-year plans (Burt, 2006).

In 2010, the U.S. Interagency Council on Homelessness published the nation's first comprehensive federal strategic plan to prevent and end homelessness. The document, entitled "Opening Doors," outlined a comprehensive and ambitious plan aimed at eliminating homelessness on a national level. The goals of the plan included ending chronic homelessness in 10 years; preventing and ending homelessness for families, youth, and children in 10 years; preventing and ending homelessness among veterans in 5 years; and establishing a path to end all types of homelessness (U.S. Interagency Council on Homelessness, 2010b). Table 28-2 summarizes the nine titles of the McKinney–Vento Act, and Table 28-3 presents selected federally sponsored programs for addressing the needs of the homeless.

Private Sector

The private sector has made a concerted effort to organize communities in the battle against homelessness by forming coalitions, alliances, and memberships that champion the causes of the homeless. These organized efforts are carried out at the national, state, and local level to positively impact the problem of homelessness in communities across the nation. Table 28-4 presents a list and description of selected resources in the private sector to combat homelessness.

ROLE OF THE COMMUNITY HEALTH NURSE

Community health nurses maintain a long tradition of providing care to vulnerable populations and play a vital role in addressing the health needs of the homeless. Settings for care include shelters, clinics, soup kitchens, churches, community centers, social service agencies, and even the streets See From the Case Files I.

Trust is an essential ingredient in the development of a therapeutic relationship with the homeless. A caring, consistent relationship is more likely to engage people who are homeless into treatment. It is sometimes difficult to establish trust with clients who have experienced negative encounters with the health care system. Often, these negative perceptions are intensified by limited resources, inadequate access to care, or prejudicial views. As with other vulnerable populations, the homeless struggle with feelings of powerlessness, loss of control, and low self-esteem. Victim blaming is common.

Table 28.2 McKinney–Vento Homeless Assistance Act Titles I to IX

Title I	Statement of findings by Congress and definition of homelessness.
Title II	Establishes the Interagency Council on Homelessness, a council comprised of 15 heads of federal agencies charged with providing leadership for activities that assist the homeless.
Title III	Authorizes the Emergency Food and Shelter Program, administered by the Federal Emergency Management Agency (FEMA).
Title IV	Authorizes the emergency shelter and transitional housing programs administered by the Department of Housing and Urban Development (HUD) including the Emergency Shelter Grant Program, the Supportive Housing Demonstration Program, Supplemental Assistance for Facilities to Assist the Homeless, and Section 8 Single Room Occupancy Moderate Rehabilitation.
Title V	Requires federal agencies to make available land and buildings for states, local governments, and agencies to use to assist the homeless.
Title VI	Authorizes programs to provide health care services to the homeless, including Health Care for the Homeless Program, Community Mental Health Services Block Grant Program, and two demonstration programs providing substance abuse and mental health treatment services to the homeless.
Title VII	Authorizes the Adult Education for the Homeless Program, the Education of Homeless Children and Youth Program (administered by the Department of Education), the Job Training for the Homeless Demonstration Program (administered by the Department of Labor), and the Emergency Community Services Homeless Grant Program (administered by the Department of Health and Human Services).
Title VIII	Amends the Food Stamp Program to facilitate access by the homeless and expands the Temporary Emergency Food Assistance Program (administered by the Department of Agriculture).
Title IX	Extends the Veterans Job Training Act.

Source: United States Department of Housing and Urban Development (HUD). (2007). ***McKinney-Vento Act***. Retrieved from http://www.hud. gov/offices/cpd/homeless/lawsandregs/mckv.cfm

Table 28.3 Federally Sponsored Programs for the Homeless

The U.S. Interagency Council on Homelessness	The U.S. Interagency Council on Homelessness coordinates the federal response to homelessness and creates a national partnership with public and private sectors to reduce and end homelessness in the United States. The council is responsible for reviewing the effectiveness of federal initiatives and programs to assist the homeless, promoting better coordination of services between programs, and informing state and local governments and private sector organizations about sources of federal homeless assistance (U.S. Interagency Council on Homelessness, 2010a).
Substance Abuse and Mental Health Services Administration	The Center for Mental Health Services, a center of the federal Substance Abuse and Mental Health Services Administration (SAMSHA), supports programs to assist the homeless mentally ill to access primary care, substance abuse and mental health services, legal assistance, entitlements, and other supportive services. The center develops models for delivering mental health services to the homeless that programs can then adopt and use. It also provides funding to states to deliver mental health services (SAMHSA, 2010).
Center for Mental Health Services	The Center for Mental Health Services operates the Homeless Resource Center, which maintains a comprehensive data base of information and resources for homeless service providers and those caring for marginalized populations (SAMSHA, n.d.).
Projects for Assistance in Transition from Homelessness (PATH)	PATH is a grant program created under the McKinney Act to support the delivery of services to persons with severe mental illnesses, including those who are homeless or at risk of becoming homeless. SAMSHA provides technical support to states and local agencies providing care through the PATH program (SAMHSA, 2008).

(Continued)

Table 28.3 Federally Sponsored Programs for the Homeless *(Continued)*

Health Care for the Homeless (HCH)	The HCH program (a provision of the McKinney Act) awards grants to community-based organizations that seek to provide quality, accessible health care to the homeless. The HCH program is administered by the U.S. Department of Health and Human Services (USDHHS). HCH projects are required to provide primary health care, substance abuse services, emergency care, outreach, and housing assistance. Many HCH projects also provide dental care, mental health treatment, supportive housing, and other services (NCH, 2009e).
The U.S. Department of Housing and Urban Development (HUD)	HUD provides funding for supportive housing for low-income families, as well as low-income individuals with disabilities, and low-income elderly. Funds can be used for housing development or rental assistance (to cover the difference between what a resident can afford to pay and the cost to operate the project). Grants are also provided to public housing agencies to rehabilitate or replace dilapidated public housing structures. Persons applying for public housing face a long waiting period, sometimes as long as 10 y (NCH, 2009d).
The White House Office of Faith-based and Neighborhood Partnerships	The White House Office of Faith-based and Neighborhood Partnerships promotes partnerships with faith-based and community organizations to more effectively serve individuals, families, and communities in need. The Office provides information on federal grants that are available to faith-based and community organizations to address the needs of the homeless (USDHHS, n.d.).

Table 28.4 Private Sector Initiatives to Combat Homelessness

National Coalition for the Homeless (NCH)	The National Coalition for the Homeless is a national network of persons committed to preventing and ending homelessness. This coalition consists of homeless activists, service providers, persons who have experienced homelessness or are presently homeless, and others who are concerned with the plight of the homeless. The coalition works to address issues related to homelessness through activities that promote civil rights and economic, health care, and housing justice. Activities of the coalition include organizing community events to raise awareness and promote the rights of the homeless, advocating for health policy that protects the homeless, educating the public on facts related to homelessness, and providing research and technical assistance. The NCH also supports local and statewide homeless and housing coalitions (http://www.nationalhomeless.org).
The National Center on Family Homelessness	The National Center on Family Homelessness is a 501c3 nonprofit organization that seeks to end family homelessness in the United States through the development of innovative programs and services that provide long-term solutions for family homelessness and through education of service providers, policy makers, and the public (http://www.family homelessness.org).
National Coalition for Homeless Veterans	This coalition seeks to end homelessness among veterans through public policy, collaboration, and building community capacity (http://www.nchv.org).
National Alliance to End Homelessness	This national membership organization seeks to mobilize leaders in business, nonprofit agencies, service providers, political leaders, and citizens to end homelessness through research, education, and public policy reform (http://www.endhomelessness.org).
Commission on Homelessness and Poverty, American Bar Association	This commission works with local and state bar associations and other organizations to develop pro bono programs to address the legal needs of the poor and homeless (http://www.abanet.org/homeless).
National Low Income Housing Coalition	The National Low Income Housing Coalition is a national membership organization dedicated to ending the housing crisis in America. A major priority of the coalition is to promote legislation that provides funding for the production of rental housing for people with extremely low incomes (http://www.nlihc.org).

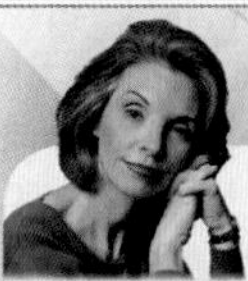

From the Case Files

Using the Nursing Process to Reach Out to Homeless Women and Children

Sheila Hendricks, a public health nurse for the Manchester City Health Department, and her colleagues were brainstorming ideas for how to reach the growing population of homeless women and children in their jurisdiction. They arranged a meeting with the director of a local rescue mission in the area. The mission provided emergency shelter to 100 homeless women and children each night. The women were allowed to remain at the shelter for 30 days provided they actively sought employment, social services, or educational opportunities. Families typically left during the day to seek jobs or other forms of assistance and returned in the evening for shelter. The community health nurses negotiated with the rescue mission to establish an on-site nursing clinic twice a week that would provide health education, screenings, and referrals on a drop-in basis. The hours of clinic operation were 4 PM to 8 PM to accommodate client schedules.

Assessment

After the clinic was in operation for 2 weeks, the following priority health issues began to emerge:

- Inadequate maternal and child nutrition
- Lack of primary health care services for women and children (i.e., immunizations, screenings, treatment for upper respiratory tract infections, dermatological problems, asthma, hypertension)
- Depression
- High rate of reported sexually transmitted infections and HIV due to history of violence, survival sex, and injection drug use
- Untreated addiction disorders

Plan

The following diagnoses were developed (in order of priority):

Impaired access to health and social services related to lack of insurance, scarce community-based resources, and lack of transportation

Ineffective family coping related to untreated addictions, mental health issues, and history of intimate partner violence

At risk for injury related to untreated addictions and mental health disorders, history of intimate partner violence, and hazards of street life

Altered nutrition less than body requirements related to lack of resources to purchase nutritious foods, addictions disorders, and chronic health issues

After assessing priority needs and establishing relevant diagnoses, the nurses developed a plan of care for this population. The priority goal was to promote access to care by linking clients to essential health and social services. The rationale for establishing this goal as a top priority was that if clients were able to access needed services, the other diagnoses could potentially be addressed (e.g., need for counseling, health care, housing, education).

Implementation

A nurse practitioner was engaged from the health department to provide primary care services to the women and children at the shelter including screening and treatment for sexually transmitted infections and treatment of common acute and chronic health conditions. Conditions requiring more extensive follow-up were referred to the local federally funded Health Care for the Homeless clinic. A social worker from the local social service agency was recruited to visit the mission on a monthly basis to assist clients to apply for housing and public assistance programs. Clients were referred to the local community mental health center for counseling related to addictions and violence issues. The nurses conducted health education programs and one-on-one counseling on topics such as parenting, coping, healthy eating, basic hygiene, and safety. They also offered health screenings for blood pressure, diabetes, HIV, and tuberculosis and provided referrals to the health department clinic for cancer screenings (i.e., mammograms, colorectal screening).

Evaluation

After the clinic had been in operation for 90 days, preliminary evaluation data revealed the following:

Sixty-five women and twenty-eight children had frequented the clinic over the past 3 months. All 65 women received health promotion teaching and a resource packet for further reference.

Eighty percent of clients who required referrals to outside agencies were successful in accessing care.

Twenty-five women and fifteen children were under the care of the nurse practitioner for acute or chronic health conditions.

Ten cases of latent TB infection were identified through TB testing, and these clients were referred to the City Health Department TB clinic for follow-up treatment.

Seven abnormal PAP smears were identified, and eight clients were diagnosed with sexually transmitted infections.

Fifteen clients were found to be HIV positive, and clients with positive screenings were referred to the City Health Department or the local Health Care for the Homeless Clinic where treatment was initiated.

Forty women applied for social service benefits. Most of these clients are still awaiting the receipt of benefits.

Some members of society perceive the homeless as responsible for their own fate. It is not uncommon to hear people speak about the homeless in derogatory terms or to suggest that the solution to the problem of homelessness is to simply "get a job."

Behaviors that would ordinarily be considered lawful in the privacy of one's home become criminal activity when they are exhibited in public. For example, the homeless can be arrested for loitering, sleeping, urinating, or drinking alcohol in public. These behaviors can trigger a criminal record; thereby jeopardizing future employment or housing opportunities. In some states, men can be incarcerated for failing to pay child support (NHCHC, 2001). Consider a man who is laid off from a low-wage job. He is unable to pay child support and is arrested. His violation generates a criminal record and compromises his ability to secure employment in the future. He becomes trapped in a cycle of poverty and homelessness that is difficult to escape.

Every nurse encounters new situations with prior assumptions, biases, and preunderstandings. When considering work with the homeless, it is important to clarify one's own beliefs and values about poverty, homelessness, addictions, and mental disorders. What has been your experience with the homeless? Have you ever observed a homeless individual asking for money or holding up signs at a busy intersection? What thoughts and feelings do encounters such as these provoke? Have you ever volunteered at a soup kitchen or food pantry, fed a group of homeless people, or donated food or clothing? Have you had the opportunity to get to know a homeless individual? Do you have a personal experience with homelessness or poverty? If so, how has it affected your understanding of what it means to be poor or homeless? See Perspectives: Voices From the Community.

It may be helpful to interview people who work with the homeless or to visit clinics, shelters, or other settings where the homeless congregate or access services. How are homeless people treated? What is a typical day like for someone who is homeless? How often do homeless persons hear their names? How often are they looked in the eye when addressed by others? How often are they touched in a way that is therapeutic, respectful, and affirming? By reflecting on your personal values and by allowing yourself to get closer to the people and places that are a part of the experience of homelessness, you will gain a deeper understanding of the homeless condition and be better equipped to serve those suffering from homelessness.

To effectively address the multifaceted problems associated with homelessness, a comprehensive and holistic approach is needed. As such, the community health nurse is responsible for implementing primary, secondary, and tertiary preventive measures to prevent homelessness or to assist those who are homeless to obtain needed services.

Primary Prevention

Primary prevention includes advocating for affordable housing, employment opportunities, and better access to health care to prevent the downward spiral into homelessness. Strategies for preventing homelessness may include financial counseling to assist clients to better manage their money, assistance in locating sources of legal or financial aid to prevent eviction (i.e., loans or grants for emergency funds to help pay for rent, utilities, etc.), or assistance in accessing social services, temporary housing, or health care to avoid a housing, health, or family crisis (Anderson & McFarlane, 2011).

Health education that addresses primary prevention may focus on positive parenting skills, violence prevention, anger management, coping skills, healthy eating, or principles of basic hygiene. Immunization programs

PERSPECTIVES: VOICES FROM THE COMMUNITY

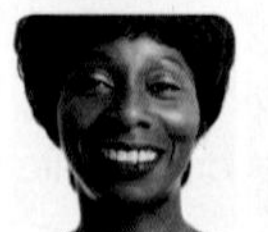

A Nurse's Viewpoint on Working with the Homeless

When I first decided to visit the homeless men's shelter, I was scared to death. Here I was, a veteran nurse with over 20 years experience in community health, and I was afraid. Afraid of what? I couldn't tell you. I suppose I harbored the stereotypes and negative images that most of us associate with homeless addicts. I remember passing this shelter years ago, looking out at the men hanging out on the street corner, and thinking to myself "Please God, don't let my car break down!" I remember thinking, "I would never step foot in a place like that."

Well, I believe God has a sense of humor. He was equipping me for a work I could never have imagined. My views about homelessness were challenged to the core when I peered into the faces of those men, heard their stories, and began to feel their pain. Theirs were stories of broken lives and lost hope but also of courage in the face of suffering and the will to survive in the midst of great adversity. These men were as diverse as their stories. They were from all walks of life. They possessed incredible gifts and talents. They were musicians, artisans, businessmen, writers, and poets. They had families who loved them and families who left them. Left because they could not continue to watch them die a little each day and be destroyed themselves in the process.

So here I am. Doing what I can to bring hope and healing. The irony is I came to bring hope and yet I am the one who is being healed. Healed in the broken areas of my life. Healed in my narrow view of life and my internal prejudices. I am so grateful to God for giving me this unique opportunity. It is a great privilege to serve these men.

—Rita, RN, age 42

will help to prevent communicable disease in this high-risk population. Counseling victims of intimate partner violence and helping them to locate safe shelter can also aid in the prevention of homelessness (Anderson & McFarlane, 2011). Addictions treatment is also important to prevent the likely consequences of untreated addiction: death, incarceration, institutionalization, or homelessness.

Secondary Prevention

The focus of secondary prevention measures is on the early detection and treatment of adverse health conditions. This requires a thorough assessment of client needs including the need for housing, health care, education, social services, and employment. Clients will also benefit from secondary prevention measures such as screening for communicable and chronic diseases (i.e., hepatitis, TB, STI, HIV, hypertension, diabetes, cancer).

Barriers to accessing services and the extent of community resources available to the homeless also need to be assessed (Anderson & McFarlane, 2011). Resources such as shelters, soup kitchens, medical clinics, social service agencies, and supportive housing should be readily accessible to the homeless population.

Lack of transportation can be a major barrier to accessing care. Some programs have responded to this need by adopting mobile health vans that provide care on street corners and in neighborhoods (Howe, Buck, & Withers, 2009). Clinics have also been established in shelters to facilitate client access. These clinics are often managed by nurses (D'Amico & Nelson, 2008). Nursing students also play an important role in promoting access to care for the homeless (Lashley, 2010).

The community health nurse should also consider the role of faith-based communities in providing physical and spiritual support to the homeless. Many places of worship have responded to the crisis of homelessness by offering food, shelter, counseling, medical care, and social services within the context of the faith community. Clinics have been built within faith communities to promote access to care. See From the Case Files II.

From the Case Files II

Faith-Based Outreach

As a faith community nurse working in a large church congregation, you are invited to develop an outreach program to minister to the needs of an inner city mission that is receiving financial support from the church. You begin by visiting the mission to conduct a needs assessment of its residents and to identify priority health issues. The shelter operates as a faith-based, nonprofit organization and is dedicated to serving the needs of homeless men with addictions. The shelter provides emergency overnight services and operates a 1-year, residential, faith-based addictions recovery program. Approximately 300 homeless male addicts frequent the shelter daily. Staff and residents have expressed concerns regarding a recent outbreak of boils among residents.

Assessment data reveal the following issues:

- Approximately 80% of clients have a history of injection drug use.
- Clients sleep in dormitory-style accommodations and share bathroom facilities.
- An on-site barber shop operated by the residents provides haircuts for a nominal fee.
- Clients have access to a small recreational area with donated exercise equipment.
- Laundry services are available, and residents take their clothing to the laundry on alternate days where it is washed. Laundry is typically washed in cold water, and at times the laundry runs out of detergent.

QUESTIONS

What additional data would you wish to gather to address the outbreak of boils at the shelter? How would you collect these data?

- What host, agent, and environmental factors may have contributed to the outbreak of boils?
- Discuss appropriate nursing interventions to address the outbreak. Consider the following levels of prevention: primary, secondary, tertiary.
- What advocacy role might the CHN play in addressing this issue?

Tertiary Prevention

Tertiary preventive measures attempt to limit disability and to restore maximum functioning. The goal is to provide rehabilitative care and support to clients who are already experiencing the consequences of homelessness. Often, homeless individuals suffer from chronic health conditions that have gone untreated for long periods of time. This neglect in attending to health needs results in significant disease morbidity. Treating complications of advanced disease, providing rehabilitative care, and offering counseling and support are important tertiary preventive strategies.

Case Management

At each level of prevention, the community health nurse functions as a case manager and coordinator of care to insure seamless delivery of services as people transition from one level of care to another. It is often difficult for the homeless to keep track of multiple appointments, negotiate the bureaucracy of multiple agencies and services, or maintain communication with providers through follow-up phone calls, letters, or visits. With no permanent address or phone, homeless clients encounter obstacles to adhering to recommendations

LEVELS OF PREVENTION PYRAMID

SITUATION: Promoting health and preventing illness among homeless male addicts

GOAL: To apply the three levels of prevention to avoid adverse health conditions, promptly diagnose and treat disorders, and assist the homeless male addict population to maintain or regain optimal health.

TERTIARY PREVENTION

- Provide case management of chronic health conditions.
- Advocate for expansion of counseling, rehabilitative services, and addictions treatment programs for the homeless.
- Advocate for supportive and transitional housing to enable homeless residents with addictions disorders to successfully transition back into the community.

SECONDARY PREVENTION

Early Diagnosis and Treatment

- Conduct mass screenings for diseases commonly found in homeless male population (TB, HIV, hepatitis, prostate cancer, colorectal cancer).
- Develop programs for health screening and early diagnosis and treatment in the community that are culturally sensitive and accessible to the homeless (e.g., mobile vans, faith community or shelter-based clinics).

PRIMARY PREVENTION

Health Promotion and Education	Health Protection
• Support employment and job training opportunities that assist clients to obtain jobs with livable wages and benefits. • Advocate through housing coalitions and legislative efforts to promote affordable housing, employment opportunities, and better access to health care. • Develop culturally sensitive health education programs that promote healthy coping, positive parenting, communication and relationship building, mental health, injury and illness prevention. • Promote programs that offer counseling and support to prevent continued high-risk behaviors as a result of untreated addiction.	• Advocate for legislation to protect citizens from environmental toxins and industrial wastes common to low-income areas. • Provide immunization services to prevent communicable disease transmission. • Counsel clients on proper nutrition, exercise, and basic hygiene to promote healthful lifestyles and prevent disease transmission. • Advocate for funding for nutrition programs for the homeless and for homeless shelters that would allow for the purchasing nutritious foods.

to follow up on test results or to notify their provider if symptoms persist or worsen. The community health nurse can help to bridge these gaps in service delivery and promote more effective adherence to therapeutic regimens.

Advocacy

Advocacy is a vital dimension of the community health nurse's role in working with the homeless. Advocacy entails working with different sectors of the community (including public officials, service providers, and persons living in the community) to develop innovative models for responding to the crisis of homelessness. Advocacy creates the broader system-wide changes needed to end homelessness (NCH, 2009k). The community health nurse acts as an advocate at each level of prevention to effect positive change. For example, the nurse may advocate for mental health and substance abuse services to promote mental health and prevent homelessness (primary prevention). Alternatively, he or she may advocate for legislation to fund supportive housing, health care, or social services to benefit the homeless chronically mentally ill (tertiary prevention). The community health nurse can also assume an advocacy role by becoming involved in local, state, or national coalitions or organizations devoted to protecting the rights of the homeless or by speaking out on legislation that impacts the homeless (NCH, 2009k). See Levels of Prevention Pyramid.

SUMMARY

Rising poverty and lack of affordable housing have led to a dramatic rise in homelessness. Poverty, lack of housing, domestic violence, mental illness, addictions, personal crisis, and natural disasters are factors that may predispose persons to homelessness.

Homeless families represent the fastest growing segment of the homeless population. Acute and chronic health problems plague the homeless. Conditions such as HIV/AIDS, diabetes, hypertension, addictions, and mental disorders are prevalent among the homeless and are difficult to treat because of the challenges associated with being homeless.

Both the public and private sectors have launched concerted efforts to combat the problem of homelessness through the passage of federal legislation (most notably the McKinney–Vento Homeless Assistance Act) and through the formation of national, state, and local coalitions and alliances to champion the cause of the homeless. There is still much to be done.

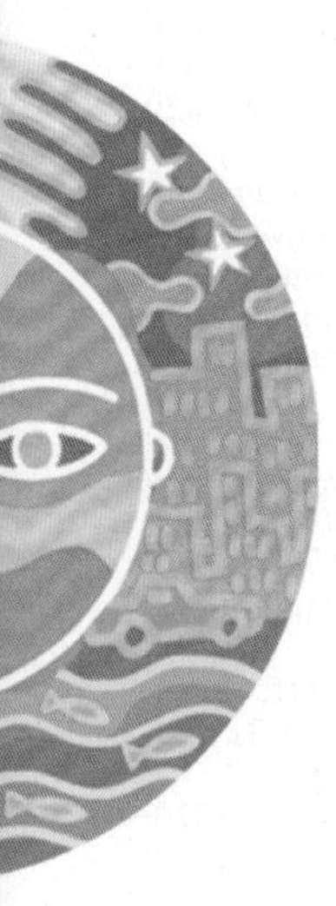

Community health nurses maintain a long and distinguished tradition of providing care to the marginalized and underserved. As such, they play a vital role in addressing the needs of the homeless in society. At the core of community nursing practice is the development of a trusting relationship. The community health nurse needs to examine his or her values and presuppositions regarding poverty and homelessness to be more effective in rendering care that is respectful, compassionate, and nonjudgmental.

The community health nurse implements primary, secondary, and tertiary preventive measures to prevent homelessness or to assist those who are homeless to obtain needed services. Primary prevention includes advocating for affordable housing, employment opportunities, and improved access to health care to prevent the downward spiral into homelessness. Secondary prevention includes screening for communicable and chronic diseases and promoting access to affordable health care and social services. Tertiary prevention includes rehabilitative and supportive care and counseling.

The community health nurse also serves as a case manager to coordinate care and to assist clients to negotiate the bureaucracy of multiple agencies and services. Finally, the community health nurse acts as an advocate to promote the rights of the homeless and to speak out on legislation impacting homelessness.

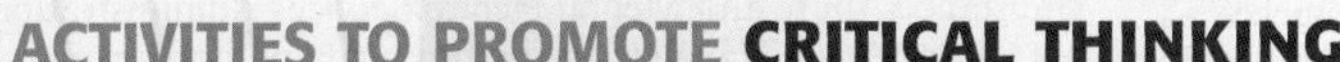

ACTIVITIES TO PROMOTE **CRITICAL THINKING**

1. Reflect in writing on the meaning of "home." Share your reflections with someone experiencing homelessness.
2. Interview a homeless person regarding the most difficult choices he or she has had to make. What were the conditions surrounding these choices?
3. Volunteer to work at a soup kitchen or homeless shelter. Observe carefully the faces, sounds, attitudes, and activities. What is it like to share in the same spaces as those who are homeless? What would it be like to be receiving rather than giving service?
4. Consider joining a local coalition to support the cause of homelessness in your community.
5. Call or write your local legislator to advocate for legislation impacting the homeless and to share your thoughts and feelings about homelessness.
6. Attend a public meeting that addresses homelessness prevention or low-income housing. Listen to the debate and consider the divergent views. What are the political, economic, and social contexts underlying these views?
7. Perform a windshield survey in a low-income community. What resources are lacking? Where is the nearest bank, school, grocery store, and health clinic? What are the conditions of the roads, homes, and other buildings? How do you feel as you drive through the community? What do you think it would be like to live there?

REFERENCES

Anderson, E., & McFarlane, J. (2011). *Community as partner: Theory and practice in nursing* (6th ed.). Philadelphia, PA: Wolters Kluwer Health/Lippincott Williams and Wilkins.

Burt, M. (2006). Testimony related to provisions of S. 1801, *The Community Partnership to End Homelessness Act of 2005*, 1–16. Retrieved from http://www.urban.org/publications/900937.html

D'Amico, J. B., & Nelson, J. (2008). Nursing care management at a shelter-based clinic: an innovative model for care. *Professional Case Management, 13*(1), 26–36.

Healthy People 2020 (n.d. a.). *Healthy People goals*. Retrieved from http://www.healthypeople.gov/2020/

Healthy People 2020 (n.d. b.). *Oral health*. Retrieved from http://www.healthypeople.gov/topicsobjectives2020/overview.aspx?topicid=32

Howe, E. C., Buck, D. S., & Withers, J. (2009). Delivering health care on the streets: Challenges and opportunities for quality management. *Quality Management in Health Care, 18*(4), 239–246.

Lashley, M. (2010). Something to smile about. *Community Works Journal*. Retrieved from http://www.communityworksinstitute.org

National Alliance to End Homelessness. (2010a). *Chronic homelessness*. Retrieved from http://www.endhomelessness.org/content/article/detail/1623

National Alliance to End Homelessness. (2010b). *Youth*. Retrieved from http://www.endhomelessness.org/section/issues/youth

National Center on Family Homelessness. (2010). *Children*. Retrieved from http://www.familyhomelessness.org/childfren.php?p=ts

National Center on Family Homelessness. (2009). *State Report Card on Child Homelessness: America's Youngest Outcasts*. Retrieved from http://www.homelesschildrenamerica.org/pdf/rc_full_report.pdf

National Coalition for the Homeless. (2006). *McKinney-Vento Act*. Retrieved from http://www.nationalhomeless.org/publications/facts.html/

National Coalition for the Homeless. (2008). *Homeless youth*. Retrieved from http://www.nationalhomeless.org/publications/facts.html/

National Coalition for the Homeless. (2009a). *Domestic violence and homelessness*. Retrieved from http://www.nationalhomeless.org/publications/facts.html/

National Coalition for the Homeless. (2009b). *Education of homeless children and youth*. Retrieved from http://www.nationalhomeless.org/publications/facts.html/

National Coalition for the Homeless. (2009c). *Employment and homelessness*. Retrieved from http://www.nationalhomeless.org/publications/facts.html/

National Coalition for the Homeless. (2009d). *Federal housing assistance programs*. Retrieved from http://www.nationalhomeless.org/publications/facts.html/

National Coalition for the Homeless. (2009e). *Health care and homelessness*. Retrieved from http://www.nationalhomeless.org/publications/facts.html/

National Coalition for the Homeless. (2009f). *HIV/AIDS and homelessness*. Retrieved from http://www.nationalhomeless.org/publications/facts.html/

National Coalition for the Homeless. (2009g). *Homeless families with children*. Retrieved from http://www.nationalhomeless.org/publications/facts.html/

National Coalition for the Homeless. (2009h). *Homeless veterans*. Retrieved from http://www.nationalhomeless.org/publications/facts.html/

National Coalition for the Homeless. (2009i). *Homelessness among elderly persons*. Retrieved from http://www.nationalhomeless.org/publications/facts.html/

National Coalition for the Homeless. (2009j). *How many people experience homelessness?* Retrieved from http://www.nationalhomeless.org/publications/facts.html/

National Coalition for the Homeless. (2009k). *How you can help end homelessness*. Retrieved from http://www.nationalhomeless.org/want_to_help/index.html#a

National Coalition for the Homeless. (2009l). *LGBT homeless*. Retrieved from http://www.nationalhomeless.org/factsheets/lgbtq.html

National Coalition for the Homeless. (2009m). *Mental illness and homelessness*. Retrieved from http://www.nationalhomeless.org/publications/facts.html/

National Coalition for the Homeless. (2009n). *Rural homelessness*. Retrieved from http://www.nationalhomeless.org/publications/facts.html/

National Coalition for the Homeless. (2009o). *Substance abuse and homelessness*. Retrieved from http://www.nationalhomeless.org/factsheets/addiction.html

National Coalition for the Homeless. (2009p). *Who is homeless?* Retrieved from http://www.nationalhomeless.org/publications/facts.html/

National Coalition for the Homeless. (2009q). *Why are people homeless?* Retrieved from http://www.nationalhomeless.org/publications/facts.html/

National Coalition for the Homeless. (2010a). *Foreclosure and homelessness prevention*. Retrieved from http://www.nationalhomeless.org/factsheets/PPR/2010/5%20-%20Foreclosure%206-10-10.pdf

National Coalition for the Homeless. (2010b). *Hate crimes and violence against people experiencing homelessness*. Retrieved from http://www.nationalhomeless.org/publications/facts.html/

National Coalition for the Homeless. (2010c). *HUD McKinney-Vento programs*. Retrieved from http://www.nationalhomeless.org/factsheets/PPR/2010/6%20-%20HMV%206-10-10.pdf

National Coalition for the Homeless. (2010d). *Universal health care*. Retrieved from http://www.nationalhomeless.org/factsheets/PPR/2010/9%20-%20Universal%20Health%20Care%206-10-10.pdf

National Health Care for the Homeless Council. (n.d.). *The basics of homelessness*. Retrieved from http://www.nhchc.org/Publications/basics_of_homelessness.html

National Health Care for the Homeless Council. (2001, June). Single males: The homeless majority. *Healing Hands, 5*(3), 1–6. Retrieved from http://www.nhchc.org/healinghands.html

National Low Income Housing Coalition. (2010). *Out of reach 2010: U. S statistics*. Retrieved from http://www.nlihc.org/oor/oor2010/OOR_US-Fact-Sheet.pdf

Song, J., Wall, M., Ratner, E., Bartels, D. M., Ulvestad, N., & Gelberg, L. (2008). Engaging homeless persons in end-of-life preparations. *Journal of General Internal Medicine, 23*(12), 2031–2045.

Substance Abuse and Mental Health Services Administration (n.d.) *Homelessness resource center facts*. Retrieved from http://www.nrchmi.samhsa.gov/Channel/View.aspx?id=18

Substance Abuse and Mental Health Services Administration. (2008). *Intro to PATH*. Retrieved from http://pathprogramarchive.samhsa.gov/

Substance Abuse and Mental Health Services Administration. (2010). *Center for Mental Health Services*. Retrieved from http://www.samhsa. gov/about/cmhs.aspx

United States Conference of Mayors. (2009). *Hunger and homelessness survey*. Retrieved from http://www.usmayors.org/pressreleases/uploads/USCMHungercompleteWEB2009.pdf

United States Department of Education. (2004). *McKinney-Vento Homeless Education Assistance Improvements Act of 2001*. Retrieved from http://www2.ed.gov/policy/elsec/leg/esea02/pg116.html

United States Department of Health and Human Services. (n.d.). *The Center for Faith-Based and Neighborhood Partnerships*. Retrieved from http://www.hhs.gov/fbci/index.html

United States Department of Housing and Urban Development (HUD). (n.d. a). *Facts about the homeless*. Retrieved from http://www.hud.gov/utilities/pring/print2cfm?page=80$∩@http%3A%2Fwww%2Eh/

United States Department of Housing and Urban Development (HUD). (n.d. b). *Homelessness: Programs and the people they serve—Highlights report.* Retrieved from http://www.huduser.org/publications/homeless/homelessness/highrpt.html/

United States Department of Housing and Urban Development (HUD). (2007). *McKinney-Vento Homeless Assistance Act.* Retrieved from http://www.hud.gov/offices/cpd/homeless/lawsandregs/mckv.cfm

United States Department of Housing and Urban Development (HUD). (2010). *The 2009 annual homeless assessment report.* Retrieved from http://www.hudhre.info/documents/5thHomelessAssessmentReport.pdf

United States Interagency Council on Homelessness. (2010a). *Interagency Council on Homelessness.* Retrieved from http://www.ich.gov/

United States Interagency Council on Homelessness. (2010b). *Opening doors: Federal strategic plan to prevent and end homelessness.* Retrieved from http://www.ich.gov/PDF/OpeningDoors_2010_FSPPreventEndHomeless.pdf

thePoint: Everything You Need to Make the Grade!

thePoint Visit http://thePoint.lww.com/Allender8e for selected readings, study aids for all learning styles, and more!

CHAPTER

29

Issues with Rural, Migrant, and Urban Health Care

"No city should be too large for a man to walk out of in a morning."

—*Cyril Connolly (1903–1974),* British critic

KEY TERMS

Built environment
Critical access hospitals
Federally qualified health centers
Frontier area
Ghettos
Health professional shortage areas (HPSAs)
In-migration
Medically underserved areas (MUAs)
Medically underserved population
Metropolitan statistical area
Micropolitan statistical area
Migrant farmworkers
Migrant streams
Out-migration
Patterns of migration
Population density
Rural
Rural health clinics
Seasonal farmworkers
Social justice
Telehealth
Urban
Urban health
Urbanized area (UA)
Urban cluster (UC)
Urban health penalty
Urban planning

LEARNING OBJECTIVES

Upon mastery of this chapter, you should be able to:

- Define the terms *rural, frontier, migrant,* and *urban*.
- Discuss the population characteristics of rural residents.
- Describe five barriers to health care access for rural clients.
- Describe the migrant lifestyle.
- Identify at least three health problems common to migrant workers and their families.
- Discuss barriers and challenges to migrant health care.
- Identify common health disparities found among rural and urban populations.
- Propose intervention strategies at the aggregate or community level to assure a healthier *built environment* in both rural and urban areas.
- Explain the concept of *social justice* and how it relates to public health nursing in rural and urban areas.
- Compare and contrast the challenges and opportunities related to rural and urban community health nursing practice.

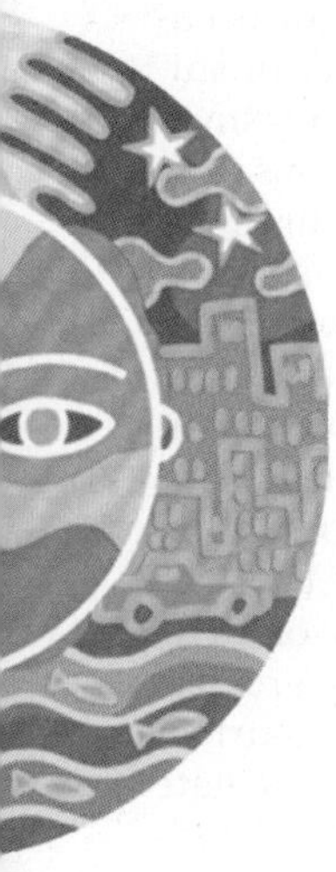

About half the population live in what is known as the suburbs, but the remainder live in one of two diametrically opposed areas: rural or urban. There is a good chance that many of you reading this book live in either very densely populated, bustling urban areas or in sparsely populated, somewhat isolated rural areas. Community health nursing in urban and rural areas requires not only general public health nursing knowledge and skills but also a unique understanding of how these distinctive environments affect the health of the populations living there. Where you live can and does markedly affect your health outcomes, with rural and urban areas having distinctive problems and issues, as described by van Dis in a seminal article (2002). These differences are much more than just the ability to shop at "Wal-Mart versus Pottery Barn" (p. 108). Both rural and urban clients have health disparities and disadvantages, although they may be dissimilar in nature.

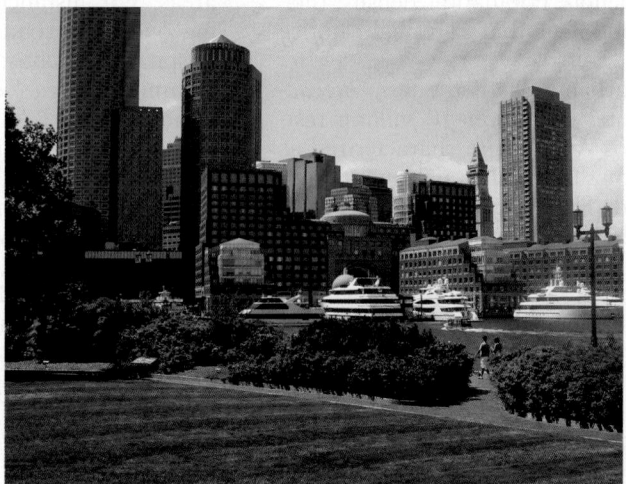

Boston Park Harbor. Source: USA.gov.

Rural nursing practice offers many opportunities. Nurses are respected community members—their judgment and opinions count. Rural nurses are key members of the health care team. They can make a difference in the lives of their neighbors, friends, and community. Rural public health nurses (PHNs) often struggle with helping clients gain access to quality health care and the inherent transportation problems found in isolated areas. The challenges are many, but the rewards are great.

Urban PHNs often specialize in particular areas of interest. They deal with different types of problems, such as homelessness, overcrowding, bioterrorism threats, and violent crime. They are often called upon to advocate for their most vulnerable clients, and they develop collaborative relationships with other professionals. Urban community health nursing can also be very rewarding and satisfying.

This chapter addresses the special health needs and concerns of rural, migrant, and urban clients and the ways in which a community health nurse can address those needs. After reading the chapter, you may come to appreciate the many advantages that rural nurses enjoy and consider rural nursing as a practice choice, or you may find that being a PHN in an urban area offers you more opportunities for specialization and networking. Either way, your contributions can improve the health of populations living at both extremes.

DEFINITIONS AND DEMOGRAPHICS

Depending on one's geographic location, professional discipline, agency or institutional affiliation, or other frame of reference, the term *rural* has different and specialized meanings. Moreover, rural populations and characteristics have changed significantly over many years. These differences and their implications are described in this chapter.

Definitions of "Rural"

The term *rural* means different things to different people. It is helpful to be aware of the precise meaning of the term as it is used in a particular agency, community, or piece of legislation because differences in semantics can affect public policy regarding rural communities. For example, federal dollars are often distributed to communities based on rural or urban status.

The U.S. government provides several definitions of rural. These can seem confusing and complicated, but it is important to understand the terms and how they are used in federal programs and grant funding. The U.S. Census Bureau (2010) identifies **urban** as all "densely settled core of census tracts and/or census blocks that meet minimum population density requirements....(it) must encompass at least 2,500 people at least 1,500 of which reside outside institutional group quarters" (para. 2). Two types of urban areas are described—an **urbanized area (UA)** or an **urban cluster (UC)**. A UA consists of densely settled territory with a population of 50,000 people. A UC has a population less than 50,000 but more than 2,000. Past descriptions have relied on a specific measure of density. **Population density** refers to the number of persons per square mile—urban areas are much more densely populated than rural areas. The U.S. Census definition of *rural* is all territory, population, and housing units located outside UAs and UCs. Some counties may include both rural and urban designations, as these designations do not follow municipal boundaries but rather denote population density (like the dense grouping of buildings that you might notice from an airplane).

A consideration in urban areas is the term *megacity*; this is an urban center with over 10 million residents. New York and Los Angeles are characterized as megacities, as are London, Tokyo, Rio de Janeiro, and others around the world (Hayes, 2011). Public health issues are intensified with larger population areas; issues with communicable disease, poverty, inadequate housing, and unemployment become even more magnified with larger populations. Since the 2000 Census, the U.S. Office of Management and Budget (OMB) reclassified the United States into metropolitan and micropolitan statistical areas. This nomenclature identifies a **metropolitan statistical area** as a core-based statistical area (CBSA) associated with at least one UA that has a minimum population of 50,000. **Micropolitan statistical areas** are CBSAs associated with at least one UC of no less than 10,000 and no more than 50,000 people (U.S. Census Bureau, n.d.). Both metropolitan and micropolitan statistical areas comprise the central county or counties containing the core, also included are adjacent outlying counties that have a high degree of social and economic integration with the central county (based on the number of people who commute to work). With such a broad definition, micropolitan statistical areas can include both rural and urban areas. Before 2003, the OMB defined urban and rural in terms of metropolitan and nonmetropolitan counties. By making these changes, the number of people living in what used to be considered nonmetropolitan areas decreased.

The U.S. Department of Agriculture (USDA) rural–urban continuum examines metropolitan and nonmetropolitan areas on the basis of counties, and this provides different data apart from census reports. State and federal agencies recognize county-level jurisdictions and governments and depend upon employment, income, and population data that are available on an annual basis (USDA, 2008). Many states have offices of rural health or other agencies dealing with issues specific to rural populations.

For the purposes of this chapter, **rural** is defined as *communities with fewer than 10,000 residents and a county population density of less than 1,000 persons per square mile*. This definition of rural is arbitrary because rural clients do not merely consider population density or community size when defining their *ruralness*. They have a multitude of reasons for defining their community as rural, such as distance from a large city, major occupations in the area (e.g., agriculture), or number of students in the local schools. If you have access to a small community, ask some of the residents the reasons why they consider their community to be urban or rural.

The term **frontier area** is used to designate sparsely populated rural places that are isolated from population centers and services, but specific definitions vary (Rural Assistance Center [RAC], 2012b). A common definition of a frontier area is one with six or fewer persons per square mile, but others include not only population density but distance and travel time to market-service areas. For instance, 60 miles or 60 minutes of driving on paved roads to the nearest 75-bed (or greater) hospital can constitute a frontier area. Rural–urban commuting area (census data) is also used to designate remote areas (RAC, 2012). It is estimated that 3 million people (4% of population) live in frontier areas that comprise 56% of the U.S. land areas. States with more than 10% of their population in a frontier area include Idaho, Nebraska, Maine, Arkansas, Oklahoma, Alaska, Arizona, Montana, Wyoming, New Mexico, Colorado, North Dakota, and South Dakota (National Center for Frontier Communities, 2009).

Health issues of concern to rural areas may be of even greater concern to frontier areas. Sparsely populated areas may be less able to attract health care professionals. The term **health professional shortage areas (HPSAs)** defines urban or rural geographic areas, population groups, or facilities with chronic shortages of medical, dental, or mental health professionals. The federal government determines which areas are HPSAs. Over 59 million people live in areas that have been designated as HPSAs for primary care, and 90.3 million live in mental health HPSAs (Fig. 29-1). In **medically underserved areas (MUAs)**, residents experience a shortage of health services; these areas are determined by the federal government using a score based on the shortage of primary care physicians, high infant mortality rates, high percentage of the population living below the poverty level, and a high proportion of residents over age 65. A **medically underserved population (MUP)** includes those with economic and cultural/linguistic barriers to primary health care services (Health Resources and Services Administration [HRSA], n.d. a).

Population Statistics

The number of persons living in urban areas of the United States tripled since the mid-1800s, to almost 60 million in 2000, and grew 10.8% from 2000 to 2010 to represent 33% of the total population. California, Arizona, and Texas showed the largest growth in suburbs of large metropolitan cities. During the same period, rural population growth was 4.5% with 46% to 60% of rural counties losing residents (Dougherty, 2011). An all time high of 51% of the population live in the suburbs. Only 16% of the U.S. population is characterized as rural, the lowest ever. The primary cause for this shift is thought to be children leaving home for larger cities with better employment opportunities. Rural areas are caught in a

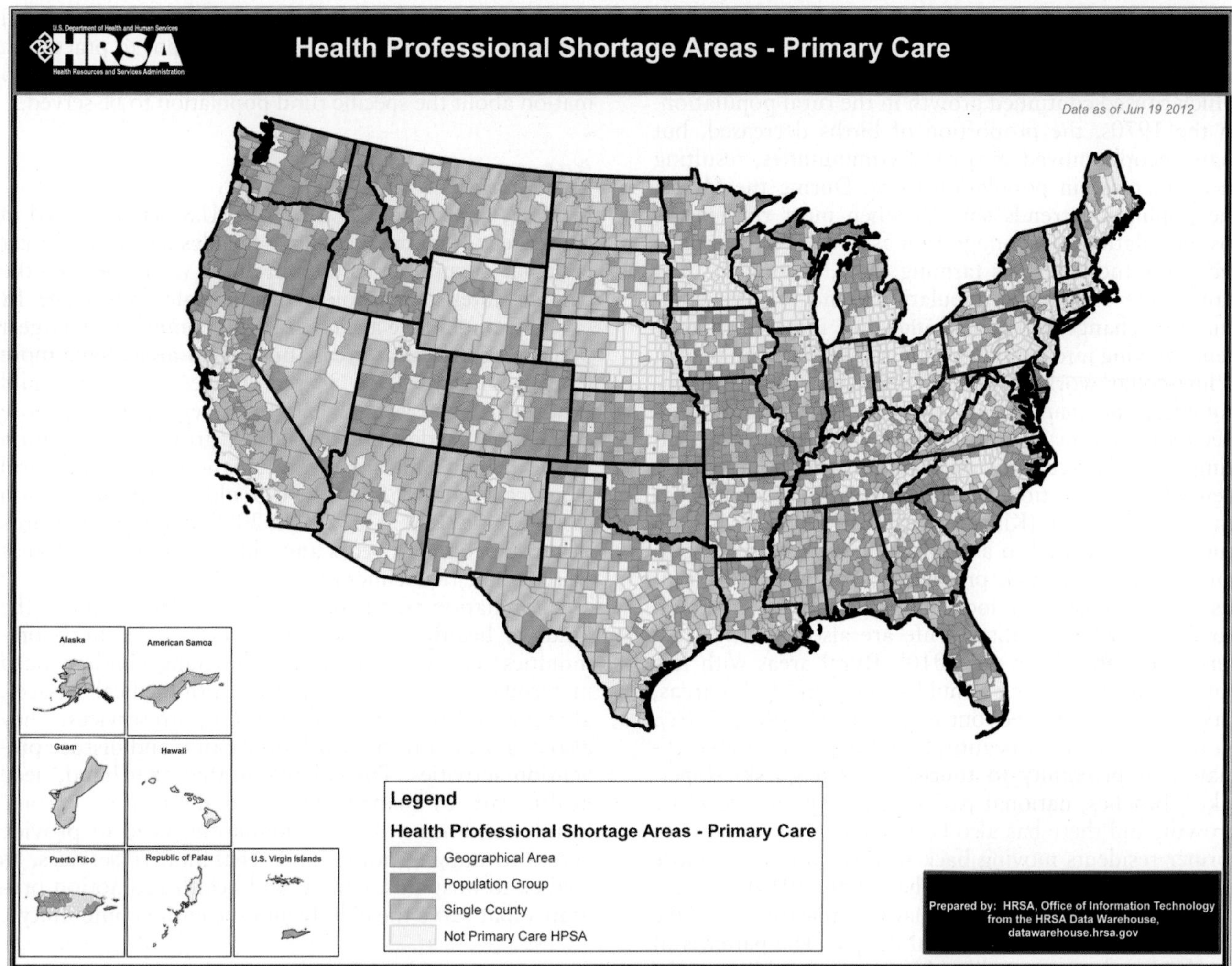

FIGURE 29-1. Health professional shortage areas—primary care.

vicious cycle, due to individuals moving away to find jobs and businesses reluctant to relocate to rural areas because of a smaller pool of potential workers. Great Plains states are at risk of losing the most population, with Appalachia, West Texas, Arkansas, and Mississippi also losing substantial portions of their populations (Nusca, 2011).

Poverty and joblessness are common among rural Americans. More part-time employment is found among rural workers (21%), and states with a high proportion of rural population often don't provide unemployment benefits for these workers (Shattuck, 2009). Rural residents are more likely to work for small companies that pay lower wages and don't offer health insurance; there are also more unemployed workers. Rural areas have high rates of uninsured and public insurance coverage (Medicaid, Medicare). There is also a higher percentage of elderly and those living in poverty, along with higher rates of chronic illness and reported poor to fair health. Rural residents are less likely to receive recommended preventive services, and they make fewer visits to health care providers. They also have fewer physicians (9% of total), and of the 2,000 rural hospitals, 75% of them have 50 or fewer beds; most are designated *critical access hospitals* (CAHs) as they have 25 or fewer beds (Agency for Healthcare Research and Quality [AHRQ], 2012; Rural Health Research and Policy Centers, 2009).

Rural areas have a slightly higher fertility rate than urban areas (Johnson & Lichter, 2012). However, this population growth related to births (termed *natural increase*) is offset by the loss of rural youth moving to more urban areas for education, jobs, and marriage (Nusca, 2011). This has been characterized as leading to a "brain drain" from rural areas, often leaving older adults or those with less education and income remaining. However, birth rates for both rural and urban areas have now "converged at below replacement levels" (Kirschner, Berry, & Glasgow, 2009, para. 4).

Changing Patterns of Migration

Population changes in rural areas are usually related to natural increase through births or through **out-migration**, the process of residents moving out of rural communities and into urban places (McGranahan, Cromartie, & Wojan, 2010). When America was a more rural country, there was more natural increase than out-migration, which caused continued growth in the rural population. In the 1970s, the proportion of births decreased, but many people moved into rural communities, resulting in an increase in population there. During the 1980s, the population trends shifted, when most rural areas lost population to out-migration as a result of economic recession and a serious farming crisis. During the first half of the 1990s, the population trend in rural communities changed to **in-migration**, an increase in residents moving into rural communities from urban places. White-collar workers were affected by changing technologies, and many young professionals with families elected to live in more rural settings. Since the beginning of the 21st century, more rural counties have experienced out-migration, and rural towns in some areas have disappeared (Kilkenny, 2010). The lack of in-migration is related to a decrease in retirees moving to rural areas along with problems recruiting professionals and managers for local manufacturing companies. Poverty and low quality of life are also causative factors (McGranahan et al., 2010). Rural areas with few natural amenities, such as mild winters and forest areas, have also experienced out-migration (Mather, 2008). Rural counties with beautiful landscapes, desirable climates, or proximity to tourist areas (e.g., ski slopes, lakes, beaches, national parks) have experienced more growth, and there has also been some remigration with former residents moving back to raise families in more rural environments (McGranahan et al., 2010).

Population trends have many implications for the health services needed by rural people. The patterns of rural migration change like shifting sand, adding to the challenge of planning resources for rural communities.

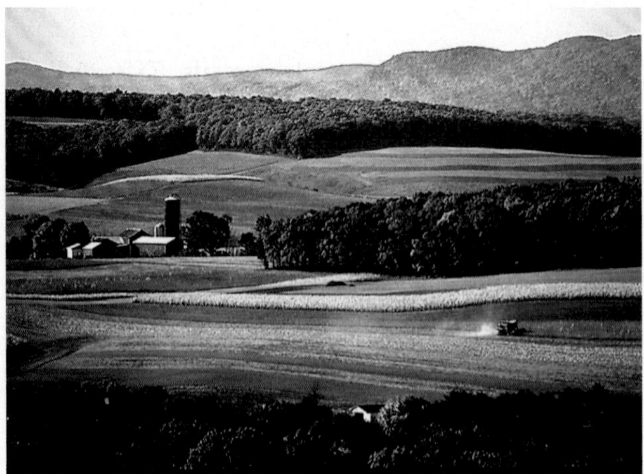

A farm in rural Pennsylvania. Source: USDA, Agricultural Research Service.

POPULATION CHARACTERISTICS

The following information is meant to describe, not stereotype, rural clients. Each rural community is unique, as are its residents. The PHN must determine whether the population characteristics discussed fit a specific rural community. The nursing student who plans to practice in the international arena will need to seek out relevant information about the specific rural population to be served.

Age and Gender

In 2008, approximately 22.7% of U.S. females lived in rural areas. The proportion of females age 35 and over is higher in rural areas than in urban areas, or even the United States as a whole. Those females below age 18 (17.5%) and above age 65 (14.6%) comprise the largest percentages in rural areas, but urban areas have more females in the 18- to 34-year range (Maternal Child Health Branch [MCHB], 2010). Elderly persons, those age 65 and older, are the fastest growing population in the United States in every location, including rural America. About 15% of the U.S. older adult population resides there (RAC, 2012a). In 2000, close to two thirds of those people 75 years and older living in rural areas were female (Kirschner et al., 2009).

Population trends have a direct relationship to the kinds of health services that are needed in rural communities. Growing families with young children need maternity, pediatric, and family health medical services, along with dental care and mental health services. They also can benefit from health promotion and disease prevention activities. The elderly, on the other hand, need health care to manage increased number of chronic health conditions. Rural communities need to provide access to nursing homes and rehabilitative services, as well as to hospitals, clinics, and health promotion programs that serve the elderly and the entire community.

Race and Ethnicity

Rural areas have historically had less racial diversity than urban areas. However, that is rapidly changing. Racial and ethnic groups have historically been concentrated in certain areas of the country—for example, Blacks in the rural South and American Indians in the rural Southwest and West, as well as Mexican Americans in the border states of the Southwest (Kirschner, Berry, & Glasgow, 2006; Kirschner et al., 2009; McGranahan et al., 2010). But these patterns are changing. Rapid Hispanic growth areas are found in the Midwest and Southeast (see Figs. 29-2 and 29-3) (Johnson, & Lichter, 2008). The Hispanic population in nonmetropolitan areas has doubled since 1980, and in some rural areas (e.g., Midwest, South), the Hispanic population disproportionately consists of young males (National Advisory Committee on Rural Health and Human Services [NACRHHS], 2008).

Higher birth rates could signal faster growth of this population, and this might lead to a need for changing health policies and practices. For instance, in rural counties with a high elderly population and established caseloads of chronic disease patients, an influx of younger Hispanic populations may require a shift in policies and resources to include more pediatric and obstetric care (Kirschner et al., 2009). All of these changes influence geographic patterns of health status.

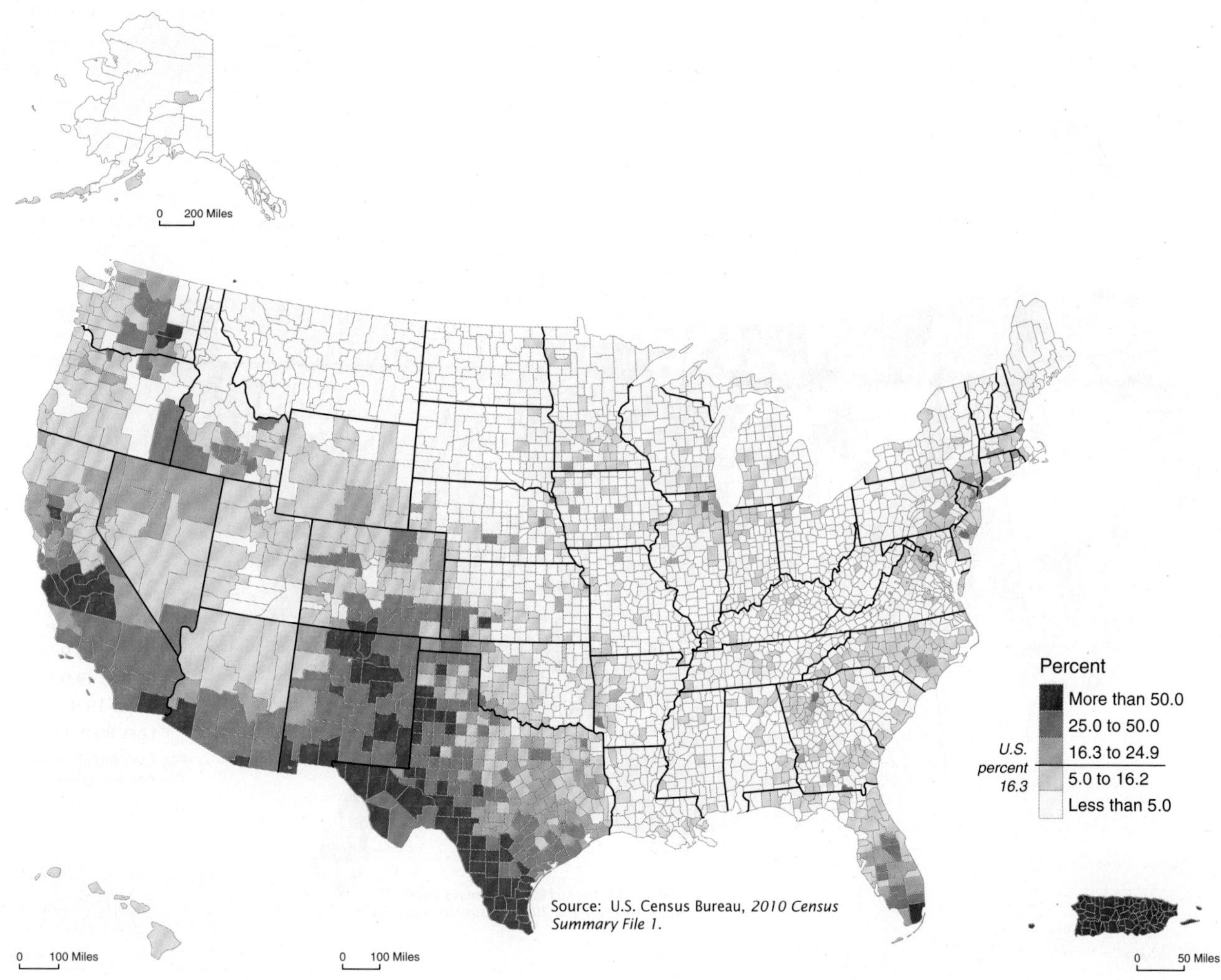

FIGURE 29-2. Hispanic or Latino population as a percent of total population by county, 2010.

Education

Rural clients in the United States have historically had lower educational attainment than those in urban areas. However, the gap is beginning to close for high school completion. In 2009, 81.7% of those living in nonmetro (rural) areas over age 25 had completed high school, while 85.2% of those in metropolitan areas did. The gap for those with college or professional degrees worsened over the last two decades from 9.5% to 12.6%, with lower levels for those in rural areas (USDA, 2011).

Rural Hispanics have the lowest percentage of educational attainment—45% never finished high school and only 7% graduated from college. However, in counties with rapid growth of Hispanic populations, enrollment in K–8 schools has grown by over 500% (Saenz, 2008; Kandel, & Parrado, 2006.).

Lower levels of education are associated with poverty, especially in rural areas. Rural schools provide education to some of this country's poorest children. The poverty rate in the 800 poorest rural school districts is similar to the rate in large urban districts, and 19% of all schoolchildren attend majority-rural districts. Many of these children have long bus rides that take time away from homework, and the districts also have higher transportation costs (Southern Poverty Law Center, 2010). Rural clients have little access to higher educational facilities, such as community colleges or universities close to home. Travel to urban areas for educational pursuits adds to the burden of obtaining additional education beyond high school.

Income, Housing, and Jobs

Some rural communities are home to some very wealthy residents, many of them landowners, business owners, farmers, or ranchers. On the average, however, the income of people in rural communities is lower than that of persons living in urban communities. This is reflected in higher rates of unemployment and lower per capita income; nonmetro (rural) income was only 71% of per capita metropolitan income in 2006 (McGranahan et al., 2010; Miller, 2009). In 2007, the U.S. unemployment rate was 4.6%, but for those living in nonmetropolitan areas, it was 5.1%, with a large number of rural

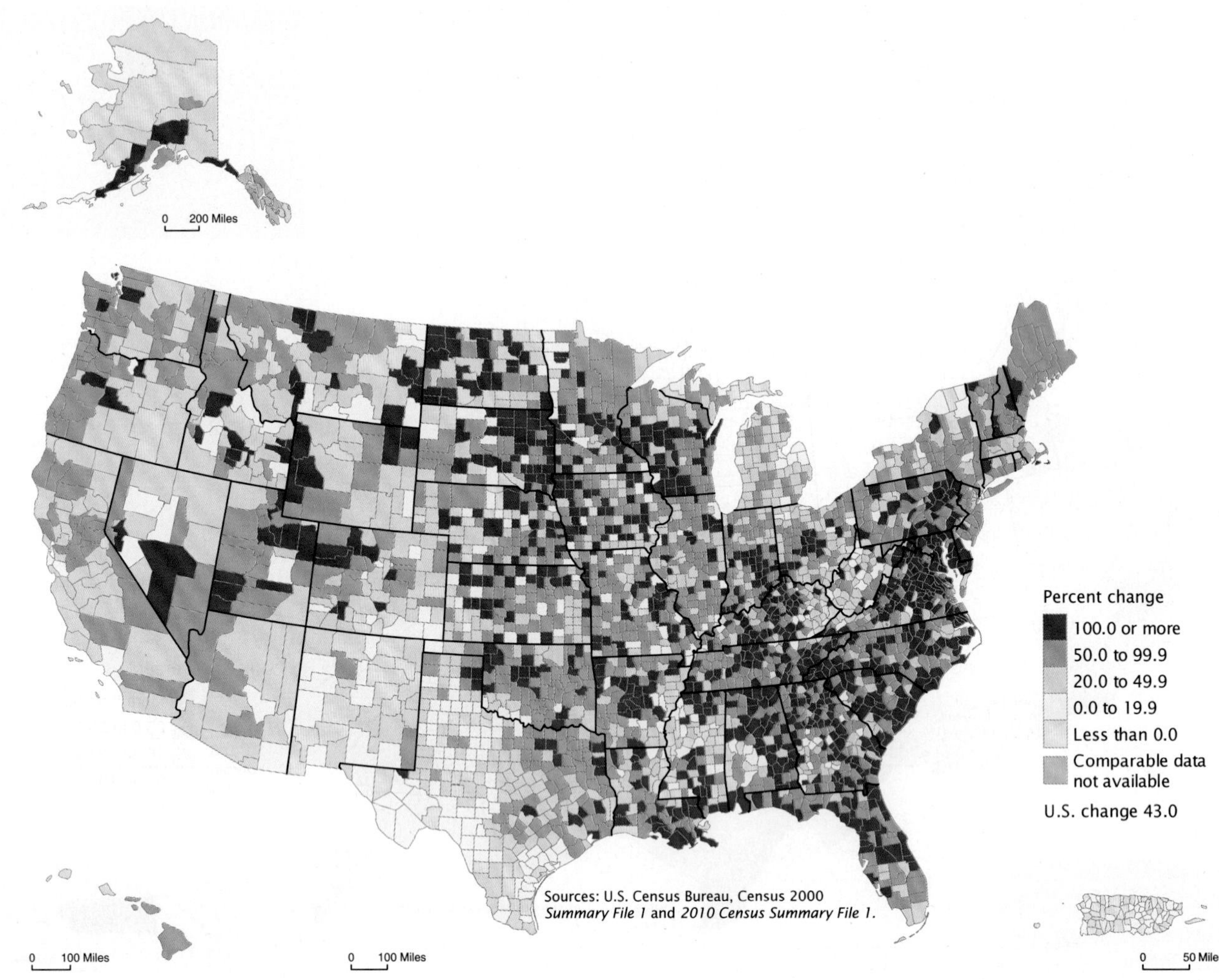

FIGURE 29-3. Percent change in Hispanic or Latino population by county: 2000 to 2010

areas at 7% (Miller, 2009). Persistent poverty, defined as 20% or more of the population living in poverty for over 30 years, is more common in rural counties than in urban ones. Of the 386 counties with this designation, 340 of them are in nonmetropolitan areas, and a large number are in the South (USDA, 2011). In 2008, more urban women lived in poverty than rural females, especially those in the 18- to 34-year age group. Over age 65, slightly more rural than urban females live in poverty (MCHB, 2010). In 2003, over one third of rural poor were children. Currently, rates of child poverty remain higher for rural children than urban children (21% and 18%, respectively). The poverty rate among rural older adults is also growing, as is debt among farmers despite government subsidy programs. In a good number of low-income rural communities, a notable amount of income may derive from federal support through health and social services such as Medicare, Medicaid, Temporary Aid to Needy Families (TANF), and food stamps (Food Security Learning Center, 2010; Kilkenny, 2010). Also, the percentage of working poor in rural areas is higher than in urban areas (Slack, 2010). A large survey of farmworkers found that 22% reported use of needs-based services by someone within their household, with 15% using Medicaid, 11% with WIC, and 8% getting food stamps. Only 1% had TANF benefits (National Center for Farmworker Health [NCFH], 2009a). See Figure 29-4, Poverty Rates by Residence.

Living in a rural area, however, has a number of economic advantages. The cost of land is lower than in urban areas; therefore, housing costs are also lower, and rural areas did not experience the wide price swings as the housing bubble burst in the mid-2000s (Bishop, 2009). The median cost of homes in remote rural areas is less than half that in urban areas. But the cost of goods is often similar to costs in urban areas, or may be higher, due to transportation expenses (Kilkenny, 2010). Taxes are usually less, and restrictions on land use are not as stringent. Less expensive land is advantageous to businesses, such as manufacturing, which may need large parcels of land. However, transportation costs are higher, and rural median housing values grew faster than urban areas since 2006 (Bishop, 2009). Earlier growth corresponded with rural in-migration but posed several problems. For cash-strapped families whose house values rose, subprime mortgages allowed them to trade equity for cash, and foreclosure rates skyrocketed. In Minnesota, for instance, rural county foreclosures outpaced foreclosures in

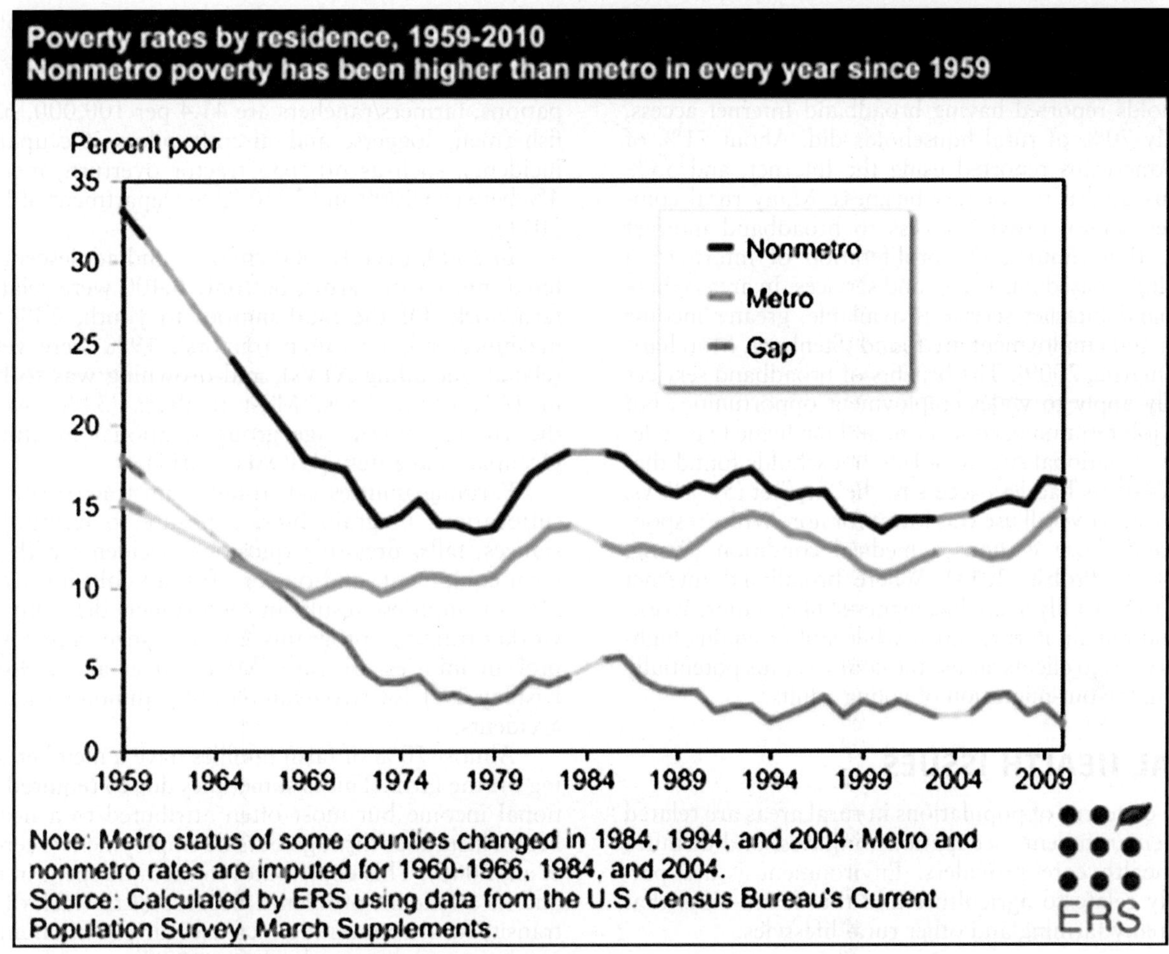

FIGURE 29-4. Poverty rates by residence, 1959 to 2010. Retrieved from http://ers.usda.gov/Briefing/IncomePovertyWelfare/povertygeography.htm#graph. Source: USDA Economic Research Service, 2011.

metropolitan counties (Oakes, 2008). Low-income families who are renters may find it difficult to find affordable housing, even when housing supply is good. While rural housing costs for the most part are lower, over one third of rural renters spend 30% of their monthly incomes on housing costs; this compares to 20% for homeowners. Most low-income housing in rural areas consists of single-family homes, not large apartment complexes, and manufactured homes comprise 15% of rental units. Older housing is also common, and units are often substandard and in need of repair. Rural renters are twice as likely to live in substandard housing than urban renters (Housing Assistance Council [HAC], 2009).

Some government assistance is available to help low-income renters. The USDA offers rent subsidies to low-income elderly or disabled residents of multifamily housing units through Section 521 (HAC, 2008). Section 8, a rental voucher program administered by the U.S. Department of Housing and Urban Development (HUD), is targeted to very low-income families who can choose from privately owned rental housing (USDHUD, 2012b). However, funds for this program are limited and applicants may wait several years for approval. Both programs supplement participants' rental costs above 30% of their income.

The United States is unique in that it feeds its population with a small proportion of workers committed to food production and still exports food products to the rest of the world. Although many people equate farming with rural life, only 4.4% of nonmetropolitan employment is directly related to agriculture (Research and Training Center: Rural, 2008). When compared with urban areas, rural communities typically offer fewer job options. Types of rural work, such as crop agriculture, manufacturing, and forestry, vary by locale, and these employment opportunities have been diminishing along with concomitant decreases in population and the shift from a goods-based to a service-based economy. Two thirds of all rural employment is now in the service sector, often in jobs that assist retirees. Although there is more manufacturing in the South, manufacturing has decreased overall, while health and social service sector jobs have increased substantially. White-collar jobs have increased; examples of white-collar occupations include professional, management, and sales, as well as technical/administrative support (NACRHHS, 2008).

Although the use of the Internet for commerce is now very common in urban and suburban areas, the *rural digital divide* still exists. In 2007, 84% of urban households reported having broadband Internet access, but only 70% of rural households did. About 71% of rural Americans reported using the Internet, and 55% of farms used it to conduct business. Many rural communities cannot provide access to broadband Internet service, thus limiting the proliferation of information technology–based businesses and services. In areas where broadband Internet service is available, greater income growth and employment are found (Stenberg, Morehart, & Cromartie, 2009). The benefits of broadband services not only apply to wider employment opportunities but also to job retraining, education, and medicine (e.g., telehealth). A national survey of U.S. households found that rural residents had less access to the Internet (59.7% vs. 69.4%), and overall use was lower for non-White respondents and those without a medical condition (Wang, Bennett, & Probst, 2011). Where broadband Internet services are readily available, higher-skilled remote workers could remain in rural areas while still providing high-tech services to clients across the country, thus potentially reducing the out-migration of young adults.

RURAL HEALTH ISSUES

Health concerns of populations in rural areas are related to the environment, occupations, injuries, and distance from health care providers. Environment issues particularly relate to agriculture and the health risks that accompany farming and other rural lifestyles.

Agriculture and Health

Although farming is not characteristic of all rural areas, where agricultural production occurs, both direct and indirect effects on health can exist. In an important classic book about this, Merchant, Coussens, and Gilbert (2006) note pesticides and fertilizers can affect water, air, and soil, and dust created from plowing for crops can affect the air quality. An "estimated 70% of antibiotics are used for nontherapeutic purposes in intensive livestock production," placing workers at risk for developing antibiotic-resistant infections (p. 4). Occupational exposures to windblown soil, organic dust, pesticides, mycotoxins, ammonia, animal dander, and hydrogen sulfite are only some of the air quality issues in rural areas (Lee et al., 2010). In Iowa, for instance, it is estimated that for every pound of corn harvested, 2 pounds of soil are "exported" (p. 7). Livestock growth-producing agents, along with radon, pesticides, and fertilizers, can contaminate ground water. Many rural residents depend on their own well water for drinking, and water quality is monitored only sporadically by well owners and then usually only for "coliform bacteria and nitrates" (p. 19). About 30% of rural residents obtain drinking water from very small water systems, without the monitoring and regulations associated with large urban water suppliers.

Agricultural-related morbidity and mortality are relatively high. Agriculture (grouped together with fishing and forestry) now ranks above mining in the rate of fatal occupational injuries (26.8 vs. 19.8 per 100,000) and it increased 9%. When examining rates for specific occupations, farmers/ranchers are 41.4 per 100,000, behind fishermen, loggers, and aircraft pilots. Occupational incidents, such as off-road tractor overturn, increased 4% between 2009 and 2010 (U.S. Department of Labor, 2011).

In 2009, over 16,000 children and adolescents suffered injuries on farms, but only 3,400 were related to farmwork. Of the fatal injuries to youth, 23% were machinery-related (often tractors), 19% were vehicle-related (including ATVs), and drowning was to blame in 16% of fatalities. Most fatalities (34%) were in the 16- to 19-year age group (National Institute for Occupational Safety [NIOSH], 2011).

Farming injuries can result from tractor rollovers, suffocations in grain bins, exposure to harmful substances, falls, fires or explosions, accidents with other farm equipment, and on- or off-road collisions. About 5% of injuries result in permanent disability, and worker-training programs to recognize hazards and prevent injuries are rare (Merchant et al., 2006). See Display 29.1 for two examples of common agricultural accidents.

Almost 70% of farm families have a member working off the farm. This is sometimes due to required additional income but most often attributed to a need for health insurance through outside employment (Merchant et al., 2006). This contributes to the time spent in travel and its attendant problems. Because of the lack of mass transit, rural commuting increases air pollution and the incidence of injury or death from traffic accidents.

The Built Environment in Rural Areas: Relationship to Health

Even with the advances of medicine and genomics, and the staggering percentage of our gross domestic product (GDP) spent on health care, scientists feel that we will not be able to significantly improve our overall health and quality of life without addressing how we plan our living spaces.

Substantial scientific evidence gained in the past decade has shown that various aspects of the built environment can have profound, directly measurable effects on both physical and mental health outcomes, particularly adding to the burden of illness among ethnic minority populations and low-income communities. Lack of sidewalks, bike paths, and recreational areas in some communities discourages physical activity and contributes to obesity; in those low-income areas that do have such amenities, the threat of crime keeps many people inside. Income segregation—the practice of housing the poor in discrete areas of a city—has also been linked with obesity and adverse mental health outcomes. Low-income and/or ethnic minority communities—already burdened with greater rates of disease, limited access to health care, and other health disparities—are also the populations living with the worst built environment conditions (Hood, 2005).

The **built environment** consists of the development of housing, highways, shopping areas, and other

DISPLAY 29.1 AGRICULTURAL ACCIDENTS

Farm Tractor Accident

Tractor accidents are common causes of death among rural youth working in agriculture. Rollover accidents are most common. However, they

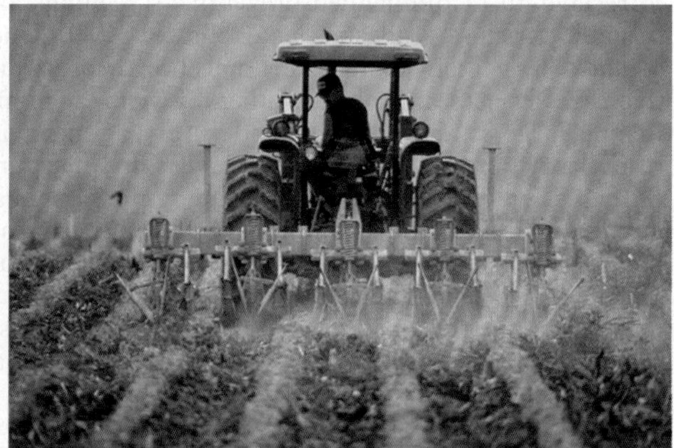

can also happen when you least expect it. Close to 7:30 one evening, a father, driving a large farm tractor with an enclosed cab and pulling a disc, had his two young boys with him (ages 3 and 5) while he was plowing a field behind the family home in rural Wisconsin. On a sloping hill, his tractor hit a bump and the 3-year-old suddenly slammed against the door handle and fell out of the tractor cab onto the ground. The father was unable to stop the large tractor before the rear tire ran over his son. Emergency personnel gave CPR to the boy at the edge of the field, and he was transferred to a nearby hospital. But he was pronounced dead less than an hour later (Gazette Staff, 2011). What was probably an enjoyable past time for this family became a sudden tragedy.

Tractor Versus Moving Vehicle

Tractor accidents are common on farms, but tractors are also often involved in traffic accidents that can lead to injuries and deaths. One example occurred in a rural New York county in 2011. Shortly before 1 PM, a car driving behind a slow-moving farm tractor that had a pesticide spray rig attached at the rear decided to pass the tractor near a curve in the road. A van carrying 14 people, including 13 from a nearby Amish community on a local farm tour, had to swerve to miss the car and ended up smashing into the tractor, the van resting underneath it. Sadly, five individuals died at the scene of the accident, and ambulances/helicopters transported nine others to local hospitals. The tractor driver was injured and stated that this was the worst accident he had seen, although drivers often passed him while he was driving his tractor on the roads to get from one field to another. The driver of the car was later charged with homicide (WHAM, 2011). This type of incident occurs frequently in agricultural areas, as drivers are often frustrated at the slow pace of agricultural equipment, and roads may be narrow.

Sources: WHAM, channel 13. (2011, July 20). *Five killed in Yates Co. tractor crash*. Retrieved from http://www.13wham.com/news/local/story/yates-county-crash/tqRkB_kSVU-gsI1t5_Y3Mw.cspx; Gazette Staff. (2011, April 8). Boy dies in farm tractor accident. *The Janesville Gazette*. Retrieved from http://gazettextra.com/weblogs/latest-news/2011/apr/08/boy-dies-farm-tractor-accident/ (Photo source: USDA Agricultural Research Service.)

man-made features added to the natural environment. As populated areas expand, stresses are placed on natural habitats, water supplies, and air quality. The built environment is inextricably related to health.

Urban sprawl is a concern in some rural areas, as people move from urban centers to more suburban environments. Urban encroachment into agricultural areas creates problems with air and water pollution, access to health care, and heat islands. *Heat islands* occur when green areas are exchanged for asphalt, resulting in temperature and ecosystem changes that can extend to more rural areas (Merchant et al., 2006; U.S. Environmental Protection Agency [EPA], 2011). Ozone levels are often highest just outside the city, because "ozone is formed relatively slowly by the action of sunlight on oxides of nitrogen and hydrocarbons" (p. 72). Urban sprawl also causes problems with water pollution and the availability of water. Encroachment of housing areas into natural habitats or farmlands can lead to wider human exposure to pesticides, herbicides, and other hazards such as mosquito-borne illnesses. Mass transit is not often available in suburban areas and almost never found in rural areas. Opportunities for health-promoting behaviors are often more limited in rural areas. Deteriorating (or no) sidewalks can be a barrier to walking in rural areas. Exercise or fitness facilities, bike paths, jogging trails, and other incentives for physical activity are also often lacking in rural communities. Obesity is prevalent in rural areas, and the physical environment, along with diet, plays a role in this epidemic (Merchant et al., 2006). A survey of rural residents from Arkansas, Missouri, and Tennessee found that frequent eating out, especially at buffets, fast-food restaurants, and cafeterias, along with perceptions of the community as not a pleasant area for physical activity were associated with higher rates of obesity (Casey et al., 2008).

Rural roads are another concern because they are often narrow, without streetlights, and poorly maintained. About 60% of traffic fatalities occur on rural roads and highways, with the highest rates on two-lane roads (Transportation Research Board of the National Academies, 2011). Slow-moving farm equipment traveling on these roads, along with speeding and failure to use safety restraints, has led to injury-related non–farm vehicle crashes according to one Iowa study (Peek-Asa et al., 2007). Researchers in North Dakota implemented a pilot program in two rural counties to "heighten awareness and safety on rural roads," but their interventions yielded "little effect on overall seat belt use" (Huseth, Vachal, Benson, & Lofgren, 2011, para. 1).

Self, Home, and Community Care

Historically, self-management of health care problems has been the most common way for rural people to cope with illness. This can be viewed as a type of strength, or it may be seen as a limitation. A rural mental health professional recently noted that the "culture of rural states" is often "one of self-sufficiency, traditional values, and patriarchal social structures" (Merchant et al., 2006, p. 41). Rural residents are often viewed as hardworking, traditional, hardy, self-reliant, and resistant to accepting help or services from outside agencies regarded by them as welfare-type programs. Many rural clients are considered individualistic, independent, and resourceful. They often take care of illnesses or injuries on their own, or have a supportive network to help them get their health needs met. Small communities commonly have strong social networks, but this type of familiarity may lead to problems with privacy and confidentiality, as well as stigma regarding mental health or substance abuse treatment.

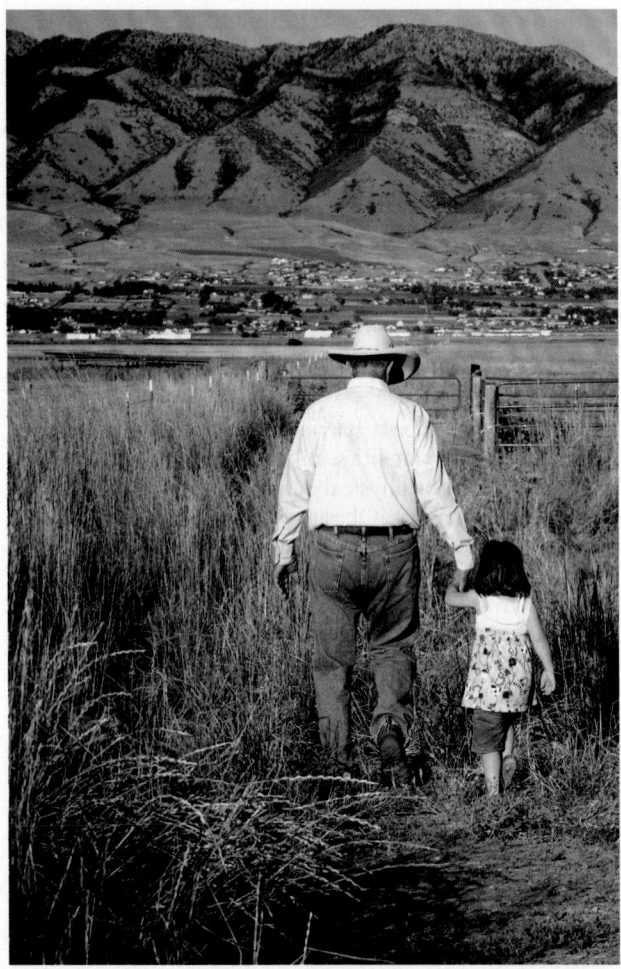

Life in a rural area may seem idyllic, but there are some significant risks of a rural lifestyle. (Private author photo with Permissions of Tamara Harris, Tobey Roos, & Richard Wosnik.)

Because cost, travel, weather, and distance are barriers to obtaining health services from formal health care providers, rural clients may employ a variety of folk treatments and home remedies before consulting a nurse or a physician; such clients tend to visit providers at a much later stage than do people in urban areas. Rural residents have fewer visits to health care providers than their urban counterparts and are less likely to receive all recommended preventive screenings and services (Krishna, Gillespie, & McBride, 2010). They are also less likely to receive home health or palliative care services and physical therapy visits at home. In one large study of urban and rural patients with respiratory illness during the last year of life, rural residents, when compared to urban counterparts, had an increased likelihood of admission to long-term care facilities (Goodridge, Lawson, Rennie, & Marciniuk, 2010). They are also more likely to report poor or fair health (one in three adults), to have chronic diseases such as diabetes, and to die from heart disease than are residents of urban areas (AHRQ, 2011; Krishna et al., 2010). Rural residents receive care in a less timely manner than urban residents and utilize physicians who are more likely to provide care that is outside their specialty areas. Compared with hospitals that are less rural, CAHs have been found to have significantly higher patient mortality rates and worse processes of care for patients having heart failure, acute MIs, and pneumonia (Joynt, Harris, Orav, & Jha, 2011). A longitudinal cohort study from Canada noted that rural patients recently diagnosed with heart failure had fewer physician office visits in the first year, higher rates of hospitalization, and more ED visits (Gamble et al., 2011).

The low population density in rural areas makes service delivery more difficult, especially for those with special health needs such as the elderly, the disabled, and others (AHRQ, 2011). Laditka, Laditka, and Probst (2009) found that rural adults and older adults had 45% to 90% greater rates of hospitalization for ambulatory care–sensitive conditions in their study of eight U.S. states. Suicide rates in rural areas, especially the rural West, can be as much as three times those in urban areas. Over twice the rate of anxiety and depression has been found in rural women, as opposed to urban women. And less than half of rural community clinics or primary care settings accurately diagnosed depression in their patients. Over 85% of the rural population resides in a mental HPSA (Smalley et al., 2012).

Home health care (HHC) is particularly difficult in sparsely populated areas, both for patients and nurses. Locating addresses in very rural areas often takes additional skills. (See Display 29.2 for the story of a home health nurse trying to locate a client's home.) The benefits of HHC are worthwhile; it allows people to stay at home, supports their hardiness, and compensates for the long distance between home and formal health care. An examination of differences in use of HHC between rural and urban adults found that rural residents received fewer number of provider days, even when predisposing

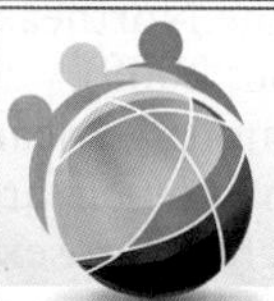

DISPLAY 29.2 LOCATING A RURAL HOME HEALTH CLIENT

The following written (verbatim) directions were given by a discharge planner to a case manager (home care nurse) when making a referral for Mary, a 67-year-old woman who lived 37 miles from the hospital:

> Drive on the gravel road east of town until you get to the third set of mailboxes. Then, turn left; drive up the road until you see the old church; cross the broken bridge toward the river. Mary lives on the third farm. Her house has some trees and a fence around it. (p. 222)

It took the home health nurse over 2 hours to drive about 30 miles on the narrow country roads after the morning rain. The nurse had to stop four times to ask residents for additional directions and hints for finding Mary's house. It was finally located, hidden in a large group of trees. The total travel time for this visit was about 4 hours.

From Bushy, A. (2003). Considerations for working with diverse rural client systems. *Lippincott's Case Management, 8*(5), 214–223.

conditions were taken into account (McAuley, Spector, & Van Nostrand, 2009).

Access to Acute Care

Rural hospitals have a high risk for financial problems and closures, thus leaving rural patients stranded without services nearby and forcing them to drive long distances for inpatient care. The Medicare Rural Hospital Flexibility Program encouraged states to form rural health networks, improve emergency medical services, and improve the financial performance of rural hospitals by designating them CAHs. **Critical access hospitals** are rural hospitals, located a minimum of 35 miles from the next hospital, or 15 miles if the terrain is mountainous or the only routes are on secondary roads (RAC, n.d.c). One intention of this designation was to reduce the number of rural hospital closures by providing cost-based Medicare reimbursements, which differ from the prospective payments given to larger hospitals. Most CAHs are nonprofit, have limited lengths of stay and bed capacity, and are heavily dependent on Medicare and Medicaid funding (Holmes & Pink, 2011).

Major Health Problems

Among major health problems affecting individuals in rural areas are cardiovascular disease (CVD), diabetes, and human immunodeficiency virus (HIV). Geography, economics, and rural lifestyle factors may account for the higher rate of these major health problems.

Cardiovascular Disease

When it comes to CVD, geography may play a role. Geographic concentrations of CVD and other diseases vary from one rural location to the next, possibly related to inadequate health care, distance from care, environmental exposures, infectious disease in the area, and other factors. These multidimensional elements interact in such a way to cause cardiovascular mortality statistics to vary among regions and ethnic groups. However, one recent national cohort study found "geographic variation in inflammatory biomarkers among otherwise healthy women that cannot be completely attributed to traditional clinical risk factors or lifestyle characteristics" (Clark, Coull, Berkman, Buring, & Ridker, 2011, para. 3).

CVD is a leading cause of death in the United States, and the total direct and indirect costs of CVD and stroke were estimated at over $503 billion in 2010 (American Heart Association, 2010). Regional variations have been noted in prevalence of CVD and stroke, as well as heart failure readmissions (Cook & Lauer, 2011). A national study found increased stroke mortality in the South (stroke belt), and many researchers are focusing on the possible underlying risk factors related to geographical variations (Cook & Albert, 2009; Cushman et al., 2008).

Rural residents may ignore early cardiovascular symptoms and give little heed to preventive interventions such as exercise and low-fat diets. Other risk factors, such as smoking and poverty, affect cardiovascular health. Adults in rural counties are most likely to smoke and use smokeless tobacco, and they are more likely to be in the presence of smokers at home and work (Vander Weg, Cunningham, Howren, & Cai, 2011). Rural residents are also more likely to be obese than urban counterparts (Wallace, Young-Xu, Hartley, & Weeks, 2010).

In addition, rural areas usually have less high-tech health care equipment available, which may affect outcomes for patients with cardiovascular emergencies. However, a study examining national data over an 8-year period found no statistical differences in quality of care and outcomes between rural and urban patients when facilities participated in Get With the Guidelines-Coronary Artery Disease Program (Ambardekar et al., 2010). Another study noted that many urban and rural patients admitted for MI did not receive guidelines recommended treatments, but those admitted to isolated and small rural hospitals had lower rates of beta-blockers and aspirin prescriptions upon discharge (Baldwin, Chan, Andrilla, Huff, & Hart, 2010). PHNs can work with health care providers to assure proper medication administration and cardiac aftercare, as well as follow-up on lifestyle changes for clients.

Diabetes

Rural populations are disproportionately affected by diabetes; the prevalence is generally greater in rural areas (7.9% vs. 6%), and this is even more pronounced among Hispanics and Blacks (Krishna et al., 2010; Zhang, Wang, & Huang, 2009). Causes for these differences are not always well understood, but may be due to less exercise, higher rates of smoking, and greater incidence of obesity in rural populations, all of which put them at a higher risk for type 2 diabetes. Rural areas have been cited as promoting obesity on a population level because of fewer opportunities for walking, as residents spend a great deal of time commuting to work or driving to essential services, and rural residence was positively correlated with BMI, distance to retail food, and commute times (Jilcott et al., 2010).

Rural populations also face greater barriers in diagnosis, treatment, and follow-up care. Some compliance issues with prescribed medication regimens may relate to the lack of health insurance and low-income levels in rural areas but could also be due to lower health literacy and education levels. Other problems with accessing care may involve transportation and weather. The lack of appropriate services, such as certified diabetes educators or endocrinologists, is also common in rural America; expensive, up-to-date technologies requiring technical expertise are not readily available in most rural areas (NACRHHS, 2008). Basic follow-up with podiatrists for diabetic foot care, ophthalmologists for retinal health, nutritionists, and health educators, as well as laboratory blood tests, can be extremely complicated for rural individuals who may have to travel great distances to access these services (Krishna et al., 2010). Programs targeted specifically to rural areas, usually provided by additional grant funding and personnel, have demonstrated success in reducing weight and improving physical activity. A Montana study of adults with diabetes and CVD exhibited an 83% completion rate, and 65% of those met the physical activity goal of 150-minutes per week. A 7% weight loss was achieved by 62% of completers (Vadheim et al., 2010). PHNs, especially in rural and frontier areas, often provide follow-up for diabetic clients who may be unable to regularly access their health care providers due to problems with distance or transportation. Home visits to check on their diet/exercise, blood glucose monitoring, and foot care are important safeguards for this population.

Human Immunodeficiency Virus Infection

Human immunodeficiency virus or HIV, the virus that causes acquired immunodeficiency syndrome (AIDS), was first identified among the urban U.S. population in the early 1980s. The Centers for Disease Control and Prevention (CDC) estimates that more than 1.1 million U.S. residents have HIV, and 34,247 were diagnosed with AIDS in 2009. In 2008, almost one-half million people were living with AIDS (CDC, 2011). About 5% to 8% of all HIV cases in the United States were among rural populations in the early 1990s, with 56,209 diagnosed with AIDS by 2007. In the South, there are rising incidences of new cases and deaths from AIDS; in 2006, 67% of new cases were in the rural South. The 2007 rate of AIDS in the South was 9.2 per 100,000, the Midwest was only 2.5, the West 3.9, and the Northeast 5.6 (Rural Center for AIDS/STD Prevention, 2009).

Also, 50% of rural AIDS cases are among African Americans, and young African American women are the fastest growing group infected through heterosexual exposures. In all racial/ethnic groups in rural areas, men have the highest rate of AIDS at 9.1 per 100,000 (almost three times that of women), and more than 50% are exposed through sexual contact with men. Injection drug use accounts for 20% of male AIDS cases, and over 50% of rural HIV infections are only diagnosed within the year after advancing to AIDS. While there have been no significant differences between rural and urban populations in numbers of sexual partners, rates of unprotected sex, and being tested for HIV, rural residents were found to be less likely to change sexual behaviors or condom use in response to the AIDS epidemic (Rural Center for AIDS/STD Prevention, 2009).

Early diagnosis and treatment of HIV/AIDS are issues that must be faced by all rural communities. Physicians, nurses, and other health practitioners need to be educated about the changing face of the disease. Because relatively few cases of HIV/AIDS may be present in any one rural community, specialized services are often not available, and it can be a challenge to stay up-to-date with the newest treatment protocols (National Rural Health Association [NRHA], 2008). Each state health department has resource persons who can provide information to health professionals in rural communities about the HIV/AIDS epidemic and current treatment protocols. A study of HIV testing and other treatment services in rural counties in the South found that 53% of health departments responding to the survey provided HIV testing, and 48% had HIV treatment sites. Clients had to travel an average of 50 miles to reach these services, which was considered a barrier, but facilitators included rapid HIV testing, integrating HIV testing into other services, and establishment of free/easily accessible HIV testing services (Sutton et al., 2010). Communities must determine the burden of disease and tailor services to their population, while at the same time providing education and case finding. Increased community awareness may be accomplished through faith-based organizations or by having local coaches or radio personalities raise the issue of HIV/AIDS; after-school service learning programs for youth may be helpful in reducing adolescent sexual risk-taking behaviors. Free HIV testing made available where rural populations gather (e.g., regional athletic events, colleges, health centers, church congregations) or high-risk groups gather (e.g., adult or gay bookstores, bars) has been found to be effective. Testing incoming and outgoing prisoners, and providing condoms, can also reach a high-risk population. Many health departments offer services through Ryan White CARE Act grant funding; these may include comprehensive care clinics or PHN case management services, as well as education/prevention. Medications delivered by mail, rather than picked up in small local pharmacies, may help with confidentiality for HIV/AIDS clients (Rural Center for AIDS/STD Prevention, 2009).

It may be difficult for a person to seek diagnosis or treatment from a rural health practitioner. Confidentiality is an issue of concern, as is lack of anonymity. People with HIV/AIDS may fear the stigma of HIV/AIDS and the rejection that is often associated with it. They may have concern for their jobs or their position in the community if their diagnosis is divulged, and they frequently fear that health care workers will break confidentiality rules (NRHA, 2008). Instead, rural people may choose to seek out HIV/AIDS testing through an urban health care facility where they know no one. Returning to the community can be devastating because of the lack of needed support services and the fear of sharing their diagnosis with others.

Another issue that may arise is that of urban residents with rural roots who return to their home communities as their illness worsens. These people seek family support and can overwhelm their caregivers, especially if the caregivers do not seek support for themselves. Community health nurses are in a good position to assist families with any health issues and can offer to facilitate connections to other social, spiritual, financial, and health care providers. A recent study of HIV-positive women found that satisfaction with social support and coping that focused on managing HIV disease were the best predictors of adherence to medication regimens (Vyavaharkar et al., 2007). A review of research on HIV medication compliance revealed that taking more than 10 pills per day was associated with higher odds of nonadherence than twice daily versus once daily medication administration (Atkinson & Petrozzino, 2009).

Access to Health Care

Insurance, Managed Care, and Health Care Services

Health insurance in today's market is costly, especially for individual purchasers. Some people, therefore, forego health insurance for themselves and their families. As noted earlier, rural workers are less likely to be offered health insurance through their employers, often because they are either self-employed or due to the size or type of employers (AHRQ, 2012; Rural Health Research and Policy Centers, 2009). Depending on their income, people may or may not be eligible for Medicaid or State Children's Health Insurance Programs (S-CHIPs). Even people who are eligible for government health assistance may not apply because of their belief that it is a sign of weakness to accept a handout.

Historically, a traditional fee-for-service model delivered health care in rural and urban communities (see Chapter 6). However, it is challenging for rural providers to deliver the cost-effective, complex health care that rural persons need via solo or small group practices. Rural patients often utilize family practice clinics. The managed care model, which attempts to control costs and improve health care delivery, has slowly diffused into rural communities. One reason for the sluggishness is that rural practitioners are reluctant to become part of organizations that negotiate to reduce their payments, as many of them already see a disproportionate number of Medicaid/uninsured patients that impact their bottom line (Texas Rural Health Association, 2010). Another reason is the low population density, making this type of health care insurance less profitable. However, more states are moving to Medicaid managed care models, and Medicare offers this option to beneficiaries. This puts rural residents at a disadvantage, as they may have poor access to services due to distance and travel time.

Building provider networks in rural communities is both time- and effort-intensive because rural providers are often inexperienced with managed care organizations (MCOs). The federal government provides support for **rural health clinics** in areas designated as underserved and nonurban (RAC, n.d.). Specialized *migrant clinics* may also be located in rural areas with large migrant worker populations. Many of these are **federally qualified health centers** that provide care to underserved populations through Medicare, Medicaid, or a sliding fee scale (RAC, n.d.). Because only 9% of physicians work in rural areas (where 21% of the population resides), midlevel practitioners, such as physician assistants (PAs) and nurse practitioners (NPs), are often employed in these clinics (AHRQ, 2012). Also, specialists are most often found in metropolitan areas; rural areas are devoid of most of the smaller-specialty physicians, and the population has difficulty accessing these services.

Rural areas are characterized by a lack of core health care services (e.g., primary care, hospital care, emergency medical services, long-term care, mental health and substance abuse counseling services, dental care, public health services). A national survey of CEOs from rural hospitals found that over 75% reported physician shortages, most commonly family practice (58.3%) and internal medicine (53.1%). Other shortages were noted for physicians specializing in psychiatry, general surgery, neurology, pediatrics, cardiology, and OB-GYN. Over 73% reported shortages of registered nurses, and over half needed pharmacists. Thirty-five percent reported a need for NPs (MacDowell, Glasser, Fitts, Nielsen, & Hunsaker, 2010). Population health services in rural areas may be covered by a combination of public health departments, physicians in private practice, and local hospitals, as well as various community agencies. In some rural or frontier areas, state health departments may offer services, as no local infrastructure may be present (Meit, Harris, Bushar, Piya, & Molfino, 2008). Many rural residents depend heavily on public health department services.

Forty percent of local health departments (LHDs) serve small towns (populations under 10,000) and rural areas. These LHDs are less likely than larger health departments to provide environmental health services, but they often provide many of the other services (e.g., primary prevention, health services, epidemiology/surveillance) found in larger health departments (National Association of County and City Health Officials [NACCHO], 2007). Many rural public health agencies are small and isolated, with a need for connections with other agencies in the region or state.

PHNs serve in a variety of capacities—often wearing many hats. Rural public health departments generally have lower public funding for programs and services and must guard against fragmentation of resources/programs. They also experience difficulty competing against urban agencies in access to grant funding and recruiting specialized staff. Transportation costs and adequate provision of a variety of services are other issues faced by rural public health departments, and all of these issues affect the health of the populations served. However, one study comparing willingness to respond to emergency situations revealed that rural health department workers were significantly more likely to respond than urban workers (Barnett et al., 2012). In all response scenarios provided (weather-related, pandemic influenza, radiological "dirty" bomb, anthrax), rural workers were more willing to respond and report to the health department; the lowest response from both groups was found for a "dirty" bomb scenario (78.7% rural, 73% urban).

Barriers to Access

In rural areas, numerous access barriers to health care exist. The physical distance between place of residence and location of health care services can be considerable. Weather and geographical barriers may also be a factor. Rural clients may be referred to a distant urban medical center for cancer therapy or other sophisticated care. Members of the population may be frustrated if they travel to a faraway site for care and do not have their problem resolved. Rural clients must be advised before they travel to make sure that the health care provider is not behind schedule or unable to see them; see From the Case Files I for a hard lesson learned by one PHN student.

Transportation can also be an issue, especially for people who do not drive or who lack dependable vehicles. Almost 33% have transportation disadvantages, with those earning between $20,000 and $50,000 spending 30% of their income on a car and the costs related to driving it (American Public Health Association [APHA], n.d.). Unpredictable weather adds to potential barriers for rural clients. Snow, ice, wind, flash floods, and rain can make travel dangerous, even over short distances. Parents may decide not to risk driving on poorly maintained roads to get their children immunized or to have their own hypertension evaluated. Elderly people may choose to delay health care when long travel times, especially in isolated rural areas, are involved. As the seriousness of a condition increases, however, people often reverse their decisions (Basu & Mobley, 2007), and travel in emergency situations can be life-threatening, not only because of the emergency itself but also because of the distance involved to get the ill or injured person to the nearest health care facility. According to a

From the Case Files I

A Lesson in Rural Transportation

I live in a relatively large city of 450,000 people. When I started my community health nursing rotation, I was assigned to a rural county public health department in an adjoining county over 50 miles from my house. To make matters worse, when I got there for my first clinical day, my professor told me that I was assigned to see clients in an isolated community another hour away from the health department! There was nothing but farmland between the county seat and this small, forgotten oil town. This small town didn't even have sidewalks, much less a fast-food restaurant! After I got over my frustration about traveling such long distances, I began to visit some of my families and started to actually enjoy my time with them. They were so appreciative and open to my suggested interventions. I really seemed to be making a difference. One older gentleman, Armando, was a diabetic who spoke very little English. He lived with his wife of 50 years, who spoke almost no English. Their children had moved away in order to go to school and get better jobs. His diabetes was not well controlled, and the rural health clinic FNP suggested that he see a specialist (actually an internist) in the county seat. I helped him make arrangements with the doctor for an early afternoon visit and made sure that he could catch the county bus that ran between the smaller communities and the county seat. When I came back for a follow-up visit the next week, I was shocked to learn that Armando's appointment had been pushed back to 4:30 PM because of the doctor's involvement in hospital emergencies, and by the time Armando was finished with his appointment, the county bus service had ended. Armando, with no money and no one to call for a ride, began walking back to his home—over 52 miles away! About halfway home, a farm truck driver gave him a lift to the large cotton farm a few miles from his home. You can imagine my horror and embarrassment when I learned of this ordeal. I never realized how difficult it was for rural people to get to their medical appointments. I always had a car and could drive wherever my gas budget could take me. I thought that the bus would not be a problem, but I learned my lesson. Now, I make sure that the physician's office understands the patient's circumstances and the importance of getting them back to the bus stop in time to make the last bus.

Andrea, Senior Nursing Student

classic study by Branas, McKenzie, and Williams (2005), almost 47 million rural Americans do not have access to either level I or level II trauma centers within an hour's driving time, leaving them at higher risk for death from injuries. However, almost 43 million urban Americans can access 20 or more trauma centers (level I or level II) within an hour's time. Hsia and Shen (2011) found that 31% of those in rural areas had difficult access to trauma centers in their analysis of a national survey.

Limited choice of health care providers is a barrier for some rural residents. Fewer physicians, nurses, dentists, and other providers work in rural areas (AHRQ, 2012). Those with special needs often must travel to urban medical centers to get required care. One seminal study of disabled adults noted that they found their local rural physicians to be less familiar with their conditions, thus requiring these disabled patients to "teach" their health care provider. They also described rural public transportation as often unreliable and inaccessible in an important study by Iezzoni, Killeen, and O'Day (2006). A literature review revealed that rural residents have diverse types of disabilities, yet have barriers to accessing needed care. Children/adolescents, mentally ill, working adults, the elderly, and those with HIV/AIDS were populations of interest, and rural health care providers were often found to be lacking in training and experience necessary to treat some of the more complex medical needs of these clients. The authors also noted the need for regional specialized care services, telehealth, better training and networking for local primary care physicians, and the use of case managers and trained local paraprofessionals to bridge the gap in care (Lishner, Richardson, Levine, & Patrick, n.d.). As Medicare payments to primary care physicians are reduced and often late, there is a real threat to rural disabled and elderly clients, as some physicians either limit the number of Medicare clients they will serve or close their offices in rural areas (Disabled World, 2010). As mentioned earlier, concerns about confidentiality or provider expertise sometimes cause clients to seek care from even more distant providers, but as the options for health care continue to shrink, rural clients may have few choices available locally. Those persons with disabilities who are also uninsured (more common in rural populations) have significantly more access barriers to care than those without disabilities (Iezzoni, Frakt, & Pizer, 2011).

New Approaches to Improve Access

The *Healthy People 2020* document mandates improvements in access, health education, health screening, immunizations, and disease morbidity for the United States. Creative ways of delivering these and other services to rural clients need to be explored. Access to care is a social justice issue: clients who live in rural areas should receive quality health care, regardless of where they choose to live.

Faith-based nursing has been a staple in rural areas, as well as with some urban communities, but is gaining momentum as more formal interventions are developed (see more on faith-based nursing in Chapter 31). Even informal support from other church members and friends may provide a compassionate environment for needed behavioral changes such as healthy diet and increased physical activity (Kegler et al., 2012). Church communities may also provide assistance and relief to caregivers in rural areas, especially when more formal services are unavailable or geographically distant (Greene, Perkins, Scott, & Burt, 2011). A formal study comparing community-based and church-based 10-week educational interventions for overweight African American females living in rural South Carolina found statistically significant reductions in weight and systolic blood pressure for both groups. However, the church-based group also had significant reductions in diastolic blood pressure and BMI, as well as improved physical activity and health care provider communication (Parker, Coles, Logan, & Davis, 2010). Researchers noted that social interaction, facilitated by group education and discussion, could actually be as vital to success as the didactic information about weight control and diet.

One approach that has been successful in numerous rural areas is the use of *mobile clinics*. These clinics bring health care providers to remote places for health screenings, immunizations, dental care, mental health visits, and other services. Mobile health clinics are frequently staffed by NPs and can improve access to health care for low-income residents. They often are available to residents on evenings and weekends and offer culturally sensitive and bilingual outreach, as well as care for uninsured clients. They may be helpful in overcoming access problems for vulnerable populations (Isler, Miles, Banks, & Corbie-Smith, 2012).

School-based clinics can improve access for schoolchildren (and sometimes their families) but may be less prominent in rural areas (see more on school-based clinics in Chapter 30). Only 27% are in rural areas and 16% in suburban areas, with the majority in urban areas. These clinics provide available, community-based, affordable, and culturally acceptable care to well and sick children. Often, grant-supported, school-based clinics facilitate the receipt of health education and primary care by children who are otherwise without easy access to health services (National Conference of State Legislatures, 2011). An evaluation of school-based clinics in Ohio found improvement in services to African Americans, with better access and cost benefits (Guo, Wade, Pan, & Keller, 2010).

Telehealth, another approach to increasing access to care, provides electronically transmitted clinician consultation between the client and the health care provider. This option is especially useful for connecting home health nurses with their patients who need close monitoring at home. It is also useful for patient and professional health education, public health applications, and health administration. Specialty health care also may be accessed, with patients and providers connected via two-way audiovisual transmission over telephone lines or the Internet, thus obviating the need for patients to leave their residences. Streaming media, video conferencing, and store-and-forward imaging are just some of the applications commonly utilized (HRSA, n.d.). Clients can also be assessed quickly by interactive communication from physician offices, hospitals, and other sites. Telehealth technology may decrease visits to emergency departments and hospitalizations, and an Arkansas health department found it helpful in providing diabetes education to patients in remote areas (Balamurugan et al., 2009). Dermatology consultations were accomplished through telemedicine consultations for farmworkers with skin diseases at rural clinics in North Carolina, and 13% of diagnoses were changes, along with 21% of recommended treatments (Vallejos et al., 2009). Grants and other funding are available to promote the use of this technology (HRSA, n.d. b).

Healthy People 2020 Goals

The four overarching goals of *Healthy People 2020* are to:

(1) Attain high-quality, longer lives free of preventable disease
(2) Achieve health equity, eliminate disparities, and improve the health of all groups
(3) Create social and physical environments that promote good health for all
(4) Promote quality of life, healthy development, and healthy behaviors across all life stages (USDHHS, 2012, para. 5)

Because of the unique health issues facing rural America, *Rural Healthy People 2010: A Companion Document to Healthy People 2010* was developed. Using surveys, literature reviews, and other methods of data collection and analysis, top priorities for rural health were identified. The document also highlighted current knowledge on rural health and identified best practices, as well as called for further research on rural health promotion (Bellamy, Bolin, Nelson, & Gamm, 2011). This process is being repeated to create a rural health companion document to *Healthy People 2020*. Certainly, there are data to substantiate continued problems with access to health care and insurance, as well as emergency services, in rural areas. And there is a higher rate of CVD and diabetes, along with obesity and tobacco use among rural populations (National Rural Health Association, n.d.). The *Healthy People 2020* document notes specific differences in oral health and social determinants of health related to geography. A national survey (n = 688) conducted between 2010 and 2011 listed the initial top ten priorities for *Rural Healthy People 2020* as (1) access to quality health services, (2) diabetes care, (3) mental health care, (4) nutrition and weight status, (5) heart disease/stroke, (6) substance abuse, (7) physical activity/health, (8) care for older adults, (9) cancer, and (10) maternal/infant/child health (Bolin & Bellamy, n.d.). However, funding cuts have prevented the broadened surveys first proposed, and the authors hope to gain further input from additional stakeholders.

Problems more commonly seen in rural areas include oral health and cigarette/smokeless tobacco use. Sixty percent of rural counties are considered professional shortage areas for dental health, and more dentists are over age 55 in rural areas (42% vs. 38% in urban). Rural populations are less likely to have an annual dental examination. They are also more likely to have tooth or gum disease, often because of higher rates of cigarette and smokeless tobacco use (Kronkosky Charitable Foundation, 2011). Oral health in rural areas is affected by the shortage of dentists and access issues (Fisher-Owens et al., 2008).

Smoking prevalence in rural areas is higher than in urban areas, and smokeless tobacco use is twice or three times higher in rural areas. Alcohol dependence is more common in rural than suburban areas (Borders & Booth, 2007; Kronkosky Charitable Foundation, 2011). Prevalence of illicit drug use is similar, but access to substance abuse services is better in urban areas. The vast majority (80%) of rural residents live in counties without detoxification facilities (Kronkosky Charitable Foundation, 2011). Latino, American Indian, and Asian rural adolescents have more chronic illnesses than do adolescents in other racial/ethnic groups (Wickrama, Elder, & Abraham, 2007).

Children who have special health care needs and who live in rural areas are less likely to be have their health care provided by a pediatrician and more likely to have unmet health care needs due to unavailability of services or transportation problems (Skinner & Slifkin, 2007). Research has demonstrated that rural residence is a risk factor for obesity and overweight in children and women (Lutfiyya, Lipsky, Wisdom-Behounek, & Inpanbutr-Martinkus, 2007). And rural areas frequently have deficient physical education programs in schools, but residents have greater inactivity and calorie consumption (Kronkosky Charitable Foundation, 2011).

Cancer disparities are found in rural populations. For example, cervical cancer rates for rural women are statistically higher than for women living in urban areas (Bernard, Coughlin, Thompson, & Richardson, 2007). Survival rates for cervical cancer are also lower in nonmetropolitan areas, especially so for rural Black women who had a 50.8% 5-year survival rate compared with 60.2% for those in metropolitan areas (Singh, 2012). Rural women are less likely to receive screening mammograms and Pap smears than urban women. Rural populations also have a lower proportion of colonoscopies to screen for colorectal cancer and to have a physician examine them (South Carolina Rural Health Research Center, 2009). Rural PHNs need to consider the *Healthy People 2020* objectives and *Rural Healthy People 2020* priority areas as guides for improving the health status of clients in rural communities.

MIGRANT HEALTH

You may never have seen migrant workers, yet you are a direct beneficiary of their labor. Have you ever thought about the people who harvest the fruits and vegetables that you eat? What would happen to the complex system of agricultural production and distribution if workers were not available to pick crops at peak harvest times? Have you ever thought about exactly who these people are, where they come from, where they live, or what their health is like? Migrant farmworkers are an integral part of the farming community in the United States and across the world. The agricultural industry relies heavily on migrant workers to harvest the almost endless array of fresh produce that appears year-round in supermarkets across the United States as fresh, frozen, and canned fruits and vegetables (Benson, 2010). More than 3 million seasonal and migrant farmworkers provide labor for the $28 billion vegetable and fruit crops of the United States (NCFH, n.d. b). Many of these workers are unauthorized or illegal immigrants to the United States, often from Mexico. A study of Canadian migrant workers, a country with a seasonal agricultural worker program offering higher wages and shorter time periods away from home and family (up to 8 months), found that 100% of those leaving Mexico on their first entry into Canada were legal temporary workers. In contrast, only 18% of those leaving for the United States were entering legally as workers with an H2A (work program) visa (Massey & Brown, 2011). The vast majority entered this country in an unauthorized manner. Because Canada recruited temporary workers from Mexico under a formal agreement, their workers were over age 18 (usually 22 to 45 years), had agricultural experience, and had no prior criminal records. Mexico also stipulated that they have some education (third to ninth grade) and be in a stable relationship (married or common law). Because of this program, with benefits to both countries and the temporary workers, Canada has a low proportion of workers becoming permanent residents and a more "circular flow" with repeat migrations. In the United States, undocumented workers often stay for longer periods of time due to tighter controls on border crossing making repeated migrations more difficult than before 9/11 (Massey & Brown, 2011, p. 119).

Despite their importance to American agriculture, migrant workers are rarely visible members of our society. They go unnoticed beyond the fringes of the camps and farms to which they travel to pursue their livelihood. Most come to the United States from other countries (78%), and of those, about 75% are from Mexico; most have been in the United States 10 years on average. The average age is 33.5 years, and 79% are males; only 58% are married, and of the 51% who are parents, 66% do not have their children with them. Approximately 42% of farmworkers are considered migrant (traveling 75 miles to obtain farm jobs), and many travel to multiple farm sites within a year. Most (34%) worked in fruit and nut crops, and 69% find employment through family and friends. Only 2% are salaried, with the majority paid low hourly wages or by the piece; one quarter of them work over 50 hours per week, and another quarter work <35 hours a week. California, Florida, Texas, North Carolina, Michigan, Washington, Tennessee, and Oregon currently have the highest number of migrant farmworkers (NCFH, 2009). They come with the hope of improving their impoverished lives. Some are legal residents, but most are undocumented aliens and live in fear of deportation. All endure backbreaking, menial labor for low wages and are often deprived of basic rights to safe working conditions, adequate sanitation/housing, health care, and a quality education for their children.

MIGRANT FARMWORKERS: PROFILE OF A NOMADIC AGGREGATE

Maintaining a low public profile, migrant workers are, for the most part, marginalized from mainstream society. They remain unseen, unheard, poorly understood, and excluded from many programs that provide health care assistance for low-income people. The migrant worker is a kind of disenfranchised person, for whom no one wants to take responsibility. Yet the needs of these workers are great. They are plagued with different, more complex, and more frequent health problems than the general population (Formichelli, 2008; Migrant Clinician's Network, n.d. a). Common ailments include infectious diseases (e.g., tuberculosis [TB], parasites), gastrointestinal disorders, dermatitis due to pesticide exposure, emotional distress and depression, vision and eye problems, cancer, and chronic illnesses, such as asthma, bronchitis, diabetes, and hypertension. They are plagued by poverty, poor nutrition, substandard housing conditions, extended working hours, and grueling, often unsafe, working conditions. Their demographics, socioeconomic conditions, and lifestyle resemble those of a Third World country despite the fact that they live and work in one of the most prosperous nations on Earth. Although migrant families are in dire need of health resources, various economic, cultural, and language barriers prevent this aggregate from accessing available health services. Only 8% of migrant farmworkers have full health insurance paid by employers, and 5% of those working seasonally have coverage (NCFH, 2009). A study found that less than 10% of Mexican immigrants (documented and undocumented) who were in the United States <10 years reported ever going to an emergency department for care, compared with 20% of native-born Mexican Americans and Whites (King, 2007).

Migrant workers live and work in areas where health care practitioners are generally in short supply. In a large national study of farmworkers, only 52% had used U.S. health care services within the last 2 years, and barriers include lack of health insurance, fear of immigration consequence, low English proficiency, and access to transportation (Hoerster et al., 2011). Among Latino immigrants, common barriers include communication problems, difficulty proving financial eligibility, and long waiting periods for gaining access to health care services. They often used traditional cultural remedies (e.g., herbal medications, traditional healers) and often blended both traditional and U.S. health care practices (Ransford, Carrillo, & Rivera, 2010). An 18-month ethnographic study of indigenous Triqui migrant workers followed them from Oaxaca, Mexico, to central California and on to the northwest area of Washington as they harvested crops. Interviews were conducted with them, and the health care providers who worked in the clinics serving them. Holmes (2009, p. 873) found that "social and economic factors in health care and subtle cultural factors... keep medical professionals from seeing the social determinants of suffering," and this leads them to inadvertently blame the patients. It was noted that the "structure and culture" of health care was often the cause of barriers to more effective multicultural health care. This demonstrates that it is essential to understand the history, demographics, environment, culture, and health care needs of the migrant worker, so that PHNs can better assist them in protecting their health and the health of all citizens.

Historical Background

Both historically and internationally, farmers have rarely been able to permanently employ the large workforces needed to harvest their crops. Throughout the 19th century, however, the small, family-owned farms typical in the United States got through the harvest by using schoolchildren, neighbors, and local day laborers. As time went by, this became more and more difficult to accomplish. During the decade ending in 1929, over half a million Mexicans migrated to the United States, many drawn to work in seasonal agriculture. With the Great Depression, many of the small, independently run farms went bankrupt, and citizens were concerned about scarce employment opportunities. Because of this, state and federal governments were lobbied by civic groups to "round up Mexican Americans indiscriminately ... and to 'repatriate' them to Mexico" (University of California, 2012, para. 5.). Within a few years, the outbreak of World War II caused an increased need for food production and additional workers, as many U.S. workers joined the military. To keep abreast of the demand for produce, the larger surviving farms turned to migrant labor for help. The Emergency Labor Program—known as the Bracero Program—was enacted in 1942 to permit temporary Mexican immigration to provide needed workers for American agriculture and industry (University of California, 2012). Between 1942 and 1964, more than 4 million Mexican workers participated in this program, leaving their families behind and coming to work in Californian fields. When this program ended, workers continued to cross the border to seek employment, often bringing along their families. Employers hired needed undocumented workers from Mexico, as well as Central and South America.

Living apart from society, the plight of migrant farmworkers was largely ignored until exposure on a 1960 television documentary—Edward R. Murrow's *Harvest of Shame*—created a national outcry. This led to the passage of the Migrant Health Act of 1962, which addressed the specific health needs of migrant workers for the first time in U.S. history. This act authorized delivery of primary and supplementary health services to migrant farmworkers (NCFH, n.d. b). Federally funded migrant health clinics serve areas in the United States where significant number of migrant farmworkers gather. In 2004, these clinics served more than 675,000 seasonal and migrant farmworkers, a number far below the estimated 3+ million farmworkers thought to be in this country (King, 2007). Services may be provided seasonally, on a temporary basis, or year-round. Staffing usually includes doctors, nurses, NPs, PAs, outreach workers, social workers, and dental and pharmacy workers, along with health educators. Transportation may also be a component in some areas. Primary and preventive health care services are provided to migrant workers and their families throughout more than 500 clinic sites (see Internet Resources found on thePoint for a map of your state). However, funding is often inadequate, and many clinics are not sufficiently staffed or operated to meet the health needs of migrant farmworkers and their dependents. Most migrant health centers receive funding from a variety of sources, including Medicaid in some instances. Additionally, although these clinics exist throughout the United States, large geographic regions are not served well or at all. Other services, such as *promotora programs* that employ Hispanic lay health workers or nursing voucher programs providing NP services at participating clinics and nurse referrals to specialists, are available in some areas (Formichelli, 2008). Migrant workers in areas without migrant clinics or other targeted services must rely on LHDs and emergency rooms for health care, or they may simply go without needed care.

The current H2A program for temporary agricultural workers permits employers to file paperwork, demonstrating a need for temporary workers that cannot be met by U.S. workers, and then workers from approved countries can apply for a visa. It allows them to work for up to 1 year in the United States, and they may bring spouses and children under age 21 under a companion visa program (H4) that does not permit them to work (U.S. Department of Homeland Security, 2012). Only a small percentage of workers and employers utilize this program, approximately 1% in the last national survey. In the same survey, 53% of farmworkers were described as unauthorized to work, 25% were U.S. citizens and 21% were legal permanent residents (U.S. Department of Labor, 2010).

Demographics

Because migrant farmworkers constitute a mobile population with shifting composition, it is difficult to precisely determine their number or origins. Estimates of the number of migrant workers vary also because of the influx of illegal and undocumented workers. A large number of seasonal and migrant farmworkers permanently reside in the United States, and 48% are either U.S. citizens or have permanent resident status (Migrant Clinicians Network, n.d.). Most of the estimated 3 to 5 million migrant farmworkers tend to be either newly arrived immigrants, with few connections, or established legal residents with limited opportunities and skills, who rely on farm labor for survival (NCFH, n.d. a). In addition to male workers, who make up the majority, you may also see mothers bring infants and young children to work with them, and the children spend their days strapped to their mother's back or playing among the pesticide-laden fields.

Seasonal farmworkers generally live in one geographic location and are principally employed in agriculture (51% or more of their time), whereas **migrant farmworkers** meet that classification while moving to find agricultural work throughout the year, usually from state to state, and establishing temporary residences (Larson, 2000). Some live apart from their families, forming groups of single men; others travel with their entire families. The average migrant farmworker spends from June to September doing seasonal harvesting, with about 8 weeks on the road traveling from farm to farm for work, and is then unemployed unless other work, such as hauling or canning, is found. Days begin before dawn and work continues for 12 hours or longer. Farmworkers cannot be paid for overtime, as federal laws exclude this category of work, and 15 states don't require workers' compensation (Barbassa, 2010). The main reason migrant workers immigrate is to find work, and most migrant farmworkers end up in areas where they already have social networks, such as family or acquaintances from their own areas of Mexico (Cohen, 2010).

As an illustration of the working conditions and wages in the tomato fields of Florida, pickers work "10 to 12 hours a day picking tomatoes by hand, earning a piece-rate of about 45 cents for every 32-pound bucket" (Schlosser, 2007, para. 1). An average workday consists of picking, carrying, and unloading about 2 tons of tomatoes. In Florida, abuses of migrant farmworkers have included nonpayment of wages and forcing workers into debt, chaining workers in trailers at night, and charges of slavery. The U.S. Department of Justice has prosecuted roughly "a half a dozen cases of slavery" in the last decade (Schlosser, 2007, para. 4). Families working in the cotton fields of Texas and other states report working long hours, and children as young as 11 may work alongside adults (Coursen-Neff, 2011).

Migrant Streams and Patterns

Migrant farmworkers usually have their permanent residence, or *home base*, in states with a traditionally high number of immigrants, like California, Texas, Florida, New York, or Illinois (King, 2007). From their home base, they move to locations where each new crop is ready for harvest. As they follow the harvest seasons of agricultural crops, migrant farmworkers move from place to place, usually along predetermined routes called **migrant streams** (Fig. 29-5). Some migrant farmworkers are multigenerational; that is, their families have been farmworkers for several generations, traveling the same streams for many years. It is very common for farmworkers to send money back home to family members; total migrant remittances constitute large sums of money and provide significant support for families in other countries, like Mexico (Cohen, 2010).

Three principal streams formulate the agricultural routes that migrant laborers follow. The *eastern stream* originates in Florida, where most of their time is spent, and extends up the East Coast through North Carolina, Tennessee, Kentucky, Virginia, and other states east of the Mississippi, as far as north as Ohio, New Jersey, New York, Connecticut, Massachusetts, New Hampshire, Vermont, and Maine. The *midwestern stream* begins in southern Texas or northern Mexico and fans out across the United States, ending in the northwestern and midwestern states bordering Canada, both east and west of the Mississippi. The *western stream* originates in California and moves up the West Coast to all western states and from central California into North Dakota (Formichelli, 2008). California, Florida, and Texas are regarded as *sending states*, as they are often home states with long growing seasons where migrant streams begin and end. Male workers may travel with

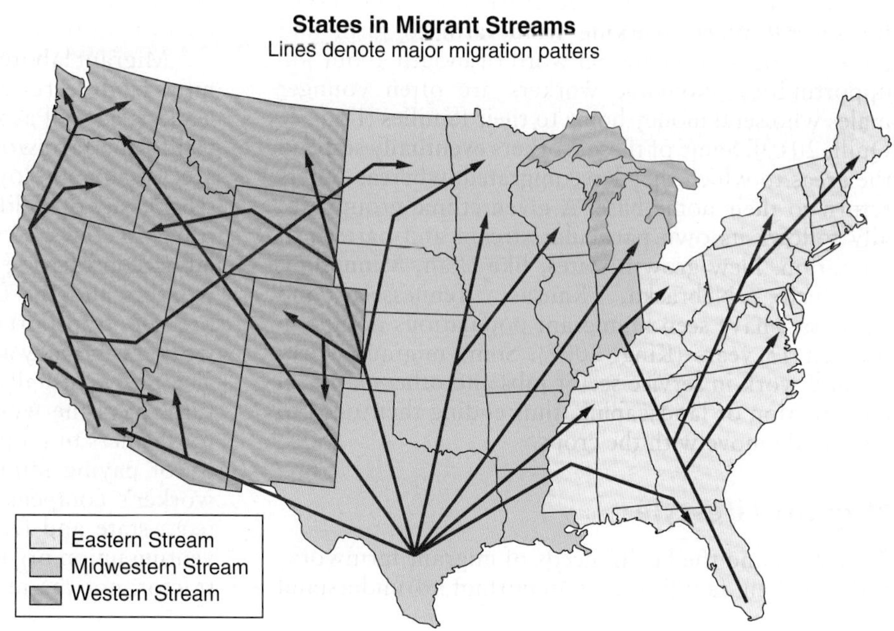

FIGURE 29-5. Migrant Streams. Source: Migrant Head Start Program, USHDHUD.

the crops and leave their families in these home states (USDHUD, 2012). Workers move from areas with cotton, tree fruits and nuts, and vegetable crops to other areas where they harvest cherries, watermelons, cantaloupes, or potatoes.

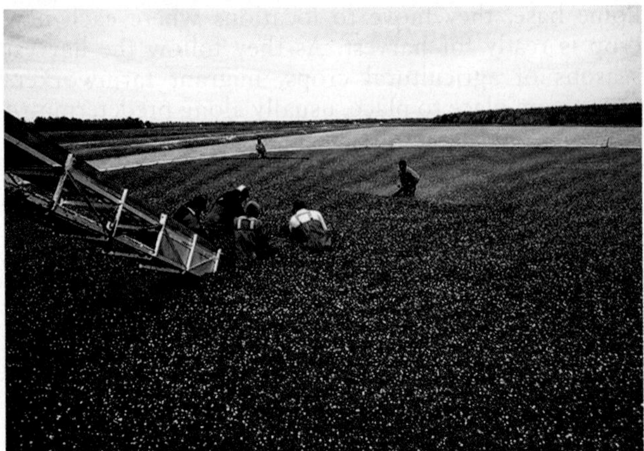

Cranberry harvest in New Jersey. Source: USDA, Agricultural Research Service.

Weather conditions and employment opportunities affect movement and patterns of migration. Because of the unpredictable nature of farmwork, the three streams are not clearly delineated, pointing to more complex patterns of movement. In addition to the migrant streams, **patterns of migration** exist, with varying lengths of stay. In a *restricted circuit*, many people travel throughout a season within a small geographic area, following the crops. *Point-to-point migration* entails leaving a home base for part of the year to travel to the same place or series of places along a route during the agricultural season, usually returning on a yearly basis. Almost 40% of seasonal farmworkers shuttle back and forth this way (Loue & Quill, 2010).

Nomadic migrant workers travel away from home for several years, working from farm to farm and crop to crop and relying on word of mouth about job opportunities. Nomadic workers are often younger males who send money home to their families (Loue & Quill, 2010). Some of these workers eventually settle in the areas to which they have migrated, whereas others return to their home base. A given ethnic group usually follows its own particular stream and pattern of migration. New growth states, like Utah, Minnesota, Wisconsin, Nebraska, Kansas, Tennessee, and Arkansas, have seen immigrant populations double in the last 15 years (King, 2007). Some migrant workers find work in service sector jobs and others labor in construction or landscaping, thus ending their need to constantly move with the crops.

Migrant Lifestyle

To understand the health needs of migrant farmworkers and their families, it is important to understand their lifestyle. Migrant workers and their families endure a transient and uncertain life, with long hours, stressful working conditions, low wages, and poor health care. Substandard housing, unsafe working conditions, and language barriers make life even more difficult (USDHUD, 2012a).

Migrant workers must confront the vagaries of an unpredictable world. Migrants typically remain in an area for only 6 to 8 weeks, working the fields 6 days a week from sunrise to sunset. Depending on weather and crop conditions, work may be plentiful 1 week and virtually gone the next. Because yearly income must be earned during the harvest season, all family members contribute to harvesting. Children are essential to the core group's economy and must help in the fields and at home (Loue & Quill, 2010). Migrant workers often drive night and day as they move from crop to crop. Typically, they travel with their children and only their most essential possessions, in aging cars, vans, and trucks. Occasionally, van loads of *solos*, or single men, migrate together. Their status is even more precarious because they lack family support systems. Male farmworkers, single or away from their families, more often engage in risk-taking behaviors of drinking alcohol, having sex with commercial sex workers, and inconsistent use of condoms (Rhodes et al., 2010).

Depending on the economy and the crop, a migrant farmworker's income varies widely. Men, women, and older children all work in the fields. Because inexpensive child care is seldom available, mothers often leave very young children alone playing in fields, where they are exposed to sun, chemicals, and dangerous machinery. Sometimes children are brought to the fields and left in cars or in cardboard boxes. Often a teenage girl or the mother of an infant may remain in the camp to babysit all the children; she is usually stranded there, because all available cars are used to take workers to the fields. There are Head Start and Migrant Head Start programs in many areas, but they can only provide services to a minority of those needing them.

Migrant laborers learn about employment opportunities from recruiters, farm labor contractors, and crew leaders, as well as from other migrants. About 33% of California farmworkers and 20% of those nationwide are usually employed through farm labor contractors (University of California, 2012). Migrant workers who travel in crews, or groups, are often employed by farm labor contractors, who act as the mediator between workers and the farmer. These contractors may also provide transportation, housing, and meals for the workers and may also supervise their work in the fields. The farmer usually pays the labor contractor, who, in turn, pays the workers. This can be viewed as a way for farmers to remove themselves from the responsibility of paying minimum wages to workers, providing worker's compensation, meeting legal responsibilities (e.g., state and federal worker safety rules), and preventing union organizing because they employ the contractor, not the individual workers. Owners may also ignore abuses, because they are not directly employing workers. The labor contractor may underreport hours of workers, or piecework, and harassment can often occur. An unscrupulous crew leader can withhold payment and keep the migrant workers in constant debt. There is often no recourse, as access to legal counsel is rare and legal aid programs funded by the federal government are prohibited from providing services to undocumented workers, and workers generally don't speak out about injustices because of fear and feelings of hopelessness. One remarkable exception is a multimillion dollar judgment awarded to five farmworkers "kept in virtual indentured servitude by their contractors" at an organic farm supplying the upscale supermarket chain, Whole Foods. The contractors charged "smuggling fees, rent, and cleaning charges" that left workers with only $2 out of their $7 hourly wage. They were threatened with violence and the contractors carried guns to ensure compliance (Goldstein, Howe, & Tamir, 2010, p. 3).

Migrant Hero

César Chavez founded the National Farm Workers Association (NFWA; later changed to United Farm Workers [UFW]), the first union in agricultural labor history to successfully organize migrant farmworkers. As a child, he traveled with his family to harvest crops, but they rarely had enough food to eat and often lived in shacks. Work was frequently scarce, wages were low, and labor contractors cheated the family out of the money they earned. Moving to California during the Great Depression, the family became part of the migrant community. Chavez attended as many as 65 different schools, and after completing eighth grade, he dropped out of school to help support his family by working full-time in the fields.

Chavez organized many successful strikes and boycotts, the most famous one being the boycott of California grapes as a protest against the indiscriminate use of pesticides by growers. This boycott lasted for longer than 5 years, and on two occasions he fasted as a protest against the use of agricultural pesticides. His efforts united people who, as individuals, had no significance in the power structure. His legacy is an example of how people can unite to build power together. He achieved great recognition, although he never had the financial trappings of success (Bardacke, 2011). Throughout his life, he ignored personal hardships to continue the struggle with union victories and losses.

HEALTH RISKS OF MIGRANT WORKERS AND THEIR FAMILIES

A community with varied and profound health needs complicated by disease and social isolation, migrant farmworkers and their families are at risk. Migrant workers, often paid piecework, labor at a fast pace, largely without breaks, in order to take advantage of the short growing season (Connor, Layne, & Thomisee, 2010). Because seasonal earnings must last the entire year, the migrant farmworker generally avoids or delays seeking health care until illness becomes debilitating. When work is primary, health is eclipsed (King, 2007). Migrant farmworkers and their families suffer illnesses caused by poor nutrition, a lack of resources to seek care early in the disease process, and infectious diseases due to overcrowding and poor sanitation. National statistics on migrant seasonal workers are sparse, with much of the data regional and only sporadically collected. Some of the statistics include:

- The life expectancy of a migrant worker is much lower than the general population, with high rates of poverty, reduced access to health care, and an inverse and increasingly powerful relationship between stressors (e.g., problems speaking English, legal status, discrimination) and mental/physical health among Mexican workers (Williams & Sternthal, 2010).
- Migrant farmworkers are more likely to come from a country with higher rates of TB (e.g., Mexico 21 vs. United States 4.6/100,000 cases of TB). Farmworkers are six times more likely to develop active TB over their lifetime than other workers, with rates between 17% and 50% commonly reported. They are also at significantly higher risk of death from TB (NCFH, 2009b).
- Migrant children are often delayed for immunizations and have an increased incidence of asthma, intestinal parasites, vitamin A deficiency, continuous ear infections, and chemical poisoning, as well as significantly higher rates of food insecurity and twice the rate of tooth decay than children in the general population (Florida Association of Community Health Centers, 2009). Almost one third of preschool migrant/seasonal farmworker children were reported to be food insecure, yet obesity was also present in these children and adults (Borre, Ertle, & Graff, 2010).
- Migrant workers have high rates of work-related conditions, such as musculoskeletal injuries, heat stress, eye injuries, hearing loss, and skin diseases, due to equipment use, exposure to chemicals, dust, and sun (Connor et al., 2010; Florida Association of Community Health Centers, 2009; May, 2009; NCFH, 2009c Quandt, Schulz, Talton, Verma, & Arcury, 2012). They often perceive that their employers are demanding and that their work is dangerous (Keifer, Salazar, & Connon, 2009). Yet, they are generally unwilling to report injuries or even complain to employers due to fear of deportation or firing. A mind-set that they must endure bad work environments as a temporary, but necessary, condition of their work life in the United States is not uncommon; they may feel that "they are undeserving of health care" (Willen, 2012, p. 807). They often continue to work while injured or ill due to

perceived difficulty leaving work and pervasive *no work, no pay* employment situations (Arcury et al., 2012; Gleeson, 2010; Hoerster et al., 2011; May, 2009).

Occupational Hazards

The hazards of agricultural employment, coupled with limited legal protection, jeopardize the health of the migrant farmworker. As mentioned earlier, agriculture (grouped with forestry and fishing) ranks first, just ahead of mining, in occupational death rate (U.S. Department of Labor, 2011). Falls, cuts, muscle strains and sprains, and repetitive motion injuries (e.g., carpal tunnel syndrome) commonly afflict migrant laborers. Migrant and seasonal farmwork typically requires stooping, long hours working in wet clothes, working with sometimes contaminated soil and water, climbing, carrying heavy loads, and exposure to the sun and the elements. Failure to perform these activities on a rigid timetable dictated by seasons and weather can result in crop loss. For instance, a shortage of workers resulted in a $1 million loss for an asparagus farmer in Michigan (Schmidt, 2012). This urgency compels farmworkers to labor in all weather conditions, including extreme heat or cold, rain, bright sun, and high humidity.

It is difficult to reach this population in order to gain a full picture of their injuries, but migrant camp health aides in Illinois and Florida surveyed 25 workers and found back pain prevalence for the past year at 35%, with about one third of workers reporting skin symptoms and also eye problems in the Florida sample. Those in Illinois reported lower proportions (24%, 16%, and 16%, respectively). Workers noted heavy lifting and work with ladders as causes of back pain and eye and skin problems most often related to fertilizer application and chemical spraying of fields/lack of handwashing facilities (Cameron et al., 2006). A California study of 654 immigrant farmworkers noted chronic disease indicators (e.g., hypertension, overweight, obesity high cholesterol) in the mostly young, male Mexican sample. Most lacked health insurance, and over their cumulative years of work, only 27% of males and 11% of females had received any work-related injury compensation (Villarejo et al., 2010).

In a small study of migrant workers, the incidence rate for work-related eye injuries was 23.8/10,000 worker years compared to a national incidence rate of 6.9 in 2009. Eye injuries (from tree branches, tools, or irritants) can cause serious problems and are seldom reported to employers. Treatment, if any, is often delayed, and penetrating or open wounds were common (Quandt et al., 2012). Extreme cold can lead to frostbite, and overexposure to the sun may result in heat stroke; farm laborers are more often at risk for these conditions. Some plants, like tobacco, pineapples, and garlic, release chemicals that are irritants or can be toxic to farmworkers who come in close contact with them (Modi, Doherty, Katta, & Orengo, 2009).

Pesticide Exposure

Migrant farmworkers are at greater risk for pesticide poisoning when fields are sprayed or during initial reentry into the field. Many migrant camps are located within large open fields or on the periphery of cropland. Overhead pesticide sprayings then endanger not only those at work in the fields but also those in the camp. If fields are not posted with warning signs, mass poisoning of farmworkers can occur: thousands of rural residents, in addition to farmworkers, have been poisoned by pesticide drift. One study of almost 3,000 cases of agricultural pesticide drift in 11 states found 47% of participants had work exposures and 14% were children under age 15. Soil fumigants comprise 45% of pesticide poisonings, and 24% are related to aerial applications (Advocate Precautionary Principle [APP], 2011). Two nurses, who as children worked alongside their families in the fields, recalled: "as the planes sprayed the fields, you could feel the drifts" and when the spray mixed with the early morning dew "the pesticide residue would be on your clothes and your skin—it looked like a white film" (Formichelli, 2008).

Contaminated water sources in the field enhance the absorption and spread of pesticides and organic compounds. EPA standards that bar entry to sprayed fields for at least 24 hours are often ignored. Pesticides can drift from the fields to contaminate food, yards, or children playing nearby. Children are at greater risk for pesticide-induced illnesses because of their higher metabolic rate, greater surface absorption, still developing organs, and possibility for chronic long-term exposure (Rauh et al., 2011). It is estimated that thousands of farmworkers suffer pesticide poisoning each year, but exact counts are not possible due to inadequate surveillance systems and reluctance of farmworkers to report injuries (Farmworker Justice, n.d.). Surveillance systems are only in place in 11 states; the Sentinel Event Notification System or Occupational Risk (SENSOR) is a means of reporting pesticide-related injuries as well as other occupational illnesses and injuries (NIOSH, 2012). Reporting of pesticide-induced morbidity and mortality is not required in every state. California has the oldest pesticide surveillance system in the United States, beginning in 1971 (California Department of Pesticide Exposure, 2010).

But, even with reporting laws, many cases are never recognized because workers do not seek medical care. Pesticide burns and rashes often go untreated because of lack of education about the dangers of pesticides and lack of available services. Migrant workers are often unaware of the hazards of pesticides. A study among adolescent Latino farmworkers found that 64.7% were traveling and working in the United

States independent of their parents, and few reported having received pesticide training; however, 21.6% of the sample reported that their current work involved mixing or applying agricultural chemicals (McCauley et al., 2006). Another study of farmworkers and pesticide applicators in Oregon fruit orchards found urine organophosphate metabolites were significantly higher for these workers than controls, and DNA damage was also significantly higher (Kisby et al., 2009). A study of North Carolina migrant and seasonal workers found that most workers had multiple detections for pesticide metabolites when tested quarterly over a 1-year period (Arcury et al., 2010). In a California study of strawberry field workers, even when wearing proper clothing/gloves and handwashing with soap, farmworkers exposed to organophosphate pesticides had significantly higher levels of exposure when compared to a national reference population sample, but there was evidence of decreased metabolite levels (Salvatore et al., 2008). Another study with strawberry harvesters found that wearing gloves reduced exposure to malathion, a powerful pesticide. However, those that ate berries had metabolites present in their urine. Wearing gloves and changing out of work clothing before returning home was found helpful in reducing exposure for their families, but additional measures were needed to reduce consumption of berries in the field (Bradman et al., 2009). An Eastern Washington state study, comparing farmworker adults and children with nonfarmworker adults and children living in close proximity to farmland, found organophosphate metabolite concentrations (urine and house dust) significantly higher among those working in the fields and their children. However, even those adults and children just living near farmland had metabolites present. Researchers found a 20% decrease in metabolite concentration for every mile of distance from farmland (Coronado et al., 2011).

One Florida study indicated that farmworkers had a rather extensive lay knowledge of pesticide exposure and that this could be combined with more required didactic training to reduce poor health effects (Flocks, Monaghan, Albrecht, & Bahena, 2007). Even though it may be required of health care providers to report pesticide poisoning, it is often misdiagnosed because the symptoms can mimic those of viral infections or heat-related illness. Symptoms of pesticide exposure include sore throat, runny nose, headache, red/swollen/watery eyes, drowsiness, itchy skin, abdominal pain, and nausea or vomiting. More severe symptoms may include sweating, salivation, blurred vision or pinpoint pupils, muscle twitching, or weakness and incontinence (especially with organophosphate or carbamate exposures). Finally, with the most severe exposures, seizures, respiratory depression, and unconsciousness or coma can occur. There are over 19,000 pesticide products registered with the EPA and more than one thousand active ingredients. Biomarkers, or signs of a specific chemical's presence in the body, are important in definitively proving exposures; however, chemical companies are not currently required to provide this information (Huber, 2011).

Only a few categories of pesticides account for more than half of the cases of acute illness; these include inorganic compounds, carbamates, pyrethroids, and organophosphates. Although the impact of acute pesticide poisoning is widely recognized, little is understood about the long-term effects of the repeated low-level exposures to which migrant farmworkers are constantly subjected. Some studies have noted memory problems, depression, neurologic deficits, miscarriages, and birth defects, along with respiratory problems and increased incidence of Parkinson's disease, as being linked to chronic pesticide exposure (McCauley et al., 2006; Wang et al., 2011; Weselak, 2008). Numerous studies have examined the link between exposure to pesticides and various neurologic problems and cancer—most often with organophosphate-based pesticides. Some pesticides have been suspected of leading to depression, suicidal ideation, and other psychological distress (Wesseling et al. 2010). Some evidence of an association between pesticide exposure and the incidence of diabetes has been found (Montgomery, Kamel, Saldana, Alvavanja, & Sandler, 2008). Non-Hodgkin's lymphoma, leukemia, prostate cancer, sarcomas, and multiple myelomas have been associated with organophosphates, herbicides, and insecticides (Cockburn et al., 2011; Colt et al., 2009; McDuffie, Pahwa, Karunanayake, Spinelli, & Dosman, 2009; Weselak, Arbuckle, Wigle, Walker, & Krewski, et al., 2008; Wiggle, Turner, & Krewski, 2009). Prenatal exposure to organophosphate pesticides has been significantly associated with attention problems in 5-year-old offspring and even stronger for male children (Marks et al., 2010).

A large body of supportive research has indicated a link between Parkinson's disease, other neurologic disorders, and pesticide exposure, and some specific pesticides (e.g., ziram, paraquat) have been implicated (Van der Mark et al., 2012; Wang et al., 2011). Display 29.3, Environmental Exposure History, is a helpful assessment tool for community health nurses working with migrant and seasonal workers to use to determine pesticide exposure. When a client presents with symptoms that may be suggestive of pesticide exposure, mnemonic prompts may help to clarify common symptoms (see Display 29.4).

Pesticide exposure can be a single event, may occur multiple times, or even be continuous. Health effects are thought to be a function of the frequency of expo sure and the dose (Montgomery et al., 2008). Most migrant workers come into contact with pesticides through their work. However, exposure to pesticides does not affect only those working in the fields. "Most farmworker housing is contaminated with a broad range of pesticides," and this exposes not only workers but also their families to pesticide-related risks. "Most workers and family members have absorbed measurable doses of pesticides" (Arcury & Quandt, 2009, p. 103). Organophosphates decrease the levels of acetylcholinesterase, found in nerve endings, and can be

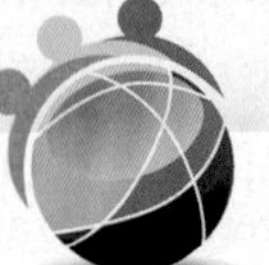

DISPLAY 29.3 ENVIRONMENTAL EXPOSURE HISTORY

Do an exposure history to:

- Identify current or past exposures
- Reduce or eliminate current exposures
- Reduce adverse health effects

Taking an Exposure History: Questions to Consider

Use the **I PREPARE** mnemonic:

I–Investigate potential exposures

- Have you ever felt sick after coming in contact with a chemical, pesticide, or other substance?
- Do you have any symptoms that improve when you are away from your home or workplace?

P–Present work

- Are you exposed to solvents, dusts, fumes, radiation, loud noise, pesticides, or other chemicals?
- Do you know where to find Material Data Safety Sheets on chemicals that you work with?
- Do you wear personal protective equipment?
- Are work clothes worn home?
- Do coworkers have similar health problems?

R–Residence

- When was your residence built?
- What type of heating system do you have?
- Have you recently remodeled your home?
- What chemicals are stored on your property?
- Where does your drinking water come from?

E–Environmental concerns

- Are there environmental concerns in your neighborhood (e.g., air, water, soil)?
- What types of industries or farms are near your home?
- Do you live near a hazardous waste site or landfill?

P–Past work

- What are your past work experiences?
- What is the longest job held?
- Have you ever been in the military, worked on a farm, or done volunteer or seasonal work?

A–Activities

- What activities and hobbies do you and your family engage in?
- Do you burn, solder, or melt any products?
- Do you garden, fish, or hunt?
- Do you eat what you catch or grow?
- Do you use pesticides?
- Do you engage in any alternative healing or cultural practices?

R–Referrals and resources (use these key referrals and resources)

- Agency for Toxic Substances & Disease Registry: *www.atsdr.cdc.gov*
- Association of Occupational and Environmental Clinics: *www.aoec.org*
- Environmental Protection Agency: *www.epa.gov*
- Material Safety Data Sheets: *www.hazard.com/msds*
- Occupational Safety and Health Administration: *www.osha.gov*
- Local health departments, environmental agencies, poison control centers

E–Educate (a checklist)

- Are materials available to educate the patient?
- Are alternatives available to minimize the risk of exposure?
- Have prevention strategies been discussed?
- What is the plan for follow-up?

Source: Agency for Toxic Substances & Disease Registry (ATSDR). (n.d.). *Environmental exposure history*. Retrieved from http://www.atsdr.cdc.gov/asbestos/medical_community/working_with_patients/docs/IPrepareCard.pdf.

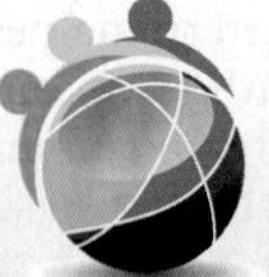

DISPLAY 29.4 MNEMONIC PROMPTS TO DETERMINE CHOLINERGIC SYMPTOMS OF ORGANOPHOSPHATE EXPOSURE

SLUDGE	DUMBBELS
Salivation	Defecation
Lacrimation	Urination
Urination	Miosis
Defecatio	Bronchorrhea
Gastric secretions	Bradycardia
Emesis	Emesis
	Lacrimation
	Salivation/seizures/sweating

The 4 Most Acute Symptoms: Bradyarrhythmias, Bronchospasm, Muscle Weakness, and Bronchorrhea.

Source: Utah Poison Control Center. (2006). Organophosphate poisoning. *Utox Update, 8*(2), 1–4.

absorbed through the skin, inhaled, or ingested. Most workers have metabolites present, and farmwork and housing close to agricultural fields are common factors associated with exposure. Drifts from sprayed fields and residues on farmworker clothing, shoes, tools, and skin, as well as food brought from the fields, are all potential sources of exposure. Vehicles can also become contaminated, as can carpets and furniture. Contaminated clothing should be kept in separate hampers and laundered separately; workers need to be encouraged to leave boots and shoes outside their homes and to change clothing and shower before eating and playing with their children. Substandard housing is also a factor.

Agricultural fields are usually located in isolated areas on the outskirts of rural communities. While in these isolated fields, migrant workers often are not provided with sanitation facilities or fresh drinking water. The Occupational Safety and Health Administration (OSHA) mandates field sanitation (at least one toilet and handwashing station) and fresh drinking water for each agricultural establishment employing 11 or more hand-labor workers on any given day (OSHA, 2011).

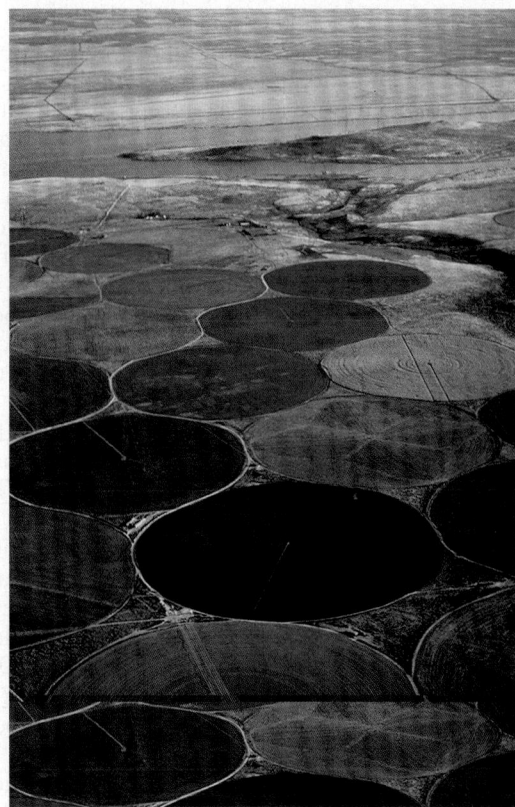

Fields in Eastern Oregon. Source: USDA, Agricultural Research Service.

Substandard Housing and Poor Sanitation

Formal demographic data on farmworker housing are often lacking. One cohort study of a farmworker population in Mendota, California (MICASA), employed door-to-door enumeration in a rural agricultural community. Almost 10% of the dwellings were classified as "back houses or unofficial dwellings," thought to have been missed during the last census (Stoecklin-Marois, Hennessy-Burt, & Schenker, 2011, p. 291). In a classic article by Cole and Crawford (1991), a vivid example of one migrant camp in Alabama highlighted workers living in a converted chicken house. An upper portion of the wall had been removed for ventilation, creating easy access for insects and birds. A dirt floor, a single light bulb, and two portable toilets located a distance away were some of the other features. Two sinks in a common living area provided the only water for the almost 60 people who lived in the chicken house. Many did not have mattresses, and because the workers were harvesting potatoes, potato baskets conveniently served as the only furniture. Such living situations still exist today. A nurse who was the child of a migrant farmworker family noted that they "lived in houses that had been condemned" and that she once "fell into a well that was covered up by grass and dirt" (Formichelli, 2008). A female farmworker, living with 13 other workers in a three-bedroom home in Watsonville, California, stated "we have to put up with this because we can't afford anything else" (Holden, n.d., p. 40). A description of dorm-style rooms in Immokalee, Florida, revealed "the shower has filthy, crumbling concrete walls—the kind that won't come clean...(and) a metal sink held by a rotting plywood counter, and the toilet often backs up, so the tiny room reeks of sewage" (p. 41).

Migrant farmworkers move frequently and often have great difficulty securing adequate housing. In the past, many growers or owners provided housing to migrant workers and their families. This practice has now become much less common, and only limited numbers of government-sponsored housing units are available for migrant workers. Housing conditions may actually be considered hazardous in some areas, and employer-owned labor camp regulations are much less stringent than Section 8 housing standards (Vallejos, Quandt, & Arcury, 2009). When private housing is available, it is often only offered at prices that outpace worker's wages. Data are scant, but a large survey of migrant workers in the eastern, midwestern, and western migrant streams conducted by the HAC revealed that over 50% of all housing units surveyed were overcrowded (only 3% of U.S. households are and 44% of mobile homes were substandard). Almost one quarter of units surveyed had at least one broken appliance or fixture, and 11% had no working stove. Between 13% and 39% of housing is owned by employers, and for those lucky enough to find employer-owned housing, over half of those units were offered without charge. Single-family homes (39%) and apartments (14%) are most commonly owned by employers, but workers and their families also are housed in barracks or dormitories, motels, and in mobile homes (Holden, n.d.; HAC, n.d.). Forty-two percent of farmworkers lived in single-family homes and 21% in apartments; fifteen percent lived in mobile homes and the same proportion in duplex/triplex housing. About 4% lived in dorms/barracks, and 2% lived in motels. Only .5% lived in tents/campsites (HAC, n.d.). The most serious housing problems were found in the Northwest region and in Florida. Over one quarter of housing units were located adjacent to agricultural fields, and more than half of these had no working shower/tub or washing machine—or both (HAC, n.d.).

Families with children occupied 65% of both severely substandard and moderately substandard units (HAC, n.d.). Structural problems, such as holes in the roof (15%), sagging frames or roofs (22%), or damage to foundations (15%), were common. Broken glass or window screens were noted in 36% of units, and peeling external paint was found in over 40% of units (Holden, n.d.; HAC, n.d.). Evidence of water damage was found in 29% of units, and 9% had exposed wiring. An examination of 183 North Carolina migrant farmworker camps in 2010 revealed 11.4 mean housing violations, with a range from 4 to 22 (Arcury et al., 2012). Bathroom violations were most common, and camps housing workers without H2A visas or posted state inspection certificates, or those examined later in the migrant season, had more violations. An example with serious consequences is Jensen Farms, a Colorado cantaloupe grower, who was fined for substandard housing provided to migrant workers in their fields and packing facility. The owner of Jensen Farms also owned the Gateway Motel, used for migrant housing during harvesting season, where workers each paid $25 per week for space in overcrowded rooms without beds (and no laundry facilities). The owner claimed that he was an "innkeeper" and did not fall within the purview for migrant and seasonal worker housing laws, but he was found out of compliance and fined $4,250. In 2011, Jensen Farms shipped out *Listeria*-contaminated cantaloupes that resulted in "the deadliest outbreak of food-borne illness in nearly 100 years" (Flynn, 2012, para. 2). While unsanitary worker housing may not be directly related to the outbreak, this may be just another indication of overall carelessness that led to unsafe farming practices.

Substandard housing is not the only concern. Crowding is also a problem, as many farmworkers, unable to find sufficient numbers of rental units, share housing—sometimes paying per-person costs. One of the few studies on migrant housing found that Minnesota seasonal vegetable workers' construction trailer barracks, housing 15 to 20 single migrant workers, rented for $90 per month per person. Cinder-block duplexes cost $40 per month per worker, and some residential hotels, lacking hot water, rented rooms for almost $600 per month. Over 75% of respondents earned <$7.50 per hour in 2006 (Ziebarth, 2006). In the HAC study, almost one third of migrant workers paid rental costs that were in excess of 30% of their gross incomes—defined as a housing cost burden (HAC, n.d.). The costs led to further crowding, as families doubled up to save expenses. In the earlier-cited Minnesota study, 21% of workers experienced "discrimination when trying to find housing" and noted that landlords "don't rent to Hispanics" or families with large numbers of children (Ziebarth, 2006, p. 349). When housing cannot be found, workers and families may have to resort to paying rent to live in garages, barns, sheds, or chicken coops, or they may be forced to stay in their cars. One Michigan farmer with 65 acres of blueberries describes the migrant workers he has employed for 7 to 9 weeks of every year for the past 25 years as "the hardest workers I know," stating that "we would not be here if it wasn't for the migrant workforce." Each year, around 90,000 migrant workers come to Michigan, but employer-provided housing only can accommodate about 22,000 of them (Schmidt, 2012, para. 3). Some economists have proposed that "permanent, but seasonally occupied, housing" may be the best investment for the least cost (Qenani-Petrela, Mittelhammer, & Wandschneider, 2008, p. 151).

Migrant Family Health

Because of frequent moves, migrant children are often educationally, socially, and physically disadvantaged. They have "some of the lowest socioeconomic and educational indicators," and their parents are frequently viewed by school personnel as difficult to reach and not involved in their children's education (Jasis & Marriott, 2010, p. 126). One explanation for their lack of participation is their extended work hours, beginning early in the morning and ending long after school hours. But some programs have been successful in reaching out to migrant parents. A community-based adult education program that improved migrant parents' self-actualization and promoted changes in interactions between parents and school personnel found that it led to improved school outcomes for migrant children (Jasis & Marriott, 2010). Migrant education programs, especially with Mexican American resource teachers as role models, have improved school completion rates (i.e., 80% completed 12th grade in 2002) and provided much-needed support (Gibson & Hidalgo, 2009).

Migrant children are often called upon by their families to stay home from school to work, care for younger children, or attend to other household chores. They may feel socially estranged, be constantly moving, and have difficulty finding health-promoting recreational activities. A large California study found significantly higher odds of developmental risk among children of undocumented Mexican parents, but not for children of documented Mexican parents (Ortego et al., 2009). This may indicate stressors related to immigration status. There has been a 45-fold increase in the number of undocumented workers taken into custody by the U.S. Immigration and Customs Enforcement (ICE) agency between 2001 and 2007. And highly publicized ICE raids have led migrant parents to withdraw their children from Migrant Head Start programs, noticeably decreasing enrollments across the country and further placing migrant children at risk for academic problems (Mather & Parameswaran, 2012).

Some research has shown that children of migrant farmworkers exhibited greater mental health problems than other children, but a review of research studies found no firm evidence for this claim and cited problems with methodologies used (Stevens & Vollebergh, 2008). Migrant college students had higher levels of depression and anxiety than their nonmigrant counterparts (55% vs. 20%) and also had higher levels of acculturative stress, in a sample of 168 college students of Mexican heritage (Mejia & McCarthy, 2010). A program available for migrant farmworkers or their children is CAMP, the College Assistance Migrant Program. An evaluation of the program found that 81% of migrant college students served within the first year continued on with a second year of study. Tutoring, counseling, and stipends are available, but no additional health services are provided (Willison & Jang, 2009).

The children of migrant farmworkers receive only fragmented health care. Health problems of migrant children include general poor nutrition, anemia, vitamin A deficiency, increased risk for respiratory and ear infections, dental problems, lead and pesticide poisoning, intestinal parasites, skin infections, TB, and delayed development (American Academy of Pediatrics, 2010).

Lack of awareness that minor symptoms, such as diarrhea or fever, may indicate a more serious underlying problem can cause delays in seeking medical attention, as can poverty and a lack of health insurance. An earache is minor, but it can lead to a major problem, such as deafness, if left untreated.

Migrant adolescents are less likely to abuse substances when they first arrive, but the likelihood increases as they remain in this country and is higher for second-generation Hispanics (The Future of Children, 2011). Overall, they are less likely to graduate from high school, because their education is often interrupted. Stress from acculturation, poor working conditions, deficient social support, and poor family functioning have been associated with greater anxiety and depressive symptoms among farmworkers in the Midwest (Hiott, Grzywacz, Davis, Quandt, & Arcury, 2008). A large study of children whose parents have been arrested, detained, and/or deported found that 50% of them had increased fear and crying episodes, and 66% had changes in sleeping and eating patterns. Over 33% were more withdrawn, clingy, anxious, angry, or aggressive (Chaudry et al., 2010).

A North Carolina study of farmworker stress found that 38% had "significant levels of stress"; the most stressful factors were identified as "difficulty finding a place to live," "not enough water to drink when I am working," "my partner is no longer with me," and being bothered "that other people use drugs" (Hiott et al., 2008, p. 36). Display 29.5 lists some stressors from the Hispanic Stress Inventory evaluation tool. Social isolation factors ranked slightly lower, but being away from friends and family was often mentioned. In this study of farmworkers, migrating mostly from Mexico, almost 42% met the classification as depressed, and over 18% had anxiety levels consistent with impaired functioning. The researchers concluded that social isolation had a stronger potential effect on anxiety, whereas poor working conditions were associated more with depression. The need for migrant workers to congregate in neighborhoods with others from their cultural background is an attempt to counter this social isolation. When surrounded by others who share their culture and speak their language, and when they can find familiar music, television, entertainment, and food, it helps to allay feelings of anxiety and depression. It is easy to understand why many migrant workers in specific migrant streams originate from the same states or communities in Mexico or other countries; it is an attempt to hold onto some semblance of their social networks as they migrate to the United States (Loue & Quill, 2010).

In the earlier-cited study by Hiott and colleagues (2008), over one third of respondents met the criteria for alcohol dependence. Alcohol use has been noted to be common among male migrant workers, and the stressors migrant farmworkers face related to their employment and acculturation put them at a higher risk for drug and alcohol abuse, as well as other high-risk behaviors (Rhodes et al., 2010). Drugs and alcohol may be used as a means of coping with separation from family and social isolation.

Problems with substance abuse may also be associated with violence. Although research on migrant children and violence is almost nonexistent, one classic article reported that 46% of children have witnessed some form of violence; 20% had witnessed a shooting and 11% had witnessed a murder (Triantafillou, 2003). Domestic violence affects migrant worker families, and children may be exposure to family violence. Kim-Godwin and Fox (2009) found intimate partner violence and alcohol use to be a serious problem in a Latino migrant population working in North Carolina. In a study conducted in Texas border counties, verbal abuse was the most frequently reported form of intimate

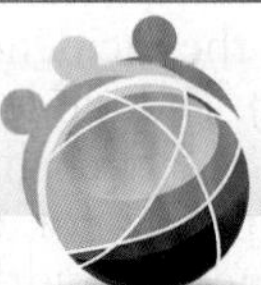

DISPLAY 29.5 EXTRAFAMILIAL AND INTRAFAMILIAL STRESSORS FOR HISPANIC ADULTS

Common Extrafamilial Stressors

Difficult interactions with others because of not being able to speak English
Feeling an expectation to work harder because of being a Latino
Feeling pressures to learn English
Difficulty finding work I want to do because I am Latino
Forced to take low-paying jobs
Continually concerned with quality of my work so that others do not consider me lazy
Being treated badly due to my poor English
Difficulty getting promotions or salary increases because I am Latino
Not having sufficient income to support my family

Common Intrafamilial Stressors

Conflicts among my family members
Physical violence among my family members
Serious arguments among my family members
Children have too liberal ideas about sexuality.
Children talk about leaving home.
Children receive bad school reports or grades.
Spouse and I disagree about how to raise our children.
Children do not respect my authority as I think they should.

Adapted from: Cavazos-Rehg, C., Zayas, L., Walker, M., & Fisher, E. (2006). Evaluating an abbreviated version of the Hispanic Stress Inventory for Immigrants. *Hispanic Journal of Behavioral Sciences, 28*, 498–515.

partner violence. Only 22% reported knowledge of a shelter where they could go to gain assistance (Kugel et al., 2009). One large California study of migrant farmworkers found a 5% prevalence of being a victim of personal violence within the past year. Males experienced violence in workplaces, or other public settings, while over 80% of self-reported violence for females was the result of domestic violence (Villarejo et al., 2010). Research on domestic violence in this vulnerable population is scant, but more than 1,000 battered farmworker women in a multicenter study were interviewed and researchers identified the typical profile as:

- Childbearing age (15–40)
- Hispanic
- Afraid of their partner
- Married or living with partner
- Drug or alcohol use by partner

The overall incidence was 20.6%. Fifty percent of abused women were pregnant at the time of the abuse (Migrant Clinician's Network, n.d. c). Nationally, just over 30% of women report sexual or physical abuse by a boyfriend or husband during their lifetime (Family Violence Prevention Fund, 2008). (See Chapter 20 for a more complete discussion of domestic violence.) What makes farmworker domestic violence so significant is the fact that these women often experience language barriers, do not have adequate access to health care, live isolated lives with little social support, and fear deportation if they report the abuse—all factors that lead them to endure their violent situation in silence. One example is a migrant woman, who shared a one-room dwelling with her husband, infant, and five single men. Her husband became increasingly violent and unpredictable. He began to beat her and the baby, and she was unable to predict what would initiate a violent attack. She finally fled when one of the men living with them also began beating her. She attributed the aggressive behavior to the powerlessness felt by the men. The Violence Against Women Act of 1994 affords protection for undocumented battered women and children by allowing them to seek legal immigration status without the help of their abusers (Migrant Clinician's Network, n.d. c). PHNs must be aware of these issues and what resources are available in the community (see Levels of Prevention Pyramid).

Infectious Diseases

As noted earlier, TB is a common infectious disease among farmworkers. Some studies find that farmworkers are six times more likely to develop active TB over their lifetime than other workers, with rates reported between 17% and 50%. Also, they are more likely to die from TB (NCFH, 2009b). Because of their migrant patterns, it is difficult to complete treatment regimens. Because of frequent moves, poor access to health care, and social isolation, it is often difficult for migrant farmworkers to be accurately diagnosed and treated. Many factors may prevent them from successfully completing a treatment regimen, and language barriers, along with cultural differences, may preclude them from fully understanding the impact of their disease on themselves and others. For instance, a Mexican migrant worker may be diagnosed with TB in California and begin treatment there but may move to Washington state to pick cherries and run out of medication before completing treatment. Moving back to California for summer work, he may again start treatment but may travel home to Mexico during the winter, only to be reinfected by an older, untreated member of his extended family.

Migrant workers are at greater risk of HIV infection for many of the same reasons. HIV-positive status may be misunderstood and, because of stigmatization and fears of deportation, may be purposely hidden from health officials. Estimated HIV rates are reported to be between 2.6% and 13%, depending on geographic area and personal risk factors like drug abuse; however, accurate national prevalence rates are almost impossible to attain (NCFH, 2011). High-risk behaviors, such as alcohol and drug abuse, sex with commercial sex workers, and inconsistent use of condoms, place male farmworkers at higher risk for HIV infection; loneliness has also been found to be strongly associated with risk factors for HIV/AIDS (Munoz-Laboy, Hirsch, & Quispe-Lazaro, 2009; Rhodes et al., 2010; Villarejo et al., 2010).

Other infectious diseases (e.g., hepatitis, enteric diseases, parasites) may commonly afflict migrant workers, often due to inadequate sanitation and hygiene facilities.

Economic Barriers and Limited Health Resources

Most migrant workers are unable to qualify for basic health and disability benefits such as Workers' Compensation, Social Security, occupational rehabilitation, and disability compensation because of undocumented status. One California survey found that between 27% of male and 11% of female migrant workers had been paid Workers' Compensation claims over the course of their work history, with the incidence increasing over time (Villarejo et al., 2010). Federal legislation passed in 2006 requires proof of U.S. citizenship (e.g., passport, birth certificate) when applying for or renewing Medicaid coverage, so undocumented workers are generally unable to qualify (Farmworker Justice, n.d.; King, 2007). As a group, migrant farmworkers have more difficulty accessing Medicaid than any other population.

Medicaid benefits have little value in the face of constant mobility, because they are not transferable from state to state. On one hand, although the low income of migrant workers meets the guidelines for state medical assistance, few families remain in one state long enough for the 30-day residency requirement. On the other hand, farmworker families may not qualify for Medicaid because, during certain months of the year, they earn more than the state's poverty limits. Ironically, migrant workers suffer from preventable and treatable diseases covered under Medicaid, but they are unable to obtain treatment. Some undocumented workers may be

LEVELS OF PREVENTION PYRAMID

SITUATION: Domestic violence in the migrant population. Research is scant; however, informal discussions occur among women and health care providers. Outreach workers sometimes possess lists of men who are abusive and their victims. Although the migrant lifestyle and experience is difficult for the entire family, women and children suffer most from family violence that the migrant way of life promotes. Isolation and subjugation to a patriarchal system usually prohibit migrant women from seeking help if they are abused. Fear of consequences and difficulty expressing negative views about husbands prevent women from speaking out (Migrant Clinician's Network. *Domestic violence in the farmworker population.* Monograph Series, n.d. c).

GOAL: Using the three levels of prevention, negative health conditions are avoided, promptly diagnosed, and treated, and/or the fullest possible potential is restored.

TERTIARY PREVENTION

Rehabilitation	Primary Prevention: *Health Promotion & Education*	Primary Prevention: *Health Protection*
• Promote family rehabilitation, with or without abuser in the home. • Encourage ways to eliminate or reduce social and geographic isolation among vulnerable women.	• Alleviate stressors of the migrant lifestyle, such as overcrowding and substandard living conditions. • Provide emotional support and educate on what constitutes abuse. • Promote self-esteem to the point where a woman can take control of her situation.	• Encourage women to contact health care providers as they migrate. • Encourage women to find appropriate lay community outreach workers for support. • Encourage migrant women to unite and create an environment that allows them to speak up and out while supporting one another against abuse.

SECONDARY PREVENTION

Early Diagnosis	Prompt Treatment
• Promptly identify an abused woman—through self-identification or by other family members or professionals—and remove her from the dangerous situation.* • Keep communication lines open, be culturally sensitive, and examine for injuries.	• Secure the victim in a safe battered women's shelter. • Assist victim to regain self-esteem.

PRIMARY PREVENTION

Health Promotion and Education	Health Protection
• Create awareness of the harsh living conditions that migrant families endure. • Advocate for improved and safe living conditions on state and national levels. • Provide adequate housing that eliminates overcrowding and offers privacy.	• Train bilingual and bicultural lay migrant women on the issues of spousal abuse and help them form support groups. • Provide opportunities for women and men to improve self-esteem which will change attitudes toward each other.

*Secondary prevention is difficult because of limited financial resources, lack of transportation, no nearby friends or relatives for support, language barriers (e.g., non-English speaking), and limited safe shelters for battered women in rural areas.

eligible for emergency Medicaid—a very limited benefit (Farmworker Justice, n.d.).

Although many are eligible for public programs such as food stamps, S-CHIP, and the Women, Infants, and Children (WIC) program, migrant farmworkers as a whole generally do not participate. They may fear immigration penalties or be totally unaware of the available benefits. Some are eligible for Social Security benefits but do not possess the ability to process their claim (NCFH, n.d. a). Workers who do not have valid Social Security numbers, but still have taxes withheld from their wages, are estimated to contribute $7 billion in Social Security taxes and about $1.5 billion in Medicare taxes—and most of them will never qualify for either Medicare or Social Security benefits (King, 2007).

Some think that undocumented workers are a drain on the U.S. economy and illegal immigration is a hot-button topic. However, a substantial amount of research demonstrates that immigrants generally pay more money into the system than they extract from it. In 2005, approximately 7% of the Texas population consisted of undocumented immigrants, and Texas spent $58 million that year for health care for undocumented immigrants. However, state revenues from undocumented immigrants exceeded what was spent on health care and education costs by almost $425 million (King, 2007). While they may earn better wages, it may come at a high personal cost. A large, longitudinal study of Mexican migrant farmworkers noted that those returning to live in Mexico have a higher prevalence of obesity, smoking, heart disease, and mental health disorders than nonmigrants. Researchers posit that migrant workers discard more traditional nutrition patterns for unhealthy behaviors (e.g., consumption of fast food, overeating), possibly due to their increased income level. Also, the stress of migration (e.g., discrimination, fear) may be associated with increased levels of depression and anxiety. They may also be returning home to Mexico for family support and to seek medical treatment for health problems (Ullmann, Goldman, & Massey, 2011).

Whatever your viewpoint on this issue, it is important to the public's health that basic health care services be available to vulnerable populations. Continued efforts must be made to conduct research assessing risks and hazards, especially those of pesticide exposure. Many government publications document the despair and isolation of migrant workers, yet very little has been done to address the living and working environments that contribute to diminished health. Although migrant workers are a mobile population and difficult to study, they are important as an integral part of our economy and because infectious disease among this population increases health risks for all (Flynn, 2012; NCFH, n.d. b; 2009c).

Unique Methods of Health Care Delivery and Primary Prevention

Because migrant health centers do not adequately meet the health needs of the entire migrant community, several innovative methods of health care delivery have been developed and implemented by community health nurses. Although changes are often minor and slow to occur in the migrant population, even minute changes are a milestone, because the migrant lifestyle does not support any type of health stability. Any progress made must be welcomed with recognition and support.

Mobile health vans staffed with bilingual community health nurses and lay workers can travel directly to migrant camps and are an effective strategy for outreach health screening and education. By going to migrant camps and delivering care where the clients live and work, especially during nonwork hours such as evenings and weekends, community health nurses increase health access and overcome barriers of culture and lack of child care. Although migrant families receive only fragmented acute care, a nurses' outreach team can succeed in encouraging migrant farmworkers to prevent illness with immunizations, good nutrition, and healthy lifestyles. A viable alternative to traditional medical clinics, the mobile nursing clinic provides primary care to an underserved population through health promotion, disease prevention, and early treatment. Mobile dental vans also provide services to migrant worker's children, often with arrangements made through school nurses, and dental care provided by dental schools or through partnerships (Mulligan, Seirawan, Faust, & Habibian, 2010). Migrant workers suffer from dental problems at a rate higher than the national average; one California study found that 36% of men had dental caries, 30% had broken or missing teeth, and 18% had gingivitis (Villarejos et al., 2010). For migrant children, over 87% of those accessing a mobile dental clinic had untreated caries (Mulligan et al., 2010).

Promotoras (i.e., lay community outreach workers), or *doulas* (i.e., usually trained childbirth assistants), have promoted health in migrant communities (Lucio et al., 2011). Some programs use *doulas* to provide classes on childbirth and other perinatal subjects in an interactive manner; these provide extensive case management services along with the traditional duties of childbirth coach. Because *doulas* and *promotoras* are generally members of the migrant community, they are readily accepted. Some *promotoras* teach parenting classes to avert child neglect/abuse; others may work with special populations to deter domestic violence or substance abuse or promote breast-feeding (Blanco, 2011). Some deal with interventions and education to control hypertension, and others facilitate early screening and treatment for cancer (Balcazar et al., 2009; Nuno, Martinez, Harris, & Garcia, 2011). One program in a rural area on the United States–Mexico border showed statistically significant improvement in reports of mammograms (two times more likely with the educational intervention from *promotoras*), and there was an even stronger result for those who had not had either mammograms or Pap smears at baseline or within the last year (Nuno et al., 2011). Some *promotoras* migrate with workers and families to provide year-round support and resources.

Information Tracking Systems

Mobility impedes continuity of care, and the inadequate system of medical record keeping for the migrant population is particularly frustrating and challenging. Data information systems are vital components for monitoring the health status of individual farmworkers as they migrate. Furthermore, these data are essential for generating research and follow-up care as well as long-range health planning. They also help justify appropriation of monies to migrant health agencies. The Migrant Clinician's Network has instituted several tracking systems (n.d. b). *TBNet* promotes the completion of TB treatment among migrant populations, and *Diabetes Track II* is geared toward those with diabetes and helps with monitoring and control. *CAN-Track* is a system for coordination of cancer care, and the newest tracking system, *Prenatal Health Network Project*, offers greater continuity for pregnant migrant women. *Heart Fax* is another system of tracking for those with CVD.

Migrant children are susceptible to medical "feast or famine" and may be either overtreated or undertreated simply because their medical histories are unknown to current providers. One now defunct method for tracking the health status of migrant school-age children was through the Migrant Student Record Transfer System (MSRTS), a computerized system that collected and maintained health and academic records for migrant children. School nurses collected data on migrant children about personal and family history; immunization status; visual, auditory, and dental problems; nutritional status; and general physical condition. Although no coordinated tracking system is now in place, states are still expected to transfer records on migrant students. However, the ability to track these children in the migratory lifestyle from work location to work location is often inconsistent and woefully lacking (Geiger, 2009). Early intervention for migrating children is not always feasible, although it has been proven to greatly improve outcomes. The creation of a national database for information on the health status of adult migrant workers has also been suggested.

MiVIA ("my way" in Spanish) is putting health records online and making them available to migrant workers and their health care providers. Workers get a photo identification card, and their records can be accessed only by the use of a personal password. They can access their medical files, medications, a medical reference guide (bilingual), and other resources, such as local clinics and doctors, public transportation, and housing online, no matter their location (Hou, 2010). The program began in California's wine country but is spreading to more distant locations.

THE ROLE OF COMMUNITY HEALTH NURSES IN CARING FOR A MOBILE WORKFORCE

Beyond barriers to health care, such as lack of health services, language, and cultural impediments; inadequate to nonexistent transportation; financial strains; underinsurance; and questionable residency status, which are by themselves formidable obstacles, the migrant lifestyle is fraught with challenges. Because of the insecurity and instability inherent in a mobile lifestyle, long-term health goals are difficult to establish and long-term follow-up of any chronic illness is doubtful. Nonetheless, community health nurses provide much-needed services using community resources, innovative thinking, tenacity, and sensitivity.

Strategies for improving the health status and resource use of migrant workers and their families include:

- Improving existing services
- Advocating and networking
- Practicing cultural sensitivity
- Using lay personnel for community outreach
- Utilizing unique methods of health care delivery
- Employing information tracking systems

Community health nurses are the major providers of migrant health services and have a crucial role in the development and management of interventions. In response to the growing need for available, accessible, and affordable health care for farmworker families, nurses are called on not only to understand the migrant lifestyle but also to help migrant families overcome the barriers to health care (see Perspectives: Voices from the Community).

An aggregate at risk, migrant workers suffer higher frequency of illness, more complications, and more long-term debilitating effects. Exacerbated by a magnitude of environmental and work stressors, the health of migrant families is also compromised by limited access to health care, mobility, language and cultural barriers, low educational levels, and few economic and political resources. Because migrant health needs are largely manageable within community settings, community health nurses are ideal health providers. Implementing health education at migrant camps, training lay health workers, and providing clinic hours to accommodate late workdays are successful interventions. Learning the language of the migrant workers and their unique cultures is also helpful in reaching this population. Community health nurses must advocate for the health of migrant workers, who have very little economic or political power, and also guide them through the complexities of a changing health care system.

In the past, male migrant workers traveled primarily in organized crews; now they may travel in family units with women and children. Added attention must be given to family members exposed to the hazards of the migrant lifestyle. Even as many migrant workers settle into communities, the cycle of poverty continues as other workers arrive from impoverished countries. With a paucity of health resources, the PHN is sometimes the only health provider who can and will care for this population.

Providing care for migrant workers presents a challenge, requiring nurses to be innovative and to go beyond the boundaries of traditional health services (see Using the Nursing Process). Although many resources

PERSPECTIVES
VOICES FROM THE COMMUNITY

"First of all, a nurse should expect the unexpected. Because of the migratory way of life...they do not always know where they will be next week or next month. Therefore we must understand that they do not always have their medical records, immunization records, or income records. Hours are very irregular, depending on what time the workers get in from the fields and what time the shifts are. Because of the distances we travel, we work anywhere from 8 to 12 hours a day. The most rewarding part of the job is bringing health services to the underserved and uninsured. The people are so gracious and appreciative of whatever services we provide."

—J. S., RN, Michigan

"Since farmworkers come to our area for only 4 months of the year, it is rare that I care for a migrant woman through her entire pregnancy. I may diagnose her pregnancy, I may see her for three or four prenatal visits, or I may meet her only once before she goes into labor and delivers her baby. I struggle with the desire to make a difference in a short period of time and with the disappointment of not being able to follow-through."

—C. K., CNM, RN, Pennsylvania

"Encourage clinicians to trust old diagnostic skills of palpation, auscultation, and careful listening. Exhaustive laboratory work or radiology studies are not likely to be welcomed by farm workers who seek relief of symptoms so that they may return to work. Be warm and interested in the whole family. If you do not speak Spanish or Creole, work with translators who understand how you work. Use translators as...vehicles to get the information out and in. Eye contact and touch are crucial. Learning to be clinically relevant as well as competently utilizing a translator is an art, and takes time and experience to hone. Learning some phrases or some of the most frequently asked questions in the language of the farm worker should be encouraged. Even the attempt to speak the patients' language will build trust and confidence. These harvesters of the nation's food are very bright and resourceful people who travel great distances and undergo severe deprivation in order to work. The nobility of this pursuit is getting short shrift in the press and legislative bodies today, but the sheer enormity of the service [that] this group of oppressed people do for the rest of us needs to be acknowledged and honored by the clinicians who will provide primary health care to them and theirs."

—W. H., RN, Michigan

"I worked as a Head Start nurse for many years in an agricultural area of California. One of my assignments was a state/county migrant farm labor housing project. I was asked to make a home visit to check on a 4-year old who hadn't come to preschool in a few days. When I arrived at the family's duplex, I found the sixth grader there, caring for all five of her younger siblings, including the 4-year old and an 8-month old baby. When I asked why she was home with all of the children, she guardedly informed me that her parents had been picked up in a raid at the tree farm where they worked and had been taken back to Mexico. The children were now alone, with no family nearby. I worked with the nun at Catholic Social Services to provide care for the children until the parents returned to the U.S. so that the children, who were all U.S. citizens, would not be placed in foster care. The parents had not been allowed to call their children before being placed on the bus to Mexico, but other workers, who were not undocumented, had seen them go and told the children about their plight. It was heartbreaking to see the fear in their eyes."

—Holly, Head Start Nurse, California

"I'm dealing right now with Hispanic women, migrant workers, who do not have any access to prenatal care, none whatsoever. What I'm doing is creative financing, a lot of begging, a lot of pleading, a lot of being nice to people I don't even want to be nice to because it means that much to me for them to get help. So I find myself in situations that are sometimes uncomfortable, but nonetheless I do it because I feel that as a nurse that's my job. Having been a farmworker myself, I would want someone to do that for my mother, and they did."

—Unidentified female nurse, Idaho Falls, Idaho

and programs exist to help migrant families, the needs are still overwhelming. By aligning with the goals of *Healthy People 2020* to improve the health of one of the most underserved populations, the community health nurse will also be improving the health of the nation as a whole.

COMMUNITY HEALTH NURSING IN RURAL AREAS

The HRSA completed the last national public health workforce study in 2005, and no PHN to population ratio was reported. However, local public health workforce data for three states were collected: Georgia, New Mexico, and New York. Urban public health worker ratios were respectively reported at 41, 16, and 30 per 100,000 population. Rural public health worker ratios were 216, 111, and 96, respectively. Differences between states were explained by varied delivery systems, and no breakdown by worker type was given (HRSA, 2005). It is difficult to estimate the total number of PHNs and to provide accurate estimates of those working in rural areas (Washington State Nurses Association, 2011). However, the average age of PHNs was reported at 46.6 years in 2005. And most rural PHNs are thought to have little education in public health, as the associate degree in nursing is often accepted by health departments in rural areas (Knudsen & Meit, n.d.). Working urban nurses with a BSN numbered 51%, while only 36% of those working in rural areas had a baccalaureate degree (Rural Health Research Center, 2007). However, rural areas promote a broad scope of PHN practice, as these nurses

USING THE NURSING PROCESS WHEN WORKING WITH MIGRANT FAMILIES

Background Data and Assessment

Elena Vasquez is a community health nurse in rural Central California. She had two migrant camps in her service area and realized that during her normal working hours she was missing the adults in the camps. She met with several farmworker families one evening and brainstormed with them. They discussed their health needs and what type of services they needed most. A similar meeting was held at the other camp. At both camps, the families were willing to work with the nurse to enhance needed health care services. The information gathered helped Elena formulate nursing diagnoses that led to innovative planning and implementation.

Nursing Diagnoses

1. Alteration in family health status related to hazardous working conditions, poverty, and mobility
2. At risk for occupational and situational injury, illness, and stress due to poverty-level working and living conditions
3. Inadequate and inaccessible health care services related to poverty, work hours, and mobility

Plan and Implementation

Elena enthusiastically approached the health department administration with the innovative ideas she was formulating. The administrator agreed to try the plan Elena proposed for 3 months if Elena could find the personnel she needed, and the results were positive.

She enlisted four other community health nurses, two social workers, and several bilingual students from the local university's community health nursing class, which used the agency as a clinical site. Each team of nurses, a social worker, and three students drove to a camp once a week on a Tuesday or Thursday evening from 5 to 9 PM (the professionals started their day at 1 PM on that day). They completed a family assessment for each family; established a health record for each person; conducted health appraisals; administered immunizations; enrolled families in the Women, Infants, and Children Supplemental Food Program (WIC); made early-evening dentist and doctor appointments and arranged transportation if needed; and held brief teaching sessions on safety, infant and child care, family planning, and any topic the people requested or Elena and her colleagues felt the families needed.

The students became as innovative as Elena. They gathered used clothing and household items from their fellow nursing students for distribution and got valuable practice teaching and delivering health care services. The volunteers' enthusiasm overflowed to the farmworkers. Some of the women planned an informal "day care" program after receiving child care classes from the nursing students. Some of the men organized a soccer team to play against the other camp on Sunday afternoons. Additional donations were solicited—toys and books for the day care program and soccer equipment for the teams.

Evaluation

The interventions were so successful that the program became a permanent service of the health department. In the following months, a nurse practitioner was added, along with a preschool teacher and students from the early elementary education program at the university. The two camps became popular with migrant workers, who stayed healthier and were more productive. In addition, the camp managers found the grounds being kept cleaner and had fewer complaints and less abuse of the cabins and shower areas. With improved health and productivity, several families were motivated to establish a permanent home in the community and not continue the migrant lifestyle.

deal with a wide variety of issues—immunizations, home health, school nursing, maternal–child health, emergency preparedness, as well as communicable disease/epidemiology. While no differences were found in regard to education level, overall perception of competency was associated with years of professional practice experience in one study of rural and frontier PHNs (Bigbee, Otterness, & Gehrke, 2010). Highest levels of competency were reported in the areas of culture, communication, and leadership/systems, while lower levels of competency were noted for basic public health, finances, policy/program planning, and analytic assessment in a study of PHN rural and frontier one-nurse offices (Bigbee, Gehrke, & Otterness, 2009). Rural health departments are often lacking in technological and communication systems, but there is an even greater need for reliable communication capability and training opportunities for rural PHNs who provide the bulk of care in rural and frontier communities (Knudsen & Meit, n.d.).

Working in a Rural Community

Like urban nurses, the proportion of rural nurses working outside hospital settings is increasing, and rural RNs are more likely to commute outside their residential areas to work in more populated areas. Many rural RNs commute to larger rural areas or urban centers to earn higher wages (Rural Health Research Center, 2007). Rural community health nurses most often grew up in rural areas or lived for a time in small communities. They frequently have extended family there. Rural PHNs are active members of their community and are highly respected professionals.

The rural community health nurse plays many roles:

1. *Advocate*: Assists rural clients and families in obtaining the best possible care
2. *Coordinator/case manager*: Connects rural clients with needed health and social services, often assisting with information on transportation

3. *Health teacher*: Provides education to individuals, families, or groups on health promotion or other health-related topics (e.g., prepared childbirth, parenting, diabetes maintenance, home safety)
4. *Referral agent*: Makes appropriate connections between rural clients and urban service providers
5. *Mentor*: Guides new community health nurses, nursing students, and other nurses new to the rural community
6. *Change agent/researcher*: Suggests new approaches to solving patient care or community health problems based on research, professional literature, and community assessment
7. *Collaborator*: Seeks ways to work with other health and social service professionals to maximize outcomes for individual clients and the community at large
8. *Activist*: With a deep understanding of the community and its population, takes appropriate risks to improve the community's health

See From the Case Files II for a day in the life of a rural PHN.

Rural community health nurses have the opportunity to use autonomy in daily practice. Nurses must rapidly assume independent and interdependent decision-making roles because of the small workforce and large workload. Rural nurses are often generalists out of necessity—as mentioned earlier (Bigbee et al., 2009). This is also true for RNs working in rural hospitals (Montour, Baumann, Blythe, & Hunsberger, et al., 2009). Rural PHNs learn to prioritize tasks quickly and work efficiently with others to get the job done. Referrals to other rural providers are facilitated because providers frequently know one another. The rural community health nurse has an advantage over urban nurses in that the rural health care system is smaller and easier to influence and change, but specialization is seldom possible and long-distance travel is generally a necessity (Bigbee et al., 2009; Cant, Birks, Porter, Jacob, & Cooper, et al., 2011; Cox, Mahone, & Merwin, 2008; Cramer, Duncan, Megal, & Pitkin, 2009).

One study examining differences between PHNs working alone and those working in multinurse offices in rural and frontier areas of Idaho found statistically significant differences in the area of "community dimensions of practice skills," indicating generalized rather than specialty skills (Bigbee et al., 2009, para. 4). However, anonymity is not easy for the rural community health nurse, who is always on duty. A trip to the grocery store on a Saturday morning may include interactions with rural clients and their families about their pressing health concerns. Rural nurses may experience role conflict, as neighbors often view them in all of their various roles—as nurse, "parent, spouse, and church member," as noted in a classic study by Rosenthal (2005, p. 43). Rural community health nurses may have confidentiality and personal/professional boundary issues that have to be addressed. However, rural community health nurses are often respected, known, and trusted by the populations they serve. Also, an

From the Case Files 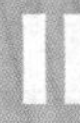

A Day in the Life of a Rural Public Health Nurse

Carol M. arrives at the Stevens County Public Health Department in rural America. She reviews her caseload for the day and begins her work. First, she telephones the principal of the local high school to let him know that she is able to speak next week to the Parent-Teacher Association about raising healthy adolescents (*health teacher*). Then, she calls the family of a hospitalized patient (*coordinator/case manager*) to plan the discharge of their family member. At 10:00 AM, Carol makes a home visit to the Wesley family. The family members explain that they have been unable to enroll for needed food stamps because they do not understand the process. Carol gives the family an informational handout with phone numbers and addresses, so that they can contact the appropriate agency (*referral agent*) and even calls her neighbor who works at the office to inform her of the need for special attention for the family (*advocate*). At lunch, Carol runs into a social worker colleague, and they discuss their concerns about the hospitalized individual with whom Carol spoke earlier in the day (*collaborator*). Both question whether the family will be able to manage the care needed for the patient without much outside support. After lunch, Carol returns to her office for a staff meeting and discusses a new charting system that she is recommending (*change agent/researcher*) for implementation by the department. At the same meeting, she agrees to work with a visiting public health nursing student during his rural practicum (*mentor*). That evening, Carol, as a concerned citizen, participates in a meeting at the town hall about issues related to local water quality. She addresses the group, giving them data and expresses concern (*activist*), then volunteers to lead others who are concerned about the issue. It is obvious that community health nurses like Carol M. often play many roles during the day. As a nursing student working in a rural community, you may have the opportunity to "try on" many of these roles.

"insider/outsider" mentality often exists in rural areas, as rural residents may tend to exclude nurses who have only lived in their communities for a short time or who want to remain less involved (Rosenthal, 2005, p. 43). This advantage makes it easier for rural PHNs to conduct research with rural populations—something that is sorely needed (Bushy, 2008).

Rural community health nurses may experience the challenge of physical isolation from personal and professional opportunities associated with urban areas. Travel to cities for basic and continuing education can be a barrier. Rural nurses may also feel isolated in their clinical practices because of the scarcity of professional colleagues. Many rural community health nurses overcome these barriers and learn to appreciate the benefits of clinical practice in a rural setting by discussing their concerns with peers through professional organizations and seeking ways to combat isolation through online education or discussion groups (Bigbee et al., 2009; McCoy, 2009; Rosenthal, 2005). See From the Case Files III for examples from nurses working in frontier areas.

The rural community health nurse often receives a salary that is lower than that of urban nurses in comparable positions (Knudsen & Meit, n.d.). However, there are benefits to rural nursing. Housing costs are usually lower than in larger cities, and long commutes to and from work on congested highways are often avoided, although rural driving can be hazardous. As a place to live and raise a family, rural communities offer a slower pace of life, open spaces, and friendly atmosphere. A study of rural hospital RNs in the Northwest found high job satisfaction among those with rural backgrounds and a preference for the rural lifestyle and indicated that these nurses enjoyed the generalist role and the autonomy and variety that it encompasses (Molinari & Monserud, 2008). The smaller system of health care in a rural community can be advantageous to the PHN. It may be easier to understand the system and initiate planned change. There are many possibilities to enhance rural nursing practice, including continuing education through distance learning or at satellite campuses, partnerships with larger medical centers, and invitations to clinical experts to provide on-site workshops (Place, Macleod, John, Adamack, & Lindsey, 2011). Grants can be written to facilitate these endeavors, and private sponsors may be approached to provide assistance. Given a smaller, more manageable community, it may be easier for PHNs to organize collaborations between private and public agencies, as well as key stakeholders within the community; collaboration is a cornerstone of public health nursing in any setting (Olson Keller, Stroschein, & Schaffer, 2011)

URBAN HEALTH

Urban health considers those characteristics of the environment as they relate to the health of the population living within large cities. According to Galea and Vlahov (2008), the factors responsible for the health of urban residents reflect three broad themes: the physical environment, the social environment, and access to health and social services. As opposed to rural areas, there may be less of a feeling of community connectedness in urban life, along with lower overall levels of trust, and weaker family and community ties. Connectedness has been shown to be a protective factor, especially for adolescent risk behaviors. Inner-city neighborhoods are

From the Case Files 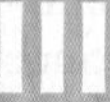

Frontier Nursing, Then and Now

As described in Chapter 2, Mary Breckinridge founded the Frontier Nursing Service in 1925, with nurse midwives providing care to clients in their own homes. Nurses traveled by horseback and on foot into the sparsely populated hollows of Kentucky (Stone, 2011). Today, nurse practitioners working in nurse-managed clinics in rural Appalachian communities in Virginia were interviewed about their practices (Caldwell, 2007) and spoke about their connections to the people and communities they serve. One said, "Here you get to know the whole family and that is rewarding…you know what is important to them…what their worries and concerns are….so you probably get closer to your patient in this area than you might outside here. It becomes an extended family, which is very rewarding" (p. 76).

Another NP described a man with severe COPD who visited her clinic. He was also a patient of another area provider, but when the NP examined the man, she noticed the gauze 4×4 he had on the back of his neck and inquired about it. The man said he "cut himself shaving." The NP pressed the man to see the wound and found that he had "cancer with the bone exposed," describing it as "the most awful thing that I had ever seen in my life. I could put my fist in there. And you could see his carotids pulsating." She told the patient how serious this was and arranged for a plastic surgeon to see him right away. He had a total neck resection and recovered completely. She reflected, "What if I had accepted his story about the sore and it being all right? It was not what he was coming to see me for……I look at more than just the chief complaint" (p. 77).

For these nurses, isolation was considered a positive aspect of their professional practice. It encouraged connection and caring relationships with their patients. (Caldwell, 2007; Stone, 2011).

often observed to have "high unemployment levels, lack of educational and jobs skills, broken families, alcohol and drug abuse, and low incomes conducive to the growth of street gangs and their culture of violence" (Vlahov, Boufford, Pearson, & Norris, 2010, p. 195). Community involvement and social networks, often deficient in densely populated areas, are components of social capital (discussed in Chapter 25), and community participation, social trust, and sense of belonging were significantly associated with positive health outcomes, such as mental and physical health (Fujiwara & Kawachi, 2008). Population turnover, racial/ethnic diversity, and poverty in urban cities are thought to contribute to the "lowered ability of individuals and communities to control crime, vandalism, and violence" (de Snyder, Friel, Fotso, & Khadr, 2011, p. 1183). Urban communities may be marked by negative social support, such as that found associated with drugs and gangs. Moreover, the social exclusion stems from the high concentration of poverty in central cities as well as high stress levels from violence and social isolation (Vlahov et al., 2007). Urban communities are made up of multiethnic and diverse racial communities, and these groups are often socially and economically separate from what one might believe to be mainstream urban communities. Poverty, especially within Black urban communities, has remained stable over time despite many social programs to address poverty and jobs (Sampson, 2009). Urban areas have been associated with *food deserts*, or areas with few or only small stores, and food insecurity has been found in urban families spending more than 30% of their income on private, rather than public, housing (Kirkpatrick & Tarasuk, 2011; Walker, Keane, & Burke, 2010). Both housing and food are more expensive in large cities.

In 2000, The Johns Hopkins University founded the Urban Health Institute as a means to bolster support among an inner-city population. This "interface between the university and the Baltimore community" was created to improve the health and wellbeing of the residents of East Baltimore (Urban Health Institute, 2012). Its mission is to promote evidenced-based interventions to solve local as well as national, health problems encountered in urban America. The New York Academy of Medicine has organized the Center for Urban Epidemiologic Studies to promote research that improves the health and wellbeing of urban populations by studying the social, biologic, and environmental influences on health (n.d.). The Academy sponsors the *Journal of Urban Health*, a publication that focuses on population-based research with low-income, disadvantaged populations living in urban areas (n.d.). But how did the health of these urban communities evolve to such a state that targeted efforts are now required? It began in the 1800s.

HISTORY OF URBAN HEALTH CARE ISSUES

Urban living has a long and checkered history in the United States. Arriving immigrants increased population density, especially in the large Eastern and Midwestern cities. Millions of immigrants arrived in the United States between the mid-1800s and the early 1900s. Because most had some family or distant relatives who had arrived here earlier, they made their ways to where these people lived, hoping to receive temporary shelter while they sought work (Dolkart, 2008). Many came with large families and roomed with other large European and Eastern European families in tenements. Others came alone or as a nuclear family without close ties to others already living here. Nonetheless, they gathered in **ghettos**, thickly populated sections of cities inhabited predominantly by members of the same minority group. This enabled them to be with people from their homeland—people who knew the same language and the same ways.

As time went on, many families left ghetto communities and found housing in smaller towns or in the beginnings of suburbs. As described in the classic work by Cutler, Glaeser, and Vigdor (1997), and more recently by Minetor (2010), the Irish left New York City in the early 20th century; then Blacks, coming from the South, moved in. Many Black families later left for outlying suburban areas, and Puerto Rican families moved in. Today, Haitian and Middle Eastern families inhabit some of the same neighborhoods. After 100 years, many of the same buildings continue to provide less than optimal shelter for a new group of immigrants. Although ghetto living provides a sense of belonging, for many it is temporary because it engenders more negatives than positives. Children and grandchildren of the original immigrants seek out a different life for themselves, away from the urban areas that are often riddled with crime, unsafe housing, and disease. Others, because of poverty, drugs, or fear of being homeless, remain in urban slum areas (Cutler et al., 1997; Dolkart, 2008; Minetor, 2010).

In a classic position paper, the American College of Physicians used the term **urban health penalty** to describe the "concentration of economic decline, job loss, and major health problems" afflicting inner-city populations experiencing health problems when healthier and wealthier residents moved to the suburbs, leaving poverty zones of economic and physical deterioration that act as determinants of health (1997, p. 485). Galea and Vlahov (2008) find urban health penalty associated with large cities where "economic inequalities in resources and opportunities" prevent subpopulations of poor from "maintaining a basic quality of life" found in mainstream society (p. 69). These unhealthy environments lead to inequality in health.

Who has been responsible for addressing the needs of these communities over the last hundred or more years? Who has been, or should have been, addressing the needs evolving among the urban communities? Two connected disciplines, urban planning and public health, have addressed these issues from the 19th century to the present. **Urban planning** worked to improve the welfare of individuals and communities by creating more healthful, efficient, attractive, and equitable places (Lerner, 2010). The activities of urban planners usually include addressing the community's needs related to transportation, housing, commercial areas, natural resources, environmental protection, and health care infrastructure (Frank & Kavage, 2008).

Public health, of course, is directed at improving human wellbeing through assessing and ensuring the delivery of services at the community level. Together, these disciplines both addressed the needs of the identified vulnerable populations. Initially, during the late 19th and early 20th centuries, these two systems were linked in promoting health by facilitating physical activity through the creation of green space. They joined together in preventing infectious diseases by ensuring healthful drinking water and sewage systems. They also protected the community from exposure to hazardous substances related to industry by monitoring land uses and instituting zoning ordinances (Boarnet & Takahashi, 2011; Crawford et al., 2010). During the middle of the 20th century, the focus of planning and public health agencies drifted apart, partly because of their successes in limiting injury and health risk caused by inappropriate mixing of land use. The target of public health agencies shifted from investigating ways to improve the infrastructure to a focus on germ theories and immunizations, challenges that were easier for physicians to address than changing environments. On the other hand, urban planning switched its energy to aiding economic development with large transportation and infrastructure. At about the same time, Rachel Carson's book *Silent Spring*, published in 1962, described the effects of pesticides on wildlife and the eventual effects on human health, thus initiating the *environmental justice movement* and focusing environmental health professionals largely on toxic chemical exposures (Mohai, Pellow, & Roberts, 2009).

According to Boarnet and Takahashi (2011), the disciplines of urban planning and public health are collaborating once again, working together to improve transportation and air quality, and addressing national health issues such as injury prevention, physical activity, health care access, energy use, and greenhouse gas emissions, along with disaster preparedness and response. This team effort is a natural partnership when addressing such concerns as physical activity and the provision of safe and accessible spaces (Jago et al., 2009). Several studies demonstrate a positive association between the presence of playgrounds/parks and green areas (grass/trees) with increased physical activity in children (Brockman, Jago, & Fox, 2011; Jago et al., 2009; Timperio et al., 2008). These joint ventures are significant in reaching those *Healthy People 2020* objectives directed at the prevention of chronic disease, injury prevention, and health promotion. Leaders at the CDC are concerned with factors that affect people and their environments and support efforts that address the improvement of both physical and social environments as related to places to live, work, and play. The CDC's *Healthy Places* describes the components involved: interaction between environment and health, poorly planned growth leading to sprawl and increased used of vehicles, and healthy community design that promotes health and wellbeing (2010).

The World Health Organization's Healthy Cities movement emphasizes health in planning and policy development. It encompasses economic and urban development and considers health inequality and urban poverty, as well as the vulnerable populations living in urban areas (WHO, 2012) (see Chapter 1 for more on Healthy Cities). Health care reform also offers opportunities to address urban health issues, especially related to health care access. Policy development to address the unique challenges of urban areas is part of public health advocacy for urban PHNs and other public health officials. And the move toward quality health care in the public health system will positively affect the health of all populations, including urban residents (Honore et al., 2011).

Urban communities must be given the opportunity to participate, particularly in activities that focus on change at the community and systems levels of prevention and public health practice. An example is the building of coalitions among key neighborhood stakeholders and agencies, as well as the individuals and families residing in those neighborhoods. Tapping into already existing neighborhood networks can facilitate health promotion efforts through capacity building and common goals that develop through collaborative partnerships. Such interventions reflect many of the key public health nursing interventions, as demonstrated in Chapter 14 through the use of the Minnesota Wheel and other models.

The *Healthy People 2020* document addresses societal determinants of health that include both physical and social environments. Notwithstanding the complexity of urban areas, particularly in large metropolitan cities, health promotion efforts and a focus on healthier environments are key components of this national health effort. Reduction of inequalities in the physical environment (e.g., transportation, parks, healthy food access) and the social environment (e.g., crime) can lead to improvement in key health indicators and aid in meeting the goals and objectives of *Healthy People 2020* (Secretary's Advisory Committee on Health Promotion and Disease Prevention Objectives for 2020, 2010). Urban development, transportation, housing, education, and agriculture must be addressed, as well as health promotion and disease prevention, in order to affect substantive change. Research and data collection is important to guide our progress.

URBAN POPULATIONS AND HEALTH DISPARITIES

The majority of the world's populace now lives in cities, which is a change from long-held rural dominance (Vlahov et al., 2007). The greatest growth of large cities around the world is among less-wealthy nations, where urban slums are developing at a rapid rate (Vlahov et al., 2010). Depending upon the classification used, more than one third of the U.S. population lives in central cities. This is the highest number since 1950 (Mather, Pollard, & Jacobsen, 2012). However, suburbs of metropolitan areas had the fastest growth, especially in the

West and the South; over half of the populace lives in *suburban areas*. More than 84% of the U.S. population lives in what are characterized as central city or metropolitan areas (Mather et al., 2012).

Although some metropolitan areas have recorded substantial population losses in central-city areas (e.g., New Orleans at 11.3%, Detroit at 3.5%), most have logged substantial gains (e.g., Atlanta had a 24% gain, Austin a 37.3% increase, a 32.1% increase in Charlotte, Orlando with 29.8%, Las Vegas and Raleigh each at over 41%) between 2010 and 2000 (Demographia, 2012).

One example of how changes in population can adversely affect large cities can be found in Detroit, Michigan. Between the 2000 and 2010 censuses, the population dropped 25% (or 237,500 people) to the lowest level since 1910. This is less than the 29% population loss experienced by New Orleans due to Hurricane Katrina. However, the total number of people was much less in New Orleans (only 140,000). The dramatic losses in Detroit pulled down the numbers for the state of Michigan, and it was the only U.S. state to show a net population loss. Auto and other industrial losses, combined with large numbers of home foreclosures, are thought to be at the root of the problem. Population loss leads to a smaller tax base and a greater proportion of poor residents, yet the city had the same maintenance expenses for sewers, water lines, and streets (Seelye, 2011). With the loss of jobs, many moved to the suburbs, and unemployment and welfare rates increased in Detroit. The poverty rate jumped from 10.4% in 2000 to 17% in 2010 (Davis, 2012).

Historically, movement to the suburbs began with the housing boom and highway expansion occurring after WWII. People moved from large cities to more suburban areas, and shopping malls and schools followed. Cars became even more essential, because public transportation did not always extend into suburban areas thereby leading to long commute times and traffic congestion. Although not all suburban areas have remained attractive and vital, an income gap persists between city and suburban residents. Poverty is two times greater in large central cities than in corresponding suburban areas (18.8% vs. 9.4%), but in total population, there were 1 million more suburban poor in 2005. This is indicative of a "suburbanization of poverty" (p. 12). Poverty rates were highest in metropolitan areas in the Midwest and South, and almost half of all large cities had significant increases in poverty rates. Only about one third of suburban areas recorded poverty rate increases. Wherever poverty rates increased nationwide, the rates of child poverty grew faster (Berube & Kneebone, 2006). As noted earlier, in 2008, more urban women lived in poverty than rural females. This was especially marked in the 18- to 34-year age group (MCHB, 2010).

Today, the declining urban situation is not confined to a few large cities. To achieve the vision of creating "social and physical environments that promote good health for all" as an overarching goal of the *Healthy People 2020* document, more must be done to promote health and prevent disease in urban areas (USDHHS, 2012, para. 5). The primary reason for health disparity, as mentioned in Chapter 25, is the disproportionate burden of certain health and social problems among different populations—in this instance, urban areas. Risks of environmental exposure to air pollution and lead, as well as consumer products (e.g., fast food, alcohol, tobacco), are greater for urban dwellers and have been shown to be significant health risks that contribute to health disparities (Olden, Ramos, & Freudenberg, 2009). Other environmental issues, such as extreme heat events where temperatures rise and lead to climate-related fatalities, have become "more frequent and intense" (Luber & McGeehin, 2008, p. 429). When examining urban form and its relationship to this weather phenomenon, Stone, Hess, and Frumkin (2010) found an increase in annual extreme heat events between 1956 and 2005, with more than twice the number of events in sprawling metropolitan areas when compared with compact metro regions. In other words, where cities grew in a more sprawling, low-density manner requiring the greater use of automobiles rather than a more concentrated high-density city, there were greater "heat-related health effects associated with ongoing climate change" (p. 1425). As with rural areas, the built environment greatly impacts urban neighborhoods.

Poor social conditions and health inequalities have been recognized in urban areas around the world. Urban slums in low- and some middle-income countries provide social exclusion for many living in poverty and threaten development (de Snyder et al., 2011). In this country, overcrowding and poor-quality housing have been found to have a direct relationship with poor mental health, developmental delay, and even to shorter stature (Vlahov et al., 2007). In a study of urban children with asthma, those living in public housing had the highest prevalence of asthma at 21.8%. Almost 69% of public housing residents reported cockroaches, while only 21% of those living in private housing had this problem. Cockroaches, water leaks, and rats were "independently associated with current asthma" status (Northridge, Ramirez, Stingone, & Claudio, 2010, p. 211). In addition to concerns about housing, hazardous waste landfill sites are often located in or near urban areas (Vlahov et al., 2007). Air pollution and noise exposure, often associated with large inner cities, have been linked to asthma, cardiovascular death, hypertension, ischemic heart disease, and hearing impairment (Vlahov et al., 2007). Continued exposure to higher sound levels found in large cities can lead to noise-induced hearing loss as well as decreased levels of work performance, increased levels of aggressive behavior, and higher rates of MI (Moudon, 2009). Lead poisoning and hazards related to asthma have been more often reported in older, larger cities (Maring, Singer, & Shenassa, 2011).

Adar and colleagues (2010) found that living in cities with higher levels of air pollution was associated with narrower retinal arteriolar diameters in the older adults (ages 46–87 years) studied. Daily increases in air pollution also had a similar effect. This led researchers to hypothesize a potential association between air pollution and CVD. Fine-particulate air pollution has been linked to increased morbidity and mortality, and researchers studied the effects of lower levels of this type of pollution over the past two decades compared to the previous two decades. They found that reductions in air pollution "accounted for as much as 15% of the overall increase in life expectancy" in the 51 metropolitan areas studied (Pope, Ezzati, & Dockery, 2009, p. 376). While overall data suggest that urban residents have better health on average than their rural counterparts, this benefit is generally greater for those at the high end of the income scale. This only magnifies the disparities in urban areas between rich and poor (Dye, 2008).

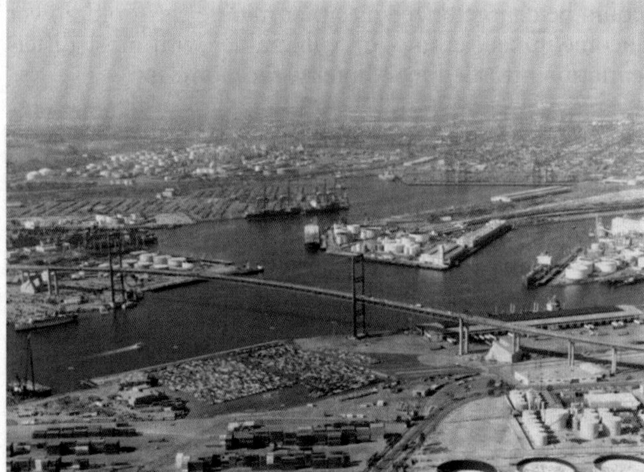

Air pollution is a common problem in metropolitan areas, as seen in this view of San Pedro in Los Angeles County. Source: California Department of Transportation.

Violence is often associated with large metropolitan cities. Kirk and Laub (2010) note that population loss from central cities is both a "cause and consequence of crime" (p. 441). The U.S. Department of Justice (Truman, 2011) revealed that the overall rate of violent crime was down 13% in 2010. Urban areas are often thought to have higher crime rates than rural ones, but no distinctions were made between rural and urban area crime in this yearly report. Jargowsky and Park (2009) found a positive association between metropolitan crime and suburbanization in a study of Uniform Crime Reports and census records. They noted that the poor were isolated in "central-city ghettos and barrios" as the middle- and upper-class city residents moved to the suburbs (p. 28). However, there are differences in levels of violence across inner-city communities (Peterson & Krivo, 2009). Social disorganization theory is thought to predict relationships between delinquency rates and neighborhood social structures and processes, and one study of Denver neighborhoods found that a consistent predictor of problem behavior among youth was a perception of limited future opportunities (Kingston, Huizinga, & Elliott, 2009). Martinez and colleagues (2008) found that illicit drug activity in Miami neighborhoods led to greater violent crime and noted that this activity was often concentrated in low-immigration and mixed ethnicity neighborhoods with fewer non-English speakers. A study of urban street gang density in Los Angeles found that urban areas with greater densities of street gangs had higher overall rates of homicide and that 90% of the variance in local homicide rates over the previous 8 years could be explained by local gang densities, high rates of unemployment and high school dropout, and greater racial/ethnic concentration/population density (Robinson et al., 2009). Fear of crime is a factor in decreased active lifestyles and, ultimately, population health (Roman & Chalfin, 2008).

Inner cities are often thought to be places with residents living in poverty in large, poorly maintained government housing projects. Dilapidated housing in central cities exposes residents to cracks in walls and ceilings, peeling paint, broken windows, leaking pipes, and pests such as cockroaches and rats. There is often limited access to adequate rental properties, and rent is often higher in large cities, making it difficult for low-income residents to find adequate housing. Nationwide, about one third of households live in rentals, but 43% of rental properties are in central cities. Most rental property in this country (80%) is considered private, with landlords not receiving any government subsidies. Rents in large metropolitan areas rose 9% between 2000 and 2005, but household incomes of renters fell 5% during that time period. As the recession began in 2008, "rent-to-income ratios were higher than they had been" since the early days of the Depression (DiPasquale, 2011 p. 58). However, landlords have not escaped financial consequences of the recession. In Chicago, 12.5% of rental properties were found to have net revenues at or below total operating costs (e.g., mortgage payments, taxes, insurance, maintenance); declining rents along with increases in insurance, energy costs, and property taxes are often to blame (Schilling, 2010). Vacancy rates in 2009 peaked at 10.6%, and rents are declining across the country (DiPasquale, 2011).

Urban poor are often forced to live in neighborhoods that do not facilitate outdoor activity or have markets that provide healthy foods, such as fresh fruits and vegetables. A study of urban retail food markets found that most corner markets do not sell low-fat dairy products or fresh produce but "conduct a lively business selling lottery tickets, cigarettes, and liquor" (Lane et al., 2008, p. 415). Researchers also noted that pregnant women living near supermarkets, regardless of their income level, had significantly fewer low birth weight babies. A study of adolescent drinking in California found that alcohol availability was significantly higher in areas with greater concentrations of lower-income minority residences and that adolescent binge drinking and driving was significantly greater when teens lived within one-half mile of alcohol retailers. The concentration of liquor stores and other alcohol outlets in disadvantaged communities contributes to teen drinking (Truong & Sturm, 2009). Low-income housing, when available, is often plagued with construction and maintenance problems and is characterized by crowding, poor quality, high population density, and attendant health problems. Over 1.3 million U.S. households are located in public housing.

Over one third of rental housing was built before 1960, and owners of multifamily rental properties that have lost tenants and income may scrimp on maintenance that decreases property values even more (DiPasquale, 2011). Homelessness is more prevalent in urban areas than in rural areas, and programs to provide consistent housing have shown promise (Hudson & Vissing, 2010; Larimer et al., 2009). See Chapter 28 for more on the homeless population.

Sociologists Wilson and Kelling first proposed the *broken window theory* in 1982, noting that if a broken window goes unrepaired, soon more windows are broken, and this sends a powerful message to residents that no one cares. Keizer, Lindenberg, and Steg (2008) tested this theory in six field experiments where neighborhoods, characterized by broken windows, litter, unreturned shopping carts, and graffiti, were studied. They found that when residents see others violating social norms or rules (e.g., disorderly or petty criminal behavior), they are then more likely to also violate norms and rules and that this is a cause for the spread of disorder.

Population density, complexity, and racial/ethnic diversity are associated with urban areas. Central cities are often home to a large proportion of poor people and those from different racial and ethnic groups (Jargowsky & Park, 2009). Less than half of all Hispanics lived in the top ten metropolitan areas in 2005, with 22% living in Los Angeles and New York. These two large cities are also home to 27% of the Asian population, with 56% living in the top ten metro areas. Over the past 15 years, there has been significant movement of Blacks to Southern metropolitan areas, but movement to other areas (e.g., Las Vegas, Phoenix, Sacramento, Minneapolis) has also occurred. Many metropolitan areas, especially in high-cost coastal areas and parts of the Midwest, have experienced losses of White residents, while other areas have shown increases; Phoenix, Atlanta, Dallas, and Las Vegas have had the greatest overall gains (Frey, 2006).

Urban poor have health problems characterized by accidental and violent injuries, as well as noncommunicable diseases (Marmot, Friel, Bell, Houweling; Commission on Social Determinants of Health, 2008). In a comparison of neighborhood characteristics in the Multi-Ethnic Study of Atherosclerosis, researchers found that distinct neighborhood features, not associated with race or ethnicity, had health modifying effects. Increased levels of smoking, depression, and not walking for exercise were found in less socially cohesive neighborhoods, while individuals living in neighborhoods with the fewest problems had less smoking, depression, and drinking (Echeverria, Diez-Roux, Shea, Borrell, & Jackson, 2008). As noted in Chapter 25, poverty makes a significant difference in health status. Goldsmith and Blakely (2010) note that political and economic forces, especially for poor city dwellers, generate poverty. Working class urban residents no longer can find industrial jobs, and a concerted effort to improve conditions in urban America is needed in the form of urban policy development.

Over the past 25 years, cities and their suburbs have become more alike, and the demographic and health profiles that were previously uniquely urban are now shared by "edge cities" and suburbs populated by poor and minority families. Political power has shifted to more affluent suburban areas, where the tax base and spending practices are greater, at the expense of these cities. Monies that once came to cities to support new resources have also declined. Hanlon (2009) studied 1,742 U.S. "inner-ring" suburbs, considered early suburban areas of large metropolitan cities. These developed just prior to or immediately after WWII and are often considered to be very similar in composition. She found, however, that this was not the case. They could be characterized as either middle class, old, lower income/mixed, ethnic, or vulnerable, with most differentiation afforded by ethnicity, race, or class.

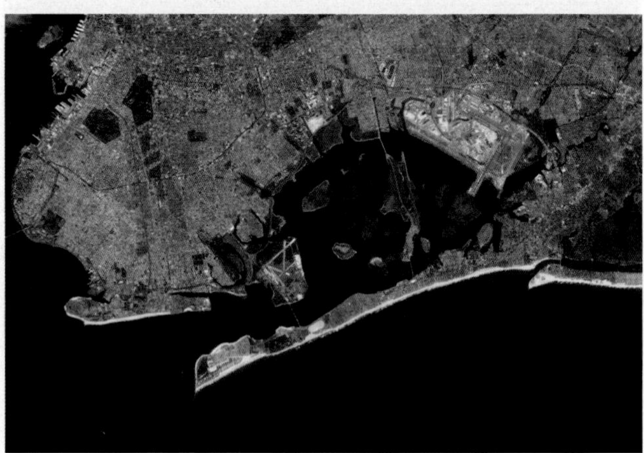

This aerial view of New York City shows Central Park and other green areas interspersed among densely populated areas, an example of good urban planning. Source: National Aeronautics & Space Administration.

Urban health disparities present a challenge that can be addressed only by the joint effort of public health and urban planning bodies. Coalitions of public health professionals, planners, builders, and architects, along with transportation engineers and government officials, are needed to promote healthy, sustainable communities (Boarnet & Takahashi, 2011). There is a move to make cities and their suburbs *sustainable communities*. These are seen as healthy places where both natural and historic resources are protected, employment is available, urban sprawl is contained, neighborhoods are safe, air pollution is minimized lifelong learning is promoted, health care and transportation are easily accessible, and all citizens have the opportunity to improve their quality of life. A federal collaborative program, the Partnership for Sustainable Communities (2009), recognizes six livability principles: (1) provide more transportation choices; (2) promote equitable, affordable housing; (3) enhance economic competitiveness; (4) support existing communities; (5) coordinate and leverage federal policies and investment; and (6) value communities and neighborhoods.

As with all good plans, the sustainable development plan requires that the recipient of the planning be involved. Democratizing the practice of urban planning is vital to its success. Communities that have been victimized through ineffective planning must be included in the decision-making process. This process will require the inclusion of the practical experience that residents bring to the table, alongside expert input. However, to ensure equitable participation and to level the discussions, the community must have access to all the necessary resources, such as technical, legal, and financial assistance. One method for achieving this is "crowdsourcing," a web-based model for citizen participation that utilizes crowd wisdom (Brabham, 2009). The health of communities must be addressed from all levels of environmental impact (individual, community, and systems). Data must be included from the various environments, such as homes, workplaces, schools, and community spaces. These approaches then bring such action in line with what is often referred to as *environmental justice*, or the marriage of environmental health and civil rights (Mohai et al., 2009). A framework to ensure such justice requires that all individuals and communities have the right to work, play, and live in environments that are safe and healthy. It also requires that polluters are punished and required to provide compensation for damages and/or renovation.

SOCIAL JUSTICE AND PUBLIC HEALTH NURSING

Justice is concerned with treating people fairly. *Distributive justice* refers to the justified distribution of burdens and benefits throughout society (see Chapter 4 for a discussion of distributive justice). In the United States, the marketplace largely determines the distribution of goods and services. Although equality is claimed as a social ideal, dramatic inequities are accepted as being determined by the law of the marketplace. In contrast, community health nursing is grounded in commitment to a just distribution of primary goods for all members of society (Falk-Raphael & Betker, 2012). The founder of American public health nursing, Lillian Wald, was in the forefront of social reform movements emphasizing just allocation of resources for the immigrant and poor laborer (Wald, 1971/1915). At the start of the 21st century, PHNs have inherited her legacy, but are we living up to it?

The hardships faced by residents in decaying urban areas are an example of social injustice. Some have called for social justice to be added to the metaparadigm of nursing (person, environment, health, nursing) for community health nursing in urban settings (Schim et al., 2006). **Social justice** occurs when a society provides for the health needs and health care issues of all people by treating people fairly, regardless of where they live or who they are. It involves an equal societal bearing of burdens and reaping of benefits, and it is a widely held view that social justice is the foundation of public health nursing. Some feel that premature death and disease or health and illness derive from the political, socioeconomic, and structural workings of society (Fahrenwald, Taylor, Kniepp, & Canales, 2007). Community health nurses who practice social justice have broad and holistic views of health; they have strong convictions that health care is a basic human right and that improving the health of communities is an example of social justice. For instance, an influenza pandemic calls for PHNs concerned with social justice to include socially marginalized and vulnerable populations (e.g., prisoners, undocumented aliens) in their planning processes. Not to do so would constitute discrimination and would be morally indefensible (Rosoff & DeCamp, 2011). Social justice deals with concepts of inclusion, participation, empowerment, and the recognition that diversity is strength—not a limitation (Racher, 2007). Social justice ensures the distribution of resources that benefits marginalized populations and holds in check the self-interest of more privileged populations. Impartiality is the goal.

PHNs must have a heightened sense of the value of cultural, racial, and socioeconomic differences and awareness that these differences are often turned into discrimination in health care services and policies. They must be determined to extend the bonds of community so that everyone has a firm place to stand and is equally entitled to health care services with a high standard of care for all.

Where is nursing's role within the concept of social justice? Social justice can be both an individual- and a population-based concept, but it is through the population lens that PHNs must focus their greatest attention. Urban health nursing directs its practice to the systems and community- or population-based level, at which both political and economic solutions must be considered. Although most nurses in urban settings continue to provide service on the individual level, nurses should step back and analyze their practice and synthesize recommendations for a plan of action at the level of community planning to better address the needs of the city or neighborhood.

For nurses, a key factor in the process is to emphasize the social justice perspective of *impartiality*, as defined originally by Barry (cited in Schim et al., 2006). This impartiality drives planning and action in a more *just* manner (i.e., as if neither side knew which position they were in: the advantageous [stronger bargaining] position or the disadvantageous [weaker bargaining] position). Thus, instead of an intervention or action being deemed *just* simply because it gives an advantage to one side or the other, it is done because its *outcome* is considered just or fair when viewed by a dispassionate outsider. The point of negotiations, then, is to get an equal share and no more. Self-interest is rationally put aside in favor of the greater good.

Therefore, although day-to-day practice usually includes individual services, the overall planning for change and improvement must occur from the perspective of the population level. From this level of practice, the construct of *person* incorporates the population level of aggregates, institutions, communities, states, and nations—not solely the individual. The concept of the *environment* at the individual level is often associated with physical and psychosocial influences. With a population focus, it incorporates economic and political structures that can influence health or illness and addresses community and global systems that must be utilized to initiate change and solutions. One area that should be considered with urban youth is working with informal neighborhood leaders, as described by Yonas and colleagues (2010). In this qualitative study, researchers found that "prominent neighborhood individuals" share information and take action, both formally and informally, to address neighborhood violence and may be an overlooked resource in developing population-focused interventions (p. 62). Engaging community stakeholders is vital to the success of urban interventions, as it is with rural ones, and faith-based nursing can also be successful there. Derose and colleagues (2010) examined this in their community-based participatory research with an urban church congregation addressing HIV/AIDS.

Like the other constructs, *health* is expanded to include a population focus that recognizes sociopolitical influences. By acknowledging the health issues encountered at the individual as well as the population level, the urban nurse can incorporate interventions that address the more dynamic societal level. In order to combine critical caring theory with public health nursing practice, PHNs contribute to creating "supportive and sustainable physical, social, political, and economic environments" (Falk-Rafael & Betker, 2012, para. 1). In reflecting on the practice of urban as well as rural community health nursing, the profession must believe that it requires more of a population focus; this is something that is often neglected throughout most of undergraduate nursing education (Fahrenwald et al., 2007).

At the same time, urban nursing practice requires cultural and racial competence in order to advocate for the communities served by nursing. Once nursing again accepts and embraces social justice as a focal concept within the practice, especially in urban and public health practices, it can challenge itself to develop more dynamic forms of advocacy and social responsibility that will not only affect its clients but shape the education and training of future nursing professionals (Fahrenwald et al., 2007). This, in turn, should lead to an enhancement of the practice and research needed to contribute solutions for addressing health disparities in all settings.

The urban nursing profession must focus, much like public health nursing, on including both primary and secondary prevention—not only at the local or community level but also include the state, national, and international levels, to enact change for the common good. The role of advocate in these practice settings must include not only the individual level but also the community or population and systems levels. An example of such actions would include advocating for adequate funding of government health systems, such as Medicare and Medicaid, and helping to ensure that all communities are safe and healthy environments in which to live and work. To connect all populations to fair and just systems "requires available, accessible, affordable, and sustainable health care that is equitably and impartially distributed without regard to personal advantage and disadvantage" (Schim et al., 2006, p. 77). Good health should not only belong to those who are blessed with the means of paying for health care, education, and safe working environments but should be a benefit for all of us living together on this planet.

Working in an Urban Setting

Urban public health nursing can be very rewarding, and many nurses are drawn to urban areas where salaries are higher and opportunities for advancement or additional education greater. In urban areas, there are a larger number of nurses, more schools of nursing, and more intensive recruitment efforts than in rural areas, although inner-city areas, much like rural settings, can have problems filling public health nursing vacancies.

Research on urban public health nursing is almost nonexistent. In a seminal study by Schulte (2000, p. 5), PHN duties in a large city in the Midwest were described as a combination of "home visiting, school assignments, clinic services, and other programs," with caseloads averaging between 90 and 140 families. Specialized positions are also common, with PHNs staffing TB and sexually transmitted diseases/infection clinics, serving assigned schools, providing staff development, or being assigned special projects such as screenings and disaster preparedness. The urban nurses in this study worked mainly with clients at or below the poverty level, and one nurse described the situation this way:

> The problems have gotten to be more. The economic situation—everything's gotten worse. The medical care is a mess—not as accessible. People are more mobile now, even more so than they were years ago... they think they left [home]... for a better place (p. 6).

Schulte (2000, p. 6) also noted that PHNs worked largely with "three interacting communities": the local physical communities to which they were assigned, the communities created by individual clients and families, and resource communities (those organized to provide services and goods to clients in need). The processes used by the urban community health nurses included:

- Forging working relationships
- Acting as a resource
- Detecting/asking the next question
- Making informed judgments
- Managing a sense of time
- Teaching
- Intervening with conditions influencing health
- Using physical dexterity

In *forging a relationship*, PHNs began with creating a "perception of presence" by identifying themselves as a PHN and passing out their card with the instruction to the client to call upon them when needed. *Acting as a resource* involves dealing with "sensitive subjects" and requires "honesty, asking direct questions, and ignoring rude behavior." *Detecting and asking the next question* "means listening to more than what is said" (Schulte, 2000, p. 7). When a client is truly heard and all information is on the table, *making an informed judgment* is then possible. *Sense of time* includes the awareness of the long-term commitment of the community health nurse to the client and the belief that results can occur, despite the lack of progress or even regression on the part of some clients. An illustration of this concept was reported by one of the PHNs in the study:

I had this one lady where I just sensed that something else was going on. She was separated from her husband, but he would come over and demand his "right"—sex—and then he'd give her money. And I kept seeing this pattern in her life. So I started getting her to talk about what kind of childhood she had ... and it came out that she had an abusive father who did the same thing—he'd rape her and then give her money. So I talked with her and then got her into counseling. I didn't see her (for awhile) and then she showed up at one of my schools and said, "You're the nurse who saw this and sent me for counseling." She told me that she went back to school, for her GED, and is now enrolled in college. It really helped change her (Schulte, 2000, pp. 7–8).

Teaching is described as an ongoing, interactive process that not only provides information about disease prevention and health promotion but also helps clients navigate the health care system. *Intervening with conditions* that affect health draws on nursing knowledge and experience and involves interceding to reduce the affect of social, political, and economic determinants of health; it involves a "mix of knowledge, experience, intuition, and sensitivity" (p. 8). *Physical dexterity* is used when completing a health assessment of a client's physical condition.

Schulte (2000) found that urban PHNs create connections through caring processes and an underlying sense of regard for their clients as human beings. Community health nurses collaborate with their clients to develop their facility for long-term health promotion and improvement of their quality of life. Their ultimate goal is to empower clients to be self-sufficient. The centrality of caring is noted in the following PHN comment:

> Public health nursing is more than a job.... When I'm out there, I care about the people, about what happens to them. I don't think I'd make a really good public health nurse if I didn't care. You get results if they know you care—they're willing to make some change. If they don't think you care at all about them, why should they take a risk for you? I think public health nursing is all about caring about people. (Schulte 2000, p. 8)

This type of caring is typical of public and community health nursing in all settings, including urban and rural health departments (Olsen Keller, Strohschein, & Schaeffer, 2011).

There are many points at which the community health nurse can make a difference in people's lives. Nurses provide services in deteriorating urban areas, with those living in poverty in all settings, and among all vulnerable populations. Nurses first need to assess themselves for their attitudes and preconceptions. Although access to care can be improved for many low-income people in urban areas, many clients simply need an advocate. The urban communities, and the poor or vulnerable people living in them, need strengthening and interventions that can be initiated by community health nurses using the nursing process as a guide.

Self-Assessment

Confronting poverty and caring for vulnerable people from diverse backgrounds, whether in rural or urban areas, necessitate reflective assessment of one's own assumptions and beliefs. Because poverty may be prevalent over a lifetime, a good number of nursing students have personal or family experience of living in poverty. However, because the stigma is so great and faultfinding so pervasive in American society, acknowledging and reflecting on this experience may well be painful. In contrast, because poverty is so hidden and frequently denied, some nursing students have lived apart from any knowledge of the human experience of poverty. They may have come to believe many of the negative stereotypes about poor people. Nursing students and practicing nurses need to ask such questions as "How have my judgments been shaped? How can I open myself to caring for those from whom most of society turns away?"

We learn from one another's stories. First, learn from your classmates, friends, and neighbors who are courageous enough to tell you their own experiences of living in poverty. Ask them and listen intently. Then, let your clients teach you. One honor that nurses have is the opportunity to work with people from all walks of life. You are particularly likely in clinical experiences in community health to meet impoverished, vulnerable individuals and families living outside the mainstream. And you can work to empower them by helping them build skills and confidence and connecting them to resources (Aston, Meagher-Stewart, Edwards, & Young, 2009). See From the Case Files IV about experiences of students through the eyes of their professors.

Improving Access

Even when government-sponsored health insurance and services are available, extensive barriers prevent many people from accessing services. The community health nurse serves as an advocate and bridge for families who need to gain access. Barriers to access associated with the clients themselves include reluctance to seek coverage because of feelings of powerlessness; being unaware that such services exist or are worthwhile; lacking resources such as a telephone, transportation, or fare for children who need to go along because no babysitter is available; being illiterate; and preoccupation with meeting survival needs and competing life priorities instead of health needs.

Barriers associated with applying for health insurance include a system that is unfriendly and complicated. Paperwork is overwhelming and may be returned for correction; presentation of paid utility bills or other statements that are not often saved may be required. Informative materials may be too difficult to understand; programs may seek to restrict enrollments by restricting information. The process may require a car, a telephone, and appointments at inconvenient times. Also, service interruptions are not uncommon, as wages vary over time. Wait times for reinstatement may be long. The nurse can intervene as a coach and guide, interpreting the system to the client and the client to the system. Likewise, the nurse can act as change agent to improve the system whenever possible.

From the Case Files IV

Examples from Community Health Nursing Instructors

Ann, a nursing faculty member at a small Roman Catholic college, had a one-to-one postclinical conference with a student and relays this conversation. The student had made many visits to an African American teen mother of two thriving children. The young mother lived in a dangerous housing project, and, although she locked him out of her second-floor apartment, her abusive boyfriend had been known to climb up the drainage pipe and over the porch roof. Sometimes, he forced open a window and beat her. The mother worked every day at a fast-food establishment; her grandmother took care of the children. After a couple of months of weekly visits, the student exclaimed, "When I read her chart, I saw her as an immoral girl—a slut—and I expected her to be a loser. Now I can't believe what I've learned about how strong she is. She just keeps fighting for herself and for her kids to survive! She's a great mom and I told her so!"

Another faculty member, Sharon, who taught community health nursing in a Midwestern school of nursing was having an informal discussion with a student who related her experience of trying to get comfortable making home visits with low-income young women. She was making brave attempts at home visits to a pregnant woman, about her age, living in the deteriorating outskirts of a major city. She thought she had established rapport and was making headway developing trust with the client. One day the client asked the student, with concern in her voice, if she had "broken off her engagement." The flustered student then had difficulty explaining the absence of her engagement ring, which she had never mentioned but the client had obviously noticed. During the previous week, she had suddenly realized she was wearing this special ring in marginal neighborhoods and thought it best to leave it at home. Of course, she thought that she had to fabricate another reason to tell the client but felt badly for being so judgmental when the client was identifying with the student and noted they had something in common.

Lynn, a new public health nursing faculty member from a large state university in the West was shocked and repulsed by the comment of one of her students during lecture one day. When discussing vulnerable populations in urban centers and rural areas, the point was made that poverty can be a generational phenomenon and that many of our clients may find it difficult to dig out of this circumstance. Social justice was discussed, along with the need for PHNs to become social activists in order to change political and socioeconomic factors that keep the status quo. One student, a Hispanic female from a middle-class family, spoke up stating "they should all get jobs at McDonalds." This spurred further discussion about population-focused versus individual-focused interventions and approaches and the need for all of us to be aware of our prejudices and stereotypical viewpoints.

Strengthening Communities

We are all connected. All of us as citizens have a stake in preventing the adverse hardships of poverty and ill health. All of society pays to support community members that do not contribute, to house those who are incarcerated, and to ignore the vulnerable. This weakens us. We fear crime in our homes, schools, businesses, and communities in general. Society, as a whole, is impacted when adults are incapable of providing nurturing environments for their children. And the alienation of many groups in society erodes our sense of community as a nation.

The common good is enhanced by strengthening community resources, including investing in people of historically low status, developing and strengthening ties within families and among people involved in neighborhood mutual support, and redeveloping neighborhood resources (see Chapter 13). Whenever possible, the PHN voices support of economic redevelopment of neighborhoods to enhance schools, housing, and employment. The community health nurse can also work to promote subsidized carpools, school-to-work transition programs, universal health insurance, and inner-city economic development programs. Reflecting community priorities and needs as well as focusing on population health are two examples of cornerstones of public health nursing (Olsen Keller et al., 2011).

Many caution well-intentioned professionals to beware when seeking solutions to vulnerability through the use of service programs alone. First, a whole population of people can become defined in terms of their problems instead of their strengths. In addition, citizens acting to help themselves within their community can be weakened when they are seen as clients requiring professional services. Finally, being dependent on multiple human services often has a disabling effect, reducing self-worth and leads to feelings of powerlessness.

Because human service interventions can have negative as well as positive effects, it is important to consider whether more community agencies are the answer to resolving community hardship. Community health planning should seriously consider an organizing process that builds community and that focuses on developing neighborhood competence to solve problems and create solutions for itself (see the discussion of community development in Chapter 15).

SUMMARY

Rural clients are a unique aggregate. Community health nurses are key to ensuring the delivery of appropriate health services to this population. There are numerous definitions of the term *rural*. In this chapter, rural is defined as communities with fewer than 10,000 residents and a county population density of fewer than 1,000 people per square mile. Between the 2000 and 2010 censuses, urban population growth was about twice that in rural areas. The elderly are a rapidly growing population in rural communities. Rural areas often have less diversity than urban cities, but that is changing in many areas. Rural clients generally have lower educational levels than urban clients, due in part to less access to higher education and lower-paying jobs. Income levels and housing costs are frequently lower than in larger cities.

Rural Healthy People 2020 initiative identifies national goals applicable to rural communities. Many at-risk populations live in these communities, where there are often fewer employment opportunities, a lack of adequate housing, and limited access to health and social services. Rural elders may have more limited alternatives for housing if they can no longer live alone. Mental health services are limited, even though the need may be great. Numerous risks are associated with agriculture. The community health nurse must help this population identify hazards and practice injury prevention.

A community health nurse needs to engage in community assessment of the rural area as a part of orientation. It is helpful to identify the strengths of the community. Rural clients are frequently resourceful and often have a supportive network of people to meet their needs.

Access to health care is an important issue in rural communities. Health insurance may not be easily available and is often not offered to self-employed and those working for smaller companies. Barriers to access include distance, weather, transportation, and limited choice of providers. Some ways to improve access in these communities are school-based clinics, mobile health vans, faith-based nursing initiatives, and use of the latest technology. University-sponsored nursing centers that could serve rural populations should be expanded.

Migrant farmworkers are an integral part of the farming community in the United States and across the world; however, they are rarely visible members of our society. As members of a community with varied and profound health needs complicated by disease, social isolation, and occupational hazards such as pesticide exposure and dangerous farm equipment, as well as substandard housing and poor sanitation, migrant farmworkers and their families often live in high-risk environments. Migrant children are often educationally, socially, and physically disadvantaged. Because migrant health centers do not adequately meet the health needs of the entire migrant community, several innovative methods of health care delivery have been developed and implemented by community health nurses, including mobile health vans and information tracking systems.

Rural community health nurses are key members of the professional community. Their roles include advocate, coordinator/case manager, health teacher, referral agent, mentor, change agent/researcher, collaborator, and activist. Community health nurses have challenges and opportunities related to their clinical practices. Confidentiality and personal/professional boundary issues may exist. Salaries for rural nurses may be lower than for nurses in urban areas. But rural community health nurses are highly respected individuals who make a difference in the communities they serve.

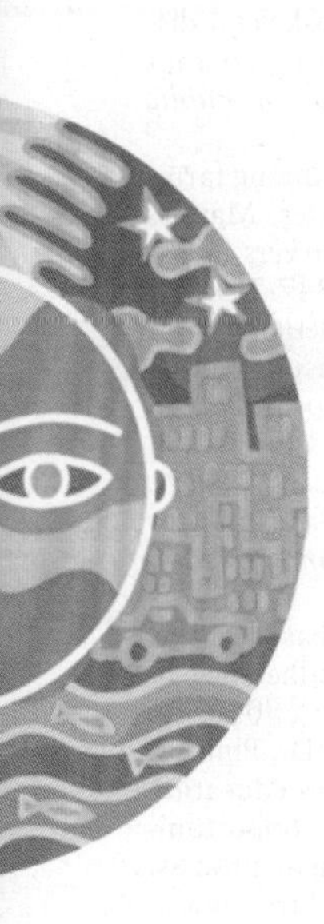

Urban health issues have existed for hundreds of years in the United States, and they continue today. Many disenfranchised and minority groups call inner cities home. Air pollution, poverty, discrimination, substandard housing, crime, and social disorganization often characterize life in urban settings. The built environment is an important consideration in urban as well as rural settings, and can contribute to greater health risks. Some large cities have had marked decreases in population and significant problems with unemployment. Although nursing services may often be delivered at the individual level, the true impact on health must be addressed at the community or population level, as well as the system level. Key to recognizing the potential impact for improvement in the health disparities that exist is the acceptance of a social justice orientation that will empower nurses to address the required changes needed within the existing social, political, and economic systems.

ACTIVITIES TO PROMOTE CRITICAL THINKING

1. Look on the Internet for six recent articles in both rural and urban newspapers relating to access to health care. After summarizing the content, identify barriers to access that are common to both and those that are different. What are the main themes relating to health and access to care?
2. Discuss with a classmate the common characteristics of rural, migrant, and urban clients. How can the public health nurse (PHN) be better prepared to meet their unique needs? What are some specific challenges facing the PHN working in a rural area? In an urban area?
3. Describe some of the benefits of rural public health nursing.
4. Compare and contrast health, living, and working concerns between migrant workers and recent immigrants. Discuss how many recent immigrants from places such as Asia, Russia, or Iraq experience the same hardships as migrant workers do. How does nomadic lifestyle affect and differentiate the needs of migrant workers and recent immigrants?
5. If you are from a rural area, interview a peer who was raised in an urban setting (or vice versa). Compare your experiences with family, school, friends, entertainment, etc.
6. Look on the Internet for examples of community needs assessment from both rural and urban areas. What are the main findings of each? How do planned interventions differ? How are they similar?
7. Debate with a classmate the need for ready access to specialist medical care and sophisticated diagnostic equipment in all communities. Is this feasible? If not, how can services best be made available to urban and rural clients?
8. Search YouTube for videos related to rural public health nursing, migrant workers, urban health, social justice, or other topics described in this chapter. Discuss key points with your clinical group and highlight the major issues.

REFERENCES

Adar, S. D., Klein, R., Klein, B., Szpiro, A. A. (2010). Air pollution and the microvasculature: A cross-sectional assessment of in vivo retinal images in the population-based multi-ethnic study of atherosclerosis (MESA). *PLoS Medicine, 7*(11), e1000372.

Advocate Precautionary Principle (APP). (2011, June 8). *NIOSH study confirms pesticide drift hazards posed by chemical pesticide applications*. Retrieved from http://apprecautionaryprinciple.wordpress.com/2011/06/08/niosh-study-confirms-pesticide-drift-hazards-posed-by-chemical-pesticide-applications/

Agency for Healthcare Research and Quality (AHRQ). (2012). *Primary Care Workforce Facts and Stats: Overview*. Retrieved from http://www.ahrq.gov/research/pcworkforce.htm

Agency for Healthcare Research and Quality (AHRQ). (2011). *National health care disparities report, 2010*. Retrieved from http://www.ahrq.gov/qual/nhdr10/Chap10a.htm

Ambardekar, A. V., Fonarow, G. C., Dai, D., Peterson, E. D., Hernandez, A. F., Cannon, C. P., et al. (2010). Quality of care and in-hospital outcomes in patients with coronary heart disease in rural and urban hospitals (from Get with the Guidelines-Coronary Artery Disease Program). *The American Journal of Cardiology, 105*(2), 139–143.

American Academy of Pediatrics. Committee on Community Health. (2010). Reaffirmed policy statement: Providing care for immigrant, homeless, and migrant children. *Pediatrics, 125*(4), e978.

American College of Physicians. (1997). Inner-city health care. *Annals of Internal Medicine, 126*(6), 485–490.

American Heart Association. (2010). Heart disease and stroke statistics—2010 update: A report from the American Heart Association. *Circulation, 121*, e46–e215.

American Public Health Association (APHA). (n.d.). *At the intersection of public health and transportation: Promoting healthy transportation policy*. Retrieved from http://www.apha.org/NR/rdonlyres/43F10382-FB68-4112-8C75-49DCB10F8ECF/0/TransportationBrief.pdf

Arcury, T. A., Grzywacz, J. G., Talton, J. W., Chen, H., Vallejos, Q. M., Galván, L., et al. (2010). Repeated pesticide exposure among North Carolina migrant and seasonal farmworkers. *American Journal of Industrial Medicine, 53*(8), 802–813.

Arcury, T. A., O'Hara, H., Grzywacz, J. G., Isom, S., Chen, H., Quandt, S. A. (2012). Work safety climate, musculoskeletal discomfort, working while injured, and depression among migrant farmworkers in North Carolina. *American Journal of Public Health, 102*(S2), S272–S278.

Arcury, T. A., & Quandt, S. A. (2009). Pesticide exposure among farmworkers and their families in the Eastern United States: Matters of social and environmental justice. *Latino Farmworkers in the Eastern United States,* doi: 10.10007/978-0-387-88347-2_5.

Arcury, T. A., Weir, M., Chen, H., Summers, P., Pelletier, L. E., Galván, L., et al. (2012). Migrant farmworker housing regulation violations in North Carolina. *American Journal of Industrial Medicine, 55*(3), 191–204.

Aston, M., Meagher-Stewart, D., Edwards, N., & Young, L. M. (2009). Public health nurses' primary health care practice: Strategies for fostering citizen participation. *Journal of Community Health Nursing, 26*, 24–34.

Atkinson, M. J., & Petrozzino, J. J. (2009). An evidence based review of treatment-related determinants of patients' nonadherence to HIV medications. *AIDS Patient Care and STDs, 23*(11), 903–914.

Balamurugan, A., Hall-Barrow, J., Blevins, M. A., Brech, D., Phillips, M., Holley, E., et al. (2009). A pilot study of diabetes education via telemedicine in a rural underserved community—opportunities and challenges: a continuous quality improvement process. *Diabetes Educator. 35*(1),147–54. Retrieved from http://www.ncbi.nlm.nih.gov/pubmed/19244570

Baldwin, L. M., Chan, L., Andrilla, C. H., Huff, E. D., & Hart L. G. (2010). Quality care for myocardial infarction in rural and urban hospitals. *The Journal of Rural Health, 26*(1), 51–57.

Barbassa, J. (2010, June 25). *Farmworkers challenge the jobless: Try our jobs*. San Francisco Chronicle. Retrieved from http://www.sfgate.com/cgi-bin/article.cgi?f=/c/a/2010/06/25/BALT1E4KUR.DTL

Bardacke, F. (2011). *Trampling out the vintage: Cesar Chavez and the two souls of the United Farm Workers*. Brooklyn, NY: Verso Books.

Barnett, D., Thompson, C., Errett, N., Semon, N., Aderson, M., Ferrell, J. et al. (2012). Determinants of emergency response willingness in the local public health workforce by jurisdictional and scenario patterns: a cross-sectional survey. *BMC Public Health, 12*, 164. Retrieved from http://www.biomedcentral.com/1471–2458/12/164

Basu, J., & Mobley, L. (2007). Illness severity and propensity to travel along the urban-rural continuum. *Health & Place, 13* (2),381–399. Retrieved from http://www.ncbi.nlm.nih.gov/pubmed/16697689

Bellamy, G. R., Bolin, J. N., & Gamm, L. D. (2011). Rural Healthy People 2010, 2020 and beyond: The need goes on. *Family & Community Health, 34*(2), 182–188.

Benson, P. (2010). *Giants in the fields: Agribusiness and farm labor politics in the United States. Anthropology of Work Review, 31*(2), 54–70.

Bernard, V., Coughlin, S., Thompson, T., & Richardson, L. (2007). Cervical cancer incidence in the United States by area of residence, 1998–2001. *American Journal of Obstetrics and Gynecology, 110*(3), 681–686.

Berube, A., & Kneebone, E. (2006, December). *Two steps back: City and suburban poverty trends, 1999-2005*. Living Cities Census Series. Washington, DC: The Brookings Institution.

Bigbee, J. L., Gehrke, P., & Otterness, N. (2009). Public health nurses in rural/frontier one-nurse offices. *Rural and Remote Health, 9*, 1282.

Bigbee, J. L., Otterness, N., & Gehrke, P. (2010). Public health nursing competency in a rural/frontier state. *Public Health Nursing, 27*(3), 270–276.

Bishop, B. (2009, January 7). When the house bubble burst, rural prices kept steady. *Main Street Economics*. Retrieved from http://www.dailyyonder.com/when-house-bubble-burst-rural-prices-kept-steady/2009/01/07/1831

Blanco, C. E. (2011). Promotoras: A culturally sensitive intervention for Hispanic breastfeeding women. *Journal of Obstetric, Gynecologic, & Neonatal Nursing, 40*(s1), s19.

Boarnet, M. G., & Takahashi, L. M. (2011). Interactions between public health and urban design. In T. Banerjee, & A. Loukaitou-Sideris (Eds.) *Companion to urban design* (pp. 198–207). New York: Routledge.

Bolin, J. N., & Bellamy, G. (n.d.). *Rural Healthy People 2020*. Retrieved from http://www.srph.tamhsc.edu/centers/srhrc/images/rhp2020#rhp2020

Borders, T., & Booth, B. (2007). Rural, suburban, and urban variations in alcohol consumption in the United States: Findings from the National Epidemiologic Survey on Alcohol & Related Conditions. *Journal of Rural Health, 23*(4), 314–321.

Borre, K., Ertle, L., & Graff, M. (2010). Working to eat: Vulnerability, food insecurity, and obesity among migrant and seasonal farmworker families. *American Journal of Industrial Medicine, 53*(4), 443–462.

Brabham, D. C. (2009). Crowdsourcing the public participation process for planning projects. *Planning Theory, 8*(3), 242–262.

Bradman, A., Salvatore, A. L., Boeniger, M., Castorina, R., Snyder, J., Barr, D. B., et al. (2009). Community-based intervention to reduce pesticide exposure to farmworkers and potential take-home exposure to their families. *Journal of Exposure Science & Environmental Epidemiology, 19*, 79–89.

Branas, C., McKenzie, E., & Williams, J. (2005). Access to trauma centers in the United States. *Journal of the American Medical Association, 293*, 2626–2633.

Brockman, R., Jago, R., & Fox, K. R. (2011). Children's active play: Self-reported motivators, barriers and facilitators. *BMC Public Health, 11*, 461.

Bushy, A. (2008). Conducting culturally competent rural nursing research. *Annual Review of Nursing Research, 26*, 221–236.

Caldwell, D. R. (2007). Bloodroot: Life stories of nurse practitioners in rural Appalachia. *Journal of Holistic Nursing, 25*, 73–79.

California Department of Pesticide Exposure. (2010). *Pesticide illness surveillance program*. Retrieved from http://www.cdpr.ca.gov/docs/whs/pisp.htm

Cameron, L., Lalich, N., Bauer, S., Booker, V., Boque, H. O., Samuels, S., et al. (2006). Occupational health survey of farm workers by camp aides. *Journal of Agricultural Safety & Health, 12*(2), 139–153.

Cant, R., Birks, M., Porter, J., Jacob, E., & Cooper, S. (2011). Developing advanced rural nursing practice: A whole new scope of responsibility. *Collegian, 18*(4), 177–182.

Casey, A. A., Elliott, M., Glanz, K., Haire-Joshu, D., Lovegreen, S. L., Saelens, B. E., et al. (2008). Impact of the food environment and physical activity environment on behaviors and weight status in rural U.S. communities. *Preventive Medicine, 47*(6), 600–604.

Centers for Disease Control & Prevention (CDC). (2010). *About Healthy Places*. Retrieved from http://www.cdc.gov/healthyplaces/about.htm

Centers for Disease Control & Prevention (CDC). (2011). *HIV/AIDS basic statistics*. Retrieved from http://www.cdc.gov/hiv/topics/surveillance/basic.htm#hivest

Chaudry, A., Capps, R., Pedroza, J. M., Castaneda, R. M., Santos, R., Scott, M. M., et al. (2010). *Facing our future: Children in the aftermath of immigration enforcement*. Washington, DC: The Urban Institute.

Clark, C. R., Coull, B., Berkman, L. F., Buring, J., & Ridker, P. M. (2011). Geographic variation in cardiovascular inflammation among healthy women in the Women's Health Study. *PLoS ONE, 6*(11), e27468.

Cockburn, M., Mills, P., Zhang, X., Zadnick, J., Goldberg, D., Ritz, B., (2011). Prostate cancer and ambient pesticide exposure in agriculturally intensive areas in California. *American Journal of Epidemiology, 173*(11), 1280–1288.

Cohen, J. H. (2010). Oaxacan migration and remittances as they relate to Mexican migration patterns. *Journal of Ethic and Migration Studies, 36*(1), 149–161.

Cole, A., & Crawford, L. (1991). Implementation and evaluation of the health resource program for migrant women in the Americus, Georgia area. In A. Bushy (Ed.). *Rural nursing* (Vol. 1. pp. 364–374). Newbury Park: Sage Publications.

Colt, J. S., Rothman, N., Severson, R., Hartge, P., Cerhan, J. R., Chatterjee, N., et al. (2009). Organochlorine exposure, immune gene variation, and risk of non-Hodgkin lymphoma. *Blood, 113*(9), 1899–1905.

Connor, A., Layne, L., & Thomisee, K. (2010). Providing care for migrant farm worker families in their unique sociocultural context and environment. *Journal of Transcultural Nursing, 21*(2), 159–166.

Cook, N. L., & Lauer, M.S. (2011). The socio-geography of heart failure: Why it matters. *Circulation: Heart Failure, 4*, 244–245.

Cook, N. R., & Albert, M. A. (2009). Regarding REGARDS: Does inflammation explain racial and regional differences in cardiovascular disease risk? *Clinical Chemistry, 55*(9), 1603–1605.

Coronado, G. D., Holte, S., Vigoren, E., Griffith, W. C., Barr, D. B., Faustman, E., et al. (2011). Organophosphate pesticide exposure and residential proximity to nearby fields: Evidence for the drift pathway. *Journal of Occupational & Environmental Medicine, 53*(8), 884–891.

Coursen-Neff, Z. (2011, November 17). *Child farmworkers in the United States: A "worst form of child labor."* Human Rights Watch. Retrieved from http://www.hrw.org/news/2011/11/17/child-farmworkers-united-states-worst-form-child-labor

Cox, K., Mahone, I., & Merwin, E. (2008). Improving the quality of rural nursing care. *Annual Review of Nursing Research, 26*, 175–194.

Cramer, M., Duncan, K., Megel, M., & Pitkin, S. (2009). Partnering with rural communities to meet the demand for a qualified nursing workforce. *Nursing Outlook, 57*(3), 148–157.

Crawford, J., Barton, H., Chapman, T., Higgins, M., Capon, A. G., & Thompson, S. M. (2010). Health at the heart of spatial planning strengthening the roots of planning health and the urban planner health inequalities and place planning for the health of people and plant: An Australian perspective. *Planning Theory & Practice, 11*(1), 91–113.

Cushman, M., Cantrell, R., McClure, L., Howard, G., Prineas, R., Moy, C. et al. (2008). Estimated 10-year stroke risk by region and race in the United States. *Annals of Neurology, 64*(5) 507–513.

Cutler, D., Glaeser, E., & Vigdor, J. (1997, January). *The rise and decline of the American ghetto.* [NBER Working Paper No. W5881]. Retrieved from http://ssrn.com/abstract=225663

Davis, K. D. (2012, January 26). Governmental fragmentation in metropolitan Detroit. *McNair Scholars Research Journal, 4*(1), article 4.

Demographia. (2012). *U.S. major metropolitan area population: 2000–2010.* Retrieved from http://www.demographia.com/db-2010usmet.pdf

Derose, K. P., Mendel, P. J., Kanouse, D., Bluthenthal, R., Castaneda, L. W., Hawes-Dawson, J., et al. (2010). Learning about urban congregations and HIV/AIDS: Community-based foundations for developing congregational health interventions. *Journal of Urban Health, 87*(4), 617–630.

de Snyder, V., Friel, S., Fotso, J. C., & Khadr, Z. (2011). Social conditions and urban health inequities: Realities, challenges and opportunities to transform the urban landscape through research and action. *Journal of Urban Health, 88*(6), 1183–1193.

DiPasquale, D. (2011). Rental housing: Current market conditions and the role of federal policy. *Cityscape: A Journal of Policy Development & Research, 13*(2), 57–70.

Disabled World. (2010, December 4). *More than one in 10 family medicine practices consider closing with continued threats to Medicare payments.* Retrieved from http://www.disabled-world.com/news/seniors/senior-health-care.php

Dolkart, A. (2008). *Biography of a tenement house in New York City: An architectural history of 97 Orchard Street.* Chicago, IL: Center for American Places.

Dougherty, C. (2011, April 11). Population leaves heartland behind. *Wall Street Journal.* Retrieved from http://online.wsj.com/article/SB10001424052748704843404576251150723518240.html?mod=WSJ_hp_MID

Dye, C. (2008). Health and urban living. *Science, 319*(5864), 766-769.

Echeverria, S., Diez-Roux, A. V., Shea, S., Borrell, L. N., & Jackson, S. (2008). Associations of neighborhood problems and neighborhood social cohesion with mental health and health behaviors: The Multi-Ethnic Study of Atherosclerosis. *Health & Place, 14*(4), 853–865.

Fahrenwald, N., Taylor, J., Kneipp, S., & Canales, M. (2007). Academic freedom and academic duty to teach social justice: A perspective and pedagogy for public health nursing faculty. *Public Health Nursing, 24*(2), 190–197.

Falk-Raphael, A., & Betker, C. (2012). Witnessing social injustice downstream and advocating for health equity upstream: "The trombone slide" of nursing. *Advances in Nursing Science, 35*(2), 98–112.

Family Violence Prevention Fund. (2008). *The facts on domestic violence.* San Francisco, CA: Author.

Farmworker Justice. (n.d.). *The dangers of pesticides for farmworkers.* Retrieved from http://www.fwjustice.org/pesticide-safety

Fisher-Owens, S., Barker, J. C., Adams, S., Chung, L. H., Gansky, S. A., Hyde, S., et al. (2008). Giving policy some teeth: Routes to reducing disparities in oral health. *Health Affairs, 27*(2), 404–412.

Flocks, J., Monaghan, P., Albrecht, S., & Bahena, A. (2007). Florida farmworkers' perceptions and lay knowledge of occupational pesticides. *Journal of Community Health, 32*(3), 181–194.

Florida Association of Community Health Centers. (2009, February 7). *Data related to farmworkers, immigrants, uninsurance, ER use and the effectiveness of community health workers.* Retrieved from http://www.fachc.org/pdf/mig_Data%20on%20farmworkers,%20immigrants,%20Uninsurance,%20ER%20and%20CHW.pdf

Flynn, D. (2012, January 21). Jensen Farms owner fined for shoddy worker housing. *Food Safety News.* Retrieved from http://www.foodsafetynews.com/2012/01/civil-fine-imposed-on-eric-jensen-over-shoddy-migrant-housing/

Food Security Learning Center. (2010). *Introduction: Rural poverty.* Retrieved from http://www.whyhunger.org/portfolio?topicId=2

Formichelli, L. (2008). A harvest of hope. *Minority Nurse.* Retrieved from http://minoritynurse.com/immigrant-health/harvest-hope

Frank, L. D., & Kavage, S. (2008). Urban planning and public health: A story of separation and reconnection. *Journal of Public Health Management & Practice, 14*(3), 214–220.

Frey, W. (2006, November). *America's regional demographics in the &llenis;00s decade: The role of seniors, boomers and new minorities.* Washington, DC: The Brookings Institution.

Fujiwara, T., & Kawachi, I. (2008). Social capital and health: A study of adult twins in the U.S. *American Journal of Preventive Medicine, 35*(2), 139–144.

Galea, S., & Vlahov, D. (Eds.). (2008). *Handbook of urban health: Populations, methods, and practice.* New York: Springer Science.

Gamble, J., Eurich, D., Ezekowitz, J., Kaul, P., Qua, H., & McAlister, F. (2011). Patterns of care and outcomes differ for urban versus rural patients with newly diagnosed heart failure, even in a universal heathcare system. *Circulation: Heart Failure,* 4(3) 317–323.

Geiger, C. T. (2009). *Educational leaders and migrant populations: Policies and issues in the state of Florida* (Doctoral dissertation, University of Florida). Retrieved from http://etd.fcla.edu/UF/UFE0024877/geiger_c.pdf

Gibson, M. A., & Hidalgo, N. (2009). Bridges to success in high school for migrant youth. *Teacher's College Record 111*(3), 683–711.

Gleeson, S. (2010). Labor rights for all? The role of undocumented immigrant status for worker claims making. *Law & Social Inquiry, 35*(3), 561–602.

Goldsmith, W., & Blakely, E. (2010). *Separate societies: Poverty and inequality in U.S. cities* (2nd ed.). Philadelphia, PA: Temple University Press.

Goldstein, B., Howe, B., & Tamir, I. (2010). *Weeding out abuses: Recommendations for a law-abiding farm labor system.* Retrieved from http://www.fwjustice.org/files/immigration-labor/weeding-out-abuses.pdf

Goodridge, D., Lawson, J., Rennie, D., Marciniuk, D. (2010). Rural/urban differences in health care utilization and place of death for persons with respiratory illness in the last year of life Rural and Remote Health 10: 1349

Greene, M., Perkins, M. M., Scott, K., & Burt, C. (2011). State responsibilities to support rural caregiving: The Georgia example. In R. C. Talley, K. Chwalisz, & K. C. Buckwalter (Eds.). *Rural caregiving in the United States: Research, practice, policy* (pp. 213–231). New York: Springer Science.

Guo, J. J., Wade, T. J., Pan, W., & Keller, K. N. (2010). School-based health centers: Cost-benefit analysis and impact on health care disparities. *American Journal of Public Health, 100*(9), 1617–1623.

Hanlon, B. (2009). A typology of inner-ring suburbs: Class, race, and ethnicity in U.S. suburbia. *City & Community, 8*(3), 221–246.

Hayes, J. C. (2011). Megacities. *Public Health Nursing, 28*(3), 201–202.

Health Resources and Services Administration (HRSA). (n.d.a.). *Shortage designation: Health professional shortage areas and medically underserved areas/populations.* Bureau of Health Professions. Retrieved from http://bhpr.hrsa.gov/shortage/

Health Resources and Services Administration (HRSA). (n.d.b.). *Telehealth.* Retrieved from http://www.hrsa.gov/telehealth/default.htm

Health Resources and Services Administration (HRSA). (2005). *Public health workforce study.* Retrieved from http://bhpr.hrsa.gov/healthworkforce/reports/publichealthstudy2005.pdf

Hiott, A., Grzywacz, J., Davis, S., Quandt, S. A., Arcury, T. A. (2008). Migrant farmworker stress: Mental health implications. *The Journal of Rural Health, 24*(1), 32–39.

Hoerster, K. D., Mayer, J. A., Gabbard, S., Kronick, R. G., Roesch, S. C., Malcarne, V. L., et al. (2011). Impact of individual-, environmental-, and policy-level factors on health care utilization among US farmworkers. *American Journal of Public Health, 101*(4), 685–692.

Holden, C. (n.d.). *Migrant health issues: Housing.* Monograph No. 8. Buda, TX: National Center for Farmworker Health.

Holmes, M., & Pink, G. (2011, April). *Risk of financial distress among critical access hospitals: A proposed model.* Flex

Monitoring Team Policy Brief No. 20. Retrieved from http://www.flexmonitoring.org/documents/PolicyBrief20_Strategies.pdf

Holmes, S. M. (2009). The clinical gaze in the practice of migrant health: Mexican migrants in the United States. *Social Science & Medicine, 74*(6), 873–881.

Honore, P. A., Wright, D., Berwick, D. M., Clancy, C. M., Lee, P., Nowinski, J., et al. (2011). Creating a framework for getting quality into the public health system. *Health Affairs, 30*(4), 737–745.

Hood, E. (2005). Dwelling disparities: How poor housing leads to poor health. *Environmental Health Perspectives, 113*(5 Student Edition), A311–A317.

Hou, S. I. (2010). Health literacy, e-health, and communication: Putting the consumer first. *Health Promotion Practice, 11*(3), 303–306.

Housing Assistance Council. (n.d.). *Farmworkers*. Washington, DC: Author. Retrieved from http://www.ruralhome.org/storage/documents/farmoverview.pdf

Housing Assistance Council. (2008). *USDA rural rental assistance program (Section 521)*. Retrieved from http://www.ruralhome.org/storage/documents/rd521ra.pdf

Housing Assistance Council. (2009). *Rural rental housing characteristics*. Washington, DC: Author.

Hsia, R., & Shen, Y. C. (2011). Possible geographical barriers to trauma center access for vulnerable patients in the United States: An analysis of urban and rural communities. *Archives of Surgery, 146*(1), 446–452.

Huber, B. (2011, June 18). *Will the EPA help farmers fight pesticide poisoning?* Retrieved from http://grist.org/industrial-agriculture/2011-06-22-public-health-advocates-urge-epa-to-require-pesticide-makers/

Hudson, C. G., & Vissing, Y. M. (2010). The geography of adult homelessness in the U.S.: Validation of state and county estimates. *Health & Place, 26*, 828–837.

Huseth, A., Vachal, K., Benson, L., & Lofgren, M. (2011). *Pilot study to assess sustained and multifaceted traffic activity on North Dakota's rural roads*. Retrieved from http://ntl.bts.gov/lib/45000/45300/45379/MPC11-233.pdf

Iezzoni, L., Killeen, M., & O'Day, B. (2006). Rural residents with disabilities confront substantial barriers to obtaining care. *HSR: Health Services Research, 41*(4), 1258–1275.

Iezzoni, L., Frakt, A., Pizer, S. (2011). Uninsured persons with disability confront substantial barriers to health care services. *Disability and Health Journal, 4*(4), 238–244.

Isler, M. R., Miles, M., Banks, B., & Corbie-Smith, G. (2012). Acceptability of a mobile health unit for rural HIV clinical trial enrollment and participation. *AIDS and Behavior*, doi: 10.10997/s10461-012-0151-z.

Jago, R., Thompson, J. L., Page, A. S., Cartwright, K., Fox, K. R. (2009). License to be active: Parental concerns and 10-11-year old children's ability to be independently physically active. *Journal of Public Health, 31*(4), 472–477.

Jargowsky, P. A., & Park, Y. (2009). Cause or consequence? Suburbanization and crime in U.S. metropolitan areas. *Crime & Delinquency, 55*(1), 28–50.

Jasis, P., & Marriott, D. (2010). All for our children: Migrant families and parent participation in an alternative education program. *Journal of Latinos and Education, 9*(2), 126–140.

Jilcott, S. B., Liu, H., Moore, J. B., Bethel, J. W., Wilson, J., Ammerman, A. S. (2010). Commute times, food retail gaps, and body mass index in North Carolina counties. *Preventing Chronic Disease, 7*(5), A107.

Johnson, K. M., & Lichter, D. T. (2008). *Population growth in new Hispanic destinations*. Carsey Institute Policy Brief No. 8. Durham, NH: University of New Hampshire.

Johnson, K. M., & Lichter, D. T. (2012). Rural natural increase in the new century: America's demographic transition. *International Handbook of Rural Demography, 3*, 17–34.

Joynt, K. E., Harris, Y., Orav, E. J., & Jha, A. K. (2011). Quality of care and patient outcomes in critical access rural hospitals. *JAMA, 306*(1), 45–52.

Kandel, W., & Parrado, E. (2006). Public policy impacts of rural Hispanic population growth. In W. Kandel, & D. Brown (Eds.). *Population change and rural society* (pp. 155–176). New York: Springer Publishing.

Kegler, M. C., Escoffery, C., Alcantara, I. C., Hinman, J., Addison, A., Glanz, K. (2012). Perceptions of social and environmental support for healthy eating and physical activity in rural Southern churches. *Journal of Religion and Health, 51*(3), 799–811.

Keizer, K., Lindenberg, S., & Steg, L. (2008). The spreading of disorder. *Science, 322*(5908), 1681–1685.

Keifer, M., Salazar, M. K., & Connon, C (2009). An exploration of Hispanic workers' perspectives about risks and hazards associated with orchard work. *Family & Community Health, 32*(1), 34–47.

Kilkenny, M. (2010). Urban/regional economics and rural development. *Journal of Regional Science, 50*(1), 449–470.

Kim-Godwin, Y., & Fox, J. A. (2009). Gender differences in intimate partner violence and alcohol use among Latino-migrant and seasonal farmworkers in rural Southeastern North Carolina. *Journal of Community Health Nursing, 26*(3), 131–142.

King, M. (2007, June 7). *Immigrants in the U.S. health care system: Five myths that misinform the American public*. Washington, DC: Center for American Progress.

Kingston, B., Huizinga, D., & Elliott, D. S. (2009). A test of social disorganization theory in high-risk urban neighborhoods. *Youth & Society, 41*(1), 53–79.

Kirk, D. S., & Laub, J. H. (2010). Neighborhood change and crime in the modern metropolis. *Crime and Justice, 39*(1), 441–502.

Kirkpatrick, S., & Tarasuk, V. (2011). Housing circumstances are associated with household food access among low-income urban families. *Journal of Urban Health, 88*(2), 284–296.

Kirschner, A., Berry, E. H., & Glasgow, N. (2006). The changing demographic profile of rural America. In W. Kandel, & D. Brown (Eds.). *The changing faces of rural America* (pp. 53–74). New York: Springer Publishing.

Kirschner, A., Berry, E. H., & Glasgow, N. (2009, January). *The changing demographic profile of rural areas*. Retrieved from http://devsoc.cals.cornell.edu/cals/devsoc/outreach/cardi/publications/loader.cfm?csModule=security/getfile&PageID=437557

Kisby, G. E., Muniz, J. F., Scherer, J., Lasarey, M. R., Koshy, M., Kow, Y. W., et al. (2009). Oxidative stress and DNA damage in agricultural workers. *Journal of Agromedicine, 14*(2), 206–214.

Knudsen, A., & Meit, M. (n.d.). *Public health nursing: Strengthening the core of rural public health*. Policy Brief. Kansas City, MO: National Rural Health Association.

Krishna, S., Gillespie, K. N., & McBride, T. M. (2010). Diabetes burden and access to preventive care in the rural United States. *The Journal of Rural Health, 26*(1), 3–11.

Kronkosky Charitable Foundation. (2011, January). *Rural healthcare research brief*. Retrieved from http://www.kronkosky.org/research/Research_Briefs/Rural%20Healthcare%20January%202011.pdf

Kugel, C., Retzlaff, C., Hopfer, S., Lawson, D., Daley, E., Drewes, C., et al. (2009). Familias con Voz: Community survey results from an intimate partner violence (IPV) prevention project with migrant workers. *Journal of Family Violence, 24*(8), 649–660.

Laditka, J. N., Laditka, S. B., & Probst, J. C. (2009). Healthcare access in rural areas: Evidence that hospitalization for ambulatory care-sensitive conditions in the United States may increase with the level of rurality. *Health & Place, 15*(3), 761–770.

Lane, S. D., Keefe, R., Rubinstein, R., Levandowski, B. A., Webster, N., Cibula, D. A., et al. (2008). Structural violence, urban retail food markets, and low birth weight. *Health & Place, 14*(3), 415–423.

Larimer, M. E., Malone, D. K., Garner, M. D., Atkins, D. C., Burlingham, B., Lonczak, H. S., et al. (2009). Health care and public service use and costs before and after provision of housing for chronically homeless persons with severe alcohol problems. *JAMA, 301*(13), 1349–1357.

Larson, A. C. (2000). *Migrant and seasonal farmworker enumeration profiles study: Washington*. Vashon Island, WA: Larson Assistance Services.

Lee, S. J., Mulay, P., Diebolt-Brown, B., Lackovic, M. J. (2010). Acute illnesses associated with exposure to fipronil—surveillance data from 11 states in the United States, 2001–2007. *Clinical Toxicology, 48*(7), 737–744.

Lerner, J. (2010, April 28). *How urban planning can improve public health*. Retrieved from http://www.miller-mccune.com/health/how-urban-planning-can-improve-public-health-11408/

Lishner, D. M., Richardson, M., Levine, P., & Patrick, D. (n.d.). *Access to primary health care among persons with disabilities in rural areas: A summary of the literature*. Retrieved from http://www.amsa.org/programs/barriers/access.pdf

Loue, S., & Quill, B. E. (Eds). (2010). *Handbook of rural health*. New York: Kluwer Academic/Plenum Publishers.]

Luber, G., & McGeehin, M. (2008). Climate change and extreme heat events. *American Journal of Preventive Medicine, 35*(5), 429–435.

Lucio, R. L., Zuniga, G. C., Seal, Y. H., Garza, N., Mier, N., Trevino, L. (2011). Incorporating what *promotoras* learn: Becoming role models to effect positive change. *Journal of Community Health, 37*(5), 1026–1031.

Lutfiyya, M., Lipsky, M., Wisdom-Behounek, J., & Inpanbutr-Martinkus, M. (2007). Is rural residency a risk factor for overweight and obesity for U.S. children? *Obesity, 15*(9), 2348–2356.

MacDowell, M., Glasser, M., Fitts, M., Nielsen, K., & Hunsaker, M. (2010). A national view of rural health workforce issues in the USA. *Rural Remote Health, 10*(3), 1531.

Maring, E. F., Singer, B. J., & Shenassa, E. (2011, April). Healthy homes: A contemporary initiative for Extension Education. *Journal of Extension, 49*(2), article 2FEA9.

Marks, A. R., Harley, K., Bradman, A., Kogut, K., Barr, D. B., Johnson, C., et al. (2010). Organophosphate pesticide exposure and attention in young Mexican-American children: The CHAMACOS study. *Environmental Health Perspectives, 118*(12), 1768–1774.

Marmot, M., Friel, S., Bell, R., Houweling, T., Taylor, S.; Commission on Social Determinants of Health. (2008). Closing the gap in a generation: Health equity through action on the social determinants of health. *The Lancet, 372*(9650), 8–14.

Martinez, R., Rosenfeld, R., & Mares, D. (2008). Social disorganization, drug market activity, and neighborhood violent crime. *Urban Affairs Review, 43*(6), 846–874.

Massey, D. S., & Brown, A. E. (2011). New migration stream between Mexico and Canada. *Migraciones Internacionales, 6*(1), 119–144.

Maternal Child Health Branch. (2010). Population characteristics: Rural and urban women. *Women's Health USA 2010*. Retrieved from http://mchb.hrsa.gov/whusa10/pdfs/w08pc.pdf

Mather, S., & Parameswaran, G. (2012). School readiness for young migrant children: The challenge and the outlook. *International Scholarly Research Network* (ISRN Education), volume 2012, article ID 847502, 9 pages., doi: 10.5402/2012/847502.

Mather, M. (2008, March). *Population losses mount in U.S. rural areas*. Population Reference Bureau. Retrieved from http://www.prb.org/Articles/2008/populationlosses.aspx

Mather, M., Pollard, K., & Jacobsen, L. A. (2012). *First results from the 2010 Census*. Retrieved from http://www.prb.org/Publications/ReportsOnAmerica/2011/census-2010.aspx

May, J. J. (2009). Occupational injury and illness in farmworkers in the Eastern United States. In T. A. Arcury, & S. A. Quandt (Eds.). *Latino farmworkers in the Eastern United States* (pp. 71–101). New York: Springer Science.

McAuley, W. J., Spector, W., & Van Nostrand, J. (2009). Formal home care utilization patterns by rural-urban community residence. *Journal of Gerontology, Series B, 64B*(2), 258–268.

McCauley, L., Anger, W. K., Keifer, M., Langley, R., Robson, M. G., Rohlman, D., (2006). Studying health outcomes in farmworker populations exposed to pesticides. *Environmental Health Perspectives, 114*(6), 953–960.

McCoy, C. (2009). Professional development in rural nursing: Challenges and opportunities. *Journal of Continuing Education in Nursing, 40*(3), 128–131.

McDuffie, H. H., Pahwa, P., Karunanayake, C. P., Spinelli, J. J., & Dosman, J. A. (2009). Clustering of cancer among families of cases with Hodgkin lymphoma (HL), multiple myeloma (MM), non-Hodgkin's lymphoma (NHL), soft tissue sarcoma (STS) and control subjects. *BMC Cancer, 9*, 70.

McGranahan, D., Cromartie, J., & Wojan, T. (2010, November). *Nonmetropolitan outmigration counties: Some are poor, many are prosperous*. Washington, DC: U.S.D.A. Economic Research Service, ERR-107.

Meit, M., Harris, K., Bushar, J., Piya, B., & Molfino, M. (2008). *Challenges, opportunities, and strategies for rural public health agencies seeking accreditation*. NORC Walsh Center for Rural Health Analysis, Policy Analysis Brief No. 13. Retrieved from http://www3.norc.org/NR/rdonlyres/EC0762D3-BF06-4B0F-B6B3-315EEC62F84A/0/PolicyBriefAccreditationJune2008.pdf

Mejia, O. L., & McCarthy, C. J. (2010). Acculturative stress, depression, and anxiety in migrant farmwork college students of Mexican heritage. *International Journal of Stress Management, 17*(1), 1–20.

Merchant, J., Coussens, C., & Gilbert, D. (2006). *Rebuilding the unity of health and the environment in rural America*. Washington, DC: National Academies Press.

Migrant Clinician's Network. (n.d.a). *The migrant/seasonal farmworker*. Retrieved from http://www.migrantclinician.org/issues/migrant-info/migrant.html

Migrant Clinician's Network. (n.d.b). *Health network*. Retrieved from http://www.migrantclinician.org/toolsource/40/health+network/index.html

Migrant Clinician's Network. (n.d.c). *Monograph series: Domestic violence in the farmworker population: Resources for clinicians*. Retrieved from http://www.migrantclinician.org/files/resource-box/DVMonograph.pdf

Miller, K. (2009). *Demographic and economic profile: Nonmetropolitan America*. Rural Policy Research Institute. Retrieved from http://www.rupri.org/Forms/Nonmetro2.pdf

Minetor, R. (2010). *A guided tour through history: New York immigrant experience*. Guilford, CT: Morris Book Publishing, LLC.

Modi, G. M., Doherty, C. B., Katta, R., & Orengo, I. F. (2009). Irritant contact dermatitis from plants. *Dermatitis, 29*(2), 63–78.

Mohai, P., Pellow, D., & Roberts, J. T. (2009). Environmental justice. *Annual Review of Environment and Resources, 34*, 405-430.

Molinari, D. L., & Monserud, M. A. (2008). Rural nurse job satisfaction. *Rural and Remote Health, 8*(4), 1055.

Montgomery, M. P., Kamel, F., Saldana, T. M., Alvavanja, M., & Sandler, D. P. (2008). Incident diabetes and pesticide exposure among licensed pesticide applicators: Agricultural Health Study, 1993–2003. *American Journal of Epidemiology, 167*(10), 1235–1246.

Montour, A., Baumann, A., Blythe, J., & Hunsberger, M. (2009). The changing nature of nursing work in rural and small community hospitals. *Rural and Remote Health, 9*(1), 1089.

Moudon, A. V. (2009). Real noise from the urban environment: How ambient community noise affects health and what can be done about it. *American Journal of Preventive Medicine, 37*(2), 167–171.

Mulligan, R., Seirawan, H., Faust, S., & Habibian, M. (2010). Mobile dental clinic: An oral health care delivery model for underserved migrant children. *Journal of the California Dental Association, 38*(2), 115–122.

Munoz-Laboy, M., Hirsch, J. S., & Quispe-Lazaro, A. (2009). Loneliness as a sexual risk factor for male Mexican migrant workers. *American Journal of Public Health, 99*(5), 802–819.

National Advisory Committee on Rural Health and Human Services [NACRHHS]. (2008). *The 2008 report to the secretary: Rural health and human services issues*. Retrieved from ftp://ftp.hrsa.gov/ruralhealth/committee/nacreport2008.pdf

National Association of County & City Health Officials (NACCHO). (2007). *Activities and workforce of small town rural local health departments: Findings from the 2005 National Profile of Local Health Departments Study*. Washington, DC: Author. CHO.

National Center for Farmworker Health (NCFH). (n.d.a). *Facts about farmworkers*. Retrieved from http://www.ncfh.org/docs/fs-Facts%20about%20Farmworkers.pdf

National Center for Farmworker Health (NCFH). (n.d.b). *Migrant health center legislation*. Retrieved from http://www.ncfh.org/?pid=186

National Center for Farmworker Health (NCFH). (2009a). *Migrant and seasonal farmworker demographics*. Retrieved from http://www.ncfh.org/docs/fs-Migrant%20Demographics.pdf

National Center for Farmworker Health (NCFH). (2009b). *Tuberculosis*. Retrieved from http://www.ncfh.org/docs/fs-What%20is%20TB.pdf

National Center for Farmworker Health (NCFH). (2009c). *Occupational health and safety*. Retrieved from http://www.ncfh.org/docs/fs-Occ%20Health.pdf

National Center for Farmworker Health (NCFH). (2011). *HIV/AIDS farmworker factsheet*. Retrieved from http://www.ncfh.org/docs/fs-HIV_AIDS.pdf

National Center for Frontier Communities. (2009). *2000 update: Frontier counties in the United States*. Retrieved from http://www.frontierus.org/2000update.htm

National Conference of State Legislatures. (2011, October). *States implement health reform: School-based health centers*. Retrieved from http://www.ncsl.org/portals/1/documents/health/HRSBHC.pdf

National Institute for Occupational Safety & Health (NIOSH). (2011). *Agricultural safety*. Retrieved from http://www.cdc.gov/niosh/topics/aginjury/default.html

National Institute for Occupational Safety & Health (NIOSH). (2012). *Pesticide illness & injury surveillance: SENSOR-pesticides program*. Retrieved from http://www.cdc.gov/niosh/topics/pesticides/overview.html

National Rural Health Association. (n.d.). *Rural health issues: Implications for Rural Healthy People 2020*. Kansas City, MO: Author.

National Rural Health Association. (2008). *About rural HIV/AIDS*. Retrieved from http://www.ruralhealthweb.org/go/left/programs-and-events/programs-and-events-overview/rural-hiv/aids-resource-center/rural-hiv/aids-resource-center

New York Academy of Medicine. (n.d.). *Urban health*. Retrieved from http://www.nyam.org/urban-health/

Northridge, J., Ramirez, O. F., Stingone, J. A., & Claudio, L. (2010). The role of housing type and housing quality in urban children with asthma. *Journal of Urban Health, 87*(2), 211–224.

Nuno, T., Martinez, M. E., Harris, R., & Garcia, F. (2011). A *promotora*-administered group education intervention to promote breast and cervical cancer screening in a rural community along the U.S.-Mexico border: A randomized controlled trial. *Cancer Causes and Control, 22*(3), 367–374.

Nusca, A. (2011, July 28). *Rural U.S. population lowest in history, demographers say*. Retrieved from http://www.smartplanet.com/blog/smart-takes/rural-us-population-lowest-in-history-demographers-say/17982

Oakes, L. (2008, January 23). Mortgage foreclosures ripple into rural Minnesota. *Star Tribune*. Retrieved from http://www.startribune.com/local/12337191.html

Occupational Safety & Health Administration. (2011). *Agricultural operations standards: Field sanitation*. Retrieved from http://www.osha.gov/pls/oshaweb/owadisp.show_document?p_table=STANDARDS&p_id=10959

Olden, K., Ramos, R. M., & Freudenberg, N. (2009). To reduce urban disparities in health, strengthen and enforce equitably environmental and consumer laws. *Journal of Urban Health, 86*(6), 819–824.

Olson Keller, L., Strohschein, S., & Schaffer, M. A. (2011). Cornerstones of public health nursing. *Public Health Nursing. 28*(3), 249–260.

Ortego, A. N., Horwitz, S. M., Fang, H., Kuo, A., Wallace, S. P., Inkelas, M. (2009). Documentation status and parental concerns about development in young U.S. children of Mexican origin. *Academic Pediatrics, 9*(4), 278–282.

Parker, V. G., Coles, C., Logan, B. N., & Davis, L. (2010). The LIFE project: A community-based weight loss intervention program for rural African American women. *Family & Community Health, 33*(2), 133–143.

Partnership for Sustainable Communities. (2009). *About us*. Retrieved from http://www.sustainablecommunities.gov/aboutUs.html#2

Peek-Asa, C., Sprince, N., Whitten, P., Falb, S. R., Madsen, M. D., Zwerling, C. (2007). Characteristics of crashes with farm equipment that increase potential for injury. *The Journal of Rural Health, 23*(4), 339–347.

Peterson, R. D., & Krivo, L. J. (2009). Segregated spatial locations, race-ethnic composition, and neighborhood violent crime. *The Annals of the American Academy of Political & Social Science, 623*(1), 93–107.

Place, J., Macleod, M., John, N., Adamack, M, & Lindsey, A. E. (2011). "Finding my own time": Examining the spatially produced experiences of rural RNs in the rural nursing certificate program. *Nursing Education Today*. In press.

Pope, C. A., Ezzati, M., & Dockery, D. W. (2009). Fine-particulate air pollution and life expectancy in the United States. *New England Journal of Medicine, 360*, 376–386.

Quandt, S. A., Schulz, M. R., Talton, J. W., Verma, A., & Arcury, T. A. (2012). Occupational eye injuries experienced by migrant farmworkers. *Journal of Agromedicine, 17*(1), 63–69.

Qenani-Petrela, E., Mittelhammer, R., & Wandschneider, P. (2008). Permanent housing for seasonal workers? A generalized peak load investment model for farm worker housing. *Journal of Agricultural and Applied Economics, 40*(1), 151–169.

Racher, F. (2007). The evolution of ethics for community practice. *Journal of Community Health Nursing, 24*(1), 65–76.

Ransford, H. E., Carrillo, F. R., & Rivera, Y. (2010). Health-seeking among Latino immigrants: Blocked access, use of traditional medicine, and the role of religion. *Journal of Health Care for the Poor & Underserved, 21*(3), 862–878.

Rauh, V., Arunajadai, S., Horton, M., Perera, F., Hoepner, L., Barr, D. B., et al. (2011). Seven-year neurodevelopmental scores and prenatal exposure to chlorpyrifos, a common agricultural pesticide. *Environmental Health Perspectives, 119*(8), 1196–1201.

Research & Training Center: Rural. (2008, February). *Small business: The changing face of rural employment*. University of Montana Rural Institute. Retrieved from http://rtc.ruralinstitute.umt.edu/SelEm/factsheets/smallruralbusinesses.html

Rhodes, S. D., Bischoff, W. E., Burnell, J. M., Whalley, L. E., Walkup, M. P., Vallejos, Q. M., et al. (2010). HIV and sexually transmitted disease risk among male Hispanic/Latino migrant farmworkers in the Southeast: Findings from a pilot CBPR study. *American Journal of Industrial Medicine, 53*(10), 976–986.

Robinson, P. L., Boscardin, W. J., George, S. M., Teklehaimanot, S., Heslin, K. C., Bluthenthal, R. N. (2009). The effect of urban street gang densities on small area homicide incidence in a large metropolitan county, 1994–2002. *Journal of Urban Health, 86*(4), 511–523.

Roman, C. G., & Chalfin, A. (2008). Fear of walking outdoors: A multilevel ecologic analysis of crime and disorder. *American Journal of Preventive Medicine, 34*(4), 306–312.

Rosenthal, K. (2005). What rural nursing stories are you living? *Online Journal of Rural Nursing and Health Care, 5*(1), 37–47.

Rosoff, P. M., & DeCamp, M. (2011). Preparing for an influenza pandemic: Are some people more equal than others? *Journal of Health Care for the Poor & Underserved, 22*(3 Suppl), 19–35.

Rural Assistance Center. (2012a). *Aging*. Retrieved from http://www.raconline.org/topics/aging/

Rural Assistance Center. (2012b). *Frontier frequently asked questions*. Retrieved from http://www.raconline.org/topics/frontier/frontierfaq.php

Rural Assistance Center. (n.d. c). *CAH frequently asked questions*. Retrieved from http://www.raconline.org/ info_guides/hospitals/cahfaq.php#whatis.

Rural Center for AIDs/STD Prevention. (2009). *HIV/AIDs in rural America: Challenges and promising strategies*. Fact sheet No. 23. Retrieved from http://www.indiana.edu/ aids/factsheets/factsheet23.pdf

Rural Health Research Center. (2007, October). *Changes in the rural registered nurse workforce from 1980–2004*. Retrieved from http://depts.washington.edu/uwrhrc/uploads/RHRC%20FR115%202Pager.pdf

Rural Health Research and Policy Centers. (2009). *Profile of rural health insurance coverage: A chartbook*. Retrieved from http://muskie.usm.maine.edu/Publications/rural/Rural-Health-Insurance-Chartbook-2009.pdf

Saenz, R. (2008). *A profile of Latinos in rural America*. Carsey Institute Fact Sheet No. 10. Durham, NH: University of New Hampshire.

Salvatore, A. L., Bradman, A., Castorina, R., Camacho, J., López, J., Barr, D. B., et al. (2008). Occupational behaviors and farmworkers' pesticide exposure: Findings from a study in Monterey County, California. *American Journal of Industrial Medicine, 51*(10), 782–794.

Sampson, R. J. (2009). Racial stratification and the durable tangle of neighborhood inequality. *The Annals of the American Academy of Political & Social Science, 621*(1), 260–280.

Schilling, J. D. (2010). *The multi-family housing market and value-at-risk implications for multi-family lending.* DePaul University, Working Paper. Retrieved from http://www.preservationcompact.org/newsletters/201006/MFHsingMarketAndVAR.pdf

Schim, S., Benkert, R., Bell, S., Walker, D. S., Danford, C. A. (2006). Social justice: Added metaparadigm concept for urban health nursing. *Public Health Nursing, 24*(1), 73–80.

Schlosser, E. (2007, November 29). *Penny foolish.* The New York Times. Retrieved from http://www.nytimes.com/2007/11/29/opinion/29schlosser.html?_r=1&scp=1&sq=Schlosser%20penny%20foolish%202007&st=cse

Schulte, J. (2000). Finding ways to create connections among communities: Partial results of an ethnography of urban public health nurses. *Public Health Nursing, 17*(1), 3–10.

Schmidt, M. (2012, February 1). *Port Sheldon Township migrant worker housing causes conflict.* Retrieved from http://www.hollandsentinel.com/news/x715341972/Port-Sheldon-Township-migrant-worker-housing-causes-conflict

Secretary's Advisory Committee on Health Promotion and Disease Prevention Objectives for 2020. (2010). *Healthy People 2020: An opportunity to address societal determinants of health in the U.S.* Retrieved from http://www.healthypeople.gov/2020/about/advisory/SocietalDeterminantsHealth.pdf

Seelye, K. Q. (2011, March 22). Detroit census confirms a desertion like no other. *The New York Times.* Retrieved from http://datadrivendetroit.org/wp-content/uploads/2011/03/NYTimes_3_22_11.pdf

Shattuck, A. (2009). *Rural workers would benefit from unemployment insurance modernization.* Carsey Institute Policy Brief No. 13. Retrieved from http://www.carseyinstitute.unh.edu/publications/IB-UI-09.pdf

Singh, G. K. (2012). Rural-urban trends and patterns in cervical cancer mortality, incidence, stage, and survival in the United States, 1950-2008. *Journal of Community Health, 37*(1), 217–223.

Skinner, A., & Slifkin, R. (2007). Rural/urban differences in barriers to and burden of care for children with special health care needs. *Journal of Rural Health, 23*(2), 150–157.

Slack, T. (2010). Working poverty across the metro-nonmetro divide: A quarter century in perspective, 1979–2003. *Rural Sociology, 75*(3), 363–387.

Smalley, K. B., Warren, J. C., & Rainer, J. P. (Eds.). *Rural mental health: Issues, policies, and best practices.* New York: Springer Publishing.

South Carolina Rural Health Research Center. (2009, June). *Rural residents lag in preventive services use: Lag increases with service complexity.* Policy Brief No. 1. Retrieved from http://rhr.sph.sc.edu/News/Final%20-%20Preventive%20Services%20Policy%20Brief.pdf

Southern Poverty Law Center. (2010). Tapping the power of place. *Teaching Tolerance, 38,* article 2. Retrieved from http://www.tolerance.org/magazine/number-38-fall-2010/tapping-power-place

Stenberg, P., Morehart, M., & Cromartie, J. (2009). Broadband Internet service helping create a rural digital economy. *Amber Waves.* Retrieved from http://www.ers.usda.gov/amberwaves/september09/features/broadband.htm

Stevens, G., & Vollebergh, W. (2008). Mental health in migrant children. *The Journal of Child Psychology and Psychiatry, 49*(3), 276–294.

Stoecklin-Marois, M. T., Hennessy-Burt, T. E., & Schenker, M. D. (2011). Engaging a hard-to-reach population in research: Sampling and recruitment of hired farm workers in the MICASA study. *Journal of Agricultural Safety & Health, 17*(4), 291–302.

Stone, S. (2011). News from the frontier. *Frontier Nursing Service Quarterly, 87*(1), 5–8.

Stone, B., Hess, J. J., & Frumkin, H. (2010). Urban form and extreme heat events: Are sprawling cities more vulnerable to climate change than compact cities? *Environmental Health Perspectives, 118*(10), 1425–1428.

Sutton, M., Anthony, M., Vila, C., McLellan-Lemal, E., & Weidle, P. (2010). HIV testing and HIV/AIDS treatment services in rural counties in 10 Southern states: Service provider perspectives. *The Journal of Rural Health, 26*(3). 240–247.

Texas Rural Health Association. (2010). *Legislative agenda for the 82nd regular session: Budget cuts.* Retrieved from http://www.trha.org/news.htm

The Future of Children. (2011, Spring). *Immigrant children.* Princeton, NJ: Author.

Timperio, A., Giles-Corti, B., Crawford, D., Andrianopoulos, N., Ball, K., Salmon, J., et al. (2008). Features of public open spaces and physical activity among children: Findings from the CLAN study. *Preventive Medicine, 47*(5), 514–518.

Transportation Research Board of the National Academies. (2011). *Research pays off: Wyoming rural roads safety program: Focusing locally on high-risk segments.* Retrieved from http://www.trb.org/Main/Blurbs/165393.aspx

Triantafillou, S. A. (2003). North Carolina's migrant and seasonal farmworkers. *North Carolina Medical Journal, 64*(3), 129–131.

Truman, J. L. (2011, September). *National Crime Victimization Survey: Criminal victimization, 2010.* U.S. Department of Justice. Retrieved from http://bjs.ojp.usdoj.gov/content/pub/pdf/cv10.pdf

Truong, K. D., & Sturm, R. (2009). Alcohol environments and disparities in exposure associated with adolescent drinking in California. *American Journal of Public Health, 99*(2), 264–270.

Ullmann, S. H., Goldman, N., & Massey, D. S. (2011). Healthier before they migrate, less healthy when they return? The health of returned migrants in Mexico. *Social Science & Medicine, 73,* 421–428.

University of California. (2012). *Hispanic Americans: Migrant workers and Braceros (1930s–1964).* Calisphere: California Cultures. Retrieved from http://www.calisphere.universityofcalifornia.edu/calcultures/ethnic_groups/subtopic3b.html

Urban Health Institute. (2012). *Welcome to the Johns Hopkins Urban Health Institute.* Johns Hopkins University. Retrieved from http://www.jhsph.edu/urbanhealth/about_us/

U.S. Census Bureau. (n.d.). *Metropolitan and micropolitan statistical areas.* Retrieved from *http://www.census.gov/population/metro/*

U.S. Census Bureau. (2010). *2010 census urban and rural classification and urban area criteria.* Retrieved from *http://www.census.gov/geo/www/ua/2010urbanruralclass.html*

U.S. Department of Agriculture (USDA). (2008). *What is rural?* Retrieved from http://www.nal.usda.gov/ric/ricpubs/what_is_rural.shtml

U.S. Department of Agriculture (USDA). (2011). *Rural income, poverty, and welfare: Poverty geography.* Retrieved from http://ers.usda.gov/Briefing/IncomePovertyWelfare/povertygeography.htm#graph

U.S. Department of Homeland Security. (2012). *H-2A temporary agricultural workers.* Retrieved from http://www.uscis.gov/portal/site/uscis/menuitem.eb1d4c2a3e5b9ac89243c6a7543f6d1a/?vgnextoid=889f0b89284a3210VgnVCM100000b92ca60aRCRD&vgnextchannel=889f0b89284a3210VgnVCM100000b92ca60aRCRD

U.S. Department of Housing & Urban Development (USDHUD). (2012a). *Common questions about migrant/farmworkers.* Retrieved from http://portal.hud.gov/hudportal/HUD?src=/states/florida/working/farmworker/commonquestions

U.S. Department of Housing & Urban Development (USDHUD). (2012b). *Housing choice vouchers fact sheet.* Retrieved from http://portal.hud.gov/hudportal/HUD?src=/topics/housing_choice_voucher_program_section_8

U.S. Department of Labor. (2010). *The national agricultural workers survey.* Retrieved from http://www.doleta.gov/agworker/report9/chapter1.cfm#summary

U.S. Department of Labor. (2011, August 25). *National census of fatal occupational injuries in 2010 (preliminary results).* News Release, Bureau of Labor Statistics. Retrieved from http://www.bls.gov/news.release/pdf/cfoi.pdf

U.S. Environmental Protection Agency (EPA). (2011). *Basic information: What is an urban heat island?* Retrieved from http://www.epa.gov/heatisld/about/index.htm

U.S. Office of Management & Budget. (2000, December 27). Standards for defining metropolitan and micropolitan statistical areas: Notice. *Federal Register, 65*(249), 82228–82238.

Vallejos, Q. M., Quandt, S. A., & Arcury, T. A. (2009). The condition of farmworker housing in the Eastern United States. In T. A. Arcury, & S. A. Quandt (Eds.). *Latino farmworkers in the Eastern United States* (pp. 37–67). New York: Springer Science.

Vallejos, Q. M., Quandt, S. A., Feldman, S. R., Fleischer, A. B., Brooks, T., Cabral, G., et al. (2009). Teledermatology consultations provide specialty care for farmworkers in rural clinics. *Journal of Rural Health, 25*(2), 198–202.

Villarejo, D., McCurdy, S. A., Bade, B., Samuels, S., Lighthall, D., Williams, D. (2010). The health of California's immigrant hired farmworkers. *American Journal of Industrial Medicine, 53*, 387–397.

Vadheim, L. M., Brewer, K. A., Kassner, D. R., Vanderwood, K. K., Hall, T. O., Butcher, M. K., et al. (2010). Effectiveness of a lifestyle intervention program among persons at high risk for cardiovascular disease and diabetes in a rural community. *The Journal of Rural Health, 26*(3), 266–272.

Van der Mark, M., Brouwer, M., Kromhout, H., Nijssen, P., Huss, A., Vermeulen, R. (2012). Is pesticide use related to Parkinson disease? Some clues to heterogeneity in study results. *Environmental Health Perspectives, 120*, 340–347.

van Dis, J. (2002). Where we live: Health care in rural vs. urban America. *Journal of the American Medical Association, 87*(1), 108.

Vander Weg, M. W., Cunningham, C. L., Howren, M. B., & Cai, X. (2011). Tobacco use and exposure in rural areas: Findings from the Behavioral Risk Factor Surveillance System. *Addictive Behaviors, 36*(3), 231–236.

Vlahov, D., Freudenberg, N., Proietti, F., Ompad, D., Quinn, A., Nandi, V., et al. (2007). Urban as a determinant of health. *Journal of Urban Health, 84*(3 Suppl), i16–i26.

Vlahov, D., Boufford, J. I., Pearson, C., & Norris, L. (Eds.) (2010). *Urban health: Global perspectives*. San Francisco, CA: John Wiley & Sons, Inc.

Vyavaharkar, M., Moneyham, L., Tavakoli, A., Phillips, K. D., Murdaugh, C., Jackson, K., et al. (2007). Social support, coping, and medication adherence among HIV-positive women with depression living in rural areas of the southeastern United States. *AIDS Patient Care STDS, 21*(9), 667–680.

Wald, L. (1971/1915). *The house on Henry Street*. New York: Dover Publications. (Originally published by Henry Hold & Co., New York.)

Walker, R. E., Keane, C. R., & Burke, J. G. (2010). Disparities and access to healthy food in the United States: A review of food deserts literature. *Health & Place, 16*, 876-884.

Wallace, A. E., Young-Xu, Y., Hartley, D., & Weeks, W. B. (2010). Racial, socioeconomic, and rural-urban disparities in obesity-related bariatric surgery. *Obesity Surgery, 20*(10), 11354–1360.

Wang, A., Costello, S., Cockburn, M., Zhang, X., Bronstein, J., Ritz, B., (2011). Parkinson's disease risk from ambient exposure pesticides. *European Journal of Epidemiology, 26*(7), 547–555.

Wang, J. Y., Bennett, K., & Probst, J. (2011). Subdividing the digital divide: Differences in internet access and use among rural residents with medical limitations. *Journal of Medical Internet Research, 13*(1), e25.

Washington State Nurses Association. (2011). *Public health and public health nursing*. Position paper. Seattle, WA: Author.

Weselak, M., Arbuckle, T. E., Wigle, D., Walker, M. C., & Krewski, D. (2008). Pre- and post-conception pesticide exposure and the risk of birth defects in an Ontario farm population. *Reproductive Toxicology, 25*(4), 472–480.

Wesseling, C., de Joode, B., Keifer, M., London L., Mergler, D., Stallones, L. (2010). Symptoms of psychological distress and suicidal ideation among banana workers with a history of poisoning by organophosphate or n-methyl carbamate pesticides. *Occupational and Environmental Medicine, 67*, 778–784.

Wickrama, K., Elder, G., & Abraham, W. (2007). Rurality and ethnicity in adolescent physical illness: Are children of the growing rural Latino population at excess health risk? *Journal of Rural Health, 23*(3), 228–237.

Wigle, D. T., Turner, M. C., & Krewski, D. (2009). A systematic review and meta-analysis of childhood leukemia and parental occupational pesticide exposure. *Environmental Health Perspectives, 117*(10), 1505–1513.

Willen, S. S. (2012). Migration, "illegality," and health: Mapping embodied vulnerability and debating health-related deservingness. *Social Science & Medicine, 74*(6), 80–811.

Williams, D. R., & Sternthal, M. (2010). Understanding racial-ethnic disparities in health: Sociological contributions. *Journal of Health and Social Behavior, 51*(S), S15–S27.

Willison, S., & Jang, B. S. (2009). Are federal dollars bearing fruit? An analysis of the College Assistance Migrant Program. *Journal of Hispanic Higher Education, 8*(3), 247–262.

World Health Organization (WHO). (2012). *Healthy Cities*. Retrieved from http://www.euro.who.int/en/what-we-do/health-topics/environment-and-health/urban-health/activities/healthy-cities

Yonas, M. A., O'Campo, P., Burke, J., & Gielen, A. C. (2010). Exploring local perceptions of and responses to urban youth violence. *Health Promotion Practice, 11*(1), 62–70.

Zhang, Q., Wang, Y., & Huang, E. S. (2009). Changes in racial/ethnic disparities in the prevalence of type 2 diabetes by obesity level among US adults. *Ethnicity & Health, 14*(5), 439–457.

Ziebarth, A. (2006). Housing seasonal workers for the Minnesota processed vegetable industry. *Rural Sociology, 71*(2), 335–357.

thePoint: Everything You Need to Make the Grade!

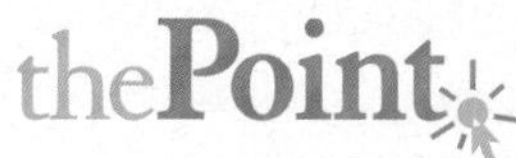

Visit http://thePoint.lww.com/Allender8e
for selected readings, study aids for all learning styles, and more!

UNIT 8

SETTINGS FOR COMMUNITY HEALTH NURSING

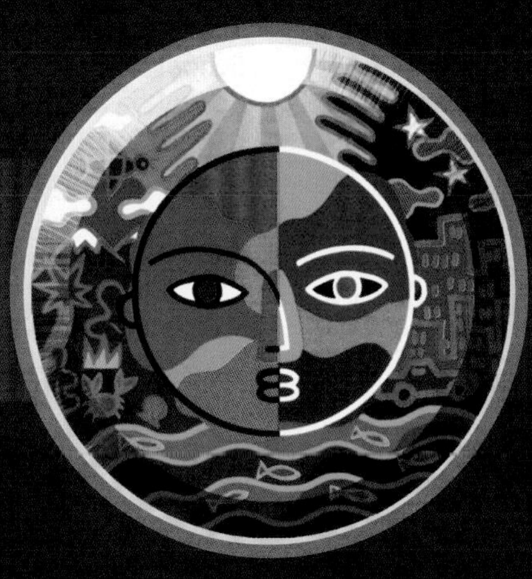

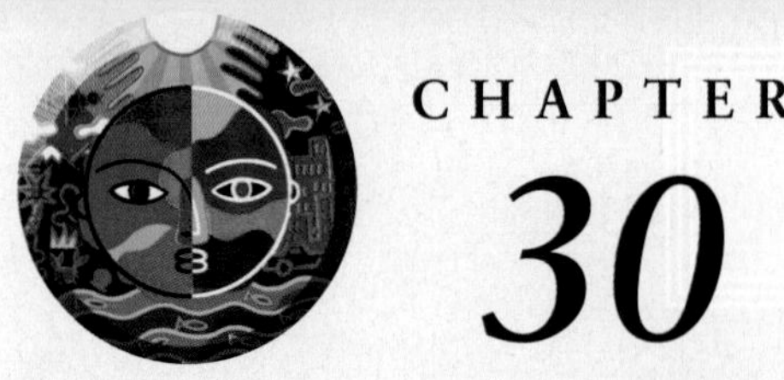

CHAPTER

30

Public Settings for Community Health Nursing

"A [community nurse] must first nurse. She must be of yet higher class and yet of fuller training than that of a hospital nurse because she has no hospital appliances at hand at all and because she has to take notes on the case for the doctor who has no one but her to report to him."

—***Florence Nightingale,*** 1876 (as cited in Edgecomb, 2001)

KEY TERMS

Corrections nurses
Indian Health Services (IHS)
Individualized education plans (IEPs)
Individualized health plans (IHPs)
Local health departments
Public health nurse
School nurse
School nurse practitioner
School-based health centers (SBHCs)
Section 504 plan
U.S. Public Health Service Commissioned Corps

LEARNING OBJECTIVES

Upon mastery of this chapter, you should be able to:

- Explain the focus of the nursing process and how public health nurses (PHNs) and other nurses working in the publicly funded sector use it to provide care in their communities.
- Describe how federal, state, and local public health infrastructures influence the population's health.
- Evaluate the potential benefits of school-based health centers (SBHCs) and discuss possible parental or community objections.
- Compare and contrast common roles and functions of PHNs, school nurses, and corrections nurses.

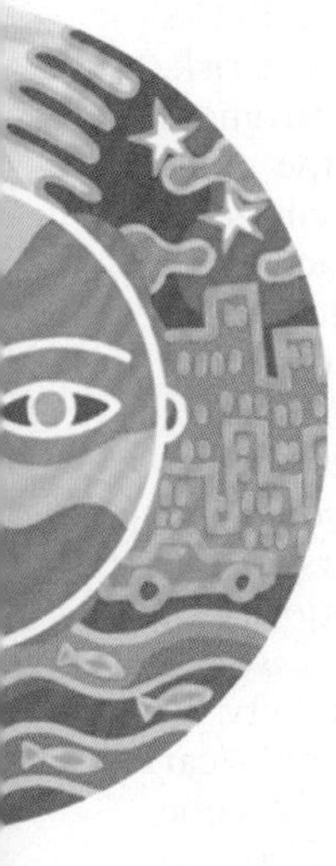

Many nursing students are not aware of the vast employment opportunities available outside the hospital in publicly funded settings. This chapter discusses several of these publicly funded health settings and the opportunities nurses can garner, particularly in services such as public health nursing, school nursing, or corrections nursing. This chapter is a practical explanation of the work of these nurses in the public sector.

Although each of these nursing opportunities differs greatly, they have several characteristics in common. First, community nurses who work in a setting supported through public funds (e.g., taxpayer-funded) still use the nursing process, but their client is a population or group of people, rather than an individual. Second, emphasis is placed on prevention of disease or disability. Third, community nurses employed in publicly funded settings work with a variety of people, usually vulnerable populations. They must be able to network and collaborate with other agencies and disciplines. For example, a nurse working in a correctional facility often collaborates with mental health workers and correctional officers. A nurse working in the public setting has many opportunities to be an advocate for individuals and the community and may serve on regional task forces or advisory boards. In addition, PHNs focus on population-based care. Nurses may perform individual care, especially correctional nurses; however, most of the focus is placed on the population as client. Finally, nurses who work in the public setting must be autonomous, flexible, creative thinkers who are self-directed and able to prioritize and use the nursing process to make educated decisions and plan care for their respective populations. Nurses who work in public settings must have the highest level of nursing, communication, problem-solving, and intellectual skills.

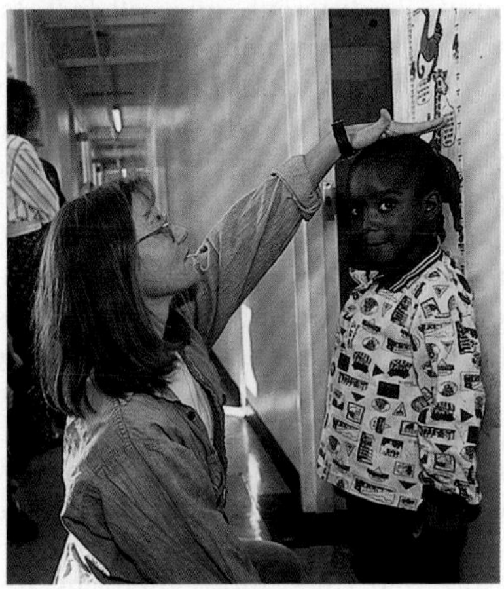

Nurses working in the public sector generally need to be very self-directed, autonomous, and creative thinkers.

PUBLIC HEALTH NURSING

A **public health nurse** is a nurse who works to promote and protect the health of an entire population (American Nurses Association [ANA], 2007a). The most recent data specify that 552,061 workers comprise the U.S. public health workforce (Gebbie & Turnock, 2006). This workforce consists of epidemiologists, nurses, environmentalists, laboratory professionals, nutritionists, dental workers, social workers, and other health care providers.

Looking at public health from a nursing perspective, approximately 7.8% of all registered nurses (RNs) work in public/community health settings (Health Resources and Services Administration [HRSA], 2010). Public or community agencies are the third largest employer of RNs, after hospitals (employing 62.2% of nurses) and ambulatory care (employing 10.5% of nurses). However, with the struggle to find adequate access to health care, along with its increased costs, more nursing care is being performed in a public or community setting. Unfortunately, you may not know of these wonderful employment opportunities available in the public sector. This section describes the role and opportunities for RNs at the local, state, and federal levels of government. The focus will be on governmental agencies, because these agencies employ the majority of PHNs.

EDUCATION

The ANA (2007a), recommends that an entry-level PHN should have a bachelor's degree in nursing. This is important because baccalaureate programs provide additional training in public health and leadership. Some states, such as California, require nurses to take additional classes and obtain certification beyond a bachelor's degree if the BSN program does not offer specific content (e.g., child abuse, public health didactic and practicum). PHNs working with specific populations, or in administration, should hold a master's degree. A PHN with a master's degree in community/public health nursing may take a national certification examination offered by the American Nurses Credentialing Center (ANCC, 2008). Many, but not all, master's programs offer dual nursing and public health degrees. The emphasis on national certification is due to an ever-increasing need to keep the population protected from health threats, such as bioterrorism (especially after September 11, 2001), emerging diseases (e.g., pandemic flu), or natural disasters (e.g., hurricane Katrina).

KEY FUNCTIONS OF THE PHN IN THE PUBLIC SETTING

Public health nursing practice consists of many areas of expertise; it

- Focuses on the health of populations
- Reflects the needs and priorities of the community

- Requires caring relationships with individuals, families, communities, and systems
- Is grounded in cultural sensitivity, compassion, social justice, and a belief in the worth of all people (e.g., vulnerable populations)
- Encompasses all aspects of health (e.g., physical, emotional, mental, social, spiritual, and environmental)
- Uses strategies to promote health that are motivated by epidemiologic evidence
- Involves individual, as well as collaborative, strategies to achieve results (Minnesota Department of Health, 2007)

In brief, the role of the PHN is to focus on the health of the public. PHNs combine their nursing and clinical knowledge of disease and the human response to it, along with public health skills, in order to accomplish their goals (ANA, 2007a; Quad Council, 2007). They apply the nursing process, not only with individuals but also with populations. PHNs are the critical link between data tracking (e.g., epidemiology) and clinical understanding of a disease or condition (McCulloch & Prieto, 2008). PHNs use the data to prioritize their interventions to stop the spread of diseases, such as measles, and also to intercede with other concerns (e.g., childhood obesity). For example, PHNs may develop a campaign for children to wear bike helmets after an increase of fatal head injuries is noted in their area. A key emphasis of the PHN is prevention, and a key focus is educating and empowering the community. Several other differences exist between PHNs and nursing in general (see Table 30.1 for a comparison).

The population that PHNs focus on can be a geographic community (e.g., a state or municipality) or a focus group (e.g., adolescents or the elderly) spanning all socioeconomic levels. To accomplish this, PHNs often work with individuals or families at highest risk, and their motive is to improve, protect, and promote the health of the entire population. One of the goals that characterize PHNs, and differentiate their goals from those of other specialty disciplines, is achieving the greatest good for the majority of people (ANA, 2007a). (See Chapter 13 for an in-depth discussion of social justice.) This requires priority planning and a basic knowledge of the community. It can also create ethical dilemmas for PHNs who may have personal and passionate issues that they would like to pursue, but which may not be the top priority for the majority of community members.

For example, many issues exist in a community. In one community, one child may have been hit by a car while riding his bike without a helmet, while at the same time, in the same community, there may be 10 births to teen moms, 20 instances of drug overdose, and an outbreak of pertussis. The PHNs in that community must prioritize which issue to address first by deciding which issue impacts the most people and what interventions will help the population thrive (ANA, 2007a). Because each community is different, once all factors are taken into account, the priorities will vary among communities. Hence, *assessment* is a critical component of public health and a key tool for the nurses who work in the public sector (Institute of Medicine [IOM], 1988) (see Display 30.1).

Another way public health nursing differs from other areas in nursing is that PHNs must actively seek out and identify potential problems and situations (ANA, 2007a). Nurses who work in a hospital setting address the issues that come to them. If a nurse works in the intensive care unit (ICU) of a hospital, she will work with her assigned patient load. PHNs, on the other hand, are out in the community identifying the problems, not waiting for problems to come to them. For example, PHNs may participate in visits to childcare centers to note any safety hazards, ensure that rules and regulations are being followed, and that children are properly immunized. These visits are part of the priority of *assurance* identified by the IOM (1988), noted in Display 30.1.

PHNs cannot perform all these activities alone. They need to collaborate with other partners and optimally use often limited resources. PHNs are in a unique situation because they work with their populations (i.e., clients) and with others to find the best solutions for a situation or problem.

Table 30.1 Comparing Public Health and General Nursing

Public Health Nursing	General Nursing
Population-based	Individual-based
Grounded in social justice	Grounded in a relationship of caring
Focuses on the greater good	Focuses on individual good (patient)
Health promotion and disease prevention	Restoration of health and function
Utilize and organize community resources	Manage resources at hand
Seek out clients in need	Take care of clients who come to them
Commitment to the community as a whole	Commitment to individual patient

Adapted from *Cornerstones of Public Health Nursing*, Minnesota Department of Health, 2007.

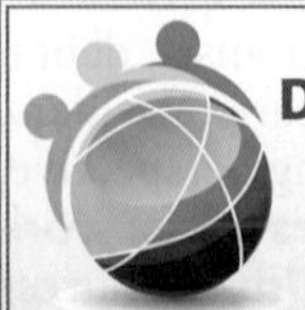

DISPLAY 30.1 THREE CORE FUNCTIONS OF PUBLIC HEALTH (IOM, 1988)

1. Assessment
2. Assurance
3. Policy Development

For instance, PHNs may notice an increase in the number of measles cases in their community. They may then work with families to identify where and how the children were exposed to the disease and with local health care providers to provide treatment and vaccinations for those at highest risk of exposure to and damage from measles. PHNs also work with school nurses and other school personnel to exclude from school attendance those children who are not adequately immunized against measles. This helps decrease the spread and potential harm due to measles. PHNs educate a variety of groups, such as parent–teacher associations (PTAs) and city or school officials, as to how measles spreads, what can be done to treat the disease, and the importance of herd immunity in protecting the public. Education thus empowers each group to be part of the solution. Finally, PHNs can work with public health officials to develop a policy for all new school entrants to receive a second booster of measles vaccine. *Policy development* is the third critical component of public health identified by the IOM (1988) (see Display 30.1).

PUBLIC HEALTH FUNDING AND GOVERNMENTAL STRUCTURES

PHNs can work at any and all levels of government. Hence, it is important to understand the organizational structure, communication, and funding streams between the federal, state, and local levels of government (see Chapter 6 for more on the structure of the public health system). At each level, all three branches of the government are involved in public health, although often the legislative and executive branches play the most important roles, and this discussion focuses on these areas.

The legislative branch (meaning Congress, state legislatures, or local councils) mandates laws or policies and decides how much of the funding in its jurisdiction will be appropriated to public health. Much of the work for public health is carried out in the executive branch of government (Fig. 30-1). Because state and local organizations can be set up in a variety of ways, nurses must check with their local health department (LHD) for specifics.

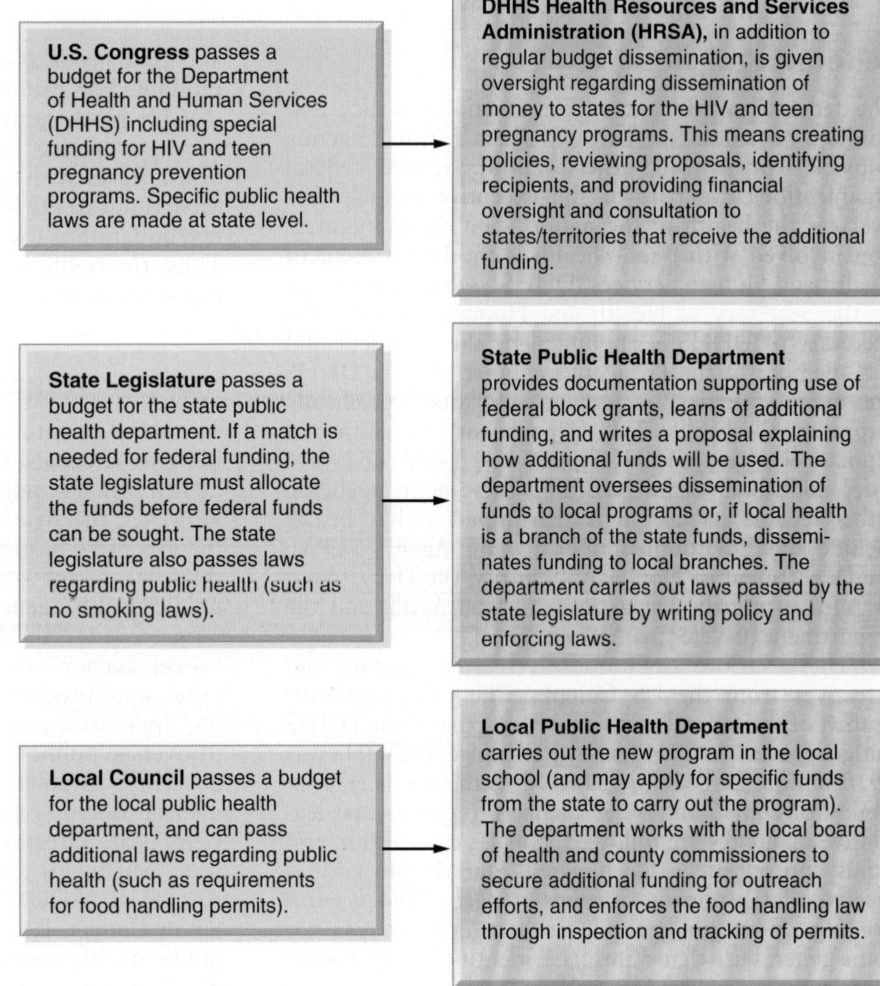

U.S. Congress passes a budget for the Department of Health and Human Services (DHHS) including special funding for HIV and teen pregnancy prevention programs. Specific public health laws are made at state level.
DHHS Health Resources and Services Administration (HRSA), in addition to regular budget dissemination, is given oversight regarding dissemination of money to states for the HIV and teen pregnancy programs. This means creating policies, reviewing proposals, identifying recipients, and providing financial oversight and consultation to states/territories that receive the additional funding.
State Legislature passes a budget for the state public health department. If a match is needed for federal funding, the state legislature must allocate the funds before federal funds can be sought. The state legislature also passes laws regarding public health (such as no smoking laws).
State Public Health Department provides documentation supporting use of federal block grants, learns of additional funding, and writes a proposal explaining how additional funds will be used. The department oversees dissemination of funds to local programs or, if local health is a branch of the state funds, disseminates funding to local branches. The department carries out laws passed by the state legislature by writing policy and enforcing laws.
Local Council passes a budget for the local public health department, and can pass additional laws regarding public health (such as requirements for food handling permits).
Local Public Health Department carries out the new program in the local school (and may apply for specific funds from the state to carry out the program). The department works with the local board of health and county commissioners to secure additional funding for outreach efforts, and enforces the food handling law through inspection and tracking of permits.

FIGURE 30-1. Examples of government organization in relation to public health.

Table 30.2 Agencies within Department of Health and Human Services

Agency	Headquarters	Responsibility and Bureaus
Health Resources and Services Administration (HRSA)	Rockville, Maryland	Medically underserved—includes Medicare/Medicaid, HIV/AIDS, maternal and child, health professions, primary health care
Indian Health Services (IHS)	Rockville, Maryland	Provides health services for Native Americans (including Alaskan Natives)
Centers for Disease Control and Prevention (CDC)	Atlanta, Georgia	Health surveillance and prevention of disease and bioterrorism
National Institutes of Health (NIH)	Bethesda, Maryland	Medical research
Food and Drug Administration (FDA)	Rockville, Maryland	Ensures safety of food, medication, medical procedures, and equipment
Substance Abuse and Mental Health Services Administration (SAMHSA)	Rockville, Maryland	Oversees prevention, diagnosis, and treatment for mental health and substance abuse
Agency for Toxic Substances and Disease Registry (ATSDR)	Atlanta, Georgia	Protects public from environmental exposures
Agency for Health Care Research and Quality (AHRQ)	Rockville, Maryland	Includes research on health care quality and effectiveness

Source: From http://www.dhhs.gov; Turnock, B. J. (2011). ***Essentials of public health*** (2nd ed.). Sudbury, MA: Jones and Bartlett Publishers.

Federal Agencies

The federal government oversees national policy and funding, provides expertise, and sets a national agenda (Novick, Morrow, & Mays, 2008). Several federal organizations are part of the executive branch that oversees the health of the nation. The main organization involved with public health is the Department of Health and Human Services (DHHS), which is overseen by the Secretary of Health and Human Services. The Secretary of DHHS is appointed by the President and is a member of the President's cabinet. Within DHHS are many agencies, including eight that specifically impact public health (U.S. Department of Health and Human Services [USDHHS], 2011a). Table 30.2 provides additional detail regarding these eight agencies. Other federal agencies that also impact public health include the Environmental Protection Agency (EPA), the Department of Homeland Security, the Department of Agriculture, the Department of Education, and the Department of Veterans Affairs.

These various organizations receive funding and directives from the US Congress (i.e., the legislative branch of the federal government) as part of the DHHS budget process. In 2011, the overall budget of DHHS was $910 billion (USDHHS, 2011b). It is the prime responsibility of DHHS and other agencies to ensure that legislative mandates are followed, policies carried out, and funds appropriately disseminated. State health entities receive a large portion of funds as part of *block grant funding*. These funds are lumped together to pay for some general use that states have identified (see Chapter 6 for more detailed information). *Healthy People 2020* and state needs assessments help set priorities for state funding. For example, the maternal and child health (MCH) block grants received by states are then used for reproductive health, child health, and immunizations. States with LHDs also disseminate a portion of these funds to the local level. In addition, state and local tax dollars are used to supplement various programs. Thus, the political leanings of state and local officials can strongly influence local health initiatives.

State Governments

The U.S. Constitution bestows states with the responsibility to safeguard the health of their citizens (Turnock, 2012). Much of public health is overseen at a state level. However, the structure of where public health fits into the executive branch of state government varies. More than half of the states have an independent state-level public health agency (Beitsch, Brooks, Menachemi, & Grigg, 2011). Another third of the states are part of a "super agency" that may include human services and other state programs (Novick et al., 2008). The governor appoints a commissioner, or leading health official, to oversee public health and serve as a member of the governor's cabinet. These cabinet members are usually medical doctors, appointed by the governor. In recent years, state directors have also included social workers (e.g., Michigan) and public health professionals (e.g., Arkansas). In 2007, Governor Phil Bredesen appointed Susan Cooper, RN, MSN, as the first nurse to serve as public health commissioner for the state of Tennessee. The first nurses appointed to director of state offices of public health were Barbara Sabol and Gloria Smith in Kansas and Michigan (Feldman, 2008).

The purpose of state agencies is to carry forth regulations and policies determined by the federal government. Examples of these programs are the Medicaid, Medicare, and State Children's Health Insurance Programs (SCHIPs). Many of these programs may have specific federal requirements, but they also allow states the ability to personalize the programs to fit the state's individual needs. An example of such a program is the MCH block grant, which provides funding and guidelines for the states. However, states determine which programs (e.g., reproductive health or children's health) will be funded and how they will be implemented.

Another example of federal leadership is the *Healthy People 2020* document that provides goals for a variety of health outcomes. States can use these outcomes, or develop additional performance measures, according to state characteristics and needs. In addition, the state agency is influenced by the state legislative body, which oversees the state budget and can pass laws specific to the state. Each state is different due to varying needs, cultures, and political environments. Examples of public health laws at a state level include immunization requirements for school entrance, seat belt safety laws, and regulations regarding parental rights concerning birth control and abortion services for teens. Other health policies that influence public health include laws to quarantine persons with communicable diseases, especially during times of outbreaks. State laws must be in place outlining legal jurisdiction of containing and reporting communicable disease; such laws often need to be updated as new threats occur. This was recently exemplified during the early 2000s when smallpox became a bioterroristic threat. State laws allowing persons to be quarantined for smallpox had expired, and new laws had to be passed in order to prepare for potential outbreaks. Without these laws in place, public health officials and law enforcement do not have the power and authority required to maintain the health of the public.

Local Public Health

Local health departments (LHDs) carry out state laws and policies (Turnock, 2012). They provide the most direct, immediate care of the population (Novick et al., 2008). For example, they may provide immunization clinics, track and treat cases of tuberculosis (TB) and other communicable diseases, and provide education on a variety of subjects (e.g., human immunodeficiency virus [HIV]/acquired immune deficiency syndrome [AIDS] prevention, smoking cessation). They often carry out programs with funding from federal and state agencies. For instance, federal funding to address asthma may be obtained through the state agency, and local agencies may organize an educational program on asthma triggers in a local business where many community members work. State and local agencies do not work alone in such endeavors, however. Collaboration is very important in addressing the public health needs of a community. Public health agencies work with private organizations, hospitals, nonprofit groups, universities, and government agencies that oversee food and housing to meet citizens' needs.

LHDs work with state health departments, some independently and some as dependent branches of the state agency. The size and services offered by a local agency also differ depending on state laws, structure, and wealth (Turnock, 2012). Close to half (45%) of LHDs in the United States have fewer than 25 employees (National Association of County and City Health Officers [NACCHO], 2010). Thus, the number of LHDs per state can vary dramatically. For example, California has only 61 LHDs, whereas Massachusetts has the most with 330 (NACCHO, 2010). Nearly all LHDs (95%) employ nurses, who make up 24% of the total public health workforce at the local level (NACCHO, 2010).

NURSING ROLES IN LOCAL, STATE, AND FEDERAL PUBLIC HEALTH POSITIONS

Nurses can work in a variety of capacities at the various levels of government, which may cover most aspects of public health (Novick et al., 2008). Generally speaking, nurses who work at the local level of public health tend to provide direct service care. For example, they often administer immunizations, monitor patients with TB, provide education to school groups, provide cancer screenings, and track communicable disease rates. Local PHNs are the eyes and ears of their communities. Many PHNs working at the local level, especially in rural or small public health departments, may have a variety of responsibilities. For instance, a PHN may be a full-time employee whose time could be split into 50% cancer screening; 25% with the Women, Infants, and Children (WIC) program; and 25% on Medicaid outreach (see Display 30.2 for an example of a PHN's day). PHNs also serve in administrative roles within agencies, as well, where they may oversee an entire bureau or program, for example, or serve as supervisors for a group of PHNs.

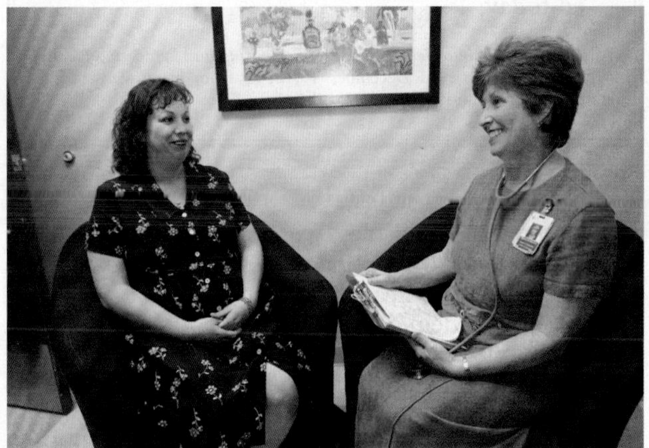

Public health nurses working for local health departments are the eyes and ears of their communities.

Within each of the governmental agencies, programs may be arranged according to a particular subject area.

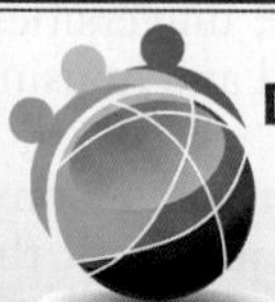

DISPLAY 30.2 A TYPICAL DAY IN THE LIFE OF A PUBLIC HEALTH NURSE

8:00 AM Staff reproductive health clinic. Provide counseling regarding family planning services, as well as breast and other cancer screenings.

10:30 AM Make a home visit to a mother and baby who is not thriving. Conduct an examination of the baby and assess the living situation. Assist the mother regarding breast-feeding, nutrition, newborn care, and parenting.

12:30 PM Attend a lunch meeting of a newly formed coalition that is concerned about the increased rate of teen pregnancy in the city. Provide statistics from community as well as firsthand knowledge of teens participating in the Women, Infants, and Children (WIC) program and the home visiting program. Offer expertise regarding how to approach the problem.

2:00 PM Investigate the case of a kindergartner who has TB. With the help of the school nurse, check immunization records of other students and staff. Contact the family to learn who else is exposed and at risk. Provide proper testing and education regarding the signs and symptoms of TB, the need for regular testing, and following the treatment regimen.

3:30 PM Staff cancer screening clinic performing Pap smears and providing counseling to women regarding risks of breast and cervical cancer. Follow up with patients from last week's clinic whose results were questionable.

5:00 PM Finish paperwork and go home knowing the community's health was positively impacted today.

Adapted from *Public Health Nursing: Promoting and Protecting Health in Colorado*. Retrieved December 19, 2011 from http://www.cdphe.state.co.us/opp/phn/PHNBrochure.pdf

For example, a PHN may work in the cardiovascular disease program, overseeing cholesterol screenings and promoting physical health and nutrition. A PHN could also work in epidemiology, tracking diseases, or be part of a community emergency response team to prepare for a natural or manmade disaster. A PHN could also work in the immunization program, promoting and tracking the immunization requirements of school-age children. The nurse may also be in charge of day care licensure requirements, traveling throughout the state and conducting inspections or writing policies. Or, the nurse could oversee a program to decrease sudden infant death syndrome (SIDS) in the state and track SIDS-related deaths. Thus, the variety of locations and programs are limitless for PHNs. The following is a brief overview of some of the main roles of nurses working at state health department and LHD. Specific options and means by which PHNs serve as advocates and change agents to protect and promote the health of all are discussed, using the nursing process as an outline. Figure 30-2 provides a practical model of how PHNs use the nursing model and public health principles in their everyday functions.

Assess

An assessment of the situation is key to any nursing care. PHNs assess the situation in a variety of ways. They observe a great deal when they are in the community and when they conduct home visits. They also assess data to identify trends. Often, nurses work with other public health personnel when assessing and tracking data, although nurses may serve as specialists in epidemiology. For example, PHNs can use morbidity and mortality statistics to determine the leading causes of death nationally and locally. They can assess communicable disease rates to identify an outbreak before it becomes too widespread. They track how many people in the community are in compliance with immunizations to keep the herd immunity high and decrease the chance of outbreaks.

PHNs use census data to determine population growth. As an example, the census indicates that the number of individuals 65 years or older will reach 1.3 billion worldwide by 2040 (Bernstein, 2009). Estimates indicate that in 2040, approximately 14% of the world's population will be over the age of 65. This is important in planning for future activities and resources. PHNs also use prevalence data to determine which ethnic groups are at higher risk than others. For example, the PHNs at the Utah County Health Department noticed an increase in sexually transmitted diseases (STDs). Upon further investigation, they learned that the greatest increases were within the Hispanic population. Through this assessment they were able to successfully target interventions for this population (Page, 2006; S. Marquez, personal communication, September 15, 2011).

Environmental risks are important to the public's health and are often assessed by nurses. For example, a PHN conducting blood tests noticed that students living in a mining community had elevated blood lead levels. This assessment information forms the basis for the nurse's intervention. Each nurse must assess his or her own community, because each has specific characteristics and needs. A community positioned next to a factory that emits fumes will have different issues than a rural community 90 miles away from any industry. At the same time, an outbreak of *Escherichia coli* in one town may identify a risk to the PHN in the neighboring town.

Diagnose

Assessment is key to diagnosing a situation or problem. For a PHN, diagnosis also includes identifying priorities

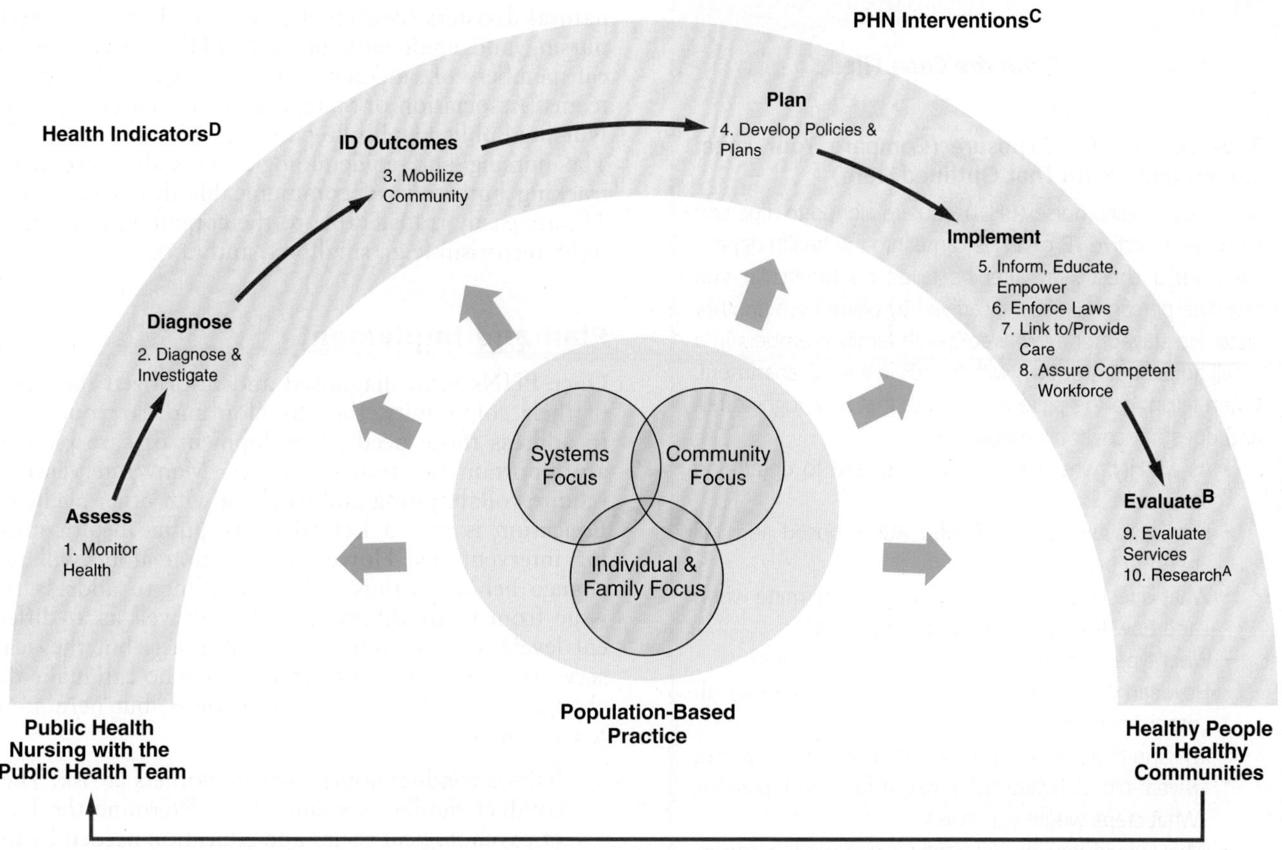

References:

(A) Public Health Functions Steering Committee. (1994, Fall). *Public Health in America.* Retrieved May 7, 2001,from the World Wide Web: http://health.gov/phfunctions/public.htm

(B) Quad Council of Public Health Nursing Organizations. (2007). *Public Health Nursing: Scope & Standards of Practice.* Washington D.C.: American Nurses Association.

(C) Minnesota Department of Health, Public Health Nursing Section. (2000). *Public Health Nursing Practice for the 21st Century: National Satellite Learning Conference; Competency Development in Population-based Practice October 5, November 2, December 7, 2000.* St. Paul, MN: Minnesota Department of Health Nursing Section. Retrieved May 7, 2001, from the World Wide Web: http://www.health.state.mn.us/divs/chs/phr/material.htm.

(D) U.S. Department of Health and Human Services. (2000). Healhy People 2010. (Vol. 1). McLean, VA: International Medical Publishing, Inc.

*Created by Los Angeles County DPH, Public Health Nursing with input from CCLHDND-Southern Region. This model serves as the basis for the CCLHDND California PHN Practice Model (05-2002).

© 2007 Los Angeles County DPH Public Health Nursing

FIGURE 30-2. Public health nursing model from Los Angeles County.

for the many concurrent issues. Nurses who work in public settings may perform skin tests or simple blood work in public clinics to determine TB exposure, or risk of high blood pressure, or other conditions (Utah County Health Department, 2008) (see From the Case Files I). Other nurses utilize microscopes to identify cases of vaginitis and cervicitis. This could all occur on the same day.

As nurses diagnose individual needs, they apply this information and watch for increased or decreased rates (e.g., of disease or injury) among the population. For instance, a nurse working in a public health clinic may notice an increase in the number of people diagnosed with diabetes. The nurse further assesses the situation to determine if it is a population need and also the degree of the problem. Another PHN may assist with newborn genetic testing. Nurses are in the perfect position to identify issues and trends early on. As more is known regarding genetic trends, the PHN can use this information to advocate policies and laws that will impact a particular population.

Constant assessment and diagnosis are tools by which PHNs identify critical situations and prioritize issues that must be addressed first. Several documents have helped PHNs prioritize issues. *Healthy People 2020*, a guide to identifying many of the nation's top priorities, is a valuable tool (USDHHS, 2010) (see Display 30.3). Public health performance standards also assist nurses in prioritizing needs (Centers for Disease Control and Prevention [CDC], 2010a; Quad Council, 2007). The IOM (2003, 2010) has also identified a need for a greater focus on informatics and genomics.

Improved medical technology has supplied immunizations that have decreased the rates of many communicable diseases. This led to the emergence of new issues and priorities for PHNs, specifically, injury prevention and the management of chronic diseases (Beitsch et al., 2011). World events have also placed additional

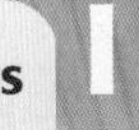

From the Case Files

Tuberculosis (TB) Exposure (Compare Your Local Government With That Outlined Here)

As a public health nurse (PHN), you are alerted to a person who has an active TB case. He came into the health department for a chest x-ray after he failed his tuberculin skin test. The person has recently arrived by plane from another state. He stayed for a few weeks with family members in a small house but now lives with friends in a small apartment. When talking to the patient, you note that he coughs often and does not cover his mouth.

- As a PHN, what steps would you take to determine exposure?
- How will you determine who was exposed and will need to be tested?
- What questions can you ask to help determine when and how the patient was exposed to TB?
- What type of education will you provide to him?
- How can you ensure that the patient is compliant with medication treatment?
- Imagine that you are the school nurse of the patient's 8-year-old daughter who has also tested positive. What steps would you take?
- What would you do differently if you were a corrections nurse and the patient was an inmate?
- What are the ethical and legal issues related to TB?

emphasis on public health roles, including the global spread of TB, bioterrorism, pandemic influenza, and natural disasters (Beitsch et al., 2011). Because of their nursing and epidemiologic skill, PHNs serve as critical members of emergency preparedness and response teams (Association of State and Territorial Directors of Nursing Public Health Preparedness Committee, 2007). The nursing and epidemiologic skills they use when tracking outbreaks of communicable diseases, such as TB, are easily transferable to the communicable agents of bioterrorism (e.g., smallpox, anthrax).

Plan and Implement

Once PHNs have diagnosed and prioritized the needs of their community, they develop and carryout plans to address those needs. Development of care plans is an important function for nurses. Many interventions require collaborating and working with other agencies. Education is also a key to many public health nursing interventions. However, education alone will not change behavior; thus, it is important to address the issue from many different angles, as well as at different levels. PHNs cannot solve all issues, but they can serve as advocates to influence those who can make the changes. The interventions are endless, but here are a few examples:

- Nurses conduct home visits to mothers at risk. They conduct family assessments to determine the level of psychological issues and education needed by the family regarding specific needs, such as responses to medication. They also help mothers receive needed psychological counseling by linking them to a local mental health agency.

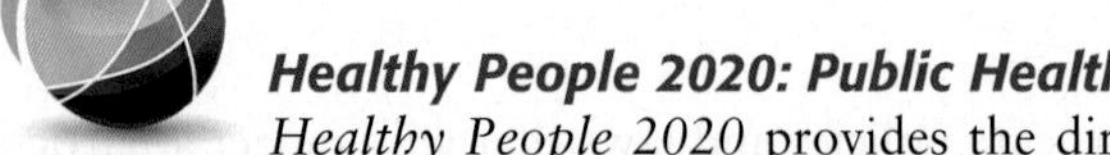

DISPLAY 30.3 *HEALTHY PEOPLE 2020*–PUBLIC HEALTH PRIORITIES

Healthy People 2020: Public Health

Healthy People 2020 provides the direction and goals for all public health nurses (PHNs). *Healthy People 2020* is used to guide prioritizing activities for PHNs. Specifically, PHNs focus on the ten leading indicators, which include:

- Access to health services
- Clinical preventive services
- Environmental quality
- Injury and violence
- Maternal, infant, and child health
- Mental health
- Nutrition, physical activity, and obesity
- Oral health
- Reproductive and sexual health
- Social determinants
- Substance abuse
- Tobacco

Healthy People 2020: School Nursing

One objective directly relates to school nurse staffing:

ECBP-5 Increase the proportion of the nation's elementary, middle, junior high, and senior high schools that have a nurse-to-student ratio of at least 1:750

Other objectives that school nurses can use to help prioritize activities include:

ECBP-2 Increase the proportion of elementary, middle, and senior high schools that provide comprehensive school health education to prevent health problems in the following areas: unintentional injury; violence; suicide; tobacco use and addiction; alcohol or other drug use; unintended pregnancy, human immunodeficiency virus

(continued)

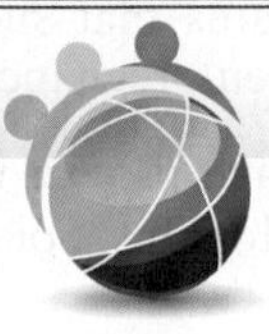

DISPLAY 30.3 *HEALTHY PEOPLE 2020*–PUBLIC HEALTH PRIORITIES *(Continued)*

(HIV)/acquired immune deficiency syndrome (AIDS), and sexually transmitted disease (STD) infection; unhealthy dietary patterns; and inadequate physical activity

ECBP-4	Increase the proportion of elementary, middle, and senior high schools that provide school health education to promote personal health and wellness in the following areas: hand washing or hand hygiene, oral health, growth and development, sun safety and skin cancer prevention, benefits of rest and sleep, ways to prevent vision and hearing loss, and the importance of health screenings and checkups
AH-6	Increase the proportion of schools with a school breakfast program
DH-5	Increase the proportion of youth with special health care needs whose health care provider has discussed transition planning from pediatric to adult health care
DH-9	(Developmental) Reduce the proportion of people with disabilities who encounter barriers to participating in home, school, work, or community activities
DH-14	Increase the proportion of children and youth with disabilities who spend at least 80% of their time in regular education programs
EH-16	Increase the proportion of the nation's elementary, middle, and high schools that have official school policies and engage in practices that promote a healthy and safe physical school environment
FP-8	Reduce pregnancy rates among adolescent females
FP-9	Increase the proportion of adolescents aged 17 years and under who have never had sexual intercourse
FP-12	Increase the proportion of adolescents who received formal instruction on reproductive health topics before they were 18 years old
IID-10	Maintain vaccination coverage levels for children in kindergarten
IID-11	Increase routine vaccination coverage levels for adolescents
IID-12	Increase the percentage of children and adults who are vaccinated annually against seasonal influenza
IID-18	Increase the proportion of children under 6 years of age whose immunization records are in fully operational, population-based immunization information systems
IVP-27	Increase the proportion of public and private schools that require students to wear appropriate protective gear when engaged in school-sponsored physical activities
MHMD-2	Reduce suicide attempts by adolescents
MHMD-3	Reduce the proportion of adolescents who engage in disordered eating behaviors in an attempt to control their weight
NWS-10	Reduce the proportion of children and adolescents who are considered obese
NWS-15	Increase the variety and contribution of vegetables to the diets of the population aged 2 years and older
OH-2	Reduce the proportion of children and adolescents with untreated dental decay
RD-5	Reduce the proportion of persons with asthma who miss school or work days
SA-3	Increase the proportion of adolescents who disapprove of substance abuse
TU-2	Reduce tobacco use by adolescents
TU-3	Reduce the initiation of tobacco use among children, adolescents, and young adults
V-2	Reduce blindness and visual impairment in children and adolescents aged 17 years and under

Healthy People 2020: Correctional Nursing

IID-27	Increase the percentage of persons aware that they have a hepatitis C infection
IID-29	Reduce tuberculosis (TB)
MHMD 7	Increase the proportion of juvenile residential facilities that screen admissions for mental health problems
MHMD-10	Increase the proportion of persons with co-occurring substance abuse and mental disorders who receive treatment for both disorders
SA-8	Increase the proportion of persons who need alcohol and/or illicit drug treatment and received specialty treatment for abuse or dependence in the past year
TU-13	Establish laws in states, District of Columbia, territories, and tribes on smoke-free indoor air that prohibit smoking in public places and worksites (13.13 correctional facilities)

- A community nurse working in risk management develops and teaches an education program about workplace safety and ergonomics. She develops policies regarding shift hours and heavy lifting.
- A school nurse serves as an advocate for a program that will assist children with special health care needs attend a clinic closer to home.
- A PHN develops a campaign for television, newspaper, and radio regarding the need to receive a flu shot. The nurse also includes incentives that target the elderly community who are at additional risk for developing complications from this illness.
- The community health nurse organizes a health clinic at local shelters providing foot care and screenings for blood pressure, diabetes, TB, and cholesterol, as appropriate.
- The school nurse works with schools to educate teens regarding birth control and the impact of teen pregnancy. She includes counseling regarding STDs. She works with the community to ensure that a variety of teen-focused activities are available for this population.
- The community outreach nurse conducts home visits to new mothers who need assistance with breast-feeding and newborn care. The nurse also contacts the housing authority to report hazardous conditions in the housing project she has visited.
- The PHN helps identify resources for families without insurance to ensure that well-child and adult screenings are performed regularly in order to reduce health care costs associated with illness.
- The school nurse organizes an immunization clinic at the local school after an outbreak of measles. The nurse also conducts classes at the school regarding communicable disease prevention and tobacco cessation.
- The PHN organizes a bicycle fair to educate the community regarding the need for bicycle helmets, in hopes of decreasing head injuries. She also works to develop public policy related to car seat usage and collaborates with local businesses in providing vouchers for discounts on car seats for low-income parents.
- The nurse, who is a paid lobbyist, works to change laws regarding smoking.
- A nurse, who is an elected member of the state legislature, sponsors a bill to increase funding for school nurses.
- After a hepatitis outbreak at a local business, the nurse conducts an assessment of the business and provides education classes and suggests policy changes to help guard against future outbreaks.

These interventions are based on evidence-based practice (EBP) (see Chapter 4). Below are some examples of EBP in public health nursing:

- Media campaigns targeting specific populations have been successfully used to educate and promote healthy behavior (Beaudoin, 2009).
- Community Guide Branch Epidemiology and Analysis Program Office (EAPO) (2009) has identified several school-based programs that successfully impact sexual activity and teen pregnancy.
    - Work-based incentive programs have proven to reduce the use of tobacco (Leeks, Hopkins, Soler, Aten, & Chattopadhay, 2010)
    - School-based programs have shown to reduce bullying and violence in schools (Farrington & Ttofi, 2009)
- Bike helmets (and legislation) have been proven to be effective in decreasing head injuries (Walter, Olivier, Churches, & Grzebieta, 2011).
- The American School Health Association has developed a toolkit to help nurses organize successful immunization programs (Boyer-Chu & Wooley, 2008).

Evaluate

The world in which PHNs work is always changing. It is crucial to constantly evaluate programs and interventions to determine if goals are reached. For example, a nurse may visit childcare facilities or senior centers to ensure that laws regarding licensure are being followed. Evaluating is often equated with assessing. PHNs also can evaluate data to determine whether various rates (e.g., infant mortality, or other health indicators) increase or decrease as a result of their interventions.

Another way that PHNs can determine if their interventions are effective is by becoming involved in research. Numerous researchers have studied the impact that PHNs have on improving population health and societal outcomes (Quad Council, 2007). The Joanna Briggs Institute (2008) found that nursing education in the emergency rooms (ERs) for adults with asthma helped to decrease future repeat ER visits and length of hospital stay. PHNs who conducted home visits to new mothers have also improved the lives of mothers and their babies. Children in the intervention group were found to have increased achievement and intellectual functioning, along with decreased aggression (Olds, 2008).

PUBLIC HEALTH NURSING CAREERS

Nurses who work at the state and federal levels tend to have consultant, or oversight-type, roles, and some nurses head programs that are specifically funded at the state and/or federal levels (e.g., HIV/AIDS, immunization programs). Some state-employed nurses may work in clinics for children with special health care needs. Some federally employed nurses may provide direct care in Indian Health Service clinics. PHNs at all levels may also be called upon to help during a disaster or communicable disease outbreak.

Among distinct opportunities at the federal level are those associated with the Department of Veterans Affairs and the Department of Health and Human Services. Agencies headed by DHHS include the National Institutes of Health (NIH), the Indian Health Service, the HRSA Services, the U.S. Food and Drug Administration

EVIDENCE-BASED PRACTICE

Public Health Nursing

This study investigated the health sources used by Chinese immigrants in the Pacific Northwest (Woodall et al., 2009). The sample was determined using zip and postal codes of areas known to have a high density of Chinese residents. A letter was sent to the homes in the area explaining the purpose of the survey. The survey was translated into both Mandarin and Cantonese and was conducted in person by trilingual interviewers (i.e., English, Mandarin, and Cantonese); 899 surveys were completed. Participants were asked where they received information regarding cancer education and prevention. Only 67% to 75% of Chinese immigrants reported obtaining health information from health care providers. Vancouver residents tended to obtain information from Chinese language television, radio, and newspapers. Seattle residents tended to receive health information from English television. Neither group used the Internet.

Nursing Implications

Results of past studies indicate Asian Americans are less likely than other racial/ethnic groups to feel that health care providers understand their experiences and values. This may be why less than three quarters of the participants relied on their health care provider for information related to cancer. Social media, especially television, seem to be sources more commonly used by Chinese immigrants. When public health nurses (PHNs) and others want to target the Chinese immigrant population, they need to remember populations in different geographic regions access information differently. In Seattle, PHNs should include the message in English television, and in Vancouver, use Chinese television, radio, and newspapers.

It is critical for a PHN to understand her population and the best mediums to reach it, as each population or community may be different. Cultural sensitivity is key to successful community outreach. Constant assessment of a community helps PHNs stay up-to-date with issues and influential media.

Reference: Woodall, E. D., Taylor, V. M., Teh, C., Li, L., Acorda, E., Tu, S., et al. (2009). Sources of health information among Chinese immigrants to the pacific northwest. *Journal of Cancer Education, 24*(4), 334–340, doi: 10.1080/08858190902854533

(FDA), the Substance Abuse and Mental Health Services Administration (SAMSHA), and the CDC.

PHNs in these agencies oversee and carryout the initiatives of *Healthy People 2020*, along with other program initiatives. Many of their functions are similar to those mentioned earlier. For example, they may oversee and develop programs, such as national surveys, that collect data used to determine priorities. Examples of these surveys include the Behavioral Risk Factor Survey (BRFS), the Youth Risk Behavior Survey (YRBS), and the National Health Interview Survey (NHIS). Federally employed PHNs may also review state funding proposals for projects and ensure that guidelines are met. They are a resource for state health department and LHD and often are called upon as consultants. Nurses working at the NIH may assist in conducting research. For example, a nurse may study the effects of applying chemotherapy directly to a tumor, instead of through intravenous or central lines (U.S. Public Health Service Commissioned Corps [USPHSCC], 2011). In addition to these opportunities, PHNs may work as clinicians for the Indian Health Services (IHS).

Indian Health Services

Indian Health Services (IHS) started from special relationships between the federal government and the Native American tribes. This relationship is based on information found in the Constitution (Article I, Section 8) and was started in 1787. Over time other treaties, policies, and laws have influenced the present structure of the IHS. The main goal of IHS is to raise the health status of all Native American Indians (IHS, 2009). It is responsible for providing health care to Native Americans (American Indians and Alaska Natives). The IHS provides services for approximately 1.9 million Native Americans in 35 states (IHS, 2009). Employment with the IHS allows a nurse to live in a variety of rural and urban settings and to work specifically with Native Americans, a vulnerable population. These nurses work and oversee health care services in clinics run by IHS. The clinics are usually focused on primary care and focus on general practice. They may work with patients who have diabetes, providing nutritional counseling and education; they may also provide immunizations, perform well-child examinations, or conduct HIV/AIDS screenings. Unique aspects of these jobs are that most clinics are located in remote areas of the country and face unique challenges. Some houses on Native American reservations may not have a telephone or consistent electricity, and these clients may have numerous special needs. This type of nursing is very challenging but can also be extremely rewarding.

Uniformed Public Health Nursing

Nurses can serve in each of the seven uniformed services of the U.S. Department of Defense (e.g., Army, Navy, Marine, Air Force), U.S. Department of Homeland Security (Coast Guard), U.S. Department of Commerce

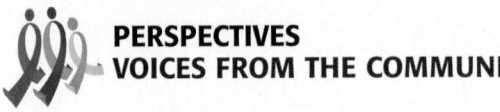

PERSPECTIVES VOICES FROM THE COMMUNITY

As an instructor of undergraduate nursing students, I want students to realize that public health nursing is a wonderful and rewarding employment opportunity. Many students often enter the nursing program not knowing much about public health nursing. They may only get minimal exposure to public health and thus do not often understand who or what is involved in public health nursing. In so doing, they miss out on a wonderful opportunity to work with a variety of people. It may be helping new moms, or working with children and adolescents, or the elderly. They may help give vaccinations or prepare for community disasters. They might teach about breast-feeding or conduct cancer-screening clinics. They are out working directly with the people, ensuring the public's health.

Public health nurses (PHNs) are able to use the science of nursing because they need to understand the pathophysiology, anatomy, human development, and disease transmission. They may not do as many hands-on procedures as hospital nurses, but they still must keep up-to-date in knowledge, as they are often teaching. In addition, they must be quick and receptive thinkers who can work independently and creatively. PHNs also are the essence of the "art" of nursing. They must understand and relate to people and grasp social systems and human behavior. They are the voice for the most vulnerable and the champion of all.

Although PHNs may not see an immediate reward for their actions, as a nurse who works in the hospital does, PHNs make a long and lasting impact not just to an individual but also for an entire society. They have the opportunity to really be a patient advocate. They do this by helping well people stay well and by preventing illness. They also help those who are sick obtain medical access. PHNs can also be involved in public policy change that can help an entire community. Public health nursing encompasses the entire art and science of nursing.

Erin M.

(National Oceanic and Atmospheric Administration [NOAA] Commissioned Corps), and the U.S. Public Health Service Commissioned Corps (USPHSCC) (NOAA, 2007; USPHSCC, 2010).

The **U.S. Public Health Service Commissioned Corps** is a group of 6,500 specially trained public health members who serve their country with the goal of protecting and promoting the health of the nation. The Corps was established in 1798, as part of an act to treat sick seamen in Marine hospitals. Over the years, the Corps expanded to oversee the health of immigrants entering the country and to assist in preventing/treating communicable disease outbreaks. Beginning in 1928, members of the Corps were assigned to work with Native Americans (in the IHS, see above) (U.S. Public Health Service Nursing Corps, 2011). The US Surgeon General oversees the Commissioned Corps, and many of its officers are stationed at other federal agencies, such as the CDC and the FDA (USPHSCC, 2010).

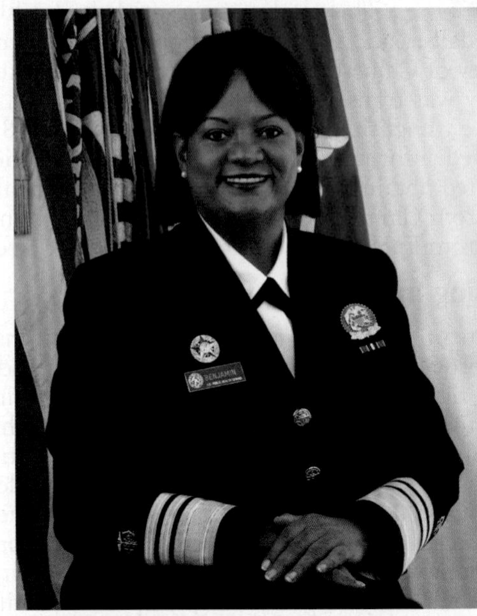

The US Surgeon General, Regina M. Benjamin, MD, MBA, oversees the Commissioned Corps, including many nurses serving in various government agencies.

Nurses are an integral part of the Corps. They provide nursing care and health care leadership around the world. Their focus is on improving health for the entire community by providing care, conducting research, or reviewing new medications. These nurses work in a variety of federal agencies, many of them listed earlier. On a daily basis, they may perform tasks similar to civilian nurses. However, as commissioned officers, they can also be deployed to protect the nation's health. For example, USPHSCC nurses were some of the first on the scene to assist in the aftermath of the 2010 earthquake in Haiti (see Display 30.4). They may also be deployed in the case of a widespread communicable disease outbreak. Their activities can be international as well, in providing expertise and support on global issues such as the Asian tsunami or the worldwide spread of HIV/AIDS.

As commissioned officers, USPHSCC nurses are compensated in addition to their regular salaries and receive veteran's benefits, health insurance, access to military base lodging and recreational facilities, and other benefits. Officers are supported with tuition and other training opportunities to further their education and advance their careers. Student tuition reimbursement and loan payment options are also available.

To qualify as a nurse in the Commissioned Corps, one must be a US citizen, <44 years old, able to pass a physical examination, possess a bachelor's or higher degree from an accredited nursing program, pass the National Council Licensure Examination (NCLEX), and hold a valid nursing license from one of the 50 states, the District of Columbia, Puerto Rico, Guam, or the U.S.

DISPLAY 30.4 UNITED STATES PUBLIC HEALTH SERVICE COMMISSIONED CORPS: HURRICANE KATRINA AND THE EARTHQUAKE IN HAITI

Here is an example from an account in the *Journal of Professional Nursing* of how nurses from the U.S. Public Health Service Commissioned Corps (USPHSCC) are called upon to help during a national crisis. The authors of the article have "regular" positions with the federal government. At the time the article was written, two authors (Debisette and Brown) worked for the Bureau of Health Professions, part of the Health Resources and Services Administration (HRSA) in the U.S. Department of Health and Human Services. The third author (Chamberlain) worked as a nurse medical evaluations officer in the Office of Commissioned Corps Support Services.

As the threat of Hurricane Katrina was imminent, the USPHSCC nurses were deployed to Louisiana; they arrived the day before the storm hit land and were some of the first to respond. In fact, nearly half of the 37-member team ($n = 15$) were nurses. The team was deployed to Baton Rouge to assist local personnel in setting up an 800-bed field hospital (including an intensive care unit) at the Pete Maravich Assembly Center at Louisiana State University. The USPHSCC nurses helped provide nursing care that included triage, treatment, stabilization, and transport to permanent facilities. They addressed the psychological, as well as physiologic, needs of the people as evacuees.

Having lost everything, the evacuees streamed into the center. Many of these evacuees, in addition to the trauma and shock associated with their losses, had special medical needs. Some needed dialysis, some were physically disabled, and some had diabetes.

USPHSCC nurses also ensured the safety and security of the people. For example, it was a USPHSCC nurse who realized that the electrical outage would create a failure of the water pump system and alerted the commanding officer. Knowing they would soon lose water, the nurses then filled bathtubs with water that was later needed for flushing toilets. The USPHSCC nurses covered gaps in care and worked long hours to ensure that the needs of everyone were met.

After working 3 weeks in the Baton Rouge area, the USPHSCC nurses traveled for 3 days with the American Red Cross and the Louisiana Department of Health and Hospitals to other parts of Louisiana to assess needs. They visited 270 shelters. They worked in teams of four (an environmental officer, a health provider trained in epidemiology, a local American Red Cross representative, and a registered nurse [RN]). Each member had specific responsibilities. The nurses assessed the ability of the shelters to address the acute and chronic health care needs of the residents, either within the shelter or by accessing local health resources. They accomplished this assignment by interviewing various shelter staff using a standardized survey tool, as well as by direct observation.

The authors concluded from their experience with Katrina:

> Nurses are often caregivers, nurturers, and advocates. In addition, they are frequently called upon to take on the roles of educators, counselors, and as evidenced here, researchers. As representatives of the USPHS, they stood with strength and courage in the face of devastation. Most of all, they [were] leaders of compassion who appreciate[d] the love, sense of community, and love for their country that emanated from the people of Louisiana in the aftermath of Hurricane Katrina. (p. 272)

From Debisette, A. T., Brown, C.R., & Chamberlain, N. (2006). A nursing perspective from United States Public Health Service Nurses. *Journal of Professional Nursing, 22*(5), 270–272.

Haitian Response

In January 2010, the United States deployed over 250 health care personnel to Haiti to assist in the aftermath of the earthquake there. This number was expected to grow to over 12,000. Members of the U.S. Public Health Service Commissioned Corps were called from around the country to join forces in providing basic medical care and checking food and water supplies.

U.S. Department of Health and Human Services, News Release (2010). Retrieved from http://www.hhs.gov/news/press/2010pres/01/20100114b.html

Virgin Islands. For more information on the USPHSCC, see the Internet Resources found on thePoint.

SCHOOL NURSING

School nurses save lives and assist in helping children so that they are able to learn and reach their greatest potential.

> School nursing is a specialized practice of professional nursing that advances the wellbeing, academic success, and life-long achievement of students. To that end, school nurses facilitate positive student responses to normal development; promote health and safety; intervene with actual and potential health problems; provide case management services; and actively collaborate with others to build student and family capacity for adaptation, self-management, self-advocacy, and learning. (National Association of School Nurses [NASN], 2007)

A **school nurse** works primarily with the students who attend the nurse's assigned schools, as well as with the families of those schoolchildren, members of the school staff and administration, health care providers, and other helping professionals within the school and community. In 2010, approximately 49.4 million school-age children attended public schools in the United States (U.S. Department of Education, 2011). These children are the parents, workers, leaders, and decision-makers of tomorrow, and their future success depends in good measure on achieving their educational goals today. Their school success is intertwined, to some degree, with the state of their health (CDC, 2011a).

Think back to your own elementary and secondary schooling. Did you have access to a school nurse? If so, how did that person influence your health and the health of your peers? If you did not have a school nurse, how do you think a school nurse might have improved your school environment or educational experience? The school nurse is a key provider of a variety of services.

HISTORY OF SCHOOL NURSING

Beginning in the mid-1800s and continuing through the early years of the 20th century, mandatory education was instituted in the United States. The early years included health services often conducted by "medical inspectors," usually physicians. In New York City, where communicable disease was rampant, inspectors sent notes home with children with the message "you are sick—go home" and citing the reason for their exclusion from school (Vessey & McGowan, 2006, p. 255). The reasons for exclusion were largely the contagious illnesses commonly found among the tenements and crowded slums of the growing city. However, parents often did not receive these notes, or couldn't read them, and because families lacked resources, most children were left untreated and simply remained out of school as truants. No efforts were made by medical inspectors to follow up on excluded children. Because these excluded children played with healthy children after school hours, the levels of contagious illness actually worsened (Vesey & McGowan, 2006; Wolfe & Selekman, 2002). As noted in Woodfill and Beyrer's classic text (1991), the absentee children promoted the spread of various communicable diseases. In 1902, the New York Board of Education contracted with Lillian Wald's Henry Street Settlement to provide a PHN to work with the families and schools to facilitate the return of healthy children to school. The nurse was Lina Rogers (she later married and added the name Struthers). She made home visits to follow up on excluded children and was assisted by other Henry Street nurses in providing care, educating families about diseases and the need for hygiene, and working with other organizations to provide needed food, shoes, and clothing (Vessey & McGowan, 2006). In the first month of the school nurse experiment, 98% of children previously excluded from school for medical reasons were treated and readmitted (Woodfill & Beyrer, 1991). The board hired 12 more school nurses, and over the next few years, other cities and states began hiring nurses to work in the schools. School nurses have historically advocated for hot lunches, breakfast programs, and the need for increased health education in schools and for families (Abrams, 2005).

School nurses continue as a specialty branch of professional nursing that serves the school-age population. More than 73,000 school nurses are estimated to be working in schools today (HRSA, 2010). However, according to the most recent (2006) School Health Policies and Programs Study (SHPPS), many school nurses oversee multiple schools, and less than half of the schools had the nationally recommended ratio of one school nurse for every 750 students (Brener, Wheeler, Wolfe, Vernon-Smiley, & Caldart-Olson, 2007). Most schools (86.3%) had at least a part-time nurse, although some schools still report not having any school nursing services.

School nurses deliver services to students from birth through age 21 years. They also work with students' families and the school community in regular and special education schools, as well as other educational settings (e.g., preschools, court, and other community schools). Studies show that having a school nurse present increases health and social services and improves absentee rates (Hill & Hollis, 2011).

The role of the school nurse has expanded over the years, along with the increase in chronic conditions and challenges in accessing health care (Engelke, Guttu, Warren, Swanson, 2008). Federal law requires school systems to provide care for children with disabilities. The Individuals with Disabilities Education Act (IDEA 1975), the Rehabilitation Act of 1973, and Title II of the Americans with Disabilities Act all mandate equal educational opportunities for all students, including children with complex medical conditions.

Legislative mandates and technology that has allowed low-birth-weight babies to survive have led to a steady increase in the number of children with special health care needs attending school (Lakdawalla, Bhattacharya, & Goldman, 2004; Nelson, 2009; U.S. Department of Education, 2011). It is now commonplace for children to attend school accompanied by feeding tubes, catheters, insulin pumps, and glucose monitors, as well as ventilators (Nelson, 2009; Wolfe & Selekman, 2002). More children with life-threatening conditions have required schools to consider "do not resuscitate" orders and provide emergency care plans (Wolfe & Selekman, p. 404).

In addition, the lack of access to health care has added extra burdens on schools as children come to school sick or miss additional days of school resulting from complications of illnesses that could have been easily treated in earlier stages. In 2010, almost 6 million children in the United States (8%) did not have health insurance (Sondick, Madans, & Gentleman, 2011). Many children can access health care services only at school (Vessey & McGowan, 2006). Results from the most recent National Health Survey indicate that 5% of children missed 11 days of school or more in the past year because of illness (Sondick et al., 2011). Children from families of lower socioeconomic status were twice as likely to miss 11 days of school or more than were children from families with higher income levels (9% vs. 4%).

School nurses are also involved in emergency preparedness and disaster planning. The NASN (2011), in their position statement on this issue, noted that school nurses are a crucial link between "local public health departments and emergency services" (para. 4). School nurse roles include prevention/mitigation, preparedness, response, and recovery. Epidemics (e.g., influenza), weather-related emergencies (e.g., hurricanes, tornadoes, earthquakes, flooding), and other sudden crises (e.g., school shootings, terrorism) are all potential issues facing school nurses. The Federal Emergency Management Institute (a division of the Department of Homeland Security and the Federal Emergency Management Administration [FEMA]) offers training courses for school administrators, school nurses, and teachers to aid them in preparing for various emergencies (see http://training.fema.gov/emiweb/emischool/). Additionally, school nurses must consider emergency evacuation plans, especially for disabled students (National Fire Protection Association, 2007) and how to best reunite students with their families.

KEY ROLES OF THE SCHOOL NURSE

To understand the role of the school nurse, one must first realize that school health, like all health programs in the community, requires a great degree of collaboration (Brener et al., 2007). School nursing services are part of a coordinated school health program that provides school health services, health education, and health promotion programs for faculty and staff.

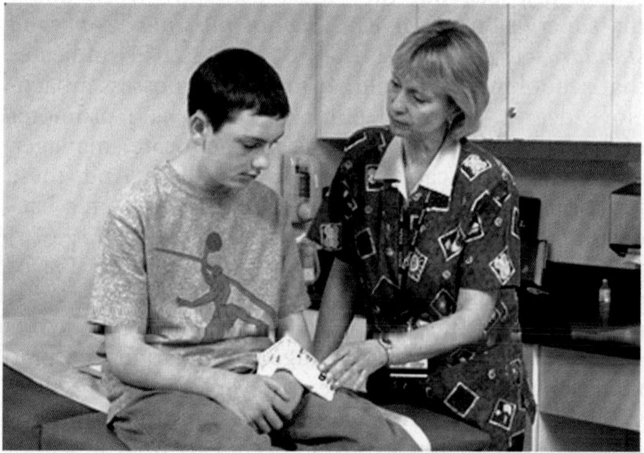

The school nurse is part of a team providing a coordinated school health program.

Liaison with the Interdisciplinary School Health Team

The nurse collaborates with counseling and psychological services, as well as physical education and nutrition services, working to provide a healthy school environment with family and community involvement (CDC, 2007). Although the school nurse plays a central role, collaboration with many other individuals is important. The coordinated school health program includes eight components and involves a variety of professionals and other people ranging from teachers, administrators, and school staff to families. The components are:

- School health services (preventive services, referral)
- Health education (kindergarten through 12th grade curricula)
- Health promotion for faculty and staff (employee health)
- Counseling, psychological, and social services
- School nutrition services
- Physical education programs
- Healthy school environment
- Family and community involvement (partnership among school, families, community groups)

Positive Working Relationship with Administrators and Teachers

The school principal influences all phases of the school health program by promoting good school health through active support of the school's health services, participation in setting health-related policies, and tapping into community resources. The principal can reinforce positive efforts within the school, ranging from the health teaching in the classroom to the cleaning activities of the custodian. Because of the principal's influential position, it is absolutely essential for the nurse and principal to maintain a positive and cooperative working relationship.

Teachers, whether they are involved in regular instruction, physical education, or special education, play a major role in school health. Because they spend the most time with students, their observations, health teaching, and personal health habits have a profound effect on student health and the quality of school health services. The school nurse and teachers must collaborate constantly, as the school nurse provides information and guidance to teachers regarding students in their classrooms with specific health conditions and concerns and teachers report on students' health concerns and behaviors.

Other health team members, such as health educators, health coordinators, psychologists, audiologists, speech therapists, occupational therapists, physical therapists, counselors, health care providers, dentists, dental hygienists, social workers, security and juvenile justice personnel, health aides, and volunteers, may also be involved, depending on the size and financial resources of the school. All team members, including students, parents, bus drivers, and custodians, have a specialized role complementary to that of the school nurse. Consultation and referral among team members are crucial to the successful implementation of the school health program (Council on School Health, 2008).

If the school system desires such services, a physician may work on a part-time consultative basis; however, fewer than 16% of school systems reported having a school physician (Brener et al., 2007). This role focuses largely on advising and consulting related to policy and medical–legal matters. A community physician may serve on a school advisory panel, acting as a liaison between the community, other health agencies, and the school. The physician or a nurse practitioner (NP) may become involved in student health appraisals, rescreenings, health problem interventions, sports physical examinations, or first aid support at sporting events.

Funding for school nursing comes from a variety of sources. School districts use support services funding for school nurses. Public health departments may also contribute funding, along with hospitals and other organizations. Federal Medicaid funding has been used to support some of the administrative and nursing services provided to children with special health care needs. Over the last 10 to 15 years, school districts have billed Medicaid for specific services provided in the school setting (e.g., case management of children with chronic illnesses such as diabetes and asthma). However, a recent ruling found that Medicaid funds were being misused and such reimbursement was stopped (USDHHS, Centers for Medicare and Medicaid, 2007). Many schools relied heavily on this funding, and as a result, school nurse positions were cut (Domrose, 2011).

RESPONSIBILITIES OF THE SCHOOL NURSE

The primary responsibilities of the school nurse are to prevent illness and to promote and maintain the health of the school community. The school nurse serves not only individuals, families, and groups within the context of school health but also the school as an organization and its membership (students and staff) as aggregates. The school nurse identifies health-related barriers to learning, serves as a health advocate for children and families, and promotes health while preventing illness and disability (NASN, 2007).

School nursing activities include care of children with special health needs, including nasogastric tube feedings, catheterization, insulin pumps, and suctioning; general and emergency first aid; vision, hearing, scoliosis, and TB screenings; height, weight, and blood pressure monitoring; oral health and dental education; immunization assessment and monitoring; medication administration; assessment of acute health problems; health examinations (especially for athletic participation or school entry); and referrals. School nurses also assess and are the frontline providers for identifying communicable diseases, such as outbreaks of H1N1 (Nelson, 2009).

Other duties that a school nurse may have include training school staff in cardiopulmonary resuscitation (CPR), universal precautions and first aid, as well as overseeing the health and wellness of school staff members. Many of these activities may be performed concurrently. See Display 30.5 for a typical day in the life of a school nurse. Each school nurse must assess and prioritize how to address the specific needs in each individual school and determine the order. This largely autonomous practice requires specific skills and training.

EDUCATION: SPECIAL TRAINING AND SKILLS OF THE SCHOOL NURSE

School nurses operate from one of two administrative bases: the school system or the public health department. In most localities, public or private school systems or districts hire school nurses, and they maintain a specialized, school-based practice. In this specialized role, the nurse can concentrate time and effort solely on the school health program and develop specialized skills in school health assessment and intervention. Today, with the emphasis on delivery of health care at community sites where clients spend most of their time (e.g., schools for children, the workplace for adults), the nurse whose specialty is school health care seems better prepared to meet the complex needs of the school-age population.

In contrast, the school nurse who operates under the board of health's jurisdiction provides services to schools as one part of generalized public health nursing services to the community. The community health nurse working through the health department usually devotes only a portion of the workday to the school; she may have additional responsibilities, such as clinic nursing and home visits. This broader base allows contact with preschoolers and their families, provides a stronger knowledge of the community and its resources, and promotes integration of in-school and out-of-school care.

Depending on the state of residence, a school nurse is usually an RN—frequently with additional education beyond the bachelor's degree in nursing, sometimes including a master's degree—who has primary responsibility for the health care of school-age children and school personnel in an educational setting. In some areas of the country, licensed practical nurses (LPNs) or licensed vocational nurses (LVNs) may be hired by school districts, but they must generally work under the supervision of an RN. *School nursing: Scope and standards of practice* (NASN & ANA, 2011) indicates that school nurses should, at minimum, possess a bachelor's degree. A school nurse functions as a promoter of health, an educator, counselor, advocate, manager, and deliverer of care (Brener et al., 2007). And, these functions require a knowledge base derived from a baccalaureate-level nursing program. Many states (39.6%) require state school nurse certification, and 29.2% of states have a policy indicating that school nurses must perform continuing education (Brener et al., 2007).

As the needs of school-aged populations become increasingly complex, some states require even more specialized training for school nurses. In California, for instance, school nurses are expected to hold a school health services credential. This credential is obtained through a postbaccalaureate program that includes a minimum of 24 semester units of course work in audiology, guidance and counseling, exceptional children, school health principles and practice, a practicum in school nursing, child psychology, and health curriculum development, in addition to other courses. However, most school nurse credential programs are now available only as part of a master's degree program. A national certification is available as well (*Careers in Focus*, 2011).

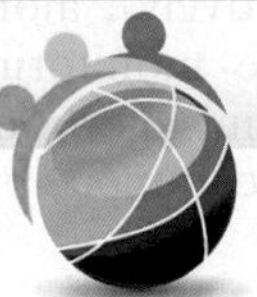

DISPLAY 30.5 A DAY IN THE LIFE OF A SCHOOL NURSE

8:00 AM The nurse begins work at her assigned middle school. A parent brings in a controlled medication (narcotic) for her son who fractured his arm the day before. The school nurse works with the parent regarding the medication protocol of the school. The nurse advises that narcotics will affect the student's concentration and ability to learn.

8:15 AM Two students come into the office to take medications (dextroamphetamine [Dexedrine] and an antidepressant for concentration and focusing).

8:20 AM First acute illness of the day! A girl has vomited and is very nervous about being in middle school. The nurse calls home to learn that the student has been to her health care provider twice this week because of anxiety. The nurse helps to calm her and talk about the situation and then walks her back to class. The nurse talks to the teacher about the student's situation.

8:45 AM Three pupils come to the nurse's office complaining of sickness. The nurse assesses them and calls the parents to explain the situation and tells them of the current illness in the school.

9:00 AM A student arrives in the office holding her nose. She was playing volleyball when she collided with another student. She is afraid her nose is broken. The nurse assesses the situation, and determines that there is a possible fracture. The student's parents are contacted, and arrangements are made for the student to visit the doctor, where the diagnosis (fracture) is confirmed and the student is treated.

9:15 AM Nurse leaves the middle school and heads for her assigned elementary school (three blocks away). She has a meeting for an individualized education plan (IEP). One student has attention deficit disorder and bipolar disorder, and so the student's parents and the educational team (which includes the school nurse) meet to determine how to best serve the student's needs while in school and set goals and objectives. The nurse's role includes educating teachers and staff about how to handle mood swings and outbursts. The nurse works with the student's health care provider regarding medications and monitors the impact of the medications. The nurse also works with the parents regarding strategies and coping skills to use at home.

10:30 AM The nurse returns to the middle school and finds six students in her office. One has a bloody nose (and is applying pressure to stop the bleeding); two collided while in physical education class (and have ice on their heads); and three have fevers and upset stomachs and are waiting for parents to arrive. The students who have head injuries are assessed for concussions and neurologic concerns. Parents are contacted regarding signs to watch for when the students return home. One of the student's parents cannot be reached, so a note will be sent home with the same information.

11:00 AM–1:00 PM Lunch time! 10 students come in for their medications. Students arrive with playground injuries to assess and monitor, and parents return calls and arrive to sign out their children.

1:00 PM The nurse receives a call from the assistant principal requesting the nurse to come to the main office. A student has been found with cigarettes and lighters. The student is given information regarding smoking and drugs. The student lives with surrogate parents who need assistance in setting limits at home and at school.

1:30 PM All immunizations have been documented and entered for the year. The nurse prints the immunization report and identifies 177 students who are not up-to-date with state requirements. The nurse will need to contact and work with the parents of these students to help them achieve compliance. Students will not be allowed to return to school until the situation is resolved.

2:30 PM The nurse attends a meeting to create a behavior modification plan for a student who is having difficulty completing assignments.

3:00 PM The school day ends.

Adapted from Weirick, K. (2003). A typical day in the life of a school nurse. *New Mexico 48*(1), 5. Retrieved from *http://www.nursingald.com/Uploaded%5CNewsletterFiles%5CNM032003.pdf*

School nurse practitioners (SNPs) are RNs with advanced academic and clinical preparation (generally certification and a master's degree in nursing), along with a guided experience in physical assessment, diagnosis, and treatment, so that the SNP may provide primary care to school-age children. Many school districts see the advantage of having an SNP on staff, rather than using the limited services of a physician. Assessment, diagnosis, treatment, and referral of injuries, communicable diseases, or other health problems can be managed more efficiently by a NP who is educationally prepared to work holistically with the school-age population and is part of the educational setting. If this arrangement is impractical, an SNP who is available to school nurses for consultation or who is employed on a part-time basis can become the impetus for comprehensive school-based health services. Some school districts utilize SNPs to provide services to teachers and staff to promote wellness or to handle job-related injuries. Some research findings cite cost savings related to SNP services, as students and staff served by them experience fewer days of absenteeism (Kerr et al., 2011).

As the population continues to become more diverse and the problems of children and their families grow in complexity, the school nurse with specialized training in school health, the education system, case management, and advanced practice nursing (e.g., NPs, clinical nurse specialists) becomes even more essential.

FUNCTIONS OF SCHOOL NURSING PRACTICE

The three main functions of school nursing practice are health services, health education, and promotion of a healthy school environment.

Health services include caring for individual students who have chronic conditions or acute situations while at the same time thinking of the entire population and tracking trends. For example, the school nurse observes an increase in the number of students diagnosed with asthma and investigates ways to help all students with asthma. One way of doing this may be to organize an *Open Airways* course (developed by the American Lung Association) to assist students in identifying triggers and managing their own care. The goal of this course would be to decrease student asthma attacks.

Health Services for Chronic Conditions

The number of children afflicted with chronic diseases is rising (Van Cleave, Gortmaker, Perrin, 2010). Commonly seen chronic problems include hay fever, sinusitis, dermatitis, tonsillitis, asthma, diabetes, seizure disorders, and hearing difficulties. In addition, acute illnesses such as stomachaches, headaches, colds, and flu are frequent complaints of school-age children. School nurses develop **individualized health plans (IHPs)** to ensure that students with special needs (e.g., chronic conditions) have these needs met. If these students attend the regular classroom, the plans may be known as **Section 504 plans**, named after the section of the Individuals with Disability Education Act that specifically allows for school accommodations with this population. For students in special education programs, nurses can coordinate IHPs with **individualized education plans (IEPs)** to develop health management goals for students. Medically fragile or technology-dependent students, who may require procedures such as suctioning or tube feeding, would have plans developed for *specialized physical health care procedures*. The five chronic conditions most often seen in school-age children are asthma, diabetes, seizures, severe food allergies, and attention deficit/behavioral disorders. A recent survey of New Jersey school nurses by Krause-Parello and Samms (2010) found that chronic conditions most often seen by the school nurse included allergies (87.3%), asthma (74.6%), ADHD (47.6%), diabetes (20.6%), and depression (9.5%). They also found that the most common procedures done by school nurses included first aid (98.4%), nebulizer treatments and inhalers (96.8% and 95.2%, respectively), along with wound care (90.5%), and glucose monitoring (87.3%). Urinary catheterizations, insulin injections, and gastrostomy tube feedings were less common, but were done by many school nurses.

Asthma

Asthma is often deemed the most common chronic disease of childhood. Although reports indicate morbidity and mortality from asthma has stabilized in the past few years, in 2010, an estimated 17% of children age 17 and younger have been diagnosed with asthma (Sondick et al., 2011). Non-Hispanic Blacks exhibit the highest asthma attack rates, and boys more often than girls reported an episode within the past year (Sondick et al., 2011). An estimated 14 million school days are missed each year because of children who suffer from asthma (Crowder, 2010). Children with asthma also tend to show comorbidities, such as depression and behavioral disorders (Blackman & Gurka, 2007). In such situations, school nurses work with students, their families, and their doctors to develop an *asthma action plan* to control, prevent, or minimize untoward effects of acute asthma episodes. Peak flowmeters can be used regularly to determine early signs of asthma problems. The activities of nurses acting as case managers have been found to decrease the number of ER visits and hospitalizations of school-age children with asthma (Magzamen, Patel, Davis, Edelstein, & Tager, 2008).

Monitoring asthma medications and teaching proper methods of inhaler use are also vital school nursing functions. Many states (88%) allow students to carry quick-acting inhalers on their person (Brener et al., 2007). It often falls to school nurses to ensure that proper protocols and training are accomplished. Researchers have shown that students with asthma do not miss more days of school, if there is a nurse available to assist with management (Millard, Johnson, Hilton, & Hart, 2009).

Diabetes

Diabetes is another common chronic illness in young people: approximately 215,000 under age 20 have diabetes. This translates into 0.26% of youth having diabetes (National Diabetes Education Program, 2011), and experts now conclude that both type 1 and type 2 diabetes mellitus are found in school-age children. It is estimated that there are 13,600 newly found youth under the age of 20 annually diagnosed with type 2 diabetes (National Diabetes Education Program, 2011). Type 2 diabetes is rising almost exponentially in adolescents, leading some scientists to frame it as a major public health crisis caused largely by obesity, sedentary lifestyle, and the predisposition of certain ethnic groups to diabetes.

Working with families and health care providers, school nurses assess and develop a care plan for students with diabetes. School nurses work closely with the family to maintain confidentiality and at the same time ensure that the school is a safe environment for the child. A multidisciplinary team approach is needed, with family, school, and physician collaboration. Training for teachers and fellow classmates is also important. Teachers are often called upon to assist students with their insulin pumps or food management. Younger children with type 1 diabetes, especially those who use insulin pumps, may need careful monitoring—something that is not always possible for the school nurse, who may not be present where and when problems arise. If the child has an insulin reaction, fellow students should be taught to quickly get the teacher (NASN, 2006). A current position of the American Diabetes Association (ADA) is that a *diabetes medical management plan* should be in place and that the "school nurse should be the primary coordinator and provider of care and should coordinate the training of an adequate number of school personnel" to assist in the care of children with diabetes (2012, p. S78). However, many school nurses do not feel comfortable delegating tasks such as administration of insulin or glucagon. Delegation has become a safety issue that has reached many state boards of nursing and legislatures (Block, 2009; Wilt & Foley, 2011). See Chapter 13 for more on this issue.

Testing blood sugar and taking insulin at school can be frustrating and can cause children to feel singled out or different from their peers. One study found that adolescents with type 1 diabetes have significantly higher rates of depression than those without diabetes (Fritsch, Overton, & Robbins, 2011). Also, some schools do not permit blood sugar testing and insulin administration in classrooms, so that school health offices are often a place of refuge for diabetic students (Winsch, 2011; Wolfe & Selekman, 2002). It is important for school nurses to understand each child's concerns and to alert teachers and school personnel to the signs and symptoms (as well as the treatment) of hypoglycemia. In addition to the obvious emergency health-related concerns for diabetic children, a classic study showed that diabetes-related severe hypoglycemia does affect memory tasks (Hershey, Bhargava, Sadler, White, & Craft, 1999). Over time, memory deficits can affect learning and progress in school.

Seizure Disorders

Seizure disorders are not uncommon in the school-age population. Epilepsy is a disorder of the brain in which neurons sometimes give abnormal signals. A person who suffers from epilepsy may have comorbidities including autism, depression, and anxiety (National Institute of Neurological Disorders and Stroke [NINDS], 2009). For almost 80% of those diagnosed, seizures can usually be controlled with medication (e.g., antiepileptic drugs specific to the pediatric population), surgical treatment, or a diet rich in proteins and fats and low in carbohydrates (a *ketogenic diet*) (NINDS, 2009).

It is important for school nurses to develop care plans to address seizure concerns during school hours. Care plans include monitoring medication compliance and teaching school staff about first aid measures for seizure victims. Children and adolescents with seizure disorders may feel embarrassed or be the victims of teasing or bullying. They may exhibit signs of school avoidance. Nurses need to work with these children and to teach all students about the disease process and the need for empathy and understanding. Similar to issues related to insulin administration for diabetic students, children with seizure disorders may have an emergency medication (Diastat) ordered by their physician. School officials may be hesitant to permit their staff to give this rectal gel to students because benzodiazepines are known to cause central nervous system depression (Valeant, 2007). The Epilepsy Foundation has advocated for its use in schools (n.d.), and school nurses are often caught between the rights of students and their parents and their state's nursing practice act.

Food Allergies

Another leading chronic condition found in school settings is severe food allergies that can lead to anaphylactic shock. Such severe allergies result in approximately 50,000 ER visits each year (Decker et al., 2008). Eight common foods account for 90% of severe food allergies. They are fish, shellfish, soy, milk, egg, wheat, peanuts, and tree nuts (e.g., cashews, walnuts). Many common foods and school supplies (e.g., play dough) can contain hidden allergens, and care must be taken to prevent exposure. School nurses coordinate and work with students and their families, along with school personnel, to raise awareness and enlist caution. They also work with families and health care providers to ensure that epinephrine via an autoinjector (EpiPen) is available for the child in case of emergencies. Epinephrine reverses the body's allergic reaction to the allergen (Dey, 2008). Many states (66%) allow students to carry an EpiPen on their person because reactions can occur very quickly (Brener et al., 2007). School nurses coordinate and ensure that proper protocol is followed. School nurses also work with teachers and lunch room personnel to alert them of the allergy, explain what can happen in a case of anaphylaxis, and provide training on how to use the EpiPen or other needed medication.

Behavioral Problems and Learning Disabilities

Other chronic childhood health problems are those of emotional, behavioral, and intellectual development. These are not always easy to detect and measure, and they can be debilitating. Although these problems are not new, awareness and concern have increased as the rates of occurrence for other life-threatening childhood diseases have diminished. Emotional or behavioral problems and learning disabilities are prevalent during childhood, with approximately one in seven children <18 years old have a special health care need (Kogan, Strickland, Newacheck, 2009).

The causes of learning disabilities and emotional behavioral problems appear to have genetic, environmental, and cultural influences. The number of children with learning disabilities in the lowest economic group is twice that in the highest group (Sondick et al.,

2011). Children who were characterized as being in fair or poor health were almost five times as likely to have a learning disability and more than twice as likely to have attention deficit hyperactivity disorder (ADHD) as children with excellent, very good, or good health status (Sondick et al., 2011). High-risk children often come from families with a high incidence of child abuse (physical and sexual) and neglect. The number of children affected by parental drug use has surpassed that of children with disabilities caused by lead poisoning, another major contributor to developmental problems in children.

ADHD is a cluster of problems related to hyperactivity, impulsivity, and inattention (Dang et al., 2007). The CDC (2010b) estimates 5.4 million school-age children between the ages of 4 and 17 have been diagnosed with ADHD. School nurses must be aware of the signs and symptoms and serve as an advocate for these children and their families. At each stage of development, those with ADHD are presented with distinct challenges. For example, children in elementary school may often have difficulty and conflict with peers, as well as problems organizing tasks. They may be more accident-prone and may have more school-related problems, such as grade retention and suspension or expulsion.

They often have problems with grooming and with handwriting, and they exhibit difficulty sleeping. ADHD is sometimes found with associated disorders, such as communication or language disorders and learning disabilities. Common comorbid conditions are depression, anxiety disorders, and conduct disorders (Dang et al., 2007).

Behavioral and emotional problems of school-age children stem from many causes. School nurses can be alert to early symptoms and refer families for counseling. Some schools are also now offering support groups for children of divorce.

Collaboration is needed between the child's family, the school, and the child's health care provider to diagnose ADHD and effectively plan appropriate interventions and educational accommodations. Teacher confirmation of ADHD-related behaviors is very important. Numerous checklists and assessment tools are available, and school psychologists typically serve as a source for additional information and resources. School nurses can assist parents in recognizing the symptoms of ADHD and obtaining appropriate treatment and follow-up (Dang et al., 2007). A multimodal treatment approach may include stimulant medication, usually methylphenidate (Ritalin or Concerta), dextroamphetamine (Dexedrine) and amphetamine (Adderall), or antidepressants (such as Wellbutrin). Other treatment includes school accommodations for learning problems and social skills training for the child with ADHD (Dang et al., 2007). Family and individual counseling, parent support groups, and training in behavior management techniques, as well as family education about the condition, are also essential features of this method of treatment.

Not all children and adolescents respond to medication, and medication dosage must be carefully monitored and titrated. School nurses can assist parents in this task. The main goal of medication for school-age children is academic improvement. If this does not occur, medication may need to be changed or discontinued. School nurses and community health nurses can work closely with school staff, parents, and physicians in determining the efficacy of treatment regimens.

Medication Administration

Medication administration for a variety of conditions is an important responsibility for school nurses (Krause-Parello & Samms, 2010). In schools where a nurse is present every day, the nurse can personally oversee medication administration. Unfortunately, many nurses cover more than one school and so other school personnel (e.g., secretaries, health aides) oversee medication administration. Over half the states have laws allowing teachers or health aides to administer medication (Brener et al., 2007). In these situations, it is ideal for school nurses to provide training and audit records to ensure that proper guidelines are followed. Multiple studies show that medication errors increase when school nurses cover multiple schools and unlicensed personnel assist in medication administration (Ficca & Welk, 2006; McCarthy, Kelly, & Reed, 2000; Richmond, 2011). Problems commonly occur with omission of doses because students fail to come to the office for medication administration. This is especially problematic with students taking insulin or antidiabetic drugs, antibiotics, and medication for ADHD.

Another issue surrounding medication administration in the school setting is regarding delegation. Each state's individual nurse practice act provides rules on delegation of nursing tasks. School nurses must understand their own state's act and the legal implications regarding their decisions. Recently, much discussion has occurred regarding the administration of Diastat gel in the school setting (NASN, 2011a). Diastat gel is often administered rectally to stop the onset of cluster seizures. However, Diastat can decrease respirations as well. School nurses have the skills and experience to properly assess such occurrences, where lay personnel, even if trained in proper administration of the medication, do not. NASN (2011a) supports only school nurses administering this medication, but parents and others have pushed the administration of Diastat by lay people.

Health Services to Prevent Illness and Injury

School nurses emphasize prevention and focus many of their efforts on prevention of communicable disease (via immunizations) and of injuries.

Immunizations

Among schoolchildren, the incidence rates of measles (rubeola), rubella (German measles), pertussis (whooping cough), infectious parotitis (mumps), and varicella (chickenpox) have dropped considerably because of widespread immunization efforts, although these communicable diseases do still occur and sometimes with serious complications such as birth defects from rubella and nerve deafness from mumps. Although the number of cases of *Haemophilus influenza* infection and hepatitis B stayed the same between 2006 and 2007, there was a decrease in the number of cases of pertussis, mumps, and hepatitis A (Maternal and Child Health Bureau, 2010).

Low immunization levels in many areas, particularly among poor populations, and increased disease rates signal the need for constant surveillance, outreach programs, and educational efforts. School nurses are deeply involved in each of these preventive activities. Health departments and schools often work collaboratively to provide immunization services. Compulsory immunization laws for school entrance, which vary among states, have enabled public health personnel to carry out these preventive services. Nearly all states (94%) have a policy of excluding students from school if they are not adequately immunized (Brener et al., 2007). Only about 17% of states require TB skin testing before entering school.

School nurses often oversee and ensure that children are in compliance with school entrance laws regarding immunizations. They may call parents directly when they note that the student is out of compliance. They may also arrange to help the student get immunized by facilitating appointments or, in some school districts, by directly providing the immunizations. The American School Health Association has developed a toolkit for school nurses and others to follow when developing successful immunization outreach programs in secondary schools where compliance is always difficult (Boyer-Chu & Wooley, 2008).

Safety

School nurses are also involved in ensuring that injury prevention efforts are encouraged. Emphasis on a healthful physical environment includes proper selection, design, organization, operation, and maintenance of the school building and playground equipment. Although no national database collects information about school injuries, it is estimated that 25% of all unintentional injuries to children happen at school (Milam & Royo, 2008).

Custodial personnel assist in the maintenance of school grounds, but school nurses must be aware of conditions and make recommendations to remedy unsafe situations. As school nurses provide first aid treatment for playground injuries, they may observe trends (e.g., a high number of injuries where faulty playground equipment or other factors influence higher injury rates) and request action. When injury trends are noted, school nurses work with maintenance departments and administration to advocate change and prevent future injury. In addition, nearly half of the states have adopted a policy directing schools to complete a report when serious injury occurs on school properties (Brener et al., 2007). School nurses also assist with physical adaptations for students with special needs (e.g., ramps, electric doors); they work to ensure safety in and around schools; and they are mindful of visual, thermal, and acoustic factors in school buildings, as well as aesthetic values. Additionally, they promote sanitation and the safety of the school bus system as well as food services.

Another area of growing concern is student safety after natural disasters or emergency situations. Recent earthquakes and potential bioterrorism events may impact schools or not permit children to return home at the end of a school day. School nurses are ideal persons to assist in disaster/emergency relief. Students do spend much of their time in school and local schools are often designated as shelters in times of disasters (NASN, 2011b). School nurses can assist in the development of emergency plans, as well as provide care and comfort to children and their families in times of emergencies.

Health Education and Health Promotion

Another main function of school nursing practice involves education and health promotion. This includes planned and incidental teaching of health concepts and

EVIDENCE-BASED PRACTICE

School Nursing

A review of the literature identified seven studies that investigated the impact of school-located influenza vaccination (SLIV) program on rates of absenteeism. Six of the articles compared schools who participated in SLIV programs with control schools. Results from all the studies indicated children who were vaccinated had fewer days of being absent.

Nursing Implications

Although school nurses often work with individual children, they also look at the school community as a whole and should conduct interventions that will benefit the whole. School nurses must also collect data and determine the effectiveness of their treatments. Finally, school nurses must also remember the goals of the institution in which they work (education) and strive to meet these goals (i.e., increased attendance) while at the same time protecting the public's health.

Reference: Hull, H. F., & Ambrose, C. S. (2011). The impact of school-located influenza vaccination programs on student absenteeism. A review of the U.S. literature. Journal of School Nursing, 27(1), 34–42. doi: 10.1177/1059840510389182 health curriculum development. In some states, school nurses even teach the regular health classes. Education may be one-on-one to help a child obtain better control over asthma or to explain to a newly diagnosed diabetic student what is occurring in his body. As an educator, the school nurse may also teach an entire class regarding a student's severe food allergy or the need for proper hand hygiene. The school nurse explains in simple terms what allergies are and helps students understand that allergies are not contagious, what to do in the case of an allergic reaction, and the importance of not sharing foods that may contain potential allergens (Green & Reffel, 2009; Wolfe & Selekman, 2002).

Because school nurses are trusted by students, students listen to them. Educational subjects are limitless, but should always apply to the specific needs of the children in the school. The nurse must use creativity and autonomy to identify and prioritize needs. A school nurse may also teach about basic first aid, nutrition, physical exercise, and seat belt safety, or provide information about careers in the health care professions.

In addition to lecture or verbal teaching, education may also be in the form of bulletin board notices, newsletters, or in-service presentations for educators and parents. These activities integrate health information with students' daily living experiences to build positive attitudes toward health and to establish sound health practices that will carry forward into adulthood.

Screenings: Opportunities for Teaching

Most local school districts provide some type of health screening services, usually through the school nurse or local health care providers. Although the goal of all screening is to promote early intervention, screening also provides the school nurse many opportunities to teach students and staff. Referral information resulting from screening results is usually given to parents, and school nurses may contact parents to encourage follow-through. Children who are not present for school screenings may not receive the benefits of these screenings (e.g., homeschooled and private school students). School nurses often help to coordinate screening resources and benefits, and they often carry out additional screenings for students who were absent when mass screenings were held.

Vision

The 2006 SHPPS noted that 93.4% of reporting school districts offered vision screening (Brener et al., 2007). School nurses often oversee routine vision screenings at periodic intervals so that vision problems that can interfere with learning may be detected and treated early (e.g., nearsightedness, farsightedness, strabismus, amblyopia). School nurses also are involved in follow-up to ensure that corrective eyewear is obtained. Local Lions Clubs may be involved in paying for area optometrists to assist with or direct screenings or to provide follow-up care.

Hearing

Hearing screenings were reported by 92% of districts (Brener et al., 2007). These mass screenings are done to detect any serious hearing deficits that may be related to recurrent ear infections or some type of sensorineural hearing loss. *Sensorineural hearing loss* involves the inner ear or the nerves leading from the inner ear. It is permanent and cannot be surgically or medically corrected (American Speech-Language-Hearing Association, n.d.).

Miscellaneous Health Screenings

Height, weight, and sometimes blood pressure and cholesterol screenings are done on a regular basis to monitor normal growth and development and allow for early intervention with populations who are especially susceptible to hypertension and heart disease.

In some areas, scoliosis screening is also done, frequently during middle school years or in fifth grade, to permit early detection and referral for medical intervention (e.g., bracing, surgery). Scoliosis may be congenital, but is often idiopathic (Lewis & Bear, 2011). Some 66% of districts reported performing scoliosis screenings (Brener et al., 2007). In Texas and some other areas of the country, acanthosis nigricans (hyperpigmentation from various causes, but sometimes a symptom of diabetes) screenings are being done to look for early markers of type 2 diabetes, especially in high-risk populations (Texas Department of Health Services, 2011).

Oral and Dental Health: Teaching and Referral

Dental caries affect more than half of school-age children and are the most common chronic disease for that age group. In 2010, about 7% of children ages 2 to 17 had unmet dental needs because their families could not afford dental care (Sondick et al., 2011). An estimated 16.3 million children do not have any dental insurance, a rate 2.6 times greater than those who do not have medical insurance (Lewis, Mouradian, Slayton, & Williams, 2007). Minority groups tend to have worst rates of dental caries. School days are lost to dental problems and dental visits, with poor children being almost twice as likely to suffer from dental caries (CDC, 2011b). The cost for dental services in 2010 was estimated to be $108 billion (CDC, 2011b).

School nurses can address dental health issues in a variety of ways. At a community level, they can educate the public about the benefits of dental fluoride treatments. They can advocate for fluoridation of drinking water, school-provided fluoride rinses or gels, and dental sealant programs. These are all cost-effective, proven methods of reducing dental caries in school-age children. At the classroom level, school nurses can provide dental education and provide toothbrushes, toothpaste, and floss to ensure that students are able to practice good dental hygiene habits. Local organizations and businesses often will donate such supplies. Many programs from the American Dental Association, the CDC, and other organizations provide resource materials.

At an individual level, school nurses can assist in finding resources for those with no dental health insurance. Finally, school nurses can successfully educate parents, especially those who are immigrants or have different cultural beliefs, regarding the importance of oral and dental health (Brown, Canham, & Cureton, 2005; Swan, Barker, & Hoeft, 2010).

Dental screenings or clinics may be conducted to determine the incidence of dental caries, especially in elementary school children, and to encourage follow-up with local dentists for necessary restorations. At the most recent national survey of schools, only 29% of districts reported performing some type of oral health screening (Brener et al., 2007).

Promotion of a Healthful School Environment

A third function of school nursing practice includes maintaining and promoting a healthful school environment. Promotion of healthful school living emphasizes planning a daily schedule for monitoring healthful classroom experiences, extracurricular activities, school breakfasts and lunches, emotional climate, discipline programs, and teaching methods. It also includes screening, observing, and assessing students to identify needs early and to report illegal drug use, bullying, suspected child abuse, and violations of environmental health standards. Health promotion also involves the nurse in supporting the physical, mental, and emotional health of school personnel by being an accessible resource to teachers and staff regarding their own health and safety.

Proper Nutrition and Exercise

Many factors can affect the school environment—heating, cooling, lighting, safe playgrounds, and policies and practices to limit bullying and social aggression or other forms of school violence. The school cafeteria and physical education activities can promote health or contribute to obesity and sedentary lifestyles.

Obesity

Obesity rates have increased for all children. Since 1980, they have doubled for children between ages 2 to 5 and adolescents (ages 12 to 19). Rates have tripled for those between ages 6 and 11 years. Approximately 12.5 million children over the age of 2 are considered obese (CDC, 2011c). In 2008, an estimated $147 billion was spent on medical care for the obese (CDC, 2011d). Obesity often begins in childhood and becomes a risk factor for cardiovascular disease and diabetes later in life. With the increase in child obesity rates, the number of children diagnosed with type 2 diabetes continues to rise, especially among youth of minority race/ethnicity. It is estimated that there are 13,600 newly diagnosed youth under the age of 20 diagnosed with type 2 diabetes annually (National Diabetes Education Program, 2011).

As children become older, families have less impact on food choices, and peers begin to have more influence. Results of the 2009 YRBS indicate that almost 88% of those surveyed ate fewer than five servings of fruits and vegetables per day during the 7 days before the survey, and 29.2% drank at least one can or bottle of soda or soft drink everyday for the 7 days before the survey (CDC, 2010c).

School nurses can do many things to assist with the obesity epidemic. They can advocate for health and physical activity classes. Resnick et al. (2009) found that a nurse-implemented, parent-directed program in the school decreased obesity among students. The 2009 YRBS revealed that 43.6% of children surveyed were not enrolled in physical education classes (CDC, 2010c). Parents are supportive of increasing physical exercise and emphasizing nutritional foods in the school setting (Murphy & Polivka, 2007; Stalter, Kaylor, Steinke, & Barker, 2010). A number of weight control programs for overweight children and adolescents are available through schools, health departments, community health centers, health maintenance organizations (HMOs), and private groups.

Undernutrition

Poor nutrition and obesity are not uncommon among adolescents, whose diets often consist of snacks with limited nutritional value interspersed among unhealthful meals. *Undernutrition* can also have serious consequences, one being an impact on the academic performance of children. Irritability, lack of energy, and difficulty concentrating are only some of the problems that arise from skipped meals or consistently inadequate nutrition (Sweeney & Horishita, 2005). Infection and illness that lead to loss of school days can affect academic progress and interfere with the acquisition of basic skills, such as reading and mathematics. Undernutrition is frequently associated with poverty and hunger, but social pressure to be thin can also spark purposeful undernutrition.

School nurses can advocate for better nutritional choices in the lunchroom and vending machines. This may include approaching the legislature to limit soft drink sales in public schools. They can also teach all grade levels regarding proper nutrition, and they can educate students and parents alike about nutritious snacks in contrast to snacks with little food value. School nurses may also work with staff to provide nutrition and exercise programs.

Eating Disorders

Eating disorders are another area of concern. Issues with body image and control are at the heart of *anorexia nervosa* and *bulimia nervosa*, common problems for adolescent girls. These diseases have emotional causes that pose complex challenges to treatment. School nurses must be aware of the signs and symptoms of eating disorders and be proactive in identifying students at risk. Scoliosis screenings are an optimal time to also observe for eating disorders, as examination of the spine allows for visualization of the body core. School nurses can work with students to develop a healthier self-concept and identify outside treatment resources (National Eating Disorders Association, 2008).

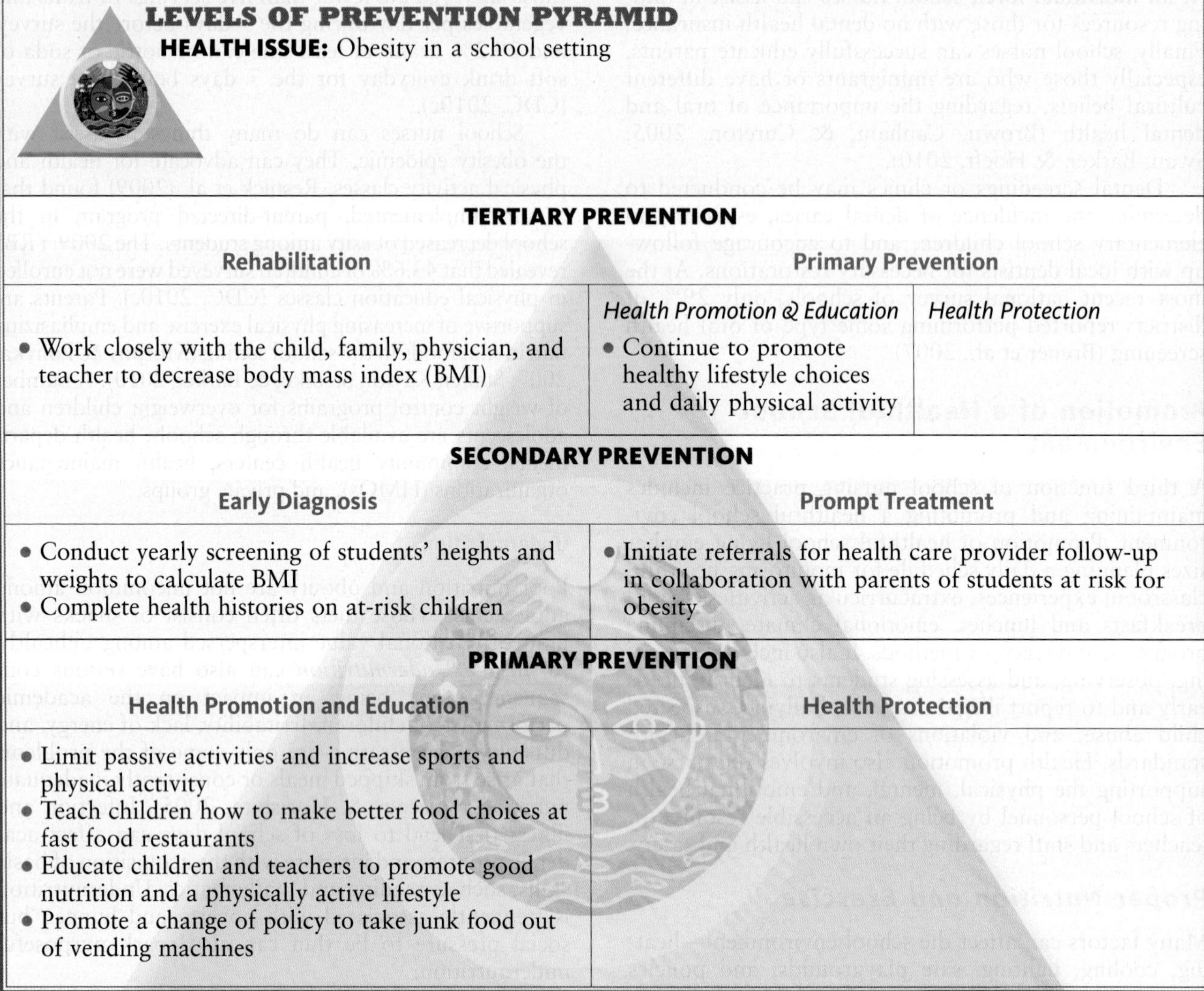

LEVELS OF PREVENTION PYRAMID

HEALTH ISSUE: Obesity in a school setting

TERTIARY PREVENTION		
Rehabilitation	**Primary Prevention**	
	Health Promotion & Education	*Health Protection*
• Work closely with the child, family, physician, and teacher to decrease body mass index (BMI)	• Continue to promote healthy lifestyle choices and daily physical activity	
SECONDARY PREVENTION		
Early Diagnosis	**Prompt Treatment**	
• Conduct yearly screening of students' heights and weights to calculate BMI • Complete health histories on at-risk children	• Initiate referrals for health care provider follow-up in collaboration with parents of students at risk for obesity	
PRIMARY PREVENTION		
Health Promotion and Education	**Health Protection**	
• Limit passive activities and increase sports and physical activity • Teach children how to make better food choices at fast food restaurants • Educate children and teachers to promote good nutrition and a physically active lifestyle • Promote a change of policy to take junk food out of vending machines		

Adolescent High-Risk Behaviors

Mortality and morbidity rates for adolescents are low overall and demonstrate considerable improvement since the early 1900s. Many of the health issues that modern adolescents face are a result of their own choices and high-risk activity; for example, sexual activity, substance abuse, injury, and violence are all high-risk behaviors in which adolescents can choose to participate or not. The effects of such choices may not be discovered for many years. From 2003 to 2006, a good number of states developed policies to address alcohol and drug use (increasing from 22% to 42%), STD prevention (up from 17.6% to 32%), suicide prevention (from 16% to 28%), and tobacco use (rising from 19.6% to 40%) (Brener et al., 2007).

Sexual Activity: Teen Pregnancy and Sexually Transmitted Diseases

Sexual activity is a sensitive issue. However, the 2009 YRBS indicates that 46% of students surveyed reported they had had sexual intercourse and 13.8% had had sexual intercourse with four or more partners in their lifetime (CDC, 2010c). Each year, about half of new STD cases in the United States occur among those between the ages of 15 and 24 (CDC, 2011e). The overall rates of syphilis, gonorrhea, chlamydia, human papillomavirus (HPV), and herpes simplex virus are climbing.

Providing STD services and HIV/AIDS education can be a daunting task. Young people with STDs are often afraid or embarrassed to seek help. Those who have been exposed to the HIV virus may not know that they are infected.

Although in some communities the school-based clinic dispenses condoms, in other areas, school nurses may be restricted in what safer-sex products they can provide. However, nurses *can* provide teens with education and with information about resources that are available outside of school property. School nurses can promote, at the local and state level, the HPV vaccine that guards against cervical cancer. They can also promote abstinence or delaying sexual initiation, as well as fostering safer-sex messages that promote the use of condoms. Sex education is effective at both delaying the onset of sexual activity and decreasing sexual activity in adolescents who are already sexually active. It is also effective in increasing safer-sex practices, knowledge of the efficacy of birth control methods, and overall sexual knowledge (Community Guide Branch EAOP, 2009).

School nurses are sometimes restricted by state and/or district policies from addressing the issues of sex education and STD (including HIV) prevention. However, they can inform students and others in the community about the existence of multimodal youth development programs and family planning programs, which are often stationed strategically in inner cities, near schools, or in school-based clinics. These agencies are empowered to provide birth control information and counseling to young people.

Substance Abuse

Substance abuse among young people was almost unknown before 1950 and rare before 1960. Now, adolescent drug experimentation and use poses serious physical and psychological threats. By the time they complete high school, 36.8% of teens report having tried marijuana, 46.3% have used tobacco, and 72.5% have consumed alcohol (CDC, 2010c). Over half (50.8%) of those who smoke have tried to quit, and 21.1% of those who have consumed alcohol tried it before they were 13 years old (CDC, 2010c).

School nurses can assist in programs targeting all substance abuse. Successful programs focus on protective factors, instead of just high-risk behaviors. The programs focus more on the root causes, or why youth choose high-risk activities. When school nurses focus on developing and advocating for protective factors that assist youth to feel part of their community (Mayberry, Espelage, & Koenig, 2009), they can help teens avoid the onset of substance abuse.

School nurses can also provide resources for smoking cessation and substance abuse programs. Pbert et al. (2011) found that school nurses are successful members of school smoking cessation programs. In addition to school-based education, programs of peer leadership and parental education/involvement and community-wide task forces have been developed to lobby for local legislation and strengthen community–school ties. School nurses can be advocates at a community level by lobbying the city council for tougher ordinances controlling advertising content and zoning (especially near schools). School nurses often work in conjunction with law enforcement officials, school district administrators, and other community agencies to ensure compliance with local regulations and prevent or delay tobacco use. Other groups, such as 4-H clubs, religious congregations, the Catholic Youth Organization, and Boy Scouts, use peer counseling to influence young people to assume responsibility for healthy lifestyles, with the goal of developing decision-making skills that lead to healthy lifestyle choices in adolescence and through adulthood. The school nurse participates in and supports existing programs in addition to counseling and referring young people who need help.

Mental Health Issues and Suicide

Depression, schizophrenia, and eating disorders may first appear during adolescence. It is estimated that 1 of 10 children suffers from a mental illness severe enough to impair them in some way (National Institute of Mental Health, 2008). Many adolescents are reluctant to seek help for emotional problems, or help may not be readily available to them. It is estimated that only one of five of those who need treatment actually receives it. Common mental health disorders in adolescence include anxiety, depression, ADHD, eating disorders, bipolar disorder, and schizophrenia (NIMH, 2008). Suicide is the third leading cause of death for young people between ages 15 and 24; it is the sixth leading cause of death in children between ages 5 and 14 (American Academy of Child & Adolescent Psychiatry [AACAP], 2008). In 2009, 20.5% of all high school students reported that they had either seriously considered or attempted suicide in the past year (CDC, 2010c). Girls attempt suicide more frequently than boys, but the actual suicide rate (those who successfully kill themselves) is higher among boys (Nock et al., 2008). School nurses must be aware of the signs and symptoms of mental illness and suicidal intentions. They can work with school psychologists, social workers, and other mental health workers to address the needs of the students. They can also provide grief counseling to peers after a student commits suicide. Recent suicides by youth have been attributed to the students being bullied. School nurses also need to be aware of the increased issues related to bullying in the schools and in cyberspace. They must watch for signs and symptoms as well as provide interventions to make people aware of and stop bullying (Dresler-Hawke & Whitehead, 2009).

Abuse

In 2009, a total of 10 children in every 1,000 had substantiated reports of maltreatment, with younger children (0 to 15 years of age) at the greatest risk (Federal Interagency Forum on Child and Family Statistics, 2011). Girls tended to be maltreated more often than boys. Black, non-Hispanic youth were also at greater risk. Most victims suffered from neglect (USDHHS, 2008). Child abuse prevention education programs can be found in many school districts as a primary preventive intervention. School nurses are required by law to report suspected or confirmed cases of abuse. In addition, school nurses can educate teachers and other school personnel regarding the signs and symptoms of abuse. Abuse can also include issues related to bullying and school violence. Eisbach and Driessnack (2010) completed a small qualitative study of school nurses and pediatric/mental health practitioners that highlighted the difficulty nurses have in dealing with this issue and their frustration with reporting abuse that often leads to subsequent inaction by authorities. It is important to be well versed in subtle signs and symptoms of maltreatment and develop strong collaborative relationships

LEVELS OF PREVENTION PYRAMID

HEALTH ISSUE: Cervical cancer community setting

TERTIARY PREVENTION	
Rehabilitation	**Primary Prevention**
	Health Promotion & Education — *Health Protection*
• Provide nursing support groups after hysterectomy and other treatment	
SECONDARY PREVENTION	
Early Diagnosis	**Prompt Treatment**
• Promote regular Pap smears • Provide Pap smear and high-risk screening counseling at local health fairs	• Provide resources of medical services available for women diagnosed with cervical cancer
PRIMARY PREVENTION	
Health Promotion and Education	**Health Protection**
• Promote healthy lifestyle choices that will decrease risk of human papillomavirus (HPV) (use of condoms, decrease tobacco use, food containing vitamin C and beta carotene) • Provide HPV vaccine at appropriate age • Educate public on risks related to cervical cancer (HPV vaccine, multiple sex partners) • Educate women to get regular Pap smears	

with social service professionals. For more information on health problems and issues concerning children and adolescents, see Chapter 22.

School-Based Health Clinics

Because of the complex and intertwined emotional, physical, and educational needs of school-age children and adolescents, a more comprehensive interdisciplinary approach to services is needed than the piecemeal approaches attempted previously. School nurses are able to do much to influence schoolchildren's health. However, often they need to refer the children to a health care provider. Yet, more parents are working and less available to take care of their children's health care needs during the day. **School-based health centers (SBHCs)** provide ready access to health care for large numbers of children and adolescents during school hours, reducing absences from school due to health care appointments. SBHCs provide a variety of services in a user-friendly manner at a convenient location.

In 2007 to 2008, there were more than 1,909 SBHCs in the United States, up from only 200 in 1990 (Strozer, Juszczak, & Ammerman, 2010). These clinics are generally established inside the schools. They are distributed in high schools (33%), middle schools (7.8%), and elementary schools (9.6%). Some clinics provide services only to schoolchildren, whereas others extend services to their families and to other neighborhood families with preschool-age children. Most centers are open full-time. Those located in middle or high schools may provide pregnancy testing and STD diagnosis and treatment, as well as birth control. However, many SBHCs do not provide contraceptive services on the school site because of school district policy or state law (Strozer et al., 2010).

SBHCs are staffed by interdisciplinary teams of helping professionals, paraprofessionals, and other staff and can include nurses, nurse practitioners, and social workers. Many hospitals, HMOs, and health departments are sponsors of these school clinics, because it is a cost-effective way to decrease visits to the emergency department and promote health, especially to underserved groups such as adolescents. Third-party billing, especially to access Medicaid funding, is increasingly more common among SBHCs, and private foundations have also been instrumental in providing financial and technical support. School nurses support the clinics by referring students who need additional attention. In some areas, school-linked health centers are utilized. These clinics are not on school property, but may be nearby or easily accessible through mass transit. Schools refer students to these centers and have established collaborative, working relationships that promote information sharing and support (Strozer et al., 2010).

Evaluation research has demonstrated that SBHCs are effective in increasing student access to health care. The majority (64%) of clients surveyed in Oregon indicated they would have not been able to receive care that day had it not been for the SBHC, and 72% said they would have missed class if the SBHC were not available (Oregon State Government, 2011). SBHCs also have been found to increase the use of contraception in sexually active teenage girls (Ethier et al., 2011).

SCHOOL NURSING CAREERS

School nurses must be able to work autonomously. They need excellent communication skills and the ability to prioritize and collaborate with many others (professional and nonprofessional). The pay for school nurses depends on location and employer (health department or school district). In some places, the wage may be lower than acute care nurses, but the health insurance and benefits package is usually quite extensive. School nurses are sometimes frustrated working in an educational setting, in which health may be a secondary priority, but their expertise is generally highly valued. In addition, school nurses may become involved with other issues in the school, such as violence prevention, that extend beyond the traditional role of the nurse.

There are many positive reasons to work as a school nurse: School nurses generally do not work on weekends, many have contracts that give them the summer off, and the daily work schedule and holidays often coincide with those of the nurse's own school-age children, thus allowing a parent to be home with children during off-school hours. Finally, for most of those employed as school nurses, it is a wonderful and rewarding experience to work with children whose eagerness and innocence can often refresh the soul. It is an opportunity to protect and heal our future leaders, who may become the ones who will eventually protect and heal the world.

PERSPECTIVES
VOICES FROM THE COMMUNITY

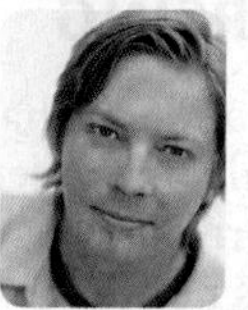

A great aspect of being a school nurse is being able to work with many different people. I like being able to work with people who aren't necessarily sick but can benefit from my help. Additionally, school nurses must become familiar with resources and people in the community and surrounding areas. By making friends and connections in multiple facilities, occupations, and the like, school nurses can involve local resources as well as specific individuals in improving the population. That is an essential aspect to recognize: nurses shouldn't be alone in working with the community; they should involve as many people as possible, because community members should be active in improving their own area.

Unfortunately, working as a school nurse takes a lot of effort and is time-consuming. Even with the work that has been done at the school, it makes me wonder just how long our interventions will last. Unlike working in a hospital, where results come in just a few days, school nurses must work tirelessly for long periods of time to see the fruits of their labors. Resources aren't as readily available as they are for other types of nursing. Being a school nurse requires learning how to get funding for projects. School nurses often don't have models to work from, as each situation may be unique. They must be innovative, resourceful, and dedicated in order to stick with a project long enough for it to be beneficial to the population.

My overall opinion on working as a community nurse has changed over the past few weeks. Being a school nurse has been hard, but rewarding. I know several students in my semester who don't really consider community nursing to be truly nursing practice. I would beg to differ; school nursing is probably the epitome of what nursing was meant to be. It is focused on service and improving the health and wellbeing of the populace. While nursing in the early days mainly dealt with fixing problems and injuries after they happened, everyone knows that an ounce of prevention is worth a pound of cure. Therefore, school nurses are doing the work that should benefit people the most. However, because their focus is on prevention, they seem to get little recognition for their work, since they are saving lives before they are endangered, they are saving teeth before they fall out, and they are saving families before they are lost. I believe their work is pivotal to the improvement of society.

Neil P., School Nurse

CORRECTIONS NURSING

Nurses who work within the criminal justice system—correctional facilities, prisons, jails, detention centers, and substance abuse treatment programs—work with clients in a range of ages from juvenile to elderly, both male and female (ANA, 2007b). The facilities in which they work can hold just a few inmates or may house over 30,000 at one time. In 2010, there were 1,605,127 state and federal prisoners (rate: 497 per 100,000 U.S. residents), a decrease of 9,228 prisoners in 2009 (Guerino, Harrison, & Sabol, 2007). The U.S. per capita rate of incarceration is the highest in the world, and approximately 15 million individuals are processed by the correctional system annually (Reznick, Comfort, McCartney, & Neilands, 2011; Walmsley, 2009). Tracking the number of nurses who work in correctional facilities is difficult. The last attempt, made in 2000, estimated the number to be 18,033 RNs (Spratley, Johnson, Sochalski, Fritz, & Spencer, 2002).

HISTORY OF CORRECTIONS NURSING

Although the correctional system of prisons and jails has been around for a very long time, it historically provided minimal, if any, health care to inmates. Prison was a punishment, and the inmates were viewed as not deserving of care that was being paid for from public dollars. The situation did not change until 1976, when the U.S. Supreme Court issued its decision regarding *Estelle v. Gamble*. The Supreme Court ruled that not providing medical services inflicted pain and denied inmates their Eighth Amendment rights. This decision led to major reforms in the corrections health system. Medical providers were hired and inmates' rights were established. These rights included (ANA, 2007b, p. 2):

- The right to access care
- The right to professional judgment
- The right to care that is ordered
- The right to informed consent
- The right to refuse treatment
- The right to medical confidentiality

Although the correctional health system is relatively new, it is under intense pressure from the courts to ensure that adequate and humane care is provided (ANA, 2007b). Several lawsuits have occurred, and unsolved issues in the correctional health care setting continue to be highlighted. Some main issues regard the provision of ethically appropriate and timely patient care for inmates. Ensuring that inmates' health needs are met—along with the growing number of inmates and the increasing intensity of their health concerns—has imposed a huge financial burden on systems that are already overtaxed. Funding for correctional health care derives from public tax dollars. Some have wondered if such care and expense should be given to incarcerated persons. This is an ethical dilemma nurses working in correctional facilities must face every day. Keeping equipment up-to-date and avoiding shortcuts can also be challenging. In an attempt to decrease costs and save money, most states utilize managed care organizations to provide some services for inmates. Correctional Medical Services (CMA, 2011) is the largest provider of prison health care in the nation. Some states may also utilize local HMOs (Russo, 2010).

Many institutions have a house clinic, medical unit, or infirmary. However, these clinics do not have the capability to provide all the services inmates may need. For example, if imaging procedures, such as magnetic resonance imaging (MRI) or computed tomography (CT) scans, are needed or specialty consultations required, inmates must go to other sources outside of the prison or jail. In these instances, most corrections' facilities use managed health care systems.

Corrections nurses work in on-site medical units housed in criminal justice facilities. These facilities can be local jails, or may be at state and federal prison. The staff members in these units focus on the individual, immediate, and ambulatory care needs of the patients. They also attend to emergency needs and may help manage chronic conditions. They often provide screenings and preventive services. Corrections nurses have the potential to assist inmates to obtain optimal health and thus save taxpayer dollars.

The challenge of corrections nursing is to maintain the fundamental nature of nursing in a challenging environment that is not primarily focused on health care and to remain nonjudgmental toward clients (ANA, 2007b). Correctional nurses may face many ethical dilemmas surrounding ensuring patient basic privacy but also maintaining personal safety. Today, corrections nurses work with a variety of clients.

Demographically, inmates differ from the general population. First, inmates have all committed some type of crime, with nearly half (52%) being violent crimes (Guerino et al., 2007). National statistics indicate a larger portion of Black (3,059 per 100,000) and Hispanic (1,252 per 100,000) male inmates than White male inmates (456 per 100,000). Males are still the majority population (93.2%) in state and federal correction facilities (Guerino et al., 2007). In addition, the inmate population is drawn disproportionately from lower socioeconomic backgrounds when compared with the general public. This increases their chances of having a long trajectory of poorer access to health care and treatment. Statistics show a greater disproportion of inmates who are chronically ill and have infectious diseases than the nonincarcerated population (ANA, 2007b).

EDUCATION

The preferred educational level for corrections nurses is a bachelor's degree. The level of skill, judgment, and autonomy needed by nurses who work in corrections is supported and developed within baccalaureate education. Some institutions may require additional coursework in criminal justice, decision-making, assessment, and administrative skills. Master's level nurses (specifically NPs) also are working in corrections, providing primary health care to inmates. National certification, through the National Commission on Correctional Health Care (NCCHC) as a certified correctional health professional (CCHP) or the American Correctional Association (ACA) as a certified corrections nurse (CCN), is available (ANA, 2007b).

FUNCTIONS OF CORRECTIONS NURSE

The prime responsibility of the corrections nurse is to restore and maintain the health of inmates by providing nursing care within correctional settings (ANA, 2007b). The work location does set corrections nurses apart as being the only nurses who enter their workplaces through metal detectors and grill gates and into a locked-down unit (FitzGerald, 2007). Yet, the knowledge and skill set of a corrections nurse overlaps the knowledge and skill sets of many other nursing specialties.

Corrections nurses use public, community, and school health nursing skills, along with skills acquired from the ER, occupational health, mental health, orthopedics, and ambulatory care specialties. Like public, community, and school health nurses, corrections nurses are autonomous and must make decisions on their own. They track and screen for communicable diseases. They assist in setting up resources so that inmates who are released can continue getting medical treatment. They also educate inmates and promote healthful lifestyles among them.

Corrections nurses often work in clinic settings, assisting the health care provider in assessing medical situations. They review sick call requests to determine what and if any action needs to be taken, and by whom (nurse or physician). They may also oversee the medical unit beds that house patients who suffer from a variety of conditions, such as neurotrauma requiring critical care or kidney disease requiring dialysis. They provide nursing care for inmates with uncontrolled diabetes, those with pneumonia needing IV antibiotics, inmates with mental health issues, or those undergoing withdrawal ("detox") from years of substance abuse (Laffan, 2005; Schoenly, 2010). They participate in administering medications, as many inmates receive a variety of medications. In addition, by law, inmates must have a physical assessment within 14 days of admittance. Corrections nurses often perform these assessments. Corrections nurses also provide assessment and assistance in occupational safety issues.

Finally, corrections nurses are called upon to assist in medical emergencies, anywhere in the facility, such as helping with an accident in a woodshop or evaluating an inmate too sick to leave his cell. If inmates need to go to a hospital or appointment outside the correctional facility, a correctional officer generally accompanies them, not the nurse. With so many responsibilities and the uncertainty of new issues, it is imperative for corrections nurses to prioritize their day (see Display 30.6). Because correctional facilities operate 24 hours a day, every day of the year, it is also vital that they also address emergency preparedness and disaster planning. *Continuity of operations plans* (COOP) are the operational guides used during disaster management in correctional facilities, and most also include Incident Command System (ICS) guidelines as outlined by the FEMA. The National Institute of Corrections publishes a guide for jail emergencies to assist corrections nurses in emergency preparedness. Taylor and Crianza (2011) provide vivid examples of natural disasters affecting a large jail system (over 10,000 inmates) and the need to plan for power, water, and telephone outages, as well as housing and moving prisoners under emergency conditions. In these situations, nursing and other staff are often asked to remain on-site for extended periods of time and while making arrangements for their own families.

Several common health concerns face corrections nurses. These concerns are mental health, drug abuse, and communicable diseases. As the inmate population grows, an increase in elderly and female inmates creates additional health concerns for correctional nurses. The following sections briefly describe some of these concerns, along with examples of what corrections nurses may do to address the issues facing them.

Mental Health Issues

The increasing number of inmates over the years may be attributed to the deinstitutionalization of individuals with mental illness in the 1970s. For example, in 1970, 368,000 beds were available for mental health services, but by 1992 only 84,000 remained (ANA, 2007b). Many people suffering from mental illness were left without assistance or support. As a result, they became homeless and, in many cases, committed crimes.

Mental health is a major concern in correctional facilities; 25% of jail inmates have been previously diagnosed with a mental illness before their incarceration (Wilper et al., 2009), with rates of mental illness of the incarcerated three to six times that of the regular population (Florida Council for Community Mental Health, 2010). Those who suffer from mental illness are three times as likely to have been physically or sexually abused in their lifetime, and 4.5% of state and federal inmates experience at least one incident of sexual victimization by staff or other inmates while in prison (Beck & Harrison, 2007). Those with mental illness tended to have longer sentences and cost more money while imprisoned due to staffing needs (Florida Council for Community Mental Health, 2010). Female, White, and young inmates tend to suffer from mental health issues more than other inmates (Glaze & James, 2010). That 74% of state inmates and 76% of local inmates with mental health concerns also suffer from substance abuse complicates the matter. Mental illness also impacts suicide rates. Between 2000 and 2007, the suicide rate in local jails (167 per 100,000) was six times higher than the rate of suicide in larger jails at 27 per 100,000 (Noonan, 2010). Inmates who committed violent crimes were twice as likely to commit suicide as those convicted of nonviolent crimes (Mumola & Karberg, 2010). One meta-analysis found a prevalence rate for traumatic brain injury (TBI) among the adult offender population of 60%, while the general population's rate is only 8.5% (Shiroma, Ferguson, & Pickelsimer, 2010). For more on mental illness and substance abuse, see Chapter 27.

Corrections nurses provide a good deal of mental health nursing care and assist in identifying undiagnosed conditions. Glaze and James (2010) found that one in every three state inmates and one in every six local jail inmates indicated that he had received mental health treatment upon admission. A postarrest diversion program, in which detainees are evaluated for mental health or substance abuse conditions, are highly recommended; one such program has reduced recidivism from 56% at prearrest to 19% for a postdiversion program (Heines, 2005; Mental Health America [MHA], 2008). A prearrest diversion program that trains police officers to identify persons with mental illness has also been successful in assisting with treatment and avoiding arrest.

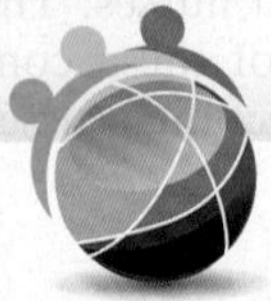

DISPLAY 30.6 A DAY IN THE LIFE OF A CORRECTIONAL NURSE

A day in my life depends on whether or not I am working at the infirmary or on the forensic unit. I will begin with the prison's infirmary.

I work 12-hour day shifts, so my day begins at 06:00 and ends at 18:30. As on any nursing unit or floor, I take report from the night shift charge registered nurse (RN). Within our infirmary, we have both a medical side and a psychiatric side where report is given. Following report, I decide with the other nurses whether or not I am going to be responsible for the medical or psychiatric patients, or the walk-ins (acute/emergency care patients). If I, for instance, take the medical side for the day, I will set up the medications and then wait for the other nurse to set up his or her medications for the psychiatric in-patients. We usually do what we call "pill line" together. Following pill line, I return to the nursing station and do my charting. Currently, we have a quadriplegic and paraplegic on our medical side who require a lot of personal care. We also have recently had several patients with MRSA (methicillin-resistant *Staphylococcus aureus*) requiring fairly extensive dressing/packing changes along with IV antibiotics. So with this in mind, following my charting, I will have officers escort the MRSA patients out to a trauma bed in order for me to perform the dressing change and/or administration of IV antibiotics (usually vancomycin) that take 1 to 2 hours to complete. Following care, these inmates return to their medical cells, and I do my usual charting. The quadriplegic and paraplegic inmates have call lights, so I have to attend to their needs when called. This may consist of feedings, diaper changes, and repositioning. Depending on the day, I will administer showers or bed baths for them. We also currently have an inmate with Parkinson's disease and comorbid psychiatric disorder and neuropathy, who also requires a great deal of care. These are the types of inmates for whom we try to get compassionate releases, so that they can be sent out to nursing homes. Unfortunately, that has not happened yet. I say that because we are not staffed for this kind of care. With this kind of patient care, I tend to remain quite busy. Fortunately for me, the other nurses are very kind and help me along the way. Usually the nurse who does the psychiatric side does not have quite the "hands-on" patient care and is usually very happy to help. In fact, we all help each other with our respective areas. Even though I am responsible for the medical in-patients, I still might take a walk-in or two and do some of the "q30-minute checks" on the psychiatric side. At the end of the day, I make sure that all my charting is done and then go on my way. There is quite a bit more actually involved, but it is difficult to explain all the situations that may develop.

On the forensic unit, I show up once again at 06:00 and take report from the night RN. On this unit I, along with our one LPN, am responsible for passing all the medications and performing all the blood sugars and insulin administrations for the diabetics in the morning, noon, and afternoon. I have to perform an extensive mental health note on all the inmates in the maximum-security unit of this building, which consists of 10 to 12 inmates on average. I then have to do a less extensive mental health nursing note on all the inmates in our B-section bottom tier, which consists of approximately 20 to 24 inmates. Following all my charting, I enter in all the diabetic care and scan all the medications passed on our electronic MAR (medication administration record). Following all of these duties, I usually make sure that all the medications are current and check for any expired critical medications that might need reordering. I may have to do some blood draws and give some shots for those inmates on forced medications. I consider this unit more of a nursing management unit rather than a hands-on patient care unit.

I decided to work at the prison for a number of reasons. First, I began my nursing career at the state hospital, and once I got sucked into the state system, I felt like working for the state throughout my career would be a very beneficial decision for me and for my family. The state offers great benefits, security, and a very good retirement. In the process of receiving my RN degree, I worked with a preceptor at the prison and enjoyed the opportunities that it offered. I really enjoyed the staff and the experience that they brought to the environment. Second, the environment was one in which I found a great deal of interest. During my clinical rotations at the prison, I was exposed to a world that many other people don't have the opportunity to experience. The prison environment certainly is not for everyone, but I felt it was for me. Once I received my RN license, I transferred from the state hospital to the prison, along with all my same benefits. Third, I love mental health nursing and that is what I am currently specializing in at the university. I am in my second year in the psych APRN program. It may sound strange that I just didn't stay at the state hospital, but I really wanted to gain the variety of medical experience the prison had to offer—on top of the mental health experience I already had. Once I graduate with my psych APRN, I plan to stay and retire after 20 years—which will only be about 12 more years—then teach perhaps until I fully retire and golf!

Travis H, Corrections Nurse

PERSPECTIVES
VOICES FROM THE COMMUNITY

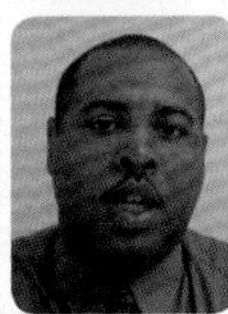

The prison is, in my opinion, a very good place to work. I believe that every student should experience nursing within corrections. I have worked floor nursing before, and working at the prison is much better. Although it can get crazy and chaotic from time to time, the atmosphere is much more laid back. Nurses at the prison seem to have a lot more autonomy than do nurses at other facilities or companies. The prison offers nurses a chance to experience many different skills. You might not gain absolute proficiency in any one skill, but you will gain many skills, and you will become very good at many of them. The nice thing is that nurses come from many different backgrounds, and so they can and will certainly help you and teach you what they know to help with your own skill base. I guarantee that if you work at the prison, you will get to see and experience things that people in normal society will never get the opportunity to see. Come to the prison, and you will get to be a medical nurse, a psych nurse, a triage nurse, an orthopedic nurse, and you can get to do the medical/psychiatric intake screenings for all the new or parole violation inmates who come to the prison on a daily basis. There is probably more, but certainly keep your minds and options open for a great and secure career.

Travis H., Correctional Nurse

Correctional nurses assist in multiple medication administrations per day to ensure that inmates receive the medications needed for their mental illnesses. They can also provide counseling regarding medication usage and assist inmates in understanding the side effects of their medication, which for some are many. Corrections nurses advocate for medication changes when they note severe side effects or a change in the mental status of inmates. Nurses can facilitate setting up medication support groups to allow inmates an opportunity to discuss concerns regarding their medications. They also can assist inmates in understanding the importance of taking their medication.

As inmates prepare to leave the institution, corrections nurses assist in finding outpatient mental health clinics and other resources that will provide support and further treatment for the inmate. Finally, corrections nurses can provide education and training to other corrections workers regarding signs and symptoms of mental illness and the impact mental health has on decision-making and the general health of a person.

Drug Abuse

Drug abuse by inmates is very high. Mumola and Karberg (2010) estimate that half of all federal prison inmates used drugs, which is a 5% increase from 1997. Female drug use increased by 11% during this same time period. All types of drug use increased, except crack cocaine, which declined from 25% in 1997 to 21% in 2004. Drug treatment programs are essential in correctional facilities. Corrections nurses can assist in identifying those in need of the treatment and assessing their willingness to participate. Of the drug users in prison, 40% of state and 49% of federal inmates had participated in treatment programs (Mumola & Karberg, 2010). Corrections nurses also provide nursing care as patients withdraw from substances while in prison. Withdrawal can cause life-threatening symptoms that need immediate medical attention.

In addition, corrections nurses can organize and provide support groups to assist inmates in staying sober and drug-free. They can advocate for the inclusion of Alcoholics Anonymous, Narcotic Anonymous, and Al-Anon services in the correctional facility. Counseling can be offered to assist inmates as they leave the facility,

EVIDENCE-BASED PRACTICE

Corrections Nursing

De Leon (2010) conducted a literature review to determine if there is substantial, empirical evidence that therapeutic communities (TCs) effectively change behavior better than other substance abuse programs. TCs are commonly used in the prison setting as treatment for drug users. An analysis of the literature indicated three subsets of evidence: case studies of single programs; comparison studies of single programs; and meta-analytic studies. In all three subsets, the evidence indicates that TCs are effective. However, additional research with a more rigorous design (such as randomly controlled trials) is needed to strengthen the argument.

Nursing Implications

It is important for nurses in any setting to know if the treatment they provide is based on evidence and is effective. It is inappropriate and unprofessional for nurses to perform activities and treatments just because it traditionally has always been done. It is also important for nurses to evaluate current treatment programs to ensure they are the most effective treatment available.

Reference: De Leon, G. (2010). Is the therapeutic community an evidence-based treatment? *International Journal of Therapeutic Communities, 31*(2), 104–128.

LEVELS OF PREVENTION PYRAMID

HEALTH ISSUE: Sexually transmitted disease (STD) in correctional facilities

TERTIARY PREVENTION

Rehabilitation	Primary Prevention	
	Health Promotion & Education	*Health Protection*
• Work closely with inmates and physician to decrease side effects of STD (i.e., cervical cancer)	• Continue to promote responsible sexual behavior	

SECONDARY PREVENTION

Early Diagnosis	Prompt Treatment
• Provide STD screening upon entering facility • Provide regular, routine STD screenings	• Provide treatment for inmates diagnosed with STDs • Promote facility policies that allow for STD screenings and early treatment

PRIMARY PREVENTION

Health Promotion and Education	Health Protection
• Teach inmates how STDs are transmitted and what can be done to stop transmission (condoms, other preventive measures) • Teach signs and symptoms of commonly occurring STDs • Teach that gonorrhea and chlamydia are often asymptomatic, and so routine screening is important for individuals at risk	

so that they do not return to prior bad habits if and when they return to areas where drug and alcohol use is rampant (MHA, 2010). Returning to this environment increases their chances of returning to substance abuse, and inmates leaving prisons or jails need to be connected to outside resources.

Communicable Disease

In correctional facilities, communicable diseases can spread quickly. A large study of state and federal prisons noted that during the 2009 to 2010 influenza season, 79% of respondents reported some level of activity while 53% reported an "outbreak" of H1N1 flu and seven deaths also occurred. Although 90% of those responding stated that they had developed some type of general disaster or influenza emergency plan before flu season, it was noted that "the lack of a consistent system of disease surveillance across prison facilities" (inmates and staff) made it difficult to determine a true baseline and quickly contain or prevent an outbreak (Potter, Schwartz, Blackmore, & May, 2011, p. 73). Utilizing the TB control model from public health, correctional facilities can "prepare for, identify, investigate, and control outbreaks of communicable diseases" such as TB, methicillin-resistant *Staphylococcus aureus* (MRSA), and influenza (Parvez, Lobato, & Greifinger, 2010, p. 238). Several communicable diseases are of great concern in the correctional community (Schwartz, 2008). These include TB, hepatitis C, and STDs including HIV/AIDS. The concern of communicable disease is not only for the health of the inmate with the disease, but the susceptibility of all inmates, and ultimately the general public (if the inmate is released while still infected). Increased rates of these diseases are due to high-risk behaviors and increased rates of abusive behaviors, including rape (CDC, 2009). Also, most US prisons prohibit distribution of condoms or sterile injection equipment (Reznick et al., 2011).

A hallmark study, conducted by the RAND Corporation, indicated that inmates were four times as likely to have active TB, nine to ten times as likely to have hepatitis C, and five times as likely to be infected with HIV as the general population (Davis & Pacchiana, 2003). Data from the end of 2006 indicated that 19,842 male and 2,138 female inmates in state prisons have HIV/AIDS (CDC, 2009). On a positive note, the rates of HIV infection have been steadily declining among inmates since 1999. The number of inmates suffering from hepatitis C varies but is estimated to be between 12% and 31% (Tan, Joseph, & Saab, 2008). Inmates are at risk for hepatitis C because of the heavy injecting drug use among prisoners. One meta-analysis indicated that hepatitis C virus is three times higher for inmates who experienced tattooing while incarcerated than those who were not, with the odds ratio for women 1.44 when compared to men (Vescio et al., 2008).

TB is widespread among prisoners and rates are much higher than in the general population. According to the World Health Organization, TB rates of inmates were 23 times higher than the general public for a variety of reasons (Baussano et al., 2010). Some have reported it as high as 50 times greater than national averages and noted that prisons are increasingly reservoirs of drug-resistant TB (O'Grady et al., 2011). Because many inmates are homeless and abuse alcohol and/or drugs, they are more susceptible to TB; to compound the problem, the closeness of living conditions in jails and prisons facilitates the quick spread of TB (Baussano et al., 2010).

Correctional nurses must track rates of communicable diseases and provide education regarding the spread and treatment of those diseases. They must provide data on the number of cases of reportable diseases to the state health department. Corrections nurses can provide preventative care by offering immunizations to inmates. In addition, they can provide the necessary treatment for TB, STDs, and other diseases and can assist in advocating for measures to decrease the spread of disease within correctional facilities.

Corrections nurses can assist institutions by providing initial screenings upon arrival of inmates and periodic screening for certain diseases. The CDC (2009) recommends routine opt-out screenings for HIV and other communicable screenings if at risk. However, screening based solely on risk may miss many inmates, and so routine screening and treatment of inmates for various communicable diseases may be beneficial and cost effective (Tan et al., 2008).

Corrections nurses can also evaluate inmates for complications, such as retinal hemorrhage and liver problems, especially in those suffering from hepatitis C (Tan et al., 2008). For chronic communicable diseases, such as HIV/AIDS, corrections nurses can facilitate and organize peer educator groups. These have been found to be successful in educating inmates on HIV/AIDS, substance abuse, and low self-esteem (Zucker, 2009). Others have demonstrated increased HIV testing in inmates and their female partners, along with better communication about HIV-related topics (Reznick et al., 2011).

Successful programs also exist to assist inmates as they prepare for release. Corrections nurses can facilitate programs that empower inmates not to return to behaviors that increase their chance of contracting HIV (Clements-Nolle et al., 2008). Corrections nurses can also identify resources for inmates suffering from TB, so that they can continue their medication and treatment upon their release.

Future Trends

Due to advances in health care, longer prison terms, and more restrictive policies, inmates are older, sicker, and remain in prison longer than they did even 20 years ago. And historically, inmates have not taken good care of themselves. Hence, a 50-year-old inmate may have the health of a typical 65-year-old in the general public (ANA, 2007b). This surge in the inmate population is creating a lack of resources and beds for the aging inmate population.

Corrections nurses can increase efforts to empower inmates to take control of their health and can provide them with resources for health care access outside the prison, so that inmates will continue their care upon release. Corrections nurses can also be advocates and lobby state and federal legislatures to allocate funding for the additional resources needed within the prison system.

The female inmate population is also increasing. In addition to women's reproductive health issues, females tend to have higher rates of diabetes, HIV, STDs, mental illness, drug abuse, and emotional issues (ANA, 2007b). Researchers have found that women in jail have a high risk of cervical cancer and increased rates of abnormal Papanicolaou (Pap) test results (Binswanger, Mueller, Clark, & Cropsey, 2011). Corrections nurses can begin providing routine cervical and breast cancer screenings for female inmates. They can also provide counseling and emotional support.

Chronic disease, such as diabetes, heart disease, and asthma, are also increasing in the incarcerated population. Corrections nurses can facilitate chronic disease clinics to educate and empower inmates to better control their chronic conditions. To this end, corrections nurses need to conduct thorough family health histories, as many health conditions tend to have a genetic component, and employ screenings to identify conditions as soon as possible, so that early intervention can decrease complications and stop disease progression. They can follow up by promoting better nutrition and exercise habits, and medication management.

Ethical and legal issues in correctional nursing often center on the patient (most often someone convicted of a crime, possibly involving violence). Caring for the patient is vital, but custody must also be maintained and safety is essential (Kent-Wilkinson, 2009). Nurses must demonstrate nonjudgmental attitudes while at the same time ensuring protection from assault. Also, correctional workers (including nurses) may be subject to lawsuits brought by inmates for *deliberate indifference*, or perceived retaliation leading to an adverse action. For instance, this may include withholding health care that could lead to increased health problems in retaliation for the inmate filing grievances or formal complaints against the worker (Johnson, 2010).

CORRECTIONS NURSING CAREERS

Corrections nurses must have good mental health and assessment skills. They must be able to communicate well and be strong nursing advocates and strong advocates for their clients. They work in an intense environment where their safety could be threatened, and they must deal with clients who may be noncompliant, combative, and manipulative. Corrections nurses must also be very flexible and knowledgeable about a variety of nursing specialties.

Salaries depend upon the state, although they tend to be generally higher than in other nursing fields. Moreover, corrections nurses usually receive extensive employee benefits and insurance packages as government employees. Despite this, nursing shortages still occur (California Department of Personnel Administration, 2009). Corrections nurses have the ability to see amazing and awe-inspiring recoveries from illnesses and injuries because they work with the same patients for a longer time than hospital-based nurses. Correctional nursing provides an opportunity to work with a vulnerable population and practice the true art and science of nursing. You use every nursing skill you have learned and advocate for a population that is in need. It is a challenging, rewarding career.

SUMMARY

Nurses who work in publicly funded settings are critical to the health and wellbeing of their communities. Public health nursing interventions are essential in keeping our nation healthy. They may not be as visible as hospital nurses, who interact with each patient in the hospital, because PHNs often work from behind the scenes. Those who come in contact with them directly know of their worth, but much of the general population remains unaware of the role and the need for PHNs. PHNs deal with a number of issues including communicable diseases, chronic diseases, injuries, STDs, and substance abuse. They work with all ages, ethnicities, socioeconomic groups, and populations. Their emphasis is on health prevention and promotion.

School nurses work with school populations including students, their families, and the school staff. They provide individual care and are the bridge between medical providers and schools. School nurses provide health care services, such as direct nursing care, first aid, and specialized health care for children with special needs. They also provide health protection measures such as immunizations and environmental assessments. Finally, school nurses provide health promotion activities including education, health screenings, immunizations, and staff wellness programs. School-based clinics are another means of providing care for the school population. Children and adolescents are important population groups for community health nurses because their physical and emotional health is vital to the future of society and because they require guidance and direction.

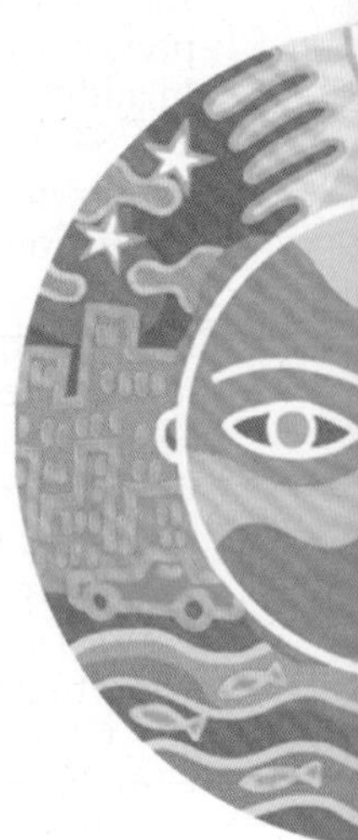

Corrections nurses work with inmates in federal, state, or local facilities, including drug treatment and juvenile detention centers. They provide individual care in facility clinics and infirmaries while also identifying and developing programs to address major health concerns of inmates, including mental illness, drug and alcohol abuse, and communicable diseases. The inmate population is growing older, staying longer, and suffering more from chronic disease. This, along with an increase in female inmates, brings additional challenges for corrections nurses.

All three nursing specialty areas impact the health of our communities. Due to the high level of nursing knowledge, communication skills, autonomy, and leadership needed for these nursing specialties, entry level should be at least a baccalaureate degree. Community nurses who work in public settings provide a valuable service needed to keep our nation healthy.

ACTIVITIES TO PROMOTE CRITICAL THINKING

1. As a government employee, a PHN must be careful not to lobby as part of her work duties. However, knowing the greatest health concerns of the population, how can PHNs serve as advocates for their clients (i.e., population) while remaining politically neutral?
2. What is the major cause of death among adolescents and children? What community-wide interventions could be initiated to prevent these deaths? Select one intervention and describe how you and a group of community health professionals might develop this preventive measure in your community. (Think outside the school setting.)
3. As a correctional nurse, you deal with people from a variety of backgrounds, social classes, and past crimes. How can your values and attitudes toward criminal activity impact your treatment of inmates? Does social class, race, age, or gender make any difference in how you feel about them?
4. One of the concerns expressed by correctional facility nurses is the antisocial behavior and manipulativeness of inmates, along with potential violence. How can a nurse working in a state prison effectively determine the health care needs of inmates?
5. Discuss possible methods of doing nutritional assessments in school-age children. What programs could be instituted to encourage healthier diets and increased exercise? What other factors might need to be considered? How could you, as a school nurse, work with schools and parents to increase physical activity and improve nutrition for school-age children and adolescents?
6. Describe possible benefits of school-based health centers (SBHCs). What are the most common misperceptions? What are frequent barriers to starting SBHCs? What steps can community health nurses take to promote community awareness and facilitate development of SBHCs in local schools?
7. Many of the chronic diseases plaguing society are attributable to people's behavior (such as eating habits, lack of exercise, tobacco use, etc.). Within your clinical group, debate the pros and cons of passing laws that restrict a person's right to behave as they wish, even if it impacts the overall population (increasing health care costs for all).
8. Most schools require that children entering school show proof of being fully immunized for a variety of communicable diseases. With a partner, discuss what would happen if schools no longer had this requirement. How else can immunizations be reinforced in the public?
9. Do you think that schools should require children with behavioral problems to be evaluated and required to take medication? Should taking that medication be a condition of their continuing enrollment? Who should pay for that evaluation and medication?
10. Many prisoners suffer from mental illness. List types of programs and/or support groups that the nurse could provide for these inmates. What about inmates not formally diagnosed with a mental illness?
11. Should inmates be required to pay for their health care (via work programs or other options) while in prison? Would it make them more accountable?
12. What are the ethical issues that nurses working in public health settings such as local health departments, schools or correctional facilities may face?

REFERENCES

Abrams, S. E. (2005). Changing times, changing needs, changing programs. *Public Health Nursing, 22*(3), 267–268.

American Academy of Child & Adolescent Psychiatry. (2008). *Fact sheet: Teen suicide*. Retrieved from http://www.aacap.org/page.ww?name=Teen+Suicide§ion=Facts+for+Families

American Diabetes Association (ADA). (2012). Position statement: Diabetes care in the school setting. *Diabetes Care, 35*(Suppl. 1), S76–S80. Retrieved from http://www.diabetes.org/assets/pdfs/schools/ps-diabetes-care-in-the-school-and-daycare-setting.pdf

American Nurses Association (ANA). (2007a). *Public health nursing: Scope and standards of practice*. Silver Spring, MD: Nursesbook.org.

American Nurses Association (ANA). (2007b). *Corrections nursing: Scope and standards of practice*. Silver Spring, MD: Nursesbook.org.

American Nurses Credentialing Center. (2008). *Public health nurse, advanced*. Retrieved from http://www.nursecredentialing.org/Certification/NurseSpecialties/AdvPublicHealth.aspx

American Speech-Language-Hearing Association. (n.d.). *Sensorineural Hearing Loss* Retrieved from http://www.asha.org/public/hearing/Sensorineural-Hearing-Loss/

Association of State and Territorial Directors of Nursing Public Health Preparedness Committee. (2007). *The role of the public health nurses in emergency preparedness and response*. Retrieved on from http://www.astdn.org/downloadablefiles/ASTDN%20EP%20Paper%20final%2010%2029%2007.pdf

Baussano, I., Williams, B. G., Nunn, P., Beggiato, M., Fedeli, U., Scano, F. (2010). Tuberculosis incidence in prisons: A systematic review. *PLoS Medicine*. Retrieved from http://www.plosmedicine.org/article/info:doi/10.1371/journal.pmed.1000381

Beaudoin, C. E. (2009). Evaluating a media campaign that targeted PTSD after Hurricane Katrina. *Health Communication,* 24(6), 515–523.

Beck, A.J., & Harrison, L. M. (2007). *Sexual victimization in state and federal prisons reported by inmates, 2007* [NCJ 219414]. Bureau of Justice Statistics Special Report. Retrieved from http://www.ojp.usdoj.gov/bjs/pub/pdf/svsfpri07.pdf

Beitsch, L.M., Brooks, R.G., Menachemi, N., & Grigg, M. (2011). Structure and functions of state public health agencies. *American Journal of Public Health, 101*(7), 1179–1186.

Bernstein, R. (2009, July 20). *Unprecedented global aging examined in new census bureau report commissioned by the National Institute on Aging*. U.S. Census Bureau News. Retrieved from http://www.census.gov/newsroom/releases/archives/aging_population/cb09-108.html

Binswanger, I. A., Mueller, S., Clark, C. B., & Cropsey, K. L. (2011). Risk factors for cervical cancer in criminal justice settings. *Journal of Women's Health, 20*(12), 1839–1845. doi: 10.1089/jwh.2011.2864.

Blackman, J. A., & Gurka, M. J. (2007). Developmental and behavioral comorbidities of asthma in children. *Journal of Developmental and Behavioral Pediatrics, 28*(2), 92–99.

Block, D. (2009). Reflections on school nursing and delegation. *Public Health Nursing,* 26(2), 112–113.

Boyer-Chu, L., & Wooley, S. F. (2008). *Give it a shot!* American School Health Association. Retrieved from http://www.ashaweb.org/files/public/Give_It_A_Shot!_Toolkit_2nd_edition.pdf

Brener, N. D., Wheeler, L., Wolfe, L. C., Vernon-Smiley, M., & Caldart-Olson, L. (2007). Health services: Results from the School Health Policies and Programs Study. *Journal of School Health,* 77(8), 464–486.

Brown, R. M., Canham, D., & Cureton, V. Y. (2005). An oral health education program for Latino immigrant parents. *Journal of School Nursing, 21*(5), 266–271.

California Department of Personnel Administration. (2009). *A comparison of total compensation of Registered Nurses in California public sector jurisdictions*. Retrieved from http://www.dpa.ca.gov/collbarg/news/Registered%20Nurses.htm

Careers in Focus: Nursing (4th ed.). (2011). New York: Ferguson (Infobase) Publishing.

Centers for Disease Control and Prevention (CDC). (2007). *Healthy Youth! Coordinated School Health Program*. Retrieved from http://cdc.gov/healthyyouth/CSHP/

Centers for Disease Control and Prevention (CDC). (2009). *HIV Testing implementation guidance for correctional settings*. Retrieved from http://www.cdc.gov/hiv/topics/testing/resources/guidelines/correctional-settings/index.htm

Centers for Disease Control and Prevention (CDC). (2010a). *National public health performance standards*. Retrieved from http://www.cdc.gov/od/ocphp/nphpsp/

Centers for Disease Control and Prevention (CDC). (2010b). Increasing prevalence of parent-reported attention-deficit/hyperactivity disorder among children—United States, 2003 and 2007. *Morbidity and Mortality Weekly Report*. Retrieved from http://www.cdc.gov/mmwr/preview/mmwrhtml/mm5944a3.htm?s_cid=mm5944a3_w

Centers for Disease Control and Prevention (CDC). (2010c). *2009 National Youth Risk Behavior Survey overview*. Retrieved from http://www.cdc.gov/healthyyouth/yrbs/pdf/us_overview_yrbs.pdf

Centers for Disease Control and Prevention (CDC). (2011a). *Health & academics data & statistics*. Retrieved from http://www.cdc.gov/healthyyouth/health_and_academics/data.htm

Centers for Disease Control and Prevention (CDC). (2011b). *Oral Health: Preventing cavities, gum disease, tooth loss, and oral cancers*. Retrieved from http://www.cdc.gov/chronicdisease/resources/publications/aag/pdf/2011/Oral-Health-AAG-PDF-508.pdf

Centers for Disease Control and Prevention (CDC). (2011c). *Obesity rates among all children in the United States*. Retrieved from http://www.cdc.gov/obesity/childhood/data.html

Centers for Disease Control and Prevention (CDC). (2011d). *Overweight and obesity economic consequences*. Retrieved from http://www.cdc.gov/obesity/causes/economics.html

Centers for Disease Control and Prevention (CDC). (2011e). *STD trends in the United States: 2010 National data for Gonorrhea, Chlamydia, and syphilis*. Retrieved from http://www.cdc.gov/std/stats10/trends.htm

Clements-Nolle, K., Marx, R., Pendo, M., Loughran, E., Estes, M., & Katz, M. (2008). Highly active antiretroviral therapy use and HIV transmission risk Behaviors among individuals who are HIV infected and were recently released from jail. *American Journal of Public Health, 98(4),* 661–666. doi: 10.2105/AJPH.2007.112656

Community Guide Branch Epidemiology and Analysis Program Office (EAOP). (2009). Prevention of HIV/AIDS, other STIs, and pregnancy: Group based comprehensive risk reduction interventions for adolescents. Retrieved from http://www.thecommunityguide.org/hiv/riskreduction.html

Correctional Medical Services, Inc (CMA). (2011). *CMS: Correctional Medical Services*. Retrieved from http://www.cmsstl.com/home.aspx

Crowder, S. J. (2010). Integrating the revised asthma guidelines into school nursing scope and standards of practice. *Journal of School Health, 80*(1), 44–48. doi: 10.1111/j.1746-1561.2009.00463

Council on School Health (2008). Role of the school nurse in providing school health services. *Pediatrics, 121*(5), 1052–1056. doi: 10.1542/peds.2008-0382.

Dang, M.T., Warrington, D., Tung, T., et al. (2007). A school-based approach to early identification and management of students with ADHD. *Journal of School Nursing, 23*(1), 2–12.

Davis, L., & Pacchiana, S. (2003). *Prisoner reentry: What are the public health challenges?* Retrieved from http://www.rand.org/pubs/research-breifs/RB6013

Dey, L. P. (2008). *About EpiPen®*. Retrieved from http://www.epipen.com/epipen_main.aspx

Decker, W. W., Campbell, R. L., Manivannan, V., Luke, A., St Sauver, J. L., Weaver, A., et al. (2008). The etiology and incidence of anaphylaxis in Rochester, Minnesota: a report from the Rochester Epidemiology Project. *Journal of Allergy and Clinical Immunology, 122*(6), 1161–1165.

Domrose, C. (2011). Unfilled school nurse positions jeopardize school healthcare. *Nurse.com*. Retrieved from http://news.nurse.com/apps/pbcs.dll/article?AID=2011109260036

Dresler-Hawke, E. K., Whitehead, D. (2009). The behavioral ecological model as a framework for school-based anti-bullying health promotion interventions. *The Journal of School Nursing, 25*(3), 195–204. doi: 10.1177/1059840509334364

Eisbach, S., & Driessnack, M. (2010). Am I sure I want to go down this road? Hesitations in the reporting of child maltreatment by nurses. *Journal for Specialists in Pediatric Nursing, 15*(4), 317–323. doi: 10.1111/j.1744-6155.2010.00259.x

Engelke, M. K., Guttu, M., Warren, M. B., & Swanson, M. (2008). School nurse case management for children with chronic illness: Health, academic, and quality of life outcomes. *Journal of School Nursing, 24*(4), 205–214. doi: 10.1177/1059840508319929

Epilepsy Foundation. (n.d.). *Diastat administration in schools: Summary of federal laws and selected cases*. Jeanne A. Carpenter Epilepsy Defense Fund. Retrieved from http://www.epilepsyfoundation.org/resources/epilepsy/loader.cfm?csModule=security/getfile&pageid=21461

Estelle v. Gamble. No. 75-929 (U.S. Supreme Court, 1976).

Ethier, K. A., Dittus, P. J., DeRosa, C. J., Chung, E. Q., Martinez, E., & Kerndt, P. R. (2011). School-based health center access, reproductive health care, and contraceptive use among sexually experienced high school students. *Journal of Adolescent Health, 48*(6), 562–565.

Farrington, D. P., & Ttofi, M. M. (2009). School-based programs to reduce bullying and victimization. Retrieved https://www.ncjrs.gov/pdffiles1/nij/grants/229377.pdf

Federal Interagency Forum on Child and Family Statistics. (2011). *America's children: Key national indicators of wellbeing, 2011*. Retrieved from http://www.childstats.gov/americaschildren/famsoc7.asp#30

Feldman, H. (2008). *Nursing leadership: A concise encyclopedia*. New York: Springer Publishing.

Ficca, M., & Welk, D. (2006). Medication administration practices in Pennsylvania schools. *Journal of School Nursing, 22*(3), 148–155.

FitzGerald, E. (2007). Inside job. *California Nurse, 103*(4), 10–19.

Florida Council for Community Mental Health. (2010). *Mentally ill inmates: Fact sheet*. Retrieved from http://www.fccmh.org/resources/docs/jails.pdf

Fritsch, S. L., Overton, M. W., & Robbins, D. R. (2011). The interface of child mental health and juvenile diabetes mellitus. *Pediatric Clinics of North America, 58*(4), 937–954.

Gebbie, K. M., & Turnock, B. J. (2006). The public health workforce, 2006: New challenges. *Health Affairs, 25*(4), 923–933. doi: 10.1377/hlthaff.25.4.923

Glaze, L. E., & James, D. J. (2010). *Mental health problems of prison and jail inmates*. (original 2006; NCJ 213600, updated 2010). Retrieved from http://bjs.ojp.usdoj.gov/index.cfm?ty=pbdetail&iid=789

Green, R., & Reffel, J. (2009). Comparison of administrators' and school nurses' perception of the school nurse role. *Journal of School Nursing, 25*(1), 62–71. doi: 10.1177/1059840508324248

Guerino, P., Harrison, P. M., & Sabol, W. J. (2007). *Prisoners in 2010*. Retrieved from http://bjs.ojp.usdoj.gov/index.cfm?ty=pbdetail&iid=2230

Health Resources and Services Administration (HRSA). (2010). *The registered nurse population: Findings from the 2008 National Sample of Registered Nurses Survey: The registered nurse population 1980–2008*. Retrieved from http://bhpr.hrsa.gov/healthworkforce/rnsurveys/rnsurveyfinal.pdf

Heines, V. (2005). Speaking out to improve the health of inmates. *American Journal of Public Health, 95*(10), 1685–1688.

Hershey, T., Bhargava, N., Sadler, M., White, N. H., & Craft, S. (1999). Conventional versus intensive diabetes therapy in children with type 1 diabetes: Effects on memory and motor speed. *Diabetes Care, 22*(8), 1318–1324.

Hill, N. J., & Hollis, M. (2011). Teacher time spent on student health issues and school nurse presence. *Journal of School Nursing, 27*(6). doi: 10.1177/1059840511429684

Indian Health Services (HIS). (2009). *Indian health service introduction*. Retrieved on from http://www.ihs.gov/PublicInfo/PublicAffairs/Welcome_Info/IHSintro.asp

Individuals with Disabilities Education Act (IDEA). (1975). 20 U.S.C. §§ 1400 et. seq., as amended and incorporating the Education of All Handicapped Children Act (EHA), 1975, P.L. 94-142, and subsequent amendments; Regulations at 34 C.F.R. §§ 300-303 [Special education and related services for students, preschool children, and infants and toddlers].

Institute of Medicine (IOM). (1988). *The future of public health*. Washington, DC: National Academies Press.

Institute of Medicine (IOM). (2003). *Who will keep the public healthy?* Washington, DC: National Academies Press.

Institute of Medicine (IOM). (2010). *Roundtable on translating genomic-based research for health: 2010 annual report*. Retrieved from http://iom.edu/~/media/Files/Activity%20Files/Research/GenomicBasedResearch/Annual%20Reports/2010_Genomics_RT_Annual%20Report.pdf

The Joanna Briggs Institute. (2008). Education interventions for adults who attend the emergency room for acute asthma. *Journal of Advanced Nursing, 62*(6), 655–656.

Johnson, D. (Summer, 2010). Professionals beware! No deliberate indifference required for this claim to find you. *CorrectCare*. National Commission on Correctional Health Care. Retrieved from http://www.ncchc.org/pubs/CC/legal_retaliation.html

Kent-Wilkinson, A. (2009). An exploratory study of forensic nursing education in North America: Constructed definitions of forensic nursing. *Journal of Forensic Nursing, 5*, 201–211.

Kerr, J., Price, M., Kotch, J., Willis, S., Fisher, M., & Silva, S. (2011). Does contact by a family nurse practitioner decrease early school absence. *Journal of School Nursing [online]*. 10.1177/1059840511422818

Kogan, M. D., Strickland, B. B., & Newacheck, P. W. (2009). Building systems of care: Findings from the National Survey of children with special health care needs. *Pediatrics, 124*(S4), S333–S336. doi: 10.1542/peds.2009-1255B

Krause-Parello, C. A., & Samms, K. (2010). School nurses in New Jersey: A quantitative inquiry on roles and responsibilities. *Journal for Specialists in Pediatric Nursing, 15*(3), 217–222.

Laffan, S. (2005). "Inside look" on correctional nursing: A unique nursing specialty. *New Jersey Nurse*. Retrieved from http://findarticles.com/p/articles/mi_qa4080/is_200501.ai_n11826429/print

Lakdawalla, D. N., Bhattacharya, J., & Goldman, D. P. (2004). Are the young becoming more disabled? *Health Affairs, 23*(1), 168–176.

Leeks, K. D., Hopkins, D. P., Soler, R. E., Aten, A., & Chattopadhay, S. K. (2010). Worksite based incentives and competitions to reduce tobacco use. *American Journal of Preventive Medicine, 38*(2S), S263–S274.

Lewis, C., Mouradian, W., Slayton, R., & Williams, A. (2007). Dental insurance and its impact on preventive dental care visits for U.S. children. *Journal of the American Dental Association, 138*(3), 369–380.

Lewis, K. D., & Bear, B. J. (2011). *Manual of school health* (3rd ed.). St. Louis, MO: Saunders.

Magzamen, S., Patel, B., Davis, A., Edelstein, J., & Tager, I. R. (2008). Kickin' asthma: School-based asthma education in an urban community. *Journal of School Health, 78*(12), 655–665. doi: 10.1111/j.1746-1561.2008.00362.x

Maternal and Child Health Bureau. (2010). Vaccine preventable diseases. In *Child Health USA 2010*. U.S. Department of Health and Human Services, Health Resources and Services Administration. Retrieved from http://www.mchb.hrsa.gov/chusa10/hstat/hsc/pages/209vpd.html

Mayberry, M., Espelage, D. L., & Koenig, B. (2009). Multilevel modeling of direct effects and interactions of peers, parents, school, and community influences on adolescent substance use. *Journal of Youth and Adolescence, 38*(8), 1038–1049.

McCarthy, A. M., Kelly, M., & Reed, D. (2000). Medication administration practices of school nurses. *Journal of School Health, 70*(9), 371–376.

McCulloch, J., & Prieto, J. (2008). *Health protection and the role of the public health nurse*. In L. Coles, & E. Porter (Eds.), *Public health skills: A practical guide for nurses and public health practitioners* (pp. 155–169). Malden, MA: Blackwell Publishing.

Mental Health America. (2008). *Position statement 52: In support of maximum diversion of persons with serious mental illness from the criminal justice system*. Retrieved from http://www.nmha.org/go/position-statements/52

Milam, K., & Royo, J. (2009). *Back to school injury statistics and safety tips*. Safe Kids North Carolina. Retrieved from http://www.ncdoi.com/media/news2/year/2009/082409b.asp.

Millard, M. W., Johnson, P. T., Hilton, A., & Hart, M. (2009). Children with asthma miss more school: Fact or fiction? *Chest, 135*(2), 303–306.

Minnesota Department of Health. (2007). *Cornerstones of public health nursing*. Retrieved from http://www.health.state.mn.us/divs/cfh/ophp/resources/docs/cornerstones_definition_revised2007.pdf

Mumola, C. J., & Karberg, J. C. (2010). *Drug use and dependence, state and federal prisoners, 2004*. [NCJ 213530, page updated 2010]. Bureau of Justice Statistics special report. Retrieved from http://bjs.ojp.usdoj.gov/index.cfm?ty=pbdetail&iid=778

Murphy, M., & Polivka, B. (2007). Parental perceptions of the schools' role in addressing childhood obesity. *Journal of School Nursing, 23*(1), 40–46.

National Association of County and City Health Officers (NACCHO). (2010). *National profile of local health departments study*. Retrieved from http://www.naccho.org/topics/infrastructure/profile/resources/2010report/upload/2010_Profile_main_report-web.pdf

National Association of School Nurses (NASN). (2006). *Diabetes in the school setting*. Retrieved from http://www.nasn.org/PolicyAdvocacy/PositionPapersandReports/NASNPositionStatementsFullView/tabid/462/ArticleId/22/Diabetes-in-the-School-Setting-School-Nurse-Role-in-Care-and-Management-of-the-Child-with-Revised-20

National Association of School Nurses (NASN). (2007). *About us*. Retrieved from http://www.nasn.org/Default.aspx?tabid=57

National Association of School Nurses (NASN). (2011a). *Medication administration in the school setting*. Retrieved from http://www.nasn.org/PolicyAdvocacy/PositionPapersandReports/

NASNPositionStatementsFullView/tabid/462/ArticleId/86/Medication-Administration-in-the-School-Setting-Revised-2011

National Association of School Nurses (NASN). (2011b). *Emergency preparedness-the role of the school nurse.*. Retrieved from http://www.nasn.org/PolicyAdvocacy/PositionPapersandReports/NASNPositionStatementsFullView/tabid/462/ArticleId/117/Emergency-Preparedness-The-Role-of-the-School-Nurse-Adopted-2011

National Association of School Nurses and American Nurses Association. (2011). *School nursing: Scope and standards of practice*. Washington, DC: Author.

National Diabetes Education Program. (2011). *Overview of diabetes in children and adolescents*. Retrieved from http://ndep.nih.gov//media/youth_factsheet.pdf

National Eating Disorders Association. (2008). *Tips for school nurses*. Retrieved from http://www.nationaleatingdisorders.org/uploads/file/toolkits/NEDA-TKE-A13-SchoolNurseTips.pdf

National Fire Protection Association. (2007). *Personal emergency evacuation planning tool for school students with disabilities*. Retrieved from http://www.nfpa.org/assets/files/pdf/fact%20sheets/evacstudentdisabilities.pdf

National Institute of Mental Health (NIMH). (2008). *Child and adolescent mental health*. Retrieved from http://www.nimh.nih.gov/health/topics/child-and-adolescent-mental-health/index.shtml

National Institute of Neurological Disorders and Stroke (NINDS). (2009). *Curing epilepsy: The promise of research*. [NIH Publication No. 07-6120]. Retrieved from http://www.ninds.nih.gov/disorders/epilepsy/epilepsy_research.htm#Section1_2

National Oceanic and Atmospheric Administration (NOAA). (2007). *About NOAA Corps*. Retrieved from http://www.noaacorps.noaa.gov/about/about.html

Nelson, R. (2009). School nurses are needed more than ever. *American Journal of Nursing, 109*(12), 25–27. doi: 10.1097/01.NAJ.0000365174.55331.e8

Nock, M. K., Borges, G., Brommet, E. J., Cha, C. B., Kessler, R., Lee, S. (2008). Suicide and suicidal behavior. *Epidemiologic Reviews, 30*(1), 133–154. doi: 10.1093/epirev/mxn002

Noonan, M. (2010). Mortality in local jails, 2000–2007. [NCJ 222988]. Retrieved from http://bjs.ojp.usdoj.gov/content/pub/pdf/mlj07.pdf

Novick, L. F., Morrow, C. B., & Mays, G. P. (2008). *Public health administration: Principles for population-based management* (2nd ed.). Sudbury, MA: Jones and Bartlett Publishers.

O'Grady, J., Maeurer, M., Atun, R., Abubakar, I., Mwaba, P., Bates, M., Kapaa, N., et al. (2011). Tuberculosis in prisons: Anatomy of global neglect. *European Respiratory Journal, 38*(4), 752–754.

Olds, D. L. (2008). Preventing child maltreatment and crime with prenatal and infancy support of parents: The nurse-family partnership. *Journal of Scandinavian Studies in Criminology and Crime Prevention, 9*(1), 2–24. doi: 10.1080/14043850802450096

Oregon State Government. (2011). *School-based health centers: 2011 fact sheet*. Retrieved from http://public.health.oregon.gov/HealthyPeopleFamilies/Youth/HealthSchool/SchoolBasedHealthCenters/Documents/FastFacts.pdf

Page, J. (2006, August 17). *Sex-disease cases soar in Utah County*. Deseret News. Retrieved from http://findarticles.com/p/articles/mi_qn4188/is_20060817/ai_n16641786

Parvez, F., Lobato, M., & Greifinger, R. (2010). Tuberculosis control: Lessons for outbreak preparedness in correctional facilities. *Journal of Correctional Health Care, 16*(3), 239–242.

Pbert, L., Druker, S., DiFranza, J. R., Gorak, D., Reed, G., Magner, R., et al. (2011). Effectiveness of a school nurse-delivered smoking-cessation intervention for adolescents. *Pediatrics, 128*(5), 926–936. doi: 10.1542/peds.2011-0520.

Potter, R. H., Schwartz, R., & May, R. (2011). The impact of the H1N1 pandemic on US prisons: Results of a national survey. *Corrections Today 73*(4), 73–74.

Quad Council. (2007). *The public health nursing shortage: A threat to the public's health*. Quad Council of Public Health Nursing.

Rehabilitation Act of 1973, Section 504. (1973). 29 U.S.C. §794 et seq., Regulations at 34 C.F.R. §104.

Resnick, E. A., Bishop, M., O'Connell, A., Hugo, B., Isern, G., Timm, A., et al. (2009). The CHEER study to reduce BMI in elementary school students: A school-based, parent-directed study in Framingham, Massachusetts. *Journal of School Nursing, 25*(5), 361–372. doi: 10.1177/1059840509339194

Reznick, O., Comfort, M., McCartney, K., & Neilands, T. (2011). Effectiveness of an HIV prevention program for women visiting their incarcerated partners: The HOME project. *AIDS Behavior, 15*, 365–375.

Richmond, S. L. (2011). Medication error prevention in the school setting: A closer look. *NASN School Nurse, 26*(5), 304–308.

Russo, K. (2010). ObamaCare prototype already exists. Retrieved from http://www.quickregister.net/links/article.php?id=80

Schoely, L. (2010). Alcohol withdrawal: Jail nurse alert. *Correctional Nurse.Net*. Retrieved from http://lorryschoenly.wordpress.com/2010/03/31/alcohol-withdrawal-jail-nurse-alert/

Schwartz, R. D. (2008). The impact of correctional institutions on public health during a pandemic or emerging infection disaster. *American Journal of Disaster Medicine, 3*(3), 165–170.

Shiroma, E., Ferguson, P., & Pickelsimer, E. (2010). Prevalence of traumatic brain injury in an offender population: a meta-analysis. *Journal of Correctional Health Care, 16*(2), 147–159.

Sondick, E., Madans, J. H, & Gentleman, J. F. (2011). *Summary health statistics for U.S. children: National health interview survey, 2010*. National Center for Health Statistics. Retrieved from http://www.cdc.gov/nchs/data/series/sr_10/sr10_250.pdf

Spratley, E., Johnson, A., Sochalski, J., Fritz, M., & Spencer, W. (2002). *The registered nurse population, March 2000: Findings from the national sample survey of registered nurses*. Washington, DC: USDHHS. Retrieved from http://bhpr.hrsa.gov/healthworkforce/reports/rnsurvey/rnss1.htm

Stalter, A. M., Kaylor, M., Steinke, J. D., & Barker, R. M. (2010). Parental perceptions of the rural school's role in addressing childhood obesity. *Journal of School Nursing. 27*(1), 70–81. doi: 10.1177/1059840510394189

Strozer, J., Juszczak, L., & Ammerman, A. (2010). 2007–2008 National school-based health care census. Washington, DC: National Assembly on School-Based Health Care. Retrieved from http://www.nasbhc.org/atf/cf/%7BB241D183-DA6F-443F-9588-3230D027D8DB%7D/NASBHC%202007-08%20CENSUS%20REPORT%20FINAL.PDF

Swan, M. A., Barker, J. C., & Hoeft, K. S. (2010). Rural Latino farmworker fathers' understanding of children's oral health. *Pediatric Dentistry, 32*(5), 400–406.

Sweeney, N. M., & Horishita, N. (2005). The breakfast-eating habits of inner city high school students. *Journal of School Nursing, 21*(2), 100–105.

Tan, J. A., Joseph, T. A., & Saab, S. (2008). Treating hepatitis C in the prison population is cost-saving. *Hepatology, 48*(5), 1387–1395.

Taylor, R., & Crianza, S. G. (2011). Lessons learned: How Harris County jail prepares for disasters. *Corrections Today 73*(4), 44–46.

Texas Department of Health Services. (2011). *Frequently asked questions: Implementation of laws on screening for Acanthosis Nigricans*. Retrieved from http://www.dshs.state.tx.us/school-health/organscreen.shtm

Turnock, B. J. (2012). *Essentials of public health*. Sudbury, MA: Jones and Bartlett Publishers.

U.S. Department of Education, National Center for Education Statistics. (2011). *Digest of education statistics, 2010* (NCES 2011-015). Retrieved from http://nces.ed.gov/programs/digest/d10/

U.S. Department of Health and Human Services (USDHHS). Centers for Medicare and Medicaid. (2007). *Medicaid program: Elimination of reimbursement under Medicaid for school administration expenditures and costs related to transportation of school-age children between home and school.* [CMS–2287–F]. Retrieved from http://www.cms. hhs.gov/MedicaidGenInfo/Downloads/CMS2287F.pdf

U.S. Department of Health and Human Services (USDHHS), Administration on Children, Youth and Families. (2008). *Child Maltreatment 2006*. Washington, DC: U.S. Government Printing Office.

U.S. Department of Health and Human Services (USDHHS). (2010). *Healthy People 2020*. Retrieved from healthypeople.gov/2020/default.aspx

U.S. Department of Health and Human Services (USDHHS). (2011a). *About Health and Human Service*. Retrieved August 24, 2011 from hhs.gov/about

U.S. Department of Health and Human Services (USDHHS). (2011b). *Department of Health and Human Services budget in brief*. Retrieved from http://www.hhs.gov/about/FY2012budget/fy2012bib.pdf

U.S. Public Health Service Commissioned Corps (USPHSCC) (2010). *U.S. Public Health Service Commissioned Corp*. Retrieved from http://www.usphs.gov/aboutus/questions.aspx#whatis

U.S. Public Health Service Commissioned Corps (USPHSCC) (2011). *U.S. Public Health Service Commissioned Corp. Profession: Nurse*. Retrieved from http://www.usphs.gov/Profession/nurse/bios.aspx#7

U.S. Public Health Service Nursing Corps. (2011). *History of Nursing in USPHSC*. Retrieved December 17, 2011 from http://phs-nurse.org/index.php/nurse-resource-manual/75-history-of-nursing-phs.html

Utah County Health Department. (2008). *PHN I/II/III*. Retrieved from http://www.utahcountyonline.org/Dept/Pers/Data/JOBData/2021.pdf

Valeant Pharmaceuticals North America. (2007). *Diastat® AcuDial™*. Retrieved from http://www.diastat.com/0-Home/

Van Cleave, J., Gortmaker, S. L., & Perrin, J. M. (2010). Dynamics of obesity and chronic health conditions among children and youth. *Journal of the American Medical Association, 303*(7), 623–630. doi: 10.1001/jama.2010.104

Vescio, M., Longo, B., Babudieri, S., Starnini, G., Carbonara, S., Rezza, G., et al. (2008). Correlates of hepatitis C virus seropositivity in prison inmates: a meta-analysis. *Journal of Epidemiology & Community Health*, 62, 305–313.

Vessey, J., & McGowan, K. (2006). A successful public health experiment: School nursing. *Pediatric Nursing, 32*(3), 255–257.

Walmsley, R. (2009). *World prison population list* (8th ed.). International Centre for Prison Studies. Retrieved from http://www.prisonstudies.org/publications/list/40-world-prison-population-list-8th-edition.html

Walter, S. R., Olivier, J., Churches, T., & Grzebieta, R. (2011). The impact of compulsory cycle helmet legislation on cyclist head injuries in new South Wales, Australia, *Accident Analysis & Prevention,43*(6), 2064–2071. doi: 10.1016/j.aap.2011.05.029

Wilper, A. P., Woolhandler, S., Boyd, J. W., Lasser, K. E., McCormick, D., Bor, D. H., et al. (2009). The health and health care of US prisoners: results of a nationwide survey. *American Journal of Public Health, 99*(4), 666–672.

Wilt, L., & Foley, M. (2011). Delegation of glucagon in the school setting: A comparison of state legislation. *Journal of School Nursing*. Pub ahead of print. doi: 10.1177/1059840511398240

Winsch, B. J. (2011). *Taking the pulse of student health needs in America: The role of school nurses in improving student health and academics*. White paper. Jefferson County Public Schools. Retrieved from http://www.jefferson.k12.ky.us/Departments/Planning/ProgramEvaluation/WebMASTER_Updates_July2011/StudentHealthNeedsinAmerica62911_BW.pdf

Wolfe, L., & Selekman, J. (2002). School nurses: What it was and what it is. *Pediatric Nursing, 28*(4), 403–407.

Woodfill, M. M., & Beyrer, M. K. (1991). *The role of the nurse in the school setting: A historical perspective*. Kent, OH: American School Health Association.

Zucker, D. M. (2009). Peer education for Hepatitis C prevention. *Gastroenterology Nursing, 32(1)*, 42–48. Retrieved from http://scholarworks.umass.edu/cgi/viewcontent.cgi?article=1002&context=nursing_faculty_pubs

thePoint: Everything You Need to Make the Grade!

thePoint Visit http://thePoint.lww.com/Allender8e
for selected readings, study aids for all learning styles, and more!

CHAPTER

31

Private Settings for Community Health Nursing

"To insure good health: eat lightly, breathe deeply, live moderately, cultivate cheerfulness, and maintain an interest in life."

—*William Londen*

KEY TERMS

Comprehensive Primary Care Center
Educational Resource Center (ERC)
Entrepreneurial nurse
Faith community nurse
Federally Qualified Health Center (FQHC)
Nurse-managed health clinic (NMHC)
Occupational and environmental health nurse
Occupational Safety and Health Administration (OSHA)
Request for proposal (RFP)
Safety-net health care provider

LEARNING OBJECTIVES

Upon mastery of this chapter, you should be able to:

- Describe the historical roots of nurse-managed health clinics.
- Identify the distinctiveness of various nurse-managed health clinic models.
- Describe funding sources for nurse-managed health clinics.
- Articulate the importance of sustainability for nurse-managed health clinics.
- Describe the evolution of faith community nursing.
- Describe and differentiate among the roles of the faith community nurse.
- Identify the steps for establishing a practice as a faith community nurse.
- Explain the role of the occupational and environmental health nurse and other members of the occupational health team in protecting and promoting workers' health and safety.
- Identify educational preparation for occupational and environmental health nurses.
- Recognize at least three adverse working conditions that impact health status.
- Discuss the opportunities for nurse entrepreneurship in community/public health practice.

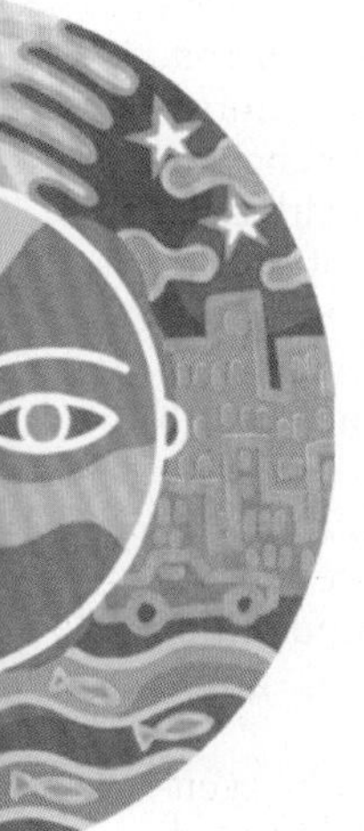

Healthy People 2020: Improving the Health of Americans (U.S. Department of Health and Human Services [USDHHS], 2010) provides clear objectives for promoting health and preventing disease for the next decade. The next 10 years will see unprecedented changes and challenges in the nation's health. As we ponder what those changes will be, the Healthy People initiative will continue to encourage collaborations across communities and sectors, empower individuals toward making informed health decisions, and measure the impact of prevention activities. Building on the Healthy People goals for the nation's health, there will be ever-increasing opportunities for community/public health nurses to make a difference in their communities. This chapter examines four distinct areas of practice in the community as potential options for your own professional road ahead. Each of these roles contributes in very tangible ways to improving the health of individuals, families, and the communities in which they live.

Chapter 30 discussed a wide variety of practice opportunities in the public sector. This chapter examines four unique private sector roles and practice environments available in the United States and in many other countries: nurse-managed health centers, faith community nursing, occupational and environmental health nursing, and nurse entrepreneurship. Nurse-managed health centers offer the opportunity for more autonomous practice and present excellent learning venues for nursing students. Many such centers are connected to academic nursing programs. Faith community nursing, begun in the mid-1980s, has gained increasing attention in many religious communities. Although the positions are frequently held by volunteers, there are increasing opportunities for paid employment. Occupational and environmental health is a specialty health practice that focuses on the health and wellbeing of the working population, including both paid and unpaid positions, and therefore covers most of the country's working adults. This role provides the vital link between nursing and sound business practices. The nurse entrepreneur role offers new venues for meeting the health care needs in communities while providing challenging and autonomous practice. Each of these areas of practice offers community health nurses an avenue to address health disparities in their communities, increase years of healthy life, and provide holistic, client-centered care to meet the current and emerging health needs in their communities, as indicated in *Healthy People 2020*.

NURSE-MANAGED HEALTH CLINICS

Nurse-managed health centers, nursing centers, or the more recent term **nurse-managed health clinics (NMHC)** are organizations that give clients access to professional nursing services. Located in or near health professional shortage areas (HPSA) and medically underserved areas (MUA) in both urban and rural communities, NMHCs are found in convenient sites where people live, work, learn, and worship. A nurse executive with an advanced degree provides oversight. Traditionally, targets of service have been those who are least likely to be engaged in ongoing health care services for themselves and their family members. Currently, NMHCs serve population groups of all ages that are both uninsured and underinsured.

Historically, the most frequently cited definition of *nursing centers* is the one developed in the mid-1980s by the American Nurses Association Nursing Centers Task Force. Display 31.1 presents a modified version of this definition. However, with an amendment to Title III of the Public Health Service Act (42 U.S.C. 241 et seq.), the Nurse-Managed Health Clinic Investment

DISPLAY 31.1 DEFINITION OF NURSING CENTER

Nursing centers—sometimes referred to as community nursing organizations, nurse-managed centers, nursing clinics, and community nurse–managed health centers are organizations that give clients and communities direct access to professional nursing services. Professional nurses in these centers diagnose and treat human responses to actual and potential health problems and promote health and optimal functioning among target populations and communities. The services provided in these centers are holistic, client-centered, and affordable. Overall accountability and responsibility remain with the nurse executive/director. Nurse-managed health centers are not limited to any particular organizational configuration. Nurse-managed health centers can be freestanding businesses or may be affiliated with universities or other service institutions like home health agencies and hospitals. The primary characteristic of the organization is responsiveness to the health needs of populations. The nurse is responsible for all-patient care and operations (Aydelotte et al., 1987; Hansen-Turton et al., 2009).

Source original citation: Aydelotte, M. K., Barger, S. E., Branstetter, E., Fehring, R. J., Lindgren, K., et al. (1987). *The nursing center: Concept and design*. Kansas City, MO: American Nurses Association.

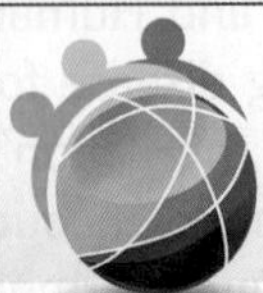

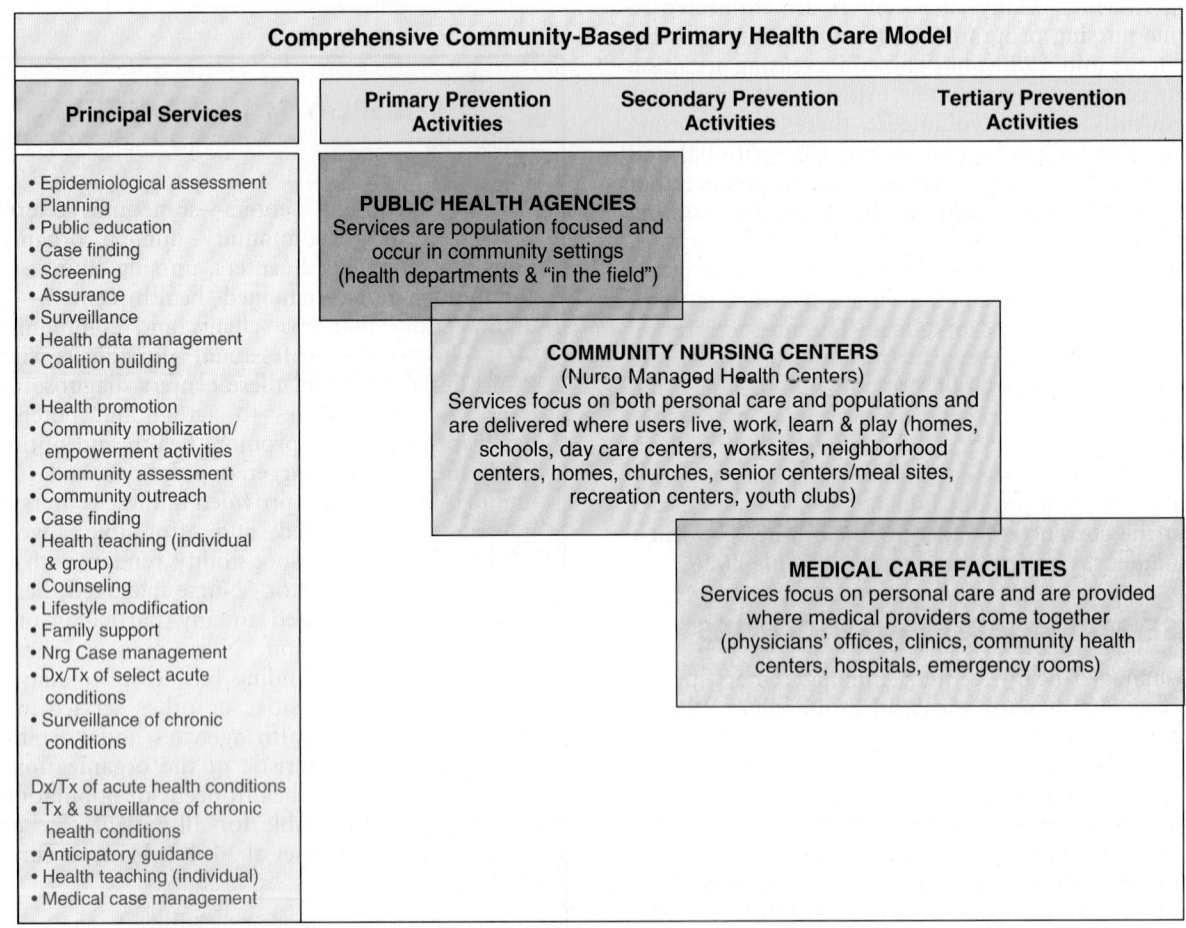

DISPLAY 31.2 DEFINITION OF NURSE-MANAGED HEALTH CLINIC

The term "nurse-managed health clinic" or "NMHC" means a nurse practice arrangement, managed by advanced practice nurses, that provides primary care or wellness services to underserved or vulnerable populations and is associated with a school, college, university, or department of nursing; federally qualified health center; or an independent nonprofit health or social services agency (United States Congress, 2009).

Act of 2009 (Senate Bill 1104/House of Representatives Bill 2754) of the 111th Congress provides a more present-day definition of NMHCs. Display 31.2 presents this definition.

While all NMHCs share the core elements of these definitions, they vary in their practice models. Services offered at NMHCs range from health promotion and wellness to conventional primary care (Hansen-Turton, Miller, & Greiner, 2009; Torrisi & Hansen-Turton, 2005). In this chapter, the terms nursing center, nurse-managed health center, and NMHC are used interchangeably to describe this model of contemporary health care.

NMHCs represent a rising movement of health centers that have emerged as vital safety-net health care providers in America's health care delivery system (Hansen-Turton & Miller, 2006). A **safety-net health care provider** is defined as a provider that by mandate or mission organizes and delivers a significant level of health care and other health-related services to the uninsured, Medicaid, and other vulnerable populations (Health Resources and Services Administration, 2005; Institute of Medicine [IOM], 2000).

NMHCs differ from other public health agencies and tertiary medical care facilities. Although some services overlap, the distinctiveness of NMHCs is found in the community orientation of the nurse-managed centers. This model is depicted by *Lundeen's Comprehensive Community-Based Primary Healthcare Model* (Lundeen, 2005) where NMHCs are referred to as community nursing centers and are the central figure in this model of health care utilized at the University of Milwaukee, Wisconsin (see Fig. 31-1).

Comprehensive Community-Based Primary Health Care Model

Principal Services

- Epidemiological assessment
- Planning
- Public education
- Case finding
- Screening
- Assurance
- Surveillance
- Health data management
- Coalition building

- Health promotion
- Community mobilization/ empowerment activities
- Community assessment
- Community outreach
- Case finding
- Health teaching (individual & group)
- Counseling
- Lifestyle modification
- Family support
- Nrg Case management
- Dx/Tx of select acute conditions
- Surveillance of chronic conditions

Dx/Tx of acute health conditions
- Tx & surveillance of chronic health conditions
- Anticipatory guidance
- Health teaching (individual)
- Medical case management

Primary Prevention Activities | **Secondary Prevention Activities** | **Tertiary Prevention Activities**

PUBLIC HEALTH AGENCIES
Services are population focused and occur in community settings (health departments & "in the field")

COMMUNITY NURSING CENTERS
(Nurse Managed Health Centers)
Services focus on both personal care and populations and are delivered where users live, work, learn & play (homes, schools, day care centers, worksites, neighborhood centers, homes, churches, senior centers/meal sites, recreation centers, youth clubs)

MEDICAL CARE FACILITIES
Services focus on personal care and are provided where medical providers come together (physicians' offices, clinics, community health centers, hospitals, emergency rooms)

FIGURE 31-1. Comprehensive community-based primary health care model. (From Lundeen, S. (1993, 2005). *Lundeen's comprehensive community-based primary health care model.* Milwaukee, WI: UW, Milwaukee College of Nursing, with permission.)

Healthy People 2020

The groundbreaking publication of *Healthy People: The Surgeon General's Report on Health Promotion and Disease Prevention* (U.S. Department of Health, Education and Welfare, 1979) focused attention on the nation's health promotion and disease prevention activities. Three decades later, *Healthy People 2020* expands on this health promotion and disease prevention initiative. The four main goals of *Healthy People 2020* are attain high-quality, longer lives free of preventable disease, disability, injury, and premature death; achieve health equity, eliminate disparities, and improve the health of all groups; create social and physical environments that promote good health for all; and promote quality of life, healthy development, and healthy behaviors across all life stages (USDHHS, 2010). Achieving *Healthy People 2020* goals requires a long-term commitment to community collaboration and partnerships among many diverse people and groups (Kinsey & Miller, 2011). NMHCs are an excellent venue to address identified Key Health Indicators to meet the goals of *Healthy People 2020*. Display 31.3 contains exemplars of *Healthy People 2020* Key Health Indicators that are applicable to NMHCs.

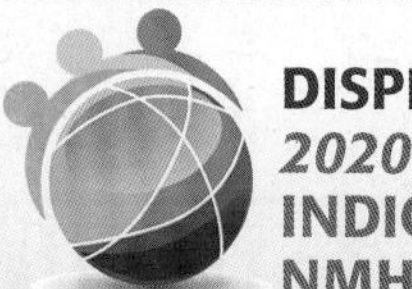

DISPLAY 31.3 *HEALTHY PEOPLE 2020* SELECTED KEY HEALTH INDICATORS EXEMPLARS FOR NMHCS

The Leading Health Indicators are organized under 12 topics. The *Healthy People 2020* Leading Health Indicators are:

Access to Health Services*
- Persons with medical insurance
- Persons with a usual primary care provider

Clinical Preventive Services*
- Adults who receive a colorectal cancer screening based on the most recent guidelines
- Adults with hypertension whose blood pressure is under control
- Adult diabetic population with an A1c value >9%
- Children aged 19 to 35 months who receive the recommended doses of DTaP, polio, MMR, Hib, hepatitis B, varicella, and PCV vaccines

Environmental Quality
Injury and Violence
Maternal, Infant, and Child Health
Mental Health
Nutrition, Physical Activity, and Obesity
Oral Health
Reproductive and Sexual Health
Social Determinants
Substance Abuse
Tobacco

History of the Nurse-Managed Model

Although today's NMHCs trace their roots to changes in national health care laws begun in the mid-1960s, the nursing model of holistic care that focuses on vulnerable populations and integrates primary care and public health dates back to the 19th century. Florence Nightingale's passion for at-risk populations, as well as her success related to health reform, provides a model for NMHCs today. Visionaries such as Lillian Wald, who founded the Henry Street Settlement, and Margaret Sanger, who initiated the first family planning clinic, are two examples of nurses providing holistic care to vulnerable populations (see Chapter 2). These nurse activists sought to resolve 20th century problems caused by immigration, urbanization, and industrialization in the United States (Beidler, 2005).

Since the late 1970s, in conjunction with the development of educational programs for nurse practitioners, faculties in schools of nursing have established nurse-managed health centers. Linkages have provided clinical sites for educating nurses at all levels and settings, as well as for faculty practice opportunities (Hansen-Turton & Miller, 2006). For example, one urban academic nursing center at Duquesne University School of Nursing in Pittsburgh, Pennsylvania, involves students and faculty in primary and secondary prevention services to the community. "Brown bag" medication review days, health fairs, safety assessments, nutrition education, computer classes, and health screenings are examples of services and special programs that undergraduate and graduate students have been engaged in for almost two decades (Hansen-Turton et al., 2009).

Today, NMHCs meet the traditional role of nurses who have historically provided compassionate health care focusing on the special needs of societies most vulnerable: the poor, the aged, those experiencing social injustice, and those living in geographic areas with limited or no access to adequate health care facilities (National Nursing Centers Consortium, 2011). Unlike traditional health care venues that provide primary care and public health services, NMHCs include community participation in program development, implementation, and evaluation (Anderko, Bartz, & Lundeen, 2005).

Nurse-Managed Health Clinic Models

There are several types of nursing centers; each has an individuality of its own that reflects the community in which it is located and the particular services it offers (Gerrity & Kinsey, 1999). Academic-based nursing centers, which are located within schools of nursing, are a common organizational structure. There are also hospital-based and freestanding community-based NMHCs that offer a mixture of primary care, health promotion, and disease prevention services (Hansen-Turton & Miller, 2006).

NMHCs meet requirements for **Federally Qualified Health Center (FQHC)** designation as defined in Section 330 of the Public Health Service Act. FQHCs are safety-net providers whereby the main purpose is to enhance primary care services in underserved rural and urban communities (USDHHS, Centers for Medicare and Medicaid Services [CMS], 2011). Hansen-Turton (2003) states that NMHCs meet all of the requirements for FQHC designation. This is an especially important designation, as it enables NMHCs to qualify for many funding sources vital to service provision that would not be available without this designation. The specific requirements are:

- be located in a MUA or serve a medically underserved population
- have a nonprofit, tax exempt, or public status
- have a board of directors, a majority of whom must be consumers of the center's health services
- provide culturally competent, comprehensive primary care services to all age groups
- offer a sliding scale fee and provide services regardless of ability to pay

The variety of nursing center models currently being used and their organizational structures demonstrates the diversity of contemporary NMHCs. Display 31.4 describes the major types of centers (wellness, specialty nursing centers, and Comprehensive Primary Care Centers) along with the various organizational structures that influence their delivery models.

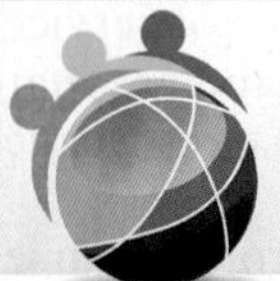

DISPLAY 31.4 NURSE-MANAGED HEALTH CENTER MODELS

Center Types:

- **Wellness Center:** provides public health as well as health promotion and disease prevention programs, focus on primary and secondary prevention strategies
- **Special Care Centers:** provide programs that target specific health conditions such as HIV or diabetes
- **Comprehensive Primary Care Center:** provides traditional primary care and public health programs

Organizational Structure:

- **Academic Nursing Center:** located within a School of Nursing
- **Freestanding Center:** independent center with its own governing board
- **Subsidiary:** part of a larger health care system, such as home health agencies, community centers, schools, and other venues
- **Affiliated Center:** legal partnership with a health care or human services organization

Adapted from: Kinsey, K., & Miller, M. E. (2011). The nursing center: A model for nursing practice in the community. In M. Stanhope & J. Lancaster, *Public Health Nursing: Population-centered health care in the community* (8th ed., pp. 461–482). Maryland Heights, MO: Mosby, Chapter 21.

Funding for Nurse-Managed Health Clinics

As NMHCs vary in their models, so too are their methods of cost-reimbursement, including the following: fee for service, sliding fees, grant support, third party payments, and cost-based reimbursement available to FQHCs (Torrisi & Hansen-Turton, 2005). Most nursing centers operational and salary budgets entail a combination of these funding sources.

In **Comprehensive Primary Care Centers**, advanced practice nurses provide primary care services. Such services are usually reimbursable under Medicaid and managed care medical insurance plans. In wellness centers, public health nurses and other interdisciplinary team members provide a range of primary and secondary prevention strategies. These services are usually not reimbursed by insurance plans but are often covered by grants and contracts (Hansen-Turton & Miller, 2006). Additionally, foundation support and private donations from community organizations and members provide fiscal support for NMHC initiatives (see From the Case Files I).

From the Case Files I

Ms. Jones is a 22-year-old mother of three small children who recently moved to an urban area. She brings her oldest child, age 6, to a local comprehensive primary care nurse-managed health clinic (NMHC) for school immunizations. During the course of the history and physical examination, the nurse practitioner becomes aware that this mother also has two younger children, aged two and three, at home. The family rents a small apartment in housing that was built in the mid-1950s. Ms. Jones reports that her mother (the children's grandmother) also resides with them. The grandmother is the child care provider, while Ms. Jones works as a local hair salon. The grandmother mother smokes 1.5 to 2 packages of cigarettes daily; Ms. Jones reports that she is a nonsmoker. Upon further questioning, the nurse practitioner learns that the 3-year-old child has a chronic cough and occasional wheezing. Ms. Jones also confides to the nurse practitioner that she recently missed two menstrual periods and is sexually active.

1. What are some possible health care needs of Ms. Jones? Her mother?
2. What screenings should be performed on Ms. Jones? Her mother?
3. What screenings should be performed on Ms. Jones' children?
4. What other interdisciplinary team members should be involved in this family's health care?
5. What are some possible referrals that would benefit this family?

It is important to distinguish between grants and contracts as funding sources for NMHCs. Funding organizations usually release guidelines regarding what initiatives they will fund. Grant guidelines are frequently termed **request for proposal** or RFP. Grants can be a source of initial start-up funding as well as to support ongoing activities (Kinsey & Miller, 2011). A proposal submitted by the NMHC to the funding organization describes how the center would meet the goals and objectives set by the funding organization. Outcomes, or the end results at a specific point in time, are increasingly becoming more important to funders. NMHCs must include measures to collect outcome data and project what outcomes will occur in their submitted proposals. Additionally, funders tend to view initiatives that include interagency collaboration in a more favorable manner. Partnering with one or more NMHCs or other community-based organizations is a strategy that provides additional strength to the proposal when it is under review by the funding organization.

Contracts are another source of funding for NMHCs. Contracts are awards establishing a binding legal procurement relationship between a funder and a recipient obligating the receiver to furnish a product or service defined in detail by the funder (National Institutes of Health, 2007). A contract has specific goals, objectives, and activities, as well as a time frame for which the activities are to be implemented and evaluated. Contracts are awarded on a noncompetitive basis and oftentimes are renewable when goals and objectives are met.

Managing the various funding streams that feed the personnel and operations budgets of a NMHC is an arduous task. To ensure that budgetary dollars are spent in the manner specified by the funding organization, meticulous record keeping and itemization of spending is another undertaking that the nurse executive or an operations coordinator of a NMHC must carry out. It is imperative that key personnel from NMHCs maintain precise records and submit accurate quarterly, semiannual, or annual reports as specified in the grant or contract award.

Sustainability of Nurse-Managed Health Clinics

Sustainability, or the ability to carry on services and health promotion activities when funding is no longer available, is one of the main challenges of NMHCs. "The challenge of sustainability" is a common dilemma that funders and grantee both face at the end of an initiative's funding period (Cutler, 2002).

NHMCs have much to offer toward resolving the national health care crisis facing vulnerable populations who are uninsured or underinsured. However, without the ability to maintain fiscal sustainability, NMHCs may fail to reach their full potential for positively influencing the future of health care (McBryde-Foster, 2005).

In the past, funders were often confronted with the task to help organizations find and secure other resources, or extend their own financial support, to ensure the continuity of services. More recently, both public and private funders are stipulating that organizations describe detailed plans for sustainability after the award period ceases in their application submitted for funding. Cutler (2002) proposes "critical sustainability questions" that can be used as a preliminary avenue of consideration for organizations such as NMHCs when completing a grant application for funding (see Display 31.5).

National Organization: The National Nursing Centers Consortium

In 1996, due to interest from several nursing center directors, staff, and community members to address all aspects of operations and to provide ongoing collaboration and continuing education, the Regional Nursing Centers Consortium (RNCC) of Pennsylvania, New Jersey, and Delaware was

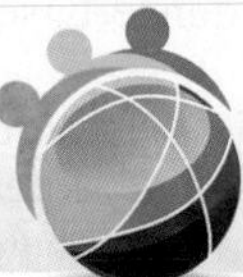

DISPLAY 31.5 CRITICAL SUSTAINABILITY QUESTIONS

When applying to a funding organization, applicants should consider the following questions:

1. Assuming acceptable results and assuming that the task will not be fully completed at the end of the grant period, is it expected that this initiative will continue beyond the period for which funding is available?
2. If so, what level of financial and other resources will be needed to continue?
3. What capacity-building measures are needed to make the initiative sustainable? How will these measures be implemented?
4. What is it about this initiative that is likely to attract interest and elicit support?
5. Who are the most likely future funders? (Be specific. If government, what level of government, what agency, what funding stream? If private, which foundation or other source?)
6. Is there a history of this entity supporting efforts (a) of this sort? and (b) of this size?
7. Would success in this effort obviate the need to spend resources on something else, and could that money be diverted to this effort? How?
8. Who within the anticipated funding organization would have to decide to fund, through what processes?

Source: Cutler, I. (2002). *End games: The challenge of sustainability* (pp. 23–24). Baltimore, MD: Annie E. Casey Foundation Publisher.

established. In the short span of 5 years, nursing centers nationwide were contacting the RNCC with inquiries related to all aspects of operations, funding, and sustainability. It became rapidly evident that the RNCC needed to expand its service area to meet the needs of NMHCs nationwide. In 2001, The National Nursing Centers Consortium (NNCC) was formed to represent NMHCs nationwide. Headquartered in Philadelphia, Pennsylvania, the NNCC expanded in 2005 to include an international focus with the addition of a NMHC in Auckland, New Zealand. The vision, mission, and goals of the NNCC are found in Display 31.6.

Best Practices of Nurse-Managed Health Centers

In contemporary health care, evidence-based practice is the process of making clinical decisions based upon the best available research evidence, clinical expertise, and client preferences in the context of available resources (Melnyk & Fineout-Overholt, 2010). NMHCs implement evidence-based practice via best practices, or the application of the best available evidence to improve practice (Youngblut & Brooten, 2001). (Chapter 4 provides an extensive overview of evidence-based practice.)

Biennially, the NNCC conducts a *Best Practice Conference* at varied national locations. This professional conference brings together nurses, staff members, funders, and political leaders to share best practices and participate in networking opportunities. Continuing education credits are available for attendance at scientific sessions. This is one exemplar of how NMHCs set standards for quality improvement and promote professional growth among members.

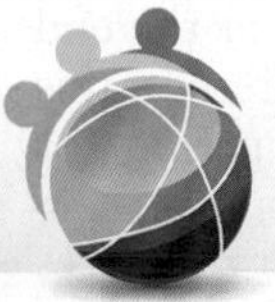

DISPLAY 31.6 NATIONAL NURSING CENTERS CONSORTIUM

Vision

To keep our nation healthy through nurse-managed health care

Mission

To advance nurse-led health care through policy, consultation, programs, and applied research to reduce health disparities and meet people's primary care and wellness needs

Goals

1. Provide national leadership in identifying, tracking, and advising health care policy development
2. Position nurse-managed health clinics as a recognized mainstream health care model
3. Foster partnerships with people and groups who share common goals

Source: National Nursing Centers Consortium (2011). *Mission, vision, goals.* Retrieved from http://www.nncc.us/about/vision.html

Nursing Research and NMHCs

NMHCs provide research opportunities, both for primary prevention and wellness initiatives. Descriptive data have been collected about client demographics, types of service provided, funding methods, and sustainability efforts. The first national collection of quality measures for NMHCs compared with national ambulatory care benchmarks is now published (Barkauskas, Pohl, Tanner, Onifade, & Pilon, 2011). The quality measures in this report were for breast cancer screening, cervical cancer screening, diabetes care, hypertension management, and smoking cessation. These authors found that quality measure findings compared favorably with national benchmarks, with high quality demonstrated for chronic disease care management. They also reported that their experience with national data collection proved to be feasible. Additional studies with multisite NMHCs designed to measure variables such as psychosocial needs, accessibility and affordability of services, and quality of life indicators are warranted.

Role of Students in Nurse-Managed Health Clinics

Undergraduate and graduate students from many disciplines play a vital part in the activities of NMHCs. These disciplines include, but are not limited to, nursing, social work, mental health, dental, nutrition, speech–language–hearing science, and public health. When students engage in NMHC activities for their clinical experience, they become aware of the distinctiveness of nurse-managed centers from other health care delivery systems, the variety of models and organizational structures that exist, and are active participants in vital nursing center activities. Most often, students are engaged in primary and secondary prevention strategies via health education, outreach, immunization, and screening programs. Roles that students fulfill are similar to the roles of their staff mentors, such as advocate, case manager, educator, and referral agent. Faculty roles in NMHC academic models involve clinical supervision and mentorship of undergraduate and graduate students assigned to the nursing center for their clinical experience (see From the Case Files II).

Future Directions for NMHCs

In 2008, the IOM appointed a committee on the Robert Wood Johnson Foundation (RWJF) Initiative on the Future of Nursing. The purpose of this committee was

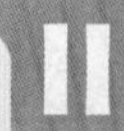

From the Case Files

Public health nurses from an academic wellness NMHC and undergraduate student nurses are conducting blood pressure and glucose screenings at a church sponsored health fair. This event is conducted on Sunday from 10 AM to 2 PM, before, during, and after church services. Approximately 50% of adults screened have hypertension and/or hyperglycemia. One African American male participant, who was asymptomatic, had severe hypertension (220/154) and was immediately transported to the nearest hospital for evaluation.

1. What are some feasible referrals that may have made for those with abnormal screening results?
2. What types of primary prevention strategies may benefit those attendees who had normal screening results?
3. What is the rationale for conducting the health fair on a Sunday?
4. In what ways do student nurses benefit from participating at a health fair?

to produce a report making recommendations for the future of nursing. This committee developed four key messages regarding the future of nursing: (1) Nurses should practice to the full extent of their education and training; (2) nurses should achieve higher levels of education and training through an improved education system that promotes seamless academic progression; (3) nurses should be full partners, with physicians and other health care professionals, in redesigning health care in the United States; and (4) effective workforce planning and policy making requires better data collection and information infrastructure (IOM, 2011). NHMCs play a vital role in the transformation of the national health care system. In NMHCs, advanced practice nurses lead interdisciplinary teams as critical safety-net providers in America's health care delivery system. Continued expansion of the NMHC model in the next decade and beyond will meet key recommendations from the IOM report on nursing's future.

FAITH COMMUNITY NURSING

Faith community nursing is one of the newest nursing specialties and one of the oldest means of health care delivery. For hundreds of years, deaconesses, sisters, and lay members of religious communities have been involved in ministering to the sick. This tradition was revitalized through the efforts of Reverend Dr. Granger Westberg. As a hospital chaplain and Lutheran minister, Westberg observed a great need for preventive and holistic health services, especially among the underserved. He estimated that one third of the illnesses his patients experienced could have been prevented, or the severity reduced, by education and health promotion (Westberg, 1990). To address these needs, he launched several church-based holistic health clinics in the 1970s, each staffed by a physician, nurse, and chaplain. These clinics provided health services to the underserved in the community for several years. The clinics eventually closed, but the experience led Reverend Westberg to recognize the unique ability of nurses to bridge the disciplines of medicine and religion and assist the client in understanding the physical and spiritual influences on health.

Spurred by the positive impact of the church-based health clinics, Westberg initiated a pilot project in 1984 in which nurses provided holistic, preventive health care for six Christian congregations in the Chicago area. These nurses were called *parish nurses*. The surrounding communities recognized the beneficial influence of the parish nurses on the six congregations. Gradually, more and more churches sought to incorporate a parish nurse into their staff. The parish nursing movement soon spread outside of Christian religious institutions and beyond the borders of the United States to Canada, Australia, and New Zealand. The International Parish Nurse Resource Center, formed in 1986, provides educational programs and resources for nurses who seek to practice as a parish nurse and for educators wishing to conduct training programs for parish nursing.

The Health Ministries Association (HMA), formed in 1989, was instrumental in developing the first *Scope and Standards of Parish Nursing Practice* (HMA, 2010). In the original standards, the term parish nurse was defined as "a registered professional nurse who serves as a member of the ministry staff of a faith community to promote health and wholeness of the faith community ..." (American Nurses Association [ANA]/HMA, 1998, p.1). The term faith community was defined as an "organization of families and individuals who share common values, beliefs, religious doctrine and faith practices ... such as a church, synagogue, or mosque ..." (ANA/HMA, 1998, p. 6). These definitions were carried over to the revised scope and standards, published in 2005, and the title of parish nurse was changed to **faith community nurse** (FCN) and the name of the specialty was changed to "faith community nursing" (ANA/HMA, 2005). Today, nurses who practice in a faith community may be referred to as a FCN, parish nurse, health ministry nurse, congregational nurse, or church nurse depending upon preference and the traditions of the faith community. No matter what title is used, a nurse who practices in a faith community is governed by the *Faith Community Nursing: Scope and Standards of Practice* (ANA/HMA, 2012).

What Do Faith Community Nurses Do?

Activities and interventions used by FCNs are as diverse as their faith communities. Authors have described key aspects of this specialty, which include meeting the emotional and spiritual support needs of the dying (Evans, 2011; Hickman, 2011) and serving as an advocate for individuals who are hospitalized, living at home, or in long-term care facilities (Hickman, 2011; Patterson, 2007). FCNs are also well positioned to address health conditions associated with stigma or embarrassment such as sexually transmitted infections and HIV (Baldwin et al., 2008) and mental health issues (Brown, 2009). The ongoing and long-term nature of the FCNs relationship with the faith community is helpful for addressing highly personal and/or stigmatized subjects as well as increasing awareness and promoting health through education.

FCNs have been instrumental in meeting the educational and health promotion needs of underserved and older adult populations. For example, Williamson and Kautz (2009) implemented a combination of "faith-placed" and "faith-based" interventions for prevention of stroke and cardiovascular disease in African American congregants. Faith-placed interventions included educational sessions, blood pressure screenings, and a commercial weight loss program. Faith-based approaches were based on scripture and included an exercise program called "Let's Get Moving; Let's Get Praising" and healthy eating education programs called "Bread of Life" and "The Body is a Holy Temple." The combination of faith-placed and faith-based programs increased awareness of stroke and heart disease and the need for diet and exercise changes in the congregation.

A review of research from 1993 to 2008 found that FCNs from diverse geographic areas and faith traditions performed consistent interventions to address health concerns that were often aligned with national health priorities (Dyess, Chase, & Newlin, 2009). In addition, many of the interventions, such as education and referral, were comparable to those used in traditional nursing practice. However, FCNs tended to engage in more health promotion interventions and to integrated spiritual and religious practices into their approaches. Earlier reviews found that caring, listening, being there, and providing health promotion and health screenings were common and effective interventions provided by FCNs (Anderson, 2004; King, 2004). In addition, providing holistic support was a major theme in the practice of FCNs (Anderson, 2004). Holistic support included actions that addressed physical, social, emotional, mental, and spiritual needs such as health education, counseling, referral to community agencies, advocacy on the client's behalf to meet needs and reduce complications, and mobilizing other members of the faith community to provide support such as visitation, meals, and transportation. Although the interventions used by FCNs do not emphasize providing direct physical care, such as medication administration, or other prescribed treatments, all registered professional nurses including FCNs share the use of the nursing process (ANA, 2004). For the FCN, implementation of a plan of care incorporates actions that fall within one or more of the seven roles of the FCN (see Display 31.7).

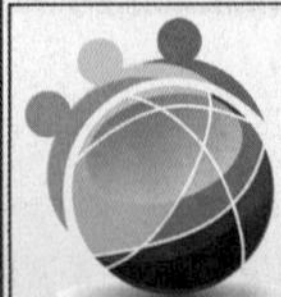

DISPLAY 31.7 ASSURING CONGREGATIONAL HEALTH AND WHOLENESS

Roles of the Faith Community Nurse

1. Health educator
2. Health counselor
3. Advocate
4. Referral agent
5. Developer of support groups
6. Coordinator of volunteers
7. Integrator of faith and health

Accountability

1. ANA scope and standards of nursing practice
2. ANA scope and standards of faith community nursing
3. Congregational standards
4. Institutional standards
5. ANA social policy statement
6. ANA code of ethics for nurses with interpretive statements
7. State nurse practice act
8. Patients rights

FCNs develop and implement a variety of health programs that address the health needs of their congregants. Many programs have been implemented that address the leading health indicators of *Healthy People 2020* such as physical activity, tobacco use, responsible sexual behavior, injury and violence, immunization, overweight and obesity, substance abuse, mental health, environmental quality, and access to health care (USDHHS, 2010). For example, the "Faith Move Mountains Program" was developed to serve the needs for cervical cancer prevention in the Appalachian Mountains (Schoenberg et al., 2009). Other programs have been created and implemented to meet specific needs of the community such as the "Welcome Home Ministries" designed to reduce recidivism for women ex-offenders, released from jail (Warner-Robbins & Parsons, 2010). The roles of the FCN (see Display 31.7) are well suited to support the development, implementation, and evaluation of these and other faith-based health programs.

Roles of the Faith Community Nurse

The goal of the FCN is "protection, promotion and optimization of health and abilities; prevention of illness and injury": and to respond "to suffering within the context of the values, beliefs, and practices of the faith community. ..." (ANA/HMA, 2012). Health promotion outcomes may be primary, directed at prevention of disease, illness, or injury; secondary, focused on early detection and appropriate intervention; or tertiary, concerned with promoting a sense of wellbeing when preventing or curing a condition may not occur. To achieve the goal of faith community nursing, seven diverse nursing roles are central to incorporate into practice.

Health Educator

A primary role of the FCN is as a health educator. Increasing awareness of health issues through health education is the foundation for health promotion and lifestyle changes. The FCN uses assessment skills to determine the health issues that may be present in the faith community and assesses the educational needs related to these issues. In the role of health educator, the FCN may provide individual and group education strategies such as providing health education materials, leading health education classes, or providing health screenings. The FCN may also develop educational displays or flyers, or write educational articles for the faith community newsletter or Web site (Patterson, 2006).

Health Counselor

When education alone is not sufficient for empowering the individual to initiate a change or seek assistance, health counseling may be indicated. In the health counseling role, the nurse seeks to understand the individual's perceptions, fears, and barriers that prevent the person from taking action. The FCN may use a five-step health counseling process described as the 5 A's: Ask, Advise, Assess, Assist, and Arrange (Agency for Healthcare Research and Quality, n.d). Using this process, the FCN asks about the person's perceptions related to a specific health concern, advises the person about the health concern and the benefits of taking health promoting actions, assesses the person's readiness to take action, offers assistance and guidance in planning ways to address the health concern, and arranges follow-up support.

Advocate

The third role of a FCN is that of an advocate, helping individuals obtain needed services or care whether in the hospital, a long-term care facility, or at home. In the advocate role, the FCN uses knowledge of the health care system and awareness of safe and effective care practices to facilitate appropriate, timely intervention. Advocacy is indicated when dealing with vulnerable populations, such as older adults, children, or the homeless, who may not have the ability to speak for themselves or may lack the knowledge or awareness of what constitutes safe, effective care (Patterson, 2007).

Referral Agent

The role of referral agent involves several related aspects. First, the nurse needs to develop knowledge of community resources and contacts. Knowledge of what is available, how the service is accessed, eligibility criteria, and limitations of the service is essential. Next, the nurse networks with and develops collaborative relationships with community leaders and agencies that provide the services. Through networking with community agencies, the FCN becomes aware of and able to easily access a variety of community resources to support the client's physical, social, financial, emotional, or spiritual needs. The nurse is able to draw upon the relationships established with agency personnel to facilitate the eventual use of these resources, when needed. The final aspect of referral involves matching the needs of the individual or group to the services available. Thoughtful referral will assist and guide the client through the health care system and connect them with needed community resources.

Developer of Support Groups

Receiving emotional support from persons who share similar experiences can provide strength, comfort, knowledge, and a sense of empowerment. When the FCN discovers a need for a support group that is not currently available in the community at large, the FCN may fulfill the role of developer of support groups. The FCN develops groups tailored to the faith community needs such as coping with loss and grief, cancer, caregiver stress, chronic illness, single parenting, addiction recovery, and more. The FCN may lead or facilitate the support groups or may train others to fulfill those positions.

Coordinator of Volunteers

The health ministry mission of a faith community typically includes a variety of services and activities to provide holistic support of the physical, social, emotional, mental, and spiritual needs of its members. Such a diverse array of services cannot be provided by the FCN alone. In the role of coordinator of volunteers, the FCN recruits, trains, and coordinates other members of the faith community. Volunteers provide or assist with a variety of services such as home, hospital, or long-term care visitations; respite care; assisting with transportation needs of home-bound individuals; calling or sending cards to ill or injured members; and assisting with health screenings. Health ministry volunteers may include nurses, counselors, physical therapists, pharmacists, and other health care providers, as well as those with no health care background.

Integrator of Faith and Health

A distinctly unique role of the FCN is as integrator of faith and health. This role emphasizes the holistic relationship between physical, social, emotional, mental, and spiritual dimensions of the person. The FCN helps the person to improve health or enhance wellness by appreciating how the dimensions of the person are interconnected and by helping the person strengthen or support the weaker aspects, as needed. The FCN assesses community's strengths and health needs and incorporates an understanding of the connection between faith and health. Using opportunities to enhance the awareness of the interaction between faith and health is central to this role.

Faith Community Nursing Practice

Models of faith community nursing practice are diverse and may be categorized according to volunteer versus salaried positions with institutional versus faith-based sponsorship. The type of practice model adopted depends upon variables such as the number of faith community members served, the existing health ministry services in place, the faith community's governance structure and financial resources, and existing health care systems in the community at large. Early in the development of faith community nursing, FCNs were typically part-time volunteers who were members of the faith community they served. This voluntary, part-time status, coupled with the newness of faith community nursing practice, has resulted in limited research on faith community nursing. Nonetheless, studies that have been conducted have validated the effectiveness of FCNs and the programs they have implemented (Brown, 2006; Brown, Coppola, Giacona, Petriches, & Stockwell, 2009; Dyess et al., 2009; Rydholm, 2006).

There are growing trends in the types of FCN delivery models used today. In larger faith communities, one trend is to include the FCN as a salaried full or part-time staff position. Smaller faith communities may join forces and pool resources to hire a full or part-time FCN to serve multiple congregations. Another trend is the formation of partnerships with organizations such as universities or hospitals, who agree to provide nursing services to the faith community. Partnerships with universities may involve individual faculty and student groups. For nursing faculty, faith community nursing can provide a flexible venue for part-time nursing practice that utilizes their skills in teaching and health promotion. Nursing students can be involved in providing service to faith communities by participating in service learning projects. The philosophy underlying service learning is that both parties benefit from the partnership; students learn and acquire needed skills, and faith communities obtain needed health education or health screenings. In one study, students were trained to provide mental health education to reduce stigma, as part of their service learning experience (Brown, 2009). The students received training to conduct mental health workshops for churches in the community. Study results found statistically significant changes in pre- and posttest scores of students and positive changes in the community's perception of mental health issues.

Regardless of the model of practice utilized, integrating the FCN position into the faith community's organizational structure is recommended (Solari-Twadell & McDermott, 2005; Westberg, 1990; Westberg-McNamara, 2006). One way this integration can be provided is through the formation of a *health cabinet* or health and wellness committee within the faith community. The health cabinet was originally described by Reverend Westberg (1990) as a way to provide health ministry for a faith community that is interested in adding a FCN to its staff. The health cabinet includes members from the faith community who are interested in promoting and sponsoring health-related activities and programs for the faith community. Members may be nurses, other health care professionals, or persons with no health care background. The FCN functions as a member of the health cabinet and receives guidance and support from the cabinet in developing, promoting, and delivering programs and services to members of the faith community.

Becoming a Faith Community Nurse

The FCN practices community nursing with a high degree of independence and autonomy. Often, the FCN deals with clients experiencing complex health care situations who may have limited resources and extensive health-related needs. Recommended educational preparation for a FCN includes a bachelor's degree in nursing with community nursing experience as part of the program (ANA/HMA, 2012) and completion of additional education such as the 36-hour *Foundations of Faith Community Nursing* course offered through the International Parish Nurse Resource Center. The *Foundations of Faith Community Nursing* course addresses the roles of the FCN and provides information on establishing, promoting, and maintaining a FCN practice. Participants gain experience in resolving complex client situations using scenarios and case studies.

Establishing a Faith Community Nursing Practice

Several steps are involved in creating a FCN position within a faith community. One of the first things to do is assess the community the nurse plans to serve, identifying the health needs of the faith community and the roles of the FCN that meet those needs. For example, a nurse might assess the demographics of the community and determine the most common health concerns and what education or health counseling needs the faith community may have. A needs assessment survey of the membership about health concerns, or topics of interest, may be conducted. Questions to explore include the following: Does the faith community need support groups for members who are experiencing the stress of illness, injury, or loss and grief?; do the members of the faith community need more information or assistance to access existing community resources?; and is there a need for health screening, respite care, or visitation for the sick or injured in their home, hospital, or long-term care facility?

Once the nurse has assessed the needs of the faith community, the next step is to identify how a FCN could help to meet those needs. The FCN uses this information to seek the support of the faith community members and staff, usually through visits with key members of the faith community, including the minister, past and present board members, and long-standing members. The nurse describes to these key members the roles of a FCN and how specific health needs of the faith community could be addressed by the services of a FCN and then solicits input from the staff and spiritual leaders of the faith community.

After key members and leaders of the faith community have verbalized support for adding a FCN to the organization's health ministry, the nurse seeks formal approval from the organization's governing body. The scope of services to be offered, time commitment expected, process of referral to the FCN, means of contacting the FCN, and other administrative aspects of the position should be negotiated before approval is finalized. The organization's bylaws, governing body, committee structure, and spiritual leader will play a part in the formal approval process and in determining where the FCN will fit in the organizational structure. The approval process may require a formal presentation of the nurse's proposal to the board members or to the faith community as a whole.

Launching a FCN practice should begin after the nurse has received educational preparation as a FCN and has received formal approval from the faith community's governing body. As a subspecialty in community health nursing, it is recommended that the FCN have educational preparation at the bachelor's level and have specific educational preparation as a FCN. A bachelor's degree in nursing provides community nursing experience, and the foundation course mentioned earlier provides knowledge of the seven roles of the FCN as well as guidance in establishing and maintaining a FCN practice. Prior to initiating services, the nurse and the faith community's administrator should assure that proper liability insurance is in effect. The FCN should carry individual professional liability insurance, and the administrator of the faith community should determine that the activities and services that will be provided are covered by the organization's insurance carrier.

If the faith community is not familiar with FCNs, the nurse will want to educate members about the roles of the FCN. The FCN can give presentations about faith community nursing to groups within the faith community, such as prayer circles, adult Sunday school, teen groups, and existing support groups. During the presentations, the FCN can discuss specific activities that will be actively pursued, such as home or hospital visitations, formation of support groups, teaching health classes, and providing health screening, health counseling, spiritual support, and referral to community resources. These presentations will provide multiple benefits for both the FCN and the members of the faith community by allowing the nurse to establish relationships with members of the faith community and by allowing members to become familiar with the FCN and the services offered.

In addition to providing presentations about faith community nursing to groups within the faith community, the nurse should consider other ways to inform members of the services provided. If the faith community publishes a newsletter or has a Web site, including a brief introduction to faith community nursing and providing some personal background and professional experience, information will be useful. The FCN may develop flyers and brochures that describe what a FCN does and the services offered. These materials may be distributed initially to new members and may be continually displayed on the community bulletin board. Business cards that provide the FCNs name, contact information, and outline FCN services may be distributed. The FCN may also write a monthly feature for the newsletter to provide health education and to keep the congregation informed of the services offered. These strategies and others will provide mechanisms for initial and ongoing marketing the FCNs services to the faith community.

Another aspect of preparation involves establishing community contacts and compiling information about community resources. The FCN should visit local health-related agencies, clinics, and hospitals and discuss services they provide and how the services can be accessed by members of the faith community. Information from community organizations, such as the March of Dimes, American Cancer Society, American Heart Association, as well as others, can provide health information and online resources for health promotion activities.

And finally, the FCN will need to decide on a method of documentation and record keeping. Documentation of the FCN activities and outcomes will provide ongoing evidence of the effectiveness of programs and interventions, which can be used to justify continuation of programs and services. Rydholm developed a format for documentation based on FOCUS charting, using the acronym DIARY (Rydholm et al., 2008). The DIARY format was specifically developed for documenting actions and outcomes related to faith community nursing. It differs from other charting formats by including the care receiver in the intervention or action stage and by including the care receiver's perceptions in the outcome or response area (see Display 31.8). Whatever method of documentation is used, the FCN will need to assure consistent documentation, confidentiality, and proper storage of the records.

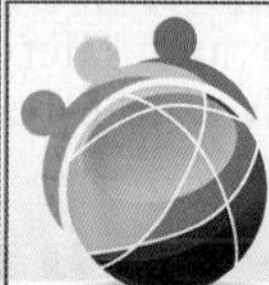

DISPLAY 31.8 DIARY DOCUMENTATION FORMAT

D = Data related to the problem
I = Interpretation of the problem
A = Actions of the care receiver and FCN
R = Response of the care receiver to the action
Y = Yield or perceived benefit/risk reduction

OCCUPATIONAL AND ENVIRONMENTAL HEALTH NURSING

Business and industry provide another group of settings for community health nursing practice. Employee health has long been recognized as making a vital contribution to individual lives, productivity of business, and the wellbeing of the entire nation. Organizations are expected to provide a safe and healthy work environment in addition to offering insurance for health care. More companies, recognizing the value of healthy employees, are going beyond offering traditional health benefits to supporting health promotional efforts. Some businesses, for example, offer healthy snacks such as fruit at breaks and promote jogging during the noon hour. A few larger corporations have built exercise facilities for their employees, provide health education programs, and offer financial incentives for losing weight or staying well. An increasing number of both large and small companies have recognized the benefits of **occupational and environmental health nurses** as part of their overall health promotion and wellness efforts.

History of the Occupational and Environmental Health Nurse

Community health nurses have a long history of involvement in occupational health. In 1895, the Vermont Marble Company hired the first *industrial nurse* in the United States to care for its employees and their families. At the time, it was an unusual demonstration of interest in employee welfare. The nursing service, which consisted mostly of home visiting and care of the sick, was free to employees and their families. Gradually that role changed. World War II showed a marked increase in employment of occupational health nurses, who practiced illness prevention and health education among employees at work.

Although occupational health nursing has been in existence since the late 1800s, the Occupational Safety and Health Act of 1970 (29 CFR 1910) led to the proliferation of occupational health nursing employment in the United States. This important legislation established the **Occupational Safety and Health Administration (OSHA)** in the Department of Labor, to ensure a safe working environment for workers in the United States. Occupational and environmental health nurses work collaboratively with others on the health and safety team to monitor employees' health and advocate for a safe work environment.

Roles of Occupational and Environmental Health Nurses

Occupational health nursing practice can be divided into three main categories: compliance, care, and health promotion. There are a number of federal and state regulations that have some health requirements. For instance, OSHA requires training and hearing tests for employees who are exposed to loud noise at the workplace (29 CFR 1910.95). The Department of Transportation requires commercial drivers to pass a physical exam before they are allowed to drive and periodically throughout their driving career (49 CFR 391). The Americans with Disabilities Act (ADA) requires employers with 15 or more employees to make reasonable accommodations for persons with disabilities (ADA, 2000), and nurses are often part of the reasonable accommodation decision-making team. In health care settings, employee health nurses are instrumental in ensuring the institution's compliance with requirements for immunizations and tuberculosis testing.

The occupational health nurse is typically the first person to evaluate an injury that occurs in the workplace. Every state has laws governing workers' compensation for occupational injuries and illnesses. Workers' compensation is generally considered no-fault insurance. In exchange for receiving free treatment and compensation for time away from work, in most states employees are banned from suing an employer for an unsafe work environment. Although some companies outsource case management for work-related injuries, many occupational health nurses manage cases to ensure the employee's optimum recovery while helping to control costs.

Occupational health nurses are in an ideal position to provide guidance, counseling, education, and coaching for employees who want to improve their health. Occupational health nurses engage in primary prevention each time they teach an employee the importance of physical activity to control weight, with every flu shot they administer, and with every safe-lifting demonstration they give. In the workplace, occupational health nurses may do cholesterol checks or body mass index (BMI) screenings as part of secondary prevention. After employees are injured or become ill, occupational health nurses may work to ensure a speedy and functional recovery, frequently helping employees work through the workers' compensation or insurance bureaucracy.

In addition to addressing the health needs of the employees, it is important for the occupational health nurse to recognize the impact of the workplace on their own personal health. For instance, there are various causes of job stress for the occupational and environmental health nurse, and there may be related personal, professional, and employer factors. The nurse may experience role ambiguity due to a lack of professional preparation or inadequate orientation and continuing education. The corporate culture and leadership may foster work overload, be nonsupportive, and have limited career opportunities for the nurse. Occupational and environmental health nurses need to apply strategies to reduce job stress and potential job strain by modeling health-affirming choices, networking with other nurses and professional organizations in the community, and setting appropriate occupational health standards.

Health Promotion Opportunities

The United States spends 16% of its gross domestic product on health care, the greatest percentage among industrialized countries (RWJF, 2009). In some countries, health care is incorporated into their social system; in the United States, employees of large companies typically get health insurance as a benefit of their jobs. As the cost of insurance increases, employers pass on some of those cost increases to workers in the form of higher premiums, copays, and deductibles (Society for Human Resource Management, 2009).

Although occupational health nurses had been advocating healthy lifestyles for several decades, US company executives only recently began to recognize the value of having healthy workers. Research supports the link between healthy lifestyle and lower health care costs indicating that healthy employees are less likely to be absent from work and more likely to be more productive when they are at work (Baker et al., 2008; Kowlessar, Goetzel, Carls, Tabrizi, & Guidnon, 2011). However, getting Americans to embrace a healthy lifestyle of physical activity, good nutrition, and sufficient rest is a challenge.

Because workers spend so much of their life at the workplace (in both hours and years), it is important to develop a culture of health at the workplace. At every encounter with an employee, whether for an occupational health exam or an injury, the nurse has an opportunity to encourage healthy choices. Occupational health nurses are learning to become health coaches as a way to assist individual employees improve their health. Health coaches use a variety of strategies and techniques to motivate individuals to set and attain goals for lifestyle improvements. Occupational health nurses partner with communications professionals to craft compelling messages that encourage healthy choices, and they may provide consultation to upper management to help ensure that benefits packages reflect the company's desire for healthful personal practices. Additionally, the occupational health nurse is in a position to influence the type of food that is offered in the company's cafeteria as well as the selection of products available in vending machines.

The Occupational Health Team

Occupational health nurses work in a team environment with a variety of other professionals. Depending on the size of the company, the occupational health team may include a safety specialist, industrial hygienist, ergonomist, physical or occupational therapist, physician, lawyer, and employee assistance counselor. Human resources, management, security, and emergency response personnel are also part of the team. The employee is central to the team and is the reason for the team's existence.

Team collaboration is essential to the success of the occupational and environmental health program, and the nurse plays a key role in ensuring adequate and appropriate communication among the members of the team. Establishing working relationships is paramount in the success of a functional and effective team (Wachs, 2005). Strong interpersonal relationship skills are extremely valuable in a team environment.

Finally, the occupational health team is not complete without the workers themselves. Employees can help identify problems and needs while contributing to decision making about health programs. Their cooperation in implementing and evaluating programs is essential for an effective health protection and promotion effort.

Settings for Occupational and Environmental Health Nursing

Occupational and environmental health nursing may be one of the most challenging and rewarding nursing specialties, affording nurses the opportunity to establish long-term relationships with their clients and address issues across the wellness–illness continuum. Unlike nursing in acute care settings and public health departments, the employer's primary mission is not typically related to health or illness. Companies exist to make a profit; occupational health and safety professionals are employed to keep workers productive and to ensure compliance with state and federal health and safety requirements.

Some nurses select occupational health nursing because they are looking for a career change away from acute care nursing. Others find that rotating shifts and working weekends and holidays are not conducive to their desired lifestyle. Still others seek fulfillment through the establishment of more long-term relationships with their clients. On occasion, nurses can move straight into occupational health when they graduate from a BSN program. Nurses who move into occupational and environmental health from an acute care setting should expect a significant learning curve to feel comfortable in this nontraditional setting. Nurses who select the field of occupational health and safety encounter experiences that differ significantly from those found in an acute care setting. To make the adjustment, the nurse should be aware of the factors that make occupational health unique. Unlike hospitals or ambulatory care centers, the workplace is a non–health care institution in which production or service (not health care) is the primary goal. The occupational and environmental health nurse participates in the organization's goals through activities that contribute to the productivity of the workforce.

In addition to learning the role of the occupational and environmental health nurse, the nurse needs to understand the parent company and become familiar with the employees' work environment and work tasks.

In many work settings, the occupational and environmental health nurse is the only health professional. In these situations, the nurse must have excellent assessment skills, not only for individuals but also for the working population served. Independent decision making is critical. Nurses in occupational settings must also have strong communication skills, including listening, speaking, and writing.

Models of practice differ depending on the philosophy and size of the company. Nurse-managed clinics are managed by registered professional nurses who employ or contract with other health professionals as appropriate (Wachs, 1997). Nurse-managed clinics may utilize occupational health nurses, a nurse practitioner or physician assistant, a physical therapist, a health educator, and a part-time occupational physician. A single-nurse unit is a common model of practice in many smaller companies. In single-nurse unit, occupational health nurses typically build strong networks of colleagues with whom they can discuss professional practice issues. Some companies use a medical model of practice in that a physician determines clinic staffing and the department's approach to clinical practice. During the early 21st century, many companies in the United States began implementing primary care clinics as a method of controlling the cost of health care. Services in primary care clinics may be extended to dependents and retirees, typically offer urgent care services, and may also provide routine health examinations in addition to the usual occupational health services needed by an employer.

Community-Based Occupational Health Nursing

Occupational health nurses work in a variety of settings. The manufacturing sector has a strong tradition of employing occupational health nurses, but utility companies, mines, retail store chains (grocery, department, home-improvement), hospitals, theme parks, banks, school systems, and government also employ occupational health nurses. Because professional nurses have a variety of skill sets, they can care for injuries, manage disabilities, counsel employees who are troubled, help workers control their chronic diseases, and encourage high-level wellness. Entrepreneurial nurses may set up an occupational health clinic in areas where many small businesses are located (e.g., industrial parks) and provide professional nursing services for employers that may not need a dedicated, full-time nurse.

Agencies external to business and industry also provide occupational and environmental health nursing services. Historically, public health nurses from visiting nurse associations made home visits to sick employees and their families. In subsequent years, public health agencies provided part-time nursing services to small companies. These services included supervising the work environment, conducting health examinations, keeping records, teaching about and counseling on health issues, providing first aid, giving immunizations, and referring workers to community resources. More recently, community health nursing services have offered health screening and health promotion programs. Furthermore, occupational and environmental health nurse consultants based in state departments of health provide consultation and continuing education programs to nurses employed in occupational health settings.

Hospital-based occupational health programs, large medical–industrial health clinics, and insurance companies also provide occupational and environmental health nursing services. These services may be in the form of direct care (rehabilitation of an injured worker) or indirect care (consultation on implementing regulations regarding record keeping or compiling health statistics).

A continuing unmet need is attending to the health of workers in smaller companies. These companies have more hazards because equipment and controls are often inadequate. They seldom, if ever, have a health professional on site. Attempts have been made by some communities to provide needed health protection services, but no sustained efforts exist. Community health nurses are in a position to accept this challenge and develop a system that will ensure ongoing service to this high-risk population.

Evidence-Based Practice and Educational Preparation

During the last two decades, a number of nursing education programs (primarily on the graduate level) have developed a specialty focus in occupational and environmental health. In addition, many continuing education programs provide occupational and environmental health nurses with updated information and skill training for identifying and assisting in the management of the physical, chemical, biologic, ergonomic, and psychosocial factors in the work environment that can affect worker health and safety.

The National Institutes for Occupational Safety and Health (NIOSH), part of the Centers for Disease Control and Prevention (CDC), is an agency established by the Occupational Safety and Health Act of 1970 [Public Law 91-596]. NIOSH is responsible for conducting research related to worker health and safety and for educating health and safety professionals to prepare them for evidence-based careers in occupational and environmental health and safety. NIOSH has established 17 **Education Resource Centers (ERCs)** to fulfill that responsibility (NIOSH, 2011). Many ERCs provide online courses, and scholarships are available (NIOSH, 2011).

Additionally, occupational health nurses may become certified in this specialty field. The American Board for Occupational Health Nurses (ABOHN) is an independent nursing specialty certification board. Founded in 1972, ABOHN is an independent not-for-profit organization that sets professional standards and conducts occupational health nursing specialty certification. ABOHN is the sole certifying body for occupational health nurses in the United States (ABOHN, 2008). This independent nursing specialty board has the stated purposes of (1) establishing standards and examinations for professional nurses in occupational health,

(2) elevate and maintain the quality of occupational health nursing services, (3) stimulate the development of improved educational standards and programs in the field of occupational health nursing, and (4) encourage occupational health nurses to continue their professional education (ABOHN, 2008).

The Effect of Work on Health

Workers in the United States generally spend more time at work than on any other activity except sleep. Thus, the work environment can have a significant impact on workers' health. The type of work that people engage in dictates the hazards they encounter. For instance, think about the work of hospital based nurses. They encounter physical hazards, such as lifting patients in bed without mechanical lifting devices. There are biological hazards associated with blood and body fluids, as well as infectious diseases. Some nurses are at risk for chemical exposures, such as those associated with operating room gases or chemotherapy. Radiation hazards may exist when working with patients undergoing radiation therapy.

Hazardous substances can get into a person's body through inhalation, ingestion, absorption, or percutaneously. Although personal protective equipment (PPE) is available to workers, some may not use PPE consistently, or the equipment may not be entirely effective. Workers exposed to chemicals may not wash their hands sufficiently before eating or smoking, thus providing an opportunity for chemicals to get into their system through ingestion or inhalation.

Employees who work in awkward positions or who do repetitive tasks that use the same muscle groups are at risk for musculoskeletal disorders (MSDs). Stressing muscles and joints repeatedly can result in inflammation and pain and can lead to serious conditions that require physical therapy and/or surgery. Employees who compound a workplace exposure with off-work activities that use the same muscle groups in similar actions will accelerate or aggravate a problem. For instance, a mechanic may work on his own car in the evenings and on the weekend, so the muscles that are used every day never really get a chance to rest and recover.

Repeated exposure to loud noise can result in a high-frequency hearing loss (Council for Accreditation in Occupational Hearing Conservation, 2011). Such hearing losses are gradual; employees may not heed advice to wear hearing protection devices, which they may consider uncomfortable or annoying. High-frequency hearing loss diminishes an individual's ability to understand what others are saying, especially in a noisy environment such as a restaurant. Research shows that hearing losses can result in social isolation with resulting depression among the elderly (Cetin, Uguz, Erdem, & Yildirim, 2010; Cohen & Turley, 2009; Lee, Tong, Yuen, Tang, & Van Hasselt, 2010). Hearing aids can provide some improvement in understanding the spoken word, but they have limitations and are very expensive (see Display 31.9).

Shift work, particularly rotating shifts, negatively impacts sleep and rest cycles (Job Accommodation Network, 2011). Insufficient sleep is associated with obesity and diabetes (Courtemanche, 2009; Seidell, 2010). Low-paying jobs may drive workers to get a second or even a third job to make ends meet. Personal stressors or balancing work and family demands, plus employer expectations at work, can have an adverse effect on worker health (see from the Case Files III).

Healthy People 2020

Occupational safety and health is one topic area found in *Healthy People 2020*. The goal of this topic area is to promote the health and safety of people at work through prevention. The intent of the ten objectives found are to prevent diseases, injuries, and deaths due to working conditions (USDHHS, 2010). The occupational and environmental health nurse plays a crucial role in assisting employees to meet *Healthy People 2020* occupational safety and health objectives.

Future Trends

A broad goal for occupational health is to promote and maintain the highest level of physical, social, and emotional health for all workers. In practice, this goal is only beginning to be realized in selected instances. Nevertheless, it is a worthy and, more importantly, an essential objective in the realization of an energized and productive working community.

However, the rapid and fundamental changes in US businesses and the economy in the 1990s and 2000s have added four critical issues that affect the practice of occupational and environmental health nursing. First, the downturn in the global economy, and in the economy of the United States specifically, has skeletonized many worksites, shut down companies, eliminated night or evening shifts, or moved companies to less expensive communities. In addition, several major scandals have eliminated employees within hours, such as with the Enron and Worldcom corporations and major banks involved in risky home loans that resulted in unprecedented housing foreclosures across the country. Second, increasing worldwide competition requires businesses to remain competitive by reducing or controlling operating costs at the lowest level possible. Third, there has been an increase in technologic hazards that require a sophisticated approach as well as knowledge of toxicology, epidemiology, ergonomics, and public health principles. Fourth, health care costs continue to escalate at faster rates than most company profits do.

Current occupational and environmental health nurse practices will continue to evolve to meet future needs. The focus is shifting from one-on-one health services to involving broader environmental, business, and research skills. One such example of this changing role was an Australian study of nurses' perceptions of their current and future roles in occupational health practice (Mellor & St John, 2007). The researchers found that wellness, management, and research were the more important activities identified. Their findings suggest that educational

DISPLAY 31.9 OCCUPATIONAL AND ENVIRONMENTAL HEALTH NURSING CARE PLAN

Evelyn Robbins has been the Occupational and Environmental Health Nurse at ABC Metals for 4 years. She works with management, the company physician (who works at ABC Metals 2 days a week), union representatives, unit foremen, individual employees, and representatives from the community businesses and neighborhoods surrounding the plant. The company employs 400 workers—380 in manufacturing, primarily an assembly line making telephone electrical boxes, and 20 management and administrative staff.

Recently, 12 employees came to the worksite clinic complaining of hand injuries that had not occurred before. Mr. Robbins treated the wounds, reported the occurrences to the foremen involved, and reported the incidents to management. In addition, she wanted to explore the cause of these injuries so that they could be interrupted. She used the nursing process in her exploration.

Assessment

- Tour the areas where the incidents occurred.
- Inquire among the foremen to determine whether there was a change in routine, equipment, employee assignment, or product being manufactured.
- Ask injured employees what they were doing when the injury occurred.
- Reassess wounds for likenesses and differences; for example, was it the right or left hand and was it on the same part of the hand in each case?

Diagnoses

- Wounds occurred in factory areas where a new piece of equipment had been installed.
- Injured employees did not receive orientation to the equipment.

Plan

- Plan to work with foremen to provide an orientation for all employees who work with the new equipment.
- Plan an orientation program (with foremen, union representatives, and one employee from each unit in the factory) for all employees before working with new equipment in the future, to prevent further injuries.

Implementation

- Implement the orientation for employees who work with the new equipment.
- Initiate the orientation program as new equipment is introduced into the factory.

Evaluation

- Have there been any new equipment–related injuries in the factory?
- Has there been any change in general safety in the factory related to the increased focus on safety with new equipment?

From the Case Files

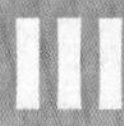

The human resources director approaches the occupational health nurse about a situation he learned about from a manager in building 2. The manager reported that an employee has been acting out during the last 2 weeks, shouting at other employees. Additionally, the employee's work product has not met quality standards on several occasions during the same time period. Another employee told the manager that she heard the employee say that he was "fed up with everyone" and was going to "put an end to it."

1. What should the occupational health nurse do?
2. Who on the team should be involved with this situation?
3. What preventive measures could be put into place as part of the team's structure to be prepared to respond to situations like this?

efforts should focus on wellness-based models of practice, research, and negotiating skills for the workplace.

Standard occupational health nurse activities include the following:

1. Supervising care for emergencies and minor illnesses
2. Counseling employees about health risks
3. Following up with employees' workers' compensation claims
4. Performing periodic health assessments
5. Evaluating the health status of employees returning to work

Emerging occupational health nurse activities include the following:

1. Analyzing trends (health promotion, risk reduction, and health expenditures)
2. Developing programs suited to corporate needs
3. Recommending more efficient and cost-effective in-house health services
4. Determining cost-effective alternatives to health programs and services
5. Collaborating with others to identify problems and propose solutions

As we move further into the 21st century, occupational and environmental health nurses and management will share the goal of developing a healthy, productive, and profitable company. A healthy company consists of healthy and productive employees, and healthy employees mean lower health care costs. Lower costs result in an increased competitive edge and higher profits. Higher profits can make more resources available to support more programs and to improve employee health.

The occupational and environmental health nurse will particularly need skills in effective communication, leadership, change management, research, business acumen, and assertiveness. These tools will be crucial for effectively interpreting the occupational health nurse's role and promoting ideas. Success of programs developed by the occupational health nurse depends on establishment of positive working relationships with the other team members. Nurses involved in occupational health have a unique opportunity to help shape the health profile of the working population. An example of this type of effort was the study by Hyeonkyeong, Wilbur, Kim, and Miller (2008) linking high job insecurity with increased risk for lower-back work-related MSDs among long-haul flight attendants. Their findings point to the need for occupational health nurses in the airline industry to be aware of the potential relationship between job tasks and work-related psychosocial factors.

The degree of the occupational nurse's influence depends on how the nurse defines the occupational and environmental health nurse role. Also, the nurse must be able to overcome the many obstacles found in the occupational setting, including restrictive company policies, misunderstanding of the nurse's role, and lack of time for innovative program development. The nurse's role in occupational health, therefore, varies considerably. It ranges from providing only emergency care for on-the-job injuries or illness to establishing comprehensive policies and programs covering health promotion, accident and disease prevention, and innovative care for disease and disability.

Occupational and environmental health nursing demands a great deal from the nurse. Individual needs in the workplace always compete for the nurse's time and take attention away from aggregate needs, often to the detriment of the latter. To maintain a proper focus on aggregate needs requires discipline and commitment—commitment based on a different mind-set and the realization that the health and productivity of workers are interrelated with the health of the community.

NURSE ENTREPRENEUR IN COMMUNITY/PUBLIC HEALTH NURSING

As you have discovered throughout this chapter, the roles and responsibilities of nurses in the community often require skill with grant writing, agency and personnel management, collaboration both inter- and intraprofessionally, fiscal management, and agency promotion. The community/public health nurse often works within an agency or organization to address unmet needs in the community with the ultimate goal of enhancing service delivery. This is true for a FCN, a nurse in a FQHC, or an occupational health nurse. These positions are often nonexistent until the nurse is able to identify a need and take the necessary steps to start a stand-alone service or to develop a role within an existing agency. There is, however, a growing trend in nursing to seek a more independent practice in health care delivery and services through entrepreneurship. In 1986, Susan Hartley of the ANA posted a letter to the editor in the American Journal of Public Health requesting information on nurse entrepreneurs with the stated goal of "developing a list of nurse entrepreneurs as part of a continuing effort to describe the delivery of nursing services" and to "gather data and resource people to support lobbying efforts to achieve payment systems for nursing" (p. 1034). This short request punctuates the growing recognition of the varied roles that nurses have and the impact of reimbursement on service delivery. As you think about your own career, can you envision yourself running a health care business, seeking a small business loan to start a venture, or having the courage to explore other professional options? Independent practice is not for everyone, and nurses are often socialized to view their role as working within a larger organization, a health department, a community clinic, and most often a hospital. At some point in your career, you may find yourself working with a nurse entrepreneur or becoming one yourself. The following discussion will give you a glimpse at the challenges and rewards of this journey.

Merriam-Webster defines an entrepreneur as "one who organizes, manages, and assumes the risks of a business or enterprise" (merriam-webster.com, 2012). By extension an **entrepreneurial nurse** is one who is willing to take on that role within a health care or social context. Common examples of nurse entrepreneurs include legal consultants, forensic nurses, owners of home health care agencies, authors, and nurse consultants in a variety of areas. For the community/public health nurse, these and many other options offer the independence to provide services in perhaps a new and innovative way. For health care to continue to respond to the changing environment, the innovators are often the ones who have the courage to test those new methods. They may fail or fall short in those efforts, but they learn from both the success and challenges and are better positioned for a successful outcome.

Steps to Becoming a Nurse Entrepreneur

One of the first steps to becoming a nurse entrepreneur is to have an idea. It doesn't have to be a new idea or even a "big" idea, but it must address an unmet need within a community. Community/public health nurses are often the first to identify the challenges and needs within a community and to explore solutions. Very often, participation in professional organizations helps to identify health care issues that can be addressed by nurses. The common refrain "why doesn't someone just (invent, build, provide, etc.)?" can often be answered by a nurse. Nurses are problem solvers, and using the nursing process, they assess the situation, identify the problem, determine a course of action, and evaluate the results. This skill can be leveraged to start a new business venture, to develop a nonprofit agency, or to create educational tools for use by other health care professionals or the general public. Whatever the health care need, nurses can and do find the solutions.

Elango, Hunter, and Winchell (2007) undertook a study of the barriers to nurse entrepreneurship through focus groups conducted by expert moderators. One group consisted of two hospital administrators, a nurse entrepreneur, an ophthalmology entrepreneur, and a dean of a nursing program with knowledge of this role. The second group included nurse practitioner students. Using a process model of entrepreneurship adapted from Bhave (1994), new venture creation was preceded by first recognizing an opportunity, overcoming challenges, and developing operational competencies. Opportunity recognition was seen as falling into three major categories, demographic trends (the aging population), opportunities in health care organizations (nursing shortage), and social trends (busy lifestyles, preventive health care, and hospital closures). Barriers to creating a new venture included legal and regulatory barriers, ethical and personal conflicts, and knowledge barriers. Operational competencies were seen as lack of management skills, minimal public awareness, and institutional support. The authors outline six suggestions to promote entrepreneurship (p. 203):

- Seek local resources to develop business skills.
- Do not be constrained by current resources.
- Build an active network within the community.
- Understand the importance of entrepreneurship.
- Mobilize professional resources at the state and national level.
- Assume an active role in public policy.

The steps outlined by Elango et al. are similar to the following five steps from the National Nurses in Business Association, Inc.:

- Review your business options and determine what you enjoy doing.
- Determine if there are enough clients (customers) for the business to make a profit doing what you enjoy.
- Obtain the knowledge needed to provide the service.
- Obtain the business knowledge needed to start and operate the business sale.
- Start and grow the business.

The president of the NNBA, Patricia Bemis, offers a number of suggestions in the development of a business plan (2006). This plan is essential to starting a business, growing a business, and obtaining financial support. At the very minimum, the business plan should include the description of the business; marketing strategies; competitive analysis, design, and development plan; operations and management plan; and financial factors. Bemis also emphasizes the need for choosing a name and the correct colors for promotional materials. She cautions that the "name of your business is not about creativity but is an integral component of your marketing strategy" (p. 1). The name should be easily spelled and pronounced, elicit a positive emotional response from the customer, and be short and to the point. The meaning of color and the important role it plays in the success of your business are included in Table 31-1. In what may seem like a frivolous topic,

Table 31.1 The Impact of Color

Color	General Impact	Business Impact
Black	Classic, authority, evil	Use it as a background color to create contrast with white text.
White	Innocence, sterility	It can be sterile and refreshing; white backgrounds with black text provide contrast; best color for Web site background
Red	Emotionally intense, strength, faster heart beat, commands attention	Boldness, in accounting associated with debt
Pink	Romantic, tranquilizing, gentleness, wellbeing	Feminine links
Blue	Color of sky and ocean, one of the most popular colors	Sanctuary, fiscal responsibility
Green	Nature, health, freedom; calming and refreshing	Status and wealth
Yellow	Cheerful, gets attention, can be overpowering if overused	Appeals to intellectual types and a good accent
Purple	Spirituality, royalty, sophistication	Upscale and works with artistic types
Brown	Solid and reliable	Suggests less importance
Gray	Authority, practicality, creativity	Portrays a traditional and conservative company
Orange	Pleasure, excitement strength and ambition	Good for highlighting information on charges and graphs

Adapted from Bemis (2006). Nurse entrepreneur: Devise and implement a great game plan. *Alternative Journal of Nursing, 11*, 1–5.

she cautions that the psychology of color and contrast is vital to your overall business plan and should be carefully selected.

Opportunities

As the health care needs of the population demand newer, better and less expensive solutions, nurse entrepreneurs are well positioned to address those needs. While there are many examples in your own communities of nurse entrepreneurship, the role of the community/public health nurse can serve as a strong base for meeting the health care challenges locally, nationally, and internationally. One example of a nurse entrepreneur is Barbara Hanna, the president and owner of a California-based home health care agency. Recognizing that local public health agencies were challenged to meet the ever-growing needs in the community, she formed a nonprofit organization *Caring Choices*. Over the past decade, this agency has joined the statewide effort to manage spontaneous responders in periods of disaster, provided an emergency food closet for needy residents, performed in-home safety checks by a registered nurse in homes with children under 5 years of age, and HIV/AIDS assistance (caring-choices.org, 2012). Garnering public and private grant funding, she has identified and addressed needed services in Northern California while leveraging scarce financial and personnel resources.

The opportunities are limitless for nurse entrepreneurship; the only missing piece is the nurse willing to take that leap, come up with an idea, explore the options, create a business plan, garner funding, and make a difference. Community/public health nurses are uniquely qualified to address the ever-growing challenges in our communities. As opportunities in one area of nursing practice recede, other avenues open up; the trick is to recognize those opportunities when they present.

SUMMARY

Healthy People 2020 guides both public and private sector nursing practice well into the next decade. Community health nurses have a number of options available to them as they seek to address the myriad health issues facing our communities. For many, opportunities may present to assume roles in a variety of nontraditional settings, including nurse-managed health centers, faith community nursing, occupational and environmental health nursing, and nurse entrepreneurship. All four roles offer the community health nurse the opportunity to address health disparities in their communities, promote healthy lifestyles, and improve the overall health and wellbeing of their respective populations.

NHMCs represent a growing movement of health centers that have emerged as vital safety-net providers in America's contemporary health care delivery system. Various nursing center models exist and are located in HPSAs or MUAs in urban and rural communities. Interdisciplinary teams of advanced practice nurses, social workers, substance abuse counselors, community health outreach workers, and students from varied disciplines provide services that generally focus on primary and secondary prevention strategies. Lundeen's Comprehensive Community-Based Primary Health Care Model demonstrates how NMHCs are distinct from public health agencies and medical care facilities. Funding sources for NMHCs include reimbursement from various organizations, sliding scale fees, grants, contracts, foundation support, and private support via gifts. Sustainability is an ongoing challenge in all NMHC models. An international organization to strengthen the capacity, growth, and development of NMHCs is the National Nursing Centers Consortium. NMHCs identify, develop, and share best practices. Nurse leaders and staff from NMHCs engage in sociopolitical activities to raise awareness of the outcomes generated by the nursing center model. These activities are implemented to raise awareness of the role of NMHCs in the health care system and to promote sustainability of the centers. Undergraduate and graduate students from various disciplines engage in all aspects of NMHC activities and augment the interdisciplinary team.

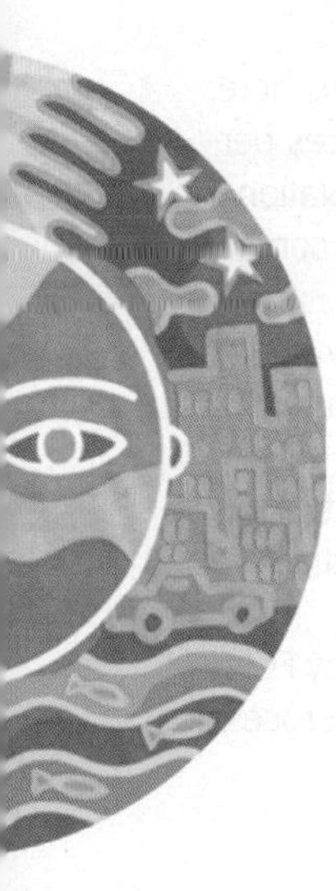

FCNs practice community nursing within a unique setting—a faith community. A FCN may provide services to a single faith community or may coordinate services for multiple communities. The FCN addresses the physical, social, emotional, mental, and spiritual needs of the faith community through the roles of health educator, health counselor, referral agent, advocate, developer of support groups, coordinator of volunteers, and integrator of faith and health.

Occupational and environmental health nursing applies the philosophy and skills of nursing, community, and environmental health to protect and promote the health of people in their workplaces. The occupational and environmental health nurse's role is evolving as business becomes more competitive and health care costs escalate at a frightening rate. That expanded role will include analyzing current trends, recommending more cost-effective and innovative in-house health services, and collaborating with other members of the multidisciplinary occupational health team, including management, to develop appropriate programs. Occupational and environmental health nurses help companies remain competitive by promoting health and wellbeing in worker populations.

The nurse entrepreneur is not a new concept. Nurses have traditionally worked within existing agencies (hospitals, clinics, or health departments), yet many have sought the autonomy of providing health-related services independently, by starting a new business venture. As community/public health nurses gain experience and confidence in starting and developing health care programs, those same skills can be utilized to identify unmet community needs, develop a business plan, seek funding sources, and start an independent business. The FCN may market his services to a number of small faith communities, a NMHC may, in addition to providing grant-based services, begin marketing services to employees of local businesses, the occupational health nurse may recognize a growing need for health education materials that could be purchased by other industries, or the nurse may leverage their specially area skills to publish educational materials or start a nonprofit agency to meet community needs. The opportunities for nurse entrepreneurship are a growing and much needed area for community/public health nurses to explore.

Each of these professional practice areas provides a unique opportunity for community health nursing practice. Escalating health care costs, increasing numbers of uninsured and underinsured, and the many gaps in services experienced by so many in our communities present an unprecedented opportunity for community health nurses. The many unmet needs in our communities can be addressed but only if there are nurses willing to take the "road less traveled" as did Lillian Wald and the other pioneers of nursing. As you ponder your options for practice, consider the challenges and the many benefits of these and the many other practice areas in your community. Perhaps you cannot envision yourself in this type of service at this point in your career. A time may come, however, when you are afforded the chance to participate in your own faith community health education efforts—or refer a client to a nurse-managed health center—or possibly collaborate with an occupational and environmental health nurse to address an emerging health issue in your community. You may even find that starting your own business or nonprofit agency affords you the independence and challenge you seek in your career.

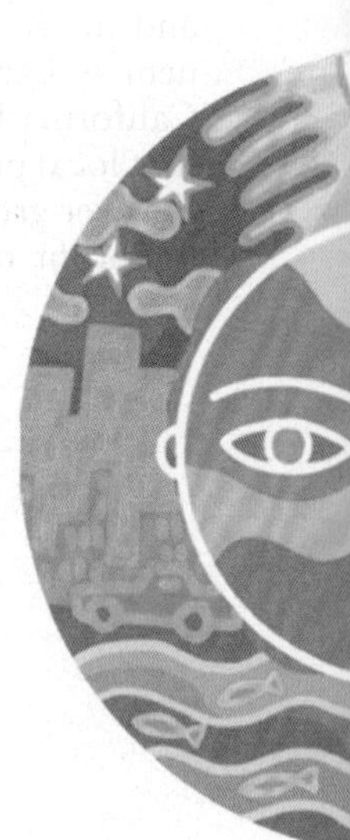

ACTIVITIES TO PROMOTE **CRITICAL THINKING**

1. You are practicing as a newly hired nurse in a NMHC. What assessments would you conduct to determine the needs for the local community that surrounds the NMHC? What sources of data (qualitative and quantitative) would be useful to you during your assessment?
2. Base upon your findings in the previous question, what public policy issues are apparent in this community? How could you, as a nurse working in this NMHC, impact public policy in the future? What key legislators would you contact? How would you accomplish this?
3. Locate a NMHC in your community. Interview a public health nurse or a nurse practitioner employed here. Ask the nurse to describe the type of NMHC model he/she works in. Ask the nurse about ***Best Practices*** performed in his/her role. If you cannot locate a NMHC in your local community, search online via the National Nursing Centers Consortium's Web site at www.nncc.us for a NMHC. Email the nurse listed as the contact person and ask him/her the questions found above.
4. This chapter covers the role of the parish nurse. Search for information about this area of community health nursing in your community. Do you know a parish nurse? If so, plan to observe his or her practice for a few hours and explore what the role entails in this faith community.
5. Use the Internet and networking to find information about faith community nursing in your community. How prevalent are FCNs in your community? Is there a local organization for FCNs? What models of practice are most commonly used in your community?
6. Contact a FCN in your area and arrange to interview or shadow the nurse. Explore the services offered by FCNs in your area. Identify the knowledge and skills needed to function effectively in the role. Discuss the process the nurse used to establish his or her FCN practice.

ACTIVITIES TO PROMOTE **CRITICAL THINKING *(Continued)***

7. Conduct a literature search to discover health programs that have been developed and used by faith communities to address the leading health indicators identified in *Healthy People 2020*. What leading indicators have the most evidence of effective health programs? Which indicators have the least evidence of effective health programs? Evaluate which health program could be adapted for use in your community.
8. This chapter covers the role of the occupational and environmental health nurse. Search for information about this specialty area of nursing in your community. Do you know an occupational health nurse? If so, plan to observe his or her practice for a few hours and explore what the role entails in this organization.
9. Think about workers that you see every day (grocery store checker, hair dresser, fire fighter, landscaper, utility lineman, etc.). What hazards are they exposed to? What are the potential health problems that they may have due to their work? What primary prevention efforts would be suitable for those workers?
10. Select an employer close to where you live or go to school. The employer may be a municipal government, a school system, or a for-profit company. If you were to provide occupational health nursing services to the workers of that employer, what information would be important to obtain before providing services? How would you obtain that information? How would you identify risks to that population? What other health care or other professionals would you include in your team approach to health care at this site?
11. Think about your clinical experiences in community/public health nursing. Are their unmet needs in the community that could be addressed through a nurse-led business? What elements would you include in a business plan? Write a one paragraph statement that you could present in obtaining a small business loan. Locate a nurse entrepreneur and discuss the challenges they met in starting their business; how were those addressed?

REFERENCES

Agency for Healthcare Research and Quality. (n.d.). *Five major steps to intervention*. Rockville, MD: U.S. Public Health Service. Retrieved from http://www.ahrq.gov/clinic/tobacco/5steps.htm

American Board for Occupational Health Nurses, Inc. (2008). Who we are and what we do. Retrieved from http://www.abohn.org/

American Nurses Association. (2004). *Nursing: Scope and standards of practice*. Silver Spring, MD: Nursesbooks.org.

American Nurses Association/Health Ministries Association. (1998). *The scope and standards of parish nursing practice*. Washington, DC: American Nurses Publishing.

American Nurses Association/Health Ministries Association. (2005). *Faith Community Nursing: Scope and standards of practice*. Silver Spring, MD: Nursesbooks.org.

American Nurses Association/Health Ministries Association. (2012). *Faith Community Nursing: Scope and standards of practice* (2nd ed.). Silver Spring, MD: Nursesbooks.org.

Americans with Disabilities Act (ADA) (2000). *A guide for persons with disabilities seeking employment*. Retrieved from http://www.ada.gov/workta.htm

Anderko, L., Bartz, C., & Lundeen, S. (2005). Practice-based research networks: Nursing centers and communities working collaboratively to reduce health disparities. *Nursing Clinics of North America, 40* (4), 747–758.

Anderson, C. M. (2004). The delivery of health care in faith-based organizations: Parish nurses as promoters of health. *Health Communication, 16*(1), 117–128.

Aydelotte, M. K., Barger, S. E., Branstetter, E., Fehring, R. J., Lindgren, K., Lundeen, S., et al. (1987). *The nursing center: Concept and design*. Kansas City, MO: American Nurses Association.

Baker, K. M., Goetzel, R. Z., Pei, X., Weiss, A. J., Bowen, J., Tabrizi, M. J., et al. (2008). Using a return-on-investment estimation model to evaluate outcomes from an obesity management worksite health promotion program. *Journal of Occupational and Environmental Medicine,50*(9), 981–990.

Baldwin, J. A., Daley, E., Brown, E. J., August, E. M., Webb, C., Stern, R., et al. (2008). Knowledge and perception of STI/HIV risk among rural African-American youth: Lessons learned in a faith-based pilot program. *Journal of HIV/AIDS Prevention in Children and Youth, 9*(1), 97–114. doi: 10.1080/10698370802175193

Barkauskas, V., Pohl, J., Tanner, C., Onifade, T., & Pilon, B. (2011). Quality of care in nurse-managed health centers. *Nursing Administration Quarterly, 35*(1), 34–43. doi: 10.1097/NAQ.0b013e3182032165

Bhave, M. P. (1994). A process model of entrepreneurial creation. *Journal of Business Venturing, 9*(3), 223–242.

Beidler, S. M. (2005). Ethical considerations for nurse-managed health centers. *Nursing Clinics of North America, 40*(4), 759–770.

Bemis, P. A. (2006). Nurse entrepreneur: Devise and implement a great game plan. *Alternative Journal of Nursing, 11*, 1–5.

Brown, A. (2006). Documenting the value of faith community nursing: Faith nursing online. *Creative Nursing, 2*, 13.

Brown, A. R., Coppola, P., Giacona, M., Petriches, A., & Stockwell, M. A. (2009). Faith community nursing demonstrates good stewardship of community benefit dollars through cost savings and cost avoidance. *Family Community Health, 32*(4), 330–338.

Brown, J. F. (2009). Faith-based mental health education: A service-learning opportunity for nursing students. *Journal of Psychiatric and Mental Health Nursing, 16*, 581–588.

Caring Choices. (2012). *Caring Choices program offerings*. Retrieved from http://www.caring-choices.org/programs.php

Cetin, B., Uguz, F., Erdem, M., & Yildirim, A. (2010). The relationship between quality of life, anxiety and depression in unilateral hearing loss. *Journal of International Advanced Otology, 6*(2), 252–257.

Cohen, S. M., & Turley, R. (2009). Coprevalence and impact of dysphonia and hearing loss in the elderly. *Laryngoscope, 119*(9), 1870–1873.

Council for Accreditation in Occupational Hearing Conservation (CAOHC) (2011). Retrieved from http://www.caohc.org/index.php

Courtemanche, C. (2009). Longer hours and larger waistlines? The relationship between work hours and obesity. *Forum for Health Economics & Policy, 12*(2), Article 2. Retrieved from http://libres.uncg.edu/ir/uncg/f/C_Courtemanche_Longer_2009.pdf

Cutler, I. (2002). *End games: The challenge of sustainability*. Baltimore, MD: Annie E. Casey Foundation.

Dyess, S., Chase, S. K., & Newlin, K. (2009). State of research for faith community nursing 2009. *Journal of Religion and Health, 49*, 188–199. doi: 10.1007/s10943-009-9262-x

Elango, B., Hunter, G. L., & Winchell, M. (2007). Barriers to nurse entrepreneurship: A study of the process model of entrepreneurship. *Journal of the American Academy of Nurse Practitioners, 19*, 198–204.

Evans, A. R. (2011). *Is God still at the bedside? The medical, ethical, and pastoral issues of death and dying*. Grand Rapids, MI: Eerdmans Publishing Co.

Gerrity, P., & Kinsey, K. (1999). An urban nurse managed primary health care center: Health promotion in action. *Family Community Health, 21*(4), 29–40.

Hansen-Turton, T. (2003). The quest for sustainability gets closer: CMS funds nurse- managed health center congressional demonstration. *Policy, Politics, and Nursing Practice, 4*, 147–152.

Hansen-Turton, T., & Miller, M. E. (2006, June). Nurses and nurse-managed health centers fill healthcare gaps. *The Pennsylvania Nurse, 61*(2) 18.

Hansen-Turton, T., Miller, M. E., & Greiner, P. (2009). *Nurse-managed wellness centers: Developing and maintaining your center. A National Nursing Center Consortium guide and toolkit*. New York, NY: Springer Publishing.

Health Ministries Association. (2010). *About HMA*. Retrieved from http://www.hmassoc.org/about_us.php.

Health Resources and Services Administration. (2005). *Medicare Part D and safety net providers*. Retrieved from http://www.hrsa.gov/medicare/modelcontract.htm

Hickman, J. S. (2011). *Fast facts for the faith community nurse: Implementing FCN/parish nursing in a nutshell*. New York, NY: Springer Publishing.

Hyeonkyeong, L. Wilbur, J., Kim, M. J., & Miller, A. M. (2008). Psychosocial risk factors for work-related musculoskeletal disorders of the lower-back among long-haul international female flight attendants. *Journal of Advanced Nursing, 61*, 492–502.

Institute of Medicine (2000). *America's healthcare safety net: Intact but endangered*. Washington, DC: National Academies Press.

Institute of Medicine (2011). *The future of nursing: Leading change, advancing health*. Washington, DC: National Academies Press.

Job Accommodation Network (2011). *Accommodation and compliance series: Employees with sleep disorders*. Retrieved from http://askjan.org/media/sleep.html

King, M. A. (2004). Review of research about parish nursing practice. *Online Brazilian Journal of Nursing, 3*(1). Retrieved from http://www.uff.br/nepae/siteantigo/objn301king.htm.

Kinsey, K., & Miller, M. E. (2011). The nursing center: A model for nursing practice in the community. In M. Stanhope & J. Lancaster (Eds.), *Public Health Nursing: Population-centered health care in the community* (8th ed., pp. 461–482). Maryland Heights, MO: Mosby.

Kowlessar, N. M., Goetzel, R. Z., Carls, G. S., Tabrizi, M. J., & Guindon, A. (2011). The relationship between 11 health risks and medical and productivity costs for a large employer. *Journal of Occupational and Environmental Medicine, 53*(5), 468–477.

Lee, A. T., Tong, M. C., Yuen, K. C., Tang, P. S., & Van Hasselt, C. A. (2010). Hearing impairment and depressive symptoms in an older Chinese population. *Journal of Otolaryngology – Head and Neck Surgery, 39*(5), 498–503.

Lundeen, S. (2005). *Lundeen's comprehensive community-based primary health care model*. Milwaukee, WI: Milwaukee College of Nursing.

Merriam-Webster.com. (2012). *Entrepreneur*. Retrieved from http://www.merriam-webster.com/dictionary/entrepreneur

McBryde-Foster, M. (2005). Break-even analysis in a nurse-managed center. *Nursing Economics, 23*(1), 31–34.

Mellor, G., & St John, W. (2007). Occupational health nurses' perceptions of their current and future roles. *Journal of Advanced Nursing, 58*, 585–593.

Melnyk, B. M., & Fineout-Overholt, E. (2010). *Evidence-based practice in nursing and healthcare: A guide to best practice* (2nd ed.). Philadelphia, PA: Lippincott Williams & Wilkins.

National Institute for Occupational Safety and Health. (2011). NIOSH Education and Research Centers (ERCs). Retrieved from http://www.cdc.gov/niosh/oep/cedirlst.html

National Institutes of Health, Office of Extramural Research (2007). *Glossary and acronym list*. Retrieved from http://grants.nih.gov/Grants/glossary.htm

National Nursing Centers Consortium (2011). *Mission, vision, goals*. Retrieved from http://www.nncc.us/about/vision.html

Occupational Safety and Health Act (29 CFR 1910). Retrieved from http://osha.gov/pls/oshaweb/owasrch.search_form?p_doc_type=STANDARDS&p_toc_level=1&p_keyvalue=1910

Patterson, D. L. (2006, March). The head is connected to the heart bone: Parish nurses as teachers. *The Clergy Journal*, 29–30.

Patterson, D. L. (2007). Eight advocacy roles for parish nurses. *Journal of Christian Nursing, 24*(1), 33–35.

Robert Wood Johnson Foundation (RWJF) (2009). Health care spending as percentage of GDP. In *Talking About Quality Part 1: Health Care Today*. Retrieved from http://www.rwjf.org/pr/product.jsp?id=45110

Rydholm, L. (2006). Documenting the value of faith community nursing: Saving hundreds, making cents—a study of current realities. *Creative Nursing, 2*, 10–13.

Rydholm, L., Moone, R., Thornquist, L., Alexander, W., Gustafson, V., & Speece, B. (2008). Community-dwelling older adults by faith community nurses. *Journal of Gerontological Nursing, 34*(4), 18–29.

Schoenberg, N. E., Hatcher, J., Dignan, M. B., Shelton, B., Wright, S., & Dollarhide, K. F. (2009). Faith moves mountains: An Appalachian cervical cancer prevention program. *American Journal of Health Behaviors, 33*(6), 627–638.

Seidell, J. C. (2010). Waist circumference and waist/hip ratio in relation to all-cause mortality, cancer and sleep apnea. *European Journal of Clinical Nutrition, 64*, 35–41.

Society for Human Resource Management (SHRM) (2009). *U.S. health care inflation to far outpace salary increases in 2010*. Retrieved from http://www.shrm.org/hrdisciplines/benefits/Articles/Pages/HealthCostForecast.aspx

Solari-Twadell, P. A., & McDermott, M. A. (2005). *Parish nursing: Development, education, and administration*. St. Louis, MO: Elsevier.

Torrisi, D., & Hansen-Turton, T. (2005). *Community and nurse-managed health centers: Getting them started and keeping them going*. Philadelphia: Springer Publishing.

United States Congress. (2009). *Nurse-Managed Health Clinic Investment Act of 2009*, S.B 1104/H.R. 2754, 111th Congress.

U.S. Department of Health and Human Services. Centers for Medicare and Medicaid Services, Medicare Learning Network (2011). *Federally Qualified Health Center: Rural health fact sheet series*. Retrieved from http://www.cms.gov/MLNProducts/downloads/fqhcfactsheet.pdf

U.S. Department of Health and Human Services. Office of Disease Prevention and Health Promotion (2010). *Healthy People 2020*. Washington, DC. Retrieved from http://www.healthypeople.gov/2020/

U.S. Department of Health, Education, and Welfare (1979). *Healthy People: The Surgeon General's report on health promotion and disease prevention*. Washington, DC: U.S. Government Printing Office.

Wachs J. E. (1997). Nurse managed occupational health centers: An overview. *AAOHN Journal, 45*(10), 477–483.

Wachs J. E. (2005). Building the occupational health team: Keys to successful interdisciplinary collaboration. *AAOHN Journal, 53*(4), 166–171.

Warner-Robbins, C., & Parsons, M. L. (2010). Developing peer leaders and reducing recidivism through long-term participation in a faith -based program: The story of welcome home ministries. *Alcoholism Treatment Quarterly, 28*, 293–305. doi: 10.1080/07347324.2010.488534

Westberg, G. E. (1990). *The Parish Nurse: Providing a minister of health for your congregation*. Minneapolis, MN: Augsburg.

Westberg-McNamara, J. (2006). *The Health Cabinet: How to start a wellness committee in your church*, Cleveland, OH: Pilgrim Press.

Williamson, W., & Kautz, D. D. (2009). "Let's get moving: Let's get praising": Promoting health and hope in an African American church. *The ABNF Journal, 20*(4), 102–105.

Youngblut, J., & Brooten, D. (2001). Evidenced-based nursing practice: Why is it important. *AACN Clinical Issues, 12*, 468–476.

thePoint: Everything You Need to Make the Grade!

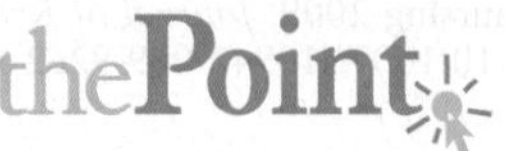

Visit http://thePoint.lww.com/Allender8e for selected readings, study aids for all learning styles, and more!

CHAPTER

32

Clients Receiving Home Health and Hospice Care

"People from all walks of life agree that someone who is sick deserves, in principle, compassion and care."

—***Paul Farmer,*** **American anthropologist and physician**

KEY TERMS

CMS (Centers for Medicare and Medicaid Services)
Community-based long-term care
Homebound
Hospice
Medicare home health benefit
Medicare hospice benefit
Medicare prospective payment system
OASIS (Outcome and Assessment Information Set)
Palliative interventions
Potentially inappropriate medications
Responsive use of self
Visiting nurse associations

LEARNING OBJECTIVES

Upon mastery of this chapter, you should be able to:

- Summarize the history and contemporary circumstances of home health and hospice care.
- Describe Medicare standards for home health and hospice programs.
- Explain family caregiver burdens of providing home care.
- Explain how Medicare reimburses home health and hospice care.
- Describe essential characteristics of home health and hospice nursing practice.
- Identify unique challenges of infection control, medication management, fall prevention, use of technology, and nurse safety during home visits.
- Contrast the goals of home health care and hospice.
- Explain the gaps in home health care and hospice and the need for a coherent community-based long-term care program in the United States.

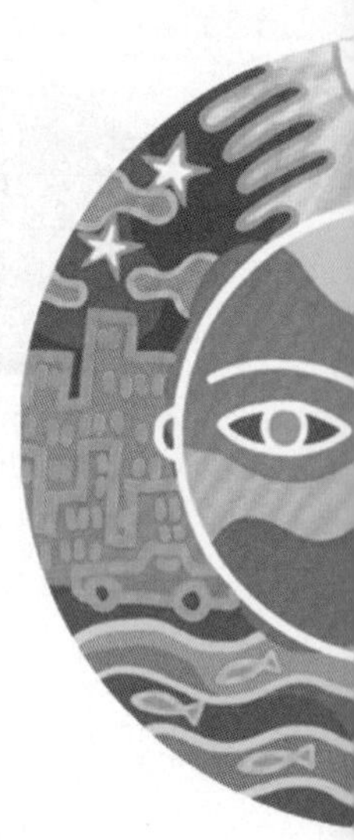

A home health nurse sits in an upscale condominium with a frail, elderly gentleman tethered to his home oxygen unit and suffering air hunger as he struggles to speak of the "good old days" when he was young, full of vigor, and taking on the world. During her next visit to a trailer park, she inspects an infected pressure sore that has become smaller and cleaner with each home visit as the client's wife carefully follows through with wound care teaching. Next, she monitors the pulmonary and cardiac status of a patient newly discharged to his aging bungalow, detecting early signs of cardiac decompensation and treating them at home in close collaboration with his physician. At that same time, her hospice nurse colleague walks into family chaos with a mother in pain and vomiting at the end of her life and then leaves with everyone calm and the patient comfortable. These are the kinds of experiences that make up the daily lives of nurses who work with home care and hospice clients. Indeed, home health and hospice programs allow nurses to practice what some see as the very heart of compassionate and highly skilled nursing care. Home health care and hospice programs are expanding and are the work settings for more and more nurses.

Home health care is discussed in the first section of this chapter, followed by an overview of hospice care. The reader is also referred to the discussions in Chapter 19 on working with families, Chapter 20 on violence in families, Chapter 24 on care of the older adult, and Chapter 26 on chronic illness.

OVERVIEW OF HOME HEALTH CARE

The need for health care at home continues to accelerate. Drastic changes in financing and more people living with complex illness have contributed to this trend. For example, early hospital discharges resulting from third-party payers' efforts toward cost containment have forced clients to return home quickly to recuperate from surgeries and severe illnesses. Likewise, a growing population survives and yet suffers from complex chronic and life-threatening illness that they struggle to manage at home. Advanced technologies such as telehealth monitoring, intravenous (IV) antibiotics, total parenteral nutrition (TPN), dialysis, and mechanical ventilation are routinely provided and maintained in the client's home. As the population ages, and particularly now that the baby boomer generation is entering their elder years, home health nursing is challenged to respond. Professional home health care agencies seek to maximize the client's level of independence and to minimize the effects of existing disabilities through noninstitutional services. Professional home health services aim to decrease rehospitalization and prevent or delay institutionalization (National Association for Home Care and Hospice [NAHC], 2010; Wajnberg, Wang, Aniff, & Kunins, 2010). The NAHC Web site provides a variety of direct services to members, including the publication *Caring* and monthly newsletters.

This section explores the evolution of home health care in the United States; describes home health agencies, clients, and personnel; and examines Medicare criteria and documentation. Finally, the unique characteristics of home health nursing are explored.

HISTORY AND POLITICS OF HOME HEALTH

Throughout human history, health care has been provided at home by family members. In the United States, the Ladies Benevolent Society in Charleston, South Carolina, made the earliest known (1813) organized effort to care for the sick poor at home (Buhler-Wilkerson, 2007). Later in the 19th century, it became possible for women to become nurses trained in the manner of Florence Nightingale, and wealthy women began to hire them as visiting nurses and to sponsor visiting nurse services. In 1893, Lillian Wald began home visiting in New York City and is famed for professionalizing visiting nursing. One of her most famous innovations was the establishment of insurance coverage for home care. Between 1909 and 1952, 100 million home visits were made to the policy holders of Metropolitan Life Insurance Company. Then, as now, the need for cost containment and therefore quick discharge were in diametric opposition to nursing goals of providing needed care at the patient's side as long as needed.

In the latter half of the 20th century, as hospitals became increasingly effective in providing acute care, more people survived to live with debilitating chronic illness and disability, and referral to home care was used to discharge those nonacute patients from the hospital (Buhler-Wilkerson, 2007). The **visiting nurse associations** (VNAs) struggled with patched-together community support until 1965, which began the era of the **Medicare home health benefit**, designed to respond to the medical needs of those convalescing from acute illness.

The Medicare home health benefit was established with certain goals in mind. It was designed to provide intermittent home visits, in which nurses and therapists would instruct clients and families in self-care. Home health nursing was clearly differentiated from longer nursing shifts in which nurses stayed in the home for several hours at a time. The period of visiting was to be brief and provide direct personal care just temporarily until patients and families could care for themselves. Neither health promotion nor long-term care was valued or reimbursed. Families were expected to manage long-term care alone. Whereas nurses had previously controlled their own practice, services under the new benefit were viewed as extensions of medical care, with physicians certifying needed services for short-term treatment of sickness.

The number of Medicare-certified home care agencies grew rapidly until enactment of the Balanced Budget Act (BBA) of 1997, which sought explicitly to reduce federal payments for home health care. To achieve this, payment to providers was changed from reimbursement for each visit to the **Medicare prospective payment system** that determined Medicare payment rates based on patient characteristics and need for services (Kulesher, 2006). The BBA resulted in a closure of 30% to 36% of the nation's Medicare-certified home health agencies and a dramatic decline in the number of patients served, with particular impact on the most vulnerable patients over 85 years old who needed intensive services. As a result, some agencies denied care to those whose complex nursing needs exceeded expected reimbursement. Both cost and number of visits declined while rates of wound healing failures, incontinence, and psychosocial problems worsened (Schlenker, Powell, & Goodrich, 2005). The long-term effect on emergency care and hospitalization, as well as diminished patient contact and increased documentation associated with these restrictive Medicare policies, was felt. This shift in service provision also impacted home health nurses, who are most satisfied when they have control over their practice and able to provide quality patient care (Ellenbecker, Boylan, & Samia, 2006).

With enactment of the Patient Protection and Affordable Care Act, many provisions are currently and will likely continue over the next decade to impact the provision of home health care. Although many of the Medicare policies for home care are unchanged, the act includes a number of new programs that if well implemented, will have a positive impact on home care. For instance, supplemental payments for rural home care providers have been reinstated for 2010 to 2015. This was done to address the lower ratio of home care professions in rural areas throughout the United States as compared to more urban areas (Centers for Medicare and Medicaid Services [CMS], 2010). New innovations included in the act are two programs that directly impact the provision of care in the home (CMS, 2012d):

- *Community First Choice Option* allows states to offer home- and community-based services to disabled people through Medicaid rather than institutional care in nursing homes.
- *Community Care Transitions Program* helps high-risk Medicare beneficiaries who are hospitalized avoid unnecessary readmissions by coordinating care and connecting patients to services in their communities.

While the new provisions can enhance the capacity of agencies to provide care, as with any change the new rules and regulations will undoubtedly be a challenge. One concerning aspect for home health care providers is the 2012 ruling by the Supreme Court (National Federation of Independent Business et al. vs. Sebelius, Secretary of Health and Human Services) that allows for states to opt out of the provision in the act to expand Medicaid services. With a growing percentage of payments for home health coming from Medicaid, this is obviously of concern to care providers and consumers of care. Home health care expenditures from Medicaid are expected to exceed Medicare payments in the coming years. How this shift in payment source and the limitation that many states may impose on Medicaid coverage is unknown at this time.

The CMS and other government Web sites provide a wealth of information for the providers of care, as well as consumers (CMS.gov; healthcare.gov). Despite the challenges, the recognition of improved outcomes and cost savings associated with home care as opposed to hospitalization and skilled nursing facility (SNF) stays is encouraging. Comparisons between these three forms of care from 2009 data showed that the average Medicare payment for 1 day of hospitalization or SNF were $6200 and $622, respectively, with a per visit cost for a home visit at $135. The cost difference is staggering, especially when considering the improved outcomes from home visiting relative to hospital admissions alone (NAHC, 2010).

Other studies provide well-grounded support of home health care services. Rahme et al. (2010) found that home care after hemiarthroplasty was associated with reduced risk of death within 3 months of discharge. Of concern in this Canadian study was the low receipt of home care (16%) at discharge. Stolee, Lim, Wilson, and Glenny (2011) conducted a systematic review to compare rehabilitation measures between home-based and inpatient rehabilitation for musculoskeletal disorders. Their findings supported home-based care with equal or improved outcomes in function, cognition, quality of life, and satisfaction with the intervention. The cost-effectiveness of home-based rehabilitation for older patients can be inferred by these findings.

It is important to be aware that a distinct difference exists between professional and nonprofessional home care services provided to clients. Professional home care is provided by professionals with licenses, certification, or specific qualifications. These professionals typically work for home care agencies with internal and external standards that guide the provision of their services. Nurses, social workers, physical therapists, occupational therapists, and home health aides are examples of professional home care practitioners. In contrast, there are home care organizations that provide nonprofessional home care and those who sell equipment for home care.

HOME HEALTH AGENCIES

The mix of Medicare-certified home health care agencies includes voluntary nonprofits, hospital-based agencies, proprietary for-profit agencies, governmental agencies, or agencies not federally certified to provide care.

Voluntary nonprofit agencies traditionally have a charitable mission and are exempt from paying taxes. They are financed with nontax funds such as donations, endowments, United Way contributions, and third-party provider payments. If nonprofit agencies make any money, they reinvest it back into the agency. Voluntary agencies are usually governed by a voluntary board of directors; they are considered community-based because they provide services within a well-defined geographic location. Whereas in the past VNAs were assured of receiving almost all of the home care referrals in their community, the proliferation of other agencies has eroded their traditional base and put them in a competitive mode. The number of nonprofit home health agencies is diminishing across the country.

Hospital-based agencies comprise about 13% of Medicare-certified agencies (NAHC, 2010). A hospital may operate a separate department as a home health agency. It may be nonprofit or generate revenue for the hospital. Hospital-based agencies are governed by the sponsoring hospital's board of directors or trustees. The referrals to such hospital-based agencies usually come from the hospital staff, and the missions of the agency and the sponsoring hospital are similar. The same is true for rehabilitation and skilled-nursing facilities with home health departments.

For-profit proprietary agencies can be governed by individual owners, but many are part of large, regional, or national chains that are administered through corporate headquarters. Proprietary agencies are expected to turn a profit on the services they provide, either for the individual owners or for their stockholders. They are required to pay taxes on profits generated. Although some participate in the Medicare program, others rely solely on "private-pay" clients. For-profit home care agencies now comprise over 60% of all Medicare-certified agencies and over 70% of all certified free-standing agencies (NAHC, 2010).

Some city and county government agencies also provide home care services. They are created and empowered through statutes enacted by legislation. Services are frequently provided by the nursing divisions of state or local health departments and may or may not combine care of the sick with traditional public health nursing services, including health promotion, illness prevention, communicable disease investigation, environmental health services, and maternal–child care. Funding comes from taxes and is usually distributed on the basis of a per capita allocation.

Many agencies providing services in the home remain outside the federal Medicare system that reimburses skilled nursing. These *noncertified* agencies are usually private and derive their funding from direct payment by the client or from private insurers. They may be governed by individual owners or by corporations. For instance, some agencies offer "private duty" shifts of registered nurses, licensed practical nurses, various therapists, or home health aides who are usually paid for "out of pocket" rather than reimbursed by insurance or Medicare. Other services include unskilled assistance in the home with homemaking or housekeeping. Some of these agencies provide live-in personal care. Some organizations provide *durable medical equipment* (DME), such as wheelchairs, commodes, beds, or oxygen. Other services provide high-technology pharmacy services.

CLIENTS AND THEIR FAMILIES

The client in home health care is not only the individual patient but also the family and any significant others. The nurse must consider how the environmental, political, economic, cultural, and religious dimensions impact the client's illness and ability to meet the goals outlined in the plan of care.

Home care recipients are predominantly White women. More than two-thirds are over age 65 (NAHC, 2010). The most common diagnoses managed at home are diabetes, chronic skin ulcer, essential hypertension, heart failure, and osteoarthritis. Most home health clients are admitted after hospitalization (48%), but an increasing number (38%) are admitted directly from the community (NAHC, 2010)

Individuals recovering from severe illness or living with debilitating chronic illness rely on family members or other sources of unpaid assistance. Almost 30% of the US population provides informal caregiving for an adult family member or friend (National Alliance for Caregiving [NAC], 2012). Two-thirds of these providers are women with an average age of 47, although people can become caregivers at any age. Frail elderly caregivers are especially vulnerable to deterioration of their own health due to their caregiving burden. Family caregiving tasks range from personal care such as bathing and feeding to sophisticated skilled care, including managing tracheostomies or IV lines. Primary caregivers are those who assume the daily tasks of care, while secondary caregivers assume intermittent responsibilities such as shopping or transportation. On average family caregivers provide 20 hours per week in the provision of care; 13% provide over 40 hours (NAHC, 2010).

These informal caregivers assume a considerable physical, psychological, and economic burden in the care of their loved one at home. When layered on top of existing responsibilities, caregiver tasks compete for time, energy, and attention. As a result, caregivers often describe themselves as emotionally and physically drained and may very much need information about resources to assist them. Likewise, the economic cost of providing home care places a significant burden on informal caregivers. Out-of-pocket expenditures include medications, transportation, home medical equipment, supplies, and respite services. These costs may be nonreimbursable and are often invisible, but they are very real to families struggling to provide care on a fixed income. While family members compassionately assume their responsibilities, their collective burden in our society as a whole is mounting. Home health nurses must continually assess the strain on caregivers as they seek to develop realistic plans of care.

HOME HEALTH CARE PERSONNEL

The largest number of home care employees are nurses and home care aides (NAHC, 2010). Registered nurses and licensed practical nurses represent just under half of full time equivalent (FTE) positions in Medicare-certified agencies. Home care aides, physical therapy staff, occupational therapists, social workers, and administrative personnel comprise the rest of the home health team. The business and office personnel of a home health agency are critical to the agency's ability to deliver services to clients. Home health nurses must acquire an understanding of the financial aspects of their clients' care and provide this information to the agency staff, so that appropriate and full reimbursement can be obtained for the services provided.

REIMBURSEMENT FOR HOME HEALTH CARE

Home health services are reimbursed by both corporate and governmental third-party payers as well as by individual clients and their families. Corporate payers include insurance companies, health maintenance organizations (HMOs), preferred provider organizations (PPOs), and case-management programs. Government payers include Medicare, Medicaid, the military health system (TRICARE), and the Veterans Administration system. These governmental programs have specific conditions for coverage of services, which are often less flexible than those of corporate payers. For a general description of these reimbursement systems, see Chapter 6. The Medicare policies for home health programs set the precedent for all other reimbursement sources and are discussed below.

Medicare Criteria and Reimbursement

Medicare is the largest single payer for home care services in the United States and has set the standard in establishing reimbursement criteria for other payers. Therefore, it is essential that home care nurses seek to understand the complex Medicare home health requirements and rules for determining eligibility for home care services. It is important to acknowledge that a person may be in dire need of care at home, yet not meet eligibility standards for home health care under Medicare. Five criteria must all be met to be eligible for reimbursement by Medicare (Display 32.1). Consider the implications of these requirements. Documentation must justify that the plan of care is medically "reasonable and necessary." The person must be under the care of a physician. He or she must be "homebound" and in need of services that Medicare narrowly defines as "skilled." A person who is "homebound" must be confined to home except for visits to the physician, outpatient dialysis, adult day center, or outpatient chemotherapy and radiation therapy. "Skilled" services are restrictively defined and include selected aspects of nursing, physical therapy, or speech therapy. Home visits must be "intermittent" and time limited. Extensive documentation is required according to Medicare specifications. All of these requirements are subject to contradictory interpretations, which can put an agency's reimbursement at risk.

The Medicare prospective payment system (PPS) pays an agency for a 60-day "episode of care." All services and many medical supplies must be provided

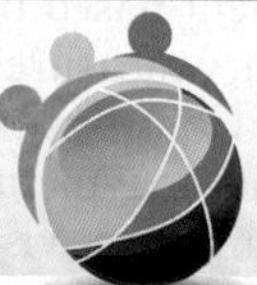

DISPLAY 32.1 MEDICARE HOME HEALTH ELIGIBILITY

1. The type of services and frequency provided must be reasonable and necessary. To determine whether this criterion is met, the client's current health status, medical record, and plan of care are evaluated. If a care plan has been ineffective with a client over a long period of time, continuation of that care plan would not be considered reasonable. Therefore, comprehensive documentation is essential to validate that the provided care was both reasonable and necessary.
2. The client must be **homebound.** This means that the client leaves the home with difficulty and only for medical appointments or adult day care related to the client's medical care.
3. The plan of care must be entered onto specific Medicare forms. The forms require very specific information regarding the client's diagnosis, prognosis, functional limitations, medications, and types of services needed. The home health nurse often has the primary responsibility for ensuring that the forms are completed appropriately.
4. The client must be in need of a skilled service. In the home, skilled services are provided only by a nurse, physical therapist, or speech therapist. *Skilled nursing services* include skilled observation and assessment, teaching, and performing selected procedures requiring nursing judgment.
5. Services must be intermittent and part-time.

under the payment amount adjusted to geographic location and determined by the patient's clinical and functional status at the start of care, as well as the projected need for services over the anticipated 60-day period (CMS, 2012a). When the patient is admitted, the patient is comprehensively assessed using a lengthy tool called the ***Outcome and Assessment Information Set* (OASIS)**. Clinical, functional, and service scores are calculated from selected OASIS items. The stated purpose of OASIS is to: "represent core items of a comprehensive assessment for an adult home care patient; and form the basis for measuring patient outcomes for purposes of outcome-based quality improvement" (CMS, 2012c). In the ongoing campaign to hold down the federal budget by diminishing health costs, home health care faces the ongoing threat of freezes or cuts in payment. For example, in the spring of 2007, the **Centers for Medicare and Medicaid Services (CMS)** proposed reduction in reimbursement, justified by their claim that patients' needs have been exaggerated in documentation submitted to them. They also required payment adjustment based on agency submission of data on selected quality measures. In 2007, the Medicare Payment Advisory Commission (MedPAC) recommended to Congress that payments be frozen and that patients co-pay for each illness visit (Markey, 2007). These proposals overlooked the reality that home health care is a cost-effective alternative to hospital and nursing home care. As home health care is restricted to save money and reduce fraud, greater amounts will need to be spent for inpatient care when people cannot cope in the absence of health care assistance at home (see Perspectives: Voices From the Community).

With the implementation of the Affordable Care Act, the provision that certification for Medicare home health services and recertification every 60 days no longer requires a face-to-face encounter by a physician and now provides for certification by a nurse practitioner, a clinical nurse specialist (CNS), certified nurse-midwife, or physician assistant (CMS, 2010). While this change will likely result in a reduction in cost for certification/recertification, home care agencies without a nurse practitioner or certified nurse specialist on staff may have to contract out for those services. Current CNS specialty certification most appropriate for home health care includes adult health, gerontological, and adult-gerontology (pending). Unfortunately, CNS certification is no longer available for home health nursing or public/community health nursing (American Nurses Credentialing Center [ANCC], 2012). The need for advanced practice nurses in these specialties will very likely increase the number of certified nurses working or contracted by home health agencies and increase the need for master's level educational preparation.

PERSPECTIVES
VOICES FROM THE COMMUNITY

It is vital to develop an expanded vision about the health care needs of frail elders and the kinds of services that are needed in the community. Sometimes, after nurses have been working in Medicare home health for a while, they may begin to identify with the Medicare guidelines. Too often, I have heard experienced home health nurses say about a patient living with severe chronic illness, "She doesn't deserve services. She doesn't have skilled needs." In contrast, I would hope knowledgeable nurses would say to families and decision makers, "She needs and deserves services, but the Medicare home health benefit will not pay for them. Our agency cannot continue to provide care because of the limits imposed on us. We'll do everything possible to find help for her, but resources are limited." This kind of insight leads to patient advocacy, development of community networks, and becoming outspoken about needed changes in health policy. Visiting nurses witness the struggles of chronically ill people living at home; we must not abandon them.

—Beth L., Nursing Instructor

Medicare Documentation

Initially, every patient must be assessed using the OASIS tool, which determines reimbursement, is integral to agency surveys and certification, and collects information used to measure quality. OASIS assessment requires combining observation and interview to determine functional status, since clients often report what they wish to be true, rather than actual ability (Godfrey, 2005). Selected quality outcomes are measured and data released on the CMS Web site (CMS, 2012b), which is accessed as "Home Health Compare" (http://www.medicare.gov/). Display 32.2 identifies selected quality measures. Note that the expectation is that of improving function, not simply stabilizing function, and consider the implications of this standard for very disabled patients.

The Medicare Plan of Care is also completed by the nurse at admission; it must be signed by the physician. It is then used to assess agency compliance with Medicare and state requirements. Obviously, great pains must be taken to assure accuracy. All follow-up services must

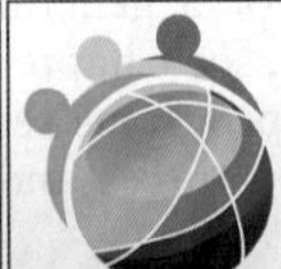

DISPLAY 32.2 SELECTED HOME HEALTH QUALITY MEASURES

Higher Percentages Are Better

- Percentage of patients who get better at walking or moving around
- Percentage of patients who get better at getting in and out of bed
- Percentage of patients who have less pain when moving around
- Percentage of patients whose bladder control improves
- Percentage of patients who get better at bathing
- Percentage of patients who get better at taking their medicines correctly (by mouth)
- Percentage of patients who are short of breath less often
- Percentage of patients who stay at home after an episode of home health care ends
- Percentage of patients with improvement in status of surgical wound

Lower Percentages Are Better

- Percentage of patients who had to be admitted to the hospital
- Percentage of patients who need urgent, unplanned medical care
- Percentage of patients with deteriorating wound status

Source: Medicare Home Health Compare Web site: http://www.medicare.gov/homehealthcompare/%28S%28nkz4x4455wefwsifxscvm545%29%29/about/overview.aspx.

match the plan of care. Likewise, OASIS identified needs and Plan of Care services must match.

HOME HEALTH NURSING PRACTICE

The practice of home health nursing has roots in community/public health nursing (see Chapter 3). The nurse provides home health nursing care to acute, chronic, and terminally ill clients of all ages in their homes while integrating public health nursing principles that focus on the environmental, psychosocial, economic, cultural, and personal health factors affecting a client's and family's health status and well-being. Home health is a unique field of nursing practice that requires a synthesis of public health nursing principles with the theory and practice of medical/surgical, geriatric, mental health, and other nursing specialties. The official journal of the Home Healthcare Nurses Association (HHNA), *Home Healthcare Nurse*, is the primary source of up-to-date nursing knowledge in this rapidly changing field of practice. The stories of home health nurses emphasize shared humanity and promotion of client autonomy (Stulginsky, 1993a, 1993b). The effective home health nurse must:

- Deliberately build trust
- Sense "where people are" and suspend judgment
- Develop a connection at the first visit
- Develop "giant antennae" to detect cues in the home
- Face persistent distractions during home visits
- Help people solve their own problems
- Keep priorities fluid
- Determine how to keep the unstable client safe until the next visit
- Thoughtfully maintain boundaries between personal and professional life
- "Make do" with limited supplies
- Face immense challenges with time management and paperwork demands
- Constantly think of personal safety in neighborhoods and homes

Nursing Practice During the Home Visit

The practice competencies of home health nurses can be illustrated with the Home Health Nursing Caregiving Wheel (Fig. 32-1).

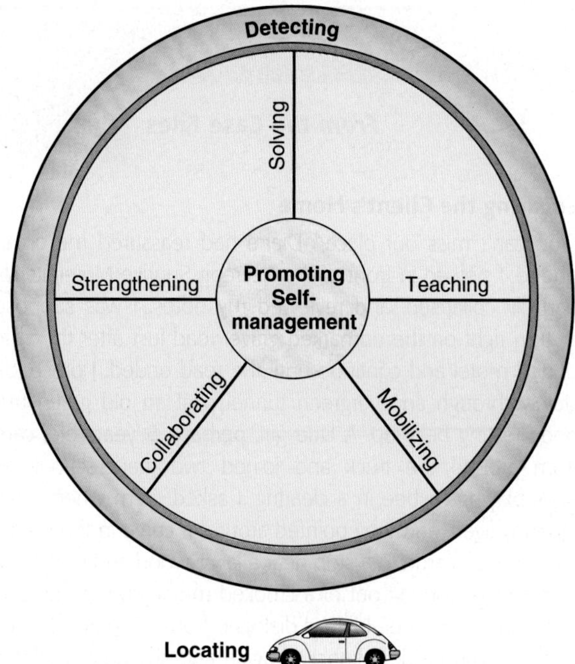

FIGURE 32-1. Home health nursing caregiving wheel.

Locating the Client and Getting Through the Door

The first step in making a home visit is finding where the person lives, which might involve telephone instructions, a map, or a global positioning system (GPS) unit. For most home health nurses, locating clients involves driving their own cars to the home. Sometimes nurses drive agency cars, and occasionally transportation may involve a bus, subway, boat, or airplane. Directions and household identification can be unclear. In rural areas, tracking down clients can involve vague instructions involving barns, bridges, trees, and other colorful local landmarks (see From the Case Files for an example). When families are unstable, clients may not be staying in households designated on the nurse's paperwork. They may have moved in with relatives or friends or back home alone, despite major care needs. Locating is especially challenging when neighbors or even family members live in fear, for whatever reason.

Even when the wheels stop at the correct household, there is the challenge of getting through the closed door and making the connection. *Always remember that you are a guest in the home.* Respect and attentive listening are the foundation. Agendas must be laid aside initially as the nurse focuses on the concerns and realities of both client and family. SmithBattle, Drake, and Diekemper (1997) describe **responsive use of self** as the process expert nurses use to come to understand the lives of vulnerable clients in the community. Assumptions and stereotypes are overturned in the process of discovering how clients live, what they believe, and who comprises their family and community.

Other nursing approaches that build the initial therapeutic nurse–client connection include helping with immediate problems that the family identifies. Start where they want in ways that make sense to them. Emphasize positives to the extent possible, rather than telling people what they are doing wrong and need to change. Autonomy should be respected, and the family should be empowered by actions recognizing that they are in charge of their lives. At the same time, the nurse must be up front and truthful regarding the medical and nursing problems that need resolution. For example, a nurse might say, "You might lose your foot if we cannot work together to figure out a plan of care that works. Let's think together about what we can do to

***From the* Case Files**

Locating the Client's Home

"You can't miss our place," Diane had reassured me on the phone. I slowed in front of the decrepit Sunrise Motel, its roof partially collapsed, and reviewed my notes. I was supposed to turn right on the unmarked gravel road just after the abandoned motel and continue until the road ended. I proceeded slowly through an evergreen tunnel past an old green truck body resting belly up. A little girl, perhaps 5 years old, came from around the truck and joined two grade-school-aged boys playing Frisbee in a clearing. I asked them where Diane Quimby lived, and they pointed around a curve in the road. In a moment, I came to a stop near a large wood and metal shed with smoke coming out of a crooked metal pipe in the roof. I knocked. No answer. I heard dialogue from "General Hospital" coming from inside. I knocked again and shouted, "Hello! It's the nurse." "Come on in!" a loud voice responded.

I pushed open the door. There was no knob. Illuminated by one weak lamp, I could just make out a round face with wire rim glasses and a long gray-blond braid. Here was Diane, sitting on a sagging sofa facing a TV tray and watching a flickering black-and-white television. I could see a wooden table in a corner, three mismatched dinette chairs, and a couple of cots against the wall. The air was hazy with the smell of wood smoke.

Diane invited me to pull up a chair. "We're worried about your infections," I began. Diane had unstable, insulin-dependent diabetes and high blood pressure. In June, surgeons had removed her gangrenous left foot with an amputation that ended just below the left knee. Now there was an infection in the wound that had not healed despite extended use of antibiotics.

During the course of the visit, I learned that Diane had no tub or shower for bathing. She also had no money for dressings and no supplies. Since Diane's vision was impaired, her 9-year-old grandson was doing the dressing changes. Until the latest surgery, Diane worked as a cook in a local "boarding home" for frail elders. She was 66 years old and had Medicare coverage. I learned that Diane was the legal guardian for two grandchildren, ages 5 and 9.

Apply the nursing process to comprehensively identify and prioritize nursing diagnoses and propose interventions. Use the Home Health Nursing Caregiving Wheel to guide your care planning.

prevent it." Since these well-tested relational strategies for developing caring connections run contradictory to the current Medicare requirements for immediate completion of the lengthy OASIS survey tool on admission, the wise nurse needs to focus on sensitively developing initial connections as well as completion of the OASIS.

Hub of the Family Caregiving Wheel: Promoting Self-Management

Home health nursing involves home visits to promote independence rather than dependence on the home health team. Lasting health improvement is only possible when the home health nurse works with the client/family to make decisions that are truly their own. Although financial incentives push home health nurses to minimize the number of visits and duration of service, pressuring a client or family to adopt the agency agenda denies any sense of partnership and can backfire, resulting in nonadherence to the therapeutic regimen. This can place a nurse in a no-win situation.

Every effort is made to develop capacity for self-care, so that the home team can safely withdraw. Obviously, this is quite appropriate for those recovering from an episode of acute illness, but it can be quite difficult when clients are living with severe chronic illness and do not have adequate caregivers to provide needed care without outside nursing assistance. Pressures to discharge are resulting in some patients discharged from home health care agencies while unable to manage care at home; indeed, a proportion of elderly clients may be discharged from home health agencies with unresolved wound and incontinence issues (Flynn, 2007). Currently, no governmental program assures long-term care for those people unable to care for themselves. The home health nurse must work closely with agency social workers to mobilize resources to care after the agency leaves.

Rim of the Home Health Caregiving Wheel: Detecting

Nurses in the home are challenged by an extraordinarily complex environment with much to investigate and frequently many distractions to ignore. Detecting is an all-encompassing, never-ending assessment process as the nurse seeks to understand the client's health in the context of home (Zerwekh, 1991). The nurse keeps her ears and eyes "wide open." The home environment surrounds the nurse with sounds, sights, and scents that need to be comprehended in light of the client's needs. Who lives in the home? How do they interact? Who are the caregivers, and how do they care? What is the relevance of culture and religion in the life of the household? How does the physical environment impact patient safety and security? Is there drug paraphernalia in the living room? Can the bathroom tub be used? The questions are endless. Sometimes the underlying etiologies of illness can be discovered by scrutinizing the "big picture" in the home. The OASIS format provides the baselines for the first visit, and then the nursing assessment broadens with each visit as the nurse continually widens his or her lens to take it all in. Home visits reveal discoveries that can never be imagined in clinic or hospital settings. Take for example the client whose refrigerator no longer chills and whose impaired vision prevents awareness of the expanding family of roaches in the kitchen.

Spokes of the Home Health Caregiving Wheel: Collaborating, Mobilizing, Strengthening, Teaching, Solving Problems

Home health nursing competencies that radiate from the hub and contribute to promotion of self-care and family care include *collaborating* with multiple team members and *mobilizing resources* in the community that can sustain the client after discharge. The home health care nurse usually is the coordinator of all other home health team members. Working with the social worker, the nurse proposes needed connections with community services. Likewise, *strengthening* involves development of self-management or family caregiving ability. People learn that they can give injections, manage IV lines, safely take complex drug regimens, provide rehabilitation for loved ones after stroke, and perform countless other skills that they do not believe possible until a nurse shows them and they discover that they can do it themselves.

The home health nurse is constantly *teaching* clients and/or family caregivers through concrete explanation, discussion, and modeling behavior. Teaching facts is no assurance of behavior change and improved management of a health problem. Underlying factors influencing health behavior must be diagnosed and addressed. Health coaching, also called *motivational interviewing*, has demonstrated effectiveness in improving chronic disease management by getting the patient and family to be actively involved (Huffman, 2007). Instead of telling people what to do, this involves asking people how they would like to change, "What worries you the most?" Those concerns and relevant feelings must be validated, and the nurse leads the person to consider options for change. The solution develops through a mutual, participatory process. Ultimately, people are responsible for their own health decisions.

Finally, home health nursing competency requires flexibility and creativity in *solving* health care problems and the challenges of everyday living. All outcomes of care can be achieved only by adapting to the skills and resources available in the home. Although people of all socioeconomic backgrounds present with severe health problems requiring home health nursing, many families live on the margins. Inderwies (in Cohen, 2007) vividly describes her 32 years of visiting the "have-nots, cannots, and will-nots" (p. 15). By this, she refers to people living on the margins of society who have few resources, little capability, and frequent resistance to being told what to do. Their housekeeping may be terrible. Their interactions may be abusive. Witnessing lives in some homes requires an awareness of self and every effort to reach beyond preconception and judgment. Caring in the homes of those living "on the ragged edge" of society necessitates a strong commitment to discovering and honoring shared humanity (Zerwekh, 2000). Sometimes awareness of our own limitations should lead to referral to another home health nurse rather than imposing our own fear and/or anger on vulnerable clients.

Home Health Nursing Case Management

The home health nurse is the case manager for each client and responsible for coordination of the other professionals and paraprofessionals involved in the client's care.

The nurse plans visit frequency and duration. Will home visits be made twice weekly, once weekly, or every day? For how long will visits continue? As the care is provided and the client's condition improves, the home health nurse determines whether the frequency of visits should be reduced or whether the client can be discharged.

The home care nurse is the primary contact with the client's physician, collaborating on the initial plan of care, reporting changes in the client's condition, and securing changes in the plan of care.

The nurse conducts case conferences among team members to share information, discuss problems, and plan actions to affect the best possible outcomes for the client. Medicare mandates such case conferences every 60 days in home care. The nurse case manager supervises the paraprofessionals, such as home health aides, who also serve the homebound client. This may entail visiting the client at a time when the home health aide is present to observe the care provided.

The home health nurse must know who is going to pay for services from the first visit to the time of discharge from the agency. If the client does not have a source of payment for the care that is needed, the agency must determine whether the client will receive the care free of charge or at a reduced rate. Many agencies have a sliding fee scale, which means that the charge for the services is based on the client's ability to pay.

Selected Nursing Challenges in the Home

Working in the home immerses the nurse in challenges unlike anything encountered in controlled institutional environments. Some of these include infection control, medication safety, risk for falls, technology at home, and nurse safety.

Infection Control

Home health nurses frequently need to work with the family to prevent infection in clients who are debilitated and may be immunocompromised; in addition, many are now dwelling at home with invasive medical devices that make them especially vulnerable to infection. Likewise, nurses are challenged to consider how to protect the home health care team, family, and community from a client with contagious disease. In such cases, all people living in the home will need instruction. Some households have inadequate facilities to control disease transmission. There may be no access to running water, no heating unit to boil equipment, or inadequate facilities to dispose of contaminated equipment. These conditions necessitate the development of creative solutions to control infection. Complexities of the home environment require the nurse to carefully consider exactly how microorganisms are likely to exit the body, how might they be transmitted, and how are they likely to enter the body of another individual. Households cannot be organized like hospital units with isolation rooms. The nurse must decide when gloves are absolutely essential, when protecting clothing with a gown is needed, when a mask should be worn, and what environmental surfaces are likely to be contaminated and must be scrupulously cleaned. How should soiled tissues or dressings, dishes, and laundry be handled? What is realistic and can actually be carried out by client and family? As in the hospital environment, hands are the main vehicle for transmission of contagion, and hand hygiene is the main intervention that must be emphasized. To guide the nurse, home health agencies have adapted infection control policies and procedures based on the Centers for Disease Control and Prevention's (CDCs) isolation precautions for health care settings (Siegel, Rhinehart, Jackson, Chiarello, & Healthcare Infection Control Practices Advisory Committee, 2011).

Medication Safety

Home health nurses assume major responsibility for medication safety. The home health client taking multiple medications is at particular risk of multiple errors in self-administration, including incorrect medication, dose, time, interval, or route. Often doses are missed or doubled. Clients may discontinue a drug or not complete the full course. Sometimes, the drug or drugs ordered are inappropriate considering the patient's condition at home.

The home presents risks of medication errors that are different from those found in hospital or nursing home. Every visiting nurse has stories of finding drawers and cupboards filled with multiple prescriptions from multiple physicians, some current and some many years old. Polypharmacy becomes very obvious in the home setting. Clients taking at least one potentially inappropriate medication were found by Bao and colleagues to be at greater risk when they received Medicare- or Medicaid-provided services (Bao, Shao, Bishop, Schackman, & Bruce, 2011). Using data from the 2007 National Home and Hospice Care Survey, 38% of elderly home health clients were taking one or more potentially inappropriate medications and the risk for polypharmacy showed a correlated increase (Bao et al., 2011). **Potentially inappropriate medications** (PIM) are "medications that generally should be avoided among patients 65 years or older either because they are ineffective or because associated adverse effects outweigh potential benefits or a safer alternative exists" (Bao et al., 2011; Fick et al., 2003). Additional findings from the Bao et al. study were an increased risk of PIM when clients were admitted to home health care from a nursing home or other subacute facility, rather than community admission. This not only supports the need for home care but improvements to discharge planning from skilled nursing facilities.

Even if the client is well organized and taking every drug prescribed, those prescriptions may have originated from several providers over time and may have contradictory side effects. Sometimes medication errors at home include failure to clearly reconcile hospital or nursing home orders with home discharge orders. Although medication boxes can helpfully organize medications, they can also confuse new or impaired users. Distraction, visual impairment, forgetfulness, depression, and cognitive impairment are common causes of unintentional medication noncompliance. The home health nurse investigates how the medication is taken by reviewing and reconciling the current list of medications and having the patient explain and demonstrate the process he goes through. Intervention requires clear and repeated instruction, updating the medication list, charting or diagramming the schedule for medication taking, and assuring that the client or caregiver knows how to use the medication box.

Some of the reasons for intentional noncompliance are knowledge deficit, unacceptable side effects, no immediately obvious consequence when the drug is stopped, resistance to authority, perception of personal weakness if needing medication, and prohibitive cost. As the cost of prescriptions is shifted onto people living with chronic illness, drug spending goes down, with partial adherence or total discontinuation of therapy by clients who cannot afford their medication. It is not surprising to note that health then deteriorates and clients with diseases such as congestive heart failure and diabetes come to need intensive medical intervention (Goldman, Joyce, & Zheng, 2007). The home health nurse seeks to nonjudgmentally elicit reasons and mutually figure out solutions that manage medications at home and prevent intensive medical interventions.

Risk for Falls

Estimates are that one in three adults 65 years and older will fall each year, with 20% to 30% suffering moderate to severe injuries (CDC, 2012). Elders living at home have a 35% to 40% chance of falling; fear of falling is a serious problem in the aging, especially in those with debilitating illness (Stanley, Blair, & Beare, 2005). Physiological risk factors include orthostatic hypotension and cardiac dysrhythmias, dizziness, neurologic and musculoskeletal effects on gait and balance, urinary urgency, impaired hearing or vision, alcohol or drug abuse, and medication effects impairing alertness, balance, urinary frequency, and blood pressure. Clients should be observed as they move through their home and carry out activities of daily living. It is important to investigate factors that obstruct movement or threaten balance. The nurse in the home should inspect sidewalks, stairs, and surfaces outside the home; floor, rugs, electrical cords, stairs, lighting, and clutter inside the home; kitchen safety; and bathroom features including grab bars and a raised seat for the toilet and safety modifications for the bathtub. Common home modifications, such as eliminating throw rugs and loose mats and the use of nonslip bath mats, have a significant protective effect. Display 32.3 lists teaching guidelines to prevent falls.

Technology at Home

Home health nurses teach patients and their family to manage a wide array of complex technologies. Home regimens often require mini-intensive care units. In the past, the average home had a limited capacity for technology; medication was swallowed and food and fluid were consumed with the aid of fork and spoon. Now, the IV needle has evolved into venous access devices and plastic IV fluid bags can be stacked in the refrigerator and hung from the arm of a lamp. The household becomes home to dialysis, ventilators, enteric and IV nutrition, and vasopressors—the list goes on. Nurses teach clients and families to manage it all; we become the guardians and advocates of complex regimens that require multiple nursing visits. Paradoxically, our primary mission is to be guardians and advocates for the well-being of client and family. Consider the human impact when the machines and the sickbed become the center of household activities. "We can slip so easily into the struggle to keep the technological regime functioning. However, nurses and other professionals in the home are in the pivotal position to witness the impact, to document the impact, and to assist clients to construct their lives in a meaningful way, so that neither illness nor medical regimes are the only reason for being" (Zerwekh, 1995, p. 12). Sometimes, we can foster dialogue with clients and families to consider the benefits and burdens of continuing technologies. Consider four reasons why technology may be inappropriate: (1) the technology is not achieving a therapeutic purpose, (2) the therapeutic purpose can be met more simply, (3) complications of the intervention outweigh benefits, and (4) the resulting quality of life does not justify the technology.

Recent information technologies being adopted by home health care agencies significantly improve quality of client care. These include medical records available instantly on the nurse's laptop and daily telemedicine monitoring of electrocardiogram, blood pressure, oxygen saturation, and other vital measures. As the results of one study caution (Shea & Chamoff, 2012), health care providers may overestimate the value of telemedicine in self-care for chronic conditions. The findings of the study support using explicit goals and intensions with clients and to individualize instructions provided. Essentially frequency of contact did not mean quality communication.

DISPLAY 32.3 TEACHING TO PREVENT FALLS

- Discuss fear of falling as normal and then urge preventive approaches.
- Identify environmental hazards and explain need for change.
- Encourage highest possible level of physical activity considering ability.
- Explain importance of reporting health status changes that increase risk of falls.
- Explain importance of recognizing sensory changes and correcting immediately.
- Teach regular blood pressure monitoring.
- Emphasize slowing down when moving and changing positions.
- Emphasize safe footwear and foot care.
- Explore strategy for responding to a fall, including calling for help and getting up.
- Demonstrate safe body mechanics to lift heavy objects and to move immobilized family members.

Modified from Stanley, M., Blair, K. A., & Beare, P. G. (2005). *Gerontological nursing: Promoting successful aging with older adults* (3rd ed.). Philadelphia, PA: F.A. Davis, with permission.

Nurse Safety

Every home health care agency should have a carefully developed program to assure the safety of personnel traveling to homes. Many work closely with local police departments to identify the wisest process for visiting dangerous neighborhoods and isolated rural areas. Display 32.4 lists practices for safe home visiting.

THE FUTURE OF CARE IN THE HOME

In conclusion, it can be seen that present-day Medicare home health care intervenes during brief episodes of acute medical trouble, relies on family at home as caregivers, and is expected to get in and out of the home as inexpensively as possible. Consider instead the true needs of the frail elderly or severely disabled who require prolonged psychosocial support, personal care, housekeeping, promotion of health, prevention of deterioration, and early detection of medical problems. In other words, they need case management that extends over months and years. For this to happen, the United States must develop a **community-based long-term care** system. Home health care leaders look to a future of reinventing themselves by moving into new lines of business to meet these needs (Cohen, 2007). Some baby boomers will be able to afford these services by paying out of their own pockets for a network of elder management services. Most baby boomers will

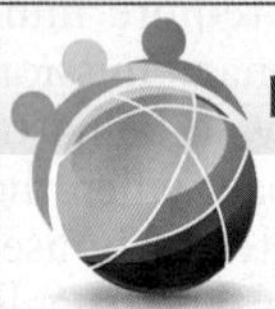

DISPLAY 32.4 SAFE HOME VISITS

- Carry a cellular phone.
- Be sure the agency knows your itinerary.
- Clarify directions before travel. Carry a map.
- Make joint visits or request security escort if safety is threatened. Refuse to visit when there is strong evidence of personal danger. Consult the police.
- Call to schedule the visit and do not go into the home without invitation.
- Dress simply without expensive jewelry. Do not carry large amounts of cash. Keep wallet or purse locked in the car.
- Wear an agency badge.
- Follow family directions about how to get by in their neighborhood and when to come in or leave their home. Patients and families usually will protect their nurse.

need the development of a national community-based long-term care benefit. The Affordable Care Act is one step in that direction, but two programs provided in the act, the Community First Choice Option and the Community Care Transitions Program, do not provide for the long-term care so often required (CMS, 2012d). They are, however, a step in the right direction. *Healthy People 2020* provides a number of objectives that support the health and well-being of home health clients and their caregivers. Refer to Display 32.5 for a list of *Healthy People 2020* objectives related to home health and hospice care (U.S. Department of Health & Human Services [USDHHS], 2010). After reviewing other categories of objectives in the full document, can you identify any that support the development of a community-based long-term care system in the United States?

OVERVIEW OF THE HOSPICE MOVEMENT

The contemporary circumstances of death in America are often dehumanizing; most people die in hospitals and long-term care institutions, surrounded by

DISPLAY 32.5 *HEALTHY PEOPLE 2020* HOME HEALTH AND HOSPICE CARE OBJECTIVES

Remember that *Healthy People 2020* has four overarching goals: (1) to attain high-quality, longer lives free of preventable disease, disability, injury, and premature death; (2) achieve health equity, eliminate health disparities, and improve the health of all groups; (3) create social and physical environments that promote good health for all; and (4) promote quality of life, healthy development, and healthy behaviors across all life stages. A vital concept for elders is that of "compressing morbidity." This means that we seek to promote healthy lives and to diminish (compress) the time they are suffering with disabling illness. Any health care system developed to provide long-term care for the elderly and those with chronic illness should maximize function and independence. How might such a system work? What role does the home care or hospice nurse have in meeting the *Healthy People 2020* objectives? Review the Healthy People objectives and see what objectives apply to home care and hospice.

These are a sample of specific *HP 2020* objectives related to home health and hospice care:

Access to Health Services:

AHS-1 Increase the proportion of persons with health insurance

AHS-2 Increase the proportion of insured persons with coverage for clinical preventive services

Dementias, including Alzheimer's Disease:

DIA-2 Reduce the proportion of preventable hospitalizations in persons with diagnosed Alzheimer's disease and other dementias

Disability and Health:

DH-11 Increase the proportion of newly constructed and retrofitted US homes and residential buildings that have visitable features

Health Communication and Health IT:

HC/HIT-4 Increase the proportion of patients who report that their health care providers always involved them in decisions about their health care as much as they wanted

Medical Product Safety:

MPS-2 Increase the safe and effective treatment of pain

MPS-5 Reduce emergency department (ED) visits for common, preventable adverse events from medications

Source: U.S. Department of Health and Human Services. (2010). *Healthy People 2020: Improving the health of Americans*. Washington, DC: U.S. Government Printing Office.

strangers. Uncertainty and denial often prevail during the final stage of life because prognoses are uncertain and many serious illnesses are now treated aggressively until the last breath. The battle against the "evil" of death seems to be the primary emphasis, with patient, family, and professionals wanting to believe that it is possible to win the final struggle. In the 21st century, fatal conditions have been turned into expensive chronic illnesses. Too often, discomfort is not relieved and treatment causes further suffering. And as the period of disability extends and the body deteriorates, social isolation develops. The modern preoccupation with action, productivity, and beauty has little interest in the process of dying. In dramatic contrast to the dehumanization of death, the **hospice** movement has developed to humanize the end-of-life experience and provide palliative care. **Palliative interventions** relieve suffering without curing underlying disease. The hospice movement has emphasized four major changes in end-of-life care: (1) Care should attend to body, mind, and spirit; (2) death must not be a taboo topic; (3) medical technology should be used with discretion; and (4) clients have a right to truthful discussion and involvement in treatment decisions (McIntosh & Zerwekh, 2006). Table 32-1 contrasts mainstream medical focus with hospice. This section explores the evolution of hospice care in the United States, describes hospice agencies, and examines Medicare criteria for hospice reimbursement. It concludes with an exploration of the unique characteristics of hospice nursing practice.

EVOLUTION OF HOSPICE CARE

In medieval Europe, hospices were refuges for the sick and dying. The contemporary hospice movement originated in England, where Dame Cicely Saunders founded St. Christopher's Hospice in 1967 (McIntosh & Zerwekh, 2006). Dr. Saunders was credentialed as a nurse, social worker, and physician. She developed a unique program based both on compassion and skillful relief of physical discomfort through around-the-clock analgesics administered by mouth. It had been previously assumed that only injections, administered sparingly, could be used for terminal pain control. The first hospice in the United States was established in 1974 in Branford, Connecticut, by Florence Wald, Dean of the Yale School of Nursing. Because even in the 1970s there was concern about saving money by shortening hospital stays and keeping people out of the hospital, hospices in the United States came to focus on providing care in the home. To that end, Congress established the Medicare hospice benefit in 1982, with the intention of keeping people at home, yet receiving comprehensive services that are less expensive than hospitalization.

Table 32.1 Contrasts Between Home Health and Hospice

Hospice	Home Health
Emphasis is on quality of life and comfort.	Emphasis is on rehabilitation and physiological stabilization.
Focus is on health of whole family.	Focus is on health of client.
Plan of care is guided by client choice.	Plan of care is determined by medical need.
Nurse is case manager until death.	Nurse is case manager until home health discharge.
Client chooses how to live last days.	Priority is given to correcting physiologic imbalances.
Intermittent visits increase in frequency as death become imminent.	Intermittent visits decrease in frequency as client stabilizes.
Nurses are expert in symptom control.	Symptom control is domain of physician with some nurses having expertise.
Sedatives and opioids are expertly adjusted to eliminate suffering.	Sedatives and opioids are used hesitantly to reduce suffering.
End-of-life disease course is managed to avoid crises.	End-of-life problems tend to be seen as medical crises.
Goal is for symptoms at end of life to be managed at home if possible.	Client is brought to hospital for unmanaged symptoms.
Spiritual care is focus of whole team.	Spiritual needs are met by own clergy.
Survivors have bereavement support.	No bereavement support is provided.

Adapted from Zerwekh, J. (2002). Home care of the dying. In I. Martinson, A. Widmer, & C. Portillo. ***Home health care nursing***. Philadelphia, PA: W.B. Saunders, with permission.

Hospice characteristics have changed over time. Initially, nearly all clients suffered from terminal cancer; presently, people with a variety of end-stage diseases are admitted. Diseases that were once rapid death sentences have now turned into chronic life-limiting diseases. With prognoses difficult to predict and denial of death a continuing issue, hospice referrals are now made very late in the disease process. Brief hospice stays make it difficult to significantly help families and clients before death occurs. Another transition in hospice is the move from charity to business (McIntosh & Zerwekh, 2006). With highly reliable Medicare payment, for-profit hospices have expanded and are competing in many communities for the hospice "market share."

HOSPICE SERVICES AND REIMBURSEMENT

As in home health care, Medicare has determined the way services are provided. The **Medicare hospice benefit** requires that a client who has a prognosis of 6 months or less must sign up for the comfort-focused hospice benefit and waive the regular hospice benefit. This mandates that the client acknowledges a terminal prognosis and chooses comforting care instead of life-extending care. When this choice is made, the hospice coordinates care in all settings, functioning both as clinical and financial case manager (McIntosh & Zerwekh, 2006). The government pays a flat rate to the hospice for each day the patient receives care. There are four payment levels: (1) routine home care with intermittent visits, (2) continuous home care when the patient's condition is acute and death is near, (3) inpatient hospital care for symptom relief, and (4) respite care in a nursing home to relieve family members. Eighty percent of care has to be provided at home or in a nursing home that has become the person's permanent residence.

Hospices coordinate home care and direct inpatient care if needed. The emphasis is on palliation, with a focus on physical, psychosocial, and spiritual comfort. A strong emphasis is placed on caring for the entire family. The hospice team includes nurse, physician, home health aides, physical and occupational therapists, social workers, volunteers, palliative medication and medical equipment specialists, and bereavement counselors. Staff meet regularly to explore together the challenges of assuring comfort at the end of life.

Volunteers fill an important need in hospice care. They act as companions to the client when the family must be somewhere else or is away for short respite. They run errands for family members, shop, organize hot meals prepared by friends and neighbors, provide child care, and perform other services as needed.

HOSPICE NURSING PRACTICE

The nurse's role is central in the hospice interdisciplinary team. The hospice nurse functions as case manager and visits the client more frequently than other members of the team. Nurses work in close collaboration with physicians to assure management of symptoms often change rapidly as the end of life nears. In addition to home visits focusing on palliation and interdisciplinary planning, hospice nurses rotate through 24-hour call 7 days a week to assure continuous availability by telephone and visits for emergent problems reported by client or family. Hospice nursing competencies and challenges are similar to those described for home health nurses, with the added expertise needed to relieve physical and emotional suffering of terminally ill people and their families. The American Nurses Association (ANA), in collaboration with other groups, has published standards of practice for hospice and palliative nursing (2007) and pain management (2005). Through the ANCC (2012), hospice nurses can receive board certification in pain management. There is no current certification for hospice or home health nursing. The practice standards and certification process provide guidance in this specialized field of nursing.

Hospice caregiving can be illustrated as a tree, strongly rooted in the process of nurses deliberately practicing self-care for themselves (Fig. 32-2). This tree has been drawn to explain the expert competencies of hospice nurses who were interviewed to capture the essence of their practice (Zerwekh, 1995, 2006). Each of the hospice nursing practices visualized by the tree diagram is briefly summarized below.

Roots of Hospice Nursing: Sustaining Oneself

Effective hospice nurses understand that to care for others, they must care for themselves. Without strong healthy roots, the tree will not thrive. *Sustaining oneself* requires deliberate effort to maintain one's own physical, emotional, and spiritual well-being. Knowing oneself, identifying sources of stress, and learning how to care for oneself are important. Expert hospice nurses keep themselves healthy by maintaining a balance between giving and receiving, letting go of predetermined agendas and idealistic hopes to achieve more than is humanly possible, being emotionally open and clear, and deliberately replenishing themselves to restore their energy (Zerwekh, 2006). "Rooted in self care, we are able to reach out with courage to the broken and terrified at the end of their lives" (p. 60). Examine the Evidence-Based Practice feature about the risk of compassion fatigue. Of note: The contemporary work environment of most nurses actually causes more stress than everyday witnessing of suffering and death (Vachon & Huggard, 2010); emphasis on productivity and finances, with limits placed on nurse empowerment and resources, can be quite disheartening. Leaders must seek to develop a caring culture that respects nurse autonomy in the face of these challenges.

The Trunk Reaching Upward: Connecting, Speaking Truth, and Encouraging Choice

Rooted in self-care, hospice nurses practice *connecting*, which refers to the centrality of relationships in

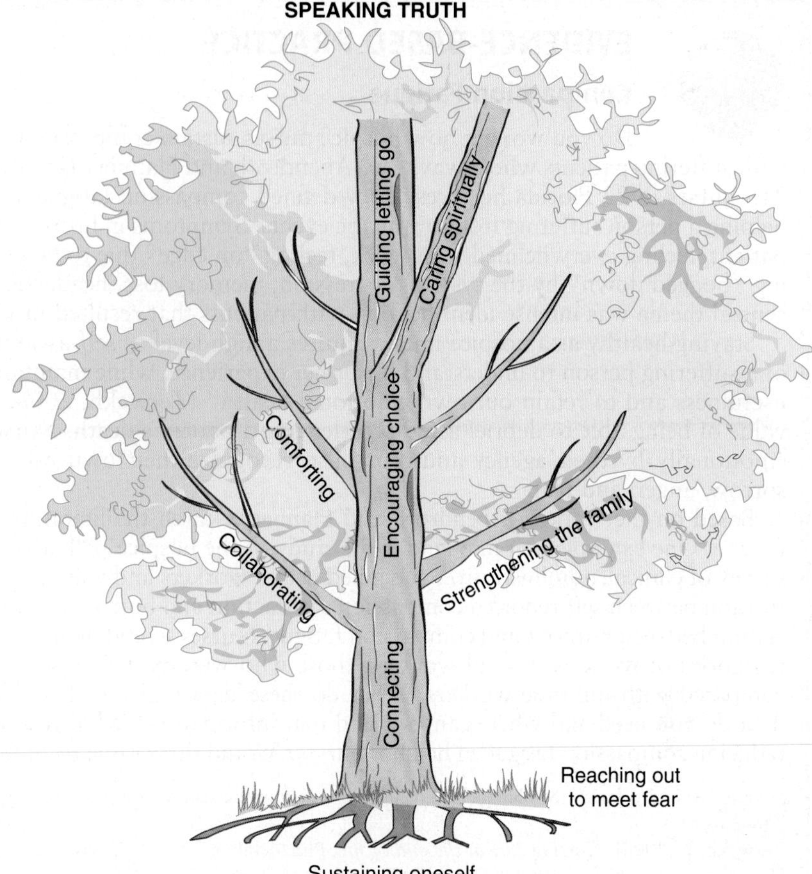

FIGURE 32-2. The hospice caregiving tree.

providing hospice care. The hospice nurse seeks to understand the emotional and spiritual distress common to the end of life, particularly the progressive experience of loss after loss. Guided by that understanding, hospice nurses emphasize attentive listening to understand each individual's unique story. This requires quieting your own thoughts to truly hear what is being expressed. Sometimes listening involves simply being present in the moment, paying attention. Having heard the client's story, it is important for hospice nurses to speak honestly when other professionals and family feel obliged to keep being cheerful and positive. Hospice nurses openly seek to speak truthfully about many issues that can be painful to discuss. *Speaking truth* is visualized as encircling the entire top of the caregiving tree. Hospice nurses bring up difficult subjects, so that the client is freed to speak about his greatest fears and concerns. Sometimes it leads to joint problem solving and *encouraging choice* through informed decision-making. After truth has been discussed and the client has made a decision, the hospice nurse often advocates for client wishes against the resistance of various authorities. Remember that these are the final decisions in a dying person's life.

Collaborating

Interdisciplinary teamwork is an essential branch on the tree. Hospice team members communicate around the table and are constantly consulting each other. The hospice interdisciplinary team members share information and work interdependently. The hospice nurse coordinates the plan of care and day-to-day efforts to provide physical and psychosocial comfort. She supervises practical nurses and nursing assistants. The physician is responsible for medical care and serves as liaison with the client's primary care physicians. Social workers, spiritual counselors, and volunteers are integral members of the hospice team. The hospice interdisciplinary team is constantly challenged to work creatively together to find solutions for complex end-of-life suffering with emotional, spiritual, and physical components.

Strengthening the Family

The death of a family member causes great disruption for all involved. When family members are in a caregiving role in the home, they experience significant personal suffering. They are vulnerable to physical and emotional illness themselves. The process of taking care involves managing the illness and all practical assistance, seeking information and resources, and preparing for death itself. Family members often are caught up with family issues and struggles with the health care system. An extremely important hospice nursing role involves strengthening family members' abilities as

EVIDENCE-BASED PRACTICE

Compassion Fatigue

Do you wonder how hospice nurses sustain compassionate practice as they work day in and day out with suffering patients who always die? Abendroth and Flannery (2006) investigated "compassion fatigue" among 216 nurses in 22 Florida hospices. They defined compassion fatigue as a traumatic stress reaction resulting from helping a person suffering from traumatic events. Symptoms in hospice nurses included being preoccupied with the patient, feeling overwhelmed with work, feeling "on edge" due to helping, losing sleep over patient's trauma, feeling "bogged down" by the system, depression, memory loss, headaches, and having "frightening" thoughts. The central theme was intense identification with patients that resulted in vicarious experiences of anxiety and pain.

Staying healthy as a hospice nurse requires a high level of self-awareness to "purposefully enter into the world of a suffering person to understand his or her experience, while maintaining enough detachment to be of practical usefulness and to retain our own emotional health" (Zerwekh, 2006, p. 50). Abendroth and Flannery note the value of being able to debrief after experiencing a patient's death. Nurses working in this area must be supported emotionally by their agency and must also recognize their own need to share stories and speak openly about sorrow, anger, and fear.

Based on the work of Abendroth and Flannery, search the literature for more current examples of compassion fatigue. One example you may find is the study of the hospice palliative care workforce in Canada using a national survey of clinical, administrative, and allied health workers and volunteers. The research demonstrated a positive correlation between self-reported compassion satisfaction and both compassion fatigue and burnout and a positive association between burnout and compassion fatigue. Nurses scored higher for Compassion Fatigue than any of the other categories of workers. For all workers, those who were part-time scored higher for compassion satisfaction when compared with full-time workers. What do these data indicate about this population of nurses? What additional data do you need and where can you find that information? What recommendations can you make with respect to reducing compassion fatigue in hospice nurses? Would these same recommendations apply to other hospice workers?

Sources: Abendroth, M., & Flananery, J. (2006). Predicting the risk of compassion fatigue. *Journal of Hospice and Palliative Nursing, 8*(6), 346–356.
Zerwekh, J. (2006). *Nursing care at the end of life*. Philadelphia, PA: F.A. Davis.
Slocum-Gori, S., Hemsworth, D., Chan, W., Carson, A., & Kazanjian, A. (2011). Understanding compassion satisfaction, compassion fatigue, and burnout: A survey of the hospice palliative care workforce. *Palliative Medicine, 0*(0), 1–7. doi: 10.1177/0269216311431311.

caregivers. Teaching caregiving requires creative teaching methods and flexibility. Often the hospice nurse is able to help family members communicate with each other, gather them together, and act as an intermediary if necessary.

Comforting

Hospice nurses develop extensive expertise in pain and symptom management. Contemporary medical/surgical nursing textbooks discuss the essentials in this field, and advanced knowledge is developed through experience, continued education, and reading. Display 32.6 lists fundamental palliative principles and Display 32.7 identifies four important components of pain relief.

Spiritual Practice and Letting Go

As death draws near, spiritual needs intensify, with the final search for meaning, reconciliation, hope, and transcendence beyond the limits of human lived experience (Dillon, Roscoe, & Jenkins, 2012; Touhy & Zerwekh, 2006). Hospice nurses recognize spiritual distress and practice spiritual caring interventions that include respect for beliefs and spiritual practices and fostering

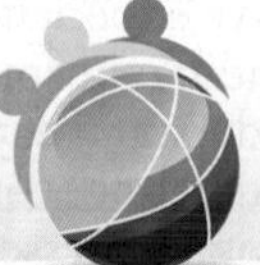

DISPLAY 32.6 FUNDAMENTALS OF PALLIATIVE CARE

- Make no assumptions about what is wrong.
- Believe the patient's report of symptoms.
- Relieve discomfort to the extent that the patient chooses and finds acceptable.
- Investigate the biologic, psychosocial, and spiritual dimensions of discomfort.
- Anticipate symptoms and relieve them before they occur again.
- Use nursing and complementary (integrative) interventions.
- Become an expert in the use of palliative medication.
- Continually evaluate the effectiveness of interventions.
- Choose the least complex and most manageable interventions that patients and families can manage themselves at home.
- Never give up. Persist in trying different palliative strategies.

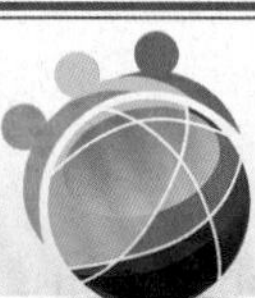

DISPLAY 32.7 ESSENTIAL COMPONENTS OF PAIN RELIEF

1. Continually assess the extent of pain and the relief afforded by interventions.
2. Schedule analgesics around the clock to maintain continuous blood levels and prevent the return of pain.
3. Use the least invasive route for analgesic administration, with oral as first choice.
4. Follow the World Health Organization (n.d.) three-step ladder:
   Step 1 for mild pain: Nonopioid (acetaminophen or NSAID) plus adjuvant such as corticosteroid, antidepressant, anxiolytic, or anticonvulsant
   Step 2 for persisting pain: Opioid and perhaps nonopioid and/or adjuvant
   Step 3 for severe pain: Strong opioid and perhaps nonopioid or adjuvant

Source: Vargas-Schaffer, G. (2010). Is the WHO analgesic ladder still valid? Twenty-four years of experience. *Canadian Family Physician, 56*, 514–517.
World Health Organization. (n.d.). *Cancer: WHO's pain ladder*. New York: Author.

reconciliation if there is a problem with estrangement from family, friends, and faith tradition. They deliberately try to keep their minds uncluttered by distracting preoccupations, so that they can listen attentively and promote life review. Cassidy (1998) states that spiritual care at the end of life involves being a companion on the dying person's journey, even when we would rather escape walking with them along the frightening path through darkness. In a qualitative meta-ethnography, Dillon and colleagues (2012) uncovered the expressed need of African Americans for hospice care that integrates and emphasizes spiritual support, not merely acceptance or tolerance. Both Cassidy and Dillon et al. challenge the hospice nurse to support that spiritual journey so needed by the dying and their family members.

Guiding letting go is a truly unique nursing practice that involves helping the client to let go of former activities and hopes, including life itself. This involves listening to intense emotions and helping the person and family find resolution. Sometimes it involves participating in a vigil at the bedside of the dying person and encouraging loved ones to say their final words of farewell.

ETHICAL CHALLENGES IN HOSPICE NURSING

The hospice nurse confronts striking ethical challenges at the end of life. "To nurse at the end of life, you need to become conscious of how value-laden the choice of medical and nursing interventions can be. We practice in the middle of an ethical minefield.... Naming and clarifying ethical issues is a prominent nursing role.... We must strengthen our voice and ask, 'Is what we are doing good for this person and family?'" (Zerwekh, 2006, pp. 180–181). Wide-ranging issues include respect or disregard for client autonomy, relief or disregard for client suffering, and avoidance of killing at the very end of life. The hospice nurse needs to develop their own knowledge of nursing and medical ethics in order to question the ethical implications of interventions and to advocate for client and family. An example of this is the widely held belief in hospice care that dehydration enhances client comfort. Cohen, Torres-Vigil, Burbach, de la Rosa, and Bruera (2012) conducted a phenomenological study with 84 caregivers and 85 clients regarding the issue of hydration of advanced cancer patients receiving hospice care. Their findings revealed that patients and their families viewed fluids as enhancing comfort, dignity, and quality of life. These findings support the need to tailor individual care based on specific patient needs and family preferences (Cohen et al., 2012). They challenge the hospice nurse to embrace ongoing professional development in order to keep abreast of best practice modalities.

THE FUTURE OF HOME HEALTH AND HOSPICE

Given a rapidly expanding population of elders living longer with challenging chronic illnesses, home health and hospice care in the home will soon need to transform into a community-based long-term care system that doesn't discharge after an acute episode or admit only at the very end of life. In response to out-of-control medical inflation, federal and state governments have sought to hold down expenses in all areas, including restrictions on home health and hospice care. However, costs keep rising in step with technologic and pharmacologic innovation and marketing. Containing costs will eventually force a shift in services from expensive institutional and high-technology interventions to community-based home services.

The entire model for service provision in the home must change to a health care delivery system that continuously serves those living with disabling and terminal illness to maximize well-being at home, anticipate and prevent crises, and minimize emergent and inpatient interventions. The Medicare definitions of homebound, medical necessity and skilled nursing must become extinct. Likewise, the current hospice admission requirement that a person must discontinue treatment in order to receive hospice services is outdated (see Evidence-Based Practice 32.2). Reception of hospice services should be based on client choice and the reality of a terminal diagnosis. A sustainable, affordable approach to care in the home will require ongoing case management to coordinate and manage resources with incentives that control cost while assuring quality of life and comfort.

EVIDENCE-BASED PRACTICE

There is a paucity of peer-reviewed studies of children and hospice care in nursing publications. One factor that may explain the lack of studies is the relative infrequent use of hospice by families of dying children. Despite the availability of hospice care for children, surveys have demonstrated that a small proportion of children who fit the criteria for hospice care actually receive services. Hospice plays an important role in supporting the child and family in the areas of medical, social, spiritual, and psychological support. The value of this service and underutilization justify research in this area.

The demonstrated effectiveness of hospice care and the low level of use led researchers in the United States and the United Kingdom to explore the factors that may contribute to this problem. In a 2010 study, Neilson, Kai, MacArthur, and Greenfield explored the experiences of community-based hospice nurses in the United Kingdom in the provision of palliative care for children dying of cancer. Using one-on-one interviews with 30 community nurses, the researchers used a grounded theory approach for data analysis in this qualitative study. The nurses identified difficulty developing and maintaining knowledge and skills as impacting their perceived competency. Another issue identified by the nurses was the need for afterhours care and the lack of financial support for these services. Hesitancy to provide services based on the level of training provided to the nurses and funding issues were both seen as important barriers to hospice care with this population.

The issue of barriers to hospice use with children was also explored by Sanchez Varela et al. (2012). In this North Carolina study of hospice organizations, the researchers used quantitative methods to determine the factors contributing to underutilization of hospice services. Factors included lack of trained pediatric nurses, pediatric pharmacy, pediatrician consultation, coordination of care, as well as inconsistent communication between care providers. Other factors of importance were limited referrals and the wishes of the family to continue with curative therapy, which could preclude qualification for hospice services.

Although the studies were conducted in separate countries, similar needs emerged from both studies. Most important to nursing practice is the limited access to ongoing education and the lack of consistent professional experiences with these children and their families. Both of these factors were seen as contributing to underutilization of services. What can be inferred from these findings is that efforts to maintain a trained hospice workforce with specialized skill in working with children, ongoing opportunities to develop and maintain skills, and wider use of hospice in this population are needed. The identified value of hospice services and the findings of these studies support ongoing research into methods to increase use of these services and the infrastructure to create and maintain a trained workforce.

References: Neilson, S., Kai, J., MacArthur, C., & Greenfield, S. (2010). Exploring the experiences of community-based children's nurses providing palliative care. *Paediatric Nursing, 22*(3), 31–36.

Sanchez Varela, A. M., Deal, A. M., Hanson, L. C., Blatt, J., Gold, S., & Dellon, E. P. (2012). Barriers to hospice for children as perceived by hospice organizations in North Carolina. *American Journal of Hospice & Palliative Medicine, 29*(3), 171–176. Doi: 10.1177/1049909111412580.

Community resources will need to be mobilized to develop interdisciplinary and volunteer teams. Clients and family caregivers will need education and supportive networks. Homemaking and personal care will be the bedrock to keep people at home as long as possible. Nurses, nurse practitioners, and home visiting physicians will need to have the diagnostic and therapeutic resources to monitor physiologic status and intervene in the home. Telehealth and home monitoring will be essential. Yet care must be taken to "limit the amount of personnel and materials in the home to avoid trespassing on the family's daily life" (Munck, Sandgren, Fridlund, & Martensson, 2012, p. 1). The focus must change from doing everything possible to prolong physiologic survival to promoting meaningful and comfortable lives. Nurses will have an active role in this process.

SUMMARY

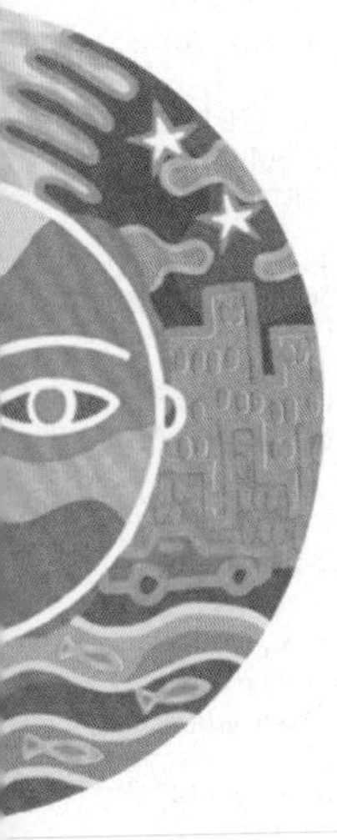

Community/public health nurses have an important role in working with elders who receive home care or hospice services. As the population continues to age, the need for nurses to work with older adults where they live, as they are discharged from acute care settings earlier and earlier and, if they are terminally ill, during their final months and days, will only increase.

There are many types of home care agencies: voluntary, proprietary, hospital-based, official, homemaker, and hospice. Care is provided by formal and informal caregivers. Professional staff members, such as nurses, social workers, therapists, and certified nursing assistants, work in collaboration with family members and, in some situations, with friends and neighbors.

Hospice is a fairly new concept in the United States but has a longer history in England. Medicare covers hospice care without the restrictions experienced by nonhospice home care clients. Hospice programs provide holistic care to clients during the last months of life. Many programs are home-based, and they often are a service offered by a home health agency. In addition to in-home hospices, inpatient hospices exist; these can be located in a freestanding building, in part of a SNF, or in a section of an acute care facility. The focus of hospice care is not aimed at cure, and it employs holistic caregiving practices that involve family members, professionals, and volunteers.

The nurse provides direct physical nursing care both in home health care and with hospice clients. In addition, the nurse teaches clients, family members, and volunteers; supervises; and case manages. Assessing clients to determine health status and eligibility for additional services and acting as a client advocate occur with both groups of clients. Determining the frequency and duration of services occurs in home care. With both home care and hospice clients, the nurse must become familiar with the requirements of documentation to promote continuity of care and ensure reimbursement.

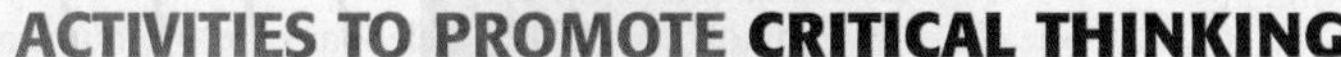

ACTIVITIES TO PROMOTE **CRITICAL THINKING**

1. Search the Internet for home health and hospice agencies in your city or town. Select two agencies and compare the employment opportunities of each. How do these job descriptions and the published pay ranges compare to hospitals in your area? What are the benefits of working in home health and hospice? Will the agency hire new graduates, or do they require prior acute care experience?
2. John S., age 58 years, was recently diagnosed with liver cancer following years of heavy alcohol consumption. At the urging of his physician, his wife contacted the local hospice agency for assistance. You have been assigned this case. When you arrive at John's house, his wife tells you that he refuses to see you and is continuing to drink alcohol. She is very distressed and begins to cry. How would you handle this situation? What are some of the issues inherent in this case?
3. Review your personal health insurance policy or that of a family member. What coverage, if any, is provided for home health or hospice care? What restrictions are stated in the coverage—total reimbursement, source of care, length of service? Do you think this will be adequate to meet your or your family member's needs? What other options might be available to help defray the cost of this type of care?

REFERENCES

American Nurses Association/American Society for Pain Management Nursing. (2005). *Pain management nursing: Scope and standards of practice*. Silver Spring, MD: Nursebook.org.

American Nurses Association/Hospice and Palliative Nurses Association. (2007). *Hospice and palliative nursing: Scope and standards of practice*. Silver Spring, MD: Nursebook.org

American Nurses Credentialing Center. (2012). *ANCC certification center*. Retrieved from http://www.nursecredentialing.org/Certification.aspx

Bao, Y., Shao, H., Bishop, T. F., Schackman, B. R., & Bruce, M. L. (2011). Inappropriate medication in a national sample of U.S. elderly patients receiving home health care. *Journal of General Internal Medicine, 27*(3), 304–310. doi: 10.1007/s11606-011-1905-4

Buhler-Wilkerson, K. (2007). No place like home: A history of nursing and home care in the U.S. *Home Healthcare Nurse, 25*(4), 253–259.

Cassidy, S. (1988). *Sharing the darkness: The spirituality of caring*. London, England: Darron, Longman and Todd.

Centers for Disease Control and Prevention. (2012). *Falls among older adults: An overview*. Retrieved from http://www.cdc.gov/homeandrecreationalsafety/Falls/adultfalls.html

Centers for Medicare and Medicaid Services. (2010). *Patient Protection and Affordable Care Act*. Retrieved from https://www.cms.gov/Regulations-and-Guidance/Legislation/LegislativeUpdate/downloads/PPACA.pdf

Centers for Medicare and Medicaid Services. (2012a). *Home health PPS*. Retrieved from http://www.cms.gov/Medicare/Medicare-Fee-for-Service-Payment/HomeHealthPPS/index.html

Centers for Medicare and Medicaid Services. (2012b). *Home health quality initiative*. Retrieved from https://www.cms.gov/Medicare/Quality-Initiatives-Patient-Assessment-Instruments/HomeHealthQualityInits/index.html?redirect=/HomeHealthQualityInits/14_HHQIOASISUserManual.asp

Centers for Medicare and Medicaid Services. (2012c). *Outcome and Assessment Information data set (OASIS)*. Retrieved from http://www.cms.gov/Medicare/Quality-Initiatives-Patient-Assessment-Instruments/OASIS/Background.html

Centers for Medicare and Medicaid Services. (2012d). *What's changing and when?* Retrieved from http://www.healthcare.gov/law/timeline/

Cohen, B. (2007, January). Best of care: Most difficult of circumstances. *Caring, 26*(1), 13–23.

Cohen, M. Z., Torres-Vigil, I., Burbach, B. E., de la Rosa, A., & Bruera, E. (2012). The meaning of parenteral hydration to family caregivers and patients with advanced cancer receiving hospice care. *Journal of Pain and Symptom Management, 43*(5), 855–865. doi: 10.1016/j.jpainsymman.2011.06.016.

Dillon, P. J., Roscoe, L. A., & Jenkins, J. J. (2012). African Americans and decisions about hospice care: Implications for health message design. *The Howard Journal of Communication, 23*, 175–193. doi:10.1080/10646175.2012.667724.

Ellenbecker, C. H., Boylan, L. N., & Samia, L. (2006). What are home healthcare nurses are saying about their jobs. *Home Healthcare Nurse, 24*(5), 315–324.

Fick, D. M., Cooper, J. W., Wade, W. E., Waller, J. L., Maclean, J. R., & Beers, M. H. (2003). Updating the Beers criteria for potentially inappropriate medication use in older adults: results for a U.S. census panel of experts. *Archives of Internal Medicine, 163*(22), 2716–2724.

Flynn, L. (2007). Managing the care of patients discharged from home health: A quiet threat to patient safety? *Home Healthcare Nurse, 25*(3), 184–190.

Godfrey, S. (2005). Conquering the dilemma of improving function. *Home Healthcare Nurse, 23*(11), 703–706.

Goldman, D. P., Joyce, G. F., & Zheng, Y. (2007). Prescription drug cost sharing: Associations with medication and medical utilization and spending and health. *Journal of the American Medical Association, 298*, 61–69.

Home Healthcare Nurses Association. (2012). *About HHNA*. Retrieved from http://www.hhna.org/About/

Huffman, M. (2007). Health coaching: A new and exciting technique to enhance patient self-management and improve outcomes. *Home Healthcare Nurse, 25*(4), 271–276.

Kulesher, R. R. (2006). Impact of Medicare's prospective payment system on hospitals, skilled nursing facilities and home health agencies: How the balanced budget act of 1997 may have altered service patterns for Medicare providers. *The Health Care Manager, 25*(3), 198–205.

Markey, C. (2007). What might the 110th Congress have in store for home health and hospice care in 2007-2008? *Home Healthcare Nurse, 25*(5), 343–344.

McIntosh, E., & Zerwekh, J. (2006). Hospice and palliative care. In J. Zerwekh (Ed.). *Nursing care at the end of life: Palliative care for patients and families*. Philadelphia, PA: F.A. Davis.

Munck, B., Sandgren, A., Fridlund, B., & Martensson, J. (2012). Next-of-kin's conceptions of medical technology in palliative homecare. *Journal of Clinical Nursing, 21*, 1868–1877. doi: 10.1111/j.1365-2702.2012.04123.x.

National Alliance for Caregiving. (2012). *About Alliance research*. Retrieved from http://www.caregiving.org/research/about-our-research

National Association for Home Care and Hospice. (2010). *Basic statistics about home care*. Retrieved http://www.nahc.org/facts/10HC_Stats.pdf

Neilson, S., Kai, J., MacArthur, C., & Greenfield, S. (2010). Exploring the experiences of community-based children's nurses providing palliative care. *Paediatric Nursing, 22*(3), 31–36.

Rahme, E., Kahn, S. R., Dasgupta, K., Burman, M., Bernatsky, S., Habel, Y., et al. (2010). Short-term mortality associated with failure to receive home care after hemiarthroplasty. *Canadian Medical Association Journal*, 182(13), 1421–1426. doi:10.1503/cmaj.091209.

Sanchez Varela, A. M., Deal, A. M., Hanson, L. C., Blatt, J., Gold, S., & Dellon, E. P. (2012). Barriers to hospice for children as perceived by hospice organizations in North Carolina. *American Journal of Hospice & Palliative Medicine, 29*(3), 171–176. doi: 10.1177/1049909111412580.

Schlenker, R. E., Powell, M. C., & Goodrich, G. K. (2005). Initial home health outcomes under prospective payment. *Health Services Research, 40*(1), 177–193.

Shea, K., & Chamoff, B. (2012). Telehomecare communication and self-care in chronic conditions: Moving toward a shared understanding. *Worldviews on Evidence-Based Nursing*, 109–116. doi: 10.1111/j.1741-6787.2012.00242.x.

Siegel, J. D., Rhinehart, E., Jackson, M., Chiarello, L., & Healthcare Infection Control Practices Advisory Committee. (2011). 2007 *Guideline for isolation precautions: Preventing transmission of infectious agents in healthcare settings* 2007. Atlanta, GA: Centers for Disease Control and Prevention. Retrieved from http://www.cdc.gov/hicpac/2007IP/2007ip_part4.html

Slocum-Gori, S., Hemsworth, D., Chan, W., Carson, A., & Kazanjian, A. (2011). Understanding compassion satisfaction, compassion fatigue, and burnout: A survey of the hospice palliative care workforce. *Palliative Medicine, 0*(0), 1–7. doi: 10.1177/0269216311431311.

SmithBattle, L., Drake, M. A., & Diekemper, M. (1997). The responsive use of self in community health nursing practice. *Advances in Nursing Science, 20*, 75–89.

Stanley, M., Blair, K. A., & Beare, P. G. (2005). *Gerontological nursing: Promoting successful aging with older adults* (3rd ed.). Philadelphia. PA: F.A. Davis.

Stolee, P., Lim, S. N., Wilson, L., & Glenny, C. (2011). Inpatient versus home-based rehabilitation for older adults with musculoskeletal disorders: A systematic review. *Clinical Rehabilitation, 26*(5), 387–402. doi: 10.1177/0269215511423279.

Stulginsky, M. N. (1993a). Nurses' home health experience: Part I: The practice setting. *Nursing and Health Care, 14*(8), 402–407.

Stulginsky, M. N. (1993b). Nurses' home health experience: Part II: The unique demands of home visits. *Nursing and Health Care, 14*(9), 476–485.

Supreme Court of the United States. (2012). *National Federation of Independent Business et al. v Sebelius, Secretary of Health and Human Services*. Retrieved from http://www.supremecourt.gov/opinions/11pdf/11-393c3a2.pdf

Touhy, T., & Zerwekh, J. (2006). Spiritual caring. In J. Zerwekh (Ed.). *Nursing care at the end of life*. Philadelphia, PA: F.A. Davis.

U.S. Department of Health and Human Services. (2010). *Healthy People 2020: Improving the health of Americans*. Washington, DC: U.S. Government Printing Office.

Vachon, M., & Huggard, J. (2010). The experience of the nurse in end-of-life care in the 21st century: Mentoring the next generation. In B. R. Ferrell, & N. Coyle (Eds.). *Oxford textbook of palliative nursing* (3rd ed.). New York, NY: Oxford University Press.

Vargas-Schaffer, G. (2010). Is the WHO analgesic ladder still valid? Twenty-four years of experience. *Canadian Family Physician, 56*, 514–517.

Wajnberg, A., Wang, K. H., Aniff, M., & Kunins, H. V. (2010). Hospitalizations and skilled nursing facility admissions before and after the implementation of a home-based primary care program. *Journal of the American Geriatric Society, 58*, 1144–1147. doi: 10.1111/j.1532-5415.2010.02859.x.

World Health Organization. (n.d.). Cancer: *WHO's pain ladder*. Retrieved from http://www.who.int/cancer/palliative/painladder/en/

Zerwekh, J. (1991). Tales from public health nursing true detectives. *American Journal of Nursing, 91*(10), 30–36.

Zerwekh, J. (1995). High-tech home care for nurses. *Home Healthcare Nurse, 13*(1), 9–14.

Zerwekh, J. (2000). Caring on the ragged edge: Nursing persons who are disenfranchised. *Advances in Nursing Science, 22*, 47–61.

Zerwekh, J. (2002). Home care of the dying. In I. Martinson, A. Widmer, & C. Portillo. *Home health care nursing*. Philadelphia, PA: W.B. Saunders.

Zerwekh, J. (2006). *Nursing care at the end of life*. Philadelphia, PA: F.A. Davis.

thePoint: Everything You Need to Make the Grade!

thePoint — Visit http://thePoint.lww.com/Allender8e for selected readings, study aids for all learning styles, and more!

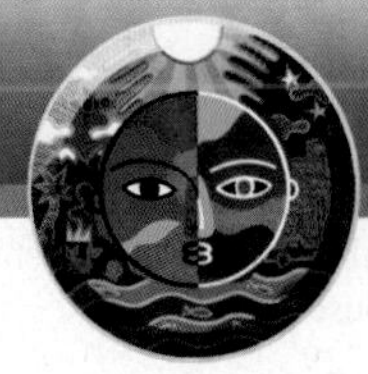

INDEX

Note: Page numbers followed by "*d*" indicate display material, "*f*" indicates figures, "*b*" indicates boxed material, and "*t*" indicates tables.

E

J

K

L

Q

R

T

U

V

W

Y